CLINICAL LABORATORY MICROBIOLOGY
A PRACTICAL APPROACH

Karen M. Kiser, MA, MT(ASCP) PBT^{CM}

Professor Emeritus, Clinical Laboratory Technology
St. Louis Community College at Forest Park
St. Louis, Missouri

William C. Payne, MS, MT(ASCP)

Assistant Professor of Clinical Laboratory Science
Arkansas State University–Jonesboro
College of Nursing and Health Professions
Department of Clinical Laboratory Science
State University, Arkansas

Teresa A. Taff, MA, MT(ASCP)SM

Program Director and Laboratory Manager of Clinical Laboratory Science
St. John's Mercy Medical Center
St. Louis, Missouri

Pearson

Boston Columbus Indianapolis New York San Francisco Upper Saddle River
Amsterdam Cape Town Dubai London Madrid Milan Munich Paris Montreal Toronto
Delhi Mexico City Sao Paulo Sydney Hong Kong Seoul Singapore Taipei Tokyo

Library of Congress Cataloging-in-Publication Data

Kiser, Karen M.
   Clinical laboratory microbiology / Karen M. Kiser,
     William C. Payne, Teresa A. Taff.
     p. ; cm.
   Includes index.
   ISBN-13: 978-0-13-092195-6
   ISBN-10: 0-13-092195-5
 1. Diagnostic microbiology.   I. Payne, William C.
II. Taff, Teresa A.   III. Title.
   [DNLM: 1. Microbiological Techniques.   QW 25
K605c 2011]
   QR67.K57 2011
   616.9'0475—dc22

                   2010000455

Notice: The authors and the publisher of this volume have taken care that the information and technical recommendations contained herein are based on research and expert consultation, and are accurate and compatible with the standards generally accepted at the time of publication. Nevertheless, as new information becomes available, changes in clinical and technical practices become necessary. The reader is advised to carefully consult manufacturers' instructions and information material for all supplies and equipment before use, and to consult with a healthcare professional as necessary. This advice is especially important when using new supplies or equipment for clinical purposes. The authors and publisher disclaim all responsibility for any liability, loss, injury, or damage incurred as a consequence, directly or indirectly, of the use and application of any of the contents of this volume.

Publisher: Julie Levin Alexander
Publisher's Assistant: Regina Bruno
Editor-in-Chief: Mark Cohen
Development Editors: Cynthia Mondgock and Marion
  Waldman, iD8 Publishing Services
Associate Editor: Melissa Kerian
Assistant Editor: Nicole Ragonese
Director of Marketing: David Gesell
Executive Marketing Manager: Katrin Beacom
Marketing Specialist: Michael Sirinides
Marketing Assistant: Judy Noh
Managing Production Editor: Patrick Walsh
Production Liaison: Christina Zingone
Production Editor: Karen Berry, Laserwords Maine
Senior Media Editor: Amy Peltier

Media Project Manager: Lorena Cerisano
Manufacturing Manager: Ilene Sanford
Manufacturing Buyer: Pat Brown
Art Director: Christopher Weigand
Cover Designer: Kevin Kall
Manager, Visual Rights and Permissions: Zina Arabia
Manager, Visual Research: Beth Brenzel
Manager, Cover Visual Research and Permissions:
  Karen Sanatar
Image Permissions Coordinator: Debbie Latronica
Composition: Laserwords Maine
Printing and Binding: Webcrafters, Inc.
Cover Printer: Lehigh Phoenix
Cover Image: CDC/Cynthia Goldsmith

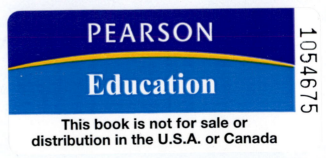

This book is not for sale or distribution in the U.S.A. or Canada

1054675

10 9 8 7 6 5 4 3 2 1

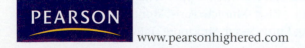

www.pearsonhighered.com

ISBN-13: 978-0-13-092195-6
ISBN-10: 0-13-092195-5

DEDICATION

This book is dedicated to my family—Jay, Cindy, and Jessica, my twin sister Carole, my parents Arthur and Elizabeth Meier—and my teachers, mentors, and students.

Karen M. Kiser

I dedicate this book to my parents, Kenneth and Mary Ann Garrison, and all of the students, clinical laboratory educators, and microbiologists who have entered my life.

Terry Taff

I dedicate this book to my family—Penny, Christy, April, Steve, and Dorian—my mother, Rose, my siblings, my students, and my mentors and fellow educators.

Bill Payne

CONTENTS

FOREWORD

Clinical Laboratory Microbiology is part of Pearson's Clinical Laboratory Science series of textbooks, which is designed to balance theory and practical applications in a way that is engaging and useful to students. The authors of and contributors to *Clinical Laboratory Microbiology* present highly detailed technical information and real-life case studies that will help learners envision themselves as members of the health care team, providing the laboratory services specific to microbiology that assist in patient care. The mixture of theoretical and practical information relating to microbiology provided in this text allows learners to analyze and synthesize this information and, ultimately, to answer questions and solve problems and cases. Additional applications and instructional resources are available at www.myhealthprofessionskit.com

We hope that this book, as well as the entire series, proves to be a valuable educational resource.

Elizabeth A. Zeibig, PhD, MT(ASCP), CLS(NCA)
Clinical Laboratory Science Series Editor
Pearson Health Science

Vice Chair & Associate Professor
Department of Clinical Laboratory Science
Doisy College of Health Sciences
Saint Louis University
St. Louis, MO

PREFACE

Clinical Laboratory Microbiology is a textbook with a practical approach to diagnostic microbiology written for all levels of students including medical laboratory scientists (MLS) (previously known as clinical laboratory scientists and medical technologists) and medical laboratory technicians (MLT) (previously known as clinical laboratory technicians). This book should also serve as a helpful bench reference for practicing laboratory professionals. Other professionals such as pathology residents, physician assistants, and nurse practitioners will find the information useful.

Our contributors have used their extensive knowledge and experience to write chapters that are interesting, readable, understandable, and practical. Most of the activities are classroom tested. The information is presented in a visually rich format that should help the student learn the content necessary to pass a national certification exam and meet entry-level performance expectations. This book also has a companion web site. An eTextbook is available to those who prefer an online format rather than a hard copy.

ORGANIZATION OF THE BOOK

Organization of the material is a critical component of learning. The learner must be able to file the new information away so that the facts can be retrieved accurately as needed. The sequence of presentation is also important in building layers of knowledge that can foster the understanding of the material needed to solve problems. With this in mind the authors divided the book into five parts. The first part is an introduction to diagnostic microbiology. It condenses pertinent material from general microbiology that is useful in understanding the work of a clinical microbiology laboratory. Part One includes information on the development of clinical microbiology, taxonomy and classification, the bacterial cell, the host's encounter with microbes, and safety.

Most of the requests submitted to clinical microbiology laboratories are for routine culture. Part Two, Routine Specimen Processing, provides an overview of each component needed to meet that request. This part covers specimen collection, cultivation of microorganisms, presumptive identification, final identification, immunological tests, and susceptibility testing. This part ends with a chapter on emerging technologies in an effort to make learners aware of what the future may hold. Change is inevitable and the learner must not only be aware of potential change but be willing to prepare for that change.

Physicians must make separate requests for certain microbiology analysis. These special requests usually use different media, processing methods, or require additional safety precautions in order to carry out the request. The authors have placed these in their own section. Part Three, Special Specimen Processing, covers acid-fast bacilli cultures, fungal cultures, ova and parasites, and viral, *Chlamydia*, and *Rickettsia* specimens.

The fourth part is devoted to clinically significant isolates. Each group of organisms' taxonomy, morphology, useful tests, and identification is described. Virulence factors and an overview of each microbe's infectious diseases are also discussed in each chapter.

Part Five takes a body system approach to the analysis of infectious disease. This is a logical approach as specimens for microbiology culture are collected and processed for clinically significant isolates based on the site of infection. The chapters are written so the anatomy and physiology of each body site is reviewed and commensal flora (if any), diseases, and laboratory diagnosis is described. Laboratory diagnosis follows the typical bench workflow and includes body site–specific information related to specimen collection, setup and incubation, workup, and interpretation of growth. Antibiograms are included in both Parts Four and Five when appropriate. Separate chapters on opportunistic infections and nosocomial infections highlight the importance of these topics. It ends with a chapter on global threats. The world is so interconnected that one can no longer consider an infectious disease as isolated. Any infectious disease could be detected in a clinical microbiology laboratory if the patient has traveled to or emigrated from another country. Soldiers may also bring home unusual microbes when returning from active duty.

THIS BOOK SUITS ALL LEVELS OF LEARNING

Recognizing that MLT and MLS programs around the country have different employer needs, prerequisites, and curriculums, the organization of this book should provide the flexibility needed for use in college courses and clinical rotations. MLT programs do not all have general microbiology courses as prerequisites, so Part One should be particularly useful. MLS students would benefit from a review of these same topics to ease their understanding of the material and prepare for the general microbiology section on the national certification examination. Parts Two and Three should be read by all students regardless of their level of practice. Parts Four and Five could easily be read in a different order or chapters selected for reading as desired. MLT programs do not all have anatomy and physiology courses as prerequisites so the overview of structure and function for each body system should aid in the student's understanding of the material presented in Part Five. Part Five should also support the clinical instruction provided in a health care setting.

The material presented in the chapters in Parts Four and Five cover the most commonly encountered microbes and diseases first then end with the more unusual isolates and their diseases. MLT instructors should be able to easily guide their students to what they need to focus on for their curriculum and the needed entry-level knowledge. Those programs that are articulated can use the same book and distinguish what has been covered in previous courses. MLT and MLS graduates should still find the book helpful while on the bench or pursuing further education. The checkpoints, learning opportunities, and case studies in each chapter should be tackled by all students in order to promote deeper learning of the material.

UNIQUE PEDAGOGICAL FEATURES

The subject of microbiology can be a challenge to learn because it is so different from other subjects a student has taken. The best approach to help overcome this obstacle to learning is to tie new information to familiar experiences (e.g., Chapter 1 provides a historical perspective of clinical microbiology); provide repetition so comfort with the material is increased and facts are transferred from short-term memory to long-term memory; frequently assess the learner's knowledge so they know what they don't know; and provide real-world problems to answer the question, "Why am I learning this?" These problems also help students learn how to think like a microbiologist, practice problem solving, and risk failure without repercussion. The 3 P's—practice, practice, practice—help to develop a more knowledgeable and confident learner. The book's pedagogy was designed to incorporate these best practices for learning.

This book has many pedagogical features that aid the student in learning the material. Each chapter begins with a chapter outline to provide the framework for the students to organize the information in their memory. Chapter objectives are provided to clarify what content the learner should grasp when completed. Instructors should feel free to modify or add to these objectives in order to meet their classroom needs. Key terms are listed, bolded, and defined in the text. These terms should foster understanding as well as build vocabulary needed to communicate with other microbiologists and health care providers. Each chapter begins with an introduction that stimulates interest and provides an overview of the chapter content. Each chapter ends with a summary of the important points covered in the chapter. Features unique to this book include:

- Taxonomy with a pronunciation guide
- The use of "Checkpoints!" throughout the chapter allows the student to assess learning, develop test-taking skills,

and promote retention. Answers are provided in the appendix.
- Real World Tips that reinforce the importance of what they are learning.
- Graphic organizers such as timelines and concept maps help visual learners grasp the content. Flow charts model the decisions that are part of identification of an unknown microorganism.
- Learning Opportunities and Case Studies provide questions that aid the student in processing the material and applying what they have learned. Answers are provided on www.myhealthprofessionskit.com
- Websites related to the chapter content are indicated.

Sprinkled throughout the chapters are photos, figures, tables, and boxes that should be especially helpful to visual learners. The images show the microorganism's microscopic morphology and growth characteristics. Photos may also demonstrate equipment and tests used in an organism's identification as well as their infectious diseases. Figures, tables, and boxes will help the student organize the information and better understand concepts.

A COMPLETE TEACHING AND LEARNING PACKAGE

The book is complemented by a variety of ancillary materials designed to help instructors be more effective and students more successful.

- The Instructor's Resource Manual is a guide is designed to equip faculty with necessary teaching resources regardless of the level of instruction. Features include suggested learning activities for each chapter, lecture outlines, and classroom discussion questions.
- Test Bank includes over 600 questions to allow instructors to design customized quizzes and exams using our award-winning TestGen 7.0 test-building engine. The TestGen wizard guides you through the steps to create a simple test with drag-and-drop or point-and-click transfer. You can select test questions either manually or randomly and use online spell-checking and other tools to quickly polish your test content and presentation. You can save your test in a variety of formats both locally and on a network, print up to 25 variations of a single test, and publish your tests in an online course. For more information, please visit: www.pearsonhighered.com/testgen.
- PowerPoint Lectures contain key discussion points, along with color images, for each chapter. This feature provides dynamic, fully designed, integrated lectures that are ready to use and allows instructors to customize the materials to meet their specific course needs. These ready-made lectures will save you time and ease the transition into use of *Clinical Laboratory Microbiology*.

PEARSON
myhealthprofessionskit™

MyHealthProfessionsKit is an online study guide that is completely unique to the market. It provides an array of assessment quizzes that have been developed within an automatic grading system that provides users with instant scoring once users submit their answers. Each student's quiz results can be emailed directly to the educator, if desired, as part of a homework assignment.

This resource also includes the answers to the Learning Opportunities, answers to the Case Study questions, chapter references, additional learning materials, and a glossary of key terms.

Select Clinical Laboratory Science, find this book, and then click to log on. To obtain a login name and password, please register using the scratch-off access code on the inside front cover of this book.

ACKNOWLEDGMENTS

No project like this book can occur without the help and encouragement of many others. We thank our contributors for sharing their knowledge and expertise. We thank our reviewers whose suggestions and encouragement inspired us to continue writing. Thanks to those who helped provide photos for the project, especially Remel, Inc., Indiana Pathology Images, Tom Barkman, and Brian Emberton. We thank Marion Waldman and Cynthia Mondgock for their helpful suggestions, support, and assistance in putting the book together. We also thank Beth Zeibig for giving us the opportunity, Mark Cohen and Melissa Kerian for their patience and gentle prodding, and Pearson Health Science for publishing this text.

Karen would like to thank her daughter, Cindy, who encouraged her to add in historical tidbits, and the rest of her family for their support, patience, and tolerance. Yes, she promises to clean up the pile of notes and books soon. She would like to thank her parents who sacrificed in order to provide their twin daughters with the opportunities they never had. Finally, thanks to her students who inspired her to be the best teacher she could be. Remember that if it walks and quacks like a duck, it probably is a duck.

Terry would like to thank her parents, Kenneth and Mary Ann Garrison, for nurturing her love of science with the many Christmas gifts of chemistry sets, a microscope and slides sets, and anatomy models. Thanks for knowing when to let her struggle and when to help out. Last but not least, thanks to the many past (and future students) who have survived one of Terry's microbiology tests and lived to tell the tale. Remember when you hear hoof beats, think horses not zebras.

Bill would like to thank all those who offered support and encouragement for this grand undertaking, especially his family. Additionally, he thanks the faculty and mentors who were instrumental in his becoming a microbiologist and proficient in his craft. He is also grateful to past and present students who inspired him with their love of learning.

REVIEWERS

Beth W. Blackburn, BS, MT
Orangeburg–Calhoun Technical College
Orangeburg, South Carolina

JoLynne Campbell, PhD, CLS(M)
Wichita State University
Wichita, Kansas

Russell F. Cheadle, BS MT(ASCP)MS
University of Rio Grande
Rio Grande, Ohio

Susan Cockayne, PhD
Brigham Young University
Provo, Utah

James E. Daly, MT(ASCP), MEd, BS
Lorain County Community College
Elyria, Ohio

Cheryl G. Davis, MS, CLS(NCA)
Tuskegee University
Tuskegee, Alabama

Daniel P. deRegnier, MS, MT(ASCP)
Ferris State University
Big Rapids, Michigan

Evelyn Glass, MS, MT(ASCP)
Navarro College
Corsicana, Texas

Rochelle Glymph, MT(ASCP)
Howard University
Washington, DC

Jeffrey S. Josifek, MS, CLS(NCA)
Portland Community College
Portland, Oregon

Hal S. Larsen, PhD, MT(ASCP)
Texas Tech University Health Sciences Center
Lubbock, Texas

Ana M. Linville, BASC
University of Texas at Brownsville
Texas Southmost College
Brownsville, Texas

Karen S. Long, MS, CLS(NCA), MT(ASCP)
West Virginia University
Morgantown, West Virginia

Bridgit Moore, MT(ASCP), CLS(NCA), MSHP
McLennan Community College
Waco, Texas

Susan R. Morton, MT(ASCP), NCA(CLS), MA
Coastal Carolina Community College
Jacksonville, North Carolina

Kim Moultney, MA
Arapahoe Community College
Littleton, Colorado

Ruth A. Negley, MEd, MT(ASCP)SM, CLS(NCA)
Harrisburg Area Community College–Gettysburg Campus
Gettysburg, Pennsylvania

Peter P. O'Brien, MBA, MT(ASCP), CLS(NCA)
Jackson State Community College
Jackson, Tennessee

Lauren Roberts, MS, MT(ASCP)
Arizona State University
Tempe, Arizona

Rodney Rohde, MS, SV(ASCP)
Texas State University–San Marcos
San Marcos, Texas

Rosemarie Romesburg, PhD, MT(ASCP)
Pierpont Community and Technical College
Fairmont, West Virginia

Lynn C. Schaaf, MS, MT(ASCP)
Community College of Philadelphia
Philadelphia, Pennsylvania

Diane Schmaus, MA, MT(ASCP)
McLennan Community College
Waco, Texas

Jeremy Spinney, MT(ASCP)
Kellogg Community College
Battle Creek, Michigan

Scott Wright, MS, CLS(M), (NCA)
Weber State University
Ogden, Utah

CONTRIBUTORS

Hassan Aziz, PhD
Armstrong Atlantic State University
Savannah, Georgia
Chapters 5, 32, 39

Brandon M. Bianski, BS
Loma Linda University
Loma Linda, California
Chapter 2

Cara Calvo, MS, MT(ASCP), SH(ASCP)
University of Washington Medical Center
Seattle, Washington
Chapters 6, 8

Marcia A. Firmani, PhD, MSPH, MT(ASCP), CLS(NCA)
University of Wisconsin, Milwaukee
Milwaukee, Wisconsin
Chapters 12, 42

Jenny Francis, BS, MT(ASCP)
Lima Memorial Hospital
Lima, Ohio
Chapter 6

Mona Gleysteen, MS, MT(ASCP), CLS(NCA)
Lake Area Technical Institute
Watertown, South Dakota
Chapter 34

Rochelle Glymph, MT(ASCP), CLS(NCA)
Howard University
Washington, DC
Chapter 16

Lora M. Green, PhD
Loma Linda University
Loma Linda, California
Chapter 2

Daila S. Gridley, PhD
Loma Linda University
Loma Linda, California
Chapters 10, 20, 21

Joy T. Henderson, MA, MT(ASCP), CLS(NCA)
St. John's Mercy Medical Center
St. Louis, Missouri
Chapters 22, 37, 41

Mark S. Johnson, PhD
Loma Linda University
Loma Linda, California
Chapter 3

Karen M. Kiser, MA, MT(ASCP), PBT^{CM}
St. Louis Community College at Forest Park, Retired
St. Louis, Missouri
Chapters 1, 4, 7, 8, 17, 18, 19, 36

Donald C. Lehman, EdD, MT(ASCP)
University of Delaware
Newark, Delaware
Chapter 15

Ruth Masterson, MT(ASCP)SM
Saint Francis Medical Center
Cape Girardeau, Missouri
Chapter 33

Lisa A. Morici, PhD
Tulane University
New Orleans, Louisiana
Chapters 25, 27

William C. Payne, MS, MT(ASCP)
Arkansas State University–Jonesboro State University
Jonesboro, Arkansas
Chapters 9, 11, 13, 14, 16, 29, 30, 31, 35

Jaya Prakash, MD, SM(NRM)
National University of Health Sciences
Lombard, Illinois
Chapters 13, 26

Masih Shokrani, PhD, MT(ASCP)
Northern Illinois University
DeKalb, Illinois
Chapter 31

Teresa A. Taff, MA, MT(ASCP)SM
St. John's Mercy Medical Center
St. Louis, Missouri
Chapters 11, 23, 24, 38, 40

Ken Baker Waites, MD
University of Alabama at Birmingham
Birmingham, Alabama
Chapter 28

ABBREVIATIONS

2-SP – 2-sucrose phosphate
A – acid
A – Adenine
A549 – Human lung carcinoma
ABC – ATP binding cassette
ABPA – Allergic bronchopulmonary aspergillosis
Abs – Antibodies
ADCC – Antibody-dependent cell-mediated cytotoxicity
AFB – Acid-fast bacilli
AIDS – acquired immunodeficiency syndrome
ALA – Delta-aminolevulinic acid
ALT – Alanine aminotransferase
ANP – Pro-atrial natriuretic peptide
APC – Antigen presenting cells
APW – Alkaline peptone water
ARDS – Acute respiratory distress syndrome
ASC – Active surveillance cultures
ASM – American Society of Microbiology
ATCC – American Type Culture Collection
ATP – adenosine triphosphate
ATTS – Ambient temperature transport system
BA – Blood agar
BAD – bacterial antigen detection
BAL – Bronchoalveolar lavage
BB – Bronchial brush
BBB – blood-brain barrier
BGMK – Buffalo green monkey cell
BCSA – *Burkholderia cepacia* selective agar
BCYE – Buffered charcoal yeast extract
bDNA – Branched DNA
BGAL – β-galactosidase
BHI – Brain heart infusion agar
BHKICP6LacZ – Baby hamster kidney cell line
BSC – Biological safety cabinet
BSE – Bovine spongiform encephalopathy
BSL – Biosafety level
BTA – Biological threat agents
BTK – Bruton tyrosine kinase
BUN – blood urea nitrogen
BV – bacterial vaginosis
BW – Bronchial wash
C – Cytosine
C´ – Complement
CA – Chocolate agar
CAAT – Cross-agglutinin adsorption test
cAMP – cyclic AMP
CA-MRSA – Community-acquired methicillin-resistant *Staphylococcus aureus*
CAP – Community-acquired pneumonia

CAUTI – Catheter-associated urinary tract infections
CCFA – Cycloserine–cefoxitin–fructose and egg yolk agar
CCHF – Crimean-Congo hemorrhagic fever
CDC – Centers for Disease Control and Prevention
cDNA – Complementary deoxyribonucleic acid
CF – Cystic fibrosis
CF – Complement fixation
CFU – Colony forming unit
CGD – Chronic granulomatous disease
CHG – Chlorhexidine gluconate
CHP – Calcineurin B homologous protein
CIN – Cefsulodin–irgasan–novobiocin agar
CJD – Creutzfeldt-Jacob disease
CLED – Cystine-lactose-electrolyte-deficient
CLIA – Clinical Laboratory Improvement Amendments
CLSI – Clinical and Laboratory Standards Institute
CMA – Cornmeal agar
CMBCS – Continuous-monitoring blood culture systems
CMS – Centers for Medicare and Medicaid Services
CMV – Cytomegalovirus
CNA – colistin-naladixic acid
CNA – Columbia Colistin-Nalidixic acid agar
CNS – central nervous system
CNS – Coagulase negative *Staphylococcus*
CO_2 – Carbon dioxide
COOH – carboxyl group
COPD – Chronic obstructive pulmonary disease
CPE – Cytopathic effect
CRE – Carbapenem-resistant *Enterobacteriaceae*
CRP – C-reactive protein
CSF – Cerebrospinal fluid
CSS – Classical surveillance (monitoring) system
CSTE – Council of State and Territorial Epidemiologists
CTA – Cystine trypticase agar
CTM – Chlamydial transport medium
CVID – Common variable immunodeficiency
DAEC – Diffusely adherent *E. coli*
DAP – Diaminopimelic acid
DAT – Direct antigen testing
DFA – Direct fluorescent antibody
DGI – Disseminated gonococcal infection
DGS – DiGeorge syndrome
DHHS – Department of Health and Human Services
DIC – Disseminated intravascular coagulation
DMSO – Dimethyl sulfoxide
DNA – Deoxyribonucleic acid
DOT – Directly observed therapy
DRSP – Drug-resistant *Streptococcus pneumoniae*
ds – Double strand

Dsb – Disulfide bond
DTM – Dermatophyte test medium
EA-D – Early antigen diffuse
EAEC – enteroaggregative *E. coli*
EAggEC – Enteroaggregative *E. coli*
EA-R – Early antigen restricted
EB – Elementary bodies
EBNA – Epstein-Barr nuclear antigen
EBV – Epstein-Barr virus
EDTA – Ethylenediamine tetra-acetic acid
EEE – Eastern equine encephalitis
EF – Edema factor
EHEC – enterohemorrhagic *E. coli*
EI – entry inhibitors
EIA – enzyme immunoassay
EIEC – enteroinvasive *E. coli*
ELISA – enzyme-linked immunosorbent assay
ELVIS – Enzyme-linked virus inducible system
EM – Erythema migrans
EM – Electron microscopy
EMB – Eosin methylene blue agar
EMEM – Eagle's minimal essential medium
ENT – Ear, nose, and throat
env – Envelope
EPEC – enteropathogenic *E. coli*
ESBL – Extended spectrum beta-lactamase
ESR – Erythrocyte sedimentation rate
ETEC – enterotoxigenic *E. coli*
F – Fertility
FDA – Federal Drug Administration
FES – Formalin-ethyl acetate
FISH – fluorescent in-situ hybridization
FITC – Fluorescein isothiocyanate
FOS – Fastidious organisms supplement
FTA-ABS – Fluorescent treponema antibody adsorption test
FUO – Fever of unknown origin
G – gas
G – Guanine
GAE – Granulomatous amoebic encephalitis
gag – Group specific antigen
GBS – Group B *Streptococcus*
GC – Gonococcus
GGA – gamma-glutamylaminopeptidase
GI – Gastrointestinal
GLC – Gas liquid chromatography
GMS – Gomori Methenamine Silver
GN – Gram-negative broth
GNB – Gram-negative bacilli
GNDC – gram-negative diplococci
GNR – Gram-negative rod
GPCCL – Gram-positive cocci in clusters
H_2O_2 – Hydrogen peroxide
H_2S – Hydrogen sulfide
H – Flagellar antigen
HA – Hemagglutinin

HAART – Highly active antiretroviral therapy
HACEK group – *Haemophilus parainfluenzae, Aggregabacter aphrophilus* (formerly known as *H. aphrophilus*), *Aggregabacter actinomycetemcomitans* (formerly known as *Actinobacillus actinomycetemcomitans*), *Cardiobacterium hominis, Eikenella corrodens*, and *Kingella kingae*
HAI – Hospital-acquired infection
HA-MRSA – Hospital-acquired methicillin-resistant *Staphylococcus aureus*
HAP – Hospital-acquired pneumonia
HAV – Hepatitis A virus
HBc – Hepatitis B virus core antibody
HBcAg – Hepatitis B core antigen
HBeAg – Hepatitis B core protein
HBsAG – Hepatitis B virus surface antigen
HBSS – Hank's balanced salt solution
HBV – Hepatitis B virus
HCV – Hepatitis C virus
HCW – Healthcare workers
HDV – Hepatis D virus
H & E – Hematoxylin and eosin stain
HE – Hektoen Enteric agar
HEV – Hepatis E virus
HGV – Hepatis G virus
HEPA – High-efficiency particulate air
HHV-6 – Human-herpesvirus-6
Hib – *Haemophilus influenzae* type b
HIV – Human immunodeficiency virus
HLAR – High-level resistance to aminoglycosides
hMPV – Human metapneumovirus
HNK – Human neonatal kidney
HPLC – High-performance liquid chromatography
HPS – Hantavirus pulmonary syndrome
HPV – Human papilloma virus
HRP – Horseradish peroxidase
Hs27 – Human foreskin fibroblast
HSV – Herpes simplex virus
HTLV – T-cell leukemia virus
HUS – Hemolytic uremic syndrome
I – Intermediate
IB – indoxyl butyrate
ICBN – International Code of Botanical Nomenclature
ICT – Immunochromatographic test
ICU – Intensive care unit
ICTV – International Committee on the Taxonomy of Viruses
IDSA – Infection Diseases Society of America
IEM – Immune electron microscopy
IF – Immunofluorescence
IFA – Indirect immunofluorescent assay
IFN – Interferon
IgA – Immunoglobulin A
IgG – Immunoglobulin G
IgM – Immunoglobulin M
IL – Interleukin

IM – Infectious mononucleosis
IMA – Inhibitory mould agar
IMViC – Indole, Methyl-red, Voges-Proskauer, citrate
INH – Isoniazid, isonicotinic acid hydrazide
IS – Insertion sequences
IV – Intravenous
JCAHO – Joint Commission on Accreditation of Healthcare Organizations (now known as The Joint Commission)
JEMBEC – John E. Martin Biological Environmental Chamber agar
IUD – intrauterine device
K – Alkaline
K – Capsular antigen
KCN – Potassium cyanide
KIA – Kligler's iron agar
KOH – Potassium hydroxide
KPC – *Klebsiella pneumoniae* carbapenemase
KSHV – Kaposi sarcoma-associated herpesvirus
LA – latex agglutination
LBRF – louse borne relapsing fever
LCMV – Lymphocytic choriomeningitis virus
LF – Lethal factor
LGV – Lymphogranuloma venereum
LIA – lysine-iron-agar
LIS – Laboratory information system
LKV – Laked blood–kanamycin–vancomycin
LOS – Lipooligosaccharide
LPCB – Lactophenol cotton blue
LPF – Low power field
LPS – Lipopolysaccharide
LR-VRE – Linezolid-resistant, vancomycin-resistant *Enterococcus*
LT – Heat-labile toxin
mAb – Monoclonal antibody
MB – Multibacillary
MAC – MacConkey agar
MAC – *Mycobacterium avium* complex
MAP – *Mycobacterium avium* subspecies *paratuberculosis*
MAT – Microagglutination test
MBC – Minimum bactericidal concentration
MDRO – Multi-drug resistant organism
MDR-TB – Multi-drug-resistant TB
MHA-TP – Microhemagglutination
MHC – Major histocompatibility complex
MIC – Minimum inhibitory concentration
Micro-IF – Microimmunofluorescence
MMR – Measles, Mumps, Rubella
MOMP – Major outer membrane protein
Mono – Monocyte
MOTT – Mycobacteria other than tubercle bacilli
MPO – Myeloperoxidase
MRC-5 – Human embryonic lung
MRI – Magnetic resonance imaging
Mr/Lu – Mink lung cells
mRNA – Messenger RNA

MRSA – methicillin-resistant *Staphylococcus aureus*
MSA – Mannitol salt agar
MSDS – Material safety data sheet
MSSA – Methicillin-sensitive *Staphylococcus aureus*
MTB – *Mycobacterium tuberculosis*
MUG – 4-methyllumbelliferyl-beta-D-glucuronide
NAD – Nicotinamide adenine dinucleotide; V factor
NADP – Nicotinamide adenine dinucleotide phosphate
NAG – *N*-acetyl glucosamine
NALC – N-acetyl-L-cysteine
NAM, *N*-acetyl muramic acid
NASBA – Nucleic acid sequence-based amplification
NAT – nucleic acid testing
N/C – nuclear material-to-cytoplasm ratio
NC – No change
NCCLS – National Committee for Clinical Laboratory Standards
NF – Nonfermenter
NFB – Nonfermenting bacilli
NGU – Nongonococcal urethritis
NH3+ – amine group
NICU – Neonatal intensive care unit
NIOSH – National Institute for Occupational Safety and Health
NK – Natural killer cells
NKT – Natural killer T lymphocyte cells
NLF – nonlactose fermenter
NNIS – National Nosocomial Infections Surveillance
NNRTI – nucleoside/nucleotide reverse transcriptase inhibitors
NOS – No organisms seen
NP – Nasopharyngeal
NPA – Nasopharyngeal aspirate
NPEC – Nephropathogenic *E. coli*
NRTI – nonnucleoside reverse transcriptase inhibitors
NTM – Nontuberculosis mycobacteria
NVS – Nutritionally variant streptococci
O – Somatic antigen
OF – Oxidation-Fermentation
OIF – Oil immersion field
OME – Otitis media with effusion
ONPG – *o*-nitrophenyl-β-D-galactopyranoside (substrate)
ONPG – ortho-nitrophenyl-β-galactosidase (enzyme)
OSHA – Occupational Safety and Health Administration
OTB – Orthotoluidine blue
PA – Protective antigen
PABA – Para-aminobenzoic acid
PAD – phenylalanine deaminase
Pap – Papanicoalaou preparation
PAS – Para-aminosalicylic acid
PAS – Periodic acid-Schiff
PB – Paucibacillary
PBB – Protected bronchial brushing
PBP – Penicillin-binding protein
PCP – *Pneumocystis jiroveci* (formerly *P. carinii*) pneumonia

PCR – Polymerase chain reaction
PCT – Procalcitonin
PDA – phenylalanine deaminase
PDA – Potato dextrose agar
PEA – Phenylethyl alcohol agar
PEP – Phosphoenolpyruvate
PI – protease inhibitors
PICC – Peripherally inserted central catheters or Pic line
PID – Pelvic inflammatory disease
pLDH – *Plasmodium* lactate dehydrogenase
PMC – Pseudomembranous colitis
PMF – Proton motive force
PMK – Primary monkey kidney
PMN – Polymorphonuclear leukocyte
PNA – Peptide nucleic acid
PNA FISH™ – Peptide nucleic acid fluorescence in situ hybridization
pol – Polymerase
PPD – Purified protein derivative
PPE – Personal protective equipment
PPLO – Pleuropneumonia-like organisms
PRAS – Pre-reduced anaerobically sterilized
PRO – proline aminopeptidase
PT – Proficiency testing
PTS – Phosphotransferase system
PVA – Polyvinyl alcohol
PYR – L-pyrronlidonyl-β-naphthylamide
PYR – pyrrolidonyl arylamidase
PZA – Pyrazinamide
QA – Quality assurance
R – Resistant
RAST – Radioallergosorbent test
RAT – Rapid assimilation test for Trehalose
RBAP – Reduced blood agar plate
RBC – Red blood cells
Redox – Oxygen reduction potential
RES – Reticuloendothelial system
RFFIT – Rapid fluorescent-focus inhibition test
RFLP – Restriction fragment length polymorphism
RIA – Radioimmunoassay
RIBA – Recombinant immunoblot assay
RID – Radial immuno diffusion
RMP – Rifampin
RNA – Ribonucleic acid
RPR – rapid plasma reagin test
RSU – Rapid sucrose urea test
RSV – Respiratory syncytial virus
RT – Reverse transcriptase
RT-PCR – Reverse transcriptase polymerase chain reaction
RT-PCR – Real-time polymerase chain reaction
RVFV – Rift Valley Fever virus
S – Sensitive/Susceptible
SAB – Sabouraud's dextrose agar
SABHI – Sabouraud dextrose with brain heart infusion agar

SAF – Sodium acetate-acetic acid-formalin
SARS – Severe acute respiratory syndrome
SARS-CoV – SARS-Coronavirus
SBA – sheep blood agar plate
SBE – subacute bacterial endocarditis
SBPA – Saprophytic bronchopulmonary aspergillosis
SCC – Staphylococcal cassette chromosome
SCID – Severe combined immunodeficiency
SDA – Sabouraud dextrose agar
SEC – Squamous epithelial cell
SEG – Segmented neutrophil
SLE – St. Louis encephalitis virus
SLE – Systemic lupus erythematosus
SMAC – Sorbitol MacConkey agar
SMX – Sulfamethoxazole
SNA – *Staphylococcus* not *S. aureus*
SNP – Single nucleotide polymorphism
SNV – Sin nombre virus
SOD – Superoxide dismutase
SPG – Sucrose glutamate phosphate
SPS – Sodium polyanethol sulfonate
sRBC – Sensitized red blood cells
SS – Salmonella-Shigella agar
ss – Single strand
SSI – Surgical site infection
SsRNA – Single-stranded ribonucleic acid
ST – Heat-stable toxin
STD – Sexually transmitted disease
STEC – Shiga-toxin *E. coli*
T – Thymine
TA – Tracheostomy and endotracheal aspirations
Taq – *Thermus aquaticus* polymerase
TB – Tuberculosis
TBRF – tick borne relapsing fever
TSA – Trypticase soy agar
TCA – Trichloroacetic acid
TCA – Tricarboxylic acid cycle
TCBS – Thiosulfate citrate bile salts sucrose agar
TCH – Thiophene-2-carboxylic acid hydrazide inhibition
TD – Traveler's diarrhea
Th1 – Helper T lymphocyte type 1
Th2 – Helper T lymphocyte type 2
Thio – Thioglycolate broth
TIGR – The Institute for Genomic Research
TM – Thayer-Martin agar
TMP – Trimethoprim
TNF – Tissue necrosis factor
TORCH – *Toxoplasmosis*, Other [usually Hepatitis B, HIV, Enterovirus, and Varicella (VSV)], Rubella, Cytomegalovirus (CMV), and Herpes simplex virus
TPHA – *Treponema pallidum* hemagglutination assay
TRITC – Tetramethylrhodamine isothiocyanate
tRNA – Transfer RNA
TSB – Trypticase soy broth

TSE – Transmissible spongiform encephalopathies
TSI – Triple sugar iron agar
TSBY – Trypticase soy blood agar supplemented with 0.5% yeast extract, hemin, and menadione
TSS – Toxic shock syndrome
TTC – triphenyltetrazolium chloride
U – Uracil
URI – Upper respiratory infection
UTI – Urinary tract infection
UV – Ultraviolet light
UVGI – Ultraviolet germicidal irradiation
VAP – Ventilator-associated pneumonia
VCA – viral capsid antibodies
VDE – Vancomycin-dependent *Enterococcus* spp.
VDRL – Venereal Disease Research Laboratories
VEE – Venezuelan equine encephalitis
VHF – Viral hemorrhagic fever
VISA – Vancomycin intermediate *Staphylococcus aureus*
VP – Voges-Proskauer
VRE – Vancomycin-resistant *Enterococcus*

VRSA – Vancomycin-resistant *Staphylococcus aureus*
VSV – Varicella virus
VTEC – verotoxin *E. coli*
VTM – Viral transport medium
VZV – Varicella zoster virus
WAS – Wiskott-Aldrich syndrome
WB – Western blot
WBC – White blood cell
WD – Working distance
WEE – Western equine encephalitis
WHO – World Health Organization
WNV – West-Nile virus
wt/vol – Weight per volume
X factor – heme
XDR TB – Extensively drug resistant tuberculosis
XLA – X-linked agammaglobulinemia
XLD – Xylose-lysine-deoxycholate agar
YAC – Yeast artificial chromosome
YE/YEPA – Yeast-extract phosphate agar

PART I
INTRODUCTION TO
DIAGNOSTIC MICROBIOLOGY

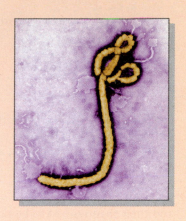

1

Development of Diagnostic Microbiology

Karen M. Kiser

■ LEARNING OBJECTIVES

Upon completion of this chapter, the learner should be able to:

1. Identify the contributions made by Leeuwenhoek, Pasteur, Koch, Lister, Ehrlich, Jenner, Fleming, and Mullis to modern diagnostic microbiology.
2. State the germ theory of fermentation.
3. State the germ theory of disease.
4. Summarize Koch's postulates.
5. Discuss the role germ theories and Koch's postulates play in current investigations of emerging infections.
6. Evaluate a current case study and relate the information to historically significant events.

KEY TERMS

acute	genomic	pestilence
attenuated	indigenous	plagues
bioinformatics	infectivity	proteonomics
chemotherapy	inoculation	pure cultures
contamination	morbidity	virulent
crystallographic	mortality	x-ray diffraction
derivatives	pandemic	zoonoses
epidemic	pasteurization	

▶ INTRODUCTION

To appreciate the modern diagnostic microbiology laboratory, we must travel back in history and examine its roots. Microbiology is a relatively young science that developed in the nineteenth century. Scientists of the day were searching for practical solutions to problems with fermentation and disease. Established scientists did not readily accept early discoveries, and their theories had to be proven and defended. Time has vindicated their conclusions. Many of the procedures performed in modern laboratories today are similar to those developed in the 1800s.

Yet arrogance has fostered some of the problems facing medicine today. Many patients and physicians believed that the right antibiotic could cure any infection. The result of overuse of antibiotics is multi-drug-resistant microorganisms, dubbed "super bugs." Again, a view of history helps us to understand the origins of these problems, as well as possible solutions.

The newer molecular diagnostic methods have developed only within the last 20 years. The speed of diagnosis and implications for epidemiology and treatment with these new techniques are amazing. Only by examining the timeline related to the development of microbiology as a science can we marvel at the lightning speed of development of today's techniques for diagnosing and treating infectious disease.

In this chapter, we explore the role of infectious disease in history. We discuss significant discoveries that promoted the development of diagnostic microbiology. Finally, we present the contributions of those who laid a foundation for our current molecular techniques.

▶ INFECTIOUS DISEASES IN HISTORY

In ancient civilizations before the birth of Christ, disease was believed to be a punishment sent by God. Many philosophers of this time believed that disease was caused by invisible animals.

EARLIEST RECORDED CASES

The first recorded case of infectious disease may have occurred circa 3180 B.C. The account reports a great **pestilence**, or deadly outbreak of a disease, in Egypt during the reign of the First Dynasty, Emperor Shemsu. No description is given to define this pestilence (Beck, 2000). Translation of an Egyptian medical papyrus, dated to around 1500 B.C., provides a list of diseases and their treatments. Table 1-1✪ shows a sample of diseases and treatments, as recorded in the papyrus. Microorganisms are now known to cause many of these diseases (Hunderfund, 1987).

Near the end of the Trojan War, circa 1190 B.C., the Greek army was largely destroyed by an **epidemic** that may have been the bubonic plague. An epidemic is an incidence of disease cases that is much higher than normally expected (Beck,

✪ TABLE 1-1

Select Ancient Diseases and Their Treatment

Ancient Disease	Treatment
Roundworm	Drink preparation from bark of the pomegranate root, soaked in water
Burn wounds	Prevent infection by rubbing burn with a frog warmed in oil
Abscess	Anoint with blood of dove, goose, swallow, or vulture
Leprous spots	Apply cooked onions, in mixture of sea salt and urine, to spots
Herpes on face	Apply dressing made from inner part of the castor-oil tree and red lead
Gangrene	None available

2000). Similarly, the body of Pharaoh Ramses V, who died in 1157 B.C., shows evidence of pustules on his face, neck, and shoulders. This may be the earliest evidence of smallpox (Kiple, 1997).

According to Roman historian Livy (Titus Livius), **plagues**, or diseases with a high death rate or widespread prevalence, struck ancient Rome in 790, 710, and 640 B.C. (Beck, 2000). In 430 B.C. a terrible plague, known as the Plague of Athens, wiped out one-third of the city and probably contributed to the defeat of the Athenian empire (Cartwright & Biddiss, 1972). Some believe the plague to be measles, and others typhus fever (Beck, 2000).

WORLDWIDE EPIDEMICS

Changes in humankind's lifestyle created favorable conditions for the epidemics that followed. Humans started out as wanderers. They lived in small groups and set up temporary camps to hunt and gather food. They didn't stay in one spot long enough to foul the water, accumulate waste, or attract rodents and insects to carry disease. Their food sources were wild game, native plants, and berries. As the human population increased and food became more scarce, humans became farmers and city dwellers. They lived in permanent sites, in more crowded conditions, which resulted in contamination of water and streets with human and animal waste as well as trash. These settlements attracted microbe-carrying rodents and insects. Animals were raised for food. Grain was grown and stored. The conditions for **zoonoses,** or infectious diseases in humans whose source is an animal; food-borne illness; and person-to-person spread of infectious disease, was in place. Table 1-2✪ lists microorganisms associated with wild and domesticated animals that may be a source of infection.

Conditions That Facilitate Epidemics

At the end of the Ice Age, some 10,000 years ago, humans began to cultivate the land and domesticate the growth of grain and animals. As mentioned previously, as the population

✪ TABLE 1-2

Animals and Their Associated Organisms

Infectious Disease	Animal Host	Microorganism
Anthrax	Cows, horses, sheep, goats, hogs, dogs, cats, hens, wild animals, and birds	*Bacillus anthracis*
Diphtheria	Cows, dogs, cats, hens	*Corynebacterium diphtheriae*
Influenza	Wild water fowls	*Influenzae A virus*
Plague	Rats, monkeys, other animals	*Yersinia pestis*
Tuberculosis	Cattle, rabbits, deer, antelopes, llamas, seals, other wild and domesticated animals	*Mycobacterium bovis*
Malaria	Birds	*Plasmodium falciparum*
Pertussis	Dogs and other animals	*Bordetella bronchiseptica*

increased, humans began to live in densely populated cities. The more daring humans explored their world, carrying with them microbes as well as their knowledge and skills. New lands were cultivated and cities created.

Cities were crowded with people. Bathing was not a high priority. Waste from people and animals was deposited in close proximity to the water sources and used to fertilize crops. Garbage littered the landscape, creating an ecological niche for vectors of disease such as rats and mosquitoes. **Indigenous** people, or original inhabitants of a region or country, were exposed to new microbes brought by the explorers.

The village barber often administered medical care. A common treatment for disease was "bleeding" or "blood-letting." The barber-surgeon lanced an external vein (commonly on the forearm) and drained some of the patient's blood into a shaving bowl. This often weakened an already weakened host (Seigworth, 1980). Those who cared for the sick moved from one patient to another without washing their hands. The setting was perfect for an infectious disease outbreak.

Human Toll

History records a number of worldwide epidemics. Figure 1-1 ■ provides a timeline of selected outbreaks and events important in history. The Black Death caused an estimated 100 million deaths during the Plague of Justinian in 542 A.D.

Twenty-five percent of the population of the Eastern and Western Roman empires died, and this loss of life may have been responsible for weakening the Roman and Persian armies enough to allow the expansion of Islam by Muslim military forces. Figure 1-2 ■ depicts a plague scene in the city of Naples in 1656 as painted by Micco Spadaro. This plague marked the beginning of the Dark Ages and is credited for killing 25 to 50% of the population in Europe and the Middle East (Kiple, 1997).

Explorers transported smallpox to the new world, which may have contributed to the conquest of the Aztec civilization as well as other native Indian cultures (Kiple, 1997). In 1875, measles killed 40,000 of Fiji island inhabitants, according to the Fiji colonial governor. Soldiers recruited from farms were susceptible to measles, and there were outbreaks of infectious disease in military camps during the Civil War, Spanish American War, and World War I. Vaccination dramatically reduced this problem (Kiple, 1997).

Other microorganisms devastated armies engaged in combat. Typhus took such a heavy toll on Napoleon's army during the invasion of Moscow that a withdrawal was necessary. Typhoid caused more deaths than bullets during the Spanish American War. The 1918 influenza epidemic is believed to have killed 30 million individuals in 6 months compared to more than eight million soldiers who died during the four years of World War I (Kiple, 1997).

Some of these early epidemics may have been the result of bioterrorism. The second **pandemic** of Black Death may have been brought to Europe, in the mid 1300s, by survivors of the siege of Kaffa, a seaside city in what is now known as the Ukraine. A pandemic is a disease that attacks the inhabitants of a continent, country, or region. Commanders of the Tartar army ordered plague-ridden corpses to be catapulted over the wall before the Tartars retreated. The survivors of the siege returned to Italy, probably carrying infected rats in their ships, leaving trails of outbreaks at every port they visited (Karlen, 1995). In America, during the French and Indian War, the English provided Native Americans loyal to

A Quote in Time

"I had a little bird
and its name was Enza
I opened the window
and Influenza"

(Kiple, 1997)

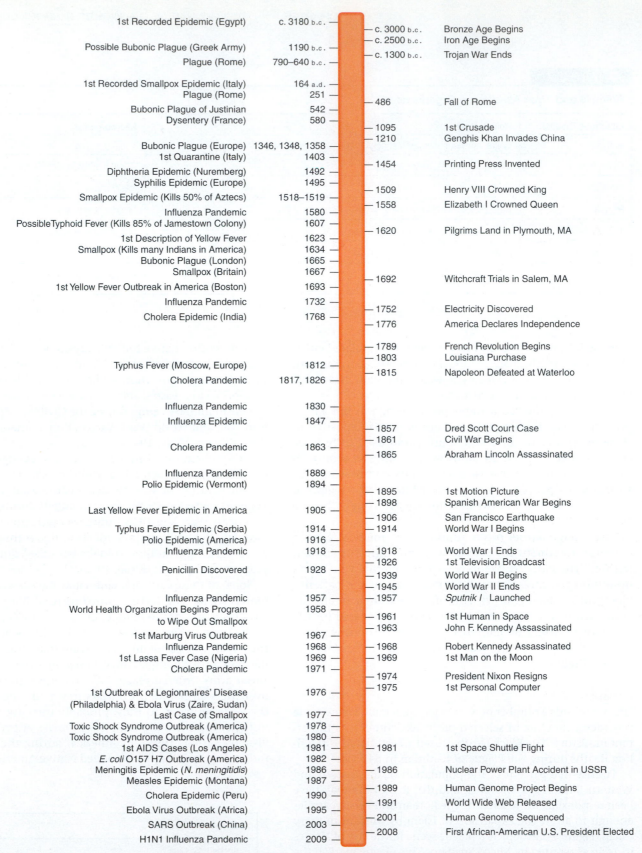

Outbreaks		Historical Events	
1st Recorded Epidemic (Egypt)	c. 3180 b.c.	c. 3000 b.c.	Bronze Age Begins
		c. 2500 b.c.	Iron Age Begins
Possible Bubonic Plague (Greek Army)	1190 b.c.	c. 1300 b.c.	Trojan War Ends
Plague (Rome)	790–640 b.c.		
1st Recorded Smallpox Epidemic (Italy)	164 a.d.		
Plague (Rome)	251		
Bubonic Plague of Justinian	542	486	Fall of Rome
Dysentery (France)	580		
		1095	1st Crusade
		1210	Genghis Khan Invades China
Bubonic Plague (Europe)	1346, 1348, 1358		
1st Quarantine (Italy)	1403	1454	Printing Press Invented
Diphtheria Epidemic (Nuremberg)	1492		
Syphilis Epidemic (Europe)	1495	1509	Henry VIII Crowned King
Smallpox Epidemic (Kills 50% of Aztecs)	1518–1519	1558	Elizabeth I Crowned Queen
Influenza Pandemic	1580		
PossibleTyphoid Fever (Kills 85% of Jamestown Colony)	1607	1620	Pilgrims Land in Plymouth, MA
1st Description of Yellow Fever	1623		
Smallpox (Kills many Indians in America)	1634		
Bubonic Plague (London)	1665		
Smallpox (Britain)	1667	1692	Witchcraft Trials in Salem, MA
1st Yellow Fever Outbreak in America (Boston)	1693		
Influenza Pandemic	1732	1752	Electricity Discovered
Cholera Epidemic (India)	1768	1776	America Declares Independence
		1789	French Revolution Begins
		1803	Louisiana Purchase
Typhus Fever (Moscow, Europe)	1812	1815	Napoleon Defeated at Waterloo
Cholera Pandemic	1817, 1826		
Influenza Pandemic	1830		
Influenza Epidemic	1847		
		1857	Dred Scott Court Case
		1861	Civil War Begins
Cholera Pandemic	1863	1865	Abraham Lincoln Assassinated
Influenza Pandemic	1889		
Polio Epidemic (Vermont)	1894		
		1895	1st Motion Picture
		1898	Spanish American War Begins
Last Yellow Fever Epidemic in America	1905	1906	San Francisco Earthquake
Typhus Fever Epidemic (Serbia)	1914	1914	World War I Begins
Polio Epidemic (America)	1916		
Influenza Pandemic	1918	1918	World War I Ends
		1926	1st Television Broadcast
Penicillin Discovered	1928	1939	World War II Begins
		1945	World War II Ends
Influenza Pandemic	1957	1957	Sputnik I Launched
World Health Organization Begins Program	1958		
to Wipe Out Smallpox		1961	1st Human in Space
		1963	John F. Kennedy Assassinated
1st Marburg Virus Outbreak	1967		
Influenza Pandemic	1968	1968	Robert Kennedy Assassinated
1st Lassa Fever Case (Nigeria)	1969	1969	1st Man on the Moon
Cholera Pandemic	1971		
		1974	President Nixon Resigns
1st Outbreak of Legionnaires' Disease	1976	1975	1st Personal Computer
(Philadelphia) & Ebola Virus (Zaire, Sudan)			
Last Case of Smallpox	1977		
Toxic Shock Syndrome Outbreak (America)	1978		
Toxic Shock Syndrome Outbreak (America)	1980		
1st AIDS Cases (Los Angeles)	1981	1981	1st Space Shuttle Flight
E. coli O157 H7 Outbreak (America)	1982		
Meningitis Epidemic (N. meningitidis)	1986	1986	Nuclear Power Plant Accident in USSR
Measles Epidemic (Montana)	1987		
		1989	Human Genome Project Begins
Cholera Epidemic (Peru)	1990	1991	World Wide Web Released
Ebola Virus Outbreak (Africa)	1995		
		2001	Human Genome Sequenced
SARS Outbreak (China)	2003	2008	First African-American U.S. President Elected
H1N1 Influenza Pandemic	2009		

Key: c. = circa; b.c. = before Christ; a.d. = anno Domini (in the year of our lord).

■ **FIGURE 1-1** Outbreaks throughout time: a historical perspective.

4

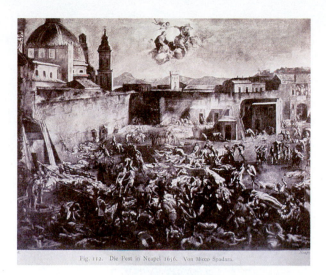

■ **FIGURE 1-2** Die Pest in Neapel 1656. Plague scene in city.
Courtesy of the National Library of Medicine.

the French with smallpox-laden blankets. "Native Americans defending Fort Carillon sustained epidemic casualties which directly contributed to the loss of the fort to the English" (Eitzen et al., 1999). See ∞ Chapter 31 for more about viral diseases, including smallpox. See ∞ Chapter 21 to learn more about *Yersinia pestis*, the cause of plague. The impact of infectious disease was felt not only by the general population, but by famous figures in history as well. Neither royalty nor peasant was immune to microbes.

FAMOUS FIGURES AFFLICTED BY INFECTIOUS DISEASE

Henry the Eighth was afflicted with smallpox and malaria. He also had a leg ulcer that never healed. Some historians think these ulcers were a result of syphilis, but one believed it to be the symptom of osteomyelitis (Lacey, 1998). Henry's daughter, Elizabeth I, raised fears over the matter of succession when she was diagnosed with smallpox and gastroenteritis and became critically ill (Weir, 1998). See ∞ Chapter 30 for more information on malaria. ∞ Chapters 35 and 39 discuss gastroenteritis and osteomyelitis.

> **A Quote in Time**
>
> Ring around the rosy
> A pocketful of posies
> "Ashes, Ashes"
> We all fall down!
>
> This simple nursery rhyme may have been a reference to the signs and symptoms of the plague epidemic during the dark ages.

> **A Quote in Time**
>
> Momento te Esse Mortalum. "Remember You Are Mortal."
> *(Captain William Hutson's tombstone, King's Chapel, Boston 1680)*

The Salem witch trials may have been a result of ergot poisoning. Eating bread and other food made from grain infested with *Claviceps purpurea* results in ingestion of the fungal toxin. The bewitched behavior of the children and young women, making the accusations of witchcraft against others, resembles some of the symptoms associated with the convulsive form of this illness (Kiple, 1997).

George Washington had a mild disfigurement from smallpox. Figure 1-3 ■ illustrates the skin pustules associated with smallpox. Washington died in 1799 after suffering from either tonsillitis or diphtheria (Schwarz, 1999). ∞ Chapter 33 provides more information on these respiratory infections. Table 1-3✪ lists other historical figures afflicted by infectious disease.

Early scientists began to question the origin of these diseases. Their search for answers resulted in the science of microbiology.

► EARLY CLUES OF MICROBIAL EXISTENCE

The invention of the microscope was the catalyst for the development of bacteriology. Until this invention, bacterial organisms were not visible to the naked eye because they were too small. What was visible was rotten food, cloudy liquids, open sores, and unexplained deaths.

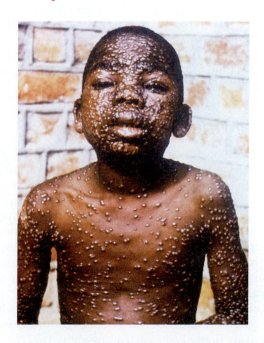

■ **FIGURE 1-3** Smallpox.

✪ TABLE 1-3

Historical Figures and Infectious Diseases

Historical Figure	Significance in History	Infectious Disease
Franklin D. Roosevelt	32nd President of the United States	Polio
William McKinley	25th President of the United States	Gunshot wound infection
Marcus Aurelius	Roman emperor and philosopher in 160 A.D.	Plague of Galen (smallpox?)
Doc Holliday	American gunfighter in the Old West	Tuberculosis
Willie Lincoln	3rd son of Abraham Lincoln	Typhoid fever
Jane Seymour	Queen of England, in the 1500s, and the 3rd wife of Henry the VIII	Purpueral fever
Walter Scott	Scottish author	Polio
Stephen Crane	American author	Tuberculosis
Howard Taylor Rickets	Credited with discovery of the family *Rickettsiaceae*	Typhus

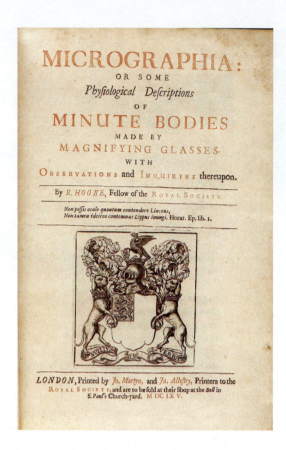

■ **FIGURE 1-4** Robert Hooke's *Micrographia*.
Courtesy of the National Library of Medicine.

EARLY MICROSCOPES

The inventor of the first microscope is unknown, but microscopes were available in the early 1600s. Hans Jansen is usually given credit for the invention in the year 1590. This early microscope contained two lenses in three sliding tubes. It was said to have a magnification of 3× when fully closed and 9× when fully opened. It was 2 inches in diameter and 18 inches long when fully opened (Jones, 1995). Giovanni Faber coined the term *microscope* in 1625. Chérubin d'Orleans designed the first binocular microscope in 1667 (Beck, 2000). The modern microscope is described in ∞ Chapter 8.

ROBERT HOOKE

Robert Hooke had a variety of interests, including physics, mechanics, astronomy, chemistry, geology, and biology. These interests led him to invent telescopes and microscopes. Hooke published a best-seller, *Micrographia* (Figure 1-4 ■), in 1665. It included specific instructions for making a single-lens, hand-held miniature microscope like that used by Antoni van Leeuwenhoek. Hooke also described the first microbe, a fungus or "hairy mould." His description was accompanied by engravings derived from his detailed drawings. The characteristics as depicted resemble *Mucor*.

A later publication, *Microscopium,* in 1678 described his microscopic techniques. A recent discovery of his writings, referred to as "Hooke Folio," dated November 1677, confirmed Leeuwenhoek's findings (Gest, 2007).

ANTONI VAN LEEUWENHOEK

Antoni van Leeuwenhoek (Figure 1-5 ■) was an amateur microscope builder who took up microbiology as a hobby. In 1677 he observed bacteria, which he called "little animals," in water. He is often called the father of microbiology because in 1684 he described the shapes of microscopic organisms seen in tooth scrapings. ∞ Chapter 3 describes microbial shapes observed in today's laboratory. Letters to the Royal Society of London communicated his microscopic observations (Brock, 1989). He did not ponder where these organisms came from or their relationships to disease. It was approximately 200 years before the origins and disease-producing characteristics of microorganisms were described in detail.

THEORY OF SPONTANEOUS GENERATION

For two centuries, scientists believed that microscopic forms of life arose spontaneously from nonliving material. This theory of spontaneous generation was upheld by the observation that broth left in an open container for over 24 hours developed a cloudy appearance.

Lazaro Spallanzani in 1799 designed a series of experiments in which he demonstrated that some microbes are more

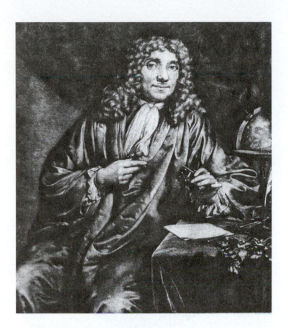

■ **FIGURE 1-5** Antoni van Leeuwenhoek/
Jan Verkolje pinx. 1686.
Courtesy of the National Library of Medicine.

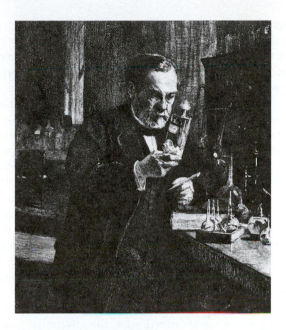

■ **FIGURE 1-6** Louis Pasteur.
Courtesy of the National Library of Medicine.

sensitive to heat than others and are easily killed. Some hardy microbes required boiling for at least one hour before they were killed. Spallanzani also demonstrated that the numbers of microbes in the broth were proportional to the size of the openings in the stoppers used to close the flasks. He theorized that either germs in the air reseeded the mixture after boiling or the air enhanced the growth of germs that remained after boiling. Spallanzani's work provided a framework for Louis Pasteur's experiments related to spontaneous generation (Brock, 1989).

Louis Pasteur

Louis Pasteur, a French chemist (Figure 1-6 ■), believed that microorganisms occurred on dust particles in the air. When these microbe-covered particles fell into broth, they reproduced rapidly, which caused the broth to appear cloudy. Pasteur designed an experiment to test this hypothesis.

Theory Disproved. To prove his hypothesis, Pasteur heated a broth to destroy the microbes and then plugged the opening of the flask with cotton. This exposed the broth to air but trapped any dust particles in the cotton. After several days at room temperature, the broth was free of **contamination** and remained clear. Pasteur found that contamination introduces microorganisms into a body site or onto a surface that previously did not contain the microorganism. This disproved the theory of spontaneous generation and proved that life must arise from preexisting life. Pasteur's experimental finding was published in 1861 (Brock, 1989). Pasteur's ability to sterilize liquid and prevent aerial contamination by microbes paved the way for future exploration of infectious disease causes.

✓ **Checkpoint! 1–1
(Chapter Objective 1)**

Which of the following men disproved, by experimentation, the theory of spontaneous generation?

    A. Antoni van Leeuwenhoek
    B. Robert Koch
    C. Joseph Lister
    D. Louis Pasteur

► LINKING MICROBES TO DISEASE

GERM THEORIES

Before his work on spontaneous generation, Pasteur developed the germ theory of fermentation. His study of the crystalline structure of chemicals using **crystallographics** led him to study the process of fermentation. The crystalline structures were **derivatives**, or chemical compounds produced from another compound, of the amyl alcohols. He published his first paper on fermentation in 1857 (Brock, 1989). Before his work, the theory of Justis Liebig was widely accepted. Liebig believed that fermentation was the result of adding a decaying substance (a ferment) to a fermentable substrate, which caused the substance to decay. He believed that fermentation was the origin of contagious disease. However, Liebig did not back up his theory with experimental evidence. Pasteur designed experiments to solve the problem of "sour" wine. He created fermentable material using yeast water, sugar, and chalk. To this mixture he added some of the gray substance that forms during alcoholic fermentation. The day after Pasteur added the gray substance, he observed evidence of fermentation and identified the principal product of fermentation as lactic acid. Under the microscope he observed organisms and became convinced that these organisms caused the fermentation. This theory—that a microbe will produce a specific change in the substance on which it grows—is the underlying principle of biochemical testing used to identify unknown microorganisms today and is known as the germ theory of fermentation. To learn more about the biochemicals used in modern laboratories, see ∞ Chapter 9. Pasteur later recommended heating the wine slightly, just below boiling, to prevent formation of this organism-containing material. This technique became known as **pasteurization,** which involves heating a liquid to a temperature that destroys bacteria (not spores) but doesn't change the liquid, and then cooling the liquid for storage.

Pasteur's work on the germ theory of fermentation, spontaneous generation, and silkworm diseases (his recommendations of ways to identify healthy silkworms helped restore silk production in France) led other scientists to consider that microorganisms could cause disease through similar processes. Pasteur also contributed to the germ theory of disease, which proposes that a specific infectious disease is caused by a specific type of microorganism. In 1862 Pasteur published a paper supporting the germ theory of disease. His later discoveries of bacteria and his work with vaccines also lent support to the germ theory of disease. Pasteur regularly advised prevention of the introduction of organisms as a way to control the microbes' effects. This is the basis of asepsis and sterilization. Table 1-4✪ lists the dates of discovery of some of the microorganisms covered in this text.

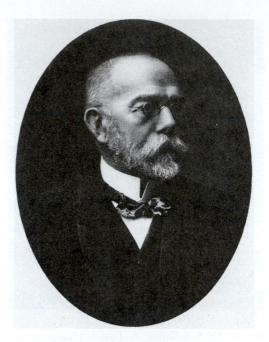

■ **FIGURE 1-7** Robert Koch.
Courtesy of the National Library of Medicine.

In 1876 a German physician named Robert Koch (Figure 1-7 ■) published the results of his work with the bacillus of anthrax (Brock, 1989). He inoculated mice with the bacillus and its spores. He observed the spore-forming bacillus in microscopic preparations of the animals' blood and spleen. He also observed the formation of bacilli from spores alone. He observed the development of anthrax symptoms and ultimately death when using a pure culture of *Bacillus anthracis*. He concluded that only this species of *Bacillus* was capable of causing this disease. This finding provided the first proof that the germ theory of disease was valid. In the previous year Ferdinand Cohn had coined the term *bacillus* and proved the heat resistance of spore-forming bacilli. Koch's experiment also confirmed Cohn's results.

SOLID MEDIA

By 1881, Koch had switched his attention to tuberculosis (Brock, 1989). From this work refinement in bacteriological techniques resulted. Koch was frustrated working with liquid cultures and recognized the importance of **pure cultures,** or isolation of a single organism. He initially tried potato slices as a medium for growing bacteria but learned that not all pathogenic bacteria would grow. He developed a solid medium by adding gelatin to the liquid broth. This liquid broth was poured onto plates, into tubes, and onto microscope slides and the gelatin present allowed it to solidify for study. Koch succeeded in gaining growth of colonies. Unfortunately, this medium could not be incubated at temperatures higher than 30°C because it would liquefy. Fannie Hesse, the wife of one of Koch's laboratory assistants, suggested the use of agar, a gelatinous material obtained from seaweed, as a solidifying

✪ TABLE 1-4

Select Infectious Agents and Their Dates of Discovery

Year	Microorganism	Discoverer
1876	*Bacillus anthracis*	Robert Koch
1879	*Neisseria gonorrhoeae*	Albert Neisser
1880	*Staphylococcus, Streptococcus, Pneumococcus*	Louis Pasteur
1882	*Mycobacterium tuberculosis*	Robert Koch
1883	*Corynebacterium diphtheriae*	Edward Klebs, Fredrick Loeffler
1892	*Clostridium perfringens*	William Welch, George Nuttal
1894	*Yersinia pestis*	Émile John Yersin, S. Kitasato
1900	*Coccidioides immitis*	W. Ophuls, H.C. Moffett
1903	*Leishmania donovani*	William Leishman
1905	*Treponema pallidum*	Fritz R. Schandinn, Erich Hoffman
1918	*Brucella abortus*	Alice Evans
1977	*Legionella pneumophila*	Joseph McDade, Charles Shepard
1982	Prions	Stanley Prusiner

agent for culture media. She had used it with jams and jellies following a recipe passed from her mother. Agar quickly replaced gelatin because agar remained solid at higher temperatures. Tables 7-1 and 7-2 in ∞ Chapter 7 lists examples of ingredients used in today's media.

KOCH'S POSTULATES

In 1882, as a result of experiments defining the etiology of anthrax and tuberculosis, Koch outlined the steps needed to prove that a specific organism caused an infectious disease (Ochoa & Corey, 1997). These became known as Koch's postulates, and they are as follows:

- The same organism must be found in all cases of a given disease;
- The organism must be isolated and grown in pure culture from the infected host;
- The organism, from pure culture, must reproduce the disease when inoculated into a susceptible animal; and
- The organism must be isolated in pure culture from an experimentally infected animal.

DEVELOPMENT OF ADDITIONAL TOOLS

In 1887 Richard Julius Petri improved on Koch's culture technique by replacing the glass plates covered with a bell jar with a double dish. The upper dish was slightly larger and served as a lid to cover the culture medium (Brock, 1989). This modification, called the petri dish, is still used today.

The contributions of Hans Christian Gram and Paul Ehrlich in the development of staining methods made it easier to see microbes. Paul Ehrlich developed the acid-fast stain in 1882 (Brock, 1989). He wanted to evaluate Koch's work with the tubercle bacilli for its use in diagnosis and treatment. Unfortunately, Koch's staining method required 24 hours. By using a different dye and acid as a decolorizer, Ehrlich sped up the procedure to between 45 and 60 minutes. He noted the resistance of this organism to acid and recognized the possible negative implications for the use of acid for disinfection and sterilization. Ehrlich's experiment was the first time a staining procedure used the acid-fast property of tubercle bacilli to help characterize them. The current method of acid-fast staining uses the same principle but different reagents.

Hans Christian Gram developed the Gram stain in 1884 (Brock, 1989). Gram wanted to be able to visualize bacteria in tissue. The method he developed not only provided that capability but also allowed for differentiation of bacteria not decolorized by alcohol from those that were decolorized. ∞ Chapter 3, "The Bacterial Cell," discusses the role of bacterial cell structure in the staining reaction. ∞ Chapter 8 describes the use of the Gram stain in presumptive identification of microorganisms. Both the Gram stain and acid-fast stain procedures

are still used today for the same purpose as originally conceived: visualizing infectious agents.

Unfortunately, these stains do not help us see viruses, so they were not much help to scientists investigating a plant disease affecting the tobacco crop, tobacco mosaic disease. The search for the cause of tobacco mosaic disease is described in the next subsection.

VIROLOGY

Tobacco mosaic disease is named for the pattern of disease it forms on tobacco plant leaves: a patchwork of light and dark areas resembling a mosaic. The plants eventually grow smaller and do not produce as much tobacco as do healthy plants (Zaitlin, 1999). The search for the cause of this disease led to the discovery of a new kind of microbe: viruses.

The first person to think that tobacco mosaic disease may have an infectious cause was Adolf Mayer in 1882 (Beck, 2000). He named the disease but was unable to isolate the causative organism. The scientist usually credited with discovering the cause of tobacco mosaic disease published his paper 10 years after Mayer proposed the disease cause.

Dmitri Ivanowski

Dmitri Ivanowski, a Russian scientist, passed the agent of tobacco mosaic disease through a filter that was believed to block the passage of bacteria. Ivanowski referred to the agent, or filtrate, as "contagium vivum fixum," or a cellular infectious agent, but didn't realize that this is a unique organism and not a bacterium. He published a paper in 1892 describing evidence of the ability of this filtrate to grow on tobacco leaves and cause the disease in healthy, new plants (Beck, 2000).

Martinus Beijerinck

In 1899, a scientist from the Netherlands, Martinus Beijerinck, recognized that a filtrate free of bacteria could still cause disease in plants. He called this agent "contagium vivum fluidum," meaning "contagious living fluid" (Brock, 1989). Many believe that this is how the term *virus* was coined. Beijerinck's insight into the nature of this new organism is astounding. He recognized that it was stable and required cell division for reproduction. He suggested that this reproductive process requires incorporation into the cell's protoplasm.

Wendell M. Stanley

It wasn't until 1935 that the virus that causes tobacco mosaic disease was isolated. An American scientist named Wendell M. Stanley crystallized a protein from tobacco plant juice prepared from plants infected with the disease. The crystallized protein not only caused typical disease but was about 1000 times more active than the juice alone (Brock, 1989). The protein's ability to invade and cause disease is known as **infectivity**.

The search for new organisms as agents of emerging diseases continues today. See ∞ Chapter 42 for information on emerging diseases. Knowledge of infectious agents and their association with specific diseases led to efforts to control these microbes.

Checkpoint! 1–2
(Chapter Objective 2)

The germ theory of fermentation states the following:
 A. *A specific disease is caused by a specific type of micro-organism.*
 B. *The same organism must be found in all cases of a given disease.*
 C. *Organisms from pure culture must reproduce the disease in a susceptible animal.*
 D. *A specific microbe produces a specific change in the substance on which it grows.*

Checkpoint! 1–3
(Chapter Objective 1)

The sequence of isolation, reinfection, and recovery of an infectious agent was developed by:
 A. *Louis Pasteur.*
 B. *Robert Koch.*
 C. *Edward Jenner.*
 D. *Joseph Lister.*

▶ EARLY EFFORTS TO CONTROL MICROORGANISMS

For nearly 100 years, the major focus of disease control was prevention of infection. Absence of infectious disease resulted from cleanliness and resistance to disease.

ANTISEPSIS

In the mid-1800s, American and European physicians concluded that doctors who handled patients in one ward were sources of infection for patients in other wards. It was suggested that physicians should wash their hands before handling patients. Most physicians, who refused to believe that they were unclean, did not embrace this practice. Two individuals are credited with providing evidence that preventing microbial contamination would reduce the rate of death: Ignaz Semmelweis and Joseph Lister.

Ignaz P. Semmelweis

Semmelweis was a physician who based his change in standard practice on personal observation. Puerperal fever was a terrible disease that took the lives of new mothers shortly after the birth of their child. Doctor Semmelweis supervised two maternity clinics. Midwives staffed one clinic, and the other clinic was used for obstetrics instruction. The one used for instruction had a death rate four times that of the other clinic. Doctor Semmelweis theorized that the student obstetricians, who did not wash their hands after leaving one childbirth and attending to another, were transferring these disease agents to mothers during childbirth from one mother to another. Semmelweis advocated the simple practice of washing hands with a chloride of lime solution between patients. The death rate subsequently plummeted. Semmelweis shared this finding with his colleagues at a lecture in 1850. However, despite clear evidence that the incidence of puerperal fever had declined in his patients, many physicians refused to change their practice and despised and hated Semmelweis because his finding suggested that they were unclean and were carriers of disease (Brock, 1989).

Joseph Lister

Joseph Lister was a British surgeon who recognized the importance of Pasteur's work on the germ theory of disease (Figure 1-8 ■). Lister suggested that open wound infections in patients were due to germs in the air around the patient. He began to spray carbolic acid in the air around his patients before surgery (Barba, 1999). This procedure, described in a paper in 1867, drastically reduced the number of deaths and laid the foundation for modern-day aseptic surgery (Brock, 1989).

The concept of preventing contamination was a significant step in the practice of medicine; however, exposure to infectious agents could not always be controlled by antiseptic methods. For many years, scientists had observed that people who

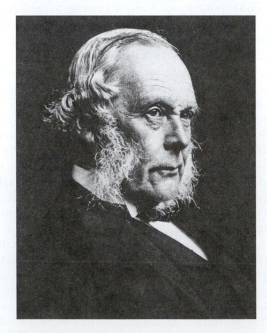

■ FIGURE 1-8 Joseph Lister.
Photo by R. A. Bickersteth. Courtesy of the National Library of Medicine.

recovered from a disease did not "catch" it again. Thus, methods that used the natural defenses of the body were developed to prevent infection.

VACCINATION

Since antiquity, smallpox has caused countless deaths and scarring. For centuries, **inoculation**, or introducing into a body the microorganism that causes a disease, was practiced in the Far East but was known to have complications. For example, sometimes people either didn't develop disease or the disease was so severe that complications of a disease (**morbidity**) or death during a specific time period (**mortality**) resulted.

Edward Jenner

In 1774, Benjamin Jesty was the first person to use cowpox to protect against smallpox. Jesty scratched pus-like material he obtained from a cow udder lesion into his family members' arms. The family later survived a smallpox epidemic (Beck, 2000). Edward Jenner, in 1796, was the first scientist to prove the validity of the procedure. He tested the observation that milkmaids infected with a mild variety of pox called cowpox did not get smallpox. He inserted cowpox into a boy's arm by making two small incisions. The boy did not develop smallpox. This and many other observations of the effectiveness of this procedure were published in his book, *An Inquiry into the Causes and Effects of the Variolae Vaccinae*, in 1798 (Brock, 1989). Many scientists consider this the first vaccination (vacca = cow) and refer to Jenner as the father of immunology.

Louis Pasteur

In 1880 and 1881, while working with the diseases fowl cholera and anthrax, Pasteur discovered that bacterial cultures could be rendered "nonvirulent" in the laboratory (Brock, 1989). Pasteur used the term **attenuated** to describe these weakened strains of microorganisms that were unable to cause disease. He injected these attenuated cultures into animals and discovered that the animals survived. He then injected the same animals with **virulent** cultures, deadly organisms that can overcome and break down a host's defenses, and he discovered once more that the animals did not die. He concluded that he had discovered a vaccine that differed from that designed by Jenner by incorporating a microscopic organism into the vaccine. Pasteur wrote, "In the vaccine of Jenner, no organism has been recognized so far" (Brock, 1989). Pasteur went on to work with vaccines and later developed a vaccine for rabies.

As important as vaccination is for controlling many infectious diseases, the body still needs time to respond to the vaccine. ∞ Chapter 4 provides details on the immune response. Were it not for the discovery of antibiotics, humankind would be susceptible to every **acute** infection, which is a severe disease process that occurs within a short time period.

CHEMOTHERAPY

For many years, doctors attempted to treat infectious diseases with chemicals. For example, syphilis was treated with mercury and arsenic; malaria was treated with quinine made from the bark of a tree. Many of these agents were toxic and caused patients' deaths. They were also not directed at a specific microorganism. Paul Ehrlich was the first to demonstrate the effectiveness of a specific chemical against a bacterial disease.

Paul Ehrlich

In the late 1800s, Paul Ehrlich (Figure 1-9 ■) published his work related to staining of cells, tissues, and bacteria. He also contributed to the field of immunology with his work on hemolysins, antitoxins, and the standardization of sera used for therapy. In 1897, he switched his attention to **chemotherapy**, the treatment of disease with a chemical. He started out searching for a chemical that could effectively treat sleeping sickness, a disease caused by a trypanosome parasite. He discovered that an arsenic compound called atoxyl worked well but was poisonous. He began to manipulate the atoxyl compound, looking for a compound that would be effective yet not harm the host. After testing 900 different compounds, he still hadn't found one. Ehrlich had his new colleague, Sahachiro Hata, test all of these arsenic compounds against the newly discovered microbe that caused syphilis. Number 606 completely cured all tested animals. Compound 606 was released as Salvarsan in 1910 and was sold worldwide. Germany, Ehrlich's home nation, became a leader in drug production, and syphilis became a curable disease. Ehrlich inspired other scientists to seek new drugs for treating infections (WGBH, 1998b).

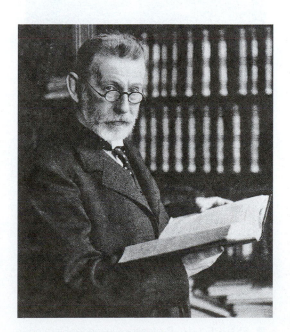

■ **FIGURE 1-9** Paul Ehrlich.
Courtesy of the National Library of Medicine.

Alexander Fleming

The discovery of penicillin was accidental in nature. Alexander Fleming (Figure 1-10) was not noted for his neatness. He was a busy man and tended to allow things to accumulate. One day in 1928, while going through a pile of old culture plates before discarding them, he noticed that *Staphylococcus* growth was inhibited by a fungal contaminant. He became curious and began to investigate. He identified the fungi as *Penicillium notatum* (WGBH, 1998a). He tested the *Staphylococcus* against other fungi but did not observe the same inhibitory effect. He also tested the fungi contaminant against other bacteria and found that it inhibited the category of bacteria known as gram positive better than those categorized as gram negative. See ∞ Chapter 8 for a discussion of the Gram stain. He also applied the contaminant to one-half of the surface of media to help select for desired organisms when processing a respiratory specimen (Brock, 1989). He presented a paper on his discovery in 1929, but it was not until World War II that any further development occurred.

In 1940 Howard Florey began clinical trials using penicillin purified by Ernst Chain. American and British troops used penicillin during World War II to prevent battlefield infections (Beck, 2000).

A Quote in Time

Alexander Fleming said, "One sometimes finds what one is not looking for."

(WGBH, 1998a

Although the puzzle of treating and preventing infectious disease was almost complete by World War II, there was still one piece missing, one more means of acquiring an infectious agent.

✓ Checkpoint 1–4 (Chapter Objective 1)

Sir Alexander Fleming:
    A. *discovered penicillin, the first antibiotic.*
    B. *developed a vaccine for smallpox.*
    C. *disproved the theory of spontaneous generation.*
    D. *proved the germ theory of disease.*

VECTOR CONTROL

In 1893, Theobald Smith and F. I. Kilbourne proved that ticks carry *Babesia microti*. Ticks transmit this organism to both animals and humans via their bite and cause babesiosis. Smith and Kilbourne provided the first description of a zoonosis and stimulated other scientists to search for additional insect carriers of disease (Baker et. al., 1999).

Major Walter Reed

In 1900, Major Walter Reed, a U.S. Army surgeon (Figure 1-11), was assigned to a team to find the cause of yellow fever. This disease killed more soldiers in the Spanish American War than were killed by the enemy. This loss of life mobilized the army to find the cause of yellow fever. There was a theory at the time that yellow fever was caused by a bacillus in

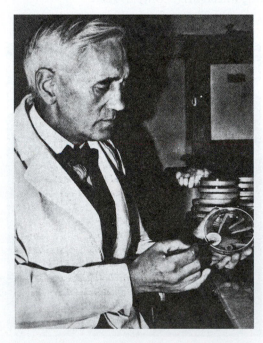

■ **FIGURE 1-10** Professor Alexander Fleming: discoverer of penicillin.
Courtesy of the National Library of Medicine.

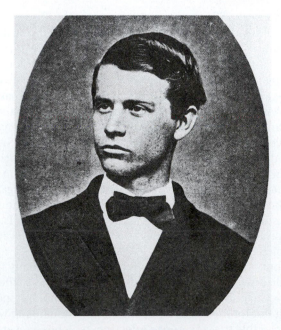

■ **FIGURE 1-11** Walter Reed in 1874.
Courtesy of the National Library of Medicine.

the hog-cholera group. Major Reed disproved that theory and then investigated another theory proposed by the Cuban physician and scientist, Dr. Carlos Juan Finlay. Finlay believed that a house mosquito carried yellow fever. Most scientists scoffed at him because even after some 100 experimental inoculations, there were no documented cases of yellow fever.

While the team was performing research in Cuba, Reed observed that it took two to three weeks for the first case of yellow fever to produce a second case. He suspected the cause of the disease was the mosquito as originally proposed by Finlay. Members of Dr. Reed's team voluntarily consented to be bitten by mosquitoes and subsequently developed the disease. Two survived and one, Dr. Jesse W. Lazear, who was in charge of the experimental mosquitoes, did not. Lazear's laboratory notes provided the key for Reed. The notes revealed that development and transmission of yellow fever involved the following scenario: A mosquito had to bite a yellow fever patient during the first 3 day of illness, and thereafter it took 12 days for the disease agent to develop in the mosquito and migrate to the mosquito's salivary gland.

Reed devised an experiment to prove that the mosquito was in fact the intermediate carrier. Two buildings were constructed. One was the "Infected Clothing Building," where volunteers spent 20 nights sleeping on sheets and pillows soiled with the blood and vomit of yellow fever victims. Not one volunteer contracted the disease. The second building, the "Infected Mosquito Building," was divided into two areas: one side with screens on the windows and no screens on the other side. The volunteers in the unscreened portion of the building, who were bitten by the mosquitoes, developed the disease. Those who were separated from the mosquitoes and protected by the screens did not develop the disease. This was the proof Reed needed. Throughout Cuba, mosquito breeding places were eliminated and homes were screened. There were no more urban epidemics of yellow fever. The scourge of yellow fever had stopped construction of the Panama Canal. Mosquito control enabled construction on the Canal to be completed. In the early 1900s, one of Major Reed's associates, Dr. James Carroll, proved that the agent that caused yellow fever in humans was a filterable virus so tiny it passed through a fine pore filter which usually trapped bacteria (Baz, no date).

Microbiology practice didn't change dramatically for about 100 years after development of techniques in the golden age of bacteriology (mid 1800s). New microorganisms continued to be discovered; new media, biochemical tests, and susceptibility methods were developed. However, the fundamental techniques continued to be used. Control methods remained the same, although the arsenal of chemotherapeutic agents increased. The groundwork for a change in methods occurred in the 1950s, when science turned its attention to the molecular world of genes and lay the foundation for modern-day **genomic** discoveries (*genomic* pertains to the complete genetic blueprint of a living organism).

▶ SOLVING THE DNA PUZZLE

The origin of molecular microbiology is in Gregor Mendel's work with peas. Mendel researched invisible "factors" (named genes in 1902), which he proposed were responsible for visible characteristics. He presented his work in 1865 and was ignored until it was rediscovered in 1900 (Terry, 2001). For the next 20 years, research revolved around chromosomes; then attention shifted to DNA.

THE DNA MOLECULE

Phoebus Levene discovered deoxyribonucleic acid (DNA) in 1929. In the 1930s, scientists used x-ray crystallography to study protein and the DNA molecule. In 1944, Oswald Theodore Avery, Colin MacLeod, and Maclyn McCarty suggested that DNA was the material that carried genetic information. Many scientists of the time were skeptical and believed the molecule was too simple for this function (Terry, 2001). By the late 1940s, the scientific community accepted that DNA is the genetic molecule, and the race was on to discover its structure and how it works.

James Watson and Francis Crick

In 1948, Linus Pauling discovered that many proteins are helical in shape and resemble a spring coil (WGBH, 1998c). James Watson and Francis Crick were impressed by this work and began to make physical models of DNA that reflected a helical structure. At the same time, another team of scientists, Maurice Wilkins and Rosalind Franklin (Figure 1-12 ■), were studying the DNA molecule using **x-ray diffraction** images,

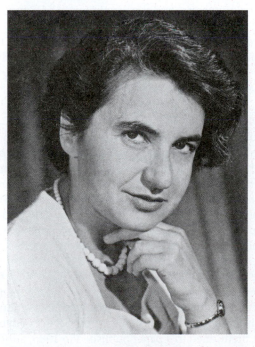

■ **FIGURE 1-12** Rosalind Franklin.
Courtesy of the National Library of Medicine.

which depend on the ability of a substance to break ionizing electromagnetic radiation into smaller pieces. Watson attended one of Franklin's lectures in 1951 in which she presented her work to date. She had found that DNA existed in two forms and deduced that the phosphate part of the molecule was on the outside. She also thought that the DNA molecule was a double helix, but she didn't believe she had enough evidence yet to publish her results. Wilkins showed one of Franklin's pictures to Watson, and it provided him with "several of the vital helical parameters" (Wright, 2001). Crick had just learned of Erwin Chargaff's findings, in the summer of 1952, regarding base pairs, which are nucleotides located on opposite complementary strands of DNA and held together by a hydrogen bond. Building on what Watson and Crick knew, they built a model of DNA and in 1953 proposed that the structure of DNA consists of two chains of nucleic acids, in the shape of a double helix, with the nucleotide bases on the inside (Beck, 2000). The scientific community immediately accepted Watson and Crick's model.

After that the function of DNA was discovered, the genetic code was broken, and scientists learned how to manipulate DNA and introduce genetic material into bacteria. It wasn't until the 1980s, however, that the tools necessary to determine genomes were developed.

POLYMERASE CHAIN REACTION

Scientists were using electrophoresis to separate molecules, and they stained the gels to make the bands more visible. In 1977, Fredrick Sanger sequenced phage DNA using restriction enzymes (Beck, 2000). Future development of molecular tools stalled until the discovery and availability of various enzymes, like DNA polymerase, and the development of computer technology.

One difficulty encountered when working with DNA, was the limited number of available molecules. The polymerase chain reaction (PCR) transformed molecular biology because it provided a means to get more copies of DNA.

Kary Mullis

Kary Mullis (Figure 1-13 ■) is an eccentric scientist who admits that the idea for PCR came to him as he was driving on a California highway to his mountain cabin in 1983 (The Nobel Foundation, 2000). The PCR procedure uses a mixture of two short, complementary strands of nucleotides to bind to a specific region of the target DNA. The four deoxynucleoside triphosphates (adenine, thymine, guanine, and cytosine) and DNA polymerase polymerize, or synthesize, a new DNA strand, which complements the target DNA. PCR uses heat to denature the target DNA into individual strands. When the temperature is lowered, a copy of each strand of the targeted DNA sequence is generated. The procedure is repeated many times, generating multiple copies of the target DNA sequence. PCR was first mentioned in a paper published in 1985, although the specific procedure was not described. In 1987 the procedure for

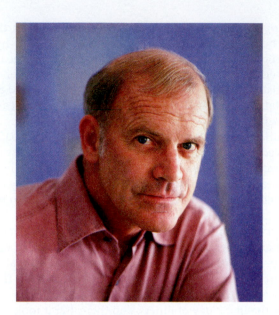

■ **FIGURE 1-13** Kary Mullis.
Photo by Mark Robert Halper.

amplifying a nucleic acid sequence of DNA was described by Mullis and Fred A. Faloona. The heat destroyed the early DNA polymerase used in the procedure during the denaturation step. DNA polymerase had to be added each time the procedure was repeated. In 1988 a thermophilic bacterium called *Thermus aquaticus* provided a heat-stable DNA polymerase (Taq polymerase) that improved the procedure and paved the way for automation (Beck, 2000).

Other tools for studying and analyzing DNA were developed in the 1980s. Procedures for genetic fingerprinting were developed by Alec Jeffries and were used for the first time in a British courtroom in 1985. An automated DNA sequencer using fluorescence was invented. A method for expressing large proteins using yeast artificial chromosomes (YACs) became available (Terry, 2001). See ∞ Chapter 9 for information on current molecular laboratory methods. The world of molecular biology was now ready to take the next step, to map and determine the genetic sequence for each living organism.

GENOME PROJECTS

In 1989 James Watson was named to head the National Center for Human Genome Research, and the Human Genome Project was launched (Terry, 2001). Other projects aimed at mapping the gene sequence of the earthworm, fruit fly, and various microorganisms were begun. In 1995 The Institute for Genomic Research (TIGR) published the genomic sequence for *Haemophilus influenzae*. This was the first complete microbial sequence published. Forty-two microbial genomes have been published since then, and more then 100 are being worked on (Nelson, Paulen, & Fraser, 2001).

The data generated from these sequencing activities spurred the development of new fields of study, such as bioinformatics and proteonomics. **Bioinformatics** is the use of computers to help make sense of accumulated biological information and was developed in response to the need to analyze vast amounts of data. **Proteonomics**, the study of proteins derived from a gene, was developed to examine the kinds of proteins produced by each gene. The first gene chip was developed in 1997 and used a combination of computer technology, PCR, and DNA chips (Terry, 2001).

New methods for medical diagnosis have also resulted. Viral loads can be monitored by assessing the amount of viral messenger RNA (mRNA) present. Fastidious and slow-growing organisms are now detected quickly using molecular techniques. Clinically relevant information provided rapidly to physicians will foster early detection and treatment of disease, lower health care costs, and decrease morbidity and mortality.

> ✓ **Checkpoint! 1–5 (Chapter Objective 1)**
>
> *The scientist who developed the procedure for the polymerase chain reaction (PCR) is:*
>   A. *James Watson.*
>   B. *Kary Mullis.*
>   C. *Francis Crick.*
>   D. *Fredrick Sanger.*

SUMMARY

In ancient times humans believed disease was caused by evil spirits. In 1677, Antoni van Leeuwenhoek used an early microscope to observe "little animals." Scientists of the day began to experiment and publish their observations. Table 1-5 summarizes key events in the development of medical microbiology.

✪ TABLE 1-5

Key Events in the Development of Medical Microbiology

Date	Development	Scientist
1665	First published description of a microbe	Robert Hooke
c. 1677	Observation of "little animals"	Antoni van Leeuwenhoek
1796	First scientifically validated smallpox vaccination	Edward Jenner
1850	Handwashing advocated to prevent spread of disease	Ignaz Semmelweis
1862	Paper published supporting the germ theory of disease	Louis Pasteur
1861	Spontaneous generation disproved	Louis Pasteur
1867	Antiseptic surgery practiced	Joseph Lister
1876	First proof of germ theory of disease with *B. anthracis* discovery	Robert Koch
1881	Bacteria grown on solid media	Robert Koch
1882	Koch's postulates outlined	Robert Koch
	Acid-fast stain developed	Paul Ehrlich
1884	Gram stain developed	Hans Christian Gram
1885	First rabies vaccination	Louis Pasteur
1887	Petri dish invented	Richard J. Petri
1892	Viruses discovered	Dmitri Iosifovich Ivanovski
1893	First description of zoonosis	T. Smith, F. I. Kilbourne
1899	Recognition of viral dependence on cells for reproduction	Martinus Beijerinck
1900	Proof that mosquitoes carry the yellow fever agent	Walter Reed
1910	Cure for syphilis discovered	Paul Ehrlich
1928	Penicillin discovered	Alexander Fleming
1953	Model of DNA proposed and built	J. Watson, F. Crick
1977	DNA sequencing method developed	W. Gilbert, F. Sanger
1983	Polymerase chain reaction invented	Kary Mullis
1995	First microbial genomic sequence published	The Institute for Genomic Research (TIGR)

Theories related to spontaneous generation of life and germs that caused disease were investigated in the early 1800s. Spontaneous generation was disproved, and the germ theory of infectious disease was proven in the mid 1800s. Efforts at controlling infections were attempted and successful, although the recommended practices were not always immediately accepted. New microorganisms were discovered as microbiological techniques were developed. The 1800s are often called the golden age of microbiology. The laboratory methods developed in the 1800s for detecting clinically relevant microbes endured for 100 years. The 1900s ushered in the use of chemotherapy to control infectious disease and the development of molecular diagnostic methods.

Today's microbiology laboratory is an eclectic mixture of traditional techniques developed in the late 1800s and the newer molecular methods. No one knows what the future will bring, but microbiology continues to be an exciting field of study.

LEARNING OPPORTUNITIES

1. On the Web (Chapter Objectives 1 and 5)

   Visit "Microbiology Timeline: Significant Events of the Last 125 Years" at http://www.asm.org/MemberShip/ index.asp?bid=16731 and review contributions made by individuals to the field of microbiology.

   Visit "The Faces of Science: African Americans in the Sciences" at https://webfiles.uci.edu/mcbrown/display/faces.html and learn about William Hinton's contribution to syphilis diagnostic testing.

   Visit "Secrets of the Dead: Crime Scene Investigations Meet History" at http://www.pbs.org/wnet/secrets/index.html. Explore the cases archive for titles such as The Mystery of the Black Death, Killer Flu, The Syphilis Enigma and Witches Curse

2. How can Koch's postulates be applied to current emerging disease investigations? (Chapter Objectives 4 and 5)

3. Take the crossword challenge on the Companion Website to check your Micro History IQ. (Chapter Objectives 1, 3, and 5)

CASE STUDY 1-1. IMPORTED PLAGUE: NEW YORK CITY, 2002 (CHAPTER OBJECTIVES 3, 5, AND 6)

Patients: 53-year-old man named Marvin and his 47-year-old wife, Mabel.

Admitting diagnosis: Marvin was diagnosed with septicemic plague, acute renal failure, acute respiratory distress syndrome, and disseminated intravascular coagulation (DIC). Mabel was diagnosed with bubonic plague.

Background: The married couple traveled from Santa Fe County, New Mexico, to New York City, where they both became ill with fever and unilateral inguinal adenopathy. Mabel was admitted and treated with antibiotics. She recovered without complications. Marvin required hemodialysis and mechanical ventilation. Both his feet were amputated. He was discharged to a long-term-care rehabilitation facility.

The couple reported that routine surveillance conducted by the New Mexico Department of Health had identified *Yersinia pestis* in a dead wood rat and fleas collected in July 2002 on their New Mexico property.

Clinical Laboratory Results

	Husband	Wife	Reference Ranges
White blood cell (WBC) count	24,700/µL (microliter)	9,500/µL	4,300–10,800/µL
Platelet count	72,000/µL	189,000/µL	130,000–400,000/µL
Blood cultures	Positive for *Yersinia pestis*	Negative	Negative
Antibodies to *Yersinia pestis*	Positive	Positive	Negative
Polymerase chain reaction	Positive for *Yersinia pestis*	Not done	

Public Health Laboratory Results

Fleas were harvested from rodents on the couple's property. The fleas were cultured for *Yersinia pestis*. Molecular testing was performed on the husband's isolate and the flea isolates. The molecular test pattern of the husband and flea isolates was indistinguishable (CDC, 2003).

1. What is the possible source of *Yersinia pestis* in this couple? What control measures should be implemented?

2. How are the germ theory of disease and Koch's postulates related to this case?

3. What year was the cause of plague discovered? In what year was culturing on solid media reported? In what year was the polymerase chain reaction discovered? How do these discoveries relate to the laboratory tests performed in this case?

4. What is the historical role of *Yersinia pestis*?

PEARSON
myhealthprofessionskit™

Use this address to access the interactive Companion Website created for this textbook. Simply select "Clinical Laboratory Science" from the choice of disciplines. Find this book and log in using your user name and password.

REFERENCES

Go to myhealthprofessionskit.com to view this chapter's references.

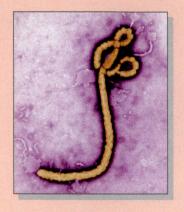

CHAPTER OUTLINE

2

Taxonomy and Classification

Lora M. Green and Brandon M. Bianski

■ LEARNING OBJECTIVES

Upon completion of this chapter, the learner should be able to:

1. Justify the importance of maintaining the taxonomic classification of plants, animals, and microorganisms.
2. Identify and relate the basic principles and approaches associated with the current taxonomic classification.
3. Describe the basic history and important events associated with taxonomic classification.
4. Identify the key individuals, along with their contributions, who helped shape the field of taxonomy.
5. Diagram the hierarchical arrangement of taxa used to classify microorganisms.
6. Explain the reasoning behind the separation of kingdoms.
7. Name the members of the six-kingdom classification system and list examples of organisms that belong to each kingdom that contains microorganisms.
8. State the definition for the terms *saprophytes* and *pathogenic.*
9. Identify and describe the factors and agents, along with their characteristics, that affect the ability of microorganisms to infect a host.
10. Compare and contrast the cellular characteristics of viruses, bacteria, fungi, and parasites.

KEY TERMS

anamorph	mutation	pathogenic
binomial	mutualism	prokaryote
dioecious	neotype	saprophytes
divergent evolution	nomenclature	schizogony
epigenetic	obligate	sporangiospore
eukaryote	opportunistic	trophozoite
hapten	parasitism	virion (virus)
hybridization		

▶ INTRODUCTION

The accurate categorization of the millions of organisms that inhabit every niche on the earth is a daunting task. The objective of taxonomy is to classify biological entities down to the unit (species) level and to devise a systematic scheme, or taxa, for cataloging these units. To write a chapter on taxonomic classification that represents a totally unique approach to the subject is nearly impossible. Nevertheless, we will try to present the information in an easy-to-read, logical format that discusses the importance, historical contributions, and rules governing taxonomic classification. Although, this textbook focuses on medically relevant microorganisms, the basics of taxonomic classification require a broader understanding of the subject, and therefore this chapter includes such general information. Whenever possible, medically relevant examples are used to illustrate particular points. After covering the basic issues of taxonomic classification, separate sections in this chapter briefly discuss issues specific to classifying viruses, bacteria, fungi, and animal parasites. To classify organisms, they must be identified and given names (**nomenclature**). Both identification and nomenclature involve systematic approaches and rules. The rules governing these approaches will be covered, and useful literature citations and websites pertaining to taxonomic classification are noted at the end of this chapter. Subsequent chapters in this book include specific details on taxonomy, identification, and nomenclature for medically important microorganisms organized into functional groupings.

▶ THE NEED FOR A TAXONOMIC CLASSIFICATION SCHEME

The science of taxonomy seems far removed from mainstream biology and medical research. The fact is that taxonomy and taxonomists, the scientists that study the identification and classification of organisms, are involved in a dynamic and important field of investigation. It has been estimated that 20 to 30 million unique organisms inhabit the earth. There are approximately 1.75 million organisms currently characterized, with an additional thousand or so being added each year. Without taxonomic classification, there would be chaos, as communication between individuals or groups would be impossible, and progress in all fields of technology, chemistry, and medicine would have been retarded by the lack of shared knowledge. To appreciate this, try to imagine a world in which objects had no specific names, and each individual or group could name any object anything they wanted to. In our world common or colloquial names are given to objects for ease of reference. However, in the fields of microbiology and clinical medicine, the need for precise, unambiguous descriptions of potential disease-causing organisms (pathogens) saves time and ultimately lives.

Taxonomic classification of organisms allows scientists and medical doctors around the world to share information using a universal language. The language chosen was Latin because it was the language of scholars when the field of taxonomy was being created. Latin was also chosen because it is an unchanging language, unlike modern languages that are fraught with conversational connotations that change the implied meaning of words with time and repeated usage. Thus, taxonomy has contributed greatly to modern civilization and afforded us longer, healthier lives through a shared understanding of the microbial world that surrounds us all.

▶ HISTORICAL CONTRIBUTIONS TO THE FIELD OF TAXONOMY

As long as humans have inhabited the earth, there has been the obvious distinction that two major groups of living things exist, namely plants and animals (Shimeld, 1999). Surely, the Neanderthals and their predecessors must have designated names for animals and knew which plants they could eat. This crude division suggested that animals were mobile and ate food, whereas plants were considered nonmobile and did not consume food. This concept was fueled because there was no knowledge of organisms that were not visible to the unaided eye. Thus, this gross categorization placed everything that was not an obvious animal into the plant category. Surprisingly, the division of all things into two kingdoms, plants and animals, persisted until relatively recently. Many scientists had recognized that bacteria, fungi, parasites, and viruses did not fit in the plant kingdom, but it was Dr. Whitaker in 1969 that formalized a reclassification by separating the plant kingdom into four separate kingdoms: plants, fungi, algae, and bacteria. This division created the five kingdom system: 1. Animalia (animals), 2. Plantae (plants), 3. Monera (bacteria), 4. Protista (mostly algae and protozoans), and 5. Mycetae (fungi). Cavalier-Smith proposed a 6 kingdom revision in 1998 consisting of Bacteria, Protozoa, Animalia, Fungi, Plantae, and Chromista (Cavalier-Smith, 1998 and Cox, 2007).

The first recorded attempts at classification note that Aristotle and others engaged in this practice as far back as 400 B.C. These were largely descriptions of plants and animals based on major morphologic or phenotypic differences. A medically relevant departure from generalized lists came about in the 2nd century A.D., when a physician, Dioscorides, described plants by their medicinal uses. His book, entitled *De Materia Medica,* was hand copied and used as the main medical reference throughout the Dark Ages, which ended about 1400 A.D.

It was not until a world-changing invention, the printing press, introduced by Johann Gutenberg around 1450 A.D., that the written word became generally accessible. This revolutionized the scientific community by allowing many people to interact around the world, spurring discussion and promoting change. Many bright scientists had parts to play in the progression of the body of knowledge we enjoy today, though they will not be mentioned here.

The modern inception of taxonomic classification was introduced by several scientists in the 1600s, including John Ray, an English naturalist (1627–1705), who applied a general scheme to describing plants and animals, and Gaspard Bauhin in 1623, who first used a two-word (**binomial**) name to classify plants. These ideas were expanded and popularized by Carolus Linnaeus (1707–1778) and are documented in his primer, entitled *Systema Naturae,* with the tenth edition published in 1758. Other contemporary taxonomists had extended the naming to include 10- to 12-word phrase type descriptions. In his texts, Linnaeus used a general name (genus, genera, plural) followed by a one-word species name strengthening the use of the binomial to classify plants and animals. Thus he is credited with the binomial and a more natural grouping for plants that allowed unknown plants to be placed into classes. Linnaeus's scheme of classification has been expanded over the decades since it was introduced, and it remains part of the systematic categorization of living organisms that is currently used.

Whenever a number of different people try to decide on a methodology or approach, there will always be arguments that sometimes result in lasting controversies. In an attempt to reconcile the different modes of classifying plants and animals, international meetings were held. A governing body was created to resolve disputes and standardize naming practices. The Zoological Record extends back to 1864 and includes systematics, taxonomy, and nomenclature and is the definitive source for this type of information. The first international botanical congress met in 1867 and constructed a set of rules called the "International Code of Botanical Nomenclature" (ICBN), which are still used today.

Another major milestone in the development of microbiological classification was brought about by the advent of the microscope. Early records from the 16th century document that pieces of crystal that were thicker in the middle and tapered at the ends were able to magnify objects. These crystals had the shape of a lentil seed and were subsequently named lenses. Their first use was as spectacles (eyeglasses). In about 1590 a Dutch spectacle maker, Zaccharias Janssen, and his son Hans experimented with lenses by placing them in tubes creating the prototype of the compound microscope and the telescope. In 1609, Galileo improved on this technology by adding a focusing device. However, the person credited with being the father of the microscope was Antoni van Leeuwenhoek, who lived in Holland (1632–1723). In his job as an apprentice in a store, he needed to count the threads in cloth, which facilitated his development of a sophisticated method for polishing lenses that allowed him to magnify items 270 times their original size. This production of fine lenses led him to construct microscopes that aided him in the biological discoveries for which he is famous. Leeuwenhoek was the first to see bacteria, red blood cells, yeast, and contaminants in water. This marked the beginning of the understanding that there was a world of microscopic living objects that had the potential to influence people's daily lives.

The invention of the printing press and the microscope were two of the most important advances that allowed scientists to share information worldwide in printed formats and to begin characterizing microorganisms into various groups and species.

 Checkpoint! 2–1 (Chapter Objective 4)

The individuals listed all contributed to advancing the field of microbiology and taxonomic classification, except:
  A. *Dioscorides.*
  B. *van Leeuwenhoek.*
  C. *Whitaker.*
  D. *Van Halen.*

▶ HISTORIC APPROACHES TO TAXONOMIC ARRANGEMENTS

Numerous approaches to taxonomic arrangements have been used throughout the years. The most common methods are artificial versus natural systems of taxonomy, phylogenic taxonomy, and numerical taxonomy.

ARTIFICIAL VERSUS NATURAL SYSTEMS OF TAXONOMY

When faced with a task of cataloging a huge number of diverse objects, several systematic approaches can be taken. These different approaches will work for taxonomic placement as long as the criteria are well defined and results in assignments that are based on objective parameters. This type of classification is referred to as an artificial system and was used for describing animals and plants in the years before Linnaeus popularized a different approach. The criterion that Linnaeus used was based on the biological properties or nature of the objects and therefore revealed more relative information about the objects than any artificial system could. This type of classification was called the natural system of taxonomic classification.

PHYLOGENIC TAXONOMY

The natural system of classification worked well until the post-Darwinian era. After Darwin published his *Origin of the Species* in 1859, the natural order based on phenotypic similarities was revised to include the relatedness between organisms. In a sense the new goal for many taxonomists of the time (and since) was to make the assignments mirror the evolutionary lineage of each organism. This type of taxonomic approach is called the phylogenetic system of taxonomy. This phylogenic system relies heavily on being able to trace the genetic history of organisms. Evolution is measured in millions of years, and the fossil record is incomplete. However, advances in determining the phylogenic lineages of microorganisms are being achieved using molecular biological methods that allow the tracking of conserved sequences of stable genes and their proteins products to estimate evolutionary time. An example of this is the ribosomal ribonucleic acid sequence, which is highly conserved across species. Comparing the sequence of the small ribosomal subunit in bacteria has allowed phylogenic relationships between seemingly unrelated bacteria to be determined. In 1977 American microbiologist Carl Richard Woese defined a new domain, or kingdom of life, the Archaea, based on his work sequencing the 16s ribosomal RNA. Dr. Woese found many species of **prokaryotes** contained 16s ribosomal RNA that more closely resemble **eukaryotes** than prokaryotes. In 1990 Dr. Woese proposed a new phylogenic tree split into three domains: the Archaea (archaebacteria), the Bacteria (eubacteria), and Eukarya (eukaryotes; Woese, 2000).

NUMERICAL TAXONOMY

The limitations of the natural and phylogenic systems gave way to an empirical system that was first described by a contemporary of Linnaeus, Michel Adanson. Adanson suggested that phenotypic similarities and differences be assigned a numeric value with all characteristics being equally weighted. The total would be calculated, and like organisms would have similar numbers. The approach was named Adansonian (numerical) taxonomy. In this system, a very large set of characteristics had to be measured (scored) to make a taxonomic assignment. In fact, the number of features was to be as large as possible and flexible so that as new features or characteristics became known, they could be added to the system. A disadvantage to this system at the time it was designed was the lack of computers to keep track and sum the scores. Currently we have the computing capacity to tabulate very large and complex sets of numbers.

▶ CURRENT APPROACHES TO TAXONOMY

In the following sections, the discussion of a species, its characteristics, and its nomenclature are discussed, it will be apparent that the current approach uses components of the natural, numeric, and phylogenic systems to categorize organisms. As such, taxonomic classification is based on phenotypic (things that can be seen, for example, morphology and/or anatomy), genotypic (genetic, gene expression), and phylogenic (evolutionarily) traits of the organisms. For microorganisms the phenotypic traits include those that are viewed microscopically. Numeric systems are often used as an additional way to subdivide groups within families or genera and will not be discussed here.

✓ Checkpoint! 2–2 (Chapter Objective 4)

Which of the following individuals is responsible for suggesting that the taxonomy of plants and animals include the relatedness between organisms as well as phenotypic similarities?

    A. *Darwin*
    B. *Linnaeus*
    C. *Woese*
    D. *All the above*

▶ THE FUNDAMENTAL UNIT OF CLASSIFICATION: SPECIES

A simple definition of a species is a population of like individuals, or for microorganisms a clonally derived population, that share a considerable set of phenotypic attributes. This shared set of characteristics must be distinguishable from those of closely related groups of individuals. This segregation and therefore species distinction works because the differences between sets of individuals or organisms are not continuous, but rather show a marked discontinuity.

Individuals or clones that make up a species are unique from all others, although there is phenotypic variation within a species. The differences result from selective pressure continually working on individuals providing genetic diversity. Taxonomists have to decide how much difference within a group is permissible before a set of changes results in the need to create a new species (or subspecies). There are differing opinions among taxonomists, with "lumpers" placing all similar groups together, in contrast to "splitters," who subdivide groups over the slightest differences.

The placement of individuals into appropriate species categories is easier for plants and animals that reproduce sexually, where genetic and evolutionary lineages can be relatively easily determined. This premise holds true as long as the individuals are free to interbreed randomly. Sharing a gene pool ensures that environmental pressures and **mutations** are dispersed throughout the population. Therefore, a population (species) may undergo change introduced by external pressures but will do so uniformly as long as there are no barriers that prevent interbreeding. Divergence in a population occurs when a physical separation segregates members of a species. Historically, these types of barriers are geographic, for example, a body of water or a mountain range. Once separated, **divergent evolution** can occur, and if a significant amount of time passes, the species will be sufficiently different so that even if reunited, they would not be capable of successful reproduction. The collective sets of genetic and hence phenotypic differences that occur as a result of isolation are the basis for species discontinuity and, in fact, establish a criterion by which a species is defined: the ability to successfully interbreed.

The criterion that works for plants and animals cannot be directly applied to microorganisms because most microbes reproduce asexually. When bacteria divide, the resulting offspring are genetically isolated from each other and hence free to undergo diversity independent from each other and from the clonal population from which they originated. Defining a species in the microbial world is complicated. The asexual reproduction of prokaryotes leads to increased diversity. Mutations and changes that occur in a haploid organism are not commingled with other organisms in the population like those of diploid, eukaryotes. This independent evolution can give rise to unique subpopulations within a relatively short period of time. For example, the growth (division) rate for a bacterium under optimal conditions is every 20 minutes; for a virus, 200 viral progeny can be produced within hours, whereas for humans, a generation takes on average 20 years. Consider that if a mutant bacterium acquires a selective growth advantage and has no growth constraints (i.e., an unlimited food supply), it can within days be clonally amplified, quickly outnumbering and outcompeting the other members of the bacterial population from which it arose. This newly emerged population may give rise to a functionally unique species of bacteria. The rapid turnover of bacteria allows mutations to accumulate, altering their genetic makeup and making it extremely difficult to track their genetic lineage. Additionally, prokaryotes are capable of direct exchange or transfer of genetic material between unrelated strains. This exchange of genetic material is in the form of plasmids, which are circular pieces of DNA that reside separately from the genomic DNA (**epigenetic** material).

The differences between microbes, plants, and animals are obviously not only their mode of reproduction. On gross phenotypic examination, most bacterial cocci look alike. Therefore, the microbial taxonomists require elaborate tests, specialized tools, and microscopes to delineate the taxa for microorganisms (see Part II, ∞ Chapters 7–13). By applying a series of tests, groups of microbes can be differentiated and categorized into discrete species or strains. Bacterial strains are equivalent to a species. The definition of a bacterial species is: a group of microbes that have similar characteristics that distinguish them from other related strains.

SPECIES CHARACTERISTICS

Ideally, the characteristics of a species would be based on a complete genotypic profile; this, however, is not the current practice. More extensive genotyping to determine species assignment will be the way of the future. However, the traditional criterion for classification uses phenotypic determinants. For the higher plants and animals, physical traits are easily recognizable. All of us can distinguish amphibians from reptiles and mammals. Microbes have few physical descriptors to aid the taxonomist in assigning them to the appropriate taxa. Microbiologists have to resort to chemical tests and microscopy that can discern properties and functional attributes of microorganisms to confirm microbial placement. Countless tests could be applied to this process. Luckily, defined sets of initial tests can relatively quickly determine the basic parameters of microorganisms and provide tentative taxonomic placement.

Some scientists will always argue the more tests the better. However, in practical terms, if an infective agent has been characterized and its drug or antibiotic sensitivity known, a patient's infection is easily eradicated. Thus basic information is often sufficient for a physician to treat a patient. The case where whole batteries of tests are necessary would be if a local disease outbreak (epidemic) or a widespread outbreak (pandemic) occurred and was caused by an unknown pathogen(s) that did not respond to known antibiotics or drugs. This would be a job for the Centers for Disease Control and Prevention (CDC). An example of such a situation is the fairly recent case that occurred in a hotel hosting a Legionnaires' convention. The majority of the guests were men over 55 years of age, many of whom drank and smoked and were thereby immune compromised (∞ Chapter 4). Many men became ill with pneumonia-like symptoms and did not respond well to typical antibiotics. Many men subsequently died of the mysterious disease. It was quickly determined that food and drinking water did not transmit the disease. It was assumed that the route of transmission was airborne exposure, although the disease did not infect individuals equally, as there were several instances where only one roommate became ill. There was an excited rush to investigate this new disease. Eventually a gram-negative rod was isolated, characterized, and found to be the same infective agent that causes a mild flulike condition called "Pontiac fever" that first occurred in the summer months near Pontiac, Michigan. It was not until the organism found its way into the moist air conditioning vents of the hotel, where uniquely susceptible hosts were staying, that the serious consequences of this bacterium become evident and spurred the investigation that discovered it was a previously unidentified bacterium. The causative agent was subsequently named *Legionella pneumophila* (Peele, 1977).

℮ REAL WORLD TIP

The number of unidentified infectious agents is difficult to estimate. Factors that influence humans coming in contact with these agents in underdeveloped countries include the clearing of ancient forests for grazing or farming of domestic livestock. A case in point is the Epon virus in the Philippines, where pig farms encroached on old forests, and the indigenous vampire bats began feeding on the pigs. The pigs became ill, and soon after pets and humans also became fatally ill. Eradication included killing hundreds of thousands of pigs, and the containment ultimately slowed the spread of this non-species-specific virus to southern Asia.

NOMENCLATURE

The rules governing taxonomic classification utilize a binomial system of nomenclature. The two word names given reflect first the genus or general category followed by the specific or species designation. Both words are italicized or underlined with only the first letter of the genus capitalized. An example from the case of Legionnaires' disease would be *Legionella* (generic name) *pneumophila* (specific name). If the genus cannot be confused with any other, then it can be abbreviated using only the first letter; common examples include *Homo sapiens* (*H. sapiens*) and *Escherichia coli* (*E. coli*). This binomial scheme is used to name all organisms. The naming of viruses is still being debated as to whether the naming should reflect functional properties or use the binomial system; however, binomials are now being more commonly used and will be discussed later in this chapter.

The criterion for naming organisms is well defined. Before a microbe can be given a species name, it must be assigned to a genus and be determined that it does not belong to a known species group. If an organism has been assigned a species (strain) designation and is later found to be identical to a previously named species, then the older name takes precedence. The same rules, however, do not apply to the naming of a genus because the designation of a genus is operationally defined and often changes as more information becomes available. In an attempt to avoid confusion, all designations that have been used to identify a microorganism are listed. An example that clarifies this idea is that *E. coli* had been placed in the genus *Bacterium* as *Bacterium coli* and in the genus *Bacillus* as *Bacillus coli*. Because these designations are synonymous, all three are listed in reference to *E. coli*. Originally, the rules included that the name of the person who first described the microbe would be placed in parentheses next to the species name. Additionally, when changes were made, the person correcting the placement was also named. This became confusing and was criticized by many scientists so that gradually individuals' names are being left off the designations.

To reduce multiple names being given to the same strain of microorganism, a reference collection of prototypic species, referred to as type strains, is maintained. The type strain can be used to determine the characteristics of a questionable microbe before a definitive assignment is made. If a type strain is lost for some reason, a search is conducted to find as close a match as possible, and a sample is added to the type collection as the **neotype** representing that particular strain of microorganism.

The complete taxonomic assignment of a species includes placement into successively larger categories of taxa. Linnaeus designated four taxa (classes, orders, genera, and species) to place plants and animals. Linnaeus was most familiar with flowers and only had a limited knowledge of animals; as such, his genera assignments were huge. These assignments have now been redistributed into several different orders and families. The current phylogenic classification includes six taxa listed here in order from specific to broad/general: species, genus, family, order, class, and phylum (or division). These major units can be further subdivided into subspecies, subgenus, subfamily, suborder, subclass, and subphylum. An additional rule of naming is that the name

of a family is formed by adding *-idae* to the end of the stem of the genus name, and *-inae* to the end of the subfamily name.

 REAL WORLD TIP

Bacterial families are noted by adding the suffix *–aceae* to the end of the genus name. For example, *Micrococcaceae* is the family while *Micrococcus* is a genus within that family.

Each successive taxa designation is broader in terms of the number of organisms it describes and therefore smaller in terms of the number of characteristics that are shared between the members. This is the hierarchical arrangement of taxonomic classification. The complete taxonomic classification for humans, a frog, a worm, and a common bacterium are shown in Table 2-1✪ (Stanier, Adelberg, Ingraham, & Wheelis, 1979). The most important grouping for microorganisms is the genus, for before any species can be designated, it has to be placed into the appropriate genus. Therefore, designations above the genus category are of little value when studying the characteristics of a particular microbe. The higher taxa serve only to show the overall placement of microbial organisms relative to other organisms (Hickman, Hickman, & Hickman, 1974).

✓ ## Checkpoint! 2–3 (Chapter Objective 5)

Arrange these taxonomic levels in order from general to specific:
- A. *Class*
- B. *Order*
- C. *Subgenus*
- D. *Family*

 TABLE 2-1

Examples of Taxonomic Classification

Taxa	Man	Frog	Worm	Bacterium
Phylum	Chordata	Chordata	Nematoda	Firmicutes
Subphylum	Vertebrata	Craniata		
Class	Mammalia	Amphibia	Chromadorea	Bacilli
Subclass	Theria			
Order	Primates	Anura	Rhabiditida	Bacillales
Suborder	Haplorrhini			
Family	Hominidae	Pipidae	Rhabitidae	*Staphylococcaceae*
Subfamily	Homininae	Xenopodinae		
Genus	*Homo*	*Xenopus*	*Caenorhabditis*	*Staphylococcus*
Species	*sapiens*	*laevis*	*elegans*	*aureus*

► TAXONOMIC CLASSIFICATION OF MICROORGANISMS

The field of taxonomic classification is being revolutionized by molecular biologic techniques. We are able to easily measure DNA, RNA, and protein, tasks that were unthought-of by Linnaeus, Adanson, and Darwin. These techniques are especially important in the characterization of microorganisms whose classification depends on separating species (strains) by functional properties. DNA base composition, nucleic acid hybridization, and protein sequences are important methodologies used in classifying microorganisms.

DNA BASE COMPOSITION

The genetic composition of all organisms, with the exception of some viruses, is deoxyribonucleic acid (DNA). DNA contains four bases, adenine, cytosine, guanine and thymine. The chemical compositions and structural differences are shown in Figure 2-1 ■.

Adenine (A) and guanine (G) are purines, and cytosine (C) and thymine (T) are pyrimidines. DNA is usually double stranded, formed by the association of a strand of bases with a complementary strand. The rules of base pairing are that an A pairs with a T and a G with a C. The molar ratio of A-T to G-C base pairs is not restricted but is constant within a species. Genetic material (chromosomes, either circular or linear) contains characteristic amounts of A-T and G-C rich regions. Base composition can be determined by relatively easy physical methods and has provided a useful tool for classifying microorganisms.

DNA can be denatured by heating. The temperature at which the two strands separate is a function of the G-C content and is referred to as the melting temperature. G-C base pairs are held together by three hydrogen bonds, whereas A-T pairs form only two hydrogen bonds (Figure 2-2 ■). Therefore, it takes more energy to separate G-C base pairs. Thus, the more G-C content, the higher the melting temperature.

In addition to the difference in temperature required to denature DNA, the nucleic acid content can be determined in several ways. The simplest way is by spectrophotometry recording the absorbance at 260 nm wavelength (A_{260} or the absorbance maxima of DNA). The A_{260} increases as the strands of DNA separate. The G-C content can also be precisely measured by density gradient centrifugation. High molar salt solutions, commonly cesium chloride (CsCl), separate strands of DNA by their density. In this way strands of DNA can be compared by their relative density in CsCl, which is a function of the G-C content.

These techniques work well for microorganisms whose DNA is mainly in their genome, but are complicated in animals and higher plants, where intracellular organelles like the mitochondria and chloroplast contain DNA that differs in its G-C content. Examples of the G-C content of different organisms are shown in Figure 2-3 ■ (Van Den Bussche, Baker, Huelsenbeck, & Hillis, 1998).

REAL WORLD TIP

Many viruses and regulatory proteins integrate with the host's genome, often with apparent randomness; however, closer inspection usually reveals that there is a motif or flanking sequence requirement for insertion. An example is the papillomaviruses, which produce proteins that recognize and bind to Adenine-Thymine rich inverted palindromic sequences (the sequence reads one way forward on one strand and the same but backward on the complementary strand) necessary for initiating viral replication.

NUCLEIC ACID HYBRIDIZATION

When denatured DNA is allowed to cool below its melting temperature, the strands go back together or reanneal. The reannealing between complementary regions of DNA is referred to as **hybridization**. It was discovered that when DNA strands from related bacteria were mixed, they could hybridize to form a doubled-stranded DNA molecule that contained one strand from each of the related bacteria and formed hybrid DNA. Conversely, when unrelated bacterial DNA strands were mixed and cooled, no hybridization occurred. Thus, this hybridization technique was an additional way to measure relatedness between bacterial strains. Inherent in the ability of two strands of DNA to hybridize with each other is that there must be a significant amount of identical DNA base sequence or homology between the strands. This idea can be expanded to conclude that, if their DNA is similar, then their genomic DNA or chromosomal DNA must be similar, and therefore not too distantly related.

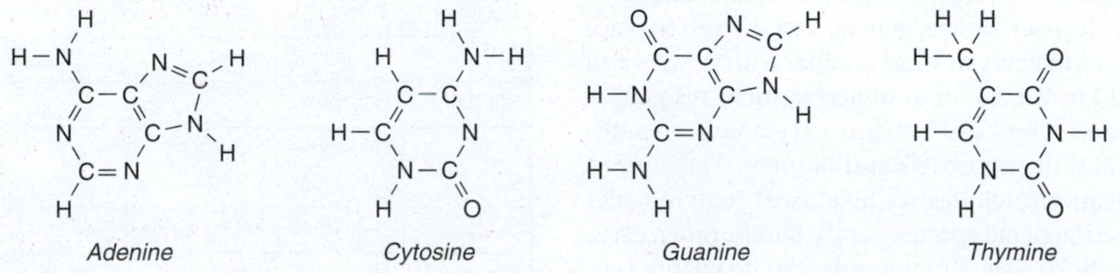

Adenine   *Cytosine*   *Guanine*   *Thymine*

■ FIGURE 2-1 Shown are stick drawings of the four deoxyribonucleic bases that make up DNA.

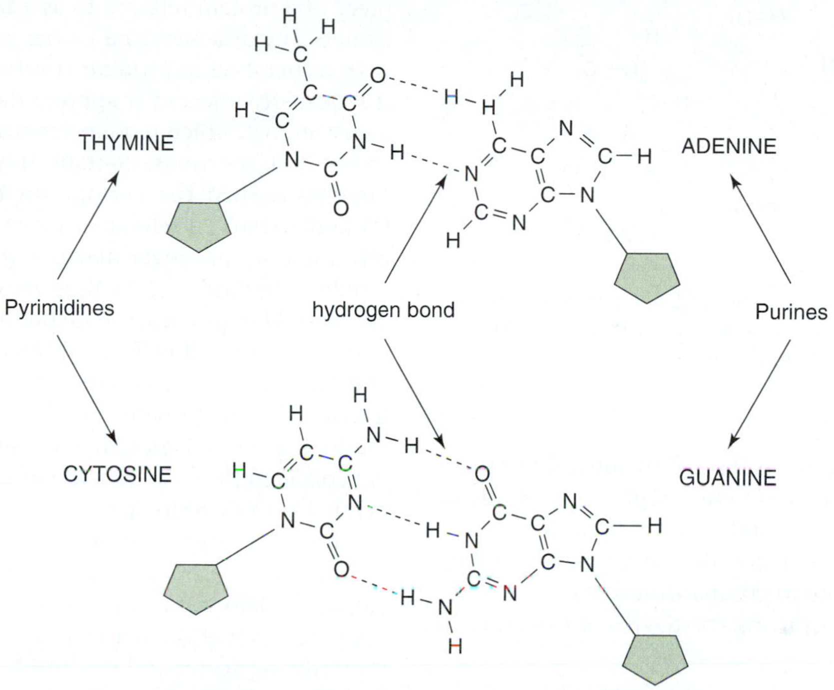

THYMINE

Pyrimidines   hydrogen bond   Purines

ADENINE

CYTOSINE   GUANINE

■ **FIGURE 2-2** Hydrogen bonding between DNA base pairs. When two strands of DNA are assembled, they associate by hydrogen bonding between the strands. Two hydrogen bonds are formed between adenine and thymine, and three hydrogen bonds are formed between cytosine and guanine.

DNA is copied or transcribed into ribonucleic acid (RNA) that is complementary to one strand of the parental DNA. RNA differs from DNA in that instead of thymine (T) RNA uses uracil (U). So the base pairing in RNA uses the characteristic G-C, but instead of A-T, the pairing is A-U, which is shown in Figure 2-4 ■. Because of the complementarity of RNA with DNA, hybrids can be formed between related strands. When RNA pairs with RNA or DNA with DNA, the association is between the same types of molecules and is referred to as homoduplex formation. When the hybrid is a mixture of DNA

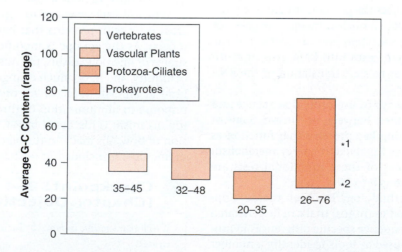

■ **FIGURE 2-3** G-C Content. The bars show the range of G-C base pair content measured in the groups indicated. The prokaryotes have the largest range. The asterisks indicate two specific bacteria. *1 (50.8) is the G-C value of *E. coli* K12, and *2 (28.6) is the value for *Borrelia burgdorferi*.

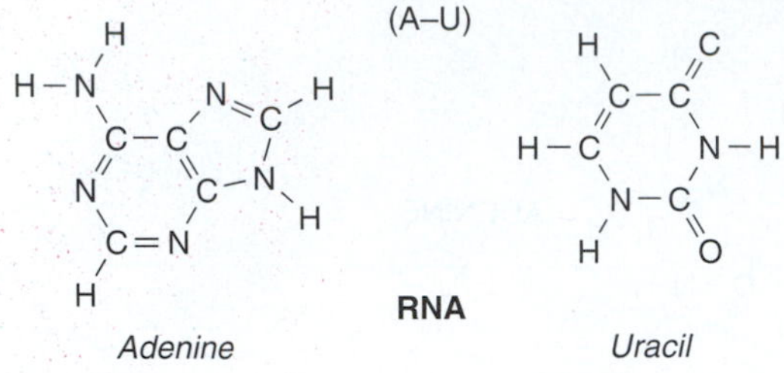

(A–U)

RNA

Adenine   Uracil

■ **FIGURE 2-4** Base differences between DNA and RNA. The bases used to make up RNA strands differ from DNA by the use of uracil (U) instead of thymine (T).

and RNA, the hybrid molecule is formed by different types of molecules and is referred to as a heteroduplex. The ability of homologous strands to form hybrids helps determine the relatedness between the strands. Typically these types of mixing experiments would be done in comparison to a known reference standard, thereby permitting the degree of similarity to be calculated.

PROTEIN SEQUENCE

The linear relationship discussed earlier, in which DNA is copied or transcribed into RNA is mirrored in the translation of the messenger RNA template (mRNA) into protein. The protein sequence directly reflects the sequence of mRNA, which in turn is a copy of the DNA. The reading of mRNA by the ribosome is done three bases at a time (codon); each codon specifies an amino acid. There is, however, a redundancy in the code so that several codons designate the same amino acid. Because of this redundancy, which occurs in the third position of the codon, many point mutations or minor changes in base composition may not affect the proteins structure or function. In prokaryotes the lack of a nuclear membrane does not permit the processing of RNA. Therefore, in bacteria as the DNA is transcribed by polymerases into RNA, it is immediately accessible to ribosomes to start translation of the RNA into protein.

There are a number of ways to use protein sequence and function to indicate relatedness between organisms. Some of these tests include identifying key proteins that function as enzymes in critical pathways involved in energy metabolism and fermentation. Examples of these functional tests are included in Part II, ∞ Chapters 8 to 10.

One very important methodology has been the development of monoclonal antibodies (mAbs) that can be generated to recognize structural or sequence specific differences in proteins. Antibodies (Abs) are used as tools to identify a number of cellular properties; some of these methods are discussed in ∞ Chapter 10. An Ab recognizes and binds to a small piece of a protein approximately three to nine amino acids in length that is called the epitope. Briefly, mAbs can be made against a total protein; however, they are usually made against a small

piece of a protein referred to as a **hapten**. The hapten is enzymatically attached to a carrier protein and usually mixed with mineral oil to form an emulsion. The protein emulsion is repeatedly injected at approximately 2-week intervals into a host animal, which is often a mouse. After immunization, the spleen from the mouse contains B-lymphocytes that make Abs directed against the epitope on the injected hapten. The immunized spleen cells are isolated and fused with a leukemia cell line that no longer makes any Abs of its own but grows rapidly. The fused cells will grow with the properties of the cancer cell but produce the Ab product from the normal fusion partner. The fused cells are diluted into wells as single cells and samples of their growth medium (supernatant) screened to check for the presence of Abs. Once Abs are detected, the producing cells are growth expanded and the antibody product collected from the supernatant. The Ab produced is monoclonal because a single immunized B-cell clone is capable of making only one type of Ab.

The other form of Ab preparation is referred to as polyclonal. A major difference in generating polyclonal Abs, versus mAbs, is that the whole protein is most often used as the immunizing agent, and the host animal is larger (goat or rabbit). Once the immunization protocol has been completed, samples of the animals' serum are tested for the presence of Abs that will bind to the immunizing protein. A medium-sized protein may contain as many as a dozen epitopes. The immunized serum contains individual Abs that bind to all the different epitopes contained within the same serum. Thus it is referred to as a polyclonal antiserum (plural-sera). The production of polyclonal antiserum in the laboratory mimics the way an individual responds to an immunization. Immunizations can be either intentional, as when they are given by a doctor to protect against disease, or naturally through exposure to infecting microorganisms. The ability of an agent (antigen) to induce an Ab response is referred to as its antigenicity.

When Abs are generated to a specific epitope, they will only cross react with proteins that have nearly the identical epitope(s). As the epitope is modified or altered as in different strains of microorganisms, the Abs bind with reduced strength or affinity, and if too much change has occurred, they will not bind at all. The topic of Ab production by individuals in response to immunization or through exposure to an infecting organism is discussed in ∞ Chapter 4, whereas a discussion of how Abs made in the laboratory aid the classification of microbes is included in ∞ Chapter 10.

✓ **Checkpoint! 2–4 (Chapter Objective 10)**

Which characteristic is shared by bacteria, fungi, parasites, and some viruses?

  A. *DNA genetic composition*
  B. *Amount of G–C content*
  C. *Melting temperature of their DNA*
  D. *Lack of the ability to act as a hapten*

▶ GENERAL FEATURES OF MEDICAL MICROBIOLOGY

Prior to discussing the specifics of viruses, bacteria, fungi, and parasites, a general description of the relevance of the host versus microbe interactions is useful. The term **pathogenic** refers to the ability of microorganisms to cause pathology (disease). Healthy individuals have natural and physical barriers that help prevent microbes from establishing an infection. Natural barriers include the immune functional capacity of an individual, which reflects their genetic background. Innate functioning would be their ability to mount an immune response and produce Abs against an infecting microorganism. Examples of physical barriers are intact skin, normal flora that covers body surfaces, enzymes, secretions, and restrictive pH. These defense mechanisms provide excellent protection. When these defenses are breached by physical trauma, chemical use (tobacco, drugs, or alcohol), or organic means (genetic susceptibility or disease), we become increasingly vulnerable to acquiring infectious diseases (see ∞ Chapter 4). Normal flora includes a variety of bacterial species that harmlessly live in our bodies and protect us by preventing other microbes from attaching to and colonizing the linings of our bodies. This is the idea of **mutualism**, also referred to as symbiosis. If this relationship becomes one sided, wherein one of the partners benefits and the other is harmed, the relationship is termed **parasitism**. Parasites burden the host, but whether the infection is tolerated and treatable or fatal often depends on the overall health of the individual prior to the infection, previous exposure to the infecting organism or related species, and genetics.

The contribution of the host to disease outcome indicates the difficulty in strictly assigning what microorganisms are **obligate** or **opportunistic** (∞ Chapter 40) pathogens. Opportunistic pathogens cause disease when the environmental conditions change, for example, from an aerobic to an anaerobic situation or location, or by the lowering of the hosts' resistance to infection. This is exemplified in the case of Legionnaires' disease, where it was the condition of the host that dictated the severity of the disease. To be considered pathogenic, the pathogen would have to always cause a disease, regardless of the number of infecting agents and the health of the host. We know from history that an absolute pathogen may not exist. Take, for example, *Yersinia pestis* (black plague); this disease caused major mortality in Europe, and albeit only small groups of people survived in the ravaged cities struck by disease, the point is they did. Scientists have now identified the mutation in a lymphocyte surface protein that prevented the immune destruction in individuals carrying this mutation. Individuals that were heterozygous (having one mutant copy and one normal copy of the gene) for the trait had a reduced severity of the illness, whereas individuals that were homozygous (having both mutant copies) did not come down with the plague. This mutation has been traced and is still expressed in the population today. It has been suggested that the mutation that allowed individuals to survive the plague may provide protection from human immune deficiency virus (HIV) in individuals that have this mutant immune cell surface protein. It appears that the mutation that prevented the immune complications of the plague is the same site the HIV virus uses to bind to and invade immune cells.

Resistance to the plague is an example of a genetically inherited trait that prevented a deadly pathogen from killing every individual that became exposed. Other factors to consider in the susceptibility of the host, for example, are the prior history of exposure to disease-causing pathogens or related strains. This idea is exemplified by the smallpox epidemic. During this deadly epidemic, milkmaids appeared to be relatively resistant to the virus. It was found that through their chronic exposure to cow pox, they developed a milder form of the pox infection, which was evident from the pox marks on their hands. This prior exposure to a related strain provided them protection from the more virulent human strain of the disease. An example of opportunistic bacteria that can be pathogenic is *Staphylococcus epidermis,* which normally resides on the skin surface and is aerobic, but is considered a facultative (when necessary) anaerobe. If, during surgery, such as joint replacement, *Staphylococcus epidermis* gets inside the body where the conditions are anaerobic, it can cause a serious infection. There are many other examples of how the host's health, history of exposure, and genetics influence susceptibility to infection, but for the sake of brevity, they will not be noted here. The point of these examples is that we come into contact with countless microorganisms, many with the potential to cause disease, but often we do not become infected because of our defense mechanisms (∞ Chapter 4) (Granato, 2003).

When we become ill and samples of body fluids are taken, the clinician or microbiologists have to decide which of the many microbes in the specimen are actually causing the disease symptoms. Part V, ∞ Chapters 32 to 39, discusses the analysis of infections in various body systems. Factors that influence the decision include proper procedures in obtaining the specimen and the proper handling of the isolate (∞ Chapter 6 and 7). If care is not taken, the sample may be inadvertently contaminated with an irrelevant organism that may cause the result to be misinterpreted. Additionally, if not properly handled, the most important microorganisms may be lost in transit to the laboratory (∞ Chapter 6 and 7). Many microorganisms require special handling to preserve them; these ideas are further discussed in Part II, ∞ Chapter 6 and 7, and Part III, ∞ Chapters 13 to 16. Any factor that changes the specimen can potentially lead to an incorrect diagnosis (∞ Chapters 8 and 9). Thus, the goal is to incubate the sample under conditions that mimic the environment of the host, thereby ensuring that the causative agent is preserved so that an accurate diagnosis can be made (∞ Chapters 7 to 13). These topics are covered thoroughly in subsequent chapters of this book. Specific information on immunologic, molecular, and susceptibility tests (∞ Chapters 9 to 11), and newly emerging techniques (∞ Chapter 12) is covered as noted in subsequent chapters of this book.

Checkpoint! 2–5 (Chapter Objective 9)

A relationship between two partners that results in the benefit to one and harm to the other is termed:

    A. *opportunistic.*
    B. *mutualism.*
    C. *parasitism.*
    D. *obligate.*

▶ PRIONS

Recently, new forms of infecting agents that are composed of protein have been identified and are referred to as "prions." These protein-based pathogens are about half the size in molecular weight of an average virus and are therefore the smallest known disease-causing agent. Little information exists regarding this class of pathogens; however, prions are known to cause scrapies in sheep and mad cow disease in cattle. This spongiform, neurodegenerative disease has been recognized in humans, with two common forms, known as kuru and Creutzfeldt-Jakob disease. The bovine form is being transmitted to humans through the ingestion of infected beef. Undoubtedly there will be an expanse of information regarding this disease and the causative agent in the near future (Watts, Balachandran, & Westaway, 2006).

▶ VIRAL CLASSIFICATION AND TAXONOMY

Viruses, like prions, would not cause disease if they were not able to gain entry into a host, as they do not encode all the necessary genes for autonomous living. Viruses exist that are capable of infecting every type of living organism, from bacteria to man. **Virions** (viruses) are usually species and tissue specific, although some nonspecific viruses infect multiple species. Factors that influence the specificity of viruses include their envelope, capsids, or surface structures that aid in attachment to the appropriate cells and introduction of their nucleic acid into the host cell(s) (Büchen-Osmond, 2007). For example, the influenza virus (Family: *Orthomyxoviridae*) causes a serious respiratory disease, and through its protein coat it binds to the epithelial cells in the lungs of humans. Interestingly, influenza was shortened to the word "flu," which has been misused to mean any viral infection. Certainly you have heard people say that they have the stomach flu. What they mean is they have an intestinal virus, as influenza always causes pneumonialike symptoms. There are now numerous examples of viruses that are species nonspecific, for example West Nile, Menangle, and Equine viruses. These cases have all been found to be transmitted from wildlife or livestock to humans via a mosquito bite.

In this section, only viruses that infect vertebrates, with emphasis placed on those infecting humans, will be dis-cussed. The taxonomy of viruses has only recently adopted the binomial scheme of classification. Designations for viruses include families and genera, with species referred to as serotypes. Higher-level taxa are not possible, as the phylogeny of viruses is not clear. The rules governing viral naming are overseen by the International Committee on Taxonomy of Viruses (ICTV).

As entities, viruses have developed unique strategies for replication and survival and are separated into families based on the type of nucleic acid in their genome, size, shape, substructure, and mode of reproduction. Within these families, the genera are subdivided largely by their antigenicity and base sequence homology. Box 2-1✪ lists the basic criterion used in the taxonomic classification of viruses. The viruses are covered in depth in ∞ Chapters 16 and 31, and as such only basic descriptions and important points will be elaborated here. Some of the more important vertebrate viruses, which can be either enveloped or nonenveloped, consisting of double-strand (ds) or single-strand (ss) DNA or RNA, are depicted in the drawings in Figure 2-5 ■ (DNA) and Figure 2-6 ■ (RNA).

✪ BOX 2-1

Characteristics Important in Classification of Viruses

    I. Hosts
       a. Vertebrates
       b. Non-vertebrates
    II. Nucleic Acid Core
       a. DNA
          1. Single-stranded (ssDNA)
          2. Double-stranded (dsDNA)
       b. RNA
          1. Single-stranded (ssRNA)
          2. Double-stranded (dsRNA)
    III. Capsid Symmetry
       a. Icosahedral
       b. Helical
       c. Complex
    IV. State of the Viron
       a. Naked
       b. Enveloped
    V. Site of Capsid Assembly
       a. Cytoplasm
       b. Nucleus
    VI. Site of Nucleocapsid Envelopment
       a. Cytoplasm
       b. Cytoplasmic Membrane
       c. Intracytoplasmic Membrane
       d. Nuclear Membrane
    VII. Reaction to Ether or Lipid Solvents
       a. Resistant
       b. Sensitive
    VIII. Number of Capsomeres
    IX. Viron Diameter (nanometers)
    X. Molecular Weight of Nucleic Acid in Viron (10^6)

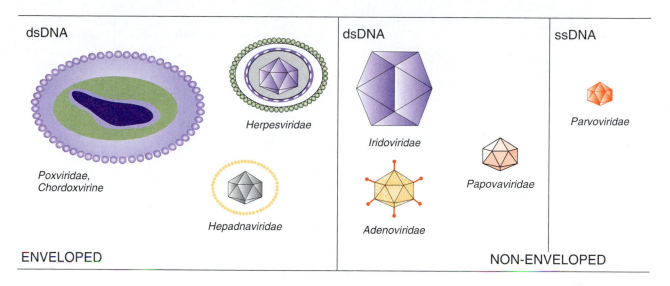

■ FIGURE 2-5 Depiction of DNA viruses that infect vertebrates. DNA viruses can be surrounded by an envelope or not protected. They come in a variety of sizes, which are portrayed on a relative scale in this drawing. The genomes of viruses can be either double (ds) or single stranded (ss).

Double-strand viruses contain both a coding copy (sense strand) that can be read by polymerases into RNA or if RNA, reverse transcribed into DNA, and a complementary strand (antisense) that is not read as a template. Single-strand viruses may contain the sense or antisense strand as their genomic material. To be successful, viruses must be able to commandeer the hosts' resources; therefore, different strategies are used by the ss and ds DNA and RNA viruses.

Some viruses become integrated into the hosts' chromosomes, where they may remain dormant; when this occurs, the virus is said to be in a lysogenic cycle where it may reside until the host cells are stressed by any number of conditions. When the viruses go into a reproduction phase and begin producing viral progeny, the stage is referred to as the lytic cycle. Subsequent paragraphs discuss some examples of common DNA and RNA viruses within the different categories depicted in Figures 2-5 and 2-6.

DNA VIRUSES

The DNA viruses are almost exclusively double-stranded, with the exception of *Parvoviridae*. Viruses in the family *Parvoviridae* are nonenveloped. The ssDNA *Parvoviridae* are very small viruses that include the genus known to pet owners as *Parvovirus*, which kills many cats and dogs. There are numerous species in the family *Parvoviridae* that infect all vertebrates. Two members of the *Erythrovirus* genus are capable of independent replication and are associated with diseases in humans. For example, Parvovirus B19 causes destruction of erythrocyte progenitor cells leading to severe aplastic anemia. Several members of the family *Parvoviridae* are dependent on coinfection with the dsDNA adenoviruses. These adeno-dependent infections in humans have not been associated with specific diseases. Viruses in this genus are not capable of

replication without the presence of the adenovirus. These ssDNA viruses exist as the sense and antisense strands packaged in separate particles and unite to form a double strand when liberated. DNA viruses in the family *Poxviridae* have genomic material with a very high molecular weight and include the genus that causes smallpox.

A medium-sized dsDNA virus of particular interest is the family *Hepadnaviridae*. These viruses, as the name suggests, infect hepatocytes, or cells of the liver, and cause hepatitis. They have a circular genome that is predominantly double-stranded DNA with a single-strand portion. Once inside the hepatocyte, the viral polymerase copies the single-stranded portion, thereby completing the double-strand circle. During infection, these viruses produce an excess of surface antigens that can be detected in the sera of infected individuals as hepatitis B surface antigen. It has been estimated that more than 300 million people are carriers of HBV.

RNA VIRUSES

The most numerous viruses that infect humans are the RNA viruses. The very small ssRNA viruses of the family *Picornaviridae* include many genera that contain important human disease-causing serotypes. The picovirus genome is a single, linear sense strand of RNA, which serves as the template for the host's ribosomes to directly translate it into protein. The assembled viral particles are approximately 27 nm in diameter and contain about 60 copies of the virus. The genus *Enterovirus'* members include, among others, poliovirus and coxsackievirus; the genus *Rhinovirus* includes the common cold virus and a variety of other viruses known to cause mild illnesses in humans. The hepatitis A virus, after significant debate, has been classified as a picornavirus and given its own genus, *Hepatovirus*.

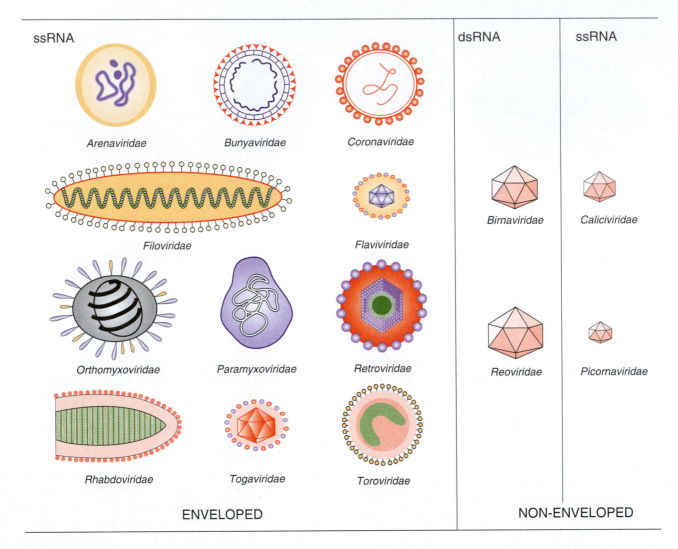

ssRNA   dsRNA   ssRNA

Arenaviridae   *Bunyaviridae*   *Coronaviridae*

Filoviridae   *Flaviviridae*   *Birnaviridae*   *Caliciviridae*

Orthomyxoviridae   *Paramyxoviridae*   *Retroviridae*   *Reoviridae*   *Picornaviridae*

Rhabdoviridae   *Togaviridae*   *Toroviridae*

ENVELOPED   NON-ENVELOPED

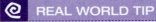 **FIGURE 2-6** Drawing of RNA viruses that infect vertebrates. RNA viruses can be protected with an external envelope or nonprotected. The RNA viruses come in a variety of sizes, which are relatively depicted here. The viral genome can be either double- or single-stranded RNA.

An example from the dsRNA nonenveloped category is the *Reoviridae,* with two genera that cause human disease: the genus *Orbivirus,* which causes Colorado tick fever, and *Rotavirus,* which causes diarrheal disease. *Rotavirus* gastroenteritis is the major nonbacterial cause of infantile diarrhea and the leading cause of infant mortality in developing countries. *Rotavirus* also infects adults that come into close contact with infants but usually causes only mild symptoms.

In the category of enveloped dsRNA viruses, two important members will be discussed: *Bunyaviridae* and *Retrovirida.* The *Bunyaviridae* family contains hundreds of members divided by biochemical, biophysical, and serological interrelationships. Members of this family are known to cause hemorrhagic fever with and without associated renal complications and have now been grouped in the genus *Hantavirus.* Cases of hemorrhagic fever have been noted in Korea, Scandinavia and eastern European countries. Only recently (1993) did an outbreak occur in the southwestern United States. The natural hosts for *Hantavirus* are rodents, and infections in humans have always been traceable to exposure of the individuals to mice, rats, and/or voles.

REAL WORLD TIP

Three years after the hantavirus outbreak in the southwest United States, an outbreak occurred in Argentina (city of Pergamino) and was found to be a different strain of the Hantavirus. A doctor treating the victims acquired the disease and traveled back to the United States for treatment. The treating physician and later his wife contracted the disease. This suggested a human-to-human transmission, which had not been thought to occur with the *Hantavirus.* A team of specialists ruled out all other modes of transmission, leaving the dangerous reality that the Hantaviruses had mutated to the point that an intermediate host was no longer required. Thus, a variant of the virus is now capable of passing directly between humans.

The family *Retroviridae* includes two genera of particular importance: the *Oncovirinae* and the *Lentivirinae*. This family of viruses are dsRNA composed of inverted dimers of linear, sense strand RNA that readily disassociates into individual strands inside the host cell. The retroviruses have a reverse transcriptase (RNA-dependent DNA polymerase) that transcribes the RNA into DNA. Replication of these viruses involves proviruses that are integrated into the host's cellular DNA. The oncogenic viruses are known to cause solid tumors (sarcomas) and leukemia, whereas, the slow-growing *Lentivirinae* are the cause of human immunodeficiency virus (HIV).

SIGNIFICANCE

As a collection of pathogenic agents, the viruses can cause harmless or fatal infections and can do so quickly or take years to manifest disease. Not too long ago, we were unable to cultivate these viruses in the laboratory. Only recently has the technology and methodology advanced sufficiently to allow us to better understand these obligatory intracellular parasites (∞ Chapter 16). The viruses are covered in detail in ∞ Chapter 31.

 Checkpoint! 2–6 (Chapter Objective 7)

Viruses belong to which of the kingdoms listed below?
A. *Plantae*
B. *Bacteria*
C. *Both A & B*
D. *None of the above*

▶ BACTERIAL CLASSIFICATION AND TAXONOMY

The kingdom Bacteria contains the prokaryotes (consisting of microorganisms, specifically bacteria, that do not contain a nucleus or a limiting membrane around their nuclear material), which as a group are the most diverse in term of habitats they colonize and extreme conditions they tolerate (Boone and Castenholz, 2001). The two major divisions or domains within this kingdom are the true bacteria (eubacteria) and archaea (archaebacteria). The archaebacteria are unique from other living organisms in the components of their cell walls and membranes. They also share characteristics with eukaryotes such as DNA (genes) that is interrupted by intervening sequences or introns. Examples of archaebacteria are found at extreme temperatures and acidity, and some produce methane gas. However, as a group, they are not medically relevant and will not be further discussed.

The eubacteria are subdivided into 27 phyla (Euzéby, 2009). Many clinically relevant species are found in 3 phyla: *Proteobacteria, Firmicutes,* and *Actinobacteria* (Boone and Castenholz, 2001). Bacteria are characteristically very small

in size (0.2 to 2 μm) compared to eukaryotic cells (these cells, which share common characteristics with fungi, have a nucleus and a limited membrane around their nuclear material), which range from 7 to 100 μm in diameter. Table 2-2✪ lists features of prokaryotes compared to eukaryotes. Bacteria do not have a true nuclear membrane but do show cellular compartmentalization, as a nucleoid is visible by electron microscopy and houses their circular chromosome. The space constraints of bacterium physically limit the amount of DNA that can be supercoiled and packed into the nuclear area. As such, bacteria have fewer genes than eukaryotic cells. The number of genes range from approximately 450 in the mycoplasma species that have lost their cell wall and are no longer free living (∞ Chapter 28), to approximately 4,300 in *E. coli* (∞ Chapter 21) (Lobry & Sueoka, 2002).

Many of the genes in prokaryotes are dedicated to housekeeping functions, energy retrieval, and metabolism. The energy requirements for most bacteria, including the medically relevant strains, are aerobic, which depend on oxygen for their respiration, or anaerobic, which obtains energy through fermentation or alternate (not oxygen) electron acceptors. Some bacteria are facultative anaerobes, in that, depending on their environment, they can respire with oxygen or by fermentation, as in the example of *Staphylococcus epidermidis*.

Bacteria are rarely found living singly, as their ability to asexually reproduce results in clonally derived colonies being formed relatively quickly. There are inherent advantages to colonial living, as the saying goes, "There is safety in numbers." A colony of bacteria can communicate through the production of soluble factors that can be received, responded to, and sent between the members of the colony. This relay of chemical information can result in bacteria sensing environmental changes and responding appropriately, thus increasing their collective survival. The exchange of information can also be through the direct exchange of plasmids that can carry antibiotic resistance genes. Additionally, the production of secreted products, like antibiotics and polysaccharides, can protect a colony from invasion. Secreted antibiotics can kill invading bacterial strains, whereas producing polysaccharides (slime) can create a physical barrier that prevents diffusion of toxins or foreign antibiotics from destroying the whole colony.

When considering bacterial traits that are important in classification, a series of defined procedures will help determine the assignment. Box 2-2✪ outlines steps in the classification of bacteria. Not all characteristics are of equal importance; the mere presence of plasmids is relatively common and therefore does not help in distinguishing one bacterium from another. However, the specific traits of the harbored plasmid, like the carrying of antibiotic resistance genes, are of potential benefit when determining the origin of seemingly related infections. An important first test that is commonly applied is the Gram stain, which is based on the structure of the bacterial cell wall (∞ Chapter 3). Gram-positive bacteria hold the crystal violet stain and become dark purple. Gram-negative bacteria do not retain the stain and are pink to red in color because of the counterstain used in the procedure. Thus a first major division separating strains of bacteria is based on their Gram staining

✪ TABLE 2-2

Characteristics of Prokaryotes Versus Eukaryotes

Feature	Prokaryotes	Eukaryotes
Size	0.2–2 µm dia	7–100 µm dia
Nucleus	no nuclear membrane	membrane-bound nucleus
Genetic material	single, circular chromosome	multiple, linear chromosomes
Cytoplasmic organelles	none	present, mitochondria, etc.
Cytoskeleton	none	present
Ribosomes	70S	80S
Cell division	binary fission	mitosis
Sexual reproduction	conjugation	meiosis
Plasma membrane	no carbohydrates, usually no sterols	includes carbohydrates & sterols
Cell walls	usually present	present in plants
Glycocalyx	capsule or slime layer	present in animal cells
Flagella	protenious, hollow, attached by a basal body	microtubular, arranged in 9+2 conformation

properties. Of course there are subsets of bacteria that are refractory to Gram stain reagents or are difficult to stain. For these strains, other tests are necessary to identify and classify them. They are discussed in depth in Part II, ∞ Chapters 8 to 11.

✪ BOX 2-2

Characteristics Important in Classification of Bacteria

I. Morphology
   a. Cell wall properties (Gram stain—positive, negative or inconclusive)
   b. Physical shape (coccus, rod)
   c. Colony morphology
II. Respiration
   a. Aerobic
   b. Anaerobic
III. Motility
   a. Tumbling behavior
   b. Smooth swinming (chemoattraction/repulsion)
IV. Metabolic properties
   a. Biotyping (biochemical reactions)
   b. Growth on different carbon sources
V. Enzymatic properties
   a. Chromogenic (color on selective media)
   b. Production of various enzymes (oxidase, collagenase)
VI. Morphological characteristics (other than shape)
   a. Flagella (single or multiple)
   b. Pili
   c. Axial filaments (spirochetes)
   d. Form endospores
VII. Nucleic Acids
   a. G-C & A-T content
   b. Ribosomal sequence (16S subunit)
   c. RNA-DNA hybridization
   d. DNA Sequence (bioinformatics)

The second-most-common characteristic to consider is the mode of respiration defined as either aerobic or anaerobic (anaerobic bacteria and anaerobic infections are discussed in ∞ Chapter 24). Thus, four distinctions can be made: gram-positive, aerobic; gram-positive, anaerobic; gram-negative, aerobic; and gram-negative, anaerobic. These criteria are typically then coupled with information regarding the shape of the bacterium. The most common shapes include: round (coccus, plural cocci), rod shaped (bacillus, plural bacilli), or spirochete shaped (helical coils). Spirochetes are unique in shape and include *Treponema pallidum,* the microorganism that causes syphilis; they are discussed as a group in ∞ Chapter 25. The most common bacteria are either cocci or bacilli, which can be organized as single bacterium or assembled into groups. Figure 2-7 ■ shows examples of the common shapes and groupings of bacteria. An example grouping of cocci is that of *Staphylococcus aureus,* which stays together in grapelike bunches and when Gram stained (positive) looks like a cluster of grapes.

By adding shape to the delineation of bacterial groupings, eight categories are formed. Figure 2-8 ■ is a tree diagram that shows the divisions based on these criteria. The majority of bacteria fall within these eight groups. The gram-negative organisms are the most numerous, in particular the gram-negative aerobic rods. All the groups include vastly different strains that are further subdivided by additional testing. Some of these distinctions are shown under the gram-negative, anaerobic rods, which includes the type of sugar fermentation (glucose) and the production of oxidase in conjunction with fermentation (see Box 2-2). Additional criteria used depends on the category of genera being considered and will be addressed in subsequent chapters; however, examples include the production of endospores, the number of flagella and/or pili, and the growth on selective media (such as Mac-Conkey agar).

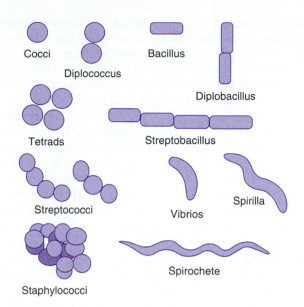

■ **FIGURE 2-7** Common shapes and groupings of bacteria. The cocci and bacilli can be single, pairs, and higher-order assemblies. The streptococci and streptobacilli are a string of bacteria, whereas the staphylococci is a cluster of bacteria. A unique shape among bacteria is the spirochete.

What should have become apparent in reading this chapter is that for all the rules, there is still considerable debate among taxonomists, including the bacterial taxonomists. Bacteria are under external stresses to undergo mutations (Lobry & Sueoka, 2002). Thus, there is no absolute or official classification scheme for bacteria. However, the scheme proposed in *Bergey's Manual of Systematic Bacteriology* is the most widely accepted system (Boone & Castenholz, 2001). The rules of bacterial nomenclature are governed by the International code for Bacterial Nomenclature, with changes and additions published in the *International Journal of Systematic Bacteriology*.

✓ **Checkpoint! 2–7 (Chapter Objective 7)**

Which of the following organisms belongs to the kingdom Bacteria?

A. *Staphylococcus epidermidis*
B. *Parvovirus B19*
C. *Hantavirus*
D. *Escherichia coli*
E. *Both A & B*
F. *Both B & C*
G. *Both A & D*

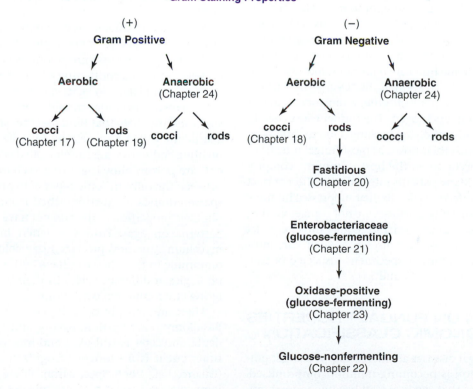

■ **FIGURE 2-8** Diagram of the eight groups of bacteria, separated by Gram stain, respiration, and shape. The division of bacteria by these three criterion results in eight functional groups. Chapters that discuss each of the specific group(s) are noted for reference.

► CLASSIFICATION AND TAXONOMY OF FUNGUS

The kingdom Fungi includes most of the clinically relevant fungi (singular, fungus) that can be in the form of yeasts or moulds. The kingdom Chromista contains 2 known human pathogens. One species in this kingdom cannot be grown on artificial medium and the other species (*Pythium insidiosum*) is a rarely isolated opportunist (Guarro et al., 1999). The study of fungi is mycology (∞ Chapter 29), which comes from the Greek word *mykes,* which means mushroom. Fungi have a significant impact on our daily lives, as they top our pizzas, raise our bread, and ferment beer and wine. They contribute to the environment, as they decompose organic matter releasing nutrients and nitrogen back into the food chain. Fungi are chemoheterotrophs, which means they require organic compounds for both their carbon and energy sources (Fromtling et al., 2003). They absorb nutrients from their environment either as **saprophytes**, living off decaying matter, or as parasites, living off living matter. They form symbiotic relationships with plants and algae and produce chemicals that kill bacteria. Most of us are alive today having survived bacterial infections with help from the mould *Penicillium notatum* that produces the antibiotic penicillin.

Over 250,000 species of fungi have been identified, of which approximately 150 species are medically relevant. At best fungi can be a nuisance and at worst deadly. Millions of people spend billions of dollars on drugs to ease symptoms of allergies due to fungal spores in the air. Fungi cause conditions such as oral and vaginal yeast infections, athlete's foot, and more serious conditions such as endocarditis and histoplasmosis, as well as many other diseases. Some fungi are poisonous, like the mushroom *Amanita phalloides,* also know as the "Death Cap," which is often mistaken for *Amanita pantherita,* a mushroom that is used as a recreational hallucinogen. The former causes death, whereas the latter is only mildly toxic. Fungi tend to form symbiotic relationships with their hosts, as most fungal infections in humans usually occur when the host is immune compromised (∞ Chapter 4). Many patients infected with HIV contract opportunistic fungal infections due to their suppressed immune systems (∞ Chapter 40). Fungal diseases are not contagious (i.e., not spread from person to person) and require direct contact with the fungal spores to contract disease. As such, care must be taken when handling sample specimens suspected of containing fungi (∞ Chapters 5, 6, 7, and 14).

INFORMATION ON FUNGAL PROPERTIES USED IN TAXONOMIC CLASSIFICATION

The numbers of fungal diseases are increasing, as a larger portion of the population is becoming immunocompromised. This increase requires that medical staff become more familiar with this growing class of potential pathogens. An initial criterion that can quickly determine whether a yeast (examples of yeasts include *Candida albicans* and *Cryptococcus neoformans*) or mould (examples of moulds include members of the genus *Penicillium* and *Histoplasma capsulatum*) has pathogenic potential is its ability to thrive at body temperature (37°C; see fungal cultures, ∞ Chapter 14). The taxonomic classification of fungus relies heavily on morphologic characteristics, most of which are unique to the kingdom Fungi. In this section, we will try to limit the discussion to the taxonomic properties of fungus that can cause mycoses (fungal infections; ∞ Chapter 29). Many yeasts and moulds were previously thought to be contaminants in biological specimens, and it was only recently that they were recognized as pathogens. Therefore, the distinction between harmless and pathogenic fungi is not absolute. The classification of fungi uses the binomial system and is governed by the International Code of Botanical Nomenclature that adopted rules for naming fungi at their meeting in Tokyo in 1993. The most recent and active code was adopted at the Sixteenth International Botanical Congress in St. Louis in 1999.

Originally fungus were placed in the plant kingdom; however, several characteristics set fungi apart from other organisms. As a group, fungi share characteristics with eukaryotes, in that they have a nuclear membrane and cytoplasmic organelles. Fungi have both a plasma membrane and a cell wall. The cell walls of fungi are different from the cell walls in plants and bacteria because they contain unique molecules, including one called chitin. Chitin is a polymer of the partially deacetylated amino sugar, *N*-acetylglucosamine, the primary molecule that makes up the exoskeleton of insects and arthropods.

Morphologic differences define the separation of fungi into yeasts and moulds. Yeast are single celled, whereas moulds are multicellular. Yeast can form colonies like bacteria when plated on selective media containing agar plates. The morphology of yeast on agar plates can be used to help differentiate species of yeast. The multicellular moulds consist of thin filamentous structures (hyphae) that bind together and branch to produce a structure called a mycelium. Mycelia may have septa segmenting and separating the elongated cells, which, when present, are porous allowing a free exchange of the cytoplasm between the cells. In some types of hyphae, the septa are very sparse. Moulds are distinguished from each other by morphologic properties, as they do not have characteristic growth patterns on agar. However, when plated on agar, their mycelium structures produce fuzzy colonies. Some fungi are dimorphic in that they can have both yeast and mould morphologies at different stages in their life cycles or under differing environmental conditions.

There are four phyla in the kingdom Fungi: Ascomycota, Basidiomycota, Chytridiomycota, and Zygomycota. The term deuteromycetes is still used and indicated a phylum at one time, but it is no longer recognized as a taxonomic rank (Guarro et al., 1999). Species from all the phyla except Chytridiomycota are known to cause diseases in humans, although infections arising from members of the phyla Basidiomycota are relatively less common. There is a continuing debate as to whether the phylum Chytridiomycota should be placed in the

✪ TABLE 2-3

Cell Wall Composition of Medically Important Fungi		
Principle Polymer	Fungal Group	Representative Genus/Species
Chitin-chitosan	Zygomycetes	*Rhizopus arrhizus*
Chitin-glucan	Ascomycetes (mycelia)	*Pseudallescheria boydii*
	Basidomycetes (mycelia)	*Schizopdyllum commune*
	deuteromycetes	*Phialophora verrucosa*
Glucan-mannan	Ascomycetes (yeast)	*Saccharomyces cerevisiae*
	deuteromycetes (yeast)	*Candida albicans*
Chitin-mannan	Basidomycetes (yeast)	*Fibrobasidiella neoformans*

kingdom Fungi or the kingdom Bacteria (Slack, Boyle, Zerr & Antoszewski, 1999).

This controversy stems from the fact that the oospores produced by the chytrids have flagella that allow their gametes to be motile, a characteristic not shared by the rest of the phyla. The placement of fungi in a kingdom of their own was largely based on the fact that they were nonphotosynthetic, had no flagellum, and had unique cell walls. The components of the cell walls differ somewhat between the members of this kingdom. Table 2-3✪ lists the unique cell wall components found in the four medically relevant phyla, including a representative genus/species from each group.

The major morphologic characteristics that are used to classify fungi are based on the type of spores produced. Spores can be produced by asexual and sexual processes, and most fungi reproduce both sexually and asexually. Members of the deuteromycetes are also referred to as fungi imperfecti, as they have no known sexual stage. The deuteromycetes contains miscellaneous fungi, and when certain members are found to have a sexual stage of reproduction, they are moved into other phyla. Examples of spores produced by the various phyla are listed in Table 2-4✪.

The formation of spores produced sexually or asexually may be associated with fruiting bodies (fructifications), which are specific structures of fungi that accompany some types of spore formation (discussed in ∞ Chapter 29). The asexual reproductive form of a mould is called the **anamorph**, and the sexual reproductive form is referred to as the teleomorph. There are two common anamorphic (asexual) structures, the **sporangiospores** and the conidia. Only members of the phyla Chytridiomycota and Zygomycota produce sporangiospores (spores protected by a sac), whereas deuteromycetes and all four phyla produce conidia type spores that are unprotected or naked spores.

There are three forms of asexual reproduction, two of which result in conidia. These are fragmentation and budding or fission. Fragmentation occurs when a piece of hyphae breaks off and replicates to form a new mould. Budding occurs when a bud is pinched off the original yeast cell and forms a daughter cell. Fission is the same process as budding except the yeast cell divides itself in half, resulting in the formation of two cells of nearly equal size. The third asexual strategy of producing spores is when the resulting spore is enclosed in a protective case referred to as a sporangium. The mould releases its sporangium into the air, which geminates later forming new moulds. Diagrammatic representations of the two anamorphic structures are shown in Figure 2-9 ■.

There are four teleomorphic structures unique to each of the phyla (deuteromycetes do not produce sexual spores). Drawings of the four types of sexual spores are shown in Figure 2-10 ■. The Chytridiomycota are a primitive aquatic fungus that produces motile oospores. The Zygomycota produces sexual spores called zygospores that are not contained within fruiting bodies that are formed when the haploid nuclei at the ends of hyphae fuse to form a diploid zygote. The zygote undergoes meiosis to form haploid cells that develop into zygospores.

Ascomycota are referred to as the "sac fungi" because their sexual spores (ascospores) are enclosed in saclike structures or asci. Meiosis occurs in the ascus between the contained ascospores. The Basidiomycota are also known as the "club fungi" in that their sexual spores (basidiospore) are formed on fruiting bodies called basidia. This phylum contains very diverse and complex fungi that includes mushrooms. Images representing the three medically relevant sexual spores are shown in Figure 2-11 ■.

✪ TABLE 2-4

Classification of Fungi by Spores		
Phyla	Sexual	Asexual
Ascomycota	Ascospores	Conidia
Basidiomycota	Basidiospores	Conidia
Chytridiomycota	Oospores	Spores & Conidia
deuteromycetes (Fungi Imperfecti)	None	Conidia
Zygomycota	Zygospores	Spores & Conidia

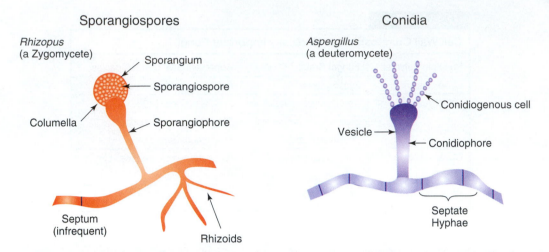

Sporangiospores

Rhizopus
(a Zygomycete)

Sporangium

Sporangiospore

Columella

Sporangiophore

Septum
(infrequent)

Rhizoids

Conidia

Aspergillus
(a deuteromycete)

Conidiogenous cell

Vesicle

Conidiophore

Septate
Hyphae

■ **FIGURE 2-9** Depiction of two kinds of asexual fungal spores.

As a group the kingdom Fungi is especially morphologically diverse with unique structures compared to the other medically relevant kingdoms. Mastery of the terminology and recognition of the various structural entities is a necessary component in identification and taxonomic placement of fungi. Fungi are an emerging medical problem as we are coming to recognize their pathological potential. The fungi are discussed in depth in ∞ Chapters 14, 29, and 40.

✓ **Checkpoint! 2–8
(Chapter Objective 8)**

Which of the following terms refer to organisms, such as fungi, that live on dead or decaying organic matter?
   A. *Conidia*
   B. *Obligate*
   C. *Saprophyte*
   D. *Epigenetic*

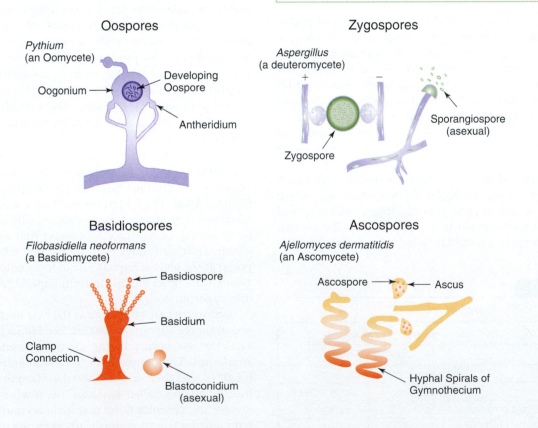

Oospores

Pythium
(an Oomycete)

Developing
Oospore

Oogonium

Antheridium

Zygospores

Aspergillus
(a deuteromycete)

+   −

Sporangiospore
(asexual)

Zygospore

Basidiospores

Filobasidiella neoformans
(a Basidiomycete)

Basidiospore

Basidium

Clamp
Connection

Blastoconidium
(asexual)

Ascospores

Ajellomyces dermatitidis
(an Ascomycete)

Ascospore   Ascus

Hyphal Spirals of
Gymnothecium

■ **FIGURE 2-10** Depiction of four different kinds of medically relevant sexual fungal spores.

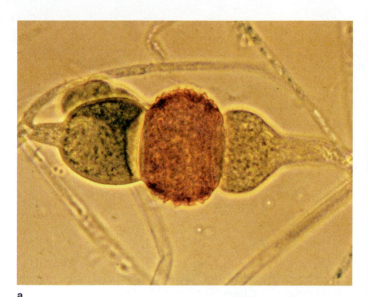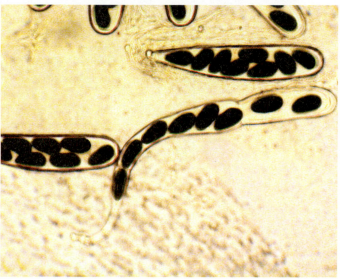

a   b

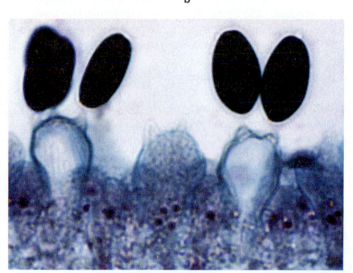

c

■ **FIGURE 2-11** Images of Sexual Spores. Panel **a.** zygospores with thick, black cell walls supported by two suspensors cells. Panel **b.** are ascospores, sexual spores enclosed in cylindrical cells called asci. Asci and ascospores are usually produced in fruiting bodies, and there are typically eight ascospores per ascus. Panel **c.** two basidiospores borne on a basidium.
These images are courtesy of George Wong, University of Hawaii.

► CLASSIFICATION AND TAXONOMY OF ANIMAL PARASITES

The microscopic, single-celled animal parasites or protozoans are placed in the kingdom Protoza, whereas the other commonly discussed group of parasites are the metazoans (round and flatworms), classified in the kingdom Animalia (Cox, 2007). The term *parasite* indicates all the members discussed in this section have developed relationships that benefit the parasite and cause harm to the host. The protozoans have a wide variety of hosts including other protozoans, animals, and humans. The metazoans have a few dozen members that are

of serious consequence to humans, and although they themselves are not microscopic, many are obligate parasites.

PROTOZOANS

The characteristics of protozoans, as a group, are that they are nonphotosynthetic, single-celled eukaryotes. They have intracellular organelles, a true nucleus, mitochondria, microtubules, etcetera, but do not associate with other cells to form organized cellular assemblies (tissues). Members of this group can be free living, with common habitats in soil and/or water. Most species of protozoans are harmless and form commensal relationships, with the remaining 20 to 30 or so species being parasites of humans.

✪ TABLE 2-5

Major Distinguishing Features of Protozoan Phyla

Phylum	Means of Locomotion	Reproduction
Apicomplexa	nonmotile when mature	sexual and asexual (alternating generations)
Ciliphora	rows of cilia	mitotic fission and/or conjugation
Microspora*	nonmotile when mature	alternating sexual/asexual
Amoebozoa	pseudopods	asexual, binary fission
Metamonada	flagella	asexual, binary fission
Parabasalia	flagella	asexual, binary fission
Percolozoa	flagella	asexual, binary fission
Euglenozoa	flagella	asexual, binary fission

*Kingdom Fungi

There are thirteen recognized phyla in the kingdom, Protozoa. Seven phyla include parasites that infect humans: Amoebozoa, Metamonada, Parabasalia, Percolozoa, Euglenozoa, Ciliophora, and Apicomplexa. The phylum Microspora is in the kingdom Fungi. The classification of protozoans into different phyla was traditionally based on their mode of locomotion and means of reproduction. The ability to use molecular methods to group the single celled eukaryotes resulted in the flagellates being divided into 4 distinct phyla. The major differences are listed in Table 2-5✪. Other considerations used for the placement of protozoans into successive taxa include physiology, morphology, and habitat requirements.

Reproduction in protozoans includes asexual reproduction by fission or **schizogony** (able to undergo multiple fission processes), sexual reproduction by conjugation, or the production of gametocytes. An additional strategy used by some protozoans is the production of cysts that encapsulates the gametes providing protection and increasing the likelihood of their surviving until they meet a suitable host.

Most of the parasitic protozoans have two or more stages in their life cycles, including a vegetative stage referred to as the **trophozoite** and a dormant stage in which they form cysts. Some species of protozoans have complex life cycles with several morphologic stages involving one or more intermediate hosts. Examples of common protozoans are listed in Box 2-3✪ (Schmidt & Roberts, 1977).

Many of the protozoan infections are transmitted by bites from arthropods in the Class Insecta that includes flies, mosquitoes, and beetles and from the Class Arachnida, or ticks. Other infections with protozoans occur by ingesting contaminated food or water and through exposure to intermediate hosts. Examples of diseases caused by protozoan infections are malaria, African and American sleeping sickness, and toxoplasmosis. Detailed discussions are covered in ∞ Chapters 15 and 30.

HELMINTHS

The metazoan helminths are also known as the "worms." Parasitic helminth infections are usually diagnosed by identification of the ova (eggs) in the feces of the host animal or, if a blood-borne parasite, identification of a particular stage in a blood sample (∞ Chapters 15 and 30). The characteristics used in taxonomic classification of the helminths include body shape, digestive system, and mode of reproduction. These basic parameters are outlined in Table 2-6✪.

✪ BOX 2-3

Common Protozoan Parasites of Humans

Phylum Sporozoea
- *Eimeria* spp. (coccidiosis)
- *Isospora* spp. (coccidiosis)
- *Toxoplasma gondii* (toxoplasmosis)
- *Cryptosporidium parvum* (cryptosporidosis)
- *Plasmodium* spp. (malaria)
- *Babesia microti* (babesiosis)

Phylum Ciliophora (ciliates)
- Class Oligohymenophorea
  - *Ichthyophthirius multifilis* (ich)
- Class Litostomatea
  - *Balantidium coli*

Phylum Microspora (microsporidia)
- *Encephalitozoon* spp.
- *Enterocytozoon bieneusi*

Phylum Parabasala
- *Trichomonas vaginalis* (trichomoniasis)
- *Dientamoeba fragilis*

Phylum Metamonada
- *Giardia lamblia* (giardiasis)

Phylum Euglenozoa
- *Leishmania* spp. (leishmaniasis)
- *Trypanosoma* spp. (African trypanosomiasis, sleeping sickness)
- *Trypanosoma cruzi* (American trypanosomiasis, Chagas disease)

Phylum Percolozoa
- *Naegleria fowleri* (meningoencephalitis)

*genus; spp = multiple species

✪ TABLE 2-6

Features of the Helminthes

Phylum (Class)	Body Shape	Digestive System	Diecious
Nematoda	round	complete	yes
Platyhelminthes	flattened	simple, saclike, or lacking	some species
Class Trematoda	leaf-shaped	simple, saclike	some species
Class Cestoda	long and segmented	lacking	no

Shape is a major factor separating members of the parasitic worms into different phylogenic categories. The roundworms, as the name reveals are round, muscular animals that are placed in the Phylum Nematoda. Listings of the most common nematodes are compiled in Box 2-4✪.

The flatworms are in the Phylum Platyhelminthes with two classes that contain human parasites, the class Trematoda that includes the flukes with their characteristic flattened leaf shape and the class Cestoda that contains the long segmented tapeworms. Box 2-5✪ contains a list of the most common Platyhelminthes.

✪ BOX 2-4

Nematoda (the Roundworms)

Class Adenophorea (Asphamidia)
- *Trichinella spiralis*
- *Trichuris trichiura*
- *Capillaria philippinensis*
- *Capillaria hepatica*

Class Secernentia (Phasmidia)
- *Enterobius vermicularis*
- *Strongyloides stercoralis*
- *Ancylostoma* spp. (hookworms)
- *Necator americanus* (hookworms)
- *Ascaris* spp. (human and pig roundworms)
- *Toxocara canis* (canine roundworms)
- *Enterobius vermicularis* (pinworms)
- *Trichostrongyloides stercoralis*
- *Anisakis* spp.
- *Onchocerca volvulus*
- *Brugia malayi* (brugian filariasis, elephantiasis)
- *Dirofilaria immitis* (canine heartworm)
- *Loa loa* (African eye worm)
- *Onchocerca volvulus* (onchocerciasis, riverblindness)
- *Wuchereria bancrofti* (bancroftian filariasis, elephantiasis)
- *Mansonella* spp.
- *Dracunculus medinensis* (guinea worm, fiery serpent)
- *Angiostrongylus* spp.

*genus; spp. = multiple species in the genus

✪ BOX 2-5

Platyhelminthes (the Flatworms)

Class Trematoda (flukes)
  Subclass Aspidogastrea
- *Aspidogaster* spp.

  Subclass Trematoda (the digenetic trematodes)
- *Dictyangium* spp.
- *Proterometra* spp.
- *Fasciola hepatica* (sheep liver fluke)
- *Schistosoma* spp. (the schistosomes or blood flukes)
- *Apocreadium* sp.
- *Paragonimus westermani* (human lung fluke)

Class Cestoda (flatworms)
  Subclass Eucestoda (tapeworms)
- *Diphyllobothrium* spp.
- *Dipylidium caninum*
- *Echinococcus granulosus*
- *Echinococcus multilocularis*
- *Hymenolepis nana*
- *Hymenolepis diminuta*
- *Taenia saginata*
- *Taenia solium*

genus; spp. = multiple species in the genus

The parasitic helminths have become specialized for life in the protective environment of the host. For example, many intestinal worms have significantly reduced digestive systems, which directly absorb nutrients digested by the host. Intestinal worms also have elaborate anchors, hooks, barbs, and/or sucker attachments for holding onto the host stomach or intestinal linings. A general feature of all parasitic helminths is the adaptation involving their reproductive systems. These worms are capable of producing extremely large numbers of eggs in an effort to ensure their survival by passage of their fertilized ova to susceptible intermediate hosts. A host by definition is the animal that houses the adult form of the parasite.

Adult worms may be **dioecious** (having separate sexes) or monecious, also referred to as hermaphroditic, meaning that one individual contains both sex organs. Sexual reproduction occurs in both cases; however, in dioecious species adult animals of both sexes are required. Adult hermaphrodites may self-fertilize, or they may copulate by exchanging eggs and sperm with other hermaphroditic animals.

The complex life cycles of many helminths involve intermediate hosts for one or more of their larval stages. Members of the class Trematoda have multiple hosts during their life cycle including at least one species of mollusk and one vertebrate. Parasitic helminth infections may be transmitted by several different mechanisms: ingestion of food or water containing an infective stage, direct penetration of the skin by an infective larval stage, and introduction via the bite from, or ingestion of, an arthropod vector. Helminth infections are more common in children due to the increased likelihood that they will ingest fecal matter from dirt, toys, or contact with other children. The best defense against the spread of parasitic helminth infections is prevention. Meat, fish, and suspect water should be thoroughly heated to destroy microorganisms. Additionally, protective clothing and shoes should be worn appropriately to reduce the amount of skin surfaces exposed, thereby minimizing sites of potential entry. Some parasites have multiple host species or spend part of their lives in soil or water, and as such, eradication is difficult. They are ubiquitous and provide a never-ending reservoir for reinfection of humans.

SIGNIFICANCE

Parasitic infections cause high rates of mortality and morbidity in third world countries. The United States enjoys a rather parasite-free existence relative to other countries due to an improved awareness of disease transmission, sanitation conditions, and our arid climate. However, several disease causing parasitic infections are pandemic. These include giardiasis and cryptosporidiosis, where infections arise from contaminated water supplies and fecal–oral contact at day-care centers. The majority of other cases seen by U.S. medical workers are species that have been contracted through international travel and/or immigration. Collectively, the majority of parasitic protozoans and metazoans have intermediate hosts and complex life cycles, facts that are important to understanding the route of transmission, treatment options, and attempts at eradication.

REAL WORLD TIP

There is evidence that the volume and speed of international travel has greatly decreased the time required for dissemination of disease and the development of a global pandemic. However, several agencies, including NASA, continually monitor the emergence and reemergence of infectious diseases as well as changes in environmental conditions that may indicate reemergence of diseases. These efforts are conducted in attempt to provide early warning to medical personnel and to provide time to prepare sufficient vaccines.

 Checkpoint! 2–9 (Chapter Objective 7)

Which of the following microorganisms is an example of a member of the kingdom Protozoa?

    A. *Staphylococcus epidermidis*
    B. *Giardia lamblia*
    C. *Enterovirus*
    D. *Legionella pneumophila*

SUMMARY

In this chapter, we came to realize that our contact with viruses, bacteria, fungus, and animal parasites does not necessarily result in infection. The majority of microorganisms form commensal or symbiotic relationships with other plants and animals, including humans. From history we recognize that the condition of the host is a factor that contributes to the pathogenesis of microbial infections, in that susceptibility to infection is increased in immunocompromised hosts and decreased in healthy individuals. Other factors that aid in resistance to contracting disease are general health, prior exposure and/or immunization, and genetics. The need for medical intervention occurs when our contact with microbes results in a parasitic relationship.

When we become infected with microbes, the microbiology laboratorian plays an important role in the diagnosis and treatment of the causative agent(s), including the oversight of specimen collection and the processing, testing, and analysis of appropriate specimens, as well as the interpretation of the results obtained. Proper treatment depends on the correct identification of the pathogenic organism(s), which is possible because of the general understanding of the characteristics and taxonomic classification of many microorganisms.

Many bright scientists have contributed to the development of the field of taxonomy over the centuries and expanded the processes used for identification and hence classification of microorganisms. These advances have improved the quality of life and increased the longevity of humans on earth. Some of the more prominent scientists that contributed to the process or stimulated thinking include Aristotle, John Ray, Carolus Linnaeus, and Charles Darwin. Additional, revolutionary contributions to the field of taxonomy and science were the printing press (Johann Gutenberg, in 1450) and the microscope (Antoni van Leeuwenhoek, 1650s).

The rules governing taxonomy are fairly rigid, although there has been a continuing debate among differing factions as to the best methods of assignment. These arguments span from the most specific (species level) to the broadest/general (kingdom) categories of taxonomic classification. International committees were assembled, with subbranches set up to deal with issues specific for the taxonomy and classification of the different phyla discussed in this chapter. These committees continue to meet on a regular basis addressing current problems, new organisms, and discrepancies associated with categorization of microorganisms in general. The controversies over categorization are worsened by the emergence of new technologies that allow infinitesimally subtle differences to be considered. Currently the capability exists to decipher the complete genotype of any organism. Where is the trade-off with respect to time and money? It is very probable within the near future that we will have eliminated the uncertainty in species assignments of microorganisms by having rapid and complete genetic sequence technology available in an instant. Thus, the field of taxonomy is in a continual state of change.

LEARNING OPPORTUNITIES

1. Why is the taxonomic classification of microorganisms important to maintain? (Chapter Objective 1)

2. Who were the key individuals that helped shape taxonomic classification, and what contributions did they make to the field? (Chapter Objective 4)

3. What were the two key historic discoveries that advanced taxonomic classification? (Chapter Objective 3)

4. Arrange the taxa used to categorize microorganisms from the smallest (most specific) to the largest (most general). (Chapter Objective 5)

5. What are the six kingdoms commonly used in the taxonomic classification of plants and animals? (Chapter Objective 7)

6. State at least one example member of each of the six kingdoms identified in question #5 that involve microorganisms. (Chapter Objective 7)

7. What is the definition of the term *pathogenic?* (Chapter Objective 8)

8. Describe two common relationships between microorganisms and their hosts that affect the ability of the microorganisms to infect a host. (Chapter Objective 9)

9. Why were kingdoms separated? (Chapter Objective 6)

10. What taxonomic approaches make up those used in current practice of taxonomic classification? Briefly describe each approach. (Chapter Objective 2)

11. What is a key cellular characteristic that differentiates fungi from bacteria? (Chapter Objective 10)

PEARSON
myhealthprofessionskit™

Use this address to access the interactive Companion Website created for this textbook. Simply select "Clinical Laboratory Science" from the choice of disciplines. Find this book and log in using your user name and password.

REFERENCES

Go to myhealthprofessionskit.com to view this chapter's references and useful websites.

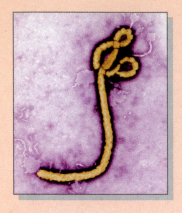

CHAPTER OUTLINE

3

The Bacterial Cell

Mark S. Johnson

■ LEARNING OBJECTIVES

Upon completion of this chapter, the learner should be able to:

1. Describe the different types of microscopes used in the microbiology laboratory setting.
2. Choose the appropriate microscope based on the morphologic information required for the identification process.
3. Describe other tools that play an important role in the isolation and identification of medically important infectious agents.
4. Predict how microbes are classified by their environmental and atmospheric requirements.
5. Describe how microbes are classified by a combination of their carbon source, energy source, and electron source.
6. Correlate the structure, composition, and function of the major external and internal components of the bacterial cell.
7. Categorize bacteria on the basis of shape or flagellar arrangement.
8. Explain how motile cells find nutrients using chemotaxis.
9. Describe prominent virulence factors that help pathogens overcome host defenses.
10. Distinguish the major structural differences between gram-positive and gram-negative bacterial cell walls.
11. Relate how structural differences in the cell wall affect the Gram stain reaction of bacteria.
12. Explain why antibiotics do not affect gram-positive and gram-negative bacteria in the same manner.
13. Describe or illustrate a typical growth curve for microbes.
14. Explain how the growth rate of microbes can be measured experimentally.
15. Describe the different mechanisms by which bacteria can be killed.
16. Describe the different methods by which microbes interconvert energy.
17. Differentiate between respiration and fermentation.
18. Relate the beneficial effects of commensal organisms as well as some of their side effects.
19. Describe the basic principles of microbial genetics and how bacterial genes are mutated and transferred.

KEY TERMS

anabolic pathway	cytoplasmic membrane	peptidoglycan
anaerobic	disinfectant	pili
aseptic	endospores	plasmids
autotrophs	fermentation	respiration
bactericidal	flagella	septic
bacteriostatic	fluorescent microscope	sterile
brightfield microscope	halophiles	teichoic acid
catabolic pathway	heterotrophs	virions
chemotaxis	lysozyme	virulence

▶ INTRODUCTION

This chapter deals with the basics of microbial cytology and physiology, as well as providing a brief look at the genetics of prokaryotic cells. The microbial world includes many organisms that are too small to be seen with the naked eye. Bacteria, an ever-present group of microorganisms, can range in size from 0.5 to 40 microns (μm) in length and exist in different shapes. They may be spherical (cocci), rod-shaped (bacilli), or helical (spirochetes). With few exceptions, they possess a cell wall that is responsible for their shape and rigidity and that allows them to exist in a hypotonic environment. When placed in a hypotonic medium, bacteria that lack cell walls lyse as water molecules in the hypotonic environment diffuse into their hypertonic cytoplasm. The composition of the cell wall also controls their ability to be stained with Gram's reagents and in addition determines whether or not they are acid fast.

Bacteria may also be surrounded by capsular material. Capsules are usually polysaccharide in nature and antiphagocytic (providing a means of defense against white blood cells of the host). Some microbes, including bacteria, possess **flagella**, structures that provide a means of locomotion in an aqueous environment.

Microbes have been able to adapt to a wide range of environmental conditions:

- Psychrophiles prefer colder temperatures (−10°C to 20°C).
- Mesophiles prefer somewhat warmer temperatures (10°C to 50°C).
- Thermophiles grow best at hot temperatures (50°C to 70°C).
- Acidophiles can survive acidic environments (a pH range from 1 to 5).
- Alkaliphiles can exist under very alkaline conditions (a pH range from 9 to 11).
- **Halophiles** are microbes that can grow (and may even require) high concentrations of salt (*Staphylococcus* species can tolerate salt concentrations as high as 10% w/v).

Bacteria may also be classified according to their susceptibility to oxygen toxicity and their need for different atmospheric components. Obligate aerobes are microorganisms that require an atmosphere in which oxygen is present. Facultative anaerobes are microorganisms capable of growing without oxygen, but usually grow better if oxygen is present. Microaerophilic organisms, such as *Campylobacter* and *Helicobacter* species, grow best when the concentration of oxygen is low (5% O_2, 10% CO_2, and 85% N_2). Anaerobes are usually defined as organisms that cannot grow in the presence of oxygen, but they actually can tolerate different levels of oxygen toxicity. There are aerotolerant anaerobes that can grow in room air if the medium is freshly made and the inoculum is quite heavy. These organisms usually produce tiny colonies because growth is very poor when oxygen is present. Moderate anaerobes can survive exposure to oxygen as long as the period of exposure is very brief. It seems that they are capable of recovering from a limited amount of oxygen toxicity. Obligate anaerobes require an oxygen-free atmosphere of carbon dioxide, hydrogen, and nitrogen. Exposure to oxygen is lethal to these organisms. Capnophiles are microbes that require an increased concentration of carbon dioxide to grow (*Streptococcus pneumoniae* and *Campylobacter* are good examples).

Microorganisms can metabolize a very wide range of substrates. Most environmental microbes have very simple nutritional requirements. They can grow quite well as long as a carbon source (such as simple sugars that provide energy) and a nitrogen source (often in the form of peptides or amino acids) are provided. Pathogenic bacteria tend to be more fastidious, and for some the growth medium must be supplemented with serum or blood.

 Checkpoint! 3–1 (Chapter Objective 4)

Organisms that are capable of growing in high concentrations of salt (and may even require an increased concentration of salt) are called:

    A. *microaerophilic.*
    B. *halophilic.*
    C. *capnophilic.*
    D. *alkaliphilic.*
    E. *mesophilic.*

▶ VISUALIZING BACTERIA

Because the human eye cannot detect objects less than 30 µm in diameter, the image of a bacterium must be magnified. The resolution, R, of a microscope is related to the wavelength of light, λ, and the numerical aperture, NA, according to:

$$R = 0.6 \, \lambda/NA \qquad \text{(eq. 3-1)}$$

The NA of a **brightfield microscope** is approximately 1.5, and the wavelength is 0.5 µm, so the resolving power is limited to about 0.2 µm [(0.6)(0.5)/(1.5) = 0.2 µm].

Although one could enlarge the image by projecting it onto a screen, it would still be impossible to resolve two objects that are separated by less than 0.2 µm. Both objects would appear as one. One could increase the resolution by decreasing the wavelength of light, but light is not visible to the eye below 0.4 µm (ultraviolet light).

To visualize an object, there must be enough contrast to see that object. To see contrast, the object must absorb or scatter some of the light. In essence, the intensity or amplitude differences of the light signal must be great enough to be perceived as contrast. Differences in the absorptivity within a microbe are generally not large enough to visualize that object. Therefore, microscopes other than the standard light microscope are commonly used to study bacteria. The phase contrast microscope enhances the refractive index differences of cell components. This instrument uses the change in the phase of light to visualize live bacteria and reveal details of their internal structure. The method relies on refractive index differences between intracellular components. Because light travels more slowly through a higher index of refraction, the phase or period of light will change relative to that of the unencumbered path, as shown in Figure 3-1 ■. Light waves that are in phase enter the cell, but fall out of phase before leaving the cell. The phase differences are then converted electronically to amplitude differences by a method developed in 1935 by Frits Zernike (1888–1966), a Dutch physicist who would receive the 1953 Nobel Prize for this invention.

The darkfield microscope makes use of light redirected from the sample against a darkfield background. Although internal components cannot be seen, it is easy to visualize the cells, which appear light against a dark background (Figure 3-2 ■).

A **fluorescent microscope** is an important tool in clinical and research labs. Fluorescent molecules are unique in that they absorb light at one wavelength and emit light at a longer wavelength. This means there is more energy absorbed than emitted by these molecules. The "missing" energy is lost as vibrational energy before the excited electrons drop to the ground state. The decay to the ground state emits light at a frequency characteristic of each fluorescent molecule. Different filters for incoming and outgoing light allow the observer or camera to visualize the fluorescence. Because most bacteria do not have naturally occurring fluorescent molecules that emit light in the visible range, exogenous stains, antibodies, or expression vectors must be added to take advantage of fluorescence microscopy. Immunofluorescence is a technique that uses a fluorescently tagged antibody to identify bacterial strains, serotypes, or other features. More recently, vectors expressing the green fluorescent protein fused to a protein of interest have been used to determine expression and/or location of the fused protein. The green fluorescent light emitted by these proteins can be visualized in live cells.

The concept of the confocal scanning microscope was invented by Marvin Minsky in 1955 and made practical in the late 1980s by Brad Amos and John White. Light is focused into a narrow beam that converges at a point on a plane. The focused light is collected through a small aperture, and scattered light is rejected. Because the viewing field is small, the microscope stage is repeatedly moved, after which images are compiled into a sharp image on that plane. Using this technique, a series of optical sections can be made through a bulk sample and reconstructed into a complete 3-D image. The appearance of this reconstruction can be quite remarkable.

The electron microscope has tremendous resolving power. This is because the relationship between resolving power and wavelength holds true for any form of radiation, and the wavelength of an electron decreases as its velocity increases. At an

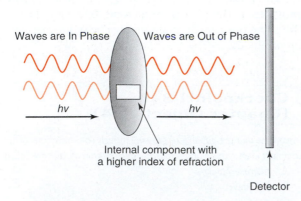

■ **FIGURE 3-1** Logic behind phase-contrast microscopy. The detector uses differences in wave phases to show contrast between parts of an image.

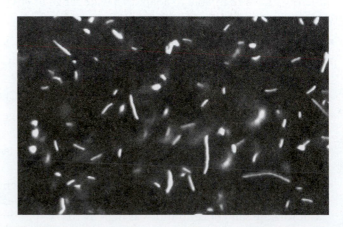

■ **FIGURE 3-2** Bacteria viewed under a darkfield microscope. Cells appear white against a dark background.

accelerating voltage of 100,000 volts, the wavelength of an electron is 0.004 nm (4 picometers). The theoretical resolution of such a microscope should be about 0.002 nm, but because of aberrations in the electron "lens," the practical resolving power is at best 0.1 nm (1 Å). Furthermore, specimen preparation, contrast, and radiation damage limit the practical resolution for biological objects to 2 nm. However, this is still 100 times better resolution than that of the light microscope.

The atomic force microscope moves like a phonograph needle. An exceptionally small tip transverses the surface, and deflection is measured with a small laser beam. The limit is approximately 0.1 Å. The scanning tunneling microscope brings a fine wire tip to within a few angstroms of a conductive surface. Electrons can "tunnel" or hop between the tip and the surface. This effect drops dramatically with distance, and small changes in position can be measured. Individual atoms can be imaged. Go to ∞ Chapter 8 to learn more about the use and care of the compound brightfield microscope. See the Companion Website for a description of the origin of bacterial cytology.

OTHER TOOLS

In addition to the microscope, the microbiologist has a new tool that allows manipulations on the microscale. Laser tweezers, now often called optical tweezers, were developed in the mid-80s by Arthur Ashkin at AT&T Bell Labs. The laser tweezers can grab a single bacterium and move it at will; even larger cells, such as sperm cells, can be moved for manipulations.

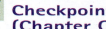

Checkpoint! 3–2 (Chapter Objectives 1 and 2)

The _____ microscope enhances the refractive index differences of cell components to visualize live bacteria and reveal details of their internal structure.

  A. phase contrast
  B. electron
  C. darkfield
  D. brightfield
  E. atomic force

► CYTOLOGY

A drawing summarizing some of the hallmarks of a typical prokaryotic cell is shown in Figure 3-3 ■. It includes features evident from an electron microscope: a capsule, cell wall, outer membrane (om), periplasmic space, peptidoglycan (pg), cytoplasmic membrane (cm), flagellum and motor, pilus and fimbriae, nuclear region, ribosomes, and inclusions (fuel stores) such as glycogen, polyphosphate, and β-hydroxybutyrate. As shown, the cell wall differs in gram-positive and gram-negative cells. The vital statistics of an *E. coli* cell are summarized in Table 3-1 ✪.

BACTERIAL SHAPES

A variety of bacterial shapes are evident. The major ones include the rod or cylindrical-shaped bacilli, the spherical cocci, and the spiral-shaped spirilla (Figure 3-4 ■). In addition, there are square and filamentous bacteria. Besides individual cellular shapes, characteristic aggregates can form, yielding different appearances (see Figure 3-4).

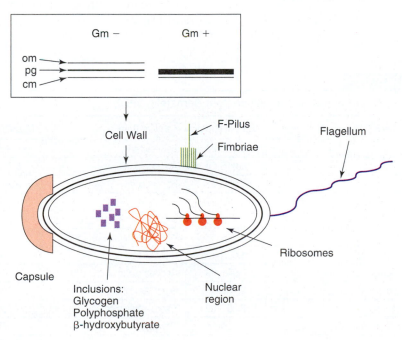

■ FIGURE 3-3 Drawing highlighting the prominent features of a bacterial cell.

✪ TABLE 3-1

Vital Statistics for an *E. coli* Cell (Values from Neidhardt & Umbarger, 1996)

Total weight	9.5×10^{-13} g
Total volume	0.9×10^{-15} liters
Water weight	6.7×10^{-13} g
Dry weight	2.8×10^{-13} g
Protein (by weight)	55%
Ribosomal RNA	16.8%
mRNA	0.8%
tRNA	2.9%
DNA	3.1%
Lipids	9.1%
Lipopolysaccharides	3.4%
Peptidoglycans	2.5%
Glycogen	2.5%
Polyamines	0.4%
Metabolites, cofactors, ions	3.5%

Checkpoint! 3–3 (Chapter Objective 7)

Bacteria that are spherical in shape are known as:

- A. *spirilla.*
- B. *bacilli.*
- C. *cocci.*
- D. *fungi.*
- E. *prions.*

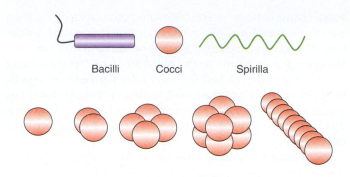

■ **FIGURE 3-4** The three primary shapes of bacteria: rods (bacilli), spheres (cocci), and spirals (spirilla). Higher organization of cells may help identify species.

BACTERIAL SIZES

Bacteria are the smallest self-contained, independent, unicellular organisms. They typically range from 1 to 1.5 μm in width and from 2 to 6 μm in length. The extremes range from approximately 0.2 μm for *Mycoplasma genitalium* to over 100 μm to 750 μm for the recently discovered *Thiomargarita namibiensis*. Uncharacterized nanobacteria as small as 50 nm in diameter have been reported, but their existence remains the subject of heated debate.

To give some perspective on the relative size of a typical bacterium, if an *E. coli* cell (2 μm) were enlarged to 1 inch, a 6-foot person (enlarged equivalently) would be 14.4 miles tall, with Mount Everest (29,028 ft) at midthigh.

The mass of a bacterium as contrasted with the mass of other well-known items is shown in Table 3-2✪. The masses are listed in Scientific Notation, where 9.11×10^{-28} is expressed as 9.11E–28.

✪ TABLE 3-2

Masses of Common Objects (Values from Bernstein, 1978)

Familiar Item	Mass in Grams	Familiar Item	Mass in Grams
Electron	9.11E–28	Bald eagle	4050
Proton	1.67E–24	Average person	6.75E+04
Carbon atom	2.00E–23	Bengal tiger	2.25E+05
Glucose molecule	5.98E–22	Blue whale	1.75E+08
Hemoglobin molecule	2.16E–19	World's diamonds (recovered)	2.50E+08
Bacteriophage	2.05E–17	World's gold (recovered)	6.00E+10
E. coli	1.00E–12	Giant oil tanker	4.00E+11
Average human cell (liver cell)	2.00E–09	Cheops pyramid	5.00E+12
Rat flea (caused the bubonic plague)	2.10E–04	Great Wall of China	1.20E+14
Honeybee	2.88E–02	Earth's total water	1.26E+24
Mouse	21	The Earth	5.97E+27
Rat	280	The Sun	1.99E+33

Note the relative weight of an *E. coli* cell is halfway (on a log scale) between an electron and a bald eagle (15 orders of magnitude greater than an electron and 15 orders less than the eagle). Impressively, the number of bacteria that would be required to equal the weight of an eagle would nearly match the number of honeybees required to equal the weight of the Great Wall of China. Nonetheless, the power of geometric growth is such that if a single *E. coli* was allowed to double every 20 min (its maximum growth rate), the weight of the organisms would reach the mass of the earth in less than 47 h (see section on growth).

THE FLAGELLAR MOTOR

Because a bacterium may weigh only a picogram, it has little inertia to overcome the viscous forces of water. On our scale, it would be like attempting to swim through wet asphalt. A bacterium traveling at 30 µm/sec coasts for about 0.04 Å when the flagellar rotation stops. This is equivalent to the space shuttle (17,000 MPH) shutting off its engine and coasting 1 mm. Motile bacteria overcome this viscous drag with a corkscrew-type rotation of their helical flagella. This motion differs from sperm motility, which does not use flagellar rotation, but a whiplike back-and-forth motion.

The motor is a small (about 40 nm across by 60 nm high) circular wheel, which is responsible for the propeller-like rotation of the flagella (for a 3-D structure, see Thomas, Francis, Xu, & DeRosier, 2006). In *E. coli,* it is reversible and is powered by proton motive force. Protons that have been translocated out of the cell into the periplasmic space by the electron transport chain (as happens in mitochondria) move back into the cell down this concentration gradient. The direction of flagellar rotation is not controlled by the proton movement, which is the same for clockwise or counterclockwise rotation. Rather, a switch on the flagellar motor controls the rotational bias. Because some bacteria are able to use a sodium ion gradient to turn the motor, it is more correct to state the energy currency for flagellar rotation is ion motive force. To conceptualize how this ion motive force is applied by the motor, think of how wind forces the rotation of a windmill. The bacterial motor generates about 10^{-18} horsepower, or about 10 hp per pound of motor. Some 1,200 protons (in *E. coli*) are required for each revolution.

Flagellar Arrangement

Not all bacteria express flagella, but those that do have a characteristic flagellar arrangement with the following definitions: monotrichous, a single-polar flagellum (Figure 3-5a ■); amphitrichous, flagella (single or in clusters) at both poles (Figure 3-5b ■); lophotrichous, a single tuft or cluster of flagella at a pole (Figure 3-5c ■); bilophotrichous, two tufts or clusters of flagella on one hemisphere (Figure 3-5d ■; e.g., magnetotactic cocci; Frankel, Bazylinski, Johnson, & Taylor, 1997); peritrichous, single flagella randomly distributed around the microorganism (Figure 3-5e ■; *E. coli*). Each flagellum requires some 50 gene products to be synthesized, but once the external structure begins lengthening, it

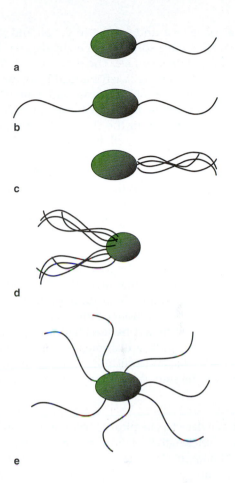

■ FIGURE 3-5 Types of flagellar arrangement in bacteria. **a.** Monotrichous. **b.** Amphitrichous. **c.** Lophotrichous. **d.** Bilophotrichous. **e.** Peritrichous.

does so in an interesting manner. The center is porous, and the monomer filament proteins migrate down this passageway to the tip, where they attach. Thus, each flagellum continues to grow, but growth is from the tip, not the base.

✓ **Checkpoint! 3–4 (Chapter Objective 7)**

Bacteria that produce a single flagellum or a cluster of flagella at both poles are termed:

   A. *monotrichous.*
   B. *amphitrichous.*
   C. *lophotrichous.*
   D. *bilophotrichous.*
   E. *peritrichous.*

Chemotaxis

Many motile bacteria have a sophisticated tracking system that allows them to find nutrients such as amino acids, sugars, and optimal concentrations of oxygen. This behavior, called

chemotaxis, is best understood in *E. coli* and *Salmonella*. These organisms have some six to eight flagella distributed randomly around their surface. The shape of each flagellum is that of a left-handed helix (a left-handed helix can be visualized by walking down a spiral staircase with your left shoulder on the inside). Therefore, if a single flagellum is rotated counterclockwise (looking from the flagellar tip toward the cell body), it pushes against the cell. If all the flagella rotate counterclockwise, they will all push toward the cell. Because the forces are not perfectly symmetric, the flagella rapidly form a tight bundle, which propels the cell forward (Figure 3-6). A clockwise rotation creates a pulling force away from the cell, the flagellar bundle separates, and the cell turns or tumbles.

Random Walk

E. coli normally swims randomly through three-dimensional space. This is called a random walk. One or 2 seconds of smooth swimming are followed by brief tumbles. In *E. coli,* smooth runs are caused by synchronous counterclockwise flagellar rotation, which causes the left-handed helical flagella to form a tight bundle. The bundle is disrupted by clockwise rotation of one or more flagella, and a turn or tumbling ensues. The new orientation for the smooth swim is random (see Figure 3-6).

Attractant and Repellent Responses

E. coli cells can detect a chemical concentration change of 1 part in 10,000 per cell length (2–3 μm) when swimming at maximum velocity (30 μm/sec). They do this by monitoring the environment in a temporal fashion (over time). This "time" factor increases sensitivity to small gradients while diminishing responses to random fluctuations (noise) in the environment. An increase in attractant or decrease in repellent is acknowledged by suppression of tumbles. An increase in repellent or decrease in attractant causes shorter runs and more frequent tumbles.

For cells to move up a concentration gradient, they must be able to compare the present attractant concentration with the recent past. In essence, they must "memorize" the local neighborhood. This memory or record is stored in the form of methyl groups on four to five glutamyl groups on the chemoreceptor. The methylation counteracts the attractant signal, "adapting" the receptor to the new attractant concentration. The adapted receptor is then poised to sense slight changes in the levels of the chemical. By monitoring the environment in this fashion, bacteria move up a concentration gradient at nearly 50% of their maximum swimming speed.

> ✔ ## Checkpoint! 3–5
> ## (Chapter Objective 8)
>
> *The sophisticated tracking system that allows microbes to find nutrients such as amino acids, sugars, and optimal concentrations of oxygen is known as:*
>
> A. *proton motive force.*
> B. *ion motive force.*
> C. *chemotaxis.*
> D. *random walk.*
> E. *gliding motion.*

PILI AND FIMBRIAE

Fimbriae and **pili** are protein projections that are thinner and shorter than flagella and are most often found in gram-negative bacteria. The terms *fimbriae* (Latin, fringe) and *pili* (Latin, hairs) are used synonymously (Brinton, 1965; Duguid & Anderson, 1967). Seven types (Type I, Type II, . . . Type VII) have been described, depending on their size and the antigens they carry. All seem to be involved in adherence or binding. The Type IV pili enables a bacterium to crawl or "twitch" across a

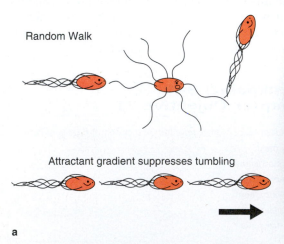

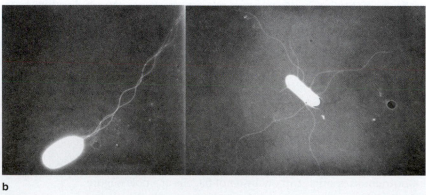

a   b

■ **FIGURE 3-6** Bacterial chemotaxis. **a.** In an isotropic environment, *E. coli* swim in a random walk pattern. The random walk pattern is inhibited by a nutrient gradient, which suppresses tumbling. **b.** Left panel: An electron micrograph shows a flagellar bundle at one end of *S. typhimurium,* resulting from the coordinated counter-clockwise rotation of flagella. Right panel: Flagella fly apart when flagella rotate in the clockwise direction, and cells tumble.
Electron micrograph taken by Graeme Lindbeck.

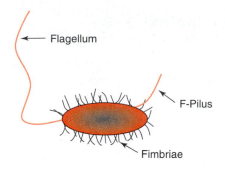

- Flagellum
- F-Pilus
- Fimbriae

■ **FIGURE 3-7** Fimbriae and the F-pilus: sticky projections used by bacteria for attachment.

smooth surface. One type (Type VII) of pili, called the "F" or "sex" pili (Figure 3-7 ■) is used to transfer DNA to other cells (conjugation). They are longer and thicker than the other types. This type is also a receptor for certain viruses, called bacteriophages (viruses that infect bacteria).

Other types can cause adherence to other bacteria or red blood cells (hemagglutination) or may be **virulence** factors. *Neisseria gonorrhoeae* is unable to cause venereal disease, *Pseudomonas aeruginosa* is unable to wreak havoc on cystic fibrosis patients, and *Streptococcus pyogenes* is unable to cause "strep" throat without specific type 1 fimbriae.

CAPSULES

Some bacteria are surrounded with a slippery slime, a sticky covering, or a mucous layer. These layers are referred to as a capsule or glycocalyx, depending on their consistency.

Capsules are uniform and condensed around the cell. The glycocalyx forms a loose meshwork of fibrils that extends outward from the cell. When this network is thick, viscous, and appears detached from the cell, it is often called a slime layer. Capsules offer protection to the bacterium and thus are important for virulence. Such capsules help resist changes in osmolarity (high salt/low salt), and they offer protection against phagocytosis. Slight changes in capsular composition change antigenicity: *S. pneumoniae* has nearly 15 serotypes. Bacteria that contain a capsule can often be identified by the type of colony they form. Those containing capsules form a smooth (S-type) colony, whereas those with capsules removed by genetic or chemical means grow as a rough (R-type) colony.

 **Checkpoint! 3–6
(Chapter Objectives 6 and 9)**

Capsules serve as virulence factors because they are:
  A. slippery when wet.
  B. sharply pointed, hairlike appendages.
  C. antiphagocytic.
  D. responsible for adherence to host cells.
  E. additional targets for antibody production.

CELL WALL

The cell wall provides the bacterium with its shape, rigidity, and resistance to osmotic pressure differences between the environment and the cytoplasm. It also acts as a sieve for molecules that are transported into the cell. Finally, it provides the supporting matrix for the capsule, pili, fimbriae, and flagella. Bacteria that lack a cell wall, such as *Mycoplasma* species, are extremely sensitive to osmotic pressure changes. Significant changes in the external environment are common. For example, the osmotic pressure difference between deionized water and 150 mM NaCl (isotonic saline) is 7.2 atmospheres. The osmotic difference between deionized water and the saturated salty water where *Halobacterium salinarium* resides is over 240 atmospheres. Because osmotic effects can be perilous, bacteria lacking a rigid cell wall are consigned to live in a restricted environment.

Inclusion Bodies

Under certain circumstances, such as a limiting nutrient or an excess of a particular nutrient, bacteria store various chemicals within the cell. For example, in the case of an overabundance of a carbon source but no available nitrogen to synthesize amino acids, the cell might store the carbon in reserve to await better times. These can accumulate, precipitate out, and form an inclusion body. These inclusions are not separated by a boundary membrane from the rest of the cytoplasm, and they may be reserves of glycogen (carbohydrate reserves), polyphosphate (or adenosine tri-phosphate reserve), and poly-β-hydroxybutyric acid (lipid reserves).

Endospores

Pasteur's findings that yeast extract remained sterile in a swan-neck flask were not reproducible by others who included hay in their infusions. John Tyndall reported that the mere presence of a bale of hay prevented sterility of the medium by boiling. In 1877, Ferdinand Cohn discovered the responsible bodies were small refractile endospores.

Genera such as *Bacillus* and *Clostridium* can form **endospores** that are resistant to extreme heat. They can be boiled for hours and still survive. The spore is formed under adverse conditions and is a complex multilayered structure that can be found within the cytoplasm of the vegetative cell or in the environment when the vegetative portion has disintegrated. Spores are protected by a peptidoglycan coat and calcium dipicolinate to stabilize its core. Spores are a major problem for the food industry. Liquids must be autoclaved at 120°C for 15 minutes or dry materials heated for several hours at high temperatures to kill spores. ∞ Chapter 5, "Safety," provides more details on autoclaves.

Checkpoint! 3–7 (Chapter Objective 6)

What structure provides the bacterium with its shape, rigidity, and resistance to osmotic pressure differences between the environment and the cytoplasm?
- *A. Ribosomes*
- *B. Capsule*
- *C. Cell wall*
- *D. Bacteriophage*
- *E. Inclusion body*

Checkpoint! 3–8 (Chapter Objective 11)

Which component of the cell wall is responsible for the ability of gram-negative bacteria to be decolorized more readily than gram-positive bacteria?
- *A. Multiple peptidoglycan layers*
- *B. Lipid-rich envelope*
- *C. Teichoic acids*
- *D. Glycoproteins*
- *E. Mycolic acids*

Gram Stain

In the 1880s, Hans Christian Gram serendipitously discovered that most bacteria could be divided into two classes by using a simple staining technique. We call these classes gram-positive and gram-negative. Those bacteria that retain a blue dye are gram-positive; those that lose the dye and turn red during the procedure are gram-negative. The difference is because of the cell wall.

Gram-positive bacteria have thick outer walls containing many layers of **peptidoglycan**, have an outer layer of **teichoic acids**, and lack lipids.

 REAL WORLD TIP

Acid-fast bacilli (*Mycobacterium)* and *Nocardia* have a cell wall structure similar to the gram-positive bacteria (small amount of peptidoglycan but no teichoic acids) and may stain weakly gram-positive. They differ from gram-positive bacteria by having an outer coat of mycolic acids, other waxes, and glycolipids. This "waxy" outer layer is hydrophobic and less permeable to reagents making the cell extremely hard to stain. For this reason the preferred staining method is the acid-fast stain, discussed in ∞ Chapter 8, "Presumptive Identification."

Gram-negative organisms have a single or a few layers of peptidoglycan and an outer lipid-rich membrane. Substances bound to the gram-negative outer membrane can readily be washed out of the organisms using alcohol or an alcohol/acetone mixture that dissolves the lipid-rich outer membrane. In the Gram stain, the dye, crystal violet, is firmly fixed to the bacterial cell wall following addition of Gram's iodine (Figure 3-8 ■). After briefly rinsing with an alcohol/acetone mixture, gram-negative cells are decolorized, but gram-positive cells retain the crystal violet dye. Another stain, safranin (which is red), is then added. This dye is taken up by the decolorized gram-negative cells; gram-positive cells remain violet. Refer to ∞ Chapter 8 to learn how the Gram stain is used in presumptive identification of an unknown microorganism.

Cell Envelope

The term *cell envelope* is an inclusive term used to describe the cell wall of a bacterium as well as ancillary features surrounding it, such as an outer membrane or capsule. The cell envelope serves several functions, but the most crucial role is to protect the cell against harsh environmental changes such as osmotic pressure. Recall that osmosis is the diffusion of molecules down a concentration gradient. A high concentration of solute on one side of a semipermeable (permeable to some but not all molecules) and a low concentration of solute on the other side sets up an osmotic gradient. Because pure water is at a concentration of 55.5M and can pass rapidly across the membrane, it is the major driving force behind osmotic pressure (Π). For an ideal solution of an uncharged solute, the osmotic pressure can be approximated by the following equation:

$$\Pi = cRT \qquad \text{(eq. 3-2)}$$

where c is the concentration of solute in moles liter^{-1}, R is 0.0821 atmospheres mol^{-1} °K^{-1}, and T is temperature in degrees

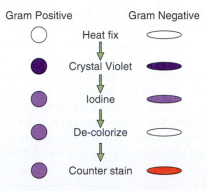

■ **FIGURE 3-8** Overall scheme for a Gram stain. Cells are adsorbed onto a slide and treated with mild heat and stained with crystal violet, which is fixed to the cell surface with iodine. The outer membrane of gram-negative cells dissolves when treated with alcohol/acetone, and these cells become decolorized as they lose the crystal violet stain. However, the thick peptidoglycan sheets of gram-positive cells retain crystal violet when treated with alcohol/acetone. When counterstained with safranin red, gram-negative cells become red, whereas gram-positive cells remain violet.

kelvin. Thus, the osmotic pressure of a 100 mM solution of sucrose relative to deionized water at 298°K would be

$$\Pi = (0.1)(0.0821)(298) = 2.5 \text{ atmospheres}$$

This is

$$(2.5) \times (14.7 \text{ psi/atm}) = 36 \text{ pounds per square inch (psi)}$$

Note: This equation gives low estimates of osmotic pressure when the sucrose concentration is above 1M because of a sequestering of six water molecules per sucrose. In essence, sucrose lowers the concentration of solvent more than expected.

Halobacterium salinarium is capable of growing in media with a 5M concentration of salts. For salts, the osmotic pressure is predicted to be twice the value expected from the mole fraction of the salt because dissociation (e.g., NaCl → Na$^+$ + Cl$^+$) doubles the solute concentration. In an ideal solution, the osmotic pressure of 5M salt relative to deionized water would be

$$\Pi = (10)(0.0821)(298) = 244 \text{ atmospheres, or } 3,596 \text{ psi}$$

In reality, bacteria are not bags of deionized water, but cells filled with some 300 to 400 mg ml^{-1} macromolecules. Because the osmotic pressure depends on the number of intracellular molecules, macromolecules that are large in size but low in number do not contribute substantially to the intracellular osmolarity. Macromolecules contribute most of their osmolar effects by their many charged groups, which bind inorganic ions of opposite charge. Additionally, the cell contains a high concentration of sugars, amino acids, and nucleotides, which if charged pull more counterions into the cell. These effects contribute to a high intracellular osmolarity, which draws water into the cell, causing outward pressure on the membrane or turgor. This turgor stretches the cell envelope and appears essential for cell enlargement and growth. Bacteria can control the turgor to a large extent by exporting or importing inorganic ions, amino acids, and neutral solutes. The cell wall also has some elasticity, so the cell volume increases or decreases, depending on an increase or decrease in turgor, respectively. Organisms without a cell wall, such as *Mycoplasma* species, are sensitive to changes in turgor and are highly susceptible to lysis.

All bacteria, with the exception of *Mycoplasma, Urea-plasma, Spiroplasma,* and *Anaeroplasma,* contain a cell wall. Chemistry aside, gram-positive cells have a thick peptidoglycan layer (cell wall) surrounding the **cytoplasmic membrane.** Gram-negative cells have a thin peptidoglycan layer and an outer membrane surrounding their cytoplasmic membrane.

Peptidoglycan Layer

The peptidoglycan layer (also known as murein or mucopeptide) is unique to the cell wall of prokaryotes and is responsible for maintaining cell shape and rigidity (like a corset or girdle). It is made in layers or sheets (like a chain-link fence). Gram-negative cells may only have one layer, but gram-positive cells may have from 15 to 50 layers. To increase integrity in gram-positive cells, each layer is cross-linked to the one beneath it. In gram-negative cells, this thin layer is cross-linked to the outer membrane. The thicker peptidoglycan layer in gram-positive cells makes them more resistant to dry locations, such as human skin. The outer membrane in gram-negative cells makes them more resistant to some antibiotics, such as penicillin.

Each sheet of the peptidoglycan layer is a polymer of the alternating sugars N-acetylglucosamine (NAG) and N-acetylmuramic acid (NAM); (Park, 1996). In *E. coli,* the average polymer length is 30 muropeptides in length. These glycan sheets are cross-linked through the N-acetylmuramic acid by a short peptide. A diagrammatic sketch is shown in Figure 3-9 ■.

The linkage between glycan monomers is through a β −(1,4) bond (Figure 3-10a ■). The peptide cross-linking is through two tetrapeptide units that are bound to the acetylmuramic acid glycan. The unusual D-amino acids and diaminopimelic acid of the tetrapeptide do not occur in proteins and are unique to the peptidoglycan. The structure of diaminopimelic acid is similar to lysine, with the addition of a carboxyl group at the amino end.

Each peptide is linked to muramic acid through an amide linkage to its carboxyl group. All mureins contain an alternating sequence of D- and L-optical isomers, but the amino acids are not universal. Cross-linking can be between adjacent tetrapeptides as well as between those of different chains. In gram-negative strains, cross-linking usually occurs between the carboxyl group of the D-alanine in position 4 of one peptide and the free amino group of diaminopimelic acid (DAP); as shown in Figure 3-10a. However, up to 20% of the cross-links in *E. coli* are not through D-alanine but through DAP residues of neighboring chains. Approximately 50% of the muropeptides are involved in cross-links, and another 5% are involved in links that hold three muropeptides together. This strong, multilayered sheet may be thought of as one large

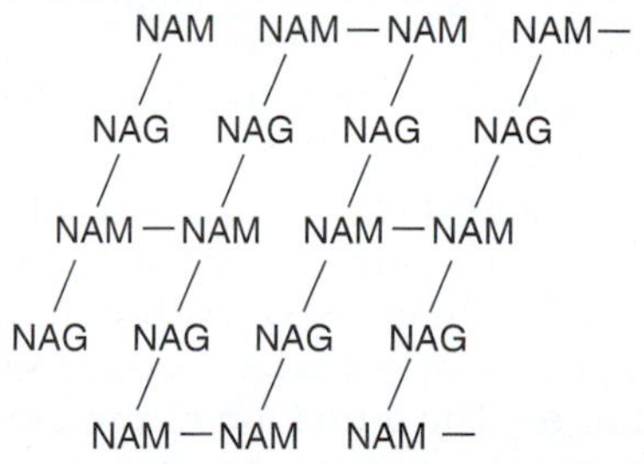

■ **FIGURE 3-9** Arrangement of peptidoglycan, with glycan sheets (NAM-NAG-NAM....) crosslinked by peptide linkages between NAM-NAM. NAM, *N*-acetylmuramic acid; NAG, *N*-acetylglucosamine.

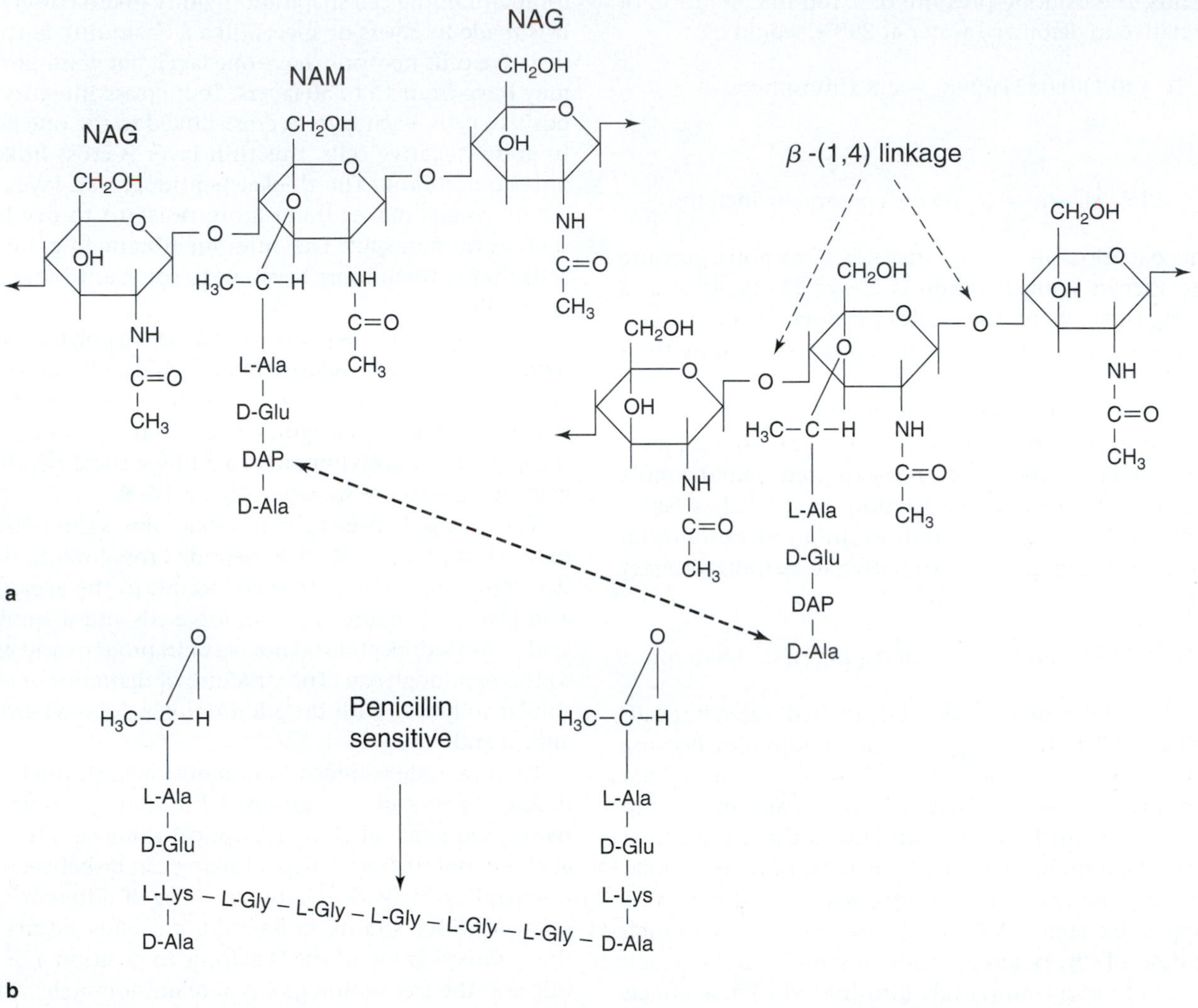

■ FIGURE 3-10 Linkages between *N*-acetylglucosamine (NAG) and *N*-acetylmuramic acid (NAM) in peptidoglycan. **a.** NAG and NAM are joined through a β–(1,4) linkage. In typical gram-negative cells (*E. coli*), neighboring glycan sheets are joined by a peptide fusion between the diaminopimelic acid and D-alanine. **b.** An additional pentapeptide links the tetrapeptide in some gram-positive cells, such as *S. aureus.* In both gram-positive and gram-negative cells, penicillin inhibits the transpeptidase responsible for forming the peptide linkage.

cross-linked molecule or sacculus (Latin, *sacculus,* meaning "little sac") that surrounds the entire cell. The typical cross bridging between two glycan sheets in gram-negative cells is shown in Figure 3-10a.

As you might guess, there are some slight differences between the peptidoglycan in gram-positive and gram-negative cells. The tetrapeptides from most gram-positive cells contain lysine rather than diaminopimelic acid. The cross-linking is different in gram-positive cells as well. In the gram-positive bacterium *Staphylococcus aureus,* for example, the cross-linkage is a pentapeptide of glycine (see Figure 3-10b ■). The formation of this cross bridge is inhibited by penicillin. ∞ Chapter 11, "Susceptibility Testing," describes how antibiotics like penicillin kill or inhibit the growth of microorganisms.

A definitive structure for the murein has yet to be determined. Although cartoons are usually drawn with the sugars in a flat plane, the mucopeptides may actually be twisted so that each strand of murein is a helix with each peptide side chain exposed approximately 90° around the helix relative to its neighbors. In this configuration, only one in every four muropeptides would be able to cross-link to a specific neighboring polymer, but it would allow for cross-linking between a total of four neighboring polymers: one above, one below, one to the left, and one to the right.

As the cell grows, glycan and peptide bonds must be broken, and new bonds must be formed. The process is highly coordinated because the cell would be lysed rapidly unless new bonds were formed before old ones were cleaved.

Teichoic Acids

The cell walls of most gram-positive bacteria also contain teichoic acids, which are acidic anionic polysaccharides

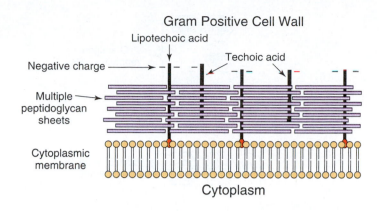

Gram Positive Cell Wall

FIGURE 3-11 Drawing showing the prominent features of a gram-positive cell wall.

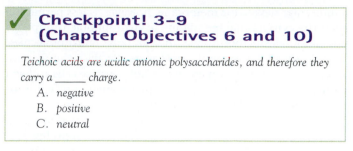
(Figure 3-11 ■). Teichoic acids contain a carbohydrate such as glucose, as well as phosphate and an alcohol. The teichoic acids are bonded to the peptidoglycan and are therefore an integral part of the cell wall. Teichoic acids can bind protons, giving the cell wall a lower pH, which decreases the rate of degradation by autolysins. Teichoic acids also bind the cations calcium and magnesium and are receptor sites for some bacteriophages. When phosphate concentrations are low, the cell replaces teichoic acids with teichuronic acids to save phosphate for ATP (adenosine triphosphate), DNA, and other important cell components.

The peptidoglycan layer of gram-positive cells is ~40 nm and comprises about 90% of the cell wall. As mentioned, it retains crystal violet in the Gram stain procedure. Besides being resistant to the alcohol/acetone treatment, another explanation for dye retention is that this layer is normally considerably hydrated. After alcohol/acetone treatment, the wall dehydrates and shrinks, trapping the primary stain–iodine complex.

Gram-Negative Envelope

The gram-negative cell envelope is far more complex than that of gram-positive cells. The peptidoglycan layer is only ~2 nm and is less than 10% of the cell wall. This layer is too thin to trap the crystal-violet complex after alcohol/acetone treatment. Teichoic acids are not present in gram-negative cell walls. Instead, these walls contain lipoproteins (lipids linked to protein molecules), which are bound to approximately 1 in every 10 mucopeptides (Figure 3-12 ■; Nikaido, 1996). Covalent binding occurs through the L-carboxyl group of the diaminopimelic acid to the epsilon amino group of the carboxy-terminal lysine of the lipoprotein. This links the peptidoglycan to the outer membrane. Additional stability between the outer membrane and the peptidoglycan might occur from outer membrane porins, which remain complexed with the peptidoglycan after detergent and heat treatment at 60°C.

OUTER MEMBRANE

The outer membrane is a second membrane that surrounds the cytoplasmic membrane (see Figure 3-12). Unlike the cytoplasmic membrane, it is rather permeable to most small molecules. The permeability is because of proteins called porins, which form channels across the membrane. These porins are large enough for molecules less than ~1,000 daltons to pass freely, but the size is strain specific. Thus, the outer membrane acts as

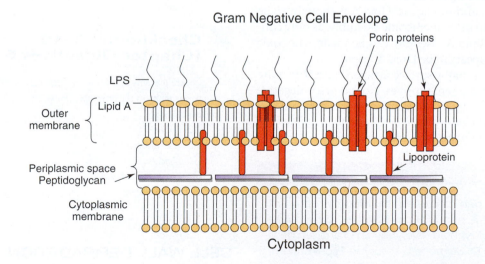

Gram Negative Cell Envelope

FIGURE 3-12 Drawing showing the prominent features comprising the cell envelope of a typical gram-negative cell.

a molecular sieve. This membrane, however, is less permeable than the cytoplasmic membrane to hydrophobic (nonpolar) and amphipathic (both polar and nonpolar ends) molecules. For this reason, some antibiotics that are effective against gram-positive cells cannot gain entry to gram-negative cells and will clearly be less effective. The outer membrane is a receptor for bacteriophages and an excellent source of antigens.

The stability of the outer membrane is conferred by cross-links to the peptidoglycan layer through the murein lipoprotein (see Figure 3-12). *E. coli* contains some 700,000 copies of this protein (Nikaido, 1996). The protein portion of the lipoprotein is bonded to the peptidoglycan layer, and the fatty acid portion associates with the hydrophobic portion of the outer membrane. The outer membrane contains two types of lipids, lipopolysaccharide and phospholipids.

LIPOPOLYSACCHARIDE

The outer leaflet (the outer layer of the bilayer) contains lipopolysaccharides (LPS), a molecule unique to gram-negative outer membranes (Raetz, 1996). It is not found in the cytoplasmic membrane. Clinically, it is important because the LPS acts as an endotoxin (*endo* means "inside," or within the cell) and an important virulence factor. When the LPS alone is introduced into animals, it causes fever and may even lead to shock and death. Thus, even after cells have been killed by antibiotics, the endotoxin can still cause problems.

The LPS has three parts: (1) a hydrophobic lipid A region, (2) a core oligosaccharide region, and (3) a hydrophilic O-antigen polysaccharide region (Figure 3-13 ■). Lipid A, which is a polar lipid, has a backbone of glucosaminyl-β-(1,6)-glucosamine bound to six or seven saturated fatty acid residues, which protrude into the outer membrane. The lipid A backbone and the neighboring region of the core contain many charged (mostly negative) groups. Mutations in *E. coli* have revealed that the O-antigen is a virulence factor required for escaping phagocytosis. Deleting the core makes strains sensitive to antibiotics, bile salts, detergents, and mutagens. Lipid A is thought to be intricately involved in outer membrane assembly, as only conditional mutants in lipid A assembly can be made. The toxic portion of the LPS appears to be Lipid A, itself.

The O-antigen is a major surface antigen, and it is quite variable even within the same species. Not all gram-negative bacteria have the O-antigen. Some that colonize mucosal surfaces such as *Neisseria gonorrhoeae* or *Haemophilus influenzae* have a short branched oligosaccharide structure.

@ **REAL WORLD TIP**

The O antigen can be used to identify different serotypes within a genus. For example, *Salmonella typhi*, the cause of typhoid fever, has an O antigen designated as Group D. *Salmonella* serotype Typhimurium, a cause of food-borne illness, has an O antigen designated as Group B.

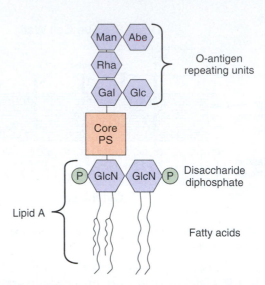

■ **FIGURE 3-13** Schematic of *Salmonella* serotype Typhimurium lipopolysaccharide layer showing the three characteristic features of an LPS layer from a gram-negative outer membrane. Lipid A, the endotoxin portion, is the most conserved, whereas the O-antigen, which is an antigenic determinant, is the least conserved. The O-antigen sugars as well as the branching structures are quite variable in different gram-negative species. Abbreviations: GlcN, *N*-acetylglucosamine; Core PS, polysaccharide core; Gal, galactose; Glc, glucose; Rha, rhamnose; Abe, abequose; Man, mannose

The negative charges of the LPS molecules bind divalent cations such as Ca^{2+} and Mg^{2+}. This noncovalent cross bridging prevents hydrophobic molecules from crossing the outer membrane. If these cations are removed by chelation or displaced by polycationic antibiotics such as polymyxins or aminoglycosides, the outer membrane becomes permeable to large hydrophobic molecules.

A summary of the cell wall characteristics of gram-positive and gram-negative cells is highlighted in Table 3-3✪.

✓ **Checkpoint! 3–10**
(Chapter Objectives 6 and 10)

_____ *are proteins that form channels across the membrane regulating permeability of the envelope. Thus, the outer membrane acts as a molecular sieve.*

    A. *Porins*
    B. *"O" antigen*
    C. *Lipid A*
    D. *Lipopolysaccharides*
    E. *Phospholipids*

CELL WALL DEGRADATION

Our tears and saliva contain **lysozyme**, an enzyme that breaks the bonds of the glycan backbone portion of the peptidoglycan

✪ TABLE 3-3

Comparison of Gram-Positive and Gram-Negative Cell Envelopes

Cell Wall Component	Gram-Positive Wall	Gram-Negative Wall
Outer membrane	Absent	Present
Periplasmic space	Absent	Present
Peptidoglycan	Thick layer	Thin layer
Peptidoglycan tetrapeptide	Usually contains lysine	All contain diaminopimelate
Peptidoglycan cross-linking	Usually via pentapeptide	Direct cross-linking
Teichoic acid	Present	Absent
Teichuronic acid	Present	Absent
Lipoproteins	Absent	Present
LPS	Absent	Present

molecule. This enzyme provides protection against bacterial invaders and is found in particularly high concentrations in egg white. It cleaves the β-(1,4) bonds between NAM and NAG (Figure 3-14 ■). If a portion of the cell wall remains after treatment with lysozyme, the cell is called a spheroplast; if none of the cell wall remains, it is called a protoplast. In these states the cell will lyse unless the osmolarity of the medium is similar to that of the cell's cytoplasm.

PENICILLIN

Cross-linking between the peptidoglycan layers is important for cell wall stability. Penicillin forms an inactive complex with transpeptidase, a key enzyme involved in cross-linking. Therefore, penicillin prevents the formation of cross bridges between the tetrapeptides of the cell wall (Figure 3-15 ■).

To add insult to the injury, several "restructuring" enzymes, called autolysins, are normally present in the cell wall. These autolysins break specific cross-linking bonds creating an equilibrium between the synthesis and breakdown of the cell wall. *Note:* A similar situation occurs in bone, where osteoblasts build bone, and osteoclasts break it down. In the presence of penicillin, synthesis is inhibited, but breakdown continues unabated. This causes cell lysis and death because of a weakened cell wall. Gram-positive bacteria such as staphylococci and streptococci are usually very sensitive to penicillin; gram-negative cells are considerably less so. Bacteria such as the *Mycoplasma*, which lack a cell wall, are totally insensitive.

Some bacteria secrete β-lactamase, which hydrolyzes and inactivates penicillin, making these bacteria more resistant to penicillin treatment. In medically related infections, this resistance is in large part because of the misuse of antibiotics. For example, if an antibiotic treatment is stopped before the infection is entirely cleared, the few surviving microbes will be those at the high end of a bell-shaped curve, excreting the highest levels of β-lactamase. These bacteria will grow and be more resistant to penicillin than the average bacterium in the original population. If the process is repeated through many cycles, a relatively resistant strain will develop. Furthermore, if the resistance is on a plasmid, it may be passed to other strains through the F-pilus. Antibiotic resistance has become the biggest challenge in controlling infection; it has become a worldwide problem, even finding its way into isolated populations such as the Aboriginals of Western Australia (Coombs et al., 2006).

✓ Checkpoint! 3–11 (Chapter Objectives 12 and 15)

Lysozyme and penicillin are capable of causing lysis because they affect _____, a key component of the cell wall.

A. *peptidoglycan*
B. *lipid A*
C. *"O" antigen*
D. *porins*
E. *phospholipids*

PERIPLASM

The region between the outer membrane and the inner membrane is called the periplasm (also, periplasmic space or periplasmic gel; see Figure 3-13). This region has an apparent high viscosity. Diffusion of proteins within this region is 0.1% and 1% of the rate expected for an aqueous and cytosolic environment, respectively. Besides a high concentration of unpolymerized

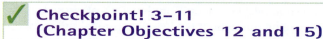

■ **FIGURE 3-14** The enzyme lysozyme degrades the peptidoglycan layer by cleaving glycan linkages.

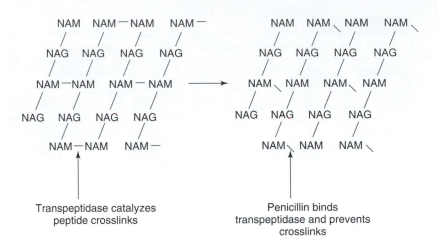

Transpeptidase catalyzes
peptide crosslinks

Penicillin binds
transpeptidase and prevents
crosslinks

■ **FIGURE 3-15** Penicillin inhibits peptidoglycan synthesis.

peptidoglycan, this region contains binding proteins that identify important nutrients. These bind to ABC transporters or chemotaxis receptors for sensing and transporting sugars, amino acids, peptides, vitamins, and ions. Also included in this region are catabolic enzymes, detoxifying enzymes, proteins for cell envelope synthesis, and some nonintegral membrane-associated proteins involved in the electron transport system. The periplasm is an oxidative environment, in contrast to the cytoplasm, which is reducing. In *E. coli,* two periplasmic pathways for disulfide bond (Dsb) formation are known. One uses DsbA and DsbB, and the other uses DsbC.

CYTOPLASMIC MEMBRANE

The inner membrane, also called the cytoplasmic membrane, is distinct and separate from the outer membrane and lies just below the peptidoglycan layer in gram-negative cells (see Figure 3-13; Kadner, 1996). This membrane is a typical lipid bilayer. Lipid bilayers are fluid, and individual phospholipids diffuse rapidly throughout the two-dimensional surface of the membrane. The phospholipids can move to the opposite side of a bacterial cell membrane in a few minutes at room temperature. Membrane proteins diffuse more slowly because of their large size. At cooler temperatures a lipid phase transition limits lateral movement in the membrane.

The cytoplasmic membrane contains the chemoreceptors, transporter proteins, and electron transport system (including the ATP synthase). When we speak of the proton motive force in gram-negative cells, we are referring to the potential across the cytoplasmic membrane.

▶ CELL GROWTH

BINARY FISSION

Bacterial growth is characterized by an increase in size as well as division into two daughter cells. This most often occurs by

binary fission. As cells grow in length (bacilli) or volume (cocci), they form a septum, then divide. The septum is an invagination of the cytoplasmic membrane and peptidoglycan. Separation occurs by cleaving the ingrown peptidoglycan (gram-positive cells) or when the outer membrane grows inward causing physical separation (gram-negative cells). Some bacteria divide by budding, where a small bleb begins as an outgrowth from the original, grows to full size, and then separates.

The arrangement of the peptidoglycan strands at the poles is unknown. Septa grow inward to form the new poles of the daughter cells. The outer membrane does not invaginate at the same time as the inner membrane and sacculus. Septation and elongation involve separate pathways because septation can be blocked without destroying elongation. Septation involves some 15 genes, 2 for cell separation, and possibly 2 more for initiation. When mutations are made in genes required for septation, the cells become temperature sensitive filament formers, and the genes are given the designation *fts.*

GROWTH MEASUREMENT

Growth is measured as an increase in the number of cells. Cell number can be determined by several means. Cultures can be counted visually under a microscope (Figure 3-16a ■), their number can be inferred from the decrease in transmitted light (because of scattered light) in a spectrophotometer (Figure 3-16b ■), they can be plated on agar and counted (Figure 3-16c ■), or the number can be estimated electronically with a Coulter counter (Figure 3-16d ■). The spectrophotometric method requires the least labor. Optical density is measured at a longer wavelength (e.g., 600 nm) where there is little light absorption by the cells.

GEOMETRIC GROWTH

One cell that divides becomes two, two becomes four, four becomes eight, and so on. The length of time between divisions

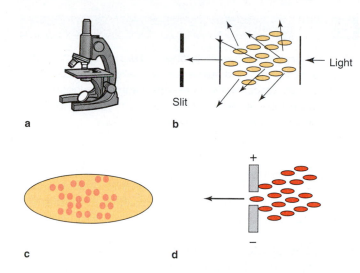

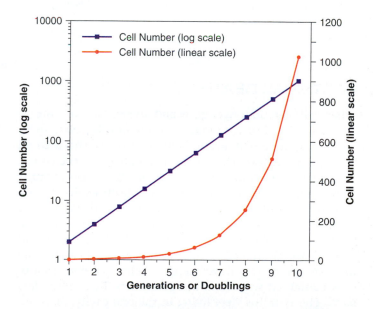

a   **b**

c   **d**

■ **FIGURE 3-16** Methods to measure cell growth. **a.** Individual cells can be counted with a microscope. This method is tedious. **b.** Cell numbers can be estimated with a spectrophotometer. Scattered light does not reach the photodetector, giving an "apparent" optical density, which is proportional to the density of cells. **c.** Dilutions of cells can be plated, and colonies that develop from single cells can be counted. **d.** A known volume (usually 100 μl) of diluted cells can be pumped through a narrow passageway and counted with a Coulter counter. The change in current from a particle passing through the narrow orifice is registered electronically and counted as a cell.

is called the doubling time or generation time. *E. coli* has a doubling time of only 20 minutes under ideal conditions (maximum aeration and rich media), so it can double as much as three times per hour! The total number of cells from the first cell follows the simple equation:

$$\text{cell number} = 2^n \qquad \text{(eq. 3-3)}$$

where n equals the number of generations. After 1 hour (three generation times), there are $2^3 = 8$ cells. After 2 hours there are $2^6 = 64$ cells. After 3 hours $2^9 = 512$ cells; 4 h, $2^{12} = 4,096$; 5 h, $2^{15} = 32,768$; 6 h, $2^{18} = 262,144$; 7 h, $2^{21} = 2,097,152$; and 8 h, $2^{24} = 16,777,216$ cells. This is quite remarkable for an 8 h day!

Clearly, if the culture began with more than one cell, say five, the equation would be:

$$\text{cell number} = 5 \times 2^n$$

Fortunately, bacteria don't grow to these huge masses because nutrients and energy sources are limiting factors for their growth.

ℯ REAL WORLD TIP

Growth in a tube of liquid culture medium is observed as turbidity (cloudiness) when compared to a clear, uninoculated tube of liquid culture medium. One must be careful to control the amount of microbial inoculum as too heavy an inoculum will also appear cloudy.

✓ Checkpoint! 3–12 (Chapter Objective 14)

How long would it take for one E. coli cell to grow to the weight of an average, 67.5 kg human?

   A. *2 weeks*
   B. *1 week*
   C. *4 days*
   D. *2 days*
   E. *1 day*

BACTERIAL GROWTH CURVE

Bacterial growth can be divided into four stages: a lag phase, an exponential or log phase, a stationary phase, and a death phase. When bacteria are transferred from one medium to another, they take some time to adapt to the new environment. The transfer is commonly from a plate or refrigerated clinical specimen. During this lag phase, the cells do not divide, but may increase in size to two- to threefold; they also actively synthesize DNA and proteins necessary for division.

After this lag phase, the exponential or log phase starts, where doubling occurs at a regular pace exemplified in the preceding example. A plot of the "logarithm of cell number" versus "time" yields a linear plot (Figure 3-17 ■). From this plot, one can determine the doubling time. The number of generations per hour is called the growth rate constant.

Exponential cells are smaller than lag-phase cells because they are dividing at a maximum rate. After essential nutrients are depleted, toxic products accumulate, or oxygen becomes limiting (cells are usually shaken at above 200 RPM

■ **FIGURE 3-17** Geometric growth of bacterial cells over 10 doublings. A semilog plot gives a straight line, and this line can be used empirically to estimate doubling time. Note that 10 doublings yields 1,024 cells from one cell. Therefore, every 10 doublings yields an increase of approximately three orders of magnitude.

for maximum aeration), the exponential or log phase ends, and the stationary phase begins.

During stationary phase, cell division rates decrease, and the rate of cell death begins to match this division. Cells begin feasting on their intracellular energy stores (glycogen, etc.), after which they begin degrading their own cellular components. The death phase becomes imminent. The death rate increases exponentially until a very low population is reached where there is equilibrium between cell growth and cell death.

 REAL WORLD TIP

If you are working with a culture that is several days old, transfer some of the growth to fresh medium to retain culture viability and avoid the death phase.

✓ **Checkpoint! 3–13 (Chapter Objective 13)**

The log phase is the period in which
   A. *cell division rates decrease and the rate of cell death begins to match cell division.*
   B. *cells do not divide, but may increase in size to two- to threefold; they also actively synthesize DNA and proteins necessary for division.*
   C. *cell numbers double at a regular pace.*
   D. *the death rate increases exponentially until a very low population is reached.*

BACTERIAL DEATH

When cells can no longer grow and divide, they are considered dead. The test is to take a culture of cells, plate them onto a nutrient medium, and look for colonies. This method is far from flawless. There is no guarantee that the conditions chosen (medium, aerobicity, anaerobicity, gas mixture, etc.) would even allow certain strains of healthy cells to grow. Modern molecular tools have revealed a surprising number of strains that have not been culturable. In one of the first such studies, PCR amplification of 16s rDNA found that ~50% of the strains from a human subgingival crevice had never been reported (Kroes, Lepp, & Relman, 1999). That is, they contained sequences not present in the protein data bank. These strains were living in the oral cavity, but once removed, they became "unculturable." Transferring samples directly to fresh media and allowing the microbes to recover enhances their survival in many cases. Cells injured by UV light or antibiotics may not grow when plated, but often can grow if allowed to recover in fresh media.

 REAL WORLD TIP

Known organisms used to check the performance of media, reagents, and stains are typically kept frozen or dehydrated. Once thawed or reconstituted the inoculum should be transferred to fresh medium twice in order to ensure accurate quality control reactions.

ANTIMICROBIAL AGENTS

When discussing antimicrobial agents, it is important to understand commonly used terminology:

- **Bacteriostatic** agents inhibit multiplication, but growth resumes when the agent is removed.
- **Bactericidal** agents kill bacteria, and their effects are irreversible. Cells cannot reproduce, even after the agent is removed.
- **Sterile** means free from all forms of life. However, as mentioned earlier, bacteria may still be present under "sterile" conditions if the criterion used for sterility is the inability to culture any organisms.
- A **disinfectant** is a chemical that kills bacteria but is too toxic to be applied directly to tissues.
- **Septic** is when pathogenic organisms are present in living tissue.
- **Aseptic** means pathogenic microbes are not present. In the microbiology lab, the use of "aseptic" techniques is a must.

KILLING MECHANISMS

Anything that damages DNA can kill cells. UV light, ionizing radiation, and chemicals can disrupt DNA integrity, prevent replication, and cause cell death. UV light induces cross-linking of neighboring pyrimidines, ionizing radiation creates breaks in single and double strands, and alkylating agents form DNA adducts or interstrand cross-links.

Agents that inhibit energy producing or biosynthetic pathways, denature protein, disrupt the cell wall or cell membrane, or oxidize free sulfhydryl groups on proteins will also kill cells.

KILLING AGENTS

Specific physical agents include heat and radiation. Because 100°C will not readily kill all spores, we use steam under 15 psi for 20 minutes at 121°C in an autoclave for sterilization. Moist air is far superior to dry heat. Sterilization using dry heat requires 160°C to 170°C for 1 hour or more. Clinical laboratory biological safety cabinets use UV light, and the food industry has used ionizing radiation for sterilization.

Chemical agents are often used in the home for killing bacteria. Poisons and respiratory inhibitors such as arsenic or cyanide are of limited use because of their toxicity for humans. Alcohols such as ethanol and isopropanol are most toxic at 70%, where they disorganize the lipid membranes and denature proteins. Phenol denatures proteins and is used as a 1% to 2% aqueous solution. Heavy metals such as mercury, copper, and silver denature proteins at high concentrations. Their high toxicity limits their use to low concentrations, where they combine with sulfhydryl groups. Oxidizing agents such as hydrogen peroxide, iodine, and chlorine inactivate cells by oxidizing sulfhydryl groups. Alkylating agents replace labile hydrogens with alkyl groups. Such agents include ethylene oxide and formaldehyde (the 37% aqueous solution is formalin). Ethylene oxide is often used for surgical instruments and is the best disinfectant for dry surfaces when rendered non-explosive with 90% CO_2. Detergents disrupt the lipid membrane of cells.

✔ **Checkpoint! 3–14 (Chapter Objective 15)**

What are the standard conditions for operation of an autoclave to sterilize instruments, media, or biohazardous waste?

  A. *100°C for 5 minutes at 14 psi*
  B. *160°C to 170°C for 15 minutes at 14 psi*
  C. *121°C for 15 minutes at 15 psi*
  D. *115°C for 21 minutes at 21 psi*

► METABOLIC PATHWAYS

Pathways that break down substrates and cellular constituents are called **catabolic pathways.** Those used to synthesize macromolecules and cell constituents are **anabolic pathways.** Those that go in both directions (catabolic and anabolic), such as the TCA (tricarboxylic acid or citric acid) cycle, are amphibolic pathways. Finally, pathways that replace intermediates drained from the TCA cycle are dubbed anaplerotic pathways.

NUTRIENT REQUIREMENTS

Cell growth requires a source of energy as well as material to build cell components. Carbon, oxygen, nitrogen, hydrogen, sulfur, and phosphorus are necessary for structure. Ions such as K^+ (potassium), Na^+ (sodium), Fe^+ (iron), Mg^{2+} (magnesium), Ca^{2+} (calcium), and Cl^- (chloride) aid catalysis or are used for membrane gradients.

MICROBIAL CLASSIFICATIONS

Microbes are classified by a combination of their carbon source, energy source, and electron source (Table 3-4). This can be quite confusing. Those that can use CO_2 for their carbon source are **autotrophs**, whereas those requiring organic molecules (such as glucose) as a carbon source are **heterotrophs.** If they can use light as an energy source, they are phototrophs, but if they require chemical energy, they are chemotrophs. If the electron source is an organic molecule, they are organotrophs, but if this source is an inorganic molecule, they are lithotrophs. Most medically relevant bacteria use organic molecules (e.g., glucose rather than CO_2) to build cellular structure, the energy stored in the bonds of these organic molecules (rather than light) as their energy source, and the organic molecules NADH (reduced form of nicotine adenine dinucleotide) and $FADH_2$ (reduced form of flavin adenine dinucleotide), rather than, e.g., inorganic Fe^{2+}, as electron donors to generate proton motive force. These classifications are summarized in Table 3-4.

► BACTERIAL PHYSIOLOGY

ENERGY PRODUCTION

Because most medically important bacteria are chemoorganotrophs (chemoheterotrophs), we will focus on chemical energy as a metabolic source. Chemical energy is stored within bonds and becomes available by "burning" the molecule as a fuel. For example, when wood is placed into a fireplace and

---

✪ **TABLE 3-4**

Classification of Microbes by Attributes of Energy, Electron, and Carbon Sources

Term Describing Physiological Type	Carbon Source	Energy Source	Electron Source
Autotroph	CO_2		
Heterotroph	Organic molecule		
Phototroph		Light	
Chemotroph		Chemical	
Organotroph			Organic molecule
Lithotroph			Inorganic molecule
Chemolithotrophic (chemototrophic)	Inorganic CO_2	Inorganic molecule	Inorganic molecule
Photolithotrophic (photoautotrophic) (photosynthetic)	Inorganic CO_2	Light	Inorganic molecule
Photoorganotrophic (photoheterotrophic)	Organic molecule	Light	Organic molecule
Chemoorganotrophic (heterotrophic)	Organic molecule	Organic molecule	Organic molecule

Adapted from Atlas, R. M. (1997). *Principles of microbiology.* Dubuque, IA: Wm. C. Brown.

burned, an enormous amount of energy is released from the wood as heat. The molecular bonds (cellulose) react spontaneously with oxygen, but these two substrates must be heated to about 900°F to overcome the activation energy. Humans too would require the same temperature to combust glucose, but avoid the requirement by using enzymes to lower the activation energy. These enzymes not only increase the rate, but also combust glucose so efficiently that the products are essentially CO_2 and water. Contrast this to a wood-burning fireplace, which emits a plume of smoke that is caused by incomplete combustion of hydrocarbons. Smokeless combustion of wood will occur, however, if the temperature is increased and an adequate supply of oxygen is supplied. To accomplish this, clean-burning incinerators have a primary chamber burner at 1,300°F and a secondary chamber burner at 1,800°F or more. This process combusts all hydrocarbons to CO_2 and water, leaving no trace of smoke.

Bacteria extract energy in precisely the same manner as humans do, but they have several more options. For **respiration**, they can use a host of electron acceptors other than oxygen, and they can use **fermentation** if respiratory electron acceptors are not available.

ELECTRON TRANSPORT SYSTEM AND RESPIRATION

Respiration involves electron flow through an electron transport chain. An electron donor starts the process, and an electron acceptor ends the process. This flow is analogous to passing a magnetic ball down a chain of increasingly powerful magnets. The energy difference between these magnets is used to perform work by moving protons from the inside of the cell to the other side of the cytoplasmic membrane. The electron transport needs two things: a source of electrons and a terminal acceptor. For higher organisms, the donor is NADH or $FADH_2$, and the terminal acceptor is oxygen. In bacteria, the varieties are astounding. A host of donors or acceptors can be used, although in aerobes, oxygen is always the acceptor of choice.

The strength of each "magnet" is measured in terms of redox potential. The more positive it is, the higher the potential. A value of "0" is given to the reduction of hydrogen. NADH holds onto electrons very poorly and has a redox potential of −320 mV, whereas oxygen binds electrons tightly, with a redox potential of +820 mV.

PROTON EXTRUSION

Electron transport systems use a combination of methods, not all of which are fully understood, to translocate protons. One clever mechanism is the arrangement of alternating organic and inorganic redox centers. Organic electron acceptors such as flavin adenine dinucleotide (FAD), flavin mononucleotide (FMN), and ubiquinone (coenzyme Q) can accept electrons and protons. Inorganic electron acceptors such as FeS (iron sulfide) centers and

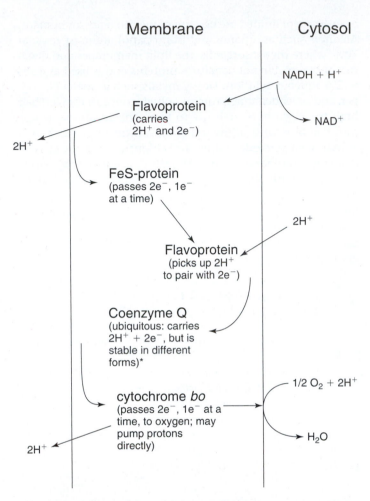

■ **FIGURE 3-18** The electron transport system in *E. coli*, with oxygen as the terminal electron acceptor. Electron transport is coupled to proton translocation, generating proton motive force. Protons can be exchanged with other cations (antiport), so that ΔpH and membrane potential are interchangeable. This system is found in the cytoplasmic membrane of bacteria. Bacteria lacking an electron transport system must waste valuable ATP to generate proton motive force.

cytochromes accept electrons exclusively. Therefore, as shown in a scheme for the *E. coli* system in Figure 3-18 ■, protons bound to $FADH_2$ must be released to reduce an FeS center. The FeS center then passes electrons to another flavin, which must take up protons if the electrons are to be accepted. The topology of the redox centers is such that these protons are released outside and picked up from the cytosolic side. Another advantage of organic acceptors is that they can hold one (semiquinone) or two electrons (hydroquinone). Thus, two electrons can be donated to an inorganic one-electron acceptor in two successive steps. Coenzyme Q is nearly universal in cytoplasmic membranes. In mitochondria it is involved in an interesting cycle known as the Q-cycle, whereby the semiquinone, without protons, takes up $2H^+$ and $1e^-$. Ultimately, two protons are extruded for each electron, which is the highest efficiency possible.

A large range of redox potentials is present in biological systems. Iron-sulfur centers show the lowest potentials (weakest ability to hold onto electrons), and copper containing redox potential shows the highest. In bacterial systems, for example, flavoproteins range from 0 to −400 mV, Fe-S proteins from +250 down to −500 mV, and iron centers from +500 to −300 mV.

PROTON MOTIVE FORCE (PMF)

Because protons are charged, their transit out of the cytoplasm yields a charged component as well as the concentration component (Gennis & Stewart, 1996; Harold & Maloney, 1996). As discussed previously, molecules move down a concentration gradient. When these molecules are charged, there is a greater driving force toward an opposite charge. Proton pumping creates a positive charge on the outside of the membrane and a negative charge on the inside of the membrane. The charge differential causes an additional drive for protons to move back into the cell. The total energy difference is therefore a sum of the electrical charge difference ($\Delta\psi$) and nonelectrical concentration difference (ΔpH) components. This total energy is called the proton motive force, which is designated by Δp. At standard temperature (25°C) and pressure, the equation, in mVolts, reduces to

$$\Delta p = \Delta\psi - 59\ \Delta pH$$

By convention, the proton motive force is negative because it is defined as the potential to move a positive charge from inside the bacterial cell or mitochondrial matrix to the outside. Initially, the Δp would be 0, but increasingly becomes more negative (harder to pump protons) as more and more protons are pumped out. The ΔpH component is defined as the inside pH minus the outside pH. Note that the proton motive force changes by 59 mV for a ΔpH of 1,118 mV for a ΔpH of 2, and so forth. If the ΔpH component is 0, all proton motive force will be in the form of the membrane potential, $\Delta\psi$.

Many salt-loving microbes, called halophiles, transport sodium ions rather than protons. In this case, the electron transport system creates a sodium motive force rather than a proton motive force. Therefore, in a universal sense, it is more correct to call the force generated by electron transport systems an ion motive force.

OXIDATIVE PHOSPHORYLATION

Oxidative phosphorylation is the process whereby the energy of biological oxidation is ultimately converted to the chemical energy of ATP. The ion motive force provides the energy source for making ATP in bacteria as well as in mitochondria. ATP synthesis occurs as a result of protons (or sodium ions) moving back into the cell through ATP synthase.

ATP SYNTHESIS

The means by which electron transport synthesizes ATP lies at the heart of chemiosmotic hypothesis. In 1961, Peter Mitchell stunned scientists studying bioenergetics by proposing a new mode of energy coupling. Previously, chemical bonds had been considered the only source for energy coupling. Thus, "substrate-level phosphorylation" had been found in the glycolytic pathway, where ATP can be generated from the 3-phosphoglycerate kinase or pyruvate kinase reactions. Today, Mitchell's hypothesis is generally accepted. In 1978, he was awarded the Nobel Prize in Chemistry for his work. The energy from the generated PMF is used directly by the enzyme ATP synthase (also known as ATPase). Interestingly, this enzyme rotates in a similar fashion to the flagellar motor, using the energy to fuse ADP (adenosine diphosphate) and P_I (a phosphate) together to form ATP.

Direct observation of a rotating F1-ATPase was reported in 1997 (Noji, Yasuda, Yoshida, & Kinosita, 1997). To demonstrate this, the group purified a mutant subcomplex of thermophilic *Bacillus* PS3. The mutant protein had 10 histidines at the N-terminus of the β subunit, which tightly bound to a nickel-coated coverslip. A cysteine residue in the γ subunit was biotinylated, and this was used to bind streptavidin. Because streptavidin has four binding sites for biotin, a fluorescently labeled biotinylated actin filament also was able to bind. The fluorescently labeled actin filament (about 2.5 µM) was large enough to visualize under a fluorescent microscope. When ATP was added to the mix, the actin filament rotated counterclockwise.

MECHANICAL ATP SYNTHESIS

More recently, scientists have been able to reverse the rotation of a purified ATP synthase and synthesize ATP mechanistically (Itoh et al., 2004). To do this, they attached a magnetic bead to the γ subunit of the ATP synthase and rotated the bead with electrical magnets.

ANAEROBIC RESPIRATION

In the absence of oxygen, the electron transport system of many bacteria can donate electrons to an alternative electron acceptor, such as fumarate and nitrate. This is called **anaerobic** respiration to differentiate it from when oxygen is the terminal acceptor. Because fumarate (+30 mV) and nitrate (+440 mV) have lower redox potentials than oxygen, they will not generate energy as efficiently. However, this pathway will generate energy more efficiently than through fermentation pathways.

METABOLIC PATHWAYS

Bacteria must be able to adapt to myriad environments, so it is no wonder that the number of potential metabolic pathways far exceeds that of mammalian cells. Figure 3-19 ■ summarizes the general approaches used by bacteria to extract energy and to build cellular material.

EMBDEN-MEYERHOF-PARNAS PATHWAY

The Embden-Meyerhof-Parnas pathway (also called the Embden-Meyerhof) is the most common glycolytic pathway from glucose to pyruvate in animals, plants, and many bacteria

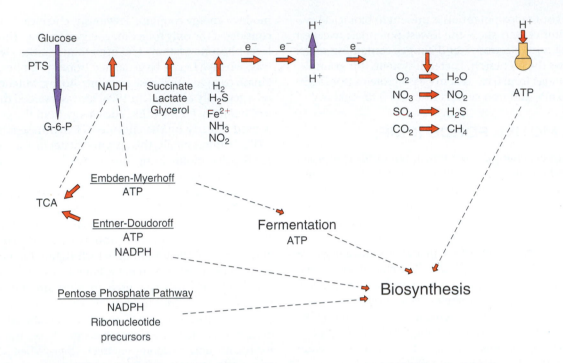

■ FIGURE 3-19 Bacteria have many pathways for generating proton motive force and energy.

(Figure 3-20 ■). In *E. coli*, 72% of all glucose is metabolized through this pathway. Four ATP molecules are produced for every glucose molecule in a process known as substrate-level phosphorylation. However, because two ATP molecules are used during the first two steps of the pathway, the net yield is only two ATP molecules. Substrate-level phosphorylation occurs during the conversion of 1,3-diphosphoglycerate to 3 phosphoglycerate, and of phosphoenolpyruvate to pyruvic acid. Two NADH molecules are formed in the glyceraldehyde-3-phosphate dehydrogenase reaction. Once formed, pyruvic acid catabolism can occur through myriad fermentation pathways as well as through the conversion to acetyl-CoA by the pyruvate dehydrogenase complex and complete oxidation to CO_2 by the tricarboxylic acid cycle.

ENTNER-DOUDOROFF PATHWAY

The Entner-Doudoroff pathway is an alternative to the Embden-Meyerhof pathway (glycolysis) for catabolizing glucose and is important for generating NADPH (nicotinamide adenine dinucleotide phosphate) and three carbon building blocks for biosynthesis under conditions where ATP is less important (Figure 3-21 ■). This pathway is found in bacteria and is not present in eukaryotic cells. The glucose-6-phosphate formed in the first step is converted to 6-phosphogluconic acid with the production of NADPH (as occurs in the pentose phosphate shunt). After dehydration, the structure is cleaved into two trioses (pyruvic acid and glyceraldehyde-3-phosphate) that can be used for biosynthesis or activated to acetyl-CoA for the TCA cycle. Notice that the energy yield is lower than for glycolysis.

PYRUVATE DEHYDROGENASE COMPLEX

Most aerobes synthesize acetyl-CoA from pyruvate through the pyruvate dehydrogenase complex. In *E. coli*, it is composed of three enzymes: 24 molecules of pyruvate dehydrogenase and dihydrolipoate transacetylase, and 12 molecules of dihydrolipoate dehydrogenase. This step results in the oxidative decarboxylation of pyruvic acid to acetyl-CoA with a yield of two ATP and four NADH molecules per pair of pyruvate molecules.

TRICARBOXYLIC ACID CYCLE

The majority of aerobic heterotrophs use the tricarboxylic acid (TCA) cycle (also called the citric acid or Krebs cycle) to generate reducing equivalents, ATP, and biosynthetic components (Figure 3-22 ■). During the cycle, acetyl-CoA is oxidized to CO_2 and water, generating 1 NADPH, 2 NADH molecules, 1 $FADH_2$, and 1 ATP. The continuation of the cycle is contingent on an electron sink for the reducing equivalents. This is supplied by the respiratory chain, which requires O_2 in animals, but, as mentioned, can also be supplied by alternative electron acceptors in many bacteria.

PENTOSE PHOSPHATE CYCLE

In *E. coli*, approximately 28% of glucose that is degraded funnels into the pentose phosphate cycle. Aside from generating NADPH for biosynthesis, this pathway is required for generating ribose, which is needed for synthesizing DNA, RNA, ATP, $NADP^+$, and NAD^+. The pathway generates

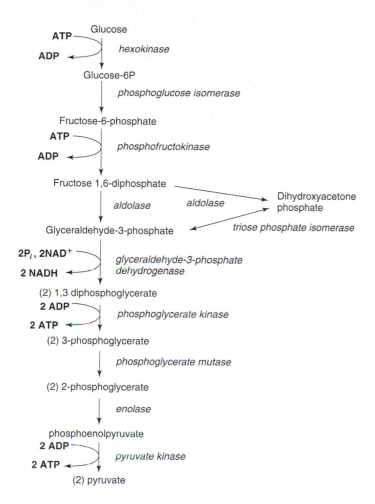

FIGURE 3-20 The Embden-Meyerhof-Parnas (glycolytic) pathway.

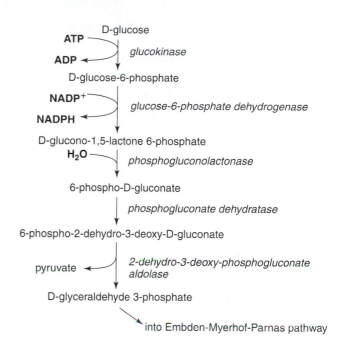

FIGURE 3-21 The Entner-Doudoroff pathway, which is an alternative to glycolysis and unique to bacteria. The D-glyceraldehyde 3-phosphate that is formed can enter the Embden-Meyerhof-Parnas (glycolytic) pathway.

ribose-5-phosphate and xylulose-5-phosphate with the following sum:

$$3 \text{ glucose-6-phosphate} + 6NADP^+ \longrightarrow$$
$$3 \text{ pentose-5-phosphate} + 3 \text{ } CO_2 + 6NADPH + 6H^+$$

Several more complex scenarios can occur from this pathway, including the complete metabolism of glucose to CO_2 with the generation of 12 molecules of NADPH.

METHYLGLYOXAL PATHWAY

Under limiting phosphate conditions, some bacteria avoid using the Embden-Meyerhof-Parnas pathway and use the methylglyoxal pathway. In this case, dihydroxyacetone phosphate is dephosphorylated to methylglyoxal, which can subsequently be converted to pyruvate and metabolized to generate ATP. Rather than generating ATP, this pathway consumes two ATP molecules.

GLYOXYLATE CYCLE

Eukaryotic cells cannot grow on acetate. Close inspection of the TCA cycle reveals why. Acetyl-CoA condenses with oxaloacetate and forms citrate. However, during the cycle, two carbons are spent in the form of CO_2 (from isocitrate dehydrogenase and α-ketoglutarate dehydrogenase), and the cycle ends up with oxaloacetate. Thus, acetate is burned as fuel, and there are no new carbons available to synthesize cellular components.

Many bacteria have a way around this dilemma. They split isocitrate by using the enzyme isocitrate lyase into succinate and malate synthase (Figure 3-23 ■). Glyoxylate can condense with acetyl-CoA to form malate. Because no carbons are lost, they can be used for synthesis of glucose through the oxaloacetate to PEP step and gluconeogenesis. This shunt across the normal TCA cycle is called the glyoxylate cycle. Recall that pathways that replenish the TCA cycle are called anaplerotic sequences. Also notice that this is a way to link the pathway of fatty acid metabolism with carbohydrate metabolism. Carbons from fatty acid can actually be converted into carbohydrates.

℮ REAL WORLD TIP

Biochemical tests that are used to identify unknown microorganisms detect by-products of metabolism (for example acid), oxidative or fermentative utilization of a carbohydrate or determine the ability of the microbe to grow in the presence of a single nutrient, such as citrate as a sole source of carbon. A positive reaction in these tests indicates the presence of these enzymes or pathways. A negative result assumes a lack of these enzymes or pathways. Understanding metabolic pathways of microbes will aid in understanding the principles of biochemical tests discussed in later chapters.

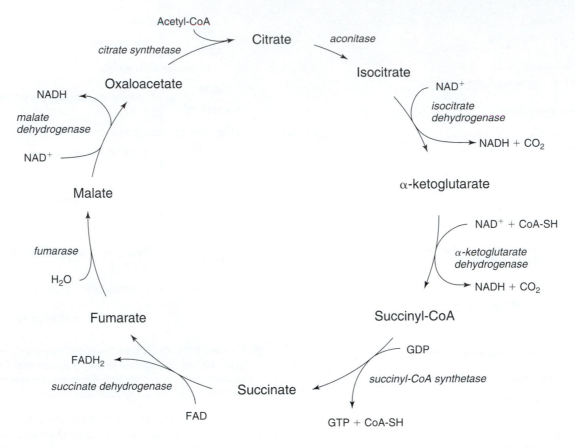

■ **FIGURE 3-22** The tricarboxylic acid cycle.

FERMENTATION

The survival of a bacterium depends on its ability to use as many resources as possible for energy. The ability to ferment allows ATP to be synthesized by substrate-level phosphorylation in the absence of respiration. Such a pathway is familiar to us because it allows humans to temporarily survive anaerobic episodes. For example, the 100-meter dash is highly anaerobic because oxygen cannot be transported to the muscles rapidly enough to accommodate the ATP needs. Fortunately, the rate of glycolysis can increase several 100-fold and meet the ATP needs for maximum power. However, there is a payoff. The efficiency is low (3 ATPs anaerobically vs. 39 ATPs aerobically for each glycogen), and the NADH synthesized during glycolysis must by reoxidized if the pathway is to continue. Without oxygen to oxidize the NADH,

the cell reoxidizes NADH with pyruvate, forming lactate. This process ultimately releases protons, which lower the pH, protonate glycolytic enzymes, compete with Ca^{++} for troponin, and stimulate pain receptors.

Bacterial fermentation processes are analogous to anaerobic metabolism in mammalian cells. In all cases, the metabolic end products are produced to reoxidize NADH, often converting a carboxylic acid to an aldehyde, or an aldehyde to an alcohol (Figure 3-24 ■).

In fermentation an organic substrate acts as the electron donor, and a product of that same electron donor becomes the electron acceptor. The oxidized products are balanced exactly by the reduced products. Coenzymes that are reduced at the beginning of the pathway are reoxidized at the end of the pathway so they are not consumed in the process.

Fermentation yields *less* ATP per mole of substrate than does respiration. Because the same molecule must serve as both electron donor and electron acceptor, complete combustion to CO_2 and water is not possible. Several types of fermentative metabolism will be familiar to you.

Homolactic fermentation is practiced by *Streptococcus, Lactococcus, Enterococcus,* and various *Lactobacillus* species. The milk industry uses this type of fermentation to sour milk and produce cheese and yogurt. Streptococci living inside our mouths stick to tooth surfaces and eat away enamel with the lactic acid

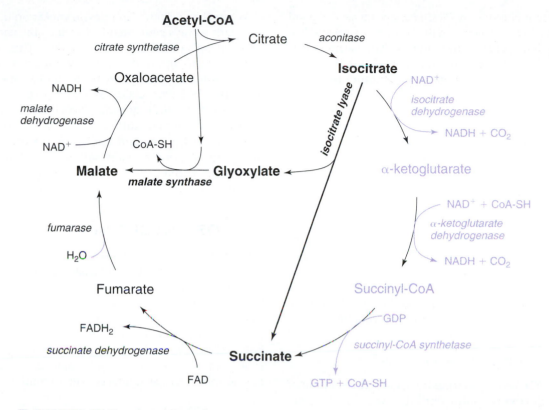

■ **FIGURE 3-23** The glyoxylate cycle.

produced by this process. *Lactobacillus acidophilus* converts milk sugar into products that don't irritate the intestine. This can aid people who are lactose intolerant.

Ethanolic fermentation occurs in many yeast strains, but is less common in bacteria. This process is used to produce beer, wine, and gasohol (gasoline and alcohol), as well as bread, which rises when CO_2 is released during fermentation.

Heterolactic fermentation uses the pentose phosphate pathway rather than the Embden-Meyerhof pathway of glycolysis.

It is called "hetero" lactic fermentation because ethanol and CO_2 are products as well as lactic acid. *Leuconostoc* species use this method to produce sauerkraut.

Propionic acid fermentation is used by *Propionibacterium*. Some of these strains can ferment lactic acid. Certain types of cheese form curds because of the lactic acid produced then *Propionibacterium* takes over. The late release of CO_2 forms the gas bubbles in Swiss cheese, and propionic acid gives it a characteristic taste.

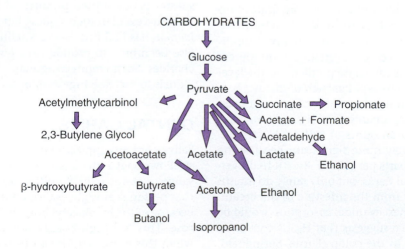

■ **FIGURE 3-24** Examples of fermentation products. Pyruvate sits at a central point in fermentation pathways.

Butyric acid fermentation by *Clostridium* yields several good organic solvents such as acetone (nail polish remover) and isopropanol, as well as butyrate and butanol. The pathway was discovered by Chaim Weizmann and allowed Britain to produce acetone for use in the manufacture of munitions during World War I.

Simple and rapid tests differentiating the end products of mixed acid fermentation (used by *E. coli*) and butanediol fermentation (used by *Enterobacter, Serratia,* and *Klebsiella*) are important as an indicator of human fecal contamination in water supplies.

RESPIRATION

The free energy for the complete combustion of glucose to CO_2 and water is -686 kcal/mol. When glucose is fermented to two molecules of the fermentation product lactic acid, the free energy is only -58 kcal/mol. Obviously, cells (such as *E. coli*) capable of both respiration and fermentation use respiration as an energy source when it is available.

MAXIMUM GENERATION OF ATP

The maximum ATP generated from the complete oxidation of a molecule of glucose is contingent on how many ATPs are generated per pair of electrons that donated to the respiratory chain. In *Paracoccus denitrificans,* electron pairs from NADH and $FADH_2$ generate 3 ATPs and 2 ATPs, respectively, yielding a grand total of 38 ATP molecules for each molecule of glucose. However, in *E. coli,* the yield from NADH and $FADH_2$ is only 2 ATPs and 1 ATP, respectively. As a result, *E. coli* produces a maximum of 26 ATPs from glucose oxidation.

GASTROINTESTINAL BACTERIA METABOLISM

The colon is populated with up to 10^{11} bacteria/mL. These bacteria live happily in a symbiotic relationship: They produce vitamin K, convert nonabsorbable carbohydrates into absorbable organic acids, and help resist colonization by invading pathogens. The human diet contains many "nondigestible" carbohydrates that become excellent carbon sources for bacteria in the colon. This can cause problems as the level of these carbohydrates rise. The rapid growth of distinct bacterial species becomes evident in the form of gases or even diarrhea. Gases produced are primarily CO_2, H_2, and CH_4, with quantitatively insignificant amounts of sulfides. That said, these sulfides are qualitatively quite significant because the nose can detect sulfides in parts per billion. Breath hydrogen correlates well with intestinal flatus, but only rarely do intestinal sulfides make their way from the intestine to the breath. Because H_2S is more toxic than cyanide, absorption would be devastating. Recent evidence suggests that H_2S is converted into safe insoluble sulfides in the colon (Furne, Springfield, Koenig, DeMaster, & Levitt, 2001).

When H_2S and other sulfides do appear on the breath, they are nearly always generated from anaerobic bacteria growing on the papilla of the back of the tongue. This can be demonstrated by gargling with 5 mL of hydrogen peroxide, which reduces sulfides from the breath for up to 8 h (Suarez, Furne, Springfield, & Levitt, 2000). Anaerobes express lower levels of catalase, the enzyme that metabolizes hydrogen peroxide. Thus far, the only proven sulfide capable of entering the bloodstream from the gut and appearing on the breath is allyl methyl sulfide, one of many sulfides found in garlic (Suarez, Springfield, Furne, & Leavitt, 1999). In this case, no amount of oral treatment will eliminate the sulfide.

LACTOSE INTOLERANCE

Most of the adult world that is not of northern European ancestry loses much of their lactase activity as they grow into adulthood. Undigested lactose makes it way to the colon, the bacteria have a feast, and diarrhea results. This is called lactose intolerance. Note that it isn't necessarily the lactose that is causing the "discomfort," but the rapid growth and metabolic products of bacteria within the colon. This is one of the most common gastrointestinal problems that a primary care physician will see, as it affects over 50 million Americans.

STACHYOSE AND RAFFINOSE

Soybeans and other legumes contain high concentrations of raffinose (0.5%) and stachyose (3.3%), two soluble oligosaccharides that humans cannot digest. These are synthesized by adding one (raffinose) and two (stachyose) galactose molecules to sucrose. The galactosyl bonds are an alpha linkage. Humans lack an enzyme to break this bond, so virtually 100% of these oligosaccharides make it to the colon, where bacteria are able to metabolize them. The bacterial growth and by-products (odorless methane, hydrogen and CO_2, and trace amounts of qualitatively significant sulfides [ppb]) have made the pinto bean industry search for ways to engineer these carbohydrate substrates out of their product. At least one entrepreneur has been successful in such a quest, but according to the *Wall Street Journal,* has had little success selling it. Some soybeans have also been bred to produce low levels of these two oligosaccharides. Such engineering may allow highly sensitive individuals to increase ingestion of these high-quality foods.

DENTAL CARIES

Saliva contains approximately 100 billion bacteria mL^{-1}. We swallow about 1 liter a day, or 100 billion bacteria. If a person's saliva contains over 1 million *Streptococcus mutans* per mL, that person is at high risk for dental caries. Sucrose is special because of the hemiacetyl bond between the glucose and fructose. This is a high-energy bond, and the energy released when this bond is split can be used by *S. mutans* (without wasting ATP) to synthesize a capsule containing sticky

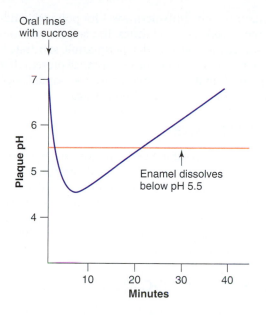

FIGURE 3-25 A Stefan curve, demonstrating the rapid drop in plaque pH after an oral rinse with sucrose. Tooth enamel begins dissolving when the pH drops below 5.5.

polymers of glucose (mutans or dextran) or of fructose (levan). This capsule allows attachment to the enamel surface. Once established on the tooth, *S. mutans* can ferment a host of carbohydrates to lactic acid. In 1940, Stefan measured the pH of plaque, after subjects rinsed with a sucrose solution. As shown in Figure 3-25 ■, the pH of plaque dropped to well below 5.5, the pH at which the enamel begins to dissolve. However, the buffering in saliva brings the pH back to neutral, and calcium and phosphate will reform the enamel. Repetitive hits with sucrose can give *S. mutans* the edge in this war. If salivary flow is compromised, caries will run rampant. Patients treated with radiation to the head or neck temporarily produce less salive and often develop several caries within a few months.

✓ Checkpoint! 3–16 (Chapter Objective 18)

Soybeans and other legumes contain high concentrations of _____ soluble oligosaccharides, which humans cannot digest. Virtually 100% of these oligosaccharides make it to the colon, where bacteria metabolize them, producing methane, hydrogen, CO_2, and trace amounts of qualitatively significant sulfides (ppb). These metabolic by-products could result in flatus.

    A. *sucrose and lactose*
    B. *raffinose and stachyose*
    C. *lactose and sucrose*
    D. *glucose and fructose*
    E. *dextran and levan*

▶ MEMBRANE TRANSPORT

MEMBRANE TRANSPORT PROTEINS

Because the lipid bilayer presents a barrier against the free diffusion of molecules into the cell, transport proteins are essential. Membrane transport proteins have peptide chains that pass through the lipid bilayer several times. This multipass topology likely enables hydrophilic molecules to escape the ravages of the lipid-rich cell membrane. Two major classes of membrane transport proteins are carrier proteins and channel proteins. Carrier proteins are also called permeases or transporters. Channel proteins usually have pores that, when open, allow solute (usually inorganic ions) to pass.

PASSIVE AND ACTIVE TRANSPORT

As discussed earlier, molecules move down a concentration gradient. Transport across a membrane and down this gradient is called passive transport. Passive transport can occur without a channel or carrier, but the rate of transport will be limited by the permeability coefficient, which is determined experimentally and is related to the size and lipid solubility of the transported molecule. The large flexibility of the bilayer lipids above the gel–liquid crystal transition creates hallways that allow small neutral molecules to penetrate. Until recently, it was thought that water diffused freely across the bilayer through these transient openings, despite water's polar character. However, we now know that there are specific transporters called aquaporins that allow water to cross the membrane almost unimpeded. However, aquaporins block protons (i.e., H_3O^+) from passing. This rapid movement of water is essential for all life, but can present problems such as rapid changes in osmotic pressure and dehydration. Desert plants must synthesize a special waxy layer to avoid dehydration.

If a molecule is present that facilitates the transport of solute across the membrane, the process is called facilitated diffusion. Facilitated diffusion can be through a pore or through a carrier molecule. Many pathogenic bacteria synthesize toxins that act as pore-facilitated transporters. These include ionophores such as the a-toxin from *Staphylococcus aureus*. Some of these transporters are antibiotics that we use against bacteria such as gramicidin A. Carrier-facilitated diffusion can also be mediated by ionophores. Valinomycin has a hydrophobic shell but an interior cavity that can chelate K^+ ions. It has a 20,000-fold preference for K^+ over Na^+. Once it binds K^+, it diffuses aimlessly through the lipid and releases the ion in a random fashion on either surface. A K^+ gradient is rapidly equilibrated.

CARRIER-MEDIATED TRANSPORT

Carrier proteins resemble enzymes. They have one or more specific binding sites for the solute (molecules) that they transport, and these binding sites can be saturated. When this happens, a V_{max} is reached. The concentration of solute transport

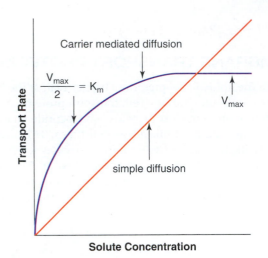

■ **FIGURE 3-26** Carrier-mediated diffusion follows a saturation profile that is similar to that of enzyme kinetics.

is maximal. This "V_{max}" is specific to each carrier. The concentration of solute that gives a rate of $V_{max}/2$ is equal to the K_m (Figure 3-26 ■).

Carrier proteins that transport a single solute in one direction are called uniporters. Other, more complex, transporters are coupled to the simultaneous or sequential transfer of another solute. If this is in the same direction, it is called symport; if these directions are opposite, it is called antiport (Figure 3-27 ■). In bacteria, the proton gradient is most commonly used, although the sodium gradient is preferentially used in halophiles.

PRIMARY AND SECONDARY ACTIVE TRANSPORT

Transporters that use ATP hydrolysis for transporting solute mediate primary active transport. Transporters that use ion gradients as discussed earlier mediate secondary active transport.

ATP BINDING CASSETTE (ABC) TRANSPORTERS

ABC transporters include over 1,000 family members. This includes uptake permeases for sugars, amino acids, inorganic

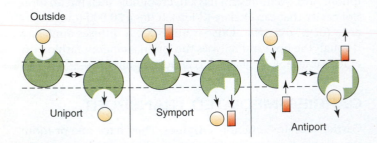

■ **FIGURE 3-27** The three types of carrier mediated transport across a membrane.

ions, vitamins, and efflux permeases for polysaccharides, LPS, lipids, heme, peptides, and drugs. In bacteria, all uptake ABC permeases are associated with a periplasmic substrate binding protein. Of note is the multidrug resistance protein that, when overexpressed, makes bacteria (as well as some cancer cells) resistant to a range of hydrophobic drugs.

ATP SYNTHASE

The bacterial ATP synthase can function in the reverse direction. That is, it hydrolyzes ATP to create proton motive force. This scenario occurs when electron donors and acceptors are limiting. Here the cell must use substrate-level phosphorylation to generate ATP, which is spent to generate proton motive force. This willingness to waste precious ATP is the cell's tribute to the importance of proton motive force for survival.

GROUP TRANSLOCATION

Only one example of group translocation is known, but it is crucial to most of the microbial world. The phosphotransferase system (PTS) is an amazing system that actively transports sugars and polyols and regulates some 20% of all bacterial genes. Over 25 PTS transporters (called permeases) are used to transport and phosphorylate the sugar (Figure 3-28 ■). The source of energy is derived from phosphoenolpyruvate (PEP; from the glycolytic cycle), which transfers its phosphate to Enzyme I, then HPr, then the Enzyme II permease complex. Enzyme II has three subunits: A, B, and C. The phosphoryl is first transferred to Enzyme IIA, then Enzyme IIB, then the incoming sugar or polyol, which is bound by Enzyme IIC. Phosphorylation of the incoming sugar or polyol is required for transport. Some of the permeases have a soluble Enzyme IIA subunit, as is shown for the glucose permease, IIA^{Glc}. Enzyme IIA^{Glc} is remarkable. When glucose is not present, it remains phosphorylated, then binds to and activates adenylate cyclase, increasing cAMP. This induces cAMP-dependent operons that code for non-PTS transport systems. In essence, the cell realizes that it no longer has the best carbon source and must induce systems to take in inferior carbon sources such as lactose. If glucose is present, the levels of phosphorylated Enzyme IIA^{Glc} drop, cAMP levels decrease, and synthesis of many genes is turned off. Furthermore, the unphosphorylated IIA^{Glc} binds other non-PTS transporters, such as the lactose permease, and inhibits transport of competing sugars. In essence, the cell is saying, "I've got it good with glucose, why waste energy synthesizing extraneous genes and transporting inferior carbon sources?" This glucose inhibitory effect is called "catabolite repression." Of PTS sugars, only glucose has this effect.

The PTS is energy efficient: the cell wastes only one ATP equivalent (PEP) to transport *and* to phosphorylate the sugar. In contrast the ATP-dependent glucose transport system requires one ATP for transport and one ATP to phosphorylate glucose.

Fluoride ion inhibits several cellular enzymes, but in particular enolase, which converts 2-phosphoglycerate to phosphoenolpyruvate. Because a good supply of PEP is required for

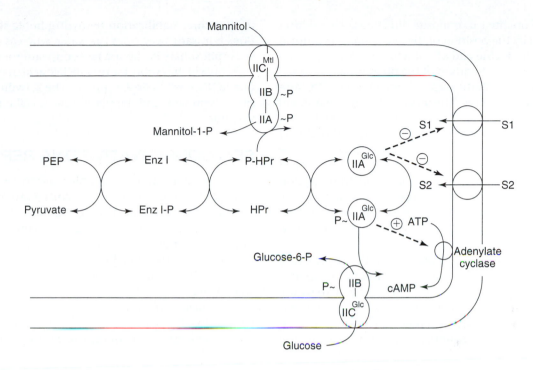

FIGURE 3-28 The phosphotransferase system (PTS). Sugars are concomitantly phosphorylated and transported by specific PTS permeases. The glucose permease indirectly regulates some 20% of all genes in *E. coli* by altering the activity of adenylated cyclase. Enz I, Enzyme I; HPr, heat stable protein; IIA^{Glc} and IIB-IIC^{Glc}, subunits of the Enzyme II glucose permease. Note that IIA^{Glc} is a soluble subunit, whereas the other two subunits are membrane bound. IIA-IIB-IIC^{Mtl}, the mannitol permease; S1 and S2 are other sugar substrates (for example, lactose), which are excluded when the glucose is transported. Nomenclature is that of Saier and Reizer (1992).

a functional PTS, fluoride will ultimately inhibit sugar transport (such as sucrose) through the PTS. This is one of two ways fluoride inhibits dental caries.

As a tribute to the importance of solute transport for survival, microbes designate a large chunk of their genome toward synthesizing transporters. A case in point is the recent sequencing of *S. mutans,* the organism that causes dental caries (Ajdic et al., 2002). Nearly 15% of its genome codes for transporters. Most of these 280 transporter genes are ATP dependent, a characteristic of organisms that lack an electron transport chain (Why do you think this would be so?). *S. mutans* has only 1 F-type ATPase (F_0F_1 ATPase), but codes for more than 60 ABC-type ATPases. About one-third of these ABC transporters are importers, whereas the rest are exporters, demonstrating the importance of ridding the cells of harmful molecules. There are 5 sugar ABC transporters and 14 phosphotransferase system (PTS) sugar transporters.

▶ BACTERIAL GENETICS

THE GENOME

A genome represents the complete set of genetic information carried by "genes" in an organism. The definition of a gene has changed throughout the years. In the early 1900s a gene was a subjective way to define heredity. These traits were eventually traced to the chromosome, and by the 1930s a gene was defined as the region of DNA coding for one enzyme or polypeptide. However, this definition falls short because not all enzymes are proteins. For example, ribozymes are RNA molecules that have catalytic function. Therefore, a better definition of a gene is the entire chromosomal segment required for a functional product.

STRUCTURE OF DNA AND RNA

The name *DNA* is short for deoxyribonucleic acid, which represents its chemical composition. This composition was known long before the helical structure was deciphered by Watson and Crick in 1953 (Watson & Crick, 1953). DNA is composed of nucleotides, which consist of a phosphate group, a 5-carbon "deoxyribose" group (missing the hydroxyl from "ribose" at carbon #2), and a nitrogenous base. The term *nitrogenous base* was originally used to describe the group as being "basic" (as opposed to neutral or acidic), as well as containing nitrogen groups. DNA includes four different bases, which include the purines, adenine and guanine (A and G), and the pyrimidines, thymine and cytosine (T and C).

For a detailed discussion of the structure of DNA, one should consult a biochemistry textbook. In brief, DNA consists of two strands that are oriented in opposite directions. These directions are defined by the position of the free hydroxyl groups at each end of a strand. One end of a strand has a free hydroxyl group from the number 5 carbon of the ribose ring (called the 5' hydroxyl, to distinguish the carbon atom it is bound to, from the carbon atoms in the base). The other end of the DNA strand has a free 3' hydroxyl group. Each nucleotide is linked to the next through a 3' to 5' linkage, leaving a single 5' hydroxyl residue at the front end, and a single 3' hydroxyl residue at the tail end free (Figure 3-29 ■); the 5' end may also be capped with a di- or triphosphate). Replication and transcription enzymes use this directionality to copy a new strand. The copied strand is synthesized in the opposite orientation. That is, the 5' end of the new strand pairs with the 3' end of the parent strand.

The association between strands is stabilized primarily through hydrogen bonding; however, hydrophobic interactions between bases of opposing strands also occur. Two hydrogen bonds stabilize adenine-thymine interactions, whereas three hydrogen bonds stabilize guanine and cytosine association. Therefore, GC-rich sequences have a higher melting temperature. Stabilization by hydrophobic stacking interactions is inward away from the water, whereas the hydrophilic sugar phosphate backbone faces outward toward the water.

RNA, which is short for ribonucleic acid, has a similar structure to DNA, with two exceptions. The 2' hydroxyl group from ribose is present, and the pyrimidine uracil is used in place of thymine.

SEMICONSERVATIVE DNA REPLICATION

In theory, there are two possible ways in which DNA could be copied. If replication were "conservative," each strand would be copied into a daughter strand, and these two daughter strands would associate, leaving the original pair intact. This is not what happens. Instead "semiconservative" replication occurs, whereby each original strand pairs with its new, freshly synthesized daughter strand. This was demonstrated elegantly in 1958 by Meselson and Stahl, who grew *E. coli* in media containing "heavy" nitrogen ($^{15}NH_4{}^+$), transferred the cells to media containing "light" nitrogen ($^{14}NH_4{}^+$), grew them for one generation, and extracted the DNA.

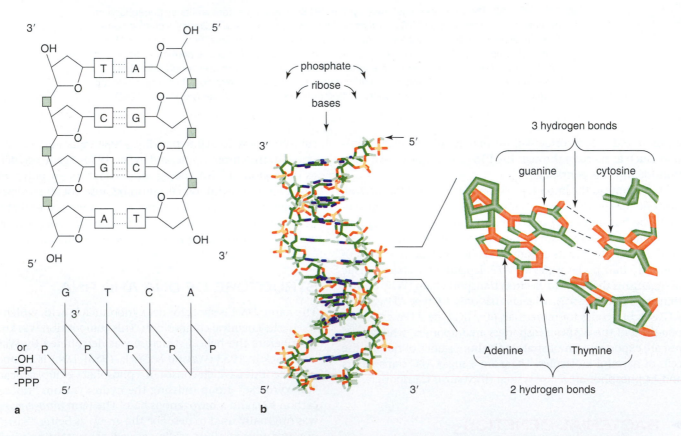

■ **FIGURE 3-29** Overall structure and base-pairing in DNA. **a.** Skeleton of four DNA base pairs. Each dotted line represents a hydrogen bond, indicating that there are two hydrogen bonds between adenine "A" and thymine "T" bases and three hydrogen bonds between guanine "G" and cytosine "C" bases. Strands are oriented in opposite directions (designated by 5' and 3' ends). The lower panel of **a** shows how the linkage is often abbreviated. Note that the 5' end may retain the 5' phosphate or be capped with -PP or -PPP. **b.** A stick cartoon figure of DNA base pairing between two DNA strands. The right panel is a tilted and magnified image of two consecutive base pairs, showing the spatial relationship and hydrogen bonding between the base pairs.

The new DNA pairs were hybrids of a heavy (parental) and light (daughter) strand, proving semiconservative replication (Meselson & Stahl, 1958).

REPLICATION

Replication in bacteria always begins at a position called the origin of replication. Because bacteria only have one origin of replication, replication proceeds until the entire genome is copied. This is different from eukaryotes, which have many sites at which replication begins and, thus, many replication forks. *Saccharomyces cerevisiae* has approximately 300 origins, whereas humans have about 20,000 origins.

Replication proceeds in an interesting way. Both strands are copied, but the DNA polymerase only synthesizes new DNA from the 5' to 3' end. Because strands pair in opposite orientations, the polymerase must proceed to the right on one strand and to the left on the other strand. To do this, one strand, called the leading strand is copied in a continuous manner, whereas the other strand, called the lagging strand, is copied in a discontinuous manner (Figure 3-30 ■). Every 1,000 to 2,000 nucleotides, the discontinuous strand is primed and copied in the back direction toward the replication fork. This segment of discontinuously copied DNA is called an Okazaki fragment, named in honor of the Tuneko Okazaki and Reiji Okazaki, who reported this in 1969 (Okazaki & Okazaki, 1969). A second hurdle in replication is that DNA polymerase requires a primer before replication can begin. This problem is overcome in the lagging strand by RNA polymerase II, which acts as a "primase," laying down a patch of RNA 4 to 15 nucleotides in length for the DNA polymerase to extend with DNA. These RNA primers must later be excised and replaced with DNA. Only one priming is required for the leading strand, but each Okazaki fragment requires a primer. For *E. coli*, this corresponds to about 4,000 primers per genome.

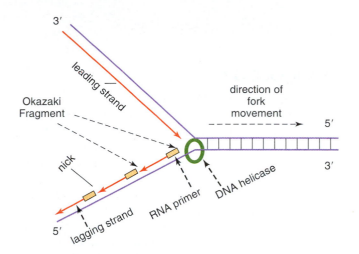

■ **FIGURE 3-30** DNA replication. The new strand is synthesized in the 5' to 3' direction. This allows only one strand (the leading strand) to be copied in the direction of the replication fork; the lagging strand must synthesize DNA fragments in the reverse direction. These are called Okazaki fragments.

segment with enough torsional strength to "melt" the local supercoiled helix and begin a process that initiates replication. The DnaB protein forms a transient complex with DnaC, which assists DnaB attachment to DNA. DnaB is a helicase that breaks the base pairing of DNA to allow room for elongation enzymes to attach to the single strands.

Most bacteria (there are a few exceptions thus far) have circular DNA and only one origin of replication. Replication, in fact, occurs in both directions, giving the appearance of the Greek letter, theta (θ). In this case, each burgeoning strand has a leading and a lagging strand that is independent of the other until the replication complexes meet.

> **Checkpoint! 3–17 (Chapter Objective 19)**
>
> *Okazaki fragments are the result of:*
>   A. *cross-linking of pyrimidines by ultraviolet light.*
>   B. *breaks in the DNA strand by ionizing radiation.*
>   C. *interstrand cross-links by alkylating agents.*
>   D. *replication of the leading DNA strand.*
>   E. *replication of the lagging DNA strand.*

E. coli has three DNA polymerases: DNA polymerase I, II, and III. DNA polymerase II is involved in DNA repair, polymerase I completes Okazaki fragments, and polymerase III is the main replicating enzyme in bacteria. The *E. coli* origin of replication is a segment of DNA containing about ~245 bp called *oriC*. Some 30 copies of protein DnaA bind to this

CODONS

Although the sequence of a bacterial protein is ultimately derived from a DNA sequence, proteins are synthesized using messenger RNA (mRNA), not DNA, as the template. DNA is first transcribed into mRNA in a process known as transcription, and the mRNA is used as a template to be translated into protein. Translation is orchestrated by ribosomes, which match specific transfer RNAs to sets of three nucleotides on the mRNA, called codons. These codons "code for" specific amino acids, which are almost universal. The code consists of 64 codons, which code for 61 amino acids, as well as three stop codons (UAA, UAG, and UGA). The AUG codon, which codes for methionine, is also the start codon. Because there are only 20 amino acids, the genetic code is redundant; more than one codon may exist for some of the amino acids.

► MICROBIAL GENETICS— BACTERIAL VARIATION

TERMINOLOGY

The genotype of an organism is defined as the genetic composition of that organism. Genes are often given mnemonics describing their functions, such as the *aer* gene, which codes for a receptor responsible for aerotaxis (oxygen taxis; Rebbapragada et al., 1997). Specific genes are designated by three lowercase letters that are italicized. If several genes are involved in the same function, they are usually distinguished by capital letters following the genotype. For example, *hisA, hisB,* and *hisC* are different genes that code for enzymes involved in histidine synthesis. Wild-type alleles are given a plus superscript (*aer*⁺), but a minus sign is not used to designate a mutant locus. Therefore one speaks of an *aer* mutant rather than an *aer*⁻ strain. Mutation sites within the same gene are given numbers in the order in which they were isolated (e.g., *hisA1, hisA2*). If there is only one gene locus, a hyphen is placed between the gene and mutant number (*aer-1, aer-2*). Other designations such as amber mutations (Am) and temperature-sensitive mutations (Ts) follow the allele number (e.g., *hisA1*(Am) *aer-1*(Ts)). A deletion is given the symbol Δ before the deleted gene or region (Δ*aer-3*).

The phenotype of an organism is an observable property, such as the ability to chemotax toward oxygen. If the phenotype is known to be controlled by a particular gene, the property is designated by the gene name. Here italics are not used, and the gene name is written with a capital letter followed by two lowercase letters, with either a plus or minus superscript to indicate the presence or absence of that property (e.g., an Aer⁻ phenotype indicates that the bacteria do not chemotax toward oxygen). Phenotypic designations are absolutely essential if mutant loci have not been mapped or identified. Other delineations, such as resistance to antibiotics, can also be used (e.g., Amp^r for ampicillin resistance). However, these phenotypic designations should be defined.

A mutation is an inheritable change in the base sequence of nucleic acid comprising the genome of an organism. There is a difference between a mutation and a mutant. A mutant is a strain that carries one or more mutations. One can map a mutation, but not a mutant, which designates a phenotype, not a genetic locus. Wild-type refers to an organism or a gene most often found in the natural setting.

SCREENING FOR BACTERIAL MUTANTS

Bacteria are haploid, so any new allele can be observed rapidly if one uses the proper screening and/or selection assays. For example, a motility mutant that reacquires the ability to swim will readily swim through tryptone semisolid agar. Using a motility plate as a screen, one can inoculate some 10 million cells in a single petri dish and select for any unusual "blebs" that might result from swimming bacteria (Watts, Ma, Johnson, & Taylor, 2004).

The easiest mutations to isolate are mutants that have selectable mutations. These mutations confer some type of advantage for the organism such as antibiotic resistance. Nonselectable mutations are more common. These do not confer an advantage, but might be easily screened if they exhibit an obvious phenotype, such as the loss of color in a pigmented organism. Less-obvious phenotypes are problematic and may require huge populations to be screened for mutations.

Mutants that require additional nutrient supplements are common, but to find these, one must first know what nutritional supplements are normal. A prototroph is defined as a wild-type strain that grows on a defined minimal medium, which is defined as the simplest number of ingredients that allow for microbial growth. For wild-type *E. coli*, this includes a sugar, salts, trace elements, and a vitamin. Using the prototroph as a standard, one can select for auxotrophs, which are mutants that cannot grow on defined minimal medium without some nutritional additive.

REPLICA PLATE SCREENING

In 1952, Esther and Joshua Lederberg developed a screening method for auxotrophic mutants (Figure 3-31 ■; Lederberg and Lederberg, 1952). As part of this screen, the pattern of bacterial colonies from one agar plate (containing complete growth medium) are transferred onto a sterile velvet cloth and replica plated onto several new plates. If the new plate contains

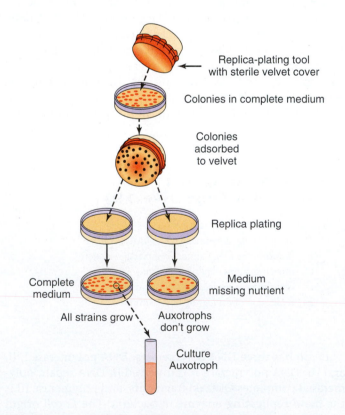

Replica-plating tool with sterile velvet cover

Colonies in complete medium

Colonies adsorbed to velvet

Replica plating

Complete medium

Medium missing nutrient

All strains grow

Auxotrophs don't grow

Culture Auxotroph

■ **FIGURE 3-31** Replica plating technique to find auxotrophic mutants.

minimal medium that is missing an essential nutrient, only the prototrophic colonies will grow. Auxotrophs will grow only on plates containing complete medium. Therefore this method distinguishes between mutants and wild-type strains based on the ability to grow in the absence of a particular biosynthetic product.

▶ MUTATIONS IN DNA

Point mutations are single nucleotide changes within DNA. These mutations can occur anywhere in the genome, but they generally have no effect on an organism unless the mutation is within a gene or in the sequences regulating gene expression. Base substitutions come in two types: (1) transitions and (2) transversions. Transitions are the most common and involve the replacement of a purine with a different purine (A and G) or a pyrimidine with a different pyrimidine (C and T). Transversions replace a purine with a pyrimidine or vice versa. As one might expect, these are less common because the difference in size between these two base classes can cause steric problems. In the author's experience, intentionally mutagenizing genes in the laboratory by random PCR or chemical mutagenesis results in approximately 80% transition mutations and 20% transversion mutations.

TYPES OF POINT MUTATIONS

Point mutations within a gene may have a range of effects, from none to extreme. Because more than one codon is used for most amino acids, a base substitution can occur that doesn't alter the amino acid residue incorporated into the protein. This type of mutation is called a silent mutation. In contrast, a point mutation that does alter the amino acid incorporated into the polypeptide chain is called a missense mutation. The missense mutation may have little effect on the protein if the characteristics of the amino acid are similar to that of the original (e.g., size, charge) or if the residue resides in an area of the protein that is not critical for structure or function. These missense mutations that *do not* change protein function are called neutral mutations. Other missense mutations can have mild or severe effects. One of the more well-known missense mutations is that responsible for sickle cell anemia, which arises from a nucleotide change in the *β-globin* gene at codon 6, converting a glutamic acid residue to a valine residue.

Some mutations have more extreme effects than simply altering an amino acid residue. For example, a mutation may convert a codon to a stop codon so that translation stops prematurely before the full polypeptide is synthesized. This type of mutation is called a nonsense mutation. Alternatively, one or two base pairs may be inserted or deleted from the coding region of a gene, yielding a shift in the reading frame for the messenger RNA. This will produce a random peptide sequence after the mutation. Such mutations are called frameshift mutations.

Sometimes a second mutation arises that corrects the defect of the first mutation. This mutation is called a suppressor mutation because it suppresses the aberrant phenotype caused by the first mutation. Suppressor mutations can be intragenic or extragenic. That is, the suppressor mutation can be within the same gene containing the primary mutation, or it can lie within a different gene. Suppressor mutations often disrupt protein function when introduced without the primary mutation, even though they restore function in presence of the primary mutation. One way in which an extragenic suppressor can correct a defect is by protein–protein complementary interactions. Here, the defect in one of two interacting proteins is corrected by a complementary defect in the other protein. This is analogous to a lock and key. The lock (first protein) is changed, so the topology of the key (second protein) must be changed for the unit to remain functional. Similarly, intragenic suppression can occur by domain–domain complementation, within a single protein. In basic research, one can use this method as a tool to show that two protein surfaces interact with each other in a biologically meaningful way.

 Checkpoint! 3–18 (Chapter Objective 19)

A point mutation that alters the amino acid incorporated into the polypeptide chain may have mild or severe effects on the resulting protein. If the characteristics of the amino acid are similar to that of the original (e.g., size, charge), or if the residue resides in an area of the protein that is not critical for structure or function, there may be little effect. This type of mutation is called a _____ mutation.

   A. *silent*
   B. *missense*
   C. *nonsense*
   D. *frameshift*
   E. *suppressor*

Causes of Mutation

The sheer number of bases and the rapid growth of microorganisms makes mutations inevitable. Mutations that develop naturally from lesions in DNA or replication errors are called spontaneous mutations. Although all organisms have mechanisms for repairing point mutations during DNA replication, some errors remain uncorrected. These errors occur at the rare frequency of 1 per 10^7 to 1 per 10^{11}. In general, DNA-based microbes have a genomic mutation rate of approximately 0.003 mutations/genome/replication.

The causes of spontaneous mutation are too involved to review here, but they can generally be divided into base mispairing, strand slippage during DNA replication, and spontaneous lesions (chemical changes).

Induced Mutations

Several means can be used to increase the rate of mutations. These include ionizing (x-rays) and nonionizing radiation (ultraviolet light), base analogs, base modifying chemicals, and intercalating agents. Using these methods, mutations can be induced at high frequency, so that there is one error per 10^3–10^6 base pairs (compared with 1 per 10^7–10^{11} base pairs for spontaneous mutations).

Multibase Mutations

In multibase mutations, deletions, inversions, or insertions occur in DNA segments. Deletions are usually not reversible and are typically caused by recombination. Recombination can also cause an inversion, whereby the orientation of a DNA segment is reversed with respect to the surrounding DNA. On the other hand, insertions are most often caused by insertion sequences (IS), which are a type of transposable element (discussed later) 700 to 1,400 base pairs in length. These insertions usually cause gene inactivation.

Recombination occurs by breaking the DNA strand and religating it in a way that causes the DNA to "cross over." The process requires homologous DNA sequences and is orchestrated by the products of the *rec* genes in bacteria. Recombination between direct repeat sequences can cause deletion, and between inverted repeats it can cause inversion mutation.

The Ames Test for Mutagenicity

The Ames test was developed in a series of papers by Bruce Ames in the early 1970s (Ames, Gurney, Miller, & Bartsch, 1972; Ames, Lee, & Durston, 1973; Figure 3-32 ■). Ames sought a way to test compounds for carcinogenicity that was less cumbersome than treating mice and rats with chemicals for long time periods. In the Ames test, bacteria are used to screen potential carcinogens. This strategy relies on the observation that the most common causes of cancer are mutations brought about by DNA damage. The Ames test has been used to test a broad spectrum of chemicals, including environmental chemicals, hair dye additives, and food coloring.

The Ames test uses a mixed culture of two *Salmonella* auxotrophs. Neither strain can synthesize histidine, so they need this amino acid for growth, unlike wild-type *Salmonella*, which can grow in media lacking histidine. One of the auxotrophic strains contains a base substitution, with the reading frame intact, whereas the other strain contains a frameshift mutation. Both of these mutations occur in the histidine operon, which is the region of the bacterial chromosome that codes for enzymes required for histidine synthesis. Therefore, these strains need a back mutation before they will be able to grow without histidine. In the Ames test, one makes the assumption that any chemical that increases the rate of back mutations (His$^+$) in these strains is mutagenic.

In the actual Ames test, the histidine auxotrophs are plated onto an agar plate that contains defined media with a small amount of histidine and the mutagen to be tested (see Figure 3-32). Some histidine is necessary because the bacteria need some time (and some opportunity) to mutate either the base substitution, or the frameshift mutation, back to wild-type. However, only bacteria that have acquired a back mutation will continue growing into a visible colony once the small amount of histidine has been used up. There will always be a small number of spontaneous mutants with buffer alone, so this value is used as a control and compared with the number of back mutants present on the plate containing the potential mutagen. The mutagenicity of a chemical is then quantitated by the increase in the number of back mutants in the treated strains.

To more closely mimic the mutagenic properties of a chemical ingested by humans, the chemical can be mixed with rat liver extract, which converts the chemical into products that would form during its metabolism in the liver.

GENE TRANSFER

Prokaryotic DNA is readily transferred between organisms, contributing to the remarkable genetic diversity of bacteria. Three distinct mechanism involved in the transfer of genetic information are (1) transformation, (2) conjugation, and (3) transduction.

Transformation

Transformation was first described in 1928 by Frederick Griffith. In this process, "naked" DNA is taken up by recipient cells and either incorporated into the chromosome or propagated extrachromosomally as a plasmid (see following section on plasmids). Cells that can accept extrachromosomal DNA or plasmids through the transformation process are called competent cells. Those cells that have received the new extracellular DNA are differentiated from those that have not by being called transformants.

Since the early experiments on natural transformation by Griffith, microbiologists have developed several artificial transformation methods to introduce DNA into cells. In the natural environment, the source of donor DNA is usually from lysed bacteria. These bacteria release considerable amounts of DNA fragments that vary in size from one to several genes. These fragments can be taken up by competent cells and either integrated into the chromosome or degraded by nucleases. The frequency of transformation is low (about 1×10^{-6} per recipient

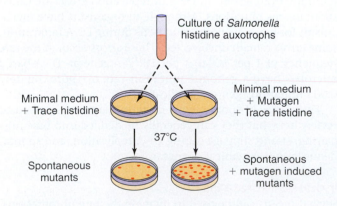

■ **FIGURE 3-32** The Ames test for mutagenicity.

Culture of *Salmonella* histidine auxotrophs

Minimal medium + Trace histidine

Minimal medium + Mutagen + Trace histidine

37°C

Spontaneous mutants

Spontaneous + mutagen induced mutants

cell or 10^{-3} when an excess of DNA is used). During DNA uptake, one of the DNA strands is degraded so only one linear DNA strand is found in the cell. It pairs with homologous DNA of the recipient cells chromosome and recombination occurs.

Artificial transformation is routinely used in the laboratory setting to introduce DNA into cells. The most common methods are heat shock and electroporation. In the heat shock method, cells are treated with a high concentration of calcium ions and then stored in the cold. DNA is added, and cells are brought up to 42°C for approximately 60 s (time is specific for strain), which causes some of the DNA to leak into the cells. Electroporation requires that cells be washed in a low ionic strength solution of glycerol-water (to keep the current low) before being exposed to a large voltage (up to 2,500 V) for a few milliseconds. This transient electric field opens small pores in the membrane and allows externally added DNA to enter the cells.

Conjugation

Conjugation is the transfer of DNA by direct contact between two living bacterial cells of opposite mating types. A donor (male) cell contains a fertility (F) factor that synthesizes the F-pilus. This pilus sticks to a recipient (female) and reels it in like a fishing line. A pore then forms in the adjoining cell membranes, and DNA is transferred from the donor to the recipient. The recipient is called a transconjugant.

The fertility factor may be chromosomal or expressed from an extrachromosomal circular plasmid. If the F-factor is on a plasmid, it codes for F-pili synthesis and the ability to form a physical union between the two cell types. One strand of the F-plasmid is nicked at the origin, and replication proceeds. It then transfers the entire plasmid to the F⁻, cell and the complementary strand is synthesized in the recipient cell (Figure 3-33 ■). The bacterial genome is not transferred, only the F-plasmid that contains the fertility factor and any associated genes that might be on that plasmid. However, the F⁻ recipient now becomes F⁺, and it now can engage in conjugation with new recipients. This process is known as F-mediated conjugation.

Approximately 1 of every 10,000 F⁺ cells integrates the F-factor into the chromosome. When the F-factor integrates into a chromosome, donor chromosomal DNA may be transferred along with the F-factor. The amount of chromosomal DNA transferred is directly related to how long the two cells remain in contact. For *E. coli,* the entire chromosome takes approximately 100 min to transfer, so this value (100 min) was used as a way to map the relative placement of genes in the *E. coli* chromosome. Because the chromosome is circular, a value of zero minutes was arbitrarily assigned to the Thr/Leu markers, and all other genes were given greater values (up to 100 min).

Donor cells that have the F-factor integrated into a chromosome have a high frequency of recombination. To designate this attribute, these cells are called Hfr (high-frequency recombination) cells. Here chromosomal DNA is transferred from the donor to the recipient. However, the F-factor is the last piece of DNA transferred, so the entire chromosome must

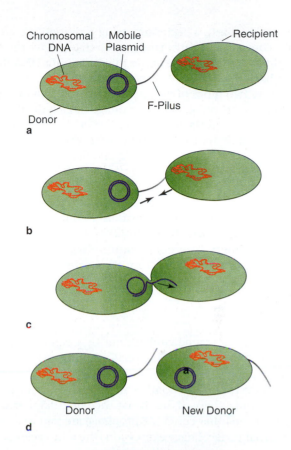

■ **FIGURE 3-33** Transfer of genetic information between bacteria by conjugation. **a.** The F-pilus attaches to a nearby cells and reels it in **b.** so that the two cells surface contact. **c.** A single strand of the plasmid is threaded into the recipient. **d.** Once the strand is copied, the recipient also becomes a donor.

be transferred and recombined into the recipient strain if the F-factor is to be inherited. This rarely happens. More typically a portion of the chromosome is transferred, so the recipient cell remains F⁻.

Transduction

The third method of genetic transfer between bacterial cells is by transduction, where the DNA is transferred with the help of a bacterial virus called a bacteriophage. When a bacteriophage infects a bacterial cell, it uses the bacterial replication machinery to make many viral DNA and RNA copies, which are repackaged into the phage head to form new bacteriophage **virions.** Sometimes, by accident, the virus picks up a segment of bacterial DNA and packages this DNA into the phage head as well as its own DNA. However, the amount of bacterial DNA that can be packaged into the virion is <1% of the bacterial chromosome.

The phage head, which surrounds the genetic material, is comprised of a protein coat. The phage attaches to a bacterium through a base plate and tail fibers and injects its genetic material into a bacterium using a springlike contraction of a contractile sheath. The bacteria that survive the viral onslaught and inherit some of the injected donor DNA (from another bacterium) are called transductants.

There are two types of bacteriophage: (1) virulent phage and (2) temperate phage. Virulent phage has a lytic life cycle that kills the bacteria (e.g., T-even phage). A temperate phage can follow lytic or lysogenic pathways (e.g., lambda phage).

Virulent Phage

Virulent phage uses the bacterium as a viral synthesis factory; they break down the bacterial chromosome and use the cell machinery to produce more phages. Up to 1,000 progeny phages are released from the bacterium as the cell lyses.

Temperate Phage

Temperate phages can be virulent, but they can also be lysogenic. In the lysogenic state, the phage genome may integrate into the bacterial chromosome as a prophage, which is replicated with the bacterial genome. This prophage is not a phage, in that it is not expressed, but it has the potential to become a phage. Bacteria that contain a prophage are said to be lysogenic for that phage. Phage expression (the lytic cycle) can be induced by factors such as UV radiation.

In the research lab, transduction is useful for introducing new mutations or genes into bacteria. In *E. coli*, P1 phage is the bacteriophage of choice to infect *E. coli* and move genes from one strain to another.

For more information, visit the Web site of the American Society of Microbiology (ASM) and the links therein. ASM members of division M study bacteriophages (http://www.asm .org/division/m/M.html).

Plasmids

Microbes often contain extrachromosomal circular DNA known as **plasmids** that code for elements that increase survival under certain conditions. These plasmids contain their own replicon, or genetic information necessary for their replication, but the other genetic information they contain is not normally essential to the host except under unusual circumstances. Examples of products expressed from these plasmids include transporters and enzymes that export or degrade xenobiotic (foreign) toxins or antibiotics. Antibiotic resistance genes on plasmids can spread rapidly between organisms by the conjugative process described previously.

Plasmids range in size from a few kilobase pairs to several hundred kilobase pairs. They can carry a few genes or hundreds of genes, but always contain an origin of replication (*ori*), which is the site at which plasmid replication is initiated. The *ori* is recognized by a trans acting initiator protein, usually called Rep, which can be encoded either by the host cell's chromosome, or the plasmid itself.

Unlike the bacterial chromosome, there can be many copies of a plasmid within a cell. The number of copies of a plasmid, called the copy number, is specific to each type of plasmid. Low copy number plasmids, like the F-plasmid and other large plasmids, are present at 1–2 copies per cell. High copy number plasmids are present at 100 copies per cell, and are generally smaller plasmids (<10 kb). Partition mechanisms help insure that a plasmid is distributed to each daughter cell during cell division. This helps maintain the stability of the plasmid in the population.

Plasmid Compatibility

If a bacterium is transformed with two different plasmids harboring different genes, only one of the two plasmids may propagate. This is most often because of interference between the replication machinery of the two plasmids, and in such a case the two such plasmids are called incompatible. Surprisingly, this incompatibility occurs when two plasmids have the same DNA replication and segregation systems, not when they have different replication and segregation systems.

Methods used in the laboratory to isolate plasmids take advantage of the small size of plasmid molecules (compared to the size of the chromosome) and/or their covalently closed, supercoiled configuration. Many commercial kits are available for plasmid DNA isolation.

Transposons

Some DNA sequences within a single cell move to different locations within a chromosome with ease. These are often called jumping genes or mobile genetic elements. The phenomenon was first observed in maize by Barbara McClintock, who won the 1983 Nobel Prize in Medicine. Such "transposable elements," named transposons, may insert into another gene and cause an insertional mutation, but the process may be reversible if it is excised cleanly. The transposon is "cut" and "pasted" into another region of DNA, using the enzyme transposase, which is often expressed by the transposon itself.

 Checkpoint! 3–19 (Chapter Objective 19)

_____ *are extrachromosomal circular DNA that code for elements that increase survival under certain conditions. They range in size from a few kilobase pairs to several hundred kilobase pairs and therefore can carry a few genes or hundreds of genes.*

   A. *Plasmids*
   B. *Bacteriophages*
   C. *Transposons*
   D. *Transconjugants*
   E. *Transformants*

SUMMARY

The modern study of microbiology began with Antoni van Leeuwenhoek in 1673, but it would be some 200 years later before observations by Pasteur, Lister, and Koch proved the relationship of microbes to disease. Several methods of microscopy are commonly used to view microbes or probe their physical architecture, including the light, phase-contrast, dark-field, fluorescent, confocal scanning, and electron microscope. The three basic bacterial shapes are rod-shaped (bacilli), spherical (cocci), and spiral (spirilla), and groups of individual cells may further associate into a higher organization. Bacteria have typical surface features that may include flagella, pili, fimbriae, and a capsule. Flagella are a means of locomotion, and the energy for this is derived by ion motive force. Motile bacteria find food, nutrients, and energy using a chemotaxis system that alters random walk behavior. Pili and fimbriae are sticky surface projections used for attachment and virulence. Capsules protect bacteria from osmotic changes, serve as a fuel reserve, and may shield bacteria from phagocytes. Intracellular precipitates can also serve as fuel sources, and these inclusion bodies may be polymers of carbon, phosphate, or β-hydroxy-butyrate. Some bacteria such as *Bacillus* species and *Clostridium* species can form heat resistant endospores, which can tolerate boiling for hours. ∞ Chapters 19 and 24 provide specific details on *Bacillus* and *Clostridium* species and their spores.

There are two major classes of bacteria, defined by the resulting color of a Gram stain. Gram-positive cells stain blue, whereas gram-negative cells stain red. The basis for this difference lies in the cell wall. Gram-positive cells have a thick peptidoglycan layer, which retains the crystal violet after alcohol/acetone treatment. Gram-negative cells, on the other hand, have a thick outer membrane, which dissolves during alcohol/acetone treatment and loses the crystal violet dye; the remaining thin peptidoglycan layer can then be counterstained with safranin red. The peptidoglycan layer is made of an alternating glycan polymer of *N*-acetylmuramic acid and *N*-acetylglucosamine. Sheets of these polymers are cross-linked through the *N*-acetylmuramic acid sugar by peptide linkages. These peptide linkages are synthesized by transpeptidases that are inhibited by penicillin. The glycan linkages can be hydrolyzed by lysozyme, an enzyme found in human tears and saliva.

The peptidoglycan layer of gram-positive cells has teichoic acid, which is an acidic anionic polysaccharide polymer. This gives the surface of such gram-positive cells a negative charge. Gram-negative cells have a much more complex cell envelope. They have both an inner and outer membrane. The outer membrane has porins that allow small-molecular-weight (<1,000 Da) hydrophilic molecules to pass. Hydrophobic molecules do not cross the outer membrane because it is surrounded by a cationic shield. This shield of cations is attracted by negatively charged lipopolysaccharides, which extend from the outer leaflet of the outer membrane. The lipopolysaccharide layer also serves as an endotoxin, so that dead cells may still cause harm. The inner membrane of gram-negative cells houses the electron transport system, ATP synthase, and transporters. The space between the membranes is the periplasm.

Bacteria grow by binary fission, and this growth can be measured using a microscope, spectrophotometer, or Coulter counter, or colonies spawned from single cells can be counted on an agar plate. There are four growth phases: lag, exponential (log), stationary, and death phases. Bacteria can be killed by chemicals, heat, or radiation, but whether an environment is free from all bacteria (sterile) depends on the definition one uses, because many bacteria cannot be cultured, even though they are living.

Unlike humans, bacteria have a vast array of potential electron donors and electron acceptors from which they can generate energy via an electron transport system. When an electron acceptor other than oxygen is used, it is called anaerobic respiration. Some bacteria do not have an electron transport system and must rely on fermentation. Fermentation is a process similar to the formation of lactic acid during anaerobic glycolysis in humans, whereby a buildup of NADH is relieved by converting pyruvate to lactate. In bacteria, numerous fermentation pathways give rise to some commercially important products, such as cheese. In the human gut, bacteria serve a symbiotic important role, producing vitamins, breaking down nonabsorbable carbohydrates into organic acids, stimulating immunity, and competing with pathogenic organisms. Too many nondigestible carbohydrates, however, can be used by bacteria in the colon to rapidly grow, causing gastrointestinal distress. This is evident with lactose intolerance and sensitivity to pinto beans. Another common problem is dental caries, which are caused by the lactic acid fermentation pathway of *Streptococcus mutans*.

Bacterial cells have specific membrane transport systems, similar to those found in eukaryotes. However, they also have transporters that involve group translocation, whereby a sugar is simultaneously phosphorylated and transported into the cell using the phosphotransferase system.

The definitions of a gene have changed over the last hundred years, from a subjective way to define heredity, to the entire chromosomal segment required for a functional product. Bacterial replication always begins at the origin of replication, and because most bacterial chromosomes are circular, they give the appearance of the Greek letter theta (θ) during replication. To copy both strands at the same time, a discontinuous strand is primed with RNA every 1,000 to 2,000 nucleotides and copied in the back direction toward the replication fork. These segments are called Okazaki fragments.

Proteins are coded by triplet sets of nucleotides on mRNA called codons. There are a total of 64 codons, 61 of which code for a total of 20 amino acids and 3 of which are stop codons. Genes are designated by uncapitalized italics, their protein products are designated without italics, and the first letter is capitalized. A phenotype is an observable property, and a strain with an altered phenotype is called a mutant. However, a mutation is different, in that it is a change in a base at the DNA level. One can map a mutation, but not a mutant. The term wild-type is used to designate an organism or gene most often found in its natural setting. The easiest bacterial mutants to isolate are those with selectable mutations, although those with nonselectable mutations can be rapidly isolated with by using the appropriate screening procedures.

Point mutations are single nucleotide changes within DNA, and these may be silent (without an amino acid residue change) or missense (the amino acid residue changes) mutations. Missense mutations that do not alter the function of the protein product are called neutral mutations. Frameshift mutations occur when one or two nucleotides (not divisible by 3) are added or deleted, altering the reading frame of the mRNA, so that a random peptide sequence is synthesized. A mutation that corrects the defect of another mutation is called a suppressor mutation, and these can either be intra- or intergenic. The sheer number of bases copied during replication makes spontaneous mutations inevitable, although the probability can be increased by UV or ionizing radiation and by certain chemicals. A simple screen for mutagens (causing mutations) is the Ames test, where histidine auxotrophs (requiring histidine for growth) are treated with potential mutagens and screened for their ability to back mutate and recover growth without histidine.

Microbes can acquire new genes via three major mechanisms. External naked DNA can be taken up by cells (transformation), DNA can be transferred directly from one cell to another with the help of fertility (F) factors (conjugation), and DNA can be transferred by a bacterial virus (bacteriophage) by transduction. Microbes commonly harbor extrachromosomal circular DNA (plasmids) that contain their own genetic information for replication, as well as other genes that may increase the cells survival. Additionally, chromosomal DNA contains mobile genetic elements (transposons), which can be excised and insert into new locations of the chromosome.

LEARNING OPPORTUNITES

1. Several microbiology students at a local university exhibited a severe cough with productive sputum. Cultures were taken and streaked on several different media. (Chapter Objectives 6, 10, 15)

   i. Isolated single colonies appeared smooth, gelatinous, and watery.

   ii. A Gram stain showed violet-colored cocci.

   iii. Discs containing antibiotics, T, U, V, W, X, Y, and Z were placed onto a plate that had a thin, homogeneous layer of the unknown organism over its surface. The following day, the plate appeared as shown below.

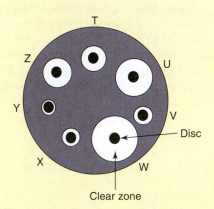

   iv. The unknown organism was streaked as a thin line onto nutrient-rich, semisolid agar. Two days later, the plate appeared as shown below:

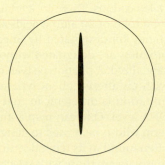

From the preceding information, draw a structure that indicates (a) the shape of the organism, (b) its minimum size, assuming that cells were visible under the light microscope, (c) the type of cell wall, and (d) any surrounding cell envelope material. Finally, (e) recommend an antibiotic shown in the first drawing to treat the infection.

2. A hospital patient contracts a bacterial infection that temporarily worsens after antibiotic therapy. You suspect that the offending agent released by the microbe is associated with the LPS. What portion of the LPS might be responsible? (Chapter Objectives 6, 9)

3. A patient presents in the ER with severe gastrointestinal distress (diarrhea, bloating, flatulence). You discover she is a German tourist who ate three bean burritos and washed them down with several milliliters of a carbonated beverage 5 hrs earlier. This was her first introduction to the burrito. Because others in her party also consumed burritos and have no symptoms, you surmise this may not be food poisoning, but the presence of some chemical constituent in the foodstuff she has consumed. What compound found in the food items consumed could be the likely cause of her gastrointestinal symptoms? (Chapter Objective 18)

4. Does an obligate anaerobe use fermentation or respiration to generate energy? Can an obligate aerobe grow in an anaerobic environment? Defend your answers. (Chapter Objectives 4 and 17)

PEARSON
myhealthprofessionskit™

Use this address to access the interactive Companion Website created for this textbook. Simply select "Clinical Laboratory Science" from the choice of disciplines. Find this book and log in using your user name and password.

REFERENCES

Go to myhealthprofessionskit.com to view this chapter's references.

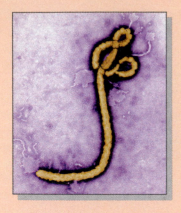

4

The Host's Encounter with Microbes

Karen M. Kiser

■ LEARNING OBJECTIVES

Upon completion of this chapter, the learner should be able to:

1. Select the portal of entry and exit that enables a microorganism to enter, spread through, and escape the human host.
2. Differentiate the characteristics of pathogenic microbes that enhance their ability to invade, spread, and cause disease in the host.
3. Distinguish the innate defenses of the host used in each body site, to include chemical and cellular processes.
4. Correlate the cardinal signs or symptoms of inflammation with the inflammatory response.
5. Relate the adaptive defenses of the host for each body site, to include chemical and cellular processes.

KEY TERMS

adhesins	fenestrated	membrane ruffling
aerosols	focus of infection	necrotic
apoptosis	immunoglobulin	opsonins
biofilm	infected	pathogenicity islands
commensal	infectious disease	quorum sensing
contagious	infectious dose	receptors
electrolytes	invasins	toxins
endogenous	local infection	zipper phagocytosis
exogenous		

▶ INTRODUCTION

When a person is **infected**, microorganisms inhabit or reside in and on the body with the potential to cause disease from womb to tomb. Survival of humans and microbes is dependent on their peaceful coexistence. If a microbe causes the death of its host, it has decreased its chances of continued existence. It has lost its food source, optimum living environment, and in some cases, the microbial community necessary to sustain its life. If humans wipe out the indigenous or naturally occurring microbes, the ability to manufacture essentials (like vitamins), break down food, and keep unfriendly and potentially pathogenic microbes at bay is diminished. When the equilibrium is lost, signs and symptoms of disease associated with a microorganism or **infectious disease** may occur.

All infectious diseases share a common pattern. There is an initial incubation period when an individual may not show symptoms but be **contagious**, which means infected individuals have the ability to transmit disease by contact with their body fluids, excretions, or feces. The development of symptoms then occurs. The symptoms provide clues as to the possible etiology or cause of infection. Finally the patient recovers, is disabled, or dies from the infectious disease.

The chain of infection requires a source or reservoir, a means of transmission, and a susceptible host. The source may be the commensal flora within our body known as **endogenous** organisms. **Commensal** microorganisms form a close relationship with humans in which one or both derive benefits without harm to either. The source may be **exogenous** or located outside the body and include other humans, animals, or insects, and environmental reservoirs such as soil or water. Means of transmission include **aerosols** or small droplets, direct contact or close and intimate contact with a microbe or its toxin, and indirect contact. Aerosols or liquid particles of varying sizes may contain microbes or their toxin. Tiny droplets hang in the air for a time and are breathed into the lungs. Large droplets fall rapidly to a surface after traveling a short distance and pose a contact risk. Contact with infectious agents can also be direct. The microbe or microbe-laden body fluid is introduced directly into the host via a cut, injection, or other type of opening. Contamination of objects with microbes may result through indirect contact if the object is inserted into the mouth or accidentally introduces an organism into a vulnerable area. A susceptible host is a person whose defense systems are less then optimal. A depressed immune state can occur because of trauma, disease, or treatment. More information on body sites possessing commensal flora is presented in Part V, "Analysis of Body Systems for Infectious Disease." A more detailed discussion of the means of transmission and what makes a person susceptible to infection is also included in information provided on each body system. ∞ Chapter 5 presents information on using personal protective equipment and good lab practice to break the chain of infection to work safely in the microbiology laboratory.

Both microorganism and host possess strategies to protect and defend themselves when an encounter occurs. This chapter will describe how microorganisms enter and exit our body sites. Factors that increase a microorganism's ability to invade the host will be discussed as well as host defense strategies. This overview of immunology is intended to provide a basic understanding of infectious disease and our defense mechanisms and is not a substitute for a more in-depth study as is provided in an immunology course or text.

▶ ENTRY, EXIT, AND SPREAD OF MICROBES

Sometimes serendipity or pure luck plays a role with microbial invaders. A microbe-laden dust particle or droplet blows into an opening, and suddenly the opportunity is there to enter the host. Other microbial invaders are mobile and capable of independently moving to the desired location. The opening must also be appropriate for the pathogen. For example, the organism that causes gonorrhea, a sexually transmitted disease, is not associated with diarrheal illness. Although it can cause rectal infections, the microorganism cannot survive the harsh conditions of the upper gastrointestinal tract.

The number of invading microbes can also determine disease development. Most diseases require a large **infectious dose**, the number of microbes required to cause an infectious disease. A few organisms can cause disease with a small number of organisms. *Shigella* spp. is an example of an organism exhibiting low-dose infectivity. Exposure to only a few organisms can result in infectious disease of the gastrointestinal tract. Refer to ∞ Chapter 21, "Enterobacteriaceae," and ∞ Chapter 35, "Gastrointestinal System," for more information on *Shigella* spp.

Microbes enter and exit the body through openings in the various body systems. If an organism gains access to the circulatory system, it can potentially spread throughout the body. Figure 4-1 ■ provides a graphic depiction of these potential entry and exit sites.

RESPIRATORY SYSTEM

A human's first encounter with microbes occurs when a baby moves down the mother's birth canal. Epithelial cells contain **receptors** or molecules on the cell's surface that are capable of binding with a microbe, drug, or other factors. The baby's mucous membrane epithelial cells of the eyes, ears, nose, and mouth pick up the mother's vaginal microbes. At birth and for the rest of our life, our respiratory system is constantly bombarded with microorganisms. Mims estimates there are 400 to 900 bacteria and mould per cubic meter in the air of our buildings. As a result, we inhale on average eight organisms per minute. Microbes exist in the droplets and particles of the air we breathe every day. It is estimated that 20,000 droplets are produced when someone sneezes (Mims, Dimmock, Nash, & Stephen, 1995). Large droplets may travel up to 3 feet then fall to the ground. They are less likely to be inhaled into the

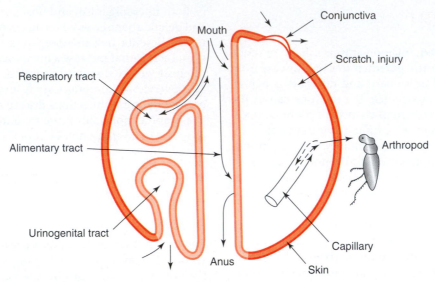

■ **FIGURE 4-1** Microbial entry and exit sites.
Reprinted from Mims' Pathogenesis of Infectious Disease. Mims, Cedric; Dimmock, Nigel; Nash, Anthony; Stephen, John, 1995. Attachment to and entry of microorganism into the body, page 10, with permission from Elsevier.

lungs. Small droplets tend to evaporate. Droplets or dust particles in the range of 1 to 4 micrometers (μm) stay suspended in the air indefinitely. These have the best chance to be inhaled and find their way deep into the alveoli of the lungs.

Nasal hairs in the nose filter the air we breathe. Ciliated epithelial cells on the mucous membranes of the respiratory system help trap larger particles and whisk them up and out of the respiratory tract. If these cells are damaged, as they often are in smokers, or excess fluid interferes with their function, gravity may allow these particles to move deeper into the lungs (Mims et al., 1995).

Our body may respond to the intrusion of our respiratory system by swallowing, coughing, or sneezing, thus forcibly expelling the microbes from our body and contributing to the organisms in the air. ∞ Chapter 33 describes the infectious diseases associated with the respiratory system.

 Checkpoint! 4–1
(Chapter Objective 1)

The portal of entrance for those organisms causing respiratory diseases such as pneumonia and the common cold is the:
   A. skin.
   B. nose.
   C. mucous membranes.
   D. blood.

GASTROINTESTINAL SYSTEM

A food-borne illness usually occurs because of contamination of our food or water with microorganisms or their toxins. **Toxins** are molecules produced by microorganisms that poi-

son the host or enhance invasion. We ingest the food and water laden with microorganisms or their toxins and enable their entry into the gastrointestinal system. Some microbes prefer the stomach, whereas others would rather to travel a little further down to inhabit the intestinal tract. Regardless of their preference, organisms that cause gastrointestinal disease or exist as commensal flora of the gut must survive the acid conditions of the stomach as well as the peristaltic or rhythmic muscular actions and secretions of the intestinal tract. At some point the toxin must be absorbed, or the disease-causing microorganism must invade the tissue lining the stomach or intestinal tract. Otherwise it will be flushed out of the body by defecation.

Colonization and invasion usually require adherence to receptors on the surface of epithelial cells via microbial adhesins. **Adhesins** are molecules on the microbes that hold fast to receptors on host cells or extracellular matrix (supportive tissues), making colonization or invasion easier. Microbes may remain on the surface of the epithelial cell causing changes in the surface of the host cell. **Invasins**, a type of adhesin molecule that activates signals in the host cell and enables bacterial entry, may allow direct entry into the cell by "**zipper phagocytosis**." Zipper phagocytosis is an invasin-directed process in which the host cell membrane is zippered around the bacterial cell as it enters. Another way is through **membrane ruffling**, a rearrangement of host cell's cytoskeleton causing its surface to protrude, enclosing bacteria into a vacuole or compartment within host cell. These processes enclose the bacteria in a cytoplasmic vacuole (Finlay & Falkow, 1997).

Microorganisms capable of penetrating the epithelial cell gain access to the subepithelial tissue. There they encounter the tissue fluid, phagocytes, and lymphatic system defenses.

Invasive microorganisms are engulfed by macrophages, and those that survive phagocytosis are then able to travel to the reticuloendothelial system (RES). The RES consists of the liver, spleen, and bone marrow. Organisms can then gain access to the bloodstream from these sites to cause systemic illness. All body sites served by circulating blood are at increased risk of infection by the invading microbe.

Some *Salmonella* spp. can cause enteric fever, which is an infectious disease characterized by a high fever because of the presence of the organisms in the blood. In a small percentage of patients infected by these *Salmonella* spp., the microbe has the ability to colonize the gallbladder, resulting in establishment of a carrier state and a source for future infections (Murray, Rosenthal, Kobayashi, & Pfaller, 2002). ∞ Chapter 21, "Enterobacteriaceae," and ∞ Chapter 35, "Gastrointestinal System," provide information about the *Salmonella* spp. causing enteric fever.

The host's response to microbial intestinal invasion or exposure to toxin is to decrease the absorption of water and electrolytes by the intestine (Davis, Mass, & Bishop, 1999). **Electrolytes** are substances whose molecules separate into ions (atoms with a positive or negative charge) when in solution. Most clinical laboratories measure sodium, potassium, chloride, and bicarbonate as part of metabolic testing panels in the chemistry department. Electrolytes function to maintain osmotic pressure, water, and acid–base balance. Decreased absorption of water and electrolytes will flood the gastrointestinal system with fluid and increase the flushing action of the intestinal tract resulting in diarrhea. The microorganisms are washed out in the fluid and exit the body in the feces. ∞ Chapter 35 provides information on infections associated with the gastrointestinal system.

Diarrhea may also result from decreasing the normal flora of the gastrointestinal tract, which allows potential pathogens to overgrow the bowel. One mechanism causing a decrease in normal bowel microorganisms is associated with the use of antibiotics and is referred to as antibiotic-associated diarrhea. The most common culprit of antibiotic-associated diarrhea is the anaerobic gram-positive rod *Clostridium difficile*. More information on this organism and its significance can be obtained in ∞ Chapter 24, "Anaerobic Bacteria."

Vomiting may also occur, resulting in expulsion from the stomach of the offending organism via the mouth. Substances released from damaged tissue or messages received from nervous system receptors located in the wall of the gastrointestinal tract, abdomen, and other parts of the nervous system, trigger the vomiting center in the brain. This in turn initiates the vomiting reflex (Nowak & Handford, 2004).

CARDIOVASCULAR SYSTEM

There are various sites of entry into the circulatory system for organisms. Openings created in skin and mucous membranes by trauma can introduce organisms directly into the bloodstream if a blood vessel is also injured. Examples of this include injuries with sharp objects, human and animal bites, accidents or violent acts, and dental extractions. Invasive medical procedures, such as indwelling intravenous catheters used for easy access to the bloodstream, also create a doorway into the cardiovascular system. A **local infection** is an infection site that is limited to one area such as a finger wound. It can spread if blood vessels are in the path. The agent may gain entry into the blood when these vessels are damaged. If the organism becomes systemic, the original site of infection is now considered the **focus of infection**, or starting point.

Microorganisms capable of penetrating the epithelial layer can enter the bloodstream via the lymphatic system. Organisms may spill over into the blood from an infected organ as may occur with pneumococcal pneumonia. The extremely vascular nature of the lungs can allow the infectious agent to seed the blood. The microorganism-laden blood then serves as the vehicle for transmission to other sites such as the central nervous system or other hosts. Once in the cardiovascular system, the microbe may invade the heart or the endothelial lining of the heart, causing lesions on heart valves or heart inflammation.

A microorganism that gains entry into the blood can freely be transported in the plasma or use white or red blood cells as a vehicle to hitch a ride to other parts of the body. To survive, the organism must be able to circumvent the actions of antibodies, complement, and phagocytic cells normally present in the circulatory system. ∞ Chapter 32 provides additional information on cardiovascular system infections.

SYSTEMIC SPREAD

The entire cardiovascular system and all body sites with blood flow are at risk of infection once a microorganism gains access to the blood. Figure 4-2 ■ illustrates the potential for the spread of infection throughout the body.

Abnormal, inflamed, quiescent, and dead tissue provides a favorable environment for the growth of circulating microbes. (Mims et al., 1995). This preference may result in a systemic infection, a life-threatening condition. Osteomyelitis may result if there is prior damage to bone. Endocarditis may result if there is previous damage to heart valves. Organs such as the brain, lungs, and kidneys may be infected, resulting in meningitis, pneumonia, or urinary tract infections, respectively. The organisms being transported through the blood may escape from the cytoplasm of the host cell and begin to multiply in the liver or spleen, blood, or endothelial cells of the vascular system.

Central Nervous System

Organisms that invade the central nervous system must cross the blood–brain barrier by invading the endothelial cells of the vessels providing blood to the brain. They may also invade the epithelial cells of the choroid plexus, tissues that lie deep within the brain and are another part of the blood-brain barrier. Microbes may enter by passing between cells, passing

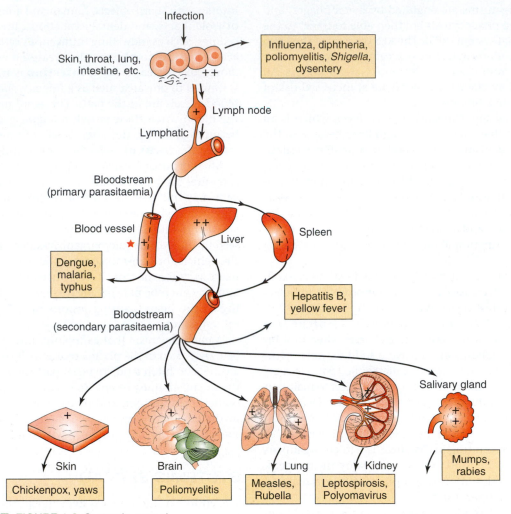

■ FIGURE 4-2 Systemic spread.

Reprinted from Mims' Pathogenesis of Infectious Disease. Mims, Cedric, Dimmock, Nigel, Nash, Anthony, Stephen, John, 1995. The spread of microbes through the body, page 114, with permission from Elsevier.

through cells, riding in leukocytes that play the part of a "Trojan horse," or spread from adjacent structures such as the ear, mastoid bones, or paranasal sinuses (Drevets, Leenen, & Greenfield, 2004). The choroid plexus, where cerebrospinal fluid (CSF) is produced, has **fenestrated** endothelium cells with a tiny opening. The pores in these cells could provide an opening needed for invasion by microbes. Viruses can enter the meninges or lining of the brain via nearby peripheral nerves (Mims et al., 1995).

The subarachnoid space, the area between the arachnoid membrane and pia mater of the brain, is the focus of many central nervous system infections. The CSF that flows in this space contains very few of the elements of host defenses such as antibodies, complement, and white blood cells. CSF does contain glucose and electrolytes, which provide a good nutritional medium for microbial growth (Nowak & Handford, 2004). Refer to ∞ Chapter 38, "Central Nervous System," for more information on infections associated with this body site.

Skeletal System

There appear to be several points of entry for organisms invading the skeletal system. Microbes infecting joints arrive in the blood and invade the synovial membrane, which lines the joint cavities. Invasion may also occur as a result of penetrating trauma or joint damage. Replacement hip and knee surgery may also allow entry of microorganisms. Organisms may spread into the bone from adjacent infected tissue. An example of this is invasion of the mastoid bone from an untreated ear infection. Prior damage to the growing ends of bones may predispose an individual to osteomyelitis. The bone marrow contained within the bones has sinusoids, which are irregular tubular spaces that take the place of blood vessels. Macrophages line these sinusoids. The organisms may grow within the sinusoids, spread to adjacent tissue, or grow within the macrophage following phagocytosis.

Prosthetic joints become coated with host proteins and provide a good surface for bacterial colonization. **Biofilm** (community of bacterial colonies covered by a layer of poly-saccharide) formation on the implant results in the inability of antibiotics to penetrate the slime layer, impaired host defenses, and provides a continuous source of infectious agents (Shirtliff & Mader, 2002). Specific information on biofilm formation and host defenses is provided in the section, "Defense Strategies," later in this chapter. More information on skeletal system infections can be found in ∞ Chapter 39.

GENITAL SYSTEM

Mucous membranes line body areas, such as the respiratory, urogenital, and gastrointestinal tracts, as well as the eyes. Mucous membranes are much more delicate then the skin. Tears in the mucous membranes of the urogenital tract may occur as the result of sexual intercourse. The insertion of a foreign object, such as a contact lens, can result in the introduction of microorganisms onto the surface of the eye. Even microbes that colonize the mucous membranes may cause problems under the right circumstances. These circumstances include childbirth, complication of pregnancy, or antibiotic treatment. Puberty and menopause play a role in the variety of microbes present in the female genital tract. The protective role of normal flora is described under "Defense Strategies," later in this chapter.

Commensal and pathogenic microorganisms of the urogenital tract can be transmitted to others via direct contact with the organism or deposition of fluids containing the organism. A sexually transmitted disease can be passed on to a partner during the sexual act. Newborns can pick up potential pathogens as they move down the mother's birth canal. Autoinoculation can occur if the organism is transferred to another site by an individual's action. For example, picking up an organism on fingers then rubbing the eye could transfer the agent from the genital area to the conjunctiva. Wiping ventrally (front to back), rather than dorsally (back to front), after defecation can transfer gastrointestinal flora into the female genital area. Organisms may also be introduced into the urethra during the sexual act, causing urethritis. Genital tract system infections are discussed in ∞ Chapter 36.

URINARY SYSTEM

There are two entrances into the urinary system. One is via the kidney or the descending route. Blood-borne pathogens may cross into the urinary system by way of the fenestrated endothelial cells of the kidney's glomerulus (Mims et al., 1995). The other entrance is by way of the urethra referred to as the ascending route.

The perineal or perirectal area is located next to the urethra on the female and is colonized with an abundance of normal flora. The anus is also nearby and is a potential source of microbes if good hygiene is not maintained. The female urethra is shorter than the male urethra, making the opening more accessible to entry by microorganisms. The incidence of urinary tract infections in males is decreased because the urethra is longer, and the normal flora present is not as prevalent as in females. If a motile infecting agent is introduced into the urethra, it is possible for it to crawl up the kidney ureter and enter the urinary system. Structural abnormalities in the urinary system, obstruction by kidney stones, or an enlarged prostate in males can prevent the bladder from completely emptying or affect the flow of urine and predispose one to infection. Once one part of the system is invaded, the entire urinary system is at risk. Organisms can also be introduced into the bladder during medical procedures such as catheterization.

The exits are the same as the entrances. If an infecting agent is able to gain access to the kidney by moving up the ureters, they may cross over into the blood circulation because of the vascular nature of the kidney. The organisms may also exit via the urethra during urination. ∞ Chapter 34 reviews infections of the urinary system.

INTEGUMENTARY SYSTEM

The integumentary system includes the skin, which lines the external surfaces of the body as well as the mucous membranes, which are continuous with the skin, or line the body cavities exposed to the external environment. Microorganisms gain entry through openings in these coverings. Openings may occur as a result of trauma, injury, or exposure to needles or sharps. Exposure to needles or sharps may be due to a medical procedure, such as venipuncture, or a personal decision resulting from body piercing, tattoos, or drug addiction. Openings may also be a result of drying conditions causing chapped hands or hangnails. Diseases may cause rashes or pustules, which create breaks in the skin. Organisms may also be introduced through the bites of insects, animals, or humans. The presence of hair on the skin can make it more difficult for motile organisms to travel across the body's surface. Shaving these areas can increase the chance of infection because of minute cuts (Mims et al., 1995). Fingers play a role in the spread of microbes when an individual scratches or rubs an irritated area of skin.

Once an organism makes it way across the skin or mucous membrane, it then gains entry to the subendothelial tissue. The gel-like nature of this layer makes it difficult for microbes to spread. Many organisms produce enzymes that help break down this barrier, allowing them to spread into adjacent organs, tissues, body cavities, or blood vessels.

Invaders may encounter the lymph system and overwhelm its defensive actions by sheer numbers. Inflammation and exercise can increase lymph flow with subsequent flushing of the invaders out of the lymphatic system and into the circulatory system. Dysfunctional phagocytes may not effectively engulf the microbes. This failure of containment by the lymph node allows microorganisms to gain access to the blood. Infections associated with the integumentary system are discussed in ∞ Chapter 37.

**Checkpoint! 4–2
(Chapter Objective 1)**

A site of infection from which bacteria and or their products spread to other parts of the body is:

    A. *a local infection.*
    B. *the focal infection.*
    C. *a primary infection.*
    D. *a mixed infection.*

▶ MICROBIAL VIRULENCE FACTORS

To cause disease, an organism must invade, multiply, secrete a toxin, or spread from its entry point. This ability to cause disease is enhanced by the possession of one or more virulence factors. Genes encoding for these virulence factors are found on plasmids, within phages, or on transposons (mobile genetic elements within the organism's DNA sometimes referred to as "jumping genes") or in clusters of genes called pathogenicity islands. **Pathogenicity islands** are groups of genes on a bacterial chromosome that code for virulence factors (Relman & Falkow, 2000; Schmidt and Hensel, 2004). Refer to ∞ Chapter 3 to review bacterial cell genetics. In certain bacteria, cell-to-cell chemical communication or **quorum sensing** determines the appropriate time to express virulence factors allowing avoidance of host defenses (Kievit & Iglewski, 2000). These virulence factors allow the organism to outwit the host defenses and invade or spread deeper into the host.

CELL WALL

An organism's cell wall structure may provide it with an advantage in its defense against the host response. Refer to ∞ Chapter 3 to review the bacterial cell wall structure. Adhesins on the bacterial cell enhance binding to tissue cells. Toxigenic microbes can take advantage of their close proximity to the host cell to deliver their toxin.

The presence of lipids in the *Mycobacterium* spp. cell wall makes them impervious to many antibiotics and disinfectants (Primm, Lucero, & Falkinham, 2004). The presence of mycolic acids in their cell wall enables them to resist the digestive effects of lysosomal enzymes and survive a white blood cell attack (van Crevel, Ottenhoff, & van der Meer, 2002). If engulfed by phagocytes, they may become an intracellular pathogen and remain unaffected by the release of chemicals from the cells granules. The white blood cell may serve as a vehicle, transporting the acid-fast organisms throughout the body, until the white blood cell dies and releases its passenger. ∞ Chapter 26 reveals more information about the *Mycobacterium* spp.

Gram-positive pathogens possess a variety of cell wall components that enhance their ability to cause disease. *Streptococcus pyogenes* (group A streptococci) possesses an M protein in its cell wall, which provides some protection against phagocytosis. The M protein appears to prevent activation of the complement pathway and also plays an important role in attachment of the organism to skin cells (Cunningham, 2000). *Staphylococcus aureus* has protein A on its cell wall that binds to the single leg of the Y-shaped IgG antibody. The single leg is also known as the Fc portion. This action renders the immunoglobulin useless for defense because it is upside down and can't bind to the bacterial cell via the antigen-binding portion (Fab) of the antibody. Refer to "Antibody and Complement Actions," later in this chapter, for a basic description of the antibody structure and to ∞ Chapter 10, "Immunological Tests," for a more detailed discussion. The bacterial cell becomes coated with this upside-down antibody preventing phagocytosis and blocking the other antibody binding sites. Some of the protein A is released into the surrounding environment, thus binding up additional antibodies and consuming complement (Mandell, Dolin, & Bennett, 2000).

Gram-negative organisms possess endotoxin in their cell wall. It is the lipid A portion of the lipopolysaccharide (LPS) located in the outer membrane of the gram-negative cell wall. It is released on lysis of the cell and causes the peripheral blood to pool, blood pressure to plummet, organs to fail, and occasionally results in death (Mims et al., 1995). The coagulation system may also be activated by LPS resulting in disseminated intravascular coagulation or DIC. DIC results in consumption of the body's blood clotting factors through clot formation and degradation. Gram-negative species also contain a periplasmic space in their cell wall. Some antibiotics are able to diffuse through the outer membrane and enter this space. Enzymes produced by bacteria, such as beta-lactamase, destroy the antibiotic, such as penicillin, before it can gain entry into the cytoplasm of the cell and carry out its inhibitory or killing effect. Refer to ∞ Chapter 11 to learn about laboratory methods used to detect these antibiotic-destroying enzymes.

EXOTOXINS

Exotoxins are chemicals manufactured and secreted by organisms. When expressed, these compounds allow the microorganism to spread, invade, and resist the host defenses. They may also play a role in helping a microbe meet its nutritional needs by breaking down complex molecules into their basic components. Host damage caused by exotoxins may be direct, such as diarrhea, or indirect, such as inflammation. Table 4-1✪ lists exotoxins and their effects on the host.

Four secretion systems are believed to be used by gram-negative bacteria. Types I and IV involve the formation of a pore or opening in the cell wall through which the toxin passes. Type II uses a molecule to help transport the toxin across the organism's outer membrane. Type III resembles a "molecular syringe" that injects the toxin into adjacent host cells (Coburn et al., 2007). Gram-positive microbes usually export proteins to the surface then release them into the external environment (Finlay & Falkow, 1997).

Exotoxins causing direct damage include spreading factors that degrade tissue or compounds that either damage cells or

⊘ TABLE 4-1

Selected Exotoxins and Their Effects on the Host

Exotoxin	Microorganism	Effect
Pneumolysin	*Streptococcus pneumoniae*	Weakens host defenses
		Promotes bacteremia
		Sensorineural deafness
Ergotamine	*Claviceps purpurea*	Ergot poisoning
Diphtheria toxin	*Corynebacterium diphtheriae*	Kills cells (epithelial necrosis, heart damage, nerve paralysis)
Tetanus toxin (neurotoxin)	*Clostridium tetani*	Spastic paralysis
		"Lockjaw"
		Respiratory failure
Alpha-toxin	*Clostridium perfringens*	Tissue necrosis (gangrene)
Cholera enterotoxin	*Vibrio cholerae*	Profuse diarrhea
Exotoxin A	*Pseudomonas aeruginosa*	Kills cells (necrotizing lesions)
Exotoxin S		Inhibits phagocytosis
Pertussis toxin	*Bordetella pertussis*	Weakens host defenses
		Increases secretions and mucus
Botulinum toxin (neurotoxin)	*Clostridium botulinum*	Flaccid paralysis
		"Double vision"
		Respiratory failure
Shiga-toxin	*Enterohemorrhagic E. coli* (e.g., O157:H7)	"Bloody" diarrhea
		Kidney failure
Toxin A (enterotoxin)	*Clostridium difficile*	"Inflammatory" diarrhea (WBC, RBC, mucus)
Toxin B (cytotoxin)		Damages cytoplasmic membrane ("cell rounding")

allow the organism to exist within a hostile environment like the stomach, intestines, or white blood cells.

Examples of spreading factors include proteinase and hyaluronidase, which break down protein and the hyaluronic acid of connective tissue. *Staphylococcus aureus* is known for its ability to spread rapidly through tissue. Streptokinase is an exotoxin that lyses clots. Streptolysins S and O lyse red blood cells as well as being antiphagocytic. Leukocidins lyse white blood cells. *Streptococcus pyogenes* (group A beta hemolytic streptococci) produces all three of these powerful exotoxins.

Listeria monocytogenes produces a phospholipase and listeriolysin, which allows it to escape from the phagosome or vacuole produced after phagocytosis. It then enters the white blood cells' cytoplasm. *Mycobacterium tuberculosis* secretes ammonium chloride that prevents lysosome fusion to the phagosome (Mims et al., 1995). Lysosomes are the white blood cell granules that contain digestive enzymes. Both of these organisms can use the white blood cell as their mode of transportation and travel throughout the body via the circulatory system. Organisms with this capability are considered intracellular pathogens. ∞ Chapter 19 provides more information on *Listeria,* and ∞ Chapter 26 details the *Mycobacterium* species.

Secretion of mucinase allows colonizing microbes to live in the mucous layer of the intestine and stomach. Some urinary tract pathogens, such as *Proteus,* produce urease. This enzyme converts urea to ammonia, which increases the pH of the urine creating more favorable conditions for growth in the urinary system (Mims et al., 1995). The urease secreted by *Helicobacter pylori* buffers the stomach acid, allowing the microbe to survive the acid's lethal effects (Covacci, Telford, Del Guidice, Parsonnet, & Rappuoli, 1999). Refer to ∞ Chapter 23 for a review of the characteristics of *Helicobacter pylori.*

The inflammatory response may be triggered by cell damage caused by exotoxins and the subsequent release of materials from the cell. The host responds with inflammation in the form of redness, pain, heat, and swelling. This may result in indirect damage of tissue. An example of this process is observed when a microorganism kills a white blood cell. Granule contents are released into the local environment, causing an inflammatory reaction in the host (Mims et al., 1995).

SPORES

The genera *Bacillus* and *Clostridium* respond to starvation and environmental stresses by forming spores. The presence of endospores allows these organisms to survive harsh environments and makes them more difficult to kill. Sporulation by *Bacillus* and *Clostridium* protects the organism's genetic material by encasing the chromosome, essential proteins, and ribosomes in multiple layers consisting of two membranes, calcium-bound peptidoglycan, and an outer coat of protein. At the end of the sporulation cycle, the bacterial cell lyses, releasing the spore. Figure 4-3 ■ demonstrates the spores of *Bacillus* species.

The DNA-containing spore lies dormant in the dust, soil, or on plants, in a manner similar to that of a plant's seed. When introduced into a suitable environment, whether by chance or trauma, the spore germinates into a vegetative cell. This process of germination is triggered by the presence of water, specific amino acids, or carbohydrates. Enzymes in the coat are activated and degrade the protein coat. This allows the entry of water causing the spore to swell and shed its coat. When RNA, protein, and DNA synthesis resumes the spore becomes a vegetative cell. The vegetative cell is capable of reproduction resulting in increased numbers of the organism in the site. Refer to ∞ Chapter 19 for more information about the *Bacillus* spore. ∞ Chapter 24 provides more information on *Clostridium* spp. spores.

Fungi produce spores as a means of reproduction. The spores are easily dispersed through the air. Systemic fungal infections usually begin with the inhalation of fungal spores into the lungs (Campbell & Stewart, 1980). Those with weakened immune systems are especially susceptible. ∞ Chapter 29, "Medical Mycology," provides additional information on fungal diseases and the use of spores to identify the specific fungus.

FLAGELLA AND PILI (FIMBRIAE)

Flagella (single: flagellum) function in locomotion of microorganisms. They are long hairlike, semirigid structures located on some bacteria. Flagella are shaped like a hook and rotate like a propeller (Madigan, Martinko, & Parker, 2000). The bacteria "run" in a straight direction when the flagella rotate to the left. The bacteria randomly "tumble" when the

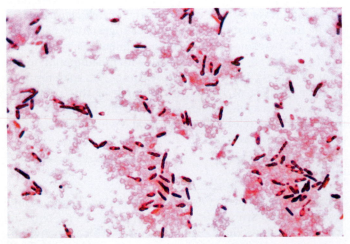

■ **FIGURE 4-3** Spores of *Bacillus* species appear as an unstained area within the cell on Gram stain.

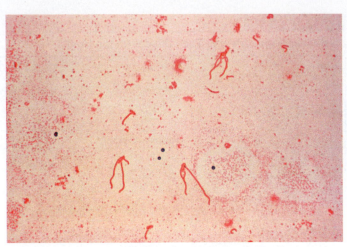

■ **FIGURE 4-4** Flagella of *Yersinia enterocolitica.*
Public Health Image Library/CDC

flagella rotate to the right. Travel toward a target is characterized by alternating "runs" and "tumbles" (Alcamo, 2001). Those bacteria that possess flagella are capable of independent movement. This is an advantage because it allows purposeful movement from one location to another and through mucus. Figure 4-4 ■ demonstrates the flagella of *Yersinia enterocolitica.*

Pili (single: pilus) or fimbriae (single: fimbria) are short hairlike structures located on gram-negative bacteria. They facilitate adhesion to body surfaces, enabling an organism to resist the defensive actions of fluid or mucus flow, thereby enhancing invasiveness. Type IV pili allows a microbe to move across a smooth surface. The pili extend and withdraw, allowing the organism to crawl in a twitching movement (Mims et al., 1995). *Neisseria gonorrhoeae* is known for its use of pili to adhere closely to the mucous membrane of the urethra and avoid the flushing action of urine. Refer to ∞ Chapter 3 to review the bacterial cell and its structures.

CAPSULE AND SLIME LAYER

A capsule is a thick layer of protein and carbohydrate tightly bound around the outside surface of the microbial cell. Not all microbes possess a capsule, but those that do are more difficult to engulf by white blood cells. The capsule also covers the organism's binding sites for antibodies and complement. This makes the defensive actions of the immune response less effective. Refer to the section on the immune response later in this chapter for more information on its defensive role. Bacteria, white blood cells, and human cells carry a negative electrical charge. Repulsion between two negatively charged cells may also play a defensive role (Alcamo, 2001). An India ink preparation demonstrating the capsule of *Cryptococcus neoformans* is pictured in Figure 4-5 ■.

A slime layer is a protective layer of loosely bound protein and polysaccharide secreted by bacterial cells. It is similar to the capsule, but its structure is thinner and not as rigid or well

■ FIGURE 4-5 Capsule of *Cryptococcus neoformans*. The structure appears as a halo around the yeast cell.

 REAL WORLD TIP

The presence of a capsule is associated with mucoid bacterial colonies. *Klebsiella* spp. are well known for their large capsule and extremely mucoid colonies on culture.

formed. It functions to protect the cell against dehydration, trap nutrients, and bind the cells together (Black, 1999).

BIOFILM

A few organisms have the ability to adhere to a surface and form a community of bacterial colonies covered by a polysaccharide coating called a biofilm. Some examples of biofilm include dental plaque on teeth and the slime formed by *Staphylococcus* spp. on indwelling intravenous and urinary catheters or other medical devices. Examples of human infections with biofilms include dental cavities, gingivitis, otitis media, endocarditis, and nosocomial infections caused by the use of contact lenses, orthopedic devices, and endotracheal tubes

Individual cells stick to a surface and move to the biofilm development site via Type IV pili. Once established, colonies are formed that grow vertically into mushroom- and cone-shaped structures. Canals between the colonies provide quorum sensing communication and circulation of nutrients or waste products. Figure 4-6 ■ provides a graphic image of a biofilm. Once the colonies reach a certain height, a polysaccharide shell is produced that covers the entire community. By forming a biofilm, organisms are able to resist antibiotics, the white blood cells, and other chemicals that may be directed at them by the host defenses. A biofilm also provides a source of infection as clumps of bacterial cells break free from the community (Schaudinn et al., 2007).

 Checkpoint! 4–3 (Chapter Objective 2)

Bacteria that produce leukocidins are considered more pathogenic because they:
   A. *destroy the host's white blood cells.*
   B. *allow the organism to spread through connective tissue.*
   C. *enhance attachment of the bacteria to body tissue.*
   D. *clot plasma to form a protective coat of fibrin.*

▶ HOST DEFENSE STRATEGIES

The host has several barriers in place to inhibit microbial invasion. These include the skin and mucous membranes. Once an organism has breached these barriers, additional actions are triggered that are designed to destroy the invaders. These active responses include the inflammatory response and the immune response. The defensive systems interact to form the innate and adaptive immunity systems.

INTEGUMENT

The integument is part of innate (natural) immunity and is the first line of defense. The integument consists of the exterior body covering of skin and the mucous membranes. When intact, they provide a barrier that is difficult to penetrate.

Skin

The skin consists of epithelial cells so tightly packed that they provide a cover that protects the host against the harsh outside environment. Pores and hair follicles dot the landscape providing shelter for residential commensal flora and some protection against the elements.

The resident normal flora helps control the microbial population by competition for food and the inhibitory effects of acidic metabolic by-products or secretions. Most of the skin is exposed to a dry environment that is constantly bombarded by the ultraviolet rays of the sun. This is not an optimum growth environment for most microorganisms. The skin areas located in the axilla and groin are moist and usually covered by clothing. These areas support a more abundant commensal flora.

At the base of the pores lie sebaceous glands that secrete sweat. The sweat's acidity and flow has a controlling effect on the microbial residents. Skin is also sloughed off regularly, removing any transient microbes.

Mucous Membranes

The mucous membranes consist of squamous epithelial cells that line the body's openings of the respiratory, genitourinary, and gastrointestinal system as well as the eye. The upper respiratory epithelial cells are ciliated, which serves to move microbes trapped in mucus up the trachea via their waving motion. After ascending the trachea they may be swallowed or pass out of the body in spit. The mucous membrane covering is more delicate than skin, less exposed to the exterior

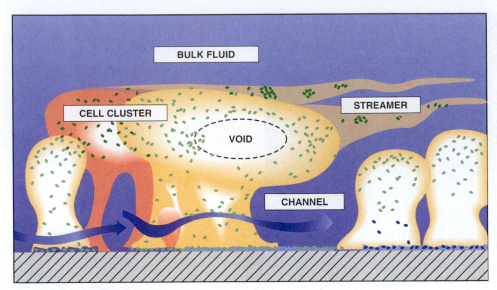

■ FIGURE 4-6 Biofilm.

Reprinted from The Center for Biofilm Engineering at Montana State University–Bozeman. Used with permission from the center.

environment, and moist. As a consequence, it is host to an abundant commensal flora. The normal flora keeps the number of pathogenic organisms under control by the same mechanisms already discussed. In addition, in the intestinal tract, normal flora participates in the host metabolic processes by generating necessary vitamins and assisting with the degradation of food.

The functions and defensive properties of the mucous membranes are enhanced by the production of secretions. Some of these secretions are acidic. Some enzymes produced are proteolytic and aid in the breakdown of food. These enzymes can damage the microbes too. Glands produce mucus, which regularly flows out of the body opening. Invading microbes get stuck in the mucus and are removed with the mucus flow.

From puberty to menopause the vaginal epithelial cells contain glycogen as a result of estrogen levels. One of the primary colonizers, *Lactobacillus* spp., utilizes glycogen. These microaerophilic gram-positive rods produce lactic acid as a metabolic by-product. This by-product creates an acid environment in the vagina, which helps to control the variety and numbers of other commensal flora. Decreased levels of estrogen in prepubescent and menopausal females create a lack of glycogen in the vaginal epithelial cells. This changes the pH of the

environment to a more alkaline one, which allows other kinds of bacteria to establish residence (Mims et al., 1995). Refer to ∞ Chapter 19 for more information on *Lactobacillus* spp.

INFLAMMATION

The second line of defense is a nonspecific or innate response to a microbial invasion. It is not targeted to a specific organism, but is a general response to any foreign agent. It does not remember the encounter or require memory of a previous exposure as occurs with antibody production. Microbial growth causing damage may stimulate the activation of macrophages and trigger inflammation, which in turn activates the immune system.

Macrophages in tissue and dendritic cells in the skin and gastrointestinal lining recognize molecules on the surface of microbes that are not found on host cells. They also recognize products released from **necrotic** cells resulting in an area containing dead, irreversibly damaged host cells and a pathological process that affects tissue and organ function. Products released include interferon, heat shock proteins, and tissue necrosis factor. These are examples of cytokines, which are a group of proteins that recruit and activate immune cells. Activated dendritic cells migrate to lymph nodes to activate lymphocytes. Cytokines released from lymphocytes activate additional macrophages and other phagocytes to respond to the infected site. Complement may attach to the cell wall of bacteria activating its alternate pathway and triggering an inflammatory response. Mast cells are tissue cells similar to basophils in the blood. They live in connective tissue located near blood vessels and, once activated, release histamine causing dilation of blood vessel. Plasma containing antibodies, complement, and blood cells flow from the vessels and into the tissues.

REAL WORLD TIP

A Gram stain of a smear from a healthy vagina reveals predominately gram-positive rods resembling *Lactobacillus* spp. A Gram stain of a smear made during a vaginal infection may reveal predominately gram-negative rods, *Staphylococcus* spp., or the cause of a sexually transmitted disease such as *Neisseria gonorrhoeae*.

Phagocytosis

The monocytes, macrophages, and neutrophils are the primary white blood cells (WBCs) involved in phagocytosis. Eosinophils kill parasites by "releasing cationic proteins and reactive oxygen metabolites into the extracellular fluid" (Delves & Roitt, 2000a, p. 39). Both eosinophils and basophils interact with IgE and are associated with allergic reactions caused by their release of inflammatory proteins.

The WBCs are produced in the bone marrow and reside in marrow storage pools until released as needed by the body. Five to eleven thousand white cells circulate in the peripheral blood. Approximately 50% to 70% of the WBCs consist of segmented neutrophils (segs), whereas 2% to 9% are monocytes (monos; Harmening, 2002). A very small percentage of the circulating WBC pool consists of eosinophils and basophils. Eosinophils reside in the tissues of the intestine and respiratory system. Basophils resemble the tissue mast cells (Mims et al., 1995). Some segs or polymorphonuclear leukocytes (PMNs) also reside in the marginal pool, where they leisurely roll across the vessel's wall at random.

The monocytes eventually leave the blood, enter the tissue, and patrol the body for foreign substances. They ultimately mature into macrophages. Some macrophages are fixed and stationary in organ systems. These include the lung macrophages or dust cells and liver histiocytes. Macrophages line the sinusoids of the spleen, lymph nodes, liver, bone marrow, and adrenal glands (Mims et al., 1995).

A microbe attempting to establish residence in a body site produces by-products as the result of growth and metabolism.

These substances signal its presence to the immune system and triggers WBC chemotaxis. Chemotaxis is also triggered by the increased concentration of chemicals released by other cells in the area such as mast cells or platelets. Products of the immune system including complement activators and cytokines also contribute to this process as well.

Chemotaxis is the directional movement of WBCs to an infected area where they are needed to attack the invader. The WBCs leave the circulatory system by squeezing between the endothelial cells in a process called diapedesis. If more cells are needed, reserve cells can quickly be released from the marginal and storage pools, increasing the number of white cells available for battle.

REAL WORLD TIP

The increase in peripheral WBCs is detected in the hematology laboratory when the total white cell count and differential are performed. An increase in segmented neutrophils is usually characteristic of bacterial infection.

The first step in the WBC ingestion process is adhesion of the microbe to the WBC. Figure 4-7 ■ illustrates the process of phagocytosis. Attachment is facilitated by **opsonins.** Opsonins, such as antibodies and complement, act like magnets attracting WBCs and enhancing phagocytosis. The foreign object or microbe is surrounded by the WBC's cytoplasm and pulled inside, creating a phagosome or vacuole. Figure 4-8 ■

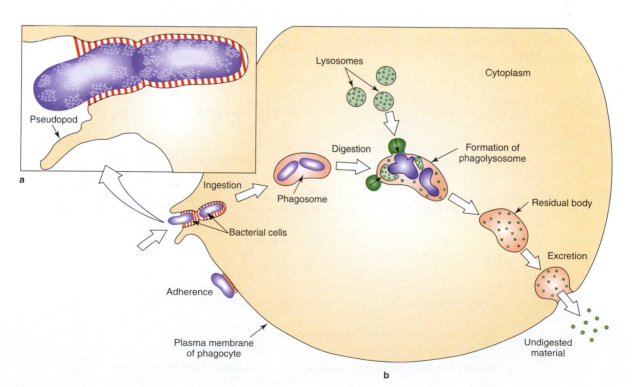

■ **FIGURE 4-7** Phagocytosis.

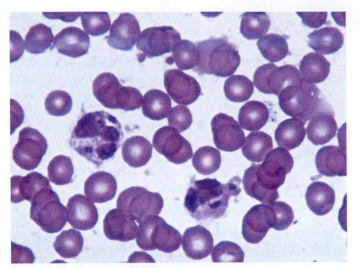

■ **FIGURE 4-8** Neutrophil with intracellular gram-positive cocci.

reveals engulfed staphylococci (gram-positive cocci in tetrads) in the cytoplasm of a PMN. The phagocytes consume oxygen as they engulf the microbe. The oxygen is used for a respiratory burst, which facilitates biochemical reactions needed for oxygen-dependent killing of microorganisms. It is called oxygen dependent because it relies on the use of oxygen to fuel the biochemical reactions. Figure 4-9 ■ provides basic information on toxic products produced as a result of the respiratory burst. The white cell's granules or lysosomes immediately adhere to the phagosome and squirt their contents inside. The pH within the phagosome falls, resulting in an acidic environment. The drop in pH, enzymes, and proteins that make up the granule contents result in oxygen-independent killing of the microbe. This fusion process results in a loss of granules, which can be observed as the white cell undergoes degranulation.

The granules contain lysozyme, which works to dissolve the cell wall of certain gram-positive microbes. Other WBC compounds include myeloperoxidase, proteolytic enzymes, B_{12} binding proteins, and lactoferrin. Membrane-associated nicotinamide adenine dinucleotide phosphate (NADP)-dependent oxidase is activated and catalyzes the oxygen-dependent biochemical reactions. These reactions produce products such as hydrogen peroxide (H_2O_2), superoxides (O_{2-}), and a bleachlike compound, all of which are toxic to many microorganisms. Antimicrobial peptides or defensins bind to the cell wall and increase its permeability, resulting in cell death (Yeaman and Yount, 2005). An iron-binding compound, lactoferrin, and vitamin B_{12} binding protein may have bacteriostatic activity by removing iron and vitamin B_{12} from the microbe's diet. Acid hydrolases act to digest the microbe after death (Miller & Britigan, 1997).

Some organisms are able to resist these actions, can stay viable within the phagocyte, and are then transported to other parts of the body, where they may continue their infection. These organisms are referred to as intracellular pathogens and include *Listeria monocytogenes, Brucella abortus,* and *Mycobacterium tuberculosis.* These intracellular pathogens use a variety of strategies to resist killing by phagocytes. They

---

ℯ ■ **REAL WORLD TIP**

Microbiologists should take note of the microbes the neutrophil has phagocytized when observed on a Gram stained smear of a clinical specimen. The observation of segmented neutrophils in a Gram stain is a key finding associated with bacterial infection. The microbes in the immediate vicinity of or in vacuoles within the neutrophil could be the potential pathogen.

$$\text{Oxygen + NADPH} \xrightarrow{\text{NADPH Oxidase}} \text{2 Superoxide (O2}^-\text{) + NADP + H}^+$$

$$\text{2 Superoxide + H}^+ \xrightarrow{\text{Superoxide dismutase}} \text{Hydrogen peroxide (H}_2\text{O}_2\text{)}$$

$$\text{Hydrogen peroxide (H}_2\text{O}_2\text{)} \xrightarrow{\text{O}_2^-} \text{Hydroxyl radical (OH·)}$$

$$\text{Hydrogen peroxide (H}_2\text{O}_2\text{)} \xrightarrow{\text{Cl}^- + \text{Myeloperoxidase}} \text{Hypochlorite (OCl}^-\text{)}$$

$$\text{Hypochlorite (OCl}^-\text{)} \xrightarrow{\text{H}_2\text{O}_2} \text{Singlet Oxygen (}^1\text{O}_2\text{)}$$

$$\text{N}_2 + \text{O}_2 \xrightarrow{\text{Nitric oxide synthase}} \text{Nitric oxide (NO)}$$

■ **FIGURE 4-9** Toxic products associated with the respiratory burst in neutrophils.
Adapted from Madigan, Michael, Martinko, John, Parker, Jack. 2000. Brock Biology of Microorganisms. Upper Saddle River: Prentice Hall, Figure 20-8.

include inhibition of WBC granule fusion, inactivation of oxidants, and escape from the phagosome.

Sometimes damage to the host can occur as a result of phagocytosis. Toxic compounds may leak out of the white cell as the phagosome is closing around the microbe (Miller & Britigan, 1997). Phagocytes unable to engulf large objects or flat surfaces coated with immune complexes release the contents of their granules into tissue spaces (Nowak & Handford, 2004). The damage done to tissue in the area of infection may cause DNA mutation and affect organ function.

Chemical Triggers

The host's immune system is alerted to the presence of pathogens by chemical signals that trigger chemotaxis. These signals include products released from bacteria, damaged tissue, complement, and cytokines. Table 4-2✪ presents a list of cytokines that assist the host in defending against microbial invasion.

Evidence points to the release of certain cytokines such as tissue necrosis factor (TNF), interleukin-1 and interleukin-8 in the stimulation of chemotaxis and inflammation (Delves &

Roitt, 2000b). The release of toxins or the presence of microbial by-products of metabolism, such as acid, may cause an irritation in the area or damage tissue and trigger the body's recognition of infection. Polymorphonuclear leukocytes and lymphocytes exhibit both a random and directional movement. They migrate toward the highest concentration of chemicals where they can phagocytose the invading microbe (Harmening, 2002). Monocytes exhibit directional movement only. Cytokines activate monocytes and help them focus on the site of infection (Mims et al., 1995).

Symptoms

Inflammatory responses result in the appearance of symptoms in the patient, which may be recognized by the physician during physical examination. Medical laboratory tests and radiologic examinations may also reflect the infectious disease process.

The basic symptoms of inflammation and infection include swelling, redness, heat, and pain. The swelling is a result of the release of plasma from the blood vessels infiltrating the

✪ TABLE 4-2

Selected Cytokines Involved in Microbial Defense

Cytokine	Source	Major Effect
IL-1	Macrophages	Activate T cells and macrophages Promote inflammation
IL-2	Helper (Th1) T cells	Activate lymphocytes, natural killer cells, and macrophages
IL-4	Helper (Th2) T cells, mast cells, basophils, and eosinophils	Activate lymphocytes, monocytes, and IgE class switching
IL-5	Helper (Th2) T cells, mast cells, and eosinophils	Differentiation of eosinophils, activated T and B cells, IgA production
IL-6	Helper (Th2) T cells and macrophages	Activate lymphocytes Acute-phase protein production
IL-8	T cells and macrophages	Chemotaxis of neutrophils, basophils, and T cells
IL-10	Lymphocytes and mast cells	Inhibition of IL-1 production
IL-11	Bone marrow stromal cells	Acute-phase protein production
IL-12	Macrophages and B cells	Production of interferon-γ Helper T type 1 (Th1) cell production
IL-17	CD4 lymphocytes	Granulocyte production via G-CSF Cytokine regulation
IL-19	Monocytes	Inhibition of IL-1 production (triggered by LPS and GM-CSF)
IL-22	T cells	Inhibition of IL-1 production Antiviral
TNF-α	Macrophages, lymphocytes, and mast cells	Promote inflammation
TNF-β	Helper (Th1) T cells and B cells	Promote inflammation
GM-CSF	Lymphocytes and macrophages	Granulocyte and monocyte production
IFN-α	Virally infected leukocytes	Antiviral
IFN-β	Virally infected cells	Antiviral
IFN-γ	Helper (Th1) T cells and natural killer cells	Activate macrophages Inhibition of Helper T type 2 (Th2) cells

IL = Interleukin; TNF = Tumor necrosis factor; GM-CSF = Granulocyte-macrophage colony stimulating factor;
IFN = Interferon; G-CSF = Granulocyte colony stimulating factor; LPS = Lipopolysaccharides.

tissue of the infected site. Lymph nodes also swell, reflecting their activity in processing microbes for a specific immune response. Red cells circulating in the blood flow out because of increased vessel permeability, causing a reddening of the area. The growth of microorganisms in the site and phagocytosis result in biochemical activity and generates pus and heat. Active destruction and swelling of the tissues presses nerves at the site, triggering the pain stimulus. The liver releases proteins as part of the acute phase response. These proteins include C-reactive protein (CRP) and fibrinogen. Proteins from muscles that are broken down during fever may provide the energy and amino acids required by actively dividing microbial cells (Mims et al., 1995). In more serious infections, tissue damage may cause organ failure, falling blood pressure, and the formation of local clots or disseminated intravascular clotting (DIC).

Medical laboratory tests reflect these changes causing higher than normal total white blood cell counts, an increased percentage of neutrophils and monocytes, increased CRP levels, and an increased erythrocyte sedimentation rate (ESR). The ESR test is a nonspecific procedure that may correlate with inflammation. With inflammation, there is increased fibrinogen, which causes the red blood cells to stick together and fall out of suspension or sediment faster. Abnormal coagulation tests detect clot formation in patients. Abnormal values for chemistry analytes reflect damage or decreased organ function. X-rays may reveal changes in the tissues or organs that result from the inflammatory response. Dead host cells, dead and dying white cells, and killed bacteria accumulate to create the creamy yellow pus associated with infection.

Checkpoint! 4–4
(Chapter Objectives 3 and 4)

When examining a Gram stained specimen smear, you note the presence of many PMNs (polymorphonuclear leukocytes). They are probably the result of the:

    A. *immune response.*
    B. *primary response.*
    C. *secondary response.*
    D. *inflammatory response.*

ADAPTIVE IMMUNE RESPONSE

The third line of defense is the adaptive immune response. Components of innate immunity interact with the components of the adaptive immunity. The adaptive response is targeted to an antigen, which can be a specific protein, carbohydrate, lipid, or nucleic acid associated with a microorganism or foreign object. It is considered specific because its focus is on the foreign invader or substance. Adaptive immunity attempts to disable or destroy the invader's disease-producing capability. It is similar to a lock and key in that the immune response usually only works against the target it was designed for, like a key that only opens the lock it was designed to open. Memory, a process by which previously encountered antigens are recognized, is also a characteristic of adaptive immunity.

When microbes enter where macrophages and dendritic cells preside, the invaders are delivered to the local lymph nodes by the lymphatic system. The battle between host and microbe continues in the lymph nodes. Lymph flow will stop if the inflammation and tissue damage is severe, thereby localizing the infection. If containment and annihilation of microbes fails, then the organisms will reproduce, and large numbers may be released into the circulation (Mims et al., 1995). Intravascular microbes are processed by antigen-presenting cells in the spleen.

Several cell types are actively involved in the adaptive immune response. The professional antigen-presenting cells include the dendritic cells located in the spleen, in lymph nodes, and near the epidermidis, monocytes/macrophages; and B-lymphocytes. These cells present the antigen to other lymphocytes, which participate in the immune response by releasing chemicals and stimulating antibody production. Memory T and B cells constitute the body's immune surveillance system.

Antigen-Presenting Cells' Response to Antigens

The major histocompatibility complex (MHC) molecules play an important role in immunity. These unique cell membrane glycoproteins are expressed on the surface of almost all human cells. Their primary function is to present antigen to T-lymphocytes for processing and recognition. T-cells are then able to determine if the antigen is "self" or foreign, based on the MHC molecule presented with it. T-cells only recognize antigen as foreign when presented with the appropriate MHC molecule found on the surface of human cells. Self-antigens are processed and presented without a MHC molecule and so are not recognized as foreign. No action is taken by the T-cells without the MHC molecule.

When an organism gains entry into a site and begins to reproduce, the inflammatory response is triggered, and neutrophils and antigen-presenting cells (APC) are attracted to the site. The APC consist of the monocytes, macrophages, and dendritic cells. They engulf the pathogen, and the organism becomes enclosed within a vesicle, where it is enzymatically broken down into short peptides. These peptides are then presented on the APC's surface along with its characteristic MHC II glycoprotein. The MHC II molecule is found on the surface of antigen-presenting cells. The antigens presented with MHC II molecules are usually those that originate outside human cells. T-lymphocytes respond to antigens associated with MCH II by releasing chemicals, undergoing clonal expansion, and stimulating B-cells to produce antibody.

MHC I molecules alert the T-lymphocytes to intracellular foreign antigens. If the pathogen is an intracellular pathogen, such as a virus or parasite, foreign peptides are presented on the infected cell's surface with the infected cell's characteristic MHC I glycoprotein. The MHC I molecule is found on the surface of nearly every somatic cell in the human body (Parham, 2005). Once determined to be a foreign peptide, the cell is destroyed. Figure 4-10 ■ depicts the antigen-presenting cells' role in defense.

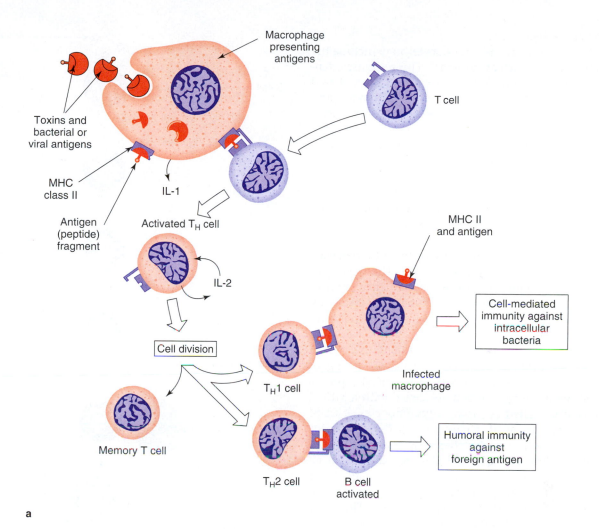

■ **FIGURE 4-10** The antigen presenting cell (APC) engulfs and processes a foreign antigen. After processing, fragments of the foreign antigen combined with MHC class I or II molecules is displayed on the APC cell surface. **a.** The MHC class II molecule presents an extracellular foreign antigen to a helper T-lymphocyte, activating it. The activated T-cell releases chemicals that trigger clonal expansion, activate macrophages and natural killer (NK) cells, and stimulate B-cells to produce antibody. **b.** The MHC class I molecule presents an intracellular foreign antigen to a cytotoxic T-lymphocyte resulting in its activation. The activated T-cell attacks and lyses the infected cell.

Lymphocyte Response

The defensive response of the lymphocytes may include the release of chemicals known as cytokines. This response establishes cell-mediated immunity. It is called cell-mediated immunity because it is activated by lymphocytes and macrophages and does not involve antibodies or complement. A second defensive response involves the production of a specific **immunoglobulin**, an antibody. Antibodies are soluble proteins designed to bind to and neutralize foreign antigen. The stimulation to produce an antibody is known as the humoral response. Antibodies are soluble in body fluids that are also known as humors, thus the term *humoral immunity*. Different types of lymphocytes participate in each kind of responsive action.

The lymphocytes are made up of two different types, each having a unique role in the immune response. The T-cells participate in cellular response, and the B-cells participate in antibody production. The role of T-cells in cell-mediated immunity and B-cells in the production of antibody are shown in Figures 4-10 and 4-11 ■.

The T-lymphocytes perform a variety of functions. Some of the T-cells circulate throughout the body, on patrol, looking for foreign substances associated with MHC I or MHC II peptides. If a host cell has a foreign antigen associated with a MHC I protein, a subclass called cytotoxic T-lymphocytes or CD8[+] cells will destroy the infected cell, recognizing that it contains an intravascular pathogen. Another subclass is the helper T-lymphocyte or CD4[+] cell. CD8 and CD4 are markers that act as receptors for the T-lymphocytes. There are two major types of helper T-cells. Type 1 helper (Th1) cells secrete interleukin-2 (IL-2) and interferon-γ (INF-γ). Type 2 helper (Th2) cells secrete IL-4, 5, 6, and 10. Refer to Table 4-3 to review activities of these cytokines.

If the helper T-cells stumble across an invader, they release chemicals that alert phagocytic cells to the danger. Helper T-cell (Th2) cytokines cause B-lymphocyte cells to transform into plasma cells, which produce the antibody that will disable the pathogen or facilitate phagocytosis. Th1 cells activate macrophages and natural killer (NK) cells facilitating cell-mediated immunity (Delves & Roitt, 2000b). The NK cell is discussed later in this chapter.

Chemicals released by the helper lymphocyte cell cause transformation of B-cells into plasma cells. Plasma cells produce the antibody. Some of the B-lymphocytes will retain their knowledge of this antigen and its corresponding antibody structure. The B-memory cells are capable of responding quicker in the production of antibody if the foreign antigen is ever encountered again.

The initial encounter with an antigen results in a primary antibody response. A subsequent exposure to the same antigen results in a secondary antibody response. Figure 4-12 ■ depicts these two responses. Notice that the secondary antibody response is quicker and results in a higher concentration of antibody. Additional T-lymphocytes use cytokines to downregulate the body's cellular response, so once the

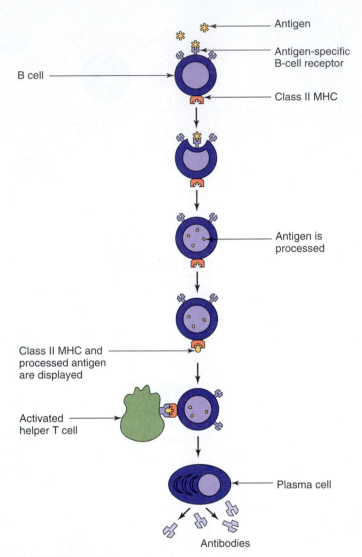

■ FIGURE 4-11 Humoral response reaction.
From 1998 Understanding Vaccines. NIH Publication no. 98-4219. National Institute Allergy and Infectious Disease.

offending organism is eliminated, it won't overreact and cause the host harm.

Another type of lymphocyte is the natural killer cell (NK). This lymphocyte defends us against intracellular pathogens such as viruses and kills certain lymphoid tumor cells (Mims et al., 1995). Cytokines activate this cell to attack MHC I associated antigens not recognized by the cytotoxic T-cells. These natural killer cells cause **apoptosis**, programmed cell death, by inserting porins or holes in the cell membrane and pouring proteolytic enzymes into the target cell. The NK cells may also bind to the target and trigger activation of apoptosis.

Natural killer T-cells (NKT) are different from the NK cell because it expresses characteristics of both the natural killer cell and the T helper lymphocyte. They appear to play a role in regulating the immune response by releasing interleukin-4

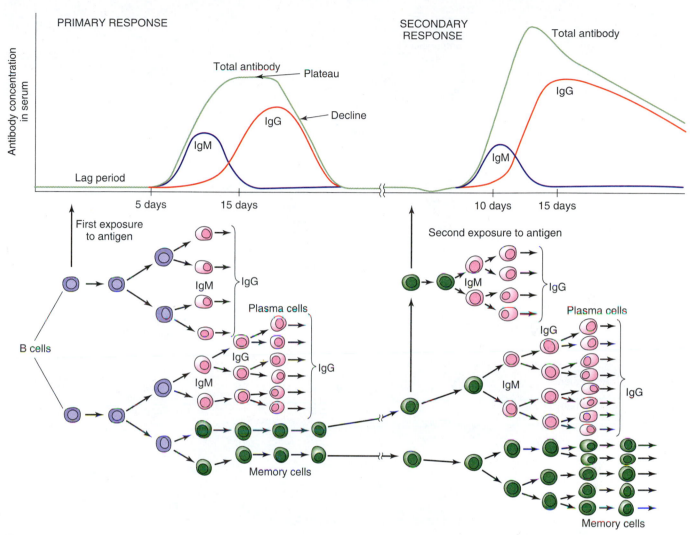

■ **FIGURE 4-12** Primary and secondary antibody response.

and interferon-gamma. See Table 4-3 for activities of cytokines. NKT cells also identify MHC-presented antigens (Delves & Roitt, 2000a, 2000b).

Antibody and Complement Actions

Antibody produced by plasma cells has a basic immunoglobulin structure in the shape of a Y. The two arms (Fab portions) of the Y bind antigen. Figure 4-13 ■ can help you visualize this structure. The single leg (Fc portion) of the Y binds to the membrane of the phagocytes, promoting opsonization and activating the complement pathway. Antibodies also coat parasites and neutralize toxins or microbes without binding to immune cells (Turgeon, 2003). Five different immunoglobulin (Ig) molecules are found in the plasma, tears, saliva, and on mucosal and B lymphocyte surfaces. The five types are IgG, IgM, IgA, IgE, and IgD. The various structures of antibodies are shown in Figure 4-14 ■.

IgG is the major circulating immunoglobulin. It is composed of a single molecule capable of binding two antigens. IgM is located on the surface of B cells, is secreted in the blood, and is a pentamer molecule capable of binding up to five times the antigens as IgG. IgM is the first type of immunoglobulin produced during an infection and indicates either a recent or recurrent infection. IgG is then produced and replaces the IgM molecules. A small amount of IgG and IgM are also found in extracellular fluids. IgA is a dimer capable of binding two times the amount of antigen as IgG when found in secretions such as the tears, saliva, breast milk, and mucus. In plasma, IgA exists as a single molecule. IgE and IgD are immunoglobulins with the same structure as IgG. IgE is present in low levels in the blood, but is concentrated in secretions especially around the respiratory and intestinal epithelial cells. It attaches to the mast cells and plays a role in allergic reactions. IgE also coats parasites, thus enhancing their

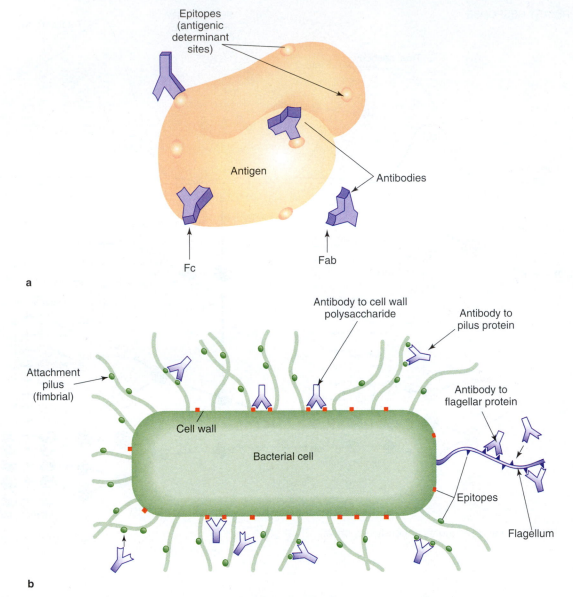

■ **FIGURE 4-13 a.** The Fab portion of the antibody binds to the epitope or antigen. **b.** Antibodies coat the microbial cell leaving the Fc portion of the molecule available to activate complement and bind to receptors on the neutrophil. This helps the phagocyte engulf the microbe.

recognition by eosinophils. IgD is found on the surface of B-lymphocytes. Both IgM and IgD serve as antigen receptors for the circulating B-lymphocytes.

Antibodies and complement have several roles in the defense of the body. Antibody may bind to antigen and trigger the complement system. The end result of the complement cascade is the formation of a membrane attack complex that damages the cell membrane causing lysis of the microbe or infected cell. Antibodies also promote and facilitate phagocytosis via opsonization. The Fab portion of the immunoglobulin molecule binds to antigens or epitopes on the microbe. Figure 4-13 illustrates this concept. Antibodies coat the microbial cell leaving the Fc portion of the

molecule available to activate complement and bind to receptors on the neutrophil. This aids the engulfment of the microbe by the phagocyte.

Activation of complement can also result in histamine release causing blood vessels to leak plasma. Complement activation can also stimulate chemotaxis, phagocytic cell buildup, foreign cell lysis, and inflammation. A depiction of the complement system is presented in Figure 4-15 ■.

Antibodies can incapacitate microbes by binding to flagella rendering them immobile. Antibodies can also fasten to pili and prevent attachment to host cells. Toxins are neutralized when antibodies attach to them. They also tie microbe to microbe forming a large mass, slowing the invasion down,

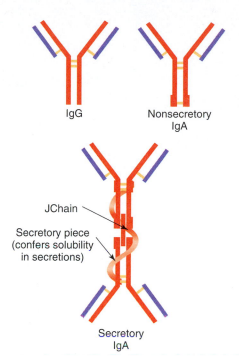

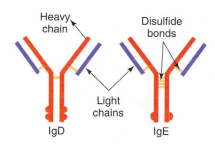

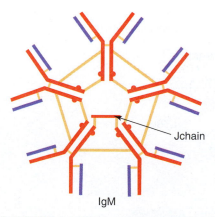

■ FIGURE 4-14 Various structures of antibodies.

and increasing opportunities for phagocytosis. Figure 4-16 ■ displays the antibodies' defensive actions.

The interaction of the individual components of the immune system is a beautifully designed protective system that helps humans survive the day-to-day encounters with the

> ✔ **Checkpoint! 4–5**
> **(Chapter Objective 5)**
>
> *The first kind of immunoglobulin produced during an infection is:*
>   A. IgG.
>   B. IgD.
>   C. IgM.
>   D. IgA.

ever-present microbe. Failure of any component can make the host susceptible to infection. Information on opportunistic infections is provided in ∞ Chapter 40. Nosocomial infections are described in ∞ Chapter 41.

SUMMARY

This chapter has presented information on the intricate defensive system that enables humans to defend themselves against pathogenic microbes and live in harmony with commensal and environmental microbes. An overview is presented in Figure 4-17 ■.

The port of entry to and exit from each body system provides opportunities both for successful invasion and defense. Microbes may enter any opening in the body and establish a thriving community. They may jump off from this initial infected site and spread deeper into the body. The innate defensive systems in each body site try to repel and prevent deeper invasion by microbes. When the innate systems fail, microorganisms may enter the bloodstream and spread throughout the body.

Microbes may possess attributes that allow them to resist the efforts of the host to control their access to the body and growth. These include the type of cell wall, the production of enzymes and toxins, the presence of certain structures like a capsule or flagella, and the ability to form a biofilm. Not all organisms possess these traits, but when they do, they are better able to cause disease.

The host defenses include both innate and adaptive immunity. Innate immunity is nonspecific with no memory of a previous encounter with a pathogen required for activation. Adaptive immunity is a specific response to a foreign microbe or their product. The host then retains memory of the encounter and the body's response. The components of the immune response include chemical, cellular, and antibody responses.

The location of the pathogen determines which component of the immune system is utilized in defensive actions. Antibodies, complement, and phagocytosis defend against extracellular pathogens located in blood, lymph, and tissue spaces. IgA antibodies and antimicrobial peptides are active against pathogens on epithelial surfaces. NK cells and cytotoxic T-cells destroy intracellular pathogens located in the cell cytoplasm. Neutrophils kill intracellular pathogens, which are enclosed in phagosomes. Each component interacts together like notes in a symphony to protect us from infectious disease.

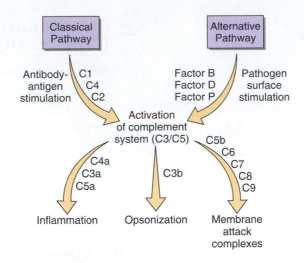

a

Bacterium — Surface antigens

Neutrophils — Blood vessel

Antibody (opsonin)

C1 — C4a

C4

C4b

Complement (C1) binds to IgG, initiating cascade

C2

C2b — C2a

C3 — C3a

CHEMOTAXIS

INFLAMMATION

Histamine

C3b — C5a

Mast cell

OPSONIZATION — C5

C5b

PHAGOCYTOSIS

C6,7

C5b67 — C8

Vascular permeability

Complement C3b

C3b receptor

Bacterium

C5b6789

MEMBRANE ATTACK COMPLEXES

LYSIS

Phagocyte

Antibody receptor

Complement lesions creating holes in cell membrane

b

■ **FIGURE 4-15** Classical and alternative complement pathways.

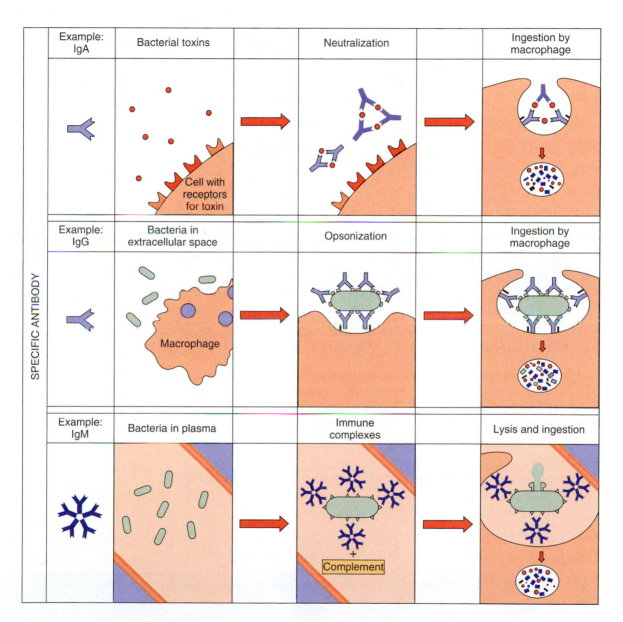

■ **FIGURE 4-16** Elimination of microbe or toxin by antibody.

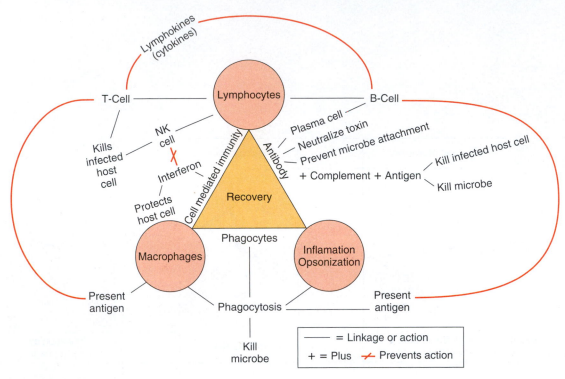

■ **FIGURE 4-17** Recovery triangle.

LEARNING OPPORTUNITIES

1. Think about a recent infectious disease (e.g., cold, strep throat, urinary tract infection) you have experienced. How does your disease mimic the events, common to all infectious diseases, presented in this chapter? What defensive actions taken by your body helped you to recover? (Chapter Objectives 1, 3, 4, 5)

2. How do microbes protect themselves against the innate host's defensive actions? (Chapter Objectives 2 and 3)

3. How do the microbes protect themselves against the adaptive host's defensive actions? (Chapter Objectives 2 and 5)

CASE STUDY 4-1. HEPATITIS B VIRUS OUTBREAK IN LONG-TERM CARE FACILITIES (CHAPTER OBJECTIVES 1, 3, AND 5)

Patients: Mabel was diagnosed with hepatitis B virus (HBV) infection in June 2003. Melvin and Mildred were diagnosed with HBV in December 2003.

Initial Report: Mabel and Melvin died from acute HBV infection. Mildred developed symptoms characteristic of acute HBV infection.

Serologic tests were run on the 158 remaining residents to determine their HBV infection status. Fifteen had acute HBV infection, 1 was chronically infected, 15 were immune, and 127 were susceptible.

Fourteen of the residents with acute HBV infection and the single chronically HBV-infected resident routinely received a fingerstick for glucose monitoring by staff at the same nursing station.

Clinical Laboratory Results:

Serologic tests:	Patients with:			
	Acute HBV	Chronic HBV	Immune	Susceptible
TB IgM antibody to HBV	Positive	Negative	Negative	Negative
Total antibody to HBV	Negative	Positive	Positive	Negative
HBV antigen	Positive	Positive	Negative	Negative

Staff members were also evaluated, and none were identified as the source of infection (Centers for Disease Control [CDC], 2005).

1. What is the portal of entry and exit for the hepatitis B virus that infected these residents?

2. Which innate defense mechanisms are relevant to this outbreak?

3. Which adaptive defense mechanisms relate to this outbreak?

4. How is an acute HBV infection distinguished from a chronic HBV infection? How does this correlate to antibody production?

CASE STUDY 4-2. SCHOOL-ASSOCIATED PERTUSSIS OUTBREAK (CHAPTER OBJECTIVES 1 AND 5)

Patients: Jessie is a 13-year-old eighth grader who attended school while ill. She was diagnosed with a pertussis infection on September 21, 2002. Her nasopharyngeal culture confirmed *Bordetella pertussis*.

Eddie is a student in the same classroom as Jessie. Her parents reported a culture confirmed case of pertussis on September 22, 2002.

Jaime, also from the same classroom, was reported as having the clinical presentation characteristic of pertussis 2 weeks earlier.

Initial Report: Investigation identified five additional people with prolonged cough illness. These included two students in the same classroom, two eighth-grade teachers, and one parent of an ill student.

Actions Taken: On September 26, the department of health notified the community of the pertussis outbreak and began control measures. A probable case

of pertussis was defined as an acute cough illness lasting 14 days or more. Control measures implemented included the exclusion of any coughing student or staff member from the school through the 5th day of antibiotic treatment. Parents of excluded students were advised to contact their health care provider for examination, to contact the department of health for culture, and to stay home and away from others (particularly infants and young children) through the 5th day of treatment. Health care providers were alerted of the outbreak.

On October 24, the department of health recommended acceleration of the vaccination schedule for infants because of the increasing number of pertussis cases. A total of 485 pertussis cases were reported to the department of health. The outbreak lasted 6 months.

Number of School Cases and Attack Rate

School Level	Number of Culture Positive Cases	Total Number of Confirmed Cases	Attack Rate
Elementary	1	27	3.9%
Middle	8	38	6.3%
High	2	48	3.0%

(CDC, 2004)

1. How did the control measures implemented by the department of health prevent further exposure to the organism that causes pertussis?

2. The usual recommended childhood vaccination for pertussis is immunizations at 2, 4, and 6 months of age. What would explain the higher attack rate in middle school students?

Use this address to access the interactive Companion Website created for this textbook. Simply select "Clinical Laboratory Science" from the choice of disciplines. Find this book and log in using your user name and password.

REFERENCES

Go to myhealthprofessionskit.com to view this chapter's references.

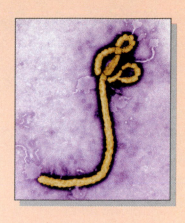

5

Safety

Hassan Aziz

■ LEARNING OBJECTIVES

Upon completion of this chapter, the learner should be able to:

1. Identify the federal agencies involved and their roles in providing a safe working environment.
2. Discuss the different types of laboratory hazards.
3. Explain the importance of safety equipment and personal protective equipment.
4. Describe the use of and apply engineering controls and work practice controls in the laboratory.
5. Classify the different biosafety levels.
6. Describe the role of the microbiologist in the detection of bioterrorism agents.
7. Discuss the laboratory's role in patient error reduction.
8. Differentiate between disinfection and sterilization, and give examples of agents/techniques used for each method.
9. Describe the purpose of standard precautions, and give examples of how they should be practiced.
10. Define nosocomial infections, and explain conditions that promote their transmission.
11. State the proper methods to manage waste in the medical laboratory.
12. Outline the components that make up a valid quality assurance program.

KEY TERMS

biohazard

biological safety cabinet (BSC)

biosafety level (BSL)

bioterrorism attack

Centers for Disease Control and Prevention (CDC)

chemical sterilization

disinfection

dry heat sterilization

engineering controls

exposure control plan

fomite

gas sterilization

hazard

high-efficiency particulate air (HEPA)

infection control committee

isolation room

material safety data sheet (MSDS)

normal flora

(continued)

KEY TERMS (continued)

nosocomial infections	risk	transmission-based
Occupational Safety	safety equipment	precautions
and Health	safety science	ultraviolet germicidal
Administration (OSHA)	standard precautions	irradiation (UVGI)
personal protective	steam sterilization	universal precautions
equipment (PPE)	(autoclave)	work practice controls
quality assurance	sterilization	

▶ INTRODUCTION

Health care professionals come in contact with body fluids that may be highly infectious. To protect both the patient and the worker, infection control measures must be enforced to minimize the spread of infection. Agencies such as the **Centers for Disease Control and Prevention (CDC)** and the **Occupational Safety and Health Administration (OSHA)** have established guidelines and regulations for health care facilities to implement to reduce the risk of spreading infectious diseases. Prior to the early 1980s and the introduction of AIDS into society, protocols were focused on protecting the patient with little or no emphasis on the health care worker's potential to become infected. The AIDS epidemic led to the development of the first protocols designed to protect health care workers, the *Guideline for Infection Control in Hospital Personnel,* published by the CDC in 1983.

SAFETY DEFINED

Safety science is the application of physical, health, and behavioral sciences to the health, safety, and well-being of people at work and in other activities. Safety is defined as an ever-changing condition in which one attempts to minimize the risk of injury, illness, or property damage from the hazards to which one may be exposed. To better understand the definition of safety, the terms *injury* and *illness* should be clarified. Injury is defined as damage to the body resulting from a single exposure to some type of energy or force; on the other hand, illness results from repeated exposures to some type of energy or force. The terms *hazard* and *risk* are interrelated. A **hazard** is defined as a condition that has the potential to produce injury and/or property damage while **risk** refers to the probability that a hazard will be activated and then produce injury or property damage (Bever, 1992).

THE OSHA ACT

The field of safety has undergone a vast transformation in the past 25 years. The early 1970's saw development of both federal and state environmental and safety legislation. The Williams-Steiger Occupational Safety and Health Act was signed into law in the late 1970s. The declared congressional

purpose of the act was to assure every working man and woman in the nation safe and healthful working conditions and to preserve human resources (Sichak, 1975). The federal law created four bodies: the Occupational Safety and Health Administration (OSHA) within the Department of Labor; the National Institute for Occupational Safety and Health (NIOSH) within the Department of Health, Education, and Welfare; the Occupational Safety and Health Review Commission within the Department of Justice; and an advisory committee for safety and health. OSHA was the enforcement arm of the OSHA Act, and NIOSH was formed to provide research and education in occupational safety and health. The Review Commission was the judicial arm that was to resolve challenges to OSHA citations and actions. The advisory committee was to provide direction for OSHA and NIOSH (Pierce, 1996).

 Checkpoint! 5–1 (Chapter Objective 1)

The agency that is considered the enforcement arm of the Occupational Safety and Health Act is:
   A. *Occupational Safety and Health Administration (OSHA).*
   B. *National Institute for Occupational Safety and Health (NIOSH).*
   C. *Occupational Safety and Health Review Commission.*
   D. *Advisory Committee for Safety and Health.*

▶ TYPES OF LABORATORY HAZARDS

The laboratory has the potential to be either a safe place or a dangerous place. The difference depends on one's knowledge of and adherence to safe laboratory practices. Many sources of potential hazards exist in the laboratory.

GLASSWARE HAZARDS

One of the most common materials used in the medical laboratory is glass. Glass is an excellent material of construction because it is relatively inexpensive, highly resistant to chemical attack, easily cleaned, and noncontaminating. Despite its advantages, glass breaks very easily. Broken glass produces extremely sharp edges that readily cut human tissue. Most glassware laboratory accidents are caused by improper use.

Glassware should be visually inspected before use to detect breaks, cracks, or chips. When glassware is broken, it should be disposed of in a sharp proof type of container so that it will not puncture the container and injure others (American Chemical Society [ACS], 1995).

 REAL WORLD TIP

Many laboratories have replaced glass phlebotomy tubes with ones made of plastic.

CHEMICAL HAZARDS

The microbiology laboratory uses hazardous chemicals on a routine basis. A hazardous chemical is one where there is significant evidence that acute exposure or chronic exposure effects may occur in exposed personnel (Nielsen, 2000). Chemical hazards may be divided into six categories: flammability, instability, reactivity, corrosivity, toxicity, and radioactivity. Any of the chemical substances in these six categories can be harmful to the human body. Learning the hazards associated with every chemical used in the laboratory and ensuring that users understand the hazards and will take the necessary precautions may seem to be a formidable task (Young, 1997a, 1997b). There are many factors influencing the toxicity of chemicals, some known and some not yet fully understood. Hence, all chemicals should be handled with respect for their potential hazards, and precautions must be taken to prevent many undesirable toxic consequences.

Chemicals must be labeled with the color and number system used by the National Fire Protection Association (NFPA). The four color sections of the diamond shaped label identify various hazards of the chemical; the blue square identifies its potential as a health hazard; the red square displays the level of fire hazard; the yellow square notes its instability or reactivity; and the white square is used to note other hazards such as radioactivity, ability to oxidize, and water reactivity. Each square contains a number from 0 to 4 to identify its level of hazard. Zero or the absence of a number denotes minimal to no hazard, 1 is slight, 2 is moderate, 3 is serious, and 4 is extreme. Figure 5-1 ■ demonstrates the NFPA label for acetone used in the gram stain procedure.

ELECTRICAL HAZARDS

The use of electrically powered equipment in laboratories has increased rapidly over the last two decades. Electrical equipment is used for operations requiring heating, cooling, mixing, and pumping, as well as for a variety of instruments used in making physical measurements. The popularity of electrical equipment is due to its convenience and relative safety. However, the use of electrically powered equipment poses a new set of possible hazards for the unaware. Electrical hazards in the laboratory include the possibility of shock, electrocution, fire, and ignition of flammable vapors and gases (Fuscaldo, Erlick, & Hindman, 1980). Shock injuries are caused by the flow of

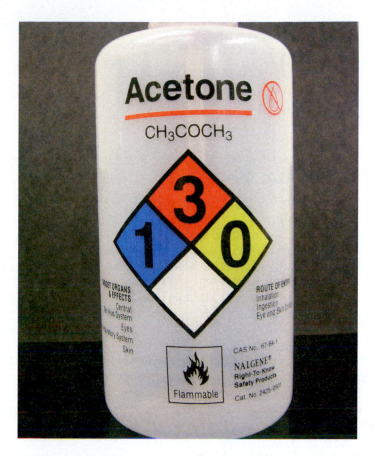

■ **FIGURE 5-1** Acetone bottle with a NFPA label. Any chemical used in the laboratory must be identified with a NFPA label to warn of its health, fire, reactivity and other risks. This acetone bottle identifies the chemical as a serious fire hazard with a slight risk as a health hazard.

electric current (amperage), not the voltage. OSHA regulations require that all electrical outlets must have a grounding connection requiring a three-pronged plug. Laboratory workers should know the location of circuit breakers and how to cut off all electrical service in case of fire or accident. All circuit breakers should be labeled properly. A good basic rule of workbench design is to use insulation. The bench itself should be made of insulating material with no accessible supporting metalwork (Pal, 1985).

 REAL WORLD TIP

Most laboratories have designated electrical outlets which are used for essential equipment. These designated outlets are often colored red. If electrical power is lost, emergency generators keep electricity flowing to these outlets ensuring continuous power and service. Once power is lost to a clinical instrument, bringing it back up can be a timely and costly process.

Checkpoint! 5–2 (Chapter Objective 2)

Electrical shock injuries are caused by:
A. *voltage.*
B. *amperage.*
C. *resistance.*
D. *capacity.*

BIOLOGICAL HAZARDS

Experimental work that involves microorganisms presents the possible hazard of infection to the individuals performing the work. Accidental infection by a pathogenic microorganism is a very real hazard in the laboratory. A **biohazard** is any bacteria, virus, fungus, protozoa, cell culture, parasite, or substance that may cause infection, allergy, or toxicity or otherwise create a hazard to human health (Fuscaldo et al., 1980). No work can be carried out using biohazardous material until a suitable and sufficient risk assessment has been carried out. Such an assessment should only be carried out by suitably qualified and experienced staff. Box 5-1 ✪ provides an example of a risk assessment for specimen processing in a microbiology department. Engineering controls are equipment or activities designed to reduce the risk of exposure to pathogens.

FIRE HAZARDS

Fire is a potential hazard in the laboratory operations. Laboratory fire hazards range from simple and relatively slow combustion of paper to the fast-burning and rapidly spreading combustion of organic solvents and occasionally to the explosive combustion of flammable gases or solids. The best way to fight a fire is to prevent it. Fires can be prevented and their severity considerably reduced by proper housekeeping and thoughtful reflection about what one is doing. This includes prompt removal of waste, separation of flammable liquids and combustible material, storage of only limited quantities of flammable material, and unobstructed aisles and exits (ACS, 1995).

RADIATION HAZARDS

Physical hazards in laboratories are generally confined to radiation in its various forms. Radiation from the portions of the spectrum that are of importance to the laboratory are visible light, ultraviolet, and infrared radiations, microwaves, and ionizing radiations (Mahn, 1991). Exposure to some radiations may be harmful to humans, depending on the intensity and duration of the exposure. Ultraviolet light, a type of nonionizing radiation, can be a hazard in laboratories because the radiation can produce tissue damage to the eyes and skin. Ionizing radiation can be hazardous to many different organs of the body. State and federal licensing regulations require that all users of radioactive materials establish adequate safety programs covering the acquisition, storage, use, and disposal of radioactive materials. The three principles of self-protection from radiation exposure are time, shielding, and distance. Radiation exposure is cumulative; thus, limiting the length of exposure at any one time is a major factor in minimizing the hazard. Some type of radiation monitoring instrument is also essential, and a trained radiation safety officer is required to maintain safe conditions at the entire facility.

 REAL WORLD TIP

Ultraviolet (UV) light is used routinely in the microbiology laboratory to disinfect the biological safety cabinets. Microbiologists can also be exposed to UV light while reading some biochemical reactions such as the ALA or porphyrin test and rapid esculin hydrolysis. The key to its safe use is to limit the microbiologist's time of exposure. Long sleeves, gloves, and approved eye protection are necessary as protective equipment.

▶ BIOSAFETY PRACTICES

Good biosafety practices require mandatory safety rules and programs. Laboratory workers must be aware of surrounding risks and should be trained in safe laboratory procedures, good biological techniques, and appropriate laboratory surveillance. The likelihood of severe injury or infections is reduced if plans for such emergencies are established and well known to all workers.

SAFETY EQUIPMENT

Medical laboratories should have a variety of equipment to be used in case an accident occurs. Each person in the laboratory must be familiar with the location of, and procedures for using, this equipment. The **safety equipment** will usually include a chemical spill kit, eyewash fountain, safety shower, fire extinguisher, fire blanket, and fire alarm system (Pal, 1985). All this equipment should be conveniently located, properly maintained, and frequently tested. The laboratory should have a plan for everyone to follow if an evacuation is ever necessary. Each individual must know the main and alternate evacuation routes as well as the procedures for accounting for each person in the laboratory (ACS, 1995). Annual competency testing must be in place to ensure every individual in the laboratory is properly trained for an emergency situation.

Laboratory areas that have special hazards should be posted with warning signs. Standard signs and symbols (Figure 5-2 ■)

✪ BOX 5-1

Task Assessment for General Specimen Processing in Microbiology

- PPE required
  - Gloves
  - Fastened Lab Coat
- Engineering Controls required
  - Biological Safety Cabinet
  - Sharps container
  - Disposable inoculating loops
  - Incinerator if disposable inoculating loops are not available

Flammable Gas

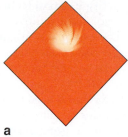

a

Danger Laser Radiation

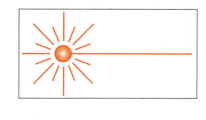

b

Radioactive Materials

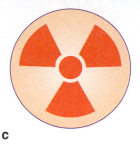

c

■ **FIGURE 5-2** Warning signs. Standard signs and symbols.

have been established for a number of special situations such as biological hazards, fire hazards (a), laser operations (b), and radioactivity hazards (c). No chemicals should be stored above eye level because of the danger of breakage or spillage involved in reaching (Federal Register, 1990).

The **biological safety cabinet (BSC)** is the principal device used to provide containment of infectious splashes or aerosols generated by many microbiological procedures. Three types of biological safety cabinets (Class I, II, III) (Figure 5-3 ■) are used in microbiological laboratories. Open-fronted Class I and Class II biological safety cabinets are primary barriers that offer significant levels of protection to laboratory personnel and to the environment when used with good microbiological techniques. The Class II biological safety cabinet, the most commonly used BSC, also provides protection from external contamination of the materials (e.g., cell cultures, microbiological stocks) being manipulated inside the cabinet. The gastight Class III biological safety cabinet provides the highest attainable level of protection to personnel and the environment (U.S. Department of Health & Human Services [USDHHS], 1995). Class III BSCs are used in laboratories, such

 REAL WORLD TIP

Do not cover the open grid at the front of the working surface of a class II BSC. Covering the grid disrupts the airflow within the cabinet and can allow aerosols to enter room.

as CDC laboratories, which work with extremely hazardous organisms such as the ebola virus.

A Class II BSC maintains negative pressure so air is constantly being pulled into the cabinet. Any aerosols created within the cabinet remain inside. Air, removed from the BSC, flows through a filter prior to exiting the facility. A BSC must be maintained and certified annually to insure proper function.

PERSONAL PROTECTIVE EQUIPMENT

Personal protective equipment (PPE) consists of gloves, masks, liquid impervious gowns, and goggles or face shield (Figure 5-4 ■). Gloves reduce the risk of cross contamination from health care personnel to patients, and patient or **fomite**, an inanimate object capable of transmitting infectious organisms from an individual to another, such as health care personnel. Emphasis on the necessity of hand washing after glove removal remains a sound practice and federal mandate. Also, it must be understood that gloves do not prevent sharp instruments from penetrating the skin. Masks and protective eyewear reduce the contamination risk to mucous membranes of the eyes, nose, and mouth. A face mask, with a HEPA filter, or respirator is necessary when working with *Mycobacterium* spp. Gowns protect clothing from contamination. Open-toe shoes or shorts should never be worn in the laboratory, and loose-fitting clothes should be avoided. The supply and repair of PPE is the responsibility of the employer.

 REAL WORLD TIP

Using gloves while reading culture plates is still optional for most laboratories. Suspected highly infectious organisms such as the dimorphic fungi, *Francisella tularensis*, *Bacillus anthracis*, and *Neisseria meningitidis* should be handled only with gloves in a BSC.

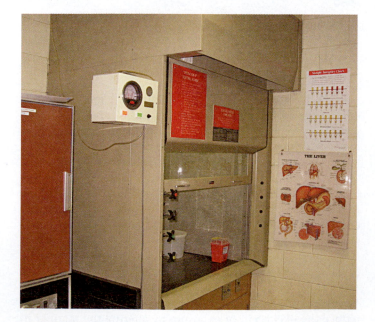

■ **FIGURE 5-3** Biological safety cabinet.

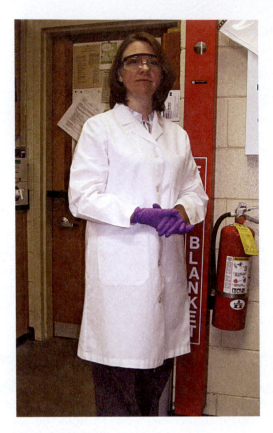

■ **FIGURE 5-4** Personal protective equipment.

 REAL WORLD TIP

Not all laboratory coats provided by employers are liquid impervious and so are not true PPE. Liquid impervious lab coats are true PPE and should be used when a spill is highly likely or the organism is highly infectious such as when processing specimens for *Mycobacterium* spp. Some laboratories have decided to use disposal liquid impervious coats for only specifically defined tasks.

 REAL WORLD TIP

Gloves used in clinical laboratories are often made of vinyl or nitrile. Latex gloves are rarely used due to the potential for latex allergies.

✓ **Checkpoint! 5–3 (Chapter Objective 3)**

Gloves are excellent personal protective equipment because they reduce the risk of contamination and prevent sharp instruments from penetrating the skin.
  A. *True*
  B. *False*

ENGINEERING CONTROLS

The objective of **engineering control** technology addresses devices that are used to isolate or remove the blood-borne pathogen hazards from the workplace. Engineering controls are based primarily on the use of adequate ventilation systems. These systems may be supplemented with **high-efficiency particulate air (HEPA)** filtration, a filter with an efficiency of at least 99.95%, that is used to separate particles from air exhaust streams prior to releasing that air into the atmosphere, and **ultraviolet germicidal irradiation (UVGI)**, which can penetrate the microbe's cell wall and inactivate tiny, airborne droplet nuclei that help transmit diseases such as measles, tuberculosis, and influenza from person to person in high-risk areas. These strategies are designed to reduce the concentration of infectious droplet nuclei in the air, prevent the dissemination of droplet nuclei throughout the facility, or render droplet nuclei noninfectious by killing the organisms they contain.

In **isolation rooms**, ventilation systems are necessary to maintain negative pressure and to exhaust the air properly. Air only moves into the room from the corridor due to the pressure created as air is exhausted out through the ventilation system. A negative pressure room is used to house individuals with tuberculosis. The negative pressure keeps the organisms inside the room. The air of a positive pressure room flows out preventing the entry of aerosolized organisms. A positive pressure room is used for individuals with immunodeficiences such as HIV.

Isolation rooms should be monitored daily when in use to ensure the pressure is maintained. Doors should be kept closed, except when patients or personnel must enter or exit the room, to maintain the appropriate pressure.

 REAL WORLD TIP

Negative pressure rooms are used in the clinical laboratory for working with easily aerosolized pathogens such as *Mycobacterium tuberculosis* and fungus.

HEPA filters can be used in ventilation systems to remove droplet nuclei from the air. These filters can be installed in ventilation ducts to filter air for recirculation into the same room or recirculation to other areas of a facility. UVGI may kill the organism contained in droplet nuclei. Because exposure to ultraviolet light can be harmful to the skin and eyes, the lamps must be installed in the upper part of rooms or corridors or placed in exhaust vents. Other controls include sharps disposal containers, needle resheathing devices, needleless vascular access systems, and biohazardous waste containers.

WORK PRACTICE CONTROLS

Work practice controls are activities that are meant to reduce the likelihood of exposure by altering the manner in which a task is performed (Centers for Disease Control and Prevention [CDC], 1999a). These controls are dependent on employee behavior. It is necessary to use good work practices in tandem with effective engineering controls and personal protective equipment to achieve the goals of this program. Work practice controls include procedures for safe and proper work that are understood and followed by managers, supervisors, and employees. Examples of some work practice controls include (1) adherence to the practice of standard precautions in all situations of occupational exposure, (2) prohibiting the recapping of needles, and (3) prohibition of pipetting or suctioning by mouth.

Employers must provide hepatitis B vaccine at no cost to any of their employees who are likely to be exposed to blood-borne pathogens. Even with work practice controls in place, accidents do occur and laboratory personnel can be exposed to hepatitis B, hepatitis C, and HIV. Policies and procedures detailing required postexposure follow-up practices include medical evaluation, laboratory testing, and provisions for confidentiality. Employees are responsible for reporting any exposure incident immediately to their supervisor. Employers are required to provide a training program at no cost and during working hours for all employees with potential for occupational exposure to blood and body fluid exposure on initial assignment and at least annually thereafter. Employers must maintain medical and training records for each employee with

actual or potential occupational exposure for a designated period of time (CDC, 1999).

 Checkpoint! 5–4 (Chapter Objective 4)

The objective of engineering control technology is to:
- A. *reduce the likelihood of exposure by altering the manner in which a task is performed.*
- B. *isolate or remove the blood-borne pathogen hazards from the workplace.*
- C. *provide employees with important guidelines for conducting work in a safe and consistent manner.*
- D. *destroy many infectious agents but not necessarily their spores.*

BIOSAFETY LEVELS

There are four **biosafety levels (BSLs)**, which consist of combinations of laboratory practices and techniques, safety equipment, and laboratory facilities. Each combination is specifically appropriate for the operations performed, the documented or suspected routes of transmission of the infectious agents, and the laboratory function or activity. Table 5-1

⊗ TABLE 5-1

The Biosafety Levels and the Agents, Practices, Safety Equipment, and Facilities Associated with Each Level

BSL	Agents	Practices	Safety Equipment	Facilities
1	Not known to consistently cause disease in healthy human adults.	Standard microbiological practices	As required for normal care of each species.	Directional air flow recommended Hand washing sink recommended
2	Associated with human disease. Hazard: percutaneous exposure, ingestion, mucous membrane exposure.	BSL-1 practices plus: Limited access Biohazard warning signs Sharps precautions Biosafety manual Decontamination of all infectious wastes	BSL-1 equipment plus: BCS I or II PPE: laboratory coats, gloves, face and respiratory protection as needed.	BSL-1 facility plus: Autoclave available
3	Indigenous or exotic agents with potential for aerosol transmission; disease may have serious health effects.	BSL-2 practices plus: Controlled access Decontamination of clothing before laundering Decontamination of all waste	BSL-2 equipment plus: Class I or II BSCs available for manipulative procedures (inoculation, necropsy) that may create infectious aerosols. PPEs: appropriate respiratory protection	BSL-2 facility plus: Physical separation from access corridors Self-closing, double-door access Negative airflow to laboratory Sealed windows
4	Dangerous/exotic agents that pose high risk of life-threatening disease; aerosol transmission, or related agents with unknown risk of transmission.	BSL-3 practices plus: Entrance through change room where personal clothing is removed and laboratory clothing is put on; shower on exiting All wastes are decontaminated before removal from the facility	BSL-3 equipment plus: Maximum containment equipment (i.e., Class III BSC or partial containment equipment in combination with full-body, air-supplied positive-pressure personnel suit) used for all procedures and activities	BSL-3 facility plus: Separate building or isolated zone Dedicated supply and exhaust, vacuum and decontamination systems

illustrates the four biosafety levels and the agents, practices, safety equipment, and facilities associated with each level.

Biosafety Level 1 represents a basic level of containment that relies on standard microbiological practices with no special primary or secondary barriers recommended, other than a sink for hand washing. Standard microbiological practices include control of access to the laboratory; washing hands, using a paper towel or knee/foot pedal to turn off the faucet, after working with hazardous material, when obviously soiled, and before leaving the laboratory; no eating, drinking, smoking, applying cosmetics, or handling contact lenses in the laboratory; no mouth pipetting; sharps handled in a safe manner; procedures performed in a manner that decreases aerosol and droplet production; work surfaces must be decontaminated after a spill or after completion of work; cultures and other infectious material decontaminated prior to disposal; a biohazard sign must be posted at the entrance to the laboratory; a program to manage pests is required; and appropriate training given regarding duties, safety precautions, exposure follow-up, and information regarding conditions that may place the individual at higher risk of infection must be provided (USDHHS & NIH, 2007).

This level is appropriate for educational training and teaching laboratories and for other laboratories in which work is done with defined and characterized strains of viable microorganisms not known to consistently cause disease in healthy adult humans. Many agents not ordinarily associated with disease processes in humans are, however, opportunistic pathogens and may cause infection in the young, the aged, and immunodeficient or immunosuppressed individuals (CDC, 1999).

Most microbiology laboratories are categorized as Biosafety Level 2, in which work is done with the broad spectrum of moderate-risk agents that are present in the community and associated with human disease of varying severity. Hepatitis B virus, HIV, the salmonellae, and *Toxoplasma* spp. are representative of microorganisms assigned to this containment level (CDC, 1999). Primary hazards to personnel working with these agents relate to accidental percutaneous or mucous membrane exposures or ingestion of infectious materials. Primary barriers should be used as appropriate, such as splash shields, face protection, gowns, and gloves. Secondary barriers such as hand washing sinks and waste decontamination facilities must be available to reduce potential environmental contamination.

Biosafety Level 3 laboratories are usually clinical, diagnostic, teaching, research, or production facilities in which work is done with indigenous or exotic agents with a potential for respiratory transmission and that may cause serious and potentially lethal infection. *Mycobacterium tuberculosis,* St. Louis encephalitis virus, and *Coxiella burnetii* are representative of the microorganisms assigned to this level (CDC, 1999). More emphasis is placed on primary and secondary barriers to protect personnel. Secondary barriers for this level include controlled access to the laboratory and ventilation

requirements that minimize the release of infectious aerosols from the laboratory.

Laboratories working with dangerous and exotic agents that pose a high individual risk of life-threatening disease, which may be transmitted via the aerosol route and for which there is no available vaccine or therapy, are considered Biosafety Level 4. Viruses such as Marburg or Congo-Crimean hemorrhagic fever are manipulated at Biosafety Level 4 (CDC, 1999). The Biosafety Level 4 facility itself is generally a separate building or completely isolated zone with complex, specialized ventilation requirements and waste management systems to prevent release of viable agents to the environment (CDC, 1999).

 REAL WORLD TIP

Most clinical laboratories are considered to be classified as Biosafety Level 2. Primary barriers such as biological safety cabinets (Class I or II) should be used when performing procedures that might cause splashing, spraying, or splattering of droplets. Biological safety cabinets also should be used for the initial processing of clinical specimens when the nature of the test requested or other information suggests the likely presence of an agent readily transmissible by infectious aerosols (e.g., *M. tuberculosis*). Examination of growth on primary media should be performed in a biological safety cabinet if growth is on chocolate agar only (until high-risk organisms, such as *Fransicella tularensis*, are ruled out) or if a Gram stain of a positive blood culture reveals gram-negative cocci, gram-negative diplococci, gram-negative coccobacillary, or no organisms seen (NOS).

 **Checkpoint! 5–5
(Chapter Objective 5)**

Laboratories in which work is done with indigenous or exotic agents with a potential for respiratory transmission and that may cause serious and potentially lethal infection belong to which safety level?
  A. BSL 1
  B. BSL 2
  C. BSL 3
  D. BSL 4

A **bioterrorism attack** is the intentional release of viruses, bacteria, fungi, or toxins to cause adverse effects on human and/or animal health and food and water supplies (CDC, 2007). These biological agents are typically found in nature, easy to produce, and relatively inexpensive, but it is possible that they could be manipulated to increase their potency to cause harm, make them resistant to current antimicrobial agents, or increase their ability to be spread into the environment (Weinstein & Alibek, 2003). Biological agents can be spread through the air, through water, in food, or through direct contact. Table 5-2✿ is an alphabetical list of bioterrorism agents and conditions associated with them.

The Center for Disease Control and Prevention (CDC) classified biological agents into three categories (A, B, and C; CDC, 2007), depending on how easily they can be spread and the severity of illness or death they cause.

✿ TABLE 5-2

Alphabetical List of Bioterrorism Agents (CDC, 2007) and Conditions (CDC, 2007)

Agent	Condition
Bacillus anthracis	Anthrax
Clostridium botulinum toxin	Botulism
Brucella species	Brucellosis
Burkholderia mallei	Glanders
Burkholderia pseudomallei	Melioidosis
Chlamydia psittaci	Psittacosis
Vibrio cholerae	Cholera Water safety threat
Clostridium perfringens	Epsilon toxin
Coxiella burnetii	Q fever
Ebola virus	Hemorrhagic fever
Escherichia coli O157:H7	Food safety threat
Nipah virus and Hantavirus	Emerging infectious diseases
Salmonella species	Food safety threat
Escherichia coli O157:H7	Food safety threat
Shigella	Food safety threat
Francisella tularensis	Tularemia
Ricin toxin from castor beans	Poisoning
Rickettsia prowazekii	Typhus fever
Salmonella species	Salmonellosis
Salmonella typhi	Typhoid fever
Shigella	Shigellosis
Variola major	Smallpox
Staphylococcal enterotoxin B	Food poisoning
Viral encephalitis alphaviruses	Venezuelan equine encephalitis, Eastern equine encephalitis, Western equine encephalitis
Cryptosporidium parvum	Water safety threat
Yersinia pestis	Plague

CATEGORY A

Example—*Yersinia pestis*
High-priority organisms or toxins that pose the highest risk to the public and national security.

- Spread or transmitted from person to person
- Result in high mortality and have the potential for major public health impact
- Can cause public panic and disrupt the social order
- Require special action to insure public health preparedness.

CATEGORY B

Example—*E. coli* O157:H7

- Are moderately easy to spread
- Result in moderate illness rates and low death rates
- Require specific enhancements of CDC's laboratory capacity and improved disease surveillance.

CATEGORY C

Example—Multidrug resistant *Mycobacterium tuberculosis*
Agents in this category are considered emerging threats for disease.

- Easily produced and spread
- Potential for high morbidity and mortality rates and major health impact.

Microbiologists may provide the first line of detection when bioterrorism agents are used. There must be a plan in place in the event of the isolation of a potential bioterrorism organism. Very few laboratories are equipped to work with most of these organisms. Microbiologists must work closely with local and state public health laboratories to ensure prompt and accurate recognition of bioterrorism agents.

 REAL WORLD TIP

In October 2001, *Bacillus anthracis* spores were intentionally delivered in letters mailed through the U.S. postal system. In all, 22 people developed anthrax, 11 developed inhalation anthrax, and 5 of those individuals died.

✓ Checkpoint! 5–6 (Chapter Objective 6)

A microbiologist isolates what he suspects to be Bacillus anthracis from a blood culture. His next step is to:
  A. *continue to work up the organism.*
  B. *review the department's policies and procedures before proceeding.*
  C. *confer with coworkers on what to do next.*
  D. *refer the organism to a reference laboratory for identification.*

SOURCES OF SAFETY INFORMATION

Laboratory workers should be advised about the potential hazards of their laboratory's ongoing work. Literature and consulting advice on laboratory safety should be readily available and accessible to those responsible for laboratory operations. **Material Safety Data Sheets (MSDS)** should be available for all chemicals in the laboratory. They are available from chemical manufacturers, suppliers, and the federal government, and they list general information, precautionary measures, and emergency information (Gerlovich, 1992). MSDSs should be kept in an organized file, and the location of that file should be posted so they can be found easily (Mahn, 1991). Most MSDS sheets are now easily accessed through the Internet.

EXPOSURE CONTROL PLAN

An **exposure control plan** requires a facility to develop a written document detailing specific needs, including exposure determination, a schedule and method of implementation for compliance, and procedures for the evaluation of exposure incidents. The plan must be accessible to all employees and reviewed and updated annually.

ACCIDENT REPORTING AND RECORD KEEPING

The prompt and proper reporting of hazards and accidents is essential for safe laboratory operations. Every laboratory should have an internal accident reporting system to help discover and correct unexpected hazards. A formal, written report stating the causes and consequences of each accident should be made. A periodic review of accident reports will often reveal problem areas or trends that need special attention.

PATIENT SAFETY ISSUES (ERROR REDUCTIONS)

Overview

Efforts to reduce medical errors, improve health care quality, and increase patient safety have been gaining national attention. A report issued in 1999 by the Institute of Medicine (IOM) presented a national agenda to address these issues and recommended strategies for change that included the implementation of safe practices at the health care delivery level. As described in the IOM report, errors most often occur when multiple contributing factors converge, and preventing errors and improving patient safety require a systems approach. This powerful report has led to changes which have shifted the focus to improving systems, engaging stakeholders, and motivating health care providers to adopt new safe practices (Institute of Medicine [IOM], 2007)

Lab's Role

Errors can occur anywhere in the testing process, pre-analytical, analytical, and post-analytical. Most errors occur in the pre-analytical phase before the specimen even reaches the laboratory's door. Errors also occur when the manufacturer's instructions are not followed and when testing personnel are not familiar with all aspects of the test system and how testing is integrated into the facility's workflow.

The laboratory must establish the number, type, and frequency of testing control materials that monitor the complete testing process. It must detect immediate errors caused by test system failures, adverse environmental conditions, and operator performance. Also, it must monitor over time the accuracy and precision of test performance that may be influenced by changes in test system performance, environmental conditions, and operator performance. Accuracy and precision are terms that should be familiar in a quality control (QC) program. Accuracy of a test is its closeness to the true value (Norusis, 1990). Precision of a result is its reproducibility (Norusis, 1990). Maintaining precision is a must for all laboratories, and it is the main purpose of the QC program.

▶ INFECTION CONTROL

Control of microorganisms is vital in the health care facility. Many microorganisms are normally found in or on the human body and are called endogenous organisms, or **normal flora**. Some endogenous organisms are colonizers, but they do not become potential pathogens unless the resistance is lowered.

DISINFECTION

Disinfection consists of various chemicals that can be used to destroy many infectious agents but not necessarily their spores. A disinfectant is selected according to the specific infectious agent known or suspected to be present, as each chemical compound has a selective germicidal activity. The most resistant to germicidal chemicals are bacterial spores, followed by acid-fast bacteria, nonlipid or small viruses, fungi, vegetative bacteria, and lipid or medium-size viruses (USDHHS & NIH, 2007b). Disinfectants are used on inanimate objects. They can be used to disinfect items made from materials that could be damaged by other cleaning techniques.

The more active a compound is, the more likely it is to have undesirable characteristics such as corrosivity. No liquid disinfectant is equally useful or effective under all conditions and for all viable agents. The most practical use of liquid disinfectants is for surface decontamination. At sufficient concentrations, they can be used as decontaminants for liquid wastes prior to disposal in the sanitary sewer (CDC, 1983). Table 5-3✪ depicts a list of liquid disinfectants used in the laboratory.

☉ TABLE 5-3

Disinfectants in the Medical Laboratory and Their Use

Disinfectant	Use
Mercurials	■ Toxic, therefore not recommended.
Quaternary ammonium compounds	■ Acceptable to control bacteria and non-lipid-containing viruses. ■ Not active against bacterial spores at the usual concentrations.
Phenolic compounds	■ Recommended for killing bacteria, including *Mycobacterium tuberculosis,* fungi, and lipid-containing viruses. ■ Less effective against spores and non-lipid-containing viruses.
Chlorine compounds	■ Active against bacteria and most viruses. ■ May be used for bacterial spores. ■ Corrosive to metal surfaces. ■ Must be made up fresh.
Iodophors	■ Recommended for general use for killing vegetative bacteria and viruses. ■ Not recommended against bacterial spores.
Alcohols	■ General use disinfectant. ■ No activity against bacterial spores.
Formaldehyde solutions	■ Used against bacteria, spores, and viruses. ■ Irritating odor. ■ Carcinogenic.
Activated glutaraldehyde	■ Limited use due to toxic properties and potential damage to eyes.
Formaldehyde-alcohol	■ Effective against bacteria, spores, and viruses.

STERILIZATION

Sterilization means all microbial life is destroyed. The purpose of sterilization is to prevent organisms from entering the body during an invasive procedure. Living tissue surfaces such as skin cannot be sterilized but can be rendered as free of organisms as possible.

Treatment necessary to achieve sterility will vary in relation to the volume of material treated, its contamination level, its moisture content, and other factors (CDC, 1983). These are general criteria and should be used for infectious agents. Proper containment and treatment at the source reduce the potential for an accidental exposure.

The four methods of sterilization are:

1. Gas sterilization
2. Dry heat
3. Chemical sterilization
4. Steam sterilization

Gas Sterilization

Gas sterilization is accomplished in a large gas oven and takes hours. It is mainly used for wheelchairs and beds. Ethylene oxide gas and paraformaldehyde are examples of gases used.

Dry Heat

Dry heat sterilization requires higher temperatures than steam sterilization and requires longer exposure times as well. It is used for items that are easily corroded such as sharp cutting instruments.

Chemical Sterilization

Chemical sterilization is a very effective method used in many laboratories when the object being sterilized is too large or too heat sensitive for autoclaving. Chemical sterilization uses the same chemical agents as chemical disinfection. However, exposure times are longer.

For surfaces such as countertops, the least expensive and most readily available chemical is a 1:10 solution of ordinary household bleach (sodium hypochlorite). However bleach is not easily rinsed, and it is only effective if the solution is mixed fresh daily. When using a chemical agent, preparation and usage instructions provided by manufacturers must be closely followed to achieve the maximum effects of the chemical.

Steam Sterilization

Steam sterilization (autoclave) is widely used in health care facilities. The autoclave uses steam under pressure to obtain higher temperatures than is achieved with boiling. Under pressure, water is converted to steam reaching a

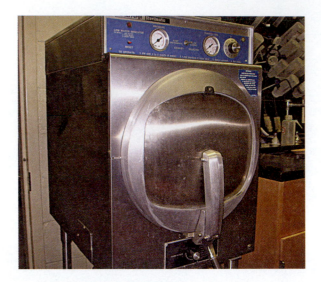

■ **FIGURE 5-5** Autoclave

temperature of 121°C. To destroy microorganisms and spores, items are autoclaved under this temperature and 15 pounds of pressure (PSI) for 15 minutes.

Every autoclave (Figure 5-5 ■) should be inspected and serviced on a regular basis to ensure the equipment is functioning properly. Quality control when using an autoclave consists of proper maintenance and proper operation. Equally important is the regular use of sterilization indicators (*Bacillus* spp. spores) and culture tests. High-density wastes or materials that insulate the agents from heat and steam penetration are not suitable for steam sterilization. Proper packaging and containment of infectious materials are crucial to achieve effective sterilization.

 REAL WORLD TIP

Liquid medium containing carbohydrates, such as phenol red sugars, cannot be sterilized with steam, chemical, dry heat, or gas. These methods destroy the carbohydrates present. The base medium is sterilized and the carbohydrate is filtered prior to addition. The filter used must have pores which are too small for the organisms to pass through so they become trapped and removed.

 Checkpoint! 5–7 (Chapter Objective 8)

An autoclave is an instrument used during:
- A. *gas sterilization.*
- B. *dry heat sterilization.*
- C. *chemical sterilization.*
- D. *steam sterilization.*

The most frequent reason for sterilization failure is the lack of contact between steam and the microorganisms (CDC, 1983).

STANDARD PRECAUTIONS

The Centers for Disease Control and Prevention (CDC) is responsible for studying pathogens and diseases in an effort to prevent their spread. As a division of the U.S. Department of Health and Human Services, the CDC issues a number of guidelines to enable health care professionals to practice responsible infection control. In 1970, The CDC developed a system of seven isolation categories for patients with infectious diseases. This system included strict isolation, respiratory isolation, protective isolation, enteric precautions, wound and skin precautions, discharge precautions, and blood precautions. In 1985, the center released the **universal precautions**, infection control guidelines designed to protect workers from exposure to diseases spread by blood and certain body fluids. They were written in response to the increased number of cases of acquired immunodeficiency syndrome (AIDS) and hepatitis B and other infectious diseases (CDC, 1988). The guidelines were revised in 1991, and a new set of guidelines was released. **Standard precautions** reflect improved recommendations intended to protect health care providers, patients, and visitors from communicable diseases (National Committee for Clinical Laboratory Standards [NCCLS], 1997). At the same time, the CDC issued a second tier of precautions called **transmission-based precautions**. These are designed for patients documented or suspected to be infected/colonized with highly transmissible or epidemiologically important pathogens for which additional precautions beyond standard precautions are needed to interrupt transmission. The three categories of transmission-based precautions include airborne precautions, droplet precautions, and contact precautions.

All occupational exposure to blood or other potentially infectious materials is regulated under the Occupational Safety and Health Administration (OSHA) Bloodborne Pathogens Standard, 29 CFR 1910.1030. Occupational exposure means reasonably anticipated skin, eye, mucous membrane, or parenteral contact with blood or other potentially infectious materials that may result from the performance of an employee's duties. The standard mandates the use of standard precautions as an approach to exposure control. According to this concept, all human blood and certain human body fluids are treated as infectious. The standard precautions concept is only one part of the overall plan to reduce exposures. Other methods of control include engineering controls, work practice controls, use of personal protective equipment, receipt of the hepatitis B vaccine, and training in exposure control. Figure 5-6 ■ and Box 5-2 ✪ summarize the standard precautions.

Standard precautions involve the use of protective barriers such as gloves, gowns, aprons, masks, or protective eyewear, which can reduce the risk of exposure of the health care worker's skin or mucous membranes to potentially infective materials. In addition, under standard precautions, it is

GLOVES

Before touching blood, body fluids, mucous membranes, non-intact skin or performing venipuncture. CHANGE gloves after contact with each patient

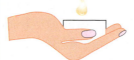
WASH

Wash hands immediately after gloves are removed. Wash hands and other skin surfaces immediately if contaminated with blood or other body fluids

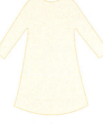
GOWN / APRON

For procedure likely to generate splashes of blood or other body fluids

MASK EYE PROTECTION

Masks and protective eyewear or face shields for procedures likely to generate splashes of blood or other body fluids

SHARPS

Dispose of needles with syringes and other sharp items in puncture-resistant container near point-of-use

DO NOT RECAP BY HAND

Do not recap needles or otherwise manipulate by hand before disposal

RESUSCITATION

Mouthpieces of resuscitator bags should be available to minimize need for emergency mouth to mouth resuscitation

WASTE / LINEN

Waste and soiled linen should be handled in accordance with disposal policy and local law

■ **FIGURE 5-6** Standard Precautions

 BOX 5-2

Standard Precautions Practices

Hand washing: Wash hands before and after potential contact with body fluids and after removing gloves.

Gloves: Should always be worn when there is potential for contact with body fluids. Change gloves after each contact with body fluid.

Masks, Eyewear, and Protective Clothing: Wear during procedures where splashing may occur.

Contaminated Waste: Dispose of waste contaminated with blood or body fluids in plastic bags tied at the top.

Sharps: Must be discarded in a nonbreakable, puncture-proof container with a lid.

Needles: Never recap needles.

Exposures: Exposures must be reported immediately

recommended that all health care workers take precautions to prevent injuries caused by needles, scalpels, and other sharp instruments or devices.

✓ Checkpoint! 5–8 (Chapter Objective 9)

Standard precautions apply only to visible blood in bodily fluids.
A. *True*
B. *False*

@ REAL WORLD TIP

Educational institutions must adhere to standard precautions and OSHA regulations. Laboratory manuals should be provided to students, and safety orientation and training must be conducted before students are allowed to perform any laboratory testing.

NOSOCOMIAL INFECTIONS

Nosocomial infections are serious problems in health care facilities. They are infections acquired by the patient while in the hospital. Hospitalized patients may be predisposed to infection because of trauma, preexisting disease, increased exposure to disease-causing microorganisms, invasive therapy, or immunosuppressive therapy. The most common nosocomial infections include surgical or traumatic wounds, urinary and respiratory tracts, and the bloodstream (CDC, 1983).

The single most important action to prevent the spread of nosocomial infections is hand washing (NCCLS, 1997). Also important is adherence to the standard precautions. Each hospital should have an **infection control committee**. Its function is to monitor and to evaluate infections occurring in the facility. The committee investigates any case of infection in an attempt to determine the cause and, thus, prevent the incident from happening again in the future. Nosocomial infections and infection control are discussed in detail in ∞ Chapter 41.

Checkpoint! 5–9
(Chapter Objective 10)

A patient acquired an infection while being hospitalized. This is considered:

    A. *nosocomial infection.*
    B. *iatrogenic infection.*
    C. *idiopathic infection.*
    D. *primary infection.*

 Checkpoint! 5–10
(Chapter Objective 11)

A phlebotomist discarded empty blood collection tubes and needles in a biohazard bag. This action is:

    A. *acceptable.*
    B. *not acceptable; needles should be recapped before disposal.*
    C. *not acceptable; needles should have discarded in a puncture-proof container.*
    D. *not acceptable; identification information on the tubes should have been destroyed.*

WASTE MANAGEMENT

Medical laboratories should have clear procedures for workers to follow to minimize the generation of waste materials. Waste materials must be handled in specific ways as designated by federal and local regulations (ACS, 1995). Biohazard waste or potentially infectious waste must be discarded directly into sealable, leakproof containers that are clearly identifiable from regular waste. Containers must be marked with the universal biohazard symbol (Figure 5-7 ■) and must be distinctly colored red or orange.

Infectious waste is described as any item that has come in contact with blood or body fluid. These items must be handled with gloves and disposed of by placing them in the appropriate biohazard containers. Sterilization and disinfection procedures are recommended when dealing with biological hazards. Needles and sharps are discarded in properly labeled sharps disposal containers. The containers must be puncture resistant, leakproof, and sealable. Each different chemical class should be kept in a separate clearly labeled disposable container. Chemicals must never be disposed into a sink or down the drain unless they are deactivated or neutralized. A chemical spill cleanup kit should be available when chemicals are involved. The kit includes absorbents and neutralizers to clean up acid, alkali, mercury, and other spills.

 REAL WORLD TIP

Biohazardous waste must never be placed with regular waste. Disposing of biohazardous materials can be very costly. Most medical facilities employ an outside agency to dispose of waste. Both parties are responsible for keeping records of all activities. Because facilities are often charged by the weight of biohazard containers, regular waste, such as paper towels, should not be placed with biohazardous waste.

▶ QUALITY ASSURANCE

DEFINED

The term **quality assurance (QA)** comprises planned and systematic actions necessary to provide adequate confidence that a structure, system, or component will perform satisfactorily in service. Quality assurance covers all activities from design, development, production, installation, and servicing to documentation. It is essential that the laboratory have a plan in place to monitor its processes, from preanalytical through postanalytical phases of testing, and make improvements.

QUALITY CONTROL

The quality control (QC) program in the microbiology laboratory requires that reagents and equipment must be monitored to ensure that they perform properly, in addition to the performance of personnel. There are two components of QC: internal and external. Internal QC consists of documenting the proper functioning of reagents and equipment at prescribed intervals and evaluating performance on split samples and within batch reproducibility studies (Isenberg, 1983). Blind specimens can also be introduced to evaluate overall performance. Continuous training and education of personnel will keep them up to date and will ensure their quality performance. The laboratory must subscribe to a proficiency testing program (external QC) to provide unbiased evaluation of personnel and testing procedures.

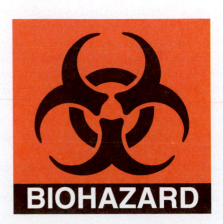

■ **FIGURE 5-7** Universal biohazard symbol

Specimen Integrity

Several types of specimens are received daily in the microbiology laboratory. All specimens should be treated as a potential source of infection. All specimens should be clearly labeled with the patient's name, age, sex, hospital number, date, and time of collection, with a fully completed "requisition form." The nature and origin of the specimen, clinical diagnosis, investigation required, and any other relevant information should be provided.

The quality of the specimen has an effect on the tests that are performed and their results. For example, a sputum specimen would be of little value if the specimen is mainly saliva; a urine specimen whose delivery to the laboratory has been delayed would give potentially false results; a clotted blood specimen would be of no use to recover any organisms present; and a dry fecal specimen would not be helpful in correct diagnosis.

Whenever possible, specimens should be collected before antimicrobial agents are administered. They should be also of sufficient quantity to permit complete examination and should be placed in sterile, sealed containers to avoid hazards to the patients and to the medical staff. A soiled outer surface of a sputum container, a leaking stool sample, and a broken or leaking blood test tube are just a few examples of a serious danger to laboratory professionals. Special specimens (e.g., cerebrospinal fluid or CSF) should be submitted to the laboratory as soon as possible and should be handled promptly on arrival to the laboratory (Isenberg, 1983).

Improperly collected specimens should be rejected. However, specimens should never be discarded until a new specimen is requested. Certain specimens, like CSF and those obtained through invasive procedures (e.g., biopsy, aspirates) are difficult to replace and, therefore, should be treated with extra care. See Table 7-5 in ∞ Chapter 7, "Cultivation of Microorganisms," for specimen rejection criteria.

The hospital should provide a central specimen processing area. This simplifies the delivery process and allows the laboratory to monitor and record all incoming specimens (Isenberg, 1983). Here, each specimen is given a laboratory accession number, and the information on the requisition form is checked. At this point, introducing the bar coding technique in identifying specimens will improve the workflow. The generated bar code must be unique to each sample and must include the sample accession number that the computer has assigned to the specimen (Nace, 1993). Therefore, all identification information will not need to be written on the specimen. It is essential that the staff processing specimens are trained to wear personal protective equipment and not be permitted to handle leaking or broken specimen containers.

Procedure Manual

Policies and procedures are important for any laboratory. The advantages of having formal policies and procedures cannot be underestimated. Written policies and procedures should clearly describe the responsibilities and testing instructions for the testing personnel. The testing procedures form the basis of training for testing personnel. These procedures should be derived from the manufacturer's instructions and should be in a language understandable to testing personnel.

To comply with regulatory requirements and to provide accurate testing, the facility must adhere to the manufacturer's current testing instructions. These instructions, as outlined in the product insert, include directions for specimen collection and handling, control procedures, test and reagent preparation, and instructions for test performance, interpretation, and reporting. In addition, certain manufacturers provide quick reference instructions formatted as cards or small signs containing essential steps in conducting a test. Quick reference instructions should be clearly posted where testing is performed (Howerton, Anderson, Bosse, Granade, & Westbrook, 2005).

New testing procedures should be reviewed and signed by the laboratory director and/or medical director before they are incorporated into the procedure manual. The manual should be updated as tests or other aspects of the testing service change and should be reviewed by the director whenever changes are made. When procedures are no longer used, they should be removed from the manual and retained with a notation of the dates during which they were in service.

Equipment

Common equipment found in the microbiology laboratory includes incubators, autoclaves, thermometers, microscopes, refrigerators, and biological safety cabinets. Periodic checks and preventive maintenance of all equipment in the laboratory should be completed. For each piece of equipment, a quality log must be maintained that records calibration checks, maintenance, upgrades, and repairs, including the date and time, procedures performed and the results, and remedial steps taken. Also, laboratories should keep the manufacturer's manuals, warranties, and so forth for the life of the equipment.

Media and Reagents

The laboratory must define criteria for those conditions that are essential for proper storage and adequate control of media and reagents. The criteria must be consistent with the manufacturer's instructions. Quality control includes the selection of satisfactory raw materials, the preparation of media according to approved formulations or specific manufacturer's instructions, and the use of well-characterized reference strains to check prepared media.

Each batch of medium prepared from individual ingredients or each different manufacturer's lot number of dehydrated medium should be tested for one or more of the following characteristics, as appropriate:

- Sterility
- Ability to support growth of the target pathogen(s)
- Ability to produce appropriate biochemical reactions

As with all other products used in testing, reagents, either purchased or prepared in the laboratory, should be clearly marked to indicate the date on which they were first opened and the expiration date, if appropriate. Each reagent should be tested to make sure the expected reactions are obtained. For example, staining procedure should be checked with known positive control specimens when the stain is prepared or a new lot number is purchased. All reagents should be tested at intervals established by the laboratory to ensure that no deterioration has occurred (CDC, 1999).

Records

"If it is not recorded, it has not been done" (Washington, 1985) says it all.

Records serve at least four purposes:

1. They document what has occurred.
2. They serve as a point of reference.
3. They aid in the recognition of trends and resolution of problems.
4. They establish the credibility of the laboratory.

Records can be paper forms manually completed, or they can be computer software where obtaining a hard copy is possible. If a bar code system is used (Nace, 1993), the computer can assign a unique accession number for each patient. Records must be retained for at least 2 years (Becan-McBride & Ross, 1989). The test record of each patient is a permanent part of the hospital record. It includes name, age, sex, identifying number, name of physician, specimen type and source, requested test, date and time of specimen received, date and time test is completed, result, and name and initials of the laboratory personnel completing the test. A final report is issued to the physician after the test is completed. The result should be reviewed for erroneous information before a final report is placed in the patient's file.

 REAL WORLD TIP

President Barack Obama wants the medical records of all Americans to be electronic by 2014. Hospitals are gearing up by installing hardware and software for using electronic medical records. By going paperless, costs will be reduced. The key will be to ensure all of the hospital computers across the U.S. are interconnected and can transfer the records securely as needed.

Proficiency Testing

Proficiency testing (PT) is an external evaluation of the quality of a laboratory's performance. When a laboratory enrolls in an approved PT program, it will receive specimens of known composition to evaluate in the same way patient specimens are routinely tested. In general, PT programs will provide five samples for each analyte or test three times per year. When testing is completed, the results must be returned to the PT program for grading during a predetermined period of time, where results are compared with the consensus answer from referee laboratories for the same specimens. With a few exceptions, the passing score is 80%.

If a laboratory receives a failing score for an analyte or test, laboratory personnel must take necessary actions to find, correct, and document any problems in the testing performance. If a laboratory fails two consecutive or two out of three PT events, the laboratory will be subject to penalties.

PERSONNEL

Clinical laboratories are organized so that personnel work together to carry out the institutional objectives effectively and efficiently (Karni, Viscochil, & Amos, 1992). A typical clinical laboratory organizational structure recognizes three major categories: laboratory director, technical supervisor, and technical personnel. The presence of a medical director (pathologist) is also recommended for definite identification (Newell, 1972). Laboratory directors assist in establishing policies and test protocols. They provide consultation services for the tests and the interpretation of results and establish all laboratory procedures and quality control practices. Also, directors ensure the proper performance of all procedures performed. Other responsibilities include budget preparation and orientation and training of new personnel and continuing education of technical and supervisory staff (Lang, 1993).

The technical supervisor assumes responsibility to implement quality control practices, to prepare daily work schedules, to maintain levels of supplies and reagents, and to help technical instruction and training. The supervisor is also responsible to be current with the procedures and equipment, to provide direct supervision of personnel, and to recommend to the director the selection, transfer, discipline, and discharge of personnel. Technical personnel are the backbone of the laboratory. They perform the required tests with minimum supervision, report results, and maintain records and equipment.

CLIA

In 1988, several media reports focused public and congressional attention on deficiencies in the quality of services provided by some of the nation's clinical laboratories. The Clinical Laboratory Improvement Amendments of 1988, or CLIA '88, resulted from congressional examination of the situation (Howerton et al., 2005). CLIA sets minimum standards designed to improve quality in all laboratory testing and includes specifications for quality control, quality assurance, patient test management, personnel, and proficiency testing. Laboratories that satisfy CLIA regulatory requirements give their patients greater confidence in the quality and reliability of the laboratory results. On January 24, 2003, the Centers for Medicare and Medicaid Services (CMS) released the latest version of the Clinical Laboratory Improvement Amendments (CLIA), termed the "Final Rules."

Competency Evaluation

Trained and competent testing personnel are essential to good-quality testing and patient care. To ensure testing procedures are performed consistently and accurately, periodic evaluation of competency is recommended, with retraining, as needed, on the basis of results of the competency assessment. Competency can be evaluated by methods such as observation, evaluating adequacy of documentation, or the introduction of simulated specimens by testing control materials or previously tested patient specimens. External quality assessment or evaluation programs, such as PT programs, are another resource for assessment.

State Licensure

States and local jurisdictions vary in the extent to which they regulate laboratory testing. Some states and localities have specific regulations for testing; some require licensure of personnel who perform testing. The person responsible for testing oversight should ensure that all state and local requirements are met. These requirements might be more or less stringent than federal requirements. When state or local regulations governing laboratory testing are more stringent than the federal CLIA requirements, they supersede what is required under CLIA.

Continuing Education

Laboratory professionals must continuously adapt to the rapidly evolving technologies in the field. Keeping up with today's constant change and innovation is a challenging task, and it is becoming a requirement by many facilities, organizations, and certification agencies.

A timetable should be prepared showing what the technical personnel must learn, the level of skill to be acquired, what job should be done, and how well and how soon (Johnson, 1972). Also, technical personnel must be familiar with the principles involved behind each test and should know its essential parts or key points.

HOSPITAL PARTICIPATION

Hospitals and medical centers are obliged to provide a safe environment for their clients, visitors, and staff. They are under a moral and legal responsibility to monitor and ensure that there is hospitalwide compliance with laws, policies, and standards for quality of patient care and facility licensure and/or accreditation.

Control of infection is the responsibility of the hospital's infection control committee, and the microbiology laboratory plays a crucial role in providing valuable information. The committee makes recommendation on the use of antibiotics, examines resistance patterns of bacteria, decides on disinfectants and cleaning agents used in the facility, devises patient isolation procedures, and monitors the applications of the rules. The committee also oversees employee health and utilizes surveillance data to determine hospital-acquired infections.

ROLE OF COMPUTERS

Computers can improve the quality and effectiveness of care and reduce cost. Most laboratories implement a laboratory information system (LIS), which is a software program that handles receiving, processing and storing information generated by medical laboratory processes. The LIS is often interfaced with laboratory instruments where patient information and test results are transmitted. Basic features of a LIS include test order entry, specimen receiving and processing, results entry, and reporting.

Personnel using the system should receive basic training in the general use of the computer and standard system software. In addition, training on confidentiality of records and information should be routine. This training must be ongoing to address the changing computer environment and enhance skills for needed specific job responsibilities.

 Checkpoint! 5–11 (Chapter Objective 12)

Which QC/QA component involves the use of external unknowns to evaluate the quality of the laboratory's performance?

 A. *Proficiency testing*
 B. *Competency evaluation*
 C. *Continuing education*
 D. *CLIA regulations*

SUMMARY

Infectious diseases often occur because of lack of education and carelessness. One must understand the importance of federal and state regulations that are set forth to protect the health and safety of patients and health care workers and limit the spread of infectious diseases. Effective infection control measures and applying standard precautions in daily operation are mandatory in health care facilities.

Patient safety, quality control, and process improvement are crucial elements of ensuring quality results. Each laboratory must implement a plan to monitor these areas. In addition, the laboratory must have a plan in place for dealing for potential bioterrorism agents.

LEARNING OPPORTUNITIES

1. Situation (Chapter Objective 2)

   a. A microbiologist notices a cracked wire on the microscope being used. What kind of laboratory hazard is this?

   b. A stool sample in a paper bag is brought to the laboratory by an outpatient. What kind of laboratory hazard is this?

2. Situation (Chapter Objective 5): A pleural fluid specimen is received in the microbiology laboratory with a request for acid-fast culture (for *Mycobacterium tuberculosis*). What biosafety level precautions should be used?

3. Situation (Chapter Objective 8)

   a. A medical laboratory technician working in a physician's office laboratory wants to wipe off the surface of the "bench" or table top prior to leaving work. Is this disinfection or sterilization? What agent might be used?

   b. A microbiologist working in a reference laboratory spills a liquid culture on the table. Protocol requires that paper towels be placed over the spill, moistened with disinfectant, and left in place for 20 minutes prior to discard. Is this disinfection or sterilization? Why?

4. Which of the following agencies has classified biological agents into three categories depending on how easily they can be spread and the severity of illness they cause? (Chapter Objective 1)

   a. Centers for Disease Control and Prevention

   b. Occupational Safety and Health Administration

   c. U.S. Department of Health and Human Services

   d. College of American Pathologists

5. A lab coat that is used as personal protection equipment must be: (Chapter Objective 3)

   a. white in color

   b. disposable

   c. impervious to liquid

   d. washed at home by the user

6. Most microbiology laboratories are categorized as: (Chapter Objective 5)

   a. Biosafety level 1

   b. BSL 2

   c. BSL 3

   d. BSL 4

7. The first line of detection of bioterrorism agents is often the: (Chapter Objective 6)

   a. attending physician

   b. phlebotomist

   c. laboratory director

   d. technical microbiologist

8. Most patient errors occur during the _____ phase of the laboratory testing process. (Chapter Objective 7)

   a. pre-analytical

   b. analytical

   c. post-analytical

9. Which of following actions is considered appropriate standard precautions? (Chapter Objective 9)

   a. the use of gloves only when specimens are visibly leaking or soiled

   b. placement of a used phlebotomy needle in the biohazardous waste

   c. using hand hygiene before and after wearing gloves and when visibly soiled

   d. all of the above

10. Nosocomial infections are most often spread by: (Chapter Objective 10)

    a. the visitors of patients

    b. poor hand hygiene of healthcare workers

    c. the excessive use of antibiotics

    d. medical devices such as intravenous catheters

11. Which of the following identifies a biohazard waste container? (Chapter Objective 11)

    a. presence of the universal biohazard symbol

    b. a red container and/or liner bag

    c. both a and b

    d. presence of the NFPA label

12. Which of the following items is considered part of a clinical laboratory quality assurance program? (Chapter Objective 12)

    a. written policies and procedures

    b. proficiency testing

    c. specimen rejection criteria

    d. all of the above

CASE STUDY 5-1. SHIGELLA OUTBREAK IN A CLINICAL MICROBIOLOGY LABORATORY (CHAPTER OBJECTIVE 4)

Patients: Six medical laboratory scientists (MLS)

Initial Report: Six clinical laboratory scientists developed symptoms characteristic of a diarrheal illness. Stool cultures grew *Shigella sonnei*.

Follow-up Results

Stool cultures were performed on four asymptomatic MLS students, completing their clinical rotations in the department, and other clinical laboratory scientists, in other departments in the laboratory, with negative results for *Shigella*. The most recent patient clinical *Shigella sonnei* isolate was compared to the outbreak isolate and determined to be different. The outbreak isolate was compared with the isolate used as a student unknown for one of the MLS students and was determined to be the same.

Risk analysis revealed a higher incidence of culture positive cases associated with instructing the MLS student, washing hands before eating or leaving the laboratory, and using the hand washing sink in the work area. The hand washing sink had faucet controls. The MLS student, who received *Shigella sonnei* as an unknown isolate, was the only person in the laboratory to routinely wear gloves. The student admitted to contaminating a finger of the glove while performing serologic typing of the unknown organism. The student also admitted to disposing of the *Shigella* suspension and washing the reusable slide in the hand washing sink rather than in the designated processing sink (Mermel et al., 1997).

1. What is the potential source of the outbreak organism?

2. What safety protocols were violated?

3. How should the MLS student have handled the laboratory accident?

PEARSON
myhealthprofessionskit™

Use this address to access the interactive Companion Website created for this textbook. Simply select "Clinical Laboratory Science" from the choice of disciplines. Find this book and log in using your user name and password.

REFERENCES

Go to myhealthprofessionskit.com to view this chapter's references.

PART II
ROUTINE SPECIMEN PROCESSING

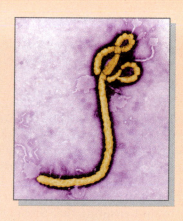

6

Specimen Collection

Cara Calvo and Jenny Francis

■ LEARNING OBJECTIVES

Upon completion of this chapter, the learner should be able to:

1. Discuss pre-analytical factors that influence the detection and recovery of microbial pathogens from specimens.
    a. Propose the effect of a pre-analytical error on specimen results.
2. Select the most appropriate container/collection device for a given specimen type, citing the advantages and disadvantages of each one.
3. Recommend the specimen of choice for a given type of infection.
4. Explain the proper specimen collection procedure and handling protocol for a given specimen type submitted to the clinical microbiology laboratory.
5. Assess the sample quality for a given specimen type according to the testing to be performed.
6. Recognize circumstances when specimens should be collected to support epidemiological and infection control activities.
7. Advise nonlaboratorians on specimen collection practices associated with postexposure incidents involving biological threat agents.
8. Evaluate and critique each of the web sites provided in the learning opportunities of this chapter.

KEY TERMS

aniline dyes	etiologic	nebulizer
aseptic	exudates	percutaneous
biological threat agents	infection control	polyvinyl alcohol
biphasic media system	mycoses	pre-analytical
epidemiology		

► INTRODUCTION

Test results reported by the clinical microbiology laboratory reflect only what has been observed following macroscopic, microscopic, biochemical, and cultural analysis. In this way, the laboratory identifies **etiologic** agent(s), those microbial organisms known to cause disease, and drugs, including antibiotics, that may be used to treat infection. The first step toward ensuring that these results are accurate and reliable begins with proper specimen collection and continues with appropriate handling and timely transport to the laboratory. The vast majority of specimens submitted are collected by patients and nonlaboratory health care personnel unfamiliar with the consequences associated with poor-quality or insufficient volume samples. Therefore, it is the responsibility of the laboratory to provide clear, concise directions to ensure that the best possible sample is collected and submitted. This chapter focuses on issues of specimen collection that affect the validity of results generated during microbiologic evaluation. The discussion will provide answers to three key questions: What is the specimen of choice for a given type of infection? When (time) should the specimen be collected? How (method) is a specimen for a given type of infection collected and handled?

► FUNDAMENTALS OF SPECIMEN COLLECTION

From the time that the physician makes a diagnosis and places an order for a microbiology culture to the time the specimen is received in the laboratory is called the **pre-analytical** phase of laboratory testing. Most errors occur during the pre-analytical phase. This means the laboratory must work diligently with physicians and other healthcare personnel to insure quality specimens are submitted for testing.

Failure to detect and recover microbial pathogens from specimens can and does result from faulty collection technique and mishandling of samples. Therefore, for a given type of infection and whenever possible, the specimen submitted to the clinical microbiology laboratory should be:

■ Collected and transported in a container that is sterile, leakproof, and preserves the viability of the pathogenic organism(s) of interest.

■ Properly identified with patient and specimen information (e.g., name, collection date) and collected in sufficient quantity to allow for complete analysis.

■ Collected before symptoms associated with the infection have subsided and before treatment is administered.

■ Collected from the site of infection using **aseptic** or sterile technique to decrease the chance that the sample will be contaminated by resident flora.

■ Sent to the laboratory without delay under conditions that minimize exposure to environmental extremes (e.g., low humidity, heat).

■ Accompanied by a request that at a minimum identifies the patient, the type of specimen submitted, the date and time of collection, the name of the physician ordering the test(s), the diagnosis, and the test or tests requested.

> ### ℮ REAL WORLD TIP
>
> National Patient Safety Goals (NPSG) have been identified by the Joint Commission to reduce patient errors. Hospitals, including the laboratories, accredited by the Joint Commission must meet specific standards including the NPSG. One goal, of the 10 total, requires the use of two patient identifiers to insure the identity of the patient who is receiving a service or treatment. These two unique identifiers must be included on all specimens, blood products, treatments and services related to the patient. Most facilities use the patient's legal name and medical record number.

CONTAINERS

A wide variety of containers and sampling devices are available to assist in collecting and transporting specimens to the clinical microbiology laboratory. Typically, the collection device and technique used to obtain a sample varies according to the testing methodology of the microbiology laboratory, the need to maintain the viability (and in the case of viral agents, infectivity) of suspected pathogens, as well as the accessibility of the sample. Additionally, the choice of what container to use is influenced by transport and safety concerns. For example, it may be necessary to submit specimens to a reference laboratory by mail or commercial shipping. U.S. federal law requires that agents of human disease or their toxins be transported in a securely closed, watertight container called a primary container that in turn is packaged in a second container. The container housing the sample must be wrapped with sufficient absorbent material to absorb the entire contents should a spill occur. Finally, the secured containers must be placed in packaging that meets specific performance requirements set forth by law.

One of the more commonly used, but perhaps least desirable, specimen collection devices is the swab. Though convenient to use, the amount of specimen that can be collected is limited. Additionally, recovery of all the material from the swab is difficult. The shaft of swabs may be wood, plastic, or wire, and the tips are covered with cotton, calcium alginate, or polyester. Swabs are typically available individually wrapped and sterile or as a component of a collection system (e.g., culturette). This type of collection system consists of a plastic tube that houses the swab, which is attached to a cap. Transport media in the bottom of the tube provides moisture for up to 72 hours (provided transport occurs under ambient temperatures) and supports the viability of the microbe(s) of interest. Refer to ∞ Chapter 7, "Cultivation of Organisms," for details on transport media formulations and uses.

Careful consideration must be given to the type of swab used to a collect specimen that will be submitted to the clinical microbiology laboratory. One reason is that some swab tip material has been shown to kill select microbes. For example, Lauer and Masters (1988) demonstrated that the glue used to attach the calcium alginate fibers to the swab shaft was toxic to *Neisseria gonorrhoeae*. Another reason is that certain types of swabs interfere with molecular-based assays (Cloud, Hymas, & Carroll, 2002). In these cases, manufacturers' recommend specific swabs should be used, and the swabs are included in the specific assay kits.

Ideally, most liquid specimens (e.g., voided urine, bronchial washings) should be collected in sterile, leakproof, screwcapped containers. When properly used, these collection vessels minimize occupational exposure to blood-borne pathogens and provide adequate volume capacity for fluid specimens. Exception is made for the aspirated contents of abscesses or fluids of sizable volume (other than urine) collected from normally sterile body sites. Aspirated material may be submitted in the syringe used to collect it as long as the needle is removed and the syringe is safely and securely sealed prior to transport to the lab. **Exudates** are body fluids excreted from infected and inflamed tissues. They are usually collected into large-volume drainage bags or bottles. These containers may be submitted "as is," provided they are appropriately labeled and sealed to prevent leakage. Specimens that are improperly identified and submitted in a leaking and/or incorrect container can and should be rejected by the lab.

Checkpoint! 6–1
(Chapter Objective 1)

Factors influencing the detection and recovery of microbial pathogens from specimens include:
- A. *transit time.*
- B. *storage temperature.*
- C. *sampling technique.*
- D. *all of the above.*

TIME OF COLLECTION

If at all possible, samples should be collected prior to administration of drug treatment. Samples collected after antibiotic therapy has begun can initially demonstrate negative culture results. When treatment is stopped, the culture may demonstrate positive results. In some cases, the lab can take countermeasures to prevent false-negative outcomes if notified that treatment was initiated. In addition, to ensure detection and/or isolation of pathogens, samples should be collected before symptoms have abated or during a time when organisms are most likely to be found in the specimen of interest. This is true

because some organisms are present in greater numbers either during the acute stage of disease (e.g., enteric or diarrheal illness and blood parasitemia) or during specific times of the day (e.g., early-morning voided urine or respiratory secretions are more concentrated). In some cases, specimens collected without regard to time of collection may prove clinically useless.

HANDLING AND TRANSPORT

Most microorganisms that cause disease in humans have optimal and specific survival requirements. Those subjected to environmental extremes or lack of energy sources die. Dead microbes cannot be isolated in culture or detected by other traditional methods used in the clinical microbiology lab. Therefore, it is very important that samples be handled and transported in a manner that ensures microbe viability. Samples are to be delivered to the lab as soon after collection as possible. If they are delayed, specimens may need to be supplemented with transport media, packaged in special environmental chambers, or stored appropriately. For example, wound specimens for anaerobic workup must be transported in a manner that protects anaerobic bacteria from exposure to oxygen. Cerebrospinal fluid must be stored at room temperature or incubated because organisms such as *Neisseria meningitidis* and *Streptococcus pneumoniae* are sensitive to cold and may be killed in refrigerated samples. Box 6-1 ✪ summarizes the appropriate storage temperature for specimens if there must be a delay prior to processing.

In all cases, due care should be taken to prevent transmission of disease caused by the microbes contained in clinical specimens. At a minimum, samples should be in leakproof containers and transported with a biohazard label prominently displayed. Specimen handlers must follow the Occupational Safety and Health Administration (OSHA) and Centers for Disease Control and Prevention (CDC) standard precautions, which require the use of personal protective equipment (e.g.,

✪ BOX 6-1

Recommended Storage Temperatures for Specimens

- Blood and bone marrow: Room temperature
- Body fluids other than blood and CSF: 4°C
- CSF: Room temperature or 35°C
- Lower respiratory: 4°C
- Specimens for viruses: 4°C
- Stool: 4°C
- Swabs or other specimens (not for the isolation of *N. gonorrhoeae*): Room temperature
- Swabs or other specimens for the isolation of *Neisseria gonorrhoeae*: Room temperature
- Tissue: Room temperature
- Upper respiratory: Room temperature
- Urine: 4°C

Checkpoint! 6–2
(Chapter Objective 2)

A swab is not the appropriate collection device to use when collecting body fluid for culture because:

   A. *it cannot be properly labeled.*
   B. *supplies are limited by manufacturers of molecular-based assays.*
   C. *the amount of sample volume that can be collected is limited.*
   D. *federal guidelines prohibit its transport across state lines.*

gloves, masks and liquid impervious lab coats) if there is a chance of exposure to disease-causing organisms.

▶ SPECIMEN TYPES

Many types of specimens are collected and submitted to the microbiology laboratory to determine the causative agent(s) of infection. Often, these specimens are collected by nonlaboratorians. To ensure recovery of pathogens from clinical specimens, it is critical that the right sample is collected correctly and properly transported to the laboratory in a timely manner.

BLOOD

Blood cultures are a very important source of diagnostic information for physicians. The presence of microbial organisms in the blood usually reflects active if not spreading infection in the tissues. Patients with bacteremia, or bacteria present in the blood, are at risk for developing septic shock, and bloodstream infections can result in death. Initiation of specific curative treatment based on blood culture findings can prove to be lifesaving. Therefore, proper collection of the blood specimen is essential.

Most blood culture collection systems are comprised of two bottles (a set). One bottle is designated as aerobic and the other as anaerobic. Each bottle contains a specific amount of liquid medium, including an anticoagulant, that promotes the detection and recovery of microbial pathogens by preventing the blood from clotting, neutralizing some antibiotics, inactivating complement, and inhibiting phagocytosis (Bartelt, 2000). The aerobic bottle is used to recover aerobes and facultative anaerobes. The anaerobic bottle is designed to support the growth of those microorganisms that do not tolerate the presence of oxygen. Importantly, when the minimum amount of blood volume for the culture set cannot be obtained, the available specimen should be inoculated into the aerobic bottle. The reason for this is that the occurrence of anaerobic bacteremia is uncommon (Wilson et al., 2001), and placing the blood into the aerobic bottle ensures maximum recovery of the most likely infecting agent.

The collection of blood for culture poses a special problem in that routine phlebotomy techniques must minimize chances of sample contamination by indigenous skin flora which are organisms that are also capable of causing disease.

REAL WORLD TIP

To maximize effort, prevent sample waste, and contribute to test sensitivity, inoculate a pediatric blood culture bottle with the small volume collected during difficult blood culture collections on adults.

In addition, because blood volume and timing are critical determining factors for establishing a diagnosis of bacteremia (Aronson & Bor, 1987), multiple specimens taken from different sites are collected in specially designed bottles like those shown in Figure 6-1 ■. Regardless of the culture system used, it is recommended that when possible, 20 mL of blood be collected from a patient older than 10 years of age and not less than 1 mL of blood per year of life from a patient younger than 10 years of age (Trevino & Mahon, 2000). Preferably, samples should be collected at the time that the patient is experiencing symptoms. It is during this time that the greatest number of organisms is found in blood circulation.

Blood culture collection begins by scrubbing the venipuncture site with 70% alcohol for at least 60 seconds. The site is allowed to air-dry. This initial cleansing is followed by application of 2% tincture of iodine (Richter, 2002). The iodine is applied to the center of the puncture site and spread outward with a swabbing motion following a concentric circle pattern. Once the iodine solution has dried, the recommended amount of blood is taken using a vacuum tube system or a butterfly or a syringe with needle and aseptically transferred using a safety transfer device to the culture bottle(s) (Dunne, Nolte, & Wilson, 1997). This requires the culture bottle tops be cleaned with 70% alcohol and dried

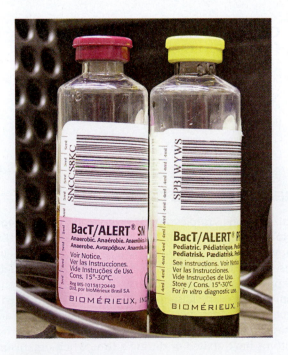

■ **FIGURE 6-1** Blood culture bottles.

before inoculation. The tops should not be cleaned with iodine because it may cause deterioration of the rubber stopper. Recent studies have shown skin "prep" kits containing chlorhexidine and alcohol to be as effective as tincture of iodine as long as the manufacturer's protocol is followed (Barenfanger, Drake, Lawhaorn, & Verhulst, 2004). ∞ Chapter 32, "Cardiovascular System," provides further information on blood cultures.

RESPIRATORY TRACT

Upper

The upper respiratory tract includes the nose and nasal cavity, the buccal cavity, the pharynx, and the larynx. The ears and eyes are connected to the upper respiratory tract via the eustachian tube and the ethmoid sinus, respectively. Infection of the tissues of the upper respiratory tract leads to the production of secretions that should be collected using a sterile swab and submitted for culture. Many types of swabs are available. The one to use is in part determined by the type of test to be done. For example, calcium alginate swabs have been shown to inhibit PCR-based assays for *Bordetella pertussis* (Wadowsky, Laus, Livert, States, & Ehrlich, 1994), the causative bacterial agent of whooping cough. However, for isolation of *B. pertussis,* the alginate swabs have been shown to perform similarly to polyester (Dacron) and cotton swabs (Cloud et al., 2002).

In cases of pharyngitis, or throat infection, the most common upper respiratory infection, material from the throat is collected by swabbing the posterior pharynx, tonsils, and adjacent areas that demonstrate inflammation and/or exudate. It is important to avoid the cheeks and tongue so the specimen is not contaminated with oral flora. The specimen of choice to diagnose infections from *Bordetella pertussis* or *Corynebacterium* includes a nasopharyngeal swab, wash, or aspirate. A calcium alginate or Dacron fiber–tipped swab on a long, thin, flexible wire is inserted into the posterior nasopharynx. The swab is rotated gently and left in place for up to 30 seconds if possible. Alternately, the nasopharynx can be flushed with sterile saline. The saline may be aspirated or allowed to drain through the nose into a sterile container. If culture media cannot be inoculated immediately, these specimens should be transported in media such as Amies with charcoal, Regan-Lowe, or casein hydrolysate solution. Specimens for *C. diphtheriae* culture and screen tests for methicillin-resistant *Staphylococcus aureus* (MRSA) can be collected on a swab. No special transport media is needed because these organisms are not fastidious. Excretions, pus, or tissue from an infected sinus can be collected by rigid endoscopy or sinus puncture and transported using a culturette system or sterile container.

An inner ear infection is also called otitis media. Samples from the inner ear should be collected using a syringe to aspirate fluid through the eardrum. If the drum has ruptured, a sterile swab can be used to collect the fluid. Otitis externa is an infection of the external ear canal, sometimes called "swimmer's ear." Samples from the external ear should be taken by firmly rotating the swab in the external canal. If any lesions are present, the crust can be removed and the exudate swabbed.

Eye cultures should be collected only by an ophthalmologist. Optimally, the specimens should be inoculated to agar plates immediately after collection. Corneal scrapings, swabs of exudate, and aspirations of intraocular fluid can help diagnose infection regardless of etiology.

Lower

Under normal circumstances, the lower respiratory tract (i.e., bronchi and lungs) is sterile. However, when infection occurs, it is important to collect the correct specimen. Two types of lower respiratory tract specimens can be submitted for culture: sputum (expectorated and induced) and bronchoscopy specimens. When collecting an expectorated sputum specimen, the patient is instructed to cough deeply to obtain a specimen from the lower tract and not postnasal fluid. An induced sputum collection is indicated when the patient has difficulty producing a sample by cough because of a lack of sputum production. In this case, the patient is instructed first to rinse the mouth with water. The patient then inhales a sufficient volume of finely aerosolized hypertonic saline produced by an instrument called a **nebulizer.** The saline induces or promotes more sputum production. Notably, because sputum specimens are subject to contamination with normal oral flora, the lab will assess sample quality using the Gram stain. The presence of numerous squamous epithelial cells indicates a poor quality specimen. See ∞ Chapter 33, "Respiratory System," for more information on collecting and processing respiratory specimens.

There are several types of bronchoscopy specimens, including bronchioalveolar lavages (BALs), bronchial washes (BWs), bronchial brushes (BBs), and transtracheal aspirates. These specimens are always collected by physicians or trained respiratory therapy personnel and may appear watery because they contain sterile saline used to flush the bronchi. These specimens, along with transtracheal aspirates, should be placed in sterile, securely capped containers and transported to the laboratory without delay.

Checkpoint! 6–3
(Chapter Objective 3)

What is the specimen of choice in cases of pharyngitis?
  A. *Expectorated sputum*
  B. *Tongue scrapings*
  C. *Swab of throat exudate*
  D. *Lesion scab*

GENITAL

Genital infections are caused by a wide variety of organisms, some of which are endogenous. However, the most common reason for collecting genital samples is to establish the presence of sexually transmitted disease (STD). Clinical history and symptoms of the patient allow the physician to deduce what type of sample needs to be collected and, in turn, which collection technique to use. ∞ Chapter 36 provides more information on genital system specimen processing.

The female lower genital tract is comprised of the vagina, cervix, and vulva. In most instances, infections of these areas may be established by swabbing the affected tissue. Aspirates as well as biopsy tissue can also be collected from the upper genital tract (ovaries, fallopian tubes, and uterus) by more invasive means. Urine is also an appropriate specimen for diagnosing genital tract infection with *Chlamydia trachomatis* by nucleic acid amplification methods in both females (Shafer et al., 2003) and males (Crotchfelt, Pare, Gaydos, & Quinn, 1998).

The urethra, prostate, and epididymis comprise the genital tract in the male. Swabbing the urethra or collecting penile exudate into a clean container are both accepted methods to obtain a sample for culture in cases of male genital infection. Bacterial infections of the prostate are commonly identified by urine culture.

STOOL

Gastroenteritis can be caused by various types of microbes, including bacteria, viruses, and parasites. However, the most common method to evaluate the cause of this illness is bacterial culture. In some cases, additional studies for toxins and parasites are needed. Depending on the patient's symptoms, the physician can order the appropriate tests to diagnose the patient.

When submitting a stool specimen, the patient should pass the specimen into a wide-mouthed, clean container, with a tight-fitting lid. Stool for bacterial culture can also be transferred into transport media containing Carey-Blair preservative, if the specimen cannot be cultured within 2 hours (Bopp, Ries, & Wells, 1999). Most commercial transport media kits have a "fill to" line on the side of the container to indicate the amount of sample to add to the vial. Overfilling or underfilling the vial can lead to inadequate preservation or dilution of organisms, thereby limiting detection and recovery of suspected pathogens. Transport media containing preservative is preferred, so that the specimen does not have to be processed immediately.

Some patients are screened to see if they harbor organisms that are of concern from an infection control standpoint (vancomycin-resistant *Enterococcus* and methicillin resistant *Staphylococcus aureus*). To submit a specimen to screen for infection control purposes, swab the rectal area of the patient and submit in a culturette. Stool can also be submitted in a sterile container or transport media containing Carey-Blair preservative. ∞ Chapter 35 provides more information on gastrointestinal system infections and specimen processing.

WOUND AND SOFT TISSUE

Wound and soft tissue cultures can be difficult to collect. The best and preferred sample is an aspirate or tissue sample, which isn't always easy to collect. If an aspirate or tissue sample cannot be obtained, then a swab sample can be collected but should be the specimen of last resort.

The area of the wound should be disinfected before sampling. If the wound is closed, the skin can be disinfected as for a blood culture. Aspirate the fluid inside the wound using a needle and syringe. If the wound is open, it should be debrided to remove the dead or dying tissue and rinsed with sterile saline. Tissue samples should be taken from the leading edge of infection, the most viable portion of tissue. If a swab has to be used, it is preferable to collect two (one for a Gram stain and one for a culture). Roll the swab over the wound, concentrating on areas of inflammation or pus. The specimens should be transported to the lab within 2 hours. Tissues are prepared for culture by mincing with sterile scissors or homogenizing with a sterile tissue grinder. Specimens for anaerobic culture should not contain squamous epithelial cells because this indicates an unacceptable specimen due to the potential presence of normal anaerobic flora. ∞ Chapter 37 provides more information on integumentary system infections. ∞ Chapter 24 discusses infections due to anaerobic organisms.

URINE

Urine cultures are most often a patient-collected sample. Therefore, thorough patient education is a must to obtain the best sample possible. Many laboratories provide patients with instructions and prepackaged supplies to facilitate easy and discrete collection. In almost all cases, a clean-voided midstream specimen is the specimen of choice. It is collected after the area around the urethral opening is gently cleansed. Urination is then initiated, and a sterile cup placed in the path of urine flow is used to collect sample. Transport tubes with a preservative (e.g., boric acid-glycerol) can be used if to the urine specimen cannot be refrigerated or processed within 2 hours of collection (Isenberg, 1998).

If the urine is collected by a long-term indwelling catheter, the urine is removed from the collection port once the port has been decontaminated. The urine should never be collected from the actual catheter collection bag because it represents pooled urine contaminated by lower urinary tract flora. A straight catheter can also be used, as long as the first part of the sample from the cath is discarded. A straight catheter is only inserted long enough to collect a urine specimen and then removed.

℮ REAL WORLD TIP

A foley urine catheter tip is not acceptable for culture. It is often colonized with normal flora of the urethra which makes it too difficult to determine the presence of potential pathogens.

Suprapubic aspirates are performed by a physician and are ideal specimens in suspected anaerobic infection. The skin above the bladder is disinfected and urine removed by aspiration. These samples should be transported in an anaerobic transport system. ∞ Chapter 34 discusses the urinary system, specimen processing and potential pathogens in detail.

CEREBROSPINAL FLUID AND OTHER BODY FLUIDS

This category of specimens consists of fluids collected from body sites normally considered to be sterile or free from indigenous flora. This includes serous fluids (pleural, pericardial, and peritoneal), synovial, cerebrospinal (CSF) and amniotic fluids. Because these specimens are collected by **percutaneous** needle aspiration or by needle puncture through the skin over the site, it is imperative that the skin is thoroughly cleaned and stringent aseptic technique used during aspiration to avoid contamination of the sample with normal skin flora.

The presence of microbes in nonurinary body fluids is usually associated with life-threatening infections requiring immediate treatment. In many such infections, fluid volumes increase, and the actual number of recoverable microbes is small because of dilution. Therefore, it is very important in these cases that as much fluid as possible be collected in sterile, leakproof containers and transported at room temperature to the lab without delay to ensure recovery of pathogens. Refer to ∞ Chapter 38, "Central Nervous System," and ∞ Chapter 39, "Skeletal System," for specific information on CSF, joint fluid, and bone marrow specimen processing.

Checkpoint! 6–4 (Chapter Objective 4)

A nursing student has called the lab requesting instruction on the proper collection of urine from a catheterized patient. What do you tell the student?
- A. *Decontaminate the catheter port and drain the urine into a labeled, sterile, screw-capped cup.*
- B. *Catheter urine samples are not accepted for culture.*
- C. *Sterilize the catheter tubing with 70% alcohol, remove urine with a 12 mL syringe, and submit to the lab as soon as possible.*
- D. *Pour at least 30 mL of urine from the catheter bag into a labeled, sterile, screw-capped cup.*

FUNGAL

Mycoses or fungal infections of clinical interest are grouped according to the site of infection. Superficial infections are limited to the uppermost layers of skin, including hair. Cutaneous mycoses are those that affect skin, hair, and nails, whereas subcutaneous infections involve muscle and connective tissues. As the name implies, systemic mycoses are infections that affect more than one area of the body and often involve connective tissues and specific organs. The diagnosis of these fungal infections is dependent on a properly collected and handled specimen. Refer to ∞ Chapters 14 and 29 for specific information on fungal infections.

The specimen of choice in superficial and cutaneous fungal infections is the diseased skin, hair, or nail tissue. Prior to collecting skin or nail material, the affected area should be carefully cleansed with 70% isopropyl alcohol and allowed to dry. The outer margins of skin lesions should be scraped with a sterile scalpel and the debris placed in a sterile container for transport to the lab. Scales from scalp lesions should be removed by scraping in a similar manner. Likewise, nails are scraped to remove keratinized material. Clippings of the infected nail(s) should also be collected. Hair should be plucked using sterile forceps. Some species of fungi fluoresce when exposed to UV light. Therefore, hairs that fluoresce under the light of a Wood's lamp should be selected and removed for culture. Alternately, hair that appears rough, scaly, or broken should be sampled. In all cases, the specimens should be transported to the laboratory in appropriately labeled sterile containers.

A variety of materials may be submitted in suspected cases of subcutaneous or systemic mycoses. The most common specimens include pus and exudate from draining lesions, blood and bone marrow, sputum and other respiratory secretions or washings as well as body fluids such as CSF, serous fluid, urine, vaginal secretions, and biopsied tissue. Importantly, the type of container used to transport these samples varies and is specimen dependent. For example, vaginal secretions should be collected and submitted on two separate swabs immersed in transport media (see ∞ Chapter 7 for details on use of transport media). With the exception of the lysis-centrifugation method, both nonautomated and automated blood culture systems use bottles containing broth media into which blood and/or bone marrow for fungal culture is inoculated. In most cases, a minimum of 5 milliliters (mL) of blood is required per bottle (adult). Pediatric bottles requiring less volume are available. Specimens are collected using aseptic technique and transported at room temperature without delay.

All other fungal specimens should be collected in screw-capped, leakproof, and sterile containers. For some, collection time is critical (e.g., blood). Clean catch first-morning-voided or catheterized urine is the preferred specimen in cases of fungal urinary tract infection. If transport delay is anticipated, urine specimens may be stored at refrigerated temperatures (2°C to 8°C). Twenty-four-hour urine and catheter-bag collections are not acceptable for fungal culture. ∞ Chapter 14 provides details on processing specimens for fungus.

PARASITOLOGY

Parasitic organisms are ubiquitous and responsible for considerable morbidity and mortality throughout the world. Diagnosis of parasitic infection is not made solely by physical examination of the patient, but in concert with information provided by the clinical laboratory. Lab test results must be accurate and reliable to aid the physician. In the clinical microbiology laboratory, identification of parasites is in large part dependent on recognition of the distinctive morphology of an organism. Therefore, it is critical that the correct specimen be obtained and submitted to the laboratory in a manner that

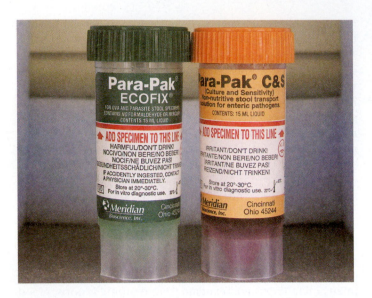

■ **FIGURE 6-2** Para-Pak collection system.

preserves morphology. Failure to do so will result in the reporting of false-negative results or at the very least misidentification of the suspected parasitic pathogen.

Fecal

Except in cases of pinworm infection, fecal specimens are examined for the presence of protozoa and helminth larvae and/or eggs. The number of specimens collected to demonstrate infection depends on a number of factors, including the severity of infection and sample quality. The usual and customary practice has been to require three stool specimens collected on alternate days because organisms are not shed in a consistent quantity on a daily basis. However, some studies have shown that examining three specimens may not be necessary, especially in low-prevalence areas (Morris, Wilson, & Reller, 1992; Valenstein, Pfaller, & Yungbluth, 1994).

Regardless of the number collected, all fecal samples should be submitted in a collection container that is clean, but not necessarily sterile, and waterproof with a leakproof lid. Commercial systems like the one pictured in Figure 6-2 ■ are commonly used.

These specimen vials come with written instructions for proper use and preservatives in case of transport delays. The preservatives formalin and **polyvinyl alcohol** (PVA) have been widely used for the preservation of helminth eggs and protozoan cysts and trophozoites. However, toxicity and safe disposal concerns have prompted the investigation of acceptable alternatives (Pietrzak-Johnston et al., 2000). Many labs now use a one-vial, nonmercuric chloride–containing collection system. Table 6-1✪ lists common fecal preservatives that are used.

Additionally, contamination of the specimen with toilet water and/or urine should be avoided. The water may contain free-living protozoa, and the urine destroys trophozoites. Sample containers should be labeled with the patient's name and the date and time of collection and then transported to the laboratory as soon as possible. The accompanying test requisition should provide the same information as well as clinical information (e.g., diagnosis, symptoms, travel history). Last, fecal specimens should be collected before the start of any drug treatments that can reduce parasite numbers. If the patient has been given barium sulfate to facilitate radiological study of the gastrointestinal tract, sample collection should be postponed for at least a week. The crystalline residue of the barium makes it difficult to visually detect intestinal parasites.

Pinworm (*Enterobius vermicularis*) females migrate at night to the perianal area to lay their eggs. Eggs rarely are found in stool. And although timing is not critical, the best time to obtain pinworm samples is in the morning before bathing. Anal swabs are used to detect the presence of pinworms. A cotton swab is rubbed over the perianal folds, but should not be inserted into the anus. The swab is then placed in a clean, dry tube, capped, and sent directly to the lab. Alternately, a strip of transparent adhesive tape is folded over a tongue depressor, sticky side out. The tip of the tape is pressed against the skin in several places around the anus. The tape is then placed sticky side down on a clean, labeled microscope slide and sent to the lab as soon as possible. Another method for collecting pinworm eggs involves the use of a smooth plastic paddle coated with tacky adhesive (Swube® Paddle, Becton, Dickinson and Company, Lincoln Park, NJ). The paddle handle is inserted through a cap of a 17 × 100 mm plastic tube

✪ TABLE 6-1

Common Fecal Preservatives

Preservative	Primary Use
Formalin, 10%	All-purpose preservative (preserves helminth eggs, larvae, and protozoan cysts) well suited for concentration and immunoassay procedures, and compatible use with acid-fast and fluorescent stains
Formalin and mercury-free fixatives (e.g., Ecofix® and Parasafe®)	Ecologically safe preservatives well suited for concentration and most immunoassay procedures and trichrome stain
Low-viscosity polyvinyl-alcohol	Preservation of morphology of protozoan cysts and trophozoites stable for several months
Merthiolate-iodine-formaldehyde	Bifunctional preservative (helminth eggs and larvae) and stain suitable for concentration procedures
Schaudinn's fixative	Preservation of morphology of protozoan cysts and trophozoites
Sodium acetate-acetic acid-formalin	Buffered preservative well suited for concentration and immunoassay procedures and compatible use with most permanent stains

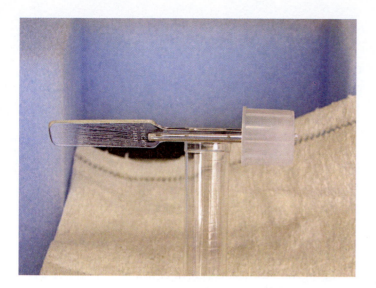

■ **FIGURE 6-3** Swube paddle.

(Figure 6-3 ■) and used in the same manner as tape. Once sampling is complete, the paddle is replaced in the labeled tube for transport to the lab. Paddle-collected specimens should be refrigerated if a transport delay of 24 hours or more is expected because the eggs remain infective and can hatch.

Urine

Urine is the specimen of choice in cases of infection by *Schistosoma haematobium*. Because the maximum numbers of eggs are shed at midday, the best specimens are collected between 10:00 A.M. and 2:00 P.M. into a sterile, screw-capped container (World Health Organization [WHO], 1991). Motile trophozoites of *Trichomonas vaginalis* may also be found in freshly voided urine, though infections by this flagellate are more frequently detected by examining material collected using a sterile cotton swab from the vagina, from the urethra, and in prostatic secretions. If a transport delay of the urine of an hour or more is anticipated, 1 mL of undiluted formalin (37%) or 2 mL of bleach can be added per 100 mL or urine to preserve *Schistosoma* eggs (WHO, 1991).

 Checkpoint! 6–5 (Chapter Objective 5)

The microbiology laboratory received a fresh stool sample in an appropriately labeled, securely capped container. The accompanying requisition identified the specimen as "stool for pinworm examination." What should be done with the sample?

A. *Examine immediately "as is" for the presence of pinworm larvae and ova*

B. *Reject as a poor-quality specimen for the testing requested*

C. *Mix with equal parts of PVA and examine for pinworm larvae only*

D. *Refrigerate until the supervisor can contact the patient for more information*

Blood, Tissue, and Sputa

Whole blood is the choice specimen to examine parasites of the blood, including *Plasmodium* spp., *Trypanosoma* spp., *Babesia* spp., and microfilariae (e.g., *Loa Loa, Wuchereria bancrofti*). Parasitemia may demonstrate periodicity depending on the organism involved. Specific timed blood collection may be necessary.

Typically, anticoagulated venous blood is adequate for the variety of diagnostic tests performed to investigate infection by blood parasites, including the examination of stained blood smears. However, common anticoagulants (EDTA, sodium citrate, and heparin) can interfere with the staining characteristics of blood and cause morphologic distortions of blood parasites, especially if there is a delay in making the smears (greater than 1 hour). For this reason, whenever possible, fresh capillary blood obtained by dermal puncture should be used to make both thick and thin smears (Figure 6-4 ■) that are allowed to air dry prior to transport to the laboratory. Thick blood smears are made by pooling two or three small drops of blood in the center of a methanol-cleaned slide and gently spreading the blood to cover an area of 2 centimeters. Thin smears are prepared in the same way as ones made in hematology for manual differential analysis.

Biopsied tissue is usually required to aid diagnosis of infections caused by parasites that do not circulate in the blood (e.g., *Trichinella spiralis*), that are rarely found in the blood (e.g., *Onchocerca volvulus*), or that are difficult to recover from other types of specimens such as sputum. Typically, these specimens are sent in appropriately labeled and sterile, screw-capped containers to pathology for fixation, embedding, sectioning, and staining. In some instances, fresh tissue may be imprinted directly onto a labeled clean glass slide prior to fixation.

Diagnosis of infection by *Paragonimus westermani* is facilitated by the microscopic examination of expectorated sputum for ova. The infective filariform larvae of *Strongyloides stercoralis* may be observed in sputum in cases of hyperinfection.

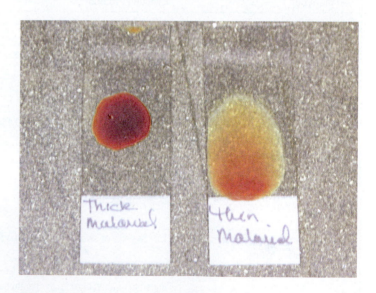

■ **FIGURE 6-4** Thick and thin malarial blood smears.

On rare occasion, the larvae of *Ascaris lumbricoides* and hookworm and the cysts of *Entamoeba histolytica* may be found in sputum. Sputum for examination in these cases should be collected in the early morning. Depending on the type of examination performed, samples may be submitted unfixed or chemically treated. For example, thick samples should be treated with 3% sodium hydroxide to reduce viscosity in preparation for microscopic examination of sediment. Sputa may also be preserved with 10% formalin and/or PVA when sediment will be used to make permanent stained slides. ∞ Chapters 15 and 30 provide additional information on processing specimens for ova and parasites and parasitic infections.

VIROLOGY

Advances in rapid diagnostic technology and the advent of routine molecular-based testing have ushered in a new era in which laboratory diagnosis of viral illness is the norm. Accordingly, the proper collection and handling of the correct specimen remains paramount. A number of factors determine what specimen to collect, as well as when and how to collect it. These factors include site of infection, viral characteristics, and method of analysis. However, as a general rule, the following approaches are recommended:

- Collect samples during the acute phase of infection. This is because the greatest number of viral particles is present early in the disease process.
- Samples collected from areas heavily populated by normal bacterial flora should be placed in antibiotic-containing transport media to reduce the numbers of bacteria

and fungi and to prevent sample drying. This is especially true of specimens taken from the upper respiratory tract and the lower genitourinary tract.

- Transport specimens to the lab immediately after collection. If transport must be delayed, refrigerate (all but blood) or leave samples at room temperature. If a delay of more than 3 days is anticipated, freeze samples at –70°C or lower (all but blood).
- Containers should be securely capped or sealed to prevent loss of sample and leakage during transportation.
- Viral lesions should be gently cleansed with sterile saline prior to sampling and the collection swab premoistened with the same.
- Vesicular fluid collected with a syringe and needle should be placed in a sterile container. The syringe and needle should be rinsed with viral transport media into the same container.
- Use of cotton-tipped or wood-shafted swabs is not recommended (Isenberg, 2004).

Table 6-2✪ summarizes collection protocols for the more common specimen types submitted for viral studies. See ∞ Chapters 16 and 31 to review viral, chlamydial, and rickettsial specimen processing and viral infections.

MYCOBACTERIAL SPECIMEN COLLECTION AND HANDLING

Mycobacteria are characterized as nonmotile, non-spore-forming, small, rod-shaped microorganisms. They are strict aerobes, and compared to most other bacteria, they are slow growing (e.g., taking more than 5 days to demonstrate colony

✪ TABLE 6-2

Viral Specimen Collection Protocols

Sample Type	Collection Protocol	Some Viruses of Interest
Blood	1–10 mL collected in anticoagulant; store at room temperature if processing delayed	Cytomegalovirus, herpesviruses, retroviruses.
Biopsy tissue	Place few grams in sterile container and add viral transport media	Cytomegalovirus, herpesviruses, adenoviruses, arboviruses
Nonurine biological fluids (e.g., CSF, serous fluid)	Minimum of 2 mL in sterile container; store refrigerated if processing delayed	Cytomegalovirus, herpesviruses, coxsackieviruses, enteroviruses
Stool	Few grams or mL (if liquid) in sterile container with viral transport media	Adenoviruses, enteroviruses, retroviruses
Swabbed genital tissue	Place swab in viral transport media	Cytomegalovirus, herpesviruses
Swabbed nasal, nasopharyngeal, or pharyngeal aspirates	Place swab in viral transport media	Rhinoviruses, adenoviruses, cytomegalovirus, herpesviruses, respiratory syncytial virus
Sputum or bronchoscopic samples	Place in sterile container	Respiratory syncytial virus, cytomegalovirus, adenoviruses
Tissue scrapings, swabbed vesicular lesion, vesicular aspirate	Place material or swabs in viral transport media	Herpesviruses, cytomegalovirus, enterovirsuses, poxviruses
Urine	Collect freshly voided urine in sterile, leakproof container; refrigerate or keep at room temperature	Cytomegalovirus, mumps and measles viruses

formation on solid culture media). Their cell walls are fortified by a thick layer of lipid that resists staining with **aniline dyes** such as those used for the Gram stain procedure and resist decolorization by acid and acid-alcohol rinses. Hence, the mycobacteria are distinguished as acid-fast bacteria. The organisms are known to cause a variety of chronic infections in humans, though pulmonary infection or tuberculosis (TB) with *Mycobacterium tuberculosis* predominates public health interest. Mycobacteria can be isolated from myriad specimens, including respiratory, body fluids, tissues, and blood. A combination of direct microscopic examination of stained smears and inoculation of solid media remains the standard and most sensitive means of detecting and recovering acid-fast bacilli from clinical material.

Sputum and bronchoscopic collections are the most commonly collected specimens sent to the laboratory to recover mycobacteria. The necessity of submitting large numbers of sputum specimens for bacteriological diagnosis of pulmonary mycobacterial infection (tuberculosis) has been questioned in recent years (Cascina, Fietta, & Casali, 2000; Nelson, Deike, & Cartwright, 1998). Nevertheless, it is recommended that at least two, first-morning, deep cough sputum or bronchoscopic samples of substantive volume be collected and submitted in separate, sterile containers. Contents should be secured with tight-fitting, screw-capped lids and labeled appropriately. If a delay in transport or processing is anticipated, these samples may be refrigerated. Likewise, other body fluids (e.g., urine, CSF), aspirates, and solid tissues should be submitted in sterile, securely capped containers. Timed or pooled urine samples are generally not acceptable specimens because they are more likely to be contaminated with normal urethral flora and contain few if any mycobacteria.

Mycobacterium avium complex (MAC) is recognized as causing severe opportunistic infections in those with AIDS (Horsburgh, 1999). The specimens of choice in these cases include fresh stool and blood (Talbot, Reller, & Frothingham, 1999). The stool should be collected in clean, wide-mouth containers and immediately submitted to the lab for processing. Prolonged transport warrants keeping the sample frozen.

Mycobacteria require complex culture media; therefore, routine blood culture systems are not adequate for the recovery of these bacteria from the blood. Culture methods in common use generally fall into three categories. The first category includes those methods where blood is directly inoculated into bottles containing liquid culture medium (e.g., BacT/ALERT MB, BioMerieux, Durham, NC). The second category includes methods in which the blood is collected into an evacuated tube (e.g., ISOLATOR 10, Wampole Laboratories, Cranbury, NJ) containing anticoagulant and chemicals that lyse the blood cells. Following centrifugation, the blood sediment is inoculated onto solid culture media. The Septi-Chek method (BD, Franklin Lakes, NJ) is a **biphasic media system** because it uses both solid and liquid media. Blood is decontaminated and concentrated prior to inoculation into 7H9 liquid media. A solid media slide is screwed into the top of the culture bottle, which is periodically inverted to allow the liquid media to coat the solid media. Regardless of the culture method used, the blood samples are collected using aseptic technique and should be collected prior to the start of drug treatment. See ∞ Chapter 13, "Acid-Fast Bacilli Cultures," and ∞ Chapter 26, "*Mycobacterium* Species," to read about specimen processing and infectious diseases associated with the mycobacteria.

ANAEROBIC

Anaerobes are normal flora of the human body. By definition, all grow in the absence of oxygen, though some are more oxygen tolerant than others. Consequently, infections involving anaerobes can and do occur at any body site, especially those where exposure to oxygen is minimal. Based on this information, it is apparent that not all specimen types are appropriate for anaerobic culture (Table 6-3✪).

Anaerobic specimens should be collected and transported as quickly as possible to the lab in a manner that preserves the moist anaerobic atmosphere of the original site of infection. Although sterile screw-capped, containers or sealed syringes can be used to transport specimens for anaerobic culture, specially designed transport systems are preferred. These systems are comprised of a tube, vial, or similar oxygen-free container that contains prereduced, anaerobically sterilized media (PRAS). Examples of different types of anaerobic transport systems are shown in Figure 6-5 ■. ∞ Chapter 24 provides additional facts about anaerobic bacteria and their diseases.

✪ TABLE 6-3

Anaerobic Specimens

Appropriate	Inappropriate
Purulent material and drainage from soft tissue wounds (e.g., bite wound)	Skin surface swabs
Biopsy tissue	Sputum
Aspirated material from abscesses	Gastric washes
Nonurine aspirated biological fluids	Voided urine
Blood and bile	Vaginal swabs
Surgical specimens	Throat or nasal swabs
Bowel contents	Stool

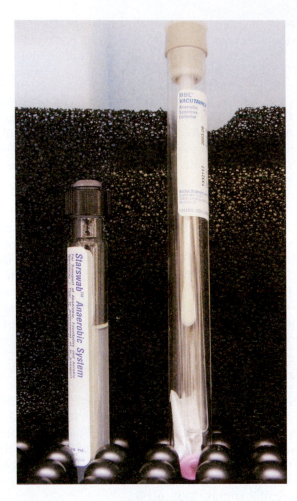

■ FIGURE 6-5 Anaerobic transport systems.

SPECIAL CIRCUMSTANCES

Traditionally, the clinical microbiology laboratory's role has been primarily a diagnostic one: detect and characterize microbial pathogens recovered from clinical specimens, and measure the pathogens' susceptibility to antimicrobial drugs. However, recent events with global impact have helped redefine this traditional role to include active investigation of the potential threat and source of infectious diseases (Snyder, 2003). Furthermore, following terrorist incidents early in the twenty-first century, the Centers for Disease Control and Prevention (CDC) developed a program that provides for a unified public health response to criminal acts in which microbial pathogens and toxins are used (Sewell, 2003). As part of the response network, clinical microbiology laboratory personnel are expected to be knowledgeable and trained in the safe collection and handling of specimens that may contain these pathogens (Centers for Disease Control and Prevention [CDC], 2000). The following sections address sample collection and handling issues in these special circumstances.

Epidemiological and Infection Control Activity

The study and measurement of the distribution and frequency of occurrence of disease in populations is **epidemiology.**

Within a healthcare facility, such as a hospital, investigative study of infectious disease with emphasis on the prevention of disease transmission is known as **infection control.** In both instances, nonclinical, such as the environment and formites, as well as clinical samples may be collected. To effectively support epidemiological and infection control efforts without wasting resources, clinical microbiology laboratories should establish criteria consistent with those of the established infection control plan that identify circumstances when samples should be collected and, in these cases, what specimens to collect. Ideally, specimens selected should have the greatest likelihood of providing meaningful information. They must not be selected arbitrarily or collected based on ease of collection because the true source of infection may be missed. Rather, these types of specimens are selected according to established protocols. Importantly, consideration must be given to the method of sample analysis and the analytical capabilities of the clinical laboratory. For example, most clinical laboratories are not equipped to handle investigations in which the primary samples are food or pharmaceuticals. In these situations, the clinical laboratory should refer the samples to a public health or reference laboratory for workup. Alternately, clinical laboratories are well suited to investigate outbreaks of infectious diseases in which the specimens of choice are body fluids, swabbed tissues, or expectorated material. Table 6-4 lists examples of the types of samples that may be collected in support of these activities. Visit ∞ Chapter 40 to learn more about opportunistic infections.

> ✓ **Checkpoint! 6–6**
> **(Chapter Objective 6)**
>
> *The clinical microbiology laboratory receives a carton of potato salad served at a hospital dinner where several people reportedly got sick. What should the microbiology technologist do next?*
>   A. *Return the specimen to the sender as "quantity insufficient."*
>   B. *Refer the sample to the state public health lab.*
>   C. *Refrigerate the sample until further instructions are received from infection control.*
>   D. *Inoculate an aliquot of salad in an aerobic and anaerobic blood culture bottle.*

Biological Threat Agents

Biological threat agents (BTAs) are microbial pathogens and toxins that have been considered for or used as weapons of war and in the commission of terrorist acts (Isenberg, 2004). Increased threats and incidences when these agents were used in recent years prompted the development of a list categorizing the biological threat agents according to the level of threat posed. For example, agents in category A include pathogens not commonly isolated in the clinical microbiology laboratory but that pose a risk to national security because they are easily dispersed or transmitted, they are highly infectious resulting in high rates of death, and they require special actions for public health preparedness (Morse, 2001). Organisms and toxins listed in category B have potential for large-scale dissemination, but

✪ TABLE 6-4

Epidemiological and Infection Control Specimen Types

Activity	Sample Type	Microbes of Interest
Environmental surveillance	Water	*Legionella* species
		Pseudomonas aeruginosa
		Rotavirus
		Enterics
	Swabbed surfaces	*Legionella* species
		Bacillus cereus
		Pseudomonas aeruginosa
	Air	*Aspergillus fumigatus*
		Mycobacterium tuberculosis
Infection control	Hemodialysate	Gram-negative bacilli
	Intravascular devices	Staphylococci
		Gram-negative bacilli
	Employee hands/nose	Yeast (*Candida* species)
		Gram-negative bacilli
		Gram-positive cocci
		Staphylococci

they have been determined to cause less illness and death in the population of interest than those in category A. Category C agents are not considered a present public health or life risk, though they have immense potential as biological threat agents.

Local community medical care facilities, including clinical laboratories, are the first places that those exposed to BTAs go to get help. It is obvious that the clinical microbiology lab will,

 REAL WORLD TIP

CDC established the laboratory response network (LRN). This network of laboratories is able to respond to biological and chemical terrorism as well as other public health emergencies. Sentinel laboratories are large hospitals which act as the first line of defense and detection. They refer suspicious samples to larger designated laboratories. The reference laboratories are able to perform testing to detect and confirm most bioterrorism agents. They do not have to refer the organisms, other than those which are highly infectious, to CDC. The national laboratories are able to work with highly infectious agents and identify specific strains of organisms. This nationwide network provides a means of rapid detection and identification of potential threats to the health of the U.S. citizens.

in these cases, be called on to assist in the investigation. Given the deadly nature of the BTAs and the importance of providing timely and accurate test results to identify possible exposure situations and resulting disease outbreaks, it is the responsibility of clinical microbiology laboratorians to have more than a brief familiarity with sample collection and handling protocols for BTA events (Somrak & Ward-Cook, 2004). What sample to collect and when to collect is dependent on not only the type of BTA and the route of exposure but also by the amount of time that has elapsed since exposure. Table 6-5✪ summarizes the basics of specimen collection and handling in these cases.

✪ TABLE 6-5

Specimen Collection in Cases of Biological Threat Agent Exposure

Agent	Disease	Threat Category	Specimen Type	Handling Conditions
Bacillus anthracis	Anthrax	A	Swab of lesion material, stool, blood, and sputum	Transport to lab at room temperature within 2 hours of collection; refrigerate stool and sputum if transport delayed more 2 hours
Brucella species	Brucellosis	B	Serum, blood, liver, spleen, or bone marrow	Transport tissues at room temperature; deliver to lab within 2 hours following collection; serum should be stored and transported frozen at −20°C
Clostridium botulinum toxin	Botulism	A	Nasal swab, exudate, serum, food, stool, soil and water	Transport nasal swab, soil, and water at room temperature; all other samples transport refrigerated
Viruses (e.g., Ebola, Marburg)	Hemorrhagic fever	A	Serum	Transport at room temperature within 2 hours of collection or refrigerate if delay anticipated
Francisella tularensis	Tularemia	A	Sputum, throat swab, bronchoscopic washes, blood	Transport to lab at room temperature within 2 hours of collection; refrigerate respiratory samples if transport delayed more than 2 hours
Ricin Toxin	Ricin poisoning	B	Nasal swab, respiratory secretions, serum	Transport refrigerated within 24 hours of collection.
Variola major	Smallpox	A	Vesicular fluid swab, scabs, biopsy tissue	Transport refrigerated within 6 hours of collection; store frozen (−20°C to −70°C).
Yersinia pestis	Plague	A	Sputum, throat swab, bronchoscopic washes, blood	Transport to lab at room temperature within 2 hours of collection; refrigerate respiratory samples if transport delayed not more than 24 hours

Checkpoint! 6–7 (Chapter Objective 7)

A university student mailroom worker is suspected of being exposed to an aerosolized category "A" biological threat agent within the last 36 hours. The student health clinic wants to know what specimen(s) should be collected. What do you advise? (Refer to Table 6-5.)

   A. *Fresh stool and expectorated sputum*
   B. *Blood and sputum*
   C. *Nasal swab and blood*
   D. *Gastric aspirate and stool*

SUMMARY

The validity and usefulness of the information produced by the clinical microbiology laboratory is dependent on the quality of specimens submitted. This chapter discussed the basics of specimen collection with emphasis on what types of specimens are collected, when and how they should be collected, and how they should be handled. For a summary of the basics of specimen collection for the clinical microbiology laboratory, see Table 6-6✪.

In general, specimens should be collected in containers that are sterile, leakproof, and correctly identified with patient and sample information. To ensure the recovery of potential

✪ TABLE 6-6

Summary of the Basics of Specimen Collection

Specimen Source	Collection Container	Patient Preparation	Time for Transport	Notes
Blood	Blood culture media (dependent on automated analyzer type)	Scrub venipuncture area first with 70% alcohol for at least 30s; let dry completely. Next cleanse with tincture of iodine or chlorhexidine, swabbing concentrically, starting at the center of the area; let area dry completely. Do not repalpate the skin.	≤ 4 hours at RT	Disinfect tops of culture bottles with alcohol. Optimum volume is 20 mL per set (adults). Maximum of 3 sets in 24 hours (adults). Draw cultures before starting antimicrobial therapy.
Respiratory—Upper				
Throat	Swab/culturette device		≤ 2 hours at RT	Swab only posterior pharynx/ tonsils. Do not let swab touch tongue or cheeks.
Nasopharyngeal	Minitip swab (thin wire or flexible)/culturette device			Place swab into posterior nasopharynx; rotate 5 seconds.
Sinus	Sterile container or syringe			Aspirate material from sinuses
Ear (inner)	Swab/culturette device or sterile container	Clean ear canal with mild soap		Aspirate through eardrum or use swab if drum is broken
(outer)	Swab/culturette device	Disinfect skin with alcohol		Firmly rotate swab in outer canal
Eye	Swab/culturette device, syringe, or sterile container	Disinfect skin around eye		Depending on symptoms, physician may roll swab over conjunctiva, perform corneal scraping, or aspirate intraocular fluid
Respiratory—Lower				
Sputum	Sterile container		≤ 2 hours at RT	Instruct patient to collect by deep cough; do not collect postnasal fluid; may need to induce by nebulizer with the inhalation of saline
Bronchoscopy	Sterile container or Lukens trap			Bronchial lavage, wash, protected catheter brush, or tracheal aspirate
Genital—Female				
Cervix/Vagina	Swab/culturette device; transport media for GC (collect additional swab for wet prep)	Clear mucus/exudate with swab; do not use lubricant on speculum	≤ 2 hours at RT	Swab into cervix or swab secretions of vaginal canal

Summary of the Basics of Specimen Collection *(continued)*

Specimen Source	Collection Container	Patient Preparation	Time for Transport	Notes
Urethra	Swab/culturette device	Disinfect skin		Massage or swab exudate
Bartholin cyst, Cul-de-sac, endometrium	Sterile container			Aspirate of fluid or biopsy of tissue
Lesion	Swab/culturette device or sterile container	Clean with saline; unroof vesicle or crust		Aspirate or firmly rub with swab to collect exudate
Genital—Male				
Prostate	Swab/culturette device or sterile container		≤ 2 hours at RT	Prostatic massage
Urethra	Swab/culturette device; transport media for *N. gonorrhoeae*			Insert swab into urethra 2–4 cm, rotate for 2 seconds; or express discharge onto transport media
Lesion	Swab/culturette device or sterile container			Aspirate or firmly rub with swab to collect exudate
Stool	Clean container, swab/culturette device, or transport media		≤ 1 hour at RT; ≤ 24 hours in preservative at RT	Collect directly into wide-mouthed container or insert swab 2.5 cm past sphincter and rotate into anal crypts
Wound/Soft tissue Wounds Tissue	Sterile container, swab/culturette device	Disinfect skin of closed wound; debride and rinse open wound with sterile saline	≤ 2 hours at RT	Aspirate fluid from closed wound, remove tissue from leading edge of infection, or swab wound concentrating on areas of inflammation or pus
Urine				
Clean-voided midstream	Sterile container	Have patient cleanse urethral area with soap, rinse with sterile saline	≤ 2 hours at RT; ≤ 24 hours refrigerated; for delayed transport use preservative	Collect directly into container; do not stop flow of urine; move container into path of voiding urine
Catheter		Cleanse skin before insertion if using straight catheter; disinfect port before sampling		Use straight catheter or aspirate from catheter port using syringe; never collect from bag
Suprapubic aspirate		Disinfect skin over bladder		Needle aspirate directly from bladder
Nonurine body fluids	Sterile, leakproof container	Aseptic cleansing of skin	<2 hours at RT	Collected by percutaneous needle aspiration
Fungal				
Skin, hair nails	Sterile container	Cleanse skin with 70% alcohol	As soon as possible	
Body fluids, exudates, tissues	Sterile, leakproof container with media as appropriate	Use aseptic technique	As soon as possible	Urine may be stored refrigerated
Parasitology				
Feces	Clean, leakproof vial with preservative		As soon as possible	For pinworm, a swab collection should be placed in a dry, capped container
Urine	Sterile screw-capped container		As soon as possible	Transparent tape on clean labeled slide is acceptable as is a paddle collection device
Blood	EDTA blood tube	Use aseptic technique	As soon as possible As soon as possible	For feces, >1 hour transport delay, add 1 mL undiluted formalin or 2 mL bleach per 100 mL of fluid
Tissue, sputa	Sterile, screw-capped container	Unfixed or chemically treated with 10% formalin or PVA		When possible, submit thick and thin blood smears prepared from fresh capillary blood
Viral	Leakproof, sterile container or culturette with transport media as appropriate		Immediately at RT	Except for blood, specimens may be frozen at −70°C in cases of transport delays > 3 days

pathogens, transport media may need to be added, though some containers come prepackaged with appropriate media. Sufficient quantity of sample should be collected for the testing required. Specimens should always be sent to the lab as soon after collection as possible. For delays of more than a few hours, samples should be stored under conditions that mini-

mize exposure to environmental extremes such as low humidity and heat. Also, the ideal sample is collected before symptoms associated with infection have subsided, before treatment is started, and in a manner that avoids contaminating the sample with normal flora. In this way, the results will prove accurate as well as reliable.

LEARNING OPPORTUNITIES

1. Visit the following websites and explore information pertinent to specimen collection. (Chapter Objective 8)

   a. Centers for Disease Control and Prevention(CDC), National Center for Infectious Diseases, Division of Parasitic Diseases, Diagnostic Procedures at URL http://www.dpd.cdc.gov/dpdx/HTML/DiagnosticProcedures.htm

   b. Centers for Disease Control and Prevention(CDC), Bioterrorism Training and Education http://www.bt.cdc.gov/bioterrorism/training.asp#general

   c. Centers for Disease Control and Prevention(CDC), Bioterrorism Preparedness and Response Program, Laboratory Information, Shipping Specimens URL http://www.bt.cdc.gov/labissues/index.asp#shipping

   d. Kortepeter, Mark LTC, Christopher, George, LTC, Cieslak, Ted, COL, eds. *Medical Management of Biological Casualties Handbook,* 5th edition. U.S. Army Medical Research Institute of Infectious Diseases (USAMRIID), Fort Detrick, Fredrick, Maryland, 2005. Online at http://www.usamriid.army.mil/education/instruct.htm

2. Have a question about specimen collection answered by the clinical experts at American Society for Microbiology C Division URL http://www.asm.org/division/c/index.htm (Chapter Objective 8)

3. Create a specimen collection card file (Chapter Objectives 2, 3, and 4)

4. A voided urine specimen is received in the laboratory at 8:00 am. The specimen is discovered at 1:00 pm sitting behind a computer monitor at the processing bench. It had not been processed yet so the microbiologist set it up. What is the effect of the 5 hour delay on the specimen results? (Chapter Objective 1)

   a. There is no effect and the specimen can be cultured.

   b. The potential pathogens present may not grow due to the delay.

   c. Any organisms present will overgrow and it will be difficult to determine the true potential pathogen.

   d. Any normal flora of the urogenital tract present will be inhibited but the potential pathogens will continue to grow.

5. A patient calls the microbiology laboratory for directions on how to collect a stool sample for a culture for *Salmonella* and *Shigella*. You request the patient to submit a: (Chapter Objective 2)

   a. stool specimen which has been preserved in polyvinyl alcohol

   b. stool in a clean, wide mouth container with a secure lid

   c. rectal swab

   d. stool specimen in viral transport medium

6. A physician calls the microbiology laboratory for information on the collection of an anaerobic wound culture. The doctor suspects the patient has osteomyelitis of the right tibia. There is a sinus tract leading to the skin surface which has a continuous discharge of pus. You request the physician submit: (Chapter Objectives 2, 3, and 4)

   a. a bone biopsy

   b. an aerobic swab of the sinus tract drainage

   c. both an aerobic and anaerobic swab of the sinus tract drainage

   d. fluid from the joint closest to the infection

7. The rubber stopper of a blood culture bottle must be cleaned prior to specimen collection with: (Chapter Objective 4)

   a. 2% tincture of iodine

   b. 70% alcohol

   c. soap and water

   d. chlorhexidine

8. Which of the following cells is used to determine the quality of expectorated sputum and anaerobic wound specimens? (Chapter Objective 5)

   a. ciliated columnar epithelial cells

   b. white blood cells

   c. red blood cells

   d. squamous epithelial cells

9. Four patients in the oncology unit have developed pneumonia due to *Legionella pneumophila*. Which of the following specimen type/body sites should be cultured by the infection control team as a possible source of the initial infections? (Chapter Objective 6)

   a. swabs of the hands of the oncology unit healthcare personnel

   b. portions of the food served to the patients

   c. swabs of and water from the sink and faucets in the patients' rooms

   d. nasal swabs of visitors of the patients

10. A large metropolitan hospital has been designated a sentinel laboratory by CDC. The microbiology department receives a white powder from the emergency room. The powder was received in the mail at the local police station. The laboratory should: (Chapter Objective 7)

    a. try to identify the suspicious powder

    b. refer the powder to CDC for testing

    c. culture the powder for the presence of *Bacillus anthracis*

    d. refer the powder to the nearest CDC designated reference laboratory for testing

myhealthprofessionskit

Use this address to access the interactive Companion Website created for this textbook. Simply select "Clinical Laboratory Science" from the choice of disciplines. Find this book and log in using your user name and password.

REFERENCES

Go to myhealthprofessionskit.com to view this chapter's references.

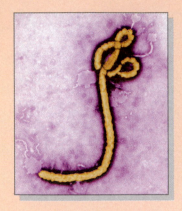

OUTLINE

7

Cultivation of Microorganisms

Karen M. Kiser

■ LEARNING OBJECTIVES

Upon completion of this chapter, the learner should be able to:

1. Distinguish between the pour plate and streak plate methods of isolation.
2. Provide examples of general purpose, selective, differential, enrichment, and transport culture media.
3. Correlate the growth pattern of bacteria on various types of culture media.
4. Identify the steps required in the preparation and storage of media.
5. Categorize organisms based on their preferred temperature for growth.
6. Classify bacteria as obligate aerobe, microaerophilic, capnophilic, obligate anaerobe, or facultative anaerobe, using growth patterns.
7. Apply rejection criteria to assess specimen suitability.
8. Select the appropriate primary media based on the specimen source.
9. Determine the order of media inoculation given a specimen.
10. Identify the correct technique for incubation of solid media.

KEY TERMS

aerotolerant anaerobe	facultative anaerobe	obligate anaerobe
agar	general purpose	psychrophile
ambient air	homogenized	purulent
anaerobic	inoculation	quantitative culture
calibrated loop	meningitis	selective
capnophilic	mesophiles	supplements
critical or panic value	microaerophilic	transport
differential	obligate aerobe	xanthochromia
enrichment		

▶ INTRODUCTION

In previous chapters, you have been asked to learn about the structure and physiology of microorganisms. This information provides you with the background needed to understand how they invade and cause disease. It also has a practical application when considering the growth needs of potential pathogens. The lab must provide the optimal growth environment by providing the organisms with the nutrients, atmosphere, and temperature they require. Lack of growth of a potential pathogen may be because of failure to provide the proper conditions for growth. The consequences to a patient could be devastating.

This chapter will outline the basic conditions used for the cultivation of microorganisms. The different forms and kinds of media will be described as well as the temperature and atmosphere of incubation. In addition, the tools and process of specimen transfer to media will be presented.

▶ MEDIA

Artificial media is designed to meet the growth needs of microorganisms of interest. All media share a basic foundation of nutrients and a solidifying agent, if desired. The best possible pH is also important for growth. Additional substances may be added to enrich the medium. Table 7-1 ✪ provides a list of nutrients commonly included in media. See ∞ Chapter 3, "The Bacterial Cell," to review information on the growth of bacterial cells.

FORMS

The three basic forms of media are liquid, solid, and semisolid. A brief description of each media form follows.

Liquid

Liquid media flows when the tube or bottle in which it is located is tilted. Organisms can grow throughout the medium and make it appear cloudy or turbid, rather then clear. Organ-

✪ TABLE 7-1	
Common Media Ingredients	
Nutrients Necessary for Growth	**Media Ingredient Supplying Nutrient**
Nitrogen, carbon	Peptone, beef or yeast extracts
Inorganic phosphate, sulfur, trace metals	Phosphate, sulfate, magnesium, calcium, iron
Growth factors	Blood, serum, vitamins, NAD (factor V), hemin (factor X)
Energy source	Carbohydrates
Protective agents	Calcium carbonate, starch, charcoal
Water	Distilled or deionized water

NAD = nicotinamide-adenine dinucleotide

isms can also grow as a pellicle or film across the surface on the liquid or as a sediment at the bottom of the tube. Some can appear as puffballs throughout the liquid. Liquid medium is used to detect small numbers of organisms in body fluids, biopsies, and other tissue samples which may not be detected on solid medium.

Solid

Solid media results when 1% to 2% **agar**, a seaweed product that solidifies liquid culture media, is added to liquid media, causing it to become firm (Koneman, Allen, Janda, Schreckenberger, & Winn, 1997). Its consistency is similar to gelatin. Like gelatin, heat is used to dissolve the agar, and the media is liquid during preparation. When the medium cools below 50°C, it begins to solidify. It may be packaged in petri dishes or tubes as slants or deeps like motility medium.

Usually the clinical specimen is placed on the surface of solid medium, so that the growth of organisms can be observed as individual colonies. These colonies can be easily used for identification and susceptibility assays, if judged clinically significant. Occasionally the specimen is added to the medium while still liquid, but still cool enough so organisms survive (45°C–50°C). This is called a pour plate, and organisms will grow throughout the solid medium as well as on the surface. This approach is good when colony counts are desired, but is difficult to use if identification is the task.

> ✔ **Checkpoint! 7–1 (Chapter Objective 1)**
>
> *The pour plate is used primarily to:*
>   A. *determine the number of colony-forming units per mL of liquid.*
>   B. *observe surface colonies for different microbial types.*
>   C. *prepare a mixed culture for long term storage.*
>   D. *enhance the growth of small numbers of microbes.*

Semisolid

Semisolid media is prepared by adding less agar (0.3%–0.5%) during preparation than the amount used in solid medium (Koneman et al., 1997). Its consistency is more like yogurt in that it is soft and will assume the shape of the container. It is usually packaged in tubes. Organisms may grow inside and on the medium, tending to stay where they are placed, unless they are motile. Semisolid medium has been used in certain biochemical tests, such as the sulfur-indole-motility tube, and in long-term storage of microbes. Figure 7-1 ■ depicts slants, deeps, and liquid forms of tubed media.

CATEGORIES

There are many different kinds of media, designed to serve different purposes. They can be categorized according to function. The basic kinds are general purpose, selective, differential,

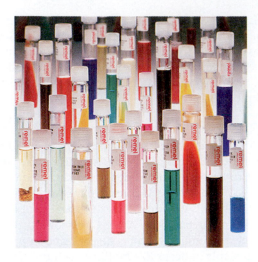

■ **FIGURE 7-1** Various forms of available tubed media. *Photo courtesy of Remel, part of Thermo Fisher Scientific.*

or some combination of these functions. Enrichment and transport media also play an important role in the detection of pathogens. Specialized media provide nutrients to grow a specific organism, whose needs are not met by the routine media. The following sections detail each of these kinds of media.

General Purpose

If the goal is to grow most organisms by meeting their basic nutritional requirements, a **general-purpose** medium designed to grow most microorganisms, or nonselective medium, is used. Some of the more fastidious microorganisms will not grow on this medium, so it's important to consider needs of the microorganism you want to grow. Adding **supplements**, which are nutritional substances that are added to media to enhance growth of microorganisms, such as sheep blood or vitamin K, can enrich general-purpose media. An example of a basic general-purpose medium is trypticase soy agar (TSA). This medium will grow most microorganisms adequately to observe growth or maintain viability. Adding 5% sheep blood to TSA to form sheep blood agar (BA), enriches the medium and more luxurious growth is obtained. An analogy would be to compare a meal of hamburger versus steak. One can survive on hamburger, but steak usually results in a happier diner.

Selective

Selective media is primary media containing inhibitory agents that select for the desired microorganisms while inhibiting the undesirable microorganisms. Various chemicals, antibiotics, and dyes are used to make the medium selective. Supplements can also be added to this media to enhance growth, but its primary purpose is selective. An example of a selective medium is Columbia colistin-nalidixic acid (CNA) agar. It contains colistin and nalidixic acid, two antibiotics that help to select for gram-positive organisms while inhibit-

ing gram-negative ones. If growth is observed on this medium, it is most likely gram-positive. These selective mediums vary in their effectiveness. Some provide total inhibition resulting in no growth of the unwanted organisms. Others just inhibit enough to result in reduced growth of the unwanted organisms, when compared to the desired organism. Sometimes the desired microorganism is inhibited too. Many times a general-purpose medium is added to the primary culture setup to ensure isolation of these strains.

Differential

Differential media allows organism growth to be distinguished using certain growth characteristics and enables the microbiologist to select for certain microorganisms of interest. Most differential mediums are also selective because they inhibit growth of certain microorganisms. An example of a differential medium is MacConkey (MAC) agar (Figure 7-2 ■). It contains bile salts and crystal violet that helps to select for gram-negative rods while inhibiting other organisms. Occasionally yeast can grow, but it is uncommon, and they have a pinpoint dry appearance. This medium also contains the carbohydrate, lactose. Those organisms that use lactose (lactose fermenter [LF]) as they grow will produce pink colonies, whereas those that do not are colorless (non-lactose fermenter [NLF]). The color change in the colony is due to a change in the pH indicator when acid by-products, from lactose fermentation, are produced. When growth occurs on the surface of MacConkey, one usually assumes they are gram-negative rods unless growth characteristics suggest otherwise (pinpoint, dry-looking colonies, for example). Table 7-2✪ provides a list of some compounds used to make media selective or differential.

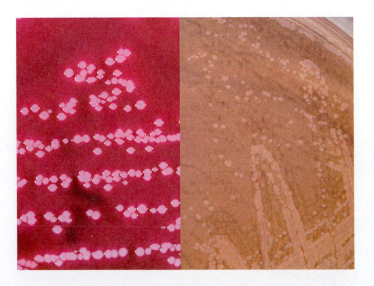

■ **FIGURE 7-2** MacConkey agar with lactose-fermenting (pink) and non-lactose-fermenting (colorless) colonies.

TABLE 7-2

Examples of Selective and Differential Media Ingredients

Ingredient Effect	Ingredients
Selective or inhibitory	Bile salts, deoxycholate, eosin
	Crystal violet, phenylethanol, NaCl
	Antimicrobial agents
	Dyes
Differential dyes or indicator	Phenol red
	Acid fuschin
	Neutral red
	Bromthymol blue
	Bromcresol purple
	Methyl red
Differential compounds	Carbohydrates, sodium thiosulfate and ferric ammonium citrate for hydrogen sulfide production, esculin

REAL WORLD TIP

Sheep blood agar can be considered a differential medium because organisms can be distinguished based on alpha, beta or gamma hemolysis.

Checkpoint! 7–2 (Chapter Objective 2)

When processing a specimen, you want to use a selective medium. You would select:
1. *Columbia colistin-nalidixic acid (CNA) agar*
2. *MacConkey (MAC) agar*
3. *Sheep blood (BA) agar*
   A. *1 & 3*
   B. *1 & 2*
   C. *2 & 3*
   D. *1, 2, & 3*

Enrichment

Enrichment broth is primary media used to enhance growth of small numbers of bacteria. Enrichment broth may also be used to encourage growth of fastidious bacteria (Isenberg, Schoenknecht, & von Graevenitz, 1979). Examples include brain heart infusion (BHI), trypticase soy broth (TSB), and thioglycolate broth (Thio).

When used to isolate fecal pathogens, enrichment media enhances the growth of the pathogens while discouraging the growth of normal bowel flora present in the specimen. Examples include gram-negative (GN) broth and selenite-F broth.

GN broth is used to select for the enteric pathogens *Salmonella* and *Shigella,* while inhibiting the normal intesti-

nal flora. Selenite broth is used to select for *Salmonella.* Inhibition may only be for a short period of time, so the procedure for each medium must be followed. In the case of GN broth, the medium must be subcultured after 6 to 8 hours of incubation for it to work effectively (Gilligan, Janda, Karmali, & Miller, 1991). Selinite-F broth should be subcultured after 12 to 18 hours of incubation (Becton Dickinson, 1988). Commonly used primary plating media, their purposes, and atmosphere of incubation are presented in Table 7-3. Box 7-1 identifies some specialty agars used in the clinical microbiology laboratory for isolation of specific pathogens.

Checkpoint! 7–3 (Chapter Objective 3)

If an organism shows healthy growth on phenylethyl alcohol agar (PEA) and no growth on MacConkey (MAC), the organism is most likely:
A. *a pathogen.*
B. *gram-positive.*
C. *gram-negative.*
D. *a lactose fermenter.*

Transport

Transport media is used to maintain the numbers and viability of organisms without an increase in their numbers during transport or while waiting for processing. It is most often used in doctors' offices and clinics where specimens may be collected but not processed. Usually the microbiology lab is off site, and there is a delay between collection and processing. Transport media (Figure 7-3 ■) is available for anaerobic as well as aerobic organisms. More delicate or fastidious organisms may not survive in transport medium. *Neisseria gonorrhoeae* is very susceptible to drying and changes in temperature. For this reason, do not refrigerate inoculated transport medium and transport as soon as possible (Koneman et al., 1997; Murray, Baron, Pfaller, Tenover, & Yolken, 1999).

Preparation and Storage

Preparation of media is similar to cooking. You follow a recipe, measure and combine ingredients, gently heat to dissolve, and dispense into appropriate containers. However, there are some important differences. When preparing media, one should use chemically clean glassware and distilled water. Weighing and measuring the ingredients should be performed carefully. Overheating the medium should be avoided.

Once the medium is prepared, it is usually sterilized by autoclaving or filtration. If an additive or supplement is used, it is added after sterilization, once the medium has cooled to 55°C to 60°C (Forbes, Sahn, & Weissfeld, 1998). Most facilities purchase media which is premade rather than making it in-house.

The media is stored in a way that prevents dehydration and deterioration. Manufacturer recommendations for storage should be followed. In general, tubed media, with loose-fitting

✪ TABLE 7-3

Commonly Used Plating Media

Medium	Atmosphere	Purpose
Sheep blood agar (SBA or BA)	CO_2 or AN	Growth of most medically significant bacteria; determination of hemolytic reactions
Chocolate agar (CA or CHOC)	CO_2	Cultivation of *Haemophilus* and *Neisseria* species
Columbia colistin-nalidixic acid agar (CNA) Phenylethyl alcohol agar (PEA)	Air or CO_2	Selective isolation of gram-positive organisms
MacConkey agar (MAC) Eosin methylene blue (EMB)	Air	Isolation and differentiation of lactose-fermenting and non-lactose-fermenting enteric bacilli
Hektoen enteric agar (HE) Xylose lysine desoxycholate agar (XLD) Salmonella-Shigella agar (SS)	Air	Isolation of *Salmonella* and *Shigella;* Differentiation of lactose-fermenting, non-lactose-fermenting, and H_2S-producing enteric bacilli
Cefsulodin-Irgasan-novobiocin agar (CIN)	Air	Isolation and differentiation of *Yersinia enterocolitica*
Campy blood agar	MA	Selective for *Campylobacter*
Mannitol salt agar (MSA)	Air	Isolation and differentiation of staphylococci
Streptococcal selective agar	CO_2 or AN	Selective for *Streptococcus pyogenes*
Thayer-Martin agar (TM)	CO_2	Selective for *Neisseria gonorrhoeae* and *Neisseria meningitidis*
Gram-negative (GN) broth	Air	Enrichment for *Salmonella* and *Shigella* in suspected carriers
Thioglycolate broth	Air	Enrichment of small numbers of bacteria and fastidious bacteria
Laked blood kanamycin-vancomycin agar (LKV)	AN	Selective for anaerobic gram-negative rods, especially *Bacteroides* and *Prevotella* spp.

CO_2 = 5%–10% carbon dioxide; AN = anaerobic; Air = ambient air; MA = microaerophilic (5% oxygen, 10% CO_2).

✪ BOX 7-1

Specialized Media for Isolation of Specific Organisms

Sorbitol MacConkey agar (SMAC)
- *E. coli* O157:H7

Thiosulfate citrate bile salt sucrose (TCBS)
- *Vibrio cholerae* and *V. parahemolyticus*

Chromogenic agar
- Available for isolation and differentiation of *Candida* spp., common urinary isolates, *E. coli* O157:H7 and MRSA

Buffered charcoal yeast extract (BCYE)
- *Legionella* spp. and *Francisella tularensis*

Bordet-Gengou agar
- *Bordetella pertussis*

Pseudomonas cepacia agar (PC)
- *Burkholderia cepacia*

Oxidative-fermentative polymyxin B bacitracin lactose agar (OFPBL)
- *Burkholderia cepacia*

Cystine-Tellurite blood agar
- *Corynebacterium diphtheriae*

Regan-Lowe agar
- *Bordetella pertussis*

V agar
- *Gardnerella vaginalis*

Cefsulodin irgasan novobiocin agar (CIN)
- *Yersinia enterocolitica*

caps, have a shorter shelf life then those with tight-fitting caps. Refrigerated media lasts longer than media stored at room temperature. Storage in bags or plastic sleeves also prolongs the shelf life of media. Tubed media with loose caps, stored at room temperature, has an expiration date of 2 weeks. If stored in the refrigerator, tubed media with loose caps has an expiration date of 4 weeks. Tubed media with tight-fitting caps may have an expiration date of 6 months. Plating media stored in plastic

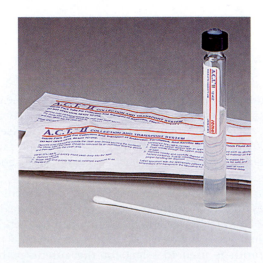

■ **FIGURE 7-3** Transport medium.
Photo courtesy of Remel, part of Thermo Fisher Scientific.

sleeves under refrigeration may have an expiration date of 4 to 10 weeks (Balows, Hausler, Herrmann, Isenberg, & Shadomy, 1991).

 REAL WORLD TIP

While most agar media is usually stored at 4°C prior to use, anaerobic media such as reducible blood agar (RBAP) is usually stored at room temperature. RBAP absorbs less oxygen when stored at room temperature than at 4°C.

Providing the proper nutrients is the first step in the cultivation of microorganisms. Growth will not occur without also providing an environment favorable for growth.

 Checkpoint! 7–4 (Chapter Objective 4)

The best way to store solid plating media to prolong shelf life is:
  A. *at room temperature at the work area.*
  B. *at room temperature in a sealed plastic bag.*
  C. *in a refrigerator, sealed in a plastic bag.*
  D. *in an incubator, sealed in a plastic bag.*

▶ ENVIRONMENT

Components of the environment that support microbial growth include temperature, atmosphere, and humidity. Each of these components is important separately and in combination for the desired outcome of microbial growth. A discussion of each of these components follows.

TEMPERATURE

The first consideration of environmental needs is the temperature. Bacteria can be divided into three categories based on their preferred temperature for growth. **Psychrophiles** prefer 0°C to 20°C (Alcamo, 2001). These organisms live in the cold regions of the world (Arctic and Antarctic) and are not associated with human infectious disease. Thermophiles prefer 40°C to 90°C for growth (Alcamo, 2001). They live in hot springs and compost heaps. Thermophiles can't grow at body temperature. Human pathogens are considered **mesophiles**, microorganisms that grow best at a temperature between 20°C and 40°C (Alcamo, 2001). A few can tolerate temperatures higher than 40°C (Madigan, Martinko, & Parker, 2000). Mesophiles that can grow in cooler temperatures are considered psychrotolerant.

The majority of microorganisms of medical interest grow best at body temperature, or 37°C. Microbiology laboratories routinely use incubators (Figure 7-4 ■) and temperature blocks

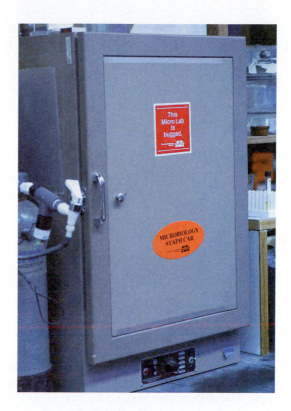

■ **FIGURE 7-4** Tabletop incubator.

(Figure 7-5 ■) set at 35°C to 37°C to incubate inoculated media. A few pathogens don't grow as well at warm temperatures. They prefer 22°C to 25°C or room temperature. Media inoculated for *Yersinia,* an intestinal pathogen, is left on the bench top or placed in an incubator at a temperature of 22°C to 25°C. A cold enrichment technique can be used to enhance the growth of *Yersinia, Listeria* and some *Campylobacter* spp. Incubation of the media or clinical specimens in a refrigerator at a temperature of 4°C to 8°C can encourage the growth of these three organisms and inhibit the growth of others. Some *Campylobacter* species,

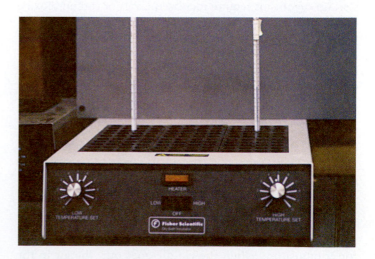

■ **FIGURE 7-5** Temp block.

another intestinal pathogen, can be selectively cultured at 42°C. It's important to know what pathogens may be isolated from a patient specimen, so the optimal temperature for growth is provided. Refer to ∞ Chapters 19, "Aerobic Gram Positive Rods," 21, "*Enterobacteriaceae*," and 23, "*Vibrio, Aeromonas, Plesiomonas, Campylobacter, Helicobacter,* and *Chromobacterium*" to learn more about *Listeria, Yersinia* and *Campylobacter.*

 Checkpoint! 7–5 (Chapter Objective 5)

Microbes that infect humans are:
- A. *psychrophiles.*
- B. *chemophiles.*
- C. *thermophiles.*
- D. *mesophiles.*

ATMOSPHERE

Temperature is not the only consideration when trying to provide the optimum environment for growth. Atmosphere is also a necessary component. Four atmospheres are often provided as culture conditions in the clinical microbiology lab. They are each described here and are known as ambient air, carbon dioxide enriched, microaerophilic, and anaerobic.

Ambient Air

Ambient air is atmosphere available without alteration of the naturally occurring gas concentration of room air. It is the same air that humans breathe. It consists of approximately 21% oxygen, 0.03% carbon dioxide, 78% nitrogen, and a mixture of other gases (Barlow Pugh, 2000). Most aerobic organisms can grow in this atmosphere, although a few may require increased levels of carbon dioxide for growth or may find the level of oxygen toxic.

Carbon Dioxide

Certain organisms require increased levels of carbon dioxide (CO_2) for growth. Most grow better in a CO_2 enriched atmosphere. Those that also require oxygen will grow in an aerobic atmosphere enhanced with 3% to 10% CO_2. Clinical microbiology laboratories have CO_2 incubators that provide an aerobic atmosphere enhanced with 5% to 10% CO_2. These incubators are connected to compressed gas cylinders that supply CO_2. When the door is closed, carbon dioxide is pumped in until the 5% to 10% concentration is achieved. The incubator will also provide the temperature needed for growth.

A candle jar (Figure 7-6 ■) may also be used to provide an aerobic atmosphere with 2% to 3% CO_2 (Isenberg et al., 1979). An unscented candle is placed near the top of a jar with a tight-fitting lid or a desiccator jar, containing the inoculated media. The candle is lit, and the lid is put on. The candle will burn, emitting CO_2, until the oxygen level falls below that required for combustion. When the candle goes out, the air in the unopened jar contains an increased level of CO_2. The oxygen

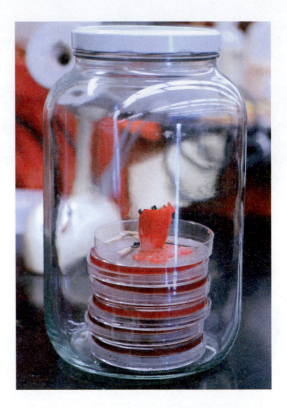

■ **FIGURE 7-6** Candle jar.

level is between 13% and 17% (Murray et al., 1999). The jar is then placed in a 35°C to 37°C incubator.

Microaerophilic

The enteric pathogen *Campylobacter* requires a **microaerophilic** atmosphere, or an atmosphere containing approximately 5% oxygen, 10% carbon dioxide, and 85% nitrogen, for growth (Koneman et al., 1997). An oxygen level greater than 6% harms these organisms. They will not grow in a candle jar because of the high oxygen level of 13% to 17% (Murray et al., 1999). To grow these organisms, the oxygen level must be decreased to lower levels. The microaerophilic atmosphere may be chemically generated or created by pumping the appropriate mixture of gases from a tank into a gas-impermeable bag, containing the inoculated media. More detailed information on *Campylobacter* is provided in ∞ Chapter 23.

Anaerobic

Microorganisms that are harmed by the presence of oxygen require an **anaerobic** atmosphere created when oxygen is removed from the environment, providing conditions for good growth. This can be done chemically or by pumping oxygen free gases into a chamber, jar, or bag. An anaerobic jar is pictured in Figure 7-7 ■.

A chemically generated atmosphere consists of hydrogen and carbon dioxide (Howard, Keiser, Smith, & Weissfeld, 1994). The hydrogen reacts with the oxygen in the jar or bag, producing water. Moisture can be observed as condensation on the

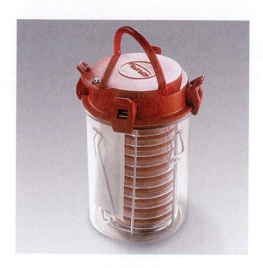

■ **FIGURE 7-7** Anaerobic jar.
Photo courtesy of Remel, part of Thermo Fisher Scientific.

side of the jar and provides early evidence that an anaerobic atmosphere has been achieved.

A mixture of gases consisting of 85% nitrogen, 10% hydrogen, and 5% carbon dioxide can be pumped into a chamber or jar to create an anaerobic atmosphere in these containers. Palladium-coated pellets catalyze the combination of hydrogen and oxygen to produce water that is removed by a dessicant.

Atmospheric Classification

Microorganisms can be classified into categories based on their atmospheric requirements. Aerobic microorganisms are those that are capable of growing in the presence of oxygen. These include obligate aerobes, capnophilic aerobes (CO_2 dependent), microaerophiles, and facultative anaerobes. Anaerobes include obligate anaerobes, capnophilic anaerobes, and aerotolerant anaerobes. Oxygen may be toxic to varying degrees to anaerobes. ∞ Chapter 24, "Anaerobic Bacteria," provides more information on specific anaerobes.

The growth pattern in various atmospheres allows one to classify an unknown organism. This is an important clue to their identity. Those organisms that grow both aerobically and anaerobically are **facultative anaerobes.** These are microorganisms able to grow with or without oxygen. Those that grow aerobically but not anaerobically are **obligate aerobes.** These are microorganisms that require 15% to 21% oxygen for growth. They grow in ambient air and carbon dioxide atmospheres. If carbon dioxide is required for growth, they are **capnophilic.** Both aerobes and anaerobes may be capnophilic. If growth occurs best in the microaerophilic atmosphere, they are microaerophiles. Microaerophiles are microorganisms that require reduced oxygen levels for growth. Whether a microaerophile grows in a CO_2 incubator or not is determined by its oxygen tolerance. For example, *Neisseria gonorrhoeae* grows well in a CO_2 incubator, but *Campylobacter* does not because the oxygen present is at a toxic level. If a microorgan-

ism only grows in the anaerobic atmosphere, it is an **obligate anaerobe**, or a microorganism that requires an oxygen-free environment for growth. If there is slight growth aerobically but good growth anaerobically, it is an **aerotolerant anaerobe**, an anaerobe that can tolerate oxygen and will show slight growth aerobically. Table 7-4 summarizes the atmospheric classification of bacteria.

As you study the microorganisms in Part 4, "Clinically Significant Isolates," pay close attention to the descriptions of their atmospheric requirements. Learn this information along with their other characteristics. This will enable you to solve the identity of unknown organisms and validate your results prior to reporting the name.

> ✓ **Checkpoint! 7–6**
> **(Chapter Objective 6)**
>
> *A microorganism that grows on media incubated in air or CO_2 but not on media incubated anaerobically is a(n):*
>   A. *capnophilic organism.*
>   B. *obligate aerobe.*
>   C. *facultative anaerobe.*
>   D. *obligate anaerobe.*

HUMIDITY

The last thing that is required for good growth of microorganisms is humidity. The humidity level should be maintained at 70%. This can be achieved by placing a container of water in the incubator, if the incubator isn't equipped with a water reservoir or humidity regulator (Isenberg et al., 1979). The container needs to be closely monitored so that it doesn't dry out or become contaminated with mould.

✪ **TABLE 7-4**

Atmospheric Classification of Bacteria

Classification	Air	CO_2	AN	MA
Aerobe:				
Facultative anaerobe	G	G	G	G
Obligate aerobe	G	G	SL to NG	G
Microaerophile	NG	V	SL to NG	G
Anaerobe:				
Obligate anaerobe	NG	NG	G	NG
Aerotolerant anaerobe	NG	SL	G	G

CO_2 = 5%–10% carbon dioxide, 13%–17% oxygen; AN = anaerobic (0% oxygen, ~5% CO_2); Air = ambient air (~21% oxygen); MA = microaerophilic (5% oxygen, 10% CO_2); G = visible growth; NG = No visible growth; SL = slight or sparse growth; V = Growth or no growth, depending on oxygen tolerance.
Source: Adapted from Table 1-1, Engelkirk, P., Duben-Engelkirk, J., & Dowell, V. R. (1992). Principles and practice of clinical anaerobic bacteriology. Belmont, CA: Star Publishing Company.

▶ **INOCULATION**

When a specimen is received in the microbiology laboratory, the time and date of receipt is stamped on the requisition on in the laboratory computer (Murray et al., 1999). The specimen is evaluated for suitability and may be rejected to ensure the safety of laboratory staff and prevent the reporting of inaccurate results (Miller, 1999). A specimen that is labeled improperly, in an unsuitable container, accompanied by an improper request, not of sufficient quantity, or received more than 2 hours after collection must be rejected. Table 7-5✪ outlines criteria that can be used to evaluate and reject an unsuitable specimen. ∞ Chapter 6, "Specimen Collection," provides specific information on collection of specimens for microbiology.

> ✓ **Checkpoint! 7–7 (Chapter Objective 7)**
>
> *An unlabeled specimen is received in the laboratory. Your best course of action would be to:*
>   A. *call the floor and request the patient's name.*
>   B. *label the specimen using the name on the requisition or information in the computer.*
>   C. *reject and request another specimen.*
>   D. *either A or B*

One must consider the specimen type to determine the need for a direct Gram stain and select the appropriate media for **inoculation**, the act of transferring a specimen from a container to a growth media. Once the proper medium is selected for the specimen type, a method of inoculation must be chosen. The kind of specimen consistency and the total number of plates or tubes to be inoculated dictate the approach taken.

DIRECT GRAM STAIN

The direct Gram stain is used to assess the quality of the specimen, determine the bacterial morphology present, and guide specimen processing. Some specimens always include a direct Gram stain when processed, whereas others require a separate order from the doctor. Table 7-6✪ provides more information on specimen sources that automatically include a Gram stain when processed.

Gram stains are examined for predominant cell type and bacterial morphology. If squamous epithelial cells are present, the specimen represents a superficially collected specimen. These specimens will typically contain commensal flora from the specimen source. Sputum with greater than 10 to 25 squamous epithelial cells per low power field (LPF) is contaminated with saliva and should be rejected. An anaerobic culture may be canceled if squamous epithelial cells are observed on the specimen's direct Gram stain. Superficial sites should not be

(text continues on p. 155)

 TABLE 7-5

Specimen Rejection Criteria

Criteria	Recommended Action
Clerical error related to inadequate or missing labels	Contact the physician or nurse. Request a new specimen. An unlabelled or mislabeled specimen must not be processed unless it is not recollectable such as a placenta or CSF. A specimen, which is not recollectable, must be identified by the ordering physician prior to processing.
Delayed transport of specimen after collection	Notify the physician or nurse. Request a new specimen. Include comment, "Specimen received after prolonged delay."
Leaking, nonsterile, or improper container	Do not process. Contact the physician or nurse. Request a new specimen. Inform supervisor if contact insists that specimen be processed. These specimens should be accepted only under exceptional circumstances. Include appropriate comment if accepted. For example, "Specimen received in improper container." Protect personnel from biohazard exposure.
Expectorated sputum specimen with >10 to 25 squamous epithelial cells/low power field (LPF)	Notify the physician or nurse that specimen is mostly saliva and not suitable for culture. Do not process. Request another specimen.
Duplicate specimens, other than blood, received within a 24 hour period	Inform the physician or nurse that only one specimen will be processed per day.
Specimen unsuitable for culture request (For example, desiccated swab, specimen in fixative other than stool for ova and parasite examination, or anaerobic culture request on cervical/vaginal specimens, urine, stool, or expectorated sputum)	Contact the physician or nurse. Request a new specimen. Inform supervisor if contact insists that specimen be processed. These specimens should be accepted only under exceptional circumstances. Include appropriate comment if accepted. For example, "These results are reported at the request of the physician and may not be accurate because the specimen was submitted in a fixative."
Quantity not sufficient	Contact the physician or nurse. Request a new specimen. If quantity is not sufficient for multiple culture requests, ask the physician to submit additional samples or to prioritize the requests.

⭐ **TABLE 7-6**

Suggested Culture Media to Isolate Potential Pathogens from Selected Specimen Sources

Specimen Source	Culture Media	"Normal Flora"	Potential Pathogens	Notes
Throat	BA or SSA	Nonhemolytic, alpha and gamma hemolytic streptococci Beta-hemolytic streptococci (not groups A, C, or G) *Staphylococcus* spp. *Haemophilus* spp. *Neisseria* spp. *Moraxella* spp. *Corynebacterium* spp. *E. coli* & other *Enterobacteriaceae* Anaerobes	Group A streptococci (*Streptococcus pyogenes*) Groups C, and G streptococci *Arcanobacterium haemolyticum*	*Corynebacterium diphtheriae, Bordetella pertussis, Neisseria gonorrhoeae, N. meningitidis,* and *Candida* spp. are identified on request. Additional media is often required. Viruses can also be the causative agents of pharyngitis.
Eye (Conjunctiva)	BA CA GS	*Corynebacterium* spp. Alpha-streptococci Coagulase negative staphylococci (CNS) *Propionibacterium* spp.	*Haemophilus influenzae* or *Haemophilus aegyptius* *Moraxella* spp. *Neisseria. gonorrhoeae* *N. meningitidis* *Staphylococcus aureus* *Streptococcus pneumoniae* *S. pyogenes* *Pseudomonas aeruginosa* *Pasteurella multocida* *Bacillus* spp.	Report *Pseudomonas aeruginosa* immediately when isolated. *Chlamydia trachomatis* is identified on request. Additional media is required. Viruses, fungi, and protozoa are also potential pathogens of the eye.
Middle Ear	BA MAC CA GS	The outer ear canal can possess the same normal flora organisms as the eye. The middle ear is normally sterile.	*Staphylococcus aureus* *Streptococcus pyogenes* *S. pneumoniae* and other streptococci *Haemophilus influenzae* *Pseudomonas aeruginosa* *Moraxella catarrhalis* Anaerobic bacteria	*Pseudomonas aeruginosa* and *Staphylococcus aureus* are known for infections of the outer ear.
Sputum, bronchial washes and other lower respiratory system specimens	BA MAC CA GS	Same as throat if the specimen passes through the upper respiratory tract at time of collection	*Streptococcus pneumoniae* *Klebsiella pneumoniae* and other *Enterobacteriaceae* *Pseudomonas aeruginosa* *Staphylococcus aureus* *Haemophilus influenzae* *Moraxella catarrhalis* *Pasteurella multocida*	Specimen quality is assessed microscopically for the presence of squamous epithelial cells which indicates the collection of saliva and not sputum. *Mycobacterium* spp., *Legionella pneumophila,* and other *Legionella; Mycoplasma* spp., viruses, and fungi are identified upon request. Additional media is required.

(continued)

✪ **TABLE 7-6**

Suggested Culture Media to Isolate Potential Pathogens from Selected Specimen Sources (*continued*)

Specimen Source	Culture Media	"Normal Flora"	Potential Pathogens	Notes
Feces/rectal swab	A moderately differential and selective enteric agar such as MAC or EMB and a highly selective and differential enteric agar such as HE or XLD is necessary. An enteric enrichment broth such as GN broth may be necessary for the detection of potential pathogens in carriers. It can also be used for EIA assay for shiga toxin producing *E. coli*. Special selective agar may be necessary for the recovery of specific pathogens such as CIN for *Yersinia enterocolitica*. e.g., BA MAC PEA HE or XLD CIN Campy BA	*E. coli* and other nonpathogenic *Enterobacteriaceae* *Pseudomonas* spp. and other non-fermenting gram negative rods Coagulase negative staphylococci *Enterococcus* spp. Alpha and gamma hemolytic streptococci Yeast Anaerobes	*Campylobacter jejuni* and other *Campylobacter* spp. *Salmonella* spp. *Shigella* spp. *E. coli*: enteropathogenic, enteroadherent, enteroinvasive, enterohemorrhagic and enteroaggregative serogroups *Vibrio cholerae* and other *Vibrio* spp. *Yersinia* spp. *Aeromonas* spp. *Plesiomonas* spp. *Listeria monocytogenes*	Demonstration of *Clostridium difficile* toxin is important but the presence of the organism in culture is not significant. Viruses and parasites are also potential pathogens. A gram stain may be used to detect the presence of white blood cells.
Urine	BA MAC PEA (if the specimen is obtained from a nephrostomy) GS (optional)	Coagulase negative staphylococci *Corynebacterium* spp. *E. coli* and other *Enterobacteriaceae* *Lactobacillus* spp. Nonhemolytic and alpha-hemolytic streptococci	*Enterobacteriaceae*: especially *E. coli, Klebsiella* spp. and *Proteus* spp. *Enterococcus* spp. *Pseudomonas aeruginosa* and other nonfermenting gram-negative rods *Staphylococcus aureus* *S. saprophyticus* *Corynebacterium urealyticum*	Voided midstream urine collected after cleansing the site is the preferred collection protocol. A calibrated loop is used to inoculate media. Greater than 100,000 CFU/mL defines a urinary tract infection. Lower CFU counts may be significant if only 1 organism and white blood cells are present. *Candida* spp., *Chlamydia trachomatis, Ureaplasma urealyticum* and *Trichomonas vaginalis* are also potential pathogens. *Corynebacterium urealyticum* and *Candida glabrata* require 2 or more days of incubation for growth. *N. gonorrhoeae* is cultured on request by adding a chocolate or Thayer-Martin agar

✪ **TABLE 7-6**

Suggested Culture Media to Isolate Potential Pathogens from Selected Specimen Sources *(continued)*

Specimen Source	Culture Media	"Normal Flora"	Potential Pathogens	Notes
Genital Ideally the physician should specify the organism of interest so the laboratory can insure the appropriate media is used. Vaginal/cervix and urethra/penis	For isolation of *Neisseria gonorrhoeae* only: GC selective agar such as TM GS For isolation of Group B streptococci only: Enriched selective broth such as LIM or Todd-Hewitt broth Routine cultures are rarely performed: BA CA MAC PEA TM GS	*E. coli* & other *Enterobacteriaceae* *S. gallolyticus* (previously known as *S.bovis*) *Enterococcus* spp. Alpha and nonhemolytic streptococci *Lactobacillus* spp. Coagulase negative staphylococci *Corynebacterium* spp. Anaerobes	*Neisseria gonorrhoeae* *Haemophilus ducreyi* Group B *Streptococcus* (*Streptococcus agalactiae*) *Candida albicans*	*Treponema pallidum*, *Trichomonas vaginalis*, *Ureaplasma* and *Mycoplasma* spp. and Herpes simplex virus are identified on request. Additional media or laboratory procedures may be required for detection. *Neisseria gonorrhoeae* and *Chlamydia trachomatis* are usually detected by molecular methods. Bacterial vaginosis is best diagnosed with a Gram stain.
Cerebrospinal fluid (CSF)	BA CA MAC (if gram negative rods are seen on direct GS) Thio (if CSF is obtained via a shunt) GS	Normally sterile	Any organism isolated should be considered significant. *Neisseria meningitidis* *Haemophilus influenzae* *Streptococcus pneumoniae* *Listeria monocytogenes* *E. coli* and other *Enterobacteriaceae* Group B *Streptococcus* (*S. agalactiae*) *Cryptococcus neoformans* *Staphylococcus aureus*	CSF should be centrifuged, prior to plating, to concentrate bacteria. A cytocentrifuged Gram stain slide provides the most sensitive means of detecting organisms on Gram stain. Do not refrigerate the specimen prior to plating. *Mycobacterium* spp., viruses, fungi, and parasites are identified on request. Additional media may be required. Normal skin flora can be significant if isolated from shunt CSF.
Superficial wound or abscess collected on an aerobic swab	BA CA (if *Haemophilus* or *Neisseria* are potential pathogens) MAC PEA GS	*Corynebacterium* spp. Alpha and gamma hemolytic *Streptococcus* spp. Coagulase negative staphylococci *Propionibacterium* spp. *Bacillus* spp.	*Staphylococcus aureus* *Streptococcus pyogenes* and other beta-hemolytic streptococci *Enterobacteriaceae* *Pseudomona aeruginosa* and other nonfermenting gram-negative rods *Enterococcus* spp. *Corynebacterium jeikeium* and other coryneforms *Actinomyces israelii*	*Mycobacterium marinum* is identified on request. Additional media required. *Actinomyces israelii* may require 2 weeks incubation for growth. Fungi, viruses, and parasites are also potential pathogens.

(continued)

⭐ **TABLE 7-6**

Suggested Culture Media to Isolate Potential Pathogens from Selected Specimen Sources *(continued)*

Specimen Source	Culture Media	"Normal Flora"	Potential Pathogens	Notes
Abscess or wound aspirate or tissue biopsy	BA CA (if *Haemophilus* or *Neisseria* are potential pathogens) MAC PEA Anaerobic media such as RBAP and LKV Anaerobic Thio GS	The same organisms seen with superficial wounds are possible.	*Staphylococcus aureus* *Streptococcus pyogenes* and other beta-hemolytic streptococci *Clostridium* spp. *Bacteroides* spp. Other anaerobes Enterobacteriaceae *Pseudomonas aeruginosa* and other nonfermenting gram-negative rods *Enterococcus* spp. *Erysipelothrix rhusiopathiae* *Corynebacterium jeikeium* and other coryneforms *Vibrio vulnificus* *Actinomyces israelii*	Cleanse skin surface prior to collection. Anaerobic transport media should be inoculated with the specimen. *M. marinum* is identified on request. Additional media required. *Actinomyces israelii* may require 2 weeks incubation for growth.
Blood	Automated detection system ■ 1 aerobic bottle ■ 1 anaerobic bottle Alternate methods ■ Lysis-centrifugation ■ Agar-slide system ■ Agar-broth system	Normally sterile	Any organism isolated should be considered significant. Coagulase negative staphylococci (CNS) *Staphylococcus aureus* *Streptococcus pneumoniae* Viridans streptococci *Enterococcus* spp. Groups A, B, and D *Streptococcus* Enterobacteriaceae *Pseudomonas* spp. *Haemophilus influenzae* *Neisseria* spp. *Bacteroides fragilis* *Clostridium* spp. Other anaerobes *Candida albicans* *Listeria monocytogenes* *Corynebacterium jeikeium* and other coryneform bacilli HACEK group	Cleanse skin surface in concentric circles prior to drawing the blood. First with 70% alcohol then 2% tincture of iodine. 1:5–1:10 blood to broth ratio is ideal. Disinfect rubber stoppers of bottles, prior to inoculation, with alcohol to avoid microbial contamination of the culture. Total volume drawn for adults should be 10–30 mL per bottle. *Mycobacterium* spp., fungi, and parasites are also potential pathogens. Lysis-centrifugation can be used for the isolation of fungi and fastidious organisms.

✪ TABLE 7-6

Suggested Culture Media to Isolate Potential Pathogens from Selected Specimen Sources *(continued)*

Specimen Source	Culture Media	"Normal Flora"	Potnetial Pathogens	Notes
Bone and joints	BA CA MAC Thio GS	Normally sterile	Any organism isolated should be considered significant. *Staphylococcus aureus* Coagulase negative staphylo-cocci *Streptococcus* spp. *Enterococcus* spp. *Pseudomonas aeruginosa* Enterobacteriaceae *Neisseria gonorrhoeae* Anaerobes	Bone biopsy and joint aspirate are the preferred specimens. Joint fluid may be inoculated into a blood culture bottles. Viruses, fungi, and *Mycobacterium* spp. are also potential pathogens.

BA = Blood agar; SSA = Strep selective agar; MAC = MacConkey agar; CA = Chocolate agar; GS = Gram stain; SS = Salmonella-Shigella agar; HE = Hektoen enteric agar; EMB = Eosin methylene blue; CIN = Cefsulodin-Irgasan-novobiocin agar; GN = Gram-negative broth; TM = Thayer-Martin agar; RBAP = Reducible blood agar; LKV = Laked kanamycin vancomycin; CFU = Colony forming units; mL = milliliter; Thio = Thioglycolate broth; HACEK Group = *Haemophilus aphrophilus* (now known as *Aggregatibacter aphrophilus*), *Actinobacillus actinomycetemcomitans* (now known as *Aggregatibacter actinomycetemcomitans*), *Cardiobacterium hominis*, *Eikenella corrodens*, *Kingella* spp.

cultured anaerobically because of contamination with commensal aerobic and anaerobic flora from skin and mucous membranes. The growth of the commensal flora creates the necessary conditions to maintain the viability of anaerobic organisms. Therefore, skin and mucous membrane surfaces contain a large number of anaerobes that frequently contaminate a wounds surface (Miller, 1999). For specific information on the growth requirements of anaerobes see ∞ Chapter 24, "Anaerobic Bacteria."

High numbers of microorganisms must be present to see them microscopically (Isenberg et al., 1979). Examination of a direct Gram stain will reveal the presence of microbes, the predominant morphology, and the presence of polymorphonuclear white blood cells. Particular attention is paid to the bacteria associated with the white blood cells (WBCs). The WBCs indicate an inflammatory response to a potential pathogen. ∞ Chapter 8, "Presumptive Identification," provides more information on the Gram stain and its use in presumptive identification. See ∞ Chapter 4, "Host's Encounter with Microbes," to review the inflammatory response.

The slide used for the direct smear can be alcohol flamed or presterilized but this is not performed in most laboratories now. The smear is prepared by rolling a swab across the slide surface or applying the specimen in a thin layer. If the swab is received in transport media or it is a single swab, it may be placed in 1 mL of broth and blended by vortexing. The broth is then used to prepare the smear and inoculate the media. The smear is fixed by either methanol fixation or heat fixation and stained. ∞ Chapter 8, "Presumptive Identification," includes the Gram stain procedure.

 REAL WORLD TIP

A cytocentrifuge should be used to prepare the gram stain slide from fluid specimens such as CSF. The instrument concentrates the specimen into a small area on the glass slide prior to staining. This instrument increases the sensitivity of organism detection by at least 100 times.

 REAL WORLD TIP

Media from new batches of uninoculated transport media should be stained to detect stainable, nonviable bacteria. The presence of these organisms may result in a false-positive Gram stain result (Isenberg et al., 1979).

SELECTION OF MEDIA

The types of media used for each specimen type are designed to isolate the potential pathogens. Table 7-6 provides suggestions for culture media that could be used for the isolation of potential pathogens from selected specimen sources. For example, the most common causative agent of "strep" throat or pharyngitis is *Streptococcus pyogenes*. Throat specimens are inoculated onto sheep blood agar because it will enhance growth and recognition of this pathogen. The microbiology laboratory uses standard operating procedures and policies to insure the appropriate media is used for inoculation for each specimen. Sometimes you will encounter a specimen type not included in a procedure. In this situation, you must consider the potential pathogens based on the body site or specimen type, as well as the commensal flora, and select the media accordingly.

The media should be examined to ensure that the surface is smooth and moist. There should not be excessive moisture that will result in a lawn of growth without isolated colonies. Aerosols may be generated if a bumpy or pitted surface is streaked. Warm refrigerated media to room temperature before use (Becton Dickinson, 1988).

 Checkpoint! 7–8 (Chapter Objective 8)

You receive a sputum specimen. It should be inoculated onto:
1. *blood agar (BA) medium.*
2. *chocolate agar (CA) medium.*
3. *MacConkey (MAC) agar medium.*
    A. *1 only*
    B. *1 & 2*
    C. *1 & 3*
    D. *1, 2, & 3*

ORDER OF INOCULATION

Once decisions are made about the choice of media, atmosphere, and tools used for specimen inoculation, one still has to determine which specimens should be processed and inoculated first and which media will be inoculated first.

Order of Specimen Processing

One should consider two things when determining the order of inoculation for specimens. Does the specimen suggest a life-threatening infectious disease and are fastidious microorganisms potential pathogens? If the specimen collected indicates an infectious disease that can quickly place a patient's life in danger, the physician will require results as quickly as possible. Examples of the types of specimen that require immediate attention are cerebrospinal fluid, pericardial fluid, amniotic fluid, vitreous fluid and blood.

Specimens that may contain delicate pathogens like *Neisseria gonorrhoeae*, which could be harmed by less-than-optimal temperature or atmosphere, should also be processed quickly. Specimens received from the intensive care unit (ICU) should also be given priority because patients in the ICU are extremely compromised and prone to infections (Miller, 1999). Those specimens received in transport media may be held longer before inoculation.

Media Order

The direct smear, if needed, should be prepared first on a glass slide which can be alcohol flamed or presterilized if desired. Solid media should be inoculated second, and broth medium, if used, last (Isenberg, 1992). The least-selective media is inoculated first

to prevent carryover of the inhibitory ingredients to other agars. Inoculate inhibitory medium with more specimen (Isenberg et al., 1979). The enriched media should always be inoculated first, then the selective and differential media. Within the group of enteric differential media, the mildly selective agar should be inoculated before the highly selective agar. The inoculation order for commonly used primary media is listed in Table 7-7 .

All media should be inoculated before streaking for isolation. Processing of specimens should be performed carefully to avoid contamination of the primary media and protect the processor from biohazardous exposure (Miller, 1999). Specimen processing and inoculation should be performed in a biological safety cabinet.

✓ **Checkpoint! 7–9 (Chapter Objective 9)**

A fecal specimen is received in the laboratory. It must be inoculated on/into blood agar (BA), MacConkey (MAC), Salmonella-Shigella agar (SS), Hektoen enteric agar (HE), cefsulodin-Irgasan-novobiocin agar (CIN), campy BA, and gram-negative (GN) broth. What is the correct order of inoculation?
    A. *BA, Campy BA, MAC, SS, HE, CIN, GN broth*
    B. *Campy BA, BA, MAC, CIN, SS, HE, GN broth*
    C. *BA, MAC, SS, HE, CIN, Campy BA, GN broth*
    D. *GN broth, BA, MAC, HE, SS, CIN, Campy BA*

INOCULATION TOOLS

A variety of inoculating tools are available for use. A description of each of these follows: inoculating loops, sterile swabs, and pipettes.

✪ **TABLE 7-7**

Inoculation Order for Commonly Used Primary Media
Blood agar (BA)
Chocolate agar (CA)
Thayer-Martin agar (TM)
Phenylethyl alcohol agar (PEA) or Columbia Colistin-Nalidixic acid agar (CNA)
Streptococcal selective agar
Campy blood agar
Mannitol salt agar (MSA)
MacConkey agar (MAC) or eosin methylene blue (EMB)
Xylose lysine desoxycholate agar (XLD)
Salmonella-Shigella agar (SS)
Hektoen enteric agar (HE)
Cefsulodin-irgasan-novobiocin agar (CIN)
Laked blood kanamycin-vancomycin agar (LKV)
Thioglycolate broth (Thio)
Gram-negative (GN) broth or other enteric enrichment broth

Source: Adapted from Isenberg, H. (Ed.). (1998). Essential procedures for clinical microbiology. Washington, DC: ASM Press. Table 1.1-8

Loops

A useful tool for specimens with a uniform consistency is an inoculating loop. Inoculating loops may be plastic and disposable or made out of nichrome or platinum wire and reusable. The choice of loop used routinely is a personal one made by laboratory management. Plastic loops are more costly and create a disposal issue, but may be deemed more convenient. Metal loops are reusable but need to be replaced when worn or melted from leaving in the incinerator too long. If a measured portion needs to be applied to the surface of the medium, a calibrated loop is used. The usual calibrations are 0.001 mL and 0.01 mL. The metal calibrated loops have a disadvantage in that they may lose their calibration with time and usage. Frequent recalibration is required. Many labs opt to use plastic disposable calibrated loops instead because of convenience.

Reusable loops are flamed for 5 to 10 seconds and cooled before streaking the specimen (Isenberg, 1998). The specimen is transferred to one section of the agar surface of each medium used and then streaked for isolation.

 REAL WORLD TIP

It is important to sterilize and then cool a nichrome or platinum wire loop prior to streaking for isolation. Use the sterile water that accumulates in the lid of the agar's petri dish to cool the loop. The sterilized loop can also be pushed into the surface of one of the agar plates to cool. If the loop is too hot, it may kill organisms or create aerosols. This can lead to false negative results because of the absence of growth and endanger the processor with exposure to aerosolized biohazardous material.

Swabs

A variety of swabs are available for specimen collection. Specimens may be received in the clinical laboratory on a swab and are transferred to the surface of the medium by rolling the swab across the surface of the first quadrant or section. Approximately a dime-sized area close to the edge of the agar plate is inoculated with the specimen. Insure all sides and the tip of the swab is used to inoculate the agar surface. Cotton swabs may also be used to transfer feces and sputum specimens to the medium surface.

Pipettes

Liquid specimens are easily inoculated onto different agar plates using a sterile plastic or glass pipette. After centrifugation, the specimen sediment is aspirated and one to two drops placed in the first quadrant of each medium. Care has to be taken that the agar plate is not inverted until the liquid is absorbed by the medium to avoid having the drop roll across the entire agar surface and potential exposure to biohazard material.

STREAKING FOR ISOLATION

Once the specimen is transferred to the surface of solid culture medium, it must be spread in a thin layer across the surface. The goal of streaking is to obtain isolated colonies. All personnel should streak in a similar manner so quantitation of growth is standardized. Laboratories can vary in using three quadrant or four quadrant streaking patterns. Quantitation of colonies can differ depending on the streaking pattern used. The number of organisms often determines if an organism should be considered part of the normal flora, a colonizer or potential pathogen. For example, in a sputum specimen, *Klebsiella pneumoniae* can be a colonizer of the upper respiratory track or the causative agent of pneumonia. Often the decision to workup *K. pneumoniae* depends on the quantitation of the organism on solid media. If the number of colonies of *K. pneumoniae* does not outnumber those of the normal upper respiratory tract flora present, it is probably a colonizer and not significant. If it overgrows the normal flora present, it may be a potential pathogen. See Figure 7-8 ■ for suggested streaking methods. Figure 7-9 ■ illustrates a way of streaking biplates.

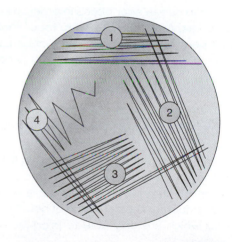

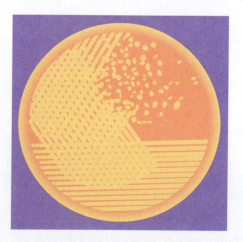

■ **FIGURE 7-8** Examples of the 4 quadrant (top) and 3 quadrant (bottom) streak plate methods of inoculation.

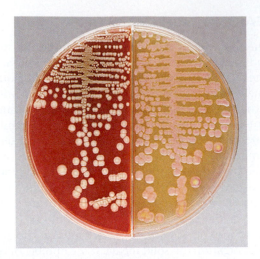

■ **FIGURE 7-9** Blood agar and MacConkey agar biplate struck with *Klebsiella pneumoniae*.
Photo courtesy of Remel, part of Thermo Fisher Scientific.

 REAL WORLD TIP

A loop is used to streak agar plates in order to achieve isolated colonies. A needle is used to touch individual colonies for performing identification tests such as a colony gram stain and biochemical and susceptibility testing.

 REAL WORLD TIP

After streaking a sheep blood agar and using the same loop, stab the agar 2 to 3 times in the area of the initial specimen placement. This creates a miniature anaerobic chamber for the detection of beta hemolytic streptococci which are only able to produce oxygen labile streptolysin O.

 REAL WORLD TIP

When streaking agar plates planted with clinical specimen, do not flame the loop between quadrants. You want to know exactly the quantity of organisms present and flaming between quadrants will dilute the number of colonies. When streaking an agar plate for an organism subculture, flame the loop just before beginning to streak the final quadrant. This will dilute the organism so individual colonies are available for testing.

All plating media is incubated "media side up" (inverted). This will prevent condensation from forming on the media surface resulting in a lawn of growth rather then isolated colonies.

 Checkpoint! 7–10 (Chapter Objective 10)

The reason for incubating solid plating medium in the inverted position (media side up) is to:

    A. *prevent contamination of the medium.*
    B. *prevent loss of moisture from the medium.*
    C. *check on solidity of the medium.*
    D. *prevent water condensation on the agar surface.*

DISTINCTIVE TECHNIQUES

Most specimens are simply inoculated onto the surface of media and incubated under optimum conditions for the growth of expected pathogens. A few specimens either require special manipulation prior to inoculation or the inoculation technique is different. These include cerebrospinal fluid (CSF) and other body fluids, urine, cultures for *Neisseria gonorrhoeae* (GC) only, acid-fast cultures, and tissue or bone specimens. A discussion of each follows.

Culture of Cerebrospinal Fluid (CSF) and Other Body Fluids

CSF is collected from patients suspected of suffering from **meningitis**, an inflammation of the membranes covering the central nervous system. This is one of the few microbiological specimens that should be handled "stat." Stat is Latin for *statim* which means immediately. A positive result is a **critical or panic value**, which is a laboratory result that indicates a life-threatening situation and requires immediate action of a physician, so it is imperative to detect and isolate any pathogen that may be present.

Examine the specimen and note any cloudiness, blood, or **xanthochromia**, a yellow coloration, as well as any other unusual color. Xanthochromia is due to the bilirubin present after the lysis of red blood cells. The specimen is centrifuged (1,500 x g for 15 minutes) prior to preparation of direct smears and inoculation of media if the volume is greater than 1 mL (Murray et al., 1999). This will concentrate the bacteria in the sediment and increase the chances of isolating even small numbers of organisms. It is important the specimen not be refrigerated if there is a delay before processing. This specimen may contain *Neisseria meningitidis* or *Streptococcus pneumoniae* that autolyse in unfavorable conditions. The specimen should be incubated at 35° in CO_2 or left at room temperature until it can be processed. ∞ Chapter 18, "Gram-Negative Cocci," and ∞ Chapter 38, "Central Nervous System," provide more information on pathogens associated with central nervous system infections.

Other body fluids may be received in the microbiology laboratory for culture. These include synovial or joint fluid and peritoneal fluid. Examine the specimen and if **purulent** (pus, formed as a result of inflammation, is present), inoculate the primary media directly (Forbes et al., 1998). If clear, centrifuge as described earlier for CSF. Synovial fluid and peritoneal fluid may be inoculated into blood culture bottles at bedside (Bobadilla, Sifuentes, & Garcia-Tsao, 1989; Von Essen & Hölttä, 1986). For more information on the infectious diseases associated with positive body fluid cultures see ∞ Chapter 32, "Cardiovascular System," ∞ Chapter 33, "Respiratory System," and ∞ Chapter 39, "Skeletal System."

Urine Culture

Quantitative cultures, a procedure that measures or estimates the number of colonies, are performed on urine specimens. The total colony count aids in the determination of the significance of the isolates. The most common technique is the use of a **calibrated loop**, an instrument providing a standardized measurement of the specimen. The most common volume for routine culture is 0.001 mL. Swirling gently mixes the urine. The calibrated loop must be held vertically and dipped into the urine just below the surface (Clarridge, Pezzlo, & Vosti, 1987). If the angle of the urine loop is held at more or less than a 90° angle, the amount of specimen picked up by the loop can be increased by up to 150% which will affect the results. It is then transferred in a single line down the center of the plate. Streaking for isolation is then performed in one direction perpendicular to the inoculation line across the entire surface of the agar plate as seen in Figure 7-9. Another technique is to transfer a measured portion of the urine to the first quadrant, in a straight line or V pattern. Streak all quadrants for isolation, as described earlier in this chapter (Isenberg, 1992). ∞ Chapter 34, "Urinary System," presents information on infections associated with the urinary system.

 REAL WORLD TIP

A urine specimen is usually inoculated onto sheep blood agar and MacConkey agars. After inoculation of the sheep blood agar, remember to redip the urine loop into the specimen before inoculation of the MacConkey agar. If this is not done, there will be significantly less colonies on the MacConkey agar than on the sheep blood agar. Colony counts are very important for a urine culture. The number of colonies present determines if a urinary tract infection exists.

Neisseria gonorrhoeae (GC) Only Culture

A positive culture for *Neisseria gonorrhoeae* (GC) has public health significance related to the control of sexually transmitted diseases. It is important to detect even small numbers of this strict pathogen. To facilitate its isolation the swab is rolled across the surface of chocolate agar or *Neisseria* selective agar in a zig-zag ("Z" or "W") pattern (Carlson, Haley, Tisei, & McCormack, 1980; Faur, Weisburd, Wilson, & May, 1973). This should ensure the transfer of the entire specimen from the swab. Streak for isolation using the routine streak pattern described earlier. Information on genital tract system infections can be found in ∞ Chapter 36. ∞ Chapter 18, "Aer-

obic Gram-Negative Cocci," provides information on the identification of *N. gonorrhoeae*.

 REAL WORLD TIP

Most laboratories no longer perform routine cultures for the isolation of *Neisseria gonorroheae*. The use of molecular diagnostic methods directly on genital swabs eliminates the potential negative effects of prolonged transportation and other environmental factors.

 REAL WORLD TIP

JEMBEC is an agar media and transport system in one used for the isolation of *Neisseria gonorrhoeae*. This small rectangle Thayer-Martin like agar plate has a small hole in which a carbon dioxide generating tablet is placed. The agar is then placed into a gas impermeable plastic bag and sealed. This system is used when there will be a delay in transportation. It works well for transporting cultures for *N. gonorrhoeae* from physician offices and STD clinics.

Acid-Fast Cultures

Acid-fast cultures are collected when the physician suspects tuberculosis (TB) or other TB-like organisms. Specimens are inoculated onto special media designed to grow the acid-fast members of the genus *Mycobacterium*. Those specimens that contain commensal flora are processed to decontaminate and concentrate the specimen. These procedures are usually performed in a separate area of the laboratory under conditions that protect laboratory personnel from aerosols. Review ∞ Chapter 13, "Acid-fast Bacilli Cultures," and ∞ Chapter 26, "*Mycobacterium* Species," for details of specimen processing and identification of acid-fast bacilli.

Cultures of Tissue or Bone

The microorganism causing an infectious disease may be embedded in the tissue or reside in the marrow of bone. When these specimens are received in the microbiology laboratory, they must be **homogenized**, emulsifying the specimen into a smooth mixture, prior to inoculation onto the appropriate media. A mortar and pestle, sterile scalpel, or manual or motorized grinder can be used for this purpose.

This activity should be performed under a biosafety hood, as aerosols may be produced. The specimen may be moistened with a small amount of sterile broth. The tissue is minced or ground until a smooth consistency is obtained.

Quantitative cultures may be requested on tissue specimens from burn patients. The number of organisms present per gram of tissue may predict the onset of septicemia and help determine if skin grafts will be successful. The specimen is weighed and then blended in a measured volume of broth or saline until a smooth consistency is obtained. The homogenate is diluted 1:10, 1:100, and 1:1000 and inoculated on the surface of media with a calibrated loop (.01 or .001 mL). The colony-forming unit or CFU/gram of tissue is calculated from the weight of the tissue and dilution (Simor, Roberts, & Smith, 1988). This procedure is painful for the patient and demanding on microbiology personnel.

A noninvasive quantitative swab culture has been shown to correlate with deep tissue biopsy results (Bowler, Duerden, & Armstrong, 2001). The specimen is collected on an alginate-tipped swab. When the swab is transferred to a diluent, it will dissolve, releasing the microorganisms. This diluent, containing organisms, is serially diluted and plated as described earlier. More information related to infections involving tissue and bone can be found in ∞ Chapter 39, "Skeletal System," and ∞ Chapter 40, "Opportunistic Infections."

SUMMARY

This chapter provided information on the way in which the clinical microbiology lab provides the conditions necessary for the growth of microorganisms. Successful growth is achieved with selection of appropriate growth media and incubation environments. Basic information on specimen processing was also presented.

Growth medium exists in liquid, solid, and semisolid form and contains the nutrients required by bacteria for growth. The form selected is determined by the purpose of the medium used for cultivation of microorganisms. For example, if one wants to enhance the growth of small numbers of bacteria, a liquid medium is best. If one wants to isolate the different kinds of bacteria as individual colonies, a solid medium is best.

Different kinds of primary media are available to assist in the growth and isolation of potential pathogens. General-purpose media provides just the basic sustenance required by most microorganisms for growth. The more fastidious organisms will grow poorly, if at all, on this medium. Enriched media provides a better growth medium for most organisms, resulting in better growth with colonies that are more easily visualized. Those organisms with special dietary requirements may not grow on enriched media, requiring their own specially formulated media. Selective media is used for specimens with commensal flora to aid in the isolation of specific types of pathogens. For example, CNA is used to isolate gram-positive bacteria. Differential media is usually selective as well, while aiding the differentiation of types of bacteria. For example, MAC is used to select for gram-negative rods while distinguishing the lactose fermenters from the nonlactose fermenters. Enrichment media is used to enhance the growth of small numbers of bacteria or fastidious bacteria. Today enrichment media is only used when small numbers of bacteria are clinically significant, as with meningitis, or to detect carriers of gastrointestinal pathogens, such as *Salmonella*. Transport media is used to maintain the viability of microorganisms during transport of the patient's specimen and if processing might be delayed.

Environmental conditions used to incubate media are an important consideration. Humidity levels must be monitored so media does not dry out. Certain microorganisms have specific requirements of temperature and atmosphere for promotion of growth. Most pathogens grow best at body temperature, so equipment is usually set at 37°C. Some pathogens require warmer or cooler temperatures for growth, so multiple incubators, set at 42°C, 25°C, or 30°C, should be available. Refrigeration may also be used for cold enhancement of growth.

Organisms may be classified as aerobes or anaerobes, based on their oxygen need for growth. Aerobes prefer oxygen, and anaerobes can be harmed by oxygen. Differences in oxygen and carbon dioxide (CO_2) concentration differentiate atmospheres and provide optimal growth conditions for different aerobes. Aerobes may be obligate, capnophilic, microaerophilic, or facultative. Obligate aerobes grow best with oxygen. Capnophiles require higher levels of carbon dioxide than is normally in the atmosphere. Microaerophiles require reduced levels of oxygen for growth. Those organisms that can grow either with or without the presence of oxygen are considered to be facultative. Different atmospheric conditions are provided in the laboratory using appropriate equipment. For example, a CO_2 environment can be provided by using a candle jar or by infusing carbon dioxide into an incubator connected to a tank of CO_2 gas.

Specimen processing is part of the preanalytical phase of laboratory testing. One must assess the specimen to determine its suitability for culture. If multiple specimens are processed, the correct order of inoculation must be determined. This decision is influenced by knowledge of the life-threatening nature of the infectious disease associated with the specimen type and the fastidious nature of the potential pathogens. Those specimens from a patient whose life is endangered or specimens containing delicate pathogens are inoculated first. Appropriate primary media must be selected based on the body site and be inoculated in an order that will allow retrieval of the pathogens, if present. In general, the least-selective media is inoculated first. Streaking for isolation (solid media) is performed in a manner that will ensure isolated colonies and standardized quantitation.

Certain specimens require special processing approaches. These include CSF and other body fluids, urine, GC, AFB cultures, and cultures of tissue or bone. Special processing may include centrifugation, grinding, or mincing the specimen. Some specimens require the use of quantitative loops or a special streaking technique.

Decisions made and techniques used during this preanalytical phase will have an enormous effect on the ability of the microbiology laboratory to detect the causative agent of an infectious disease. The welfare of the patient and ability of clinicians to determine the correct diagnosis depend on our knowledge and skills.

LEARNING OPPORTUNITIES

1. Suppose you are processing a specimen that has been inoculated onto blood agar (BA), chocolate agar (CA), Columbia colistin-nalidixic acid agar (CNA), and Mac-Conkey (MAC). Which media will grow a gram-positive organism? Which media will grow a gram-negative organism? (Chapter Objective 3)

2. How is the bacteria's environment, provided by the lab, the same as our body? How is the environment provided by the lab different? (Chapter Objectives 3, 5, and 6)

3. Imagine you are setting up the new microbiology cultures. The following specimens arrive in the laboratory at the same time:

   ▪ Sputum with a diagnosis of pneumonia

   ▪ CSF with a diagnosis of meningitis

   ▪ Urine with a diagnosis of urinary tract infection (UTI)

   ▪ Abscess for anaerobic culture

   Prioritize the work and explain your reasoning. (Chapter Objective 9)

PEARSON
myhealthprofessionskit

Use this address to access the interactive Companion Website created for this textbook. Simply select "Clinical Laboratory Science" from the choice of disciplines. Find this book and log in using your user name and password.

REFERENCES

Go to myhealthprofessionskit.com to view this chapter's references.

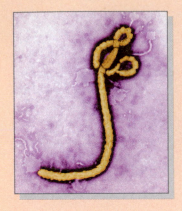

8

Presumptive Identification

Cara Calvo and Karen M. Kiser

■ LEARNING OBJECTIVES

Upon completion of this chapter, the learner should be able to:

1. Identify the uses for brightfield, darkfield, phase, and fluorescence microscopy.

2. Describe the appearance of microorganisms viewed with brightfield, darkfield, phase, and fluorescence microscopy.

3. Relate the parts of a compound light microscope to their function.

4. Explain the use of Köhler illumination when examining patient specimens with a compound light microscope.

5. Communicate proper use, care, and maintenance of a microscope.

6. Resolve common problems associated with microscope usage.

7. Describe the use of Gram stain, acid-fast stains, and fluorochrome dyes to presumptively identify microbes.

8. Accurately interpret Gram stain reactions to facilitate the presumptive identification of microbial pathogens.

9. Identify bacteria and fungi observed in stained smears made from clinical material based on characteristic microscopic morphology and arrangement.

10. Correlate distinctive colony morphology with colony growth on various media to establish a presumptive identification.

11. Differentiate alpha, beta, and gamma hemolysis on a sheep blood agar plate.

12. Integrate knowledge learned in previous chapters with information presented in this chapter to categorize clinically relevant microbes according to their microscopic morphology, unique colony characteristics, and rapid test results.

KEY TERMS

acid-fast

alpha hemolysis

beta hemolysis

chromogens

colony

contrast

diagnostic microbiology

direct smear

differential stain

fluorescence

fluorochromes

gamma hemolysis

Gram stain

mordant

pathogenic

plate reading

pleomorphic

presumptive
 identification

resolution

sensitivity

simple stain

specificity

swarming

working distance (WD)

▶ INTRODUCTION

Diagnostic microbiology is the medical science concerned with isolating, identifying, and quantifying **pathogenic** or disease-causing microbes found in clinical specimens. Previous chapters introduced the concepts underlying the biology of these organisms, the collection techniques used to ensure recovery of viable organisms from various types of samples, and the conditions suitable for their in vitro (growth in a standardized, artificial environment) cultivation. The aim of this chapter is to explain how the clinical microbiology laboratory is able to quickly generate reliable, preliminary or **presumptive identification** of suspected pathogens found in these samples.

Before we discuss the use of stains to aid the microscopic examination of clinical samples, the kinds of microscopy used in the laboratory, the compound microscope's parts and function, plus usage are reviewed. Next, we look at how culture techniques coupled with plate reading methodology help differentiate related groups of organisms one from another and provide clues to the identity of microbial pathogens. Last, a survey of rapid, easily performed test methods is presented. Other more complex procedures that may be used to definitively identify suspected pathogens are covered in greater detail in later chapters of this text.

▶ PRESUMPTIVE IDENTIFICATION

Clinical microbiology laboratorians are charged with the responsibility of identifying infectious disease agents as quickly and accurately as possible. In the past, clinical microbiologists depended on laborious test procedures and technically complex assays to produce clinically useful results. Several days to weeks might pass before sufficient data was available to identify the bacterial, fungal, viral, or parasitic agent causing an infection. However, advances in technology and the addition of automated instruments have much improved the timeliness with which pathogen identifications are made and the culture results reported without sacrificing accuracy and pre-

cision. Often, the laboratory is able to provide a preliminary identification after microscopically observing a stained preparation of clinical material and/or after **plate reading.** This is the process of characterizing colony morphology and growth patterns on primary culture media. Rapid, presumptive identification of a pathogenic microbe can also be made using biochemical tests or commercially available identification kits. Results are available in a matter of minutes to a few hours.

The ability to properly use a microscope is a critical skill required by all laboratory professionals. Developing this skill requires knowledge of the parts of the microscope, correct illumination, care, and patience. In addition, the three P's are needed: practice, practice, practice!

▶ MICROSCOPY

The purpose of a microscope is to magnify an object that cannot be seen with the naked eye. The microscope should enlarge the specimen image, provide image **resolution** or isolate the image details, and provide **contrast** or make the details visible to the eye or camera (Abramowitz, 2003).

A light microscope that uses a bulb or daylight to illuminate the specimen is the most common microscope used in the clinical laboratory. The two kinds of light microscopes are stereoscope and compound. The stereoscope provides a three-dimensional (3-D) image of the object being examined. It is used to magnify larger, 3-D objects like colonies. The compound microscope has several lenses that allow the user to examine thin samples. A compound microscope provides a virtual image that is backward and upside down when compared to the actual image (Abramowitz, 2003).

CATEGORIES OF MICROSCOPY USED IN MICROBIOLOGY

Many kinds of microscopy are available in the clinical laboratory. The most common is brightfield microscopy, but fluorescent, phase, and darkfield microscopy can also be used to examine patient specimens. Electron microscopy plays an important role in virology and research, but is rarely used in clinical laboratories.

Brightfield

The term brightfield refers to the appearance of the object being examined in contrast to a white background. Light from a bulb or mirror passes through the specimen, allowing the viewer to see an enlarged, dark image of the specimen in a bright field of view. Brightfield microscopy is used to examine microorganisms and cells in stained and unstained preparations. Viruses cannot be seen using brightfield microscopy.

Fluorescent

Fluorescent microscopy is used to screen specimens for acid-fast bacilli, fungi, and bacteria. Fluorescence is also used in direct detection of microorganisms using immunologic and molecular methods. ∞ Chapter 9, "Final Identification," and ∞ Chapter 10, "Immunological Tests," provide information on these techniques. The specimen is stained with fluorescent compounds or **fluorochromes** that, when exposed to specific, high-energy, shorter wavelengths of light, are excited and emit a bright light. This emitted light is a lower-energy, longer wavelength light of a different color. The color of the light is dependent on the fluorochrome stain and the excitation wavelength of light used. Xenon or mercury bulbs are typically used as the light source to generate the required wavelength, such as ultraviolet light. Excitation filters are used to select high-energy light at the required wavelength for the fluorochrome. A dichromatic beamsplitter filter is used to separate light into two colors. A dichroic mirror is a used to reflect small specific ranges of colors. It reflects the high-energy light and passes on the lower energy or emitted light to the viewer. Barrier filters are used to remove stray light and pass on the desired emitted fluorescence (Foster, 1997). These filters are usually enclosed in blocks or cubes. Specific filter combinations are required for each application.

Light from the source passes through the excitation filter, and only the desired high-energy light is reflected by the dichroic mirror onto the specimen. The fluorochrome stained specimen emits a low-energy, longer wavelength light that passes through the dichroic mirror and barrier filter to the viewer. Fluorescent objects appear as a bright light against a dark background. Figure 8-1a ■ depicts the light path through fluorescent filters. Figure 8-1b ■ demonstrates detection of *Mycobacterium tuberculosis* in a sputum sample using a fluorochrome stain.

Commonly used fluorochrome stains include auramine O (yellow-orange fluorescence), calcofluor white (bright, apple-green fluorescence), and acridine orange (orange fluorescence). Table 8-1✿ lists typical excitation and barrier filter requirements for these commonly used fluorescent stains. Figure 8-2 ■ shows the wavelengths of light used in microscopy.

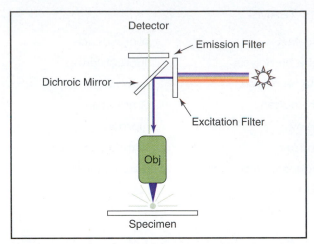

a

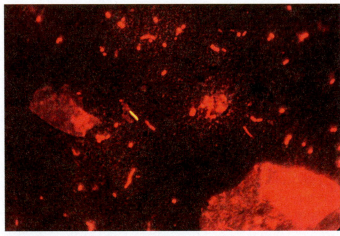

b

■ **FIGURE 8-1 a.** Light path through fluorescent filters. *From http:// enwikipedia.org. Author: Jennifer C. Waters.* **b.** A single *M. tuberculosis* bacillus in a sputum smear is stained using fluorescent auramine with acridine orange counterstain. *Public Health Image Library/CDC*

Darkfield

Darkfield microscopy uses reflected light to highlight the edges of the organism. Figure 8-3 ■ illustrates the light path of a brightfield microscope (a) compared to a darkfield microscope (b). The organism appears as a highlighted object against a dark background. The appearance is similar to a negative obtained in black-and-white photography. It is primarily used to examine skin and mucosal lesion specimens for spirochetes characteristic of syphilis (Centers for Disease Control and Prevention [CDC], 1994).

Phase Contrast

Phase contrast microscopy uses a filter, usually green, to select for one wavelength of light. The filtered light causes the object to appear darker with greater contrast against the background. Specimens are not stained. Phase contrast microscopy can be

✪ TABLE 8-1

Fluorescent Stains

Fluorochrome	Fluorescence	Excitation Light	Excitation WL	Barrier WL
Auramine O	Yellow-orange	Blue	460	515
Acridine orange	Orange	Blue	490	515
Calcofluor white	Apple green	Violet	440	500–520
Fluorescein isothiocyanate (FITC)	Apple green	Blue	490	515

WL = wavelength

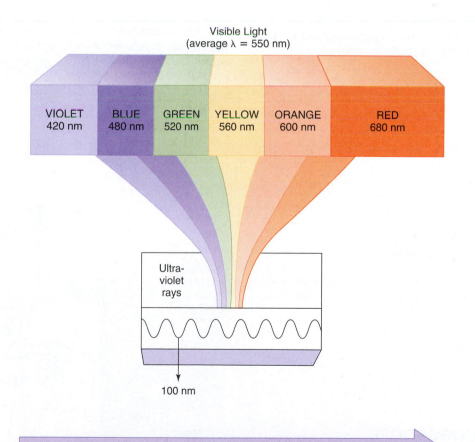

■ FIGURE 8-2 Wavelengths of light used in microscopy.

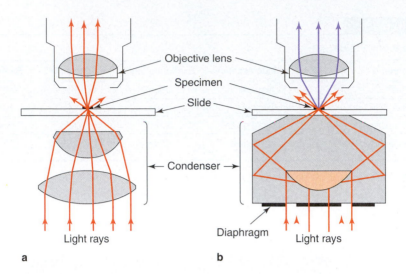

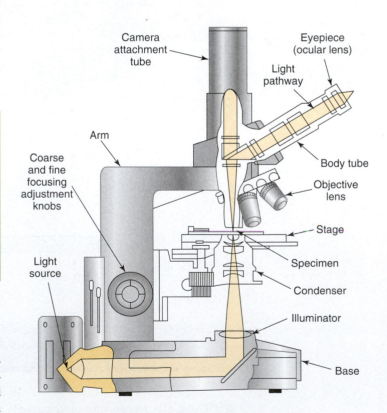

■ **FIGURE 8-3** A comparison of the illumination in brightfield (a) and darkfield (b) microscopy.

used to examine specimens for fungi, parasites, and bacteria (Forbes, Sahm, & Weissfeld, 2007; Foster, 1997).

Electron

Electron microscopes are complex and only used for specialized needs found in virology or research. Electron microscopes bombard the specimen with electrons and imprint the image on a fluorescent screen like a "TV screen." The image is magnified 100,000 times showing a 3-D image and details of internal structure not visible by any other means (Forbes et al., 2007).

 Checkpoint! 8–1 (Chapter Objective 1)

When using this form of microscopy to examine an unstained "wet prep," spirochetes appear highlighted against a dark background. You are using:

  A. *brightfield microscopy.*
  B. *ultraviolet microscopy.*
  C. *electron microscopy.*
  D. *darkfield microscopy.*

PARTS OF A MICROSCOPE AND THEIR FUNCTION

To use and maintain the microscope competently, an understanding of their parts and what they do is needed. The brightfield microscope will be used most often and will be covered in this section. A brightfield microscope consists of a tube with lenses at either end, a stage for the specimen, controls to pro-

vide and concentrate light, and controls to focus the specimen image. Figure 8-4 ■ pictures the path of light through a compound light microscope. The major parts of the compound microscope are also labeled.

■ **FIGURE 8-4** The compound light microscope.

Lenses

A compound microscope has two sets of lenses mounted on the body tube. The ocular lens is nearest the eye and located in the eyepiece. The ocular lens magnifies the real image of the specimen to create a virtual image. The usual magnification of the object is 10 times (10×) its original size. The ocular lenses slip into the eyepiece and may fall out if the scope is turned over. A binocular microscope contains two ocular lenses. The eyepiece is adjustable to the width of the user's eye pupils by pushing or pulling the eyepiece or rotating a dial near the eyepiece. One or both eyepieces may be focused to adjust for differences in fields of vision. A micrometer may also be placed into an eyepiece to help measure objects in the field of view.

The objective lenses are screwed into a rotating nosepiece, on the other end of the body tube, nearest the specimen. Objective lenses gather light and create a real image. There may be three or four objective lenses: scan, low power, high power, and oil immersion. The scanning objective magnifies the specimen image four times (4×), low power magnifies 10 times (10×), high power magnifies 40 to 50 times (40×, 45×, or 50×), and oil immersion magnifies 95 to 100 times (95× or 100×) its original size. The total magnification can be calculated by multiplying the magnifying power of the ocular lens by the magnifying power of the objective lens.

Checkpoint! 8–2
(Chapter Objective 2)

The total magnification of an object when using the oil immersion lens (100×) is:
  A. *100*
  B. *10*
  C. *1,000*
  D. *10,000*

Each objective lens is engraved with markings that provide information on magnification, numerical aperture, mechanical tube length (usually infinity), and coverslip thickness. Review Figure 8-5 ■ to see an example of the objective markings. The numerical aperture number indicates the light-gathering and resolving power of the objective. The greater the number, the greater the resolution and the closer the objective needs to be to the specimen being examined. This distance between the specimen and the bottom of the objective lens is the **working distance (WD).** If oil is required to collect enough light, it will be noted on the objective. Figure 8-6 ■ depicts the role that immersion oil plays in preventing the loss of light. The thickness of the coverslip is important to note. If a coverslip is too thick or too thin, the image may be hazy or blurry. A coverslip number of zero (0) indicates that no coverslip is needed. A minus sign (–) indicates that the objective can be used with or without a coverslip (Foster, 1997).

Rotating the nosepiece until it clicks allows the user to align the selected objective lens in the light path over the specimen

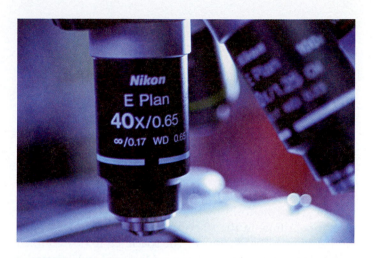

■ FIGURE 8-5 Objective lens markings. 40× indicates magnification, 0.65 is the numerical aperture number, ∞ represents the mechanical tube length, usually infinity, and 0.17 is the coverslip thickness.

to be examined. Do not move the nosepiece by grasping an objective and using it to swing in place. This will loosen the objective. The oil immersion lens should only be used with one drop of immersion oil. This drop of oil will come into direct contact with the lens, preventing light scatter and ensuring sufficient light to focus the object being studied. Be careful not to drag the 40 or 45× objective through immersion oil on a slide when moving the nosepiece to use the 100× objective.

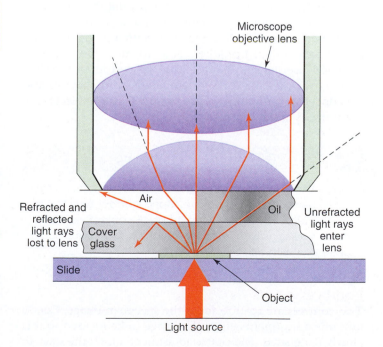

■ FIGURE 8-6 Immersion oil.

Stage

The stage is a platform used to hold a slide containing the specimen. A hole in the stage allows light to shine through the specimen to be examined. The specimen to be examined is placed over the hole in the stage. Most clinical laboratories use a mechanical stage that easily allows movement of the slide for thorough examination of different areas of the specimen. The movement of the object is opposite the actual object's movement. The mechanical stage controls may be mounted either on top or below the stage.

Substage Condenser and Iris Diaphragm

The substage condenser concentrates and focuses the light through the specimen, providing sharp contrast and a clear image. It is mounted underneath the stage near the light source. The substage condenser control is also beneath the stage and allows the microbiologist to raise and lower the substage condenser.

    The iris diaphragm is a part of the substage condenser apparatus and allows the user to control the intensity of light and the light path. Closing the condenser aperture restricts the beam to light traveling straight up. Opening the condenser aperture allows light at different angles to be gathered by the condenser (Foster, 1997). Condensers with a numerical aperture of greater then 1 require that a drop of oil be placed on the condenser lens in contact with the bottom of the slide (Abramowitz, 2003). The substage condenser apparatus also has condenser centering screws to ensure that the object being examined is in the center of the field.

REAL WORLD TIP

Open the iris diaphragm about one-third its diameter when using the 10× objective. Open it about two-thirds its diameter when using the 40 or 45× objective. Keep the iris diaphragm fully open when using the 100× objective with oil.

Focus Controls

Two controls are used to focus the specimen image. Coarse and fine adjustments allow the image to be focused so it is clearly delineated. The coarse adjustment allows the stage to move up and down quickly for general focusing. The fine adjustment moves the stage up and down very slowly so

the object can be delicately focused. The coarse adjustment and fine adjustment knobs are located on the arm of the microscope.

Light Source and Controls

The light source is usually a tungsten-halogen bulb that provides high-intensity white light. It is located in the base of the microscope, sending light up through the substage condenser. The bulb is turned on and off with either a switch or a rheostat control. The rheostat control also controls the intensity or brightness of the light. If electricity is unavailable, a mirror can be mounted on the base allowing natural light to provide the illumination needed.

REAL WORLD TIP

When changing the bulb of a microscope, do not handle it with your fingers. Use a tissue to handle the new bulb. The oil from your fingers can cause the bulb to explode.

Base and Arm

The "skeletal" system of the microscope is the base and arm. The microscope rests on the base. The base also contains the light source, a neutral density filter, a blue filter, and sometimes the on–off switch or rheostat control. The field diaphragm is a ring around or just behind the light opening. The field diaphragm controls glare, haze, and the size of the lit area in the field of view (Foster, 1997). The blue filter changes a yellow light to a more natural white light. The neutral density filter decreases the brightness of the background (Abramowitz, 2003). The stage, nosepiece, body tube, eyepiece observation tube, and various controls are attached to the arm.

USING THE MICROSCOPE

Successful microscopy requires patience, proper illumination, and careful examination of the specimen. With practice, the steps required to perform this skill will become automatic. The microscope must be kept clean and maintained so it is available to examine patient specimens when needed. Users must also pay attention to how they sit at the microscope to avoid musculoskeletal problems. Proper illumination and image focus can help prevent eye fatigue and headaches.

Ergonomics

A variety of medical problems have been reported by microscope users. They include problems with the back, headaches, shoulders, arms, neck, wrists, hands and fingers, eyestrain, the legs, and feet. Poor posture and positioning are the main risk factors (Carr, Fellers, & Davidson, 2008). Newer ergonomically designed microscopes attempt to address these issues, but may not be available in every laboratory.

A neutral body posture is required to effectively work at a microscope for long periods. This neutrality can be obtained by sitting erect, with feet firmly on the floor and forearms parallel to the floor. Frequent breaks are encouraged. Box 8-1✪ provides some basic ergonomic guidelines for microscopy.

Focusing the Image

Turn on the bulb and set the light intensity to a comfortable level. Place the specimen to be examined on the stage, and center the specimen in the middle of the path of light. Align the scan or low-power objective in the path of light. Adjust the eyepiece so you see one circle of light. Close your nondominant eye or the eye using the focusing eyepiece, and turn the coarse adjustment knob until the image is clear. Fine-focus if needed. If a focusing eyepiece is available, close your dominant eye or the eye using a fixed eyepiece and turn the eyepiece focus ring until the object is in focus.

✪ BOX 8-1

Basic Ergonomic Guidelines

Eyes
- Place eyepieces just below the eyes.
- Eyes should look down at 30- to 45-degree angle.
- Adjust eyepiece focus so both eyes are focusing on object.
- Remember to blink your eyes so the surface of the eye does not dry out.
- Wear your glasses if you have astigmatism.

Neck
- Try not to bend your neck forward too much.
- Neck should bend no more then 10 to 15 degrees.

Back
- Sit erect.
- Support lower back.

Arms and Wrist
- Place upper arms perpendicular to the floor.
- Place forearms parallel to floor.
- Keep elbows close to the body.
- Keep wrists straight.

Legs
- Feet should rest on floor or foot rest.
- Backs of thighs should be supported by chair.

Breaks
- Take 5- to 10-minute break every hour.
- Exercise during break (stretch, bend, flex, rotate).

⊚ REAL WORLD TIP

You can determine your dominant eye by forming a triangle with your fingers and choosing an item 20 to 30 feet away to look at. Start with the triangle in your lap, raise it quickly, and look through the triangle at the object. Close the right eye, and if the object does not move, your left eye is dominant. If the object moves, you are right-eye dominant (Foster, 1997).

Recenter the object, rotate the nosepiece so the next higher power objective lens is in the light path, and turn the fine adjustment knob until the image is clear. Recenter the object in the field, rotate the nosepiece so the next higher power objective lens is placed in the light path, and fine-focus until the image is clear. Place a drop of immersion oil on top of the specimen prior to clicking the oil immersion objective into place. Remember that as you focus up and down, you are seeing one layer of the specimen at a time. With higher magnification, you are seeing a thinner layer (Richards, 1958).

Most current microscopes are parfocal, which means that once an image is focused under low power, only fine adjustment is needed to focus under higher magnifying powers.

Illumination

Lighting the object properly is one of the most important steps performed prior to looking at the specimen. If it is not done well, the object may not be visible at all or lack the sharp contrasts needed to identify microorganisms and cells. The light should be bright, glare-free, and evenly dispersed in the field of view (Abramowitz, 2003).

There are several ways to control the light. The rheostat control turns the light on and controls the intensity of light radiated from the bulb. The rheostat control should be set at the lowest wattage possible to provide sufficient illumination. The substage condenser, field diaphragm, and iris diaphragm play a role in adjusting Köhler illumination.

Köhler illumination requires only a few seconds of time to ensure adequate resolution and uniform illumination of the object to be studied. Figure 8-7 ■ illustrates the field of view for each step of the process. Adjust the eyepiece width and ocular lens focus prior to setting Köhler illumination. Start by rotating the low-power (10×) objective into place, and focus on a large object such as a cell. Make sure the object is in the center of the microscope field. Close the field diaphragm, and partially close the iris diaphragm. Make sure the focused object is in the center of the dark circle. Use the centering screws to adjust, if needed. Adjust the substage condenser until a polygon surrounding the object is sharply delineated. A red and blue halo should be observed.

If one observes a soft yellow light, the substage condenser is too high. If a soft magenta or blue halo is observed, the substage condenser is too low. Only slight adjustment of the substage condenser is needed to correct the illumination of the object in its plane of observation.

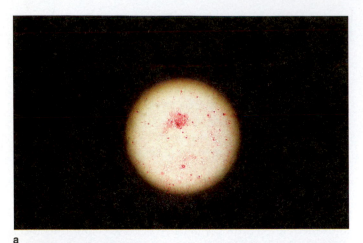

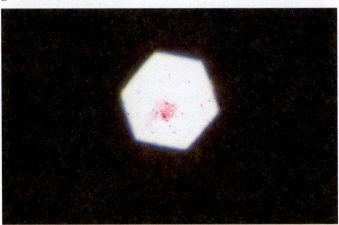

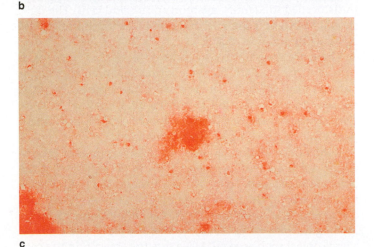

■ **FIGURE 8-7** **a.** Fields of view related to Köhler illumination steps (focused object is in the center of the field, field diaphragm is closed, and iris diaphragm is partially closed). **b.** Fields of view related to Köhler illumination steps (polygon surrounding the focused object; notice the red and blue halo). **c.** Fields of View related to Köhler illumination steps (final appearance of object with field diaphragm open).

Open the field diaphragm until you can't see the polygon in the microscopic field. Open the iris diaphragm until the object is most visible. If there is too much glare, close the iris diaphragm slightly. If the object is difficult to see, open the iris diaphragm slightly. These steps may be needed with each objective (Gill, 1997). Remember that filters and the rheostat control can also be used to adjust the intensity of light.

Care of the Scope

The microscope is an essential piece of equipment used daily in the microbiology laboratory. Dust, dirt, and oils are its enemy. Keeping it clean and maintained will enable it to be used a long time.

Basic daily care of the microscope includes turning the light off and keeping the scope covered when not in use. Never leave the oil immersion lens sitting in oil when not in use. Clean the oil off the oil objective lens and stage when finished. If the microscope is put away in a cabinet, rotate the nosepiece till the scan or low-power objective lens is in place. Carry the microscope carefully with one hand on the base and the other hand on the arm.

REAL WORLD TIP

Clean the oil objective after each use. Allowing the oil to remain on the objective can eat at the cement which holds the glass lens in place and eventually loosen it.

Optical surfaces should be dusted, lenses and eyepieces cleaned with lens cleaner, and the body, filters, and light cover wiped with a soft cloth once a month. Twice a year the microscope should be taken apart, cleaned, and reassembled by a factory authorized, trained person (Isenberg, 1992).

REAL WORLD TIP

Lens paper should be used to wipe oil off the lenses. Paper towels and Kimwipes may scratch the lenses (Isenberg, 1992). If the lens is still dirty, moisten a cotton swab or lens paper with lens cleaner and wipe with a concentric, circular motion, from the center.

✓ Checkpoint! 8–5 (Chapter Objective 4)

Before putting the microscope away in a cabinet, it is important to:
  A. *wipe the objective lens off with a paper towel.*
  B. *leave the 100× objective immersed in oil.*
  C. *rotate nosepiece so the scan objective is in place.*
  D. *rack the stage up.*

Basic Troubleshooting

A good microscopist is able to deal with minor issues that arise to ensure competent examination of a patient's specimen. Many of these issues are related to poor Köhler illumination adjustment or dirt, mascara residue, and dust. Problems frequently encountered include the inability to focus the object, light issues, background appearance, or foreign objects in the field of view.

If you are having problems seeing the specimen image, check that the lenses and eyepiece are clean. Rotate the eyepiece and objectives. Move the slide and substage condenser. Clean the part that is causing the foreign object to streak, move, or disappear (La Trobe University, 1996). Check Köhler illumination, the iris diaphragm setting, and rheostat control. You may need to click the objective in place or tighten the objective. You may need to wipe off excess oil or add oil. If you were able to focus the image on lower powers but not high power or oil, check that your slide is right side up. Table 8-2 ✪ provides more

✪ TABLE 8-2

Basic Microscopy Troubleshooting

Problem Related to	Possible Cause	Possible Fix
Light		
No light	No power	Plug in or turn on
		Reset circuit breaker
		Open field diaphragm
		Increase rheostat control
		Replace or repair electrical cord
	Bulb burnt out	Replace bulb
Flickering light	Loose bulb or plug	Tighten connection
	Broken wire	Replace or repair electrical cord
Not enough light	Dirty bulb	Clean prior to putting in
	Incorrect Köhler illumination	Correct Köhler illumination; remove filters
Too much light	Rheostat too high	Lower rheostat; close iris diaphragm
	No neutral density filter	Use neutral density filter
Base warm	Rheostat too high; not enough light	Lower rheostat; check alignment of parts and cleanliness
Bulb burns out quickly	Wrong bulb	Replace with correct wattage bulb
Can't see because of glare	Dirt or debris	Clean condenser lens; close field diaphragm slightly
Background		
Yellow-orange graininess	Condenser too high	Lower condenser by 1–2 mm
Field partially darkened	Part of neutral density filter in field	Move filter in or out of light path
Yellow-orange light	No blue filter	Place blue filter in light path
	Low voltage	Turn rheostat control higher
	Field diaphragm not centered	Center field diaphragm
Dimly lit	Condenser too low	Raise condenser by 1–2 mm
Crescent-shaped dark area on either side of field	Objective not in place	Click objective into place
Objects		
Particles stay in focus when the specimen is moved	Dirt or debris	Clean filters or top of light opening
Shiny objects in field	Holes in neutral density filter coating	Replace neutral density filter
Unable to focus object	Too much or too little oil	Clean objective
	Too much or too little light	Open or close the iris diaphragm
	Loose objective	Tighten objective
	Slide or coverslip too thick	Check that only one coverslip is used
		Check thickness of coverslip
	Check for fingerprints	Clean objective, slide, or coverslip
Image hazy or blurry image	Too much or too little oil; dried oil	Clean objective
	Too much fluid	Reduce fluid between slide and coverslip
Double image	Incorrect eyepiece setting	Adjust eyepiece to user's pupil distance; focus eyepiece.
Object disappears when switching from one objective to another	Object is not centered	Recenter object before switching to next power.
	Slide is upside down	Place slide with specimen side up on stage

specific information on troubleshooting commonly encountered problems.

 REAL WORLD TIP

One of the two most common problems encountered when using a microscope is the inability to find material on the slide to focus on at 10×. Focus on the frosted edge of the slide first. This will place you on the same optical plane as the material. Move to the area of the original material and you should be able to find it even if it is scanty. The second most common problem encountered is the inability to find the material on 100× even though it is visible on 10×. This most often is due to the slide being placed on the stage upside down.

▶ MICROSCOPIC MORPHOLOGY OF MICROBES

The microscopic examination of stained smear preparations made from clinical samples is rapid, cost effective, and one of the initial steps toward a presumptive identification. At the very least, the information provided by examining stained smears made from specimens can support decisions regarding the quality of the sample, as well as media selection and approaches to the cultivation of microorganisms.

STAINING

On occasion, the examination of an unstained wet mount preparation is sufficient to presumptively identify a microbial pathogen. To make a wet mount smear preparation, the specimen is mixed with a drop of sterile water or saline on a clean glass slide and coverslipped. Note: Water should not be used to examine the trophozoite or active, feeding form of protozoa, as they may be lysed by hypotonic environments. If the sample is liquid, the water or saline is omitted. This type of preparation has the advantage of allowing viable, motile organisms to be viewed. Table 8-3 ❂ summarizes a few of the more common techniques used to examine unstained, wet preparations.

In the section on microscopy it was explained that, to be visible, cells and other microscopic matter, which are intrinsically colorless, must contrast with the field of view background. Contrast is often achieved by using a stain. Stain solutions are composed of a solvent and one (**simple stain**) or more colored molecules called **chromogens.** These electrochemically active molecules interact with cells and noncellular material through ionic bonds. As a result, the cells or material are dyed or stained with the color of the chromogens.

Stains are classified as acidic or basic. The chromogen of an acidic stain has a net negative charge, whereas the chromogen of a basic stain has a net positive charge. This means that when an acidic stain is applied to slide preparation containing cells, it bonds with the positively charged structures like cytoplasmic organelles, but when a basic stain is applied, it bonds with negatively charged cellular components like chromatin.

❂ TABLE 8-3

Common Technique Used to Examine Unstained Clinical Material

Technique and Common Use	Procedure
Brightfield light microscopy: Saline wet prep Detect the presence and motility of *Trichomonas* species in vaginal exudates Detect the presence of parasites in fecal specimens Differentiate yeast cells from bacteria.	A small amount of specimen is mixed with a drop of sterile saline on a glass slide and overlaid with a coverslip. Using the 10× objective and reduced light, examine for flagella and an undulating membrane used for purposeful, directional movement or parasitic forms or budding yeast cells.
Brightfield light microscopy: Iodine wet prep Detect and differentiate parasites in fecal specimens	A small drop of specimen in mixed with a drop of iodine solution on a glass slide and overlaid with a coverslip. Using the 10× objective and reduced light, examine for parasitic forms and their internal structures.
Brightfield light microscopy: KOH prep Detect fungal elements (e.g., hyphae) in skin, hair, and nail clippings	A small aliquot of specimen is immersed in a drop of 10% potassium hydroxide (KOH) on a clean glass slide, coverslipped, and incubated for 20–30 minutes at room temperature. Using the 40× objective and reduced light, look for fungal elements (e.g., hyphae).
Brightfield light microscopy: India ink Detect the capsule of the yeast, *Cryptococcus neoformans*, in CSF.	A drop of liquid specimen is mixed with a drop of ink on a clean glass slide and coverslipped. Using 10× objective, examine the slide and confirm suspect findings using 40× objective. Organisms appear bright and shiny against a charcoal gray to black background.
Darkfield microscopy Visualize motile treponemal spirochete bacteria retrieved from syphilitic lesions.	Lesion fluid is placed on a clean glass slide and a coverslip placed over the fluid. Organisms appear bright and shiny against a black background.

⭐ TABLE 8-4

Examples of Methods to Prepare Smears for Staining

Clinical Specimen Type or Consistency	Smear-Making Technique
Liquid	Use a sterile pipette, inoculating loop, or syringe to transfer one drop of well-mixed liquid onto the surface of a clean, labeled slide. Use a sterile applicator stick or a loop to spread the liquid over the surface of the slide to a uniform thickness covering an area no more than two-thirds of the area of the slide. Alternately, a cytocentrifuge can be used to concentrate a liquid specimen onto a clean glass slide. This has proven to be 100 times more sensitive in the detection of organisms compared to placing one drop of the liquid specimen directly on a slide.
Soft formed (i.e., feces) or mucoid (i.e., sputum) or specimen collected with a swab (culturette)	Immerse a sterile swab in the soft-formed specimen to saturate. Roll the swab right and left to deposit specimen onto the slide surface and spread to a uniform thickness covering an area no more than two-thirds of the area of the slide.
Biopsied tissue	Pick up a small piece of tissue with heat-sterilized forceps and gently touch the tissue to the surface of a clean slide several times but in adjacent areas in the center of the slide. Alternately, the tissue can be emulsified with an aliquot of sterile broth medium and a drop of the emulsion used to make a smear.
Colony growth from solid plate media	Place a drop of sterile saline onto a clean glass slide. Touch a well-isolated colony using an inoculating loop, needle, or sterile applicator stick. Emulsify the colony into the liquid before spreading to a uniform thickness on the slide.

As a general rule, simple stains have limited use in the diagnostic microbiology laboratory. They provide enough contrast to identify physical features of microscopically viewed material, for example, size, shape, and arrangement. However, **differential stains**, made of two or more chromogens, further enable the microscopist to differentiate cellular components within a single cell and to detect fine structural differences among various cell types present in a single specimen.

Most stain methods require the material of interest to be fixed to a clean glass slide (i.e., a smear preparation is made). The smear may be made from a patient specimen (**direct smear**) or from microbial growth in culture. Specimen type or consistency often dictates the technique used to make a smear. Table 8-4⭐ highlights some methods used to prepare smears for staining according to specimen type or consistency. Once a specimen is transferred to a clean glass slide, it is allowed to air dry thoroughly prior to staining.

REAL WORLD TIP

Heat and chemical methods are both acceptable techniques to fix (adhere) the sample material to the surface of a glass slide; however, dry heat coupled with 95% methanol fixation preserves cell morphology, enhances visualization of internal cell structures, and is very useful for examining bloody material.

REAL WORLD TIP

Overheating or forcing a prepared smear to dry by placing it over an incinerator or open flame can damage and distort human and bacterial cells.

A wide variety of stains is used in the diagnostic microbiology laboratory. Table 8-5⭐ lists the more commonly used simple and differential stains. Additional information regarding the Gram stain, the acid-fast stains, and fluorochromes follows.

In 1884, Hans Christian Gram, a Danish physician and bacteriologist, published a staining method (Gram, 1884) that today remains the most commonly used stain in microbiology laboratories. Gram's stain allows most bacteria to be segregated into two groups, gram positive and gram negative, on the basis of the physical and chemical properties of their cell walls (Davies, Anderson, Beveridge, & Clark, 1983). Notable exceptions include bacteria that do not have a cell wall (e.g., *Mycoplasma pneumoniae*), obligate intracellular organisms (e.g., *Chlamydia* species), and acid-fast bacteria (e.g., *Mycobacterium tuberculosis*).

Today, **Gram stain** reagent compositions and staining times vary from the original published procedure, but the underlying principle and interpretation remains the same. An aqueous solution of crystal violet dye is applied to an air-dried, heat-fixed smear. Following a water rinse, Gram's iodine is added to the smear. This **mordant** chemically enhances the bonding of the alkaline crystal violet dye to the acidic microbial cell walls by combining with the dye to form an insoluble complex. Next, an alcohol or acetone reagent is used to decolorize or rinse away unbound dye-iodine complex. A water rinse follows to stop the

REAL WORLD TIP

The most critical step in the performance of a Gram stain is decolorization. Too much alcohol or acetone and all organisms, even gram positives, will lose the crystal violet-iodine complex. Too little and gram-negative organisms will retain the complex. Determining how much decolorizer to use is an acquired skill that can be achieved with practice.

✪ **TABLE 8-5**

Common Simple and Differential Stains Used in the Diagnostic Microbiology Laboratory

Stain(s)	Other Name	Use
Lugol's iodine	N/A	Enhances visualization of nuclei and cytoplasmic structures in protozoan trophozoites and cysts and cestode, nematode, and trematode ova on wet preps
Methylene blue	Tetramethyl thionin	Simple, basic stain enhances contrast when microscopically examining body fluids; dye in differential stains (e.g., Wright's, Ziehl-Neelsen)
Methyl violet 10B (Crystal Violet)	Hexamethyl pararosanilin	Simple, basic primary stain in Gram stain
Safranin	Dimethyl safranin	Simple, acidic counterstain in Gram stain
Nigrosin, water soluble	Acid black 2	Simple, acidic stain optimizes visualization of microbial capsules
Gram stain	N/A	Primary microbiology stain used to differentiate most bacteria into two groups: those that retain the basic dye (crystal violet) following a decolorizing rinse with acid-alcohol and appear blue-purple in color (gram positive) and those that do not and appear red-pink (gram negative), the color of the counterstain safranin
Kinyoun; Ziehl-Neelsen (AFB or acid-fast bacilli stains)	N/A	Alternate common differential microbiology stain used to visualize bacteria with mycolic-acid rich cell walls (*Mycobacterium* spp.) that are resistant to staining
Wright's Giemsa	N/A	A differential stain enhancing detection and visualization of intracellular organisms (e.g., malarial parasites) and white blood cells in fecal smears
FITC	Fluorescent isothiocyanate	A fluorochrome label attached to monoclonal antibodies for detection of specific microbial pathogens
Acridine orange	N,N,N′,N′-tetramethylacridine- 3,6-diamine	A fluorochrome stain demonstrating preferential binding to nucleic acids. It can confirm the presence of bacteria and yeast in blood and body fluids when the numbers of organisms are low.
Auramine-O (basic yellow-2) or Rhodamine B	N/A	These fluorochromes, which preferentially bind mycolic acid, are acid-fast bacilli (AFB) stains.
Calcofluor white	N/A	A fluorochrome stain that enhances visibility of fungi and bacteria in biopsied tissue and blood cultures.

decolorization. The last step is the addition of a counterstain, safranin, a red-colored dye. Gram-positive organisms, with thick cell walls composed of peptidoglycan and teichoic acid, resist decolorization and appear purple in color due to retention of the crystal violet and iodine complex (Figure 8-8).

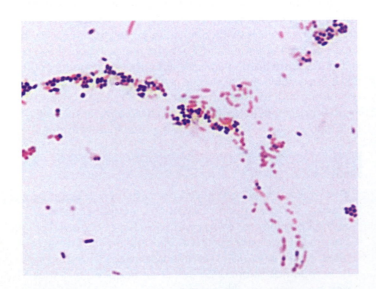

■ **FIGURE 8-8** Gram-stained smear of gram-positive cocci and gram-negative bacilli.

Gram-negative organisms have thin cell walls of peptidoglycan overlaid by lipopolysaccharide. When treated with the decolorizer, these organisms readily lose the crystal violet-iodine complex and are colorless; however, they retain the safranin counterstain and therefore appear red in color (Figure 8-8).

Gram stain results are validated through the use of control slides. These can be purchased from commercial vendors or made using bacteria of known Gram stain reactivity (e.g., *Escherichia coli*—gram-negative and *Staphylococcus epidermidis*—gram-positive).

 Checkpoint! 8–6 (Chapter Objective 7)

The following results were obtained for the Gram stain control slides: The control slide with E. coli demonstrated pink rods, and the control slide with S. aureus demonstrated purple cocci. What is the correct interpretation of these Gram stain results?
A. E. coli is gram positive and S. aureus is gram negative
B. E. coli is gram negative and S. aureus is gram positive

Another common stain used in the diagnostic microbiology laboratory is the **acid-fast** stain. Some organisms, such as mycobacteria, have a cell wall rich in mycolic acids. These compounds are composed of long chains of fatty acids, which give the cell wall a waxy character. This wax coating enables the organism to resist staining as well as decolorization when rinsed with acid-alcohol. Two different acid-fast stain procedures have been developed: the Ziehl-Neelsen method (Lamana, 1946; Neelsen, 1883) and the Kinyoun method. Both use carbolfuchsin as the primary stain, but the Ziehl-Neelsen requires that the slide, once flooded with stain, be heated to steaming. The heat facilitates stain penetration of the waxy cell wall of an acid-fast microbe. The high concentration of phenol in the Kinyoun stain eliminates the need for heating. Thus, the Kinyoun method is referred to as the "cold" method (Forbes et al., 2007). After 5 minutes, the slide is washed with deionized water. Excess water is drained, and then the slide is destained with 3% acid-alcohol (95% ethanol and 0.5% hydrochloric acid) for several minutes. The slide is rinsed and drained again, counterstained with methylene blue or brilliant green for several minutes, and rinsed one last time before being allowed to air dry. Acid-fast organisms stain red to magenta against a blue or green background (Figure 8-9 ■), depending on the counterstain used (Isenberg, 2005).

Positive and negative control slides are run each time an acid-fast stain is performed and before new lots of reagents are put into use. *Escherichia coli* may be used as the negative control, and *Mycobacterium tuberculosis* ATCC 25177 is the recommended positive control.

When fluorochrome dye molecules are exposed to ultraviolet radiant energy (excitation light), they become energized. As these molecules return to their normal energy state, they re-emit radiant energy (emission light) in the visible light spectrum. This activity is referred to as **fluorescence.** Auramine O and rhodamine B are two fluorochrome stains used to detect acid-fast

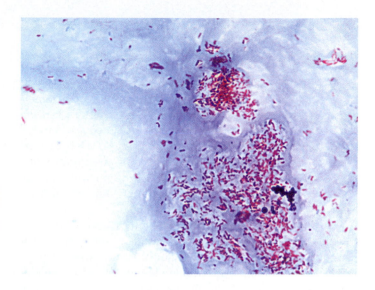

■ **FIGURE 8-9** Acid-fast bacilli (Kinyoun stain) observed in a sputum smear.

organisms. The use of fluorescent stains requires the use of a fluorescent microscope. Refer to the microscopy section in this chapter for additional information on fluorescent microscopy. The observable color of these stains depends on the wavelength of the emitted radiant energy and is unique to each fluorochrome. Typically, acid-fast organisms stained with auramine O or auramine-rhodamine demonstrate a yellow to orange-red fluorescence against a dark background, depending on the filters used.

MORPHOTYPES

In addition to stain reactions, cellular size, shape, and arrangement provides helpful information in making a presumptive identification of bacterial and fungal microbes. There are three common shapes observed in bacteria. Cocci are spherical, bacilli are rod shaped meaning they are longer than they are wide, and spirochetes are spiral shaped. Variations of these basic morphologies are also observed. For example, very short bacilli may be described as coccobacilli. Yeasts typically appear as round to oval-shaped cells and may demonstrate smaller, ellipsoidal protrusions (buds) during asexual reproduction. They are much larger in size than cocci.

 REAL WORLD TIP

Some microbiologists use the word *rod* to describe rectangular shaped organisms. Others prefer the word *bacilli*. Either description is accurate. Microbiologists also often use abbreviations to save time when recording Gram stain reactions. Gram-negative rods are often documented as GNR while gram-positive cocci in clusters are recorded as GPCCL.

Cell size is an obvious morphological characteristic of microbes that can be used to help identify them. Most bacteria of clinical interest have diameters in the range of 0.2 to 2.0 microns and lengths that range from 1 to 6 microns (Winn et al., 2006). Mycoplasmas are considered to be among the smallest bacteria with diameters measured in nanometers (Domermuth, Nielsen, Freundt, & Birch-Andersen, 1964). *Escherichia coli,* a bacillus of average size, has been measured at 1.5 to 3.5 μm (length) with a diameter range of 0.70 to 0.85 microns (Pierucci, 1978). The largest known bacteria are sulfur oxidizers. They can reach diameters of 160 to 750 microns and are visible to the naked eye (Schulz, Brinkhoff, Ferdelman, Hernandez Marine, Teske, & Jorgensen, 1999).

Many microorganisms can be presumptively identified by the presence of intracellular inclusions unique to their genera. For example, some gram-positive bacilli of clinical interest (e.g., *Bacillus* and *Clostridium* species) are known to produce endospores. These are metabolically inactive structures containing DNA and ribosomes and ensure that the bacteria will survive when food and other environment resources are limited. Their size, shape, and intracellular position are criteria frequently used to identify and differentiate spore-forming bacteria. For example, *Clostridium tetani,* a rod-shaped, gram-positive obligate anaerobe, develops a large, round, terminal spore (i.e., located at the end of the cell) as it ages. In contrast, *Bacillus* species produce small, oval-shaped subterminal (i.e., located toward but not at the center of the cell) spores under aerobic conditions.

Corynebacteria, small, club-shaped gram-positive bacilli, produce intracellular metachromatic granules on Loeffler's medium. The granules are energy reserves and stain blue to purple with methylene blue. They may be microscopically observed in smears made from culture (Widra, 1959).

> **REAL WORLD TIP**
>
> Some *Bacillus* species strains (gram-positive bacilli) can be confused with nonfermentative gram-negative bacilli (NFB) because they stain gram negative, do not exhibit typical *Bacillus* spp. colony morphology, and may not sporulate. Spore formation may be encouraged by inoculating an atypical colony onto triple iron sugar agar (TSI) and incubating it for several days. Subsequent observation of spores on a smear indicates the organism is not an NFB because these organisms do not form spores (Bartelt, 2000).

In addition to intracellular structures, extracellular bacterial structures can be detected. Some organisms produce a capsule. This polysaccharide layer lies outside the cell wall. It is a protective layer that prevents phagocytosis or engulfment by white blood cells. The presence of a capsule often makes the organisms more virulent or pathogenic meaning they can cause disease more easily. Stains do not adhere to the surface of the capsule and so it appears as a clear halo around the organism on Gram stain.

ARRANGEMENTS

Another characteristic that is used to presumptively identify microbes is cell arrangement. Cellular arrangement is the manner in which microbial cells distribute themselves in the space they occupy. These arrangements are dependent on the number of planes in which the cells divide and whether the daughter cells separate from the parent cell once division is complete. Tzagoloff and Novick (1977) studied the geometry of *Staphylococcus aureus* cell division and found that these organisms divide in three alternating perpendicular planes, and the sister cells remain attached to each other after cell division. This explains the characteristic "grapelike" clustering arrangement exhibited by these bacteria. Similarly, streptococci commonly divide in a single plane and sister cells remain attached. As a result, these bacteria are characterized and presumptively identified because they form chains of variable lengths, especially if grown in broth culture (Figure 8-10). In 1956 Kuhn and Starr described a unique type of cell division observed in a species of *Arthrobacter* that resulted in random angular arrangements (**pleomorphic**) of bacterial cells described as "V-forms," "palisades," "chinese letters," "log jam," "picket fence," and "coryneforms." Today, these terms are universally used to describe the microscopic cellular arrangement common to *Corynebacteria*

> **REAL WORLD TIP**
>
> Sometimes it may be difficult to determine the characteristic Gram stain morphology and arrangement of an organism. Growing the organism in a liquid medium such as thioglycolate broth can help. Organisms from a liquid medium or clinical specimen provide the most characteristic Gram reaction, microscopic morphology, and arrangement.

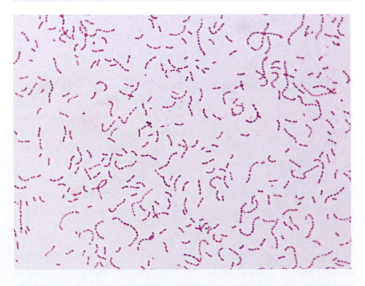

■ **FIGURE 8-10** Gram-stained smear of streptococci demonstrating chain arrangement following growth in broth culture. The organisms may be aging because they appear slightly gram variable. The characteristic arrangement still suggests streptococci.

TABLE 8-6

Microscopic Profiles of Some Clinically Important Bacteria

Gram Stain Reaction	Organism(s)	Morphology	Arrangement
Gram-positive	*Staphylococcus aureus*	Large round cocci	Clusters ("grapelike")
	Rothia mucilaginosa (previously known as *Stomatococcus mucilaginosus*)	Large round cocci	Tetrads
	Streptococcus pyogenes	Small oval cocci	Chains
	Streptococcus pneumoniae	Small oval cocci	Diplococci (lancet shape)
	Bacillus anthracis	Large spore-forming bacilli	Single and chains
	Corynebacterium species	Small club-shaped bacilli	Pleomorphic, pallisading diphtheroids (resembling the Gram stain of *C. diphtheriae*)
	Listeria monocytogenes	Small bacilli	Single
	Lactobacillus species	Medium to long bacilli	Chains
Gram-negative	*Neisseria* species	Small cocci	Diplococci ("coffee-bean")
	Haemophilus species	Small coccobacilli to long bacilli	Pleomorphic
	Escherichia coli	Small plump bacilli	Single, chains
	Proteus species	Small bacilli	Single
	Pseudomonas aeruginosa	Large bacilli	Single, chains
	Campylobacter species	Medium curved bacilli	Single

species. Pleomorphic is most commonly used to describe the many forms of *Haemophilus* spp. In cerebrospinal fluid, *Haemophilus influenzae* is recognized by its wide variation in morphology, which ranges from coccobacilli to long thin filamentous bacilli. Other arrangements that may also be seen in bacteria include tetrads (cells divide in two, perpendicular planes) and diplococci (two cells). Table 8-6 ✪ profiles the microscopic morphology of some bacteria of clinical importance to humans.

 Checkpoint! 8–7 (Chapter Objective 8)

While reviewing a Gram-stained smear the technologist observed a few, small, gram-negative cocci arranged like "coffee beans" in pairs. Based on this information, the likely presumptive identification is:

A. *Neisseria species.*
B. *Campylobacter species.*
C. *Staphylococcus aureus.*
D. *Streptococcus pyogenes.*

► **GROWTH REQUIREMENTS**

Another important step toward a presumptive identification is interpreting organism responses to changes in their environment by manipulating the conditions of cultivation.

SELECTIVE MEDIA

A standard approach to the presumptive identification of microbes is to correlate observed morphologic and metabolic characteristics with expected ones. In ∞ Chapter 7, "Cultiva-

tion of Microorganisms," it was explained that various kinds of media are used to meet the growth needs of the microorganisms of interest. More important, the use of selective media enhances presumptive identification strategies because this type of media supports the growth of certain bacteria and eliminates others. For example, growth on CNA (colistin-nalidixic acid agar) or PEA (phenylethyl alcohol agar) indicates the organism is gram-positive. Likewise, growth of yellow-colored colonies on mannitol salt agar, a selective and differential media, is presumptive evidence of *Staphylococcus aureus*. MacConkey agar (MAC) is best known for its ability to select for gram-negative rods and further differentiate them based on their ability to use lactose for metabolism.

 REAL WORLD TIP

Organisms which grow on sheep blood agar will also grow on chocolate agar. The opposite of this statement is not true. *Haemophilus* spp. will only grow on chocolate, which contains the factors released from lysed red blood cells that it needs to grow.

ATMOSPHERIC REQUIREMENTS

Noting the environmental conditions under which the growth occurred is also a clue to the presumptive identification of the organism isolated. For example, anaerobic bacteria should not be considered in an identification scheme when growth occurs on primary culture plates incubated in ambient or room air. Similarly, *Campylobacter* spp. (thermophilic, microaerophilic, and capnophilic) would not be considered in an identification scheme if no growth occurs on a Campy blood agar plate incubated at 42°C with decreased oxygen and increased carbon dioxide.

▶ COLONY MORPHOLOGY

In a nutrient-rich, solid media environment bacterial cells will not only survive, they also reproduce. As the numbers of cells increase, visible evidence of growth appears in a form known as a **colony.** Colonies develop physical characteristics (e.g., size, shape, and color) that are genetically determined, but colony morphology is also influenced by the culture environment: temperature, oxygen and carbon dioxide levels, and humidity. Likewise, in broth and semisolid media, microorganisms, as they increase cell numbers, distribute themselves in distinctive patterns. In addition, as the microorganism increases in numbers, changes in media color and clarity can occur. These changes are associated with metabolic processes unique to specific microbes. When correctly interpreted and described, all these colony morphologies can aid a presumptive identification.

SIZE

Size is determined by the diameter of a colony. In practice, colony size is described in relative terms: pinpoint (less than 1 millimeter), small (about the size of a pin head), medium, and large. Figures 8-11 ■ and 8-12 ■ illustrate the concept of relative colony size.

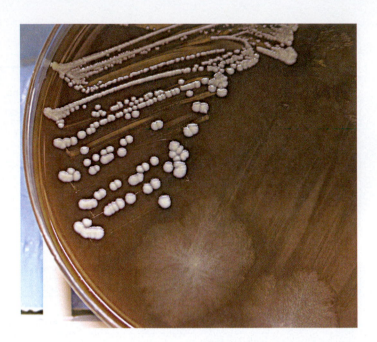

■ **FIGURE 8-12** Relative colony size: very large, spreading, gray-colored colonies adjacent to small, round, white colonies.

SHAPE

Terminology used to describe the geometric form of a colony on solid media varies, but the general features that are universally assessed include (a) form as in round, oval, amorphous (no definitive form), or filamentous with finger-like projections; (b) margin (edge of the colony) as in smooth, undulate (wavy), lobate (lobes), fringed or filamentous; and (c) elevation (colony height) as in flat, convex or domed, umbonate with a raised center, and umbilicate or cratered where the cen-

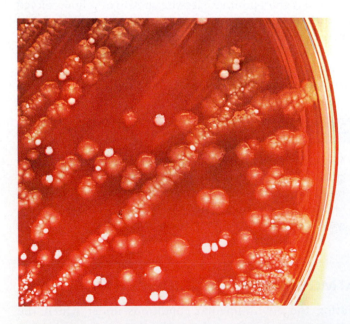

■ **FIGURE 8-11** Relative colony size: larger gray colonies of a gram-negative rod mixed with smaller white colonies of a gram-positive cocci.

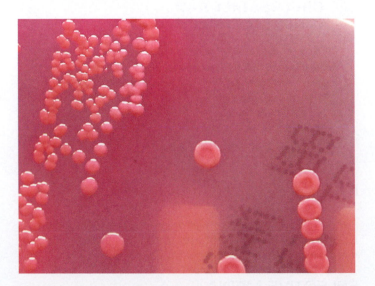

■ **FIGURE 8-13** *Escherichia coli* grown on MacConkey agar. The colony form is round, the margin is smooth, and the elevation is umbilicate.

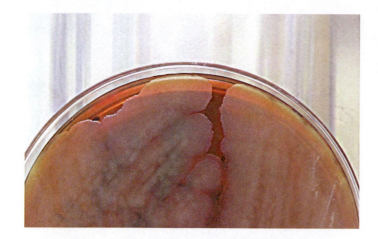

■ FIGURE 8-14 *Bacillus* species grown on trypticase soy agar with 5% sheep blood. The colony form is irregular, the margin is undulate, and the elevation is raised.

ter of the colony is lower than the colony edges. Figures 8-13 ■, 8-14 ■, and 8-15 ■ show a number of diverse colony shapes of bacteria grown on solid agar media.

Microorganisms display a wide variety of growth patterns when cultivated in broth. Figure 8-16 ■ illustrates the characteristic growth of different bacteria in thioglycollate broth.

Perhaps the most common but unique colony morphology phenomenon that clinical microbiologists encounter is **swarming.** Swarming is defined as an organized form of multicellular translocation across the surface of solid media. Swarming is reported by Senesi et al. (2002) to be a strategy developed by some bacteria to ensure their rapid expansion in their natural environment. As a result, swarming bacteria are able to establish infection in a host. Figure 8-17 ■ shows swarming as exhibited by *Proteus mirabilis,* a common urinary tract pathogen.

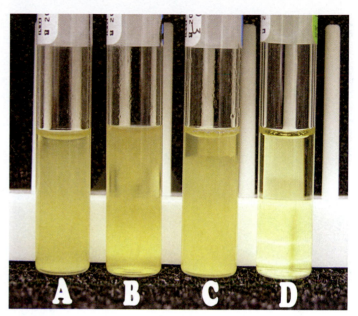

■ FIGURE 8-16 Patterns of growth of different bacteria in thioglycollate broth. a. A facultative anaerobic gram-negative bacilli showing homogenous growth throughout the media. b. A facultative anaerobe gram-positive cocci showing growth throughout the media but with more growth toward the top. c. An anaerobe gram-positive bacillus showing growth toward the bottom of the tube. d. Tube D is an uninoculated media control.

APPEARANCE

Colony texture, pigment production, and density are the appearance factors that are assessed whenever size and shape are determined. Colony texture refers to the relative moisture

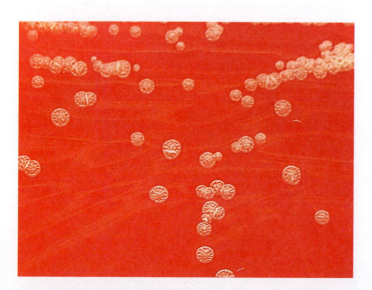

■ FIGURE 8-15 *Staphylococcus* spp. grown on trypticase soy agar with 5% sheep blood. The colony form is round, the margin is smooth, and the elevation is umbonate.

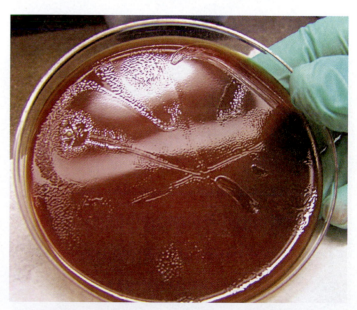

■ FIGURE 8-17 *Proteus mirabilis* swarming on trypticase soy agar with 5% sheep blood.

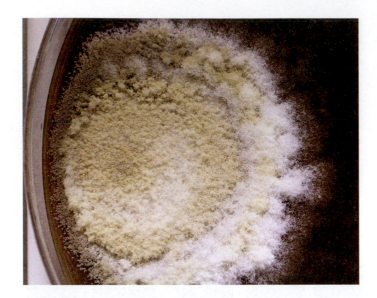

■ **FIGURE 8-18** Dry texture of an unknown contaminating mould colony growing on chocolate agar.

content of a colony. Figures 8-18 ■, 8-19 ■, and 8-20 ■ show examples of colonies that are dry, moist (shiny), and mucoid (shiny and slimy) in appearance.

> **REAL WORLD TIP**
>
> Examine all blood plates in a well-lighted area, tilting the plates back and forth to clearly see all of the features of small colonies. Young yeast colonies may be mistaken for *Staphylococcus* species except that yeast may produce short protrusions that look like fringe from the margins of individual colonies.

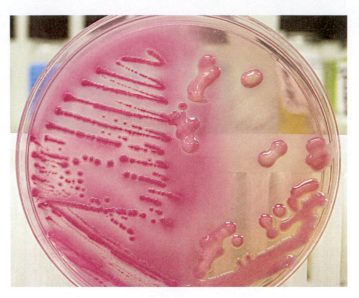

■ **FIGURE 8-20** Mucoid colonies of *Klebsiella pneumoniae* (right) compared to the dark dry colonies of *E. coli* (left) on MacConkey agar.

Some bacteria produce pigments that impart unique color to the microbial colony and diffuse into the surrounding media coloring it. The type and color of pigment produced is often unique to the organism, making pigment production useful in identifying bacteria. Figures 8-21 ■ and 8-22 ■ show the pigment production of two different organisms: *Micrococcus luteus* (lemon yellow), a gram-positive cocci and *Pseudomonas aeruginosa,* a gram-negative bacillus (blue-green). Other pigment colors that may be noted are coral, orange, black, and red.

Density is an optical property displayed by microbial colonies. Terms used to describe density include opaque (light

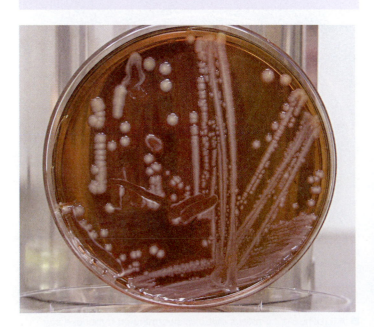

■ **FIGURE 8-19** Moist colonies of *Enterobacter aerogenes* on trypticase soy agar with 5% sheep blood.

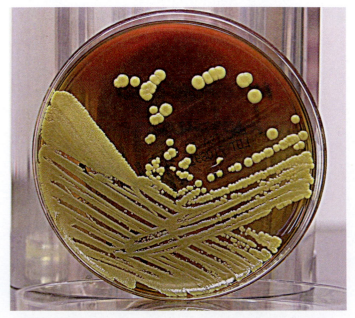

■ **FIGURE 8-21** *Micrococcus luteus* showing lemon yellow–pigmented colonies on trypticase soy agar with 5% sheep blood.

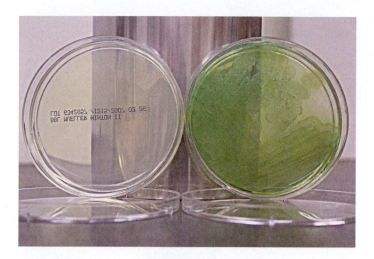

■ **FIGURE 8-22** *Pseudomonas aeruginosa* demonstrating blue-green pigment on Mueller-Hinton agar (right) compared to an uninoculated plate (left).

won't shine through), translucent (light will shine through with difficulty), and transparent (light shines through). In a study by Enos-Berlage and McCarter (2000), *Vibrio parahaemolyticus,* a gram-negative, saltwater bacterium, colonies showed both opaque and translucent phenotypes. The researchers concluded that the opaque colony cells contained higher levels of polysaccharide and were less tightly packed then the translucent colony cells. Figures 8-23 ■ and 8-24 ■

 **Checkpoint! 8–8
(Chapter Objective 9)**

True or False: Growth of two colony types on BAP, one colony type on MAC, and one colony type on PEA strongly suggests a presumptive identification of a gram-negative and a gram-positive organism.

A. *True*

B. *False*

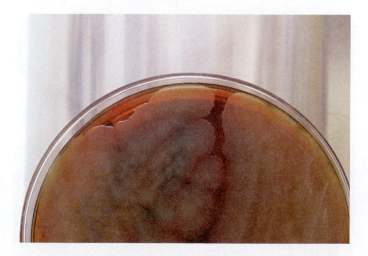

■ **FIGURE 8-23** Opaque colonies of *Bacillus* spp. on trypticase soy agar with 5% sheep blood.

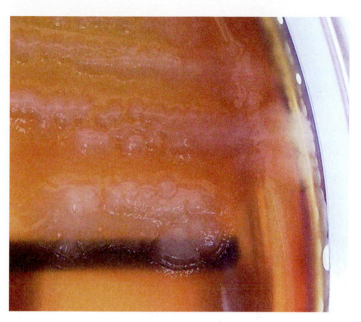

■ **FIGURE 8-24** Translucent colonies of an unknown gram-negative bacillus on trypticase soy agar with 5% sheep blood.

show examples of opaque and translucent colonies much like Enos-Berlage and McCarter described.

HEMOLYSIS

Many bacteria produce exotoxins referred to as hemolysins that destroy red cells and hemoglobin. Visible evidence of this destruction is called hemolysis. Hemolysis on blood agar is used to preliminarily identify and to guide additional testing to differentiate a number of clinically important bacteria including *Listeria monocytogenes* (Fujisawa & Mori, 1994), *Staphylococcus aureus* (Boerlin, Kuhnert, Hussy, & Schaellibaum, 2003), and *Clostridium perfringens* (Buchanan, 1982).

Hemolysis is also one of the characteristics most commonly used to identify and differentiate streptococci. Original work by Todd in 1938 showed that group A streptococci (*Streptococcus pyogenes*) produces two hemolytic exotoxins. One he called streptolysin-O because it is oxygen labile and is apparent only under anaerobic conditions (the metabolite is neutralized by oxygen), and the other he named streptolysin-S because it is oxygen stable, which is apparent when the plate

 REAL WORLD TIP

Streptolysin O is only seen under anaerobic conditions. When plating clinical specimens, develop the habit of stabbing the sheep blood agar in the primary area of inoculation after streaking. Stabbing the agar creates a mini anaerobic chamber. If streptolysin O is present, an area of enhanced hemolysis will appear around the stab mark.

is incubated in ambient air (it is not neutralized by oxygen and therefore active even when oxygen is present).

Several types of hemolysis are recognized on blood agar. **Alpha hemolysis** (Figure 8-25 ■) appears as a green discoloration of the media immediately adjacent to the colony of bacteria secreting the exotoxin. The red blood cells in the agar are partially lysed. This hemolysis type is best seen around colonies of *Streptococcus pneumoniae*.

Figure 8-26 ■ illustrates **beta hemolysis.** It is recognized as a zone of clearing underneath and around the bacterial colony due to complete lysis of the red blood cells. This is the hemolysis type produced by both *Streptococcus pyogenes* and *Streptococcus agalactiae*. Some gram-negative bacilli also produce beta hemolysis on blood agar, including *E. coli* and *Pseudomonas aeruginosa*.

Gamma hemolysis or non-hemolytic is used to indicate the absence of hemolysis or no change in the agar. Figure 8-27 ■ illustrates gamma hemolysis. *Enterococcus* species are usually gamma hemolytic.

Checkpoint! 8–9 (Chapter Objective 10)

While evaluating the bacterial growth on a BAP inoculated with exudates from a tissue wound, the technologist noted a clearing of the area around several small translucent colonies. This type of hemolysis is called:

    A. *alpha.*
    B. *beta.*
    C. *gamma.*
    D. *delta.*

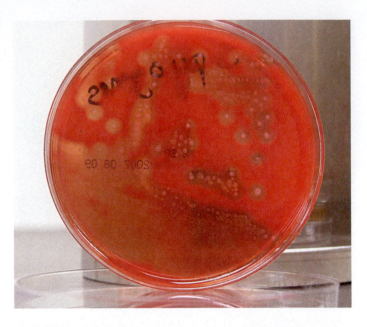

■ **FIGURE 8-26** Beta hemolysis of colonies of *Streptococcus pyogenes* on trypticase soy agar with 5% sheep blood.

 REAL WORLD TIP

Reflected light from overhead lighting makes it difficult to detect and interpret hemolysis on blood agar plates. To resolve this problem, hold the agar plate up so the light passes through the plate (transmitted light).

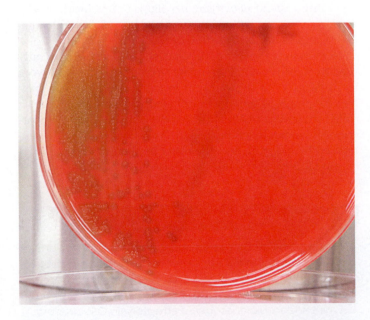

■ **FIGURE 8-25** Alpha hemolysis of colonies of *Streptococcus pneumoniae* on trypticase soy agar with 5% sheep blood.

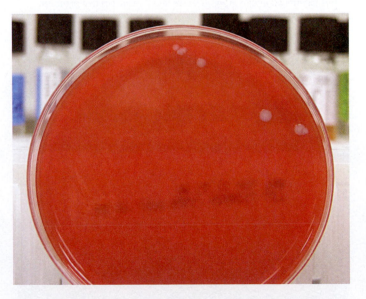

■ **FIGURE 8-27** Gamma hemolysis of *Staphylococcus epidermidis*.

▶ RAPID TEST METHODS FOR ORGANISM IDENTIFICATION

We began this chapter by emphasizing the importance of timely and accurate reporting of microbial identification. Techniques focused on microscopic and macroscopic examination of microbial morphology as an aid to presumptive diagnosis have been reviewed. In practice however, a systematic approach leading to definitive identification only begins with phenotypic evaluations. It continues with the use of a variety of biochemical test methods that are meant to be used in conjunction with those that rely on morphologic assessment. This chapter ends with a brief overview of the most commonly used rapid test methods in support of presumptive identification. The Clinical and Laboratory Standards Institute (CLSI) has created guidelines for minimum identification requirements for some common clinical isolates. This reduces the time to results, which can lead to better patient care. Box 8-2 ✪ provides examples of criteria used to rapidly identify some of the more commonly isolated potential pathogens.

✪ BOX 8-2

Examples of Rapid Identification of Commonly Isolated Potential Pathogens

E. coli
- Beta hemolytic, wet, gray colony
- Dry, dark lactose fermenter
- Spot indole positive

Pseudomonas aeruginosa
- Blue-green pigment production
- Grapelike odor
- Nonlactose fermenter
- Oxidase positive

Proteus mirabilis
- Swarmer on sheep blood agar
- Nonlactose fermenter
- Oxidase negative
- Spot indole negative

Proteus vulgaris
- Swarmer on sheep blood agar
- Nonlactose fermenter
- Oxidase negative
- Spot indole positive

Streptococcus pneumoniae
- Gram-positive cocci in pairs and short chains
- Alpha hemolytic, umbilicated or mucoid colonies
- Catalase negative
- Soluble in bile

Enterococcus species
- Gram-positive cocci in chains
- Catalase negative
- Esculin/PYR +/+

The majority of these methods are designed to detect enzymes that microbes use to metabolize and grow. Additionally, inhibitory profiles are used to measure the capacity of the organisms to survive exposure to various agents that otherwise kill the organisms.

CATALASE

During respiration, many microbes produce potent oxygen radicals and by-products that are toxic to cells. One of these toxins is hydrogen peroxide, H_2O_2. To neutralize this toxin, organisms produce an enzyme, catalase, that converts the hydrogen peroxide to water and molecular oxygen. In addition, white blood cells use peroxides to kill engulfed organisms. Organisms which produce catalase may be able to survive inside the white blood cells.

A number of aerobic and anaerobic bacteria (Hansen & Stewart, 1978) produce catalase, including *Staphylococcus* species, *Listeria monocytogenes*, *Bacillus* species, and *Bacteroides fragilis*. The catalase test is performed by placing a bacterial colony on a clean glass or plastic slide and adding a drop of 3.0% hydrogen peroxide reagent to cover it. A positive test result, indicating the test organism makes catalase, presents as effervescent bubble production, similar to that of carbonated soda. This reaction is observed in Figure 8-28 ■.

@ REAL WORLD TIP

Red blood cells contain catalase. False-positive catalase results can occur if a piece of the sheep blood agar is removed with the colony. To determine if the agar is causing the positive reaction, place a piece of it on a slide and drop the hydrogen peroxide reagent onto it. If the reaction is less than that of the organism, the organism can be considered catalase positive. False positive results can also occur if an iron-containing needle is used to place the organism into a drop of reagent.

COAGULASE

Staphylococcus aureus produces two forms of the enzyme, coagulase, which catalyzes the conversion of fibrinogen to fibrin, which results in either a clot or agglutination. Bound coagulase or clumping factor is attached to the bacteria's cell wall. Extracellular coagulase or free coagulase is secreted by *S. aureus* into its environment. Free coagulase enzyme complexes with a coagulase reacting factor, found in plasma, which coverts fibrinogen to fibrin.

A slide coagulase test is performed using rabbit plasma and a saline suspension of the test organism. A drop of the suspension is placed on a slide and mixed with a drop of rabbit plasma. Clumps or agglutination appear if the organism possesses clumping factor. A control with only the organism and saline

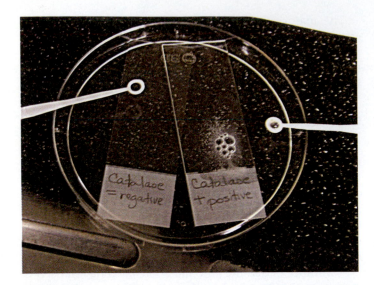

■ **FIGURE 8-28** Catalase test. Visible bubbles indicate a positive test.

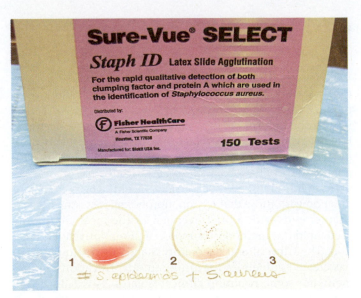

■ **FIGURE 8-29** Slide latex agglutination test. Agglutination of reagent latex particles indicates a positive test (number 2 well).

suspension must be performed in tandem with the plasma testing to ensure any agglutination present is not due to auto-agglutination. Organisms taken from salt containing media, such as mannitol salt agar, have a tendency to autoagglutinate in saline. Because not all *S. aureus* strains test positive for clumping factor, all negative slide tests must be confirmed by the tube coagulase test. Chapter 17, "Aerobic Gram-Positive Cocci," provides photographs of both the slide and tube coagulase test.

In the tube coagulase test, a few colonies of test organism are emulsified in 0.5 mL of rabbit plasma in a test tube. The tube is incubated at 35°C for 4 hours. The presence of a jellylike clot is a positive reaction. After 4 hours, a negative tube test is further incubated overnight at room temperature. Some *S. aureus* strains produce very little free coagulase so only a weak clot is formed. Other strains can produce staphylokinase, a fibrinolysin, which can lyse any clot formed. Incubation at room temperature can reduce the production of staphylokinase.

Commercial latex agglutination tests have replaced the slide and tube coagulase tests because they are rapid, convenient, technically simple, and cost effective (Jungkind, Torhan, Corman, & Bondi, 1983). A number of test kits are available from various manufacturers, but the principle of analysis is the same. On a plastic test card, a few test colonies are emulsified with latex particles coated with antibodies against protein A, a cell wall protein unique to *S. aureus,* and fibrinogen. The test card is gently rotated for a few seconds then observed for agglutination (Figure 8-29 ■). Agglutination indicates the organism produces bound coagulase (clumping factor) and/or possesses protein A.

SPOT INDOLE

Tryptophanase is an enzyme that breaks down the amino acid tryptophan into indole, pyruvic acid, and ammonia. The spot indole test is used to detect indole production on colonies

grown on sheep blood or chocolate agars. This test is used to presumptively identify *Escherichia coli* isolated from a primary culture plate. Other organisms positive for indole include *Vibrio* species, *Aeromonas hydrophila,* and *Pasteurella multocida.* Significantly, most enteric gram-negative rods are not indole positive with the notable exceptions of *Proteus vulgaris* and *Klebsiella oxytoca.*

To perform the test, a test colony is smeared across a white piece of filter paper saturated with Kovac's or Ehrlich's test reagent. The chemical name of the indole reagent is para-dimethylaminobenzadehyde. The appearance of a red-pink color indicates a positive test (Figure 8-30 ■).

ℓ REAL WORLD TIP

A direct spot indole test can be performed on colonies grown on sheep blood and chocolate agars. These two media contain tryptophan. The test cannot be performed on colonies from MacConkey. The fermentation of carbohydrates inhibits the production of tryptophanase and lactose fermenting colonies already appear pink, which is the same color as a positive indole reaction.

ℓ REAL WORLD TIP

Indole can diffuse into the agar and be carried by swarming *Proteus* spp. A mixed culture of *E. coli* and *P. mirabilis* will result in a false positive spot indole reaction for *P. mirabilis* due to the production of indole by *E. coli.* Only pure isolates must be spot tested for indole production.

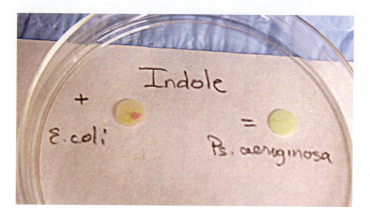

■ **FIGURE 8-30** Spot indole test. Red color indicates a positive test.

OXIDASE TEST

Cytochrome c oxidase is an enzyme that facilitates the transfer of electrons to oxygen in aerobic bacterial respiratory transport systems. The oxidase reagent substitutes as the electron acceptor and changes from colorless to purple. The reagent is biochemically known as tetramethyl-para-phenylenediamine dihydrochloride. The spot oxidase test is most commonly performed to presumptively identify *Pseudomonas aeruginosa*, *Neisseria* species, *Campylobacter* species, and *Pasteurella multocida*.

The test is performed by smearing a test colony, using a wooden stick, across a piece of filter paper saturated with test reagent. Using a needle or loop can cause false positive reactions. A swab can substitute for filter paper and be used to touch the colony to be tested. The reagent can also be dropped directly on the colony on agar but it will kill the organism. Insure a subculture of the organism is made prior to direct testing. The appearance of any purple color, within 10 to 30 seconds, indicates a positive test (Figure 8-31 ■). Organisms

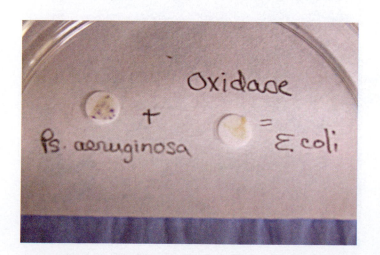

■ **FIGURE 8-31** Spot oxidase Test. Purple color indicates a positive test.

should not be tested from media with carbohydrates such as MacConkey agar. The fermentation of carbohydrates can inhibit the oxidase reaction.

> **@ REAL WORLD TIP**
>
> Do not place the filter paper saturated with oxidase reagent directly on the bench top. The bleach used to clean the countertop will cause a false positive reaction when it touches the reagent.

ESCULIN HYDROLYSIS

The ability to hydrolyze esculin is most often used to identify *Enterococcus* species. The rapid version of this test uses a paper disk impregnated with esculin. The organism is placed in a straight pencil line down the center of the disk using a wooden stick. After 15 minutes incubation, the disk is viewed under an ultraviolet light. Intact esculin fluoresces bright white under UV light while its breakdown product esculitin appears black. A positive test produces a black line where the organism hydrolyzes esculin. Esculin is often combined with the substrate L-pyrronlidonyl-β-naphthylamide (PYR) on the same disk for two tests in one. *Enterococcus* species is esculin and PYR positive.

PYR HYDROLYSIS

A variety of gram-positive and gram-negative organisms produce the enzyme L-pyrroglutamylaminopeptidase whose substrate L-pyrrolidonyl-β-naphthylamide (PYR) is hydrolyzed to α-naphthylamine. However, this test is primarily used to presumptively identify *Enterococcus* species and *Streptococcus pyogenes*. Consequently, positive results of this test must be correlated with the test organism's Gram stain reaction, colony morphology including type of hemolysis if present, and catalase reaction.

Several commercial PYR test kits are available, but the methodologies are similar. A reagent paper disc containing PYR is moistened with deionized water, then a colony of the test organism is smeared onto the disc. A color-developing reagent (cinnamaldehyde) is added after a brief incubation at room temperature. Any red color that develops indicates a positive test (Figure 8-32 ■).

BILE SOLUBILITY

The autolysis of *Streptococcus pneumoniae* is accelerated with the addition of bile salts. A solution of 10.0% sodium deoxycholate can be dropped directly on colonies on agar. Be careful not to forcefully wash away the colony when the drop is placed. Bile soluble colonies disappear within 30 minutes. It can also be performed in a test tube using a heavy inoculum

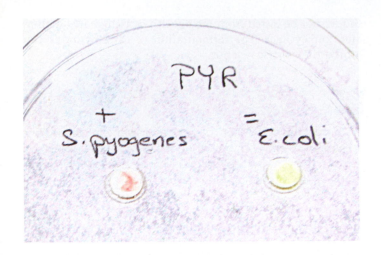

■ **FIGURE 8-32** PYR test. Red color indicates a positive test.

of the suspected organisms in the reagent. A control tube with saline and organism must be included. After incubation for 3 hours at 35–37°C, the organism reagent tube is compared to the saline control tube. Positive bile solubility appears as clearing of the tube with sodium deoxycholate when compared to the saline control tube, which remains turbid.

INHIBITORY PROFILES

The challenge in diagnostic microbiology is to design a test system that can consistently and accurately identify the pathogen of interest, which is known as **sensitivity**, and can distinguish nonpathogens, which is known as **specificity**, to eliminate them from consideration as agents of disease. Testing a microbe's ability to grow in the presence of inhibitory agents, including antibiotics, is a time-honored approach to presumptive identification. It was explained in ∞ Chapter 7, "Cultivation of Microorganisms," that inhibitory agents and antibiotics are used as ingredients in selective media. Using selective media allows the clinical microbiologist to screen for the organism(s) of interest to the disadvantage of the other microbes that may be present in the specimen. This is what contributes sensitivity to the time-honored approach of microbe identification. Using selective with differential media and including antibiotic susceptibility testing is what makes the test system specific. To clarify, consider the following examples.

Streptococcus pneumoniae is a frequent lower respiratory tract isolate of clinical importance. Presumptive identification is therefore imperative. This gram-positive cocci is known to produce an umbilicated or mucoid alpha-hemolytic colonies on sheep blood agar. They must be distinguished from the clinically insignificant alpha-hemolytic streptococci (Isenberg, 2005). Columbia colistin-nalidixic acid (CNA) and phenylethyl alcohol (PEA) agars are selective media that allow growth of gram-positive organisms and inhibit the growth of most gram-negative ones. Both are routinely used to isolate staph-

ylococci and streptococci from polymicrobial specimens. The presumptive identification of this pathogen is strengthened when optochin is used as a test directly on the sheep blood agar of cultures of respiratory specimens (Kellogg, Bankert, Elder, Gibbs, & Smith, 2001). *Streptococcus pneumoniae* growth is inhibited by this chemical. Specifically, a standardized paper disk impregnated with ethylhydrocupreine hydrochloride (optochin) is placed onto an inoculated 5% sheep blood agar plate that is incubated at 35°C for 18 to 24 hours in 5% CO_2. A clearly defined zone of inhibition (14 to 16 mm or greater depending on the disk size used) indicates a susceptible result (Figure 8-33 ■).

Additional examples of inhibitory profiling that aid presumptive identification of bacteria include

- Growth of lemon yellow–colored colonies on mannitol salt agar, strongly suggesting that the organism is a pathogenic staphylococci (*Staphylococcus aureus* or *Staphylococcus saprophyticus*)
- Growth in the presence of the antibiotics trimethoprim and sulfamethoxazole, strongly suggesting the organism is a gram-positive pathogenic streptococci (either *Streptococcus pyogenes* or *Streptococcus agalactiae*)
- Growth in broth or solid media containing urea as the sole carbon source and subsequent hydrolysis of the urea to ammonia as evidenced by a color change of the media to a brilliant pink, strongly suggesting that the organism may be *Proteus* species or *Helicobacter pylori*

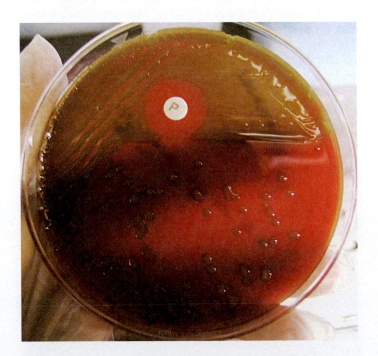

■ **FIGURE 8-33** Optochin susceptibility test on sheep blood agar. A zone of growth inhibition (≥14 mm) around the 5 µg optochin disk affirms the presumptive identification of the gram-positive, alpha-hemolytic, catalase-negative *Streptococcus pneumoniae*.

✓ Checkpoint! 8–10 (Chapter Objective 11)

A small, gram-negative cocci demonstrating a "coffee bean" arrangement on smear tested positive for oxidase and catalase. The organism grew well on CHOC agar incubated at 35°C in 5% CO$_2$, but did not grow on BAP with 5% sheep blood. Based on all available information, the presumptive identification of the organism in question should be reported as:

    A. *Staphylococcus aureus.*
    B. *Escherichia coli.*
    C. *Listeria monocytogenes.*
    D. *Neisseria species.*

SUMMARY

This chapter presented the principles and practices underscoring the presumptive identification of microbes of clinical interest. The initial step toward a laboratory diagnosis of infection usually begins with the microscopic examination of specimen.

There are five kinds of microscopy used in a clinical microbiology laboratory. Brightfield and fluorescent microscopy are commonly used. Darkfield and phase contrast are less commonly used. Electron microscopy is rare in clinical settings but more common in research settings.

The compound light microscope is the most commonly used microscope. Knowledge of the parts and their function allow the user to make the necessary adjustments to ensure adequate specimen illumination, resolution, and contrast.

When using a microscope, a neutral body position and frequent breaks are important to avoid injury. The user should take time to ensure that the eyepieces are adjusted for their eyes. Proper Köhler illumination adjustment is required for adequate specimen resolution and contrast. The object should be brought into focus using the coarse adjustment knob first, then the fine adjustment knob. Remember to recenter the object of interest prior to changing objectives. A drop of immersion oil is usually required when using the 100× objective. When the microscopic work is finished, oil should be removed, the power turned off, and the microscope covered.

The fine art of microscopy is a critical skill needed by laboratorians. Developing this skill requires knowledge of microscopy, practice, and patience. The ability to troubleshoot basic problems ensures accurate and timely results.

The use of various stains aids detection and characterization of microbes. Gram stained smears are assessed to determine the Gram reaction (i.e., positive or negative) and to describe the cellular morphologies and arrangements that characterize and distinguish organisms. Microscopic evaluation yields much important information, but subsequent evaluation of culture growth (e.g., colony size, shape, and growth distribution) is an equally important step toward making a presumptive diagnosis. Nevertheless, the presumptive identification of a microbial pathogen is not complete without consideration of rapid test data. Many of these methods focus on establishing a microbe's metabolic capabilities by detecting key enzymes used for growth, as well as probing the microbe's ability to survive challenges by inhibitory agents. Confidence in a presumptive diagnosis rests on completing a bacterial profile developed from information provided by microscopic evaluation, colony growth assessment, and biochemical testing.

LEARNING OPPORTUNITIES

1. Examine the following figure and answer the following questions (Chapter Objective 2).

    a. What is the magnification power of objective A (left) and objective B (right) in the image provided?

    b. Which objective requires usage of a drop of immersion oil?

    c. Which objective has the higher numerical aperture?

    d. Which objective will be closer to the specimen being examined?

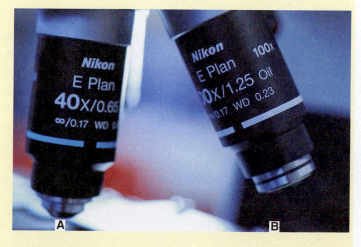

2. List the steps required to achieve proper Köhler illumination (Chapter Objective 3).

3. Situation (Chapter Objective 5):

   a. You are trying to examine a stained urine specimen smear under oil immersion but are unable to clearly define the object of interest. What do you do?

   b. When examining a specimen you notice foreign objects in the field of view. What do you do?

4. Visit the ASM Microbe Library at http://www.microbelibrary.org/ASMOnly/details .asp?id=1095 and review the Gram stain tutorial.

5. Challenge your Gram stain interpretation skills. Visit the slide show at http://www.meddean.luc.edu/lumen/DeptWebs/microbio/med/gram/slides/slide1s.htm

6. Visit and interact with a microbiology blog about various microorganisms: American Society for Microbiology—Small Things Considered: The Microbe Blog at http://schaechter.asmblog.org/

7. Use a virtual bacteriology laboratory. This site will familiarize you with the science and techniques used to identify different types of bacteria based on their DNA sequence: Howard Hughes Medical Institute Bioactive Labs: The Virtual Bacteria ID Lab at http://www.hhmi.org/biointeractive/vlabs/bacterial_id/index.html

8. Create a microbe profile database: For each of the organisms discussed in this chapter, write its presumptive profile on a 4 × 6 index card. Use colored cards to organize profiles according to family, genera, etc.

9. A positive blood culture is Gram stained and reveals no organisms. The microbiologist uses acridine orange on the same blood culture and now sees bright orange coccobacilli on a black background. What type of microscope did he use to view the acridine orange stained specimen? (Chapter Objectives 1 and 2)

   a. brightfield

   b. fluorescent

   c. darkfield

   d. electron

10. You have placed a Gram stained slide on the stage of a brightfield microscope. Once you have it focused using the 10× objective, you place a drop of immersion oil on the slide and move the 100× objective in place. You focus the field of view using the: (Chapter Objective 3)

    a. fine adjustment

    b. coarse adjustment

    c. rheostat

    d. iris diaphragm

11. You are able to focus on a Gram stained slide using the 10× objective. After placing immersion oil on the field of view, it will not focus using the 100× objective. What is one explanation for this problem? (Chapter Objective 6)

    a. Too much light is coming through the iris diaphragm.

    b. The wrong oil was used.

    c. The 100× objective is loose and needs to be tightened.

    d. The slide is upside down.

12. A microbiologist views pleomorphic gram-negative coccobacilli in the cerebrospinal fluid from a 1-year-old female. Based on this Gram stain reaction and microscopic morphology she suspects: (Chapter Objectives 7, 8, and 9)

    a. *Neisseria meningitidis*

    b. *Corynebacterium* spp.

    c. *Haemophilus influenzae*

    d. *Streptococcus pneumoniae*

13. An umbilicated colony isolated from a lower respiratory specimen demonstrates lancet-shaped gram-positive diplococci which are susceptibile to optochin. This organism will also be: (Chapter Objectives 9, 10, 11, and 12)

    a. alpha hemolytic

    b. beta hemolytic

    c. gamma hemolytic

    d. alpha prime hemolytic

14. A urine culture demonstrates large, wet, gray, beta-hemolytic colonies on sheep blood agar and dark, dry lactose fermenters on MacConkey agar. The microbiologist establishes that the organism on the sheep blood agar is catalase positive, oxidase negative and spot indole positive. These results correlate with: (Chapter Objectives 9, 10, 11, and 12)

    a. a pure culture of *Proteus mirabilis*

    b. a mixed culture of organisms and the indole test cannot be trusted

    c. a pure culture of *E. coli*

    d. a mixed culture of *Staphylococcus* spp. and an indole positive *E. coli*

PEARSON
myhealthprofessionskit™

Use this address to access the interactive Companion Website created for this textbook. Simply select "Clinical Laboratory Science" from the choice of disciplines. Find this book and log in using your user name and password.

REFERENCES

Go to myhealthprofessionskit.com to view this chapter's references.

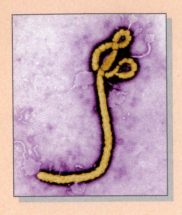

9

Final Identification

William C. Payne

■ LEARNING OBJECTIVES

Upon completion of this chapter, the learner should be able to:

1. Interpret biochemical reactions used in the identification of microorganisms recovered from clinical specimens.

2. Relate the appropriate use of each biochemical test.

3. Correlate the principles of the biochemical tests used to their reactions.

4. Describe the materials and methods used in these biochemical tests.

5. Determine the proper incubation conditions (time, temperature, and atmosphere) for setting up the biochemical tests used in the identification process.

6. Relate the appropriate reagents and the proper amounts added prior to reading the biochemical tests as well as the proper sequence when adding the reagents.

7. Determine any limitations or potential errors associated with the interpretation of biochemical or immunologic tests and molecular testing.

8. Differentiate potential pathogens based on biochemical tests.

9. Discuss commercially available systems used in the identification of microorganisms.

10. Summarize the principle, methodology, and utility of the various techniques used in molecular diagnostics.

11. Restate the principle, methodology, and utility of immunologic tests used to identify microorganisms recovered from clinical specimens.

KEY TERMS

antibiotics	fermentation	opportunists
antibody	fluorogenic substrates	phenotypic criteria
antigens	immunologic techniques	polymerase
chromogenic substrates	molecular diagnostics	plasmid
conventional substrates	molecular techniques	saprophyte
denaturation	nucleotides	serologic techniques

▶ INTRODUCTION

Microbes (bacteria, viruses, fungi, and parasites) have adapted to a very wide range of habitats, including soil, aquatic environments, and the human body. In their association with humans they have the potential to exert a profound influence on human health. Many harmless microorganisms colonize areas of the human body where they benefit from humans as a source of nutrients, warmth, and moisture. They may or may not provide any useful return to their human host, but neither do they pose a significant threat of disease. These organisms may be referred to as **saprophytes**, or nonpathogens. Other microbes have earned a fierce reputation as agents of disease because they are capable of evading host defenses and invading host tissues. These organisms are referred to as pathogens.

Many of the organisms that colonize humans become a normal part of an individual's flora and are beneficial because they compete with pathogens for nutrients and space, and they keep the immune system stimulated so it is primed to ward off infection. Some microbes cause disease, but only when favorable circumstances permit, such as instances when the host's immune system is weakened, or when an individual's normal flora is eliminated by the use of broad-spectrum **antibiotics**, or compounds synthesized by microbes, which exert an inhibitory or lethal effect on the growth of other microorganisms. These organisms are referred to as **opportunists.**

When an individual exhibits the signs and symptoms of an infectious disease, physicians rely on clinical microbiologists to isolate, identify, and determine the antimicrobial susceptibility patterns of the microbe or microbes causing the infection. Specimens from the patient are sent to the microbiology laboratory for cultures and susceptibility testing. Organisms that have been isolated are evaluated. Those deemed to be clinically significant or a potential pathogen must be identified. There are a number of reasons why identification is important. Knowing the identity of a microorganism allows one to

- Distinguish harmless microbes from pathogenic microbes
- Characterize an outbreak of disease and determine the source
- Verify the authenticity of pathogenic strains as a follow-up to the results of a preliminary report or for quality control purposes

- Determine the appropriate antimicrobial therapy because misidentification can lead to inappropriate therapy and treatment failure

Accurate identification of the causative agent of an infectious disease is important in the prevention, control, and treatment. The best identification methods are those that are rapid, sensitive, accurate, and available in kit form or automation. Methods for confirming the identity of microorganisms will be discussed in this chapter. This includes the consideration of:

- **Phenotypic criteria**—physical and metabolic characteristics that can be readily observed (colony size, shape, and color; presence or absence of hemolysis; pigment production; staining characteristics; etc.).
- Physiological characteristics (motility, spore formation, capsule production, etc.).
- Biochemical reactions (carbohydrate utilization, amino acid degradation, enzyme production, etc.).
- **Molecular techniques**—identification of microbes by an analysis of the structure and function of various molecular components found within microorganisms (DNA, RNA, proteins, etc.).
- **Immunologic/serologic techniques**—the qualitative or quantitative analysis of antibodies in the host's serum or microbial **antigens**, large proteins or polysaccharide molecules that elicit an immune response, in patient specimens (sputum, blood, cerebrospinal fluid, urine, or tissues).

▶ CONFIRMATORY BIOCHEMICAL TESTS

Preliminary testing must be performed to give some direction on the choice of biochemical tests that would be beneficial in determining the final identification of microorganisms isolated from clinical specimens. In most cases the investigative process begins with a staining procedure, which provides the means to record some description of the microscopic morphology of the test organism. The Gram-stain method is one of the most important staining techniques in microbiology. For the majority of the bacteria encountered in the clinical laboratory, determining the Gram reaction and morphotype (cocci or bacilli) is the logical starting point for the identification process to begin in earnest, and few microbiologists will proceed without benefit of the Gram stain results.

The Gram reaction, which is designated as gram-positive or gram-negative, is determined by the composition of a microorganism's cell wall. However, some bacteria, such as mycobacteria and spirochetes, do not stain well with the Gram reagents, and in such cases other staining methods can provide the preliminary information required to begin the final identification process. An acid-fast stain is used to determine the ability of organism's cell wall to resist decolorization of a carbol fuchsin or fluorescent stain by an acid-alcohol decolorizer. This stain is used in the identification of *Mycobacterium* species and a modified acid-fast stain for *Nocardia* species and some coccidian parasites (*Cryptosporidium parvum, Cyclospora cayetanensis,* and *Isospora* species). Spirochetes, such as *Treponema, Leptospira,* and *Borrelia* species, benefit from methenamine silver staining or Giemsa staining, respectively. See ∞ Chapter 8 for a review of presumptive identification of isolates.

Once the microscopic morphology of a microorganism has been established, any combination of biochemical tests may be used in the final identification process. Individual microbiology laboratories or commercial identification system manufacturers may use different biochemical characteristics to determine the identity of an unknown organism. Often flowcharts found in microbiology texts use different step by step procedures to outline the identification process (differing in terms of the biochemical tests selected). The basis of the identification process is comparing the biochemical and physiological characteristics of unknown organisms with that of organisms that have already been classified. Tables, charts, and computer databases are the means most often used to accomplish this task.

Checkpoint! 9–1 (Chapter Objective 8)

The Gram reaction of a microorganism (whether it is gram-positive or gram-negative) is determined by the composition of its:

A. *cytoplasmic (or cell) membrane.*
B. *genome (RNA or DNA).*
C. *cell wall.*
D. *capsule (polypeptide or polysaccharide).*

COMMONLY USED BIOCHEMICAL TESTS

All living cells produce enzymes. Enzymes are indispensable to multicellular organisms and unicellular organisms because they are the driving force behind all metabolic processes. They are responsible for catabolism, the breakdown of macromolecules into their basic subunits (i.e., protein hydrolysis into peptides and amino acids) and anabolism, the production of macromolecules from their molecular subunits (i.e., the synthesis of starches from monosaccharides or the production of

nucleic acids from nucleotide subunits). The ability of a bacterium to produce certain enzymes can be exploited in the identification process. In most cases, enzymatic tests are easy to perform and provide rapid results. The enzymatic characterization of microorganisms makes use of the fact that many enzymes are constitutively present and therefore rapidly detectable (Bascomb & Manafi, 1998).

Many of the biochemical tests used to identify microorganisms demonstrate the ability of test organisms to degrade specific substrates such as carbohydrates, amino acids, nucleic acids, proteins (such as gelatin), and other organic molecules. Amino acid degradation involves processes such as deamination, decarboxylation, and dihydrolization. Enzymatic degradation may result in the production of acidic or alkaline by-products, which can be detected by the use of pH indicators such as phenol red, brom cresol purple, and brom thymol blue.

Other biochemical tests involve the ability of an organism to grow in the presence of a single nutrient or carbon source or the ability to grow in the presence of one or more inhibitory substances such as antimicrobial agents (optochin, bacitracin, colistin, vancomycin, etc.), certain dyes (crystal violet, for example), bile salts, or increased NaCl (salt) concentrations. In some cases physiological characteristics can be useful, such as the ability to grow under different atmospheric conditions (aerobic, capnophilic, microaerophilic, or anaerobic) or different temperature ranges psychrophilic (0°C–20°C), mesophilic (20°C–40°C), or thermophilic (40°C–75°C) organisms. For most pathogenic bacteria, the optimal temperature for growth is 35°C to 37°C. ∞ Chapter 7, "Cultivation of Microorganisms," presents additional information on the techniques used to obtain environmental conditions that result in microbial growth.

In the following sections, the underlying biochemistry, the proper techniques of performing, the usefulness, and the interpretation of many of the most commonly used biochemical tests will be discussed.

The Catalase Test

The catalase test is used to determine if an organism produces the enzyme catalase. This enzyme catalyzes the breakdown of a hydrogen peroxide molecule (H_2O_2) into molecules of water and oxygen:

$$2\,H_2O_2\ \rightarrow\ 2\,H_2O + O_2\ \text{(bubbles)}$$

The catalase test is very easy to perform, and the results are seen almost immediately as effervescent bubbles. See ∞ Chapter 8, "Presumptive Identification," for more information on the catalase test.

This test is often used in the identification of gram-positive cocci. It serves to differentiate *Staphylococcus* and *Micrococcus* species (catalase positive) from *Streptococcus* species (catalase negative). It is also useful in the identification of gram-positive rods. *Corynebacterium* species, *Bacillus* species, and *Listeria monocytogenes* are all catalase positive. *Erysipelothrix rhusiopathiae* and *Lactobacillus* species are catalase negative. ∞ Chapters 17 and 19 provide additional information about gram-positive cocci and gram-positive rods.

Bacillus species and *Clostridium* species are both large, spore-forming gram-positive rods. *Bacillus* species and some aerotolerant species of the genus *Clostridium* grow on the aerobic blood agar plate. These organisms will look very similar when a Gram stain of the organisms is observed, but a catalase test will easily distinguish between the two genera, as *Bacillus* species are catalase positive and *Clostridium* species are catalase negative. ∞ Chapter 24 provides more information about anaerobic bacteria.

Catalase tests may also be performed to identify acid-fast bacilli. The semiquantitative catalase test and heat-stable or 68°C catalase test is described in ∞ Chapter 26, "*Mycobacterium* Species."

 REAL WORLD TIPS

Enterococcus species are very closely related to the streptococci and are typically considered to be catalase negative. However, some *Enterococcoccus* species, and in particular *E. faecalis*, may produce a small trail of bubbles when tested for catalase, and this may be a source of confusion for the novice microbiologist. Not only is the quantity of effervescence quite small, but it also tends to be somewhat delayed. This is not considered to be a positive catalase test.

The Oxidase Test

The cytochrome oxidase test can be instrumental in the identification of gram-negative bacilli and cocci. Cytochrome-*c* oxidase is an enzyme found in specific bacteria such as *Neisseria* species, *Pseudomonas* species, and bacteria in the *Vibrionaceae* family, which includes *Vibrio, Aeromonas* and *Plesiomonas* species. In contrast, gram-negative bacilli in the family *Enterobacteriaceae* are oxidase negative. The oxidase test is also important in the identification of nonfermenting gram-negative bacilli such as *Moraxella, Burkholderia, Alcaligenes, Elizabethkingia* (all oxidase positive), *Acinetobacter* and *Stenotrophomonas* (both oxidase negative). ∞ Chapter 8, "Presumptive Identification," provides additional information about the oxidase test. Oxidase reagent–impregnated disks, slides, strips, and swabs are commercially available.

The modified oxidase test is used in the identification of catalase-positive, gram-positive cocci. It is used in the differentiation of *Micrococcus* species, which generate a positive reac-

 REAL WORLD TIPS

■ Only fresh oxidase reagent that is colorless should be used. Old reagent that has been exposed to room air may have a light purple color.

■ Atmospheric oxygen can change the color of the reagent, producing a false positive, so the test must be read within the time limit appropriate for the reagent used.

tion, and *Staphylococcus* species, which generate a negative test. ∞ Chapter 17 provides more information on the modified oxidase test and its role in the identification of gram-positive cocci.

The Coagulase Test

The coagulase test determines whether an organism is capable of clotting plasma using the enzyme coagulase. It is used to differentiate the pathogenic, coagulase-positive *Staphylococcus* species from the coagulase-negative staphylococci. Coagulase-positive staphylococci include *S. aureus*, a pathogen isolated from humans, and *S. intermedius* and *S. hyicus*, animal isolates that are rarely recovered from humans. Other *Staphylococcus* species, such as *S. epidermidis* and *S. saprophyticus*, do not produce the coagulase enzyme and are referred to as coagulase negative staphylococci (CNS). The reagent used in this procedure is rabbit plasma containing EDTA as the anticoagulant. Two tests can actually be used to determine the ability of an organism to produce the enzyme. A positive slide test is detected by clumping or agglutination of the organism. A positive tube test presents as a jelly-like clot. The coagulase test is discussed in ∞ Chapter 8, "Presumptive Identification." Chapter 17, "Aerobic Gram-Positive Cocci," provides photographs of the reactions of the coagulase slide and tube tests.

In the clinical laboratory, isolation of an organism whose Gram morphotype is gram-positive cocci in clusters is suggestive of a *Staphylococcus* or *Micrococcus* species. If the organism is catalase test positive and coagulase test positive, many institutions might consider this sufficient evidence to report the identity of the organism as *S. aureus*, particularly if the typical colony morphology (golden-yellow pigmented, smooth, raised colonies surrounded by a zone of beta hemolysis) is present. ∞ Chapter 17 presents additional information on the identification of gram-positive cocci.

 REAL WORLD TIPS

■ Because a significant number of *S. aureus* strains may not produce clumping with the slide coagulase test, but will produce clot formation with the tube coagulase test, a negative slide coagulase test must be confirmed with the more accurate tube coagulase test.

■ Do not shake the tube coagulase tube when checking for a clot. This will cause a breakdown of the clot that will not reform with additional incubation and result in a false-negative result.

■ Citrated plasma (rabbit or human) is not recommended for the coagulase test because contamination with citrate-using organisms, other than *Staphylococcus aureus*, may yield false-positive results. Consumption of the citrate (the anticoagulant) will lead to coagulation or clot formation (Murray, Baron, Jorgensen, Landry, & Pfaller, 2007).

✔ Checkpoint! 9–2 (Chapter Objective 2)

The catalase test is very useful:
  A. *for the identification of gram-positive bacteria (cocci and rods).*
  B. *for the identification of gram-negative bacteria (cocci and rods).*
  C. *to differentiate members of the family Enterobacteriaceae from those of the family Vibrionaceae.*
  D. *to differentiate Staphylococcus aureus from coagulase negative staphylococci such as S. epidermidis.*

✔ Checkpoint! 9–3 (Chapter Objective 1)

A positive slide coagulase test is seen as:
  A. *clumping of the test organism suspension.*
  B. *a smooth suspension of the test organism.*
  C. *the generation of a purple color.*
  D. *the generation of bubbles (effervescence).*

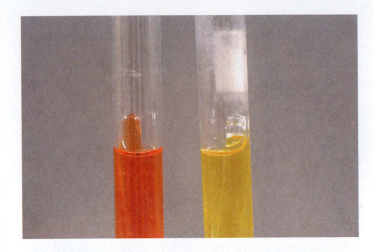

■ **FIGURE 9-1** The right tube shows gas production from fermentation. The Durham tube traps gas produced during fermentation, displacing the medium. A positive result for gas will show a bubble in the tube. The right tube also shows phenol red carbohydrate fermentation broth. Organisms able to ferment the carbohydrate produce acid products, converting the phenol red pH indicator from a red-orange color to a yellow color. Gas may or may not be produced, dependent on the strain of organism isolated. A positive reaction, therefore, is generation of a yellow color. Gas production can be detected with inclusion of a Durham tube.

Carbohydrate Fermentation Broths

Carbohydrate **fermentation** involves the utilization of carbohydrates as an energy source in the absence of atmospheric oxygen. A large number of carbohydrates can be fermented. Bacteria are usually only capable of fermenting certain carbohydrates. The ability of a particular microbial species to ferment specific carbohydrates can be a useful tool in the identification process.

Carbohydrate utilization can result in the generation of different by-products, including organic acids (formic, lactic, pyruvic, butyric, succinic, etc.) and gases such as CO_2 and H_2. The production of acid by-products lowers the pH of the surrounding medium, and this can be detected by pH indicators (phenol red or Andrade's) incorporated into the media. Gas production may be detected in broth medium through the use of a small tube (Durham tube), which has been placed upside down and immersed within the liquid. When gas is generated in the fermentation process, it is trapped and appears as a bubble within the inverted Durham tube (Figure 9-1 ■).

To perform the procedure, the broth, which contains a single carbohydrate source, is inoculated with the test organism and allowed to incubate at 35°C, in ambient air, for 24 to 72 hours. Longer incubation may be needed to confirm a negative result. Any biochemical test that contains a pH indicator must be incubated in ambient air. Incubation in a carbon dioxide atmosphere creates carbonic acid, which can cause a false positive reaction. If the organism is able to ferment the carbohydrate in phenol red carbohydrate broth, it will produce acid products that convert phenol red from a red-orange color to a yellow color. Gas may or may not be produced, depending on the strain of organism isolated. A positive reaction, therefore, is generation of a yellow color and possibly bubbles because of gas production. A negative reaction is no color change (red-orange) or the development of a deep red color

because of utilization of peptones, which produces alkaline by-products (see Figure 9-1).

 REAL WORLD TIP

A control tube, with no carbohydrates present, must be included when testing for carbohydrate fermentation or oxidation. The control tube must remain negative (no color change) for any results to be considered valid. This ensures the organism does not react with any ingredient other than the carbohydrate present.

Oxidative-Fermentative Tests

A single carbohydrate, sterilized by filtration, is aseptically added to a semisolid basal medium (such as Hugh-Leifson OF medium) at 45°C to 50°C while the medium is still liquid. The final concentration of the carbohydrate should be 0.5% to 1.0%. The incorporation of a small concentration of agar to the medium produces the semisolid consistency at room temperature, retards diffusion of atmospheric oxygen throughout the medium, and concentrates the acids produced. Brom cresol blue is often present in the medium to act as a pH indicator because it is more sensitive for the detection of acid by-products than other pH indicators. Phenol red or brom cresol purple may also be used.

Different metabolic pathways used by microorganisms will produce different patterns of carbohydrate utilization, either oxidative or fermentative. Fermentative and oxidative utilization of a variety of carbohydrates results in the production of acidic by-products. Oxidative pathways require oxygen, whereas fermentation of carbohydrates can proceed under anaerobic conditions. The incorporation of pH indicators allows the detection of peptone or amino acid utilization (alkaline by-products) as well as catabolism of carbohydrates (acid production).

Oxidative pathways produce less acid by-products then fermentative pathways. As a result, the acid by-products can be hidden by the resulting alkalinity of peptone utilization, causing a false-negative result. Hugh-Leifson OF medium specifically addresses this problem by lowering the peptone concentration and raising the carbohydrate concentration. More acid should be produced relative to alkaline by-products produced because of peptone utilization, allowing a true positive result to be visible.

To perform the test, two tubes of oxidation-fermentation (OF) medium are inoculated for each carbohydrate tested. One tube is overlaid with sterile mineral oil, which acts as a barrier to atmospheric oxygen, producing the anaerobic conditions that induce fermentation of the carbohydrate source. This is called the closed tube. The other tube is called the open tube because it is not overlaid with oil. This allows oxygen to diffuse into the medium in the upper portion of the tube. If the test organism is known to be a nonfermenter (oxidizer), only the open tube (without oil) needs to be tested.

Fermenters are able to produce acid in both tubes because fermentation can occur with or without oxygen. Oxidizers only produce acid in the tube exposed to air. No acid is produced anaerobically by oxidizers. If the organism is unable to utilize the carbohydrate, it is a nonoxidizer (Figure 9-2 ■).

OF test media are used to differentiate major groups such as the *Enterobacteriaceae* (fermenters) from other gram-negative bacilli specifically the nonfermenters, such as *Pseudomonas* species. It can also be used to distiguish *Staphylococcus* species, which are fermenters, from *Micrococcus* species, which are nonfermenters or nonoxidizers. In addition, this medium can be used to identify oxidative microorganisms.

ONPG Test for β-Galactosidase

Two enzymes are required for organisms to utilize the carbohydrate lactose: β-galactoside permease and β-galactosidase. Permease transports lactose into the bacterial cell, where it is available for metabolism. Without permease, the bacterial cell has to wait for mutant cells to produce permease and then lactose can diffuse into the cell. This process takes longer (more then 48 hours) to use the carbohydrate. These so-called late lactose users have delayed positive lactose results. Once lactose is inside the bacterial cell, β-galactosidase hydrolyzes it, forming galactose and glucose. Rapid lactose fermenters have both enzymes. Non-lactose fermenters are deficient in both enzymes.

The ONPG test uses a colorless compound, ortho-nitro-phenyl-β-D-galactopyranoside, to detect β-galactosidase, indicating the ability to utilize lactose. To perform the test, a heavy

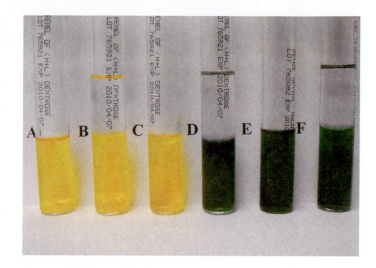

■ FIGURE 9-2 Oxidation-Fermentation Test. Oxidizers only produce acid in the tube exposed to air. No acid is produced anaerobically by oxidizers. Fermenters are able to produce acid in both tubes because fermentation can occur with or without oxygen. Tubes A and B demonstrate an organism that is a glucose fermenter (acid production under aerobic conditions and acid production under anaerobic conditions [oil overlay]). Tubes C and D show a glucose oxidizer (acid production in air; no acid production anaerobically [oil overlay]). Tubes E and F demonstrate a nonoxidizer (no acid production in air; no acid production anaerobically [oil overlay]).

inoculum prepared from growth on lactose-containing medium, is emulsified into the ONPG broth and incubated 20 minutes. If colorless after 20 minutes, reincubate and read at 1, 2, 3, and 24 hours, stopping when a positive reaction is observed. Yellow is a positive result that indicates the formation of ortho-nitrophenol (a yellow compound) and galactose (Figure 9-3 ■). A negative result is colorless after 24 hours of incubation. ONPG

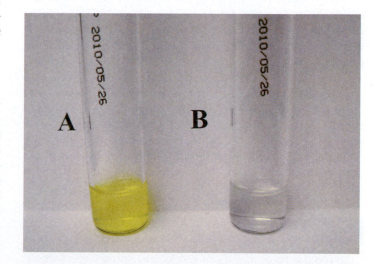

■ FIGURE 9-3 ONPG. A positive reaction is noted by a yellow color as seen in tube A compared to a negative reaction in tube B.

disk, tablets, and broths are available commercially. This test is also included in many of the commercial multitest and automated identification systems discussed later in this chapter.

 REAL WORLD TIP

The ONPG test is not a substitute for lactose fermentation because only β-galactosidase is measured.

Triple Sugar Iron Agar (TSI)

Triple sugar iron agar (TSI) is primarily used to differentiate the *Enterobacteriaceae* and screen for enteric pathogens based on carbohydrate fermentation and hydrogen sulfide production. TSI contains basal nutrients for bacterial growth, phenol red indicator, compounds to detect hydrogen sulfide, and three carbohydrates: 0.1% glucose (dextrose), 1.0% lactose, and 1.0% sucrose. Lactose and sucrose are complex carbohydrates and exist in a 10-fold greater concentration then glucose. Glucose, a simple carbohydrate, is usually used first and metabolized quickly due to its limited amount. An organism that is able to metabolize lactose and/or sucrose will not exhaust the supply of these carbohydrates due to their larger concentrations.

TSI is a slant agar with two reaction chambers: the aerobic slant and the anaerobic deep or butt. This configuration allows oxidation of carbohydrates in the slant and fermentation of carbohydrates in the tube bottom or butt. If the organism is only able to metabolize glucose, it will run out of the simple sugar within the incubation period and begin to break down proteins for energy. If it has the ability to metabolize lactose and/or sucrose, it will not exhaust these sugars within the incubation period and will not need to metabolize proteins. Kligler's iron agar (KIA) is similar to TSI but lacks sucrose.

TSI is inoculated using a needle and a single colony. Stab the butt once then streak the slant, in a zig-zag motion, while exiting the tube. Incubate for 18 to 24 hours at 35°C to 37°C in ambient air with a loose cap. The results must be read no earlier than 18 hours and no later than 24 hours for accurate interpretation.

The reactions of the slant and butt are recorded as acid or A (yellow), alkaline or K (red), or no change or NC. The reaction of the slant is recorded first and the butt second (e.g., acid/acid or A/A). Gas production, a by-product of fermentation (CO_2 and H_2), is observed in the butt as a crack or split in the medium, a gas bubble, or dislocation of the medium from the bottom or side of the tube. It is recorded by adding a G or circling the butt reaction (e.g., acid/acid with gas or A/AG).

 REAL WORLD TIP

Leave the lid of the TSI or KIA loose. Some organisms produce a lot of gas from carbohydrate fermentation and the tube can explode if the lid is tightened.

Hydrogen sulfide production is detected as a black precipitate in the medium. An organism, which can produce hydrogen sulfide, generates H_2S gas from sodium thiosulfate in the medium. An acid environment is required for an organism to produce hydrogen sulfide. The H_2S gas reacts with ferric ions (Fe^{3+}) from ferric ammonium citrate to form a black precipitate, ferrous sulfide (FeS).

$$\text{Bacteria + acid environment + sodium thiosulfate} \rightarrow H_2S \text{ gas} \uparrow$$
$$H_2S \text{ gas} + Fe^{3+} \rightarrow \text{FeS (black precipitate)} \downarrow$$

The presence of a black precipitate is recorded by adding H_2S to the recorded slant and butt reactions (e.g., acid/acid with gas and H_2S or A/AG, H_2S). Sometimes so much black precipitate is produced that the acid reaction in the butt cannot be observed. When working with a member of the family *Enterobacteriaceae,* always assume an acid butt exists if an organism produces hydrogen sulfide.

 REAL WORLD TIP

KIA and TSI are less sensitive in the detection of hydrogen sulfide than other detection media such as SIM.

 REAL WORLD TIP

KIA is more sensitive than TSI in the detection of hydrogen sulfide. The presence of sucrose in the TSI slant tends to suppress the enzyme for hydrogen sulfide production. So an organism may be positive for H_2S, using KIA, but be negative on TSI slant.

The following are valid TSI reactions (Figure 9-4 ■) for gram-negative bacilli:

- Alkaline (red)/acid (yellow) or K/A indicates a glucose only fermenter, peptones used.
- Acid (yellow)/acid (yellow) or A/A indicates a glucose fermenter that also ferments either lactose or sucrose or both.
- Alkaline (red)/alkaline (red) or K/K indicates a nonfermenter, peptones used, creating an alkaline reaction.
- Alkaline (red)/no change (NC) or K/NC indicates a nonfermenter, peptones used.
- No change in color from an uninoculated tube or NC/NC, but growth is visible on the slant, indicates a nonfermenter.
- Record the presence of gas and/or H_2S (black precipitate) as described earlier.

If a yellow slant with no change in the butt is observed in a TSI, check to make sure the butt was stabbed. If the tube was inoculated correctly, it could be a gram-positive organism. Gram stain the growth on the slant and recheck colony morphology and catalase test results.

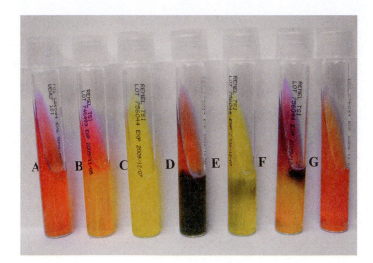

■ **FIGURE 9-4** TSI reactions. Tube A: K/NC is characteristic for nonfermenters such as *Pseudomonas* species. Tube B: K/A is observed with nonlactose fermenters such as *Shigella* species. Tube C: A/A is observed with organisms that ferment glucose and lactose or sucrose or all three sugars. This is characteristic for organisms such as *E. coli.* Tube D: K/A H_2S is usually seen with *Proteus* species. Tube E: A/A H_2S G is observed with organisms such as *Citrobacter freundii.* Note the subtle H_2S production. It can be suppressed with the fermentation of sucrose. Tube F: K/A moustache of H_2S. This reaction is characteristic for *Salmonella typhi.* The organism only produces a small amount of H_2S at the point where the deep and slant meet. Tube G: The last tube in the series is uninoculated for comparison.

 REAL WORLD TIP

All *Enterobacteriaceae* ferment glucose so the TSI reaction will always exhibit an acid butt. If a member of the family *Enterobacteriaceae* is also a lactose fermenter (LF) on MacConkey then it will always exhibit an acid/acid TSI reaction. So if one knows a member of the *Enterobacteriaceae* is a lactose fermenter on MacConkey, then you can deduce its TSI reaction will be A/A.

 REAL WORLD TIP

Proteus vulgaris, *Serratia marcescens*, and *Yersinia enterocolitica* produce A/A reactions on TSI but K/A reactions on KIA. This is due to their ability to ferment glucose and sucrose but not lactose. Since KIA has no sucrose, the only reaction possible for these organism is K/A.

The Urease Test

The urease test is used to detect the presence of the enzyme urease. Urease is capable of splitting urea into ammonia and carbon dioxide.

$$(H_2N_2)_2C{=}O \rightarrow CO_2 + H_2O + 2\ NH_3$$

The ammonia molecule reacts with a water molecule to produce ammonium (NH_4OH), which is alkaline and raises the pH of the surrounding medium. This is indicated by the color change of the medium to a pink or red color when phenol red is used as an indicator.

To perform the test, the urease broth or agar is inoculated with a pure colony of the test organism. After an incubation period of 18 to 24 hours at 37°C in ambient air, urease positive organisms, such as *Proteus* species, can rapidly change the color of the test medium to a pink or red color within a few hours. A weak positive reaction can be observed when only the slant turns pink. Some organisms give a delayed reaction and may require as long as 4 to 5 days to give a detectable positive reaction. Negative reactions are seen as no color change. A rapid urease test can be performed by using a heavy inoculum and reading the result after 4 hours of incubation. If negative, the test is reincubated for a total of 18 to 24 hours and read again. See Figure 9-5 ■ for positive, weak positive, and negative urea agar reactions. This test is useful in the identification of *Proteus* species as well as *Helicobacter pylori.* These organisms generate rapid urea-positive results.

 Checkpoint! 9–4 (Chapter Objectives 1 and 3)

Carbohydrate fermentation results in the formation of _____, which leads to the generation of _____ when phenol red is used as the pH indicator.

    A. *alkaline by-products; a yellow color*
    B. *alkaline by-products; a pink-to-red color*
    C. *acid by-products; a purple color*
    D. *acid by-products; a yellow color*

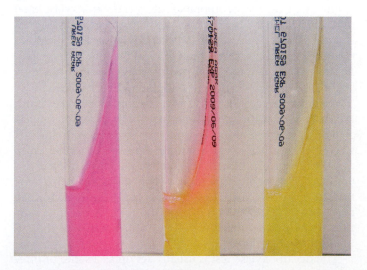

■ **FIGURE 9-5** The urease test. The test organism on the left is positive (development of a bright pink color). The middle tube demonstrates a weak positive reaction, while the tube on the right is negative.

Checkpoint! 9–5 (Chapter Objectives 5 and 7)

A phenol red carbohydrate tube, containing lactose, is inoculated with a pure culture of Proteus mirabilis. After 24 hours of incubation at 35°C to 37°C, in a carbon dioxide environment, the expected result would be:

A. *a yellow color.*

B. *an invalid reaction.*

C. *no color change.*

D. *a red color.*

Amino Acid Degradation Tests

Biochemical tests that determine the ability of an organism to deaminate, dihydrolyze, or decarboxylate certain amino acids can be used in identification schemes. There are about 20 different amino acids, and bacteria usually metabolize specific ones. The most commonly used amino acids are ornithine, lysine, arginine, phenylalanine, and tryptophan. The basic amino acid structure is shown. The side chain (R) is different for each amino acid.

$$
\begin{array}{c}
R \\
| \\
NH_3{}^+ - CH - COOH
\end{array}
$$

Decarboxylase enzymes cleave the carboxyl groups (COOH) from amino acids, converting them to amines that are alkaline metabolic by-products. Testing requires the broth media be overlaid with sterile mineral oil because anaerobic conditions are required for the process. Examples of decarboxylase tests include lysine and ornithine. With brom cresol purple as the pH indicator, a positive reaction is seen as the generation of a purple color indicating the creation of alkaline conditions. A negative reaction is seen as a yellow color because of fermentation of glucose, which is incorporated into the decarboxylase basal medium (Figure 9-6). The glucose is fermented by the organism, usually a member of the *Enterobacteriaceae,* and the pH of the broth is dropped to less than 4.5 and the tube turns yellow. At this pH the decarboxylase enzymes are induced and then act on the amino acid present and the tube turns purple.

Arginine dihydrolase is also an anaerobic process (i.e., broth media is overlaid with sterile mineral oil) involving amino acid degradation. This involves a two-step process. In the first step of this biochemical reaction, arginine is converted to ornithine. The ornithine is then acted on by ornithine decarboxylase, producing an amine, which raises the pH. Therefore, the process generates alkaline conditions. A positive reaction is the production of a purple color. A negative reaction is the production of a yellow color because of the fermentation of glucose.

The decarboxylase test is usually set up as a series of three tubes: arginine, lysine, and ornithine. A control tube, containing glucose but no amino acid, must also be included. The control tube must turn yellow to indicate the organism has used the glucose present to drop the pH so the amino acid

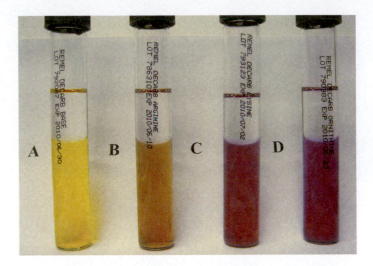

■ **FIGURE 9-6** The decarboxylase test. **Tube A:** The base tube is valid. It must be yellow to demonstrate the organism fermented the glucose present. **Tube B:** Arginine is negative and appears as a dirty yellow gray color. **Tubes C and D:** Lysine and ornithine are positive as noted by the purple color. The development of a purple color is because of the presence of alkaline by-products when brom cresol purple is used as the pH indicator.

enzymes will be induced. The inoculating needle must be sterilized between inoculation of the tubes. This prevents the carryover of amino acids from tube to tube. The tubes are incubated for 18 to 24 hours at 35°C in ambient air. Reading the tubes before 18 hours will result in false negative results because all of the tubes will be yellow.

 REAL WORLD TIP

The decarboxylase test must be modified to test nonfermenting bacilli such as *Stenotrophomonas* species. This group of organisms cannot ferment glucose, so both the control (a tube without amino acid) and a negative result show no change from an uninoculated tube. ∞ Chapter 22 discusses the use of the modified decarboxylase test for nonfermenters.

REAL WORLD TIP

Forgetting to place oil on the decarboxylase tubes can result in false positive reactions. The organisms may deaminate proteins under aerobic conditions. With an overlay of oil, any alkaline reaction present is due to decarboxylation only.

Phenylalanine deamination is a reaction that requires oxygen; therefore, a solid agar slant is the medium used. The enzyme phenylalanine deaminase (PAD) breaks the bond between the amine group ($NH_3{}^+$) and the rest of the amino acid molecule, phenylalanine, to yield phenylpyruvic acid.

The phenylpyruvic acid is detected by the addition of 10% ferric chloride. A positive reaction is seen by the immediate production of a green color on the slant (Figure 9-7 ■). A negative reaction is seen as a yellow color on the slant because of the addition of the ferric chloride, a reagent with a yellow color. A positive reaction is unstable and can fade with time.

The tryptophan deaminase (TDA) test, as seen in Figure 9-16, is very similar to the phenylalanine deaminase test and is often substituted for this test in miniaturized and automated identification systems. The tryptophan deaminase test utilizes a broth medium. The reagent used to detect the biochemical reaction is the same as that used in the phenylalanine deaminase test, 10% ferric chloride. A positive reaction is seen by the generation of a brown color. If the medium remains yellow after the addition of ferric chloride, the test result is negative.

Lysine Iron Agar (LIA)

Lysine iron agar (LIA) is used to differentiate the *Enterobacteriaceae* and screen for enteric pathogens such as *Salmonella* and *Shigella* species. This medium detects decarboxylation or deamination of lysine and hydrogen sulfide production. LIA is a tubed, solid, slant medium, and results are recorded in a manner similar to TSI (i.e., slant/butt). To inoculate the medium, select a single, pure colony with a sterile needle, streak the slant, and stab the bottom twice.

The lysine deamination reaction (red) is observed in the slant, and the lysine decarboxylation reaction (purple or alkaline) is seen in the butt. Hydrogen sulfide production is indicated by a black precipitate. A purple slant and yellow butt is negative for decarboxylation and deamination. The following are valid LIA reactions (Figure 9-8 ■) for gram-negative bacilli:

■ Alkaline (purple)/acid (yellow) or K/A indicates a negative result for decarboxylation and deamination of lysine (e.g., *Citrobacter*).

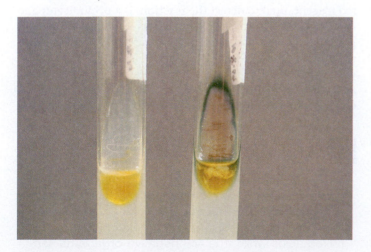

■ **FIGURE 9-7** The phenylalanine test. The test organism on the right is positive (development of a green color). The test organism on the left is negative.

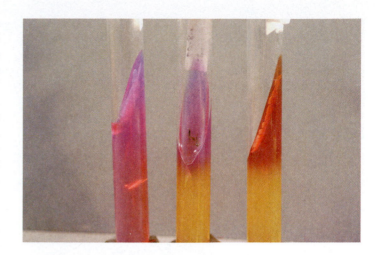

■ **FIGURE 9-8** Possible LIA reactions for fermenting gram-negative rods: K/K (left), K/A (middle), and R/A (right).

■ Alkaline (purple)/alkaline (purple) or K/K indicates decarboxylation of lysine (e.g., *E. coli* and *Enterobacter*).

■ Red (red)/acid (yellow) or R/A indicates deamination of lysine (e.g., *Proteus*, *Providencia*, and *Morganella*).

■ Record the presence of H_2S (black precipitate) with the butt reaction (i.e., K/K, H_2S). In LIA, production of hydrogen sulfide only occurs in an alkaline environment so assume the lysine decarboxylation is also positive (e.g., *Salmonella* and *Edwardsiella*) if the butt reaction is obscured by the black precipitate.

@ REAL WORLD TIP

To ensure valid results and interpretation of LIA, double-check that the slant has growth and the bottom of the tube was stabbed prior to recording results.

IMViC Tests

The indole (Figure 9-9 ■), methyl-red (Figure 9-10 ■), Voges-Proskauer (Figure 9-10), and citrate (Figure 9-11 ■) tests make up the IMViC tests. The indole, methyl-red, and Voges-Proskauer tests are inoculated with a pure, single colony or one or two drops of an organism suspension in saline. Citrate is a solid medium and requires a light inoculum of the slant.

The indole test often uses SIM medium, which also detects hydrogen sulfide production and motility. Kovacs' or Ehrlich's reagent is used to detect indole after the breakdown of the amino acid tryptophan. ∞ Chapter 8, "Presumptive Identification," summarizes the principle and use of the test. Figure 8-30 demonstrates a rapid spot indole test.

The methyl red-Voges-Proskauer (MR-VP) test is run as two tests in one broth tube. Organisms that metabolize glucose produce pyruvic acid. The MR-VP test determines how the organism further degrades pyruvic acid. There are two possible pathways: the pyruvic acid is converted to low pH mixed acids or converted to acetoin (acetyl-methylcarbinol). Most of

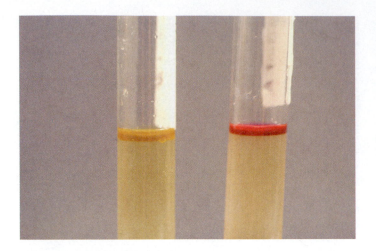

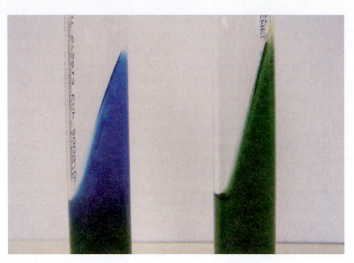

■ FIGURE 9-9 The indole test. The tube on the right shows a positive test (formation of a red ring). The tube on the left shows a negative reaction (no red ring).

■ FIGURE 9-11 Citrate test. The tube on the left demonstrates a positive reaction (blue), while the tube on the right is negative. Remember growth without a color change is also considered a positive reaction.

the *Enterobacteriaceae* use one pathway or the other. It is rare for an organism to use both pathways. *Hafnia alvei* and *Proteus mirabilis* may use both pathways.

$$\text{Glucose} \rightarrow \text{pyruvic acid} \nearrow \text{Acetyl-methyl carbinol (acetoin) (MR=VP+)} \searrow \text{Mixed acids at a pH} < 4.4 \text{ (MR+VP=)}$$

A two mL MR-VP broth is inoculated with a pure colony. The tube is incubated for 18 to 24 hours at 35°C in ambient air. After incubation, 1 mL is removed for the VP test. The remaining 1 mL is reincubated for an additional 24 hours for the methyl red test. The VP test requires the addition of 0.6 mL of 5.0% alpha naphthol and 0.2 mL of 40% potassium hydrox-

ide (KOH). The order of the reagents is critical. If the reagents are reversed, KOH can react with peptones present and present with a false positive reaction.

Alpha naphthol reacts with acetoin to create diacetyl which then reacts with KOH to produce a pink color after 10 to 20 minutes (Figure 9-10). A negative reaction remains colorless. After 1 hour, the two reagents can react to form a copper color, which is a negative reaction. A positive VP reaction differentiates *Klebsiella*, *Enterobacter*, *Serratia* and *Pantoea* species from other genera in the family *Enterobacteriaceae*.

The remaining broth is tested, after 48 hours incubation, for the methyl red reaction. The MR test determines if pyruvic acid is broken down into low pH mixed acids. Organisms that are MR positive can overcome the natural buffering system and maintain these acids at a pH of 4.4 or less. The methyl red reagent, used to detect the reaction, is a pH indicator and is more acidic than other pH indicators. It detects changes in pH ranges lower than other pH indicators. A positive MR is red after addition of the MR reagent (Figure 9-10). This indicates a pH of 4.4 or less. An orange reaction is inconclusive and must be retested. A yellow reaction is due to a pH of 6.0 or greater and is considered negative.

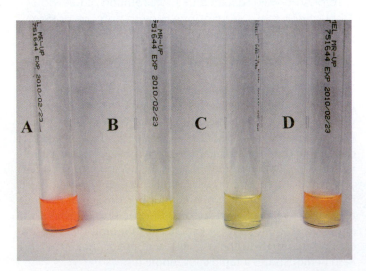

■ FIGURE 9-10 The methyl-red-Voges Proskauer (MRVP) test. **Tube A:** *E.coli* is MR positive. **Tube B:** *Enterobacter cloacae* is MR negative. **Tube C:** *E. coli* is VP negative. **Tube D:** *E. cloacae* is VP positive. The MR test must be performed after 48 hours incubation, while the VP test is performed after 24 hours incubation.

REAL WORLD TIP

All *Enterobacteriaceae* ferment glucose and, at 24 hours incubation, all members of the family present with a positive MR reaction. After 48 hours, true MR positive organisms are able to maintain the low pH mixed acids while true MR negative organisms cannot. Testing the MR reaction too early may present with a false positive reaction.

The citrate test determines if an organism is capable of using sodium citrate as the sole source of carbon for metabolism and growth. The agar slant contains citrate and ammonium phosphate. Organisms that can use citrate can also extract nitrogen from the ammonium salt to produce ammonia, which is alkaline. The brom thymol blue indicator is green and turns blue with alkaline byproducts (Figure 9-11). The tube is inoculated lightly on the slant and incubated at 35°C in ambient air for 18 to 24 hours. Flame sterilize prior to inoculation of this tube with organism. This prevents the carryover of glucose or nitrogen from other tubes. This can create a false positive reaction. A heavy inoculum leads to dead organisms that release enough carbon and nitrogen to create a false positive reaction. Growth on the slant but no color change is still considered a positive reaction because the organisms are using the carbon and nitrogen to grow but have not had enough time to turn the pH indicator blue.

Motility

Motility can be observed by three methods: flagella stain, hanging drop of bacterial suspension, or semisolid medium. Determination of motility by a flagellum stain or the hanging drop method can be cumbersome and difficult to interpret. The flagellum stain is rarely performed in most clinical microbiology laboratories and often reserved for large reference laboratories. In the hanging drop method, a drop of 18 to 24 hour bacterial suspension is placed on the center of a cover slip. A small drop of water is placed in the four corners of the cover slip. A glass slide with a depressed center is placed over the slide and both are rapidly flipped over and read under a microscope using the 40× objective. If a depressed slide is not available, a ring of petroleum jelly can be built up on a regular glass slide to create a depression. Brownian movement is the random movement of organisms due to collisions with molecules in the liquid. This can be confused with the purposeful, directional movement of motile organisms.

Tubed medium must possess less than 0.4% agar to demonstrate motility. The sulfur-indole-motility (SIM) tube is often used to demonstrate motility. A straight sterile needle is used to stab the agar to about one half its depth. Do not move the needle from side to side as the agar is being stabbed. After overnight incubation at 35°C in ambient air, motility is seen as fuzziness or haziness away from the line of inoculation (Figure 9-12 ■). A nonmotile organism will demonstrate growth only

 REAL WORLD TIP

Motility medium with triphenyltetrazolium chloride or TTC is an easier way to determine motility. TTC is a colorless dye that turns red with organism growth. Motility away from the stab line of inoculation is easier to view due to the red dye (Figure 9-12). One potential problem with this medium is that some organisms may be inhibited by the dye, causing a false negative reaction.

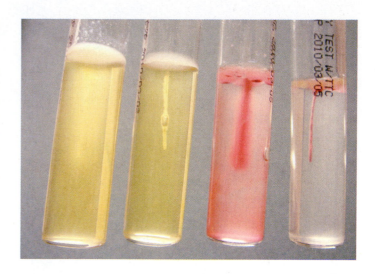

■ **FIGURE 9-12** Motility test. The tube on the far left demonstrates a motile organism as seen by the haze of growth away from the stab line. The middle left tube is nonmotile. The middle right tube shows a motile organism using motility medium with the dye, TTC. It is much easier to interpret than the tube on the far left. The tube on the far right is nonmotile.

within the stab line. *Klebsiella* and *Shigella* species are the nonmotile genera of the family *Enterobacteriaceae*. *Yersinia* species and *Listeria monocyotogenes* are only motile at room temperature. The use of two motility agar tubes, one incubated at 25°C and one at 35°C, are necessary for their identification. One tube can be used if the negative motility tube is incubated at room temperature after 48 hours incubation at 35°C.

Nitrate Reduction

Nitrate is reduced to nitrites by all members of the family *Enterobacteriaceae*. Other organisms are able to further reduce nitrites to nitrogen gas (N_2). The nitrate broth is inoculated and incubated for 24 hours, at 35°C in ambient air, prior to testing. After incubation, 5 drops of each of the two reagents is added. Reagent A is alpha-naphthylamine and reagent B is sulfanilic acid. These two reagents react with nitrite to form a red color within 1 to 2 minutes. If the organism is able to reduce nitrate to nitrogen gas, then nitrites are not available to react with the two reagents and the broth remains colorless. A colorless broth will also occur if the organism did not reduce nitrates at all.

A negative (colorless) nitrate test requires further testing to determine if the organism did not reduce nitrates or reduced them to nitrogen gas. A pinch of zinc dust is added to the broth and observed for a color change. Zinc is able to reduce nitrate to nitrite. If the organism reduced nitrate to nitrogen gas, then there are no nitrates present and the addition of zinc dust will have no effect. This is considered a positive test. If nitrates were not reduced then zinc will reduce them to nitrites. Nitrites will then react with the two reagents present, and the tube will turn red. Figure 9-13 ■ depicts all of the nitrate tube reactions.

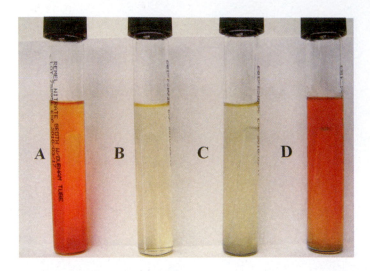

■ **FIGURE 9-13** Nitrate test. Tube A: The *Enterobacteriaceae* are able to reduce nitrates to nitrites as demonstrated by the red color after addition of reagents. Tube B: No color change after addition of nitrate reagents requires further testing. Either the organism reduced nitrate beyond nitrites or did not reduce it at all. Tube C: No color change after the addition of zinc is a positive reaction. Zinc is able to reduce nitrates to nitrites. If no nitrates are available there is no color change. Tube D: A red color after the addition of zinc indicates a negative test. The unreduced nitrates were reduced by zinc and then reacted with the reagents to cause the red color.

@ REAL WORLD TIP

For the nitrate test, red after addition of reagents A and B is positive, but red after the addition of zinc dust is negative.

The IMViC reactions can be used to group *Enterobacteriaceae* into probable genera. H_2S production, decarboxylation and deamination reactions, and results for lactose fermentation can enhance presumptive identification to genus. The microbiologist can correlate this presumptive identification to genus with Gram stain results, colony morphology, screening test results, and final identification to species and judge the accuracy prior to finalizing the report to the physician. If results do not correlate, then a search for a possible error (either recording or reading) or mistaken identity can occur. Table 9-1 ✪ summarizes commonly used tests for identification of bacteria. Figure 9-14 ■ suggests a scheme for presumptive identification to a genus using IMViC, H_2S, decarboxylation, and deamination test results. Refer to ∞ Chapter 21, "*Enterobacteriaceae*," for more information on each genus and specific tests to identify to species.

Susceptibility to Antibiotics or Chemicals

A bacterial isolate's susceptibility to a particular antimicrobial agent or chemical can also be useful in the identification process. Antibiotic or chemical impregnated disk or nutrient broth into which the antibiotic or chemical has been incorporated can be used. Impregnated disks are often employed when a solid agar medium is to be used. A zone of inhibition around the disk would indicate susceptibility. Growth up to the edge of the disk or small zone sizes demonstrates resistance and may be considered a negative reaction. Some disk tests (e.g., optochin) require measurement of the zone size for interpretation. A broth medium is used for automated identification systems. Inhibition of growth (a clear broth) after 18 to 24 hours of incubation would indicate susceptibility. Turbidity would indicate resistance.

- Gram-positive bacteria are usually susceptible to vancomycin, an antimicrobial agent that acts on the cell wall. Gram-negative bacteria are, for the most part, resistant. *Lactobacillus, Leuconostoc,* and *Pediococcus* species are gram-positive organisms that are resistant to vancomycin. Certain gram-negative bacteria, such as *Elizabethkingia, Moraxella,* or *Acinetobacter* species, may be susceptible to vancomycin, and a zone of inhibition may be exhibited. Vancomycin susceptibility helps to establish the Gram "status" of organisms, particularly anaerobes, with uncertain Gram stain results.

- Gram-negative bacteria for the most part are susceptible to colistin (polymyxin E) and polymyxin B. Gram-positive bacteria are frequently resistant. Colistin and polymyxin B can be used to help establish the Gram reactivity of an organism, especially anaerobes.

- Group A streptococci (*Streptococcus pyogenes*) are susceptible to bacitracin (Figure 9-15 ■). Some strains of group C and group G streptococci may also exhibit inhibition. Most group B streptococci (*Streptococcus agalactiae*) and most other strains of beta hemolytic streptococci are resistant and do not exhibit a zone of inhibition. Bacitracin is described in ∞ Chapter 17, "Aerobic Gram Positive Cocci."

- *Streptococcus pneumoniae* is susceptible to optochin. Other alpha hemolytic streptococci, enterococci, and viridans streptococci are usually resistant and do not exhibit inhibition. ∞ Chapter 17, "Aerobic Gram Positive Cocci," discusses the optochin test. Figure 8-33 demonstrates a susceptible optochin test.

∞ Chapter 8, "Presumptive Identification," and ∞ Chapter 11, "Susceptibility Testing," describe the use of inhibitory profiles

✓ Checkpoint! 9–6 (Chapter Objective 6)

Which reagent(s) is (are) used to detect the end product of the Voges-Proskauer test?

    A. 10% ferric chloride
    B. 5% alpha naphthol and 40% KOH
    C. Kovac's or Ehrlich's
    D. methyl red

✪ **TABLE 9-1**

Commonly Used Conventional Tests

Test Procedure	Purpose of the Test Procedure	Reagents Added	Positive Reaction	Negative Reaction
Catalase test	To detect the presence of the enzyme catalase	Hydrogen peroxide	Evolution of bubbles	No effervescence
Oxidase test	To detect the presence of free or extracellular oxidase enzyme	Tetramethyl-*p*-phenylenediamine	Development of purple color within 30 seconds	No color development or delayed reaction
Tube coagulase (incubated at 35°C–37°C for 4 hrs)	To detect the presence of free or extracellular coagulase enzyme	None	Formation of a clot	No clot formation
Carbohydrate fermentation (incubated at 35°C–37°C for 18–24 hrs or longer)	Tests the ability of an organism to utilize a carbohydrate source for energy production	None (Phenol red is incorporated into the medium as a pH indicator)	Medium changes to a yellow color (acid production) and in some cases produces gas (bubbles)	No color change or production of a red color (alkaline by-products)
Urease test (incubated at 35°C–37°C for 18–24 hrs or longer)	Detects the presence of a urease enzyme, which catalyzes the breakdown of urea into ammonia and CO_2	None (phenol red is used as a pH indicator)	Production of a pink to red color	No color change
Indole test (incubated at 35°C–37°C for 18–24 hrs)	To determine if an organism has the ability to produce indole as a by-product of tryptophan metabolism	Kovacs' reagent	Production of a red ring at the surface of the medium	No red color
Citrate test (incubated at 35°C–37°C for 18–24 hrs)	To determine if an organism is capable of utilizing citrate as the sole source of carbon for metabolism and growth	None (bromthymol blue is used as a pH indicator)	Production of a blue color as a result of alkaline metabolic by-products or growth on slant	No growth on slant and no color change
Methyl red test (incubated at 35°C–37°C for 48 hrs)	To demonstrate the ability of an organism to produce and maintain stable acid by-products as a result of glucose metabolism	Methyl red indicator	Bright red color of the broth after addition of the methyl red indicator	A yellow color is seen in the broth
Voges-Proskauer test (incubated at 35°C–37°C for 18–24 hrs)	To demonstrate the ability of an organism to produce a neutral by-product (acetoin) as the result of glucose metabolism	40% potassium hydroxide and 5.0% alpha naphthol	Pinkish-red color of the broth	Yellow color of the broth (copper color may occur after mixing reagents)
Ornithine and lysine decarboxylase and arginine dihydrolase (incubated at 35°C–37°C for 18–24 hrs)	To demonstrate the ability of an organism to decarboxylate an amino acid to form an amine with resulting alkalinity (MacFaddin, 2000)	Bromcresol purple is incorporated into the medium as a pH indicator	Turbid purple to a faded-out gray-purple	Clear yellow color
Tryptophan or phenylalanine deaminase test (incubated at 35°C–37°C for 18–24 hrs)	To demonstrate the ability of an organism to produce indole and pyruvic acid as a result of tryptophane metabolism	10% Ferric chloride	Immediate formation of a brown color (TDA) or green color (PAD)	Clear yellow color
Hippurate hydrolysis (incubated at 35°C–37°C for 18–24 hrs)	To detect the presence of the enzyme hippuricase	Ninhydrin reagent	Formation of a deep purple color	No color change
Esculin hydrolysis (incubated at 35°C–37°C for 18–24 hrs)	To demonstrate the ability of an organism to hydrolyze esculin to esculetin and glucose	None	Formation of a black to dark brown color	No color change
Bacitracin susceptibility (incubated at 35°C–37°C for 18–24 hrs)	To determine if beta hemolytic streptococci are inhibited by bacitracin	None	Inhibition of bacterial growth in the presence of bacitracin	Growth of the organism in the presence of bacitracin
Optochin susceptibility (incubated at 35°C–37°C in carbon dioxide for 18–24 hrs)	To determine the ability of optochin to inhibit the growth of an organism	None	Inhibition of bacterial growth in the presence of optochin. Zone of inhibition must be measured for accurate interpretation.	Growth of the organism in the presence of optochin
ONPG test (incubated at 34°C–37°C for 20 min–24 hrs)	Determine the ability of an organism to ferment lactose by detecting the presence of β-galactosidase	None	Production of a yellow color	No color change (colorless)

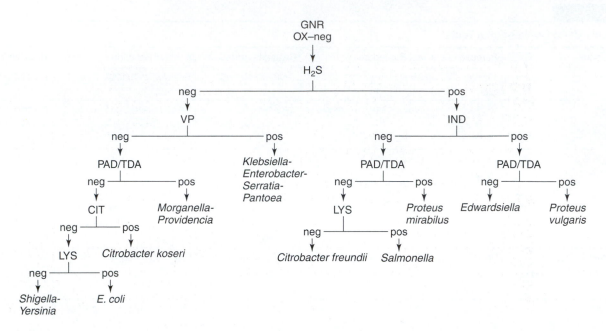

FIGURE 9-14 Presumptive identification of clinically significant *Enterobacteriaceae* to genus. GNR = gram-negative rod; OX = oxidase; pos = majority of strains are positive; neg = majority of strains are negative; H₂S = hydrogen sulfide; IND = indole; VP = Voges-Proskauer; PAD/TDA = phenylalanine or tryptophane deaminase; CIT = citrate; LYS = lysine decarboxylase; ORN = ornithine decarboxylase.
*Providencia (IND pos, CIT pos, ORN neg); *Morganella* (IND pos, CIT neg, ORN pos); *Proteus* (*P. mirabilis*—IND neg, ORN pos; *P. vulgaris*—IND pos, ORN neg; *P. pennari*—IND neg, ORN neg).

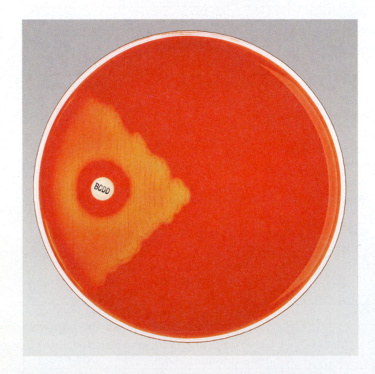

FIGURE 9-15 Bacitracin disk with group A streptococci. Group A streptococci (*Streptococcus pyogenes*) are susceptible to bacitracin. This is indicated by a zone of growth inhibition around the disc.
Photo courtesy of Remel, part of Thermo Fisher Scientific.

in presumptive identification. ∞ Chapter 17 describes the use of susceptibility disks to identify gram-positive cocci. ∞ Chapter 24 describes the use of high-potency disks (colistin, vancomycin, and kanamycin) to initially group anaerobic bacteria for identification.

✓ **Checkpoint! 9–7 (Chapter Objective 8)**

Susceptibility to _____ is commonly used in the identification of the etiologic agent of group A strep infections (Streptococcus pyogenes).
  A. *bacitracin*
  B. *optochin*
  C. *vancomycin*
  D. *colistin*

COMMERCIALLY AVAILABLE MULTITEST SYSTEMS

The **conventional substrates** found in plated and tubed media described earlier have been miniaturized and packaged as multitest systems that contain biochemical tests and can be used in the identification of various medically important microorganisms. These commercially available multitest systems may use microtubes or microtiter plates containing dehydrated substrates that are reconstituted by adding a suspension of the test organism. Substrate impregnated discs may also be added to the wells of a microtiter plate to which the suspen-

✪ TABLE 9-2

Commonly Used Multitest Systems for the Identification of Gram-Negative Rods

Multitest Systems	Manufacturer	Purpose
API 20E	bioMérieux	Identification of *Enterobacteriaceae* and nonfermenting gram-negative rods
API Rapid 20E	bioMérieux	4-hour identification of *Enterobacteriaceae*
API 20 NE	bioMérieux	24- to 48-hour identification of non-*Enterobacteriaceae* gram-negative rods
BBL Enterotube II	Becton Dickinson	Rapid identification of *Enterobacteriaceae*
BBL Oxi/Ferm Tube II	Becton Dickinson	Rapid identification of gram-negative oxidative-fermentative bacteria
BBL Crystal Enteric/NF ID Kit	Becton Dickinson	Identification of clinically significant aerobic gram-negative bacteria in the *Enterobacteriaceae* family and more frequently isolated glucose nonfermenting bacilli
RapID ONE	Remel	19 substrates for the identification of oxidase negative *Enterobacteriaceae*
RapID NF Plus	Remel	17 substrates for the identification of oxidase positive enteric organisms and nonfermenting gram-negative bacilli
MicroScan System	Dade Behring	Identification of *Enterobacteriaceae* and other gram-negative bacilli
Vitek System	bioMérieux	Identification of commonly encountered gram-negative bacilli

sion of the test organism is applied. The organisms metabolize the substrates over an 18- to 24-hour incubation period, and the reaction can be read visually with the results being recorded on report sheets. Alternatively, rapid test systems, which can provide identification of microbes in less than 4 to 6 hours, often use **chromogenic substrates.** Chromogenic substrates are synthetic compounds that are colorless and can be converted to colored compounds by preformed enzymes found in bacteria. Because the biochemical processes are carried out by preformed enzymes that are excreted into the environment, growth of the organism during testing is not a requirement for test results. The identification of slow-growing organisms can require a significant investment in time when the organism must grow in the medium to metabolize the substrate. The use of preformed enzymes that are readily excreted into the growth medium and begin the metabolic process immediately represents a significant saving in terms of time.

The use of **fluorogenic substrates** represents another advance in the identification process. A wide range of synthetic substrates, based on conjugates of carbohydrates, amino acids, and peptides with the fluorogen, 4-methylumbelliferone (4MU), are commercially available. Enzymatic cleavage of these substrates yields a brightly fluorescing compound that is readily detected when long-wave ultraviolet illumination is used. No developing reagents are required with this methodology (Maiden, Tanner, & Macuch, 1996).

Once the test results are generated, a computer database is often referenced in the identification process, whether conventional substrates, such as carbohydrates, amino acids, urea, citrate, or chromogenic/fluorogenic substrates are used. Tables 9-2✪ to 9-5✪ list commonly used multitest systems for identification.

API (bioMérieux, Hazelwood, MO) has developed several multitest identification systems designed to assist in the identification of microbes isolated in the clinical laboratory.

✪ TABLE 9-3

Commonly Used Multitest Systems for the Identification of Gram-Positive Bacteria

Multitest Systems	Manufacturer	Purpose
API Staph	bioMérieux	Overnight identification of *Staphylococcus* and *Micrococcus* species
RapID EC Staph	bioMérieux	2-hr identification of commonly occurring staphylococci
API 20 Strep	bioMérieux	Identification of *Streptococcus* and *Enterococcus* species
API Coryne	bioMérieux	Identification of *Corynebacterium* species
BBL Crystal Gram Positive ID Kit	Becton Dickinson	Identification of clinically significant gram-positive organisms in 18 hours
BBL Crystal Rapid Gram Positive ID Kit	Becton Dickinson	Identification of clinically significant gram-positive organism in 4 hours
RapID STR	Remel	14 substrates for the identification of beta-hemolytic and viridans streptococci
RapID CB Plus	Remel	18 substrates for the identification of *Corynebacterium*, *Actinomyces*, and other irregular gram-positive coryneform bacteria
MicroScan System	Dade Behring	Gram Positive Breakpoint Combo Panel for the identification of gram-positive bacteria
Vitek System	bioMérieux	GPI card for the identification of gram-positive bacteria

✪ TABLE 9-4

Multitest Systems for the Identification of *Neisseria* and *Haemophilus* Species and *Moraxella Catarrhalis*

Multitest System	Manufacturer	Purpose
API NH	bioMérieux	Allows identification of *Neisseria* and *Haemophilus* species and *M. catarrhalis* in 2 hours
BBL Crystal Neisseria/Haemophilus ID Kit	Becton Dickinson	Identification of clinically significant *Neisseria, Haemophilus,* and other fastidious organisms in 4 hours
RapID NH	Remel	13 substrates for the identification of *Neisseria, Haemophilus, Moraxella,* and *Kingella* species
MicroScan System	Dade Behring	HNID panel for the identification of fastidious gram-negative cocci and coccobacilli
Vitek System	bioMérieux	NHI card for the identification of fastidious gram-negative cocci and coccobacilli

✪ TABLE 9-5

Multitest Systems for the Identification of Anaerobes

Multitest System	Manufacturer	Purpose
API 20 A	bioMérieux	24-hour identification of anaerobes
RAPID ID 32 A	bioMérieux	4-hour identification of anaerobes
BBL Crystal Anaerobe ID Kit	Becton Dickinson	Identification of clinically significant anaerobes in 4 hours
RapID ANA II	Remel	18 substrates for the identification of anaerobic gram-negative rods, gram-positive rods, and cocci in 4 hours
MicroScan System	Dade Behring	Rapid anaerobe identification system for anaerobes
Vitek System	bioMérieux	Vitek Anaerobic Identification (ANI) card for the identification of anaerobes

Microtubes with dehydrated substrates are reconstituted by adding a bacterial suspension. After an 18- to 24-hour incubation, the reactions are read and recorded (Figure 9-16 ■). An organism identification code is generated by first assigning a point value of 1, 2, or 4 for each positive reaction and a 0 for each negative reaction on the forms provided. (Each commercial system has their own approach for assigning these numbers, so follow the manufacturer's instructions.) The numbers for each group of biochemical tests are added together to generate the code profile. For example, look at the API 20E® test results of the bottom strip in Figure 9-16. The ONPG, the first microtube, is positive (assign a 1); ADH, the second microtube, is negative (assign a 0); and LDC, the third microtube, is positive (assign a 4). These three numbers are added together to form the first digit of the code profile, a 5. The code profile generated, using the API 20E form for recording positive and negative results, is 5215773. The code profile is matched to a database to establish identification (Forbes, Sahm, & Weissfeld, 2002).

A number of identification kits can be used to identify facultative gram-positive cocci such as the MicroScan GP (Figure 9-17 ■) and Rapid GP panels (Dade Behring Inc., West Sacramento, CA) and the Vitek GPI Card. Others are specific for streptococci such as the API 20 Strep, RapID STR (Innovative Diagnostics, Atlanta, Ga.), Rapid ID Strep (bioMérieux), and Strep-Zym. These products contain enzymatic and sugar fermentation tests with incubation times of 4 to 24 hours. The BBL Crystal Gram-positive ID Panel (Becton Dickinson) includes 121 gram-positive taxa and requires an overnight incubation; the BBL Crystal Rapid Gram-Positive ID Panel requires a 4-hour

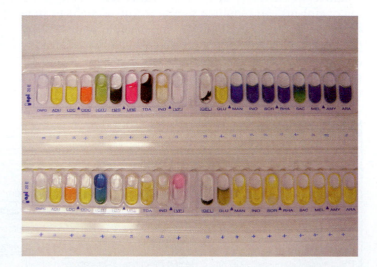

■ **FIGURE 9-16** API (bioMérieux, Hazelwood, MO) has developed several multitest identification systems designed to assist in the identification of microbes isolated in the clinical laboratory. Microtubes with dehydrated substrates are reconstituted by adding a bacterial suspension. After an 18- to 24-hour incubation, reagents are added, and the reactions are read and recorded. The top API 20E test strip is inoculated with *Proteus mirabilis*. The bottom API 20E test strip is inoculated with *Klebsiella pneumoniae*.

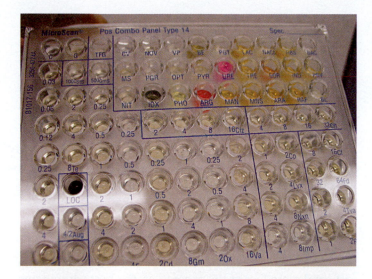

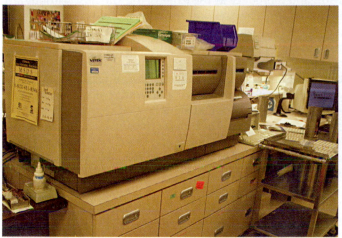

■ **FIGURE 9-17** GramPos ID panel (MicroScan). The gram-positive identification panel allows gram-positive organisms to be identified and susceptibility testing to be performed on the same microtiter plate. *Staphylococcus aureus* was inoculated to this panel and incubated for 18 hours in a non-CO_2 incubator at 37°C.

incubation period and identifies frequently isolated gram-positive bacteria, including *Aerococcus, Lactobacillus, Micrococcus, Pediococcus, Staphylococcus, Streptococcus,* corynebacteria, as well as species of *Bacillus, Gardnerella, Leuconostoc, Listeria;* and other gram-positive bacteria (Bascomb & Manafi, 1998).

The HNID® system (Dade Behring) is designed for rapid identification of *Neisseria* species, *Haemophilus* species, *Moraxella catarrhalis,* and *Gardnerella vaginalis.* In addition, biotyping of *H. influenzae* and *H. parainfluenzae* may be performed, as well as detection of beta-lactamase production.

This test system uses both conventional and chromogenic tests to identify fastidious gram-negative cocci and bacilli. The HNID® panel is rehydrated and inoculated from an organism suspension equivalent to a #3 MacFarland turbidity standard. The test system is incubated for 4 hours, after which changes in pH and utilization of certain substrates or other biochemi-

cal reactions are interpreted for identification. A rapid acidimetric method is used for the detection of the enzyme beta-lactamase (Dade Behring, 2001). Other test systems for the identification of *Haemophilus* and *Neisseria* species include RapID NH system (Innovative Diagnostic Systems, Atlanta, GA) and the Vitek NHI card (bioMérieux).

Multitest systems have also been developed for the identification of anaerobes. These include the RapID ANA II (Innovative Diagnostic Systems), the An-IDENT system (bioMérieux-Vitek, Inc., Hazelwood, MO), and the Vitek Anaerobe Identification (ANI) Card (Koneman, Allen, Janda, Schreckenberger, & Winn, 1997).

AUTOMATED IDENTIFICATION SYSTEMS

The plated and tubed media, which form the basis of manual identification methods, have been miniaturized so they can be used by the various commercially available automated identification systems used in microbiology laboratories. Automated identification systems have found widespread acceptance in clinical laboratories and offer greater accuracy and an increased speed of identification over manual methods. The MicroScan Walkaway (Dade MicroScan Inc., West Sacramento, CA) and the Vitek 2 System (Figure 9-18 ■) are two very popular automated identification systems. Both have used conventional panels with instruments that can read and interpret panel results, perform antibiotic susceptibility testing, and print results without human intervention. Additionally, speed has been improved by the use of fluorogenic substrates, allowing results to be generated with as little as a 2-hour incubation period. A computer-assisted algorithm is used to determine the final identification. The Vitek 2 system uses disposable cards containing fluorogenic substrates (Bascomb & Manafi, 1998). The MicroScan Walkaway can use a 96-well microtiter plate containing conventional substrates or fluorogenic substrates (Figure 9-19 ■).

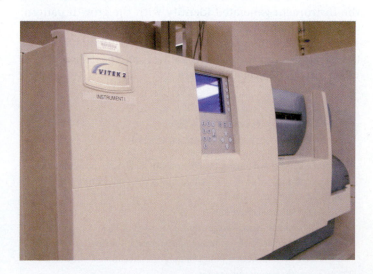

■ **FIGURE 9-18** Vitek 2 automated identification and susceptiblity system (bioMérieux, Hazelwood, MO).

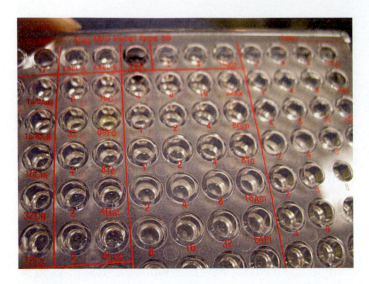

■ **FIGURE 9-19** Negative MIC (MicroScan). Determination of the MIC of a gram-negative rod using the MicroScan automated test system. Pictured is a microtiter plate, which can be used in the MicroScan Walkaway (Dade MicroScan Inc., West Sacramento, CA).

Obviously, a major convenience of automation is that it releases the microbiologist to perform other duties while the instrument effectively and reliably carries out the functions of identifying microbes and identifying susceptibility patterns. In addition, these instruments can be interfaced with laboratory information systems, so reporting results could be carried out automatically. Institution-specific reports on isolates and antibiotic resistance can also be generated and used by infectious disease for epidemiologic purposes. As marvelous as these automated systems are, a good microbiologist must still determine that the identity makes sense prior to reporting the results. Errors and unusual results are detected by correlating the instrument-generated identity with the growth pattern, Gram stain results, colony morphology, key test reactions, and susceptibility antibiogram. It is important to question the identity and follow up with additional tests or repeat suspect tests when a lack of correlation exists.

✓ **Checkpoint! 9-8**
(Chapter Objective 9)

Both the Vitek 2 system and the MicroScan Walkaway are automated systems that use a(n) _____ to determine the final identification of the isolated infectious agent.

   A. octal code conversion

   B. computer-assisted algorithm

   C. disposable cards containing fluorogenic substrates

   D. 96-well microtiter plate containing conventional substrates or fluorogenic substrates

---

▶ MOLECULAR DIAGNOSTICS

Molecular diagnostics involves the use of nucleic acids (genomics) and proteins (proteomics) to diagnose and monitor human diseases and is one of the fastest growing segments of the diagnostics market. During the 60s and 70s, human knowledge of biological processes reached the point that it became possible to devise techniques based on processes occurring at the cellular and molecular level. This allowed the development of tests that exhibited great specificity. Because of this specificity, the tools and techniques of molecular diagnostics are quite precise and operate in known, predictable ways.

NUCLEIC ACID (DNA/RNA) PROBES

Infectious agents usually coexist in a parasitic relationship with, and reproduce at the expense of, the host without any useful return. They rely on the host for nutritional support and in the process destroy host tissues as they proliferate. Effective treatment of infectious agents requires the rapid isolation and identification of those organisms capable of causing disease. The clinical signs and symptoms of an illness are often not specific enough to make a definitive diagnosis because many disease states exhibit signs and symptoms that are very similar to each other. The quicker diagnostic information can be conveyed to the physician, the greater the chances of the correct diagnosis and the quicker effective therapy can be initiated.

Conventional diagnosis is based on the isolation and culture of the infectious agent, which can be a process that is time consuming. For some of the microorganisms that can be cultured, the incubation period may be very prolonged. For example, *M. tuberculosis* requires as long as 4 to 8 weeks for growth of mature colonies. In addition, other problems are associated with conventional diagnosis:

- To culture an infectious agent, the microorganism must be viable when it is placed on or into the appropriate culture media. Unfortunately, all infectious agents are not able to be cultivated. Some microorganisms cannot be grown in artificial media (hepatitis B virus, rotaviruses, *Mycobacterium leprae*, etc). Other organisms are fastidious in their nutritional requirements, making them difficult to grow (*Haemophilus ducreyi*, *Bartonella* species, *Abiotrophia* species, etc.).

- Other microorganisms are too dangerous to culture in the routine clinical laboratory. Biosafety level 4 agents such as Lassa, Marburg, and Ebola viruses must be sent to a P-4 containment facility. Some organisms are dangerous because of the possibility of laboratory acquired infections through exposure and accidental inoculation (*Brucella* species, *Salmonella typhi*, *Francisella tularensis*, etc.).

- Once a microorganism has been recovered and grown in sufficient quantity, the identification process comes into play. Identification relies primarily on biochemical characteristics. The determination of an organism's biochemical characteristics requires pure cultures and may yet require additional testing before definitive identification is accomplished. *Salmonella* and *Shigella* species, for example, require serologic testing for confirmation. Unfortunately, problems with cross-reactivity can erode confidence in serologic procedures as confirmatory tests.

Based on the knowledge gained in the last decades of the 20th century, the development of molecular diagnostics seems to hold great promise in solving the problems associated with the isolation and identification of infectious agents. ∞ Chapter 3, "The Bacterial Cell," reviews the basic structure of DNA and its role in microbial genetics.

Nucleic Acid Synthesis

Both DNA and RNA chains are produced in cells by copying a preexisting DNA strand, according to the rules of Watson-Crick pairing. The template is the DNA from which the new strand (DNA or RNA) is copied. The copy preserves all the information (base sequence) found in the template and has a complementary sequence (not an identical one).

template DNA	5'-ATGCCAGCTCATTATC-3'
DNA strand copy	3'-TACGGTCGAGTAATAG-5'
template DNA	5'-ATGCCAGCTCATTATC-3'
RNA strand copy	3'-UACGGUCGAGUAAUAG-5'

In the overwhelming majority of cases, a preexisting strand of DNA is copied into a new strand of DNA or RNA in cells (plants, animals, protozoa, bacteria, etc.), but in some viruses, RNA molecules (strands) are produced by copying preexisting RNA molecules. In an unusual turn of events, retroviruses produce a new strand of DNA by copying a preexisting RNA molecule. In other words, instead of the flow of information being this:

$$DNA \rightarrow RNA \rightarrow protein$$

Retrovirus (an RNA virus) must perform an extra step:

$$RNA \rightarrow DNA \rightarrow RNA \rightarrow protein$$

All RNA and DNA synthesis proceeds in one direction, from the 5' to the 3' end.

template DNA	5'-ATGCCAGCTCATTATC-3'
DNA strand copy	← 3'-GAGTAATAG-5'

Nucleotides (molecules that make up RNA and DNA) used in the construction of nucleic acid chains are 5'-triphosphates (containing three phosphate groups) of the ribonucleotides (in the case of RNA) or deoxyribonucleotides (in the case of DNA). The alpha phosphate of the incoming nucleotide is attached to the 3' hydroxyl of the ribose (or deoxyribose) of the preceding residue to form a phosphodiester bond.

Special enzymes called **polymerases** elongate RNA or DNA strands by the addition of nucleotides to the 3' prime end of the strand. An accurate copy of a nucleic acid by a polymerase always requires a template. DNA polymerases are the enzymes that copy DNA to make new strands of DNA, in a process called replication. RNA polymerases are the enzymes that copy RNA from DNA in a process called transcription. Bacterial cells have one type of RNA polymerase that synthesizes messenger (mRNA), ribosomal (rRNA), and transfer (tRNA) RNA molecules.

Nucleic Acid Technology

Each infectious agent (bacteria, fungi, parasite, or virus) carries a unique genetic code. Genetic information is stored and transmitted in the form of nucleic acid polymers. Deoxyribonucleic acid (DNA) carries the genetic "blueprints" of a microorganism and its progeny or descendents. Viruses are the exception because they are capable of transferring genetic information to successive generations through either DNA or RNA molecules.

Infectious disease requires the presence of foreign DNA or RNA in host tissues. Because each organism contains unique nucleic acid sequences, molecular biotechnology appears to be the ideal mechanism to discriminate between microbial and human nucleic acid sequences. Nucleic acid probe technology uses labeled or tagged nucleic acid segments (DNA or RNA) to detect the presence of microorganisms in a patient specimen or to identify a particular microorganism that has already been isolated in pure culture but has not been identified. The label is a molecule that allows the nucleic acid segment to be visualized. DNA segments have been the most popular choice for creating nucleic acid probes. It is even possible to make a DNA probe using a strand of RNA (such as the genome of RNA viruses) as the template. In this case, the DNA probe is synthesized using enzymes called reverse transcriptases (or RNA-dependent DNA polymerase). These enzymes are able to synthesize complementary DNA from the viral RNA. The source of reverse transcriptase enzymes is retroviruses.

PREPARATION OF NUCLEIC ACID PROBES

The first step in preparing a DNA probe is to isolate a segment of the DNA strand for which the nucleotide base sequence is known. This requires cutting the DNA strand into small segments. Restriction endonucleases, enzymes obtained from unique bacteria, are capable of cutting DNA strands at a particular site containing a specific nucleotide sequence. For example: an endonuclease that recognizes the sequence "G (guanine) A (adenine) T (thymine) C (cytosine)" will make cuts wherever that particular sequence occurs along the strand. The end result is a combination of fragments of differing sizes obtained by cleavage wherever "G A T C" sequences are located. Gel electrophoresis is then used to sort the fragments on the basis of size and surface charge. The desired fragment is then inserted into a carrier such as plasmids and viruses and cloned by host cells. Alternatively, an amplification technique, such as the polymerase chain reaction, can be used to make multiple copies of the desired fragment.

The Use of Plasmids as Cloning Vectors

One way to clone, or create an exact replica of, the desired fragment is to insert it into a carrier such as a bacteriophage, a virus that infects bacteria. By inserting the DNA fragment into the viral genome, the process of viral multiplication within the bacterial host cell multiplies the DNA segment.

In many cases the cloning vector, a means of transmitting genetic material, is a **plasmid**, a circular strand of extrachromosomal DNA found in the cytoplasm of certain bacteria. Plasmids are used because of their ability to multiply to large numbers once they have entered or been placed in the cytoplasm of its bacterial host cell. To insert the DNA fragment into the vector or cloning vehicle, the plasmid is cut with the same endonuclease used to produce the target DNA fragments. The annealing process (joining the DNA fragment with the plasmid DNA) is carried out using enzymes called ligases, which restore the covalent bonds between strands of DNA. The endonucleases and ligases used to cut and anneal the DNA strands are both obtained from bacterial sources.

Once the DNA fragment has been inserted into the plasmid and the plasmid taken up by the bacterium, the bacterium is subcultured to fresh medium to propagate, or reproduce, the altered plasmid with its foreign piece of DNA. The plasmids are then released from the bacterial cells by lysis. The DNA fragment can be removed from the plasmid using the same endonuclease used to insert it. It is then purified by electrophoresis in an agarose gel.

Radiolabeling the Nucleic Acid Probe

One method of labeling the nucleic acid probe is to add a radioactive isotope to the DNA fragment. This allows the DNA fragment to be detected. The advantage of using radioisotopes is due to their sensitivity. Even very tiny quantities of the radioisotope can be detected. There are, however, some disadvantages:

- Special radioactivity counting equipment is required.
- Personnel must be trained and licensed in the use of radioactive compounds.
- There may be some variability in activity because radio-labels are added using enzymatic reactions.
- Radioactive decay leads to a decrease in activity.
- Disposing of radioactive material after its use is a problem.

Now that the probe has been prepared and labeled, the labeled probe must be separated into separate strands to be used. **Denaturation** or separation of the two strands is accomplished with detergents, enzymes, NaOH (sodium hydroxide), or heat.

A successful probe is one that will hybridize or combine with either DNA or RNA of the target organism but does not hybridize with nucleic acids from other organisms that may be present in the sample.

Nonradioactive Markers to Label Probes

Radioactive labels such as ^{32}P (phosphorus) and ^{35}S (sulfur) are the most sensitive methods for detecting hybridization. They are not the most practical. Radioactive probes require repeated synthesis, need special safety precautions, are time consuming and are technically difficult. For these reasons, radioactive labels have not been practical for clinical laboratories. Non-radioactive markers have been developed that have overcome these obstacles.

Biotin, a water-soluble vitamin, can be incorporated into the DNA molecule without destroying its ability to hybridize with complementary DNA strands. The biotin molecule possesses a structural analogue of thymine, deoxyuridine, which can be incorporated into DNA in place of a thymine nucleotide and serve as a marker.

If the probe finds a segment on the target DNA that is complementary, it will hybridize with the target DNA from the test organism. The positive reaction (hybridization) may be detected by adding avidin conjugated with an enzyme such as alkaline phosphate.

Avidin is a protein found in egg white. It binds very strongly to biotin. Each avidin molecule has four binding sites for biotin, so it is extremely sensitive. The enzyme-conjugated avidin will attach itself to the biotin bound to the nucleic acid probe. Chromogenic substrates (colorless compounds that can be converted to a colored compound) can then be added. The chromogen is converted to a colored compound by the enzyme conjugated to the avidin. The appearance of the colored compound indicates the presence of the biotin-labeled nucleic acid probe (McInnes, Dalton, Vize, & Robbins, 1987).

Fluorescein is a fluorescent molecule. It can be attached or conjugated to an **antibody**, a large molecule that is glycoprotein in nature and produced by B lymphocytes following an antigenic stimulus. The fluorescein-antibody conjugate is used to visualize the presence of the biotin-labeled nucleic acid probe in place of the enzyme-labeled avidin. The antibody specificity is directed against biotin, the molecule that has been incorporated into the DNA probe. The fluorescein-conjugated antibody attaches to the biotin molecules in the DNA probe. Hybridization of the probe to the DNA of the target organism is detected by fluorescence of the fluorescein-labeled antibody under ultraviolet light. New electronics capable of producing images at extremely low levels of light can be coupled with computer-assisted image analysis to enhance detection. With this capability, it has been predicted that systems could be developed that are capable of detecting a single microorganism gene within an infected cell.

How DNA Probes Work

Nucleic acid probe technology was originally developed to detect microorganisms in clinical specimens or to confirm the identity of organisms that have been isolated in pure culture. In the first step, cells are disrupted and the DNA strands separated out. The DNA is then denatured, meaning the double strand is separated into single strands using enzymes, detergents, or heat. The single-stranded DNA is fixed to a solid surface. The labeled probe is added and allowed to react with material on the solid support. If complementary sequences are present, the probe anneals or combines with the target DNA bound to the support medium. The support medium is washed to remove unbound DNA and nonspecifically bound DNA.

Radiolabeled nucleic acid probes can be detected using photographic film. A dark spot on the photographic film indicates where the radiolabeled probe, bound to the target DNA, is located. Another method of determining whether the labeled probe is present is to measure counts per minute using an instrument capable of detecting radioactive decay (particles).

Identifying the presence of a biotin-labeled probe depends on the type of avidin conjugate. If the avidin is enzyme labeled, a chromogen is added and the color measured. If the avidin uses a fluorescein-conjugated antibody directed against biotin, then ultraviolet light can be used.

Sensitivity and specificity of probe technology are diminished when applied to certain specimens such as stool and sputum. Unacceptable nonspecific binding to extraneous materials in the specimen tends to occur. This, in many cases, has made the use of probe technology unsuitable for identifying organisms directly from clinical specimens that contain large amounts of cellular material. However, nucleic acid probes have been found to be most useful in confirming the identity of microorganisms isolated from such specimens. Table 9-6 ✪ provides a listing of nucleic acid probes in use in the clinical laboratory today.

The Modified Approach of Gen-Probe

Gen-Probe, a major biotechnology company in San Diego, CA, devised probe technology that uses a DNA probe to detect complementary strands of ribosomal RNA. The advantage to this is not immediately obvious until one realizes that there is only one copy of complementary DNA per cell, but thousands of ribosomal RNA segments in the same cell. Organisms may contain more than 10,000 ribosomes, and consequently there are an equal number of ribosomal RNA molecules. Additionally, RNA molecules are already single stranded and therefore ready to hybridize without the necessity of incorporating a denaturation step.

Another key difference in Gen-Probe technology is the fact that their system does not use a solid support system. Gen-Probe has devised what is called an in-solution approach. Hybridization occurs in solution after the cells have been lysed. The resulting DNA probe–RNA hybrids will then bind to the mineral hydroxyapatite. Hydroxyapatite does not bind a nonhybridized probe. Any nonhybridized nucleic acid molecules would then be washed away. The hydroxyapatite is spun into a pellet by centrifugation (Kohne, 1986).

✪ TABLE 9-6

Examples of Current Uses for Nucleic Acid Probes
(Market for probe technology = $1 billion)

Gen-Probe

Mycobacterium tuberculosis	Group A streptococci	Blastomyces dermatitidis
Neisseria gonorrhoeae	Group B streptococci	Histoplasma capsulatum
Chlamydia trachomatis	Enterococcus species	Coccidioides immitis
Haemophilus influenzae	Streptococcus pneumoniae	
Staphylococcus aureus	Campylobacter species	
Listeria monocytogenes		

Gene-Trak

Listeria monocytogenes, Salmonella species, S. aureus, E. coli

Dynagene

HIV 1	Streptococcus pyogenes
Hepatitis B virus	Vancomycin resistance in Enterococcus
Chlamydia trachomatis	species (Van A/Van B genes)
Neisseria gonorrhoeae	

AdvanDx

Candida albicans, Enterococcus faecalis, E. coli, Pseudomonas aeruginosa, Staphylococcus aureus

PNA Probes

AdvanDx, of Woburn, MA, uses peptide nucleic acid (PNA) probes with fluorescence in situ hybridization (FISH) for rapid identification of microorganisms from blood cultures. PNA molecules lack the usual sugar phosphate backbone of DNA. Their backbone is an uncharged, neutral "pseudopeptide." The same Watson-Crick base pairing rules for hybridization are followed for complementary RNA and DNA targets, but they bind more readily and tightly (Oliveira, Procop, Wilson, Coull, & Stender, 2002). ∞ Chapter 14, "Fungal Cultures," shows a yeast identification from a positive blood culture using PNA FISH in Figure 14-21.

Tests for Infectious Diseases

The fact that the human immunodeficiency virus (HIV) has three unique genes, *GAG, POL,* and *ENV,* which are part of the viral genome, makes probe technology an ideal way to detect the presence of the virus in clinical specimens because the presence of genes unique to HIV lends specificity to the assay. These HIV-specific genes provide targets for probe technology that will not be found in other families of virus.

POLYMERASE CHAIN REACTION (PCR)

A single copy of a nucleic acid is often undetectable by conventional hybridization methods. Using PCR, a single copy of a nucleic acid target is multiplied to 10^7 (10 million) or more copies, greatly improving sensitivity because multiple targets can readily be detected. Polymerase chain reaction (PCR) is a combination of complementary nucleic acid hybridization and nucleic acid replication. It is the most widely used target nucleic acid amplification method.

The polymerase chain reaction (Figure 9-20 ■) process begins with denaturation of the target nucleic acid. Heating the sample to 94°C accomplishes two objectives: disruption of the organism releasing the nucleic acids and denaturation of DNA into single strands. Chemical or enzymatic methods are also available. For RNA targets, denaturation is not required.

Step 2 involves primer annealing. Primers are short sequences of nucleic acid (oligonucleotides 20 to 30 nucleotides long) that specifically hybridize (anneal) to a nucleic acid target (essentially functioning like a probe). The abundance of available gene sequence data allows the design of primers specific for a number of microbial pathogens: genus-specific primers, species-specific primers, primers for virulence factors or primers for antibiotic-resistance genes. Pairs of primers are needed. One primer anneals to a specific site of one target strand of the DNA. The other primer anneals to a specific site on the opposite end of the other complementary DNA strand. The annealing process is conducted at 50°C to 58°C or more.

The annealing of primers to the target sequence allows extension of the primer-target duplex, via DNA polymerase, which adds nucleotides to the 3′ end of each primer. *Taq* polymerase, an enzyme obtained from thermophilic bacteria, catalyzes primer extension at 72°C. This enzyme can withstand

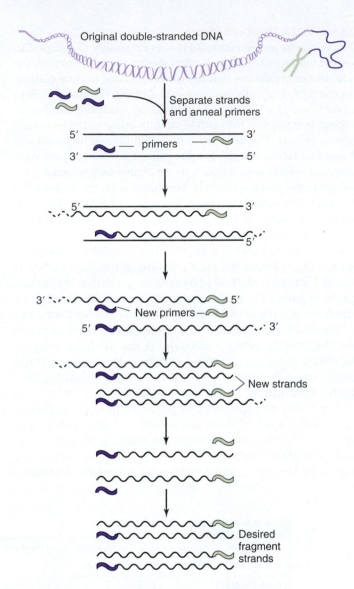

■ **FIGURE 9-20** Illustration of the polymerase chain reaction (PCR).

the 94°C temperature used in the denaturation step. All the components required for each reaction step, the target nucleic acid, the primers, the buffers, the deoxynucleotides are placed into the reaction vessel because all three reactions, denaturation, annealing, and extension, occur in the same tube. An instrument known as a thermal cycler, holds the reaction vessel and carries the PCR mixture through each reaction step at the precise temperature and for the optimal duration. The number of double-stranded fragments is doubled with each cycle. In 30 to 40 minutes, which allows 30 to 50 repetitive cycles, 10^7 to 10^8 target copies are generated. The specific PCR amplification product (each target nucleic acid copy) is referred to as an amplicon.

Detection of the target nucleic acid strand can involve the use of radioactive, colorimetric, fluorometric, and chemiluminescent signals to detect a probe hybridized with the amplicon.

A variation of traditional PCR is real-time PCR. This method performs the amplification and detection steps at the same time generating a faster result. A thermal cycler with precision optics (Figure 9-21 ■) monitors fluorescence emitted from sample cells. Fluorescence increases as amplified product binds the fluorescent dye. A computer monitors the data during every cycle and generates an amplification plot for each product detected. If the temperature that the target nucleic acid strand separates or "melts" away (resulting in a drop in fluorescence) is plotted on the *x*-axis and the fluorescence is plotted on the *y*-axis, a "melting curve" can be analyzed increasing the specificity of detection. The temperature peak of each melting curve is different for each product detected (Murray et al., 2007). Real-time PCR can be used for identification, quantification (e.g., HIV viral load) and multiplex analysis (e.g., respiratory infectious diseases).

RESTRICTION FRAGMENT LENGTH POLYMORPHISMS (RFLPS) OR DNA FINGERPRINTING

Restriction fragment length polymorphisms (RFLPs) or DNA fingerprinting is a two-step process incorporating enzymatic digestion and electrophoresis of DNA fragments. This technique allows definitive identification of microbial pathogens but is less exacting than nucleic acid sequencing. Enzymatic digestion of DNA is accomplished using any number of endonucleases (which recognize a specific nucleotide sequence or restriction site). It catalyzes the digestion of the nucleic acid strand at that site, causing a break. The number and size of fragments depend on:

- The length of the nucleic acid strand (the longer the strand the greater the number of restriction sites).
- The nucleotide sequence of the strand (governs how often the restriction site occurs).
- The particular enzyme used (governs where the cut will be made). Enzymatic digestion of a strand whose nucleotide sequence provides several recognition sites for endonuclease A, but only a few for endonuclease B, will produce more fragments with endonuclease A. In addition, the size of the fragments produced will depend on the number of nucleotides between each of endonuclease A's recognition or restriction sites on the nucleic acid being digested.

Target DNA may be produced using PCR or cultivation of the organism. Separation of fragments after digestion is through electrophoresis in agarose gel (Figure 9-22 ■). DNA fragments are separated according to differences in size, with smaller fragments migrating faster and farther than large fragments. This results in the formation of nucleic acid bands (containing fragments of roughly the same size). Ethidium blue, a fluorescent dye, is used to stain the nucleic acid bands. Photographs of the stained gels can then be kept for a permanent record. The patterns obtained are called restriction patterns, and differences between microorganism restriction patterns are known as restriction fragment length polymorphisms.

Microbiologists performing molecular procedures must follow good laboratory practices to maintain nucleic acid integrity and avoid contamination from the environment and other patient specimens. Gloves should be worn. Splashing can be avoided by pulse spinning prior to opening the reaction tube and using screw caps rather then snap caps. Cross contamination can be prevented by only opening one specimen at a time. Work surfaces should be cleaned with bleach.

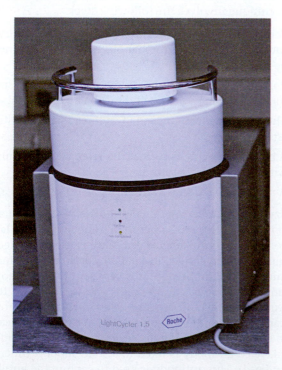

■ FIGURE 9-21 Real-time PCR instrument (Roche's LightCycler).

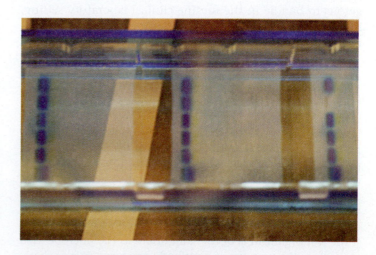

■ FIGURE 9-22 Gel electrophoresis

Checkpoint! 9–9
(Chapter Objectives 7 and 10)

Unacceptable nonspecific binding to extraneous materials tends to occur with _____ when certain specimens, such as stools and sputum, are tested. This leads to diminished sensitivity and specificity and limits the use of this technology for direct specimen testing.

    A. *nucleic acid probe technology*

    B. *the polymerase chain reaction (PCR)*

    C. *DNA fingerprinting (restriction fragment length polymorphisms, or RFLP)*

    D. *Southern blotting*

Checkpoint! 9–10
(Chapter Objective 10)

_____ are capable of cutting DNA strands at a particular site containing a specific nucleotide sequence. These enzymes obtained from bacteria are useful in techniques such as nucleic acid probe production and DNA fingerprinting.

    A. *Polymerases*

    B. *Ligases*

    C. *Restriction endonucleases*

    D. *Isomerases*

▶ IMMUNOLOGIC TESTS

IMMUNOASSAYS

Immunoassays involve the use of antibody-antigen reactions to detect one of the reactants. The specificity of antibodies lends a definite advantage to the use of this technology. Because these reactions take place in a very short time period, the results may be produced rapidly. Specificity, sensitivity, and short turnaround times are reasons this technology is very popular. For organisms that are slow growers, those that cannot be cultured on artificial media, and those that are too dangerous to handle in the routine clinical laboratory setting, identification may be accomplished using immunologic techniques that are rapid and specific.

Type-Specific Antibody

Type-specific antibody can be used to identify or serotype microorganisms. Injecting suitable animals, such as rabbits or goats, with killed organisms, which have been rendered harmless but continue to be antigenic, will induce the animal to produce polyspecific antibody that will react with antigens present on the cell wall of the organism. If a suspicious test organism is isolated in the clinical laboratory setting, a saline suspension of the organism can be made and mixed with the type-specific antibody. The preparation is rotated by hand or on a mechanical rotator and examined within a specified time. If the test organism is of the same strain as the microbe used to produce the type-specific antibody, the formation of aggregates, referred to as clumping or agglutination, should occur. If the test organism is not the correct species or serotype, then

aggregates do not form, and a smooth suspension remains. The agglutination process usually occurs within 1 minute. Longer times may lead to nonspecific agglutination as evaporation concentrates the proteins in the antisera.

In some cases this agglutination reaction may not be readily apparent. Another approach is to use type-specific antibody, which is attached to latex particles. Addition of these antibody coated latex particles to a saline suspension of the test organism will result in coagglutination of the latex particles and the test organism. Alternatively heat or enzymatic digestion can be used to remove antigens from the cell wall of the test organism. This extraction solution can be mixed with antibody-coated latex particles, and a positive reaction would be agglutination of the latex particles. A smooth suspension would be indicative of a negative reaction.

Antibody-coated latex particles can also be used to test body fluids such as blood (serum or plasma), pleural fluid, urine, or vesicular fluid for the presence of viruses or capsular antigen. This approach has proved to be useful to identify the presence of herpes simplex virus in vesicular fluid from herpes simplex virus type 1 and type 2 lesions, cytomegalovirus in urine, and the capsular antigen of *Haemophilus influenzae* type b, *Neisseria meningitidis, E. coli* K1, *Streptococcus pneumoniae,* and *Cryptococcus neoformans* from cerebrospinal fluid

Immunofluorescent Assays

Direct fluorescent assays (DFA) are used to detect the presence of foreign antigen in patient specimens such as secretions, body fluids, and tissues. This foreign antigen from invasive microorganisms can be detected using fluorescent-labeled antibody specific for antigens of the pathogenic organism. The DFA technique involves the following steps:

- Patient specimen is added to the slide, allowed to dry, and then fixed (formalin, methanol, ethanol, or acetone may be used as a fixative).

- Polyclonal or monoclonal fluorescent antibody (specific for the antigen) is added and incubated on the slide.

- The slide is washed, mounted, and read with an ultraviolet microscope.

- A positive reaction is seen as fluorescence of the microbe within a dark background.

- A negative reaction is seen as a lack of fluorescence.

Enzyme immunoassay (EIA) is another technique used to detect infectious agents. Rather than using fluorescent-labeled antibody, an enzyme-labeled antibody is used to detect the presence of foreign antigen in a patient specimen. This method is particularly useful because it is very sensitive (able to measure antigen in the picogram range) and very specific. It does not require the use (and expense) of an ultraviolet microscope and can be read either macroscopically or microscopically. It is also amenable to automation using a microplate reader.

Unlabeled antibody is fixed to a solid support (microtiter well or bead). This antibody is used to capture the antigen of the test organism. The patient specimen is added and incubated to allow an antigen-antibody reaction to occur. The system is then washed to remove unbound antigen. An enzyme conjugated antibody is added, followed by an incubation period and washing. The substrate for the enzyme, a chromogen, is added, and the enzyme attached to the antibody converts the colorless chromogen to a colored compound (Figure 9-23 ■). This constitutes a positive reaction, which can be visually measured or measured by a spectrophotometer, and indicates that the organism in question is present within the patient specimen (sputum, blood, urine, or other body fluids and secretions). A lack of color development is a negative reaction indicating the organism is not present.

Monoclonal Antibodies

Monoclonal antibodies are those produced by a single B cell line or clone. The antibody specificity is directed against a single epitope or antigenic determinant. Epitopes are specific

regions in the structure of an antigen to which an antibody attaches. Antigens are composed of numerous epitopes. Polyclonal antiserum contains elements directed against any number of different epitopes, and cross reactivity is possible between antigens of closely related species that might share similar epitopes. The production and use of monoclonal antibodies are described in ∞ Chapter 10, "Immunological Tests."

SUMMARY

The identification process begins with an initial assessment of bacterial growth on some type of growth medium. With experience, microbiologists often learn to recognize microbes by observing the physical appearance of colonies on different media. Colony size, pigment production, hemolysis, and colony morphology (raised, flat, umbilicate, rough, smooth, mucoid, etc.) are suggestive of certain microbes. For example, exudate from a surgical or traumatic wound may be subcultured to various media, including a blood agar plate. If the predominant organisms are seen to produce small, transparent colonies with large zones of beta hemolysis, an experienced microbiologist will suspect this organism to be group A streptococci or more specifically, *Streptococcus pyogenes*. The next step would be to Gram stain the organism to make sure the gram morphology is consistent with *S. pyogenes*, small gram-positive cocci. Next, a catalase test would be performed, and if the organism is catalase negative, this is also consistent with *S. pyogenes*. At this point any number of options are available to identify the isolate:

- Direct serotyping of colonies can be done from a saline suspension. In the case of a beta-hemolytic streptococci or enterococci, cell wall antigens could be extracted enzymatically and the solution mixed with antibody-coated latex particles. If the antibody is specific for group A streptococci, a positive reaction, agglutination, would be sufficient evidence to report the organism as group A streptococci.
- Additionally conventional tubed and plated media or reaction disks could be used for biochemical testing such as PYR, esculin and hippurate hydrolysis, bacitracin and optochin susceptibility, urease production, and carbohydrate fermentation.
- Another option would be to choose a commercially available multitest system such as API 20 Strep or RapID STR. These would be read visually and a numerical profile generated. The numerical profile of the unknown organism can be compared to those given in an identification code book or database.
- A third option is to use one of the automated test systems such as the Vitek 2 System or the MicroScan Walkaway. Most large medical institutions or acute care facilities have made an investment in an automated multitest system because results can be obtained quickly and reliably.

Remember that a good microbiologist will always correlate the final identification to test results, antibiogram, colony morphology, and Gram stain prior to reporting results. If the

  Checkpoint! 9–11 (Chapter Objective 11)

_____ *are used in the identification of infectious agents and do not require the use of radioactive isotopes, scintillation counters, fluorescent labels, or fluorescent microscopes, yet the use of antibodies to detect antigens unique to the test organism confers sensitivity and specificity.*

A. *Direct fluorescent antibody techniques*
B. *Indirect fluorescent antibody techniques*
C. *Latex agglutination tests*
D. *Enzyme immunoassays*

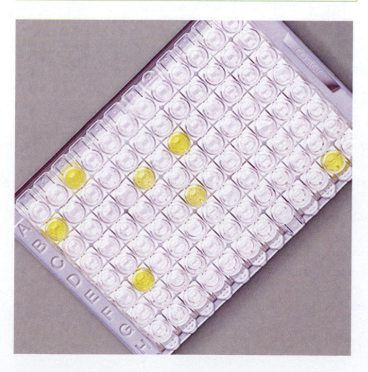

■ **FIGURE 9-23** Enzyme immunoassay (EIA) showing positive (yellow) and negative (colorless) reactions.
Photo courtesy of Remel, part of Thermo Fisher Scientific.

correlation makes sense, then the final report is generated. If there is little or no correlation, then the microbiologist should search for the reason why. The isolate could be unusual and misidentified by the commercial kit database or automated instrument. It may be a mixed culture rendering the test results worthless. Test results could be erroneous because of a clerical error or performance error. Correlation and follow-up are necessary to ensure accurate results.

LEARNING OPPORTUNITIES

1. On the Web:

   See animations of PCR, gel electrophoresis, sequencing, and other molecular techniques at the Biology Animation Library.

   http://www.dnalc.org/ddnalc/resources/animations.html

   Identify an unknown bacterium from the base-pair sequence using ribosomal DNA, at the Virtual Bacterial ID Lab.

   http://www.hhmi.org/biointeractive/vlabs/

2. The following table lists some commonly isolated members of the family *Enterobacteriaceae* and some biochemical tests that could be used in the identification process. Use this information to answer the questions that follow the table. (Chapter Objectives 4, 5, 6, 8, and 9)

Isolate	Ind	Cit	Ure	VP	H$_2$S	Orn	Lys	Arg	TDA	Glu	Lac	Suc
E. coli	+	0	0	0	0	+	+	0	0	+	+	V
Shigella boydii	0	0	0	0	0	0	0	0	0	+	0	0
Salmonella typhi	0	0	0	0	+	0	+	0	0	+	0	0
Edwardsiella tarda	+	0	0	0	+	+	+	0	0	+	0	0
Proteus vulgaris	+	0	+	0	+	0	0	0	+	+	0	0
Proteus mirabilis	0	+	+	0	+	+	0	0	+	+	0	0
Klebsiella pneumoniae	0	+	+	+	0	0	+	0	0	+	+	+
Enterobacter cloacae	0	+	+	+	0	+	0	+	0	+	+	+

Ind = indole; Cit = citrate; Ure = urease; VP = Voges-Proskauer; Orn = ornithine; Lys = lysine; Arg = arginine; H$_2$S = H$_2$S production; TDA = tryptophane deaminase; Carbohydrate fermentation; Glu = glucose; Lac = lactose; Suc = sucrose; + = majority of strains are positive; 0 = majority of strains are negative; V = variable (some strains are positive, some are negative)

a. Will glucose fermentation differentiate any of the microorganisms listed in the table?

b. The production of arginine dihydrolase will differentiate _____ from the other isolates. How is this test performed?

c. Will lactose fermentation differentiate the isolates that produce H$_2$S as a metabolic by-product?

d. What biochemical tests will differentiate the two *Proteus* species?

e. Which isolate is biochemically inert (metabolically inactive) when the biochemicals listed are used?

f. Which isolates are Voges-Proskauer positive? What reagent(s) is (are) added to generate a result?

g. What combination of tests will differentiate the Voges-Proskauer positive isolates?

3. You observe the following biochemical reactions on a catalase-positive, oxidase-negative, gram-negative rod: indole = red; methyl red = red; Voges-Proskauer = colorless; citrate = green; TSI = K/AG; LIA = R/A; urea = pink after 4 hr; ornithine decarboxylase = purple (Control is yellow). (Chapter Objectives 3, 8, and 9)

   a. What does the TSI result tell you about this organism? What colony morphology would you expect on MacConkey?

   b. What does the LIA tell you about this organism? What other biochemical tests would you expect to be positive?

   c. What is the presumptive genus of this organism?

PEARSON
myhealthprofessionskit™

Use this address to access the interactive Companion Website created for this textbook. Simply select "Clinical Laboratory Science" from the choice of disciplines. Find this book and log in using your user name and password.

REFERENCES

Go to myhealthprofessionskit.com to view this chapter's references.

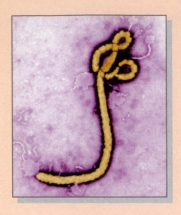

OUTLINE

10

Immunological Tests

Daila S. Gridley

■ LEARNING OBJECTIVES

Upon completion of this chapter, the learner should be able to:

1. Identify and describe the major cells and soluble substances (cell-mediated and humoral immunity) involved in three major functions of the immune system.
2. Identify the major organs, cells, and processes involved in immune responses and their functions.
3. Identify and describe the basic characteristics of antigen–antibody reactions.
4. Identify and describe the applications of monoclonal antibodies.
5. Categorize laboratory assays according to whether they involve precipitation, agglutination, complement, or a marker such as a fluorescent dye, radionuclide, or enzyme immunoassays.
6. Discuss the basic principles behind the presented tests.
   a. Interpret results.
   b. Determine potential sources of errors.
7. Interpret a set of antigen or antibody tests.
8. Determine the type(s) of antibodies that are typically present in microorganism-related disease states.
9. Analyze case studies, propose solutions where appropriate, and determine the roles that immunologic cells and/or substances play.

KEY TERMS

affinity	cross-reactivity	immunogen
antibody	cytokine	monoclonal antibodies
antigen	epitope	paratope
aviditiy	heterophile antigen/	polyclonal
cell-mediated	antibody	specificity
complement	humoral	titer

▶ INTRODUCTION

This chapter presents a brief overview of the major components of the immune system and describes the basic functions of the two classical branches, innate and acquired. Defense mechanisms that operate against bacteria, viruses, and other infectious agents are also discussed. The basic principles and procedures involved in immunological tests commonly used in clinical laboratories (precipitation, agglutination, complement-mediated reactions, immunofluorescence, radioimmunoassays, and enzyme-linked immunosorbent assays) are described.

▶ WHAT IS IMMUNOLOGY?

The basic concepts of immunology were originally proposed by microbiologists studying resistance to infectious agents many decades ago. Since then, numerous contributions have been made over the years by biochemists, physiologists, molecular geneticists, pathologists, and investigators in other disciplines. The collective efforts by these individuals have resulted in tremendous progress in unraveling the intricate and very complex mechanisms of immune function.

The immune system maintains a harmonious balance between the internal and external environment via three basic functions: (1) defense against infectious agents as well as inanimate materials that enter the body; (2) homeostasis, which is characterized by removal of dead or dying cells and other worn-out components; this function also includes the destruction of cells that accidentally reach unnatural sites in the body; and (3) surveillance, the removal of cells that have mutated or become altered by other means (McPherson, 2001b). Immune responsiveness can be modified by a variety of factors. Indeed, no two individuals respond with exactly the same degree of intensity. In some cases, inheritance of certain genes, or lack thereof, can lead to immunodeficiency diseases. More subtle genetic variations also exist that influence the degree of responsiveness to a particular agent. Age is another important modifying factor. It is well known that the very young and very old have less than optimal immune function, rendering them more susceptible to infection than young adults. Metabolic factors include variations in certain hormones. For example, persons with low levels of adrenal or thyroid hormones are more prone to infection than those who produce normal amounts. Stress, overcrowding, poor sanitation, and poor diet are additional factors that can increase the risk for infection.

ANTIGENS

An **antigen** is any substance that has potential to stimulate the immune system. An antigen capable of inducing a measurable immune response is also known as an **immunogen.** A vast number of potential sources of antigens exist, including structural components of bacteria, bacterial toxins, viruses,

fungi, pollens, transplanted tissues, and blood cells received during transfusion. Proteins are excellent antigens in that they tend to provoke the strongest immune responses. However, there are some exceptions like gelatin, which has an unstable three-dimensional structure. Complex carbohydrates (polysaccharides) are moderately immunogenic. Examples include lipopolysaccharides (LPS) and capsules produced by bacteria and oligosaccharides, which determine the ABO blood groups. Lipids are poor immunogens, although a significant response can be waged when they are coupled to a large protein. Nucleic acids (DNA/RNA) are very poor immunogens, although the ability to respond is present, as exemplified by patients with autoimmune diseases such as systemic lupus erythematosus.

MAJOR COMPONENTS OF IMMUNE SYSTEM

Historically, the immune system has been divided into two major branches. **Cell-mediated** immunity is made up of the T and B lymphocytes, natural killer cells, macrophages, and granulocytes. **Humoral** immunity consists of **antibodies** (soluble protective Y-shaped proteins produced by the B cells) and the family of proteins that make up the **complement** (C') system. Both systems act together to recognize and attack foreign antigens. The cell-mediated branch is governed by the T lymphocytes, which have receptors. Once the receptors are activated, they directly attack foreign substances and secrete protein and glycoprotein substances called **cytokines**, which communicate with other immune cells and help regulate their functions. Humoral immunity consists of antibodies (IgG, IgA, IgM, IgD, and IgE) as well as complement. However, because of the highly complex and interactive network of cells, tissues, organs, and soluble factors, it is difficult to classify any one particular immune response as being only humoral or only cell-mediated.

The thymus and bone marrow, as the major sites of T and B lymphocyte maturation, respectively, are the primary (central) organs. Because the T cells are critical in immune regulation, they are often referred to as the "master" cells. The thymus, in turn, is referred to as the "master gland" of the immune system because it is the major site of T cell maturation. Secondary lymphoid organs include the spleen, lymph nodes, tonsils, appendix, Peyer's patches, and adenoids. In addition to the T and B cells, other participating cell types include natural killer (NK) cells, neutrophils, monocytes, macrophages, eosinophils, basophils, mast cells, and platelets.

RESULTS OF IMMUNE ACTIVATION

In healthy individuals, an antigen is usually cleared rapidly from the body. The route by which the antigen gains entrance determines the most likely site where it will be presented to the appropriate cells so that effective immune activation will take place. Antigens that enter via the blood usually activate immune cells in the spleen; those that lodge in the skin or subcutaneous tissues activate immune cells in the lymph nodes, and those that enter through the gastrointestinal and respiratory tracts activate immunocytes residing in mucosa-associated lymphoid tissues.

Deficiency in one or more of the major components of the immune system can result in serious diseases such as severe combined immunodeficiency disease, X-linked infantile agammaglobulinemia, and congenital thymic aplasia. However, immune responsiveness is not always free of risk for pathological consequences. Some individuals develop hypersensitivity reactions after inhalation, ingestion, or contact with an allergenic substance. Autoimmune diseases such as systemic lupus erythematosus, rheumatoid arthritis, and type 1 insulin-dependent diabetes mellitus occur when the immune system attacks endogenous or "self-" antigens. Go to the Companion Website for a brief review of immunology.

Numerous benefits have been gained through an increased knowledge of immune mechanisms. Among the greatest, if not the most significant, is immunization against infectious agents. Millions of lives have been saved and many millions more have been spared debilitating diseases such as polio and smallpox. Immunization of domestic and farm animals has brought increased economic benefits and increased safety from microbes with the potential to be transmitted to humans. Tremendous efforts are now ongoing to develop vaccines against human immunodeficiency virus type 1 (HIV-1; e.g., the cause of acquired immunodeficiency syndrome [AIDS]) and infectious agents that could be used for bioterrorism. In other cases, products of the immune system such as cytokines are being genetically engineered for possible use in therapy for a variety of pathological conditions (Massey & McPherson, 2001).

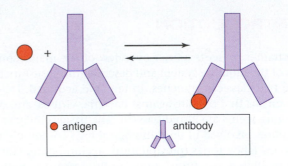

■ **FIGURE 10-1** Reversibility of antigen–antibody reactions. The interaction of antibody and antigen does not result in the formation of a new molecule because the binding is noncovalent (i.e., there is no sharing of electrons). Instead, it is a freely reversible reaction that can proceed back and forth numerous times. The length of time that the two reactants stay together depends on the microenvironment and the strength of the binding.

is reversible (Figure 10-1 ■). Antibodies have remarkable **specificity;** they are able to distinguish between very small differences in the primary structure, in the spatial conformation of the immunogen, and/or in a combination of both. The **epitope** or portion of the antigen to which the antibody attaches consists of a small contiguous sequence of subunits (amino acids or monosaccharides). In addition, the spatial folding or configuration of an antigen can bring into close proximity subunits that make up an epitope for one molecule of antibody. For most antigens, the 3-D structure is the determining factor of whether or not an antibody will bind.

The terms *affinity* and *avidity* are related, but not identical. **Affinity** refers to the strength of a single bond between the **paratope** (the part of the antibody that binds to the antigen) and the epitope. The higher the affinity, the more likely the antigen–antibody bond will remain intact. On a molecule-to-molecule basis, IgG has the greatest affinity compared to all other isotypes. The strength of the binding is expressed as the equilibrium constant (K) in the following formula: K = [bound antibody (Ab) and antigen (Ag) complex]/[Ab] × [Ag]. The square brackets indicate the concentrations of the two reactants. The antibodies generated in vivo, or in the body, against a complex antigen with a number of epitopes differ in their affinity for that antigen. The affinities of antibodies binding to a single antigen have a random, rather than bell-shaped or Gaussian, distribution. Furthermore, antibodies produced in a secondary response to a T-dependent antigen have a higher average affinity than those produced during the primary response. Although the mechanisms for this phenomenon are not entirely clear, the increase in average affinity ("affinity maturation") is associated with B cell switching from IgM to IgG production and an increased mutation rate in the V region. In contrast, **avidity** (functional affinity) refers to the strength of multivalent binding (i.e., the cumulative strength of all bonds between the antigen and antibody molecules present in a specimen, e.g., avidity of the serum). IgG, IgD, IgE, and monomeric

---

✓ Checkpoint! 10–1 (Chapter Objective 1)

What are the three major functions of the immune system?

   A. *Agglutination, precipitation, surveillance*
   B. *Surveillance, defense, complement activation*
   C. *Defense, homeostasis, surveillance*
   D. *Agglutination, defense, complement activation*
   E. *Homeostasis, complement activation, agglutination*

 ANTIBODY METHODS

GENERAL PROPERTIES OF ANTIGEN-ANTIBODY BINDING

Three characteristics hold true for virtually all antigen–antibody reactions: (1) antibody recognizes the three-dimensional (3-D) shape and/or primary sequence of antigen; (2) the bonds that hold the two together are weak (i.e., they are noncovalent), there is no electron sharing, and hence the two reactants never become one molecule; and (3) the interaction

IgA have two identical binding sites. Dimeric IgA has 4 binding sites. IgM, with 10 potential binding sites, has the greatest avidity, but only 5 sites usually bind with the antigen simultaneously. This is because of steric hindrance or crowding, which is the natural repulsion between electron clouds on large molecules. In other words, each Fab (antigen binding fragment) region can interfere with the binding of its neighboring Fab regions. The multivalence of antibodies and antigens leads to a synergistic increase in the overall strength of the binding. In other words, the overall binding strength is always greater, usually manyfold greater, than the arithmetic sum of individual bonds.

Four forces hold antigen and antibody together: (1) an electrostatic or ionic force comes into play when oppositely charged ions such as NH_3^+ and ^-COO are brought close together; (2) hydrogen bonding is a force because of interaction between electropositive and electronegative atoms such as O^- and H^+; (3) hydrophobic force is related to the expulsion of water molecules between hydrophobic amino acids such as isoleucine and valine as they approach one another; and (4) Van der Waals force involves randomly oscillating electrons that create dipoles or natural gaps maintained between positive and negative charges. All these forces are weak, but if the two reactants are close enough together, they favor antigen–antibody binding rather than not binding. A number of factors affect the strength of these forces, including the concentrations of antibody and antigen, pH, ionic strength of the medium, temperature, and the nature of the solvent. In general, the closer the two reactants are to each other in a medium that has a physiologic pH of 7.4, little or no interfering ions or other factors, and a temperature of 37°C, the greater is the strength of the binding.

Checkpoint! 10–2 (Chapter Objective 3)

On a molecule-to-molecule basis, which class of antibody has the highest affinity for antigen?
  A. *IgG*
  B. *IgA*
  C. *IgM*
  D. *IgD*
  E. *IgE*

SPECIFICITY AND CROSS-REACTIVITY

Specificity refers to the ability of an antibody to differentiate between the epitope that induced it and other antigenic determinants. Thus, antibody binds best to the antigen that induced its production. **Cross-reactivity** refers to the ability of an antibody, specific for one antigen, to react with a second similar yet unrelated antigen. For this to occur, the second antigen must have an identical or similar epitope as the inducing antigen. Cross-reactivity, thus, is a measure of relatedness between two different antigens. We make use of cross-reactivity every day. For example, the toxoid used for immunization

against tetanus is made by chemically modifying the toxin produced by *Clostridium tetani*. In the immunized individual, antibodies induced by the toxoid will bind to and neutralize the bacterial toxin, should the person ever become infected. **Heterophile antigens** have epitopes that are found on widely differing forms of life. In other words, the antigenic determinants of some plants, animals, and microorganisms can be very similar in structure to those in humans. For example, red blood cells (RBCs) of humans with blood group A and a pneumococcal capsular polysaccharide possess the same epitope; cells from humans with blood group B have an epitope found on certain serotypes of *E. coli*. Conversely, antibodies that bind to antigens not responsible for their production are known as **heterophile antibodies.** An example is the screening test for Epstein-Barr virus, the cause of infectious mononucleosis, which detects human IgM antibodies that bind to antigens on sheep or horse erythrocytes.

 REAL WORLD TIP

After a throat infection with *Streptococcus pyogenes*, antibodies are produced against the organism's M protein. The M protein shares epitopes with human heart tissue. Antibodies produced against the organism cross-react with myocardial cells causing rheumatic fever. Because rheumatic fever can occur 2 to 4 weeks after infection, the organism may no longer be present in the throat. Serologic diagnosis must be used to detect the antibodies produced against the organism and its many exotoxins. Antibodies used for diagnosis include antistreptolysin O, anti-DNase B, anti-NADase, antistreptokinase, and antihyaluronidase. Increased antibody titers or levels are present for up to 2 months after infection.

MONOCLONAL ANTIBODIES

Monoclonal antibodies (MAb) are produced by a genetically engineered single B cell to produce a single kind of antibody. The technique for monoclonal antibody production, first described by Köhler and Milstein in 1975, created a revolution in immunology and has also had a dramatic impact on many biomedical sciences. It allows for production of virtually unlimited quantities of antibodies that are chemically, physically, and immunologically homogenous. Unlike **polyclonal** sera, which is because of activation of many different B cells, in monoclonal sera all the MAbs are directed against a single epitope and thus are highly specific. Because normal B lymphocytes survive for only a few days outside the body, large amounts of MAbs are generated by first creating a hybridoma (i.e., a myeloma cell—malignant B cell) fused with an activated normal B cell. The myeloma partner gives the hybridoma the property of "immortality," whereas the B cell provides the single antibody. MAbs have numerous applications, especially with flow cytometry. Uses include crossmatching before organ transplantation, quantification of CD4$^+$ T helper and CD8$^+$ T cytotoxic cell levels in AIDS patients, immunohistologic analyses of tissue biopsies, and in specific and rapid diagnosis of bacterial, viral, and other infections. In vivo applications of MAbs are still relatively few; most preparations approved by the Food and Drug Administration have been for cancer detection and treatment.

PRACTICAL ASPECTS

It was initially challenging to translate the basic knowledge of immunology into tests that are useful in the practice of medicine. Today, numerous immunologic evaluations are routinely performed on a wide array of cells, tissues, and biological fluids to assist in diagnosis, prognosis, and optimal therapy design. Most assays described here use many of the recently elucidated principles of basic immunology. However, correct interpretation is not always as easy as it may seem because of differences in developmental, genetic, and environmental aspects among individuals (Pincus & Abraham, 2001). Furthermore, false positives and false negatives are always possible because no test is 100% foolproof.

To observe or measure antigen–antibody interactions, a secondary phenomenon (something in addition to antibody binding to antigen) must occur. These measurable consequences include, but are not limited to, precipitation, agglutination, complement fixation, and labeling antibody or antigen with a marker such as a fluorescent dye, radionuclide, or enzyme. The sensitivity of laboratory tests based on these measurable consequences can vary greatly. In general, the most sensitive assays are those that use a marker to indicate that an antigen–antibody reaction has taken place. In many assays commonly used in clinical laboratories, the **titer** or the reciprocal of the highest dilution at which there is a detectable result of an antibody (or antigen) is the reported end result (Table 10-1✪).

Analysis of paired sera (acute [during the disease state] and convalescent [after recovery from the disease state]) is often needed to establish a specific diagnosis. Ideally, the first specimen should be collected as early as possible after infection, whereas the second specimen should be collected approximately 10 to 21 days (average of ~14 days) later. A fourfold rise in antibody titer between the acute and convalescent sera against the suspected microbe indicates that it has recently infected the patient.

PRECIPITATION

Basic Principles

In precipitation reactions, both the antibody and antigen are soluble. Cross-linking of the two results in an increasingly larger lattice, which eventually becomes insoluble and exits the solution in the form of a precipitate. The proportion of antibody and antigen to each other is critical for a detectable

✪ TABLE 10-1

Example of Antibody Titer in Serum

Serum (Antibody) Dilution								
undiluted	1:2	1:4	1:8	1:16	1:32	1:64	1:128	1:256
–	–	+	++	+++	++	+	–	–
prozone		zone of equivalence					postzone	

The patient's serum was tested for the presence of antibodies against a soluble antigen. Serial twofold dilutions were made of the serum, and the amount of antigen was kept constant throughout. –: no precipitate; +: slight precipitate; ++: moderate precipitate; +++: heavy precipitate. The results show that the antibody titer is 64 (i.e., the highest dilution of serum at which there is still a positive reaction). The lack of precipitate at "undiluted" and 1:2 is because of excess antibody for the amount of antigen that is present (prozone); the lack of precipitate at 1:128 and 1:256 occurred because the antibody in the serum has now been diluted too much for the amount of antigen that is there (postzone). A positive reaction is detected within the zone of equivalence, where the amount of antibody and the amount of antigen are within optimal concentrations in relation to each other.

precipitate to form. If there is too much antibody for the amount of antigen (prozone) or if there is too much antigen for the amount of antibody (postzone), the results will be negative. In the zone of equivalence, the proportions of antibody and antigen are equivalent in relation to each other or, at the very least, are within the range in which a visible precipitate can form. These concepts are illustrated in Table 10-1.

✓ Checkpoint! 10–3 (Chapter Objective 3)

A serum sample from a patient with a respiratory tract infection is tested for antibodies against Streptococcus pneumoniae. A positive reaction is obtained only when the serum is diluted 1:16 or higher. Lack of a precipitate at dilutions less than 1:16 is because of a phenomenon known as _____.

    A. *zone of equilibrium*
    B. *prozone*
    C. *zero zone*
    D. *postzone*
    E. *zone of negativity*

Common Laboratory Tests Involving Precipitation

Precipitin Ring Formation. In this test, solutions containing antigen and antibody are carefully layered one on top of the other to avoid mixing of the two reactants. This procedure is often performed in a test tube. During incubation, the antigen and antibody diffuse toward each other and form a ring or band of visible precipitate at the zone of equivalence. The size and intensity of the band reflect the quantity of the precipitated immune complex. From left to right in Figure 10-2 , antigen and antibody molecules in the layered solu-

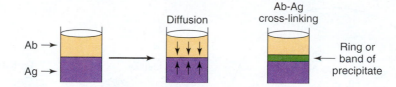

■ **FIGURE 10-2** Precipitin band formation test. After antibody is carefully layered over a suspension of antigen, both reactants diffuse toward each other. A band of precipitate forms when the amounts of the two reactants are within the zone of equivalence with respect to each other.

tions are shown diffusing toward one another. When the proportions of the two reactants reach appropriate concentrations in relation to each other, a visible precipitate forms, usually at or near the interface between the solutions. This test was used in studies performed by Rebecca Lancefield to determine the specific M cell wall protein present in strains of beta hemolytic *Streptococcus* spp. She used antiserum with antibody to a specific M protein layered on top of a suspension of the organism in a capillary tube. If the antibody and antigen were homologous, then a visible layer formed between the two.

℮ REAL WORLD TIP

The precipitin ring formed at the interface can be easily disrupted when moved. The layer may be difficult to see, depending on the amount of antigen present. This test does not provide a means to quantitate the results.

Nephelometry.

Nephelometry involves the measurement of light scattered from the main beam of a transmitted light source (Figure 10-3 ■). The precipitate formed by antigen–antibody complexes produces increased reflection that can be measured. Light rays from a laser or other high-intensity light source are collected in a focusing lens and passed through the sample tube containing antigen and antibody. Light passing through the tube and emerging at a 70° angle is collected by another lens and focused into an electronic detector. The signal is converted to a digital recording of the amount of turbidity in the sample and can be mathematically related to either antigen or antibody concentration. This automated technique is useful for measurement of serum antibodies and complement components when large numbers of samples must be analyzed. However, the equipment is relatively expensive, and the test tubes must be optically very clear and have no scratches, bumps, or fingerprints, as these may give erroneous results. In addition, if the serum has a high lipid content or the blood has hemolyzed, an inaccurate result may be obtained. Today, many nephelometers will automatically subtract the background reading of the patient's serum.

Ouchterlony (Double-Diffusion) Assay.

The Ouchterlony test is based on the principle in which both antigen and antibody diffuse through a semisolid agar medium to form stable immune complexes at the point of equivalence, which can be visualized. It is a double diffusion method because both reactants are moving through the medium at the same time. Small wells are punched in the agar, and antigen and antibody samples are placed in opposing wells. Both reactants diffuse toward one another in a moist chamber for 12 to 24 hours, as shown in Figure 10-4a ■. The three classic reaction patterns (identity, partial identity, and nonidentity) are depicted in Figure 10-4b ■. This test can be used for semiquantitative analysis once the specificity of the two reactants has been determined (Figure 10-4c ■). Double-diffusion assays can be used with all biological fluids. They are virtually 100% specific in detecting the appropriate antibody or antigen, whichever is unknown. However, they are of low sensitivity, have a relatively long incubation period, and require a considerable amount of laboratory time.

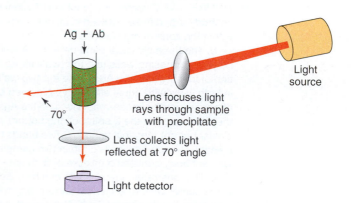

■ **FIGURE 10-3** Basic components of a nephelometer. Nephelometry is an automated procedure that quantifies the amount of serum antibody (Ab) against a specific antigen (Ag). A soluble preparation of a known antigen is mixed with the patient's serum in an optically clear test tube by inversion. A precipitate forms if the serum contains antibody that can bind to the antigen. The amount of light reflected at a 70° angle by the precipitate is detected and mathematically converted into the concentration of the antibody.

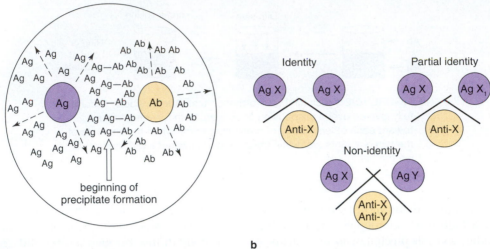

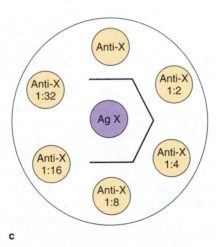

■ FIGURE 10-4 Ouchterlony (double-diffusion) test. **a.** In this test, both the antigen (Ag) and the antibody (Ab) diffuse outward in all directions from wells cut in agar. A band of precipitate forms within the zone of equivalence.

b. The three classical band patterns. A smooth, continuous, curved band of precipitate between opposing wells (the top two with Ag X and the bottom one with anti-X) indicates a reaction of identity (i.e., the Ags in the top two wells are identical and the anti-X can bind to the Ag X in both wells with equal efficiency). A curved band with a spur sticking out indicates a reaction of partial identity (cross-reactivity; i.e., the Ags in the top two wells are partially identical because they both contain the X epitope); the bottom well contains the X antibody that reacts with the similar but not identical antigens. Two bands that cross each other indicate a reaction of non-identity. The top two wells contain two completely different antigens (Ag X and Ag Y); the well with antibody contains a mixture of both anti-X and anti-Y.

c. Demonstrates how this test can be used for semiquantification of antibody. Ag X is placed in the center well, whereas the surrounding wells contain twofold dilutions of serum known to contain antibody against Ag X. The curved, smooth, unbroken band of precipitate that forms gets progressively less dense as the antibody dilution increases, until it is no longer visible. Thus, the titer of anti-X can be determined. The titer of the anti-X is 8 or the reciprocal of the highest dilution at which there is still a detectable reaction. An Ag can be semiquantified in the same manner by reversing the wells which contain the Ag and antibody.

The Ouchterlony assay must be set up with care. Irregular patterns of precipitation may occur because of overfilling of wells, irregular hole punching, or unlevel incubation. Other factors that can affect the results include drying out of the gel, inadequate time for diffusion, and fungal or bacterial contamination of the gel substrate.

Radial Immunodiffusion (RID).

In radial immunodiffusion, an antigen diffuses concentrically through a medium that contains antibody. RID is a single-diffusion method because only one reactant moves through the medium, whereas the other is fixed in the medium. First, an antibody is homogenously incorporated into molten agar, which is then allowed to harden. Wells are then cut in the agar. One well is filled with the test sample, whereas additional wells are filled with solutions containing known concentrations of the antigen (i.e., standards), which will be precipitated by the antibody. After 24 to 48 hours, the diameters of the circular precipitates formed around the wells containing the known concentrations of the antigen are used to make a standard curve. The diameter of the precipitin ring produced by the test sample is proportional to the concentration of the antigen, which can be determined from the standard curve. This assay is widely used for quantification of a variety of serum proteins, including antibodies and complement components.

Radial immunodiffusion has been replaced by the more sensitive ELISA method. Sources of errors include underfilling or overfilling the wells. If rheumatoid factor is present in the sample, it can react with IgG and create a false precipitin ring.

Zone Electrophoresis.

A number of tests use electrophoresis or the separation of antigens and antibodies using an electric current. The use of an electric current speeds up the diffusion and sharpens the precipitin bands. A description of zone electrophoresis is included here because proteins in a mixture are often separated electrophoretically before further steps are performed. The separation of proteins by this method is based on their size and surface charge, resulting in different rates of migration in an electrical field. Different types of optically clear, inert support media can be used (e.g., agarose, paper, or cellulose acetate strips). Serum or other biological fluid is placed at the origin, and an electrical current is applied using an alkaline buffer. Five bands are obtained with normal serum: albumin, α1-globulin, α2-globulin, β-globulin, and γ-globulin (Figure 10-5 ■). Albumin travels fastest toward the

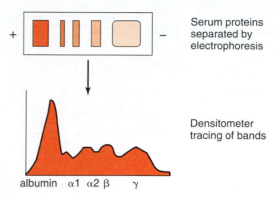

Serum proteins separated by electrophoresis

Densitometer tracing of bands

albumin   α1 α2 β   γ

■ **FIGURE 10-5** Zone electrophoresis. In this procedure, serum is dispensed onto an optically clear, inert support media (e.g., agarose gel or cellulose nitrate) and an electrical current is applied. Proteins migrate at different rates in an electrical field and hence are physically separated. The support media is then passed through a densitometer that measures the density of each migrated protein and also generates a curve. The diagram shows a typical curve with multiple peaks that are obtained with normal serum. Albumin migrates fastest toward the anode (positive pole), whereas the γ-globulin fraction that contains antibodies is closest to the cathode (negative pole).

anode (positive pole), whereas the γ-globulin fraction, which contains antibodies, remains closest to the cathode (negative pole). The strips are then stained for protein and scanned in a densitometer. Scanning converts the band pattern into peaks. This procedure is useful in diagnosis of immunoglobulin-secreting myelomas, Waldenstrom's macroglobulinemia, and hyper- and hypogammaglobulinemias.

Multiple myeloma is malignancy involving plasma cells. The cells produce an abnormal amount of immunoglobulin. A large spike will appear in the γ-globulin band if only one immunoglobulin is produced. IgG is the most common immunoglobulin observed. A large broad band will appear in the γ-globulin band if multiple abnormal immunoglobulins are produced (i.e., IgG and IgA).

Immunoelectrophoresis.

This technique combines electrophoretic separation, diffusion, and immune precipitation. As shown in Figure 10-6 ■, a well and trough are cut in a gel, usually agarose. The patient's serum is dispensed into the well, and the electrical current is turned on. After migration is completed, the current is turned off, and an antibody preparation is then dispensed into the trough. The separated proteins and the antibodies diffuse outward and form bands of precipitate

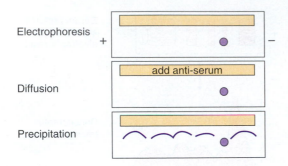

■ FIGURE 10-6 Immunoelectrophoresis. This procedure combines electrophoresis, diffusion, and precipitation. A well and trough are cut in a slab of agar gel. Serum is placed in the well, and the electrical current is turned on to separate the proteins. After turning the current off, antiserum is dispensed into the trough, and diffusion is allowed to take place. Bands of precipitate form at the zone of equivalence, where the antigen and antibody concentrations are within the optimal range in relation to each other. The bottom panel of the diagram shows the five bands of precipitate typically seen with normal serum.

at the zone of equivalence. Both identification and approximate quantification can be accomplished for proteins in serum, urine, cerebrospinal fluid, and other biological fluids. This technique is less widely used now than in the past, having been replaced by immunofixation, immunoblotting procedures, and latex agglutination tests, which are easier to interpret.

Counterimmunoelectrophoresis. This test is performed in agar gels in which the pH is such that the antigen and antibody have opposite electrical charges. Application of an electrical current then forces the antigen and antibody to migrate toward each other. This procedure is much faster than the Ouchterlony assay, because of application of an electric current, with incubation time being reduced to about 1 to 2 hours. Furthermore, the sensitivity is increased by as much as 20-fold.

Rocket Electrophoresis. Another variation employing an electrical field is called "rocket electrophoresis." In this case, the pH of the gel is selected so that antibodies remain immobile in the gel, and the antigen has a negative charge. The band of precipitate that forms has the appearance of a nose of a rocket, the height of which is proportional to the antigen concentration. The concentration of the antigen in the test sample can be interpolated from a standard curve. The two reactants can be reversed so that quantification of antibody can also be done by this method.

Western Blot. Several versions of tests use immunoblotting. The Western blot, designed for detection of specific proteins, is similar to the Southern blot, which measures DNA, and the Northern blot, which measures RNA. Its main uses are

for identification of serum proteins in difficult diagnostic problems and in which results of more routine tests are equivocal. The test is widely used as a confirmatory test for antibodies against infectious agents such as HIV-1, the AIDS virus. As shown in Figure 10-7 ■, antigens are first separated by electrophoresis using standard polyacrylamide gels. The current is turned off, and the gel is placed onto a nitrocellulose membrane. The separated proteins are then electrophoresed a second time (i.e., "blotted") into the membrane. The nitrocellulose traps the proteins so that they will not immediately begin migrating once the electrical current is turned off (hence more definitive bands are obtained than in gels). The patient's serum, along with positive and negative controls, is then dispensed onto the nitrocellulose. Precipitin bands form if the serum contains antibodies capable of binding to one or more of the antigens. However, the amount of precipitate is often very small. To overcome this limitation, the membrane is overlaid with an antihuman antibody, which is labeled with an enzyme or a radionuclide such as ^{125}I. Binding of the second antibody to the first is detected by either adding a colorless substrate, which is converted to a colored product by the enzyme (a chromogen), or by autoradiography. This technique is highly specific, but requires careful quality control and is time consuming. Western blot kits with antigen-impregnated membranes and positive and negative control sera are now commercially available for certain antibodies (e.g., anti-HIV).

ℯ REAL WORLD TIP

A diagnosis of HIV-1 infection can be devastating to the patient, causing emotional turmoil and, in some cases, thoughts of suicide. A reliable confirmatory test, such as the Western blot, can rule out (or rule in) HIV-1 infection.

ℯ REAL WORLD TIP

The electric current can serve as a potential source of error in the electrophoresis procedure. If the current is applied in the wrong direction, the sample will move in the wrong direction. If too weak a current is used, separation of the bands may not occur. If too strong a current is used, the proteins will be denatured.

Flocculation Tests. The term *flocculation* refers to the fleecy, tuftlike, or wool-like precipitate that appears under certain conditions. The fine, granular precipitate may be viewed either macroscopically or microscopically. Historically, the VDRL (Venereal Disease Research Laboratory) test has been among the most commonly used flocculation tests. It can be done on serum from patients suspected of being infected with

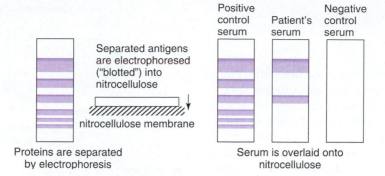

Positive control serum
Patient's serum
Negative control serum

Separated antigens are electrophoresed ("blotted") into nitrocellulose

nitrocellulose membrane

Proteins are separated by electrophoresis

Serum is overlaid onto nitrocellulose

■ **FIGURE 10-7** Western blot for serum antibodies. This test is frequently used as a confirmatory test for antibodies against HIV-1. In this case, proteins of the virus are first separated in a polyacrylamide gel by applying an electrical current. The current is then turned off, the gel is placed onto a nitrocellulose membrane, and the electrical current is once again turned on. This second application of an electrical field ("blotting") forces the separated proteins into the nitrocellulose membrane. After again turning off the current, the patient's serum is added. If it contains antibody that binds one or more of the viral antigens trapped in the membrane, immune complexes will form. Detection of the complexes is often facilitated by adding an antihuman antibody that is labeled with an enzyme or a radionuclide such as ^{125}I. Binding of the labeled antibody is detected by either adding a colorless substrate that is converted to a colored product by the enzyme or by autoradiography.

Treponema pallidum, the etiologic agent of syphilis. Infection frequently induces the production of reagin, an antibody that binds to cardiolipin. In a positive test, cardiolipin-lecithin-coated cholesterol particles come out of solution as a flocculent precipitate, which is visualized with a microscope. Because *T pallidum* antigens are not involved, the assay has a high incidence of false positives. Nevertheless, it has been a useful

screening test for syphilis over a number of decades. Today it is the test of choice for cerebrospinal fluid to determine central nervous system involvement. The commercially available RPR (Rapid Plasma Reagin) test, which comes with all needed ingredients and positive and negative controls, has replaced the VDRL in many clinical laboratories. As in the VDRL test, the antigen is cardiolipin-lecithin-cholesterol, but the solution also contains charcoal particles, which allow for macroscopic visualization of the flocculated precipitate on a specially treated cardboard card. The RPR is more rapid and easier to perform than the VDRL test. It is used primarily on serum for testing.

 REAL WORLD TIP

Syphilis is a sexually transmitted disease caused by *Treponema pallidum*. The organism cannot be grown in culture, so serologic methods are needed for diagnosis. The nontreponemal tests, VDRL and RPR, are used to screen for syphilis. They detect reagins, which are antibodies against cardiolipin rather than antibodies produced against the organism itself. Both tests lack specificity and are prone to false-positive reactions. Age, pregnancy, malignancy, systemic lupus erythematous (SLE), and viral infections can cause false-positive reactions. Confirmatory testing using treponemal tests that detect antibody directed against the organism itself must be used. Confirmatory tests are not subject to as many false positives and are more sensitive but more difficult to perform.

✓ **Checkpoint! 10–4 (Chapter Objective 7)**

A test is performed on a patient's serum to determine the titer of antibodies against the Epstein-Barr virus (EBV, the cause of infectious mononucleosis). A positive reaction is obtained at serum dilutions of 1:2, 1:4, 1:8, and 1:16, whereas a negative result is obtained at 1:32, 1:64, and 1:128. Based on this information, what is the titer of the anti-EBV antibody?

A. 2
B. 16
C. 32
D. 64
E. 128

► AGGLUTINATION METHODS

BASIC PRINCIPLES

When antibodies cross-link with cells or particles, they clump together or agglutinate. Tests involving agglutination are generally more sensitive than precipitation reactions because the endpoint is more easily detectable. Cross-linking of cells or commercially manufactured particles (e.g., latex and bentonite beads) by antibody directed against surface antigens leads to readily visible clumping. The concentrations of the two reactants in relation to each other is important, although less so than in precipitation reactions. On a molecule-to-molecule basis, IgM antibodies are the best agglutinators because they are the largest and have 10 potential binding sites (Fab), more than any other isotype. The actual number of binding sites that attach is usually less than the 10 potential binding sites in each IgM molecule because each physically interferes with the binding of neighboring Fab regions. Figure 10-8 ■ shows antigen-coated particles cross-linked by antibody; large macroscopic aggregates will form as more bonds are formed. Many particulate antigens (including RBC and other cells) have a net negative surface charge when suspended in saline. This negative surface charge causes a diffuse layer or "cloud" of positively charged ions to accumulate around the cells and most commercially available particles. This results in what is known as the zeta potential, the main factor that determines the repulsion effects between two adjacent particles (Figure 10-9 ■). Thus, agglutination may not occur even when antibody specific for the antigen is present. The zeta potential is effectively reduced by addition of serum albumin or by pretreatment of cells with enzymes such as trypsin. The end result is that the repulsion force created by the zeta potential is overcome to the extent that agglutination is possible.

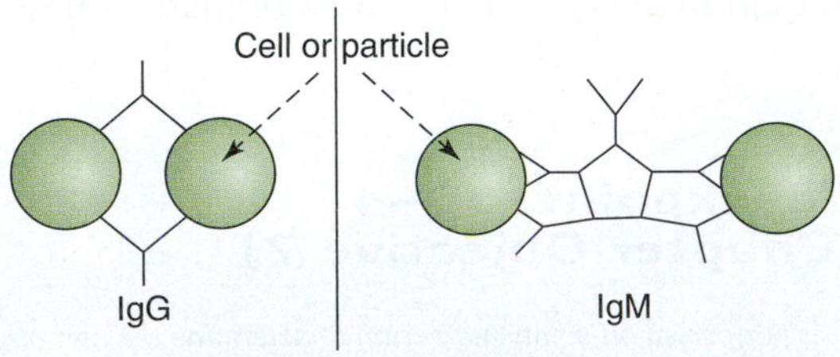

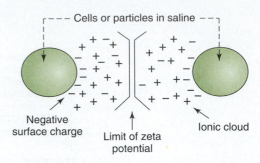

■ **FIGURE 10-9** Zeta potential. Cells and many commercially made beads or particles have a net negative surface charge when suspended in saline. Consequently, positively charged ions gather around and create an electrical or zeta potential that increases the distance between them. Antibody specific for the antigen is thus unable to span the distance, and a false negative occurs. Addition of serum albumin or pretreatment of cells with enzymes such as trypsin will reduce the repulsion and allow agglutination to occur.

COMMON LABORATORY TESTS INVOLVING AGGLUTINATION

Agglutination of Bacteria and Other Microbes

Many bacteria, when combined with the appropriate antibody, will form small clumps within a matter of a few minutes. The clumps are best visualized using a light source (e.g., a light box). Bacteria isolated from patients can be identified in this manner using commercially available antibodies. Conversely, serum from patients can be tested to detect antibodies against specific commercially available bacteria. Agglutination tests for antibodies against *Francisella tularensis*, *Brucella* species, and *Salmonella typhi* are included in panels referred to as "febrile agglutinin" tests. Occasionally, cross-reactive bacteria are used to detect antibodies against agents that are difficult to culture. A prime example of this is the Weil-Felix test in which *Proteus* species are used to detect antibodies against *Rickettsia*. In addition, certain isolates, such as *E. coli*, as well as other members of the *Enterobacteriaceae* family, can be serotyped based on their capsular (K), somatic or cell wall (O), and flagellar (H) antigens. Some of these antigens are associated with pathogenicity and virulence. For example, *E. coli* serotype O157:H7 is frequently implicated in hemorrhagic colitis and hemolytic uremic syndrome. Strains of *Salmonella typhi*, which possess the Vi antigen (a specific type of K antigen), are more virulent than their counterparts that do not express it. Antibodies against other microbes such as *Toxoplasma gondii*, *Leishmania*, and *Plasmodium* can also be detected by agglutination. Tests involving agglutination of bacteria and other microbes can be performed either in test tubes or on slides.

■ **FIGURE 10-8** Comparison of IgG and IgM agglutination efficiency. As shown in the diagram, IgG is a relatively small molecule that has only two sites that can bind to an antigen. In contrast, pentameric IgM is significantly larger and has 10 potential binding sites. Hence, on a molecule per molecule basis, IgM is much more efficient at binding and holding two cells or particles together compared to IgG, as well as all other isotypes. According to some estimates, the strength of a bond between IgM and an antigen is approximately 750 times greater than that between IgG and an antigen.

Agglutination Using Particles Coated with Antigen or Antibody

In these assays, soluble antigen or antibody is attached to inert particles such as latex or bentonite beads. In the case of bound antigen, antibodies in a test sample will cause the particles to agglutinate if they are specific for the antigen. For example, latex beads coated with thyroglobulin will agglutinate if autoantibodies against the hormone are present, thus aiding in the diagnosis of lymphocytic thyroiditis (Hashimoto's disease). Particles with attached antigens are also used to detect antibodies against infectious agents such as *Trichinella spiralis,* *Histoplasma capsulatum,* and *Cryptococcus neoformans.* In contrast, particle-bound antibodies can be used to detect antigen. This latter approach is the basis of the RA (rheumatoid arthritis) test, which detects rheumatoid factor in serum. These types of assays, although simple and rapid, are relatively insensitive and costly.

REAL WORLD TIP

Salmonella spp. can be serotyped based on the somatic (O) antigen in their cell wall. The somatic antigen can be masked by the capsular (K) antigen. The somatic antigen is heat stable, whereas the capsule antigen is heat labile. Antibody against a specific somatic antigen can be attached to a plastic bead. If a suspected *Salmonella* spp. does not serotype by latex agglutination, it may be because of the presence of a capsule. Boiling the organism suspension will destroy the capsule. The organism can then be retested to determine its somatic antigen present by latex agglutination.

REAL WORLD TIP

Many laboratories use latex agglutination to identify *Staphylococcus aureus*. Latex beads are coated with fibrinogen to detect clumping factor and IgG to detect protein A. Methicillin-resistant *S. aureus* (MRSA) may possess a capsule that can mask clumping factor and protein A and present with a false-negative result. A new generation of latex tests has now added antibodies to the mixture to also detect the capsular antigens of MRSA.

Hemagglutination Tests

Agglutination of RBCs is known as hemagglutination. Several different versions fall under this general designation. Active hemagglutination involves antigens that are actively expressed by the RBC itself (i.e., they are an integral part of the cell). In the direct version, washed RBCs are mixed with an antibody. For example, IgM against the ABO antigens is mixed with the cells to determine blood group prior to blood transfusion or organ transplantation. Direct hemagglutination tests are also used to obtain titers of anti-A, anti-B, cold hemagglutinins (IgM antibodies that react best at temperatures between 4°C and 25°C or room temperature, rather than at 37°C), and for heterophile antibodies that agglutinate sheep or horse RBCs in patients suspected of having infectious mononucleosis. Indirect hemagglutination tests detect antibodies, usually IgG, that bind to RBCs, but by themselves cannot cause agglutination. In these cases, a second antibody specific for human immunoglobulin is added to induce agglutination. In passive hemagglutination, a soluble antigen is first adsorbed to RBCs (i.e., the antigen is not an integral part of the cell itself). RBCs will spontaneously adsorb many different substances. If a particular substance does not adsorb well, the cells can be treated with tannic acid, chromium chloride, or another agent so that adsorption becomes possible. Substances that spontaneously adsorb to RBCs include antigens of *E. coli, Yersinia,* and *Toxoplasma,* antibiotics such as penicillin, the endotoxin of *Mycoplasma pneumoniae,* bovine serum albumin, DNA, and many viruses. The microhemagglutination test for *T. pallidum* (MHA-TP) is among the most commonly used assays involving a soluble antigen adsorbed to erythrocytes. Another version in which agglutination of RBCs is used is known as hemagglutination inhibition. This approach is used primarily for semiquantitation of antibodies against influenza virus. The underlying basis is that antibodies against the hemagglutinin molecule on the surface of the virus will prevent RBC agglutination.

▶ COMPLEMENT METHODS

BASIC PRINCIPLES

As mentioned earlier, the proteins that make up the complement system are present in the blood circulation in inactive form. Once activated, they interact with each other in a specific sequence. If one or more of the major components is missing, below normal level, or nonfunctional, the biological consequences of complement activation will not occur. Antigen–antibody complexes in solution, as well as on the surface of cells, can activate complement when either IgG or IgM are involved. An end result in the case of RBCs is that they lyse. This phenomenon is useful in the clinical laboratory setting and can be used to measure antibody, as well as the integrity of the complement pathways (Dodd & Sims, 1998).

COMMON LABORATORY TESTS INVOLVING COMPLEMENT

Complement Fixation Test

During activation, complement components become consumed or "fixed" to antibodies that are bound to antigen. The amount of complement that is used up is proportional to the concentration of the antibody (Kaufman, Sekhon, Moledina,

Jalbert, & Pappagianis, 1995). The assay described here is performed to detect and semiquantify antibody. There are two major stages in this procedure. First, a known antigen is mixed with the patient's serum, which has been depleted of complement by heating for 30 minutes at 56°C; a known amount of complement in the form of guinea pig complement is added. Complement is not species specific. If the serum contains antibody that is specific for the antigen, it will bind and activate (fix) complement. In the second stage, sheep RBCs coated with IgG are added as the indicator; these are known as "sensitized" RBCs (sRBCs). If the sRBCs lyse, it is considered a negative test because it indicates that the patient has no antibodies against that particular antigen (i.e., complement has not been fixed or consumed by antigen–antibody in the first stage). On the other hand, if the sRBCs do not lyse, it is a positive reaction; the patient has antibodies against the antigen (i.e., complement has been fixed by antigen–antibody in the first stage and is no longer available for interaction with the sRBCs). Positive and negative reactions are illustrated in Figure 10-10 ■. Complement fixation is the underlying principle of the Wasserman test, which is used as a reference for new assays developed to assist in diagnosis of syphilis. The test is also used for identification and quantification of antibodies against *Mycoplasma pneumoniae, Bordetella pertussis, Coccidioides immitis, Histoplasma,* and many viruses. However, the assay is technically difficult, and many controls are necessary to ensure the test is working properly.

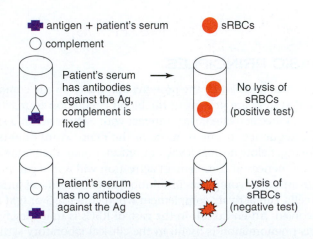

■ FIGURE 10-10 Complement fixation test. This test is used to detect and quantify antibody against a predetermined antigen. The underlying principle is based on the fact that complement (C') components are used up or "fixed" when the complement cascade is activated. In the first stage, the known antigen is mixed with the patient's serum (heat-inactivated), and a known amount of complement is added. If the serum contains antibody specific for the antigen, it will bind to it and activate complement. In the second stage, sheep red blood cells coated with IgG ("sensitized" sRBCs) are added. No lysis of the sRBCs is a positive reaction (patient has antibodies against the antigen; was fixed in first stage). Lysis of the sRBC, indicates a negative reaction (patient has no antibodies against the antigen; complement was not fixed in first stage).

Assays for Complement

A relatively simple measure of complement activity is to quantify the amount of serum that results in lysis of 50% of sheep erythrocytes sensitized with IgG in a standard preparation as determined by the total complement hemolytic activity test (CH_{50}). This can be carried out in test tubes or in wells of microtiter plates. Another method is to incorporate the sRBCs into agar gels, dispense the patient's serum into wells cut in the agar, and then measure the zone of hemolysis around the wells. The procedures for quantifying individual complement components often involve highly sensitive tests that include a marker such as a radioactive nuclide or enzyme (described later). Because the level of a particular complement component does not indicate that it is functionally active, mixtures of all necessary components, except the one under investigation, can be incubated together with sRBCs. If the activity of the component of interest is defective, the sRBCs will not lyse.

 Checkpoint! 10–5 (Chapter Objective 7)

Which of the following is the correct interpretation when sheep red blood cells lyse in the complement fixation test?

A. *The patient's serum is deficient in at least one of the major complement components.*
B. *The patient's serum has antibodies against the antigen.*
C. *The patient's serum is deficient in C3.*
D. *The patient's serum has no antibodies against the antigen.*
E. *The patient's serum has an excessive amount of all major complement components.*

► IMMUNOFLUORESCENCE METHODS

BASIC PRINCIPLES

Fluorescence is the emission of light of one color (i.e., wavelength) when a dye is irradiated with light of a different color. Fluorescent compounds are easily bound to free amino groups on antibodies and then used as markers to indicate that an antigen–antibody reaction has taken place. Among the most commonly used dyes in clinical laboratories are fluorescein isothiocyanate (FITC, greenish-yellow) and tetramethylrhodamine isothiocyanate (TRITC, reddish-orange).

 REAL WORLD TIP

It takes experience to use a fluorescent microscope. The technologist must be able to separate out fluorescence because of a true signal from background fluorescence because of other substances present in the sample tested.

COMMON LABORATORY TESTS INVOLVING IMMUNOFLUORESCENCE

Immunohistochemistry

These tests are especially suitable for detection of antigens in various tissues (immunohistochemistry) and on cell surfaces. A fluorescence microscope is needed to visualize the reaction. There are both direct and indirect versions of these tests (Figure 10-11 ■). In the direct test, a fluorescence-labeled antibody is directly applied to cells or sections of biopsy specimens on slides. In the indirect test, an unlabeled antibody is added first (or may already be there in the case of certain autoimmune diseases), and the fluorescent antibody is added second. The second antibody binds to the first antibody so that the antigen-antibody1-antibody2 complex can be visualized. This latter technique has an advantage over the direct procedure in which the same secondary antibody can be used to detect a variety of primary antibodies and also tends to give brighter fluorescence. These types of assays are extensively used to detect autoantibodies and sometimes provide support for a specific diagnosis based on the pattern of fluorescence. The technique can also be used to detect infectious agents in tissues and exudates, as well as antibodies against a variety of microbes. A classic example of this latter application is the test for antibodies against *Treponema pallidum*. In this assay, killed bacteria are incubated with the patient's serum; a second fluorescence-labeled antihuman antibody is then added.

Flow Cytometry

Flow cytometry with a fluorescence-activated cell sorter can analyze individual cells and isolate them on the basis of their surface antigens, size, and/or granularity. Antigens can be detected on the cells after labeling them with fluorescence conjugated antibodies. The number of fluorescent cells, as well as the ratio of fluorescent-to-nonfluorescent cells can be determined with much greater efficiency, speed, and accuracy than by manual counting. Many models are now capable of analyzing 1,000 cells or more per second. A mixture of cells suspended in highly pure saline is passed through a very small orifice, one cell at a time. Each individual cell is hit for a fraction of a second by a laser beam of a certain wavelength. If the cell has fluorescent antibody attached to it, it will give off color of a different wavelength and be counted separately from the total number of cells passing through the orifice. If the labeled cells are to be separated from the mixture, the machine can be set to deliver an electrical charge to the drop of saline containing the cell so that it will be diverted as it passes between electrically charged plates and collected in a container different from the one collecting unlabeled cells. Flow cytometry techniques can be used to quantify many different leukocyte populations in specimens of blood, virtually all other biological fluids, and bone marrow. Identification of lymphocyte subpopulations, based on clusters of differentiation (CD) molecules expressed by T helper and T cytotoxic cells, is often performed in this manner to follow patients infected with HIV-1. Flow cytometers are powerful tools with numerous other applications, including determination of cell maturation and activation, cell cycling, phagocytosis, NK cell cytotoxicity, and presence of intracellular cytokines (Keren, McCoy, John, & Carey, 2001).

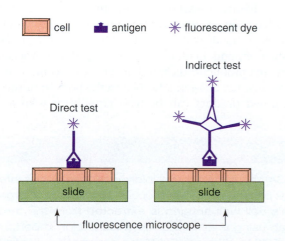

■ **FIGURE 10-11** Immunofluorescence. Fluorescent dyes can be attached to antibodies and visualized under a fluorescence microscope. When added to cells or tissues fixed to a slide, these antibodies may be used to detect antigens on the surface of bacteria, as well as histological sections. In the direct test, the primary antibody has the fluorescent label, whereas in the indirect test the primary antibody is added first (or it may already be there, as in the case of some autoimmune diseases), and then a labeled secondary antibody is added next.

> ⓔ **REAL WORLD TIP**
>
> Flow cytometry requires a single cell suspension for analysis. Solid tissues cannot be used because they are clumps of cells that scatter too much light as they flow past the laser beam and emit too much fluorescence.

Radioimmunoassays (RIA)

Radiolabeling of either antibody or antigen (the usual case) with radionuclides such as ^{131}I (iodine) or ^{125}I greatly increases test sensitivity and specificity. This technique is used to quantify very small quantities of substances such as hepatitis B antigen, insulin, progesterone, and carcinoembryonic antigen. The underlying principle of the classical radioimmunoassay (RIA) is competition of radiolabeled and unlabeled antigen for the same limited amount of antibody. A standard curve is first made by adding varying amounts of unlabeled antigen to a mixture containing a constant amount of antibody and a constant amount of radiolabeled antigen. After the reaction has taken place, the amount of unbound radiolabeled antigen is equivalent to the amount of unlabeled antigen that was added, as shown in Figure 10-12 ■. Thus, when a predetermined volume of a patient's serum is substituted for the unlabeled antigen, the amount of antigen (unlabeled), if present in the serum, can be obtained from the standard curve. Precipitation

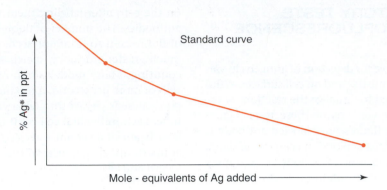

Ag unlabelled Ag* radiolabelled	Percentage of Ag* in precipitate	Percentage of Ag* in supernatant
10 Ab + 20 Ag*	100%	0%
10 Ab + 20 Ag* + 6 Ag	70%	30%
10 Ab + 20 Ag* + 12 Ag	60%	40%
10 Ab + 20 Ag* + 18 Ag	10%	90%

■ **FIGURE 10-12** Classical radioimmunoassay (RIA). In this test, a radiolabeled and a nonlabeled antigen compete for the same limited amount of antibody. A standard curve, similar to that shown in the diagram, is constructed. Thus, when a certain volume of the patient's serum is added to the antibody/radiolabeled antigen mixture, the antigen in the serum (if present) competes with its radiolabeled counterpart. After counting the amount of radioactivity in the precipitate and a supernatant, the concentration of the antigen in the serum can then be obtained from the standard curve.

of the complexes, which are often in very small quantities, can be accomplished by the addition of a second antibody or an agent such as ammonium sulfate or polyethylene glycol. However, solid-phase RIA tests are now available, which simplify the separation of antigen–antibody complexes from free antigen. In these versions, either the antigen or antibody is covalently bound to a solid surface such as Sephadex, polystyrene, or cellulose beads. A variation known as the radioallergosorbent test (RAST) makes use of a solid-phase material to which antigen is attached. The RAST is used to measure the amount of IgE in a patient's serum that has been generated in response to an antigen (allergen), including some that is derived from infectious agents. In the second stage of the assay, the IgE attached to antigen is detected by addition of radiolabeled antibody, which binds to IgE. Major disadvantages of these procedures include problems with use and disposal of radioactive waste, short half-life of radionuclides, and relatively high cost of equipment and reagents.

Enzyme-Linked Immunosorbent Assay (ELISA)

The enzyme-linked immunosorbent assay (ELISA) is used routinely for screening patient sera for many different antibodies and can also be used to detect antigens. This test is very popular in that it is highly sensitive, safe, economical, simple to perform, and versatile, and it requires minimum instrumentation. The assay is most often performed using plastic 96-well

microtiter plates (Figure 10-13 ■). Antigen is adsorbed to the bottom of wells, and the patient's serum is then added. During incubation, antibody specific for the antigen will bind. Anything not bound is washed off, and an antihuman antibody conjugated to an enzyme is added. If the first antibody is there, the second antibody will bind to it. Again, everything unbound is washed off, and a colorless substrate is added. Appearance of a colored product indicates that the serum contained antibody against the antigen adsorbed to the bottom of the well. The colored product can be read visually or with a spec-

> **ⓔ REAL WORLD TIP**
>
> ELISA can be used to rapidly diagnose throat infections because of *Streptococcus pyogenes*. The organism's cell wall antigen is extracted from the throat swab using enzymes or chemicals prior to performing ELISA. Although ELISA is very specific, it can be insensitive (false negative) if low numbers of organisms (antigens) are present, which may occur early in the infectious process. It is recommended that two swabs be collected from the patient. If the ELISA direct test is negative, then the second swab can be used for a traditional culture.

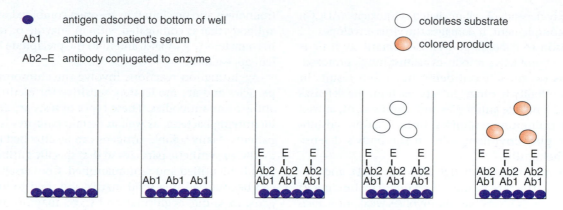

● antigen adsorbed to bottom of well

Ab1   antibody in patient's serum

Ab2–E   antibody conjugated to enzyme

○ colorless substrate

● colored product

■ FIGURE 10-13 Major steps in an enzyme-linked immunosorbent assay (ELISA). These tests are usually performed in 96-well microtiter plates. The diagram illustrates the series of steps that would be performed (i.e., the events taking place in a single well). A known antigen (Ag) is first adsorbed to the bottom of the well, and the patient's serum is added next. If the serum has antibody (Ab1) against the Ag, it will bind; anything not bound is washed off. A second antihuman antibody conjugated with an enzyme (Ab2-E) is then added. If Ab1 is present, Ab2 will bind to it; again, anything unbound is washed off. Finally, a substrate for the enzyme is added; if Ab2-E is there, the enzyme breaks down the substrate to yield a colored end product. ELISA plate readers very rapidly determine the optical density (O.D.) of each well. The concentration of Ab1 in the patient's serum is interpolated from a standard curve.

trophotometer. The concentration of the antibody can be determined by including a series of standards along with the test sample. ELISA kits are now commercially available that assist in rapid diagnosis of diseases involving infectious agents such as HIV-1, respiratory syncytial virus, influenza, β-hemolytic *Streptococcus* group A, *Giardia lamblia, Cryptosporidium parvum,* and many others (Kaufman et al., 1995).

 ### Checkpoint! 10–6 (Chapter Objective 6)

What is the basic principle of the classical radioimmunoassay?
  A. *Lysis of radiolabeled erythrocytes*
  B. *Agglutination of radiolabeled leukocytes*
  C. *Fusion of radiolabeled and unlabeled plasmacytes*
  D. *Clumping of radiolabeled antigen–antibody complexes*
  E. *Competition between radiolabeled and unlabeled antigen for a limited amount of antibody*

SUMMARY

The immune system is critical in maintaining a balance between the internal and external environment (Sompayrac, 2003). Antigens recognized as foreign or different from normal self initiate immune responses that involve complex actions and interactions among various organs, cells, and soluble substances. The primary lymphoid organs are the thymus and bone marrow. Cells of the immune system include T and B lymphocytes, monocyte-macrophages, neutrophils, eosinophils, basophils, mast cells, and platelets. Antibodies are globular proteins secreted by activated B lymphocytes that bind specifically to the antigen that induced their production. Complement consists of a family of proteins that interact with antigen–antibody complexes and cell membranes to assist in antigen elimination.

Immunologic defenses against infectious agents consist of both innate and acquired immunity. In some instances one is more important than the other in controlling infection, although there is overlap. The most important defenses against bacteria are the phagocytic abilities of neutrophils and macrophages, antibodies, and complement activation. Phagocytic cells can kill engulfed bacteria through O_2-dependent and -independent mechanisms. Antibodies can neutralize potent toxins such as those that cause diphtheria and tetanus. Antibodies and certain complement breakdown products (C3b) also facilitate phagocytosis by binding to bacteria, a process known as opsonization. When either IgG or IgM form a complex with an antigen on the surface of bacteria, complement activation causes them to lyse.

Immune attack against viruses is induced primarily by proteins that protrude from the virus itself or from the virus-infected cell. Factors important in controlling viral infections are interferon, natural killer (NK) cells, cytotoxic T lymphocytes, and antibodies. Cytotoxic T cells eradicate virus-infected cells by binding to viral peptides presented to them by an antigen-presenting cell (APC) in the groove of a major histocompatibility complex (MHC) class I molecule. In addition, because nearly all cells of the body express class I molecules and are also capable of degrading viral proteins to some extent, a virus-infected cell can act as the APC, as well as the target. Antibody can neutralize viral infectivity, block uncoating, opsonize cells, and mediate antibody-dependent cell-mediated cytotoxicity (ADCC); together with complement, it damages the virus envelope.

In comparison to bacteria and viruses, relatively little is known regarding protective responses against fungi, protozoa, and helminths (worms). T cell deficiency often results in increased susceptibility to fungal infections. Immune defenses against protozoa include antibodies and complement, as well as cell-mediated immune responses. Inflammation, eosinophils, and IgE play dominant roles in the body's defense against many helminths.

The five isotypes of antibody (IgG, IgA, IgM, IgD, and IgE) are based on the structure of their H chains. The binding of antibody to antigen is reversible and involves weak, noncovalent forces (electrostatic or ionic, hydrogen bonding, hydrophobic, and Van der Waals). The term *affinity* refers to the strength of a single bond between the paratope of the antibody and its complementary epitope on the antigen. *Avidity* refers to the overall binding strength between multivalent antibody and multivalent antigen. Each antibody is specific for the epitope that induced its production. However, one antibody can bind to more than one antigen if the antigens have identical or related epitopes (i.e., the antibodies cross-react). MAbs are used extensively in clinical laboratory tests. Large amounts are produced by commercial companies that make hybridomas for this purpose. An important advantage of MAbs over polyclonal antibodies is their high specificity.

Numerous antigen–antibody tests are used to help establish an accurate diagnosis, determine prognosis, and design optimal therapeutic regimens. The titer of an antibody or antigen (i.e., the reciprocal of the highest dilution of antibody or antigen at which there is still a detectable reaction) is an often-reported end result. In precipitation, and to a lesser extent also in agglutination reactions, the proportion of antigen and antibody in relation to each other is important. A false negative may occur if the patient's serum has too much antibody for the amount of antigen present (prozone).

Precipitation reactions in liquids or gels can be used to identify and quantify both antibodies and antigens. Tests based on precipitation include precipitin ring formation, nephelometry, Ouchterlony, and radial immunodiffusion. Electrophoretic separation of proteins, together with a precipitation reaction, is used in immunoelectrophoresis, counterimmunoelectrophoresis, and rocket electrophoresis. In the Western blot test, elec-trophoresis and precipitation are often combined with a second antibody that is conjugated with an enzyme or radionuclide. In some tests (e.g., VDRL and RPR) the precipitate has a flocculent appearance.

Agglutination reactions involve the clumping of cells or particles and are moderately sensitive for identifying either antigens or antibodies. These types of tests are also useful in identifying bacteria, as well as certain parasites isolated from patients. Many soluble antigens can be attached to cells such as RBC or synthetic particles so that specific antibodies can be readily identified and semiquantified. Conversely, antibodies can be attached to a solid matrix and used to identify antigens. In saline, agglutination by IgG may not occur unless serum albumin is added or cells are pretreated with an enzyme.

Tests that include fluorescent dyes, radionuclides, or enzymes have very high sensitivity. Cells (and tissues) labeled with fluorescent dyes such as FITC and TRITC can be analyzed under a fluorescence microscope or by flow cytometry. Use of a flow cytometer greatly increases the accuracy and speed of evaluation compared to manual counting. Radioactive labels have long been used to determine that an antigen–antibody reaction has taken place. The classical RIA is based on competition between nonlabeled and radiolabeled antigen for the same limited amount of antibody. Molecules present in very low concentrations can be quantified in this manner. ELISAs are solid-phase immunoassays in which an enzyme-anti-immunoglobulin complex is used to indicate the presence of specific antibodies. There are also variations of these tests by which an antigen can be identified and its concentration determined. Quantification is done by colorimetric evaluation after addition of a substrate for the enzyme. ELISAs are among the most commonly used tests.

Many variations exist in the specific test procedures discussed in this chapter. Laboratory techniques for detecting antigens and antibodies have become increasingly more sensitive and accurate, especially over the last decade. The range of antigens that can be detected and quantified has also increased dramatically. Advances in computer and other technologies have automated many procedures so that results can often be obtained very rapidly. Collectively, these improvements have significantly enhanced the quality of health care and should continue to do so in the future.

LEARNING OPPORTUNITIES

1. Identify the master cell of the cell-mediated immune system and the soluble substance it secretes. (Chapter Objective 1)

Master Cell	Soluble Substance
a. B cell	Immunoglobulin
b. T cell	Cytokine
c. Neutrophil	Complement
d. NK cell	Interferon

2. Which of the following organs/body sites is the source of the cells that produce antibodies? (Chapter Objective 2)

   a. Thymus

   b. Spleen

   c. Lymph nodes

   d. Bone marrow

3. Antibodies produced after a throat infection with *Streptococcus pyogenes* can react with cardiac tissue of the same individual. This is an example of: (Chapter Objective 3)

   a. a heterophile antibody

   b. a monoclonal antibody

   c. specificity

   d. avidity

4. Flow cytometry is an example of detection of cell antigens by _____ antibodies. (Chapter Objective 4)

   a. polyclonal

   b. heterophile

   c. monoclonal

   d. cross reacting

5. An agglutination test differs from a precipitation test because the former: (Chapter Objectives 5 and 6)

   a. creates cross-linking between antigen and antibody

   b. has an end result that is a visible reaction

   c. depends on the concentration of antigen and antibody

   d. makes use of a carrier particle for the antibody

6. A very tired 18-year-old freshman male college student developed a sore throat and fever during the week of final exams. The symptoms continued to worsen over the next few days. When his throat became so sore and swollen that he could not swallow or eat well, he went to the college infirmary. It was noted that the patient had a fever, a petechial rash on the palate, and swollen cervical lymph nodes (lymphadenopathy). A routine throat culture was done, but revealed only normal flora. A blood test indicated a high white blood cell count with 20% of the lymphocytes having an atypical appearance, suggesting polyclonal stimulation. Blood tests for Epstein-Barr virus (EBV), the cause of infectious mononucleosis, were ordered. A positive result (i.e., agglutination) was obtained in the heterophile antibody test, which mixes the patient's serum with horse red blood cells. The diagnosis of infectious mononucleosis was confirmed using EBV capsid antigen.

   Which antibody was most likely detected in the heterophile antibody agglutination test? (Chapter Objectives 8 and 9)

   a. IgG

   b. IgM

   c. IgA

   d. IgE

7. What role do T cells play in the resolution of this disease? (Chapter Objectives 2 and 9)

    a. Tc cells kill virus infected cells.

    b. Th cells secrete cytokines, which produces more Tc cells.

    c. T cells produce immunoglobulins.

    d. Both a and b

8. A 6-year-old female complains of a sore throat. Her pediatrician notes that her throat is slightly red and collects two throat swabs. She orders a rapid ELISA test for detection of *Streptococcus pyogenes*. In the laboratory, one swab is used to inoculate a sheep blood agar. The second swab was treated with enzymes to extract the group A streptococcal antigen, and then a rapid ELISA test for *Streptococcus pyogenes* was performed. The ELISA test yields a negative result, and the inoculated sheep blood agar is incubated. After 24 hours, very light growth of *Streptococcus pyogenes* is identified from the throat culture.

    How can the difference between the ELISA result and the culture result be explained? (Chapter Objectives 6 and 9)

    a. The child had not had time to produce IgG needed for the ELISA test.

    b. The enzyme extraction destroyed the antigen detected by the ELISA test.

    c. The ELISA reaction is probably a false negative because of a low number of organisms.

    d. The child is possibly immunosuppressed, so the ELISA test will not react properly.

9. This case involves a 26-year-old male who volunteers in an HIV clinic. He was accidently stuck with a used needle. The needle had been used on a patient who is HIV negative but has chronic hepatitis B. At his last physical 1 year ago, he had received the hepatitis B vaccination series of three doses given over a 6-month period. The results are as follows: Hepatitis B surface antigen—negative, Hepatitis B core IgM antibody—negative, Hepatitis B surface IgG antibody—positive.

    The physician interprets the results as: (Chapter Objectives 7, 8, and 9)

    a. susceptible to the Hepatitis B virus, but it is not present at this time

    b. immune to the Hepatitis B virus

    c. infected with the Hepatitis B virus

    d. false positive for the Hepatitis B surface IgG antibody result

REFERENCES

Go to myhealthprofessionskit.com to view this chapter's references.

11

Susceptibility Testing

William C. Payne and Teresa A. Taff

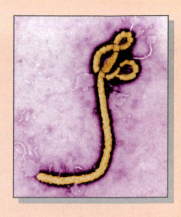

■ LEARNING OBJECTIVES

Upon completion of this chapter, the learner should be able to:

1. Discuss criteria used to select an appropriate antibiotic for therapy.
2. Summarize the major classes of antibiotics.
    a. Describe the origin, mode of action, and spectrum of activity for each.
    b. Provide examples of each class.
    c. Associate adverse effects with each.
    d. Select antibiotics appropriate for treatment of specific organisms.
3. Explain how a bacteriostatic antibiotic eliminates an organism compared to one that is bactericidal.
    a. Categorize antibiotics as either bacteriostatic or bactericidal.
4. Describe the resistance mechanisms found in bacteria.
    a. Differentiate intrinsic and acquired resistance.
        i. Discuss the means of acquisition of resistance mechanisms.
    b. Provide examples of each.
5. Explain the goal of antibiotic susceptibility testing.
6. Determine the role of the Clinical and Laboratory Standards Institute (CLSI) in the clinical microbiology laboratory.
7. Relate the importance of standardization of susceptibility testing.
    a. Identify standardized factors in place.
        i. Predict the outcome if a standardized factor is altered.
8. Compare the methods used for susceptibility testing.
    a. Describe the inoculation, required medium, incubation, reading, and interpretation of each.
    b. Discuss advantages, disadvantages, limitations, and potential sources of errors for each.

9. Define minimum inhibitory concentration (MIC).

 a. Read and interpret the results of an antibiotic susceptibility test.

10. Describe special procedures and methods necessary to detect unique resistance mechanisms.

 a. Correlate each with specific organisms or resistance mechanisms.

 b. Discuss the inoculation, required medium, incubation, reading, and interpretation of each.

 c. Edit susceptibility results as necessary.

11. Compare the minimum bactericidal concentration (MBC) and serum bactericidal tests.

 a. Describe the relationship between the MIC and MBC of an organism.

 b. Discuss the principle and performance of each method.

12. Summarize the process of ensuring the accuracy of susceptibility testing.

13. Relate the necessity for review of susceptibility testing results prior to reporting.

 a. Detect and resolve unusual resistance profiles.

14. Assess the importance of resistance surveillance.

15. Describe the communication of susceptibility results.

16. Verify the necessity for quality control and validation of antibiotic susceptibility testing.

17. Discuss methods available for assay of antimicrobial agents.

KEY TERMS

analogue

antibiogram

antibiotic

bactericidal

bacteriostatic

beta-lactamase

competitive antagonist

heteroresistance

minimum bactericidal concentration (MBC)

minimum inhibitory concentration (MIC)

mode of action

peak concentration

penicillinase

pharmacokinetics

plasmids

porin

selective toxicity

spectrum of activity

synergy

trough concentration

▶ INTRODUCTION

Clinical microbiologists play a pivotal role in prevention, control, and surveillance of infections. The scope of practice for this profession includes all aspects involved in the diagnosis and investigation of bacterial, viral, fungal, and parasitic infections.

The first step in investigating the cause of infectious diseases is isolating microorganisms from clinical specimens such as blood, other body fluids, and tissues. Once a microorganism is isolated, it must then be identified. Pathogenic organisms, which are responsible for much of the sickness and death suffered by humans, must be differentiated from commensal organisms, which may colonize the same areas of the body without harming the host. In severe infections some type of therapeutic agent will likely be prescribed to assist the immune system in eradicating any microbes that are determined to be the cause of a patient's illness. Because of the relatively recent emergence of multi-drug-resistant strains of microbes, several different antimicrobial agents may have to be tested to evaluate their effectiveness in treating an infectious disease. In this chapter, the different classes of antimicrobial agents and the manner in which these agents affect microbes is explored. In addition, the **spectrum of activity** or the range of susceptible organisms for each class is discussed. An antibiotic's range can be very narrow and organism specific or broad and extensive. The chapter also reviews mechanisms of resistance and includes a discussion of the methods used to determine the susceptibility of a microbe to a particular antimicrobial agent. Go to the Companion Website to review a brief history of antimicrobial therapy.

An **antibiotic** (Greek; *anti,* against + *biosis,* life) is a substance, produced by fungi or bacteria, that inhibits the growth of other microorganisms. Such substances are of value to microorganisms that compete for space and nutrients in an ecological niche containing a wide variety of microbes. Soil is an excellent example of this type of diversity because as many as one billion microbes encompassing some ten thousand different species may be recovered from a small sample of earth. As a matter of fact, many of the antibiotics that have been discovered are naturally occurring or chemically altered metabolic by-products produced by soil organisms.

 ## Checkpoint! 11–1 (Chapter Objective 2)

Antibiotics are substances produced by _____ and _____, which inhibit the growth of other microorganisms.
   A. *Ben and Jerry*
   B. *bacteria and fungi*
   C. *fungi and viruses*
   D. *viruses and parasites*

▶ THE IDEAL ANTIBIOTIC

Whether or not a newly discovered or developed antimicrobial agent will be useful depends on a number of factors. If the ideal antibiotic were discovered or designed, it would possess the following properties:

- The compound exhibits **selective toxicity.** That is to say it exerts detrimental or lethal effects on the etiologic agent of disease without inducing adverse affects on the host. Compounds have been discovered that interfere with essential metabolic pathways used by certain infectious organisms. They do not, however, interfere with the metabolism of host cells, which therefore remain unaffected. Provided these compounds kill or inhibit the growth of the offending organism without causing undue harm to the host, they can be said to exhibit selective toxicity.

- The compound is useful in treating diseases caused by a number of different types of microbes not only gram-positive and gram-negative bacteria, but mycobacterial species, fungal species, parasites, and viruses, as well. In other words, a wide range of microorganisms are included in the spectrum of activity. In reality, microbes differ greatly physiologically, so this attribute is not easy to achieve.

- The host does not develop hypersensitivity or allergic reactions to the compound. Almost any foreign matter that is ingested, inhaled, or injected into the body has the potential to elicit an immune response. Anaphylaxis, a hypersensitivity reaction, is potentially lethal if the reaction is sufficiently severe and medical attention is not readily available. The ideal antibiotic is devoid of allergenic properties so symptoms such as allergic skin rashes, gastrointestinal upset, and symptoms associated with anaphylaxis, such as vasodilation, bronchoconstriction, and edema, are not experienced.

- Organisms do not develop resistance to the antimicrobial agent. Mutation and selective pressures within health care facilities do not lead to the emergence of infectious agents that are unaffected by administration of the compound. Mechanisms of resistance, including the production of drug-inactivating enzymes, alteration of drug targets, and alterations in the mechanism of drug uptake, do not occur.

- There are no problems with toxicity at serum or plasma drug concentrations necessary to eliminate microorganisms from the blood and tissues. In other words, if high serum concentrations of the antimicrobial agent are needed to eradicate the microbe, there are no adverse effects on host cells.

- The antimicrobial agent is water soluble, so it is readily absorbed into the blood. In addition, none of the various substances found in plasma or the gastrointestinal system inactivate the drug.

- The compound is not readily secreted by the kidneys nor metabolized by the liver, allowing sufficient plasma levels to be maintained. It is not necessary to administer the drug numerous times or at frequent intervals. The patient remains compliant and takes the entire dosage prescribed.

- The therapeutic agent penetrates well into tissues and even crosses the blood–brain barrier. This makes treatment of abscesses and central nervous system infections more effective.

- The cost is minimal, so the patient can afford it financially.

Unfortunately, the ideal antimicrobial agent has yet to be discovered or developed. Clinicians must deal with the same type of criteria, such as toxicity, the emergence of resistant strains, allergic reactions, maintenance levels, and other factors, when prescribing antimicrobial agents for the treatment of infection.

▶ THE NEED FOR ANTIMICROBIAL SUSCEPTIBILITY TESTING

Although some organisms exhibit predictable susceptibility patterns to antimicrobial agents, it is impossible to predict, with any certainty, the effectiveness of a drug in treating infections caused by different microbes. Some species are capable of developing resistance to commonly used therapeutic agents. This makes it necessary to conduct susceptibility tests, the results of which must be communicated to the clinician. The following sections of this chapter deal with the most commonly used antimicrobial agents, their spectrum of activity, side effects, **mode of action** or how they affect organisms, mechanisms of resistance, and methods used in susceptibility testing.

▶ A REVIEW OF THE BACTERIAL CELL WALL

Antibiotics can attack several different structures on a bacterium. A review of the cell walls of gram-positive and gram-negative organisms is necessary to understand their modes of action.

Gram-positive cell wall synthesis occurs in three phases. The first step involves the production of *N*-acetyl glucosamine (NAG) and *N*-acetyl muramic acid (NAM), the subunits of an essential cell wall component called peptidoglycan. Next, these carbohydrate subunits are linked together to form long chains. In the last stage, these long peptidoglycan chains are cross-linked by peptide units or short chains of amino acids by transpeptidase enzymes. This forms a lattice that holds the thick gram-positive cell wall together. Figure 11-1 ■ demonstrates a cross section of gram-positive cell wall.

The gram-negative cell wall is actually made up of two thin layers with a periplasmic space separating the two. The outer lipopolysaccharide membrane has channels or **porins**, which allow small molecules, such as sugars, amino acids, and antibiotics, to enter and exit the cell. The periplasmic space can contain enzymes that degrade antibiotics before they are able to attack the inner peptidoglycan layer. Figure 11-2 ■ identifies the structures present in the gram-negative cell wall.

▶ COMMONLY USED ANTIMICROBIAL AGENTS

ANTIBACTERIAL COMPOUNDS

The ability of an antibacterial agent to render bacteria harmless can occur through a variety of mechanisms. The drug may interfere with the ability of a bacterium to manufacture cellular

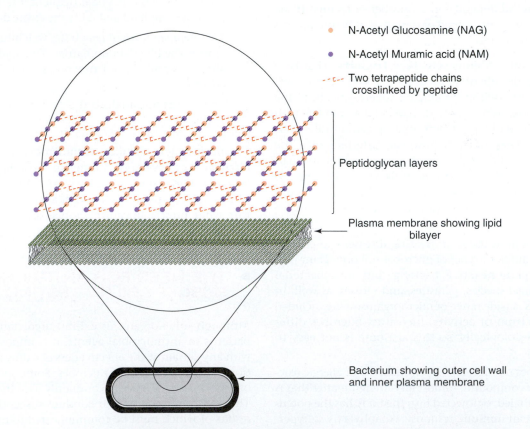

■ **FIGURE 11-1** Gram-positive cell wall. The cell wall of a gram-positive bacterium is made up of cross-linked peptidoglycan chains. Antibiotics can disrupt the gram-positive cell wall at different points in its synthesis.
From http://en.wikipedia.org/wiki/File:Gram-positive_cellwall-schematic.png. Credit: Twooars.

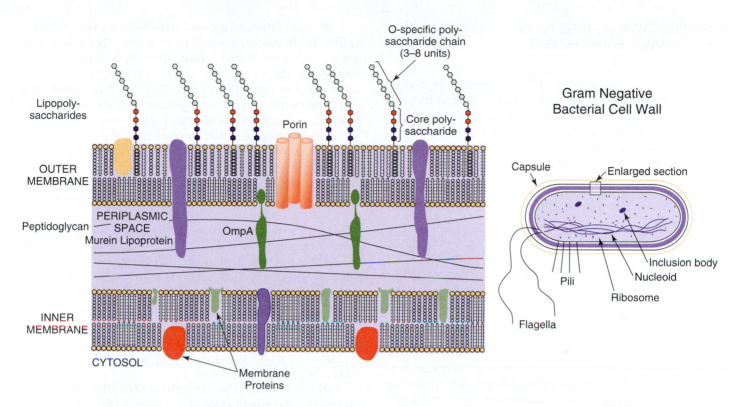

O-specific poly-saccharide chain (3–8 units)

Gram Negative
Bacterial Cell Wall

Lipopoly-saccharides

Porin

Core poly-saccharide

OUTER MEMBRANE

Capsule

Enlarged section

PERIPLASMIC SPACE

Peptidoglycan

Murein Lipoprotein

OmpA

Inclusion body

Pili

Nucleoid

Ribosome

INNER MEMBRANE

Flagella

CYTOSOL

Membrane Proteins

■ **FIGURE 11-2** Gram-negative cell wall. The gram-negative cell wall is thinner than that of the gram-positive. Most antibiotics used in the treatment of gram-negative organisms enter through the porin channels in the outer membrane.
From http://en.wikipedia.org/wiki/File:Gram_negative_cell_wall.svg. *: From Jeff Dahl.*

components essential for its survival, therefore having their greatest effect on bacteria undergoing cell division. For example, one or more steps in the synthesis of the cell wall may be inhibited or the agent may interfere with protein synthesis by attaching to portions of the ribosome. An antibiotic may also affect permeability of the cell membrane leading to leakage of cellular contents and death to the bacterium. Other drugs may interfere with nucleic acid replication or synthesis. One mode of action can be to prevent separation of the complementary DNA strands. These compounds may be structurally similar to nucleic acid subunits, so they are incorporated into newly formed strands. This renders the new strands ineffective in carrying a meaningful code. Some therapeutic agents act as an **analogue** or substitute for compounds vital to metabolic processes of the cell, such as precursor substances, and so interfere with certain metabolic pathways necessary for the cell to survive.

Antimicrobial agents may be **bacteriostatic** or **bactericidal.** Agents that have an inhibitory effect on bacterial growth but do not necessarily kill the organism are called bacteriostatic. Because metabolically inactive organisms may survive, cellular and humoral host defenses must also be relied on to eradicate the invading microorganism. Bactericidal agents are able to exert lethal effects on microorganisms. In the fol-

lowing section, antibiotics are discussed according to their mode of action.

 REAL WORLD TIP

Physicians often use brand names, such as Bactrim or Septra, when requesting antibiotic susceptibility results. Microbiologists usually identify antibiotics by the generic name, such as trimethoprim-sulfamethoxazole. To provide excellent customer service, one option is to create a chart in the microbiology laboratory that cross-references the brand names of antibiotics with their generic name.

 Checkpoint! 11–2 (Chapter Objective 3)

An antibiotic that has a lethal effect on a microorganism is known as:

    A. *an analogue.*

    B. *a porin.*

    C. *bacteriostatic.*

    D. *bactericidal.*

ANTIBIOTICS AFFECTING CELL WALL SYNTHESIS

β-Lactams

The β-lactams are among the oldest antibiotics in use. All members of this class contain a beta-lactam ring in its structure. Figure 11-3 ■ demonstrates the beta-lactam ring common to this group of antibiotics. They are considered bactericidal because they inhibit cell wall synthesis. Most microorganisms cannot exist without a cell wall. Table 11-1✪ summarizes the antibiotics affecting cell wall synthesis by their spectrum of activity and specific mode of action.

Penicillins

Chemical Properties.   The basic structure of penicillin is a thiazolidine ring, a beta-lactam ring or penem, and a side chain. The beta-lactam ring is the square in the center of the molecule seen in Figure 11-3. The form of penicillin that was first used was actually a mixture of structurally related compounds of which penicillin G (benzylpenicillin) was the most effective. Unfortunately, penicillin G is acid labile, and the highly acidic environment of the stomach makes it necessary to administer the drug by deep intramuscular injection. Luckily, another form of penicillin, penicillin V (phenoxymethylpenicillin), has increased resistance to gastric acid inactivation and can be administered orally. They are called the natural penicillins because they were among the first antibiotics found in nature.

Penicillin is known for hypersensitivity as its major side effect. Allergic reactions can range from a mild rash to hives to anaphylaxis.

Spectrum of Activity.   Penicillin is effective against staphylococcal strains, which are unable to produce an enzyme that can destroy it, but these strains are few and far between now. It tends to have a very narrow spectrum of activity but is still useful in the treatment of gram-positive organisms other than *Staphylococcus* spp. The alpha and beta hemolytic streptococci, other than penicillin resistant *S. pneumoniae*, have remained relatively susceptible. It is also effective against some gram-negative organisms such as *Neisseria meningitidis*, *Pasteurella multocida*, and *Eikenella corrodens*, as well as some anaerobes such as *Fusobacterium* spp., *Prevotella* spp., *Actinomyces* spp., and *Peptostreptococcus* spp. It is still useful in the treatment of spirochete infections such as syphilis and pharyngitis caused by *Streptococcus pyogenes*.

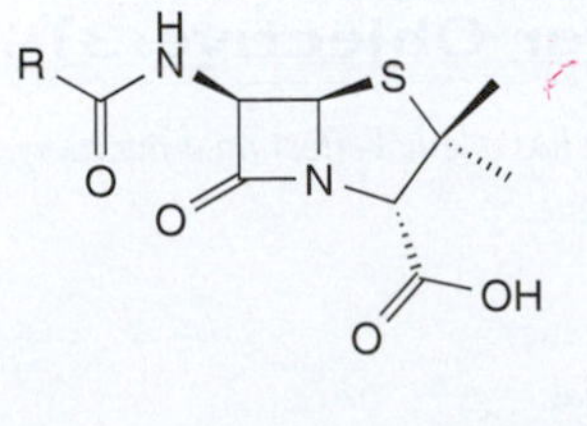

■ **FIGURE 11-3** Basic chemical structure of penicillins. The center square is the beta-lactam ring.

In the early days of its use, penicillin was very effective against *Staphylococcus aureus,* but now strains are able to produce an enzyme called **penicillinase**, a type of **beta-lactamase.** This substance is capable of destroying the antibacterial effect of penicillin by breaking the beta-lactam ring present in its structure. Other organisms have also acquired the ability to produce beta-lactamase. These include some strains of *Neisseria gonorrhoeae, Enterococcus* spp., *Haemophilus* spp., *Moraxella catarrhalis, Bacteroides* spp., and *Prevotella* spp., as well as some members of the *Enterobacteriaceae.*

When this phenomenon was discovered, drug companies began investigating ways to render the penicillin molecule resistant to the action of penicillinase enzyme. Chemical changes were made in the side chain structure, which, by adding bulk to the molecule, rendered beta-lactamase ineffective. As a result, the semisynthetic penicillins were created. These penicillinase-resistant penicillins, such as methicillin, nafcillin, oxacillin, and dicloxacillin, were subsequently introduced to the market. They possess bulky side chains that prevent the beta-lactamase of *Staphylococcus* spp. but not necessarily those of gram-negative rods, from attacking their beta-lactam ring. They are used primarily for treatment of *Streptococcus* spp. and methicillin-susceptible *Staphylococcus* spp.

It should be noted that the natural pencillins lack activity against the majority of gram-negative rods. Once again chemical changes were made to the basic penicillin molecule to increase their spectrum of activity, and more semisynthetic penicillins were created. The addition of an alpha-amino group into the benzyl chain led to the creation of the aminopenicillins, which include ampicillin and amoxicillin. They have an extended spectrum of activity against some gram-negative rods such as non-beta-lactamase-producing *Haemophilus* spp. and *Enterobacteriaceae* such as *E. coli, Salmonella* spp., and *Shigella* spp. They are also effective against *Enterococcus* spp., other gram-positive organisms, and *Neisseria meningitidis*.

The introduction of an alpha-carboxyl group into the benzyl chain created the carboxypenicillins such as ticarcillin and carbenicillin. This group of antibiotics has a spectrum of activity similar to the natural penicillins and aminopenicillins. They also exhibit an extended spectrum of activity and are effective against even more gram-negative rods, including the *Enterobacteriaceae* and *Pseudomonas* spp.

The addition of ureido or piperazine rings created ureidopenicillins, which include mezlocillin and piperacillin. This group exhibits a spectrum of activity similar to that of the carboxycillins with extended activity against *Pseudomonas* spp. and most of the *Enterobacteriaceae* as well as anaerobes.

Mode of Action.   Penicillins are able to inhibit the activity of bacterial enzymes essential for peptidoglycan synthesis. These enzymes are often referred to as penicillin-binding proteins (PBPs). Inhibition of cell wall synthesis leads to activation of membrane-associated autolytic enzymes, which destroy the cell wall and ultimately result in cell death.

REAL WORLD TIP

Neisseria spp. and *Moraxella catarrhalis* may be difficult to differentiate from other *Moraxella* spp. A penicillin disk can be used to differentiate the two groups. A lawn of organism is created on a blood agar plate. A 10-unit penicillin disk is placed in the center, and the medium is incubated overnight at 35°C to 37°C in CO_2. The next day, a Gram stain is prepared from the edge of the zone of inhibition. *Neisseria* spp. and *M. catarrhalis* will retain their gram-negative diplococci morphology, whereas other *Moraxella* spp. display as long gram-negative threads.

✓ Checkpoint! 11–3 (Chapter Objective 2)

What structure within the penicillin molecule is destroyed by beta-lactamase?

- A. *Penem*
- B. *Side chain*
- C. *Thiazolidine ring*
- D. *Ureido or piperazine rings*

✪ TABLE 11-1

A Summary of the Antibiotics Affecting Cell Wall Synthesis

Antibiotic	Spectrum of Activity	Mode of Action

Natural penicillins
■ Penicillin V
■ Penicillin G
	■ Gram-positive organisms other than *Staphylococcus* spp.
	■ Some gram-negative organisms
	  ■ *Neisseria meningitidis*
	  ■ *Pasteurella multocida*
	  ■ *Eikenella corrodens*
	■ Non-beta-lactamase-producing anaerobes
	■ *Treponema pallidum*
		Inhibits activity of bacterial enzymes essential for peptidoglycan synthesis (penicillin-binding proteins)

Penicillinase-resistant penicillins ■ Methicillin ■ Nafcillin ■ Oxacillin ■ Cloxacillin ■ Dicloxacillin	■ *Streptococcus* spp. ■ Methicillin-sensitive *Staphylococcus* spp.	Same as the natural penicillins
Aminopenicillins ■ Ampicillin ■ Amoxicillin	■ Non-beta-lactamase-producing *Haemophilus influenzae* ■ *Enterobacteriaceae* ■ Gram-positive organisms such as *Enterococcus* spp. ■ *Neisseria meningitidis*	Same as the natural penicillins but can penetrate the outer membrane of some gram-negative organisms
Carboxycillins ■ Ticarcillin ■ Carbenicillin	■ Activity similar to natural penicillins and aminopenicillins ■ *Pseudomonas* spp. ■ Most *Enterobacteriaceae* ■ Anaerobes	Same as the natural penicillins but can penetrate the outer membrane of some gram-negative organisms and has a higher affinity for penicillin-binding proteins
Ureidopenicillins ■ Mezlocillin ■ Piperacillin	■ Activity similar to the carboxycillins	Same as the natural penicillins

Beta-lactam + Beta-lactamase inhibitor
■ β-lactamase inhibitors
  ■ Clavulanic acid
  ■ Sulbactam
  ■ Tazobactam
	■ Beta-lactamase producing *Staphylococcus* spp.
	■ Beta-lactamase producing gram-negative rods
		Same as the natural penicillins once the beta-lactamase inhibitor neutralizes the effect of beta-lactamase

(continued)

⊛ TABLE 11-1

A Summary of the Antibiotics Affecting Cell Wall Synthesis (*continued*)

Antibiotic	Spectrum of Activity	Mode of Action

Cephalosporin generation
■ 1st
  ■ Cefazolin
  ■ Cephalexin
■ 2nd
  ■ Cefuroxime
  ■ Cefaclor
  ■ Cefoxitin (a cephamycin)
■ 3rd
  ■ Ceftazidime
  ■ Cefixime
  ■ Ceftriaxone
■ 4th
  ■ Cefepime
■ 5th
  ■ Ceftobiprole
	1st generation
	■ Some gram-positive such as beta-lactamase-producing *Staphylococcus aureus*
	■ Some gram-negative bacteria such as *E. coli*
	2nd generation
	■ Greater activity against gram-negative rods
	■ Greater activity against anaerobes such as *Bacteroides fragilis*
	3rd generation
	■ Greater activity against gram-negative bacteria, including *Pseudomonas aeruginosa*
	■ Increased resistance to beta-lactamase enzymes
	■ Treatment of meningitis caused by *Neisseria meningitidis, Haemophilus influenzae,* and *Streptococcus pneumoniae*
	4th generation
	■ Gram-negative rods that are resistant to 3rd-generation cephalosporins
	5th generation
	■ *Pseudomonas aeruginosa*
	■ Methicillin-resistant *Staphylococcus aureus* (MRSA)
	■ Penicillin-resistant *Streptococcus pneumoniae*
		Same as the natural penicillins

Carbapenems ■ Imipenem ■ Meropenem ■ Doripenem ■ Ertapenem	■ Gram-positive organisms ■ Gram-negative organisms, including *Pseudomonas aeruginosa* ■ Anaerobes	Same as the natural penicillins
Monobactams ■ Aztreonam	■ *Pseudomonas aeruginosa* and other gram-negative rods	Same as the natural penicillins
Glycopeptides ■ Vancomycin Lipoglycopeptide ■ Teicoplanin ■ Daptomycin	Glycopeptides ■ Methicillin-resistant *Staphylococcus aureus* ■ Other gram-positive bacteria Teicoplanin ■ MRSA ■ *Enterococcus faecalis* ■ Penicillin-resistant *Streptococcus pneumoniae* Daptomycin ■ MRSA ■ Vancomycin-resistant *Enterococcus* spp. ■ Vancomycin-intermediate and -resistant *Staphylococcus aureus*	Vancomycin forms a complex with the terminal end of the peptides, which cross-link the peptidoglycan chains. Daptomycin acts on the cytoplasmic membrane to cause the loss of essential ions such as potassium.

β-Lactam/β-Lactamase Inhibitors.   Some beta-lactams can be administered in conjunction with a beta-lactamase inhibitor. This combination restores activity to the beta-lactam in some beta-lactamase-producing organisms. The beta-lactamase inhibitor and the beta-lactam are said to act in **synergy.** The combined inhibitory action of the two compounds is greater than either one can produce individually.

One example of a beta-lactamase inhibitor is clavulanic acid, which is an agent originally derived from *Streptomyces clavuligenes.* Other beta-lactamase inhibitors include sulbactam and tazobactam. The beta-lactamase inhibitors themselves have little, if any, antibacterial activity. They bind to the β-lactamase of the *Staphylococcus* spp. and render it ineffective. Some are also able to inactivate those produced by some gram-negative rods.

Ampicillin/sulbactam is used for treatment of beta-lactamase-producing methicillin-susceptible *Staphylococcus aureus, Haemophilus influenzae,* most anaerobes, and some gram-negative rods. Sulbactam, on its own, is effective against *Acinetobacter* spp. Amoxicillin/clavulanic acid is effective against beta-lactamase producing *Haemophilus influenzae,* methicillin-sensitive *Staphylococcus aureus, Moraxella* spp., and penicillin-resistant anaerobes. Piperacillin/tazobactam is used as therapy for infections caused by *Pseudomonas aeruginosa,* the *Enterobacteriaceae, Enterococcus* spp., and anaerobes. Ticarcillin/clavulanic acid has a spectrum of activity similar to piperacillin/tazobactam but is slightly less effective against *Pseudomonas aeruginosa* and *Enterococcus* spp.

Cephalosporins

Chemical Properties.   The cephalosporins are metabolic by-products of a fungus known as *Acremonium.* These compounds are similar in structure to the penicillins in that both possess a beta-lactam ring. However, cephalosporins differ by possessing a dihydrothiazine ring instead of the thiazolidine ring found in the pencillins. Figure 11-4 ■ demonstrates the structure of a cephalosporin. The presence of the beta-lactam ring unfortunately confers the same vulnerability to beta-lactamases as seen with penicillin. The addition of a methyl group to the beta-lactam ring, producing synthetic forms of the cephalosporins, did much to provide resistance to inactivation by these enzymes.

Because of a structure similar to penicillin, those with hypersensitivity to penicillin may also show similar reactions with the cephalosporins. Other side effects include diarrhea, nausea, and inflammation at the site of intravenous infusion.

Spectrum of Activity.   The presence of two side chains, as opposed to the single side chain of the penicillins, provided the opportunity to create first-, second-, third-, and fourth-generation cephalosporins. Each generation has a broader range of activity than the one before it. The first-generation or narrow spectrum cephalosporins, such as cefazolin, are effective against some gram-positive and gram-negative bacteria but still have a comparatively narrow spectrum of activity. They are useful against some strains of *E. coli* and methicillin-susceptible, beta-lactamase-producing *Staphylococcus aureus, Streptococcus pneumoniae,* and *Streptococcus pyogenes,* but not *Enterococcus* spp.

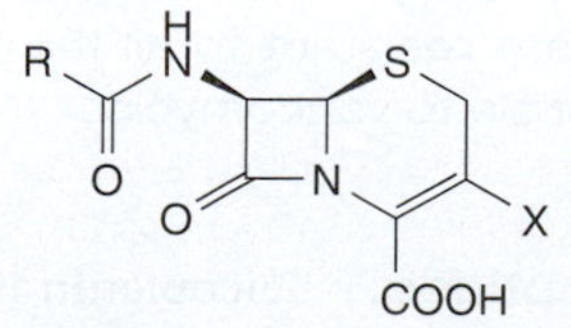

Second-generation or expanded spectrum cephalosporins, such as cefoxitin, have much greater activity against gram-negative rods, *Streptococcus pneumoniae,* methicillin-susceptible *Staphylococcus aureus,* and anaerobes including *Bacteroides fragilis.* Cefoxitin is really a member of the cephamycin group of beta-lactam antibiotics but is usually regarded as a second-generation cephalosporin.

Third-generation or broad spectrum cephalosporins, for example, ceftazidime, cefotaxime, and ceftriaxone, have a better ability to penetrate the lipid-rich outer envelope of gram-negative bacteria such as the *Enterobacteriaceae* and *Pseudomonas aeruginosa* and have greater resistance to beta-lactamases, making them the drugs of choice for beta-lactamase-producing *Neisseria gonorrhoeae.* They are also able to cross the blood–brain barrier to treat meningitis, making them effective against *Neisseria meningitidis* and beta-lactamase-producing *Haemophilus influenzae,* as well as *Streptococcus pneumoniae.* The third-generation cephalosporins can be hydrolyzed by enzymes produced by some *Enterobacteriaceae.* These resistance mechanisms will be discussed later in this chapter.

Cefepime has been described as the first of the fourth-generation or extended spectrum cephalosporins and is active against many gram-negative bacilli that are resistant to cefotaxime and ceftriaxone. It is effective in the treatment of *Bacteroides fragilis, Pseudomonas aeruginosa,* as well as strains of *Klebsiella, Enterobacter, Serratia,* and *Citrobacter* that are resistant to third-generation cephalosporins such as ceftazidime. It is more resistant to beta-lactamases than the third generation. The ability to cross the blood–brain barrier makes it useful in the treatment of meningitis.

There is now an unofficial fifth generation of the cephalosporins consisting of ceftobiprole. It has the advantage of having the spectrum of activity of the third and fourth generations. It is useful against *Pseudomonas aeruginosa,* methicillin-resistant *Staphylococcus aureus,* and penicillin-resistant *Streptococcus pneumoniae.*

Mode of Action.   The cephalosporins inhibit cell wall synthesis by binding to and inactivating penicillin-binding proteins that are responsible for the bactericidal effect of these antibiotics in susceptible bacteria. Ceftobiprole, a fifth-generation cephalosporin, can bind to the unique penicillin-binding protein, PBP2a, produced by MRSA.

Other β-Lactams

Carbapenems.   This bactericidal group of beta-lactams includes imipenem, meropenem, doripenem, and ertapenem. They have the widest spectrum of activity compared to other beta-lactams. They work against both gram-positive and gram-negative organisms. As a group they are resistant to beta-lactamase.

Unfortunately, MRSA and VRE are resistant to the carbapenems. Most of the *Enterobacteriaceae,* which are resistant to other β-lactams because of beta-lactamase production, are

■ **FIGURE 11-4** Basic chemical structure of cephalosporins (R and X represent side rings).

sensitive to the carbapenems. They are also effective against *Pseudomonas aeruginosa* as well as anaerobes. They are usually reserved for intravenous use with severe infections to prevent the development of resistance.

Monobactams.   Aztreonam is the most commonly used antibiotic of this bactericidal group. *Chromobacterium violaceum* was the original source of this antibiotic. It is now produced synthetically. It is resistant to the gram-positive beta-lactamase but susceptible to the extended spectrum beta-lactamases produced by some *Enterobacteriaceae*. It is used primarily for treatment of *Pseudomonas aeruginosa* and other gram-negative rods because of its low activity against gram-positive organisms and anaerobes.

Glycopeptides and Lipoglycopeptides

This group of antibiotics interferes with cell wall synthesis but by a different mechanism than the β-lactams. They are considered bactericidal.

Vancomycin

Chemical Properties.   Vancomycin is a very large molecule that is a complex 1.5 kD tricyclic glycopeptide (Figure 11-5 ■) derived from *Amycolatopsis orientalis* (formerly *Nocardia orientalis*). It is the only glycopeptide marketed for clinical use in the United States. Vancomycin can be administered intramuscularly, intravenously, or orally. Because it is poorly absorbed if given orally, this route would not be effective for treating wound infections. High concentrations can accumulate in the stool, making it an effective treatment for pseudomembranous colitis, a toxigenic disease attributed to *Clostridium difficile*.

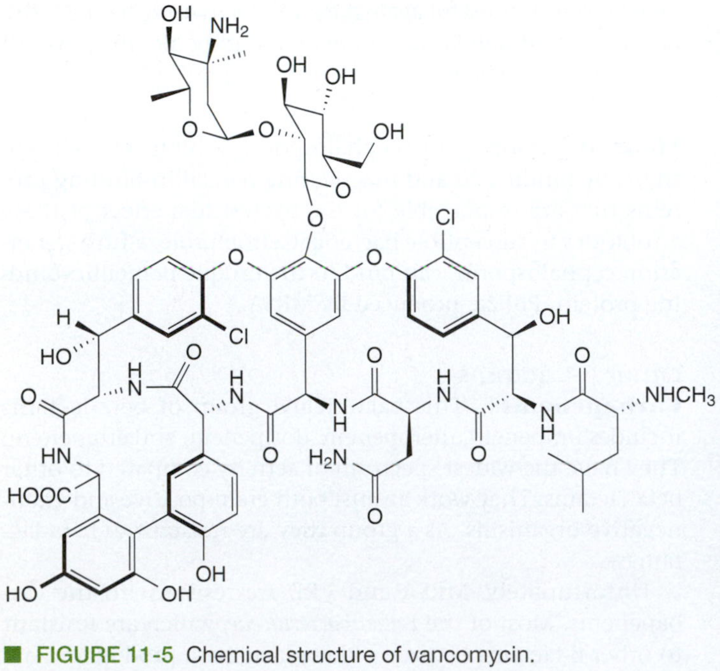

■ **FIGURE 11-5** Chemical structure of vancomycin.

Side effects of therapy with vancomycin include inflammation at the intravenous infusion site, ototoxicity, and nephrotoxicity. Rapid infusion can lead to "red man" syndrome, which produces flushing of the face and chest with hypotension and hives.

Spectrum of Activity.   Vancomycin was introduced as a therapeutic drug more than 40 years ago to treat staphylococcal infections that failed to respond to penicillin but quickly fell into disuse with the development of methicillin to treat penicillin-resistant *Staphylococcus aureus*. It was only a short time before strains of *S. aureus* became resistant not only to penicillin but also to methicillin. Vancomycin has become the drug of choice to treat infections caused by methicillin-resistant *S. aureus* (MRSA) as well as other gram-positive bacteria, including the streptococci, such as penicillin-resistant *S. pneumoniae, Clostridium* spp., *Listeria* spp., *Bacillus* spp., and *Actinomyces* spp. Some strains of *Enterococcus* spp. have now acquired vancomycin resistance because of its increased use.

It has recently been noted that clinical failure rates as high as 45% have been associated with vancomycin when used alone in the treatment of serious MRSA infections such as bacteremia and pneumonia. For this reason, combination therapy, such as vancomycin and rifampin, has been proposed to combat this problem. Most species of gram-negative bacteria are resistant to vancomycin because the large molecule cannot penetrate the outer membrane of these organisms. This means gram-negative organisms have a built-in resistance to it, so its use is automatically ineffective in treating infections caused by these organisms.

Mode of Action.   Vancomycin affects bacterial growth by inhibiting cell wall synthesis. It does this by forming a complex with the terminal end (the D-alanyl-D-alanine amino acyl residues) of the peptide cross-links composed of five amino acids (L-alanine-D-glutamic acid-l-lysine-L-D-alanine-D-alanine). Penicillin inhibits cell wall synthesis by binding to the transpeptidase enzymes (PBP) that produce the peptide cross-links. In contrast, vancomycin binds to the peptide cross-bridge itself and prevents it from binding to the active site of the transpeptidase enzymes and, in this manner, interferes with cross-linking of the peptidoglycan chains.

> ℮ **REAL WORLD TIP**
>
> Because the mode of action of vancomycin is different than that of the β-lactams, organisms such as MRSA, which are resistant to all the β-lactams, are usually susceptible to vancomycin.

Other Glycopeptides.   Teicoplanin is a relatively new lipoglycopeptide that has limited FDA aproval for use in the United States. It is effective against gram-positive organisms such as MRSA, penicillin-resistant *Streptococcus pneumoniae*, and *Enterococcus faecalis.* Daptomycin is a lipoglycopeptide, which is a derivative of a glycopeptide. It is very effective against gram-positive organisms, including MRSA and vancomycin-resistant *Enterococcus* spp. It is currently reserved for treatment of vancomycin-intermediate and -resistant *Staphylococcus aureus* (VISA/VRSA).

ANTIBIOTICS AFFECTING THE CELL MEMBRANE

Polypeptides

This group of antibiotics damages the cytoplasmic membrane of organisms. Table 11-2✪ summarizes the polypeptides based on their spectrum of activity and mode of action.

Bacitracin

Chemical Properties.   Bacitracin is a complex of at least nine cyclic peptide antibiotics consisting of peptide-linked amino acids as seen in Web Figure 11-6 ■. It is a by-product of the bacterial species *Bacillus licheniformis* (a member of *B. subtilis* group).

Spectrum of Activity.   Bacitracin is primarily effective against gram-positive bacteria, including beta-lactamase-producing staphylococci and a few gram-negative bacteria such as gonococcus and meningococcus.

Mode of Action.   Bacitracin has the ability to inhibit synthesis of the cell wall by preventing the addition of peptidoglycan, a major component of the cell walls of gram-positive bacteria. This is a result of interference with the final dephosphorylation step in cycling the phospholipid carrier that transfers peptidoglycan to cell. It also causes damage to the organism's cell membrane.

This antibiotic is used topically to treat open skin infections, such as dermal ulcers, cuts, scrapes, burns, or cases of eczema that have become infected, as well as eye infections. Although it is seldom used internally because of its propensity to cause nephrotoxicity, it can be administered intramuscularly to treat infants with pneumonia and empyema caused by staphylococci.

℮ REAL WORLD TIP

Bacitracin is an antibiotic used primarily as a topical antibiotic and usually sold in concentration of 500 units. It can be used in the laboratory to presumptively differentiate *Streptococcus pyogenes* from other beta-hemolytic streptococcus. *S. pyogenes* is sensitive to low concentrations (0.04 units) of bacitracin, whereas other beta-hemolytic *Streptococcus* spp. are usually resistant.

Polymyxins

Chemical Properties.   The polymyxins are a group of cyclic polypeptide antibiotics originally derived from *Bacillus polymyxa.* These bactericidal compounds contain both lipophilic and lipophobic groups with a smaller peptide ring, peptide chain, and a long chain fatty acid, as seen in Web Figure 11-7 ■. Polymyxin B and E, also known as colistin, are the only ones approved for clinical use because of the significant toxicity of other polymyxins.

Spectrum of Activity.   The polymyxins, particularly polymyxin B, are used to treat infections caused by gram-negative bacteria and have little effect on gram-positive bacteria and anaerobes. *Proteus, Providencia,* and *Neisseria* species are resistant. Polymyxin B has proved especially useful in the treatment of *Pseudomonas aeruginosa* infections. Nephrotoxicity and neuromuscular problems or neurotoxicity are possible consequences of use. Polymyxin B is used primarily to treat ear, eye, skin, and mucous membrane infections where local absorption is poor.

℮ REAL WORLD TIP

Polymyxin E, also known as colistin, is commonly used to determine when the Gram reaction of the isolate is uncertain. By applying filter paper discs impregnated with vancomycin or colistin to an inoculum on a blood agar plate, the Gram reaction may be deduced. Gram-negative organisms are inhibited by colistin, whereas gram-positive organisms are inhibited by vancomycin.

✪ TABLE 11-2

Antibiotics Affecting the Cell Membrane

Antibiotic	Spectrum of Activity	Mode of Action
Bacitracin	■ Gram-positive organisms including beta-lactamase-producing *Staphylococcus* spp. ■ Some gram-negative organisms such as *Neisseria gonorrhoeae* and *N. meningitidis*	Prevents the addition of peptidoglycan to the cell wall and disrupts the cell membrane
Polymyxins B and E (colistin)	■ Gram-negative bacteria, including *Pseudomonas aeruginosa*	Disruption of phospholipid constituents of cell membrane causing the intracellular contents to leak out of cell and leading to death

Mode of Action.   The polymyxins bind to the outer surface of the cell membrane affecting phospholipid of the cell membrane. The cell's integrity is disrupted, which leads to increased cell permeability. In this manner, they act similar to the action of detergents, causing intracellular contents to leak out, killing the cell.

 Checkpoint! 11–4 (Chapter Objective 2)

Which of the following is seldom administered orally because of the potential for systemic toxicity such as nephrotoxicity? The principle use of this antibiotic is as a topical agent to prevent skin, eye, and wound infections.

A. *Bacitracin*
B. *Colistin*
C. *Vancomycin*
D. *Daptomycin*

ANTIBIOTICS AFFECTING PROTEIN SYNTHESIS

Protein Synthesis

Proteins are essential for almost all biological processes. They form important structural components of both eukaryotic and prokaryotic cells and, in the form of enzymes, are responsible for most of the biological activities of cells. According to the central dogma of molecular biology, there is a flow of information through DNA, RNA, and proteins in the form of template-directed synthesis. DNA forms the template on which messenger RNA (mRNA) is synthesized in a process called transcription, and mRNA forms the template through which proteins are synthesized by a process called translation. Translation of the genetic code, carried in mRNA, is brought about through an intermediary molecule, transfer RNA (tRNA). Transfer RNA decodes the base sequence of mRNA and translates that into the amino acid sequence of proteins, which in turn determines their function within the cell.

$$\text{DNA} \xrightarrow{\text{Transcription}} \text{mRNA} \xrightarrow[\text{tRNA}]{\text{Translation}} \text{protein}$$

The complex interaction of mRNA, tRNA, and amino acids does not take place in free solution within the aqueous environment of the cell's cytoplasm but occurs within the confines of an intracellular structure called a ribosome. The ribosome itself is composed of individual RNA molecules of differing lengths (called ribosomal RNA or rRNA) plus varying numbers and types of proteins. Structurally, the rRNA and proteins of ribosomes are assembled into two subunits, a large subunit and a small subunit. The two subunits are designate in terms of Svedberg units, a measure of the rates of sedimentation when they are centrifuged. The length of the rRNA molecules and the number of proteins in each subunit is different in prokaryotic and eukaryotic cells, and as a consequence the sizes of the subunits differ. The ribosomes of prokaryotic cells are composed of a 50S (Svedberg units) and a 30S subunit creating a 70S ribosome, whereas the large subunit of eukaryotic cells is 60S and the small subunit is 40S, creating an 80S ribosome. The differences that exist between the ribosomes of prokaryotic cells, such as bacteria, and the ribosomes of eukaryotic cells, such as mammalian cells, allows antibiotics to exhibit selective toxicity for bacteria. Table 11-3✪ compares the ribosomes of prokaryotes and eukaryotes. Table 11-4✪ summarizes the antibiotics that inhibit protein synthesis.

Aminoglycosides

The aminoglycosides are considered bactericidal. They inhibit the organism's ability to synthesize proteins vital for growth.

Chemical Properties.   The aminoglycosides are a group of structurally related antibiotics that contain two or more

---

✪ TABLE 11-3

Comparison of Prokaryotic and Eukaryotic Ribosomes: (S = Svedberg units)			
Prokaryotic Ribosome (70S)		Eukaryotic Ribosome (80S)	
Large subunit (50S)	Small subunit (30S)	Large subunit (60S)	Small subunit (40S)
1.6×10^6 MW	0.9×10^6 MW	2.8×10^6 MW	1.4×10^6 MW
23S rRNA	16S rRNA	28S rRNA	18S rRNA
(~2900 nucleotides)	(~1540 nucleotides)	(~4800 nucleotides)	(~1900 nucleotides)
5S rRNA		5S rRNA	
(~120 nucleotides)		(~120 nucleotides)	
		5.8S rRNA	
		(~160 nucleotides)	
32 proteins	21 proteins	50 proteins	33 proteins

⊙ TABLE 11-4

Protein Synthesis Inhibitors

Antibiotic	Spectrum of Activity	Mode of Action

Aminoglycosides
▪ Gentamicin
▪ Tobramycin
▪ Amikacin
▪ Spectinomycin
	▪ Gram-negative bacteria
	  ▪ *Pseudomonas aeruginosa*
	  ▪ *Acinetobacter* spp.
	  ▪ *Enterobacteriaceae*
	  ▪ *Yersinia pestis*
	  ▪ *Francisella tularensis*
	▪ Gram-positive bacteria
	  ▪ Methicillin sensitive *Staphylococcus aureus*
	▪ *Mycobacterium* spp.
	▪ *Neisseria gonorrhoeae*
		Binds irreversibly to the 30S ribosomal subunit preventing translation of mRNA

Tetracyclines
Glycylcyclines
▪ Tigecycline
	▪ Gram-positive bacteria
	▪ Gram-negative bacteria
	▪ Intracellular organisms
	  ▪ *Rickettsia* spp.
	  ▪ *Ehrlichia* spp.
	  ▪ *Mycoplasma* spp.
	  ▪ *Chlamydia/Chlamydophila* spp.
	  ▪ *Brucella* spp.
	▪ Spirochetes
	▪ MRSA
	▪ VRE
	▪ *Acinetobacter baumannii*
		Binds irreversibly to the 30S ribosomal subunit preventing attachment of transfer RNA

Macrolides
▪ Erythromycin
▪ Azithromycin
▪ Clarithromycin
	▪ Gram-positive bacteria
	  ▪ *Staphylococcus* spp.
	  ▪ *Streptococcus* spp.
	▪ Gram-negative bacteria
	  ▪ *Moraxella catarrhalis*
	  ▪ *Neisseria* spp.
	  ▪ *Haemophilus* spp.
	  ▪ *Bordetella pertussis*
	▪ Intracellular organisms
	  ▪ *Rickettsia* spp.
	  ▪ *Mycoplasma* spp.
	  ▪ *Chlamydia/Chlamydophila* spp.
	  ▪ *Legionella* spp.
	  ▪ *Bartonella* spp.
	▪ Atypical *Mycobacterium* spp.
		Binds to the 50S ribosomal subunit inhibiting elongation of the polypeptide chain

(continued)

⊘ TABLE 11-4

Protein Synthesis Inhibitors (*continued*)

Antibiotic	Spectrum of Activity	Mode of Action

Chloramphenicol	■ Gram-positive organisms
	  ■ MRSA
	■ Gram-negative organisms
	  ■ *Neisseria meningitidis*
	  ■ *Haemophilus influenzae*
	  ■ *Enterobacteriaceae*
	■ Anaerobic organisms
	■ *Chlamydia* spp.
	■ *Mycoplasma* spp.
	■ *Rickettsia* spp.
		Binds to the 50S ribosomal subunit inhibiting elongation of the polypeptide chain

Clindamycin	■ Methicillin-sensitive *Staphylococcus aureus* ■ Penicillin-sensitive *Streptococcus pneumoniae* ■ Viridans *Streptococcus* ■ Group A *Streptococcus* ■ Anaerobes	Binds to the 50S ribosomal subunit inhibiting elongation of the polypeptide chain
Streptogramins ■ Quinupristin/Dalfopristin	■ Vancomycin-resistant *Enterococcus faecium* ■ Penicillin-resistant *Streptococcus pneumoniae* ■ Vancomycin-intermediate or -resistant *Staphylococcus* spp.	Binds to two different sites on the 50S ribosomal subunit inhibiting elongation of the polypeptide chain
Oxazolidinone ■ Linezolid	■ MRSA ■ Vancomycin-resistant and -sensitive *Enterococcus* spp. ■ Penicillin-sensitive and -resistant *Streptococcus pneumoniae*	Binds to the 50S subunit where it meets the 30S subunit to prevent the formation of the 70S complex
Mupirocin	■ Gram-positive organisms ■ MRSA	Binds to tRNA synthetase to inhibit protein synthesis

amino-sugars linked by glycoside bonds to an aminocyclitol ring nucleus as seen in Web Figure 11-1 ■. In streptomycin the aminocyclitol ring is streptidine and in all others 2-deoxy-streptamine. The polycationic nature of this class of antibiotics makes them very soluble in water and poorly soluble in lipids. Despite the fact that these drugs are water soluble, they are poorly absorbed from the gastrointestinal tract and rapidly excreted by the kidneys. The route of administration is usually intramuscular or intravenous, but side effects include nephrotoxicity and irreversible ototoxicity caused by damage to the cells of the inner and middle ear. Neomycin is particularly toxic, so it is not used systemically. It is commonly used topically for the treatment of skin and mucous membrane infections, burns, and wounds.

Naturally occurring aminoglycosides include:

- The first aminoglycoside, streptomycin, was isolated in 1943 from *Streptomyces griseus*
- Tobramycin, kanamycin, and neomycin were isolated from *Streptomyces fradiae*

- Gentamicin, a fermentation by-product of *Micromonospora purpurea*, is the most widely used antibiotic in this class
- Sisomicin, which was also isolated from a species in the genus *Micromonospora*

The semisynthetic aminoglycosides include:

- Netilmicin, a derivative of sisomicin
- Amikacin, a derivative of kanamycin

ⓔ REAL WORLD TIP

The spelling of the generic name of an aminoglycoside can tell its origin. Those that are derived from *Streptomyces* species end with the suffix "-mycin," whereas those derived from *Micromonospora* species end with the suffix "-micin."

Spectrum of Activity.   The aminoglycosides inhibit both gram-negative and gram-positive bacteria, but they are used primarily to treat infections caused by aerobic gram-negative bacteria. This is because less toxic agents are readily available as effective agents for gram-positive bacteria. Uptake of aminoglycosides into the bacterial cell is through an energy-requiring, carrier-mediated transport system, and for this reason they are much less effective against anaerobic bacteria that have less energy available.

These drugs are commonly used in the treatment of severe infections of the abdomen and urinary tract, bacteremia, endocarditis, and other serious gram-negative bacillary infections. They are bactericidal against a wide range of gram-negative bacilli, including *Pseudomonas* spp., *Acinetobacter* spp., and the *Enterobacteriaceae*. In combination with the beta-lactams or vancomycin, they work synergistically. The beta-lactams act on the cell wall and facilitate penetration of the aminoglycosides into the cell. They often work well against methicillin-sensitive *Staphylococcus aureus*. One aminoglycoside, tobramycin, is the drug of choice for treating *Pseudomonas aeruginosa* infections in cystic fibrosis patients. It can be aerosolized to reach deep into the lungs.

Gentamicin is useful in the treatment of unusual pathogens such as *Brucella* spp., *Yersinia pestis,* and *Francisella tularensis.* Spectinomycin is effective against *Neisseria gonorrhoeae.* Amikacin is usually reserved for gram-negative organisms that are resistant to gentamicin and tobramycin. Certain mycobacterial infections, in particular tuberculosis, usually respond well to the administration of streptomycin.

Mode or Action.   The aminoglycosides attach to the bacterial cell membrane and are drawn into the cell via protein channels called porins. Review Figure 11-2 to observe the location of porins in the cell wall of gram-negative organisms. Most sources of information attribute the bactericidal effect of these drugs to their ability to bind very tightly and irreversibly to structural components of the 30S ribosomal subunit. This binding of the drug to the ribosome prevents attachment of the mRNA, which in turn prevents translation. In addition, aminoglycosides may cause misreading of the genetic code, which results in the formation of nonsense proteins (Forbes, Sahm, & Weissfeld, 2007). In either case, protein synthesis is effectively shut down, a condition leading to cell death. Some researchers have proposed that initially the

bactericidal effect can be attributed to the ability of the polycationic aminoglycoside molecules to create fissures in the outer cell membrane leading to the leakage of cellular contents (Gonzales & Spencer, 1998).

Tetracyclines
The tetracyclines inhibit protein synthesis. They are bacteriostatic and so are used less often because of the bactericidal effect of the beta-lactams.

Chemical Properties.   A group of structurally related compounds referred to as the tetracyclines includes chlortetracycline, oxytetracycline, tetracycline, demeclocycline, methacycline, doxycycline, and minocycline and tigecycline. These antibiotics consist of four fused six-membered rings forming a hydronaphthacene nucleus and various side chains that can be substituted to produce different antibacterial compounds as noted in Web Figure 11-2 ■. These drugs are amphoteric, able to form salts with both strong bases or acids, and are readily absorbed after oral administration. Dairy foods; antacids containing aluminum, calcium, or magnesium; and compounds containing minerals such as iron decrease the absorption of tetracyclines, so administration with an empty stomach is best.

The new glycylcyclines have the core structure of a tetracycline with substitutions that make them effective against a broad range of organisms. They are not affected by resistance mechanisms used by organisms against tetracycline. Tigecycline is the first glycylcycline released for use. It is only available for intravenous administration.

REAL WORLD TIP

Tigecycline has been called the "tiger" of the tetracyclines.

Spectrum of Activity.   The tetracyclines are used to treat a broad spectrum of bacterial infections, but unfortunately plasmid-mediated resistance is common. Alpha and non-hemolytic streptococci, other gram-positive bacteria, gram-negative bacilli, intracellular organisms such as rickettsiae, *Ehrlichia* spp., *Mycoplasma* spp., and *Chlamydia/Chlamydophila* spp. as well as spirochetes are usually susceptible to tetracyclines. Beta-hemolytic streptococci are not usually treated with these drugs because up to 25% are resistant when tested in vitro. Tetracyclines are primarily used to treat urinary tract infections, Rocky Mountain spotted fever, primary atypical pneumonia, *Vibrio* spp. infection, shigellosis, Lyme disease, psittacosis, trachoma, lymphogranuloma venereum, brucellosis, anthrax, and cases of syphilis that are resistant to penicillin. Doxycycline can be used for chemoprophylaxis of malaria caused by chloroquine-resistant *Plasmodium falciparum*. Other protozoal diseases, such as amoebiasis, are known to respond well to the administration of tetracyclines. Aside from the systemic uses for tetracyclines,

REAL WORLD TIP

Most microbiology laboratories employ cascade when reporting the susceptibility testing results of the aminoglycosides. Tobramycin is only reported if gentamicin tests as resistant. In turn, amikacin is reported only if tobramycin is resistant. This controls the use of tobramycin and amikacin to prevent unnecessary resistance from developing. It also helps control costs by promoting the use of gentamicin, which is the least expensive of the three aminoglycosides.

topical ointments and creams containing meclocycline have been used to control acne.

Tigecycline is useful for gram-positive and gram-negative infections, especially those that are caused by multi-drug-resistant organisms. It is effective against MRSA, vancomycin-resistant *Enterococcus* spp., and *Acinetobacter baumannii,* but not *Pseudomonas aeruginosa.*

Administration of tetracyclines and glycylcyclines nearly always alter intestinal flora because of its broad spectrum of activity. Oral administration may cause nausea, vomiting, and diarrhea and may also be associated with the development of pseudomembranous colitis and candidiasis. Tetracyclines should not be given to children less than 12 years of age and pregnant or nursing women because administration has been associated with permanent staining of the teeth and abnormal bone growth.

Mode of Action.   The tetracyclines and glycylcyclines bind reversibly to the 30S subunit of the ribosome. This inhibits attachment of the aminoacyl-tRNA to the acceptor site on the mRNA-ribosome complex, effectively shutting down protein synthesis.

Macrolides

The macrolides are very large molecules that inhibit protein synthesis. As a group, they are considered bacteriostatic.

Chemical Properties.   The macrolides are composed of a macrocyclic lactone (macrolide) ring attached to two sugar structures. They differ in the number of carbons in the macrolide ring, in the chemical substitutions on structures attached to various carbons, and in their amino and neutral sugars. This group of antibiotics is valuable because of their ability to enter and concentrate in phagocytic cells.

Erythromycin is derived from *Streptomyces erythreus.* Oleandomycin, spiramycin, and josamycin are also naturally occurring antibiotics. Azithromycin, clarithromycin, and dirithromycin are semisynthetic compounds. Telithromycin is a derivative of erythromycin, which is part of a new class of antibiotics called the ketolides.

Erythromycin may be administered topically, intramuscularly, intravenously, and orally. Azithromycin (Web Figure 11-3) may be administered orally and intravenously, whereas clarithromycin and dirithromycin are only administered orally. Macrolides are absorbed well by the gastrointestinal tract and diffuse readily through most body tissues but do not cross the blood–brain barrier because of their size. Erythromycin is inactivated rapidly by the acid environment of the stomach, but the newer macrolides are resistant to acid inactivation. These drugs are concentrated by the liver and excreted in urine and bile unchanged.

Historically, the macrolides are relatively safe antibiotics. They may promote pseudomembranous colitis because of the overgrowth of toxin producing *Clostridium difficile.* Most complaints are related to the gastrointestinal tract. Side effects may include an upset stomach.

Spectrum of Activity.   The macrolides have proven to be effective in treating infections brought on by gram-positive cocci such as streptococci and staphylococci, some gram-negative bacteria such as *Neisseria* spp. and *Haemophilus* spp., spirochetes, *Mycoplasma* spp., *Chlamydia/Chlamydophilia* spp., and rickettsiae. They have the ability to penetrate white blood cells and so are effective against intracellular pathogens such as *Legionella* spp. and *Rochalimaea* spp, previously known as *Bartonella* spp.

Historically, erythromycin has been important in combating pediatric infections such as bronchitis and atypical pneumonias, but its limited gram-negative spectrum has hampered its use to treat ear infections. Newer macrolides have enabled clinicians to treat otitis media and sinusitis more effectively.

Azithromycin appears to have greater activity against gram-negative organisms, but especially *Moraxella catarrhalis* and *Haemophilus influenzae.* It is less effective against gram-positive organisms than erythromycin. Clarithromycin works better against gram-positive organisms than erythromycin. Telithromycin show improved activity against gram-positive organisms, especially those that are erythromycin resistant.

These antibiotics are considered to be the drugs of choice for treating *Bordetella pertussis, Mycoplasma pneumoniae,* and *Legionella* spp. They are also used in the treatment of anaerobic infections, sexually transmitted diseases such as gonorrhea and syphilis resistant to penicillin, soft chancre, and the etiologic agents of nongonococcal urethritis. These agents have been shown to exhibit activity against atypical mycobacterium such as *Mycobacterium scrofulaceum, M. avium-intracellulare complex, M. kansasii,* and *M. chelonei.*

Mode of Action.   Macrolides bind to the 50S ribosomal subunit and inhibit the transfer of the growing peptide chain from the peptidyl or donor site to the amino acid at the aminoacyl or acceptor site of the ribosome. Transpeptidation and consequently the process of protein synthesis is shut down.

✓ **Checkpoint! 11–5 (Chapter Objective 2)**

Which class of bacteriostatic antibiotics is often used to treat intracellular infections because it can penetrate and concentrate in phagocytic cells?

A. *Glycopeptides*
B. *Macrolides*
C. *Aminoglycosides*
D. *Glycylcyclines*

Chloramphenicol

Chloramphenicol is a bacteriostatic antibiotic that is no longer used routinely in the United States. It has been replaced by more effective and safer antibiotics such as the beta-lactams.

Chemical Properties.

Chloramphenicol, which is presently produced by chemical synthesis, was originally isolated from *Streptomyces venezuelae*. This lipid soluble compound is slightly soluble in water and contains a nitrobenzene ring, as noted in Web Figure 11-4 ■. It can be administered topically to treat eye, ear, and skin infections; orally; or intravenously, but because of poor absorption it is not administered intramuscularly. Chloramphenicol is rapidly and completely absorbed by the gastrointestinal tract and diffuses well into tissues and body fluids. It readily crosses the blood–brain barrier and the placenta.

Serious side effects, principally bone marrow depression leading to anemia, leukocytopenia, and thrombocytopenia have been observed following the use of this antibiotic. A rare, fatal complication, aplastic anemia, is another hazard associated with its administration. Careful monitoring of the peripheral blood may be appropriate. The antibiotic is metabolized in the liver, so those with poor liver function can reach toxic levels. Recent studies have shown that a chloramphenicol metabolite produced by bacteria in the intestinal tract, dehydrochloramphenicol, may be responsible for DNA damage and carcinogenicity associated with the development of leukemia or lymphoma.

Spectrum of Activity.

Chloramphenicol is active against gram-positive and gram-negative bacteria, anaerobic bacteria, *Chlamydia/Chlamydophila*, *Mycoplasma*, *Ehrlichia*, and *Rickettsia* spp. *Neisseria meningitidis*, *Haemophilus influenzae*, and most of the species in the family *Enterobacteriaceae* are susceptible to this drug. It is effective against MRSA but not *Pseudomonas aeruginosa*. It has been used to treat typhoid fever and other serious *Salmonella* infections, meningitis caused by strains of *Haemophilus influenzae* resistant to ampicillin, meningococcus infection, serious *Bacteroides fragilis* infections, and rickettsial infections resistant to tetracycline. More recently, in the United States and Europe, the use of chloramphenicol has largely been replaced by the use of third-generation cephalosporins and quinolones that do not have the same tendency for toxicity of the bone marrow.

Mode of Action.

With the exception of streptococci, where it is bactericidal, chloramphenicol is a bacteriostatic antibacterial agent capable of inhibiting protein synthesis. Because of its lipid solubility, it is thought that this compound diffuses into the cell through the cell membrane where it binds reversibly to the peptidyltransferase component of the 50S ribosomal subunit. Because the drug prevents peptide bond formation and therefore the process of chain elongation, the synthesis of new proteins is effectively stopped. Chloramphenicol and erythromycin compete for the same ribosomal subunit, and therefore, the two medications could conceivably have an antagonistic effect on each other if given concurrently. Because both antibiotics compete for the same target site, the combination of the two would not be as effective as if taken individually.

Other Protein Synthesis Inhibitors

Clindamycin.

Clindamycin is usually a bacteriostatic antibiotic that belongs to the lincosamides class. It differs from the macrolides based on its structure. It can be bactericidal in some situations. It binds to the 50S ribosome and inhibits protein synthesis in the same manner as the macrolides and chloramphenicol. It may compete with these antibiotics if given together. It is useful for methicillin-sensitive *Staphylococcus aureus*, penicillin-sensitive *Streptococcus pneumoniae*, viridians *Streptococcus*, group A *Streptococcus*, *Actinomyces* spp., and anaerobes. The use of this antibiotic can lead to pseudomembranous colitis. It can cause a shift in the normal gastrointestinal flora, allowing *C. difficile*, which is resistant to the antibiotic, to grow and produce toxin.

 REAL WORLD TIP

Clindamycin is effective in the treatment of infections caused by community-acquired methicillin resistant *Staphylococcus aureus*, provided the patient has not had previous erythromycin therapy. If the isolate tests as erythromycin resistant and clindamycin sensitive, further testing is needed because erythromycin can induce resistance in clindamycin. The "D" test is used to detect inducible clindamycin resistance and discussed later in this chapter in the "Special Methods and Procedures" section.

Streptogramins.

The streptogramins are actually a combination of antibiotics such as quinupristin and dalfopristin. The two antibiotics are bacteriostatic and work synergistically to bind to different sites on the 50S ribosome and inhibit protein synthesis. They are known for their effectiveness against vancomycin-resistant *Enterococcus faecium* but not vancomycin-resistant *E. faecalis*. *E. faecalis*, the more common of the two species, is intrinsically resistant due to its ability to pump out the antibiotic. They are also effective against penicillin-resistant *Streptococcus pneumoniae* and vancomycin-intermediate or -resistant *Staphylococcus* spp. Side effects of this intravenous antibiotic combination include irritation at the infusion site and joint and muscle pain.

Oxazolidinone.

Linezolid is the first bacteriostatic antibiotic in this group. It inhibits protein synthesis by a unique mechanism by preventing the 30S and 50S ribosome subunits from connecting to form the 70S complex. It does not appear to be affected by resistance mechanisms that affect other antibiotics that inhibit protein synthesis. It is effective against gram-positive organisms such as MRSA and vancomycin-resistant and -sensitive *Enterococcus* spp. It is bactericidal against penicillin-resistant and -sensitive *Streptococcus pneumoniae*. Unfortunately, resistance has now been reported. It has been used for treatment of mycobacterial infections.

Mupirocin.   This topical antibiotic can be bacteriostatic or bactericidal, depending on the concentration used for treatment. It appears to inhibit protein synthesis by binding to tRNA synthetase. This unique target does not appear to allow for cross-resistance. It is an effective antibiotic against gram-positive cocci, especially MRSA. It is used to eliminate colonization of the nose by *Staphylococcus aureus*. It can also be used to treat superficial skin infections caused by *Staphylococcus* and *Streptococcus* spp.

ANTIBIOTICS AFFECTING NUCLEIC ACID SYNTHESIS

DNA Replication

Before a cell can undergo mitosis, it must first duplicate its genetic material. In this process, called DNA replication, the original (parent) DNA strand acts as a template for the synthesis of a complementary (daughter) strand. The first step in DNA synthesis is unwinding or denaturation of the double-helix structure so replication may be carried out on each strand simultaneously and bidirectionally. A variety of enzymes are required for the replication process.

- Helicase enzymes are responsible for unwinding the DNA helix. Unwinding the DNA helix increases coiling ahead of the replication fork, a condition called supercoiling.

- Topoisomerases are enzymes that cut one or both of the DNA strands to relieve the increased tension of unwinding the DNA helix and subsequently reseal the cut ends.

- DNA gyrase is a topoisomerase enzyme that cuts DNA strands, allowing uncoiling to occur, and then reseals and recoils the strands.

- DNA polymerases are enzymes that replicate complementary strands of DNA.

DNA cannot replicate without RNA. DNA creates a model of the amino acids it needs by making a strand of mRNA. Messenger RNA attaches to the ribosome and assembles amino acids as dictated by the DNA. RNA polymerase is used in the synthesis of transfer RNA. Transfer RNA (tRNA) collects amino acids from the cell's cytoplasm and carries them back to mRNA for inclusion. A long chain of amino acids is then made according to the DNA's orders for its replication.

Antibiotics that affect DNA synthesis may do so by inhibiting the action of any one of these enzymes. RNA and its associated enzymes can also be inhibited so proteins cannot be made. Whatever the mechanism, the end result is the cessation of cell division, the eventual killing and eradication of the invading organism, and resolution of the infection process. Table 11-5✪ summarizes the antibiotics that affect DNA and RNA.

Quinolones

The quinolones are considered bactericidal. They act on DNA gyrase and other topoisomerases to interfere with DNA replication. In gram-positive organisms they attack topoisomerase IV while they act on DNA gyrase in the gram-negative organisms. Some of the newer quinolones may affect both enzymes in the same organism.

Chemical Properties.   The quinolones possess a two-ring quinolone (naphthyridine) nucleus with different side chain substitutions (Web Figure 11-5 ■). In the 1980s a new class of quinolones, called the fluoroquinolones, were created by the addition of a fluorine atom to the number 6 position of the quinolone ring, which increased the spectrum of activity against gram-negative bacteria. The current list of quinolones includes ciprofloxacin, norfloxacin, levofloxacin, ofloxacin, pefloxacin, moxifloxacin, and gemifloxacin.

These water-soluble drugs are well absorbed from the gastrointestinal tract, regardless of the presence of food; however, the presence of bivalent cations (for example, Mg^{2+}) is known to reduce activity. Once absorbed, the quinolones are widely distributed, penetrating well into tissues and body fluids. They can cross the cell membrane and so are capable of penetrating phagocytes. This makes them effective against intracellular pathogens such as *Brucella, Listeria, Salmonella,* and *Mycobacterium* spp. Administration may be orally or through injection.

There has been speculation that the fluoroquinolones may have adverse effects on human cells. Resistance can also develop rapidly with use. They are often reserved for serious infections in the hospital setting. Gastrointestinal disorders have been reported. Arthralgia, joint swelling and erosion of the cartilage have also been reported. They have been implicated in spontaneous rupture of the Achilles tendon. Trovafloxacin has been pulled off the market because of the potential for severe hepatoxicity. It can only be used if its benefits outweigh the risks.

Spectrum of Activity.   Most of the quinolones are effective in the treatment of infections caused by gram-negative bacteria such as the *Enterobacteriaceae, Haemophilus* spp., *Neisseria* spp., and *Moraxella catarrhalis*. The fluoroquinolones are broad-spectrum antibiotics and are effective against both gram-positive and gram-negative bacteria such as *Staphylococcus* spp. and *Pseudomonas aeruginosa*.

Ciprofloxacin, a fluoroquinolone derivative of nalidixic acid, is useful in the treatment of a wide range of infections including pneumonia, bone infections, diarrhea, skin infections, and urinary tract infections. It is particularly effective against gram-negative bacilli such as salmonellae, shigellae, *Campylobacter* spp., *Neisseria* spp. (except *N. gonorrhoeae*), and *Pseudomonas* spp. It is moderately effective against gram-positive bacteria such as *Streptococcus pneumoniae* and *Enterococcus* spp. Ciprofloxacin is recommended as the initial therapy for the treatment of anthrax, and then may be switched to benzylpenicillin, amoxicillin, or doxycycline if proven to be susceptible.

The fluoroquinolones show activity against *Mycobacterium* spp. They also exhibit activity against *Legionella pneumophila, Mycoplasma* spp., *Chlamydia/Chlamydophila* spp., and *Ureaplasma*

✪ TABLE 11-5

Nucleic Acid Inhibitors

Antibiotic	Spectrum of Activity	Mode of Action

Quinolones
■ Fluoroquinolones
	Gram-negative organisms
	■ *Enterobacteriaceae*
	■ *Haemophilus* spp.
	■ *Neisseria* spp.
	■ *Moraxella catarrhalis*
	■ Gram-positive organisms
	■ Gram-negative organisms
	  ■ Including *Pseudomonas aeruginosa*
	■ *Mycobacterium* spp.
	■ Intracellular organisms
	  ■ *Legionella pneumophila*
	  ■ *Mycoplasma* spp.
	  ■ *Chlamydia/Chlamydophila* spp.
	  ■ *Ureaplasma* spp.
		Inhibits DNA gyrase in gram-negative organisms and topoisomerase IV in gram-positive organisms
		Newer quinolones may affect both enzymes

Rifampin	■ *Mycobacterium tuberculosis*
	■ *M. avium* complex
	■ *Neisseria meningitidis* carrier state
	■ *Staphylococcus* spp.
	  ■ Including MRSA
	■ *Streptococcus spp.*
	  ■ Including multi-drug-resistant *Streptococcus pneumoniae*
	■ Intracellular organisms
		Inhibits DNA-dependent RNA polymerase

Metronidazole	■ Anaerobes ■ Microaerophilic organisms ■ Protozoa	Creates breaks in DNA strands

Nitrofurantoin	■ Urinary pathogens
	  ■ Gram-positive organisms
	  ■ Gram-negative organisms
		Targets protein and enzyme synthesis as well as direct damage of DNA

spp. Some of the newer quinolones are now much more effective against *Streptococcus pneumoniae* and *Staphylococcus aureus*.

Because norfloxacin is rapidly excreted and concentrated in urine, it is used almost exclusively to treat acute and chronic urinary tract infections caused by susceptible gram-negative rods such as *E. coli, Proteus, Enterobacter,* and *Klebsiella.* It is not effective for *Pseudomonas* and gram-positive cocci.

Mode of Action. The targets of the quinolones are the enzyme DNA gyrase, a type II topoisomerase, and topoisomerase IV, another type II enzyme, which are essential for DNA replication. These drugs inhibit subunits of the gyrase and topoisomerase IV enzymes, which are responsible for making a nick in the DNA strand. The enzymes nick and rejoin the DNA template during replication, allowing DNA to uncoil for replication and to recoil so it may be repacked into the daughter cell. It has been also been shown that another antibacterial action of the quinolones is to increase double-stranded DNA breakage.

Rifamycins
Chemical Properties. Rifampin is a semisynthetic derivative of rifamycin, an antibiotic produced by *Streptomyces mediterranei.* It consists of a large aromatic ring with aliphatic

bridges, as seen in Web Figure 11-6 ■. This drug is usually given orally because it is readily absorbed in the gastrointestinal tract and widely distributed throughout the body, including cerebrospinal and other body fluids, as well as tissues.

Spectrum of Activity.

The most important use of rifampin is the treatment of tuberculosis in combination with other drugs. It exhibits bactericidal action against intracellular and extracellular *Mycobacterium tuberculosis* and may also be prescribed for the treatment of *Mycobacterium avium* complex (MAC) in patients with HIV infection. It is always used in combination with other antibiotics because if used as a single treatment agent for *Mycobacterium* spp., resistance can develop quickly.

Rifampin is an effective treatment for asymptomatic cases of the meningococcal carrier state to eliminate *Neisseria meningitidis* from the nasopharynx. It is not recommended for acute meningococcal infection because of the rapid emergence of resistance to the medication. It does not penetrate the outer membrane of all gram-negative organisms effectively.

Because of its ability to concentrate well inside cells, it is effective against intracellular pathogens. Using combination therapy has been shown to be useful against *Staphylococcus* spp. including MRSA, *Streptococcus* spp. including multi-drug-resistant *S. pneumoniae, Haemophilus influenzae, Campylobacter jejuni,* and *Chlamydia/Chlamydophila* spp.

Side effects include hepatoxicity, gastrointestinal disorders, and skin rashes. It can stain the bodily fluids, such as tears, urine, and sweat, orange. Although this is not a harmful effect, it can disturb the patient unless informed of the side effect.

Mode of Action.

In susceptible cells, this medication inhibits the DNA-dependent RNA polymerase, which initiates the chaining formation of mRNA. It does not interfere with the RNA polymerase activity in human cells. Rifamycins are known to interact with drugs used to treat AIDS patients such as ketoconazole, an antifungal agent, and daprone, an antibiotic used for prophylaxis against *Pneumocystis jiroveci* pneumonia.

℮ REAL WORLD TIP

Novobiocin is a bactericidal antibiotic that inhibits DNA synthesis by targeting DNA gyrase and topoisomerase. It is effective against gram-positive organisms, especially MRSA and *Clostridium difficile.* It is no longer available in the United States because of a high rate of hypersensitivity reactions.

Staphylococcus saprophyticus is intrinsically resistant to novobiocin. It can be used in the laboratory as an identification test to differentiate *S. saprophyticus* from other *Staphylococcus* spp. in urine cultures.

Other DNA Synthesis Inhibitors

Metronidazole.

The active form of this bactericidal antibiotic may cause breaks in DNA strands. Activation of metronidazole occurs under anaerobic conditions, which makes it very potent for use against anaerobes and microaerophilic organisms. It is also effective against protozoa such as the flagellates and amoebas. It is used in the treatment of bacterial vaginosis and pseudomembranous colitis caused by *Clostridium difficile.* Adverse effects include gastrointestinal disorders, headache, and a lingering metallic taste. It can increase the effect of warfarin, which in turn will increase prothrombin times, a coagulation laboratory test.

Nitrofurantoin.

This antibacterial antibiotic concentrates very well in the urine. It may have several targets involved in protein and enzyme synthesis, such as altering ribosomal proteins as well as direct damage of DNA. It is effective against most gram-positive organisms, including *Staphylococcus* spp. and *Streptococcus* spp., as well as gram-negative organisms, such as *E. coli* and *Klebsiella* spp., which cause urinary tract infections. Its most common side effect is gastrointestinal disorders.

ANTIBIOTICS AFFECTING METABOLIC PROCESSES OR ACTING AS COMPETITIVE ANTAGONISTS

Analogues of Para-Aminobenzoic Acid (PABA)

Mode of Action.

Folic acid is a B vitamin that is required for DNA synthesis. Para-aminobenzoic acid (PABA) is a precursor molecule used by bacteria in the production of folic acid. In other words, PABA is an intermediary compound found in the synthesis of folic acid. When **competitive antagonists** or molecules similar in structure to substances essential for cellular metabolism are present, they compete with PABA for combining sites on the enzymes required for folic acid synthesis. For example, the enzyme, dihydropteroate synthetase, which catalyzes the conversion of dihydropteridine to dihydropteroate, reacts with sulfonamides, structural analogues of PABA, in place of PABA. As a consequence, these drugs inhibit the production of folic acid and secondarily DNA synthesis. If DNA replication does not occur, then cell division is not possible. PABA analogues would be bacteriostatic agents rather than bactericidal. Adverse reactions include hypersensitivity reactions, nausea, vomiting, and diarrhea. Table 11-6 ✪ summarizes the antibiotics that inhibit folic acid synthesis.

Folic Acid Synthesis Inhibitors

- Sulfonamides are primarily used to treat urinary tract infections. Susceptible organisms include the *Enterobacteriaceae*, especially *E. coli, Haemophilus influenzae, Staphylococcus aureus, Streptococcus pyogenes, S. pneumoniae,* and *Neisseria gonorrhoeae.* It is usually used in combination with another folic acid inhibitor, trimethoprim.

⊗ TABLE 11-6

Metabolic Processes Inhibitors or Competitive Antagonists

Antibiotic	Spectrum of Activity	Mode of Action

Sulfonamides	■ Urinary isolates
	  ■ Gram-positive organisms
	  ■ Gram-negative organisms
		Inhibits folic acid synthesis

Para-aminosalicylic acid (PAS)	*Mycobacterium tuberculosis*	
Sulfones	■ *Mycobacterium leprae* ■ *Pneumocystis jiroveci* ■ *Toxoplasma gondii*	

Trimethoprim
■ Usually used in combination therapy with the sulfonamide, sulfamethoxazole
	■ Gram-positive organisms, including community-acquired MRSA
	■ Gram-negative organisms
	  ■ *Legionella* spp.
	  ■ *Stenotrophomonas maltophilia*
	  ■ *Burkholderia cepacia*
	■ *Pneumocystis jiroveci*	

- Para-aminosalicylic acid (PAS) is used in treatment of *Mycobacterium tuberculosis* but only in combination with other drugs.

- Sulfones, such as dapsone, are used in the treatment of leprosy, a disease caused by *Mycobacterium leprae*. It has also been useful in the treatment of *Pneumocystis jiroveci* pneumonia (PCP), a fungal infection commonly seen in AIDS patients, as well as *Toxoplasma gondii*.

- Trimethoprim (TMP), a diaminopyrimidine, also targets the folic acid pathway by blocking the final step in the conversion of PABA to folic acid. Because it inhibits a second step in folic acid synthesis, it is usually used in combination with sulfamethoxazole (SMX) for a synergistic effect to treat urinary infections. TMP-SMX is effective against most gram-positive cocci and gram-negative rods, except for *Pseudomonas aeruginosa*. It is also effective in the treatment of community-acquired MRSA infections and *Pneumocystis jiroveci* pneumonia in immunocompromised individuals. *Stenotrophomonas maltophilia* and *Burkholderia cepacia*, although often multi-resistant, remain susceptible to TMP-SMX. It is also effective against *Legionella* spp., community-acquired MRSA, and *Streptococcus pneumoniae*.

✓ Checkpoint! 11–6 (Chapter Objective 2)

A synergistic effect is best illustrated by the antibiotic:
- A. *sulfonamide.*
- B. *para-aminosalicylic acid.*
- C. *dapsone.*
- D. *trimethoprim-sulfamethoxazole.*

MISCELLANEOUS ANTIBIOTICS

Antimycobacterial Agents

Strains of *Mycobacterium tuberculosis* (MTB) can easily develop resistance when single-agent therapy is used. To prevent the rapid development of resistance combination, therapy must be given for long periods of time. Antibiotics often used in combination include isoniazid, rifampin, ethambutol, and pyrazinamide. Multi-drug-resistant MTB now requires the use of alternative agents such as the aminoglycosides and quinolones, which are less effective. The alternative choices are becoming limited, and resistant MTB is becoming a worldwide threat.

Isoniazid.   Isoniazid, isonicotinic acid hydrazide (INH), as seen in Web Figure 11-7 , is an antibiotic that is used primarily in the treatment of tuberculosis in combination with other drugs. The exact mechanism by which it inhibits the growth of *Mycobacterium tuberculosis* is not well known. It is possible that it interferes with the synthesis of mycolic acids, an essential component of the mycobacterial cell wall. This drug is bactericidal for growing cells only and is effective for intracellular bacteria. It can injure liver cells, causing hepatitis.

Ethambutol.   This bacteriostatic antibiotic works to inhibit formation of the mycolic acid cell wall. One significant adverse effect is optic neuritis. The optic nerve becomes inflamed, and vision can be impaired.

Pyrazinamide.   Pyrazinamide (PZA) is a bactericidal agent whose mode of action is not well known. It probably decreases the pH so the environment is not conducive for the growth of *Mycobacterium tuberculosis*. Vomiting and nausea are common side effects.

Antifungal Agents

Amphotericin B.   Amphotericin B inhibits organisms whose cell membranes contain sterols, such as eukaryotic and some prokaryotic cells. Bacteria lack sterols. The antibiotic has a higher affinity for and selectively targets the fungal cell membrane sterol, ergosterol, compared to the human cell membrane sterol, cholesterol. It disrupts the cell membrane of yeast and moulds, causing intracellular potassium, magnesium, sugars, and metabolites to leak out of the cell and leading to death. It is used most often for the treatment of invasive infections caused by moulds such as *Aspergillus* spp. and yeasts such as

Candida spp. and *Cryptococcus* spp. This antifungal agent is associated with nephrotoxicity, nausea, and vomiting but is still considered the drug of choice for invasive fungal infections.

 REAL WORLD TIP

Although most invasive infections caused by *Candida* spp. can be treated with amphotericin B, *C. lusitaniae* is intrinsically resistant to it.

Flucytosine.   Flucytosine appears to interfere with DNA synthesis and RNA transcription. It is used to treat infections caused by *Candida* spp., *Cryptococcus neoformans,* and *Aspergillus* spp. This agent may depress the bone marrow and affect renal and liver function.

Azoles.   This group of antifungal agents prevents sterol synthesis, which in turn causes the organism's membrane to leak. Azole agents in use include ketoconazole, itraconazole, fluconazole, and voriconazole. They are used in the treatment of infections caused by *Candida* spp., *Cryptococcus neoformans,* *Coccidioides* spp., *Histoplasma* spp., *Paracoccidioides* spp., and *Blastomyces* spp. They are also effective against *Aspergillus* spp., *Epidermophyton* spp., *Microsporum* spp., and *Trichophyton* spp. Adverse effects include hepatitis, nausea, headache, hair loss, and visual disturbances.

Caspofungin.   This antifungal agent inhibits the production of several cell wall molecules so its integrity is disturbed. It is active against *Candida* spp. and *Aspergillus* spp. There are only minor side effects with its use. *Cryptococcus neoformans* is intrinsically resistant to this antifungal agent.

Griseofulvin.   This antifungal agent binds to keratin precursor cells in hair and nails so they become highly resistant to fungal invasion. It is used primarily for the dermatophytes: *Microsporum* spp., *Epidermophyton* spp., and *Trichophyton* spp. Common side effects include nausea, diarrhea, and headache.

▶ ANTIBIOTIC RESISTANCE MECHANISMS

GENERAL CONSIDERATIONS

Early in this chapter it was stated that the inability of bacteria to become resistant to the deleterious effects of an antibiotic would be a very desirable property if one were to develop the "ideal" antibiotic. Unfortunately, bacteria and other organisms have developed ways to ward off the harmful effects of antimicrobial agents, and as a consequence, the eradication of infectious agents has not been achieved. Bacterial antibiotic resistance has instead become a substantial problem. A

few years ago the evolution of "superbugs," or strains of microbial agents too powerful to be controlled by antibiotics, began to be a very real possibility. Another problem associated with the emergence of resistant strains has been the necessity to use more toxic or more expensive alternative drugs. In the following section, the mechanisms by which bacteria may develop resistance to infection are discussed.

NATURAL OR INTRINSIC ANTIMICROBIAL RESISTANCE

Inherent or intrinsic resistance is defined as resistance that is naturally occurring and, therefore, present in most strains of a certain microbe, even before the advent of antibiotic usage. For example, although most genera in the family *Enterobacteriaceae* are susceptible to the polymyxins, the *Proteus-Providencia-Morganella* group, *Serratia,* and *Edwardsiella* appear to be inherently resistance to polymyxin B and E (colistin). This phenomenon is evident in most strains of these species when susceptibility testing is performed, independent of the source of isolation.

Another example is the inherent resistance of anaerobes to aminoglycosides as a result of the lack of an oxidative electron transport system. The oxidative electron transport system, through which aerobes and facultative anaerobes are able to obtain energy, is required for the uptake of aminoglycosides. Because these drugs cannot gain access inside the anaerobic cell, its target, the ribosome remains inaccessible. In essence, the absence of a suitable transport system renders the anaerobic bacterium impermeable to the antibiotic.

It should be noted that intrinsic resistance patterns can be used in the phenotypic identification of organism. For example, novobiocin resistance is used in the differentiation of *Staphylococcus saprophyticus* from other coagulase negative staphylococci. *S. saprophyticus* is resistant to novobiocin, whereas most other coagulase negative staphylococci are susceptible and will exhibit a zone of inhibition around a novobiocin-impregnated filter paper disc. Table 11-7✪ summarizes some of the more commonly recognized intrinsic resistance patterns produced by organisms.

ACQUIRED OR MUTATIONAL RESISTANCE

Acquired resistance refers to instances where previously susceptible infectious agents develop resistance as the result of exposure to an antimicrobial agent. In other words, the use of an antibiotic supplies selective pressure for the emergence of resistant strains.

Chromosomal mutations can occur spontaneously in any population of living organisms and, if beneficial, may provide a selective advantage to those possessing the new trait. In the case of antibiotic resistance, mutations can occur during the

✪ TABLE 11-7

Intrinsic Resistance Patterns That May Be Used to Confirm an Organism's Identity

Organism	Antibiotic/Class	Intrinsic Resistance Mechanism
Aerobes	Metronidazole	Cannot reduce the antibiotic to an active form
Anaerobes	Aminoglycosides	Antibiotic cannot cross cell membrane
Enterococcus faecalis	Quinupristin-dalfopristin	Ability to pump out the antibiotic
Enterococcus faecium	β-lactams	PBP with a decreased affinity to bind antibiotics
Gram-positive organisms	Aztreonam	PBP with a decreased affinity to bind the antibiotic
Gram-negative organisms	Vancomycin	Antibiotic cannot cross the outer membrane
Klebsiella spp.	Penicillin, carbenicillin, and ticarcillin	Production of β-lactamases
Leuconostoc, Pediococcus, and *Lactobacillus* spp.	Vancomycin	Lacks the target for binding the antibiotic
MRSA	β-lactams	PBP with a decreased affinity to bind antibiotics
Proteus, Providencia and *Neisseria* spp.	Polymyxins	Antibiotic cannot bind to outer membrane
Pseudomonas aeruginosa	Penicillin	Production of an inducible beta-lactamase
Pseudomonas aeruginosa	Trimethoprim/sulfamethoxazole	Ability to pump out the antibiotic
Pseudomonas aeruginosa and *Proteus* spp.	Tetracycline	Ability to pump out the antibiotic
Stenotrophomonas maltophilia	Imipenem	Production of β-lactamase

period an individual is undergoing antibiotic treatment. This allows resistant bacteria to overcome the activity of the antimicrobial agent and outgrow the susceptible cells. A new population of resistant bacteria then emerges under the influence of this selective pressure. Changes brought about by chromosomal mutations that result in antimicrobial resistance include:

- Target site modification such as a change in penicillin binding proteins, which can lead to resistance to the beta-lactam antibiotics such as penicillins.

- Reduced permeability, which results in altered porin channels or decreased active transport or influx across the cell wall and so a decreased uptake of the drug.

- The ability to bypass inhibited metabolic pathways such as the overproduction of dihydrofolate reductase, an enzyme required for folic acid synthesis, which is the target for the antibiotic trimethoprim.

- Activation of efflux systems. Efflux pumps are proteins found in the cell membrane. They actively transport drugs and other chemicals out of the cell, preventing the accumulation of an effective intracellular concentration of the antimicrobial agent.

- Production of an enzyme that can degrade or modify the antibiotic.

- Any combination of the preceding resistance mechanisms.

These acquired resistance mechanisms can occur because of mutation or the acquisition of **plasmids**, which are small bits of extrachromosomal DNA capable of encoding bacterial resistance and virulence factors such as exotoxins. DNA resistance plasmids released by a bacterium may be picked up by another bacterium, even those that are not genus or species related.

Bacteria can transfer resistance genes by other mechanisms. After death, bacteria release their DNA. Other organisms may come in contact with the free fragments DNA, absorb them, and incorporate them into their own DNA. This is known as transformation. Bacteriophages are viruses that infect bacteria. They are able to transfer DNA from one organism to another in a mechanism known as transduction. During conjugation, bacterial cells are able to transfer DNA via cell to cell contact. Bacteria are promiscuous and can conjugate with organisms outside their genus.

Transposons have also been implicated in the transfer of antibiotic resistance. They are also known as jumping genes because they can spread across a wide range of bacterial species and jump from plasmid to plasmid, plasmid to chromosome, and chromosome to plasmid. These mobile segments of DNA contain genes that encode proteins that confer antibiotic resistance as well as proteins required for the gene itself to be transposed into the host's genome. Transposons can be inserted into chromosomes or plasmids in areas where no homology exists. Detection of bacteria with chromosomes that have undergone transposition can be accomplished by culturing them in the presence of an antibiotic that normally inhibits growth of the bacteria. The bacteria that possess the transposon will be capable of sustaining growth and cell division in the antibiotic enriched growth medium. Bacteria that have not incorporated the antibiotic-resistance DNA are unable to grow. Tn-9 has been identified as an *E. coli* transposon that contains a gene that encodes not only resistance to chloramphenicol but also the protein required to integrate the transposon into the *E. coli* genome.

Checkpoint! 11–7
(Chapter Objective 4)

Which of the following acquired-resistance mechanisms involves viruses that transfer DNA from one organism to another?

A. *Transformation*
B. *Conjugation*
C. *Transduction*
D. *Transposons*

MECHANISMS OF ANTIMICROBIAL RESISTANCE

Four mechanisms of antimicrobial resistance have been recognized: modification of the target, enzymatic inactivation of the antimicrobial agent, decreased permeability or uptake of the agent as well as the ability to actively pump out the agent, and last, any combination of these mechanisms (Rice, Sahm, & Bonomo, 2003).

Modification of the Target

As discussed previously, the mode of action for some antimicrobial agents is binding to specific target sites on a microbe. In turn, some functions, essential to the life processes of the cell, are inhibited to the point that cellular activity ceases and the microbe dies. Depending on the target bound by the drug, cell wall synthesis may be inhibited, protein synthesis may cease, cell membranes may be damaged to the extent that cell contents may be lost, DNA replication may be inhibited, or enzymes required for some vital biochemical pathway may be shut down.

If the original target of the antimicrobial agent is altered in some manner, it may reduce or prevent binding to the extent the antimicrobial agent is ineffective. These alterations, which confer resistance, may be accomplished by chromosomal mutations or through the action of plasmids or transposons.

Examples of chromosomal aberrations which confer resistance include

■ Alterations of the penicillin-binding proteins (PBPs) involved in cell wall synthesis. These altered PBPs do not bind to beta-lactam antibiotics sufficiently to inhibit cell wall synthesis. Bacteria then develop resistance to beta-lactam antibiotics such as penicillins or cephalosporins. This can be observed in methicillin-resistant *Staphylococcus* spp., vancomycin-resistant *Enterococcus* spp., and *Streptococcus pneumoniae.*

■ Mutational alterations in the subunits of DNA gyrase enzymes. Because DNA gyrases are the target of quinolone activity, these changes lead to resistance to the inhibition of growth by fluoroquinolones.

■ Alterations in outer membrane proteins (porins). Decreased uptake of the antimicrobial agent prevents adequate accumulation of the drug to the point that it is rendered ineffective.

■ Alterations to the enzyme, RNA polymerase, which render the drug rifampin ineffective.

■ Alterations to the ribosomal subunits prevent binding of streptomycin to the ribosome. Mutation of the *rpsL* gene in *E. coli* is a good example of this process. This gene encodes a ribosomal protein, S12, which becomes one of the components of the ribosome. Normally streptomycin inhibits protein synthesis by forming a complex with S12. The production of an abnormal S12 protein, as a result of mutations to the rpsL gene, would prevent binding of streptomycin to the ribosome and therefore confer resistance. Other ribosomal modifications can be found in *Neisseria gonorrhoeae, Staphylococcus aureus, Pseudomonas aeruginosa, Enterococcus faecalis,* and *Mycobacterium tuberculosis.* Alterations lead to the emergence of streptomycin-resistant strains.

Examples of plasmid or transposon conferred resistance include

■ A plasmid mediated resistance to macrolides, such as erythromycin, occurs through encoding of an enzyme, which methylates a component of the 50S ribosomal subunit. Because macrolides inhibit protein synthesis by binding to the 50S ribosomal subunit, these antibiotics are rendered ineffective.

■ Trimethoprim resistance is associated with acquisition of a plasmid, which encodes production of a dihydrofolate reductase enzyme resistant to the effects of trimethoprim.

■ A plasmid-encoded dihydropteroate synthetase is responsible for resistance to sulfonamide antibiotics. This enzyme also affects the folic acid pathway.

■ Transposon associated vancomycin resistance, such the *Van*A phenotype carried by the 11-kb transposon Tn 1546, has been detected in enterococci. In addition, transfer of high-level glycopeptides (vancomycin) resistance has been accomplished between *Enterococcus faecalis* and *Staphylococcus aureus* in the laboratory setting. There is reason to believe that this could occur in nature, and perhaps this may be the mechanism behind recent reports of strains of vancomycin-intermediate and vancomycin-resistant *S. aureus.* It is a well-established fact that resistance genes may be passed on to other strains within a species and even between species in other genera. The dissemination of resistance genes may allow pathogenic bacteria to develop resistance to multiple antibiotics, especially under the selective pressure of excessive use of antimicrobial agents.

■ The *mec*A gene is carried on a mobile genetic element and is the mechanism behind the emergence of strains of methicillin-resistant *S. aureus* (MRSA). This gene encodes a new penicillin binding protein that has a low affinity for methicillin, a penicillinase-resistant penicillin, as well as all the other beta-lactams. This new PBP (a β-lactamase-resistant transpeptidase) exhibits little or no ability to bind to methicillin, rendering the antibiotic ineffective in inhibiting cell wall synthesis and therefore of little use in the treatment of infections caused by these strains of *S. aureus.*

Inactivation of an Antimicrobial Agent

Genes may encode enzymes that are capable of converting an active antimicrobial agent to an inactive form and thereby conferring resistance. One of the best examples of this phenomenon is the production of enzymes that have the capacity to hydrolyze the beta-lactam ring of beta-lactam antibiotics such as penicillins, cephalosporins, and imipenem. Once the beta-lactam ring has been destroyed, the antibiotic is no longer able to bind to PBPs and inhibit cell wall synthesis. These enzymes may be encoded by chromosomal or plasmid-mediated genes.

Staphylococcus spp. is well known for its ability to produce beta-lactamase, but gram-negative bacteria also commonly have chromosomally mediated genes for β-lactamases capable of destroying the activity of cephalosporins. A notable example of this is the chromosomally encoded cephalosporinase, designated AmpC, produced by nearly all members of the family *Enterobacteriaceae* and strains of *Pseudomonas aeruginosa.* Rare isolates of *Enterobacter cloacae, Serratia marcescens,* and all strains of *Stenotrophomonas maltophilia* have evolved a chromosome gene for β-lactamases known as imipenemases, which confers resistance to imipenem.

Many different varieties of plasmid mediated β-lactamases have also been found in the periplasmic space of gram-negative bacteria. Enzymes, such as TEM-1, are responsible for resistance to penicillins such as ampicillin, carbenicillin, piperacillin, and ticarcillin with additional hydrolytic activity effective against a few of the first-generation cephalosporin antibiotics such as cephalothin. Originally the activity of these enzymes was not extended to the broad-spectrum second- and third-generation cephalosporins. Eventually, however, isolates of *Klebsiella pneumoniae, Proteus mirabilis, Enterobacter cloacae, Serratia marcescens, Escherichia coli,* and *Citrobacter freundii* acquired plasmid-mediated extended-spectrum β-lactamases that conferred resistance not only to first-generation cephalosporins but now also to broad-spectrum ephalosporins such as cefamandole, cefotaxime, ceftazidime, ceftizoxime, and ceftriaxone.

Other plasmid mediated enzymes, such as the chloramphenicol acetyltransferase encoded by the plasmid R387 from *E. coli,* confer resistance to classes of antibiotics. As the name implies, chloramphenicol acetyltransferases transfer an acetyl group from acetyl coenzyme A to the primary hydroxyl on C6 of chloramphenicol, preventing the antibiotic from binding to the ribosome. These enzymes have been found in a wide variety of organisms, including gram-positive and gram-negative bacteria and anaerobes.

 REAL WORLD TIP

Staphylococcus spp., *Haemophilus influenzae, Moraxella catarrhalis, Neisseria gonorrhoeae,* and some anaerobic gram-negative rods excrete their beta-lactamase into their environment, whereas gram-negative rods, such as *Klebsiella* spp., *E. coli,* and *Stenotrophomonas maltophilia* retain theirs in their periplasmic space. A chromogenic cephalosporin test will rapidly detect the beta-lactamase produced by organisms that excrete it but not those that retain it internally.

Decreased Permeability, Decreased Uptake, and Increased Efflux

Before antimicrobial agents can exert detrimental effects on their target species, they must first gain entrance into the interior of the organism. Many microbes have developed mechanisms capable of blocking the entry of drugs into the cell. Mechanisms of resistance may include lack or modification of an active transport system, modification of the antimicrobial agent to prevent transport, creating permeability barriers or pumping the agent out.

Gram-negative bacteria, by virtue of the nature of their lipid rich, outer membrane surface, have what might be called an innate resistance to some antibiotics that are effective against gram-positive bacteria. Many antibiotics are simply incapable of adsorption onto and penetration of the outer membrane of gram-negative bacteria because of its high lipid content. Vancomycin resistance seen in gram-negative bacteria is a good example of this mechanism because the large antibiotic molecule is unable to penetrate the outer membrane of these organisms.

Another reason for decreased uptake in gram-negative bacteria is a change in the number or character of porin channels. Water-filled channels, composed of proteins called porins, allow the diffusion of molecules across the outer membrane of gram-negative bacteria. Because beta-lactamases and aminoglycosides must pass through the porin channels to reach the penicillin-binding proteins and ribosomes, respectively, altered porin channels lead to diminished levels of these drugs. *E. coli* provides a good example of this. This organism produces two or more types of porin channels, OmpF and OmpC. Changes in one or both of these porins through mutation lead to decreased susceptibility to β-lactam antibiotics.

Decreased levels of an antibiotic can also be a result of an increased efflux of the drug. This is often associated with the ability of many bacteria to pump substances out of the interior of the cell and back into the environment. The net result of this increased efflux is to prevent the accumulation of sufficient levels of an antimicrobial agent to the extent that it is unable to affect the growth of the targeted microbe.

This phenomenon is associated with the low-level resistance of *P. aeruginosa* to a wide variety of antimicrobial agents as a result of an efflux system. Another example is the presence of the *msr*A gene found in both *S. aureus* and coagulase-negative staphylococci. This gene encodes a transport protein that confers inducible resistance to 14- and 15-member macrolides. In a similar manner, an *mre*A (macrolide resistance efflux) gene performs much the same function for a strain of *Streptococcus agalactiae*.

Combination of Mechanisms

Some microbes are capable of using several different mechanisms that can confer resistance to an antibiotic. Beta-lactam antibiotics may be ineffective to treat *Neisseria gonorrhoeae* infections because strains can arise that not only are able to produce a beta-lactamase, but may also have the capability to alter their PBPs or possess outer surfaces impermeable to beta-lactams.

Checkpoint! 11–8 (Chapter Objective 4)

Which of the following resistance mechanisms is used by methicillin-resistant Staphylococcus aureus?
   A. *Modification of the antibiotic target*
   B. *Inactivation of the antimicrobial agent*
   C. *Decreased permeability*
   D. *Both A and B*

▶ SUSCEPTIBILITY TESTING METHODS

INTRODUCTION

When penicillin was introduced, it was hailed as a miracle and considered to be the drug of choice to treat staphylococcal infections. Unfortunately, the miracle would be short-lived. From 1946 until the end of the decade *Staphylococcus aureus* could be successfully treated with penicillin. By 1950 about 80% of the strains of *S. aureus* in the hospital environment were no longer responsive to penicillin because of the appearance of beta-lactamase enzymes, which rendered the bacterium resistant to the effects of the drug. During the 1960s a semi-synthetic, broad-spectrum penicillin, called methicillin, became available for use against penicillin-resistant *S. aureus* strains. Shortly thereafter, strains of *S. aureus* emerged that were resistant to methicillin. These methicillin-resistant *S. aureus*, or MRSA, created a problem that remains today.

The saga has continued. The glycopeptide antibiotic vancomycin has become the drug of last resort to treat MRSA. It was greatly feared that eventually strains of vancomycin-resistant *S. aureus*, or VRSA, would arise in the United States. The prediction materialized in June of 2002, as a strain of VRSA (MIC $\geq$ 32 µg/mL) was isolated from a catheter exit site on a 40-year-old diabetic with vascular disease and chronic renal failure in Michigan. This was the first confirmed case of VRSA

in the United States. Tests revealed this strain was not only resistant to vancomycin but also to teicoplanin and oxacillin.

It is not possible to predict the extent an organism will be susceptible to the vast arsenal of antibiotics at our disposal because resistant strains seem to be constantly emerging under the selective pressure of antimicrobial therapy. Drug dynamics, microbial activity, and host response are also factors in the struggle between humans and microbes. There has been no clear winner in the war when microbes are pitted against antimicrobial agents.

Once a potential pathogen has been isolated, identification and susceptibility testing are usually performed. Susceptibility testing has become the means to measure the response of microorganisms to antimicrobial therapy.

The Clinical and Laboratory Standards Institute (CLSI) is a nonprofit organization that produces standards for medical testing in the health care community. The CLSI subcommittee on antimicrobial susceptibility testing develops the standards, methods, quality control parameters, and interpretive criteria for susceptibility testing used in most microbiology laboratories. This document is revised annually to ensure the detection of emerging resistance.

SELECTION OF ANTIMICROBIAL AGENTS FOR TESTING

Because it is impractical to test every potential pathogen against every antimicrobial agent, decisions must be made to determine which agents should be tested against which organisms. Often this decision is made by a team consisting of the microbiology laboratory, infectious disease specialists, and the pharmacy. This group may review data such as the cost and toxicity of antimicrobial agents as well as emerging resistance patterns within the facility. CLSI provides annual recommendations of antimicrobial agents to include for testing and reporting. Suggested groupings are provided for first choice agents, alternative or supplemental agents, and urinary agents based on the organism being tested. Each antibiotic in every class does not need to be used in testing. Often a representative antibiotic is tested, then the results for the others in the class can be considered equivalent. An example would be the use of cephalothin to predict the results of the first-generation cephalosporins.

CLSI takes into account intrinsic resistance when suggesting agents for testing and reporting. For example, the listing for the *Enterobacteriaceae* does not include vancomycin as a suggested agent for testing because all gram-negative organisms are intrinsically resistant to vancomycin. The large-molecule agent cannot pass through their cell wall. The documents include information on resistance mechanisms and the agents that are affected. They also take into account the agents that have the ability to pass through the blood–brain barrier, if the organism is isolated from CSF, as well as those that concentrate in the urine. The CLSI susceptibility documents contain a wealth of information. Even though it only makes recommendations for clinical practice, it has become the bible for clinical microbiology laboratories that perform susceptibility testing.

 REAL WORLD TESTING

Reading a CLSI document can be intimidating because of the vast amount of information present. The footnotes provide valuable detailed information and must not be overlooked. The susceptibility documents are released annually. A designated individual in the microbiology laboratory must review them thoroughly for updates on release.

METHODS

Susceptibility testing has evolved into something very complicated because of dwindling resources, the demand for high quality and patient safety, as well as rapidly emerging resistance mechanisms. Deciding when to perform susceptibility testing depends on the clinical significance of an organism isolated, its predictable susceptibility pattern, and the availability of standardized methods for testing an isolate. Very few organisms are left that do not require routine susceptibility testing. *Streptococcus pyogenes, Streptococcus agalactiae,* and *Neisseria meningitidis* are predictably susceptible, and testing is rarely required. Testing is occasionally required for *Haemophilus influenzae, Neisseria gonorrhoeae, Moraxella catarrhalis,* and anaerobes. All other organisms require routine susceptibility testing because of their ability to acquire resistance mechanisms.

In this section, we examine the standardized methods used to gauge the inhibitory effect of antimicrobial compounds. These include disk diffusion, which uses antibiotic impregnated disks, broth dilution, in which the antibiotic is suspended in a solution, agar dilution, in which the antibiotic is incorporated into the agar, variations of these manual methods, and automated commercial systems.

 REAL WORLD TIP

If there is no standardized susceptibility method or interpretative standards available for an organism such as *Staphylococcus saprophyticus,* susceptibility testing should not be performed. The physician may need to consult with the infectious disease specialist for guidance.

Some terms dealing with susceptibility testing need to be introduced at this point:

- **Minimum inhibitory concentration (MIC)** is the lowest concentration of an antimicrobial agent that visibly inhibits the growth of an organism.

- **Minimum bactericidal concentration (MBC)** is the lowest concentration of an antimicrobial agent that results in the death (greater than or equal to 99.9%) of the test organism.

- **Synergistic effect** is the greater antimicrobial activity resulting from a combination of individual agents as opposed to the expected sum of the effects of either acting alone.

- **Peak concentration** is the amount of medication in the blood that represents the highest level of a drug during an administration cycle.

- **Trough concentration** is the minimal level of a drug during an administration cycle. Traditionally trough levels are obtained at a specified period of time, such as 30 minutes, before administration of the next dose of drugs.

- **Susceptible** or **sensitive** is an interpretive category that indicates an organism that is inhibited by the recommended dose or achievable level, at the site of infection, of an antimicrobial agent.

- **Intermediate** represents an organism that may require a higher dose of antibiotic for a longer period of time to be inhibited. The physician must weigh the benefits of treatment versus the side effects of the antibiotic used. This interpretive category also allows for a buffer zone, between susceptible and resistant, to prevent minor changes from making a major difference in interpretation.

- **Resistant** indicates an organism that is not inhibited by the recommended dose or achievable level, at the site of infection, of an antimicrobial agent. It may also indicate the presence of resistance mechanism in the organism.

Diffusion Methods

In the 1960s, Drs. Bauer, Kirby, Sherris, and Truck standardized an antibiotic susceptibility method known as disk diffusion. This provided microbiologists with a method that gave reliable and reproducible results. It still bears the nickname "Kirby-Bauer" today.

A standardized bacterial inoculum is applied to the entire surface of a Mueller-Hinton agar plate prior to the sterile application of thin paper disks impregnated with the antimicrobial agents to be tested. The plates are incubated at 35°C in ambient or room air and, after 16 to 18 hours, are examined for areas where growth of the organism is inhibited by the antibiotic. The diameter of this clear area around each disk, called a zone of inhibition, is measured using a ruler or dial caliper. Zones of inhibition surrounding the disks are interpreted using zone size ranges, established by antibiotic manufacturers and CLSI, for individual antimicrobial agents to determine which are most suitable for use in antimicrobial therapy.

The zone of inhibition is the result of a concentration gradient created by diffusion of the antimicrobial agent into the solid agar growth medium. Because the antibiotic diffuses out of the disk faster than it diffuses through the agar, the highest concentration will occur in the area immediately surrounding the impregnated disk with the concentration decreasing as the distance from the disc increases. Eventually, a point is reached where the amount of antibiotic in the agar is insufficient to inhibit growth of the test organism, as seen in Figure 11-6 ■. Because the antibiotic diffuses out like the spokes of a wheel, the zone of inhibition is circular. The diameter, measured in millimeters, is related to the minimal inhibitory concentration of the drug for that organism. The results are qualitative with no numeric value and are recorded as susceptible, intermediate, and resistant. Disk agar diffusion breakpoints, the values that determine the interpretive categories of susceptibility, have been determined by plotting the zone diameters against the MICs derived from the testing of a large number of strains of various species.

It should be noted that the disk agar diffusion test is not applicable for slow-growing organisms, such as *Mycobacterium* spp., moulds, or anaerobic bacteria. Fastidious organisms such as *Haemophilus influenzae*, *Neisseria* spp., and *Streptococcus pneumoniae* require modifications of the disk diffusion procedure and are discussed in the "Special Methods and Procedures" section of this chapter.

The current testing procedure is standardized for urinary and systemic antibacterial agents and rapidly growing aerobic or facultative bacteria only, such as *Staphylococcus* spp., *Enterococcus* spp., *Enterobacteriaceae*, *Pseudomonas aeruginosa*, *Acinetobacter* spp., *Burkholderia cepacia*, *Stenotrophomonas maltophilia*, and *Vibrio cholerae*. Antibiotic disk manufacturers and CLSI supply interpretative standards for disk diffusion susceptibility testing in the form of charts or tables listing the different antimicrobial agents and their corresponding zone

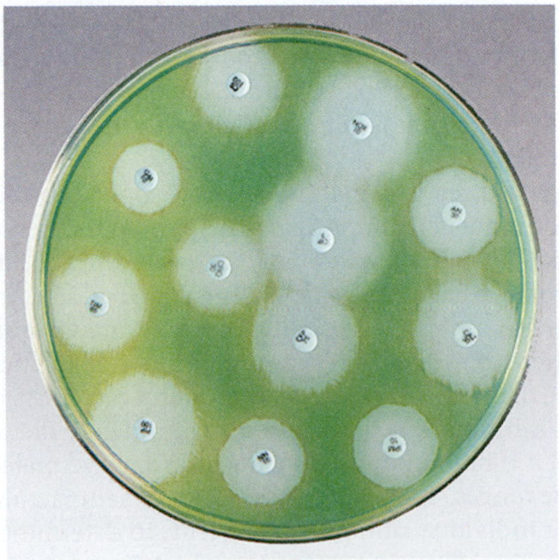

■ **FIGURE 11-6** Disk agar diffusion susceptibility testing of *Pseudomonas aeruginosa* on Mueller-Hinton agar. Note the zones of inhibition surrounding the antibiotic impregnated discs indicating susceptibility of the test organism.
Photo courtesy of Remel, part of Thermo Fisher Scientific.

diameter interpretive standards expressed in millimeters (mm). Quality control strains of *Escherichia coli*, *Staphylococcus aureus*, and *Pseudomonas aeruginosa* must be tested on a regular schedule to ensure that the test results are both accurate and reproducible.

Standardized Factors.   Many technical factors are known to influence zone diameters and must be standardized to maintain the precision and accuracy of the procedure. The concentration of the antibiotic or chemotherapeutic agent is controlled by the disk manufacturer who impregnates 6 mm disks with accurately determined amounts assayed by methods established by the Food and Drug Administration (FDA). The zone of inhibition is associated with a specific concentration of the drug having the ability to inhibit a critical density of test organisms. The concentration of the drug in the agar is affected by the rate of diffusion, whereas the concentration of the organism is affected by the inoculum density and the rate of growth. The disks, often sold in a cartridge of 50, must be kept refrigerated or frozen until used. They have to sit at room temperature, in a closed container with a desiccant, 1 to 2 hours before use. Disks that have reached the manufacturer's expiration date must be discarded.

The inoculum density is a critical factor in the disk diffusion test. The inoculum may be prepared by suspending colonies from an 18- to 24-hour agar plate into broth or saline. This method is easier and works well into the workflow for most microbiology laboratories. The colonies may also be placed into a broth medium and incubated at 35°C until the appropriate density is achieved if a fresh isolate of organism is not available. It is important to use organisms in the log phase of growth. After 18 to 24 hours, organisms begin dying and will reduce the number of live organisms in the inoculum density.

An inoculum equal to 1.5×10^8 CFU (colony-forming units) per milliliter (mL) is necessary. This is easily obtained by using a density standard for comparison to create the appropriate inoculum. McFarland standards, made from the precipitation of barium chloride and sulfuric acid or latex beads, are a range of tubes with varying turbidities. The inoculum tube is compared to the 0.5 McFarland tube, and saline or broth is added until the turbidity of the inoculum equals that of the standard tube. Figure 11-7 ■ demonstrates the range of McFarland standard tubes used in most microbiology laboratories. A small spectrophotometer offers a more convenient, faster, and reliable means to verify the turbidity of an inoculum.

REAL WORLD TIP

A 0.5 McFarland standard should yield an absorbance of 0.08 to 0.1 at 625 nm wavelength using a spectrophotometer with a 1 cm light path.

Once the inoculum is at the appropriate density, there should be no more than a 15-minute delay before it is plated onto the agar plate. Extending the time to inoculation may

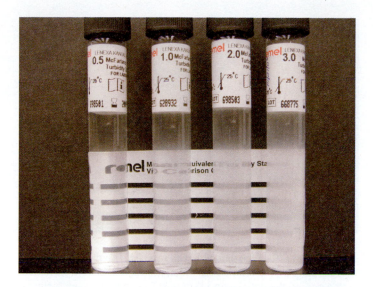

 FIGURE 11-7 McFarland standards. This array of McFarland tubes displays the variety of turbidity standards used in the microbiology laboratory. The black-lined comparison card, behind the tubes, provides a visual means for easier comparison of the turbidity of the standard and inoculum.

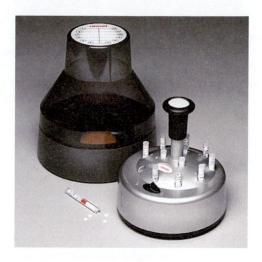

 FIGURE 11-8 Antibiotic dispenser. This dispenser allows for storage and delivery of up to eight different antibiotics. The device is placed on top of the inoculated agar plate, and the large handle in the center is pressed down. This releases one of each of the eight disks, at the appropriate distance from each other and the agar's edge, onto the agar surface. Sterile forceps are then used to gently tap each disk to ensure it adheres to the agar surface when the plate is inverted for incubation.
Photo courtesy of Remel, part of Thermo Fisher Scientific.

allow the organisms to continue cell division and may falsely reduce the diameter zones. A sterile swab is dipped into the inoculum, and excess liquid is expressed. The swab is used to create a solid lawn of growth in three directions across the entire surface of the agar. Once done, the swab should be run around the edge of the agar, where it meets the plastic petri disk. The plate should sit for a few minutes to allow excess moisture to be absorbed, but there should be no more than a 15-minute delay in placement of the antibiotic disks. Extending the time to placement of the disks allows the organisms to get a head start on growing, and results may appear falsely resistant.

After placement of the disks, the agar plate is inverted and incubated at 35°C in ambient air. If the plate is not inverted, moisture can collect on the lid, rain down onto the disks, and diffuse the antibiotic across the surface of the agar. The disk diffusion agar plate is incubated for 16 to 18 hours. If read prior to 16 hours, the results may be falsely susceptible. Reading after 18 hours, unless recommended by CLSI, usually results in false resistance.

> **REAL WORLD TIP**
>
> The generation time of some organisms can be as little as 20 minutes. If the inoculum broth or inoculated agar plates sits for more than 20 minutes, the number of bacteria present may have doubled, and this will affect the susceptibility results negatively.

> **REAL WORLD TIP**
>
> When using the disk diffusion test, *Staphylococcus* spp. is incubated for a total of 24 hours if it appears sensitive to oxacillin and vancomycin at 16 to 18 hours of incubation. Oxacillin- and vancomycin-resistant *Staphylococcus* spp. are slow growing. This is also true for vancomycin-sensitive *Enterococcus* spp., which require additional incubation time to detect.

The use of a 150 mm Mueller-Hinton agar plate allows the placement of multiple antibiotic disks. No more than 12 disks should be placed 24 mm, from disk center to disk center, from each other and from the edge of the agar. A 100 mm agar plate will accommodate up to 5 disks. Once the antibiotic disk touches the agar surface, the antibiotic begins to diffuse, and it cannot be moved. Most laboratories use a disk dispenser for storage and dispensing of antibiotics disks. Figure 11-8 ■ shows a self-tamping antibiotics disk dispenser.

Alteration of any of the standardized factors can have a negative effect on the disk diffusion results. The standardized factors ensure the results obtained are accurate, reliable, and reproducible. If the inoculum is too light, a longer period of time is required to reach the critical density. The antibiotic will diffuse farther, and the zone sizes are larger. Results can be interpreted as falsely susceptible. Conversely, if the inoculum is too heavy, the critical density of the microorganism is reached before diffusion of the antibiotic is sufficient. The antibiotic zone will be smaller. In this case, results can be incorrectly interpreted as falsely resistant. Figure 11-9 ■ demonstrates the effect of a heavy inoculum on susceptibility test results.

The rate of diffusion can be affected by agar concentration and hence the solidity of the agar medium. An agar concentration between 1.5% and 2.0% is within the range of acceptability. This concentration allows the free diffusion of the drug into the medium.

The activity of certain antibiotics, such as penicillin, can be adversely affected by pH, and this has a significant effect on zone sizes. An acceptable pH range is 7.2 to 7.4. For this reason, fermentable carbohydrates, which could lead to the production of metabolic acids, must be omitted from the formulation of the agar growth medium. Mueller-Hinton is the recommended agar for the disk diffusion susceptibility method. If the pH of the Mueller-Hinton agar is too low, it can lead to false resistance with the aminoglycosides, erythromycin, and clindamycin and false susceptibility with tetracycline and penicillin. Figure 11-10 ■ illustrates the difference in zone diameters that can occur when the agar pH is too low. A pH greater than 7.4 displays false susceptibility with the aminoglycosides, erythromycin, and clindamycin.

In addition, susceptibility plates should not be placed in an incubator under conditions of increased carbon dioxide concentration. CO_2 reacts with water on the surface of the medium, creating carbonic acid, which decreases the pH:

$$H_2O + CO_2 \rightarrow H_2CO_3 \rightarrow H^+ + HCO_3^-$$

The resulting carbonic acid may negatively affect the activity of some antibiotics, as noted in the previous paragraph.

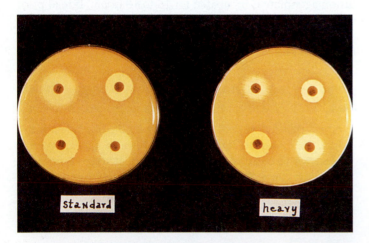

■ **FIGURE 11-9** Disk diffusion with heavy inoculum. The disk diffusion agar plate on the left was plated using an inoculum equal to a density of 1.5×10^8 CFU (colony-forming units) per milliliter (mL), whereas the agar plate on the right was done using a heavier inoculum. Note the smaller zone sizes on the heavy inoculum agar plate compared to the corresponding zones on the agar plate on the left. Using an inoculum with turbidity greater than the recommended 0.5 McFarland may create zone diameters, which are interpreted as falsely resistant.
From Public Health Image Library (PHIL), CDC/Gilda L. Jones.

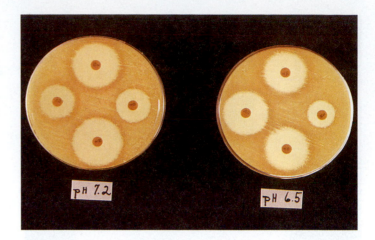

■ **FIGURE 11-10** Disk diffusion with low pH. The disk diffusion agar plate on the left has the recommended pH of 7.2, whereas the one on the right has a pH of 6.5. The same four antibiotic disks were placed on each agar plate in the same location for comparison. Note the dramatic difference in zone diameters for the antibiotics at 9 o'clock and 3 o'clock on both agar plates. When the agar pH is too low, the zone sizes for the aminoglycosides, erythromycin, and clindamycin will become smaller, as seen in the disks at 3 o'clock. The zone sizes for tetracycline and penicillin will be larger as noted at 9 o'clock.
From Public Health Image Library (PHIL), CDC/ Gilda L. Jones.

The thymidine or thymine level of the Mueller-Hinton agar can affect the susceptibility results of the sulfonamides and trimethoprim. Thymidine and thymine compete with sulfonamide and trimethoprim for the same sites in the synthesis of folic acid. This negates the bacteriostatic action of this group of antibiotics, and they appear falsely resistant. Commercial Mueller-Hinton agar is made with as little thymidine as possible.

℮ REAL WORLD TIP

New lots of Mueller-Hinton agar should be tested for appropriate thymidine levels using *Enterococcus faecalis* and trimethoprim-sulfamethoxazole. If the thymidine levels are acceptable, *E. faecalis* will exhibit a zone of inhibition with a diameter of greater than 20 mm. If the levels are too high, then there will be no zone of inhibition.

The levels of cations, such as calcium, magnesium, and zinc, can affect the results of carbapenems, tetracycline, and the aminoglycosides with *Pseudomonas aeruginosa*. High levels of zinc will cause false resistance against the carbapenems. Magnesium and calcium are antagonists of the aminoglycosides.

Low concentrations will create false susceptibility, whereas high concentrations will lead to false resistance. Daptomycin presents with false resistant zones with low concentrations of calcium, whereas high concentrations may create false susceptible zones.

Even the amount of agar in the plate has to be considered, as the depth of the agar can affect zone sizes. A uniform depth of approximately 4 mm is recommended because thinner plates lead to increased zone sizes, which may be falsely interpreted as susceptible, whereas deeper depths are associated with zones of decreased diameters and may be interpreted as falsely resistant. It stands to reason that the antibiotic would diffuse along two planes, radial, spreading outward from the disk like the spokes on a bicycle wheel, through the medium as well as downward into the agar and therefore would be affected by the depth of the agar.

Zone sizes tend to increase, depending on the incubation temperature. Diffusion of the antibiotic increases as the temperature rises because the viscosity of the agar decreases. There may be false susceptibility of organisms to certain antibiotics with increased temperatures, particularly antibiotics that affect DNA replication and protein or cell wall synthesis. In both cases, the end result would be inappropriately larger zone sizes. One should also consider the possibility that lower temperatures could decrease the rate of growth and therefore prolong the time required to reach a critical density of organism. This, too, could result in larger zone sizes in the same manner as a light inoculum does. It is plausible that stacking too many sensitivity plates could have the effect of prolonging growth because the center plates would take a longer time to reach the correct incubation temperature.

Reading a disk diffusion susceptibility test takes some experience and skill to master. The agar plate must be inspected to ensure the growth is adequate and appears as a solid lawn of growth of one organism. The agar plate is held inverted over a black surface. Using overhead light and the unaided eye, measure the diameter of the obvious margin of the zone of inhibition, including the disk, using a ruler or a sliding caliper. The result is recorded in millimeters (mm). Ignore the swarming of *Proteus* spp. over the zone of inhibition of some antibiotics.

 Checkpoint! 11–9 (Chapter Objective 7)

The disk agar diffusion technique is being used to determine the antibiotic susceptibility of E. coli isolated from a urinary tract infection. Forty minutes elapses between the time the inoculum is applied to the surface of the Mueller-Hinton agar plate and the application of the discs impregnated with antibiotics. What effect might this have on the interpretation of zone sizes?

A. *No effect*
B. *Potential for false resistance*
C. *Potential for false susceptibility*

 REAL WORLD TIP

- The disk diffusion test for *Staphylococcus* spp. and oxacillin and vancomycin, as well as *Enterococcus* spp. and vancomycin, is read much more closely than the traditional method. The lid of the agar plate is removed, and the agar plate is held, agar side up, to a light source (transmitted light) to look for individual colonies that may be present in the zone of inhibition around the disk. The presence of one colony may mean the organism is resistant.

- The incidence of vancomycin-resistant *Staphylococcus* spp. (VRSA) in the United States has been very low to date. The presence of even one colony of *Staphylococcus* spp. in the zone of inhibition for vancomycin may mean the organism is a potential VRSA. Further testing of the resistant colony is essential to ensure it is not a contaminant. Reporting VRSA has major consequences for the patient and facility and should be done only after rigorous testing.

DILUTION METHODS

Tube broth dilution, microtube or microtiter tray dilution, and agar dilution tests can be used quantitatively to obtain MICs, as well as qualitatively to obtain sensitive, intermediate, or resistant results. In all of these, twofold serial dilutions of the antimicrobial agent are made. The test organism is added to the different concentrations of the drug, and after an appropriate incubation period, each dilution is examined for growth, which is indicated by turbidity of the growth medium. If the organism is susceptible, growth of the test organism will be inhibited at a particular concentration, which is usually expressed in micrograms per milliliter (μg/mL). These methods are standardized for most of the same factors as the disk diffusion method. Table 11-8✪ summarizes examples of standardized factors for both disk diffusion and dilution methods and the effect if any are modified.

Macrodilution and Microdilution

The MIC is the lowest concentration of antimicrobial agent that inhibits in vitro growth of the microbe and is interpreted as the concentration of the last tube or microtiter well, in the broth method, or agar plate where visible growth cannot be detected (National Committee for Clinical Laboratory Standards [NCCLS], 2003). The MIC numeric value as well as an interpretation of sensitive, intermediate, or resistant is reported to provide the physician quantitative results. The objective of determining an MIC is to achieve antibiotic serum levels that inhibit growth of the pathogen at both peak, or highest, level of antimicrobial agent in vivo, and trough, or lowest, level of antimicrobial agent in vivo,

✪ TABLE 11-8

Examples of Standardized Factors Used in Disk Diffusion and Broth Dilution Methods and the Effect of Changes

Standardized Factor	Effect of Change
Inoculum equal to 0.5 McFarland	■ Too heavy = potential for false resistance ■ Too light = potential for false susceptibility
Less than 15-minute delay to inoculation of testing medium	■ >15 minutes delay = potential for false resistance
Less than 15-minute delay to application of antibiotic disks	■ >15 minutes delay = potential for false resistance
Depth of agar (4 mm)	■ Too shallow = potential for false susceptibility ■ Too deep = potential for false resistance
Incubation time (16–18 hours)	■ <16 hours incubation = potential for false susceptibility ■ >18 hours incubation = potential for false resistance
Incubation atmosphere (ambient air)	■ Incubation in CO_2 = potential for false resistance

pH (7.2–7.4)	■ Decreased pH
	  ■ Potential for false resistance with clindamycin and aminoglycosides
	  ■ Potential for false susceptibility with tetracycline, penicillins, macrolides, and quinolones
	■ Increased pH
	  ■ Potential for false susceptibility with clindamycin and aminoglycosides
	  ■ Potential for false resistance with tetracycline, penicillins, macrolides, and quinolones

Thymidine or thymine level	■ Increased levels = potential for false resistance with trimethoprim-sulfamethoxazole
Cation concentration (Mg^{++}, Ca^{++}, and Zn^{++})	■ Increased Mg^{++} and Ca^{++} content = potential for false resistance with aminoglycosides and tetracycline ■ Decreased Mg^{++} and Ca^{++} content = potential for false susceptibility with aminoglycosides and tetracycline ■ Increased Zn^{++} content = potential for false resistance with carbapenems ■ Increased Ca^{++} content = potential for false susceptibility with daptomycin ■ Decreased Ca^{++} content = potential for false resistance with daptomycin

concentrations in the dosing cycle. The goal of the clinician is to achieve and maintain an antibiotic level at least two to four times the MIC value at the site of infection. In urinary tract infections, such as cystitis, urine rather than serum levels should be used.

Many of the standardized factors used for the disk diffusion susceptibility test apply to the broth dilution test as well. Mueller-Hinton broth is used as the base medium for the antimicrobial agents. One major difference is the density of the inoculum used. For macro tube dilution, a twofold serial dilution of each antimicrobial agent is prepared in 13×100 mm test tubes with a minimum volume of 1 mL. The potential pathogen is used to create an inoculum, in broth or 0.9% saline, equal to a 0.5 McFarland standard or 1.5×10^8 CFUs (colony-forming units) per milliliter (mL). This inoculum is then diluted again 1:150 so there is now 1×10^6 CFU/mL. One milliliter of the inoculum is added to each tube of the serial dilution of the antimicrobial agent. This results in a final organism density of 5×10^5 CFU/mL.

In the microdilution version, serial dilutions of the antimicrobial agent are made in a microtiter tray with a minimum volume of 0.1 mL. The initial inoculum, equal to a 0.5 McFarland standard, is diluted 1:10, and 0.0005 mL of the final inoculum is inoculated into each well. The final organism density, in each well, is 5×10^5 CFU/mL.

After inoculation of the tubes or microtiter well, a drop of the final inoculum is struck onto a sheep blood agar plate. This serves as a quality control measure. It provides a visual means to ensure adequate growth and purity of the organism tested. It is often known as the CFU or colony-forming unit agar plate.

In the macrodilution method, growth appears as turbidity. In the microdilution method growth usually appears as a button in the bottom of the well. The lowest concentration of antimicrobial agent that visibly inhibits growth is the MIC. If there is growth in a series of tubes or wells and one, unexpectedly, displays no growth, ignore this skip. If there are multiple skips in a series, do not report the results for this antimicrobial agent. Figure 11-11 ■ demonstrates a microtiter MIC panel with serial dilutions of multiple antimicrobial agents.

Broth dilution is useful in establishing criteria for new antibiotics not standardized for disk agar diffusion testing and

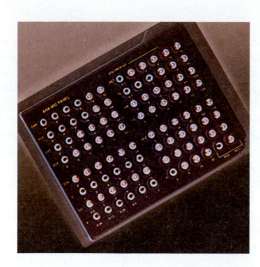

■ FIGURE 11-11 Microtiter broth susceptibility method. This microdilution MIC method uses a microtiter tray for the serial dilutions of multiple antibiotics. Reading each agent from left to right, the first well or lowest concentration visibly displaying inhibition of growth is the MIC. In the lower right wells of the microtiter, note the sterility control well as well as a positive control well to ensure the organism grows using this method.
Photo courtesy of Remel, part of Thermo Fisher Scientific.

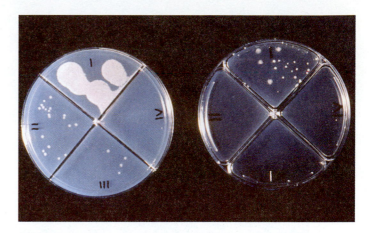

■ FIGURE 11-12 Agar dilution. In this agar dilution susceptibility method, assume the lowest concentration of the antimicrobial agent is present in quadrant I and increases in quadrants II, III, and IV. The agar plate on the left should be reported using the antimicrobial agent concentration present in quadrant IV as the MIC value. The agar plate on the right is reported using quadrant II as the MIC value.
From Public Health Image Library (PHIL), CDC.

determining susceptibility to antibiotics, such as the polymyxins, which diffuse poorly in agar. There is the added advantage of looking at the effect of combinations of particular antimicrobial agents to evaluate the possibility of synergistic or antagonistic effects.

Agar Dilution

Dilutions of an antimicrobial agent can be incorporated into individual agar plates to determine an organism's MIC. Agar dilution methods are valid for use with slow growers such as fungi and mycobacteria and anaerobes. If a separate plate is used for each antimicrobial agent dilution, multiple organisms can be spotted onto each. The final organism density on each plate should be 10^4 organisms per spot. The MIC is interpreted as the lowest concentration that visibly inhibits the organism. Ignore agar plates that show only one colony present. Figure 11-12 ■ illustrates an example of an agar dilution susceptibility method.

COMBINATION OF DIFFUSION AND DILUTION

The gradient diffusion method, or Etest, is a variation of the disk diffusion test that provides quantitative rather than qualitative values. It is often called an MIC on a stick. It is used for rapidly growing aerobes and facultative aerobes. It can also be used for anaerobes as well as fastidious organisms such as *Haemophilus* spp., *Neisseria* spp., and *Streptococcus pneumoniae*. The agar and suspension medium as well as inoculum turbidity, incubation atmosphere, and time can differ for anaerobes and fastidious organisms. Many of the standardized factors in

place for disk diffusion are also used for the gradient diffusion method.

In this method, a plastic-coated strip contains a gradient or gradually increasing concentration of an antimicrobial agent on the side that makes contact with the inoculated agar. An interpretation scale is printed on the side facing up from the agar. If a 150 mm agar plate is used, several strips can be arranged like the spokes on a wheel on the agar surface to allow as many as five different antimicrobial agents to be tested on one plate.

After incubation, the end result is an elliptical zone of inhibition relative to the concentration of the antimicrobial agent along the strip. The value of the MIC can be determined by reading the interpretative scale at the place the zone of inhibition intersects the strip. Reading and interpreting results for this test can be tricky for some organisms and antibiotic combinations. Refer to the manufacturer's package insert for a detailed interpretation of results. Results have been shown to correlate well with standard agar dilution methods. Figure 11-13 ■ demonstrates a vancomycin Etest strip tested against *Staphylococcus aureus*.

 Checkpoint! 11–10 (Chapter Objective 8)

Which of the following methods provides a quantitative MIC value using an agar base?

    A. Macro broth dilution
    B. Micro broth dilution
    C. Gradient strip
    D. Disk diffusion

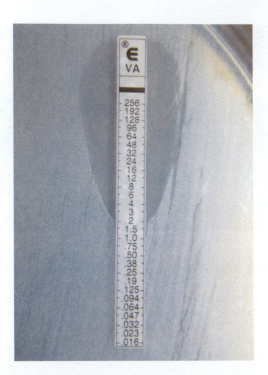

■ **FIGURE 11-13** Gradient strip. This isolate of *Staphylococcus aureus* demonstrates a vancomycin MIC of 2 μg/mL using the gradient diffusion method. Ignore the tiny band of inhibition extending from the 2.0 to 1.0 value on the right hand side of the strip. The MIC is determined by connecting the two ends of the ellipse where they meet the strip with an imaginary line. If the line falls between two dilutions, round the MIC up to the higher dilution.

COMMERCIAL AUTOMATED SUSCEPTIBILITY TESTING SYSTEMS

The disk and gradient diffusion as well as broth and agar dilution susceptibility tests are standardized to ensure accurate and reproducible results. There is still a human factor involved in setting up, reading, and interpretation which is more difficult to standardize. Although costs are often reasonable for these methods, they can be labor intensive.

There is now instrumentation available that can measure, record, and review the zone sizes of disk diffusion results. Interpretation of results is done based on software that uses CLSI recommendations. It can recognize unlikely results and potential resistance mechanisms. Some instruments have the ability to use the disk diffusion results to predict the MIC value.

Automated broth dilution systems have been available for about 30 years. These instruments are able to detect growth in microvolumes of broth with various dilutions of antimicrobial agents. Results may be available in as soon as 6 hours because of the small volumes used for testing. Detection is photometric, turbidimetric, or fluorometric, depending on the system. Most instruments are able to perform identification as well as susceptibility testing.

Automated systems tend to be very expensive, but the increased reproducibility, decreased labor costs, and potential for rapid results can outweigh the cost. These systems are still meant for rapidly growing organisms, so traditional disk diffusion and broth dilution tests are still needed for other organisms. The automated systems have software, with rules and algorithms, that interprets the results based on published recommendations. The software can verify that the results of bacterial identification and susceptibility testing correlate. It makes recommendations when the results do not make sense. For example, it will flag *Klebsiella pneumoniae* when it tests as susceptible to ampicillin. This is highly improbable because of *K. pneumoniae*'s ability to produce beta-lactamase, which destroys ampicillin.

Most microbiologists have a difficult time trying to remain current on all the CLSI recommendations as well as common and emerging resistance mechanisms and their detection. The use of this susceptibility testing interpretation software is a major advantage of automated systems. These systems have shown difficulty detecting some resistance mechanisms, but the manufacturers have done a reasonable job keeping up with emerging resistance mechanisms and their detection.

The antimicrobial agent panels available cover the range of agents in use in most facilities. The manufacturers can create unique panels for institutions, but they tend to be too costly for most to purchase. There is often a delay in the addition of new antimicrobial agents. The use of another method is usually needed if the physician requests testing against the latest agent not available on the manufacturer's antimicrobial panel.

▶ SPECIAL METHODS AND PROCEDURES FOR DETECTING RESISTANCE

Special methods and procedures may be needed to detect resistance in some organisms, depending on the susceptibility testing techniques used. Before use, automated commercial systems must be tested and challenged to ensure they can detect resistance mechanisms. If the automated instrument cannot detect all known resistance mechanisms, then supplemental testing must be performed.

Staphylococcus spp., *Enterococcus* spp., and now more and more gram-negative rods have acquired resistance mechanisms, which may not be easily detected with traditional testing. CLSI provides guidelines for special procedures for the detection of resistance beyond the traditional susceptibility testing.

@ REAL WORLD TIP

Dr. Paul Schreckenberger says much of microbiology is now mental microbiology. Testing, such as antibiotic susceptibility testing, is often easy to set up, but it is now much more difficult to know if the answer is correct (Schreckenberger, 2008).

MINIMUM BACTERICIDAL CONCENTRATION

As a follow-up to finding an organism's MIC to an antimicrobial agent, the minimal bactericidal concentration (MBC) or killing level can be determined. The MBC can be obtained by subculturing to an agar-based medium all of the dilutions where there is no visible growth. After a visual inspection, an aliquot (10 or 100 μL) is taken from each MIC tube or well not showing visible growth and is spread across the entire surface of a separate agar plate. Following incubation, examine the MBC plates for growth or lack of colony growth for each dilution subcultured. The absence of growth indicates the level of antibiotic was bactericidal, whereas the appearance of colonies on the agar surface indicates the level was bacteriostatic.

Usually the MIC and MBC are within one to two dilutions of each other, but there have been cases where an organism exhibits an MBC that is significantly higher than the MIC. This is a situation that may have therapeutic implications, as the organism may be developing a tolerance for that drug. Indications for this test include serious infections in immunocompromised individuals who require higher levels of antimicrobial agents to fight infection as well as serious infections located in sites that are difficult to reach with antimicrobial agents such as osteomyelitis and meningitis.

SERUM BACTERICIDAL TEST

The serum bactericidal test, also known as the Schlicter test, was developed to measure the serum bactericidal activity of an antibiotic in cases of systemic infection such as infective endocarditis. In this method, the patient's bacterial pathogen is isolated in culture. The patient's blood is drawn at the peak level of the antimicrobial agent, which is about 30 to 60 minutes after a dose is given. The trough level is drawn about 15 to 30 minutes before the next dose. Each serum is serially diluted, and a standardized amount of the patient's organism is added.

The serum titer level that prevents growth of the pathogen can be determined as well as the effect of antibiotic combinations. In making an interpretation of the test results, the endpoint is the lowest dilution of the patient's serum that will kill 99.9% of the organisms present. A peak serum level of >1:64 and a trough level of >1:32 is considered appropriate for treatment of bacterial endocarditis. This test is rarely used because of the presence of so many uncontrollable variables. It is usually performed by reference laboratories.

BETA-LACTAMASE

Beta-lactamase is a very common resistance mechanism used by many different bacteria. Hundreds of beta-lactamases have been identified in gram-positive and gram-negative organisms. These beta-lactamases have the ability to affect the penicillins, cephalosporins, carbapenems, and monobactams, depending on the organism. Most clinical laboratories perform routine beta-lactamase testing on *Staphylococcus* spp., *Moraxella catarrhalis*, *Neisseria gonorrhoeae*, *Haemophilus* spp., and *Enterococcus* spp. Testing for beta-lactamase production in the *Enterobacteriaceae* and other gram-negative rods can be a problem for automated commercial systems. It has become a complicated process to understand and incorporate in the clinical laboratory and is discussed later in this chapter.

There are three recognized methods of detection of beta-lactamase by *Staphylococcus* spp., *Moraxella catarrhalis*, *Neisseria gonorrhoeae*, *Haemophilus* spp., and *Enterococcus* spp. The acidimetric method involves a penicillin solution with a pH indicator such as phenol red. If the organism produces beta-lactamase, the solution changes from red to yellow. Penicillin is broken down into penicilloic acid, which creates an acid environment and changes the color of the pH indicator. It is used for testing *Staphylococcus* spp., *Haemophilus* spp., and *Neisseria gonorrhoeae.*

The iodometric method is based on the organism's ability to break down penicillin in a starch solution. Often the solution is dried onto filter paper. If the organism is able to break down penicillin, penicilloic acid is produced. An iodine solution is added to the filter paper after it has been inoculated with organism. If penicilloic acid is present, it combines with the iodine and there is no color change. If the organism is beta-lactamase negative, the iodine combines with the starch to create a purple color. This method is rarely used in clinical laboratories today. It can be used to test *Neisseria gonorrhoeae.*

Most facilities use the chromogenic cephalosporin or nitrocefin method for detection of beta-lactamase. Nitrocefin is a cephalosporin, containing a beta-lactam ring, which has the unique ability to change colors. When the beta-lactam ring of nitrocefin is broken, it turns pink. Figure 11-14 ■ demonstrates two organisms that are beta-lactamase positive by the chromogenic cephalosporin or nitrocefin method.

The test is usually used on *Haemophilus* spp., *N. gonorrhoeae*, *Moraxella catarrhalis*, *Enterococcus* spp., and *Staphylococcus* spp. If a *Staphylococcus* spp. isolate does not test positive on initial testing, it is recommended that it be retested after exposure to oxacillin or cefoxitin. Some strains require exposure to a beta-lactam to induce the production of beta-lactamase. Induction can be done in a broth or from the growth at the edge of a disk diffusion test. The test is read immediately for most organisms, but should be held up to an hour for *Staphylococcus* spp. Automated commercial susceptibility systems have incorporated

 Checkpoint! 11–11 (Chapter Objective 11)

Which of the following statements is true for both the serum bactericidal test and the minimum bactericidal concentration test?

A. *Both are a measure of the bactericidal level of an antibiotic.*

B. *Both involve the use of a patient's peak and trough serum for testing.*

C. *Both use an endpoint equal to 99.9% kill of the organisms present.*

D. *Both are an extension of the minimum inhibitory concentration test.*

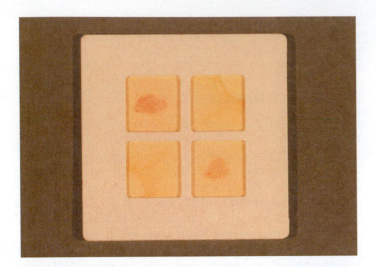

■ **FIGURE 11-14** Nitrocefin test. This chromogenic cephalosporin or nitrocefin test demonstrates two organisms that are beta lactamase positive. They are located in the upper-left and lower-right squares. The pink color is because of the color changing or chromogenic cephalosporin. When its beta-lactam ring is broken because of the presence of beta-lactamase, it turns pink.

beta-lactamase into their panels, and testing at the bench for *Staphylococcus* spp. is rarely done.

STAPHYLOCOCCUS AUREUS

Detection of Oxacillin Resistance

Methicillin-resistant strains of *Staphylococcus aureus* (MRSA) have become a significant problem in the hospital setting and more recently in the community setting because of their increasing frequency as the cause of serious invasive infections leading to sepsis, endocarditis, and other life-threatening illnesses. The hospital-acquired strains are usually multiresistant, whereas the community-acquired strains tend not to exhibit multiresistance. Both strains flourish even in the presence of a beta-lactam antibiotic because the penicillin-binding proteins (PBP) of the organism have been altered because of acquisition of the *mec*A gene. The beta-lactam antibiotic lacks the sufficient affinity for the altered PBP called PBP2a. They are resistant to all beta-lactams antibiotics, including the cephalosporins and carbapenems. These organisms must be challenged with non-beta-lactam agents, such as the glycopeptide vancomycin, which act to interfere with cell wall synthesis in a different manner (Forbes et al., 2007).

Two other mechanisms may be responsible for MRSA. One possible method proposed is the overproduction of beta-lactamase. With enough enzymes, even the penicillinase-resistant penicillins can be destroyed (Chambers, 1997). Another potential means is because of strains that do not contain the *mec*A gene. They can have modified PBP genes that do not bind as well with the beta-lactams or the strains have the ability to over-

produce PBPs (Chambers, 1997). Both mechanisms are rare but may account for borderline or low-level methicillin resistance.

Resistance can be difficult to detect. All the organisms tested may possess the gene for resistance, but only a few may display it when tested. This is known as **heteroresistance.** A small volume of inoculum is used for testing, and so the number of organisms exhibiting resistance is even smaller. These organisms tend to grow more slowly and better at temperatures ≤35°C. They can potentially be overgrown when tested on rapid automated commercial systems. Currently agar- and broth-based methods and nucleic acid amplification tests can detect MRSA.

Oxacillin. Oxacillin resistance is best determined by broth-dilution methods or an agar screen. Automated commercial systems must be validated to ensure the detection of MRSA. The most commonly used agar screen involves the use of Mueller-Hinton agar with 4% NaCl and 6 μg of oxacillin per milliliter. The organism inoculum is standardized to match the turbidity of a 0.5 McFarland standard. Using a sterile swab, spot inoculate the agar with the suspension. The agar is incubated for a full 24 hours at 33 to 35°C in ambient air. It can be held up to 48 hours. Growth of more than one colony on the agar medium is a sign of methicillin resistance, whereas no growth is an indication of susceptibility to methicillin.

REAL WORLD TIP

The oxacillin agar screen cannot be used to detect resistance in coagulase negative *Staphylococcus* spp. There is 6 μg of oxacillin in the agar screen. Coagulase negative *Staphylococcus* spp. is considered resistant at a level of >0.5 μg/mL for oxacillin.

Cefoxitin. Cefoxitin can be used to predict resistance because of the presence of the *mec*A gene in both *Staphylococcus aureus* and coagulase-negative *Staphylococcus* spp., even with heteroresistance. Cefoxitin is able to strongly induce the expression of the *mec*A gene much better than the beta-lactams (Swenson, Skov, & Patel, 2007). It can be performed using a 30 μg cefoxitin disk for the disk diffusion test or done using a broth dilution method. Interpretation of the results differs for *Staphylococcus aureus* and coagulase-negative *Staphylococcus* spp. Refer to the CLSI guidelines for details for interpretation. Cefoxitin can be used alone to accurately determine oxacillin resistance or as a backup test if oxacillin results show borderline resistance. Commercial automated methods are accurate for prediction of resistance because of the *mec*A gene, but not all manufacturers include cefoxitin in their panels (Swenson et al., 2007).

Latex Agglutination. This method detects MRSA, which possess the *mec*A gene, but not those that appear as oxacillin resistant because of hyperproduction of beta-lactamase or other modified PBPs. The basis of the test is a monoclonal antibody against the product of the *mec*A gene—PBP2a. A heavy inoculum is required. The PBP2a is extracted with the use of reagents and heat. The test can be used for testing coagulase negative *Staphylococcus* spp. They must first be induced to produce PBP2a by performing disk diffusion with oxacillin prior to testing. Colonies growing closest to the disk are used for testing. Although it has been shown to be a good test, all the required manipulation delays results for the patient.

Chromogenic Agar.

Direct specimens, often nasal and perianal swabs, can be inoculated onto a specialized agar. Chromogenic agar is selective and differential for MRSA. The addition of an antibiotic such as oxacillin or cefoxitin selects for methicillin resistant organisms. A chromogenic or color changing substrate specific, for *Staphylococcus aureus,* is also incorporated. MRSA then creates pigmented, such as mauve or denim blue, colonies that are easily differentiated from other organisms that may grow. The agar plates are read at 24 hours and again at 48 hours if no suspicious colonies are present. These agars have been shown to be cost effective, but results may not be available for 48 hours. Most facilities use chromogenic agar to cost effectively screen surveillance specimens for MRSA from hospitalized patients. Susceptibility testing is usually not performed on surveillance cultures. The key information is the presence of MRSA. Patients harboring MRSA must remain in isolation. Those with negative surveillance cultures can be removed from isolation and thereby save the facility money.

Nucleic Acid Detection.

Another method for detecting MRSA is to identify the presence of the gene responsible for methicillin resistance, the *mec*A gene. This can be accomplished through the use of molecular diagnostics on colonies or directly on specimens. Molecular methods, such as PCR, detect the staphylococcal cassette chromosome (SCC). This mobile piece of DNA carries the *mec*A gene. Real-time PCR or polymerase chain reaction can be used to amplify the gene encoding resistance to increase sensitivity and specificity. Although molecular methods tend to be expensive, they can provide results from direct specimens much faster than traditional testing using colonies. The increased cost in testing is often offset by the savings in infection control measures. Additional information on molecular diagnostics can be found in ∞ Chapter 9, "Final Identification."

Detection of Inducible Clindamycin Resistance

Hospital-acquired strains of MRSA are usually erythromycin and clindamycin resistant. Many community-acquired strains are usually susceptible to clindamycin, so it is still a viable option for treatment of skin and soft tissue infections. Erythromycin, a macrolide, and clindamycin, a lincosamide, have similar modes of actions on bacteria. They both inhibit protein synthesis.

Erythromycin resistance is because of two possible genes. The *msr*A gene allows the organisms to pump the antibiotic out. This resistance mechanism is known as efflux. The *erm*

gene creates an enzyme that can also lead to resistance. Erythromycin resistance because of the *erm* gene can trigger a resistance enzyme for clindamycin as well. The resulting clindamycin resistance is either always present or is only induced with exposure to erythromycin. When an MRSA isolate is erythromycin resistant and clindamycin susceptible, further testing is needed. Without testing, it is not known if the clindamycin result is valid because the organism may never have been exposed to erythromycin (induced).

The "D," or disk approximation, test determines if erythromycin resistance can induce resistance to clindamycin. The edge of an erythromycin disk is placed 15 to 26 mm away from the edge of a clindamycin disk on a Mueller-Hinton agar plate inoculated with the suspect *Staphylococcus* spp. After incubation, examine the appearance of the edge of the clindamycin zone closest to erythromycin. If erythromycin induces clindamycin resistance, a flattened zone will appear in the area between the two disks and the clindamycin zone will look like a "D." Figure 11-15 ■ illustrates an organism that demonstrates inducible clindamycin resistance. Clindamycin should not be used to treat an infection caused by an inducible *S. aureus* strain. Inducible strains have a higher risk for mutations, which can lead to resistance in the presence of either antibiotics (Hindler, 2004).

The "D" test is valid for use with all *Staphylococcus* spp. It can be used for both oxacillin-susceptible and -resistant strains of *S. aureus* as well as coagulase negative *Staphylococcus* spp.

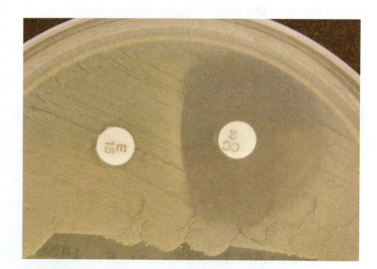

■ **FIGURE 11-15** Inducible clindamycin resistance test. This "D" test demonstrates an MRSA that possesses inducible clindamycin resistance. Note the flattened edge closest to erythromycin (E). The entire clindamycin (CC) zone of inhibition resembles a "D." This organism is erythromycin resistant because of the presence of the *erm* gene. Its presence triggered the inducible *erm* gene for clindamycin. The organism should be reported as clindamycin resistant regardless of the MIC value obtained. Without the "D" test, this organism would have been falsely reported as clindamycin susceptible.

Detection of Vancomycin Resistance

Vancomycin is a critical antibiotic for treatment of serious MRSA infections. Because of the increased use of this glycopeptide, resistance has emerged. There have been seven reported cases of vancomycin-resistant *Staphylococcus aureus* (VRSA) since 2002. Each case had a history of infection or colonization with MRSA and vancomycin-resistant *Enterococcus* spp. (VRE) and had received prior vancomycin therapy. The VRSA isolated were MRSA, which became resistant because of acquisition of the *van*A gene from VRE.

Vancomycin intermediate *Staphylococcus aureus* (VISA) are also rare but still an emerging issue. These organisms possess a vancomycin MIC in the range of 4 to 8 µg/mL. They often appear as pinpoint colonies that do not look like a typical *S. aureus*. ∞ Chapter 17, Figure 17-10, provides an image that demonstrates the difference in colony size of VISA compared to *S. aureus*. Once removed from vancomycin, on subculture, the colonies resemble a typical *S. aureus* colony and become vancomycin susceptible again.

Detection of VISA and VRSA is not valid using disk diffusion because the disk zones cannot differentiate VISA from susceptible strains. Methods such as the gradient diffusion or Etest, broth dilution, agar dilution, or automated commercial systems that have been validated and provide a MIC value are recommended to detect VISA and VRSA. A vancomycin screen agar should be used in tandem with routine validated and nonvalidated susceptibility testing. A brain heart infusion (BHI) agar containing 6 µg/mL of vancomycin is recommended. Any growth on the agar is a possible VISA or VRSA. The use of a magnifying glass is recommended for inspection of the agar surface.

VISA is able to grow in the range of 4 to 8 µg/ml of vancomycin. One weakness of the agar screen is that it is not able to detect VISA with an MIC of 4 µg mL. This explains the reasoning behind running the screen plate with an MIC method. Any growth on the vancomycin agar screen requires further testing to determine if the organism is a VISA or VRSA. Even if the vancomycin screen does not grow, any susceptibility method used that provides an intermediate or resistant vancomycin value must also be retested.

The susceptibility of the organism is retested using a validated MIC method to determine the exact level of resistance. The identification of the suspect isolate is reconfirmed. Once confirmed as a possible VISA or VRSA, the organism is saved for future testing as well as sent to the state public health laboratory. The laboratory must notify infection control, the physician, and the Centers for Disease Control and Prevention (CDC) of the isolation of possible VISA/VRSA (CDC, 2006).

ENTEROCOCCUS SPP.

Detection of Glycopeptide (Vancomycin) Resistance

In the mid 1980s the first vancomycin-resistant *Enterococcus* spp. (VRE) was reported. They acquired this trait because of the acquisition of plasmids that encode for the resistance. There are currently six types of resistance associated with *Enterococcus* spp. These include the genes *van*A, *van*B, *van*C, *van*D, *van*E, and *van*G. *Van*A and *van*B are the two most common types associated with VRE. *Van*A demonstrates a high level of resistance to both vancomycin and teicoplanin, a lipoglycopeptide. *Van*B shows variable resistance to vancomycin but is susceptible to teicoplanin. Both can be transferred to other organisms via plasmids. The first VRSA isolated in the U.S. was from a patient with an infection caused by MRSA, VRE, and *Klebsiella oxytoca*. The VRSA probably acquired the *van* gene from the VRE.

*Van*D, *van*E, and *van*G can be transferred to other organisms as well. *Van*D displays variable resistance to vancomycin and teicoplanin. *Van*E and *van*G show low-level resistance to vancomycin and are susceptible to teicoplanin. *Van*C is an intrinsic gene that is always present but cannot be transferred to other organisms. It is found in *Enterococcus gallinarum*, *E. casseliflavus*, and *E. flavescens*. They exhibit a low-level resistance to vancomycin and are teicoplanin susceptible.

Enterococcus faecalis is the most common species isolated in the clinical laboratory. It accounts for up to 80% of isolates, whereas *E. faecium* makes up of about 15%. It is important to differentiate *E. faecalis* and *E. faecium* from *E. gallinarum*, *E. casseliflavus*, and *E. flavescens*. The three former are naturally vancomycin resistant and do not pass their gene, whereas the first two species can acquire and pass the resistance genes. Detection of vancomycin resistance in *Enterococcus* spp. is important for infection control measures. The goal is to place carriers on isolation to prevent passing the organisms possessing the transferable vancomycin resistance genes from person to person.

The vancomycin agar screen uses a BHI agar with 6µg/mL of vancomycin. It is inoculated with a 0.5 McFarland suspension of *Enterococcus* spp. and incubated for a full 24 hours in ambient air at 35°C before interpretation. Any growth, even one colony, is suspicious for vancomycin resistance. The organism should be tested with an MIC method and identified. If the isolate identifies as *E. casseliflavus*, *E. gallinarum*, or *E. flavescens*, it is not an infection control issue. These organisms cannot transfer their resistance gene to other organisms. Refer to ∞ Chapter 17, "Gram-Positive Cocci," for information on the phenotypic differentiation of the *Enterococcus* spp. If an automated commercial system has been validated for the detec-

---

✓ Checkpoint! 11–12 (Chapter Objectives 8 and 10)

One issue with use of the 6 µg/mL vancomycin screen agar for detection of VISA is:

A. *it must be held for 48 hours before results are available.*

B. *the organisms are able to grow in the range of 4 to 8 µg/mL and could be missed.*

C. *it is not validated for use with VISA.*

D. *it does not detect vancomycin resistance because of acquisition of the vanA gene.*

tion of VRE, it can be used and the agar screen eliminated. The gold standard for detection is the use of molecular diagnostics for the presence of the *van* gene.

REAL WORLD TIP

Vancomycin-dependent *Enterococcus* spp. (VDE) have appeared because of the increased use of vancomycin. They have acquired the ability to use vancomycin for cell wall synthesis. On disk diffusion, they are easily recognized because they do not grow on routine media except in the area around the vancomycin disk. Rather than being inhibited by the drug, they are stimulated to grow.

Detection of High Level Aminoglycoside Resistance

Enterococcus spp. are intrinsically resistant to low levels of aminoglycosides. They are often treated with a synergistic combination of a cell wall antimicrobial agent, such as ampicillin or vancomycin, and an aminoglycoside that can overcome the low level resistance. The cell wall agent punches a hole in the organism's cell wall, and then the aminoglycoside can enter and bind with the ribosomes. *Enterococcus* spp. now have the ability to acquire plasmids that encode for high-level resistance to aminoglycosides (HLAR) at levels >2000 µg/mL. These strains are not treatable using the synergistic combination of antimicrobial agents and are an infection control concern.

If the automated commercial susceptibility system has been validated for high-level aminoglycoside resistance, it is appropriate to use. Some facilities may select to use a cost-effective agar screen for detection of HLAR in *Enterococcus* spp. Agar dilution plates, disk diffusion, and broth dilution methods are available. Gentamicin and streptomycin are the best antibiotics to use for testing *Enterococcus* spp. High-level aminoglycoside resistance is being detected, so unique antibiotic levels are used for testing. The disk diffusion tests gentamicin at 120 µg/mL and streptomycin at 300 µg/mL. The agar and broth dilutions both test gentamicin at 500 µg/mL and streptomycin at 1000 µg/mL and 2000 µg/mL, respectively.

The agar dilution method uses an organism suspension equal to the turbidity of a 0.5 McFarland standard. The disk diffusion and broth dilution methods require the same inoculums used for routine susceptibility testing discussed earlier in this chapter. Growth in the presence of either high-level antibiotic, in the agar and broth dilutions methods, indicates HLAR. The disk diffusion zones of inhibition must be >10 mm to be considered susceptible. Those in the range of 7 to 9 mm zone are considered inconclusive and must be verified by another method. A zone of ≤6 mm for either antibiotic is considered resistant to high-level aminoglycosides. All test methods should be incubated at 35°C in ambient air for a full 24 hours before interpretation.

STREPTOCOCCUS PNEUMONIAE

Detection of Penicillin Resistance

There is an increasing level of resistance to penicillin appearing in *Streptococcus pneumoniae*. The use of a penicillin disk screen can provide valuable information without having to perform a full susceptibility test. A 1 µg/mL oxacillin disk is used to screen for resistance to penicillin. It is more sensitive than penicillin in picking up resistance. A Mueller-Hinton agar with sheep blood is the base medium. The isolate inoculum is prepared as for any disk diffusion method. It is incubated for 16 to 18 hours at 35°C in a CO_2 environment. Although most susceptibility tests should not be incubated in a carbon dioxide environment, some *S. pneumoniae* cannot survive without it. This method has been standardized using this medium and atmosphere.

Isolates that demonstrate a zone of inhibition >20 mm can be considered susceptible to penicillin. Those with a zone of <20 mm require further testing. Although oxacillin is more sensitive in picking up resistance, it is almost too sensitive. Those that exhibit a zone of <20 mm can still be penicillin resistant, intermediate, or susceptible. An MIC method, such as gradient diffusion, is needed to verify the result and is used for reporting. Because of the increase in penicillin resistance among *S. pneumoniae,* some facilities have forgone the penicillin screen and proceed to the MIC method.

STREPTOCOCCUS SPP.

Detection of Inducible Clindamycin Resistance

Just as *Staphylococcus* spp. can exhibit inducible clindamycin resistance with exposure to erythromycin, so can beta hemolytic *Streptococcus* spp. The procedure is similar to that of the *Staphylococcus* spp., but a Mueller-Hinton with sheep blood agar is used. The erythromycin and clindamycin disks are placed only 12 mm apart, edge to edge, compared to 15 to 26 mm for the *Staphylococcus* procedure. If the organism displays a flattened edge on the clindamycin zone, so that it resembles a "D," it is considered resistant to clindamycin.

GRAM-NEGATIVE RODS

The gram-negative rods, including the *Enterobacteriaceae* and nonfermenters, have developed hundreds of beta-lactamases, many more than gram-positive organisms, which has led to multiresistant organisms. They have proven to be an infection control nightmare in the hospital setting. Most of the genes responsible are located on chromosomes and can always be on (constitutive) or induced with exposure to antibiotics. Those that are induced may be difficult to detect in the laboratory if the organism has not been previously exposed to the appropriate antibiotics. As a group, they can be resistant to most of the cephalosporins, monobactams, and expanded spectrum penicillins. This leaves few options for treatment. The addition of plasmid mediated enzymes has now only added to the multiresistance of these organisms. Organisms can possess multiple beta-lactamases making their detection an even bigger challenge in most clinical microbiology laboratories. The frequencies with which these multiresistant organisms are appearing make them as frightening as the appearance of the first vancomycin-resistant *Staphylococcus aureus*. Table 11-9 ✪ summarizes the three most significant beta-lactamases that should now be detected in the clinical laboratory.

The beta-lactamases of gram-negative rods can be classified based on their function. Class A beta-lactamases hydrolyze the penicillins, which include the aminopenicillins and penicillinase stable penicillins. They can be inhibited by clavulanic acid. This class of beta-lactamases is the most common. They tend to be plasmid mediated and can be spread among different genera of organisms. The beta-lactamase produced by *Staphylococcus* spp. and *Enterococcus* spp. belong to this class. It also contains the extended spectrum beta-lactamases (ESBL). The ESBLs are discussed in detail later in this chapter. The newest beta-lactamase to appear in class A is the carbapenemases. These are also discussed later in this chapter.

Class B beta-lactamases require a metal ion, such as zinc, to hydrolyze all beta-lactams, including the carbapenems. They can be inhibited in the presence of EDTA, which chelates the metal ions. They are not inhibited by beta-lactamase inhibitors such as clavulanic acid. The only beta-lactam that may be effective is aztreonam. These powerful enzymes can be found on the chromosome of *Stenotrophomonas maltophilia*. Plasmids coding for these enzymes have now been acquired by *Pseudomonas aeruginosa*, *Acinetobacter* spp., and a few *Enterobacteriaceae*. Organisms possessing class B beta-lactamase are often resistant to the fluoroquinolones and aminoglycosides.

The class C beta-lactamases have been found in most of the *Enterobacteriaceae*. It includes the chromosomal AmpC enzyme, a cephalosporinase, which is discussed later in this chapter. Often this class requires exposure to a beta-lactam to induce production of the enzymes. They are not inhibited by the beta-lactamase inhibitor clavulanic acid but sometimes by tazobactam. This class tends to respond to imipenem.

Class D beta-lactamases are not as common as the others. They can be present in *Pseudomonas aeruginosa*, *Acinetobacter baumannii*, and rare *Enterobacteriaceae*. They can show activity against the carbapenems, cephalosporins, penicillins, and oxacillin. They are resistant to beta-lactamase inhibitors.

ESBL

The extended-spectrum beta-lactamases (ESBLs) have the ability to destroy the carboxypenicillins (ticarcillin and carbenicillin), ureidopenicillins (piperacillin and mezlocillin), and aztreonam, as well as the cephalosporins other than cefoxitin. They are usually susceptible to the carbapenems (imipenem, meropenem, doripenem, and ertapenem), the cephamycins (cefoxitin), and the beta-lactamase inhibitors (clavulanic acid,

✪ TABLE 11-9

A Comparison of the Three Most Significant Gram-Negative Rod Beta-Lactamases

Beta-Lactamase	Resistant Antibiotics	Susceptible Antibiotics	Indicator Antibiotic(s)	Additional Testing Necessary	Associated Organisms	Recommended Changes to Antibiotic Results	Other
Extended spectrum beta-lactamase (ESBL)	Carboxypenicillins, ureidopenicillins, aztreonam, cephalosporins other than the cephamycin—cefoxitin	Carbapenems, cephamycins (cefoxitin), beta-lactamase inhibitors	Resistance to ceftazidime, cefotaxime, ceftriaxone, cefpodoxime, cefepime, or aztreonam	ESBL screen	*E. coli, K. pneumoniae, Proteus mirabilis,* other *Enterobacteriaceae*	Change all penicillins, cephalosporins, and aztreonam to resistant	Plasmid mediated
AmpC	1st-, 2nd-, and 3rd-generation cephalosporins, aztreonam, beta-lactamase inhibitors	Carbapenems, 4th-generation cephalosporin—cefepime	Resistance to cefoxitin and susceptible to cefepime	Cefoxitin induction test	*Serratia* spp., *Providencia* spp., *Citrobacter freundii, Enterobacter* spp., *Morganella morganii, Aeromonas* spp., and *Pseudomonas aeruginosa*	No changes to susceptibility testing results, but notify physician of potential for antibiotic therapy failure	Inducible enzyme that can be induced by cefoxitin, imipenem, and ampicillin
Carbapenemase (*Klebsiella pneumoniae* carbapenemase [KPC] or Carbapenem resistant *Enterobacteriaceae* [CRE])	Penicillins, cephalosporins, carbapenems, and aztreonam	Some beta-lactamase inhibitors	Resistance to carbapenems	Hodge test	*Klebsiella* spp., *E. coli,* and other *Enterobacteriaceae*	Change all beta-lactams to resistant	Plasmid mediated

tazobactam, and sulbactam). In addition, they tend to be resistant to the fluoroquinolones and aminoglycosides.

ESBLs were created because of a mutation in the plasmid genes that code for common beta-lactamases, TEM-1, SHV-1, and OXA-1, present in the *Enterobacteriaceae*. Because it is located on a plasmid, it has the potential to be transferred to other organisms. *E. coli* and *Klebsiella* spp. are well known for their ability to produce ESBLs, but now they can be found in *Proteus mirabilis* as well as *Enterobacter* spp., *Serratia* spp., and other *Enterobacteriaceae*. CLSI recommends routine testing of *E. coli*, *Klebsiella* spp., and *Proteus mirabilis* for the presence of ESBL.

The antibiotics ceftazidime, cefotaxime, ceftriaxone, cefpodoxime, cefepime, and aztreonam can act as markers or indicators on the susceptibility testing results for ESBL-producing organisms. All are usually resistant. CLSI provides detailed guidelines for detection of ESBL. Because the beta-lactamase of these organisms is susceptible to clavulanic acid, it can be used as part of the screening process. Both disk diffusion and broth dilutions methods are provided by CLSI. They use ceftazidime and cefotaxime alone and in combination with clavulanic acid. In the disk diffusion method, an increase of >5 mm of the zone of inhibition of the antibiotic plus clavulanic acid indicates an organism that produces ESBL. Figure 11-16 ■ demonstrates detection of an ESBL-producing organism using the disk diffusion method. In the broth dilution a threefold increase in the MIC of the antibiotic plus clavulanic acid is also indicative of an ESBL-producing organism. In both methods, clavulanic acid restores the inhibitory action of the antibiotics. Automated commercial susceptibility systems for the detection of ESBL must be approved by the FDA and validated by the facility before use. Any organism that is shown to produce ESBL, with either antibiotic used for screening,

requires all the penicillins, cephalosporins, and aztreonam be reported as resistant regardless of the initial results.

Checkpoint! 11–13 (Chapter Objective 10)

Which of the following antibiotics would not *be changed to resistant on review of the results of an ESBL-producing organism?*

   A. *Aztreonam*
   B. *Cefotaxime*
   C. *Piperacillin-tazobactam*
   D. *Ceftriaxone*

AmpC

The AmpC enzymes are cephalosporinases and usually located on the organism's chromosome. They are inducible, which means the organism must be exposed to the appropriate antibiotics before they produce high levels of the enzymes. Once induced, the AmpC enzymes act on the first-, second-, and third-generation cephalosporins, the penicillins, and aztreonam, but not the carbapenems and the fourth-generation cephalosporin, cefepime. Organisms are best induced to produce the AmpC enzymes by the presence of cefoxitin, imipenem, and ampicillin. These enzymes are usually associated with *Serratia* spp., *Providencia* spp., *Citrobacter freundii*, *Enterobacter* spp., *Morganella morganii*, *Aeromonas* spp., and *Pseudomonas aeruginosa*.

 REAL WORLD TIP

Dr. Paul Schrekenberger uses the acronym "SPACE" to remember the most common organisms associated with the production of AmpC enzymes (Schreckenberger, 2008).

The AmpC enzymes differ from ESBL in several ways. They are not usually produced by the same organisms. They are not affected by the beta-lactamase inhibitors like ESBL. Once activated, the AmpC susceptibility results can resemble those of an ESBL, but when the ESBL screen is performed, it is negative. The AmpC enzymes act on cefoxitin unlike ESBLs.

The indicator or marker antibiotics for the potential of AmpC enzymes' production include susceptibility to cefepime and resistance to cefoxitin. A disk diffusion method using cefoxitin, cefotetan, or cefmetazole as the inducing antibiotic has been proposed (Sundin, 2009). The suspect organism is tested against cefoxitin as the AmpC inducing antibiotic and ceftazidime as the detection antibiotic. It is set up similar to the *Staphylococcus* "D" or induction test. If the organism produces Amp C enzymes, the cefoxitin will induce production of high levels of the enzymes. There will be no zone around the cefoxitin disk. The zone around ceftazidime is blunted or "D" shaped similar to the zone observed in the *Staphylococcus* spp. clindamycin induction test. This is because of the presence of the AmpC enzymes acting on ceftazidime. Figure 11-17 ■ demonstrates an AmpC induction test in the organism that produces the enzyme.

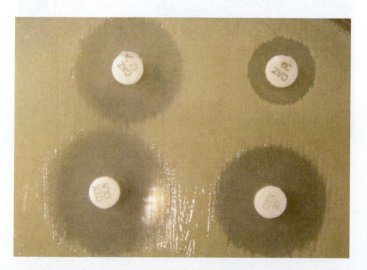

■ **FIGURE 11-16** ESBL screen. This *Klebsiella pneumoniae* demonstrates the ability to produce ESBL. The antibiotics cefotaxime (CTX) and ceftazidime (CAZ) are used alone and in combination with clavulanic acid (CLA). Note the increase in the zone size with the addition of clavulanic acid. The beta-lactamase inhibitor has restored the inhibitory effect of the antibiotic.

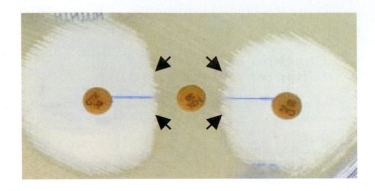

■ **FIGURE 11-17** AmpC induction test. AmpC must be induced to detect its presence in high levels. Cefoxitin is a good inducer of high levels of the AmpC enzyme. In this disk approximation test, the organism being tested produces AmpC in response to the presence of cefoxitin (FOX). In turn, the enzyme hydrolyzes the antibiotics ceftazidime (CAZ) and cefotaxime (CTX). This appears as a blunting or D shape in the zones of inhibition closest to the area where the enzyme is produced.
From Qin, X., Weissman, S. J., Chesnut, M. F., Zhang, B., & Shen, L. (2004). Kirby-Bauer disc approximation to detect inducible third-generation cephalosporin resistance in Enterobacteriaceae. *Annals of Clinical Microbiology and Antimicrobials, 3, 13. Retrieved May 5, 2009 from http://www.ann-clinmicrob.com/content/3/1/13.*

Currently there are no CLSI guidelines for the detection and reporting of these organisms. It is recommended the organisms listed earlier be reported with the original susceptibility results, but the physician should be notified of the potential for development of inducible resistance with therapy (Schreckenberger, 2008).

Carbapenemases

The carbapenems: imipenem, ertapenem, doripenem, and meropenem, are often reserved for serious infections with drug-resistant gram-negative rods. A plasmid has been discovered that now accounts for an enzyme producing resistance to all penicillins, cephalosporins, carbapenems, and aztreonam. It can be inhibited by the beta-lactamase inhibitors, clavulanic acid and tazobactam. This makes it very difficult to treat because there are few antibiotics left that are effective. Currently tigecycline is one of the few antibiotics available for therapy.

It was first discovered in *Klebsiella pneumoniae,* and so the name *Klebsiella pneumoniae* carbapenemase (KPC) has been used. Its presence began, and is more prevalent, in the coastal U.S. states, especially New York, but has not been shown to be widespread in every state to date. Its presence may be greater than believed because laboratories may not be performing the test to detect its presence.

The plasmid has been found rarely in other *Enterobacteriaceae. Klebsiella pneumoniae* appears to be the most common pathogen, but it has also been found in *E. coli.* The name carbapenemase-resistant *Enterobacteriaceae* (CRE) is now used to describe the

organisms that exhibit the enzyme. Because resistance is caused by a plasmid, it has the potential to be transmitted to other organisms, which makes this an infection control issue.

Because it is inhibited by clavulanic acid, a carbapenemase-producing organism may resemble an ESBL producer. It is suggested that any ESBL-positive *K. pneumoniae* or *E. coli* be further tested for the presence of carbapenemase (Sundin, 2009). Ertapenem is the indicator or marker antibiotic for detection of the enzyme. Other carbapenems may appear intermediate or susceptible because the enzyme seems to prefer ertapenem over the others. Any *Enterobacteriaceae* that displays resistance to any carbapenem should be suspicious for carbapenemase.

The modified Hodge test can be used to confirm a suspected carbapenemase-producing *Enterobacteriaceae.* Using the disk diffusion method, a suspension of *E. coli* is prepared and plated onto a Mueller-Hinton agar. One ertapenem or meropenem disk is placed in circle in the center of the agar. Using a loop and three to five colonies of the suspected organism, a straight line is drawn, on top of the *E. coli,* from the edge of the testing disk then out to the edge of the agar plate. After incubation, an organism that produces the enzyme will hydrolyze the carbapenem present. With the antibiotic destroyed, the *E. coli,* which is normally susceptible to the carbapenem, is able to grow up to the disk in the area of the carbapenemase-producing isolate. Figure 11-18 ■

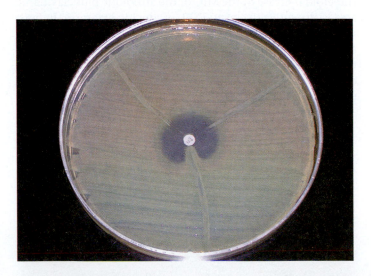

■ **FIGURE 11-18** Hodge test. The Hodge test is used to confirm carbapenemase-producing organisms. Imipenem (IMP) is used here as the carbapenem for testing. A lawn of *E. coli* ATCC 25922 is created, and three suspect organisms were drawn in a line, on top of it, from the edge of the imipenem disk to the agar plate's edge. After incubation, the *Klebsiella pneumoniae,* located at 6 o'clock on the agar plate, demonstrates a positive result. The organism produces carbapenemase, which in turn destroys the imipenem in the area of its growth. The *E. coli* is now able to grow where the antibiotic has been destroyed. The *E. coli,* located at 10 o'clock, and the *K. pneumoniae,* located at 2 o'clock, are not enzyme producers, and the growth of the *E. coli* remains inhibited by the imipenem.
Photo by Laura Knoll, MA, MT(ASCP), CLS(NCA).

illustrates a positive Hodge result and two negative results. Once a carbapenemase-producing organism has been confirmed, all beta-lactams should be reported as resistant.

 REAL WORLD TIP

- Gram-negative rods can acquire any of hundreds of beta-lactamases. They can also exhibit other resistance mechanisms. To make things more complicated, organisms can possess multiple resistance mechanisms making testing and detection difficult. Gram-negative rods can possess and express both AmpC enzymes and ESBL. If this occurs, then treat the susceptibility results as for an ESBL producer (Schreckenberger, 2008). Confirmation of carbapenemase production trumps all other resistance mechanisms detected. All beta-lactam antibiotics should be reported as resistant for carbapenemase-producing organisms (Schreckenberger, 2008).

- Hand hygiene is essential for the prevention of the spread of carbapenemase-producing organisms as well as other multi-drug-resistant organisms. Nurses wearing artificial fingernails have been implicated in nosocomial outbreaks (Gupta et al., 2004).

FASTIDIOUS ORGANISMS

Although susceptibility testing is usually reserved for rapidly growing organisms, CLSI has modified procedures for some fastidious and slow-growing organisms. These include *Streptococcus pneumoniae, Haemophilus influenzae, Neisseria gonorrhoeae,* and *N. meningitidis,* as well as *Helicobacter pylori* and other organisms. The base medium, incubation atmosphere and time, and other standardized factors are adapted to ensure the growth of each organism. Details on the procedures and interpretation criteria can be found in CLSI documents.

 REAL WORLD TIP

It is very important to remember that if there is no standardized procedure or interpretative criteria listed for an organism in the CLSI documents, then it cannot be tested. A good example is vancomycin susceptibility testing for *Staphylococcus aureus.* An MIC method is valid for detection of vancomycin resistance, but there are no interpretive criteria for *S. aureus* using a disk diffusion method. A microbiologist can test *S. aureus* against vancomycin by disk diffusion, but the results cannot be reported because they cannot be interpreted.

ANAEROBES

Anaerobes can possess resistance mechanisms. Anaerobic susceptibility testing should not be performed routinely but is important when an anaerobic infection does not respond to therapy. Agar dilution, broth microdilution, and gradient strip methods are currently in use. The atmosphere for incubation is critical to ensure the survival and growth of anaerobic organisms. Results can take up to 48 hours.

FUNGI

As the isolation of yeasts and moulds increase in immunocompromised individuals, the need for antifungal susceptibility testing becomes critical. CLSI offers procedures and interpretive guidelines for yeasts and moulds. A broth dilution method is most often used and may require incubation of up to 4 days before interpretation. Disk diffusion can now be used for testing *Candida* spp.

MYCOBACTERIUM SPP.

Susceptibility testing for *Mycobacterium tuberculosis* is critical for detection of multi-drug-resistance strains. Testing is usually performed in specialized laboratories. An agar-based susceptibility test can be performed using decontaminated and concentrated specimens that demonstrate acid-fast bacilli. Results can take up to 3 weeks.

Automated systems can now provide "rapid" susceptibility testing results for *Mycobacterium* spp. Depending on the system used, actively growing cultures may be used or decontaminated and concentrated specimens that demonstrate acid-fast bacilli. Results may be available in 3 to 8 days after inoculation.

▶ MOLECULAR TESTING

Detecting the genes responsible for resistance can be done using molecular methods such as polymerase chain reaction (PCR) assays. Detection of the *mec*A gene for oxacillin resistance in *Staphylococcus* spp. is now available for clinical laboratories. These methods, performed directly on clinical specimens, provide results faster than growing the organism and then performing traditional susceptibility testing. The detection of the presence of a resistance gene, in molecular testing, does not mean the gene is turned on or expressed. Mutations in the organism's genetic code for resistance may also prevent its detection with PCR primers in use.

▶ QUALITY ASSURANCE OF ANTIBIOTIC SUSCEPTIBILITY RESULTS

Using standardized methods for antibiotic susceptibility testing should provide accurate and reliable results. The results must correlate with the organism's identification and make sense.

Review of the susceptibility results prior to release is an important part of the quality assurance process in the laboratory. The use of automated commercial susceptibility systems and laboratory information systems can make the process easier.

Susceptibility data review should be done as soon as possible after the results are available. This allows time for corrective action of errors found without delaying results for the physician. A three-tier review should be utilized. The microbiologist reading out the susceptibility results has the important position to detect unusual or unlikely resistance patterns. The bench microbiologist must ensure all results correlate with the organism isolated from the patient's culture. The microbiology supervisor or manager tracks and monitors the competency of the staff microbiologists to ensure the effectiveness of the first two tiers of review.

Most automated commercial susceptibility systems possess software that can detect unlikely or unusual patterns, but this does not release the microbiologist from performing a thorough review of the results. Table 11-10 summarizes susceptibility testing patterns that demonstrate unlikely or unusual results. Detection of unlikely or unusual susceptibility patterns can prevent the patient from being subjected to ineffective or inappropriate therapy. It also allows for immediate notification of the infection control and others if it is valid.

Once an issue has been detected on susceptibility testing results, then the microbiologist must resolve the problem. Items to be considered in the resolution of unlikely or unusual susceptibility results may include

- Clerical and transcription errors
- Susceptibility panel and identification system not inoculated with same organism
- Reading errors such as misreading diameter of zone of inhibition or air bubble or dry well in susceptibility panel
- Inoculum used was contaminated and not a pure isolate
- Policies and procedures not followed
- Organism identification is incorrect
- Incorrect antibiotics tested
- Incorrect interpretive criteria used
- Potential intrinsic or acquired resistance mechanism present

Resolution of unlikely or unusual susceptibility results may require repeat testing of either the antibiotic panel or organism identification. A review of previous patient results may determine whether the results have been detected previously.

✪ TABLE 11-10

Examples of Susceptibility Testing Patterns That May Require Further Evaluation

Organism	Suspicious Susceptibility Pattern
Staphylococcus spp.	■ Vancomycin intermediate or resistant ■ Clindamycin susceptible and erythromycin resistant
Enterococcus faecalis	■ Ampicillin resistant ■ Quinupristin-dalfopristin susceptible
viridans *Streptococcus*	■ Vancomycin intermediate or resistant ■ Penicillin intermediate or resistant
Beta hemolytic *Streptococcus*	■ Penicillin intermediate or resistant ■ Clindamycin susceptible and erythromycin resistant
Enterobacteriaceae ■ Especially *Klebsiella pneumoniae* and *E. coli*	■ Carbapenem resistant ■ Potential carbapenemase
E. coli *Klebsiella pneumoniae* *Proteus mirabilis*	■ Ceftazidime, cefotaxime, ceftriaxone, cefpodoxime, or aztreonam resistant ■ Potential ESBL
Serratia spp. *Providencia* spp. *Citrobacter freundii* *Enterobacter* spp. *Morganella morganii* *Aeromonas* spp. *Pseudomonas aeruginosa*	■ Cefoxitin resistant and cefepime susceptible ■ Potential AmpC
Klebsiella pneumoniae	■ Ampicillin susceptible
Pseudomonas aeruginosa	■ Gentamicin, tobramycin, and amikacin resistant ■ Gentamicin and/or tobramycin susceptible and amikacin resistant
Stenotrophomonas maltophilia	■ Carbapenem susceptible ■ Trimethoprim-sulfamethoxazole resistant

---

✔ Checkpoint! 11–14 (Chapter Objective 13)

Which of the following organism/susceptibility patterns requires further investigation because of the potential for unlikely or unusual results?
  A. *E. coli resistant to imipenem*
  B. *Klebsiella pneumoniae resistant to ampicillin*
  C. *Enterococcus faecalis resistant to quinupristin-dalfopristin*
  D. *Staphylococcus aureus erythromycin resistant and clindamycin resistant*

 REAL WORLD TIP

The use of continuing education and proficiency testing can improve antibiotic susceptibility testing and reporting in the clinical laboratory.

Additional testing, such as the Hodge test for carbapenemase confirmation, or alternative testing may be necessary to confirm resistance mechanisms.

▶ ANTIBIOTIC RESISTANCE SURVEILLANCE

Monitoring the emerging resistance of the organisms encountered in a medical facility can provide valuable information. An **antibiogram** is an annual document that organizes an institution's antibiotic susceptibility data for its most commonly isolated organisms by antibiotic. It can be further divided by services, such as the intensive care unit or surgery, or specimen types, such as blood cultures, within the facility. The information allows the pharmacy to monitor inappropriate and excessive antimicrobial used. Physicians use the information to determine appropriate therapy before the patient's own organism data is available. Table 11-11✪ provides an example of an institution's antibiogram. CLSI provides guidelines for the cre-

> **ⓔ REAL WORLD TIP**
>
> If an organism's identification is available but not the susceptibility report, the microbiologist can use the institution's antibiogram or current literature to provide the physician with viable options for treatment.

ation of a valid antibiogram. Its use prevents skewed data because of duplicate isolates in multiple cultures from a patient.

▶ COMMUNICATION OF ANTIBIOTIC SUSCEPTIBILITY RESULTS

Agar and broth dilutions and gradient strip results are usually reported with the organism's MIC in µg/mL for each antibiotic and its interpretation based on CLSI interpretive criteria. Disk diffusion results are reported only as an interpretation (S, I, R). The report should account for cross resistance. If *Staphylococcus* spp. produces beta-lactamase then penicillin, ampicillin, and other beta-lactams should both be noted as resistant.

With the assistance of the pharmacy and infection control physicians, the susceptibility report is often set up so the less expensive antibiotics are listed first. Most reports use cascade reporting. This suppresses results based on other results. When gentamicin is susceptible, then tobramycin and amikacin are suppressed. This guides the physician to use the less-expensive and less-toxic gentamicin.

The age of the patient dictates if tetracycline is reported. When an individual is 12 years of age or younger, then the tetracycline results should be removed. Tetracycline can stain teeth and cause abnormal bone growth. The specimen type can also determine which antibiotics are to be reported. Nitrofurantoin should only be reported on urine isolates. Certain antibiotics can be suppressed to prevent their use. The

✪ TABLE 11-11

An Example of an Institution's Antibiogram

Organism (# tested)	Ampicillin	Ampicillin/Sulbactam	Aztreonam	Cefazolin	Ceftazidime	Ceftriaxone	Clindamycin	Gentamicin	Levofloxacin	Nitrofurantoin	Rifampin	Tobramycin	Trimethoprim/Sulfamethoxazole	Tetracycline	Vancomycin
Methicillin-resistant *Staphylococcus aureus* (MRSA; 700)							46	98		100	98		95	95	100
Staphylococcus not *S. aureus* (SNA; 550)							58	66		100	95		65	89	100
Vancomycin-resistant *Enterococcus* spp. (VRE; 365)	24								99	44					
S. pneumoniae (170)						90	80		99				58		
E. coli (1020)	60	68	98	92	97	98		91	86	99			98	98	
K. pneumoniae (435)	2	78	93	91	93	93		98	92	74			94	92	
P. aeruginosa (425)			76		83			84	80			93			

Note: The number in each column indicates % sensitive isolates.

vancomycin results should be suppressed for vancomycin-susceptible *Enterococcus* spp. and thus prevent selective pressure for resistant strains.

QUALITY CONTROL AND VALIDATION OF ANTIBIOTIC SUSCEPTIBILITY METHODS

CLSI documents provide recommended guidelines, testing frequencies, and interpretive criteria for susceptibility methods used in clinical laboratories. New methods and antibiotics require 20 or 30 consecutive days of testing against specific strains of bacteria. The testing organisms are strains that provide a reliable and consistent susceptibility pattern of results. These organisms are obtained from the American Type Culture Collection (ATCC). This nonprofit organization maintains collections of molecular genomes, cell lines, and microorganisms. ATCC strains are also used in the clinical microbiology laboratory to perform quality control on identification methods, reagents, and media.

When quality control results do not fall within the required interpretive criteria, immediate resolution is required. Often the first step in resolution of susceptibility quality control issues involves repeating the testing with a new subculture of the ATCC strain of organism and antibiotic(s) involved. If this does not resolve the issue, then all aspects of the susceptibility process must be reviewed for potential errors. The results of the antibiotics involved should not be reported for patients until the quality control issues are resolved.

When a new susceptibility method is implemented, the clinical laboratory must perform method validation. This means the method must be challenged to ensure it performs accurately in the laboratory setting. This also includes testing the method to ensure precision and accuracy. Organisms with known susceptible, intermediate, and resistant results are run to evaluate the method's precision. This would account for potential random errors associated with preparation of the organism inoculum, pipetting, and other manual steps in the process. Patient organisms are also tested in parallel on both the new and previously used methods to ensure the accuracy of the new method.

Checkpoint! 11–15 (Chapter Objective 16)

Quality control of antibiotic susceptibility testing and method validation are essential to ensure the:

 A. *competency of the microbiologist.*
 B. *accuracy and precision of the methods and instruments.*
 C. *appropriate antibiotics are being tested.*
 D. *physicians' customer satisfaction.*

ASSAYS OF ANTIMICROBIAL AGENTS

A more precise determination of the concentration of an antibiotic in body fluids has become necessary as a result of the use of antimicrobial agents that exhibit toxicity, for example, the aminoglycosides and vancomycin. In this manner the levels of a particular medication may be more carefully monitored to guard the health of the patient from unwanted side effects such as kidney damage. MICs and MBCs are in vitro measurements of a particular drug, which may or may not adequately represent the true in vivo concentrations that are subject to pharmacokinetics. **Pharmacokinetics**, the study of drugs and drug metabolites in body fluids, tissues, and bodily excretions, incorporates data on trough and peak levels of therapeutic drugs. Samples to determine the trough serum concentration are drawn 30 minutes before administration of the next dose. Peak concentration samples are drawn after the dose is given. Samples drawn to determine peak levels must be timed to coincide with when anticipated highest levels should occur. This will be influenced by the route of administration, and it is generally accepted that intravenous injection leads to peak levels within 30 minutes, whereas intramuscular and intradermal injections peak within 90 minutes of administration. Excretion of a particular drug by the kidneys and metabolism by the liver will directly affect attainable levels and are important reasons that it may be desirable to accurately measure the amount of drug that is actually present in body fluids such as serum or plasma. With this information, it can be ascertained whether or not effective drug levels are attained in vivo. A discussion of assay methods is presented in this section.

Agar Diffusion Method

The agar diffusion method is a microbiological assay wherein an overnight broth culture of the test organism is added to approximately 20 mL of melted Mueller-Hinton agar that has been allowed to cool to 50°C. At this temperature, the agar solution is hot enough to remain in a liquid state and yet cool enough that the test organism will suffer no ill effects when it is mixed into the growth medium. The molten solution containing the test organism is then poured into a 150 mm petri dish and allowed to solidify. Filter paper disks are impregnated with specified concentrations of the antibiotic mixed into antibiotic-free serum. These discs are placed on the surface of the agar. These standardized concentrations of the antibiotic to be measured will be used to construct a curve from which the unknown concentrations in a particular body fluid can be determined. The serum, or other body fluid to be tested, is added to other filter paper disks, which are also added to the surface of the agar. The plate is incubated for 15 hours at 35°C. The zone sizes around the disks containing graduated concentrations of antimicrobial agent are measured and plotted on a graph against the known concentrations. The zone sizes obtained from the disks containing the body fluid are measured, and the concentration of the antimicrobial agent can now be interpolated from the graph. The greatest disadvantage of this method is the fact that growth of the organism delays reporting the results until the next day.

Immunoassays

Radioimmunoassay (RIA) and enzyme immunoassay (EIA) are two techniques that have the distinct advantage of being extremely sensitive, precise, and rapid means of measuring the quantity of antimicrobial agent in a body fluid.

In the competitive radioimmunoassay, radiolabeled gentamicin competes with unlabeled gentamicin in the patient's serum for binding sites on an antibody, specific for gentamicin, which is attached to a solid surface. Any unbound gentamicin is washed from the assay vessel, and the amount of labeled gentamicin bound to the antibody can be measured. In this test procedure, the amount of radiolabeled gentamicin bound to the antibody is inversely proportional to the amount of unlabeled gentamicin in the patient's serum.

Enzyme immunoassays use a sandwich method in which antibody to the antimicrobial agent is bound to a solid surface. When the body fluid is added to the assay vessel, any of the drug present presumably attaches to the binding site of the antibody. After unbound antimicrobial agent is washed away to prevent a false-positive reaction, a second antibody, which is enzyme labeled, is added. This antibody attaches to the antimicrobial agent, which is now sandwiched between the two antibodies. A chromogenic substrate for the enzyme is then added to the assay. This chromogenic substrate is degraded by the enzyme into an end product that is a colored compound. At a specified time the reaction is stopped and the amount of color development is proportional to the amount of antimicrobial agent in the body fluid.

 **Checkpoint! 11–16
(Chapter Objectives 11 and 17)**

Which method is used to measure the level of an antibiotic in serum to prevent toxicity?

   A. Disc agar diffusion test
   B. Minimal inhibitory concentration testing
   C. Serum bactericidal test
   D. Radioimmunoassay

SUMMARY

Antimicrobial susceptibility testing is routinely performed on organisms isolated and identified as the etiologic agent of bacterial infections and increasingly for fungal infections. This is a direct result of the emergence of organisms resistant to the effect of antimicrobial agents. Antibiotics that are effective in resolving the infection should exhibit little or no toxicity to the host, have a wide spectrum of activity, be readily absorbed

and maintained at therapeutic levels, and be cost effective. These would fit the criteria of an ideal candidate for antimicrobial therapy.

Since the discovery of penicillin in the early part of the 20th century, many different antimicrobial agents have been discovered, and it is hard to imagine the age of modern medicine without these important drugs. Antimicrobial agents are designed to inhibit the growth of microbes or bring about their destruction.

Antibiotics may act in several different ways. Agents, such as penicillins, cephalosporins, vancomycin, and others, affect cell wall synthesis. Bacitracin and the polymyxins affect the cell membrane, allowing cell contents to leak out of the cell. Other antimicrobial agents such as the aminoglycoside, tetracycline, macrolide antibiotics, chloramphenicol, and others affect protein synthesis. Proteins are structure components of cells and enzymes, which are essential for biochemical activities within the cell and are therefore indispensable. Quinolones, such as ciprofloxacin and norfloxacin, and others interfere with nucleic acid synthesis, while the sulfonamides and trimethoprim interfere with folic acid metabolism. Both actions will have a deleterious effect on bacterial growth and proliferation.

Susceptibility testing can be performed by different methods, but the two most popular methods are the disk agar diffusion method and broth dilution procedures. The disk diffusion method is approved only for rapidly growing aerobic and facultative anaerobic bacteria such as staphylococci, streptococci, and the *Enterobacteriaceae*. With this technique, the test organism is applied to the surface of a Mueller-Hinton agar plate in a manner that would produce a confluent lawn of growth. The suspending medium (broth or saline) of the inoculum must have time to be absorbed before antibiotic impregnated discs are applied to the agar surface. After incubation at 35°C to 37°C in a non-CO_2 incubator, the antibiotic will have diffused into the agar medium, creating a concentration gradient, and the inoculum will have had time to proliferate. A zone of inhibition will be seen around those antibiotics able to affect the growth of the test organism. This zone of inhibition is measured and is related to the minimal inhibitory concentration (MIC), a reflection of the effectiveness of the antibiotic.

Broth and agar dilution methods use serial dilutions to determine the minimal inhibitory concentration of an antimicrobial agent. A suspension of the test organism is added to serial dilutions of the antimicrobial agent and allowed to incubate under appropriate conditions. The lowest concentration that visibly inhibits growth of the test organism constitutes the MIC and provides useful information concerning the level of antimicrobial agent (dose) that should be effective in eradicating the infection. The gradient diffusion test provides an MIC value with the ease of use of a disk diffusion method.

A major problem in the treatment of infectious diseases has arisen over the past few decades. That problem is the emergence of microbes that have developed resistance to commonly used antimicrobial agents. Several mechanisms of antimicrobial resistance have been recognized: modification of the antimicrobial agent's target, enzymatic inactivation of the antimicrobial agent, decreased permeability or uptake of the agent, ability to bypass inhibited metabolic pathways, activation of efflux systems and any combination of these mechanisms. The emergence of microbes resistant to antimicrobial agents has not only made the treatment of infectious diseases much more challenging for clinicians, but has also added the task of detecting microbial resistance to the scope of practice of microbiologists.

LEARNING OPPORTUNITIES

1. Which of the following criteria is probably the last to be considered by a physician when selecting an antibiotic for treatment of an infectious agent? (Chapter Objective 1)

   a. Potential side effects

   b. Potential for development of resistance mechanisms

   c. Availability of a generic form of the antibiotic

   d. Site of the infection

2. Categorize each of these resistance mechanisms as either intrinsic (I) or acquired (A). (Chapter Objective 4)

   a. Vancomycin resistance in gram-negative rods _____

   b. Vancomycin resistance in *Lactobacillus* spp. _____

   c. Vancomycin resistance in *Enterococcus faecalis* _____

   d. Aminoglycoside resistance in anaerobes _____

   e. Extended spectrum beta-lactamase production in *E. coli* _____

   f. Metronidazole resistance in aerobes _____

3. Antibiotic susceptibility testing is performed to determine: (Chapter Objective 5)

   a. the effectiveness of an antibiotic against an organism

   b. the presence of intrinsic resistance mechanisms

   c. if an organism is capable of expressing resistance mechanisms

   d. the spectrum of activity of an antibiotic

4. The Clinical and Laboratory Standards Institute (CLSI) is a nonprofit organization that develops standards for: (Chapter Objective 6)

   a. susceptibility methods

   b. quality control methods

   c. interpretive criteria

   d. all of the above

5. The disk diffusion test on the left in the following figure was set up using the standardized procedure. The procedure for the disk diffusion test on the right in the figure was altered in some manner. Which altered standardized factor could account for the smaller zone sizes? (Chapter Objective 7)

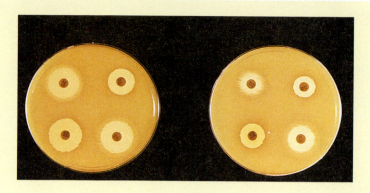

From Public Health Image Library (PHIL), CDC/Gilda L. Jones.

   a. Media depth too thin

   b. Less than a 15-minute delay in placement of the disks

   c. Less than 16 hours of incubation

   d. Inoculum heavier than the 0.5 McFarland standard

6. Using the following figure, interpret the minimum inhibitory concentration of this *Streptococcus pneumoniae* isolate tested against vancomycin. The organism's vancomycin MIC, in µg/mL, is: (Chapter Objective 9)

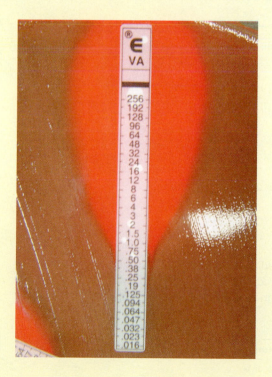

   a. 1.00

   b. 0.75

   c. 0.50

   d. 0.38

   e. 0.25

7. Measure and interpret the gentamicin disk diffusion test in the following figure against *E. coli*. (Chapter Objective 8)

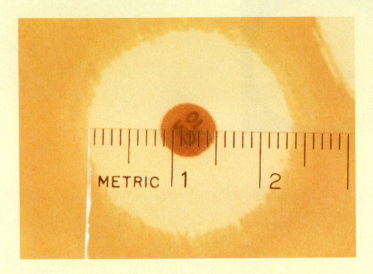

From Public Health Image Library (PHIL), CDC/Gilda L. Jones.

Interpretive Criteria for Disk Diffusion Using Gentamicin *Zone sizes to the nearest whole milliliter (mm)*		
Resistant	Intermediate	Susceptible
≤15	14–19	>20

a. What is the diameter of the zone of inhibition measured in millimeters?

   a. 2.4 mm

   b. 17 mm

   c. 24 mm

   d. 28 mm

b. Interpret the disk diffusion result of this organism against gentamicin.

   a. Susceptible

   b. Intermediate

   c. Resistant

8. A 12-year-old male was admitted with a draining abdominal wound after surgery for removal of his appendix. The drainage was cultured and revealed heavy growth of *Staphylococcus aureus*. The automated broth dilution susceptibility testing results included

Antibiotic	MIC (µg/mL)	Interpretation
Beta-lactamase	Not applicable	Positive
Penicillin	4	R
Cefazolin	2	S
Clindamycin	0.5	S
Erythromycin	16	R
Oxacillin	16	R
Vancomycin	0.5	S

a. What potential resistance mechanism(s) is/are suspected based on these results? (Chapter Objective 13)

b. On further testing, the organism gave the results in the following figure. How do you interpret this result?

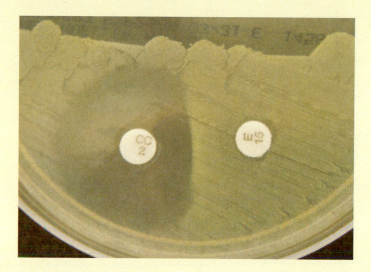

a. Positive ESBL screen

b. Positive Hodge test

c. Positive for inducible erythromycin resistance

d. Positive for inducible clindamycin resistance

c. How should the original susceptibility report be modified based on the results in question 8b and any other possible resistance mechanism(s) present? (Chapter Objectives 10 and 13)

9. Review of susceptibility results, as a quality control measure, would detect unlikely or unusual susceptibility patterns. Which of the following demonstrates an unlikely or unusual susceptibility pattern that requires further investigation? (Chapter Objective 12)

a. *Streptococcus pyogenes*, which is erythromycin susceptible and clindamycin susceptible

b. *E. coli*, which is resistant to ceftazidime and aztreonam

c. *Stenotrophomonas maltophilia*, which is susceptible to trimethoprim-sulfamethoxazole

d. Viridans *Streptococcus*, which is penicillin susceptible

10. The following antibiotics were tested against a *Staphylococcus aureus* isolate:

Penicillin

Oxacillin

Erythromycin

Clindamycin

Cefazolin

Vancomycin

The organism is beta-lactamase positive and possesses the *mec*A gene. Based on these results, list the antibiotic(s) that will be rendered ineffective by this organism. (Chapter Objective 13)

11. An 80-year-old female, admitted with renal failure, developed pneumonia after 5 days in the hospital. An expectorated sputum culture revealed significant growth of *Klebsiella pneumoniae*. The organism provided the following disk diffusion susceptibility results:

Antibiotic	Zone Size in Millimeters	Interpretation
Aztreonam	14	R
Ceftriaxone	25	S
Cefoxitin	21	S
Imipenem	22	S
Cefotaxime	29	S
Ceftazidime	14	R

a. Which resistance mechanism do you suspect in this organism, based on these results? (Chapter Objectives 10 and 13)

a. AmpC

b. Carbapenemase

c. ESBL

d. None

b. What additional testing is necessary to confirm your suspicions? (Chapter Objective 10)

a. No further testing is necessary

b. ESBL screen

c. Hodge test

d. AmpC induction screen

c. On further testing, the organism produced the following disk diffusion susceptibility results:

Antibiotic	Zone Size in Millimeters
Cefotaxime with clavulanic acid	34
Ceftazidime with clavulanic acid	30

Based on these results, which antibiotic(s) in the original report should be reported as resistant, regardless of the original result? (Chapter Objectives 10 and 13)

12. An institution's antibiotic resistance surveillance is best monitored by using: (Chapter Objective 14)

a. an antibiogram

b. a daily review of all the patients' susceptibility reports

c. the pharmacy's weekly antibiotic usage reports

d. the input of the staff microbiologists

13. Effective communication of antibiotic susceptibility results includes: (Chapter Objective 15)

    a. the use of cascade reporting

    b. suppression of tetracycline results on an individual under the age of 12 years

    c. suppression of nitrofurantoin on nonurinary isolates

    d. all of the above

    e. both a and b

14. A 51-year-old male was admitted with fever of unknown origin (FUO). The patient has a history of cardiovascular problems. Several years ago his primary physician noted a heart murmur, and he was subsequently diagnosed with valvular stenosis as a result of narrowing of the mitral valve. Presently the patient's symptoms include general malaise, chills, easily fatigued, and a temperature of 39°C. His serum chemistry results are unremarkable, but hematologic findings reveals a white blood cell count of 16,200/mm^3.

    Blood cultures were performed and all yielded growth of *Enterococcus faecalis*. It was now evident that this patient was suffering from bacterial endocarditis because of a vegetation residing on his mitral valve. The organism proved to be vancomycin susceptible and does not produce beta-lactamase.

    Which of the following antibiotics should provide effective treatment of this infection? (Chapter Objective 2)

    a. Gentamicin

    b. Vancomycin

    c. Ampicillin

    d. Nitrofurantoin

15. A 7-year-old male was admitted in acute respiratory distress. The patient's parents stated that he seemed to suffer from infections far more frequently than most children. When he began to suffer frequent nosebleeds and bruised very easily, he was taken to a pediatrician, who diagnosed him with acute lymphocytic leukemia. Since his initial hospitalization, he has been aggressively treated to eradicate as many leukemic white blood cells as possible, but unfortunately one of the consequences of the chemotherapy has been the development of a profound leucopenia.

    His latest symptoms include fever, chills, cough, shortness of breath, hemoptysis, and chest pain. Chest radiographs revealed a few opacities (light areas) of variable size located in the upper areas of the lungs, consistent with tuberculosis. Sputum specimens were sent for mycobacterial cultures as well as routine and fungal cultures. No mycobacteria were seen on smears or recovered in the mycobacterial cultures, and only normal upper respiratory flora was isolated on the routine cultures. After 3 days, fungal growth was noted on the fungal culture consistent with a mould. It was identified as *Aspergillus fumigatus*. The same mould was recovered on a subsequent culture.

    Which antifungal agent should be considered to treat this invasive infection? (Chapter Objective 2)

    a. Fluconazole

    b. Amphotericin B

    c. Griseofulvin

    d. Isoniazid

PEARSON
myhealthprofessionskit

Use this address to access the interactive Companion Website created for this textbook. Simply select "Clinical Laboratory Science" from the choice of disciplines. Find this book and log in using your user name and password.

REFERENCES

Go to myhealthprofessionskit.com to view this chapter's references.

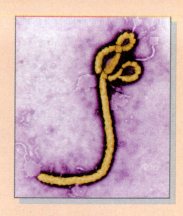

12

Emerging Technologies

Marcia A. Firmani

■ LEARNING OBJECTIVES

Upon completion of this chapter, the learner should be able to:

1. Describe emerging genomic and postgenomic scientific fields, including:
   a. toxicogenomics
   b. pharmacogenomics
   c. metabolomics
   d. bioinformatics
2. Define microarrays and biochips, and explain how they are being used to diagnose various medical conditions.
3. Define DNA vaccines and discuss their principle and purpose.
4. List the major methods used to administer DNA vaccines.
5. Distinguish the advantages and disadvantages of DNA vaccination compared to conventional immunization methods.
6. Relate how the field of epidemiology has become adapted to the genomic era.

KEY TERMS

biochip	metabolomics	pharmacogenetics
bioinformatics	molecular epidemiology	toxicogenomics
DNA vaccine	microarrays	
genetic epidemiology	pharmacogenomics	

▶ INTRODUCTION

The clinical laboratory has evolved over the past 50 years into a complex, technology-driven endeavor. The principal tasks of the clinical laboratory include diagnosing and screening diseases, monitoring health and therapeutic response, and measuring deviations from normal physiology in humans. The current scientific understanding is being reoriented toward genomic knowledge, technologies, and practices. We have now entered the genomic era, which is bringing forth the newest and most powerful science and technology available. Molecular Koch's postulates have been proposed to evaluate a gene's role in a bacteria's ability to cause disease (Falkow, 2004). The various fields of inquiry that have been made possible by emergent technologies are reshaping the scientific field. Moreover, emerging technologies in the clinical diagnostic laboratory are becoming more and more useful. The introduction of genetic technologies into the clinical field opens up a wide range of possibilities that will not be exclusively determined by the technologies but also by how they are utilized. The new technologies can support efforts to better understand the pathways of the human body and the ways in which these pathways affect human health and illness.

▶ GENOMICS

Genomics is the study of the functions and interactions of all the genes in a genome (Guttmacher & Collins, 2002). The application of genetic and genomic technologies has begun to transform clinical practices within many health-related fields. These technologies provide new models and techniques for studying genetic traits, environmental exposures, and gene-environment interaction in the production of human health and illness (Shostak, 2003). However, the data generated through genomic technology is highly complex, which has led to the emerging field of systems biology. The systems biology approach uses the power of mathematics, engineering, and computer science to analyze and integrate genomic data to create working models of entire biological systems (Spivey, 2004). The various "omics" that have contributed to our increased understanding of biology and have been incorporated into genomic technology include toxicogenomics, pharmacogenomics, and metabolomics. Moreover, the vast amount of data generated from genomic-based studies has led to the emergence of the field of bioinformatics.

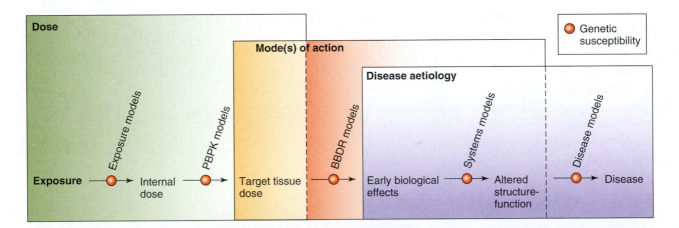

■ **FIGURE 12-1** The sequence of events between initial exposure to a toxicant and final disease outcome are shown from left to right. Note that genetic susceptibility (red dot) influences every level of toxicologic analysis. After exposure, the ADME (absorption, distribution, metabolism, and excretion) systems of the body control local concentrations of a chemical stressor in various body compartments. This is affected by genetics through the involvement of specific alleles encoding various transporters and xenobiotic (foreign substance)-metabolizing enzymes, among others. Mathematical models such as exposure models, physiologically-based pharmacokinetic (PBPK) and biologically-based dose response (BBDR) models can be used to approximate these processes. PBPK models are a set of differential equations structured to provide a time course of a chemical's mass–balance disposition (wherein all inputs, outputs, and changes in total mass of the chemical are accounted for) in preselected anatomical compartments. BBDR models are dose-response models that are based on underlying biological processes. Once the target tissue is exposed to a local stressor, the cells respond and adapt or undergo a toxic response; this process can be modeled with systems toxicology approaches. Finally, the disease outcome itself can be mimicked by genetic or chemically induced models of particular diseases. The colored boxes show the type of toxicologically relevant information that can be obtained from each set of model.

Reprinted by permission from Macmillan Publishers Ltd: Waters, M. D., & Fostel, J. M. (2004). Toxicogenomics and systems toxicology: Aims and prospects. Nature Reviews Genetics, 5, *936–948.*

TOXICOGENOMICS

Toxicogenomics is the study of gene expression and gene production involved in adaptive responses to toxic exposures. Toxicology, or the study of poisons, focuses on the substances and exposures that cause adverse effects to living organisms. The rapid accumulation of genomic-based data has catalyzed the application of gene-expression analysis to understanding the mechanisms of chemicals and other environmental stresses on biological systems, which have facilitated the emergence of the field of toxicogenomics (Figure 12-1 ■). The three principal goals of toxicogenomics are to understand the relationship between environmental stress and disease susceptibility, to identify useful biomarkers of disease and exposure to toxic substances, and to elucidate the molecular mechanisms of toxicity (Waters & Fostel, 2004).

Consequently, integrating data derived from "omics" technologies can contribute to the development of a toxicogenomics knowledge base (Figure 12-2 ■) and the development of systems toxicology as it relates to molecular-expression profiling (Waters & Fostel, 2004).

PHARMACOGENOMICS

Pharmacogenomics is the study of the various genes that determine drug behavior. **Pharmacogenetics** refers to the study of inherited differences in drug metabolism and response (Ito & Demers, 2004). Many factors determine drug responses, including gender, nutritional status, kidney and liver function, concomitant diseases and medications, and the disease being treated. In addition, it has become clear

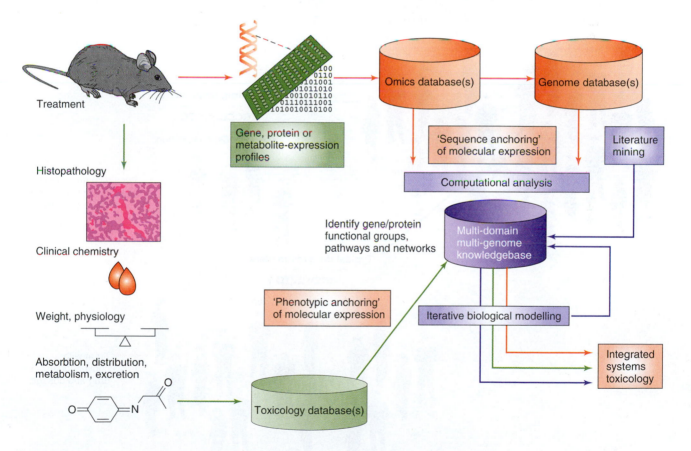

■ FIGURE 12-2 A framework for systems toxicology. This figure indicates the paths from the initial observation (rat in upper left) to an integrated toxicogenomics knowledge base (blue cylinder), and on to systems toxicology (bottom right). The "-omics" data stream is shown by the clockwise path from rat to knowledge base; and the "traditional" toxicology approach is shown in the anticlockwise path. The knowledge base will integrate both data streams, along with literature-based knowledge and, by virtue of iterative modeling, will lead to a systems toxicology understanding. The framework involves phenotypic anchoring (to toxicological endpoints and study design information) and sequence anchoring (to genomes) of multidomain molecular-expression data sets in the context of conventional indices of toxicology and the iterative biological modeling of the resulting data.

Reprinted by permission from Macmillan Publishers Ltd: Waters, M. D., & Fostel, J. M. (2004). Toxicogenomics and systems toxicology: Aims and prospects. Nature Reviews Genetics, 5, 936–948.

that genetic factors can modify drug responses (Schmitz, Aslanidis, & Lackner, 2001). For example, patients with the same diagnosis may respond differently to a chemotherapeutic agent because of allelic differences (Figure 12-3 ■). In fact, many genetic variants have been identified that interfere with certain drugs. Hence, the genetic constitution of an individual is relevant for both the efficacy and safety of a given drug regimen, which is the central topic of pharmacogenomics. The practice of pharmacogenetics involves genotyping patients and treating those who would be poor drug responders with a drug other than the conventional drug or with a different dosage than usual (Prows & Prows, 2004). The ultimate goal of pharmacogenetic research is to determine which drug and drug dosage will be most effective in a patient so that the drug can be prescribed safely at the beginning of treatment.

METABOLOMICS

Metabolomics is the evaluation of tissues and biofluids such as urine, blood plasma, and saliva for metabolite changes that may result from environmental exposures or from disease. Because metabolites, including carbohydrates, amino acids, and lipids, are the by-products of processing food into energy, metabolomics has the potential to determine what has actually happened inside a cell.

BIOINFORMATICS

Bioinformatics is a multidisciplinary field comprising molecule biology, genetics, mathematics, and computer science. Bioinformatics is a rapidly emerging field that bridges the gap between biological knowledge and clinical therapy. For exam-

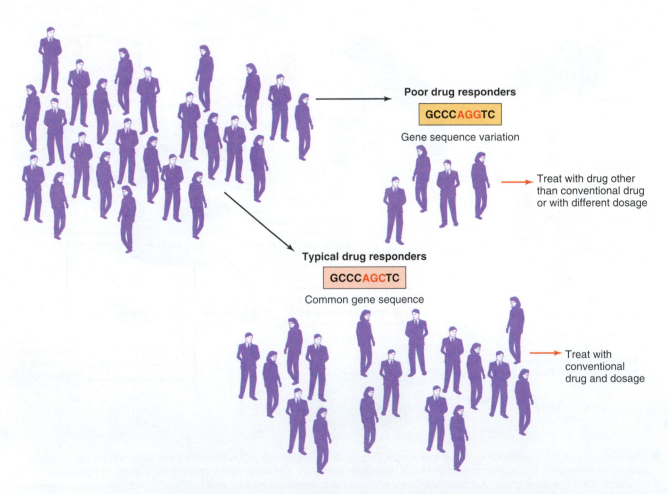

■ **FIGURE 12-3** Pharmacogenetics is the study of genetic differences in the alleles associated with individual variability in a drug response. Patients with the same diagnosis respond differently because of allelic differences. In this example, the normal gene sequence is GCCCAGCTC, but the mutation gene sequence is GCCCAGGTC. The AGC in the sequence of the normal gene codes for serine, but the AGG in the mutation gene's sequence codes for arginine. The substitution of arginine for serine in the drug-metabolizing enzyme molecule will cause the enzyme to be less effective or ineffective; this person is considered a "poor drug responder." The practice of pharmacogenetics involves genotyping patients and treating those who would be "poor drug responders" with a drug other than the conventional drug or with a different dosage.
From Prows, C. A., & Prows, D. R. (2004). Medication selection by genotype. American Journal of Nursing, *104(5), 60–70.*

ple, bioinformatics may be used to combine genomic technologies with the development of drugs designed to work against specific molecular targets (Desany & Zhang, 2004). Because of the enormous amount of data generated from the advanced genomic technologies available today, the speed of data generation exceeds that of interpretation. Consequently, large volumes of genomic and postgenomic data have become challenges in computational science. Hence, the drawback of high-throughput data generation is developing methods to aid in the understanding of all the data. Therefore, the integration of large and disparate data sets provides an opportunity for gene-level distinctions to be made between the different biological states that the data represents. This approach to bioinformatics and associated methodologies can be applied across a range of technologies to facilitate the rapid identification of new target leads for further experimental validation (Desany & Zhang, 2004). Clinical informatics is the development of methodologies to improve biomedical research and clinical care by integrating experimental and clinical information systems. As bioinformatics moves from constructing raw biomolecular data into their biological functions and clinical importance, quality clinical information will become the critical component of further progress. For example, patient biomolecular information may some day be included in an electronic medical record as the most predictive clinical information for diagnostics, therapeutics, and prognostics. Consequently, integration of bioinformatics and clinical informatics systems will be one of the primary challenges in the next decades (Kim, 2002).

Checkpoint! 12–1 (Chapter Objective 1)

Which of the following emerging genomic fields is the study of gene expression and gene production involved in adaptive responses to toxic exposures?

A. *Genetic epidemiology*
B. *Molecular epidemiology*
C. *Toxicogenomics*
D. *Bioinformatics*

▶ GENOMIC TECHNOLOGIES

Because of the influx in the amount of DNA sequence information, numerous technologies have been developed and improved on so that the vast genomic data available can be more readily utilized. Currently, we are entering an era where new types of experiments are possible because of enhanced technologies, such as high-density arrays and the development of DNA vaccines.

MICROARRAYS

DNA microarrays were introduced commercially in 1996. Since that time, microarrays, or **biochips**, have revolutionized how scientists explore cellular functions that are associated with

medical disorders and are paving the way to faster, more accurate diagnoses of many medical conditions and tailoring therapies to a specific individual.

Several types of **microarrays** exist, but all are capable of studying genetic material obtained from various tissue samples. Biochips consist of a lawn of single-stranded DNA molecules (probes) that are tethered to a chip that is often no larger than a thumbprint. Because DNA is the material that forms the more than 30,000 genes in human cells, scientists are capable of studying which genes or sequences in a sample are involved in a particular phenotypic process or disease manifestation (Figure 12-4 ■). Instead of detecting and studying one gene at a time as the conventional genomic technology allows, DNA microarrays can track thousands or tens of thousands of specific DNA or RNA sequences simultaneously on a single chip (Lockhart & Winzeler, 2000).

In microarray technology, each probe (genes or shorter DNA sequences) sits on an assigned spot within a checkerboard-like grid on a chip and are detected by a scanner because the DNA or RNA molecules from the sample carry a fluorescent tag or some other type of measurable label. Once a chip has been scanned, a computer converts the raw data into a color-coded readout (Figure 12-5 ■). Not only can investigators determine the presence of a gene or sequence in a sample, but they can also detect the expression or activity levels of those genes (Figure 12-6 ■).

Carefully designed arrays have the potential to determine the precise cause of infection or disease in a patient. In addition, gene-detecting microarrays could identify an individual's genetic propensity to a variety of disorders. Biochips can do this by revealing an individual's single nucleotide polymorphisms (SNPs) and thus predict the person's likelihood of

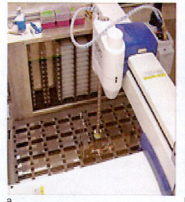
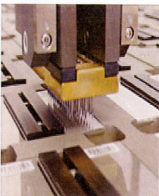

a   b

■ **FIGURE 12-4** Microarray instrumentation. Robots at the Institute for Genomic Research print gene chips—glass slides with up to 60,000 spots of unique single-stranded DNA molecules. When tissue samples are analyzed, fluorescently labeled RNA attaches to the DNA; the brightness of each spot corresponds to the amount of RNA—the expression level—of a particular gene. The robots work much like a desktop inkjet printer filled with DNA.

From J. Hasseman, The Institute for Genomic Research.

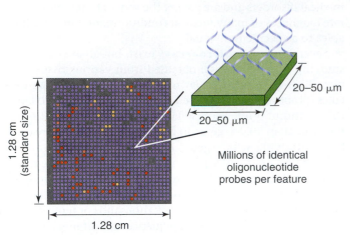

Millions of identical
oligonucleotide
probes per feature

1.28 cm (standard size)

20–50 µm

20–50 µm

1.28 cm

Up to ~ 400 000 features per microarray

■ **FIGURE 12-5** Gene expression analysis using microarrays. Oligonucleotides are synthesized on a "chip" to act as probes on the microarray surface. Approximately 30 oligonucleotides represent the partial sequence of one gene. Fluorescently labeled cDNA is hybridized to the microarray to allow expression level comparisons of up to 15,000 genes in the test sample. *Illustration courtesy of Affymetrix, Santa Clara, CA.*

acquiring Alzheimer's disease, diabetes, specific cancers, and so on. The people at greatest risk would then be able to receive close monitoring, intensive preventive care, and early intervention. Refer to Box 12-1✪ for an overview of microarrays.

✪ BOX 12-1

Microarray Overview

- DNA microarrays, also known as DNA chips, gene chips, or biochips, can track tens of thousands of molecular reactions in parallel on a wafer (chip) that is about the size of a thumbprint. The chips can be designed to detect specific genes or to measure gene activity in tissue samples.
- Microarrays are a valuable tool for scientists studying the roots of cancer and other complex diseases, for infectious diseases pathogenesis, and for drug researchers. Microarrays are also being studied as rapid diagnostic and prognostic tools.
- The research and diagnostic information provided by biochips and protein arrays may eventually enable physicians to provide highly individualized therapies and intervention strategies (Friend & Stoughton, 2002).

However, there is a downside of such knowledge, including increased anxiety and discrimination by employers and insurance agencies. In addition, several roadblocks need to be addressed before microarray technology becomes a standard technology in the clinical setting, such as lowering the cost of chips, scanners and other equipment. Moreover, the technology may not be feasible because of the need of specialized equipment and the appropriate training and skills to perform the technique. Box 12-2✪ summarizes the major applications of microarrays.

■ **FIGURE 12-6** Gene expression analysis in two tissue samples using spotted DNA microarray. RNA extracted from samples 1 and 2 is labeled with red or green fluorescent dyes. The dye-labeled RNA populations are mixed and hybridized to the microarray, on which cDNA has been spotted from thousands of genes, each spot representing one gene. The RNA from each sample hybridizes to each spot in proportion to the level of expression of that gene in the sample. After hybridization, the red and green fluorescent signal from each spot is determined, and the ratio of red to green reflects the relative expression of each gene in the two samples. For example, the gene TEP1 is shown to be expressed at a higher level in sample 2 than in sample 1. *Reprinted by permission from Macmillan Publishers Ltd: Brown, P. O., & Botstein, D. (1999). Exploring the new world of the genome with DNA microarrays. Nature Genetics, 21(1 suppl.), 33–37.*

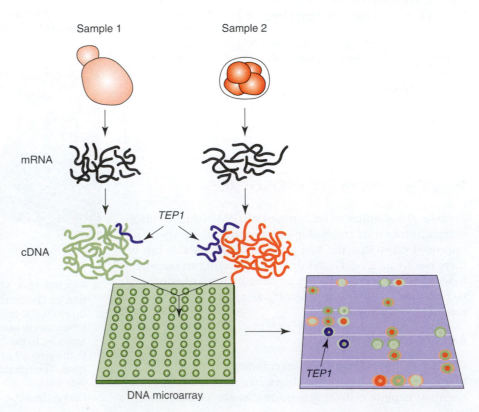

Sample 1

Sample 2

mRNA

cDNA

TEP1

DNA microarray

TEP1

⚙ BOX 12-2

The Major Applications of Microarrays Fall into Three Groups

I.   **Gene expression profiling**—RNA extracted from a complex sample (such as body tissues or fluids or bacterial isolates) is applied to the microarray. The result reveals the level of expression of tens of thousands of genes, effectively all the genes in the genome, in that complex sample. This result is known as a gene expression "profile" or "signature."

II. **Genotyping**—Genomic DNA, extracted from an individual's blood or saliva, is amplified by the polymerase chain reaction and applied to the microarray. The genotype for hundreds or thousands of genetic markers across the genome can be determined in a single hybridization. This approach has considerable potential in risk assessment, both in research and clinical practice.

III. **DNA sequencing**—DNA extracted from an individual's blood is amplified and applied to specific "resequencing" microarrays. Thousands of base pairs of DNA can be screened on a single microarray for mutations in specific genes whose normal sequence is already known. This greatly increases the scope for precise molecular diagnosis in single gene and genetically complex diseases (Aitman, 2001).

From Altman, Timothy J. Science, medicine, and the future: DNA microarrays in medical practice. *British Medical Journal*, 2001.

✓ Checkpoint! 12–2 (Chapter Objective 2)

Microarrays can be used to do all of the following, except:
   A. *identify genes or DNA sequences.*
   B. *identify single nucleotide polymorphisms.*
   C. *analyze gene expression levels.*
   D. *determine the date and time that an individual will be afflicted with a disease.*

DNA VACCINES

DNA vaccines consist of antigen-encoding bacterial plasmids that are capable of inducing antigen-specific immune responses when inoculated into a suitable host (Manoj, Babiuk, & van Drunen Little-van den Hurk, 2004). Specifically plasmid DNA or recombinant viral vectors are encoded with proteins from pathogens, allergens, or tumors that can be injected into the host in an attempt to be used as a prophylactic or therapeutic treatment for infectious diseases, allergies, and cancer. In addition, plasmids encoding normal human proteins are being tested as vaccines and treatments for autoimmune diseases (Liu et al., 2004). This type of vaccine has been intensively studied in the past decade.

Successful vaccines should be able to induce strong immune responses that are long-lasting and provide protection against different strains of the same pathogen. DNA vaccines are

⚙ BOX 12-3

Advantages of DNA Vaccines Compared to Live, Killed, or Subunit Vaccines

1. DNA vaccines are simple to design and inexpensive to manufacture.
2. DNA vaccines possess a built-in adjuvant (an immune system stimulant).
3. DNA vaccines are safer than live vaccines because there is no risk of infection.
4. Immune responses induced by DNA vaccines are generally of long duration in mice.
5. DNA vaccines induce strong antibody and cellular immune responses in neonates.
6. In contrast to live vaccines, antibody responses are not produced against naked DNA (Manoj et al., 2004).

Adapted from Manoj, S., Lorne, B. A., van Druden Little-van den Hurk, S. (2004). Approaches to enhance the efficacy of DNA vaccines. *Critical Reviews in Clinical Laboratory Sciences, 41*(1), 1–39.

advantageous (Box 12-3⚙) in that they can induce strong cellular immune responses, are relatively easy to design and construct, are chemically stable, and are less costly to produce (Nagata, Aoshi, Uchijima, Suzuke, & Koide, 2004). In addition, this methodology affords the opportunity to construct multivalent vaccines. For example, DNA vaccines allow integration of several antigens into the plasmid or the ability to administer a mixture of plasmid vectors (Ivory & Chadee, 2004). Consequently, DNA vaccines are considered a promising alternative to attenuated live vaccines in the field of infectious diseases. The development of multivalent vaccines consisting of several antigens is a novel approach to create a broad range of protection against different pathogenic strains and stages. However, there are limitations of DNA vaccines. For example, DNA vaccines have not been capable of inducing robust antigen-specific immune responses in large animals. In addition, the humoral responses produced are often not strong enough to confer protection from infection (Manoj et al., 2004). Unlike conventional vaccines, such as subunit or killed, which only depend on the host to induce an immune response to antigens, DNA vaccines depend on the host to first produce the antigen and then induce specific immune responses. Hence, efficient transfection into the host cell must first occur for DNA vaccines to produce sufficient quantities of the antigen, which can be a problem.

✓ Checkpoint! 12–3 (Chapter Objective 3)

DNA vaccines elicit an immune response from a suitable host by administering:
   A. *foreign microbial antigens.*
   B. *antigen-encoding bacterial plasmids.*
   C. *genetically engineered antigens.*
   D. *attenuated pathogens.*

The limitations of DNA vaccination emphasize the need for enhanced efficacy and delivery systems. Some of the major immunization methods used for DNA vaccine delivery are intramuscular injection, gene gun bombardment of DNA-coated gold particles into the epidermis, intradermal immunization, and topical application. Moreover, several carrier-mediated DNA vaccine methods have been reported such as liposomes, microparticle encapsulation, and attenuated bacteria.

Pathogens and cancer remain the leading causes of death worldwide. The development of vaccines to prevent diseases for which no vaccine currently exists, such as AIDS or malaria, or to treat chronic infections or cancer as well as improve efficacy and safety of existing vaccines, is a high priority (Moron, Dadaglio, & Leclerc, 2004). Consequently, numerous studies have demonstrated that injection of plasmid DNA coding for certain genes results in the induction of humoral and cellular immune responses against the respective gene product. This vaccination approach covers a broad range of possible applications, including the induction of protective immunity against microbial pathogens, and opens new perspectives for the treatment of cancer. In addition, DNA immunization is a promising immunotherapy against allergy (Hartl, Weiss, Hochreiter, Scheiblhofer, & Thalhamer, 2004).

✓ ### Checkpoint! 12–4 (Chapter Objective 4)

DNA vaccines can be administered by:
1. *gene gun bombardment.*
2. *topical application.*
3. *intramuscular injection.*
   A. *1 only*
   B. *2 only*
   C. *1 and 2*
   D. *1, 2, and 3*

▶ ## EPIDEMIOLOGY IN THE GENOMIC ERA

Epidemiology is the study of the distribution and determinants of health-related states or events in specified populations and the application of this study to control health problems (Last, 1995). However, the field of epidemiology has recently emerged into the genomics era and has an increasingly important role in the conduct of population-based research to assess the utility of genomic information in improving health and preventing disease (Gwinn & Khoury, 2002). In recent years, epidemiology has evolved into a field that uses systematic applications of epidemiological methods to assess the impact of genetic variation in disease occurrence (Khoury, Millikan, Little, & Gwinn, 2004).

GENETIC EPIDEMIOLOGY

Genetic epidemiology is the intersection between the fields of genetics and epidemiology. Genetic epidemiology integrates traditional epidemiological methods with concerns of human genetics to assess the interactions involved in the etiology and progression of disease (Khoury, Beaty, & Cohen, 1993). This field has been rapidly emerging because of advances in molecular biology.

MOLECULAR EPIDEMIOLOGY

Molecular epidemiology uses molecular biological techniques and biomarkers in epidemiological studies to assess individual exposure, doses, preclinical effects, risks, and susceptibility to harmful substances or disease.

As demonstrated in Table 12-1 ✪, human genome epidemiology plays an important role in the continuum from gene discovery to the development and application of genomic information for diagnosing, predicting, treating, and preventing disease (Khoury, Little, & Burke, 2004). Many genomic tests being developed will predict the risk of common diseases in otherwise healthy people to guide decisions about preventive or therapeutic strategies (Khoury, 2003). Consequently, an epidemiological approach is fundamental to evaluating genomic tests, including those intended for population screening and disease prevention (Khoury, McCabe, & McCabe, 2003).

SUMMARY

Considering that diseases are associated with genetic mutations resulting in defective protein development and production, it is not surprising that a genomic revolution has emerged. Genome sequencing has initiated the growth of new technologies, such as DNA microarrays, to transform medicine and afford opportunities to scrutinize genes. Several omics-based technologies, often referred to as postgenomics, have already

---

✪ **TABLE 12-1**

Human Genome Epidemiology

Genomic Discovery	Epidemiologic Impact on Genomics
Gene discovery	Epidemiologic approaches to sound study design: selection, representativeness, and generalizability
Gene characterization	Epidemiologic measures of risk; measurement of gene–environment interaction; methods for validation and adjustment for extraneous factors
Genomic testing	Epidemiologic evaluation of sensitivity, specificity, and predictive values of genetic tests; decision analysis using epidemiologic measures

Adapted from Table 1 of Khoury, M. J., Milliken, R., Little, J., & Gwinn, M. (2004). The emergence of epidemiology in the genomics age. *International Journal of Epidemiology, 33*, 936–944. Reprinted by permission of Oxford University Press.

begun to affect disease diagnosis and drug development by identifying new targets and methods of validation. Current applications for genomics include molecular medicine, health risk assessment, evolution and human migration, and DNA forensics (Buehler, 2005). Consequently, genomics has evolved novel methods for genetic analysis, which has generated new insights into biology and medicine because of the potential of finding cures for human diseases (Buehler, 2005).

LEARNING OPPORTUNITIES

1. Visit these websites: (Chapter Objectives 1 and 2)

   a. Perform a microarray experiment in a virtual biotechnique laboratory at http://learn.genetics.utah.edu/units/biotech/microarray/.

   b. Explore the National Center for Biotechnology Information at http://www.ncbi.nlm.nih.gov/About/primer/index.html to learn more about emerging technologies described in this chapter.

2. Situation: You are investigating an epidemic of rheumatic fever that occurred in 1997. You wonder whether this epidemic is related to the 1980 epidemic (Potera, 2002). How would you go about investigating these two outbreaks using emerging technologies to determine a linkage? (Chapter Objectives 1 and 6).

PEARSON
myhealthprofessionskit™

Use this address to access the interactive Companion Website created for this textbook. Simply select "Clinical Laboratory Science" from the choice of disciplines. Find this book and log in using your user name and password.

REFERENCES

Go to myhealthprofessionskit.com to view this chapter's references.

PART III
SPECIAL SPECIMEN PROCESSING

13

Acid-Fast Bacilli Cultures

Jaya Prakash and William C. Payne

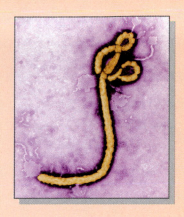

OUTLINE

■ **LEARNING OBJECTIVES**

Upon completion of this chapter, the learner should be able to:

1. Relate the different levels of mycobacteriology laboratories.

2. Evaluate safety issues that are pertinent to mycobacteriology.

3. Discuss optimal conditions and methods for specimen collection, transport, and storage for acid-fast bacilli (AFB) cultures.

4. Differentiate staining methods for AFB based on principle, procedure, advantages, and disadvantages of each.

5. Correctly interpret the results of AFB smears.

6. Discuss procedures used in processing specimens for AFB to include direct inoculation versus digestion and decontamination, neutralization, and concentration.

7. Relate the different methods for digestion, decontamination, and concentration of specimens for AFB culture to include reagent purpose.

8. Select appropriate procedures or methods based on specimen type.

9. Relate methods used to isolate and cultivate AFB to include the different types of media used, the advantages and disadvantages, and conditions for incubating cultures.

10. Select AFB culture media for each specimen type.

11. Presumptively identify *M. tuberculosis* complex.

12. Summarize the identification of mycobacteria including biochemical, molecular, liquid chromatography, and sensitivity tests.

KEY TERMS

acid-fast

digestion–
   decontamination

Kinyoun stain

Mantoux test

nonphotochromogens

photochromogens

rapid growers

scotochromogens

tuberculosis

Ziehl-Neelsen stain

▶ INTRODUCTION

Individuals working in the mycobacteriology section of a clinical laboratory must be able to isolate mycobacteria from a variety of clinical specimens. Mycobacteria, also called **acid-fast** bacilli (AFB), are different from other bacteria because their cell walls are rich in lipids and, in particular, waxy substances. This property makes them resistant to the effects of harsh environmental pressures such as acidity, alkalinity, and desiccation. It also makes working with these organisms more dangerous than working with more fragile infectious agents. For this reason, the isolation and identification of these organisms requires methods of specimen collection, handling, and processing that are quite different from those used with the gram-positive and gram-negative bacteria routinely isolated. As with other organisms that are "out of the ordinary," a significant amount of experience and expertise is required to interpret test results (Table 13-1). This is because of the fact some of these organisms take extraordinary periods of time to become mature colonies. Patience, organization, documentation, and communication skills are also needed for accurate and clinically relevant results. Procedures common to all three levels of mycobacteriology services are found in this chapter. Those methods unique to Level 3 services are found in ∞ Chapter 26, "*Mycobacterium* Species."

Some of these organisms, *Mycobacterium tuberculosis* in particular, are transmitted by the airborne route and may be extremely difficult to treat. Therefore, laboratory safety is of the utmost importance when dealing with mycobacteria and clinical specimens that may contain them.

✪ TABLE 13-1

Levels of Mycobacteriology Services

Service Provided	Level 1	Level 2	Level 3
Acid-fast smears	Yes	Yes	Yes
Culture	No	Yes	Yes
Identification of *M. tuberculosis* complex	No	Yes	Yes
Identification of other mycobacteria	No	No	Yes
Mycobacterium species susceptibility testing	No	No	Yes

Source: Adapted from Della-Latta & Weitzman, 1998.

✓ Checkpoint! 13–1 (Chapter Objective 1)

A laboratory that performs acid-fast smears, culture, and identification of M. tuberculosis *complex is providing:*

A. *level 1 services.*
B. *level 2 services.*
C. *level 3 services.*
D. *level 4 services.*

▶ LABORATORY SAFETY

Mycobacterium tuberculosis is the primary cause of **tuberculosis**, an infection of the lungs and other organs, in humans. It is a highly infectious pathogen that is transmitted primarily through inhalation of airborne respiratory droplets. For this reason, laboratory safety is best accomplished by preventing aerosol production. Biosafety level (BSL) 2 precautions are a must, not only to guard laboratory workers from the real possibility of disease transmission within the laboratory setting, but also to prevent contamination of samples from uninfected patients. This would, of course, lead to a false-positive result. The proper use of biological safety cabinets; personnel protective equipment such as gowns, gloves, and respiratory masks; centrifuges with safety carriers; and germicides is required. All work, including preparing smears for staining, processing patient specimens, setting up cultures, isolating mycobacteria on growth media, as well as biochemical and susceptibility testing, should be performed within the confines of a biological safety cabinet (BSC). The BSC should be large enough to hold all the necessary equipment for processing specimens and setting up cultures (Figure 13-1 ■). When working with cultured organisms or clinical specimens from known or highly suspected extensively drug-resistant tuberculosis (XDR TB) patients, BSL 3 precautions are necessary (CDC, 2008a).

Even when work is done under the protection of a BSC, it is important to wear protective apparel (liquid impermeable gowns that fasten securely from behind, masks, and gloves). Germicides such as 5% phenolic compounds, 3% to 8% formaldehyde solutions, sodium hypochlorite solutions, and 70% ethanol are recommended to decontaminate work areas before and after processing. Work may be performed on a towel moistened with disinfectant that is discarded once work is completed. Paper towels wet with disinfectant are used to wipe off the outside and lip of tubes after decanting the contents.

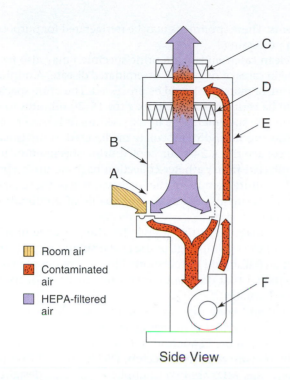

Room air

Contaminated air

HEPA-filtered air

Side View

■ **FIGURE 13-1** Class 2 Biological Safety Cabinet (BSC). **a.** Front opening. **b.** Sash. **c.** Exhaust HEPA filter. **d.** Rear plenum. **e.** Supply HEPA filter. **f.** Blower.
From the Centers for Disease Control and Prevention (CDC).

Mycobacteria have cell walls containing waxy compounds. Consequently, inserting material containing these organisms into an open flame or incinerator may produce spattering and the danger of producing infectious aerosols. A sand flask, containing a layer of washed sand that is covered by a layer of a germicidal solution, can counteract this danger and should be kept inside the working area of biologic safety cabinets. Inoculating loops and wires should be immersed in the sand flask where large clumps of infectious material can be cleaned off prior to their introduction into open flames or incinerators. See Table 5-1 in ∞ Chapter 5, "Safety," to review biosafety level practices.

Another element of safety in working with AFB is skin testing of personnel using tuberculin purified protein derivative (PPD). This procedure can determine exposure to *Mycobacterium* species and seroconversion, a delayed-type hypersensitivity reaction. This is important for individuals who are at risk of exposure to *M. tuberculosis* and is especially important for individuals who work in the mycobacteriology section of the microbiology laboratory. Tuberculin skin testing should be performed annually.

The **Mantoux** or tuberculin PPD skin test involves the injection of five tuberculin units (0.1 mL of antigen) just under the epidermis of the inner surface of the forearm. A tuberculin syringe with a 27 gauge needle is used for the injection. The small bump, seen at the injection site, disappears shortly as the liquid is absorbed. A positive skin test is the result of a

delayed-type hypersensitivity reaction, and therefore the test should be read after 48 to 72 hours have elapsed. A health care professional trained to read TB skin tests carefully evaluates the injection site for signs of a positive reaction. This individual examines the site visually and palpates the site. Erythema or redness at the injection site is not abnormal, but evidence of induration (feeling firm or hardened to the touch) and swelling are indications of exposure and seroconversion. The size of the raised area is determined using a ruler, and the measurement in millimeters is recorded. The absence of a raised area (0 mm) is a negative skin test. A raised area of 5 mm or more is considered to be a positive skin test in individuals who are immunosuppressed (such as individuals with AIDS), those exposed to individuals with active TB, and those with radiographic evidence (the presence of fibrotic lesions on chest x-rays, which is consistent with past TB infection). A raised bump measuring 10 mm or greater is a positive skin test for individuals recently arrived in the United States from countries where TB is endemic, persons injecting illicit drugs, persons in high-risk environments (crowded conditions), persons employed in mycobacteria laboratories, and children under the age of 4. Persons with raised areas 15 mm or greater are considered positive (About.com, 2007).

 Checkpoint! 13–2 (Chapter Objective 2)

What procedure is used to demonstrate exposure to mycobacteria and seroconversion?

    A. *A significant rise in antibody titer*
    B. *Radiographic evidence (fibrotic lesions in the lungs)*
    C. *The tuberculin PPD skin test*
    D. *Coughing and the production of sputum*

▶ SPECIMEN COLLECTION

Specimens for mycobacterial cultures should be collected in sterile, leakproof, nonwaxed, disposable containers. Collection methods should bypass, as much as possible, areas known to contain contaminating microbes. Skin and mucous membranes are colonized with microorganisms that will quickly outgrow the slow-growing mycobacteria, rendering their recovery much more difficult if not impossible. Consider the number of organisms present in a stool sample. Swabs are not acceptable because they contain insufficient material, and if organisms are few in number, they may become entrapped among the fibers. Stool specimens are only acceptable in AIDS patients where *Mycobacterium avium* complex (MAC) organisms may occur in sufficient numbers to be recovered. Patient specimens can be stored at 2°C to 8°C if they cannot be immediately processed.

Sputum is the specimen collected most often to diagnose respiratory illnesses caused by *M. tuberculosis* and other respiratory pathogens. Clinicians must instruct patients to cough very deeply to obtain the thick exudate (sputum) produced in the lower respiratory tract. Sputum is brought up the trachea and through the oral cavity and deposited into an appropriate sterile container. It is important that the specimen be sputum and not saliva, a watery secretion from the salivary glands found in the mouth and oropharynx. For adequate evaluation of the infectious process; three specimens should be collected over a period of 3 consecutive days (Harvell, Hadley, & Ng, 2000; Nelson, Deike, & Cartwright, 1998). Additional specimens may be accepted after consultation with the patient's physician. Specimens should contain 5 to 10 mL of material and should not be pooled specimens. Twenty-four-hour pooled specimens introduce the risk of increased bacterial contamination and are not acceptable. An aerosolized, sterile, 10% solution of sodium chloride may be used to induce sputum production in patients unable to produce acceptable quantities of sputum. Although induced sputum may have a watery appearance and may be mistaken for saliva, it is an acceptable specimen for the diagnosis of tuberculosis. Induced sputum should be labeled as such to avoid confusion with specimens that are largely saliva. Other specimens that are frequently collected on patients unable to produce sputum include bronchial washings, bronchoalveolar lavage, and transbronchial biopsy material collected using more invasive procedures such as bronchoscopy.

Gastric lavage is another option for patients unable to produce acceptable sputum specimens. Respiratory secretions produced in the lower respiratory tract are moved up the trachea by the action of ciliated epithelial cells, which line the upper respiratory tract. This respiratory exudate is either swallowed reflexively or spit out, normal human behaviors that help to prevent particles and organisms trapped in mucus from entering the bronchi and lungs. Three samples collected over a period of 3 consecutive days is the norm for processing gastric lavage specimens (Cernoch, Enns, Saubolle, & Wallace, 1994). Early morning specimens collected before the patient has eaten are the preferred specimen. Although AFB is resistant to the effects of acid environments, they are not totally impervious to degradation by stomach acid. Consequently, specimens should be processed immediately, or a sodium carbonate buffer solution should be added to neutralize the hydrochloric acid in stomach contents if processing within 4 hours cannot be accomplished. Phenol red, a pH indicator, can be incorporated into the buffer to indicate neutralization (phenol red is yellow at a low or acid pH and pink to red at a neutral or alkaline pH).

Patients must fast for at least 8 hours before an early morning specimen is taken. To collect material from a gastric lavage, the patient's oropharynx can be anesthetized with a topical anesthetic to relax the gag reflex. The patient then swallows a gastric tube as sterile water is sipped to ease the delivery of the tube into the stomach. Also, 20 to 30 mL of sterile water can be instilled by mouth or by injection through the tube. A 50 mL syringe attached to the tube is used to aspirate stomach contents. These specimens may be refrigerated for purposes of batch processing.

A clean catch midstream urine specimen may also be submitted in cases of suspected disseminated disease. A minimum of 40 mL of material should be processed. The urine specimen should be centrifuged at 3000 x g for 15–20 minutes to concentrate the specimen. The urinary sediment is used to make acid-fast smears and to inoculate media used in the isolation of mycobacteria. A 24-hour pooled urine specimen or material collected from catheter collection bags are unacceptable for AFB culture because of the increased risk of bacterial contamination (many organisms are capable of proliferating at room temperature).

To evaluate ulcerative lesions for the presence of AFB, a biopsy of the leading edge of the lesion should be performed. This material should be transported to the laboratory in a sterile container that does not contain preservatives or fixatives such as formalin.

Blood and bone marrow specimens may be collected for AFB cultures in cases of disseminated disease. The Isolator lysis system (Wampole Laboratories, Cranbury, NJ) and BACTEC 13A blood culture bottles (Becton, Dickinson and Company, Cockeysville, MD) are two examples of systems designed to isolate mycobacteria from blood specimens. Many automated systems have developed media for direct inoculation of blood and bone marrow. Consult manufacturer specifications regarding culture of blood and bone marrow specimens. Sodium polyanethol sulfonate (SPS) is the anticoagulant contained in blood culture bottles. Collection in evacuated tubes containing SPS or heparin is an acceptable alternative, but the use of EDTA anticoagulated tubes is prohibited. It should be noted that microorganisms can be trapped in clotted blood, and therefore coagulated blood is not acceptable. SPS may also be added to other body fluids that may clot such as pleural and pericardial fluid.

 Checkpoint! 13–3 (Chapter Objective 3)

The appropriate sputum collection procedure to establish the presence or absence of acid-fast bacilli (AFB) in the lower respiratory tract is:

    A. *three specimens collected over a period of 3 consecutive days.*
    B. *three specimens collected 1 hour apart.*
    C. *a pooled specimen collected over a 24-hour period.*
    D. *the first morning specimen before any food is eaten.*

▶ MYCOBACTERIAL STAINS

Information gathered by the microscopic examination of AFB smears prepared from material sent for acid-fast cultures can provide useful information to clinicians. The result of examining an AFB smear is not as sensitive as the results of a culture, but may provide a relatively rapid presumptive diagnosis.

Persons with a negative smear should be cultured before being considered negative for tuberculosis. Care should be taken to avoid contamination of negative specimen smears with AFB positive specimen smears. Nontuberculosis mycobacteria (NTM) exist in the environment, including in tap water, so filtered or sterile water should be used in staining procedures (Graham, Warren, Tsang, & Dalton, 1988).

The reaction of mycobacteria to the Gram stain is variable. Because of the waxy components found in the cell wall of these bacteria, permeability to the Gram staining reagents is highly variable, with some organisms appearing to be gram positive, some having a beaded appearance, and in some cases the organism may not stain at all with the crystal violet and safranin dyes. The very substances that make these organisms difficult to stain with Gram stain reagents, the waxes and mycolic acids of the cell wall, also confer resistance to decolorization with acid–alcohol solvents. This property of being "acid-fast" is not a property native to most other microbial life forms, although certain coccidian parasites, such as *Cryptosporidium* and *Cyclospora* species, and some nonmycobacterial organisms such as *Nocardia* species, and *Rhodococcus* species, exhibit varying degrees of acid-fastness.

 REAL WORLD TIP

When performing acid-fast stains, it is important to remember that all mycobacteria (*Mycobacterium leprae*, for example) are not acid fast to the same degree as *M. tuberculosis*.

Staining direct smears (material that has not been concentrated) is suitable for specimens from normally sterile sites and that do not contain contaminating bacteria (i.e., biopsy specimens). Two to three drops of the specimen are placed on a clean glass slide and spread evenly over an area of 1 to ½ inch. The smear is allowed to air dry and is then fixed by one of the following methods:

- The use of an electric slide warmer set at a temperature between 65°C to 75°C for a period of 2 hours (alternatively 80°C for 15 minutes).
- Passing the air-dried smear through the blue flame of a Bunsen burner three or four times, taking care not to overheat (or char) the specimen. The CDC does not recommend this method of heat fixation (CDC, 2008a) because Bunsen burners are rarely used in microbiology laboratories and can create aerosols.
- Immerse the air-dried smear in absolute methanol for 1 minute. The methanol should not be reused for other slides to avoid cross-contamination with other specimens. Alternatively, a methanol fixative spray may be used.

 REAL WORLD TIP

Viable AFB may still be present after heat fixing, so handle smears carefully using gloves and discard the slide in a biohazard sharps container (Della-Latta & Weitzman, 1998).

Concentrated smears may be prepared from specimens in which few organisms are likely to be present, for example, body fluids that are normally sterile. In this case, the specimen can be centrifuged in screw topped containers and the sediment used to prepare the smear. Specimens likely to contain contaminating organisms can also be concentrated following a digestant–decontamination process. For pleural fluids that may have clotted, sputolysin or dithiothreitol may be used as a digestant to dissolve the clot before smear preparation.

A 5% sodium hypochlorite solution (undiluted household bleach) can be used as a decontaminant to kill all organisms present, including AFB. An equal amount of bleach is added to the specimen and allowed to sit 15 minutes before processing (CDC, 2008a). In this manner, the smears can be prepared on the open bench. The clinician should be alerted to the fact the specimen is no longer useful for AFB cultures because all organisms have been killed.

CARBOL FUCHSIN–BASED STAINS

The carbol fuchsin reagent of the **Ziehl-Neelsen stain** renders acid-fast organisms a red color. The Companion Website provides the Ziehl-Neelsen staining procedure. The application of heat and the incorporation of phenol (carbolic acid) into the staining solution allows the primary stain to penetrate the waxy cell wall of mycobacteria. Once stained, the AFB retain the fuchsin stain and resist decolorization with an acid–alcohol decolorizing agent (3% hydrochloric acid in 95% ethanol). Objects that are not acid fast (most other bacteria, fungal elements, organic debris, and body cells) are decolorized and subsequently stained blue by the methylene blue counterstain (Figure 13-2 ■). Smears are examined using the oil immersion lens. At least 300 fields should be examined before reporting the smear result as negative (Huebner, Good, & Tokars, 1993).

The **Kinyoun stain** has higher concentrations of basic fuchsin and phenol, which delivers greater penetration of the dye into the cell wall. This eliminates the need for heating the smear. With the Kinyoun staining procedure, 3% sulfuric acid in 95% ethanol is used as the decolorizing agent. ∞ Chapter 8, "Presumptive Identification," provides a photo of a positive Kinyoun stain (Figure 8-9). The Kinyon stain procedure is available on the Companion Website. A modification of this stain is used to stain organisms that are partially or weakly acid fast, such as *Nocardia* species, *Rhodococcus* species, and coccidian

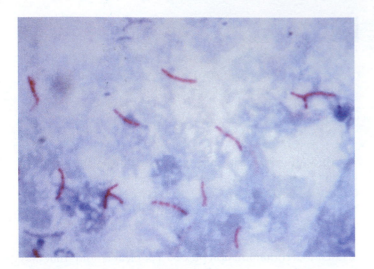

■ **FIGURE 13-2** Positive Ziehl-Neelsen stained smear.
Public Health Image Library (PHIL)/CDC and Dr. George P. Kubica

parasites. In the modified Kinyoun stain, the decolorizer is a 1% sulfuric acid solution. The Ziehl-Neelsen method is preferred over the Kinyoun method because of its higher sensitivity in detecting positive acid-fast bacilli (Somoskövi et al., 2001).

FLUOROCHROME STAINS

Fluorescent dyes are also used in staining AFB. Dyes such as auramine and rhodamine or a combination of both are popular. These fluorescent dyes are able to penetrate the cell wall and remain in the cell walls of AFB after decolorization. Potassium permanganate is used to quench nonspecific fluorescence and provide a dark background for better contrast. With these dyes, AFB fluoresce, absorbing ultraviolet light, and emitting visible light that the human eye perceives as a yellow, red, or orange color, depending on the exact nature of the fluorescent dye or combination used (Figure 13-3 ■). The appearance

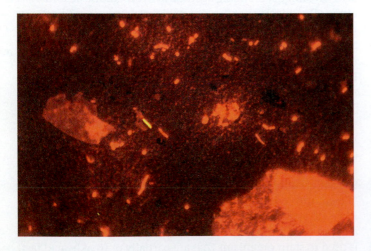

■ **FIGURE 13-3** Positive fluorochrome stained smear. Note the single yellow acid fast bacillus.
Photo courtesy of the Centers for Disease Control and Prevention (CDC).

of brightly lit objects against a dark background provides better visual acuity than that obtained with the carbol fuchsin stains.

Smears can be scanned (250×), which provides a larger field of vision than the oil immersion field. This allows smears to be examined more quickly because 30 fields rather then 300 are examined before reporting as negative for AFB. The high-power objective (450×) is used to confirm the bacilli morphology of a positive smear. The fluorochrome staining procedure can be found on the Companion Website.

Fluorochrome stained smears should be read immediately or stored at 2°C to 8°C in the dark to avoid fading of fluorescence and a false-negative result. The rapid-growing mycobacteria may not fluoresce (Master, 1995). Organic debris may sometimes fluoresce, causing a false positive with the auramine-rhodamine stains, and for this reason it is recommended that positive smears stained with these fluorochromes be restained and confirmed with the Ziehl-Neelsen stain or reexamined by a second person. Positive results should be reported to the clinician in charge of the patient (Box 13-1⊙).

🄮 REAL WORLD TIP

Wipe the oil immersion lens off after each positive AFB smear to avoid cross contamination of subsequent smears and a false-positive result (Cernoch et al., 1994).

🄮 REAL WORLD TIP

All positive acid-fast smears and cultures for *Mycobacterium tuberculosis* must be reported as soon as possible. Most facilities consider them to be critical results. Rapid communication to the physician, state and local health agencies can help prevent the spread of the organism.

▶ SPECIMEN PROCESSING

Normally sterile specimens, such as tissues specimens (lung tissue for example), biopsy material, and body fluids (blood, bone marrow, spinal fluid, etc.) do not require decontamination to eliminate contaminating bacteria. However, tissue specimens should be ground aseptically with a sterile mortar and pestle designed for tissue grinding, or some other type of tissue homogenizer should be used. A small amount of sterile physiologic saline or 0.2% bovine albumin may be added prior to grinding, and the material can then be inoculated directly to both liquid and solid mycobacterial media. Body fluids should be concentrated by centrifugation. When centrifuging body fluids, safety carriers with screw caps must be used in

✪ BOX 13-1

Examination and Interpretation of AFB Smears

A minimum of 5,000 to 10,000 organisms per mL must be present in the specimen to be detected by smear examination.

For carbol fuchsin stains, three lengthwise passes and nine width-wise passes are required (equivalent to about 300 fields) to examine the smear. This usually requires about 15 minutes. Count and record the number of AFB seen per field.

For fluorochrome stains at least three lengthwise passes (at 250× magnification this is equivalent to at least 30 fields; at 450× magnification this is equivalent to about 70 fields) is required to examine the smear adequately. This usually takes about 2 to 3 minutes to accomplish. Count and record the number of AFB seen.

Quality control smears should be used each time AFB smears are performed: A negative control is a gram-negative bacilli such as *E. coli*, and the positive control is *M. tuberculosis*.

Interpretation:
- 0 AFB seen in all the fields examined is recorded as: No AFB seen.
- 1 to 2 on the entire slide is recorded as: doubtful results and should be confirmed with another specimen.
- 1 to 9 per 100 fields using the oil immersion lens and 2 to 18 per 50 fields using the low-power objective (450×) should be reported as 1+.
- 1 to 9 per 10 fields using the oil immersion lens and 4 to 36 per 10 fields using the low-power objective (450×) should be reported as 2+.
- 1 to 9 per field using the oil immersion lens and 4 to 36 per field using the low-power objective (450×) should be reported as 3+.
- Greater than 9 per field using the oil immersion lens and >36 per field using the low-power objective (450×) should be reported as 4+.

Source: Adapted from Della-Latta & Weitzman, 1998.

case the specimen processing container should break. The safety carriers should only be opened in a biological safety cabinet. The sediment obtained after centrifugation is used to prepare smears and to inoculate media.

Sputum (both expectorated and aerosol induced), bronchial washings, gastric lavage, skin lesions, wound aspirates, urine, and stool specimens (AIDS patients only) may contain contaminating organisms that colonize mucous membranes of the upper respiratory, gastrointestinal, and urogenital tracts, as well as mucus. These rapidly growing organisms can quickly overgrow any mycobacteria in the specimen. For this reason, it is necessary to use some **digestion–decontamination** procedure prior to inoculation of media. The most commonly used reagent for processing acid-fast specimens is an *N*-acetyl-L-cysteine (NALC) and sodium hydroxide solution (4% NaOH). NALC is the mucolytic agent that liquefies mucus and organic debris. Sodium hydroxide, a strong alkali, is the decontaminant that kills the contaminating bacteria. As mentioned pre-

viously, the high lipid content of the mycobacterial cell wall makes them more resistant than other organisms to the effect of the alkaline decontaminant solution. It should be noted, however, that overexposure to NaOH is toxic to mycobacteria as well. A phosphate buffer is usually added after the decontamination step to dilute the bactericidal activity of NaOH. Sometimes a bovine albumin solution is also added to further buffer and detoxify the specimen. The NALC-NaOH digestion and decontamination procedure is available on the Companion Website.

A similar procedure can be followed using only 2% to 4% NaOH instead of NALC–NaOH. It does not produce good results with excessively mucoid sputum specimens and may kill most of the tubercle bacilli. Other methods have also been used for working with AFB specimens that may contain contaminating microorganisms:

- Zephiran-trisodium phosphate (Zephiran or benzalkonium chloride is a detergent)
- Dithiothreitol (Sputolysin) with 2% NaOH
- Cetylpyridinium chloride with NaCl
- 5% oxalic acid treatment may be used when *Pseudomonas* species are found to be contaminating the specimen
- 4% sulfuric acid

 REAL WORLD TIP

The use of individual reagents and pipettes for each specimen helps prevent cross contamination of AFB negative specimens with AFB positive specimens.

 Checkpoint! 13–4 (Chapter Objective 4)

When the Ziehl-Neelsen stain is properly used to stain AFB, they should:
  A. *appear to be red in color against a blue background.*
  B. *appear to be blue in color against a red background.*
  C. *appear as small blue colonies with a fried egg appearance.*
  D. *appear to be brightly lit against a dark background.*

 Checkpoint! 13–5 (Chapter Objective 6)

The most popular digestant–decontaminant solution for processing specimens that may contain contaminating organisms is:
  A. *Sputolysin.*
  B. *cetylpyridium chloride.*
  C. *sulfuric acid.*
  D. *N-acetyl-L-cysteine and NaOH.*

Checkpoint! 13–6 (Chapter Objective 7)

Which of the following ingredients is a mucolytic agent?
A. *N-acetyl-L-cysteine*
B. *trisodium phosphate*
C. *M/15 phosphate buffer*
D. *sodium hydroxide*

Checkpoint! 13–7 (Chapter Objective 8)

All of the following specimens generally require decontamination except:
A. *sputum.*
B. *clean voided urine.*
C. *gastric aspirates.*
D. *cerebrospinal fluid.*

▶ ISOLATION OF ACID-FAST BACILLI

It is recommended that liquid medium be used for primary culture along with inoculation of a Lowenstein-Jensen slant, an egg-based medium (Tenover et al., 1993). Agar-based solid media can also be added to isolate mycobacteria and observe colony morphology. Media must be formulated to provide the nutritional requirements of these slow-growing bacteria with a highly complex cell wall composition. Medium containing heme should be added if the patient is deficient in cellular immunity or *M. haemophilum,* a rare fastidious skin pathogen, is suspected. Chocolate agar can be used if incubated at 32°C (Males, West, Bartholomew, 1987). See ∞ Chapter 26, "*Mycobacterium* Species," for more information about *M. haemophilum.*

In addition to the proper nutrients, antibiotics and other inhibitory substances may be incorporated into the basal media to inhibit the growth of contaminating microorganisms in specimens from areas of the body that are colonized with other microorganisms.

EGG-BASED MEDIA

Egg-based media contains whole egg, potato flour, salts, glycerol, and malachite green (0.025%), a dye that inhibits the growth of contaminating bacteria. Although most media is sterilized using steam under pressure, egg-based media is dispensed as slants and sterilized by flowing steam in a process called inspissation. The heat coagulates the egg protein creating a solid medium. Egg-based media are an excellent growth medium because of their capacity to neutralize toxins. However, a major problem with egg-based media is liquefaction, a process in which contaminating bacteria, such as pseudomonads and *Proteus* species, which secrete proteolytic enzymes, convert the solid slants to a thick soup. Examples of egg-based media include the following:

- Lowenstein-Jensen (LJ) medium (Figure 13-4a ■) is the most popular egg-based medium and includes modifications (LJ-Gruft, which contains penicillin and nalidixic acid, LJ with pyruvic acid, and LJ with iron).

- Wallenstein medium is formulated much like LJ medium, but contains a higher concentration of malachite green. This medium is an excellent medium for recovery of non-tuberculous mycobacteria, especially *M. avium* complex (Forbes, Sahm, & Weissfeld, 2002).

- Petragnani is another medium with a relatively high concentration of malachite green, making it more inhibitory than LJ medium and better able to discourage the growth of contaminating organisms.

- American Trudeau Society medium (ATS) contains less malachite green than LJ medium, making it less inhibitory and more likely to grow contaminating bacteria.

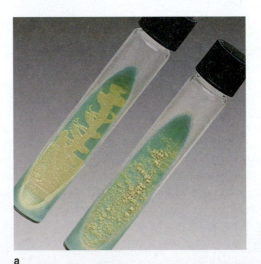

a

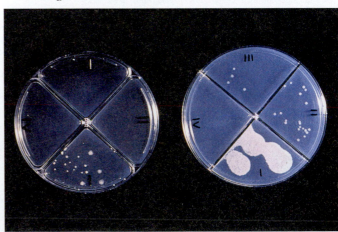

b

■ **FIGURE 13-4 a.** Lowenstein-Jensen Medium with *M. avium* (left) and *M. tuberculosis* (right). *Photo courtesy of Remel, part of Thermo Fisher Scientific.* **b.** Susceptibility test using 7H10 agar. *Photo courtesy of the Centers for Disease Control and Prevention (CDC).*

AGAR-BASED MEDIA

Agar-based media are chemically defined, containing salts, vitamins, oleic acid, albumin, glycerol, dextrose, and malachite green. Because these media are transparent, microscopic observation of growth is possible making growth detection quicker. Microcolony morphology may be used for presumptive identification. Excessive exposure to heat and light should be avoided to prevent the breakdown of oleic acid into formaldehyde, which is inhibitory to microorganisms, including the mycobacteria. Examples of agar based media include:

- Middlebrook 7H10 and Middlebrook 7H10 selective
- Middlebrook 7H11 and Middlebrook 7H11 selective (differs from 7H10 by the addition of an enzymatic hydrolysate of casein)

Antibiotics may be added to both egg-based and agar-based media to make them selective. This prevents contaminating bacteria, which may survive the decontamination process, from overgrowing the mycobacteria. Specific concentrations of antibiotics can be added to agar-based media and used for susceptibility testing (Figure 13-4b ■). An X-factor strip can be added to 7H10 agar to provide the hemin required for growth of *M. haemophilum* (Vadney & Hawkins, 1985).

LIQUID MEDIA

The use of liquid media increases the recovery of organisms when they are few in number because organisms grow better in liquid than on solid media. Examples of broths designed to grow mycobacteria include

- Middlebrook 7H9, 7H12, and 7H13 broths (do not expose to excessive heat and light)
- BACTEC 12B
- Dubois Tween albumin broth

OTHER TB MEDIA

Septi-Chek AFB system (Becton, Dickinson and Company, Sparks, MD) is a biphasic medium that contains modified Middlebrook 7H9 broth and a three-sided paddle with chocolate agar, modified 7H11 agar, and LJ medium. Growth of *Mycobacterium* species can be observed on the three-sided paddle.

Commercial systems include:

- Mycobacterial Growth Indicator Tube (Becton, Dickinson, Sparks, MD) or MGIT is a fluorescence-based system that uses Middlebrook 7H9 broth as the growth medium. Oxygen depletion because of growth of mycobacteria is detected by fluorescence (Figure 13-5 ■) after exposure to an ultraviolet light source. Fluorescence can be detected manually or by an instrument. Most clinical specimens,

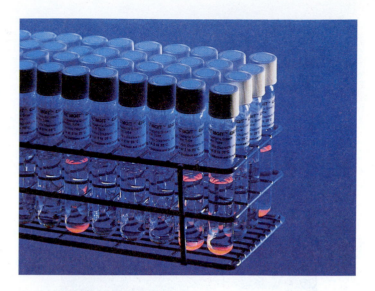

■ **FIGURE 13-5** Positive MIGT tubes are detected based on fluorescence.
Courtesy of and © by Becton, Dickinson and Company.

other than blood and urine, can be processed (Della-Latta & Weitzman, 1998).

- BACTEC 460 TB (Becton, Dickinson)—a radiometric system. Gases in the system are periodically sampled to detect radiolabeled CO_2, a by-product of mycobacterial growth. BACTEC 12 B bottles are used for most clinical specimens. BACTEC 13A bottles are used to culture blood and bone marrow specimens.

- BACTEC 9000 MB (Becton, Dickinson)—another fluorescence-based system that detects growth through oxygen consumption. Middlebrook 7H9 is the growth medium. Myco/F sputa bottles are used to culture most specimens. Myco/F-lytic bottles are used to culture blood and bone marrow.

- ESP II Mycobacteria System (AccuMed International, Westlake, OH) detects pressure changes that occur within the sealed bottle. These pressure changes are the result of mycobacterial metabolism leading to gas production or consumption (Metchock, Nolte, & Wallace, 1999). ESP Myco medium is suitable for culture of blood and bone marrow.

- MB BacT/Alert (Organon Teknika, Durham, NC) is another automated system designed for detecting mycobacterial growth. Microorganisms present in the growth medium (Middlebrook 7H9 supplemented with pancreatic digest of casein, bovine serum albumin, and catalase) use substrates producing CO_2 in the process. In the presence of the CO_2, the color of the gas-permeable sensor at the bottom of the bottle changes from a dark green to a lighter green or yellow color. The instrument, which monitors the bottles every 10 minutes, is able to detect the color change (Ang, Mendoza, Bulatao, & Cajucom, 2007) The BacT/Alert 3D (Figure 13-6 ■) can be used for processing blood and bone marrow.

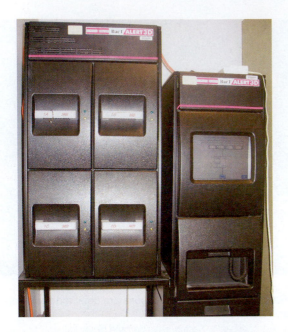

■ **FIGURE 13-6** BacT/Alert 3D.

Many of these systems have been FDA approved for susceptibility testing. A specific concentration of a single drug is incorporated into the growth medium. A bottle containing the antibiotic and one without antibiotic is inoculated with a standardized inoculum. Growth is detected as described earlier.

Inoculate solid and broth medium with two drops of inoculum. Follow the manufacturer's instructions for commercial systems regarding inoculum amount. Most mycobacteria responsible for human infection grow well at 35°C to 37°C, with the exception of *M. marinum* and *M. ulcerans,* which grow best at 25°C to 30°C. If chocolate agar or 7H10 with an X-factor strip is used instead of 7H10 plus hemin to grow *M. haemophilum,* it should be incubated at 30°C to 32°C (Males et al., 1987; Vadney & Hawkins, 1985). An atmosphere of increased CO_2 (5%–10%) is recommended for culturing mycobacteria and is required for the growth of *M. tuberculosis.* Cultures should be examined within the first 3 to 5 days after incubation, then twice a week for the first 4 weeks and then weekly for the next 4 weeks (Della-Latta & Weitzman, 1998). Follow the manufacturer's instructions for commercial systems regarding examination for growth.

✓ **Checkpoint! 13–8 (Chapter Objective 9)**

The most popular egg-based medium used for the growth of mycobacteria is:

A. *Lowenstein-Jensen medium.*
B. *Wallenstein medium.*
C. *Petragnani medium.*
D. *Middlebrook 7H10.*

▶ **PRESUMPTIVE IDENTIFICATION OF MYCOBACTERIA**

Examination of the macroscopic or colony morphology of isolates growing on solid media is the initial step in identifying mycobacteria. The presence of pigmentation should be readily apparent (pale yellow brown, yellow, orange, etc.). Using a hand lens, it should be noted whether the surface of the colonies is smooth, rough, or dry and granular in appearance. The edge or margin of the colony may be circular or irregular. The size of colonies and whether they are elevated or flat are also criteria to be considered. The consistency of the colonies produced may be another consideration and may be ascertained when the colony is removed from the surface of the agar with an inoculating loop or needle. Consistency can be:

■ Butyrous (butterlike)
■ Viscid (sticky)
■ Mucoid (slimy)
■ Friable (dry and brittle)

When transparent media such as the Middlebrook agar is inoculated the 10× objective may be used to examine the surface of the media for early growth by inverting the plate, placing it on the stage of the microscope, and focusing through the bottom of the plate and the agar medium itself. Two microcolony types may be observed. Those that resemble *M. tuberculosis* are corded similar to rope, and those that resemble *M. avium and M. intracellulare* have dense centers that resemble fried eggs. Advantages of microcolony examination include early detection of positive or mixed cultures, selection of a single probe for identification rather then several, and the addition of susceptibility testing to detect drug resistance. Using this technique *M. tuberculosis* colonies can be detected on average in 7 days in acid-fast stain positive cultures (Welch, Guruswamy, Sides, Shaw, & Gilchrist, 1993). Suspect colonies should be stained and confirmed as acid-fast bacilli.

Cord formation can also be observed in acid-fast stains of positive liquid medium. Virulent strains of *M. tuberculosis* complex grow as tight, ropelike or serpentine cords (Figure 13-7 ■), whereas avirulent TB and other mycobacteria grow in a more haphazard, detached manner. Some NTM produce loose bundles and clumps or pseudo cords. Inexperienced microscopists should ensure that "the long axis of the bacteria is parallel to the long axis of the cord" before reporting as positive for cording (McCarter, Ratkiewicz, & Robinson, 1998). If too few organisms are observed in the smear, reincubate the medium before considering it negative for cord formation.

Based on certain physiologic characteristics (pathogenicity, rate of growth, and pigment production), mycobacteria can be categorized into one of the following five Runyoun groups, *M. tuberculosis* complex, photochromogens, scotochromogens, nonphotochromogens, or rapid growers (Figure 13-8 ■).

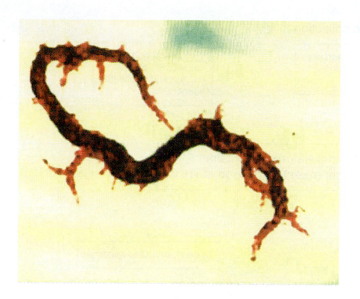

■ **FIGURE 13-7** Serpentine cord formation typical of *M. tuberculosis* complex.

Photo courtesy of Bruce A. Hanna, PhD.

The *M. tuberculosis* complex includes *M. tuberculosis*, *M. bovis*, *M. africanum*, *M. microti*, and *M. carnetti*. *M. tuberculosis* produces buff-colored, dry, corded, colonies with a flat periphery and a "cauliflower-like" center (Figure 13-9 ■). Members of the *M. tuberculosis* complex are slow growers, requiring 4 to 8 weeks to produce mature colonies on egg-based media.

Photochromogens are slow growers that produce smooth, buff-colored or lightly pigmented colonies on egg-based media when incubated in the dark. When the tube is exposed to light, a yellow to orange-yellow pigment is produced. This phenomenon is referred to as photoreactivity.

Scotochromogens are also slow growers. They produce smooth, yellow to orange pigmented colonies (Figure 13-10 ■) when grown in the dark. The color deepens on exposure to light using a 60 watt bulb for 1 hour.

Nonphotochromogens grow slowly. These organisms may produce buff-colored or lightly pigmented colonies, but the pigmentation does not deepen with exposure to light.

Rapid growers are mycobacteria that produce mature colonies within 7 days of incubation.

Table 13-2✪ differentiates the most commonly isolated *Mycobacterium* species.

The goal of mycobacteria laboratories should be to generate clinically relevant results. These are rapid and accurate test results that can be used by physicians to contain and treat tuberculosis. The current standard requires specimens to be received by the laboratory within 24 hours of collection, an acid-fast smear result within 24 hours after specimen receipt, detection of positive cultures within 14 days after specimen receipt, identification reported within 21 days, and susceptibility results reported within 30 days (Shinnock, Iademaraco, & Ridderhof, 2005). Methods for identification of mycobac-

teria are discussed in the next section. More detailed information on molecular methods is provided in ∞ Chapter 9, "Final Identification." The mycobacteria chapter (∞ Chapter 26) will provide specific information on conventional biochemicals used for AFB identification.

▶ OTHER METHODS OF IDENTIFICATION

Although physiologic criteria are used to assign isolates to a particular subgroup as described in the previous section, identification to the genus-species or complex level requires a more sophisticated approach.

CONVENTIONAL BIOCHEMICALS

Biochemical tests can be performed to identify an acid-fast bacilli isolate. Niacin accumulation, nitrate reduction, and 68°C catalase testing can identify 96% of *M. tuberculosis* isolates (Table 13-3✪); however, 3 weeks are required after initial isolation to produce results (Huebner et al., 1993). Compare this time to biochemical tests used to identify rapidly growing organisms such as staphylococci, streptococci, and enteric gram-negative rods that are usually read within 18 to 24 hours. A detailed discussion of biochemical tests used to identify acid-fast bacilli is found in ∞ Chapter 26, "*Mycobacterium* Species." Refer to the chapter for additional information.

Traditional methods for the identification and susceptibility testing of mycobacteria often require a substantial investment in time and labor before results can be reported to the clinician. Fortunately other test methods that are much more rapid were devised in the 1970s, and more recently, molecular methods, such as nucleic acid tests, hold the promise of direct detection of mycobacteria in clinical specimens themselves, eliminating the need to grow these organisms.

GAS LIQUID CHROMATOGRAPHY (GLC) AND HIGH-PERFORMANCE LIQUID CHROMATOGRAPHY (HPLC)

High-resolution gas chromatographic analysis of fatty acids can allow the prompt identification and reporting of results. GLC and HPLC are used to generate fatty acid profiles based on the presence of mycolic acids, substances that are found in a limited number of bacterial genera. *Corynebacterium*, *Nocardia*, *Rhodococcus*, and *Mycobacterium* all contain mycolic acids as part of their cellular makeup. Mycolic acids are a major component of the lipid content of mycobacterial cell walls. These long-chain fatty acids differ in the number of carbon atoms (60 to 90 for mycobacteria) and functional groups and generally vary with the species.

For GLC, not only mycolic acids, but also the whole lipid component of the cell wall is analyzed. The pattern of peaks

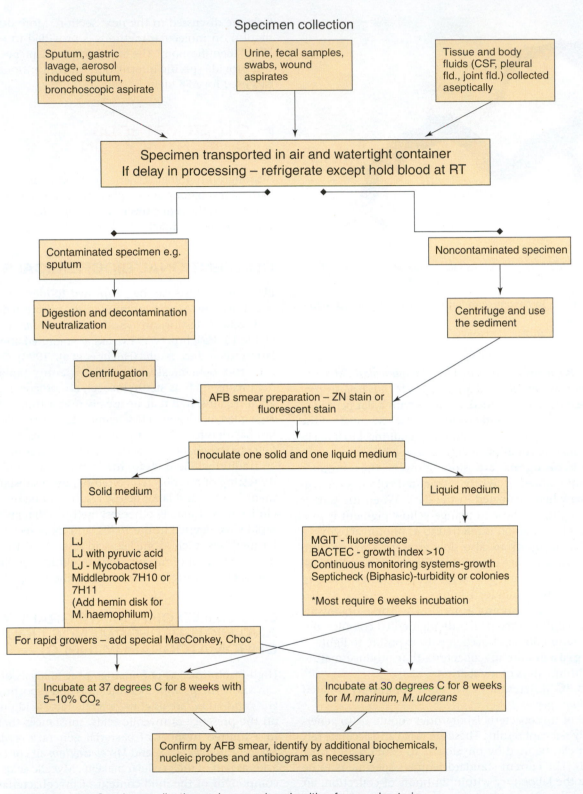

■ FIGURE 13-8 Specimen collection and processing algorithm for mycobacteria.

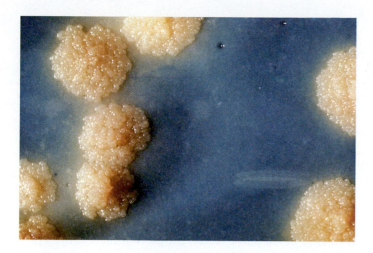

■ **FIGURE 13-9** *M. tuberculosis* colony. They are often described as rough and buff.
Photo courtesy of the Centers for Disease Control and Prevention (CDC)/Dr. George Kubica.

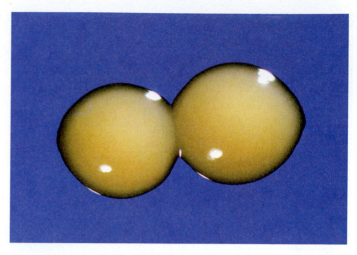

■ **FIGURE 13-10** Scotochromogen colony.
Photo courtesy of the Centers for Disease Control and Prevention (CDC)/CDC Connects.

with varying heights allows the test organism to be identified to the species level or to be placed into groups of related species. With HPLC analysis, mycolic acids are separated on the basis of their polarity and carbon chain length. Each species is characterized by a pattern that varies in the number, position, and height of the peaks (Tortoli, 2003).

MOLECULAR TESTING

Direct sample testing from clinical specimens using nucleic acid amplification tests, such as the Gen-Probe and Roche assays, is limited to sputum, tracheal aspirates, and bronchoscopy specimens. The preparation for molecular testing requires the same digestion–decontamination procedures as are used in preparing smears and inoculating cultures. The resulting sediment is used for molecular testing as per the instructions provided by the kit manufacturer. Molecular testing is capable of identifying mycobacteria that are difficult to speciate because of relatedness, a condition that biochemical tests alone cannot always meet.

The Amplicor Mycobacterium Tuberculosis Test (Amplicor, Roche Molecular Systems, Branchburg, NJ) relies on DNA amplification for the diagnosis of pulmonary tuberculosis. The Amplified Mycobacterium Tuberculosis Direct Test (AMTDT, GenProbe, San Diego, CA) uses a slightly different approach,

that of ribosomal ribonucleic acid (rRNA) testing. The sensitivities of Amplicor and AMTDT have been reported as 98% and 100%, respectively, for smear-positive specimens and 50% and 46%, respectively, for smear-negative specimens in comparison to cultures (Lebrun, Mathieu, Saulnier, & Nordmann, 1997).

Culture confirmation may be accomplished using 16S rRNA sequencing. This methodology relies on the identification of "signature sequences." The AccuProbe assay (GenProbe) is a commercially available test kit that can be used to identify isolates from a solid culture medium or a broth culture such as *M. tuberculosis*, *M. avium*, *M. intracellulare*, *M. gordonae*, or *M. kansasii* based on species-specific sequences found within the bacterial genome.

DNA sequencing is another method used to identify isolates. These methods are highly accurate and rapid, but are also labor intensive and expensive. The isolate must first be disrupted to release the bacterial DNA. The polymerase chain reaction is used to amplify the 16S rRNA gene, and the species-specific nucleic acid sequence of the unknown isolate is compared with known signature sequences to identify the isolate.

Restriction fragment length polymorphism (RFLP) analysis, another labor-intensive procedure, can be used to study the epidemiology of different strains of *Mycobacterium tuberculosis*. RFLP, more commonly known as DNA fingerprinting,

⊘ TABLE 13-2

Important Species of Mycobacteria				
M. tuberculosis Complex	Photochromogens	Scotochromogens	Nonchromogens	Rapid Growers
M. tuberculosis	*M. kansasii*	*M. gordonae*	*M. avium* complex (MAC)	*M. fortuitum*
M. bovis	*M. marinum*	*M. scrofulaceum*		
M. africanum				

TABLE 13-3

Identification of *M. tuberculosis*	
Acid-fast smear	Positive (tight, serpentine cording)
Colony	Buff, dry, corded, flat periphery, "cauliflower-like" center
Niacin	Positive (yellow)
Nitrate	Positive (pink to red)
68°C Catalase	Negative (no bubbles)

✔ Checkpoint! 13–9 (Chapter Objective 11)

Mycobacterium tuberculosis can be presumptively identified with observation of:

1. *slow-growing buff colonies.*
2. *corded colonies.*
3. *photopigmentation.*
   A. *1 & 2*
   B. *1 & 3*
   C. *2 & 3*
   D. *1, 2, & 3*

is the technique used to study nosocomial and community outbreaks. Isolates proliferate on an appropriate growth medium, and the organism's DNA is subsequently extracted. The DNA is then digested using a restriction endonuclease, which cuts the nucleic acid strand at specific locations called restriction sites. The end result is the formation of DNA fragments of differing sizes. The DNA fragments are separated electrophoretically using agarose gels. The RFLP patterns of isolates are then compared. Isolates that demonstrate identical banding patterns would be the same strain of *M. tuberculosis* (Metchock et. al., 1999). See ∞ Chapter 9, "Final Identification," to review molecular techniques.

✔ Checkpoint! 13–10 (Chapter Objective 12)

Which methodology is more accurate at identifying mycobacterial isolates?

   A. *Acid-fast staining*
   B. *Photoreactivity*
   C. *Molecular testing*
   D. *Biochemical tests*

SUMMARY

The mycobacteria are a significant cause of morbidity and mortality. The most widely known disease associated with the mycobacteria, tuberculosis, has been known since antiquity. Hippocrates, the Greek physician known as the founder of

medicine, described the disease some 400 years before the birth of Christ. In the 19th century sanatoriums were established to treat individuals who had contracted "consumption," one name by which tuberculosis became widely known. During the 20th century much progress was made in the diagnosis and treatment of tuberculosis, and the fear of "consumption" was greatly lessened until the end of the century, when multidrug-resistant strains appeared, and the reemergence of tuberculosis as a major public health menace seemed possible again, even in industrialized countries.

The importance of the clinical laboratory in the diagnosis and treatment of tuberculosis could hardly be overstated. Because the disease is spread through inhalation of droplet nuclei containing the organism, safety in working with specimens and isolates depends on the prevention of aerosol production, working under negative pressure, and the use of biological safety cabinets, high-efficiency particulate air (HEPA) filters, personal protective equipment, and effective germicides.

Sputum is the specimen used most often for the evaluation of pulmonary tuberculosis. The patient should be instructed to cough deeply to collect the thick exudate from the lower respiratory tract. Sputa, gastric and bronchial lavages, urines, and other specimens likely to contain contaminating microorganisms should be processed with a digestant–decontaminant solution, the most popular of which is N-acetyl-L-cysteine (NALC)–NaOH. Normally sterile specimens, such as cerebrospinal fluids, other body fluids, and tissue specimens, usually do not need to be decontaminated. Body fluids should be concentrated by centrifugation and the sediment used to inoculate suitable media. Tissue specimens should be disrupted by grinding aseptically with a small amount of sterile saline or broth.

Smears, which can provide a rapid presumptive diagnosis, can be stained by either of two staining methods. With carbolfuchsin stains, such as the Ziehl-Neelsen stain, acid-fast bacteria retain the red color of the fuchsin dye because of the high concentration of lipids, particularly the waxy mycolic acids. The high lipid content allows the cell wall of mycobacteria to resist decolorization with an acid–alcohol decolorizer. Other organisms and body cells are decolorized and stained blue by the use of the methylene blue counterstain.

Fluorochrome stains use fluorescent dyes such as auramine, rhodamine, or a combination of both. These fluorescent dyes penetrate the cell wall of mycobacteria and remain after decolorization. For this reason, acid-fast organisms appear to be brightly lit against a darkened background. Other cellular material is decolorized, and any nonspecific fluorescence is quenched by the use of a potassium permanganate solution.

Commercially available media is available for the cultivation of AFB. There are solid and liquid media, both of which can be made selective by the incorporation of antibiotics and other inhibitory substances such as malachite green. Media designed for mycobacteria include the following:

- Lowenstein-Jensen slants, the most commonly used egg-based medium, which contains whole egg, potato flour, salts, glycerol, and malachite green.
- Middlebrook 7H10 and 7H11, chemically defined, agar-based media, which is poured into petri dishes. Because the medium is transparent, microscopic examination of colony morphology is possible, and in many cases growth occurs sooner than what is seen with egg-based media.
- Liquid media, such as Middlebrook 7H9 and Dubos-Middlebrook Tween albumin broths are available. These liquid media increase recovery when the numbers of organisms are few, as is typical of tissue specimens and body fluids.

Because mycobacteria are slow-growing organisms, traditional methods of identification, which rely on biochemical tests such as niacin production, tellurite reduction, and catalase production, can be time consuming. Many *Mycobacterium* species are very closely related and may be difficult to speciate with traditional methods. Rapid identification and susceptibility results for *M. tuberculosis* are needed to contain and adequately treat the patient with tuberculosis. *M. tuberculosis* is a slow-growing, buff-colored, corded, colony that is niacin and nitrate positive; 68°C catalase negative. Virulent MTB's serpentine, corded morphology can be observed on acid-fast bacilli grown in liquid medium.

Recent advances now make it possible to identify some of the more important *Mycobacterium* species with molecular testing. These methods are highly accurate, rapid, and becoming increasingly more popular, because their use permits positive patients to be identified and isolated from other patients and the general public before the TB organism can spread. Not only are molecular methods such as gene amplification techniques, DNA sequencing, RFLP assays, and 16S rRNA sequencing of benefit in the identification of mycobacteria at the genus-species level, but they will also likely be of use in the identification of drug-resistance strains. Consult ∞ Chapter 9, "Final Identification," for more information on molecular diagnostics.

LEARNING OPPORTUNITIES

1. What is the appropriate method for collecting sputum specimens? (Chapter Objective 3)

2. Describe the appearance of *Mycobacterium* species when the auramine-rhodamine fluorescent stain is used to detect the presence of acid-fast bacilli (AFB) in clinical specimens. (Chapter Objective 5)

3. What substances in the cell wall of the mycobacteria confer resistance to decolorization with acid–alcohol solvents used in the Ziehl-Neelsen, Kinyoun, and fluorescent stains? (Chapter Objective 4)

4. List two commercially available systems that can be used to isolate AFB directly from blood specimens. (Chapter Objective 10)

PEARSON myhealthprofessionskit™

Use this address to access the interactive Companion Website created for this textbook. Simply select "Clinical Laboratory Science" from the choice of disciplines. Find this book and log in using your user name and password.

REFERENCES

Go to myhealthprofessionskit.com to view this chapter's references.

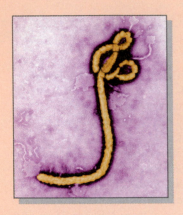

OUTLINE

14

Fungal Cultures

William C. Payne

■ LEARNING OBJECTIVES

Upon completion of this chapter, the learner should be able to:

1. Define the five types of mycoses categorized according to the body systems affected.

2. List major pathogens according to body systems they are most likely to affect.

3. Apply safety measures designed to protect laboratory workers who work in the mycology section of the microbiology laboratory.

4. Choose the appropriate method for processing specimens in order to detect the presence of fungal elements and isolate fungi.

5. Differentiate direct examination methods.

6. Relate the expected results for each direct examination method.

7. Determine the appropriate direct examination method, based on the specimen type.

8. Describe media designed to cultivate various species of fungi.

9. Select media appropriate for isolating different fungal species based on the specimen type, body system affected, or pathogens that are likely to be isolated.

10. Determine the appropriate incubation temperature, incubation period, and atmospheric requirement for isolating fungi on different fungal media.

11. Correlate macroscopic or colony morphology of fungi such as hyaline moulds, dematiaceous moulds, and yeasts.

12. Describe the fungal elements associated with moulds and yeasts.

13. Correlate microscopic morphology with major fungal pathogens.

14. Summarize additional approaches to the identification of fungi to include biochemical, molecular, and susceptibility tests.

15. Presumptively identify *Candida albicans, C. glabrata,* and *Cryptococcus neoformans.*

KEY TERMS

Note: Additional key terms can be reviewed in Chapter 29, "Medical Mycology."

ascospores	condiophore	septate hyphae
aerial mycelium	dematiaceous hyphae	sporangiophore
arthroconidia	germ tubes	sporangiospores
aseptate hyphae	hyaline hyphae	sporangium
basidiospores	hyphae	true hyphae
blastoconidia	phialides	vegetative mycelium
conidia	pseudohyphae	zygospores

▶ INTRODUCTION

The fungi, as a group, include organisms such as moulds, yeasts, and mushrooms. Most fungi serve a very beneficial role in nature by contributing to the breakdown of organic debris and thereby returning nutrients to the soil. However, some species are known to be important pathogens, the cause of disease in both animals and plants (i.e., rusts, smuts, and rots). Several fungal species pose a significant threat to the health and well-being of humans, making them important medically.

Fungal infections in humans are not uncommon, and their increased incidence corresponds with the increasing number of immunocompromised or immunosuppressed individuals. Most fungal infections are chronic, such as athlete's foot and vaginal yeast infections, but some fungi are capable of causing acute infections that can be life threatening. The serious nature of the disease is often related to the tissues affected. As a matter of fact, fungal infections, or mycoses, are often categorized according to the body systems they affect (Table 14-1✪), for example:

- Superficial mycoses, a term referring to fungal infections affecting the outermost layers of skin, the stratum corneum. The stratum corneum is primarily squamous epithelial cells, which are rich in the protein keratin. This skin layer, which lacks nerves and vasculature, is composed of dead skin cells that are constantly being shed.

- Cutaneous mycoses, a term referring to fungal infections that penetrate layers of skin as deep as the dermis. The dermis is the layer of skin that contains blood vessels, nerve endings, sweat and sebaceous glands, and hair follicles. Because this layer is innervated and has a blood supply, these infections are often associated with sensations of itching, burning, and pain, as well as an inflammatory response.

- Subcutaneous mycoses refers to infections caused by fungal species that are able to invade the deeper layers of connective tissue that underlie the skin. Tissues such as fascia and even bone may be involved. The fungi associated with subcutaneous mycoses are often saprophytes found in soil and decaying vegetation. They gain access into the body through traumatic implantation of fungal elements into the subcutaneous tissues via thorns and splinters.

- Respiratory mycoses are fungal infections brought about by inhalation. The respiratory tree, including the lungs, may be invaded. Such illnesses are characterized by symptoms suggestive of respiratory infections such as, fever, cough, shortness of breath, chest pain, and in very serious cases, hemoptysis (blood in the sputum). These symptoms can be identical to those seen with other respiratory pathogens such as bacteria and viruses. The failure of the symptoms to subside with the administration of broad-spectrum antibiotics can be an important clue that the etiologic agent may be fungal. Knowing that a patient resides in an area where certain fungal species are endemic may add further support to the initial diagnosis.

- Systemic (disseminated) mycoses are fungal infections that spread from the initial focus of infection (such as the respiratory tract) to involve multiple organ systems. Symptoms are often nonspecific and are dependent on the affected organs. Because disseminated disease is more common in patients who have weakened immune systems, the prognosis can be very poor, and immediate intervention may be necessary. Leukemia, lymphoma, transplantation, long-term antibiotic therapy, diabetic ketoacidosis, and other debilitating conditions predispose individuals to disseminated mycoses. Even organisms that are not usually considered to be fungal pathogens, such as the Zygomycetes or *Aspergillus* species pose a significant threat.

✪ TABLE 14-1

Clinical Classification of Fungal Infections

Classification	Etiologic Agents	Disease
Superficial mycosis (skin and hair)	Malassezia furfur	Pityriasis versicolor
	Phaeoannellomyces werneckii	Tinea nigra
	Trichosporon beigelii	White piedra
	Piedraia hortae	Black piedra
Dermatophytosis (skin, hair, nails)	Microsporum species	Athlete's foot, nail infections, hair infections, ringworm, favus, etc.
	Trichophyton species	
	Epidermophyton floccosum	
Subcutaneous mycosis (subcutaneous tissues)	Cladosporium carrionii	Chromoblastomycosis
	Fonsecaea pedrosoi	Chromoblastomycosis
	Phialophora verrucosa	Chromoblastomycosis
	Rhinocladiella aquaspersa	Chromoblastomycosis
	Pseudallescheria boydii	Mycetoma
	Madurella mycetomatis	Mycetoma
	Acremonium	Mycetoma
	Alternaria species	Phaeohyphomycosis
	Bipolaris species	Phaeohyphomycosis
	Curvularia species	Phaeohyphomycosis
	Exophilia species	Phaeohyphomycosis
Systemic mycosis (multiple organ systems)	Blastomyces dermatitidis	Blastomycosis
	Histoplasma capsulatum	Histoplasmosis
	Paracoccidioides immitis	Paracoccidioidomycosis
	Coccidioides immitis	Coccidioidomycosis
	Sporothrix schenckii	Sporotrichosis
	Penicillium marneffei	Infects immunocompromised patients
Zygomycosis	Rhizopus species	Zygomycosis
	Mucor species	Zygomycosis
	Absidia species	Zygomycosis
Yeasts (monomorphic, nonfilamentous fungi)	Candida species	Variety of infections: cutaneous, fungemia, systemic (disseminated)
	Cryptococcus species	
	Rhodotorula species	
	Trichosporon species	
	Malassezia species	
Opportunistic mycosis (often considered contaminants)	Aspergillus species	Opportunistic mycoses
	Penicillium species	
	Paecilomyces species	
	Scopulariopsis species	
	Fusarium species	
	Acremonium species	
	Geotrichum species	
	and others	
Pneumocystosis	Pneumocystis jiroveci (formerly P. carinii)	Pneumocystosis (a diffuse interstitial pneumonia)

A number of antifungal agents are available, and if the fungus is susceptible, their administration should provide relief from the effects of the fungal infection. Obviously, it must first be ascertained that the cause of the infection is actually fungal in nature. As previously stated, fungal, bacterial, viral, and even some parasitic infections may elicit many of the same symptoms, making the true etiology of the infection difficult if, not impossible, to elucidate without the more concrete proof provided by the results of a culture. The results of a culture, for those organisms that are cultivable, are still accepted as the gold standard of the diagnostic process. The sensitivity and specificity of other methods, such as staining procedures and immunologic methods are measured against the results of the fungus culture. In this chapter direct examination techniques as well as other routine procedures used in the clinical laboratory for isolating, culturing, and presumptively identifying yeast will be explored. ∞ Chapter 29, "Medical Mycology," provides specific information on the identification and diseases of fungal pathogens.

► LABORATORY SAFETY

Because moulds are transmitted primarily through inhalation or through breaks in the skin, it is important to follow procedures that reduce the risk of exposure to fungal spores, which may be airborne and result in implantation of fungal elements into the tissues. The safety rules outlined in Box 14-1 ✪ should be followed when working with specimens for fungus cultures and working with fungal (i.e., mould) isolates. Yeast can usually be worked with in the same way as bacterial colonies. See ∞ Chapter 5 to review laboratory safety guidelines.

✪ BOX 14-1

Laboratory Safety in the Mycology Laboratory

1. Never attempt to sniff a fungal colony.
2. Use a biological safety cabinet when working with moulds and systemic yeast.
3. All media, reagents, and specimens should be autoclaved or incinerated before disposal.
4. Petri dishes should not be used for cultures unless sealed with oxygen and CO_2 permeable enclosures.
5. Bench tops should be disinfected daily.
6. Test tubes should have screw-type caps.
7. Immunocompromised personnel should not work in mycology.
8. When using scalpels, tweezers, and needles, exercise care! Avoid puncture wounds.
9. Transfer and work over disinfectant-soaked towels.

**Checkpoint! 14–1
(Chapter Objective 1)**

Certain fungi are able to invade the deeper layers of connective tissue that underlie the skin, causing fungal infections known as _____. Trauma, caused by thorns and splinters, implants fungal elements into the body of the host, allowing these organisms to proliferate in host tissues.

    A. *superficial mycoses*

    B. *cutaneous mycoses*

    C. *subcutaneous mycoses*

    D. *respiratory mycoses*

    E. *systemic (disseminated) mycoses*

▶ SPECIMEN COLLECTION

Many specimens collected for fungal cultures are collected the same as for bacteriological culture. ∞ Chapter 6, "Specimen Collection," presents information pertinent to specimen collection in microbiology. All specimens submitted to the clinical microbiology laboratory should be collected aseptically and placed in a sterile, leak proof container and transported as soon as possible. Policies and procedures should be in place to establish minimum volume requirements and criteria for frequency of testing as well as specimen rejection. The specimen must be properly labeled with at least two patient identifiers, such as medical record number and date of birth, in addition to the patient name. The specimen source is essential information that must be included. As with bacteria, determining the significance of fungi may be dependent on the specimen source.

Skin and nails should be disinfected with 70% alcohol prior to collecting the specimen. The affected nails should be clipped and sent to the laboratory along with any debris under the nail. The skin surface should be scraped at the edge of the lesion. Ten to 12 hairs with the shafts intact should be collected for fungal culture.

If an oral yeast infection is suspected, the patient should rinse the mouth with saline prior to the lesions being swabbed. Expectorated sputum, bronchial alveolar lavage, and other deep respiratory specimens are acceptable for culture. Corneal scrapings are usually inoculated directly to a sterile slide and media by the physician at the patient's bedside.

Sterile fluids such as cerebrospinal fluid and other body fluids are useful for culture. A minimum of 2 mL is required. As with bacterial body fluid infections, the more fluid submitted, the better the chance of recovery. Cerebrospinal fluid can be used for latex agglutination testing for the detection of *Cryptococcus neoformans.*

Blood and bone marrow can be collected using bedside inoculation of media bottles from an automated blood culture system. Automated systems have proven effective to recover yeasts. Moulds may not be detected due to their slow growth. Medical devices such as intravenous catheters can become colonized with fungi. Removal and culture of the catheter tip, as well as concurrent blood cultures, may reveal the infecting organism. Serum can be used for the antigen detection of *Cryptococcus neoformans* and *Histoplasma capsulatum.*

Abscesses and wounds are also acceptable for culture. Aspiration of the sample is much better than merely swabbing the wound surface. If a swab must be used, several should be submitted to ensure adequate specimen. Tissue is ideal to demonstrate invasive fungi. Formalin must not be used for transport. If drying of the specimen is a concern, sterile saline can be added to the sterile transport container.

Urine is collected as for bacterial culture. A first morning clean-catch specimen is adequate; catheterized urine is also acceptable. A 24 hour urine collection is not acceptable for fungal culture.

▶ PROCESSING SPECIMENS

Some specimens collected for fungal culture require processing prior to inoculation to culture media. Other specimens are inoculated to culture media in the same manner as bacterial cultures.

Flecks of blood, pus, or caseous (cheese-like) material in sputum should be selected for culture. Liquefaction with a mucolytic agent such as N-acetyl-L-cysteine without sodium hydroxide and centrifugation of the liquified sputum specimen helps in recovery of *Pneumocystis jiroveci* (formerly *P. carinii*) (Murray, Baron, Jorgensen, Pfaller, & Yolken, 2003). Sputum and vaginal specimens should be Gram stained and subcultured to appropriate fungal media. Yeast may colonize the upper respiratory and urogenital tracts and consequently may be seen on the Gram stain and may grow on cultures as part of an individual's resident mucosal commensal flora.

Urine should be refrigerated until processed. Yeast can cause urinary tract infections and will grow on routine media such as sheep blood agar. Because urinary tract infections are defined by the number of organisms isolated, urine fungal cultures are plated as for a routine bacterial urine culture using a calibrated loop. The quantity isolated determines if the yeast isolated are significant or colonization.

Body fluids such as spinal fluid should be concentrated by centrifugation or filtration. The sediment is used to make a smear for Gram staining and for subculturing to fungal media. The supernatant may be used for serologic tests. Morris, Smith, Mirrett, and Reller (1996) suggested that CSF should not be cultured for fungi if the cell count and chemistry results are normal (i.e., clear, less then five WBCs, and normal protein concentration) for immunocompetent patients because abnormalities should be present if meningitis is present. Barenfanger, Lawhorn, and Drake (2004) noted that the cryptococcal antigen test and/or bacterial cultures can replace fungal cultures as long as chronic meningitis is not suspected, patients are not immunodeficient, and *Candida* or *Cryptococcus* is suspected as the major cause of fungal meningitis.

REAL WORLD TIP

Histoplasma capsulatum, Coccidioides immitis, Blastomyces dermatitidis, Aspergillus fumigatus, and *Rhizopus* spp. may not survive a delay in processing. If these organisms are suspected, the specimen should be processed as soon as possible (Isenberg, 2004).

Tissues should be minced or ground and plated to fungal media. If a Zygomycete is suspected as the etiological agent, the tissue should be minced because grinding destroys their fungal elements. The tissue pieces are planted on the agar surface. *Histoplasma capsulatum* is isolated best from ground tissue (Murray et al., 2003).

Automated blood culture systems can be used for the isolation of yeast especially for *Histoplasma capsulatum* and *Cryptococcus neoformans.* Filamentous fungi are isolated best using a lysis-centrifugation system (Isolator from Wampole Laboratories, Cranbury, NJ). Soap in the collection vial lyses the red and white cells and the tube is then centrifuged to create a sediment, which is inoculated onto agar plates. Bone marrow specimens can also be processed using the lysis-centrifugation method.

Hair can be viewed under an ultraviolet light, prior to processing, to look for fluorescence due to the presence of *Microsporum* and *Trichophyton* spp. Hair and nails should be cut, using sterile scissors, into small pieces prior to inoculation to media. Hair, skin, and nails are applied directly to the agar surface and pressed into the agar.

A dissecting scope should be used to examine exudates, pus, and drainage for the presence of granules. If granules are present, half the specimen should be washed with sterile distilled water, centrifuged, and crushed with a sterile glass rod prior to inoculation of media. Granules should also be selected from the unwashed specimen and crushed between two slides for microscopic examination. Box 14-2 ✪ summarizes the processing requirements for commonly collected specimens cultured for fungus. Special procedures that provide direct, rapid detection of fungi in specimens are also listed.

► **DIRECT EXAMINATION**

Most fungal species, yeasts being the major exception, require several days or even weeks for mature growth to be attained. If the fungal infection is acute, it is important that the causative agent be identified as quickly as possible so treatment may be initiated promptly. Direct examination of the clinical specimen may provide information that allows some form of therapy to be instituted long before the final results of the culture are delivered. Examination of a Gram stain or

potassium hydroxide preparation can provide enough detail to distinguish whether the etiologic agent is a mould or a yeast species and in the case of the dimorphic moulds (yeast forms at 35°C to 37°C, and mould forms at 22°C to 25°C), the morphologic characteristics of the tissue phase can be quite distinctive. If **hyphae** or long branching filaments are observed, suspect a mould; with single or budding cells, suspect a yeast-like fungi.

Compared to identification schemes for bacterial species, relatively few biochemical tests are useful in the identification of moulds. A detailed study of the morphologic features of an isolate is often crucial to the identification of a fungal species, and this is especially true of the moulds.

✪ BOX 14-2

Specimen Processing

Sputum and vaginal specimens: Gram stain and subculture to appropriate fungal media.

Urine cultures: Plate to routine and fungal media using a calibrated loop as for a routine bacterial urine culture.

Body fluids: Body fluids such as spinal fluid should be concentrated by centrifugation. The sediment is used to make a smear for Gram staining and for subculturing to fungal media. The supernatant may be used for serologic tests.

Tissues: Tissues should be minced or ground and plated to fungal media.

Blood: Automated blood culture systems can be used for the isolation of yeast. Filamentous fungi are isolated best using a lysis-centrifugation system (Isolator from Wampole Laboratories, Cranbury, NJ).

Special Procedures:

- India ink preparations of cerebrospinal fluid can be examined for the presence of encapsulated yeast.
- Latex agglutination tests can be used on serum and CSF to detect the polysaccharide capsular antigen of *Cryptococcus neoformans.*
- Potassium hydroxide preparations can be used in the examination of skin, nails, and hair.
- Gram stain procedure and calcofluor white can be used to evaluate materials from mucous membranes and body fluids, including urine.
- Periodic acid-Schiff, methenamine silver, hematoxylin and eosin, and calcofluor white stains can be used in the examination of tissue sections.
- Direct fluorescent antibody techniques can be used to detect the presence of fungal antigens in clinical specimens.
- Peptide nucleic acid (PNA) fluorescent in-situ hybridization (FISH) is a rapid and specific means to detect and identify yeast in blood cultures.
- Nucleic acid amplification to detect fungal pathogens in clinical specimens is available in some reference laboratories.

GRAM STAIN

Fungal elements typically stain as gram positive without any special modification of the Gram stain procedure. In specimens such as sputa, vaginal smears, or stool smears, oval or round, budding yeast, or **blastoconidia**, and tubelike structures, or **pseudohyphae**, and **true hyphae** can be seen quite well, even when examined using the high power lens (45×). In cases of candidiasis, the gram-positive blastoconidia and pseudohyphae (Figure 14-1 ■) typical of *Candida* species can be distinguished readily from the other cellular forms such as epithelial cells, white blood cells, and bacteria that are normally seen in vaginal smears, sputums, and other clinical specimens. In cases of urinary tract infections and fungemia, fungal elements may be seen in Gram stained smears made from urinary sediment and material aspirated from the bottles of positive blood cultures. Gram-positive **arthroconidia** or barrel- or rectangular-shaped hyphal fragments may be seen in Gram stained sputa in cases of geotrichosis, a rare infection associated with lesions of the mouth, intestines, and lungs.

Remember that yeast can be part of the normal microbiota of mucous membranes, and their presence can be the result of colonization, and not necessarily indicative of an invasive process. On the other hand, yeast and moulds or any other microbe should not be present in normally sterile sites such as tissues and body fluids (spinal fluid, blood, etc.). The presence of fungal elements in clinical specimens of this type is always considered to be significant.

POTASSIUM HYDROXIDE PREPARATION

A 10% solution of potassium hydroxide, KOH, is very useful in the examination of specimens such as extremely viscous

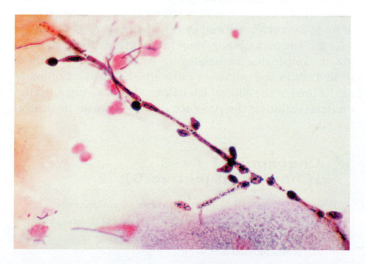

■ **FIGURE 14-1** Gram stain of vaginal smear in which the oval blastoconidia and long tubular pseudohyphae of *Candida albicans* can be seen. The pseudohyphae resemble a string of sausages due to the pinched constrictions between the cell walls.
From Centers for Disease Control and Dr. Stuart Brown.

 Checkpoint! 14–2 (Chapter Objective 5)

The _____ of fungi resists digestion with potassium hydroxide.
A. cytoplasmic (cell) membrane
B. cell wall
C. nucleus
D. ribosomes
E. mitochondria

sputum specimens or keratinized tissues such as skin, hair, and nails. Potassium hydroxide digests the protein, keratin, which is found in skin, hair, and nails. The process of clearing these tissues allows fungal elements to be visualized more easily. The chitinous cell wall of fungi resists digestion with KOH, but with time, even the fungal cell walls may appear to dissolve.

This method of direct examination has proved to be especially useful in cases of dermatophytosis such as athlete's foot and ringworm and in cases of pityriasis versicolor, superficial phaeohyphomycosis, vaginal candidiasis, thrush, and systemic mycoses. Appropriate specimens include skin scrapings, nail scrapings, and tissue samples (such as biopsies). Once the keratinized tissues have been cleared, the hyphal elements will more readily be seen.

Material from the clinical specimen is added to a 1 × 3 inch glass slide followed by the addition of a drop or two of KOH. The preparation is allowed to incubate for one hour at room temperature before examination with the low power (10×) and high dry objectives. The process may be hastened by the application of heat, such as passing the slide through the flame of a Bunsen burner or placing it on a heat block. Care should be taken that the solution is not allowed to boil. With time, the fungi present are also destroyed by the KOH.

INDIA INK PREPARATION

India ink, a dark liquid substance originally made from lampblack and water, is used to visualize the hyaline capsules of *Cryptococcus neoformans*. India ink is a colloidal suspension of carbon particles in an aqueous solution that, in actuality, does

 REAL WORLD TIP

Red and white blood cells may also be present in clinical specimens and may confuse the novice mycologist. It is helpful in such cases to remember that human body cells will not be encapsulated, they do not have a cell wall, nor will they produce buds as yeast cells do. These characteristics, as well as the fact that red and white blood cells can be lysed by the addition of KOH, can be useful in distinguishing body cells from fungal cells.

not stain fungal elements. It does, however, provide a dark background that outlines the polysaccharide capsular material surrounding mucoid strains of the yeast, *C. neoformans*. If the light focused on the specimen by the substage condenser is properly adjusted, it will pass through the preparation, and the capsule will appear as a clear halo surrounding the blastoconidia. Figure 14-2 ■ demonstrates the capsule of *C. neoformans*, in CSF, using india ink. A positive India ink result is considered diagnostic for cryptococcal meningitis. As a word of caution, some cryptococcal strains may not be encapsulated.

 REAL WORLD TIP

Caution: Excess India ink may render the preparation too opaque for the encapsulated yeast to be seen.

Clinical specimens, such as spinal fluid or sputum, may be added to a glass slide in cases of suspected cryptococcosis. A small amount of India ink is added to the specimen and mixed to make an emulsion. A coverslip is applied, and the preparation is carefully examined with the low power and high dry objectives under conditions of reduced illumination.

PERIODIC ACID-SCHIFF (PAS) STAIN FOR FUNGUS

The periodic acid-Schiff stain (Figure 14-3 ■) can be invaluable in examining skin scrapings and tissue sections. The carbon-to-carbon bonds found in the carbohydrate constituents of the fungal cell wall are oxidized by the periodic acid to form aldehydes. Aldehyde groups are then able to combine with the basic fuchsin dye to form a magenta-colored complex. Human body cells that lack the chitinous cell walls possessed

■ **FIGURE 14-2** India ink can be added directly to cerebrospinal fluid and examined under the microscope for the presence of *Cryptococcus neoformans*. The large capsule of the yeast appears as a halo around the cell against a dark background.

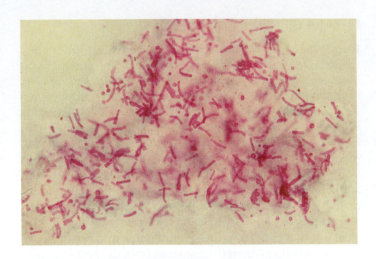

■ **FIGURE 14-3** *Malassezia furfur*, the causative agent of pityriasis versicolor, a superficial fungal infection, seen in a skin scraping stained with the periodic acid-Schiff (PAS) stain. It resembles spaghetti and meatballs.
From Centers for Disease Control (CDC) and Dr. Lucille K. Georg.

by fungi are decolorized by the metabisulfite solution. Fungal elements stain a rose red color, whereas the background is decolorized to a light pink color.

GOMORI METHENAMINE SILVER (GMS) STAIN

The methenamine silver stain is another special stain that is used to demonstrate the presence of fungal elements in the tissues. The chitinous components of the fungal cell wall are oxidized to produce aldehyde groups, which react with silver nitrate to form metallic silver. Fungal elements such as yeast cells, hyphae, and *Pneumocystis jiroveci* (previously known as *P. carinii*) will be outlined in black, whereas the internal parts of fungi are anywhere from a deep rose color to black (Figure 14-4 ■). The background should stain green. The GMS stain may be invaluable in diagnosing *Pneumocystis* pneumonia (PCP) because the organism cannot be cultured on ordinary media used in the clinical laboratory. Diagnosis usually relies on demonstrating the presence of the organism in clinical material.

✓ **Checkpoint! 14–3 (Chapter Objective 6)**

When _____ is used for direct examination of patient specimens, fungal elements will be a rose red color, whereas the background, which is decolorized, will be a light pink color.

    A. *potassium hydroxide*
    B. *the periodic acid-Schiff stain*
    C. *the Gomori methenamine silver stain*
    D. *the Giemsa stain*
    E. *the Gram stain*

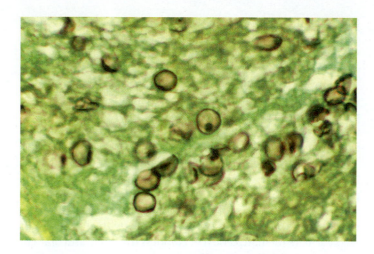

■ **FIGURE 14-4** *Pneumocystis jiroveci* seen in the lung tissue of an AIDS patient. This tissue section, showing the cyst but not the internal nuclei, was stained using the methenamine silver stain.
From Centers for Disease Control (CDC) and Dr. Edwin P. Ewing, Jr.

GIEMSA STAIN

The Giemsa stain is often used in the detection of *Histoplasma capsulatum* in bone marrow smears. In cases of disseminated histoplasmosis, small intracellular yeast forms can be seen within the cytoplasm of phagocytic cells. In patients infected with the human immunodeficiency virus (HIV) that has progressed to full-blown AIDS, the organisms may even be seen in peripheral blood smears stained with the Wright stain. *Pneumocystis jiroveci* (previously known as *P. carinii*) may also be detected in lung impression smears using the Giemsa stain (Figure 14-5 ■).

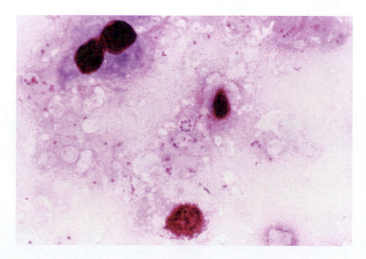

■ **FIGURE 14-5** *Pneumocystis jiroveci* seen in rat lung tissue. This impression smear was stained using the Giemsa stain. This stain demonstrates the eight nuclei, seen in the center of the micrograph, within the cyst but not the cyst wall itself.
From Centers for Disease Control (CDC) and Dr. Mae Melvin.

ACID-FAST STAINS

Acid-fast stains, such as the Ziehl-Neelsen stain and the modified Kinyoun stain, can be used to detect the presence of ascospores in yeast cultures. **Ascospores**, or sexual spores contained in a saclike structure called an ascus, will be stained red by the basic fuchsin dye, whereas blastoconidia will be stained blue (methylene blue is used as the counterstain). See the Companion Website and ∞ Chapter 13, "Acid-Fast Bacilli Cultures," to review the procedures for acid-fast stains.

THE SPORE STAIN

The spore stain, which utilizes malachite green, may also be used to demonstrate the presence of ascospores. In this case the ascospores will be stained green, and blastoconidia are stained red by sodium safranin, the counterstain.

CALCOFLUOR WHITE STAIN

Calcofluor white (Figure 14-6 ■) is a dye that binds specifically to cellulose and chitin. It is used in mycology to examine tissues, sputum, body fluids, skin scrapings, and corneal scrapings for the presence of fungal elements. Because calcofluor white is a fluorescent dye, examination of clinical material requires the use of a fluorescent microscope equipped with the correct ultraviolet light filters. This fluorescent dye absorbs ultraviolet light, which is invisible to the human eye and releases visible light that can be detected when examining a

@ **REAL WORLD TIP**

The calcofluor stain can be combined with KOH to enhance the detection of fungi in clinical specimens (Isenberg, 2004).

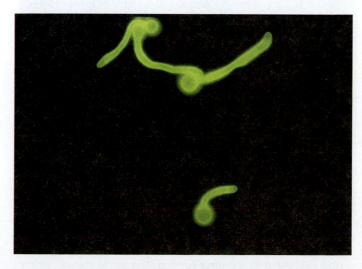

■ **FIGURE 14-6** Calcofluor white stain showing *C. albicans* germ tubes.
From Centers for Disease Control (CDC) and Dr. Brian Harrington.

clinical specimen containing fungal elements. Because calcofluor white does not bind to background material, the fungal elements appear to fluoresce brightly, whereas the background remains darkened.

FLUORESCENT ANTIBODY STAINS

Fluorescent compounds can be coupled to antibody molecules. These fluorescent-labeled antibodies are then used to detect fungal elements in tissue specimens or body fluids. In this procedure, material from the clinical specimen is added to a 1 × 3 inch glass slide, it is allowed to dry, and the preparation is then fixed. Methanol and acetone are popular fixatives. Reagent antisera containing the fluorescent-labeled antibodies is added to the slide, which is incubated at the appropriate temperature and for a specified time period. The slide is washed to remove unbound antibodies. A drop of mounting medium is added to the slide as well as a coverslip, and the preparation is examined using a fluorescent microscope. If the corresponding fungal species is present, fluorescent fungal elements will be observed against a dark background (Figure 14-7). If the corresponding fungus is not present, there is no fluorescence (a negative reaction). The use of fluorescent antibody stains is simple, sensitive, and very specific.

LATEX AGGLUTINATION

Latex agglutination tests are popular because they are easy to use, sensitive, and have a short turnaround time. This technique has largely replaced India ink preparations in the detection of encapsulated yeast that can be found in cerebrospinal fluid (CSF) in cases of disseminated *Cryptococcus neoformans*.

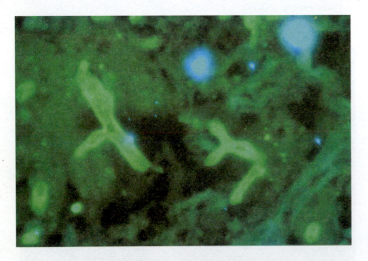

■ **FIGURE 14-7** Zygomycosis is a systemic infection seen primarily in immunocompromised patients. The etiologic agent of this infection was *Rhizopus arrhizus*. This tissue section, which has been stained with a fluorescent antibody stain, demonstrates the root-like rhizoids that are characteristic of the group. *From Centers for Disease Control (CDC) and Dr. William Kaplan.*

Latex agglutination is much more sensitive and can provide evidence of infection in cases where blastoconidia are few in number and would escape detection using india ink or the organism is non-encapsulated.

A drop of spinal fluid is mixed with the suspension of latex particles coated with antibody to the capsular antigen. If the polysaccharide capsular material is present in the clinical specimen, the antigen–antibody reaction is seen as clumping or agglutination of the latex particles.

When fungal elements are observed under the microscope, it is important to note morphological characteristics that may provide clues to the identity of the fungus. One may observe spherules, septate cells, or hyphae of moulds. Record whether the hyphae is broad, short or long, septate (with cross walls) or aseptate, dark (dematiaceous) or colorless (hyaline), and branching (45° or 90°). When yeastlike organisms are observed, record the presence of pseudohyphae, single or multiple budding, size (large or small), and shape (cigar-shaped or broad base). Note the presence of a capsule and whether the yeast is intracellular or extracellular.

One would suspect *Coccidioides* if spherules are observed. Broad, aseptate hyphae might indicate Zygomycosis. Chromoblastomycosis fungi may have dark, branched, septate hyphae or dark, round septate cells. If colorless septate hyphae that branch at a 45° angle are seen, suspect *Aspergillus*. Dermatophytosis fungi may present as colorless, branched, septate hyphae with arthroconidia. *Histoplasma capsulatum* is intracellular, and *C. neoformans* or *Rhodotorula* may have a capsule. Cells with multiple budding suggest *Paracoccidioides*. Large cells with a broad base are suspicious of *Blastomyces*. *Sporothrix* has small, cigar-shaped cells. Pseudohyphae are characteristic of *Candida* or *Saccharomyces*. Additional microscopic features used to identify fungal isolates will be presented later in this chapter (Campbell & Stewart, 1980; Hazen, 1998; Larone, 1995).

> ✓ **Checkpoint! 14–4**
> **(Chapter Objective 7)**
>
> *Potassium hydroxide preparations are useful in the diagnosis of:*
>   A. *dermatophytosis.*
>   B. *vaginal candidiasis.*
>   C. *superficial phaeohyphomycosis.*
>   D. *thrush.*
>   E. *All of the above*

▶ FUNGUS CULTURE MEDIA

Fungi are primarily environmental organisms. As a rule, environmental organisms must be able to survive harsh condition, such as temperature extremes, acid and alkaline environments, and periods of time when nutrients may scarce. The nutritional needs of fungi are very simple, and consequently fungi usually do not require special nutrients or a complex list of added ingredients. Primary isolation media must only provide a carbon source, usually glucose, and a nitrogen source such as peptones or amino acids. Therefore, fungi are capable of growing on most types of laboratory media. If necessary, blood may be added as enrichment. Fungi grow well on nutrient agar, tryptic soy agar, blood agar, and chocolate agar, the same types of media that are commonly used to isolate bacteria. However, some media are designed specifically to grow fungi. These media may be used because they are inhibitory, are designed to discourage the growth of bacteria or saprophytic fungi in non-sterile body sites or specimen types, or are differential, producing phenotypic characteristics (such as pigments) that allow certain species to be identified more readily.

SABOURAUD DEXTROSE AGAR (SDA)

This medium contains refined peptones and glucose (dextrose) at a concentration of 4% (w/v). The high sugar concentration of this medium, as well as the acid pH (5.6), creates an environment that tends to inhibit the growth of most bacterial species. Moulds and yeast grow very well on Sabouraud dextrose agar, making it an excellent growth medium for the isolation and cultivation of most fungal species (Figure 14-8 ■).

SABOURAUD DEXTROSE AGAR, EMMONS MODIFICATION

This medium is a modification of Sabouraud dextrose agar in which the glucose concentration has been reduced to 2% (w/v) and has a slightly more acidic pH. The lower sugar concentration and higher pH encourages the growth of fungi, especially *Blastomyces dermatitidis,* but unfortunately that of

bacteria as well. For this reason, an antibiotic, chloramphenicol, must be added for the growth of gram-negative and gram-positive bacteria to be inhibited. Cycloheximide, a fungicidal substance, is also added to inhibit the growth of saprophytic (rapid growing) fungi, such as *Penicillium, Aspergillus, Rhizopus,* and the dematiaceous fungi. Pathogenic fungi, such as *Histoplasma capsulatum, Blastomyces dermatitidis, Coccidioides immitis, Sporothrix schenckii,* and the dermatophytes can grow freely without interference from contaminating microbiota (normal flora) of the skin and mucous membranes. Unfortunately, *Cryptococcus neoformans,* an opportunistic yeast that is associated with serious pulmonary and central nervous system illnesses, is inhibited by cycloheximide and will not grow on this medium. Inhibitory media, such as Sabouraud dextrose agar, inhibitory mould agar, and birdseed agar are better suited for the isolation and cultivation of *C. neoformans.*

BRAIN HEART INFUSION (BHI) AGAR

Brain heart infusion (BHI) agar is a growth medium that is frequently used in the cultivation of fastidious microorganisms, especially yeasts. It is often enriched with sheep blood. It is used to cultivate fungi and is the medium recommended for the conversion of dimorphic fungi. When incubated at 37°C, the mould phase of dimorphic fungi can be converted to the yeast or tissue phase. Antibiotics can be added to make it a selective medium.

SABOURAUD DEXTROSE WITH BRAIN HEART INFUSION AGAR (SABHI)

This is a growth medium used for the isolation and cultivation of pathogenic fungi, especially yeast (Figure 14-9 ■). It is usually supplemented with 5% sheep blood as an enrichment. Chloramphenicol and cycloheximide may be added as

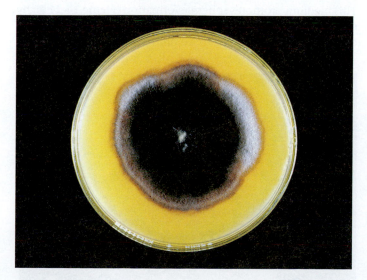

■ **FIGURE 14-8** *Curvularia geniculata,* one of the dematiaceous fungi, can be seen growing on Sabouraud dextrose agar. Note that the surface growth is dark. The reverse or underside of the colony is also black.
From Centers for Disease Control and Prevention (CDC).

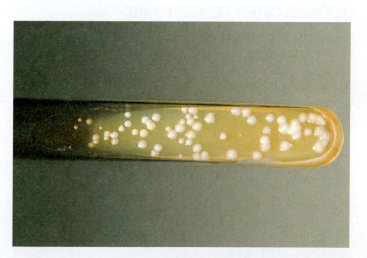

■ **FIGURE 14-9** *Cryptococcus neoformans* growing on a SABHI agar slant. The slightly mucoid colonies are characteristic.
From Centers for Disease Control (CDC) and Dr. William Kaplan.

Checkpoint! 14–5 (Chapter Objective 8)

What properties of Sabouraud dextrose agar make the medium inhibitory to the growth of most bacteria?
  A. *Low pH (5.6) and high glucose concentration*
  B. *High pH (10.0) and high sucrose concentration*
  C. *Addition of bile salts*
  D. *Incorporation of inhibitory dyes*
  E. *Increased salt concentration (10% NaCl)*

Checkpoint! 14–6 (Chapter Objective 9)

Cryptococcus neoformans produces a brown or black pigment (melanin) when grown on:
  A. *Sabouraud dextrose agar*
  B. *Sabouraud dextrose agar, Emmons modification*
  C. *inhibitory mould agar*
  D. *brain heart infusion agar*
  E. *birdseed agar*

inhibitory agents. It is not recommended for the conversion of dimorphic fungi.

INHIBITORY MOULD AGAR (IMA)

This medium is used in the recovery of pathogenic fungi from clinical specimens that may have contaminating bacteria of skin and mucous membranes (gram-positive and gram-negative bacteria). This medium contains chloramphenicol but not cycloheximide.

YEAST-EXTRACT PHOSPHATE AGAR (YEPA)

This medium is used to isolate the dimorphic fungi, *Blastomyces dermatitidis* and *Histoplasma capsulatum,* from specimens that may contain commensal flora. After inoculation with the specimen, a drop of concentrated ammonium hydroxide is added to an uninoculated area of the agar surface. The ammonium hydroxide inhibits bacteria and other fungi.

DERMATOPHYTE TEST MEDIUM

Hair, nails, and skin scraping can be directly inoculated to this medium. If a dermatophyte grows, it will turn the medium from yellow to red and may provide a presumptive identification. Colony pigmentation cannot be evaluated on this medium, but other macroscopic and microscopic characteristics can be studied.

BIRDSEED (GUIZOTIA ABYSSINICA SEED) AGAR

This medium, which is also known as niger seed or caffeic agar, is used in the isolation of *C. neoformans* from clinical specimens. *C. neoformans* produces phenoloxidase which breaks down the niger seed. It is detected as a brown pigment (melanin) when isolated on birdseed agar. Yeasts belonging to other genera, such as the *Candida* species, do not produce the brown color.

CHROMAGAR™ CANDIDA

This chromogenic selective medium is used to isolate and differentiate the more common yeast of the genus, *Candida.* Beckton, Dickinson and Company (BD), of Franklin Lakes, NJ, created this agar, and it is now widely used in microbiology laboratories. Other companies have created their version of this chromogenic agar. *Candida albicans, C. tropicalis,* and *C. krusei* can be presumptively identified using colony color. *C. albicans* forms light to medium green colonies. *C. tropicalis* forms dark blue to blue gray colonies, and *C. krusei* produce flat colonies with pink centers. Testing to confirm identification is recommended. *C. dubliniensis* may be distinguished from *C. albicans* by its dark green colony (Jabra-Rizk et al., 2001). Further testing on a potential *C. dubliniensis* isolate is recommended. Other yeasts produce light to dark pink colonies. A patient with a mixed yeast infection can also be detected on this medium. Figure 14-10 ■ represents a mixed yeast culture grown on CHROMagar™.

CONVERSE MEDIUM

This medium promotes spherule formation (Figure 14-11 ■) by *Coccidioides immitis* when incubated at 40°C under an increased concentration of CO_2. The tissue phase of *C. immitis* consists of

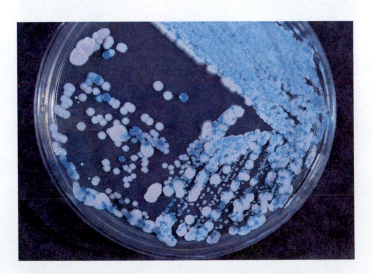

■ **FIGURE 14-10** A mixed culture of yeast growing on chromogenic agar.

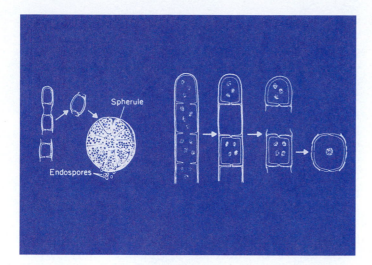

■ FIGURE 14-11 Spherule with endospores is the form of the dimorphic fungi, *Coccidioides immitis*, found in the tissues and when it is cultured using Converse medium.
From Centers for Disease Control (CDC) and Dr. Errol Reiss.

large, round, double-walled spherules containing endospores. *C. immitis* does not produce the tissue or yeast phase on BHI agar enriched with sheep blood, as the other dimorphic fungi do, even when incubated at 35°C. Conversion of *C. immitis* from the mould phase (thick-walled arthroconidia that alternate with disjunctor cells) to the yeast tissue phase (spherules with endospores) requires the use of Converse medium.

CORNMEAL AGAR

Cornmeal agar with Tween 80 is used to promote the characteristic microscopic morphology of yeasts especially chlamydoconidia production in *Candida albicans*. The organism is inoculated onto a section of the agar and then covered with a coverslip. After 24–72 hours incubation at room temperature, the area is examined under the 10× and 45× objectives of the microscope.

POTATO DEXTROSE AGAR

This medium is used to promote the sporulation of moulds. Once the organism is grown, slide culture preparations are made and stained with lactophenol cotton blue (LPCB) to view its microscopic morphology.

Primary culture medium should include inhibitory media, in addition to selective media, if the specimen was collected from a nonsterile site. Enriched media should be included to grow fastidious, dimorphic fungi. If *Malassezia furfur* is suspected, blot the surface of the medium with sterile olive oil to provide the fatty acids needed for growth. Medium specifically designed to grow a particular fungus, such as a chromogenic agar for yeasts, may also be added to the primary culture setup (Murray et al., 2003). Table 14-2✪ lists fungal culture media used for the isolation and identification of fungi.

✪ **TABLE 14-2**

Fungal Culture Media

Use	Medium
Isolation of saprophytic and pathogenic fungi	Sabouraud dextrose agar (SDA)
	Brain heart infusion (BHI) agar
	Sabouraud dextrose with brain heart infusion (SABHI)
	Potato Dextrose or Potato Flake agar
Isolation of pathogenic fungi	SDA, Emmons modification
	BHI with antibiotics
	BHI enriched with sheep blood agar
	Inhibitory mould agar (IMA)
	Yeast-extract phosphate (YEPA) agar
	Dermatophyte test medium
Identification of fungi	Cornmeal with tween 80 agar
	Cornmeal with dextrose agar
	Urease test medium
	Yeast fermentation broth
	Yeast nitrogen base agar
	Niger seed or birdseed agar
	Chromogenic agar
	Rice medium
	Potato dextrose agar
	Tomato juice agar
Conversion of dimorphic fungi from the mould phase to the tissue or yeast phase	BHI enriched with sheep blood (incubated at 37°C)
	Converse medium (incubated at 40°C)

∞ Chapter 29, "Medical Mycology," describes the use of specific fungal media to identify isolates.

Fungal cultures should be incubated at 30°C if available, 25°C if not available, in ambient air. Media used for identification, such as Converse medium, may have different incubation temperatures and atmospheres. The agar plates should be sealed with gas impermeable tape or placed in a gas impermeable bag in order to prevent contamination of the environment and other culture plates. Cultures should be examined every 2 to 3 days for the first 2 weeks, then once a week for 3 weeks. Cultures should be held for 4 weeks if the specimen is skin or nails or up to 6 to 8 weeks if dimorphic fungi are suspected (Labarca, Wagar, Grasmick, Kokkinos, & Bruckner, 1998).

Quantitation of yeast and moulds is problematic. They are larger than bacterial cells so using the same quantitation methods (1+, 2+ or light growth, moderate growth, and so forth) does not accurately count them. Yeast may be considered significant if they are the predominant organism when compared to the normal flora present. If it is a sterile body site, yeast should always be considered significant. Depending on the body site, knowing if the yeast isolated is *C. albicans* or not may be sufficient for the physician.

Moulds are more difficult when determining significance. They can be found in the environment and may contaminate specimens as well as agar plates. Often histopathology is used in conjunction with fungal culture results. Factors to consider which may help determine the significance of the presence of a mould as a potential pathogen include:

- The presence of an invasive mould in stained tissue sections
- The presence of mould structures on direct specimen stains
- Isolation from a sterile body site/specimen type
- Isolation of the same mould species from multiple specimens of the patient
- Isolation of a mould on multiple agar plates in a culture
- The individual is immunocompromised or immunosuppressed
- The individual is on broad spectrum antibiotics
- Clinical signs and symptoms of patient leads physician to suspect fungus
- Growth of specific organisms such as the dimorphic fungi *Histoplasma capsulatum*

Checkpoint! 14–7 (Chapter Objective 10)

What medium and environmental conditions are required to promote spherule formation by Coccidioides immitis?

A. Sabouraud dextrose agar at 25°C
B. Sabouraud dextrose agar at 37°C
C. Converse medium at 40°C with increased CO₂
D. brain heart infusion agar at 37°C in ambient air
E. brain heart infusion agar at 42°C

▶ IDENTIFICATION OF FUNGAL SPECIES

This section introduces the identification process for fungal species. Colony morphology and microscopic morphology of fungi will allow either preliminary or final identification of the isolate. Final identification of certain fungi may require additional tests. ∞ Chapter 29, "Medical Mycology," will present more specific information on identification and diseases of medically significant fungi.

MACROSCOPIC (COLONY) MORPHOLOGY

The identification of fungal species often begins by taking note of the morphologic characteristics of surface growth. Filamentous fungi, the moulds, are composed of tubelike structures referred to as hyphae. Masses of hyphal elements that extend below the surface of a growth medium, the **vegetative mycelium**, allow a mould colony to adhere tightly to the growth medium. The term *vegetative* may also be used to describe hyphae capable of forming asexual reproductive structures. Growth that extends above the growth medium and that supports reproductive structures, the **aerial mycelium**, provide mould colonies with characteristics such as topography, texture, and color. Topography describes the contour of the colony surface and is often depicted as flat, folded, raised, wrinkled, irregular, or heaped. The manner in which the texture of a colony is described is very subjective, but terms used include *smooth, glabrous, chalky* or *powdery, suedelike, lacelike, fuzzy, velvety,* and even *fluffy* or *cottony.* Color, which is just as subjective as texture, may be described as white, yellow, red, blue-green, dark green, gray, tan, brown, beige, and black.

The reverse or underside of a mould colony may be described using the same colors as just listed. Most descriptions of mould texture and color refer to growth observed on Sabouraud dextrose agar (SDA) or potato dextrose agar (PDA). For example, moulds, such as *Aspergillus* and *Penicillium* species, often have a surface that is green or blue-green in color with a velvety or cottony texture. The reverse of these hyaline moulds is often described as being white or nonpigmented. The dematiaceous moulds usually have a black, dark gray, dark green, or brown colored surface, with a velvety or suedelike texture. The reverse is usually black or darkly pigmented. On Sabouraud dextrose agar, yeasts form discrete, white to tan-colored colonies with a smooth surface and a butyrous consistency (like soft butter). Some yeast species such as *Rhodotorula rubra* may form pink or coral-colored colonies. *Cryptococcus neoformans* may produce mucoid colonies because the blastoconidia are frequently surrounded by a polysaccharide capsule. Figure 14-12 ■ shows the macroscopic morphology of *Fusarium fujikuroi*. Table 14-3✿ summarizes the macroscopic morphology of select fungi.

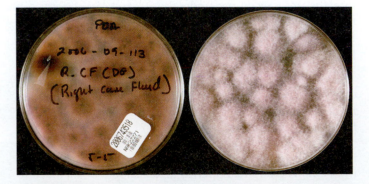

■ **FIGURE 14-12** Macroscopic morphology (surface and reverse) of *Fusarium fujikuroi* growing on potato dextrose agar. The fuzziness on the colony surface is due to aerial mycelia extending up from the surface. The growth into the agar seen on the plate's reverse side is the vegetative mycelia.
From Centers for Disease Control (CDC)/Mark Lindsley, Sc.D. D(ABMM), Lynette Benjamin, and Shirley McClinton.

✪ TABLE 14-3

Macroscopic Morphology of Select Fungi (Pathogens and Nonpathogens)

Mould	Texture	Color of Surface	Color of Reverse
Aspergillus species	Velvety or cottony	Green, yellow, black	White
Penicillium species	Powdery	Bluish-green	White
Paecilomyces species	Powdery or velvety	Yellowish brown	Off-white to brown
Scopulariopsis species	Powdery	Light brown	Tan to brown
Fusarium species	Cottony	Pink to violet	Light in color
Rhizopus species	Cottony	Gray or yellowish brown	White (nonpigmented)
Hortaea (previously known as *Phaeoannellomyces*) *werneckii*	Moist or velvety	Greenish black to black	Black
Microsporum canis	Coarsely fluffy	White	Deep yellow
Fonsecaea pedrosoi	Velvety	Dark green, gray, or black	Black
Coccidioides immitis (mould phase)	Cottony	Gray or tan to brown	White to gray
Rhodotorula species	Moist, sometimes mucoid	Pink to coral	Not applicable
Candida albicans	Creamy or pasty	Cream colored	Not applicable

MICROSCOPIC MORPHOLOGY

Although the macroscopic morphology of fungal species is able to give a general idea of the identification of a fungal isolate, the microscopic morphology of fungi, especially when fungal structures remain intact, can nearly be definitive. Microscopic morphology is especially important in the identification of moulds. Biochemical testing is not the primary means of identification as for bacteria and yeasts.

An experienced mycologist can, at a minimum, identify the genus of commonly isolated moulds (i.e., *Aspergillus* species, *Penicillium* species, *Fusarium* species, *Phialophora* species). The stained tissue sections, demonstration of the yeast or tissue phase of the systemic fungi in situ, may be unique enough that microscopic morphology can presumptively identify the invading organism to the genus-species level (i.e., *Coccidioides immitis, Blastomyces dermatitidis, Paracoccidioides brasiliensis*). Scotch tape or "tease" preparations can be made from the aerial mycelium of mould colonies, stained with lactophenol cotton blue, and examined microscopically. Slide cultures (Figure 14-13 ■) using a medium that stimulates the production of conidia, such as potato dextrose agar, can provide the microscopic morphology details that are required for identification purposes.

Fungal elements that can readily be seen using the low-power and high-power objectives include:

- Blastoconidia, mother and daughter cells resulting from asexual reproduction (budding) of yeast cells (Figure 14-1).
- Pseudohyphae, structures formed by elongation of blastoconidia that fail to separate after the budding process (Figure 14-1). Pseudohyphae can be differentiated, from true hyphae, by the pinched cell wall constrictions between adjoining cells. They can look like a string of sausages.

- **Germ tubes**, elongated structures produced by elongation at the apical end of tubular extensions from the parent cell (Figure 14-6). Germ tubes are the initial stage of the development of true hyphae.
- **Hyaline hyphae**, hyphal elements that are nonpigmented (Figure 14-14 ■).
- True hyphae, tubelike structures that grow by elongation with the formation of cross walls called septa. True hyphae are also known as septate hyphae (Figure 14-15 ■).
- **Septate hyphae**, hyphae that contain septa at fairly regular intervals (Figure 14-15).
- **Aseptate or non-septate hyphae**, hyphae that are sparsely septate. Cross walls are few and far between as seen in Figure 14-16 ■.

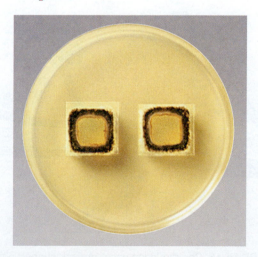

■ **FIGURE 14-13** Slide culture with PDA growing *Aspergillus niger.*
Photo courtesy of Remel, part of Thermo Fisher Scientific.

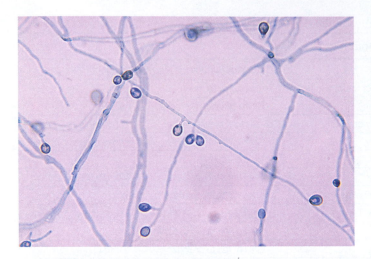

■ **FIGURE 14-14** Microscopic morphology of *Pseudallescheria boydii*, one of the many causes of eumycotic mycetomas. The stain used was lactophenol cotton blue (LPCB). The stalk-like conidiophore holds the large oval conidia. Note the hyaline septate hyphae.
From Centers for Disease Control (CDC).

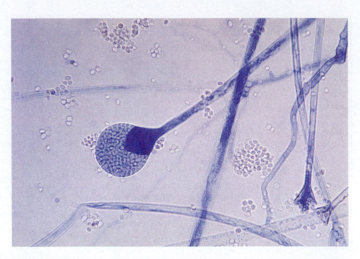

■ **FIGURE 14-16** The stalk-like sporangiophore holds the rounded sporangium, which is filled with sporangiospores. This organism is *Mucor* species and displays aseptate hyphae.
From Centers for Disease Control (CDC)/Lucille K. Georg.

■ **Dematiaceous hyphae**, hyphal elements that are darkly pigmented (Figure 14-17 ■)

■ **Conidia**, fungal elements that are the result of an asexual reproductive process. Conidia are borne on the tips of aerial mycelia and may easily be dispersed by the wind. Some fungi produce large conidia or macroconidia as well as smaller conidia or microconidia (Figure 14-18 ■).

■ **Phialides**, tubular or flask-shaped cells that produce conidia (Figure 14-15).

■ Arthroconidia, conidia formed by fragmentation of true hyphae (Figure 14-19 ■).

■ Aerial mycelia, hyphae that extend above the surface of a growth medium to bear the fruiting or reproductive structures of moulds (Figure 14-12).

■ Vegetative mycelia, hyphae that extend below the surface of a growth medium to absorb nutrients (Figure 14-12).

■ **Ascospores** (Figure 14-20 ■), **basidiospores**, and **zygospores**, fungal elements that are formed as the result of sexual reproduction and can go on to form another organism.

■ **Condiophore**, aerial mycelium that bears conidia (Figure 14-14).

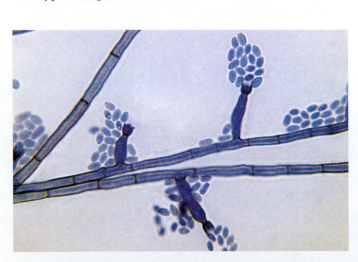

■ **FIGURE 14-15** Conidia-laden vase- or flask-shaped phialides of *Phialophora verrucosa*. This organism shows true septate hyphae.
From Centers for Disease Control (CDC)/Libero Ajello.

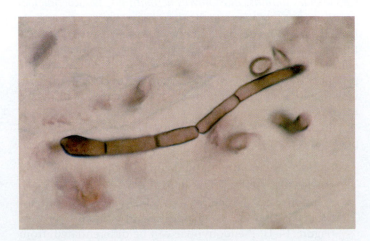

■ **FIGURE 14-17** Pigmented or dematiaceous septate hyphae of *Exserohilum rostratum*.
From Centers for Disease Control (CDC)/Dr. Libero Ajello.

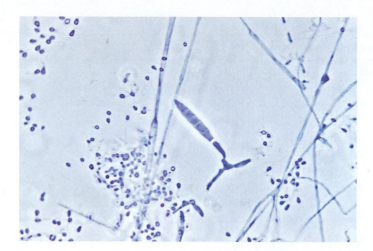

FIGURE 14-18 The single large finger-shaped macroconidium and small oval microconidia of *Microsporum persicolor* are visible. *From Centers for Disease Control (CDC)/Dr. Arvind A. Padhye.*

- **Sporangiophore**, aerial mycelium that bears the sporangium (Figure 14-16).

- **Sporangium**, saclike structure containing sporangiospores (Figure 14-16).

- **Sporangiospores**, asexual spores contained within the sporangium (Figure 14-16).

In the identification of yeast, cornmeal agar with Tween 80 is useful for promoting and determining their microscopic morphology. Boxes 14-3✪ through 14-6✪ and Table 14-4✪ summarize the microscopic morphology of various fungi.

The addition of certain tests, such as urease production, production of germ tubes and chlamydoconidia, pigment pro-

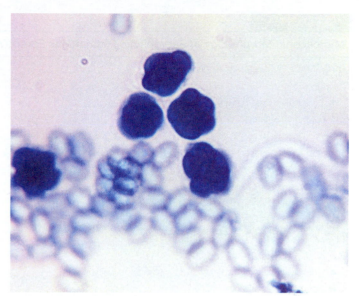

FIGURE 14-20 Ascospore (small egg-shaped structures) and asci (larger dark blue structure) of *Talaromyces flavus*. *From Centers for Disease Control (CDC)/Lucille Georg.*

duction, hair perforation, carbohydrate assimilation, and carbohydrate fermentation, make definitive identification possible. Some examples of useful characteristics include:

- Production of a water-soluble red pigment by *Trichophyton rubrum* when grown on cornmeal agar supplemented with 1% glucose.

- Hair perforation by *Trichophyton mentagrophytes*.

- Production of germ tubes by *Candida albicans* when a light inoculum is incubated in bovine serum at 37°C for up to 3 hours.

- Production of a urease enzyme by *Cryptococcus neoformans*.

- Production of phenoloxidase (an enzyme that converts caffeic acid to melanin) by *Cryptococcus neoformans*.

Molecular diagnostics hold the promise of exciting new ways to identify fungal species directly from specimens. Techniques such as polymerase chain reactions, nucleic acid probes,

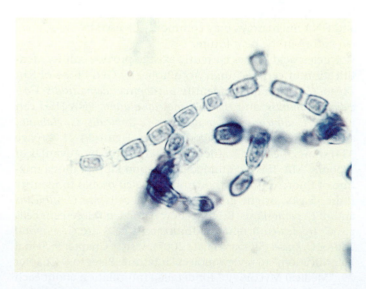

FIGURE 14-19 Rectangle-shaped arthroconidia of *Coccidioides immitis*. *From Centers for Disease Control (CDC)/Dr. Hardin.*

> ✓ **Checkpoint! 14–8 (Chapter Objective 11)**
>
> *Dematiaceous moulds are characterized by:*
>   A. *the production of a water-soluble red pigment.*
>   B. *aseptate hyphae, which range in diameter from 5 to 15 microns.*
>   C. *septate hyaline hyphae with a diameter of 3 to 6 microns.*
>   D. *darkly pigmented hyphae producing colonies with a dark surface and black reverse.*
>   E. *rhizoids.*

⊛ BOX 14-3

Microscopic Morphology of Saprophytic Filamentous Fungi (Moulds)

ZYGOMYCETES (aseptate hyphae)

Absidia
- Sporangiophores between rhizoids on stolon (internodal)
- Pear-shaped sporangium

Mucor
- Sporangiophores arise directly from mycelium (branched or single)
- Round sporangium, no rhizoids or stolons

Rhizopus
- Unbranched sporangiophores arise opposite rhizoids
- Stolons connect to rhizoids

HYALINE SAPROPHYTES (septate hyphae)

Aspergillus fumigatus
- Single row of flask-shaped phialides on upper half of vesicle
- Conidiophores smooth

Aspergillus flavus
- Double row of phialides cover entire vesicle
- Echinulate conidiophore (rough, pitted, spiny)

Aspergillus niger (begin as white wooly colonies and then turn black)
- Double row of phialides cover entire vesicle
- Conidiophores smooth

Penicillium
- Elongated phialides with chains of round conidia

Paecilomyces
- Elongated phialides bear chains of conidia (oval shaped)
- Conidia may be rough or smooth, and pigmented or hyaline

Scopulariopsis
- Large, thick-walled, lemon-shaped conidia
- Become echinulate with age

Fusarium
- Microphialoconidia: one- to two-celled and occur in groups or singly
- Macrophialoconidia: two- to five-celled (rough or smooth) and are sickle shaped

Chrysosporium
- Short conidiophores poorly differentiated from mycelium
- Single round to club-shaped conidia (rough or smooth)

Sepedonium species
- Large, round, thick-walled macroconidia that may be smooth or rough
- May occur singly or in clusters

Acremonium
- Unbranched tapering conidiophores
- Closely packed balls of elliptical shaped conidia

DEMATIACEOUS SAPROPHYTES (septate hyphae)

Alternaria
- Chained conidia that contain horizontal and vertical septa

Cladosporium
- Short chain of dark, one- to four-celled conidia from forked shield cells

Curvularia
- Large four- to five-celled dark conidia
- Central cell enlarged resulting in boomerang shape

Bipolaris
- Dark cylindrical four- to five-celled poroconidia usually in clusters

Nigrospora
- Short fat conidiophores
- Black conidia, single, oval-shaped, smooth-walled

⊛ BOX 14-4

Microscopic Morphology of Superficial Fungi

Hortaea (previously known as *Phaeoannellomyces*) *werneckii*
- Yeast portion contains only dark one- to two-celled blastoconidia
- Mould portion has blastoconidia in large clusters along septate hyphae

Malassezia furfur ("spaghetti and meatballs" morphology)
- Thick, round to oval cells in clusters with short angular hyphae

Piedraia hortae
- Dark thick-walled, septate hyphae with swellings
- Asci-containing ascospores may be present

Trichosporon beigelii (*T. cutaneum*)
- Hyaline hyphae with blastoconidia and arthroconidia
- Look for arthroconidia on direct exam

and DNA microarrays may commonly be used in the clinical laboratory in the near future.

Nucleic acid probes currently exist to provide culture identification of certain fungi. AccuProbe, by Gen-Probe of San Diego, CA, can rapidly identify *Blastomyces dermatitidis, Coccidioides immitis,* and *Histoplasma capsulatum.* PNA FISH can identify *C. albicans, C. parapsilosis, C. tropicalis, C. glabrata,* and *C. krusei* in positive blood cultures. Figure 14-21 ■ (page 334) shows the Yeast Traffic Light PNA FISH™, by AdvanDx of Woburn, MA. It is a culture identification kit that uses a mixture of fluorescein and rhodamine-labeled probes to identify these yeasts. Bright green fluorescent cells are *C. albicans* and/or *C. parapsilosis.* Bright yellow or golden fluorescent cells are *C. tropicalis.* Bright red fluorescent cells are *C. glabrata* and/or *C. krusei* (Shepard et al., 2007). Visit ∞ Chapter 9, "Final Identification," to review molecular testing. Refer to ∞ Chapter 29, "Medical Mycology," for detailed information about each fungus and their associated diseases.

Methods for susceptibility testing of fungi include broth dilution (macrodilution and microdilution), agar dilution, and

★ BOX 14-5

Microscopic Morphology of Dermatophytes

Microsporum audouinii
- Rare irregularly shaped macroconidia; thick rough walls and two to nine cells
- Rare club-shaped microconidia, occurring singly along septate hyphae

Microsporum canis
- Numerous macroconidia—rough, thick-walled, spindle-shaped; 6 to 15 cells
- Few one-celled, club-shaped microconidia
- Septate hyphae

Microsporum gypseum
- Numerous macroconidia—rough, thin-walled, elliptical shape; four to six cells
- Few single-celled, club-shaped microconidia
- Septate hyphae

Epidermophyton floccosum
- Numerous macroconidia—smooth, thin-walled, club-shaped; two to four cells
- No microconidia
- Septate hyphae

Trichophyton mentagrophytes (ectothrix hair invasion)
- Granular colonies
- Numerous pencil-shaped, smooth, thin-walled macroconidia; five to eight cells
- Round microconidia in grapelike clusters
- Septate hyphae

Trichophyton rubrum (ectothrix)
- Smooth-walled, pencil-shaped macroconidia; three to eight cells
- Numerous club-shaped microconidia borne singly along the septate hyphae
- Produces a deep red pigment

Trichophyton schoenleinii (endothrix)
- Favic chandeliers are the most prevalent feature
- No macroconidia under routine conditions
- Microconidia formed on rice
- Septate hyphae

★ BOX 14-6

Microscopic Morphology of Fungi Causing Subcutaneous Mycoses

Cladosporium carrionii
- Branching chains of conidia
- Shield-shaped cell at base of chain
- Dark, septate hyphae

Phialophora verrucosa
- Flask-shaped phialides with cup-shaped collarettes
- The conidiophores may be single or multiple, lateral or terminal, and bear easily disrupted masses of oval conidia
- Dark, branched, septate hyphae

Fonsecaea pedrosoi
- Polymorphic fungus: may be three types of anamorphs
  a. Cladosporium type—conidia in branched chains
  b. Phialophora type—conidia produced in flasklike phialides
  c. Rhinocladiella type—conidia formed along sides of irregular club-shaped conidiophores (resemble bent knee)
- Dark, branched, septate hyphae

Scedosporium apiospermum
- Hyaline, septate hyphae with simple long or short conidiophores
- Unicellular oval conidia single or in groups

Sporothrix schenckii—dimorphic fungus
  25°C—mould phase with conidiophore having conidia in rosette formation
  37°C—yeast phase with round, oval, or fusiform budding cells called "cigar bodies"

---

agar diffusion methods (disk and E-test). Variations of the microdilution method include a colorimetric method (fungal growth causes a color change) and a spectrophotometric method (measuring turbidity with a spectrophotometer). Refer to ∞ Chapter 11, "Susceptibility Testing," for information on sensitivity testing methods.

IDENTIFICATION OF YEASTS

Yeasts are routinely isolated from sputum as part of the normal flora of the oral cavity and may be seen on Gram stains used to determine the quality of a specimen (saliva vs. true sputum) submitted for culture and susceptibility testing. Yeast, such as *Candida albicans*, grows readily on most nutritive and enriched agars used in the isolation of bacteria. It is not unusual to find colonies of yeast on blood and chocolate agars in cultures of patients colonized with yeast as well as patients suffering from invasive infections.

Yeast may cause urinary tract infections, and the number of yeast isolated on a blood agar plate, used to detect the presence of urinary pathogens, should be quantitated in the same manner as bacteria. Low numbers of yeast may be considered skin or urogenital contaminants and therefore may not be significant. If any of the systemic fungi are isolated from urine, they should be considered significant, as their presence may reflect a disseminated fungal infection.

Body fluids, such as cerebrospinal fluids, should be concentrated by centrifugation. Gram stained slides are best prepared from fluid concentrated onto a glass slide by cytocentrifugation. The sediment can also be used to make Gram stains and inoculate media. In cases of cryptococcosis, the sediment can be used to make an India ink preparation. The supernatant may be used for serologic tests such as latex agglutination tests for the capsular antigen of *Cryptococcus neoformans*.

✪ TABLE 14-4

Microscopic Morphology of the Systemic Fungi

Systemic Fungi	Tissue (Yeast) Phase at 35–37°C	Mould Phase at 22–25°C
Blastomyces dermatididis	■ Large spherical yeast (8 to 12 μm) with thick walls ■ Blastoconidia attached to parent cell by a broad base	■ Small oval smooth walled conidia borne on short lateral hyphae-like conidiophores
Coccidioides immitis	■ Large round thick walled hyaline spherules (30 to 60 μm) filled with one-celled hyaline endospores (2 to 4 μm)	■ Alternating one-celled thick walled barrel shaped arthroconidia and disjunctor cells
Histoplasma capsulatum	■ Small oval yeasts (2 to 5 μm) resembling *Candida glabrata*	■ Round tubercule one-celled macroconidia ■ Microconidia are small (2 to 5 μm) one-celled smooth walled and borne on hyphae-like conidiophores
Paracoccidioides brasiliensis	■ Multiple budding blastoconidia around large one-celled hyaline thick walled cells ■ Blastoconidia are variable in size and arranged radially around the parent cells attached by narrow tubular denticles ■ Often described as a "pilot's or ship's steering wheel"	■ Hyphae are typically sterile ■ Fresh isolates produce one celled hyaline conidia
Sporothrix schenckii	■ Conidiophores with conidia in a rosette formation	■ Round, oval, or fusiform budding cells called cigar bodies
Penicillium marneffii	■ Indistinguishable in size and shape from *H. capsulatum*	■ Typical *Penicillium* spp. ■ Morphology

Hematoxylin and eosin, periodic acid-Schiff (PAS), and Gomori's methenamine silver stains, as well as calcofluor white can be used to detect the presence of blastoconidia and pseudohyphae in tissue sections and biopsy material. A potassium hydroxide preparation may be used to digest sputum, nail and skin scrapings to detect fungal elements.

To identify yeast isolated from clinical specimens, cornmeal agar with Tween 80 is often used to demonstrate the microscopic morphology of yeast species. Blastoconidia, arthroconidia, chlamydospores (Figure 14-22 ■), pseudohyphae, and true hyphae can be evident, depending on the species of yeast isolated.

Identification tests can include:

■ Germ tube test—rabbit, bovine, sheep, or human serum are inoculated with a small amount of the test organism. The test tube is incubated at 35°C for 2 to 3 hours. A small quantity of the test medium is examined for the presence

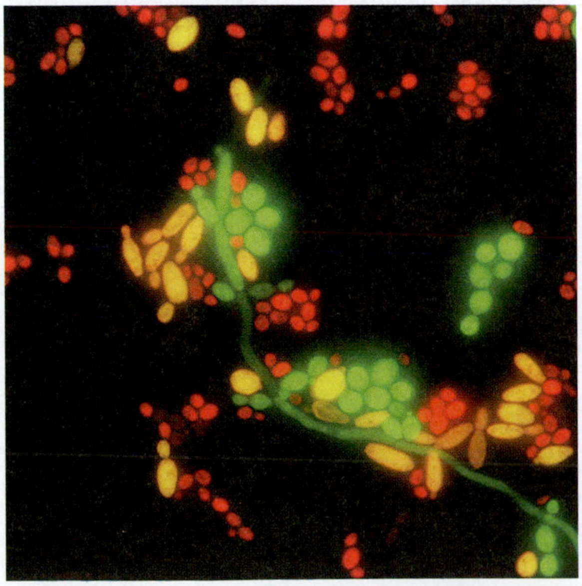

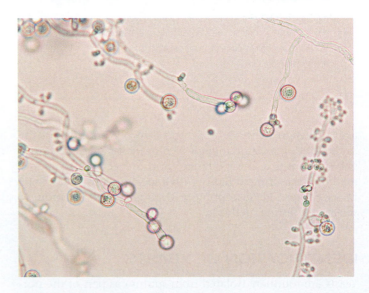

■ **FIGURE 14-21** Yeast Traffic Light PNA FISH™.
From AdvanDx.

■ **FIGURE 14-22** Thick-walled, terminal chlamydospores, pseudohyphae, and blastoconidia of *C. albicans.*

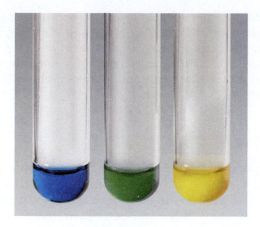

■ **FIGURE 14-23** Positive (yellow) and negative (blue, blue-green, or green) reactions for Rapid Trehalose Assimilation Broth.
Photo courtesy of Remel, part of Thermo Fisher Scientific.

of tubelike structures (Figure 14-6) with parallel walls extending from the blastoconidium. No constriction at the point of origin from the blastoconidium should be seen. A direct germ tube can be performed on positive blood cultures by adding 10 to 20 μL of the bottle contents to serum and incubated as described (Sheppard, Locas, Restieri, & Laverdiere, 2008).

■ Assimilation tests—determination of the ability of yeasts to utilize a carbon or nitrogen source, most often under aerobic conditions. A positive reaction is seen as growth in the medium (turbidity, formation of a pellicle at the surface of the medium, or growth at the bottom of the tube). The rapid assimilation test for trehalose (RAT) is used to identify *C. glabrata*. It turns yellow when positive (Figure 14-23 ■).

■ Fermentation—the anaerobic utilization of carbohydrates producing ethanol and CO_2 (bubbles in the Durham tube indicate the presence of CO_2 gas).

■ Urease production—the breakdown of urea produces alkaline by-products that cause the pH indicator to turn bright pink.

RAPID IDENTIFICATION OF YEAST

The Clinical and Laboratory Standards Institute, or CLSI provides guidelines for the rapid identification of three of the most commonly isolated yeasts. Using colony morphology, microscopic morphology, and simple tests, an experienced microbiologist can identify *Candida albicans, C. glabrata,* and *Cryptococcus neoformans* (Table 14-5✪).

   C. albicans presents with colonies that have pointy projections resembling stars or "feet" and are germ tube positive. *C. dubliniensis* may have similar colonies as *C. albicans* and are also germ tube positive. *C. dubliniensis* will not grow at 45°C, whereas *C. albicans* will (Pinjon, Sullivan, Salkin, Shanley, & Coleman, 1998). See ∞ Chapter 29, "Medical Mycology," for more information on *C. dubliniensis. C. tropicalis* may also appear to have "feet" with longer incubation but are germ tube negative. Rapid kits that test for L-proline aminopeptidase (PRO) and β-D-galactosaminidase (BGA) are available commercially. Figure 14-24 ■ shows an example of a commercial enzyme test system, BactiCard Candida. The kits provide results faster then the 2-hour germ tube. *C. albicans* is positive for both enzymes.

   C. glabrata forms pinpoint colonies on blood agar and appears as small, oval yeast cells without pseudohyphae. This yeast is able to ferment or assimilate trehalose in a few hours. RAT has been described previously and is available commercially.

✓ **Checkpoint! 14–9 (Chapter Objective 12)**

Yeast reproduces asexually by budding. In some cases, the daughter cells separate from the mother cells, but in other cases the two cells remain loosely attached and elongate producing structures that resemble "a string of sausages." The technical term for these fungal structures is:

   A. *true hyphae.*
   B. *pseudohyphae.*
   C. *arthroconidia.*
   D. *conidiophores.*
   E. *sporangiophores.*

✪ **TABLE 14-5**

Rapid Identification of Yeast

Yeast	Colony	Wet Preparation	Rapid Test
Candida albicans	Starlike or exhibiting "feet"	Oval, budding yeast	Germ tube positive Chlamydoconidia positive PRO and BGA positive
C. glabrata	Very tiny or pinpoint	Small, budding yeast No pseudohyphae	RAT positive
Cryptococcus neoformans	Mucoid	Large, round yeast	Urease positive Caffeic acid disk positive

PRO = L-proline aminopeptidase; BGA = β-galactosaminidase; RAT = rapid assimilation trehalose

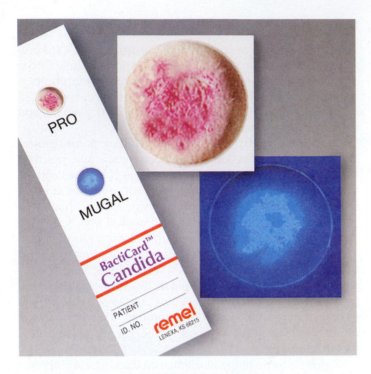

■ FIGURE 14-24 BactiCard Candida showing positive results for L-proline aminopeptidase (PRO) and β-galactosaminidase (MUGAL).
Photo courtesy of Remel, part of Thermo Fisher Scientific.

The colony of *C. neoformans* is usually mucoid, and the yeast cell appears large and round microscopically. A capsule may be observed in the wet preparation. The suspicious colony should be screened with a rapid urea and if positive tested with a caffeic acid disk. The caffeic acid disk tests for the enzyme phenol oxidase, and *C. neoformans* is positive (brown pigmentation on disk) for this enzyme (Figure 14-25 ■).

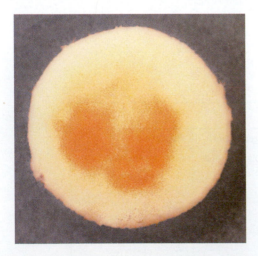

■ FIGURE 14-25 Caffeic Acid Disk with a positive reaction for *Cryptococcus neoformans*.
Photo courtesy of Remel, part of Thermo Fisher Scientific.

Standard methods should be used to confirm the identity when the isolate is recovered from blood, sterile tissue, or body fluids and for cases that have legal implications or epidemiologic importance. This approach provides "clinically relevant results in a timely manner" and will aid antifungal therapy (Baron, 2001).

SUMMARY

The importance of diagnostic laboratories being able to demonstrate, isolate, and identify pathogenic fungi has greatly increased with the growing number of immunocompromised individuals. Many fungal species that have been considered to be nonpathogens and only isolated on culture media as a result of contamination by spores carried to and fro in air currents now have to be taken into consideration as etiologic agents of disease because they may be found in tissues and body fluids of individuals with weakened immune systems. Clinical laboratory personnel must be familiar with the following:

- Safety measures used to protect individuals who work with fungal cultures
- The type of specimens needed to demonstrate fungi and to isolate them from clinical materials
- Procedures for direct microscopic examination of specimens that may contain fungi (for example, staining techniques that allow fungal elements to be visualized in tissues and body fluids)
- Culture procedures used to isolate fungi (fortunately, most procedures are simple and no elaborate or expensive equipment is required)
- Stains that allow the mycologist to study the microscopic morphology of fungi that have been cultured in vitro (using slide culture techniques)
- The macroscopic appearance of the organism when grown in culture
- The microscopic appearance of the organism when grown in culture

Superficial fungal infections rarely, if ever, pose a serious threat to the health and well-being of individuals and are primarily of concern for cosmetic reasons. Treatment options are available, and if the presence of the organism can be proven and the identity can be ascertained, patients subject to this illness may find relief when the appropriate therapy is applied.

Even individuals who are immunocompetent may acquire dermatophytic mycoses, and these diseases, although not life threatening, can be inflammatory and discomforting (burning and itching). Dermatophytes, the causative agents of athlete's foot and ringworm, are widespread, and because some have adapted to humans as a native host, they are stubborn pathogens. Treatment options are available, and the sooner dermatophytes are discerned to be the cause of a patient's pain and misery, the sooner effective treatment may be administered.

Subcutaneous mycoses, respiratory mycoses, and disseminated mycoses represent illnesses that can be a cause of significant morbidity and mortality. The correct diagnosis may allow the patient to experience symptomatic relief or may be lifesaving. Direct examination techniques may provide enough information for rapid intervention on the part of the clinician—much sooner than the results of a culture may be rendered. Where direct evidence may be lacking, it may be the final results of a fungal culture that allow the correct diagnosis to be made so antifungal therapy may be instituted.

Different direct examination methods and a description of what a mycologist can expect to see on examination were presented in this chapter. Knowing what to expect can help the novice mycologist determine the direct examination method that will provide the most relevant information.

To isolate fungal pathogens, the mycologist must be aware of the different types of fungal media and what organisms they are designed to support or inhibit. It is also important to comprehend the appropriate environmental conditions that will facilitate the growth of various fungi. This chapter contains information that allows individuals who become familiar with this material to make decisions about the appropriate medium and environment to isolate fungi that are commonly encountered in the clinical laboratory setting.

To correctly identify the species of fungi that may be recovered from clinical specimens, a mycologist must be familiar with the macroscopic (or colony) morphology and the microscopic morphology of the various fungal species. Pictorial representations (line drawings and photographs) as well as the descriptions of the different fungal elements and species presented in this chapter will aid students and the novice mycologist in their quest to make knowledgeable decisions on the correct identity of fungi recovered from clinical specimens on a routine basis. ∞ Chapter 29, "Medical Mycology," presents greater detail on specific fungi and their diseases.

LEARNING OPPORTUNITIES

Many Web sites offer a wealth of additional information on fungi. Some examples are listed here.

http://www.merck.com/mmhe/sec17/ch197/ch197a.html

http://www.nlm.nih.gov/medlineplus/fungalinfections.html

http://www.doctorfungus.org/

http://www.medmicro.wisc.edu/resources/imagelib/mycology/index.html

1. A patient is seen by her physician because of erythematous, itchy, scaly skin lesions that recently appeared on her forearms and abdomen. The patient is an animal lover who owns several cats and dogs. Skin scrapings are sent to the laboratory in a sterile, clean, dry container for direct examination.

   a. What method of direct detection will clear the skin cells and facilitate the detection of fungal elements that may be present?
   (Chapter Objectives 5, 6, and 7)

   b. Describe the appearance of dermatophytic fungi in skin lesions.
   (Chapter Objectives 6 and 12)

   c. The surface of the isolated mould is white and coarsely fluffy, whereas the reverse is deep yellow. Microscopically numerous macroconidia and few microconidia were observed. What is the most likely cause of this patient's symptoms?
   (Chapter Objectives 11 and 13)

   d. Describe how you would work safely with fungal specimens and fungal isolates like this one. (Chapter Objective 3)

2. *Histoplasma capsulatum* is a mould that is endemic to the Ohio and Mississippi River valleys. It can cause diseases ranging from asymptomatic to acute, fulminant, respiratory infections.

   a. Describe three types of media that can be used to isolate this organism from a body site likely to be colonized by other microbes such as bacteria.
   (Chapter Objective 9)

   b. Describe the microscopic appearance of the mould phase seen when the organism is cultured on a nutritive type medium such as SDA at room temperature. (Chapter Objective 13)

  c. Describe the microscopic appearance of the organism when it is cultured on brain heart infusion agar supplemented with blood and incubated at 37°C. (Chapter Objective 13)

3. *Pneumocystis jiroveci* (formerly known as *P. carinii*), an organism once considered to be a protozoan parasite, causes disease in the immunocompromised host. It cannot be grown in artificial media, and diagnosis is based on the clinical presentation (signs and symptoms), radiography (x-rays), and histological examination of affected tissues (the lower respiratory tract).

  a. What methods of direct observation can best be used to demonstrate the presence of the organisms in host tissues? (Chapter Objective 13)

  b. Describe the microscopic appearance of the organisms in tissue specimens. (Chapter Objective 4)

CASE STUDY 14-1 (CHAPTER OBJECTIVES 2, 11, 12, 13, AND 15)

A sputum specimen from a 54-year-old female suffering from systemic lupus erythematosus is submitted to the laboratory for a routine culture and susceptibility testing. She is heavily immunosuppressed to control her symptoms associated with lupus.

Examination of a Gram stained smear made from the sputum specimen revealed the presence of numerous pus cells, moderate gram-positive cocci in pairs and short chains, occasional gram-negative rods, and many blastoconidia with pseudohyphae. The specimen is subcultured to a blood agar plate, a chocolate agar plate, a phenylethyl alcohol agar plate, and a MacConkey agar plate. After 24 hours, growth typical of the normal upper respiratory tract flora is recovered. After 48 hours of incubation, small, white, smooth, colonies with a "spiderlike" appearance are seen to be the predominant organism. A Gram stain reveals that the organism is yeast. Figure 14-26 ■ shows the germ tube result that occurred within 3 hours.

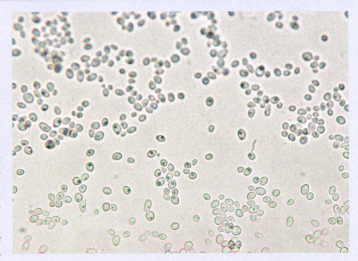

■ FIGURE 14-26

1. What is the genus and species name of this yeast?

CASE STUDY 14-2 (CHAPTER OBJECTIVES 2, 11, 12, 13, AND 14)

Lung tissue from a migrant worker living in Arizona is submitted to the microbiology section of the laboratory. A section of tissue stained with the periodic acid-Schiff stain is also sent. Examination of the stained tissues reveals the presence of spherules (30 to 70 microns in diameter) with endospores (2 to 5 microns in diameter).

After 5 days of incubation at room temperature, fungal growth is seen on the Sabouraud dextrose agar supplemented with chloramphenicol and cycloheximide. By 10 days the surface of the mould colony is white with a cottony texture. The reverse is also white.

Growth is taken from the mould culture, placed on a slide containing lactophenol cotton blue, and examined with the low power and high dry objectives. Septate, branched hyphae with thick-walled, barrel-shaped arthroconidia are seen. The arthroconidia alternate with thin-walled, empty joiner cells.

1. What is the genus and species name of this mould?

2. What test can provide rapid, culture identification of this mould?

3. What further testing should be used to confirm the identity of this mould?

PEARSON
myhealthprofessionskit™

Use this address to access the interactive Companion Website created for this textbook. Simply select "Clinical Laboratory Science" from the choice of disciplines. Find this book and log in using your user name and password.

REFERENCES

Go to myhealthprofessionskit.com to view this chapter's references.

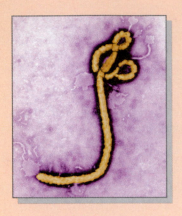

15

Ova and Parasites

Donald C. Lehman

■ LEARNING OBJECTIVES

Upon completion of this chapter, the learner should be able to:

1. Identify criteria for rejection of a specimen for an ova and parasite examination.
2. Determine optimal specimens for the recovery and detection of parasites.
3. Describe procedures for collection, preservation, and transportation of clinical specimens and the advantages and disadvantages of each.
4. Explain the necessity for collection of peripheral blood samples at periodic times of the day for some blood-borne parasites.
5. Describe the purpose, advantages, and disadvantages of saline and iodine direct and concentrated wet mounts and stained smears.
   a. Differentiate the two most common fecal concentration methods in use.
6. Describe the calibration of an ocular micrometer and the measurement of an object using a calibrated microscope objective.
7. Discuss stains used for detecting parasites to include their purpose and interpretation.
8. Select procedures for the recovery, detection, and identification of parasites.
   a. Outline the purpose, reagents used, and interpretation.
9. Discuss alternate methods for diagnosis of parasitic infections/infestations.

KEY TERMS

amastigote	karyosome	protozoa
buffy coat	larvae	stippling
cyst	microfilaria	trophozoite
formalin	parasite	trypomastigotes
gravid	polymerase chain	
helminth	reaction (PCR)	

▶ INTRODUCTION

Parasitic diseases are a major cause of morbidity and mortality throughout the world; however, inhabitants of the tropics and subtropics suffer most from these types of diseases. The World Health Organization (WHO) estimates that 350,000,000 to 500,000,000 people are infected with malaria annually, and 10% of all deaths in Africa are because of this disease (World Health Organization [WHO], n.d.a). It is also estimated that 2 billion people worldwide have intestinal roundworm infection (WHO, n.d.b), and it is not uncommon for an individual to have more than one parasitic disease at a time.

Parasitic diseases are less prevalent in developed countries because of good sanitation procedures that help limit the transmission of intestinal parasites. In addition, the United States and Europe lie within the temperate zone, so the winters are generally harsh enough to interfere with the life cycle of parasites that have a developmental stage outside the human host. Also, several parasites require species-specific arthropod vectors for transmission, and in some cases these vectors are not present in the United States. However, with worldwide travel increasing, numerous opportunities exist to acquire a parasitic infection. Each year, approximately 10 million Americans travel abroad.

A **parasite** is an organism that lives at the expense of, or harms, its host. Bacteria, viruses, and fungi can meet this broad definition. However, generally in the clinical laboratory "parasite" refers to eukaryote organisms: **protozoa** (one-celled organisms) and **helminths** (wormlike animal). Some protozoa are nonpathogenic and have a commensal relationship with the host, where the protozoa benefit and the host is neither harmed nor helped. In this chapter, the more important procedures used to diagnose parasitic infections in the United States will be discussed. ∞ Chapter 30, "Parasitology," provides details on the identification of parasites.

▶ SPECIMEN COLLECTION AND TRANSPORT

The laboratory diagnosis of parasites has classically been based on direct observation of the parasite, either macroscopically, as in the case of the larger helminths, or microscopically. Parasites range in size from intracellular forms measuring about 1 μm up to tapeworms measuring 30 feet in length. More recently, rapid molecular biology kits have become available and are now being used in laboratories. Although generally not as reliable, some parasitic diseases can be diagnosed by the detection of antibodies to infectious agents. As with any sample submitted to the clinical laboratory, specimens for parasites must be properly collected, labeled, and transported to ensure quality results.

INTESTINAL SPECIMENS

Some of the more prevalent parasitic infections involve the gastrointestinal tract. In the United States, a recent study found *Blastocystis hominis* to be the most common intestinal para-

☢ TABLE 15-1

Incidence of Intestinal Parasites in the United States

	*Number (% of Patients Positive)
Ascaris lumbricoides	14 (0.5)
Blastocystis hominis	662 (22.8)
Chilomastix mesnili	5 (0.2)
Cyclospora cayetensis	14 (0.5)
Cryptosporidium parvum	121 (4.2)
Dientamoeba fragilis	12 (0.4)
Endolimax nana	46 (1.6)
Entamoeba coli	50 (1.7)
Entamoeba histolytica/E. dispar	68 (2.3)
Entamoeba hartmanni	7 (0.2)
Giardia lamblia	19 (0.6)

*A total of 2,896 patients were tested; 90 patients had multiple infections. Data adapted from Amin, O. (2002). Seasonal prevalence of intestinal parasites in the United States during 2000. *American Journal of Tropical Medicine and Hygiene, 66*(6), 799–803.

site, present in 22.8% of the 2,896 patients examined (Amin, 2002; Table 15-1 ☢). *Cryptosporidium parvum* was the second-most-common parasite, detected in about 4% of the patients. A total of 916 patients were infected with one or more intestinal parasite. Other important intestinal parasites include *Giardia lamblia, Cyclospora, Entamoeba histolytica, Dientamoeba fragilis*, microsporidia, and a number of helminths. Abdominal discomfort and diarrhea are the most common symptoms of intestinal parasitic infection.

A fresh stool specimen is often the preferred specimen; rectal swabs do not contain sufficient material for testing. The fecal sample should be collected into a clean, dry, widemouth container free of water and urine. Water may contain free-living parasites that could be misidentified as clinically significant species, and the low pH of urine can harm some parasites by stopping motility or distorting their morphology. Samples should be collected before a barium enema; barium obscures the microscopic detection and cannot be removed during the concentration procedure. A stool sample containing barium will have a gray chalky appearance and should be rejected. Barium is used to provide contrast for x-rays of the intestine. It can take up to ten days to clear barium from the intestinal tract. Other substances that can interfere with the detection of

---

✔ **Checkpoint! 15–1 (Chapter Objective 1)**

A stool sample, containing barium, should be rejected for an ova and parasite examination because the contrast material:
  A. *fluoresces and provides a false positive result.*
  B. *resembles some parasites.*
  C. *kills parasites.*
  D. *obscures parasites.*

intestinal parasites include mineral oil, antibiotics, anti-diarrhetic agents, anti-nausea agents, and medical testing dyes.

The number of fecal specimens to be submitted is somewhat controversial. Historically, three specimens collected on separate days at least 1 day apart is recommended. These samples are usually analyzed separately. Collecting multiple samples is considered important because several species of intestinal protozoa are passed intermittently in the stool. It has been suggested that the third specimen be collected after administering a laxative. The laxative can have a flushing or purging action that may lead to more organisms passing in the stool. Alternatively, multiple specimens from the same patient could be pooled and analyzed as a single specimen. The advantage of this is the time saved in processing a single specimen. However, small numbers of parasites could be missed because of a dilution effect.

Some studies have reported that 71% to 91% of pathogenic protozoa present in a stool sample could be found by examination of a single specimen (Branda, Lin, Rosenberg, Halpern, & Ferraro, 2006; Hiatt, Markett, & Ng, 1995). Therefore, only if the first sample was negative, would a second one be analyzed. If multiple stool samples are received on the same patient, they could be saved in a preservative pending the results of the first sample. This would be more cost effective than analyzing three specimens initially. A rejection criterion many hospital laboratories use is not to analyze stool samples for ova and parasites (O & P) on patients who have been hospitalized more than 3 days. It is unlikely that gastrointestinal tract infections are because of intestinal parasites in these individuals.

The laboratory should receive fresh specimens within 30 minutes of collection. This is often not often possible or practical for most individuals requiring an ova and parasite examination. If a time delay is expected between collection of the fecal sample and processing, fixatives should be used. Fixatives generally fall into one of two categories: those that can be used for wet mount examinations and concentration procedures and those that can be used for permanent stained smears. The patient should be given detailed instructions and preservatives for home collection. A number of preservatives are available; no preservative is perfect for all situations (see Table 15-2). It is sometimes necessary to use two different preservatives for each stool sample.

✪ TABLE 15-2

Some Commonly Used Fecal Preservatives

Preservative	Comment
5% to 10% Formalin	Good for stool concentration procedures, but does not preserve trophozoites well. Does not preserve parasites well for permanent stained smears.
Sodium acetate-acetic acid-formalin (SAF)	Preserves parasites for both concentration and permanent stained smears and does not contain mercury. Has a poor adhesive quality for permanent stains.
Schaudinn's fixative	Used to fix fresh fecal material for permanent staining; not recommended for concentration procedures. Excellent preservation of cysts and trophozoites. Contains mercury.
Polyvinyl alcohol (PVA)	Excellent preservation of cysts and trophozoites and adhesive quality for permanent smears. Although it can be used for concentration procedures, it is not recommended. Contains mercury.

℮ REAL WORLD TIP

Fresh stool specimens should be transmitted to the laboratory as quickly as possible. Liquid specimens should be preserved within 30 minutes of passage not receipt in the laboratory. Liquid stool specimens are more likely to contain protozoan trophozoites, the motile feeding stage, that can disintegrate easily. Semiformed stool should be preserved within one hour. Semiformed stool can contain both trophozoites and cysts, the hibernation stage. Formed specimens can wait for preservation within the day of receipt. Formed stool are more likely to contain protozoan cysts that are hardier and can survive longer without preservation. If any delay in transport is expected a preservative should be used.

Formalin or formaldehyde has probably been the most widely used fixative. It works well for concentration procedures and most immunoassays but not for the **polymerase chain reaction (PCR)**, a technique used to amplify and detect organism DNA. Formalin does not, however, preserve parasite morphology for permanent stained smears. A 5% solution of formalin is recommended for preserving protozoa, and a 10% solution is recommended for helminths because the lower concentration may not kill helminth ova. In fact, unless the 10% formalin is heated to 60°C, ova can continue to develop. If a laboratory does not want to have two different concentrations available, a 5% solution makes a good general-

✔ Checkpoint! 15–2 (Chapter Objectives 2 and 3)

What is the most common specimen collection method used to detect intestinal parasites?

    A. *One pooled sample over a 24-hour period*
    B. *Two samples collected the same day examined separately*
    C. *Three samples collected 1 day apart examined separately*
    D. *Three samples collected 1 day apart pooled together*

purpose concentration (Garcia, Shimizu, & Deplazes, 2003). Most commercially prepared formalin preservatives are 10%. To preserve parasite morphology, sodium phosphate buffers are often added to formalin solutions to maintain a neutral pH (neutral formalin).

Schaudinn's fixative, which contains 95% ethanol, mercuric chloride, and distilled water, is used for fresh specimens collected in house and works well for permanent stained smears. However, the mercuric chloride is toxic and can cause chemical disposal problems. Polyvinyl alcohol (PVA), a plastic resin, is often added to Schaudinn's fixative as an adhesive. When fecal material is smeared onto a microscope slide, the PVA is responsible for adhesion. PVA makes the fecal suspension more viscous and less suitable for concentration procedures. A low-viscosity PVA (Meridian Diagnostics, Inc., Cincinnati, OH) is available. Stool samples are generally mixed with fixatives in a ratio of one part stool to three parts fixative.

Sodium acetate-acetic acid-formalin (SAF) can be used in a single-vial system preserving specimens for both concentration procedures and permanent stained smears. SAF does not contain mercury so it is safer, but parasite morphology will not be quite as sharp as fixation with mercuric chloride. SAF does not have good adhesive qualities; therefore, albumin-coated slides are recommended for permanent stained smears. When SAF is used as a fixative for stained smears, iron hematoxylin stain gives better results compared to the trichrome stain.

Because of the toxicity of mercury and formalin, a number of less-toxic single-tube substitutes have been developed: ECOFIX (Meridian Diagnostics, Inc., Cincinnati, OH), PARASAFE (Scientific Devices Laboratory, Inc., Des Plaines, IL), and Proto-fix (Alpha-Tec Systems, Inc., Vancouver, WA). Although Proto-fix does not contain mercury, it does contain formaldehyde. ECOFIX contains zinc-based PVA and is used with the ECOSTAIN (Meridian Diagnostics, Inc.) modification of the trichrome stain. The PARASAFE procedure, using ethanol bis-carbonyl compounds, was reported to have a darker background compared to the other two methods after trichrome staining (Jensen et al., 2000). Zinc-based fixatives do not always reveal internal structures of protozoa as clearly as mercury-based PVA. When used for stained smears, ECOFIX and

Proto-fix are acceptable alternatives to PVA. PARASAFE is less satisfactory for the identification of *Entamoeba histolytica/ E. dispar, Entamoeba coli,* and *Chilomastix mesnili.* Compared to formalin for concentration procedures, ECOFIX was less sensitive (Fedorko et al., 2000).

Other specimens from the intestinal tract, including duodenal aspirates, endoscopy specimens, and biopsied material, can be submitted. These specimens are collected in the hospital and should be transported to the laboratory as quickly as possible. Duodenal aspirates are more likely to contain motile protozoa; they should be held at room temperature until examined.

 Checkpoint! 15–3 (Chapter Objective 3)

What compound in the preservative Schaudinn's fixative is responsible for fixation and toxicity?
- A. *Acetic acid*
- B. *Formalin*
- C. *Mercury*
- D. *Zinc sulfate*

BLOOD SPECIMENS

A number of parasites can be detected in blood, such as *Plasmodium, Babesia, Trypanosoma,* and the **microfilaria,** the larval stage of some nematodes. The **buffy coat,** a layer of white cells found between plasma and red blood cells following centrifugation of whole blood, Knott's concentration preparations, and thick and thin smears are used in detecting blood parasites. Smears can be prepared directly from fingersticks, blood collected in blood collection tubes by venipuncture, or from buffy coats. EDTA is the preferred anticoagulant. To detect **stippling** or granules in the erythrocyte seen with some *Plasmodium* spp., smears should be made from blood samples within 1 hour of collection. Some parasites, particularly the microfilariae, exhibit periodicity and migrate through the bloodstream at specific times of day. It may be necessary to collect one specimen in the morning (10:00 a.m.) and another sample late in the evening (10:00 p.m.) depending on the blood parasite suspected. It is important that the collection time is recorded on the tube of blood.

 Checkpoint! 15–4 (Chapter Objectives 2 and 4)

Blood samples are collected in the morning and evening to diagnose infections caused by:
- A. *microfilariae*
- B. *Plasmodium species*
- C. *Babesia species*
- D. *Trypanosoma species*

REAL WORLD TIP

Duodenal contents can be collected by using a gelatin capsule containing a coiled string and weight. The end of the string, extending from a small hole in the top of the capsule, is taped to the patient's face and the capsule is swallowed. The capsule dissolves and, after about four hours, the string reaches the duodenum. Mucus and parasites adhere to the string. The string is removed; the mucus is stripped and examined for parasites.

OTHER BODY SPECIMENS

Urogenital tract specimens can be submitted to the laboratory for the detection of *Trichomonas vaginalis*. This is probably the most common parasite in the United States, and it is most noted for causing vaginitis. Vaginal discharge can be collected via a swab, which is placed into a transport medium or tube containing about 1 mL of sterile saline. The InPouch TV system (Biomed Diagnostics, San Jose, CA) combines a wet mount preparation and a culture method to detect *T. vaginalis* (Figure 15-1 ■). The top portion of the InPouch TV functions as a slide and is examined under a microscope. The InPouch TV system can be used for vaginal and urine specimens. The sample is kept at room temperature and quickly transported to the laboratory.

A 24-hour urine collection may be used to detect the ova of *Schistosoma haematobium*. A single urine specimen may be collected between 12 noon and 3 p.m. The ova are excreted in highest concentrations during these hours. Urine should be centrifuged and the sediment examined for the presence of parasites.

Lower respiratory tract samples may also contain parasites. Some intestinal helminths migrate through the body and pass through the lower respiratory tract as part of their life cycle, whereas some parasites, such as the lung fluke *Paragonimus westermani,* preferentially infect the lungs. These organisms can sometimes be detected in sputum samples. *Cryptosporidium*, microsporidia, *Pneumocystis jiroveci* (previously *P. carinii*) (Stringer, Beard, Miller, & Wakefield, 2002), a fungus with a morphology resembling parasites, and *Entamoeba histolytica* can be found in lower respiratory tract specimens. Blood-tinged areas should be selected for testing. Viscous specimens can be treated with a mucolytic agent and centrifuged to concentrate parasites.

Biopsied material of muscle, liver, intestinal, brain, skin, and lung tissue can also contain parasites. Often only a small amount of material is collected via a biopsy and may not be representative of the diseased tissue. Material to be examined by light or electron microscopy should be immediately placed into fixative. A portion of the biopsy may be placed in formalin if histologic stains for identification of parasites are requested. If a culture for protozoa has been requested, the tissue sample should be placed into a sterile container containing a small amount of sterile paper or a sponge moistened with sterile water.

► SPECIMEN PROCESSING

Processing specimens for the detection of parasites includes macroscopic examination, direct microscopy, concentration of the specimen followed by microscopic examination, cultures, and molecular biology assays. The procedures used depends on the type of specimen and the parasites suspected. The specimen should be processed immediately if a fixative is not used.

INTESTINAL SPECIMENS

The microscopic examination of a stool specimen is often referred to as an ova and parasite (O & P) examination. Figure 15-2 ■ provides a flowchart for processing and examination of stool specimens for parasites. When the laboratory receives a fresh stool specimen that has been collected in house, the date and time of collection and the consistency of the sample should be noted. Typically, stool samples can be categorized as liquid, soft, or formed. Soft is the appearance of normal stool specimens. The presence of gross amounts of blood or mucus should also be reported. Adult worms or tapeworm proglottids may be present.

Fresh, liquid stools are more likely to contain motile **trophozoites**, the active, feeding stage of a protozoa. Formed stool is more likely to contain **cysts**, the stage of a protozoan's life cycle offering resistance to unfavorable conditions. A direct wet mount should be performed on all fresh liquid stools to detect trophozoites. Motile **larvae** (singular larva), a young parasite form that has a markedly different morphology compared to an adult, and ova may also be observed in fresh specimens. Preservatives kill but maintain the morphology of protozoa; therefore, direct wet mounts are not usually performed on preserved specimens. To prepare a wet mount, a

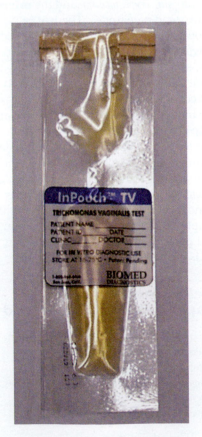

■ FIGURE 15-1 InPouch TV system.

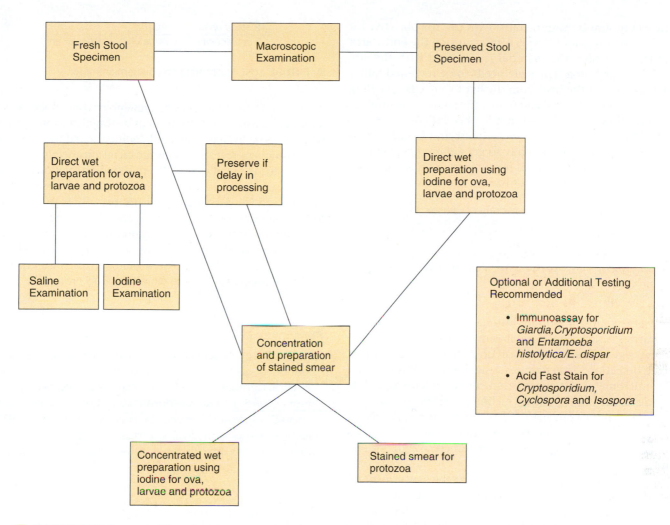

■ **FIGURE 15-2** Suggested flowchart for processing and examination of stool specimens for parasites

small amount, approximately 2 mg, of fecal material is suspended in a drop of saline on a microscope slide. If blood or mucus is present, it should be selected for microscopic examination because parasites are often in higher numbers in these materials. A 22 × 22 mm coverslip is placed over the suspension; some prefer a larger coverslip. The suspension should be thin enough to be able to just read newspaper text through it. If the suspension is heavier than that, smaller parasites will be obscured. If the suspension is too light, the examination will not be sensitive enough to detect organisms.

To prevent drying of the material during examination, the coverslip can be sealed with clear nail polish or vaspar, a mixture of petroleum jelly and paraffin. Because the sample is unstained, it is important to increase the contrast by reducing the amount of light passing through the sample; otherwise, protozoa can easily be missed. This is best done by raising the condenser to the highest level and adjusting the light by narrowing the aperture on the substage diaphragm. Some microscopes do not have a substage diaphragm, so it is necessary to lower the condenser.

✓ **Checkpoint! 15–5**
(Chapter Objective 5)

Direct wet mounts on fresh, liquid feces are performed primarily to detect:
   A. *cysts.*
   B. *motile trophozoites.*
   C. *red blood cells.*
   D. *white blood cells.*

 REAL WORLD TIP

Vaspar is made by melting equals parts of paraffin and petroleum jelly. Heat the mixture slowly; remember paraffin is flammable if overheated.

The wet mount is examined first with the 10× objective for large helminth eggs and larvae. After scanning the entire area under the coverslip, the material is reviewed with the 40× objective for protozoa. The slide needs to be reviewed rather quickly to prevent the heat from the light source from killing the parasites. It is more difficult to identify some of the trophozoites once they are no longer motile. It is difficult to use the oil immersion objective on a wet mount and is not recommended. It can be done carefully to get a more detailed look at suspicious objects. Intestinal protozoa seen on wet mounts should be confirmed with a permanent stained smear.

 REAL WORLD TIP

Gently tapping on the coverslip of a wet mount can cause suspicious objects to roll over and provide a better view.

One of the most important criteria for identifying intestinal parasites is size. Therefore, it is necessary to calibrate the 10×, 40×, and 100× objective lenses on all microscopes used for parasite detection. This requires a stage micrometer and an ocular micrometer. A stage micrometer is a microscope slide with lines etched in the glass. The lines on the stage micrometer are generally 10 µm apart. An ocular micrometer is placed in one eyepiece. Using the 10× objective, focus on the lines etched into the surface of the stage micrometer. Align one end of the ocular micrometer with one end of the stage micrometer. Then look for the first two lines, one on the ocular micrometer and the other on the stage micrometer, that coincide with each other. To determine the distance between two lines on the ocular micrometer for the 10× objective, divide the number of stage units by the corresponding number of ocular units, then multiply by 10 (the distance in µm between the lines on the stage micrometer). For example, if 12 stage units corresponded to 10 ocular units, divide 12 stage units by 10 ocular units, then multiply by 10 ocular units/stage units (Figure 15-3). The result is 12 µm for each ocular unit. To determine the size of an object viewed with the 10× objective, simply multiply the number of ocular units by 12 to find the size in µm. The procedure must be repeated for the 40× and 100× objectives.

$$\frac{12\ stage\ units}{10\ ocular\ units} \times \frac{10\ \mu m}{1\ stage\ unit} = \frac{12\ \mu m}{1\ ocular\ unit}$$

■ **FIGURE 15-3** *Calibrating an ocular micrometer.*

Some intestinal parasites can resemble white blood cells. In addition to using motility to help distinguish protozoa from white blood cells, stains are used. Iodine-stained wet mounts of fresh specimens reveal cytoplasmic inclusions helpful in identifying protozoa. Lugol's and D'Antonio's iodine solutions are commonly used. Gram's iodine, used in bacteriological stains, should not be used for visualizing parasites because it is too strong. Iodine stain is helpful in visualizing and identifying the internal structures of cysts but will kill trophozoites. Examining specimens stained with an iodine solution can also reveal helminth ova and larvae. Methylene blue, a vital stain, can be used on wet mounts to help detect white blood cells and protozoa.

 REAL WORLD TIP

Iodine is a commonly used stain for microscopic examination of wet mounts of stool specimens. Although several formulations of iodine can be used, it is important to use a fresh preparation. Lugol's iodine stock should be diluted 1:5 with distilled water prior to use. Iodine stocks and dilutions must be stored in a dark brown bottle. The dilutions lose potency after about 2 weeks.

Because intestinal protozoa are relatively small and are often present in low numbers, they can easily be missed on direct examination. Therefore, concentration procedures are an important part of diagnostic parasitology. Sedimentation and flotation are two categories of concentration procedures. In the flotation procedure, a solution with a high specific gravity is used causing parasites to rise to the surface and the debris settles in the bottom of the tube. In sedimentation methods, solutions with low specific gravity are used, and the parasites are found in the sediment.

The most commonly used concentration procedure is formalin-ethyl acetate sedimentation (FES). Kits, such as the Fecal Parasite Concentrator Kit (Remel, Lenexa, KS) and CONSED (Alpha-Tec Systems, Inc.), are available. In the FES procedure, the specimen is first filtered through two layers of gauze; the filtrate is then suspended in about 10 mL of saline or water. The suspension is centrifuged at 500 X *g* for approximately 10 minutes. There should be about 1 mL of sediment. The pellet is resuspended in saline or water and centrifuged again. Washing continues until the supernatant is relatively clear.

Once the supernatant is clear, it is poured off, and the pellet is resuspended in 9 mL of a buffered 5% to 10% formalin solution. If it is a fresh specimen, the sample should set at room temperature for about 10 minutes to kill parasites that

✓ **Checkpoint! 15–6 (Chapter Objective 6)**

When calibrating an ocular micrometer, you find that five stage units correspond to 20 ocular units. You subsequently measure a cyst with a diameter of 10 ocular units. What is the diameter of the cyst in µm?

   A. 120
   B. 40
   C. 25
   D. 10

may be present. If it is a preserved specimen, the parasites have already been killed by the preservative, and it is not necessary to wait. Next, 3 mL of ethyl acetate is added, and the sample is mixed vigorously for about 30 seconds. Hemo-De, a terpene-based, nontoxic, biodegradable substitute, can be used in place of ethyl acetate. The sample is then centrifuged at 500 X *g* for 10 minutes. Four layers should result: (1) a top layer of ethyl acetate or Hemo-De, (2) a plug of debris, (3) a formalin solution, and (4) sediment. Any parasites present should be in the sediment. A wooden applicator stick is inserted into the tube to dislodge the debris plug from the inside of the tube, and the supernatant is poured off, leaving about 1 mL of formalin to resuspend the pellet. An iodine wet mount of the sediment should be examined. A saline wet mount is not necessary because any parasites present are killed and will no longer exhibit motility.

The sedimentation concentration procedure has several stopping points in the procedures. It causes less distortion of parasite and is very good at removing fatty substances from stool. Most facilities choose to use the sedimentation concentration procedure due to its ease of performance and consistency of results.

The zinc sulfate flotation procedure works well for detecting protozoan cysts and some helminth ova. This procedure generally produces cleaner wet mounts than sedimentation methods. A 33% aqueous solution of zinc sulfate is prepared. For fresh, unpreserved stool specimens, the specific gravity of the zinc sulfate solution is determined by a hydrometer and adjusted to 1.18 by adding more zinc sulfate or distilled water. Most parasites have a specific gravity of 1.05 to 1.15 and so float. Some operculated ova (those with lids) and infertile *Ascaris lumbricoides* ova are not concentrated well because their specific gravity is greater then 1.20 and they sink.

A small portion of a fresh stool sample is mixed in a solution of 5% or 10% neutral formalin and left at room temperature 30 minutes to kill any parasites that might be present. The stool sample is then filtered through two layers of gauze into a 15 mL conical centrifuge tube until 0.5 to 1 mL of sediment is obtained. The sediment is resuspended into about 15 mL of 0.85% saline. The mixture is centrifuged for 10 minutes at 500 X *g*. The sample should be washed again if the supernatant is not clear. Once the supernatant is clear, decant the supernatant and suspend the sediment in a solution of zinc sulfate. The sample is centrifuged for 2 minutes at 500 X *g*. Without removing the tube from the centrifuge, a small volume of the surface film is removed with either a heated and cooled bacteriological loop or a Pasteur pipette and placed onto a microscope slide. A drop of iodine can be added, and then a 22 × 22 mm coverslip is placed over the suspension.

Formalin-preserved specimens can be used if the specific gravity of the zinc sulfate solution is adjusted to 1.20. The higher specific gravity solution can distort the appearance of some ova and is not recommended. If zinc-sulfate is the only method used for concentration of stool specimens then both the surface film and pellet should be examined, which increases

turnaround time. The flotation concentration method has no stopping points in the procedure. Once completed, slides must be read immediately. At 30 minutes, cysts begin to disintegrate and, at one hour, all parasites begin to sink.

Because of their similarities and small size, it is often difficult distinguishing the protozoa on wet mounts. Stained smears allow for detection of the small protozoan parasites. It is also easier to see the detailed internal structures of protozoans to insure accurate identification. It creates a permanent record that can be reviewed later if questions arise and is probably the most important procedure for the diagnosis of intestinal parasites. For these reasons, a permanent stained smear is recommended on all stool samples for O & P examination.

 REAL WORLD TIP

Parasite infections can elicit the production of eosinophils. The breakdown products of eosinophils are called Charcot-Leyden crystals. The crystals are long and thin with pointed ends similar to a toothpick. They may be present in wet mounts as well as stained smears.

 Checkpoint! 15–7 (Chapter Objective 5)

What is the primary reason for performing a stained fecal smear?
  A. *Evaluating the quality of the specimen*
  B. *Detecting intestinal helminth ova*
  C. *Distinguishing intestinal larvae*
  D. *Distinguishing pathogenic protozoa from nonpathogens*

Fecal material for staining must first be treated with a fixative. The fixative helps the specimen adhere to the microscope slide. For fresh specimens, fecal material is spread onto a microscope slide, and before the material dries, the slide is fixed with Schaudinn's fixative for 30 minutes. Stool samples placed directly in Schaudinn's fixative with PVA should be fixed for at least 30 minutes. The suspension should then be well mixed and a portion poured onto a paper towel for 3 minutes to absorb excess PVA. Material from the paper towel is used to make smears. The prepared slides should be dried for several hours at 37°C or overnight at room temperature before staining.

 REAL WORLD TIP

Use a long wooden applicator stick to prepare a stool smear for staining. Dip the stick into the fixed specimen then roll it across a glass slide from edge to edge so it creates an area about the size of a postage stamp. Do not make the slide too thick or it will flake off during the staining procedure.

SAF-preserved specimens are mixed and filtered through two layers of gauze into a 15 mL conical centrifuge tube. The sample is centrifuged for 1 minute at 500 X *g*, and the supernatant is decanted. The material is smeared onto a microscope slide coated with albumin to increase the adhesiveness. The smear is allowed to air-dry for at least 30 minutes.

Iron hematoxylin is the classic fecal parasitology stain. When performed properly, this stain produces well-defined inclusions and nuclei. The stain procedure is available on the Companion Website. Unfortunately, this stain does not always produce consistent results and is subject to variations in preservatives, stain concentrations, and staining times. Because of its ease of use, the Wheatley's modified trichrome stain is commonly used for permanent smears. The procedure is available on the Companion Website. A modified acid-fast stain is used for detecting *Cryptosporidium, Cyclospora,* and *Isospora* in fecal material. The acid-fast stain is routinely used in bacteriology to visualize the mycobacteria. To detect intestinal parasites, a weaker decolorizer—1% sulfuric acid—is used instead of acidified ethanol.

After staining the smear with either iron hematoxylin or trichrome stain, the smear can be permanently mounted with resin medium and a coverslip. After the resin has dried for one hour at 37°C or overnight at room temperature, the smear can be examined. The smear can be examined with the 10× objective for helminth ova and larvae but most facilities do not use this practice. Ova and larvae often stain so dark that they can be easily overlooked. A thorough and complete examination of the stained slide using the 100× objective (oil immersion) is required.

Protozoa stained with the iron hematoxylin stain will have a bluish-gray cytoplasm with dark purple nuclear membranes and **karyosomes** (a clump of nuclear chromatin). The background is often gray to blue. With the trichrome stain, the cytoplasm typically stains a light blue-green with dark purple-red nuclear membranes and karyosomes. The trichrome background stains green. Acid-fast stained fecal smears do not need to be permanently mounted with a coverslip; after completely air-drying, they can be examined with the 100× (oil immersion) objective for *Cryptosporidium, Cyclospora,* and *Isospora.* In the acid-fast stain, cysts of *Cryptosporidium* and *Cyclospora* will retain the carbol fuchsin, the primary stain, and appear as pink to red circles or ovals, approximately 4 μm and 8 μm, respectively. *Cyclospora* tend to stain less uniformly. *Isospora* species will appear as a large clear oval structure with one or two pink circles inside it.

Microsporidia are obligate intracellular, spore-forming protists; approximately 140 genera and over 1,200 species have been described from every major animal group. *Microsporidium* infection is most often associated with immunocompromised patients, particularly patients with human immunodeficiency virus infection. The diagnosis of intestinal microsporidiosis is often initiated by light microscopy examination of fecal specimens for spores. A small amount of unconcentrated fecal material is smeared onto a microscope slide. Concentration procedures used for other intestinal parasites fail to concentrate *Microsporidium* spores due to their small size. However, the FES

and flotation concentration procedures will remove some fecal debris resulting in cleaner preparations that may make it easier to see microsporidium spores. Unfortunately, the concentration procedures may also cause the loss of *Microsporidium* spores resulting in false-negative results.

The microsporidia cannot be detected with routine fecal stains. Many spores are acid-fast positive; however, because of the small size of the spores, identification is difficult with this stain. A modified trichrome stain can be used, in which one of the stains, chromotrope 2R, is used at 10 times the normal concentration, and the staining time is increased to 90 minutes (Weber-green modified trichrome stain for *Microsporidium*). Some prefer a different counterstain—aniline blue (Ryan-blue modified trichrome stain for *Microsporidium*)—instead of fast green. Heated stains may decrease the staining time and may also improve the sensitivity of the staining: 37°C for 30 minutes or 50°C for 10 minutes (Weber & Canning, 2003). The spores of microsporidia will appear as pinkish ovals measuring 1 μm to 4 μm; unfortunately, a number of objects in stool specimens may also have this appearance. Even with staining, because of their small size, microsporidia can be easily missed. The use of quality control slides is imperative. A number of other stains have been developed for detecting *Microsporidium.* Cytological stains of duodenal and ileal tissue collected by endoscopy is a very sensitive method of diagnosing intestinal microsporidiosis. Electron microscopy can be used; this method is very specific, but because of the small volume of tissue examined, it is not as sensitive as other methods.

 Checkpoint! 15–8 (Chapter Objective 7)

What stain is most frequently used to detect Cryptosporidium, Cyclospora, and Isospora in fecal material?
  A. *Modified acid-fast*
  B. *Gram's*
  C. *Methylene blue*
  D. *Trichrome*

EXAMINATION FOR PINWORM

Unlike other intestinal helminths, pinworm or *Enterobius vermicularis* is not typically diagnosed by microscopic examination of fecal material. The **gravid** (containing ova, developing embryos, or larvae) female worm migrates out of the anus, generally at night, to deposit ova on the perianal skin folds. The ova can be collected by using a piece of cellulose tape wrapped around a tongue depressor so that the sticky side is facing outward. Specimen collection is done first thing in the morning before the infected individual gets out of bed. The tape is applied to several perianal regions. The tape is then sent to the laboratory for microscopic evaluation. A swab coated with vaspar can be prepared and used as well. Plastic paddles with a sticky covering, stored inside a plastic tube, are commercially available (Scientific Device Laboratory, Des

Plaines, IL; Figure 15-4). The plastic paddle can be viewed directly microscopically. Care should be taken when working with specimens for pinworm examination. The ova are alive and infectious within hours of being deposited.

Checkpoint! 15–9 (Chapter Objective 8)

Which of the following is the most sensitive specimen for the diagnosis of pinworm?

A. *Stool specimen*
B. *Perianal material*
C. *Duodenal aspirate*
D. *Rectal swab*

BLOOD SPECIMENS

Requests for blood smear examinations for blood-borne parasites should be considered a STAT (to be done immediately) procedure, with both positive and negative results called to the physician as soon as possible. Infection with the malaria parasite, *Plasmodium falciparum*, can be fatal.

Stained blood smears are generally considered the reference method for diagnosing blood-borne parasites. Electron microscopy has been reported to be helpful in distinguishing *Plasmodium* from *Babesia* but is not practical for most facilities. Procedures for processing blood samples must be readily available so medical laboratory scientists on the evening shift can process and examine the stained blood smears. However, it

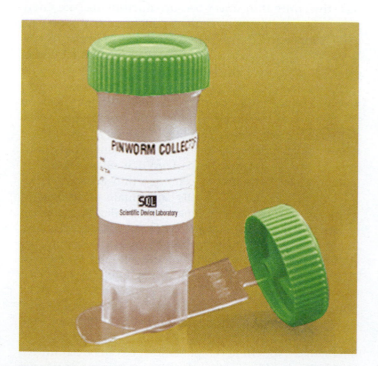

■ FIGURE 15-4 Pinworm collector (SDL).
Courtesy of Scientific Device Laboratory.

may be necessary for the blood smears to be reviewed the next morning by a pathologist or experienced parasitologist.

 REAL WORLD TIP

Automated hematology analyzers present with abnormal results for an individual with malaria. The results are not specific enough to diagnose malaria due to the low incidence of the infection in the United States. Other countries, with a higher rate of incidence, have greater experience and success in interpreting results and diagnosing the infection from automated analyzer results.

Parasites can be detected in whole blood and buffy coats. Concentration procedures can increase the sensitivity of detecting blood parasites. Although it is sometimes possible to find motile microfilariae and trypanosomes in blood wet mounts, stained smears are more often used. The Giemsa stain is the preferred stain for blood smears, although the Wright's stain, used in hematology, is acceptable. Whole blood is used to create both thick and thin smears for microscopic examination. The red blood cells in the thick smear are lysed, whereas the red blood cells in the thin smear are fixed to prevent their lysis. Because a larger volume of blood is examined with the thick smear, it is more sensitive than the thin smear. However, because the red blood cells are lysed, it is more difficult to identify some parasites, so the thick smear is less specific.

Thick and thin smears can be made on separate slides or on the same slide (Figure 15-5). To create a thick smear, a drop of blood is placed on one end of a microscope slide. If the thick smear is too thick, the material will flake off during staining. A thin smear can be made on the remaining area of the slide. For a thin smear, a drop of blood is placed on the slide and spread across the surface of the slide using the edge of another microscope slide; smears are made in the same manner as those for a white blood cell differential in hematology. The feathered edge results in one layer of red blood cells. This is ideal for observing the details of the red blood cells and organisms.

Several smears should be made on each blood sample. Once the thick and thin smears have air-dried, the thin smear is fixed in absolute methanol for 1 minute before staining with

Checkpoint! 15–10 (Chapter Objective 8)

Thick smears, for detection of Plasmodium species, are:

A. *prepared from peripheral blood.*
B. *lysed to release the parasites from the red blood cells.*
C. *more sensitive than thin smears.*
D. *All of the above*

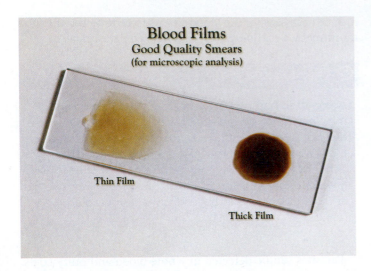

Blood Films
Good Quality Smears
(for microscopic analysis)

Thin Film

Thick Film

■ **FIGURE 15-5** Example of a thick and thin blood film.
Public Health Image Library/CDC and Steven Glenn, Laboratory and Consultation Division

the Giemsa stain. If the thick and thin smears are on the same slide, it is important not to allow the methanol to come in contact with the thick smear.

Giemsa stain is commercially available as a stock solution. Working solutions are made by mixing 1 part of the stock solution with 10 to 50 parts of phosphate buffer (pH 7.0 to 7.2); fresh working solution should be prepared daily. The staining time is determined by the dilution. Generally, with a 1:20 dilution, the staining time is 20 minutes; with a 1:30 dilution, the staining time is 30 minutes, and so on. However, these are only guidelines; each laboratory must determine which dilution and staining times work best. A 1:50 dilution stained for 50 minutes generally works best for thick smears, whereas less-dilute stains for a shorter staining time seem to work better for thin smears.

After fixing the thin smear, the entire slide is submerged in Giemsa stain covering both the thick and thin smear. After staining, the red blood cells should appear pale red, and white blood cells should have a pale purple cytoplasm with purple nuclei. Eosinophilic granules will stain bright red, and neutrophilic granules will be pink-purple. *Plasmodium* spp. will have a blue cytoplasm, and the nuclear dots will stain red to red-purple. Other blood-borne parasites, such as *Babesia* and trypanosomes, will stain similar to *Plasmodium*. The sheath of the microfilariae often does not stain with the Giemsa stain, but will appear as a halo around the organism. Their nuclei will be clearly visible.

Wright's stain is an alternative to the Giemsa stain. Wright's stain is commercially available in a ready-to-use liquid form, or as a powder that must be dissolved in absolute methanol and filtered before use. Stain prepared from powder must also be diluted in phosphate buffer (pH 6.6 to 6.8) similar to the Giemsa stain. Because Wright's stain contains methanol, the thin smear does not need to be fixed. However, before staining, the red blood cells in the thick smear must be lysed by

submersion into distilled water. If thick and thin smears are on the same slide, it is important not to let the distilled water come in contact with the thin smear.

After lysing the red blood cells in the thick smear, the slide is submerged in Wright's stain solution. The optimal staining time must be determined for each lot of stain. Staining with Wright's stain is generally inferior to Giemsa stain, and the thick smear is prone to stain precipitation. The red blood cells appear with light tan to reddish cytoplasm, and white blood cells have light blue cytoplasm with dark blue nuclei. Eosinophilic granules are bright red, and neutrophilic granules are pink or light purple. The *Plasmodium* spp. and the other blood-borne parasites have a pale blue cytoplasm with red nuclear dots. As with the Giemsa stain, the sheath of the microfilariae often does not stain, but their nuclei will be clearly visible.

ℯ REAL WORLD TIP

Once an individual is diagnosed with malaria, it is important to determine the level of infection to ensure therapy is effective. It is calculated as a percentage by counting the number of infected red blood cells per 100 red blood cells.

The stained thick smear should first be scanned on low power, the 10× objective, to not miss the larger microfilariae. Then the oil immersion lens (1,000× total magnification) should be used to examine about 100 fields. The thin smear should also be examined first on low power. It is important to scan the entire thin smear because microfilariae are rarely present in large numbers. Particular attention should be paid to the periphery of the smear because the microfilariae tend to be pushed to the edge when the smears are made. A minimum of 200 to 300 fields on the thin smear should be carefully examined with the oil immersion lens. If suspicious objects were seen on the thick smear, then considerably more fields on the thin smear should be examined. Because people review slides at different speeds, it is better to look at a minimum number of fields than to use a minimum amount of time; however, it usually takes an experienced medical laboratory scientist 15 to 20 minutes to examine a thin smear.

Peripheral mononuclear cells can contain **amastigotes**, which are a form of trypanosome without a flagellum and can be seen in *Trypanosoma cruzi* and *Leishmania* species infections. Mononuclear cells and **trypomastigotes**, a form of trypanosome with an undulating membrane and kinetoplast located posterior to the nucleus, can be found in buffy coat preparations. Blood for buffy coat preparation is collected by venipuncture with an anticoagulant such as EDTA or sodium citrate. Whole blood can be transferred to a Wintrobe sedimentation tube and centrifuged at 100 X *g* for 30 minutes. Alternatively, the entire venipuncture tube can be centrifuged for 100 X *g* for 15 minutes, and a Pasteur pipette or transfer pipette is used to transfer the buffy coat to another tube for centrifugation again. After centrifugation, the mixture will separate into three layers: plasma layer on top, a buffy coat layer containing the white blood cells, and packed red blood cells on the bottom. The buffy coat should be examined directly by adding a drop of the buffy coat to a drop (0.5 mL) of saline on a microscope slide. The blood is mixed in the saline, and a coverslip is added. The blood should be examined with the 10× objective looking for motile microfilariae and trypanosomes. Some of the buffy coat material should be used to make stained thin smears.

The quantitative buffy coat (QBC; Becton Dickinson, Sparks, MD) procedure uses microhematocrit centrifugation to concentrate blood parasites. Blood samples are centrifuged in glass capillary tubes precoated with the fluorescent stain acridine orange. The tubes are placed into a special holder, immersion oil is applied, and the sample is examined microscopically. Although the QBC procedure is easier to perform and requires less experience than microscopic examination of Giemsa stained smears, it does require specially prepared tubes, a microhematocrit centrifuge, and a fluorescent microscope. When compared to microscopic examination of Giemsa stained smears, the QBC procedure had a sensitivity of 88% to 98% (Lema et al., 1999).

If microfilariae are suspected, a number of different concentration techniques can be used. Some procedures, such as the Knott concentration procedure and the gradient centrifugation technique, use a series of centrifugation steps. The membrane filtration technique uses a filter with 5 μm pores and is very efficient.

OTHER SPECIMENS

Bone marrow aspirates can be used to detect *Plasmodium, Trypanosoma,* and *Leishmania* that may not have been seen on peripheral blood smears. Bone marrow material should be stained with the Giemsa stain. Aspirates of cysts and abscesses may contain amebae; these specimens may require concentration by centrifugation.

Genital specimens for *Trichomonas vaginalis* should be immediately examined microscopically at 400× for motile trophozoites. The trophozoites of *T. vaginalis* are about the size of white blood cells and possess four anterior flagella and an undulating membrane. It is important to examine the specimen quickly while the trophozoites are motile; this makes it easier to distinguish them from white blood cells. Never store the sample at 4°C; this will kill the trophozoites. Samples submitted in the InPouch TV are directly examined. If the initial microscopic examination is negative, the specimen is pushed into the bottom pouch, which contains a broth for cultivation. Direct microscopic examinations have a sensitivity of only 63%, whereas cultures have a sensitivity of about 94% (Beverly, Venglarik, Cotton, & Schwebke, 1999). Diamond's medium is also available for the cultivation of *T. vaginalis.*

T. vaginalis can also be detected by examining vaginal material stained with the Gram stain. Some individuals report better staining of *T. vaginalis* if basic fuchsin is used as the counterstain instead of the standard safranin. *T. vaginalis* can be identified on Pap smears and material stained with acridine orange. Direct immunofluorescent and enzyme immunoassay (EIA) tests are also available.

Because some microsporidia cause systemic infections, they can be detected in many different clinical specimens. Besides fecal material, microsporidia can be found in fluids such as urine, sputum, bronchoalveolar lavage fluid, and cerebrospinal fluid, as well as tissue samples. Microsporidia can cause infections in a variety of tissue sites including the intestinal tract, eye, lower and upper respiratory tract, and urogenital tract. Samples are fixed in formalin for histologic examination and glutaraldehyde for electron microscopy. The material can be stained with some of the same stains discussed previously for intestinal microsporidia.

P. jiroveci can be detected in induced sputum and bronchoalveolar lavage specimens. Preparations are made with a cytocentrifuge, and the fungi can be visualized with a number of stains such as methenamine silver, orthotoluidine blue (OTB), or Giemsa. OTB metachromatically stains precystic and cystic stages of *P. jiroveci* and other fungal cell walls reddish violet. Giemsa stains nuclear and cytoplasmic structures of all *Pneumocystis* stages.

Cyst and abscess aspirates may need to be treated with streptokinase to break down the tissue, red and white blood cells. The specimen should then be centrifuged to concentrate the parasites. Wet mounts and stained smears can be prepared and examined. Tissue biopsies are used to prepare impression smears. The tissue surface is pressed against a glass slide numerous times and stained. The tissue can be sectioned for histologic staining. A muscle biopsy may be submitted for the diagnosis of trichinosis. The specimen is pressed between two glass slides to create a thin layer for review for the encysted larvae. A parasitology textbook should be used as a resource for detailed procedures for the processing and examination of specimens other than fecal.

▶ IMMUNOLOGIC AND MOLECULAR BIOLOGY ASSAYS

The world of diagnostic microbiology has changed significantly with the development of molecular biology assays. These assays typically detect either nucleic acids (DNA or RNA) or proteins (antigens). The nucleic acid assays often use an amplification step, such as PCR, followed by a probe to detect the amplified target sequence of nucleotides. Antigen detection assays are based on an immunologic reaction between an antigen and an antibody. Most antigen detection kits are based on enzyme immunoassay (EIA) or direct fluorescent antibody (DFA) methodologies.

Several commercial molecular biology kits are available for a number of parasites. The advantage of using molecular biology assays is the quick turnaround time. The disadvantages are the cost and the fact that the kits only detect one or two organisms. With microscopic examination, a number of different parasites can be detected at once by an experienced medical laboratory scientist. Therefore if only a molecular biology assay is performed, a significant parasitic infection could be missed. In the United States, *Cryptosporidium* and *Giardia lamblia* are two of the most important and common intestinal parasites, so many laboratories have adopted kits for these organisms. Examples include enzyme immunoassay (EIA) kits for *Cryptosporidium*: ProSpec T (Alexon-Trend, Ramsey, MN), Premier (Meridian Bioscience, Cincinnati, OH), and RIM Cryptosporidium (Remel, Lenexa, KS); EIA kits for *G. lamblia*: ProSpec T Premier and RIM Giardia; and an EIA kit that detects both *Cryptosporidium* and *G. lamblia*: ProSpec T. Meridian also makes a DFA kit for detection of both of these parasites. The Triage parasite panel (BIOSITE Diagnostics, San Diego, CA) detects *C. parvum, G. lamblia,* and the *Entamoeba histolytica/E. dispar* complex. Molecular biology kits have a reported sensitivity between 66% and 100% and specificity from 92% to 100% (Garcia, Shimizu, & Bernard, 2000; Gonin & Trudel, 2003; Pillai et al., 1999; Sharp, Suarez, Duran, & Poppiti, 2001).

Molecular biology assays are also very useful in distinguishing the pathogenic *E. histolytica* from the nonpathogenic *E. dispar*. These two species are morphologically indistinguishable. Failure to distinguish them can result in unnecessary treatment. Isoenzyme analysis of cultured ameba is the reference method; however, this test is technically demanding and is not routinely performed by clinical laboratories. At least four EIA-based kits are available for the detection of *E. histolytica/E. dispar* complex, and three kits are specific for *E. histolytica*.

Several molecular biology kits are available for detecting *T. vaginalis* such as the Affirm VP$_{III}$ (Micro-Probe/Becton-Dickinson; Franklin Lakes, NJ), a DNA probe assay that also detects *Gardnerella vaginalis* and *Candida* spp. Recently the Affirm Ambient Temperature Transport System (ATTS) was released, allowing the processing of specimens for up to 3 days after collection (Brown, Fuller, Daris, Schwebke, & Hillier, 2001). The Quick-Trich (PanBio InDx, Baltimore, MD) is a latex agglutination assay for *T. vaginalis*. Before a laboratory adopts any molecular biology assay, it must consider the how long it takes for results, cost-effectiveness, and accuracy of the assay.

Several molecular biology assays are available for detecting *Plasmodium falciparum*. The ParaSight-F (Becton-Dickinson) and the NOW ICT Malaria test (Binax, Portland, ME) are dipstick antigen-capture immunologic assays based on the detection of histidine-rich protein 2 secreted by *P. falciparum*. The NOW assay is a rapid immunochromatographic test (ICT) that also detects an antigen common to all four species of malaria: *P. falciparum, P. vivax, P. ovale,* and *P. malariae*. When compared to microscopic examination, the NOW ICT had a sensitivity of 100% for *P. falciparum* and a specificity of 96.2% (Wongsrichanalai et al., 2003). For *P. vivax* the sensitivity was 87.3% and the specificity was 97.7%. In a similar study, the sensitivity for *P. falciparum* was 70% with a specificity of 99% (Fernando, Karunaweera, Fernando, Attanayake, & Wickremasinghe, 2004). A prototype ParaSight F+V assay detecting both *P. falciparum* and *P. vivax* is being field-tested (Forney et al., 2003). The OptiMAL Assay (Flow Incorporated, Portland, OR) is an immunologic detection system for *Plasmodium* lactate dehydrogenase (pLDH). Currently, this assay is only for research and development; it has not yet been approved for diagnostic use. In field studies it has a sensitivity of 79.3% and a specificity of 99.7% (Kolaczinski et al., 2004). The OptiMAL may be better for follow-up after treatment because of the earlier disappearance of pLDH compared to the antigens used in other assays.

These malarial immunologic tests have the advantage of being easy to perform and interpret and not requiring as much expertise as examining a stained blood smear. However, the immunologic assays are much more expensive than diagnosis by microscopic examination, and this may be a barrier for widespread use in many countries where malaria is endemic (Fernando et al., 2004). The immunoassays are generally considered very sensitive and specific, although rheumatoid factor positive specimens can give false-positive results (Mishra, Samantaray, Kumar, & Mirdha, 1999). PCR assays have been reported to detect as few as four parasites per microliter (Tham, Lee, Tan, Ting, & Kara, 1999).

Checkpoint! 15–11 (Chapter Objective 9)

Which of the following is able to distinguish E. histolytica from E. dispar?
  A. Antigen detection assays
  B. Serologic testing
  C. Number of nuclei in cyst
  D. Size of trophozoites

▶ SEROLOGIC ASSAYS

During the course of infection by parasites, individuals form a number of different antibodies, although many of these antibodies are not protective. It is difficult to diagnose most parasitic diseases by serologic tests, possibly because of the selection of the wrong antigen, variable antibody response in different patients, and cross-reactions of antibodies. For these reasons and because the tests are generally technically demanding, few clinical laboratories offer serologic testing for parasitic diseases. The Centers for Disease Control and Prevention provides serologic testing for a number of parasites.

REAL WORLD TIP

Some parasites can be cultured on specialized medium. *Naegleria fowleri*, a pathogenic cerebrospinal fluid parasite, can be cultured on nonnutrient agar using *Escherichia coli* as a food source. Very few laboratories perform parasite cultures.

SUMMARY

This chapter provides information on the transportation, processing, and examination of clinical specimens for the diagnosis of parasites. As with any microbiological specimen, quality results depend on receiving a quality specimen. For stool specimens in particular, this involves the use of a preservative. Although formalin and mercury-containing solutions like PVA are generally excellent preservatives, their use has decreased lately because of toxicity. Although fecal material and blood are the two specimens most people think of, parasites can be found in almost any body sample.

The laboratory diagnosis of parasitic infections is often based on the microscopic examination of clinical specimens. The specimen can be directly examined or examined after a concentration procedure. The formalin-ethyl acetate sedimentation and the zinc sulfate flotation procedures are the concentration procedures most frequently used on stool specimens. Wet mounts of stool samples are an excellent way to diagnose intestinal helminth infections by detecting ova, larvae, and adult worms, whereas permanent stained smears are valuable in diagnosing intestinal protozoa infections. Iron hematoxylin and trichrome are the preferred stains. The blood-borne parasites are diagnosed by the examination of peripheral blood specimens or occasionally bone marrow aspirates. Blood smears are stained with either the Giemsa or Wright's stains.

Molecular biology assays have started to become an integral part of diagnostic parasitology. A number of kits are available to detect some of the more prevalent intestinal parasites, along with *T. vaginalis* and *Plasmodium*. These assays are based on a variety of techniques including EIA, immunofluorescence, and nucleic acid probes. Molecular biology assays have the advantage of shorter turnaround times and require less expertise; however, they tend to be expensive and can only detect one or two parasites at once. Unlike with bacteria, cultivation techniques are not commonly used in diagnosing parasites. In addition, because of antigen variation and cross-reactivity, serologic assays are not very valuable.

LEARNING OPPORTUNITIES

1. You have been asked to develop a protocol for detecting intestinal parasites. What are some important considerations? (Chapter Objectives 2, 3, and 8)

2. Why are fecal samples not the best specimen for diagnosing pinworm infection? (Chapter Objectives 2 and 8)

3. What are the advantages and disadvantages of using a thick smear compared to a thin smear for the diagnosis of blood-borne parasites? (Chapter Objectives 5 and 8)

4. What procedures are available for diagnosing vaginitis caused by *Trichomonas vaginalis?* (Chapter Objectives 8 and 9)

PEARSON myhealthprofessionskit™

Use this address to access the interactive Companion Website created for this textbook. Simply select "Clinical Laboratory Science" from the choice of disciplines. Find this book and log in using your user name and password.

REFERENCES

Go to myhealthprofessionskit.com to view this chapter's references.

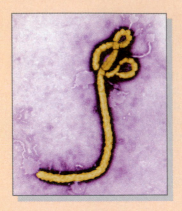

16

Viral, Chlamydial, and Rickettsial Specimens

Rochelle Glymph and William C. Payne

■ LEARNING OBJECTIVES

Upon completion of this chapter, the learner should be able to:

1. Provide instructions for proper collection of a given type of viral specimen, including timing, selection, procedure, collection devices and containers, and requirements for viral transport medium.

2. Describe viral transport medium, including its use, the constituents, and their purposes.

3. Verify proper transport of viral specimens, including interim storage and mailing.

4. Provide instructions for preparation (initial processing) of a given type of specimen for virus isolation.

5. Distinguish primary cell cultures, diploid cell lines, and established cell lines.

6. Provide instructions for isolating viruses in traditional monolayer cell cultures, including inoculation, incubation, maintenance, and monitoring during incubation.

7. Describe detection and confirmation of viral isolates in traditional monolayer tube cell cultures.

8. Describe shell vial and microwell centrifuged enhanced isolation methods, including inoculation, incubation, and reading and interpretation of results.

9. Distinguish co-cultured cells, cryopreserved monolayer cells, and transgenetic (transformed) cells used for virus isolation.

10. Relate methods of direct detection of viruses in specimens, including test application and evidence suggesting presence of virus.

11. Summarize serodiagnosis of virus infections, including application and specimen collection and analysis.

12. Describe collection, transport, storage, and preparation of specimens for diagnosis of infection caused by *Chlamydia/Chlamydophila* and *Rickettsia*.

13. Describe detection of *Chlamydia/Chlamydophila* and *Rickettsia* in clinical specimens.

KEY TERMS

cell cultures

cell lines

cytopathogenic effect
  (CPE)

monolayer

nucleic acid probes

passaging

polymerase chain
  reaction (PCR)

propagation

refeeding

► INTRODUCTION

Specimens for diagnosis of viruses, *Chlamydiaceae* and *Rickettsia* command special attention. The infections being diagnosed are often serious, possibly life threatening, and therefore timely and accurate diagnosis is vital for specific treatment and patient management. Although *Chlamydiaceae* and *Rickettsia* are bacteria, the basic approaches for specimen collection and analysis are more similar to those for viruses. The distinctive intracellular nature of these organisms calls for special attention to specimen collection and analysis for reliable diagnosis.

These agents of infection will most likely be revealed when special guidelines for specimen collection and transport are followed, and the most appropriate diagnostic methods are selected and performed.

The optimal specimen contains infected host cells and viable organisms. Because of their fragile nature, viability must be preserved until the specimen is processed. These agents don't grow on artificial media; therefore, isolation requires living host cell systems. Gram stain and biochemical tests have no role in their laboratory diagnosis. Identification is based on cytohistologic, serologic, and molecular approaches.

This chapter describes collection, transport, and analysis of specimens for reliable diagnosis of viruses, *Chlamydiaceae,* and *Rickettsia*. It is important to note that the basic guidelines for specimen collection presented in ∞ Chapter 6 and the basic principles of cultivation presented in ∞ Chapter 7 are relevant for these organisms; however, some are superseded by more specific guidelines and approaches. The basic principles and procedures of immunologic tests explained in ∞ Chapter 10 and the molecular tests explained in ∞ Chapter 9 will not be repeated in this chapter. Rather, the application of these methods and the evidence suggesting the presence of these agents of infection will be presented. Information on the biological characteristics, disease, and clinical manifestations of the medically important viruses, *Chlamydiaceae,* and *Rickettsia* is provided in ∞ Chapter 31, which covers intracellular organisms, and will not be addressed in this chapter.

Because viruses, *Chlamydiaceae,* and *Rickettsia* are three distinctive groups of infectious agents, each will be discussed separately.

► VIRAL SPECIMENS

A variety of body tissues and fluids are useful for the diagnosis of viral infection, and the proper selection, collection, and transport of these specimens is of critical importance for accurate laboratory diagnosis. Because no single method will reliably diagnose infection, diagnosis is traditionally accomplished by performing cultural methods in conjunction with noncultural methods. The basic analytical approaches for identification of viruses in clinical specimens include isolation in living cells; direct detection of viral inclusions, antigens, and nucleic acids; and the detection of viral antibodies.

SAFETY

Biosafety level (BSL) 2 or 3 practices should be followed when collecting and analyzing specimens for viral diagnosis. Refer to ∞ Chapter 5, "Safety," to review these guidelines.

 REAL WORLD TIP

Most viruses encountered in a clinical microbiology laboratory usually only require BSL 2 safety practices. It is rare for most laboratories to attempt isolation of the SARS coronavirus (BSL3) or Ebola virus (BSL4).

COLLECTION AND TRANSPORT

Optimal results can only be obtained from specimens of optimal quality. Every specimen for virus detection should be carefully selected and collected using aseptic techniques and the appropriate collection devices and containers. Specimens should contain as much virus as possible, particularly for viral isolation, and should be transported in conditions that will maintain virus viability until processing. Specific guidelines for specimen collection and transport must be observed to ensure the specimen is of optimal quality.

Time of Collection

The best time to collect specimens for virus isolation is during the acute phase of illness, usually in the initial 3 to 5 days after the onset of symptoms. Virus shedding is optimal during this time, and specimens will be most productive. After 5 days, virus shedding begins to decline rapidly. As a result, specimens collected 7 or more days after onset will most likely yield negative culture results, even when infection exists. In patients with disseminated or persistent infections, virus shedding does not decline rapidly, and specimens will remain productive beyond 7 days. These infections can be life threatening, so specimens should be collected as early as possible for timely diagnosis and treatment. Autopsy specimens should be collected as early as possible following death.

 REAL WORLD TIP

There is a seasonality to some viruses. Over 200 viruses show an increase in infection rates during the late fall, winter, and early spring. Influenza, parainfluenza, and respiratory syncytial viruses are well-known winter viruses. Rotavirus is considered the winter vomiting and diarrhea virus. Outbreaks of aseptic meningitis due to enteroviruses peak in summer and fall. The newest epidemic virus, novel influenza A H1N1, is a virulent strain introduced to a susceptible population. This explains how it is spreading even during summer months when influenza viruses are normally absent.

Specimen Selection

The best specimen is the tissue involved. Specimens collected from the site of the actual infection represent the active disease process and permit maximum detection. Multiple body sites are involved in patients with disseminated infections such as generalized, systemic, congenital, or perinatal infections and in immunodeficient or immunosuppressed patients. In these cases, each affected site should be sampled. Viruses disseminate via the blood and cerebrospinal fluid (CSF); therefore, blood, and in most cases cerebrospinal fluid, should always be collected. Viruses enter the body through the respiratory and gastrointestinal tracts and exit in the respiratory secretions (i.e., adenoviruses, influenza, measles, coronaviruses), urine (cytomegalovirus, human herpes virus 8 [Santos-Fortuna & Caterino-de-Araujo, 2005], measles, mumps) and feces (enteroviruses, adenoviruses, noroviruses, rotaviruses). It is appropriate to select specimens from the points of entry and exit, depending on the clinical diagnosis and the virus suspected. Table 16-1 summarizes specimen selection based on the clinical syndrome and the viruses suspected.

 REAL WORLD TIP

Viruses require living cells to reproduce so it essential that specimens contain human cells in order to ensure recovery of the viruses.

Collection Materials

All collection devices and containers must be sterile. Specimen containers should have a secure closure and be leakproof, nonbreakable, and capable of withstanding freezing and thawing. Only swabs with tips made of Dacron, rayon, or other polyester fibers and shafts made of plastic or aluminum are appropriate. Calcium alginate and cotton fibers are toxic for many viruses and should be avoided. Calcium alginate is especially toxic for the herpes simplex viruses. Wooden shafts should be avoided because they are inhibitory for viruses.

 REAL WORLD TIP

The microbiology laboratory must provide healthcare workers detailed procedures for collection of specimens for viral testing. It is also necessary to ensure that the proper collection devices are available for use. Physicians and other healthcare workers often select a swab as their preferred collection device, but it is often one of the worst for viral testing.

Collection Methods

The method of collection depends on the site of infection and the type of clinical material. Aspirates, washings, scrapings, swabs, voided specimens, and biopsy and autopsy tissues are appropriate for analysis. Aspirates, washings and scrapings are better than swabs; however, swabs are collected more often because they are easier and more convenient to collect and less intimidating to the patient. Regardless of the collection method, it is important that the specimen contain host epithelial cells. Table 16-2 summarizes collection procedures for individual specimens appropriate for viral diagnosis.

✔ Checkpoint! 16–1 (Chapter Objective 1)

Which of the following guidelines correctly describes the proper selection and collection of a specimen for virus isolation?

    A. *Specimens should be collected during the second week of infection.*

    B. *Swabs with calcium alginate tips are preferred for collecting lesion material.*

    C. *Specimens should be selected from the site of active involvement.*

    D. *Specimens should not contain host epithelial cells.*

✪ TABLE 16-1

Specimen Selection for Viral Diagnosis

Clinical Syndrome	Common Associated Viruses	Recommended Specimen(s)
Aseptic meningitis and encephalitis	Arbovirus	CSF, brain tissue, blood
	Cytomegalovirus	CSF, brain tissue
	Enterovirus	CSF, throat swab, stool, brain tissue
	Herpes simplex virus	CSF, brain tissue, blood
	Human immunodeficiency virus	CSF, blood
	Lymphocytic choriomeningitis virus (LCMV)	Serum
	Measles	CSF, urine
	Mumps	CSF, urine, serum, mumps
	Rabies (zoonotic)	Brain biopsy
	Varicella zoster virus	CSF, brain tissue, skin lesions
Congenital & perinatal infections	Cytomegalovirus	Urine, throat swab, blood, CSF, tissue
	Enterovirus	CSF, throat, stool, brain tissue, urine
	Hepatitis B virus	Blood
	Herpes simplex virus	Vesicle, CSF, throat, brain tissue
	Human immunodeficiency virus	Blood, CSF, tissue
	Parvovirus	Amniotic fluid, liver tissue
	Rubella	CSF, throat swab, urine
	Varicella-zoster virus	Vesicle, throat
Exanthems	Herpes simplex virus	Vesicle fluid or scrapings
Vesicular lesions and rash	Varicella-zoster virus	Vesicle fluid or scrapings
	Enterovirus	Vesicle scrapings, throat swab, stool
	Measles	Throat swabs, blood
	Parvovirus B19	Serum
	Rubella	Throat swab, urine
Conjunctivitis and corneal lesions	Adenovirus	Conjunctival swab or corneal scraping
	Enterovirus	Conjunctival swab or corneal scraping
	Herpes simplex virus	Conjunctival swab or corneal scraping
	Varicella-zoster virus	Conjunctival swab or corneal scraping
Gastroenteritis	Adenovirus (types 40 and 41)	Stool
	Norovirus	Stool
	Rotavirus (primarily infants)	Stool
Urogenital tract infections		
Urinary tract	Adenovirus	Urine
	Herpes simplex virus	Urine
	BK virus (polyomavirus)	Urine
	Cytomegalovirus	Urine
Genital	Herpes simplex virus	Genital swab, vesicle swab, or fluid
	Human papilloma virus	Genital swab, lesion biopsy
Malaise syndrome/glandular	Epstein-Barr virus	Serum
	Cytomegalovirus	Blood, urine, throat
Myopericarditis, pleurodynia	Coxsackie B virus	Heart or pericardial tissue, blood, stool, throat swab
	Echovirus	

(continued)

⊛ TABLE 16-1

Specimen Selection for Viral Diagnosis (continued)

Clinical Syndrome	Common Associated Viruses	Recommended Specimen(s)
Posttransplantation syndrome Immunosuppressed or immunodeficient patients	Adenovirus	Throat swab, tissue, blood
	Cytomegalovirus	Urine, throat swab, tissue, blood, bronchial washing
	Epstein-Barr virus	Serum
	Human herpesvirus-6 (HH6)	Blood
	Herpes simplex virus	Throat swab, vesicle fluid, tissue
	Human immunodeficiency virus	Blood, CSF
	Parainfluenza virus	Nasopharyngeal (NP), throat swab, tissue, bronchial washing
	RSV	NP, bronchial washing, tissue
	BK virus	Urine
	Varicella-zoster virus	Vesicle fluid, tissue, blood
Respiratory tract infections (upper) *Influenza, pharyngitis, croup, bronchitis, bronchiolitis, rhinitis*	Adenovirus	Nasopharyngeal swab, throat swab
	Cytomegalovirus (neonates)	
	Epstein-Barr virus	Serum
	Enterovirus	Nasopharyngeal swab, throat swab
	Herpes simplex virus	
	Influenza virus	Nasopharyngeal swab, throat swab, sputum
	Lymphocytic choriomeningitis virus (LCMV)	Serum
	Parainfluenza virus	Nasopharyngeal swab, throat swab
	Respiratory syncytial virus	Nasopharyngeal swab
	Rhinovirus	Nasopharyngeal swab, throat swab
Herpangina, stomatitis, pharyngitis	Adenovirus	Throat swab, oral lesions
	Enterovirus	
	Herpes simplex virus	
Pneumonia	Adenovirus	Throat swab, NP, lung tissue, bronchial washing, blood
	Cytomegalovirus	Urine, throat swab, lung tissue, blood, bronchial washing
	Herpes simplex virus	Throat swab, bronchial washing, lung tissue, oral lesions, blood
	Influenza virus A, B	Throat swab, NP, lung tissue, bronchial washing
	Parainfluenza virus 1, 2, 3	Throat swab, sputum, NP, lung tissue, bronchial washing
	Respiratory syncytial virus	NP, bronchial washing, lung tissue
	Varicella-zoster virus	Lung tissue, bronchial washing, skin lesions, blood
Hepatitis	Hepatitis viruses	Serum

SPECIMEN TRANSPORT AND STORAGE

Specimens should contain the maximum amount of virus at the time of collection. Every attempt should be made to maintain the condition of the specimen until it can be processed. Any delay in transport and improper storage conditions may result in the loss of virus viability and may compromise recovery. Cold temperatures and transport media are used to help preserve infectivity of viruses in specimens during transport and storage (Figure 16-1 ■).

Time and Temperature

All specimens should be transported promptly to the laboratory for processing. If immediate delivery is not possible, specimens should be held at 2°C to 8°C (refrigeration temperatures, on wet ice or a cold pack) and transported to the laboratory on wet ice or a cold pack within 2 hours. One exception, anticoagulated blood, should be held and transported at ambient temperature because low temperatures will interfere with separation of the blood components.

⭐ TABLE 16-2

Collection of Specimens for Virus Detection

Specimen Type	Collection Guidelines
Swabs/scrapings, vesicle aspirate, small tissue pieces	
Swabs	*Swab with sufficient force to collect host's epithelial cells. Avoid swabs with calcium alginate tips or wooden shafts.*
Cervical	Remove exocervical mucus with swab and discard.
	Insert fresh swab at least 1 cm into the endocervical canal and rotate against the mucosa for 5–10 seconds.
	Place in 1–2 mL viral transport medium (VTM).
Conjunctival or corneal	Use flexible fine-shafted swab premoistened with sterile saline.
	Swab lower conjunctiva.
	Place in 1–2 mL VTM.
	Corneal or conjunctival scrapings should only be collected by an ophthalmologist or other trained personnel and placed in 1–2 mL VTM.
Lesion (vesicle)	Select only fresh lesions.
	Gently wipe vesicle with sterile saline to cleanse.
	Disrupt (lance) vesicle and collect fluid with swab; with same swab, collect cells from base of lesion.
	Place in 1–2 mL VTM.
Lesion (nonvesicular)	Premoisten swab with sterile saline.
	Collect cells from base of lesion.
	Place in 1–2 mL VTM.
Mucosal	Swab back and forth across involved surface.
	Place in 1–2 mL VTM.
Nasal	Insert flexible, fine-shafted swab into nostril, rotate swab, and let it rest for several seconds to absorb secretions.
	Use separate swabs for each nostril.
	Place in 1–2 mL VTM; both swabs may be placed in the same tube.
Nasopharyngeal	Insert flexible, fine-shafted swab through nostril into the nasopharynx and rotate gently a few times.
	Place in 1–2 mL VTM.
Pharyngeal (throat)	Depress tongue with a tongue blade to prevent contamination with saliva.
	Vigorously swab tonsillar areas and posterior nasopharynx.
	Place in 1–2 mL VTM.
Rectal	Insert swab 4–6 cm into rectum, and roll against mucosa.
	Place in 1–2 mL VTM.
Urethral	Express and discard exudate.
	Insert flexible, fine-shafted swab 2–4 cm into urethra, gently rotate swab 2–3 times and withdraw.
	Place in 1–2 mL VTM.
	Patients should not urinate for at least 1 hour prior to collection.
Vesicle aspirate	Wipe vesicle with sterile saline.
	Aspirate fluid with a needle and syringe.
	Immediately rinse syringe with 1–2 mL VTM.
Tissue pieces	Small pieces.
	Place in 1–2 ml VTM.
Fluids (CSF, other sterile body fluids, respiratory fluids, urine)	
Amniotic fluid	Place 5–8 mL in a sterile, leakproof container.
	No VTM.
Bronchoalveolar lavage (BAL)	Place 8–10 mL in a sterile, leakproof container.
	No VTM.

(continued)

✪ **TABLE 16-2**

Collection of Specimens for Virus Detection *(continued)*

Specimen Type	Collection Guidelines
Cerebrospinal fluid (CSF)	Place 2–5 mL in sterile, leakproof container. No VTM.
Nasopharyngeal aspirate (NPA)	Use mucus collection device, insert catheter through the nasal passages. Apply suction. Wash aspirate through tubing with 5–8 mL of VTM or sterile saline. Transfer material from trap to a sterile container. VTM is optional, but preferred.
Pericardial fluid	Minimum of 2 mL in a sterile container. No VTM.
Pleural fluid	Minimum of 2 mL in a sterile container. No VTM.
Saliva	Sample anterior floor of mouth and near Stenson's ducts. Collect 1 or 2 swabs. Place swabs in 1–2 mL VTM.
Urine	5–10 mL of midstream clean-voided urine in a sterile container. No VTM.
Solids (tissues; stools)	
Autopsy tissue	1 to 2 grams of tissue into sterile container. Add 8–10 mL VTM.
Stool	2–4 grams in a sterile container. Add 8–10 mL of VTM if transport will be delayed.
Blood	
Blood	8–10 mL in anticoagulant (EDTA, sodium citrate, or heparin); minimum of 2 mL for pediatrics. No VTM.
Bone marrow	2 mL in anticoagulant (EDTA, sodium citrate, or heparin). No VTM.

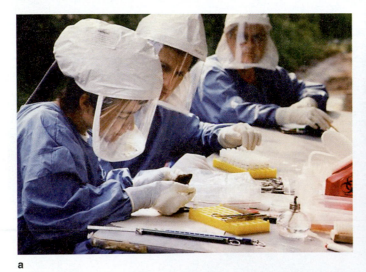

a

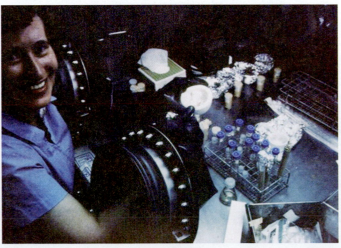

b

■ **FIGURE 16-1** Specimen Collection. **a.** Three CDC health officials inspecting specimens suspected of being connected with a Hantavirus outbreak. **b.** CDC virologist Herta Wulff, PhD, working with specimens through the sealed portals of a "glove box" during a 1975 Marburg vector investigation.
Courtesy Public Health Image Library (PHIL), Centers for Disease Control and Prevention (CDC), Atlanta, GA.

REAL WORLD TIP

Respiratory syncytial virus and cytomegalovirus are especially sensitive to delays in transport. Respiratory syncytial virus, cytomegalovirus, and varicella zoster virus are very susceptible to freezing.

Transport Media

Liquid transport media such as viral transport medium (VTM) and 2-sucrose phosphate (2-SP) are preferred for transporting viral specimens. VTM is used to provide moisture, preserve the infectivity of viruses, and control microbial contamination in specimens. It is composed of a balanced salt solution as the base, protective protein (albumin, serum, or gelatin), antibacterial and antifungal agents, and a buffering system to maintain the pH.

2-SP is a buffered sucrose solution containing transport medium and was originally designed as a chlamydial transport medium. The sucrose in the medium prevents inactivation of viruses by reducing the effect of freezing or prolonged refrigeration. This is particularly useful for the more fragile enveloped viruses. VTM, 2-SP, and other liquid transport media should be stored at –20°C for up 6 months and thawed just before use.

Amies or Stuart's semisolid transport media may be used to transport swabs for viral diagnosis. Ideally, swabs in these media should be transferred to VTM immediately on arrival in the laboratory. Stool specimens in buffered glycerol are also acceptable for viral isolation.

If the time between collection and processing may exceed 1 hour, swabs, scrapings, vesicle aspirates, stools, and tissue specimens, which are susceptible to drying or contamination by normal flora, should be placed in suitable transport medium. Transport medium is not required for blood, cerebrospinal fluid, urine, and respiratory fluids because virus viability does not diminish quickly in these specimens. Although not required, respiratory fluids should be transported in VTM to inhibit contaminating respiratory flora.

Checkpoint! 16–2 (Chapter Objective 2)

Viral transport media:
  A. *should be used to transport blood and cerebrospinal fluid.*
  B. *provides moisture and preserves viral infectivity.*
  C. *contains protein to inhibit growth of bacteria and fungi.*
  D. *may be stored at room temperature for up to 4 months.*

Storage and Shipping

Specimens that cannot be processed on arrival in the laboratory should be held at 2°C to 8°C for up to 48 hours. If a delay in processing beyond 48 hours of collection is imminent, specimens should be frozen at –70°C. However, freezing specimens before culturing is not recommended. The enveloped viruses are more fragile than the densely packaged naked viruses and may lose infectivity. Specimens that must be mailed should be snap frozen at –70°C and shipped on dry ice. All specimens shipped through the mail or by commercial courier must be packaged and labeled in compliance with federal regulatory guidelines. Table 16-3 summarizes collection, transport, and storage of the four general categories of specimens.

Checkpoint! 16–3 (Chapter Objective 3)

Which of the following viral specimens was correctly transported and stored?
  A. *Anticoagulated blood transported to the laboratory at 2°C to 8°C within 2 hours of collection.*
  B. *Specimens to be mailed were frozen at –20°C and shipped on ice.*
  C. *Viral specimens transported at room temperature.*
  D. *Specimens that could not be processed on arrival in the laboratory were held for 2 days at 2°C to 8°C.*

✪ TABLE 16-3

Specimen Transport and Storage

Specimen Type	Transport	Interim Storage
Swabs/scrapings, vesicle aspirate, small tissue pieces	Deliver to lab at 2°C to 8°C, on wet ice or a cold pack.	2°C to 8°C, refrigerator, wet ice, or cold pack. Do not freeze. Freeze at –70°C *only* if transport will be delayed >48 hours.
Fluids (CSF, other sterile body fluids, urine, respiratory)	Deliver to lab at 2°C to 8°C, on wet ice or a cold pack.	2°C to 8°C, refrigerator, wet ice, or cold pack. Do not freeze. Freeze at –70°C *only* if transport will be delayed >48 hours.
Solids (tissues; stools)	Deliver to lab at 2°C to 8°C, on wet ice or a cold pack.	2°C to 8°C, refrigerator, wet ice, or cold pack. Do not freeze. Exception; stools for rotavirus may be frozen at –70°C. Freeze all others at –70°C *only* if transport will be delayed >48 hours.
Blood and bone marrow	Deliver to lab at room temperature.	Room temperature; do not refrigerate. Process within 6 hours of collection.

REAL WORLD TIP

Storage of viral specimens at –70°C and 4°C is preferred over –20°C.

SPECIMEN ANALYSIS

Specimens accepted for viral diagnosis should be analyzed as soon as possible after collection, preferably within the initial 24 hours of collection. The standard approaches for viral diagnosis include isolation, cytohistopathology, serology (immunoassays), and molecular diagnosis. No single approach is sufficient for every case, so laboratories combine approaches for optimal viral diagnosis. The selection of methods used depends on several variables, including the type of specimen, the virus suspected, the intended purpose of the assay, turnaround time, and the capabilities of the laboratory performing the analysis.

Specimen Accessioning

All specimens received by the laboratory must first be evaluated to determine suitability for further processing. The specimen is evaluated to ensure that collection and transport guidelines have been followed and that the information required for laboratory processing is provided on the specimen label and requisition form. Information required for the laboratory record and for appropriate specimen processing and interpretation of results include patient and physician information, specimen source and type, date and time of collection, date of onset of symptoms, clinical picture including therapy, agent suspected, and tests ordered. The ordering physician should be notified immediately regarding inadequate specimens or information so that replacement specimens, additional samples, and/or required information can be provided.

REAL WORLD TIP

Patient history information such as recent travel, immune status, or recent vaccinations may be necessary to ensure timely recovery of viruses. Physicians should list specific viruses for specimen testing. Sending orders for a generic viral culture may delay results.

Specimen Preparation

The goal of specimen preparation is to concentrate the virus in the inoculum, inactivate bacterial and fungal contaminants, and eliminate or reduce toxicity. The particular protocol is determined by the type of specimen and varies among laboratories. Generally, all specimens should be vortexed in VTM for 2 minutes to release of the virus into the fluid; three to five sterile glass beads are included in the vial or tube with the VTM to facilitate release of the virus. Swabs should be expressed and discarded after vortexing. Samples that contain contaminating bacteria and fungi, blood, mucus, or other host substances

should be centrifuged. Hanks' balanced salt solution (HBSS) with antibiotics should be added to those specimens that likely contain bacteria and fungi. Specimens should be centrifuged at 3500 rpm (3000 X g) for 30 minutes at 2°C to 8°C and the virus containing supernatant used as the inoculum. Centrifugation removes debris and bacteria. The sediment can be used for direct detection methods. Anticoagulated blood should be separated by fractionation and the white blood cells obtained for testing. All processed specimens should be stored at –70°C after testing. Table 16-4✪ provides a general approach to specimen preparation for viral diagnosis.

Virus Isolation

Virus isolation is routinely performed for detection of the majority of viral pathogens. The method involves inoculation of a prepared specimen into a living host cell system, followed by a period of incubation, and examination for evidence of viral proliferation. A positive result indicates not only a viral infection, but also the presence of a viable virus in the host. No other diagnostic approach has the distinction of being able to determine virus viability.

Viral isolation systems include cell cultures, leukocyte cultures, tissue cultures, organ cultures, embryonated eggs (Figure 16-2 ■, page 364), and laboratory animals. The monolayer cell culture is the most frequently used system for isolation of viruses in diagnostic virology laboratories (Figure 16-3 ■, page 364). Other culture systems are primarily reserved for specialized and research laboratories. This section describes the traditional and advanced cell culture systems that are practical for use in a clinical virology laboratory.

Propagation of Cell Cultures. **Cell cultures** are metabolically active mammalian cells grown in vitro. Many different types of human and animal tissue may be cultured. Cell cultures are prepared by first treating the parent or donor tissue with proteolytic enzyme and/or a chelating agent to dissociate the cells. The dissociated cells are then suspended in a nutrient growth medium and dispensed into plastic or glass containers (tubes, flasks). The cells will settle to one side of the container, adhere to the surface, and proliferate, forming a **monolayer**— a confluent single layer of cells extending from the midpoint to the bottom of the container. Once the monolayer has formed, the growth medium should be removed and replaced with maintenance medium. The cell culture is then ready to be inoculated. Otherwise, it should be stored at 2°C to 8°C for 1 to 2 weeks and the maintenance medium changed every 3 to 4 days.

Cell cultures may be subcultured by a process known as serial transfer or **passaging.** The process involves gently detaching the monolayer from the container surface, harvesting and washing the cells, and suspending them in fresh growth medium. The cell suspension is then dispensed into new containers and incubated at 35°C. The newly planted cells adhere to the surface of the container and proliferate, forming a secondary cell culture. A **cell line** is established when the cell culture can be serially transferred numerous times without losing susceptibility to virus infection.

✪ TABLE 16-4

Specimen Initial Processing/Preparation

Specimen Type	Preparation
Swabs, scrapings, vesicle aspirate in VTM	Vortex for 30 to 60 seconds.
	Discard swab (optional).
Tissue samples in VTM	Prepare a 10% to 20% (wt/vol) homogenate; add 1 gram to 4 to 9 mL of VTM or HBSS with antimicrobial agents, and grind until well homogenized.
	Alternative: Add a 5 mm piece of tissue to 3 to 4 mL VTM or HBSS with antimicrobial agents and grind until well homogenized.
	Centrifuge the homogenate for 10 min at 4°C or allow homogenate to settle by gravity for 10 to 15 minutes.
	Transfer supernatant to a sterile tube for analysis.
Respiratory fluids (NPA, TA, BAL) in VTM	Remove aliquot for antigen detection or slide preparation.
	Add antimicrobial agents if not in VTM; allow BAL to stand 15 minutes.
	Vortex for 15 to 30 seconds, 60 seconds for NPA with excessive mucus; if specimen remains viscous, centrifuge for 5 minutes, discard mucous layer and vortex.
Stool	Mix 1 gram stool with 4 to 9 mL of VTM or HBSS with antibiotics in a 15 mL sterile, screw-cap, conical centrifuge tube containing 3 to 5 sterile glass beads.
	Vortex for 60 seconds.
	Centrifuge for 20 minutes.
	Transfer supernatant to a sterile tube.
	Optional: decontaminate by filtration.
Urine not in VTM	Mix thoroughly by pipetting up and down.
	Retain 3 to 4 mL and add antimicrobial agents, achieving concentration as if in VTM.
	Optional: Add a few drops of sodium bicarbonate to neutralize pH.
CSF and other sterile body fluids not in VTM	Optional: add antimicrobial agents and let stand 15 minutes.
Blood (anticoagulated)	Mix by gently inverting.
Preparation of leukocytes by the ammonium chloride method	Transfer 3 to 5 mL to a conical centrifuge tube containing 10 mL of ammonium chloride solution.
	Rock for 5 minutes at room temperature.
	Centrifuge for at 160 X g for10 minutes at 4°C.
	Remove and discard supernatant fluid.
	Suspend cell pellet in 1 mL of ammonium chloride solution and add 9 mL more of ammonium chloride to the tube; mix thoroughly.
	Centrifuge for at 160 X g for10 minutes at 4°C.
	Remove and discard supernatant fluid.
	Suspend the WBC pellet in approximately 1.2 mL of phosphate-buffered saline.

NPA = nasopharyngeal aspirate; TA = tracheal aspirate; BAL = bronchoalveolar lavage fluid; HBSS = Hanks' balanced salt solution.

REAL WORLD TIP

On subculture, scraping the cells from the cell line container surface may damage them and cause the loss of the virus. Trypsin and a small sterile rubber spatula can be used to release the monolayer and then fluorescent antibody stain can be used on the cells, or they can be passed to another monolayer.

Types of Cell Lines. Three basic types of cell lines are primary cell cultures, diploid cell lines and heteroploid cell lines (Tables 16-5✪ and 16-6✪).

Primary cell cultures are composed of cells obtained directly from mammalian tissue. The cells are mainly epithelial and have the same diploid chromosome as the parent tissue. The cells may possibly be subcultured one or two times, but with subsequent passages, the cells will alter and lose susceptibility to virus infection. Primary cell cultures will isolate most viruses, but they have a short life span and are the most expensive type of monolayer cells.

Diploid cell lines (low passage or semicontinuous) are cultures of connective tissue cells usually derived from

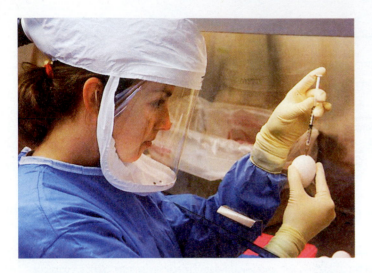

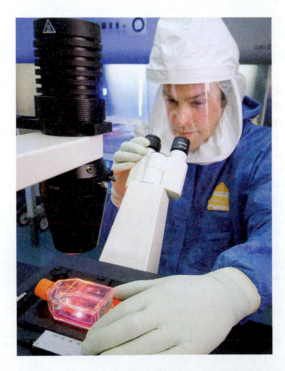

mammalian fetal fibroblastic tissue. The cells have the same diploid chromosomes as the parent tissue and may be serially transferred 20 to 50 times before the chromosomes alter and susceptibility to virus infection is lost. Diploid cell lines are the only type of cell cultures that will recover cytomegalovirus (CMV).

Heteroploid cell lines (continuous, established, immortalized) are derived from tumor, malignant, cancer, or transformed cells (Figure 16-4 ■). The cells have a heteroploid chromosome count, grow rapidly, and remain receptive to virus infection though an indefinite number of passages. Only HSV, RSV, enteroviruses, and adenovirus viruses can be isolated in heteroploid cell lines. Other viruses cannot infect or replicate in heteroploid cells lines.

Cell types differ in their susceptibility to various viruses. Because no single cell type is susceptible to all viruses, several types of cell cultures should be inoculated for virus isolation. The cell types are selected based primarily on the specimen type, virus suspected, and clinical diagnosis.

Table 16-6 summarizes characteristics of the cell lines, commonly used cell lines and the viruses that are isolated using them.

Cell Culture Media.   Cultured cells require moisture and a supply of nutrients to grow and survive. Two basic types of cell culture media, growth and maintenance media, are used to overlay the monolayer and provide moisture and a supply of nutrients to the cell culture. Both media are prepared with Eagle's minimal essential medium (EMEM) in either Hanks' or Earle's balanced salt solution with a bicarbonate buffering system. Antibiotics are added to inhibit growth of contaminating bacteria and fungi. The medium also contains a buffering system and pH indicator to control and monitor the pH in the cell culture. Serum is added to the medium to preserve cell viability. Growth medium is enriched with 10% serum and is designed to support rapid cell growth during **propagation** of the monolayer. Maintenance medium contains less than 2% serum and keeps the cells of the monolayer in a steady state of metabolism. It should be used during storage of the monolayer prior to inoculation and during incubation following inoculation with clinical specimens.

Cell Culture Systems

Several cell culture systems are available for isolation of virus. The time-honored monolayer cell culture requires technical expertise and days to weeks before results are obtained. Innovations in cell culture formats and technologies have been developed to enhance isolation of viruses from clinical specimens. The shell vial assay and microwell (cluster) plates are easier to perform and detect viruses in less time than the traditional monolayer cell cultures. Most laboratories routinely perform both the traditional monolayer cell culture and the shell vial assay for virus isolation. Cryopreserved monolayer cells, co-cultivated cell cultures, and transgenic cell cultures also improve virus detection and identification. This section

✪ TABLE 16-5

Characteristics of Cell Cultures

Cell Lines	Synonyms	Morphology Chromosome	Passages	Common Cell Lines
Primary	None	Epithelial Normal diploid	0–2	Human neonatal kidney (HNK) Rhesus monkey kidney (RMK) Rabbit kidney (RK)
Diploid	Semicontinuous Low passage Finite	Fibroblastic Normal diploid	20–50	Human embryonic lung (MRC-5 and WI-38) Human newborn foreskin (HNF)
Continuous	Established Heteroploid Transformed Immortalized	Epithelial Abnormal Heteroploid	Infinite	Human cervical carcinoma (HeLa) Human epidermoid laryngeal carcinoma (HEp-2) Human epidermoid lung carcinoma (A-549) African green monkey kidney (Vero) Baby hamster kidney (BHK-21) Mouse karyotype (McCoy) Mink lung (ML)

✪ TABLE 16-6

Cell Lines Commonly Used for Virus Isolation

Commonly Used Cell Lines		Viruses Commonly Isolated
Primary	AGMK—African green monkey kidney	HSV types 1 and 2, enteroviruses, mumps virus, RSV, rubella virus, VZV
	HNK—Human neonatal kidney	Adenovirus, BK virus, HSV—types 1 and 2, measles, mumps virus, parainfluenza virus 1–4, poxvirus
	PMK—Primary (Rhesus) monkey kidney RMK—(Primary) Rhesus monkey kidney	Enteroviruses, influenza virus types A, B and C, measles, mumps, parainfluenza types 1–4, poxvirus, rhinoviruses
	RK—Rabbit kidney	HSV types 1 and 2
	PBMC—Peripheral blood mononuclear cells CBMC—Cord blood mononuclear cells	HIV-1, HIV-2, HTLV-1, HTLV- 2,
Diploid	HLF—Human lung fibroblast MRC-5—Human embryonic lung WI-38—Human embryonic lung	BK virus, CMV, enteroviruses, HSV types 1 and 2, poxvirus, rhinoviruses, VZV
	HNF (HF)—Human newborn (fetal) foreskin	BK virus, CMV
Continuous	A-549—Human epidermoid lung carcinoma	Adenovirus, HSV types 1 and 2, influenza virus types A, B, and C, parainfluenza virus types 1–4, measles (shell vial), RSV, VZV
	BGMK—Buffalo green monkey kidney	Enteroviruses
	BHK-21—Baby hamster kidney	HSV types 1 and 2
	Graham-293—Adenovirus-transformed human kidney	Adenovirus types 40–41
	H292—Human pulmonary epidermoid carcinoma	Enteroviruses
	HeLa—Human cervical carcinoma	Adenovirus
	HEp-2—Human epidermoid laryngeal carcinoma	RSV
	ML—Mink lung	CMV (shell vial), HSV types 1 and 2

CMV = cytomegalovirus; HIV = human immunodeficiency virus; HTLV = human T-cell leukemia virus; HSV = herpes simplex virus; RSV = respiratory syncytial virus; VZV = varicella-zoster virus.

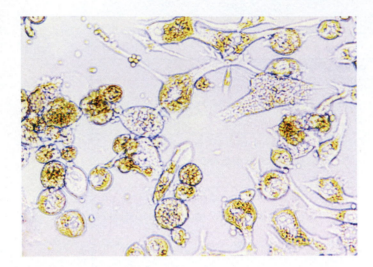

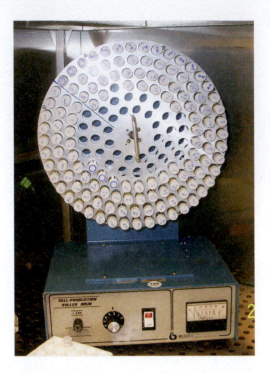

■ **FIGURE 16-4** HeLa cell monolayer infected with *Trypanosoma cruzi*, a blood and tissue protozoan parasite. HeLa cells are human cervical cancer cells that are an immortal or continuous cell line and can be used to propagate viruses and other intracellular parasites.
Courtesy Public Health Image Library (PHIL), Centers for Disease Control and Prevention (CDC), Atlanta, GA.

■ **FIGURE 16-5** Roller drum used to hold and rotate cell culture tubes.

describes the traditional and newer advancements in cell culture techniques.

Monolayer Cell Culture.

The tube monolayer cell culture is the most common format for viral isolation. The cells are cultured in a 16×125 mm glass or plastic round-bottomed, screw-capped tube with the monolayer growing on one wall of the bottom half of the tube. The cell culture is first drained of growth medium, inoculated with 0.2 to 0.3 mL processed specimen and incubated immediately at 35°C in an aerobic environment. Cell culture tubes should be positioned with the monolayer on the bottom side of the tube. A stationary rack or roller drum should be used to hold the culture tubes. The roller drum (Figure 16-5 ■) rotates and improves viral infection of monolayer, ensures constant exchange of media, and possibly improves cell metabolism. Cultures are incubated initially for 12 to 24 hours to allow the virus to settle and adsorb to the monolayer. At the end of this period, the culture medium is removed and replaced with an equal volume of fresh maintenance medium. This process is called **"refeeding"** and should be conducted once or twice each week during the incubation period. The incubation period for recovery of most viruses is 5 to 28 days. Cultures are monitored daily, or at least three times per week, for quality and microscopic changes in the monolayer. The system is observed macroscopically for visible changes in the color of the medium and microscopically at 10× magnification for evidence of viral proliferation. Table 16-7✪ summarizes processing of traditional tube cell cultures and shell vial cultures.

> **@ REAL WORLD TIP**
>
> *Mycoplasma* spp. are cell wall deficient organisms that are the scourge of cell cultures. They contaminate the cell lines and cause changes in the cells unrelated to the presence of a virus. These organisms can also affect the cells' growth and susceptibility to viruses. Commercial vendors who test and verify that their cells are free from *Mycoplasma* spp. are the best source of cell lines. Cell lines obtained from noncommercial sources should not be used until tested for the presence of the contaminant.

Viral isolates in cell cultures are most commonly detected by the presence of **cytopathogenic effect (CPE)** or hemadsorption. CPE is defined as degenerative changes in the normally smooth, flat cells of the monolayer because of proliferation of the infecting virus. To detect CPE, the monolayer should be exam-

---

 ### Checkpoint! 16–4
(Chapter Objective 6)

Isolation of viruses in the tube monolayer cell cultures involves:

  A. *inoculation of the cell culture with 1 mL of prepared specimen.*
  B. *refeeding the cell culture two times each week during incubation.*
  C. *monitoring the cell culture weekly for macro- and microscopic evidence of viral proliferation.*
  D. *incubating the cell cultures at 25°C in an anaerobic environment.*

✪ TABLE 16-7

Virus Isolation: Tube Cell Culture and Shell Vial

Tube Cell Culture	Shell Vial
Select two tubes/vials of each cell culture type; one of each type can be used as long as it has overlapping sensitivities with other cell cultures.	
Screen monolayer for confluency (near 100% monolayer), deterioration, and contamination.	Screen monolayer for confluency (slightly subconfluent preferred), deterioration, and contamination.
Decant or aspirate and discard the medium from each monolayer.	
Rinse monolayer with HBSS or phosphate buffered saline (PBS) for influenza and parainfluenza virus.	
Decant 0.2 to 0.3 mL of prepared specimen to each monolayer in the following sequence: fibroblast, primary nonsimian, transformed, primary simian (prevents cross contamination).	
Incubate in a slanted position, with the inoculum overlaying the monolayer, for 45 to 90 minutes at 35°C.	Centrifuge at 700 X *g* for 45 minutes at 22°C to 35°C.
Remove and discard inoculum.	
Refeed monolayer with 1 to 2 mL of culture medium warmed to room temperature, in the order used for inoculation.	
Incubate at 35°C in a stationary horizontal position. Medium should overlay the monolayers and not extend into the neck or caps. Tubes may also be incubated in a roller drum rotating at 12 to 15 rotations per hour.	Incubate at 35°C in an upright position.
Save specimens at 4°C for 1 day or –70°C for longer; snap freezing in an ice acetone slurry is preferred, particularly for the enveloped viruses.	
Read microscopically at 10× magnification for CPE or hemadsorption.	Read for detection of viral antigens or nucleic acid.
Results in 5 to 28 days.	Results in 24 to 48 hours.

ined through the wall of the container using an inverted microscope at 10× magnification. CPE is seen as cell rounding, swelling, shrinking, formation of clusters of cells; syncytia (giant multinucleated cells following fusion of multiple cells), cytoplasmic vacuolation, cellular granulation, nuclear or cytoplasmic inclusion formation, or loss of adherence of the monolayer. Preliminary grouping of viruses may be made based on the cell line(s) infected and the characteristic morphology of the CPE.

In some instances CPE may not be recognized in fluid cultures but may be recognized as plaque formation when the virus is cultured under a thin layer of agar instead of maintenance medium. During incubation, the agar will limit the virus spread to adjacent cells, localizing areas of cellular destruction (Figure 16-6 ■). An indicator incorporated in the medium will stain uninfected cells, but cells infected with virus will not stain and will appear as clear areas, or plaques, within the monolayer.

Some viruses infect cells without producing CPE and must be detected by other means. Hemadsorption, which refers to the specific attachment of red blood cells to virus infected cells, is the second-most-common method of detecting viral proliferation in cell cultures. Infection of the cell cultures by influenza viruses and parainfluenza viruses will result in alteration of the infected cell surface, and red blood cells will specifically attach to the virus-infected cells of the monolayer. In this method, 0.1 to 0.2 mL of a 1% suspension of guinea pig red blood cells is added to the monolayer and allowed to incubate at 2°C to 8°C for 60 minutes. The monolayer is then viewed for hemadsorption. Red blood cells adhered to the monolayer indicates viral infection. This test should be performed on cultures of respiratory and CSF specimens in particular.

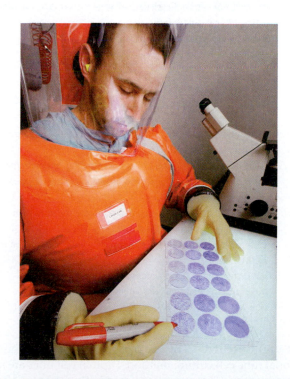

■ **FIGURE 16-6** A microbiologist in the process of counting viral plaques within fixed monolayers of cells.
Courtesy Public Health Image Library (PHIL), Centers for Disease Control and Prevention (CDC), Atlanta, GA.

REAL WORLD TIP

Viral identification based on CPE or hemadsorption is only considered presumptive. Further testing is required for definitive identification.

Viral neutralization, interference challenge, and other methods for detection of viral isolates are used in reference, research, and specialized laboratories.

Presumptive identification of the virus may be determined based on cell types that support viral replication, time to detection, and morphology of CPE. Confirmation of identification is most commonly accomplished by immunofluorescence and nucleic acid detection. Other less commonly used methods for confirmation of viral isolates include neutralization by inhibition of CPE or plaque formation using known type-specific antisera; hemagglutination inhibition, hemadsorption inhibition, indirect IFA, ELISA, immunoblotting, and complement fixation. All of these may be used to identify type-specific viruses within a group except the complement fixation test, which can only identify virus groups but not types.

REAL WORLD TIP

Some viruses, such as Epstein-Barr virus, hepatitis virus, norovirus, papillomavirus, parvovirus, and rotavirus, are not detected using cell line isolation. Nucleic acid, antigen, or antibody detection are most often used to demonstrate their presence.

Checkpoint! 16–5 (Chapter Objective 7)

Which of the following statements regarding detection and confirmation of viral isolates in cell cultures is incorrect?

    A. *CPE in cell cultures appears as cell rounding, syncytia formation, nuclear, or cytoplasmic inclusions, other degenerative changes.*

    B. *Production of CPE and hemadsorption are the most common means of detecting viral isolates in cell cultures.*

    C. *Hemadsorption is seen as red areas of cellular destruction in the monolayer.*

    D. *Confirmation of identification of viral isolates in cell cultures is most commonly accomplished by immunofluorescence or nucleic acid detection.*

Shell Vial Culture.   This is a rapid modification of the conventional tube cell culture method. Diploid cell lines are most commonly used. The monolayer grows attached to a 12 mm round coverslip contained in a 1 dram glass or plastic vial. The prepared specimen is inoculated into the shell vial, and the system is centrifuged at low speed for 1 hour to enhance infec-

tion of the monolayer and incubated at 35°C for 24 to 48 hours. Detection does not rely on CPE but rather detection of viral antigens by immunostaining with FITC-labeled monoclonal antibodies or horseradish peroxidase (HRP) or detection of nucleic acid with probes. The shell vial assay was originally developed for *Chlamydia trachomatis* and adapted for CMV. Isolation of CMV in the standard tube cell culture typically takes 10 to 30 days. The shell vial decreases detection time to 16 to 48 hours. The system has been adapted for HSV, influenza, and a variety of other viruses.

Urine, blood, respiratory, and cerebrospinal fluid specimens are appropriate for this method.

Microwell (Cluster) Plate.   This cell culture format, similar to the shell vial assay, is a centrifuge enhanced, pre-CPE detection method. Cell cultures are prepared in plastic, flat-bottomed, multiwell panels with the monolayer growing attached to the bottom of the microwells. Following inoculation of the individual microwells with the prepared specimens, the plate is covered and centrifuged at low speed for 1 hour, then incubated at 35°C for 24 to 48 hours. Individual microwells can be stained with monoclonal immunofluorescent stain and read microscopically for evidence of specific staining.

Checkpoint! 16–6 (Chapter Objective 8)

All the following apply to both the shell vial assay and microwell (cluster) plates except:

    A. *cultures are centrifuged after inoculation to enhance infection of the monolayer cells.*

    B. *viral isolates are detected by observing for production of CPE or hemadsorption.*

    C. *viral isolates may be detected within 48 hours of incubation.*

    D. *viruses may be identified based on detection of viral antigen by immunostaining.*

Cryopreserved Monolayer Cells.   Cryopreservation of cell lines aims to address the issue of availability of cell cultures in the laboratory. Cells are preserved by slow freezing and stored at subzero temperatures. All biological activity will effectively cease at temperatures below −130°C, yet cells remain stable and retain the same level of sensitivity.

Cells to be cryopreserved should be in the exponential (log) phase of growth. The cells are harvested and suspended in growth medium with 10% to 20% serum, no antibiotics, and 10% dimethyl sulfoxide (DMSO) or glycerol as a cryoprotectant to prevent cellular damage during freezing. Cells should be cooled slowly at a rate of 1°C per minute to prevent ice crystals and other damaging effects of freezing. When cells reach a temperature of −70°C, they should be transferred immediately to liquid nitrogen, where they can be stored indefinitely. Alternatively, cells may be stored for 4 months at −70°C.

Cryopreserved cells may be revived by quick thawing. As soon as they are removed from the liquid nitrogen or −70°C freezer, the cells should be gently swirled in a 37°C water bath until thawing is completed. The cryoprotectant DMSO or glycerol should be removed from the cells by washing or diluting, respectively. Cells should be allowed to incubate overnight before being dispensed into cell culture tubes or vials. Cryopreserved cells may also be purchased as ready-to-use monolayers grown in shell vials.

Co-Cultured Cells. These are two or more different cell types grown together as a single monolayer, to facilitate isolation of a wider range of viruses in a single system. Routinely culturing for every common agent of a viral syndrome may not be practical if too many individual cell lines are required. Co-cultivated cell lines allow isolation and differentiation of multiple viruses in the same test system, reducing the number of test systems required for virus isolation. The technique uses shell vials or cluster plates seeded with the mixed monolayer. Cell types selected for the mixture are those that will isolate the most common viral pathogens of the syndrome being diagnosed. Following inoculation, centrifugation, and incubation for 1 to 3 days, the monolayer is stained with fluorescein-labeled monoclonal antibodies and examined for presence of viral antigens.

Several co-cultivated cell lines are commercially available for rapid virus identification. A monolayer comprised of A549 mixed with MDCK or mink lung (Mv1Lu) cells is used to distinguish the major respiratory viruses. The system provides rapid isolation and identification of influenza A and B viruses, respiratory syncytial virus, adenovirus, parainfluenza virus (types 1, 2, and 3), and metapneumovirus. Distinguishing lesions of HSV and VZV is particularly important in immunocompetent and immunodeficient patients. A mixed monolayer of Hs27 (human foreskin fibroblast), A549 (human lung carcinoma), and MRC-5 (human embryonic lung) cells distinguishes among HSV-1, HSV-2, VZV, and CMV. A broad range of enteroviruses can be isolated in 1 to 3 days using engineered Buffalo green monkey kidney (BGMK) cell line co-cultured with A549 cells. Isolation of viruses in co-cultured cells is a rapid and sensitive method for viral diagnosis and is an excellent approach when reliable and rapid results are important.

Transgenic (Transformed) Cell Line. Through genetic engineering, a cell line can be stably altered by the introduction of foreign genetic elements. These genetically altered cells lines can then be used as sensitive cell culture systems for detecting a specific virus or virus family. Transgenic cells that facilitate virus detection are designed and engineered to detect a virus based on a virus-specific event. The basic strategy is to stably introduce genetic elements (derived from viruses, bacteria, or cellular sources) into a cell so that when the cell is infected by only a particular virus, a virus-specific event is initiated, and an easily assessable enzyme is produced.

The prototype for this emerging technology is the enzyme-linked virus inducible system (ELVIS). The system is commercially available for use in the rapid isolation and identification

of HSV types 1 and 2 from lesions and body fluids using a transformed baby hamster kidney cell line (BHKICP6LacZ). The transgenic BHK cells have been modified to include an HSV promoter (HSV-1*UL39*) and an *E. coli* LacZ reporter gene. When either HSV-1 or HSV-2 infects the cells, the promoter triggers the reporter gene, and the cell generates the enzyme β-galactosidase. The enzyme can be detected in as few as 16 hours by staining the monolayer with a chromogenic β-galactosidase substrate. HSV-infected cells stain intensely blue, whereas uninfected cells fail to stain. HSV infection of cells also results in the production of type-specific proteins. A positive culture can be typed using fluorescein-labeled monoclonal antibodies (MAbs) specific for HSV-1 and HSV-2. The specific type is detected microscopically by its fluorescence.

The original ELVIS system has been modified to allow both identification and typing of HSV types 1 and 2. The new system is the ELVIS HSV ID/Typing Test System. The staining system includes chromogenic β-galactosidase substrate, type-2 specific fluorescein labeled MAbs, and type-1 specific nonlabeled MAbs. After 1 hour of incubation, the monolayer is examined for the presence of blue cells using the light microscope. If blue cells are observed, HSV infection is indicated, and the monolayer should then be examined using fluorescent microscopy. If apple green fluorescent cells are seen, the HSV is type-2; if no fluorescence is seen, the HSV is type-1. The reaction can be confirmed using fluorescein-labeled goat antimouse antibodies, which will react with the type-1 specific monoclonal antibodies in the HSV-1 infected cells.

Checkpoint! 16–7 (Chapter Objective 9)

You are inoculating a cell culture monolayer that is comprised of two different cells lines. You are inoculating:

   A. *co-cultured cells.*
   B. *transformed cells.*
   C. *cryopreserved cells.*
   D. *transgenic cells.*

Direct Detection of Viruses

Assays for detection of virus particles, viral inclusions, viral antigens, and viral nucleic acid in clinical specimens are particularly useful for identification of viruses that do not readily grow in cell cultures. These methods are regarded as rapid methods because results are generally obtained within a few hours or the next day. They are generally less expensive and require less time and technical skill than isolation methods. The specificity is generally high, but sensitivity may be low; therefore these procedures are used in conjunction with other methods for reliable diagnosis.

Electron Microscopy (EM). The small size of viruses is beyond the resolving power of the light microscope; thus, electron microscopy is used for studying virus morphology. The major use of EM is identification of diarrhea-associated viruses, such as rotavirus, noroviruses, and caliciviruses because they are difficult or impossible to detect by other diagnostic methods. EM is also very useful in distinguishing herpes simplex virus from pox virus in lesions. Specimens are most commonly examined by a negative stain technique. Viruses appear as light particles against a dark background and can be differentiated based on size and shape.

A specimen must contain at least 10^5 to 10^6 virus particles per milliliter for viruses to be readily detected by EM, otherwise false-negative results may be obtained. Immune electron microscopy (IEM) facilitates detection of viruses in low concentrations, thereby greatly enhancing the sensitivity and specificity of EM. In this method, virus specific antibody is used to aggregate virus particles, making the viruses in the specimen easier to detect.

Although direct examination of specimens by EM is a rapid and specific method of diagnosis, it is not commonly available in clinical virology laboratories because the high cost, time consumption, and requirement for technical expertise make the procedure impractical. Figure 16-7 ■ is an electron micrograph of virus particles (typically rotaviruses or noroviruses) detected in a fecal specimen.

Cytohistopathology.   Smears of infected host tissue stained most commonly with Giemsa, hematoxylin, or other cytological stains are examined by light microscopy for presence of viral inclusions and/or morphological changes in the infected host cells. Inclusions are replicating virus particles in the cell nucleus or cytoplasm and may be characteristic of a virus group. Although detection of these characteristic inclusions and morphologic changes is not sensitive or specific, such findings can

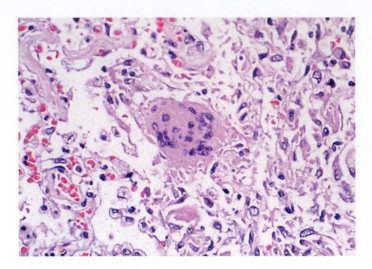

■ **FIGURE 16-8** A photomicrograph showing the histopathology associated with the SARS virus (a coronavirus). Note the characteristic CPE consisting of a multinucleated giant cell with no conspicuous viral inclusions.
Courtesy of Public Health Image Library (PHIL), Centers for Disease Control and Prevention (CDC), Atlanta, GA.

provide information useful for early presumptive identification. For example, RNA viruses typically induce intracytoplasmic inclusions, and DNA viruses are suggested by intranuclear inclusions. Intranuclear inclusions with an "owl's eye" appearance are caused by CMV. Multinucleated giant cells or syncytial cells suggest infection by HSV, VZV, RSV, and other viruses (Figure 16-8 ■). Go to ∞ Chapter 31 to see more electron micrograph and histopathology photos of intracellular pathogens.

Immunodiagnosis.   Immunologic assays performed directly on clinical material for presence of viral antigens are some of the most frequently performed methods in diagnostic virology. The various techniques employ specific monoclonal or polyclonal antiviral antibodies to detect viral antigen in specimens by direct and indirect immunostaining with fluorescent or enzyme-labeled antibodies, enzyme immunoassays, and particle agglutination.

Direct immunofluorescent (DFA) assays are rapid, highly specific methods. They are used most commonly for detecting viruses in respiratory specimens for RSV (Figure 16-9 ■), influenza viruses, parainfluenza virus, adenovirus, lesion samples for HSV (Figure 16-10 ■) and VZV, and blood for CMV. The direct method is more sensitive than the indirect method and is therefore most commonly used. In the direct method, viral antigen is reacted with fluorescein-labeled antiserum. The indirect method involves complexing the virus with unlabeled antiserum and adding fluorescein-labeled antiglobulin. The presence of fluorescent intracellular viral inclusions or syncytia is indicative of virus proliferation.

The CMV antigenemia test is a rapid and sensitive immunofluorescent assay that will detect CMV infection prior to devel-

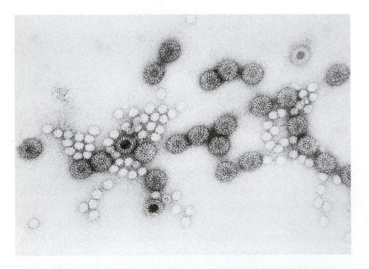

■ **FIGURE 16-7** This is an electron micrograph depicting rotavirus virions and a number of unknown 29 nanometer virus particles. "Rota" is Latin for "wheel," and the typical morphology of rotaviruses is that of a wheel with a wide hub and short spokes because of the double-shelled capsid.
Courtesy Public Health Image Library (PHIL), Centers for Disease Control and Prevention (CDC), Atlanta, GA.

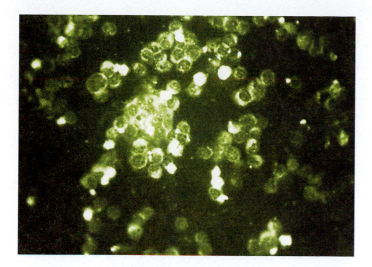

■ **FIGURE 16-9** This is a photomicrograph illustrating the detection of respiratory syncytial virus (RSV) using an immunofluorescent technique.
Courtesy Public Health Image Library (PHIL), Centers for Disease Control and Prevention (CDC), Atlanta, GA.

opment of clinical disease. The assay is semiquantitative and can also be used to estimate the likelihood of disease progression and to monitor the response to therapy. The method involves separation of peripheral blood leukocytes from the patient's blood. The leukocytes are then quantitated, smeared, and stained with fluorescein-labeled monoclonal antibodies against pp65 early matrix proteins of CMV. The stained smears are examined microscopically, and the number of fluorescent cells is determined.

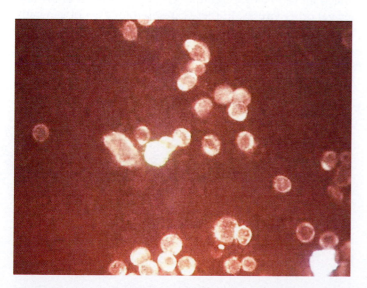

■ **FIGURE 16-10** A photomicrograph illustrating the detection of a herpes smear cell culture using an immunofluorescent technique. The use of a fluorescent-labeled monoclonal antibody allows HSV type 1 to be distinguished from HSV type 2.
Courtesy of Public Health Image Library (PHIL), Centers for Disease Control and Prevention (CDC), Atlanta, GA.

Immunofluorescent methods can be labor intensive and time consuming. They require technical expertise to grade the intensity and describe viral inclusion morphology and may present a challenge to the inexperienced laboratorian.

Enzyme immunoassays use specific antiviral antibodies labeled with enzymes to detect viral antigens present in the specimen. A color change results from the enzyme reacting with its substrate and indicates presence of viral antigen.

Enzyme immunoassay methods are especially useful for diagnosing hepatitis B virus, rotavirus, measles, rubella, and noroviruses. Immunoperoxidase staining is an enzyme immunoassay similar to immunofluorescent staining. The method uses antibodies labeled with a horseradish peroxidase. Direct and indirect methods may be performed and are similar to those used for immunofluorescent staining with an additional step—the addition of a substrate solution. The preparation is read for alterations in color using light microscopy. Viruses that may be detected by this method include herpes simplex virus, cytomegalovirus, and various other viruses.

Particle agglutination is the least technically demanding direct detection method. The method uses latex particles coated with antibody specific for the virus suspected. The specimen is mixed with the antibody-coated latex particles on a glass slide. Presence of agglutination indicates a positive reaction. The major clinical utility for this method is detection of rotavirus and other viral agents of diarrhea in stool specimens.

Molecular Techniques. Identification of viruses using molecular techniques relies on detection of a unique nucleic acid sequence within the genome of the virus in the specimen. Viruses may be detected in blood, CSF, urine, sputum and other types of specimens using molecular assays. The two types of methods available for direct detection of viral genomes are hybridization using nucleic acid probes, and genome amplification, particularly polymerase chain reaction (PCR). These methods are highly sensitive and specific, especially PCR, and their role in diagnostic virology is becoming increasingly important. These techniques are discussed in detail in ∞ Chapter 9 of this textbook. This section summarizes the specific application of nucleic acid probes and PCR to diagnostic virology.

Nucleic acid probes for direct detection of viruses are radioactively or chemically labeled DNA or RNA segments that are complementary to a unique nucleic acid sequence within the virus genome. In direct assays, the probe is introduced into the prepared specimen. If the virus suspected is present, the probe will hybridize with the complementary amino acid sequence in the viral genome. The hybridized nucleic acid is confirmed through detection of the radioactive or chemical label. The complete hybridization reaction is generally carried out in solution (liquid) phase because this process is more rapid and sensitive than solid phase.

Probes procedures require 10^4 to 10^5 molecules of the target viral nucleic acid for positive results, and therefore this method is not particularly sensitive. Sensitivity is generally no higher than isolation and antigen detection techniques that are simpler and less expensive to perform. Hence, nucleic acid probes are not widely used in diagnostic virology for direct detection. The one major diagnostic application of nucleic acid probes is the detection and typing of human papillomavirus (HPV) group by in situ hybridization in whole cells or tissue sections. The hybrids are detected microscopically. Immunohistochemical staining will also detect HPV, but probes are the only means of distinguishing among the more than 60 types.

Polymerase chain reaction (PCR) is the best developed and most widely used nucleic acid amplification method for detection of viruses. PCR involves enzymatic duplication of short DNA sequences to produce millions to billions of copies. The specific virus sequence is then detected by nucleic acid probes, electrophoresis, or other detection methods. PCR is an extremely sensitive and specific method with the capability of detecting nonreplicating viral genomes and as few as one virion in a clinical sample. Since the first practical application of PCR in 1985, many technical improvements have been made to enhance sensitivity and specificity. Two advancements with significant application in virology are reverse transcriptase PCR (RT-PCR) and real-time PCR (RT-PCR). (Both are designated in the literature as RT-PCR.)

The reverse transcriptase PCR (RT-PCR) method has been developed for detection of viral RNA. The viral genome in most RNA viruses is present only as RNA and does not undergo reverse transcription into a DNA intermediate during its life cycle. Because PCR targets DNA sequences only, RNA must be converted to complementary DNA (cDNA) for the PCR process. An enzyme, reverse transcriptase, is used to convert viral RNA to cDNA. Because a reverse transcription step is included, the method is referred to as reverse transcriptase PCR. Viruses that are commonly detected using reverse transcriptase PCR include HCV, influenza viruses (detection and typing), norovirus and rotavirus in feces, rubella virus, and enterovirus (Moe et al., 1994).

Traditionally, PCR is a two-step procedure involving the initial amplification reaction followed by a separate procedure for analysis of the amplified product. Real-time refers to production of results as they occur, rather than assessing results at the completion of the run. In real-time PCR, both amplification and detection of amplicons are completed in the same closed system. As amplicons are produced, fluorescent-labeled probes bind with them. The technique uses an instrument that records fluorescence at the end of each cycle. The sensitivity and specificity of real-time PCR is comparable to that of conventional PCR. Real-time has added advantages in that the contamination risk is lower, the method is simpler to perform, and results are obtained in 1 hour or less.

Serology

Serologic assays identify viruses based on the detection of viral antibodies in a patient's serum. For many years diagnosis of viral infections was based primarily on serology. Although the emphasis in diagnosis has shifted to viral isolation and antigen and nucleic acid detection methods, serology remains an important approach to diagnosis. Serodiagnosis is indicated when isolation of viruses is impractical or impossible, when virus shedding has ceased and is not present in the clinical sample at a level that can be detected, when antigen or nucleic acid detection methods are not available, and when the clinical significance of an isolate is questionable. Serologic assays can also be useful in providing early presumptive identification so that treatment can be initiated while waiting for isolation results. In addition, serology can be used to indicate current infection, congenital infection, and immune status.

The most reliable results are obtained when paired acute and convalescent sera are tested simultaneously. The acute phase serum is generally collected during the first week of illness, and the convalescent serum is collected 2 to 3 weeks after onset. Detection of a fourfold rise in antibody between paired acute and convalescent sera strongly supports a current infection. The identity of a virus is not determined, but instead some viruses may be eliminated. Detection of virus specific IgM in acute phase serum may also indicate current or recent infection; in newborns, detection of IgM indicates congenital infection. Detection of IgG indicates immunity or current or past infection; presence of IgG in the serum of newborns indicates maternal antibodies and not infection.

Serologic methods include complement fixation, neutralization, immunofluorescence, hemagglutination-inhibition, enzyme immunoassay, Western blot, recombinant immunoblot assay (RIBA), and others. There may be false-negative or false-positive results with serologic tests, and results should be interpreted with caution. Also, antibodies develop late in infections caused by respiratory viruses, measles, mumps, and several other viruses. In these cases, serology is not generally used for diagnosis.

 Checkpoint! 16–8 (Chapter Objective 11)

Viral serodiagnosis:

    A. *is only reliable when acute and convalescent paired sera are analyzed.*

    B. *measures viral antigens in clinical specimens.*

    C. *can be used to indicate current infection, congenital infection, and immune status.*

    D. *is the preferred approach for diagnosis or respiratory viruses.*

► ***CHLAMYDIACEAE* SPECIMENS**

Specimens for diagnosis of *Chlamydia trachomatis* should be collected from the genital tract, respiratory tract, and eyes. Specimens for the detection of *Chlamydophila pneumoniae* are collected from the respiratory tract (nasopharyngeal aspirates, throat swabs, and bronchoalveolar lavage [BAL] fluid). Specimens for the diagnosis of *Chlamydophila psittaci* include sputum, BAL, pleural fluid, blood, and tissue. Diagnostic approaches are similar to those for viruses and include isolation in cell culture, cytology, antigen and nucleic acid detection, and serology.

SPECIMEN COLLECTION AND TRANSPORT

Because these organisms are obligate intracellular pathogens, specimens for detection of chlamydiae must contain the columnar epithelial cells from the involved mucosa. Swabs, scraping, and small pieces of tissue, most commonly from endocervix, urethra, and conjunctiva, are the specimens most often submitted. Urine is appropriate only for nonculture detection tests.

Swabs are submitted more frequently, although scrapings are better. As with collection of viral specimens, swabs with calcium alginate or cotton tips and wooden shafts should not be used for chlamydiae. Purulent discharge is unacceptable because all cells present are dead. Before sampling the infection site, any mucus or purulent discharge on the mucosal surface should be cleared away with a swab and discarded. A fresh swab should be rotated over the mucosa for about 10 seconds to collect the specimen. Alternatively, a cytobrush can be used to gently scrape the mucosa. Specimens should be placed in chlamydial transport medium (CTM) at the time of collection. 2-SP and sucrose glutamate phosphate (SPG) are the most common CTMs.

Specimen Transport and Storage

To maintain the infectivity of chlamydiae, specimens should be kept cold and processed as soon as possible following collection. Specimens should be placed at 4°C or on wet ice or a cold pack and transported to the laboratory immediately. If transport is delayed, the specimen should be held at 2°C to 8°C. Ideally, transport should not be delayed beyond 4 hours. Specimens should be placed at 4°C on arrival in the laboratory. Those that cannot be processed within 48 hours should be frozen at –70°C.

Specimen Preparation

Specimens should be vortexed or sonicated in CTM for 2 minutes to release the infective elementary bodies (EBs) from intact host cells into the fluid. Swabs should be removed and discarded. Large pieces of tissue should be minced into smaller pieces or ground to a paste using CTM and a sterile tissue grinder.

✓ Checkpoint! 16–9 (Chapter Objective 12)

Specimens for detection of chlamydiae:
- A. *must contain columnar epithelial cells.*
- B. *should be collected using calcium alginate swabs.*
- C. *should be placed in Amies transport medium.*
- D. *should be held at 2°C to 8° C for up to 7 days if processing is delayed.*

ISOLATION OF *CHLAMYDIACEAE*

Isolation in traditional tube cell cultures is not routinely performed in most clinical laboratories. Although this diagnostic approach is 100% specific, the sensitivity is only 70% to 85%. The preferred means of isolation is by a centrifuge enhanced inoculation method. Both the shell vial and microwell plate are suitable assays. The standard cell line is McCoy cells treated with cycloheximide (Figure 16-11 ■). Cycloheximide inhibits the division of McCoy cells and improves isolation. This is because chlamydiae replicates best in cells that are not undergoing cell division. HeLa229, buffalo green monkey kidney, and a number of other cell lines have also been successful in isolating chlamydiae, but are not as frequently used.

Prior to inoculation, the cell culture medium is removed and discarded. The vortexed specimen is inoculated onto the monolayers of the shell vial or microwell plate and centrifuged at 1500 X *g* for 45 to 60 minutes at 35°C. The culture is then refed with culture medium containing cycloheximide and incubated at 35°C for 48 to 72 hours.

Following incubation, cell monolayers are stained and examined microscopically. Chlamydiae is identified by the presence of one or more intracytoplasmic inclusions. Inclusions are oval and large, often occupying >50% of the cell cytoplasm. Fluorescein-labeled antibody, Giemsa or iodine stains are used to differentiate the inclusions. Laboratories

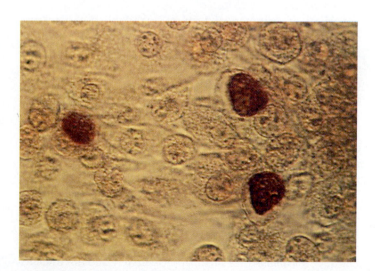

■ **FIGURE 16-11** A photomicrograph of a McCoy cell monolayer with intracytoplasmic inclusions of *Chlamydia trachomatis* stained with iodine.
Courtesy of Public Health Image Library (PHIL), Centers for Disease Control and Prevention (CDC), Atlanta, GA.

most frequently use fluorescein-labeled monoclonal antibodies to stain the monolayer. Monoclonal antibodies to identify *C. psittaci* are not commercially available. A fluorescence microscope is used to examine the entire monolayer at 200×; 400× should be used to confirm inclusions. Inclusions stain bright apple green (Forbes, Sahm, & Weissfeld, 2007).

Iodine and Giemsa stains are less sensitive than the fluorescent stain. Iodine stains inclusions light to dark brown. The glycogen in inclusion of *Chlamydia trachomatis* stains reddish brown, but the glycogen inclusions of *C. pneumoniae* and *C. psittaci* does not stain. Giemsa stains chlamydiae inclusions purple (Murray, Baron, Pfaller, Tenover, & Yolken, 1999).

DIRECT DETECTION

Direct testing of clinical samples provides rapid, presumptive identification of chlamydiae. Positive findings should be confirmed using culture or another direct detection method.

Cytological Examination

Demonstration of inclusions in stained direct smears of epithelial specimens can provide an early indication of infection. Inclusions can be detected with immunofluorescence, Giemsa, or iodine staining methods. Most laboratories routinely use immunofluorescence staining. Apple green inclusions in urethral, cervical, conjunctival, and other epithelial specimens suggest chlamydiae. The Giemsa stain is particularly useful for rapid diagnosis of acute inclusion conjunctivitis in newborns. The presence of purple intracytoplasmic inclusions in conjunctival scraping stained with Giemsa establishes identification with >90% sensitivity.

Antigen Detection

A variety of commercial tests are available for detecting chlamydiae antigens in urogenital and respiratory specimens. Methods employ monoclonal antibodies that detect group specific lipopolysaccharide (LPS), or the species specific major outer membrane protein (MOMP) of *Chlamydia trachomatis*. Immunofluorescence (IF) and enzyme immunoassay (EIA) methods are most frequently performed. Latex agglutination and other antigen detection methods are available but not frequently used. Specimens for testing by these commercial procedures should be collected and processed according to instructions by the manufacturers.

Immunofluorescence Testing (IF)

Fluorescein-conjugated monoclonal antibodies detect elementary bodies (EBs) as opposed to inclusions. The infectious EBs of *C. trachomatis* are small, approximately 300 nm in diameter, bright apple green, extracellular structures. The edges of EBs are smooth when stained with anti-MOMP antibodies. The replicating reticulate bodies will also stain and must not be mistaken for EBs. Reticulate bodies are larger than EBs and may have a peripheral halo.

Enzyme Immunoassay (EIA)

This method detects chlamydiae LPS in patients' specimens. Specimens are first treated to solubilize antigens. The antigens are then captured on beads or in the bottom of microwells and reacted with an enzyme-labeled detector system. Development of color change indicates the presence of chlamydial antigen. Because other gram-negative bacteria produce LPS, false-positive results can occur and should be confirmed by immunofluorescence testing.

Molecular Detection

Nonamplified and amplified nucleic acid tests are used for the detection of *Chlamydia trachomatis* in urogenital specimens only. The tests are highly sensitive and specific, particularly the amplified nucleic acid tests.

DNA probes are chemiluminescence-based assays that use an acridinium ester-labeled ssDNA probe that is complementary to rRNA of *C. trachomatis*. The labeled DNA-RNA hybrid emits light that is measured with a luminometer.

Nucleic acid amplification tests are the most sensitive tests for detection of *C. trachomatis* (Stanley, 2002). The PCR method is most commonly used and can detect as few as 10 elementary bodies in a specimen.

SEROLOGY

Serologic tests are most useful for diagnosing respiratory infections caused by *C. pneumoniae* and *C. psittaci* and invasive, systemic infections caused by *Chlamydia trachomatis,* such as neonatal pneumonia and lymphogranuloma venereum. Serology, however, has little value when diagnosing acute infections such as genital and ocular infections. Antibody detection methods include complement fixation (CF), microimmunofluorescence (Micro-IF), immunofluorescence (IF), and enzyme-linked immunosorbent assay (ELISA). Due to the hazards associated with isolation of *C. psittaci*, serological tests are preferred and available through CDC.

The complement fixation test is the most widely used serologic methods for diagnosis of chlamydiae infections. A single antibody titer greater than 1:64 in symptomatic patients, or a fourfold rise in antibody titer to lymphogranuloma venereum (LGV) antigens indicates current LGV infection. Because many patients seek medical attention following the acute stage, demonstration of a fourfold rise in titer between acute and convalescent paired sera is improbable. Complement fixation is not useful for diagnosing eye and genital infections or neonatal pneumonitis.

The Micro-IF test is more sensitive than the complement fixation test. LGV may be diagnosed if symptomatic patients have a single IgM antibody titer of >1:32 or a single IgG antibody titer >1:2000. Eye and genital infections may be diagnosed by demonstrating a fourfold rise in antibody titers between paired acute and convalescent sera. Seroconversion may be difficult to demonstrate in individuals who have chronic or repeat chlamydial infections. The most significant application of the Micro-IF test is confirmation of neonatal pneumonitis, and it is the method of choice in these situations.

► *RICKETTSIA* AND *COXIELLA* SPECIMENS

Biosafety level 3 practices should be used while handling specimens and during testing for rickettsiae (*Rickettsia* and *Orientia*) and *Coxiella*. Because of the biological containment specifications, most clinical laboratories only offer serologic testing. Isolation and direct detection methods are generally performed only by reference and specialized laboratories. The clinical laboratory may be required to provide guidance for specimen collection, storage, and transport to the testing laboratory and must therefore be knowledgeable of specimen requirements.

SPECIMEN COLLECTION, TRANSPORT, AND STORAGE

Specimens for diagnosing rickettsial and *Coxiella* infections should be collected as early as possible following onset of symptoms. Selection of specimens is usually limited to blood, petechial rash or eschar (lesion) biopsy, and visceral tissue. Specimens collected for isolation or direct detection should be snap frozen and shipped on dry ice to the testing laboratory. If there is a delay in transport, specimens may be stored at −70°C until they are transported. Serologic assays require paired acute and convalescent serum samples for reliable diagnosis. Table 16-8✪ summarizes general collection and handling of specimens for diagnosis of rickettsiae and *Coxiella*.

Isolation

Isolation of rickettsiae and *Coxiella* is performed only rarely in reference or specialized laboratories. The method involves inoculation of the buffy coat or plasma from heparinized blood into shell vials with Vero, MRC5, or HELF (human embryonic lung fibroblasts) cell lines and antibiotic-free medium enriched with potassium, serum albumin, and sucrose. Following 48 hours of incubation, the culture can be confirmed by indirect immunofluorescence with specific monoclonal antibody demonstrating the presence of four or more organisms. Molecular methods can also be used to detect rickettsiae and *Coxiella* in cell cultures and shell vial cultures. Even though the sensitivity of isolation methods is poor, the method should always be performed when the only specimen available is autopsy tissue.

Direct Detection

Immunohistologic and molecular detection of rickettsiae and *Coxiella* in clinical material are sensitive, specific, and rapid methods of diagnosis. Biopsy specimens of skin rash, eschar, or other tissue are examined by direct immunofluorescence staining or immunoperoxidase staining with labeled species and group specific polyclonal and monoclonal antibodies. The immunoperoxidase stain is only 70% sensitive and is only used for diagnosing Rocky Mountain spotted fever and rickettsialpox.

PCR is the most frequently performed molecular method and is more specific than the antibody-based immunohistologic detection methods. Fresh skin biopsy samples are preferred for DNA detection. Blood, the buffy coat, plasma, and occasionally paraffin-embedded tissue may also be examined for DNA of rickettsiae and *Coxiella*.

Serologic Assays

Most clinical laboratories only offer serologic testing for diagnosis of infections caused by rickettsiae and *Coxiella*. Indirect immunofluorescence is the most sensitive and specific method, and the "gold standard" for serodiagnosis. The microimmunofluorescence test (micro-IF), a modification of the immunofluorescence method, and the latex agglutination are also currently used for diagnosis. Demonstration of a rising antibody titer is important for confirming active infection, and both the conventional immunofluorescence method and

✪ TABLE 16-8

Collection, Transport, and Analysis of Rickettsiae and *Coxiella* Specimens

Specimen	Collection	Transport/Storage	Diagnostic Methods
Blood	10–12 mL heparinized (rickettsiae) EDTA or sodium citrate (*Coxiella*)	4°C for up to 24 hours Snap freeze and store at −70°C beyond 24 hours	Isolation Immunocytologic PCR
Serum	10–12 mL, clotted blood; collect acute sample at onset; collect convalescent sample 1–4 weeks later	4°C for several days −20°C or lower for prolonged periods	Serology: IFA Immunoperoxidase Latex agglutination
Skin lesion	3 mm diameter punch biopsy of a mucopapule or the margin of an eschar	Snap-frozen or fixed in formaldehyde	Immunohistologic PCR
Biopsy or autopsy tissue	Brain, spleen, lung, liver, other visceral tissue	4°C for 24 hours −70°C for delays longer than 24 hours	Isolation Immunohistologic PCR

the micro-IF methods can detect both IgM and IgG antibodies. IgM antibodies can be detected in the first week of infection, and IgG antibodies are usually detected 7 to 10 days following onset on symptoms. Both methods are reliable for distinguishing active, recent, and past infections. The latex agglutination method requires less time, and is simpler and more economical to perform, but cannot determine the immunoglobulin class and is therefore not reliable for distinguishing past or recent infections. An enzyme immunoassay and a dot immunoassay are also available but not as widely used.

Checkpoint! 16–10 (Chapter Objective 13)

Which statement is incorrect and should not be included in a laboratory protocol for diagnosis of rickettsiae in clinical specimens?

    A. *Isolation should be attempted routinely on all specimens except autopsy material.*

    B. *Examine skin rash, eschar, and other tissue by direct immunostaining.*

    C. *Perform PCR on biopsy samples, blood, buffy coat, and plasma.*

    D. *Perform indirect immunofluorescence assays on paired acute and convalescent sera.*

SUMMARY

A wide variety of specimens are useful for the diagnosis of infections caused by viruses, chlamydiae species, rickettsiae species and *Coxiella* species. These specimens can be hazardous and must be collected and handled with caution, using BSL 3 practices in most cases. Specimens should be collected early in the course of infection. Viruses in particular should be collected in the first 3 to 5 days of infection. Because viruses, chlamydiae, rickettsiae, and *Coxiella* are intracellular agents of infection, it is critical that specimens contain host material. VTM and 2-SP liquid transport media are most appropriate for viruses and chlamydiae; transport medium is typically not used for rickettsiae and *Coxiella*. Specimens should be transported to the laboratory at 2°C to 8°C, except blood, *Coxiella,* and rickettsial specimens, which are transported at room temperature. If specimens cannot be processed immediately, they should be held at 2°C to 8°C for the short term or frozen at –70°C for extended periods of time; specimens for rickettsiae and *Coxiella* should be frozen immediately if processing is delayed.

The methods used for identification differ from those of bacteria, and many require special technical expertise to perform and interpret. Isolation in monolayer cell cultures of primary, diploid, and heteroploid cell lines of mammalian tissue is the traditional method for isolation in the clinical virology laboratory. Viruses are recognized primarily by presence of CPE or hemagglutination and confirmed using immunofluorescence or nucleic acid detection in most cases. Isolation in cell cultures is the primary means for detection of viruses, but this diagnostic approach is time consuming and requires technical expertise. A number of technological advances have made detection more convenient, rapid, and less technically demanding. The use of the shell vial and microwell centrifuge enhanced inoculation, pre-CPE detection methods, decrease detection to 48 hours or less. Monolayer cells may be cryo-preserved, thereby ensuring availability of cell cultures for isolation when necessary. Cell lines may be co-cultured, reducing the number of individual cell lines needed for isolation. Transgenic cells, which have been genetically modified, permit infection by a singe type of virus, thus simplifying detection and identification.

Isolation of chlamydiae, rickettsiae, and *Coxiella* in cell cultures is not commonly performed in the clinical virology laboratory. When isolation of chlamydiae is required, shell vials with cycloheximide-treated McCoy cells are preferred. Isolation of rickettsiae and *Coxiella* is too technically demanding and thus is only performed in reference and specialized laboratories.

Direct examination of clinical specimens for presence of viruses, chlamydiae, rickettsiae, and *Coxiella* provide a rapid means of diagnosing infections. These methods identify the infectious agents primarily based on detection of the organism itself, its antigens, or unique nucleic acid sequences. The electron microscope is used to identify groups of viruses based on morphology, but this approach is not practical in the clinical diagnostic laboratory. Light microscopy is used to provide early evidence of infection based on cytohistological staining or immunostaining of clinical material demonstrating changes in host cell morphology, inclusions, or in case of rickettsiae, the organism. The sensitivity of this method is low and should only be used for presumptive diagnosis. Antigen detection methods include immunofluorescence, enzyme immunoassay, and latex agglutination. Immunofluorescence is the most sensitive and specific of these, but some methods require technical skill to perform and interpret. A microimmunofluorescence test is particularly useful for diagnosing infections caused by chlamydiae and rickettsiae. Nucleic acid detection methods, nucleic acid probes, and the polymerase chain reaction in particular have become more widely available. PCR is one of the most sensitive detection methods and is being used in the clinical laboratory with higher frequency. Reverse transcriptase PCR allows detection of RNA viruses. In real-time PCR, both amplification and detection of amplicons are completed in the same closed system. The nucleic acid sequences are detected as they are produced, and the amplicons can be identified within 1 hour.

Serologic tests for specific antibodies are most reliable when a fourfold rise in antibody titer can be demonstrated between paired acute and convalescent sera. Some infections can be diagnosed based on detection of IgM or IgG antibodies alone. The complement fixation test is one of the most reliable methods for diagnosing viruses and chlamydiae. The microimmunofluorescence method is a highly sensitive and specific method and is used for diagnosing rickettsial and chlamydial infections.

Finally, it is important to note that although the level of testing differs greatly from one facility to another, all laboratory professionals should be knowledgeable of the requirements for specimen collection, transport, and storage. Advanced approaches in isolation and molecular diagnostic techniques will most likely greatly increase the availability of more rapid and reliable diagnoses.

LEARNING OPPORTUNITES

1. Gram stain and biochemical tests have no role in the laboratory diagnosis of intracellular pathogens such as viruses, *Chlamydia,* and *Rickettsia.* Direct detection of intracellular pathogens and their identification is often based on three other different approaches. Name them. (Chapter Objective 10)

2. When is the best time to collect viral specimens? Why? (Chapter Objective 1)

3. Explain the difference between primary cell cultures and heteroploid cell cultures. (Chapter Objective 5)

4. List the different types of cytopathic effect that are observed in monolayer cell cultures as an indication of viral growth. (Chapter Objective 7)

5. One of the most popular methods of diagnosing chlamydial infections is immunofluorescence testing using fluorescein-conjugated monoclonal antibodies. Describe the microscopic appearance of elementary bodies (EBs) using this method. (Chapter Objective 13)

6. Molecular detection of *Rickettsia* in clinical material uses sensitive, specific, and rapid methods of diagnosis. What is the most frequently performed molecular method? (It is more specific than the antibody-based immunohistologic detection methods.) (Chapter Objective 13)

PEARSON
myhealthprofessionskit™

Use this address to access the interactive Companion Website created for this textbook. Simply select "Clinical Laboratory Science" from the choice of disciplines. Find this book and log in using your user name and password.

REFERENCES

Go to myhealthprofessionskit.com to view this chapter's references and useful websites.

PART IV
CLINICALLY SIGNIFICANT ISOLATES

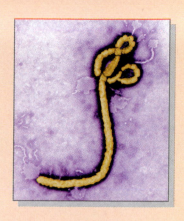

17

Aerobic Gram-Positive Cocci

Karen M. Kiser

■ LEARNING OBJECTIVES

Upon completion of this chapter, the learner should be able to:

1. Categorize the gram-positive cocci using their general characteristics.

2. Summarize the principle and purpose of each differential test used in the identification of the gram-positive cocci.

3. Identify positive and negative reactions for each differential test used in the identification of the gram-positive cocci.

4. Relate the microscopic and culture characteristics for each gram-positive coccus.

5. Determine species of gram-positive cocci using microscopic morphology, colony morphology, and biochemical results.

6. Predict the antibiotic susceptibility pattern for *Staphylococcus aureus,* group A and group B beta-hemolytic *Streptococcus, Enterococcus: E. faecalis* and *E. faecium,* and *Streptococcus pneumoniae.*

7. Describe the natural habitat, virulence factors, and clinical infections associated with gram-positive cocci.

   a. Correlate patient populations associated with infections because of gram-positive cocci.

8. Distinguish those gram-positive cocci that are clinically relevant from those that are considered normal flora.

9. Identify the purpose of the primary plating media used for isolating gram-positive cocci.

10. Correlate patient history, body site/specimen type, colony morphology, Gram stain reaction, identification and susceptibility testing results to identify an organism, assess its clinical significance, and recognize errors.

KEY TERMS

butyrous	odontogenic	superantigen
compromised	opportunistic	superinfections
contact precautions	pneumococcus	toxigenic
epidemiologic	satellite	umbilicated
immunocompromised	sequelae	

TAXONOMY

Family *Micrococcaceae* (mī'-krō-kok-ā-'sē-ē)
  Genus *Micrococcus* (mī'-krō-kok-ĕs)
  Genus *Rothia* (rŏth'-ē-ă)
    R. mucilaginosa (mū-sĭl-ŏj-ĭn-ō-sa)
Family *Staphylococcaceae* (staf'-i-lō-kok'-ā'-sē-ē)
  Genus *Staphylococcus* (staf'-i-lō-kok'-ŭs)
    S. aureus (ore-rē-us)
    S. epidermidis (e-pĭ'-der-mi-dis)
    S. hyicus (hī-ĭ-kŭs)
    S. intermedius (in-ter-mē'-dē-ŭs)
    S. lugdunensis (lŭg-dū-nĕn-sĭs)
    S. saprophyticus (sap-rō-fit'-tĭ-cŭs)
    S. schleiferi (shlā'-fair-eye)
  Genus *Gemella* (je-mel'-ă)
Family *Streptococcaceae* (strep-tō-kok'-ā'-sē-ē)
  Genus *Streptococcus* (strep-tō-kok'ŭs)
    S. agalactiae (ā-gah-lak-tēa-ī)
    S. anginosus (previously a member of the
      "*S. milleri*" group) (ăn'-jĭ-nō'-sŭs; mil-ler-eye)
    S. constellatus (previously a member of the
      "*S. milleri*" group) (kŏn'-stŭ-lŏt-ŭs)
    S. intermedius (previously a member of the
      "*S. milleri*" group) (ĭn'-tĕr-mē'-dē-us)
    S. gallolyticus (previously known as *S. bovis*)
      (găl-ō-lĭ-tĭ-kŭs; bō-vĭs)
    S. dysgalactiae (dis-gă-lak-tea-eye)
    S. pneumoniae (new-mō-nē-ī)
    S. pyogenes (pie-ahj-e-nēēz)
    viridans *Streptococcus* (veer-ĭ-danz)
  Genus *Lactococcus* (lak-tō-kok'-ŭs)

Family *Enterococcaceae* (en'-ter-ō-kok'-ā'-sē-ē)
  Genus *Enterococcus* (en'-ter-ō-kok'-ăs)
    E. casseliflavus (kay-sē-li-flā-vŭs)
    E. faecalis (fee-kay-lis)
    E. faecium (fee-see-um)
    E. gallinarum (gah-lah-nar-um)
  Genus *Vagococcus* (vā-gō-kok'-us)
  Genus *Tetragenococcus* (te-tra-jen-ō-kok'-us)
Family *Leuconostocaceae* (loo-kō-nos'-tok-ā'-sē-ē)
  Genus *Leuconostoc* (loo-kō-nos'-tok)
  Genus *Weissella* (vīs-sell-la)
Family *Lactobacillaceae* (lak-tō-bă-sil'-ā'-sē-ē)
  Genus *Pediococcus* (pē'-dē-ō-kok'-ŭs)
Family *Aerococcaceae* (ār-ō-kok'-ā'-sē-ē)
  Genus *Abiotrophia* (ā-bī-ō-trō'-phe-ă)
  Genus *Aerococcus* (ār-ō-kok'-ŭs)
  Genus *Facklamia* (făck-lām-ia)
  Genus *Globicatella* (glō-bĭ-că-tĕl-lă)
  Genus *Dolosicoccus* (do-ló-sĭ-kok'-ŭs)
Family "*Peptostreptococcaceae*" (pep'-to-strep-
  to-kok'-ā'-sē-ē)
  Genus *Helcococcus* (hel'-cō-kok'-ŭs)
Family *Carnobacteriaceae* (kar'-nō-bak-tēr-ā'-sē-ē)
  Genus *Alloiococcus* (al-loy-ō-kok'-ŭs)
  Genus *Granulicatella* (gra-nū-lĭ-că-tĕl-lă)

▶ INTRODUCTION

The aerobic gram-positive cocci are some of the most frequently isolated organisms from patient specimens. They are also members of the normal flora in most body sites covered with skin or lined with mucous membranes. The challenge, as we examine the growth from these sites, is to separate the "flowers" from the "weeds." In other words, detect potential pathogens and distinguish them from the "normal flora" by performing appropriate identification tests. This process begins by grouping them into possible genera first with screening tests, then follow with the specific test(s) to identify to genus and species.

In this chapter, general characteristics of each genus will be presented. Within each genus the morphology and useful tests for identification will be described. Key reactions that distinguish the gram-positive cocci will be detailed along with their clinical significance.

CHAPTER OVERVIEW

This chapter focuses on the clinically significant gram-positive cocci that are isolated from human specimens. New species being discovered as commensal (living in or on another without injury) organisms are isolated as causative agents of disease in compromised patients. Recent taxonomy changes have resulted in the creation of new families, reorganized genera, and new species. The challenge is to stay up to date with these new discoveries and use this knowledge to provide clinically relevant information for physicians.

► CATALASE POSITIVE

The catalase test provides helpful information and should be used to screen a colony that appears microscopically as gram-positive cocci. See ∞ Chapters 8 and 9 to refresh your knowledge of the catalase test procedure. If the tested colony bubbles, like carbonated soda, when suspended in 3% hydrogen peroxide, it is catalase positive. The possible genera include *Micrococcus* spp. and *Staphylococcus* spp. Rare strains of *Staphylococcus* spp. can be catalase negative (Koneman, Allen, Janda, Schreckenberger, & Winn, 1997). Although *Enterococcus* spp. are traditionally considered catalase negative, a rare weakly catalase-positive *Enterococcus*- or *Streptococcus*-related cocci may be encountered. Information on these organisms is presented later in the chapter.

Checkpoint! 17–1 (Chapter Objective 1)

Which of the following reactions characterize the genera Staphylococcus spp. and Micrococcus spp.?

1. Catalase negative
2. Catalase positive
3. Gram-positive cocci
4. Gram-negative cocci

   A. *1 & 3*
   B. *2 & 3*
   C. *2 & 4*
   D. *1 & 4*

USEFUL BIOCHEMICAL TESTS

The appropriate biochemical tests are selected after making a presumptive identification. This presumptive identification considers the Gram stain result, catalase result, and colony morphology. Identification of an unknown organism is the result of observing key reactions associated with a particular species.

Several biochemical tests are available to screen, identify, and distinguish the catalase-positive aerobic gram-positive cocci. Biochemical tests useful in screening for *Micrococcus* spp. include bacitracin, modified oxidase test and susceptibility to bacitracin,

furazolidone, and lysostaphin. Tests routinely used for the identification of *Staphylococcus* spp. include coagulase and novobiocin susceptibility. In addition to describing these tests, other tests which may be used to speciate the *Staphylococcus* spp. are also included in the following components of this section.

Bacitracin and Furazolidone Susceptibility

Bacitracin and furazolidone are antibiotics used to aid in the differentiation of *Micrococcus* spp. from coagulase-negative *Staphylococcus* spp. The bacitracin and furazolidone susceptibility tests consist of two commercially prepared disks, each impregnated with one of the two antibiotics. The bacitracin test (also known as Taxo A) uses a disk containing 0.04 units of bacitracin. The furazolidone (FX) disk contains 100 µg of the antibiotic. The suspected *Micrococcus* colony is streaked for confluent (solid) growth on sheep blood agar. The disks are deposited on the surface with each on one-half of the agar plate. If the organism is a *Micrococcus* spp., it will exhibit the following growth pattern on the plate: resistant (no zone of inhibition) to furazolidone and sensitive (a zone of inhibition >10 mm) to bacitracin. If the organism is a *Staphylococcus* spp., it will exhibit the following growth pattern: sensitive (zone of inhibition >15 mm) to furazolidone and resistant to bacitracin.

Modified Oxidase

The modified oxidase test detects cytochrome c enzymes and uses a 6% reagent compared to the traditional 1% oxidase reagent used to screen gram-negative rods. The traditional oxidase test is described in ∞ Chapters 8 and 9. It is modified by the addition of dimethyl sulfoxide (DMSO). The DMSO appears to enhance the uptake of reagent by the gram-positive cell wall. Several colonies, which are less than 24 hours old, are selected from sheep blood agar with a wooden applicator stick and inoculated onto the reagent-impregnated disk. The appearance of a dark blue color within 2 minutes is a positive result (Faller & Schleifer, 1981). Prepared Microdase disks, as seen in Figure 17-1 ■, are available (Thermo Fisher Scientific/Remel, Lenexa, KS). A positive modified oxidase result is characteristic of *Micrococcus* spp. Most *Staphylococcus* spp. are negative. Some rare nonhuman strains of *Staphylococcus* spp. can be modified oxidase positive.

Susceptibility to Lysostaphin

Lysostaphin is a mixture of enzymes that cut the unique crosslinks of peptidoglycan in the cell wall of *Staphylococcus* spp., making them lyse. The cell wall of *Micrococcus* spp. does not lyse in the presence of lysostaphin. The enzyme can be used as a liquid or disk. *Staphylococcus* spp. demonstrates either clearing of an organism suspension or inhibition of growth around a disk, depending on the method used. *Micrococcus* spp. remain in suspension or are resistant to the action of the enzyme. It is very important that the organisms are grown on beef peptone-based medium prior to testing. This ensures the *Staphylococcus* spp. has access to the correct amino acids necessary to build the unique cross-links of peptidoglycan in their cell wall.

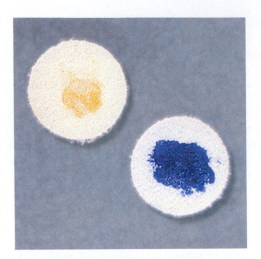

■ **FIGURE 17-1** Negative (left) and positive (right) reaction for the Microdase Disk.
Photo courtesy of Remel, part of Thermo Fisher Scientific.

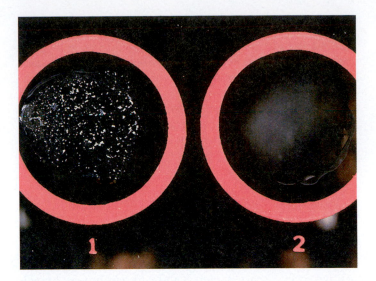

■ **FIGURE 17-2** Slide coagulase with positive (left) and negative (right) reactions.

> ℮ **REAL WORLD TIP**
>
> The lysostaphin susceptibility test provides the expected results in its name. Lysostaphin lyses *Staphylococcus* spp.

> ℮ **REAL WORLD TIP**
>
> Many laboratories do not screen catalase-positive gram-positive cocci with bacitracin and furazolidone susceptibilities, modified oxidase, or lysostaphin. Rather than maintaining all of these testing materials, it is faster and cheaper to begin with Gram stain then perform a catalase and proceed to the staphylococcal latex agglutination test to differentiate *S. aureus* from coagulase-negative *Staphylococcus* spp. *Micrococcus* spp. is very rare and is usually suspected based on its unique Gram stain of GPC in tetrads and yellow pigmented colony. Laboratory testing that can be completed the same day is preferred over testing that takes up to 24 hours before interpretation.

Coagulase

The coagulase test is used to determine the ability of a potential *Staphylococcus* isolate to clot plasma. The slide coagulase detects clumping factor or "bound" coagulase, whereas the tube coagulase detects free or "extracellular" coagulase. Not all coagulase-positive *Staphylococcus* possess clumping factor, so a negative slide coagulase must always be followed by a tube coagulase test. A positive slide test, as seen in Figure 17-2 ■, results in clumps forming in the test circle compared to the smooth suspension of a negative result. A saline control must be run in conjunction with the slide coagulase test to ensure any agglutination detected is true and not because of

autoagglutination of the organisms. The saline control should remain as a smooth suspension.

> ℮ **REAL WORLD TIP**
>
> Auto-agglutination can occur in the slide coagulase test when the colony is taken from a medium with a high salt concentration such as mannitol salt agar. Without a saline control, any agglutination present cannot be trusted because it could be a false-positive reaction.

A positive tube coagulase test is indicated by clotting of the plasma, as seen in Figure 17-3 ■. The tube coagulase is read every 30 minutes for up to 4 hours incubation to prevent a

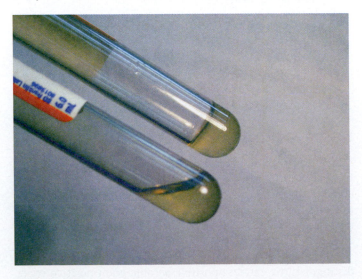

■ **FIGURE 17-3** Positive (top) and negative (bottom) tube coagulase reactions.

false-negative result because of lysis of the clot by the enzyme staphylokinase or fibrinolysin. If negative after 4 hours incubation, the tube is held at room temperature and read the next day after 24 hours. Incubation at 35°C overnight may increase the production of staphylokinase. ∞ Chapters 8, "Presumptive Identification," and 9, "Final Identification," provide more information on the coagulase test.

 REAL WORLD TIP

To improve turnaround time for patient results, it is possible to perform a tube coagulase test directly from positive blood cultures. Once a blood culture has been identified as positive with gram-positive cocci in clusters, remove about 10 mL and centrifuge at 150 X *g* for 10 minutes. This removes most of the red blood cells. Remove the supernatant and centrifuge again at 1000 X *g* for 15 minutes. This leaves a pellet of organisms. Remove the supernatant and resuspend the pellet in 1 mL of sterile saline. The remaining suspension can be used to inoculate a few drops into a tube coagulase. If a result is positive, it can be accepted, but if it is negative, the result cannot be trusted because of a procedure sensitivity of only 86%. A negative direct coagulase requires additional testing for identification (McDonald & Chapin, 1995).

Most clinical laboratories will identify a coagulase-positive *Staphylococcus* as *S. aureus*. If a source of infection is an animal exposure such as a dog bite or in a sterile body site, other coagulase-positive *Staphylococcus* spp., such as *S. intermedius*, *S. hyicus*, and *S. schleiferi*, should be considered also. Refer to "Other Coagulase-Positive *Staphylococcus*" later in this chapter.

 Checkpoint! 17–2 (Chapter Objective 3)

When you observe a clot in the coagulase tube, you record this reaction as:

   A. *negative.*
   B. *positive.*
   C. *contaminated.*
   D. *acceptable.*

Commercial Slide Agglutination Tests

Latex agglutination slide tests have replaced the slide and tube coagulase tests for routine use in detecting the ability of a *Staphylococcus* isolate to clot plasma because of its ease of use and rapid results. The commercial kits contain a reagent consisting of latex beads coated with fibrinogen that detects clumping factor or bound coagulase. Some kits also include an IgG antibody that will react with the unique protein A

present in the cell wall of *S. aureus*. A positive reaction is indicated by agglutination. Refer to Figure 8-29 in ∞ Chapter 8, "Presumptive Identification," for an example of a commercial latex agglutination test for the identification of *Staphylococcus aureus*.

False negatives can occur with encapsulated methicillin-resistant *S. aureus* (MRSA). A follow-up test using the tube coagulase is highly recommended if MRSA is suspected. Some second-generation kits now include latex beads coated with monoclonal antibodies that detect clumping factor, protein A, and specific *S. aureus* surface polysaccharides. These kits detect MRSA more reliably then the previous generation of kits (Smole, Aaronson, Durbin, Brecher, & Arbeit, 1998). Overall, the latex agglutination commercial kits have shown increased sensitivity and specificity when compared to the traditional tube coagulase. The increased cost of the kits is offset by the rapid turnaround of results compared to the tube coagulase test.

Most clinical laboratories report an organism that tests latex agglutination positive as *S. aureus*. Other *Staphylococcus* spp. can produce clumping factor and generate agglutination. *S. lugdunensis* is not reliably identified by the commercial latex agglutination kits (Kloos & Bannerman 1994). *S. schleiferi* subsp. *schleiferi* can also produce clumping factor and so produce a positive latex agglutination. Sterile body fluid isolates or clinically relevant isolates of an animal origin may require further identification to ensure an accurate identification.

 REAL WORLD TIP

Be sure to correlate colony morphology with the latex agglutination coagulase reaction obtained because other organisms, such as the urinary isolate *S. saprophyticus*, may also agglutinate generating a false-positive test result. *S. aureus* is usually beta-hemolytic, whereas *S. saprophyticus* is nonhemolytic. *S. saprophyticus* produces a negative slide coagulase test result, so agglutination does not appear to be because of clumping factor (Murray, Baron, Pfaller, Tenover, & Yolken, 1999). Urinary isolates require additional testing for confirmation of the identification.

DNase/Thermonuclease

The DNase or thermonuclease test is used to presumptively identify *S. aureus*. Both correlate well with a positive coagulase result. In cases where colony morphology resembles a *S. aureus*, white to yellow and beta-hemolytic, and the latex agglutination test or coagulase test is negative or weakly positive, the DNase test may help in its identification.

If the isolate produces deoxyribonuclease, it will denature DNA present in the medium. A positive result is indicated by a clear halo around the growth when flooded with 1N HCl (hydrochloric acid). Toluidine blue can also be used in place of HCL. Toluidine blue is a dye that remains blue in the presence of intact DNA and turns pink in the presence of nucleotides from denatured DNA. The growth on DNase agar can be flooded with 0.1% toluidine blue or the dye is incorporated in the medium. A color change from blue to rose-pink zones around the colonies is a positive result.

Organisms other than *S. aureus* can also be DNase positive. These include *Micrococcus* and *Staphylococcus epidermidis* (Hoeprich, Lachica, & Genigeorgis, 1971). Some staphylococci do not grow on DNase with toluidine blue (Becton Dickenson Microbiology Systems, 1988). A photo of the DNase test reaction can be found in ∞ Chapter 18, "Gram-Negative Cocci."

The test for thermonuclease activity is a variation of the DNase procedure. The nuclease produced by *S. aureus* is stable when heated, whereas the nuclease of other organisms, such as *S. epidermidis,* is destroyed by heat. An organism is grown in a broth for 2 to 4 hours then boiled for 15 minutes and cooled. In the laboratory, positive blood culture broth, displaying gram-positive cocci, can be boiled and tested in the same way. This provides a rapid means of identification of *S. aureus* in a patient with a potentially fatal infectious disease.

Wells are cut into DNase or thermonuclease agar containing toluidine blue. The wells are then filled with several drops of the boiled and cooled broth culture. The plate is incubated at 35°C for 2 to 4 hours. A positive result is indicated by a light pink zone around the well (Remel, 1997). A positive result for thermonuclease activity, as observed in Figure 17-4 ■, is presumptive for identification of catalase-positive gram-positive cocci as *S. aureus.* Other coagulase-positive staphylococci such as *S. intermedius* and *S. hyicus* are also positive, but they are considered rare isolates in most laboratories. Further testing may be needed in the case of an animal bite or organisms isolated from a sterile body site. *Staphylococcus epidermidis* does produce small amounts of thermonuclease, but it is heat labile and destroyed when boiled.

 REAL WORLD TIP

If a white or yellow beta-hemolytic, catalase-positive, gram-positive cocci in clusters proves to be tube coagulase or latex agglutination negative, the thermonuclease test can be used to identify the organism as *S. aureus*. Although *S. intermedius* and *S. hyicus* can also prove to be positive by the thermonuclease test (TNT), they are rare isolates in most clinical laboratories.

Trehalose-Mannitol Broth

The trehalose-mannitol broth test, as seen in Figure 17-5 ■, is a rapid carbohydrate fermentation test. Both carbohydrates are combined in one tube with a pH indicator. It is used to presumptively identify *S. epidermidis*. Other coagulase-negative *Staphylococcus* usually ferment one or both of the sugars, producing acid that turns the pH indicator yellow and indicates a positive result. *S. epidermidis* does not ferment either sugar resulting in a purple or gray purple color after 4 hours incubation on a rotary shaker (Isenberg, 1992).

Novobiocin Susceptibility

The novobiocin test consists of commercially prepared disks impregnated with the antibiotic novobiocin (NB). It is used to presumptively identify *S. saprophyticus*. Resistance to novobiocin is determined by preparing a suspension of coagulase-negative *Staphylococcus* spp. equal to a McFarland 0.5 standard. The suspected organism is streaked onto the surface of a sheep blood agar or Mueller-Hinton plate for confluent (solid) growth. A 5 µg novobiocin disk is applied to the surface. A zone of inhibition less than 16 mm indicates resistance as observed in Figure 17-6 ■. Resistance is characteristic of

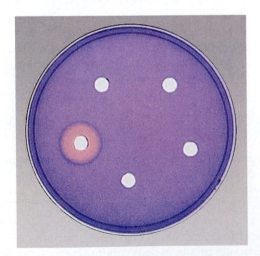

■ **FIGURE 17-4** Positive reaction (at 8 o'clock) for *S. aureus* on thermonuclease agar.
Photo courtesy of Remel, part of Thermo Fisher Scientific.

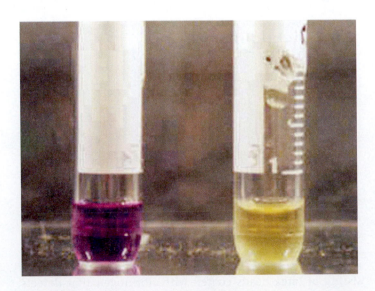

■ **FIGURE 17-5** Trehalose-mannitol broth negative (left) and positive (right) reactions.

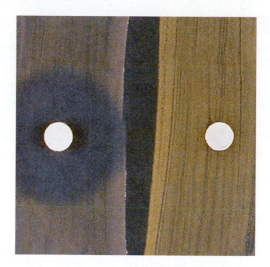

■ **FIGURE 17-6** Susceptible (left) and resistant (right) reactions for the novobiocin susceptibility test.
Photo courtesy of Remel, part of Thermo Fisher Scientific.

S. saprophyticus, a urinary isolate. This result is uncommon in other clinically relevant species and is only used on urine isolates (Murray et al., 1999).

Polymyxin B Susceptibility

Resistance to polymyxin B, an antibiotic, is helpful in the identification of clinically significant *Staphylococcus* spp. A 300-unit disk can be added to the same plate used for testing novobiocin resistance. A zone of inhibition less than 10 mm indicates resistance. Resistant human isolates include *S. aureus, S. epidermidis, S. hyicus,* and occasionally *S. lugdunensis* (Murray et al., 1999).

 Checkpoint! 17–3 (Chapter Objective 2)

Which of the following antibiotics disks can be used to differentiate S. saprophyticus from other coagulase-negative Staphylococcus spp.?

A. *Bacitracin*
B. *Furazolidone*
C. *Novobiocin*
D. *Polymyxin B*

Pyrrolidonyl Arylamidase or Pyrrolidonase (PYR)

The PYR test is used to detect the enzyme L-pyrrolidonyl arylamidase in microorganisms. The test can be performed as a broth test, agar test, or impregnated on filter strips or disks. A pink color, after the addition of the PYR reagent, is a positive result. *S. haemolyticus, S. lugdunensis, S. schleiferi* subsp. *schleiferi,* and *S. intermedius* are positive (Murray et al., 1999). The procedure can be reviewed in ∞ Chapter 8, "Presumptive Identification."

Ornithine Decarboxylase

A positive result for the ornithine decarboxylase test accurately identifies *S. lugdunensis* (Murray et al., 1999). A loopful of organism is inoculated into the medium and overlaid with oil. The organism ferments the glucose present in the medium, the pH drops, and then it produces ornithine decarboxylase. A change from gray to purple is a positive result, whereas a change to yellow is negative. A control tube without the amino acid ornithine must be inoculated at the same time as the test. This ensures the organism does not react with anything other than the ornithine present. ∞ Chapter 9, "Final Identification," provides detailed information on this biochemical test.

Voges-Proskauer (VP)

The Voges-Proskauer test detects acetoin or acetyl methyl carbinol, a by-product of glucose fermentation. A pink color after addition of two reagents indicates a positive result. This test is helpful in distinguishing the two *S. aureus* subspecies and the other coagulase-positive *Staphylococcus: S. schleiferi* subsp. *schleiferi, S. schleiferi* subsp. *coagulans, S. intermedius,* and *S. hyicus.* A positive VP reaction is characteristic for *S. aureus* subsp. *aureus* but a negative VP reaction is characteristic for *S. aureus* ssp. *anaerobius. S. schleiferi* subsp. *coagulans* is VP positive. *S. schleiferi* subsp. *schleiferi, S. intermedius,* and *S. hyicus* are VP negative and can be distinguished from *S. aureus* ssp. *anaerobius* with further testing as described later in this chapter. Refer to ∞ Chapter 9, "Final Identification," to review the Voges-Proskauer test.

Urease

Urea broth medium detects the release of ammonia because of the action of the enzyme urease on urea. The increased pH changes the color of the medium. No color change is a negative reaction while the generation of a pink to red color is positive. *S. epidermidis, S. warneri, S. saprophyticus, S. intermedius,* and *S. hominis* are positive (Murray et al., 1999). Refer to ∞ Chapter 9, "Final Identification," for more information on the urease test.

Commercial Identification Kits

Commercially available gram-positive identification kits consist of carbohydrate fermentation tests, conventional biochemical tests, or chromogenic enzyme substrate tests (Koneman et al., 1997). These kits identify *S. epidermidis* accurately but are less accurate for the other coagulase-negative *Staphylococcus* spp. (Weinstein et al., 1998). Additional testing such as ornithine decarboxylase or tests for coagulase and clumping factor may be necessary (Murray et al., 1999).

MICROCOCCUS

Micrococci closely resemble one of the commonly isolated genera, the staphylococci, and must be identified when present to avoid misidentification.

Growth Requirements

The micrococci are obligate aerobes that may be isolated from cultures of clinical specimens in routine incubation conditions of ambient air or CO_2 and 35°C to 37°C (Murray et al., 1999).

Identification

Many different genera of microorganisms are catalase positive. When a catalase-positive colony is isolated from a patient specimen, a Gram stain assists in determining possible genera. Identification of *Micrococcus* spp. is accomplished by observing the typical microscopic and colonial morphology and key biochemical reactions.

Microscopic Morphology. The micrococci are large gram-positive cocci arranged in pairs, tetrads, and clusters. Their predominant arrangement is typically tetrads (or squares of four cocci). This unique arrangement can be a clue that the organism is a *Micrococcus* spp. They can resemble *Staphylococcus* spp., so it is important to correlate the microscopic morphology with the colony characteristics.

Colony Morphology. Micrococci colonies can be very distinctive. They may present with a bright yellow, orange, pink, tan, or white pigmented colony (Forbes, Sahm, & Weissfeld, 1998). They are 1 to 2 mm and nonhemolytic with a high convex (domed) colony profile (Koneman et al., 1997). This characteristic may help to distinguish this genus from *Staphylococcus* spp. colonies, which tend to be more flattened. ∞ Chapter 8, Figure 8-21, shows the easily recognizable bright yellow colonies of *Micrococcus luteus,* the most commonly isolated species, on blood agar.

Key Biochemical Reactions. Micrococci can be distinguished from the other strongly catalase-positive, gram-positive cocci by a positive modified oxidase test result, sensitivity to bacitracin, and resistance to furazolidone and lysostaphin, as noted in Table 17-1 .

---

❷ REAL WORLD TIP

A positive modified oxidase test may not correlate with a positive traditional oxidase test. *Micrococcus* spp. provides variable results with the traditional oxidase test. They are usually weak but positive when tested with 1% oxidase reagent, tetramethyl-*p*-phenylenediamine (MacFaddin, 2000). The preferred method for detecting cytochrome c in the *Micrococcus* spp. is the modified oxidase test using the 6% oxidase reagent with DMSO.

✪ TABLE 17-1

Screening Tests for *Micrococcus* and *Staphylococcus*

Genus	Modified Oxidase	Bacitracin	Furazolidone	Lysostaphin
Micrococcus spp.	+	S	R	R
Staphylococcus spp.	−	R	S	S

+ = positive; − = negative; R = resistant; S = sensitive

✔ Checkpoint! 17–4 (Chapter Objective 5)

A yellow colony that appears as gram-positive cocci in clusters, bubbles with catalase reagent, and turns dark blue when rubbed onto a modified oxidase disk is:

  A. *Micrococcus spp.*
  B. *S. aureus*
  C. *coagulase-negative Staphylococcus spp.*
  D. *S. saprophyticus*

Clinical Significance

Micrococci are found on the skin, in mucous membranes, and in the oropharynx as normal flora (Forbes et al., 1998). They are also present in the environment (Koneman et al., 1997). Micrococci are seldom isolated from clinical specimens. When present, they are usually considered harmless. They are often an environmental contaminant. The organism may be significant when associated with infections in those who are **immunocompromised** because underlying illness or therapy has diminished their normal immune response. When isolated from sterile body sites, the physician should be consulted to determine potential clinical significance. The organism has been associated with pneumonia, meningitis, and endocarditis. It has also been isolated in cases of infection because of colonization of intravenous catheters and cerebrospinal fluid (CSF) shunts similar to another common skin organism, *Staphylococcus* spp.

STAPHYLOCOCCUS

Members of the genus *Staphylococcus* spp. are some of the most frequently isolated catalase-positive, gram-positive cocci.

Growth Requirements

Staphylococci are usually facultative anaerobes. The two exceptions to the rule include *S. aureus* subsp. *anaerobius,* which grows best under anaerobic conditions, and *S. hominis,* which grows best under aerobic conditions.

The staphylococci do not require any special conditions for growth. They grow on most nonselective medium in ambient air or CO_2, at 35°C to 37°C. They also grow on gram-positive selective agars such as Columbia colistin naladixic acid (CNA) and phenylethyl alcohol (PEA). Colonial growth should be examined after 24 and 48 hours of incubation to avoid testing mixed cultures and reporting inaccurate results (Kloos & Bannerman 1994).

Microscopic Morphology

Gram-positive cocci arranged in pairs, tetrads, short chains, and "grapelike" clusters are considered characteristic of the staphylococci. Review the characteristic Gram stain reaction and arrangement of *Staphylococcus* spp. in Figure 17-7 ■.

℮ REAL WORLD TIP

Streptococcus spp. may mimic *Staphylococcus* spp. on a smear, so it is important to correlate the microscopic results with colony morphology and screening test results. Remember the *Staphylococcus* spp. produce large, white to yellow, opaque colonies that are either beta-hemolytic or nonhemolytic and catalase positive. Colonies of *Streptococcus* spp. are usually small, gray translucent colonies that can be alpha-, beta-, or gamma-hemolytic and catalase negative.

Coagulase-Positive *Staphylococcus*

The presence of the coagulase enzyme is usually associated with *Staphylococcus aureus,* which is clinically significant in humans. Detection of this enzyme is considered the "gold" standard for identification of this potentially pathogenic organism.

◆ *Staphylococcus aureus*

Identification

Staphylococcus aureus is one of the most frequently recognized pathogens isolated in the laboratory. Identification is based on observing its characteristic microscopic and colonial morphology and key biochemical reactions.

Colony Morphology. The typical colony (Figure 17-8 ■) is 1 to 2 mm in size, opaque, round, **butyrous** with a butter-like consistency, white to golden yellow, and exhibiting a low convex (rounded) profile (Koneman et al., 1997). Most species are beta-hemolytic on sheep blood agar, although nonhemolytic colonies do exist. Orange and yellow orange colonies have also been isolated (Murray et al., 1999).

℮ REAL WORLD TIP

Aureus is the Latin word for golden.

Mannitol salt agar (MSA) is a selective and differential medium designed to select for staphylococci because of their tolerance for high salt concentration (7.5%). It also distinguishes the pathogen *S. aureus,* which ferments mannitol, from other species. On MSA, *S. aureus* will produce yellow colonies with yellow zones. Figure 17-9 ■ demonstrates the yellow colonies of mannitol fermenting *S. aureus* on MSA. Most of the other *Staphylococcus* spp. appear as opaque colonies with pink zones on MSA. Other strains such as *S. saprophyticus* and *S. haemolyticus* can also ferment mannitol, so it is no longer considered a definitive identification tool. Refer to ∞ Chapter 7 to review selective and differential medium.

℮ REAL WORLD TIP

Some *Staphylococcus* spp. colonies may be off-white and resemble the subtle gray colonies of *Enterococcus* or Group D *Streptococcus* (Koneman et al., 1997). A negative or weak positive catalase test is characteristic of *Enterococcus* and Group D isolates, whereas *Staphylococcus* spp. is strongly catalase positive. Remember, *Staphylococcus* colonies are white, and *Streptococcus* colonies are usually gray.

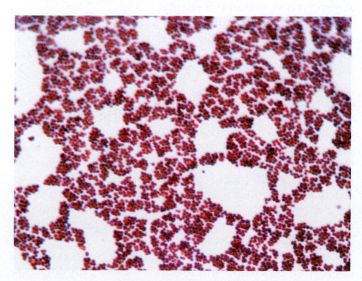

■ FIGURE 17-7 Gram stain of staphylococci.

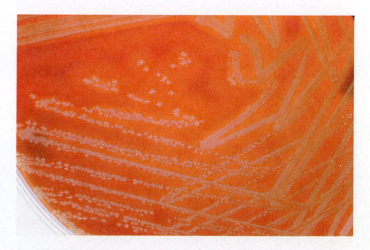

■ FIGURE 17-8 Hemolytic *S. aureus* colonies on sheep blood agar.

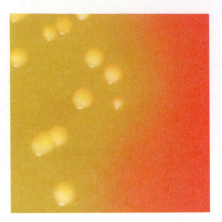

■ **FIGURE 17-9** *S. aureus* colonies on mannitol salt agar.
Photo courtesy of Remel, part of Thermo Fisher Scientific.

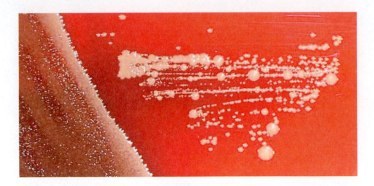

■ **FIGURE 17-10** The small-colony variants of *S. aureus* are much smaller compared to a traditional colony on sheep blood agar after 24 hours of incubation at 35°C. They could be overlooked in mixed cultures.
From Tenover, Fred C., Biddle, James W., and Lancaster, Michael V. Increasing resistance to vancomycin and other glycopeptides in Staphylococcus aureus. *Emerging Infectious Diseases, 7(21), 327–332.*

 REAL WORLD TIP

Mannitol salt agar is rarely used as an identification tool for *S. aureus* in today's laboratories. Too many other *Staphylococcus* spp. are able to ferment mannitol. It is more useful as a selective medium to isolate the organisms from body sites with normal flora such as nasal and perianal. Oxacillin or cefoxitin can be added to the medium to help isolate methicillin-resistant *S. aureus* (MRSA).

 **Checkpoint! 17–5
(Chapter Objective 9)**

Mannitol salt agar is used for:

    A. *differentiating fermenters from oxidizers.*
    B. *selective inhibition of salt-tolerant organisms.*
    C. *selective isolation of gram-positive organisms.*
    D. *selective isolation of pathogenic staphylococci.*

Small variant colonies (SVC) of *Staphylococcus aureus* can occur in patients with persistent or relapsing infections after prolonged antibiotic therapy. These small colonies are usually associated with long-term use of aminoglycosides and vancomycin. This unique colony morphology can also be isolated from cystic fibrosis (CF) patients who are on long-term trimethoprim-sulfamethoxazole (SXT) therapy. The SVC seen in CF patients are actually thymidine dependent because SXT blocks the organism's folic acid pathway.

SVC are slow growing, sometimes taking up to 6 days to appear, nonhemolytic, and nonpigmented. Because they are so slow growing, they can be easily missed in mixed cultures. They revert to regular colonies, on subculture, once removed from the presence of the antibiotic. SVC produce decreased amounts of coagulase and are mannitol negative. Figure 17-10 ■ provides a comparison of the size of small-colony variants of *S. aureus* and a traditional colony.

Key Biochemical Reactions. *S. aureus* is coagulase positive. If a negative result is obtained when using a commercial latex agglutination test, a tube coagulase test should be performed. Methicillin-resistant *S. aureus* (MRSA) have been associated with false-negative agglutination results because of the presence of a capsule that can mask the cell wall protein A. If a colony suspicious for *S. aureus,* white to yellow and beta-hemolytic, produces a negative tube or latex agglutination coagulase test, a DNase test or thermonuclease test should be performed. *S. aureus* is usually DNase and thermonuclease positive. Rarely a coagulase-positive species other than *S. aureus* may be encountered. Additional testing may be required to speciate these isolates. Refer to "Other Coagulase-Positive *Staphylococcus*" later in this chapter.

Most clinical laboratories report a catalase-positive, coagulase or commercial agglutination test positive, gram-positive cocci as *S. aureus.* Figure 17-11 ■ provides a basic scheme for *Staphylococcus* spp. identification.

Antibiogram. The typical pattern associated with susceptibility testing is resistant to ampicillin and penicillin. This is usually because of a plasmid-associated β-lactamase or penicillinase (Koneman et al., 1997). *S. aureus* isolates that are resistant to daptomycin or linezolid, intermediate or resistant to quinupristin-dalfopristin or vancomycin, or resistant to oxacillin are significant and should be reexamined to verify the purity, identity, and accuracy of susceptibility results of the isolate (Hindler, 2005; National Committee for Clinical Laboratory Standards [NCCLS], 2003).

Penicillin-binding proteins (PBP) produce enzymes that are essential in producing and maintaining the peptidoglycan layer of the *S. aureus* cell wall. Beta-lactams antibiotics, such as

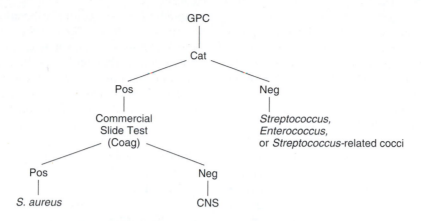

■ **FIGURE 17-11** Basic scheme for routine *Staphylococcus* identification. GPC = gram-positive cocci; Cat = catalase; Pos = positive; Neg = negative; ( ) = alternate test procedure; Coag = slide and tube coagulase; CNS = coagulase-negative *Staphylococcus*

penicillin, ampicillin, and the cephalosporins, bind to the PBP, cell wall synthesis stops, and the organism dies. Beta-lactamase or penicillinase destroys the beta-lactam ring of the beta-lactam antibiotics and the organism thrives.

To overcome the effect of beta-lactamase, penicillinase-resistant penicillins, such as methicillin and oxacillin, were created. Methicillin-resistant *S. aureus* (MRSA) found a way to evade methicillin and oxacillin by altering its PBP again. They have acquired a *mecA* chromosomal gene, which codes for a new PBP called PBP2a. This altered PBP does not bind with the beta-lactam antibiotic or penicillinase-resistant penicillins, and cell wall synthesis continues. Methicillin- or oxacillin-resistant strains of *S. aureus* (MRSA) are resistant to all β-lactams, including cephalosporins and carbapenems (Centers for Disease Control [CDC], 2007b).

S. aureus has developed significant resistance to multiple antibiotics including vancomycin. The detection of *Staphylococcus*' resistance mechanisms is very important for infection control. Its resistance mechanisms and testing procedures are discussed in detail in ∞ Chapter 11, "Susceptibility Testing."

 REAL WORLD TIP

PBP2a can be found in MRSA as well as methicillin-resistant coagulase-negative staphylococci. A latex agglutination test can detect PBP2a. This provides a rapid means to detect MRSA. Molecular diagnostics techniques also provide rapid detection as well. Both methods are faster than traditional susceptibility methods. Knowing if a patient's *S. aureus* isolate is PBP2a negative can prevent the unnecessary use of vancomycin for treatment.

 REAL WORLD TIP

MRSA were first discovered when methicillin was still being used in the United States. Oxacillin is more resistant to degradation in storage and better at detection of heteroresistance. The name MRSA has remained, but they should technically be called oxacillin-resistant *S. aureus* (ORSA) now.

 REAL WORLD TIP

Cefoxitin, used either in the disk diffusion or MIC method, is a good inducer of the *mecA* gene. MRSA are resistant to cefoxitin.

 REAL WORLD TIP

A coagulase latex agglutination positive *Staphylococcus* that is sensitive to penicillin may indicate a coagulase-positive species other than *S. aureus*. Further testing to speciate may be necessary if the patient is immunocompromised or the specimen source is an animal source such as a dog bite. Refer to Table 17-3 for differentiating biochemicals.

✓ **Checkpoint! 17–6 (Chapter Objective 6)**

S. aureus should be:
  A. *resistant to penicillin.*
  B. *resistant to methicillin.*
  C. *sensitive to penicillin.*
  D. *intermediate to methicillin.*

Clinical Significance

Pathogenesis.   Staphylococci may be isolated from most clinical specimens either as normal flora, a colonizer or a pathogen. A variety of infectious diseases are associated with *Staphylococcus aureus*. Consult Box 17-1 ✪ for a listing of specific diseases associated with the organism.

Most *Staphylococcus* spp. infections remain on the surface of the body, where it remains controlled by host defenses. Spread of the organism across the face is often because of the action of fingers transporting the microbe from one area to another (Mims, Dimmock, Nash, & Stephen, 1995). Nasal carriers may transmit the organism by aerosols (Mandell, Dolin, & Bennett, 2000). If the skin or mucous membrane is broken by disease, surgery, or trauma, *S. aureus* can enter the subendothelial tissue causing local infections. Toxins can be produced that result in skin rashes or systemic effects. If the numbers of microorganisms overwhelm the host defenses, they may gain access to the lymphatic system and bloodstream. This allows them to spread throughout the body and results in infections such as pneumonia, endocarditis, and osteomyelitis. Adhesions on the cell wall allow *S. aureus* to bind to nasal mucosal cells and proteins in the extracellular matrix of the subendothelial layer. These include fibronectin-binding proteins, clumping factor, and collagen-binding protein. These membrane-associated proteins appear to be expressed during the early log phase of growth when the bacterial cell number is low thereby promoting adhesion and colonization (Brady, Leid, Costerton, & Shirtliff, 2006). Phagocytosis by endothelial cells aids in the organism's invasiveness (Mandell et al., 2000).

Staphylococcal Defense Mechanisms.   The staphylococci produce substances that allow them to defend themselves against the host's defenses. Many of these substances are produced once the organism's numbers have increased enough to achieve colonization and establish active infection (Brady et al., 2006). The enzyme coagulase allows the organism to clot plasma. This may create a barrier or a wall around the organism that prohibits the phagocytes from approaching and engulfing it. Staphylococci may also coat themselves with the clotted plasma disguising their true identity and preventing opsonization. Some organisms possess a capsule or slime layer that provides protection from engulfment by white blood cells (Koneman et al., 1997). Formation of a biofilm can also protect the organism against antibiotics and host defenses (Brady et al., 2006).

Hemolysins produced cause membrane damage to various cell types. Leukocidins activate and then kill the responding white blood cells by causing pores to form in the cell membrane (Gillet et al., 2002). Spreading factors are enzymes produced by *S. aureus* that destroy various types of tissues. These include lipases, hyaluronidase, and deoxyribonuclease (DNase). The spreading factors once appeared to contribute to the invasiveness of *S. aureus,* but are now thought to play a role in metabolism by making nutrients available to the bacterial cell (Mims et al., 1995). The protein A in the cell wall of a *S. aureus* organism binds the Fc portion of immunoglobulins instead of the Fab sites, resulting in inhibition of opsoninization and phagocytosis. Protein A may also be released into the surrounding environment neutralizing the effectiveness of complement and antibodies (Mandell et al., 2000). The staphylococci may also act as a **superantigen** or a molecule that activates many more T cells than normal. This results in extensive growth and cytokine release causing a nonspecific and nonproductive response from T and B lymphocytes as seen with toxic shock syndrome (Mims et al., 1995). Consult ∞ Chapter 4, "The Host's Encounter with Microbes," to review the host defenses.

Toxigenic Diseases.   Some diseases are the result of **toxigenic** strains of *S. aureus*. Toxigenic strains are organisms capable of producing an extracellular poison. They can produce an enterotoxin that rapidly acts on the sympathetic nervous system (via leukotriene and histamine release by mast cells) resulting in vomiting. It may increase intestinal peristalsis resulting in diarrhea (Mandell et al., 2000). The organism grows and produces toxin in contaminated food. Ingestion of the toxin-laden food results in symptoms of food poisoning within 2 to 4 hours. Food poisoning is because of ingestion of the toxin rather than the presence of the organism. ∞ Chapter 35 describes infections of the gastrointestinal system.

The organisms associated with toxic shock syndrome (TSS) produce a toxin that overstimulates the immune system, which in turn affects various organ functions and dramatically lowers blood pressure. The patient's loss of organ function and resulting life-threatening drop in blood pressure could result in shock and death. It is most frequently associated with the use of tampons in menstruating women. It has also been seen in nonmenstruating women, children, and men when the organism grows within the tissues (as in wound infections) producing the toxin, which is absorbed into the blood stream.

✪ BOX 17-1

Infectious Diseases Associated with *S. aureus*

Folliculitis

Impetigo

Furuncles

Carbuncles

Wound infections

Scalded skin syndrome

Toxic shock syndrome

Food poisoning

Pneumonia

Bacteremia

Endocarditis

Osteomyelitis

Pyoarthritis

Meningitis

Abscesses in various organs

Antibiotic associated colitis and diarrhea

Refer to ∞ Chapter 36 to review infectious diseases of the genital system.

Another toxin called exfoliatin or epidermolytic toxin results in a sloughing off the epidermal layer. It produces scalded skin syndrome, which characteristically occurs in neonates and previously healthy children. The toxin causes the skin to blister. The blisters rupture, and the skin peels off in large sheets. ∞ Chapter 37, "The Integumentary System," provides additional information on skin infections. Table 17-2✪ provides a listing of *S. aureus* exotoxins and their actions.

Other Infectious Diseases. *S. aureus* is known to cause skin infections such as impetigo, eye infections, and systemic infections such as osteomyelitis. Its ability to colonize intravenous (IV) catheters and surgically implanted devices, such as artificial joints, has resulted in an increase in sepsis caused by this organism (Fournier & Philpott, 2005). It is a rare cause of antibiotic-associated diarrhea. Antibiotic use inhibits the normal gastrointestinal flora, allowing *S. aureus* to proliferate and produce toxins. Refer to ∞ Chapters 32, "Cardiovascular System," 35, "Gastrointestinal System," 37, "The Integumentary System," 38, "Central Nervous System," and 39, "Skeletal System," to review skin, eye, bone marrow, and other systemic infections.

S. aureus is one of three microorganisms associated with higher morbidity and mortality in cystic fibrosis patients. The doctor should be notified of their presence in the respiratory cultures of these patients (Shreve et al., 1999). It is often a small-colony variant because of long-term use of trimethoprim-sulfamethoxazole. Refer to ∞ Chapter 33, "Respiratory System," for more information about the organisms associated with cystic fibrosis patients.

S. aureus is the most frequently isolated invasive nosocomial pathogen (Fournier & Philpott, 2005). One of the most troubling characteristics of these isolates is their resistance to methicillin and the potential for development of reduced susceptibility to vancomycin. A recent study estimates the incidence of invasive methicillin-resistant *S. aureus* or MRSA infections at approximately 94,360 with 18,650 deaths (Klevens et al., 2007). Most of these infections are health care associated, but community-associated infections began emerging in 1981 (Chambers, 2001).

There are apparent differences between the health care–associated methicillin-resistant *S. aureus* (HA-MRSA) and the community-associated methicillin-resistant *S. aureus* (CA-MRSA). HA-MRSA is multi-drug-resistant, whereas CA-MRSA is susceptible to most non-beta-lactam antibiotics. The CA-MRSA isolates are more likely to possess the ability to produce a necrotic cytotoxin known as Panton-Valentine leukocidin (PVL; Klevens et al., 2007).

HA-MRSA infections include surgical wound infections, urinary tract infections, bloodstream infections, and pneumonia. These nosocomial infections occur in patients with weakened immune systems. CA-MRSA occurs in healthy individuals and may present as a "spider-bite," pimple, boil, or other skin infection (CDC, 2005). Life-threatening infections associated with CA-MRSA include necrotizing fasciitis and severe necrotizing pneumonia (Gillet et al., 2002; Miller et al., 2005). PVL is the cause of the necrosis.

Risk factors for HA-MRSA include admission to an intensive care unit, prior antibiotic treatment, surgery, and exposure to a MRSA colonized patient. Groups at higher risk for CA-MRSA include those who are younger, athletes, military recruits, prisoners, Alaska natives, Native Americans, Pacific Islanders, and men having sex with men (CDC, 2005; Davis et al., 2007). Factors increasing the chance of infection include contaminated items and surfaces, shared items such towels, crowded living conditions, poor hygiene, and breaks in the skin (CDC, 2005).

S. aureus resistant to both methicillin and vancomycin was first isolated in the United States in 2002 (Périchon & Courvalin, 2004). Vancomycin-resistant *S. aureus* (VRSA) are believed to have acquired the *van*A gene for vancomycin resistance from vancomycin-resistant *Enterococcus* spp. (VRE). A two year study reported a high prevalence of VRE/MRSA co-colonization upon admission to an intensive care unit at a tertiary care hospital. The authors believe that these patients are at higher risk of acquiring and transmitting VRSA (Furuno et al., 2005). Adherence to infection control practices such as wearing gloves and washing hands can reduce the spread of VISA/VRSA (CDC, 2003). ∞ Chapter 5, "Safety," reviews infection control practices. Consult ∞ Chapter 41 for more information on nosocomial infections.

✪ TABLE 17-2

Staphylococcus aureus Exotoxins and Their Actions

Exotoxins	Actions
Alpha-hemolysin	Lyses red blood cells
	Causes skin cell death
	Damages nervous tissue
Beta-hemolysin	Lyses red blood cells
Gamma-hemolysin	Lyses red blood cells
	Lyses neutrophils and macrophages
Delta-hemolysin	Lyses red blood cells
	Disrupts cell membranes
Toxic shock syndrome toxin-1 (TSST-1)	Reactivates bacterial cell wall–induced arthritis
	Increases lethal effect of endotoxin on susceptible host
	Causes nonspecific T-lymphocyte proliferation
	Causes fever
Staphylococcal enterotoxins (A-E, G-I)	Causes vomiting
	Causes nonspecific T-lymphocyte proliferation
	Causes fever
Exfoliative toxins (A & B)	Causes detachment and shedding of epidermis
	Causes nonspecific T-lymphocyte proliferation
Leukocidin	Lyses neutrophils and macrophages

Checkpoint! 17–7 (Chapter Objective 5)

A direct smear of pus from a surgical incision reveals polymorphonuclear leukocytes and gram-positive cocci in clusters. The colonies on sheep blood agar are beta-hemolytic, white, and butyrous. There is no growth on MacConkey agar. The organism bubbles with 3% hydrogen peroxide, displays a smooth suspension on the slide coagulase test and clots in the tube coagulase test. The organism is most likely:

   A. *Staphylococcus epidermidis*
   B. *S. aureus*
   C. *S. lugdunensis*
   D. *Micrococcus spp.*

◆ Other Coagulase-Positive Staphylococci

Staphylococcal species, other than *S. aureus*, may be coagulase positive with commercial latex agglutination tests because they possess clumping factor or bound coagulase. These include *S. lugdunensis* and *S. intermedius*. Other species, *S. schleiferi* ssp. *coagulans*, *S. hyicus*, and *S. intermedius*, may produce extracellular or free coagulase so they will be tube coagulase positive. Some of these organisms are also thermonuclease positive. They include *S. lugdunensis*, *S. schleiferi*, *S. hyicus*, and *S. intermedius*. Differentiation of these organisms should be considered on a case-by-case basis after consultation with the physician.

Identification

Most of the time identification is complete when a coagulase-positive *Staphylococcus* is detected. Physicians usually treat any coagulase-positive *Staphylococcus* as clinically significant and accept its identification by the laboratory as *S. aureus*. *S. aureus* and other coagulase-positive species can be found in farm and domesticated animals such as dogs, horses, fowl, pigs, and cattle. Further speciation may be appropriate in the case of a dog bite or exposure to other animal sources. These animal isolates are rarely isolated in humans even with frequent exposure to animals.

Colony Morphology. The colonies of other coagulase-positive *Staphylococcus* often resemble a nonhemolytic *S. aureus*. They may present as a 1 to 2 mm, white, opaque, nonhemolytic colony. *S. lugdunensis* may be weakly hemolytic and have a yellow-orange pigment after 3 to 5 days (Forbes et al., 1998). *S. intermedius* can be beta-hemolytic. These organisms may also produce yellow colonies on MSA, similar to *S. aureus*, because of fermentation of mannitol.

Key Biochemical Reactions. If a commercial coagulase latex agglutination test positive *Staphylococcus* spp. is isolated from a sterile body site or dog bite, a laboratory may perform additional tests to confirm a *S. aureus* identification. Table 17-3✪ lists key biochemical reactions for differentiating *S. aureus* from the other coagulase-positive *Staphylococcus* spp. associated with human infections. *S. lugdunensis* and *S. schleiferi* subsp. *schleiferi* are tube coagulase negative. *S. lugdunensis*, *S. schleiferi* subsp. *schleiferi*, and *S. intermedius* are pyrrolidonyl arylamidase (PYR) positive, whereas *S. aureus* subsp. *aureus* is PYR negative. *S. aureus* subsp. *aureus* is VP positive, whereas *S. intermedius* is VP negative. *S. schleiferi* subsp. *coagulans* and *S. hyicus* are nitrate positive, whereas *S. aureus* subsp. *anaerobius* is nitrate negative. *S. schleiferi* subsp. *coagulans* is VP positive, whereas *S. hyicus* and *S. aureus* subsp. *anaerobius* are VP negative (MacFaddin, 2000).

Clinical Significance

S. intermedius, *S. schleiferi* subsp. *coagulans*, and *S. hyicus* are **opportunistic** pathogens of animals and are rarely isolated from human specimens (Mahon, Lehman, & Manuselis, 2007). Opportunistic pathogens are organisms that can cause disease only in patients whose defenses are impaired. Dog bite wounds have yielded *S. intermedius* (Koneman et al., 1997).

✪ TABLE 17-3

Key Biochemical Reactions of Coagulase-Positive *Staphylococcus* spp. Commonly Associated with Human Infection

| Species | Tube Coag | CF | PYR | Heat Stable Thermonuclease | Polymyxin B Resistance | Orn | VP | Nitrate | Acid from: | |
									Treh	Mann
S. aureus ssp. *aureus*	+	+	−	+	+	−	+	+	+	+
S. aureus ssp. *anaerobius*	+	−	ND	+	ND	ND	−	−	−	−
S. schleiferi ssp. *coagulans*	+	−	ND	+	ND	−	+	+	−	v
S. hyicus	v	−	−	+	+	−	−	+	+	−
S. intermedius	+	v	+	+	−	−	−	+	+	(v)
S. schleiferi ssp. *schleiferi*	−	+	+	+	−	−	+	+	v	−
S lugdunensis	−	(+)	+	−	v	+	+	+	+	−

+ = positive; − = negative; v = variable; ( ) = delayed reaction; ND = no data; Tube Coag = extracellular or free coagulase; CF = clumping factor; PYR = pyrrolidonyl arylamidase; Orn = ornithine decarboxylase; VP = Voges-Proskauer; Treh = trehalose; Mann = mannitol

S. lugdunensis and *S. schleiferi* subsp. *schleiferi,* both potential human microbes, are tube coagulase negative, and their clinical significance is described with the other tube coagulase-negative *Staphylococcus* spp.

Coagulase-Negative Staphylococci

Coagulase-negative staphylococci (CNS) are common isolates from clinical specimens. They are frequently regarded as contaminants but may cause disease in **compromised** individuals or those whose underlying illness or therapy has diminished their host defenses. Approximately 75% of coagulase-negative staphylococci are resistant to methicillin. Infections caused by CNS are usually treated with vancomycin (Srinivasan, Dick, & Perl, 2002). One should be suspect of any coagulase-negative staphylococci whose susceptibility result indicates intermediate or resistant results for vancomycin or is not sensitive to linezolid (NCCLS, 2003). Refer to ∞ Chapter 11 to review staphylococci susceptibility testing protocols.

◆ *Staphylococcus epidermidis*

The second most commonly isolated *Staphylococcus* species is *S. epidermidis.* It represents 50% to 80% of all coagulase-negative *Staphylococcus* isolates (Koneman et al., 1997). It is also a member of the commensal flora of skin and mucous membranes lining the body's orifices. Distinguishing it from the known pathogen *S. aureus* is the primary aim of testing.

Identification

In most clinical laboratories a commercial latex agglutination test for clumping factor is used to differentiate *S. aureus* from the other species. If negative, the isolate is reported as coagulase-negative *Staphylococcus* spp. Additional testing is necessary if the laboratory needs to specifically identify *S. epidermidis.*

Colony Morphology.   The typical colony morphology of *S. epidermidis* is that of a 1 to 2 mm gray-white, opaque, nonhemolytic colony (Forbes et al., 1998). ∞ Chapter 8, "Presumptive Identification," contains a photo of *S. epidermidis* on sheep blood agar. Variations have been observed. Traditionally the lack of beta-hemolytic activity decreases the chances that one is dealing with *S. aureus.* Exceptions do occur, however, and further testing is necessary. *S. epidermidis* will grow on MSA, but the media usually remains red and the colonies are small.

Key Biochemical Reactions.   When a staphylococcal Gram stain and colony appearance is observed, it is important to screen the colony for catalase. If positive, a test to detect coagulase is performed. *S. epidermidis* is slide and tube coagulase negative. Many laboratories stop testing once the pathogen *S. aureus* is ruled out and report the isolate as coagulase-negative *Staphylococcus* spp. or *Staphylococcus* spp. not *S. aureus.* When isolated in pure culture or repeatedly from sterile body fluids and sites, especially in compromised patients, further testing may be necessary for speciation (Murray et al., 1999). Consultation with the physician is helpful in determining whether to perform further identification and susceptibility tests.

A test for acid production from trehalose-mannitol broth is useful, as *S. epidermidis* is negative and most of the other coagulase-negative staphylococci are positive. Those that may also be negative in this test can be ruled out by checking for resistance to novobiocin and polymyxin B. *S. epidermidis* is sensitive to novobiocin and resistant to polymyxin B. Figure 17-12 ■ provides a possible identification scheme for *Staphylococcus* spp. Refer to Table 17-4✪ to review key biochemical reactions that distinguish the clinically significant coagulase-negative *Staphylococcus* spp.

Clinical Significance

S. epidermidis is part of the normal flora in many body sites. Often, when isolated, it is usually suspected of being a contaminant. It resides normally on skin and is especially fond of plastic medical devices. It grows on and around indwelling intravenous and urinary catheters. It is capable of generating a slime layer or biofilm that protects it against phagocytosis and antibiotics (Koneman et al., 1997). Once it establishes residence in an indwelling intravenous catheter, it can easily gain access to the bloodstream via the catheter's insertion site. In compromised patients it may cause a variety of prosthetic (artificial) device associated and systemic infections. It is also a common cause of hospital-acquired urinary tract infections (Mandell et al., 2000). Box 17-2 ✪ provides a list of diseases associated with coagulase-negative *Staphylococcus* spp. Refer to ∞ Chapters 40 and 41 to learn more about opportunistic and nosocomial infections.

◆ *Staphylococcus saprophyticus*

Another member of the genus *Staphylococcus* that can be significant is *S. saprophyticus.* It may be necessary to identify this organism to species if a suspect colony is isolated from the urine of a female.

Identification

Colony Morphology.   The colony of *S. saprophyticus* (Figure 17-13 ■) resembles the other coagulase-negative staphylococci. It is usually a white, opaque, nonhemolytic colony approximately 2 mm in size. Some strains are very white and appear almost fluorescent white. Occasional yellow or orange colonies occur (Forbes et al., 1998). Small colonies that may or may not ferment mannitol can be observed on MSA.

Key Biochemical Reactions.   When a white, opaque, nonhemolytic colony is isolated and appears as a gram-positive cocci in a Gram stained smear, perform a catalase test. If it is catalase positive, perform a test for coagulase. If the isolate is coagulase negative, it may be reported as a coagulase-negative *Staphylococcus* spp. unless it was isolated from the urine of a female. If isolated from urine, a test for resistance to novobiocin is also performed. A catalase-positive, coagulase-

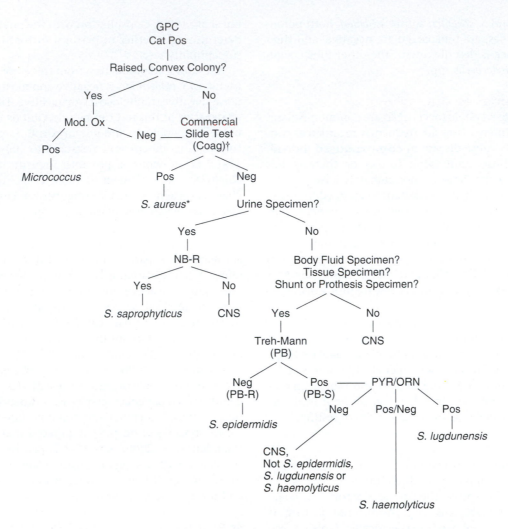

■ **FIGURE 17-12** Identification of clinically significant *Staphylococcus*. Pos = positive; Neg = negative; GPC = gram-positive cocci; Cat = catalase; Mod. Ox = modified oxidase; Coag = coagulase; ( ) = alternate test procedure; NB = Novobiocin; R = resistant; S = susceptible; CNS = coagulase-negative *Staphylococcus* spp.; Treh-Mann = trehalose-mannitol broth; PB = Polymyxin B; PYR/ORN = pyrrolidonase/ornithine decarboxylase.

†If delayed reaction (on sterile body site), rule out S. lugdunensis with PYR, tube coagulase, and ornithine decarboylase.

*If dog bite, rule out S. intermedius with PYR. If sterile body site, rule out S. schleiferi with PYR, tube coagulase, and ornithine decarboxylase.

negative gram-positive cocci that is resistant to novobiocin is presumptively identified as *S. saprophyticus*. ∞ Chapter 34 presents information on processing urine specimens.

Clinical Significance

S. saprophyticus is associated with urinary tract infections in young sexually active females (Murray et al., 1999). It is the most commonly isolated coagulase-negative *Staphylococcus* spp. from community-acquired urinary tract infections (Mandell et al., 2000). It adheres to the epithelial cells that line the urinary system. It also produces urease, which helps its invasiveness into bladder tissue (Kloos & Bannerman, 1994). When symptoms or white blood cells are present, significant numbers of coagulase-negative *Staphylococcus* spp. may require further testing to identify the organism. *S. saprophyticus* can be significant in counts <100,000 colonies/mL in infected females.

✪ TABLE 17-4

Key Biochemical Reactions of Coagulase-Negative *Staphylococcus* spp. Commonly Associated with Human Infection

Species	Tube Coag	CF	PYR	Urease	Heat Stable Thermonuclease	Novobiocin Resistance	Polymyxin B Resistance	Orn	Acid from: Treh	Mann	Aerobic Growth	Anaerobic Growth
S. epidermidis	−	−	−	+	−	−	+	(v)	−	−	+	+
S. haemolyticus	−	−	+	−	−	−	−	−	+	v	+	(+)
S. warneri	−	−	−	+	−	−	−	−	+	v	+	+
S. saprophyticus	−	−	−	+	−	+	−	−	+	v	+	(+)
S. hominis ssp. hominis	−	−	−	+	−	−	−	−	v	−	+	−
S. hominis ssp. novobiosepticus	−	−	−	+	−	+	ND	−	−	−	+	−
S. lugdunensis	−	(+)	+	v	−	−	v	+	+	−	+	+
S. schleiferi ssp. schleiferi	−	+	+	−	+	−	−	−	v	−	+	+

+ = positive; − = negative; ( ) = delayed reaction; v = variable; ND = no data; Tube Coag = extracellular or free coagulase; CF = clumping factor; PYR = pyrrolidonyl arylamidase; Orn = ornithine decarboxylase; Treh = trehalose; Mann = mannitol

A pure isolation of the organism in urine, regardless of the count, should be pursued. *S. saprophyticus* may also cause non-gonococcal urethritis in males and females and prostatitis in males. It has been rarely associated with wound and blood-stream infections (Murray et al., 1999).

✓ Checkpoint! 17–8 (Chapter Objective 5)

A urine culture, on a 26-year-old female, grew >100,000 colonies/mL of a white, opaque, nonhemolytic colony. The colony stained as a gram-positive cocci, bubbled with 3% hydrogen peroxide, did not clot plasma in the tube coagulase test, and grew up to the edge of a novobiocin disk. It should be reported as:

    A. *S. aureus.*
    B. *coagulase-negative Staphylococcus spp.*
    C. *S. epidermidis.*
    D. *S. saprophyticus.*

◆ Other Coagulase-Negative Staphylococci

Gram-positive cocci that are catalase positive and coagulase negative may be significant if isolated from sterile body sites. Some species may be multi-drug-resistant and mimic MRSA and VISA/VRSA. It may be important to speciate such organisms to document the role they play in causing infectious disease and avoid misidentification.

Identification

Colony Morphology. This group of microorganisms may be suspected when a 3 to 5 mm, cream to yellow-orange, opaque, nonhemolytic colony, which stains as gram-positive

cocci, is observed (Murray et al., 1999). The colony of *S. lugdunensis* can be very pleomorphic in size and resemble a mixed culture rather than a pure isolation. It can be white to yellow with beta-hemolysis and has a unique haylike odor. If the isolate is cultured from a nonsterile body site, identification usually stops, and it is reported as a member of the normal flora present. If isolated from a sterile body site, consultation with the physician or the laboratory standard operating procedures may be necessary to determine the level of speciation and susceptibility testing necessary.

Key Biochemical Reactions. If speciation is necessary, additional tests are required. These may include pyrrolidonyl

✪ BOX 17-2

Infectious Diseases Associated with Coagulase-Negative *Staphylococcus* spp.

Endocarditis
Bacteremia
Intravenous catheter infection
Cerebrospinal fluid shunt infection
Continuous ambulatory peritoneal dialysis associated peritonitis
Osteomyelitis
Wound infection
Vascular graft infection
Prosthetic joint infection
Urinary tract infection
Brain empyema
Breast abscess
Endophthalmitis after ocular surgery
Mediastinitis

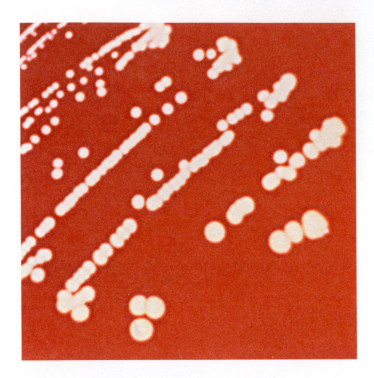

■ **FIGURE 17-13** *S. saprophyticus* on sheep blood agar.
Photo courtesy of Remel, part of Thermo Fisher Scientific.

arylamidase (PYR), ornithine decarboxylase (ORN), and tests for resistance to novobiocin and polymyxin B. See Figure 17-12 and Table 17-4 for more specific information on possible biochemical choices.

Clinical Significance

The coagulase-negative *Staphylococcus* species are usually members of the normal flora of skin but may be clinically significant when isolated from immunocompromised individuals. They are also associated with infections arising from invasive medical procedures, indwelling medical devices and systemic infections such as septicemia and endocarditis (Koneman et al., 1997).

S. haemolyticus is the second most commonly isolated coagulase-negative *Staphylococcus* spp. It is multi-drug-resistant and may have reduced sensitivity to vancomycin (Murray, Baron, Jorgensen, Pfaller, & Yolken, 2003; Srinivasan et al., 2002). Additional testing should be performed to ensure it is not confused with a vancomycin-intermediate or -resistant *S. aureus*.

The coagulase-negative *S. lugdunensis* is an infrequent isolate that can be associated with clinically significant infections. It follows an aggressive, destructive clinical course which resembles that of *S. aureus*. This may be because of its virulence factor, δ (delta)-like toxin, which resembles the δ-toxin of *S. aureus*. Endocarditis caused by this organism is accompanied by high morbidity and mortality rates of up to 70% (Frank, Reichert, Piper, & Patel, 2007).

Accurate identification of *S. lugdunensis* is important for proper treatment of the infection. Some strains of *S. lugdunensis* possess clumping factor and can be positive on some rapid agglutination tests. This may cause the microbiologist to misidentify the organism as *S. aureus*. *S. lugdunensis* can be weakly beta-hemolytic and yellow on sheep blood agar making it even more difficult to differentiate from the typical yellow, beta-hemolytic colony of *S. aureus*. In addition some strains may be resistant to methicillin and display tolerance for vancomycin (Frank et al., 2007). Most *S. lugdunensis* strains are *mecA* gene negative and beta-lactamase negative, so penicillin can be used as its drug of choice. Positive PYR and ornithine tests and negative tube coagulase will differentiate it from *S. aureus* (Tan, Ng, & He, 2008).

▶ CATALASE NEGATIVE

If a gram-positive cocci is observed on a smear of a gray or clear, translucent colony, *Enterococcus* spp., *Streptococcus* spp. or related *Streptococcus*-like genera should be suspected. The catalase test is the most helpful, easiest, and least expensive screening test used to differentiate *Staphylococcus* spp. from *Enterococcus* spp. and *Streptococcus* spp. A negative result is characteristic of *Enterococcus* spp., *Streptococcus* spp. and some of the related genera. A weak positive could still indicate *Enterococcus* spp. or one of the related genera. It is very important that the test be performed correctly to avoid false positives.

> **ⓔ REAL WORLD TIP**
>
> Accidentally picking up red blood cells from sheep blood agar along with the colony can cause a false-positive catalase reaction. Red blood cells possess the catalase enzyme. Test a piece of the agar with the catalase reagent and compare the result with that of the organism. This will help determine if the positive result is because of red blood cells from the medium or the organism.

Gram stain morphology is an essential part of the identification strategy for the catalase-negative gram-positive cocci. The best microscopic morphology and cellular arrangement is obtained from staining growth from liquid thioglycollate medium. Close attention must be paid to arrangement of the cocci. Note whether the cocci are round and arranged in clusters or tetrads consistent with *Staphylococcus* spp. Oval cocci in pairs and chains are suggestive of *Enterococcus* spp. and *Streptococcus* spp. *Streptococcus pneumoniae* characteristically appears as football-shaped cocci in pairs or diplococci. These arrangements provide preliminary clues to the possible identity of an unknown catalase-negative cocci. Some species of this group of organisms can appear gram negative if the cells are old or the patient is receiving antibiotic therapy. The Gram stain procedure and potential sources of errors are discussed in ∞ Chapter 8, "Presumptive Identification."

USEFUL BIOCHEMICAL TESTS

Several biochemical tests are available to screen, identify, and differentiate the catalase-negative aerobic gram-positive cocci. Biochemical tests useful for identification of the beta-hemolytic streptococci include the pyrrolidonase (PYR) test and the serogroup antigen test. The gamma and alpha-hemolytic streptococci are often identified using the optochin or bile solubility test, PYR test, growth in 6.5% NaCl broth, and bile esculin test. The leucine aminopeptidase (LAP) test is useful in the detection of other *Streptococcus*-related cocci, which can resemble the more commonly isolated *Enterococcus* spp. and *Streptococcus* spp. In addition to describing these tests, other tests that may be useful to speciate these organisms are included later in this chapter.

L-pyrrolidonyl Arylamidase or Pyrrolidonase (PYR) Hydrolysis Test

The PYR test is positive for the *Enterococcus* spp., *Streptococcus pyogenes,* animal associated beta-hemolytic streptococci such as *Streptococcus porcinus,* and a few of the other related streptococcus-like cocci. For accurate results ensure only well-isolated colonies or pure cultures are tested (Murray et al., 1999). The test is available as a broth, agar, or disk. The disk test is performed by rubbing some of the colony onto filter paper impregnated with the substrate, L-pyrrolidonyl-β-naphthylamide (PYR). If the organism hydrolyzes the substrate, a pink to red color occurs after the color developing reagent is added. This is a positive result. The PYR test has been combined with the esculin hydrolysis test on the same disk for the identification of *Enterococcus* spp. and Group D *Streptococcus.* ∞ Chapter 8, "Presumptive Identification," provides a photo of the PYR test and further information about it.

∞ Chapter 8, "Presumptive Identification,"

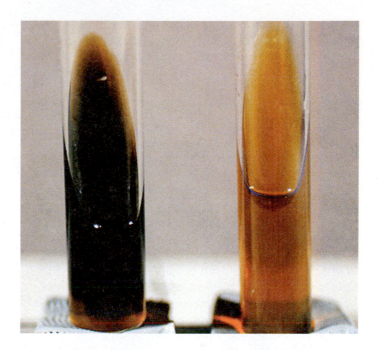

■ **FIGURE 17-14** Positive (left) and negative (right) reaction on bile-esculin agar.

the other related *Streptococcus*-like cocci. It should be used in conjunction with the 6.5% NaCl broth. It is available as a rapid disk test. In the rapid test, intact esculin fluoresces under ultraviolet light. When esculin is broken down, its by-products do not fluoresce under ultraviolet light and appear as a dark spot where the organism was inoculated. To review the rapid esculin hydrolysis test, visit ∞ Chapter 8, "Presumptive Identification."

6.5% NaCl

The 6.5% NaCl test, as observed in Figure 17-15 ■, determines an organism's ability to grow in a high salt concentration. Members of the genus *Enterococcus* spp., *Streptococcus agalactiae,* as

Bile Esculin (BE)

The BE test, as seen in Figure 17-14 ■, assesses the organism's ability to grow in the presence of 20 to 40% bile and produce the enzyme esculinase. If the organism grows on the medium, it is able to tolerate the bile present. If a black precipitate forms in the medium, the organism produces the esculinase enzyme, which hydrolyzes the esculin present. The BE test is positive for the *Enterococcus* spp., and the group D *Streptococcus, Streptococcus gallolyticus* (previously known as *S. bovis*), as well as a few of

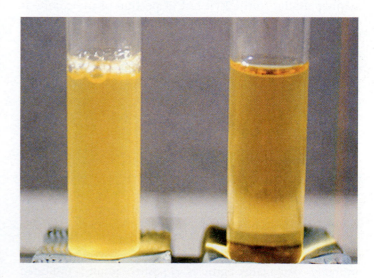

■ FIGURE 17-15 Positive (right) and negative (left) 6.5% NaCl broth.

well as some of the related *Streptococcus*-like organisms, can grow in this medium. A positive result is indicated by turbidity. A light inoculum is necessary to avoid a false positive reaction.

 REAL WORLD TIP

The BE test and 6.5% NaCl broth were once used exclusively to identify *Enterococcus* spp. Because of the increased use of vancomycin for the treatment of MRSA, vancomycin-resistant catalase-negative gram-positive cocci, such as vancomycin-resistant *Enterococcus* spp. (VRE), *Pediococcus* spp., and *Leuconostoc* spp., have emerged. These three organisms are all BE positive and show growth in 6.5% NaCl broth. *Pediococcus* spp. and *Leuconostoc* spp. are not considered an infection control issue because their resistance mechanism cannot be transferred to other organisms, whereas VRE are significant nosocomial pathogens. The LAP and PYR tests will differentiate the three organisms.

 ## Checkpoint! 17–9 (Chapter Objective 3)

The 6.5% NaCl test is considered positive when one observes:
   A. *blackening in the media.*
   B. *inhibition of growth.*
   C. *growth in the broth.*
   D. *an arrowhead or flame-shaped clearing.*

Leucine Aminopeptidase (LAP)

The LAP test (Figure 17-16 ■) detects the presence of the enzyme leucine aminopeptidase. The test is performed in a manner similar to the PYR test. A portion of the colony is rubbed onto filter paper impregnated with the substrate leucine-β-naphthylamine. Formation of a pink to red color after addition of the color developing reagent is a positive result. The color developer is the same one used for the PYR test. *Enterococcus* spp., *Streptococcus* spp., and some of the other related cocci are LAP positive. A negative result may indicate one of the other *Streptococcus*-related genera. The LAP test is often used in combination with the PYR and esculin tests.

Serogroup Antigen Tests

Commercially prepared latex kits, like that pictured in Figure 17-17 ■, are available to detect the group specific carbohydrate antigen located on the cell wall of beta-hemolytic catalase-negative cocci and non-beta-hemolytic Group D cocci. Most kits use acid or enzymes along with heat to expose the antigen on the cell wall. This extract is then reacted with group-specific antibody-coated latex particles. A positive result is indicated by agglutination. These antigens were first described in the

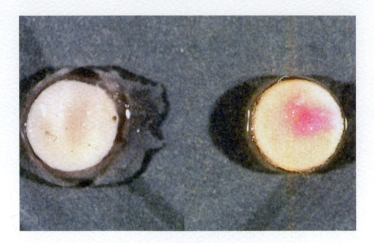

■ **FIGURE 17-16** Negative (left) and positive (right) LAP test.

1930s by Rebecca Lancefield. The most common antigens tested are Lancefield groups A, B, C, D, F, and G (Koneman et al., 1997). Commercial kits using coagglutination or enzyme-linked immunoassay methods are also available (Forbes et al., 1998).

Groups A, C, D, and G beta-hemolytic streptococci can share antigens with other species such as *S. anginosus* and *S. constellatus*. Additional testing may be necessary to confirm the identification and distinguish clinically significant isolates from normal flora (Ruoff, Hinnebusch, Glenn, & Cohen, 1999). Review the package insert of the kit in use for specific information on possible cross-reactions. Further information on this topic is provided later in this chapter.

Strep Screens

Remel (Thermo Fisher Scientific, Lenexa, KS) markets the Bacti-Card Strep, as shown in Figure 17-18 ■, which provides for quick screening of catalase-negative cocci. It includes the PYR, LAP, and esculin tests. The Visi-Spot Card, manufactured by J & S

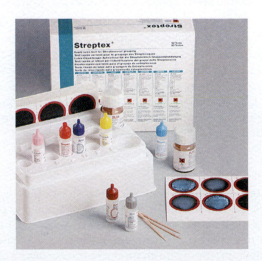

■ **FIGURE 17-17** Positive and negative results for the Streptex test kit.
Photo courtesy of Remel, part of Thermo Fisher Scientific.

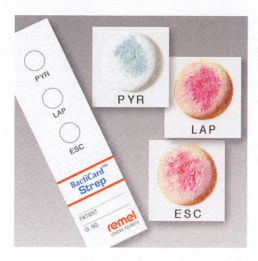

■ **FIGURE 17-18** Positive reactions for the BactiCard Strep.
Photo courtesy of Remel, part of Thermo Fisher Scientific.

Medical Associates (Framingham, MA) and available from Hardy Diagnostics (Santa Maria, CA), combines the PYR and esculin tests. The esculin test measures esculinase activity but does not test for bile tolerance as in the BE test. One can expect a BE positive organism to be esculin positive, but remember that the esculin test tells the microbiologist nothing about the organism's ability to grow in the presence of bile. Additional testing is necessary for presumptive identification. See previous descriptions of these tests in this chapter.

Bacitracin (Taxo A)

The bacitracin test is performed by placing the test disk on the surface of a sheep blood agar plate, which is either part of a direct specimen culture or a subculture of the suspected organism. The bacitracin or Taxo A disk is then placed in the center of the primary inoculated area. The disk contains 0.04 units of the antibiotic bacitracin. If this concentration inhibits the growth of the test organism after overnight incubation, a zone of no growth is observed. Any zone of inhibition is considered a positive reaction.

Historically this test was used to presumptively identify group A beta-hemolytic streptococci. It is no longer recom-

 REAL WORLD TIP

The sensitivity of the bacitracin disk can be increased by adding a trimethoprim-sulfamethoxazole (SXT) disk. *S. pyogenes* is susceptible to bacitracin but resistant to SXT. Other beta-hemolytic *Streptococcus* spp. are usually susceptible to SXT. The bacitracin and SXT disk tests require 24 hours for interpretation. The PYR test is more specific for the identification of Group A beta-hemolytic *Streptococcus (S. pyogenes)* and only takes 10 minutes for results.

mended for this purpose because groups C and G beta-hemolytic streptococci may also be inhibited by bacitracin (Forbes et al., 1998). Now the PYR and serogroup antigen tests have replaced the bacitracin (Taxo A) disk for routine use. The disk can also be used to distinguish the small beta-hemolytic colony type, *S. anginosus, S. constellatus,* and *S. intermedius* previously known as the "*S. milleri*" group, from the large-colony type, *S. pyogenes. Streptococcus pyogenes* is sensitive, and the others are resistant (Murray et al., 1999). ∞ Chapter 9, "Final Identification," summarizes the bacitracin (Taxo A) test.

CAMP Test

The name of the CAMP test is an acronym of its discoverers, Christie, Atkins, and Munch-Petersen. It detects the production of CAMP factor, a diffusible, extracellular protein (Murray et al., 2003). CAMP factor interacts with a beta-hemolysin (beta-lysin) produced by certain strains of *S. aureus*. The interaction of the two produces an enhanced hemolysis of the beta-lysin. Most laboratories use the ATCC 25923 strain of *S. aureus* as the source of beta-lysin. The result is the lysis of the medium's sheep blood cells in the area where the CAMP factor and beta-lysin meet (MacFaddin, 2000). The CAMP reaction uses a streak line of growth of a beta-lysin-producing strain of *Staphylococcus aureus* down the center of a sheep blood agar. Disks containing the beta-lysin compound are also commercially available. The unknown organism is struck at a right angle to the line of *Staphylococcus aureus* inoculum or disk. The unknown organism should be placed as close as possible to the *Staphylococcus aureus* line or disk but without touching. The test plate is incubated in ambient air at 35°C overnight. The use of a CO_2 environment for incubation can cause false-positive results with non-group B *Streptococcus* spp. (MacFaddin, 2000).

If the unknown streptococcus produces CAMP factor, beta-hemolysis is enhanced where the two organisms meet. A positive result is indicated by an arrowhead-shaped zone of complete hemolysis, as seen in Figure 17-19 ■, much wider than the zone produced by the organism itself. Production of CAMP factor is characteristic of *Streptococcus agalactiae* or group B *Streptococcus. S. iniae,* a fish pathogen and very rare human isolate, is also CAMP positive. It differs from group B by its positive PYR and VP results. *Listeria monocytogenes* is also CAMP positive, but its pattern resembles more of a shovel rather than an arrowhead. Refer to ∞ Chapter 19 for more information on *Listeria* spp. and other gram-positive rods.

 REAL WORLD TIP

The CAMP test is considered a presumptive test for the identification of group B *Streptococcus*. Its result must be used in combination with other tests for the definitive identification of this organism. The latex agglutination test using group B specific antibody is considered a definitive test.

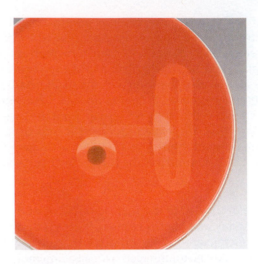

■ **FIGURE 17-19** Positive arrowhead result for the CAMP Test.
Photo courtesy of Remel, part of Thermo Fisher Scientific.

Hippurate Hydrolysis

The hippurate test, as observed in Figure 17-20 ■, can replace the CAMP test for identification of group B streptococci. It is still considered a presumptive identification test. If the unknown organism possesses hippurate hydrolase or hippuricase, it will break down sodium hippurate into benzoate and glycine. There are two methods for detection of the end products: one for benzoate and one for glycine. The detection of benzoate is determined by the persistence of a heavy precipitate. The rapid method detects glycine producing a deep purple color. Group B *Streptococcus* produces a positive reaction in both methods. Other organisms, including *Listeria* spp., *Enterococcus* spp., and *Staphylococcus* spp., are also positive. ∞ Chapter 9, "Final Identification," summarizes the hippurate hydrolysis test.

Optochin (Taxo P)

The Taxo P or optochin (pronounced ŏp-tōe-kĭn) disk contains the chemical ethylhydrocupreine hydrochloride. It is used to differentiate *Streptococcus pneumoniae* from other alpha-hemolytic *Streptococcus* spp. *S. pneumoniae* is sensitive to the chemical and produces a zone of inhibition. To perform the test, a catalase-negative alpha-hemolytic colony is inoculated onto sheep blood agar to produce a solid lawn of growth. The optochin or Taxo P disk is aseptically applied to the agar surface. The plate is incubated in CO_2 overnight. Most identification tests are not incubated in CO_2. *S. pneumoniae* is fastidious and requires CO_2 for growth, and so the test must be incubated in a carbon dioxide atmosphere.

To properly interpret the results, the zone of inhibition must be measured. If using the 6 mm disk, a zone of 14 mm or greater is considered a sensitive result (Gardam & Miller, 1998). With the 10 mm disk, a zone of 16 mm or greater is sensitive (MacFaddin, 2000). Alpha-hemolytic streptococci other than *S. pneumoniae* are not inhibited by optochin (Taxo P) and show no zone of inhibition. Suspicious isolates with smaller zones require further testing, such as bile solubility (Murray et al., 1999). ∞ Chapter 8, "Presumptive Identification," provides a photo of a sensitive optochin (Taxo P) result.

Bile Solubility

Streptococcus pneumoniae possesses an autolytic enzyme that can be activated by bile salts such as sodium deoxycholate. This results in lysis of the cell wall. The liquid reagent is dropped onto an 18- to 24-hour-old colony on agar. Bile solubility is indicated by the disappearance of the colony within 30 minutes. The area of alpha-hemolysis remains. If the tube test, as seen in Figure 17-21 ■, is performed, a slightly turbid suspension of the organism will clear with the addition of sodium deoxycholate indicating bile solubility. Approximately

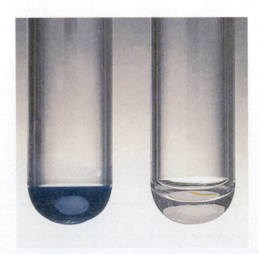

■ **FIGURE 17-20** Positive (left) and negative (right) reactions for the hippurate hydrolysis test.
Photo courtesy of Remel, part of Thermo Fisher Scientific.

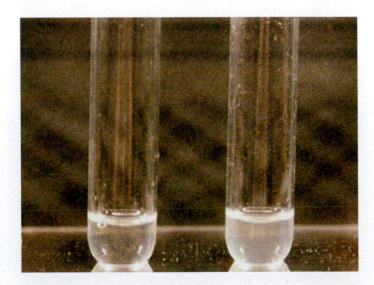

■ **FIGURE 17-21** Tube bile solubility positive (left) and negative (right) reactions.

5% to 10% of *S. pneumoniae* can be insoluble in bile, so additional testing may be required if incomplete lysis occurs.

When performing a spot bile solubility test on a colony, ensure the agar plate remains level and does not move around too much after addition of the reagent. An insoluble colony can wash away with too much movement. This creates a false solubility reaction.

Checkpoint! 17–10 (Chapter Objective 2)

A rapid test for differentiating Streptococcus pneumoniae *from other alpha-hemolytic streptococcal colonies is:*

A. *inulin fermentation.*
B. *the catalase reaction.*
C. *bile solubility.*
D. *optochin susceptibility.*

Voges-Proskauer (VP)

The VP test is used to detect acetylmethcarbinol or acetoin produced by *Streptococcus anginosus, S. constellatus,* and *S. intermedius* (all previously known as the *S. milleri* group) from glucose metabolism. In a rapid version of the traditional VP test, all the growth from an 18- to 24-hour plate is removed with a swab and inoculated into the VP broth. After 6 hours incubation at 35°C, two reagents (alpha-naphthol and sodium hydroxide with creatine) are added, and the tube is vigorously shaken. A change to a cherry red color within 15 minutes indicates a positive result. Rust or pink reactions are also recorded as positive (Facklam & Elliott, 1995). The small-colony beta-hemolytic streptococci, *S. anginosus, S. constellatus,* and *S. intermedius,* are VP positive, whereas other beta-hemolytic streptococci are negative.

The order of reagent addition for the VP test is very important. Alpha-naphthol is added first and then 40% KOH with creatine. If the reagents are added in reverse order, the reaction observed may be weak positive or false negative.

β-Glucuronidase (BGUR)

The BGUR test can be performed instead of the VP test. It detects β-glucuronidase in large-colony groups C and G beta-hemolytic streptococci. Commercially available test strips or MacConkey agar with methylumbelliferyl-β-D-glucuronide can be used. Both methods are read for fluorescence under a long-wave ultraviolet light. The BGUR test appears to be more accurate than the rapid VP test for identifying large-colony-forming beta-hemolytic groups C and G streptococci (Kirby & Ruoff, 1995). Large-colony-forming groups C and G beta-hemolytic streptococci fluoresce, whereas the small-colony-forming *S. anginosus, S. constellatus,* and *S. intermedius* (all previously known as the *S. milleri* group) are negative.

Motility and Pigment

The motility and pigment tests are used to separate the non-motile, clinically significant vancomycin-resistant enterococci (VRE) from the motile, intrinsically vancomycin-resistant enterococci, which are members of the normal flora. The clinically significant VRE have the ability to transfer their vancomycin resistance gene to other organisms, whereas the intrinsically resistant strains cannot transfer their resistance. It is very important to differentiate the two for infection control purposes. Motility test medium, incubated for 24 to 72 hours, or a direct microscopic method, after 2 hours incubation, can be used to detect motility. It is very important that the motility test medium be incubated at 25°C to 30°C. A positive result, as observed in Figure 17-22 ■, is indicated by diffusion of growth away and around the streak line where the organism was initially inoculated.

The direct microscopic method requires the inoculation of trypticase soy broth with one drop of an organism suspension after incubation for 2 hours. The wet prep is examined for cocci exhibiting rapid, darting, directional movement (Horn, Tóth, Kariyama, Mitsuhata, & Kumon, 2002). *Enterococcus faecalis* and *E. faecium* are nonmotile. *E. casseliflavus, E. flavescens,* and *E. gallinarum* are motile and are not an infection control issue because they are unable to transfer the vancomycin-resistance gene.

The colony pigment may not be visually apparent on sheep blood agar. To detect pigment production, sweep up some colonial growth on a sterile white swab and examine for a bright lemon yellow color. *E. casseliflavus* and *E. flavescens* are

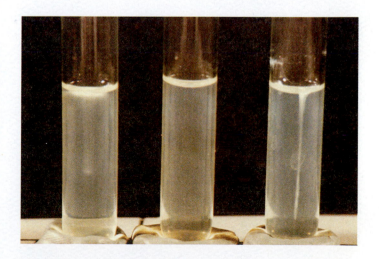
■ **FIGURE 17-22** Positive (left), uninoculated (center), and negative (right) motility test medium.

pigmented and are not an infection control concern. DNA studies indicate that *E. flavescens* and *E. casseliflavus* may be the same species (Carvalho, Teixeira, & Facklam, 1998; Murray et al., 1999).

Methyl-α-ᴅ-Glucopyranoside (MGP)

MGP is a test to detect the ability of enterococci to acidify methyl-α–ᴅ-glucopyranoside. It is used to separate the "atypical" intrinsically resistant enterococci, such as *E. casseliflavus* and *E. gallinarum,* from *E. faecium*. *E. faecium* is the most common strain of vancomycin-resistant enterococci that can potentially transfer its resistance gene to other organisms. This makes it a significant infection control issue. Misidentification of *E. gallinarum* or *E. casseliflavus* as a VRE increases costs for the hospital and patient as well as exposing the patient to unnecessary antibiotic therapy. The MGP broth is inoculated with several colonies taken from sheep blood agar. A change in the pH indicator from purple to yellow is a positive reaction as seen in Figure 17-23 ■. A positive result will differentiate the "atypical" intrinsically resistant enterococci from the negative reaction for *E. faecalis* and *E. faecium* (Carvalho et al., 1998). The MGP test is used in combination with the tests for motility and pigmentation to confirm the presence of a clinically significant, vancomycin-resistant *Enterococcus* spp. (VRE).

Vancomycin Susceptibility/Resistance

Determination of vancomycin resistance is helpful in detecting the presence of *Leuconostoc* spp. and *Pediococcus* spp. These two genera are intrinsically resistant to vancomycin but are unable to transfer their resistance to other organisms via gene transfer. A heavy inoculum is streaked onto the surface of half of a trypticase soy agar (TSA) or TSA with 5% sheep blood to create a solid lawn of growth. A 30 μg vancomycin disk is aseptically placed in the middle of the streaked area. After overnight incubation in 37°C ambient air, examine for a zone of inhibition around the disk. Any zone of inhibition is interpreted as sensitive, whereas growth to the edge of the disk is considered resistant. Most *Enterococcus* spp., *Streptococcus* spp.,

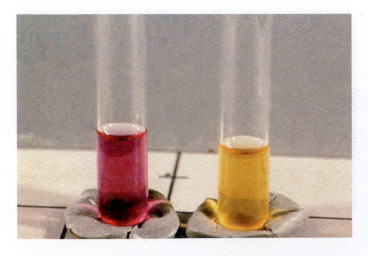

■ **FIGURE 17-23** MGP broth negative (left) and positive (right) reactions.

and some of the other related *Streptococcus*-like cocci are sensitive. *Leuconostoc* spp., *Pediococcus* spp., and occasional enterococci are resistant (Murray et al., 1999).

Staphylococcus Streak or Satellite Test

Nutritionally variant streptococci, such as *Abiotrophia* spp. and *Granulicatella* spp., will not grow on most routine agars such as sheep blood agar. These organisms must be provided with a source of pyridoxal or vitamin B_6. Pyridoxal or vitamin B_6 can be provided with a *Staphylococcus aureus* streak or disk. *S. aureus* releases these factors into the medium. A streak line of *S. aureus* is placed, in a single line, across an area inoculated with the potential nutritionally variant streptococci. If the unknown organism is an *Abiotrophia* spp. or *Granulicatella* spp., the organism will **satellite** or only grow around the around the colonies of another microbe, which supplies it with needed growth factors. An alternate method uses commercially available disks impregnated with pyridoxal to observe the satellite pattern (Murray et al., 1999).

A description of how each of the tests covered in this section is used in the identification of the catalase-negative cocci is outlined in the next section.

ENTEROCOCCUS

The enterococci are frequent isolates from clinical specimens. They exist in our environment on plants, on animals, and in the soil. The *Enterococcus* spp. were once members of the Group D streptococci. In the 1980s, they were removed from the genus *Streptococcus* based on molecular testing and also because of their potential resistance to penicillin and high-level aminoglycosides and emerging resistance to vancomycin. They colonize the body's surface and mucous membranes, especially the gastrointestinal and genitourinary systems, and have the ability to cause infectious disease. The most common isolate is *E. faecalis,* but *E. faecium* is the most frequent vancomycin resistanct isolate in the hospital setting and tends to be more resistant to antibiotics, such as ampicillin, than *E. faecalis* (Forbes et al., 1998).

General Characteristics

The enterococci are a fairly hardy group of microorganisms requiring no special conditions to obtain good growth. They are considered to be facultative anaerobes that grow well on routine supportive media and media designed to grow gram-positive organisms. They grow in ambient air or CO_2 at a temperature of 35°C.

The typical microscopic morphology of *Enterococcus* spp. is that of gram-positive cocci in chains that resemble streptococci. *Enterococcus* spp. grows as a 0.5 to 1 mm gray-white colony as seen in Figure 17-24 ■. They may be alpha-hemolytic or nonhemolytic, but rarely beta-hemolytic.

◆ *Enterococcus faecalis*

E. faecalis is the most commonly isolated species. It is a member of the normal flora in the genital and gastrointestinal systems, and can be associated with several infectious diseases.

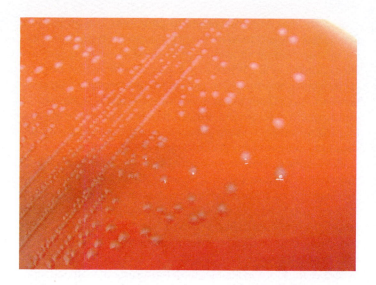

■ **FIGURE 17-24** *E. faecalis* colonies on sheep blood agar.

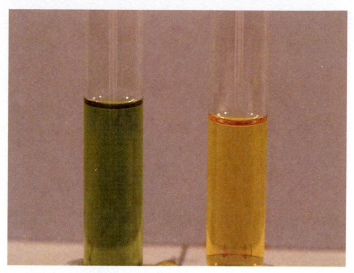

■ **FIGURE 17-25** Positive (right) and negative (left) reactions for the pyruvate test.

Identification

Most clinical laboratories routinely identify an organism as an *Enterococcus* spp. using the pyrrolidonyl arylamidase (PYR), leucine aminopeptidase (LAP), and esculin tests. Isolation from sterile body sites or exhibition of vancomycin resistance usually requires identification to species. Identification of *E. faecalis* requires correlation of typical colony characteristics and biochemical reactions to an expected sensitivity or antibiogram pattern.

Key Biochemical Reactions.

A colony resembling an *Enterococcus* spp. can be screened with the pyrrolidonyl arylamidase (PYR), leucine aminopeptidase (LAP), and esculin tests or bile esculin and 6.5% salt broth. A positive result in all of these tests is characteristic of *Enterococcus* species.

The enterococci will usually agglutinate with the group D antiserum in the serogroup antigen test. A positive test for the group D antigen is not specific for enterococci, as other species, such as *Pediococcus* spp. and *S. gallolyticus* (previously known as *S. bovis*), can also carry this antigen. Surprisingly only about 80% of *Enterococcus* spp. actually carry a detectable group D antigen. Most laboratories reserve serogroup antigen testing for identification of the beta-hemolytic streptococci.

Some other catalase-negative *Streptococcus*-like organisms that appear as chains microscopically, such as *Globicatella*, may also be BE positive, so the LAP test result is useful. The enterococci are LAP positive, whereas these other cocci may be LAP negative. The enterococci can be grouped into five groups based on reactions in mannitol, sorbose, and arginine. Group II *Enterococcus* contains the most commonly isolated human species and is characterized by positive reactions in mannitol and arginine. The other groups are members of animal gastrointestinal tracts and the environment and are rare human isolates.

Other *Streptococcus*-like organisms may mimic the *Enterococcus* spp. in both their colony morphology and biochemical reactions. *Vagococcus* spp. can be differentiated from *Enterococcus* spp. by their inability to grow at 45°C. Enterococci grow at both 10°C and 45°C. *Lactococcus* spp. may not grow or grow poorly at 45°C. *Lactococcus* spp. produce a negative result for a commercially available DNA probe for *Enterococcus* (Facklam & Elliott, 1995).

It is important to differentiate *E. faecalis* and *E. faecium* because of their difference in susceptibility patterns. *E. faecalis* is nonmotile, nonpigmented, and generates a negative methyl-α-D-glucopyranoside (MGP) result. It can be distinguished from *E. faecium* by a positive pyruvate test (Figure 17-25 ■) and a negative arabinose (Figure 17-26 ■) result. Table 17-5✪ reviews

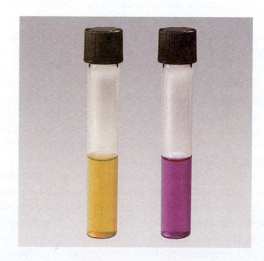

■ **FIGURE 17-26** Positive (left) and negative (right) reactions for heart infusion broth with Bromcresol Purple and 1% Arabinose. *Photo courtesy of Remel, part of Thermo Fisher Scientific.*

⭐ TABLE 17-5

Differentiation of Vancomycin Resistant *Enterococcus* spp.

Species	MOT	PIG	MGP	PYU	Arab
E. faecalis	–	–	–	+	–
E. faecium	–	–	–	–	+
E. gallinarum	+	–	+	–	+
E. casseliflavus/ E. flavescens	+	+ (yellow)	+	v	+

MOT = motility; PIG = pigment; MGP = methyl-alpha-D-glucopyranoside; PYU = pyruvate; Arab = arabinose; + = positive; – = negative; v = variable
Source: Adapted from Table 3, Carvalho et al., 1998; Table 1, Hanson & Cartwright, 1999; Table 2, Murray et al., 1999.

tests helpful in distinguishing *E. faecalis* from other vancomycin-resistant *Enterococcus* spp.

Commercial kits identify *E. faecalis* well and the other species fairly accurately. Identification may require additional tests (Bascomb & Manafi, 1998). Microbiologists should realize mistaken identification of the other species is always possible (Forbes et al., 1998).

Antibiogram. The enterococci can be potentially resistant to the beta-lactams, such as penicillin, aztreonam, cephalosporins, clindamycin, methicillin or oxacillin, trimethoprim-sulfamethoxazole, and the aminoglycosides. Because susceptibility is unpredictable, testing is necessary for these organisms.

Most enterococci are sensitive to vancomycin. Resistance is because of the presence of *van*A, *van*B, *van*D, or *van*E genes and is of **epidemiologic** importance. Epidemiology is related to factors used to control the presence or absence of a pathogen or disease in the hospital environment. These organisms must be controlled in the hospital environment because they have demonstrated the ability to transfer these genes to other organisms such as *Staphylococcus aureus*. Rectal swabs are often used to screen individuals for *E. faecalis* or *E. faecium* possessing these genes. Once isolated, pigment, motility, and MGP tests are used to rule out the isolation of *Enterococcus* spp. that possess the vancomycin gene, which can be transferred to other organisms. *Enterococcus* spp. that possess the *van*C gene demonstrate low-level resistance to vancomycin, which cannot be transferred to other organisms.

E. faecium is intrinsically resistant to the beta-lactams, especially the cephalosporins and penicillinase-resistant penicillins, low levels of aminoglycosides, clindamycin, fluoroquinolones, and trimethoprim-sulfamethoxazole. They may acquire resistance to high concentrations of beta-lactams and aminoglycosides, glycopeptides such as vancomycin and teicoplanin, tetracycline, erythromycin, fluoroquinolones, rifampin, chloramphenicol, fusidic acid, and nitrofurantoin (Cetinkaya, Falk, & Mayhall, 2000).

E. faecalis is still susceptible to penicillin and ampicillin. Beta-lactamase producers are rare but have been isolated. Tests for beta-lactamase should be performed on enterococci isolates (Gordon et al., 1992). Any *E. faecalis* isolate that displays (1) resistance to ampicillin, penicillin, or linezolid or (2) resistance to teicoplanin but not vancomycin or (3) sensitivity to quinupristin-dalfopristin should be viewed with suspicion. Identification should be confirmed, and the susceptibility test should be reviewed for potential sources of error.

Resistance to vancomycin and high-level aminoglycosides should also warrant identification of the isolate, especially if this pattern of resistance is uncommon in the institution (Miller, 2007; NCCLS, 2003). Vancomycin and high-level aminoglycoside resistance (HLAR) is becoming more and more common in the hospital environment because of the increased use of these antibiotics. ∞ Chapter 11, "Susceptibility Testing," describes methods available for determining in vitro susceptibility to antibiotics and potential sources of error associated with testing procedures.

REAL WORLD TIP

Long-term use of vancomycin creates not only VRE but also vancomycin-dependent *Enterococcus* (VDE). VDE actually use vancomycin to build their cell wall. Once removed from the antibiotic, they can revert to their original vancomycin-resistant state. This cycling back and forth makes their elimination difficult.

✓ Checkpoint! 17–11 (Chapter Objective 6)

One would expect the antibiotic susceptibility pattern of E. faecalis to be:

1. *sensitive to penicillin.*
2. *resistant to vancomycin.*
3. *resistant to penicillin.*
4. *sensitive to vancomycin.*
   A. *1 & 2*
   B. *1 & 4*
   C. *3 & 2*
   D. *3 & 4*

◆ *Enterococcus faecium*

E. faecium is the second most commonly isolated enterococci, representing 5% to 10% of the isolates but accounts for most of the vancomycin resistant strains (Mandell et al., 2000). Isolation of multiresistant strains is increasing in hospitals and is of concern because of this organism's association with nosocomial infections.

Identification

Most laboratories do not identify beyond the genus for this organism. If it is isolated from specimens collected from sterile sites or it exhibits vancomycin resistance, speciation is usually necessary. The microscopic morphology, colony morphology, and biochemical reactions for PYR, LAP, and esculin are the same as for *E. faecalis*.

Key Biochemical Reactions.   *E. faecium* shares the characteristics of the Group II *Enterococcus*. Review the characteristics for *E. faecalis*. It is also nonmotile, nonpigmented, and methyl-α-D-glucopyranoside (MGP) negative. One means to differentiate it from *E. faecalis* is by the pyruvate test. *E. faecium* is pyruvate negative, as observed in Figure 17-25. The arabinose test is also helpful in that *E. faecium* is positive as seen in Figure 17-26. Table 17-5 compares the reactions of the vancomycin-resistant enterococci for select biochemical tests.

Antibiogram.   *E. faecium* is intrinsically resistant to certain antibiotics. It is more resistant then *E. faecalis* to penicillin, ampicillin, piperacillin, imipenem, and ciprofloxacin (Gordon et al., 1992). Any *E. faecium* that appears resistant to linezolid should be checked for purity and the identification verified. Common sources of error should be reviewed to insure the accuracy of the results. Resistance to high-level aminoglycosides and quinupristin-dalfopristin may also be suspect in certain institutions if that antimicrobial pattern is uncommon (Miller, 2007; NCCLS, 2003).

◆ Other *Enterococcus*

Other species of enterococci are rarely isolated from clinically significant specimens (Jett, Huycke, & Gilmore, 1994). Identification to genus and the susceptibility report is all that is usually necessary for most specimens (Murray, 1990).

Identification

Identification to genus is routinely performed in most clinical laboratories. Identification to species may be necessary when isolated from sterile sites or if the isolate displays vancomycin resistance. The microscopic morphology, colony morphology, and results for the pyrrolidonyl arylamidase (PYR), leucine aminopeptidase (LAP), and esculin tests will identify to the genus *Enterococcus*.

Key Biochemical Reactions.   The reactions for the battery of tests used to identify to genus has been described previously in this chapter. Three species may mimic VRE but do not cause nosocomial infection or illness because their vancomycin-resistance gene is not transferable to other organisms. They are *E. gallinarum*, *E. flavescens*, and *E. casseliflavus*. DNA studies indicate that *E. flavescens* and *E. casseliflavus* are related species so only reactions for *E. casseliflavus* will be described (Carvalho et al., 1998; Murray et al., 2003).

E. gallinarum and *E. casseliflavus* share the characteristics of *Enterococcus faecalis* and *E. faecium*. It is cost effective to rule out these organisms to save the money associated with isolation of patients with VRE that have the potential to transfer the vancomycin-resistance gene. The minimum suggested differentiation tests include motility and pigment. *E. gallinarum* and *E. casseliflavus* are motile. *E. casseliflavus* produces a bright yellow pigment, whereas *E. gallinarum* does not. The methyl-α-D-glucopyranoside (MGP) test is helpful to distinguish these "atypical" strains, which are nonmotile or nonpigmented. The MGP test, as seen in Figure 17-23, is positive for *E. gallinarum* and *E. casseliflavus*. Refer to Table 17-5 for differentiation of VRE.

Antibiogram.   The antibiogram of other enterococci resembles the pattern of *E. faecalis*. However, the non-*E. faecalis* and non-*E. faecium* enterococci tend to be more resistant to penicillin and ampicillin (Gordon et al., 1992).

Clinical Significance

Enterococci are associated with community-acquired and nosocomial urinary tract infections, nosocomial wound and soft tissue infections, bacteremia, and endocarditis (Murray et al., 2003). Because they are part of the normal intestinal flora, infections of the intra-abdominal and pelvic areas are possible. Box 17-3 ✪ lists the infectious diseases associated with *Enterococcus* spp. The most common enterococci isolated are *E. faecalis*, which accounts for up to 80% of infections followed by *E. faecium*, which account for up to 15% of the remaining infections.

Vancomycin-resistant *Enterococcus* (VRE) are of concern in nosocomial infections. Many hospitals screen the rectal swabs or feces of patients for VRE using media containing 6 mcg/mL of vancomycin. Organisms that grow may be VRE. The motility and pigment tests must then be used to rule out *E. casseliflavus*, *E. flavescens*, and *E. gallinarum* from *E. faecalis* and *E. faecium*. ∞ Chapter 11 reviews screening methods for vancomycin-resistant enterococci.

The enterococci are members of the normal flora in the oral cavity and gastrointestinal and female genital tracts. It is not unusual to isolate these organisms from upper respiratory, stool, urine, and female genital specimens (Jett et al., 1994).

✪ BOX 17-3

Infectious Diseases Associated with *Enterococcus* spp.

Urinary tract infection (Nosocomial most common)

Endocarditis

Bacteremia

Intra-abdominal and pelvic infections

Wound and soft tissue infections

Neonatal sepsis

Meningitis (rare)

Respiratory tract infection (unusual and rare)

Not much is known about the virulence factors of the enterococci. Their ability to withstand the effects of broad-spectrum antibiotic treatment may contribute to their association with "**superinfections**" in patients. Superinfections are caused by a microbe that is resistant to the antibiotics used to treat an initial infection caused by another organism. Pheromone production encourages conjugation and exchange of plasmids and genes between enterococci. These plasmids code for antibiotic resistance, cytolysins, and aggregation substance. Adherence to renal epithelial cells appears to be aided by this aggregation substance. Enterococci can also adhere to heart valves. Production of protease and hyaluronidase may play a role in invasive disease (Jett et al., 1994). A retractable extracellular surface protein produced by enterococci may allow them to hide from the immune system. Extracellular superoxide is produced more often by invasive enterococci then colonizing enterococci (Mundy, Sahm, & Gilmore, 2000). Other microorganisms may enhance the growth of enterococci, but more investigation into this aspect of enterococci life is needed (Mandell et al., 2000).

Many enterococcal infections are believed to originate from the intestinal tract. Epithelial cells or leukocytes located in the intestinal tract engulf the bacteria, which adhere to the lumen. The bacteria can leave the cells and enter the abdominal region or be carried to the mesenteric lymph nodes by the phagocytes. In the lymph nodes, they can reproduce, enter the bloodstream, and spread throughout the body (Jett et al., 1994).

Patients at risk of developing an infection because of enterococci are compromised by either severe underlying disease or surgery. Often their gastrointestinal tract is colonized with the organism. Long hospital stays and prior antibiotic therapy play a role in creating the conditions for invasion. The organism may enter the blood directly from the gastrointestinal tract because of damage done to the mucosa by chemotherapy such as in cases of malignancies. Previously infected sites may be the source for direct invasion into other sterile sites. The hands of health care providers as well as medical equipment may also transfer the organism. Nosocomial portals of entry include urinary tract catheters, intravascular lines, and wounds such as decubitus ulcers or burns (Mandell et al., 2000; Sakka et al., 2008). ∞ Chapters 40 and 41 provide information on opportunistic and nosocomial infections.

Enterococcal species other than *E. faecalis* and *E. faecium* are rarely associated with infections or outbreaks and are rare isolates from clinical specimens. Some of these other *Enterococcus* species may be isolated from feces or rectal swabs used to screen for VRE. These species do not appear to transfer their resistance gene, which is usually the *van*C gene and so are not an issue for infection control.

When a patient is positive for VRE, the individual is placed in isolation or cohorted with other VRE positive patients. Limited health care workers may be allowed to work with these individuals, and **contact precautions** are used to stop transmission of these microorganisms from one person to another. Contact precautions protocol requires wearing gloves and gown with patient contact. Follow-up screening is done on VRE positive patients and their roommates. Additional screening may also be performed on patients in the area. When such patients are discharged, their rooms are thoroughly cleaned in a manner designed to rid the surfaces of enterococci and the plasmids carrying the vancomycin-resistance genes. This is an expensive process but well worth the cost if nosocomial infections are to be prevented. It is a waste of resources to put forth this effort for organisms such as *E. gallinarum* and *E. casseliflavus*, which are vancomycin resistant but cannot transfer their resistance gene. They must be ruled out when a vancomycin-resistant *Enterococcus* spp. is isolated. Refer to Table 17-5 for differentiation of these organisms.

Because identification of enterococci to species is not routine, the role of the other enterococci in infectious disease is not clearly defined. They have been isolated from clusters of infections (Murray et al., 1999) and from specimens associated with endocarditis (Murray, 1990). There have also been recent reports of infection of the central nervous system, osteomyelitis, and cholecystitis caused by these enterococci.

STREPTOCOCCUS

Another commonly isolated catalase-negative genus that must be considered along with the enterococcus are the streptococci.

General Characteristics

Most members of this genus are facultative anaerobes, but some are fastidious and require increased levels of CO_2 for growth. *Streptococcus pneumoniae* may grow best initially in an anaerobic atmosphere. The best medium for initial isolation is sheep blood agar incubated at 37°C. They will also grow on chocolate agar and gram-positive selective agar.

On Gram stain they will appear as gram-positive cocci in chains (see Figure 8-10 for an example). *S. pneumoniae* may appear as lancet or football shaped diplococci or cocci in pairs, as observed in Figure 17-27 ■. Staining growth from liquid thioglycollate broth medium or directly from the patient specimen will provide the best microscopic morphology for basing identification decisions.

**Checkpoint! 17–12
(Chapter Objective 5)**

A small, gray, gamma-hemolytic colony which appears as gram-positive cocci on the Gram stain is isolated from a decubitus wound specimen. The PYR test turns red after addition of the PYR reagent. It blackens a bile-esculin agar slant and grows in 6.5% NaCl. It is a:

    A. *group D Streptococcus.*

    B. *S. pyogenes.*

    C. *S. pneumoniae.*

    D. *Enterococcus spp.*

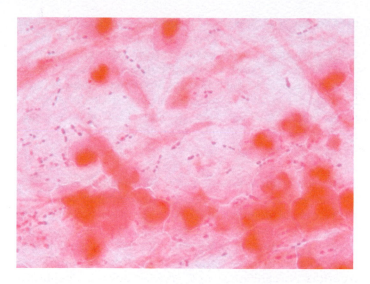

■ **FIGURE 17-27** Direct Gram stain of *S. pneumoniae* in a sputum specimen.

Hemolytic Reactions

One of the most useful first steps is to categorize isolates resembling streptococci according to their hemolytic reactions on sheep blood agar. The three categories are beta-(β)hemolytic, alpha-(α)hemolytic, and gamma-(γ)hemolytic. The beta- and alpha-hemolytic zones are produced around the colonies and may be narrow to wide. They are observed best with transmitted light shining from behind the agar plate. A beta-hemolytic organism completely lyses the red blood cells in the medium to produce a clear zone around the colony. A green zone characterizes alpha-hemolysis and is produced by the effect of peroxide on hemoglobin in the red blood cells. The appearance of greening around colonies is influenced by media composition, the type of blood used, and oxygen availability because peroxide cannot exist without oxygen (Facklam, 2002). A wide green zone is sometimes misidentified as beta because there appears to be a small zone of complete lysis surrounded by a second zone of greening. This type of hemolysis is referred to as alpha-prime or alpha′. The absence of any hemolysis is known as gamma-hemolytic or nonhemolytic. Refer to ∞ Chapter 8 to review images of alpha-, beta-, and nonhemolytic colonies. Once the hemolytic reaction is determined then appropriate tests are selected for identification.

 REAL WORLD TIP

If you are having difficulties determining the kind of hemolysis, place the plate on the stage of a dissecting microscope and carefully examine the area around the colony with low or high power. Intact red blood cells are seen with nonhemolytic (gamma) and alpha-hemolytic colonies. No red blood cells are observed with beta-hemolysis.

Beta-Hemolytic Streptococci

Colonies surrounded by a clear zone or beta-hemolysis, catalase-negative, and gram-positive cocci in pairs and chains include *Streptococcus pyogenes* (group A β *Streptococcus*), *S. agalactiae* (group B β *Streptococcus*), groups C, F, and G streptococci, and other streptococci. They can be commensal organisms but also potential pathogens. Colonies of the *Enterococcus* spp. are rarely beta-hemolytic and are usually not considered when hemolytic colonies are observed. *Enterococcus* spp. are usually gamma-hemolytic and rarely alpha-hemolytic.

◆ Group A Beta *Streptococcus* (*Streptococcus pyogenes*)

The group A beta-hemolytic streptococci are frequently isolated from clinical specimens and have the ability to produce **sequelae** after infection. Sequelae are pathologic processes that can occur after an initial infection with a microorganism. They may have long-lasting effects on a patient. It is important to quickly identify the presence of *S. pyogenes* in specimens so the physician can treat appropriately to prevent sequelae.

Identification

Identification of group A *Streptococcus* requires correlation of colony morphology with antigen and biochemical tests.

Colony Morphology.   Group A beta-hemolytic streptococci appear as large, greater than 0.5 mm, gray, and transparent to translucent colonies with a large or wide zone of beta-hemolysis on sheep blood agar (Forbes et al., 1999). The zone of beta-hemolysis is wider than the colony itself. Most will grow and form typical colonies on blood agar with trimethoprim-sulfamethoxazole (SXT) such as group A *Streptococcus* selective agar, or SSA. Figure 17-28 ■ demonstrates the wide-zone beta-hemolytic colonies typical for *S. pyogenes* on sheep blood agar.

It is important to distinguish small-colony types, which are less than 0.5 mm, from the large beta-hemolytic colony of group A. The group A antigen can be carried by other species, and they usually present as small beta-hemolytic colony types. These small beta-hemolytic colony types can be part of the normal flora and can cause infections, but are not associated with sequelae. The small beta-hemolytic colony types are members of the microaerophilic *Streptococcus* spp. (previously known as the *S. milleri* group) and are discussed later in this chapter and in ∞ Chapter 24, "Anaerobic Bacteria."

The beta-hemolytic reaction of *S. pyogenes* is the result of production of two hemolysins. Streptolysin S is stable in an environment with oxygen. Streptolysin O is labile or destroyed by oxygen. Strains of *S. pyogenes* exist that produce only Streptolysin O. Surface hemolysis would not be visible with these organisms, resulting in an inability to detect their presence. This false-negative culture result could have serious consequences if the patient develops one of the autoimmune sequelae because of a lack of treatment. Placing a cut in the first quadrant of the blood medium after inoculation, placing a

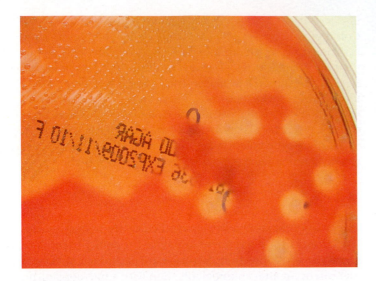

■ **FIGURE 17-28** The colonies of *S. pyogenes* display a translucent gray colony with wide-zone beta-hemolysis on sheep blood agar. The beta-hemolytic zone is typically wider than the colony itself.

coverslip over the first quadrant inoculum, or incubation in an anaerobic atmosphere will enhance visibility of the beta-hemolysis produced by this strain of *S. pyogenes* (Bourbeau, 2003).

 MEMORY TOOL

Use the hemolysin letter to help remember their oxygen susceptibility. Streptolysin **S** is oxygen **S**table. Streptolysin **O** is destroyed by **O**xygen.

 Checkpoint! 17–13 (Chapter Objective 4)

After streaking a sheep blood agar plate with a throat swab, the purpose of stabbing the inoculum into the agar (or placing the plate in an anaerobic jar) is to:

    A. *clean off the inoculating loop.*
    B. *obtain isolated colonies of respiratory flora.*
    C. *provide reduced oxygen tension for better growth.*
    D. *enhance the beta-hemolytic activity of the pathogen.*

Key Biochemical Reactions.   In addition to its negative catalase reaction, *Streptococcus pyogenes* is positive for pyrrolidonyl arylamidase (PYR) and the group A antigen. The microaerophilic streptococci, *S. anginosus, S. constellatus,* and *S. intermedius,* can also be group A antigen positive, but are PYR negative and usually presents with a smaller colony compared to *S. pyogenes.* The Taxo A or bacitracin test was once

used routinely to identify *S. pyogenes*. Other species may be susceptible to bacitracin (Taxo A), so it is not considered as definitive a test as it once was. Antigen testing is routinely used in most laboratories. Molecular diagnostics testing using DNA probes or real-time PCR is employed in some laboratories for rapid detection of *S. pyogenes* directly from throat specimens (Bourbeau, 2003). Refer to Figure 17-29 ■ for an algorithm for the identification of beta-hemolytic *Streptococcus* spp.

Antibiogram Pattern

S. pyogenes is universally sensitive to penicillin, the cephasporins, and vancomycin. Routine susceptibility is not usually performed unless isolated from a significant body site such as blood, treatment failure, or the physician is considering the use of erythromycin or other macrolide that has the potential for resistance. In some settings, rather than performing and reporting susceptibilities on *S. pyogenes* isolates, a published susceptibility, determined by review of pertinent literature, is reported. With all the emerging resistance of organisms, *S. pyogenes* has remained one of the few organisms that is susceptible to many antibiotics.

Resistance to macrolides, such as erythromycin, has been documented (Forbes et al., 1998). According to CLSI any beta-hemolytic *Streptococcus* spp. that is not sensitive to ampicillin, penicillin, third-generation cephalosporin, linezolid, or vancomycin should be viewed with suspicion. The isolate should be checked for purity and correct identification, and technical errors must be ruled out. If the results are confirmed the isolate should be saved and sent to a reference laboratory for verification.

Clinical Significance

S. pyogenes may be isolated from the throat, eyes, superficial wounds, abscesses, blood, and other sterile body fluid specimens. Isolation of this organism from a specimen may be considered a "panic or critical value" in some microbiology labs. A "panic or critical value" is a laboratory result that indicates a life-threatening condition that requires immediate attention of a physician. Some laboratories have reduced their panic or critical value list to ensure only those with life-threatening consequences are included. Isolation of *S. pyogenes* from a throat specimen may not be considered a panic value, but its isolation from a wound specimen may be critical because of the potential for necrotizing fasciitis.

Pathogenesis.   *S. pyogenes* produces numerous enzymes and exotoxins that allow them to spread through tissues and cause the clinical syndromes associated with group A infections. Table 17-6✪ provides a list of *S. pyogenes* exotoxins and their actions. Some streptococcal pyrogenic exotoxins, which cause fever and redness with infection, may also act as a superantigen causing a massive nonspecific and nonproductive response from T cell lymphocytes (Cunningham, 2000). Refer to ∞ Chapter 4, "The Host's Encounter with Microbes," to review host defenses.

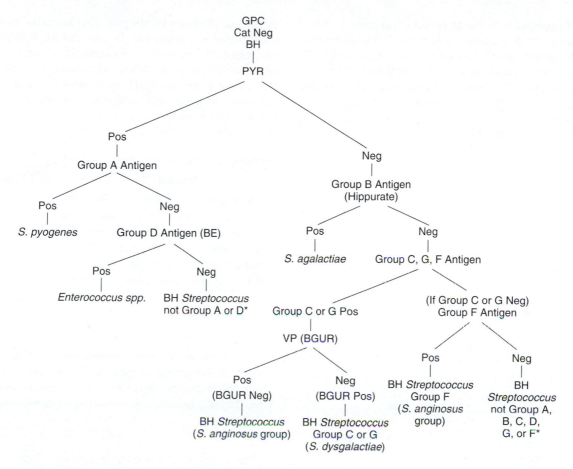

■ **FIGURE 17-29** Identification of beta-hemolytic *Streptococcus*.
BH = beta-hemolytic; GPC = gram-positive cocci; Cat = catalase; Pos = positive; Neg = negative;
PYR = pyrrolidonase; BGUR = B-glucuronidase; ( ) = alternate test.
May need to rule out nonhuman isolates.

✪ TABLE 17-6

S. pyogenes Exotoxins and Their Actions

Exotoxins	Actions
Plasminogen-plasmin-binding proteins	Enhance invasion or movement through tissue
Glyceraldehyde-3-phosphate and Enolase	Activates collagenases and proteases
Streptokinase	Dissolves fibrin clots
Streptococcal pyrogenic exotoxins	Causes nonspecific T-lymphocyte proliferation
	Causes fever and hypotension
	Enhances endotoxic shock
	Triggers inflammatory response
	Activates collagenases and proteases
	Causes rash, strawberry tongue, and skin shedding of scarlet fever
C5a peptidase	Inactivates complement product (C5a)
	Inhibits chemotaxis
Streptolysins S and O	Causes lysosomes to release contents into cytoplasm, thus killing the phagocyte
	Lyses red blood cells
	Damages membranes of cells
	Inhibits white blood cell chemotaxis

Virulence factors such as the M protein and capsule, illustrated in Figure 17-30 ■, provide some protection from phagocytosis. The M protein and lipoteichoic acid, in the cell wall, aid in adhesion to body surface cells. Certain M proteins (types 1 and 3), characteristically seen in invasive infections, appear to interact with endothelial cells and monocytes, causing the release of tissue factor, which results in the activation of the coagulation system and the formation of clots. Direct injury to the endothelium by streptolysin O or other exotoxins may also trigger coagulopathy (Bryant, 2003). Biofilm formation may result in antibiotic treatment failure and recurring infection (Baldassarri et al., 2006). Immunoglobulin-binding proteins may cause anti-IgG antibodies to be generated and deposited in heart and kidney tissue, causing damage. This leads to the sequelae associated with some group A streptococcal infections (Cunningham, 2000).

ⓔ REAL WORLD TIP

There are more than 100 different M serotypes. Immunity to group A *Streptococcus* is serotype specific. Once an individual has an infection with one M serotype, they are still susceptible to infection with the remaining M serotypes. This helps explain why there is no vaccine available for *S. pyogenes*.

ⓔ REAL WORLD TIP

Individuals, especially children, can carry *S. pyogenes* without exhibiting symptoms. They usually carry an avirulent form of the organism with decreased protein M. Carriers are usually not at risk of spreading disease to others.

The ability to adhere is the main factor that determines the capacity of group A streptococci to cause disease. They are able to attach to host tissues strongly enough to resist the local defenses of the host such as mucus and salivary flow. Previous damage to the host tissues' outer surface may assist with attachment to epithelial cells and colonization by group A streptococci. *S. pyogenes* also appears to have the ability to invade epithelial cells. Internalization of group A streptococci within cells involves proteins such as M protein, fibronectin-binding proteins, and small peptides. They induce ingestion of the streptococci and cytoskeletal rearrangement within the cytoplasm during invasion. Streptococcal fibronectin and fibronectin-binding proteins join to receptors on the epithe-

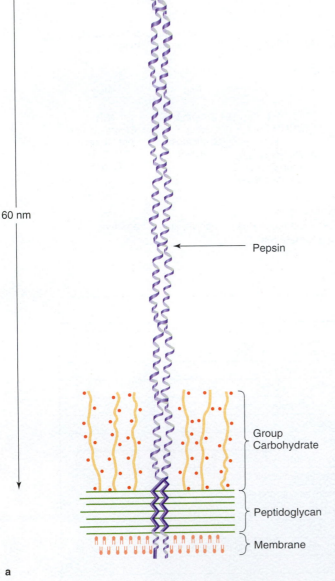

60 nm

Pepsin

Group Carbohydrate

Peptidoglycan

Membrane

a

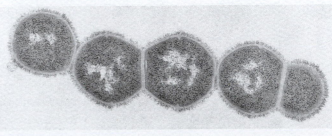

b

■ **FIGURE 17-30 a.** M protein model. **b.** Electron microscope photo of group A streptococci.
Courtesy of the Laboratory of Bacterial Pathogenesis and Immunology, The Rockefeller University, New York, New York.

lial cells and also trigger invasion. This may be the mechanism behind the persistence of streptococcal infections that allows the organism to evade the host defenses. This internalization process may enhance invasive disease or containment of the infecting microbe by the host. Virulence factors and the site of invasion may determine the outcome of internalization. Molecules that resemble those on host's cells may play a role in development of the poststreptococcal sequelae (Cunningham, 2000).

Infectious Diseases.   *S. pyogenes* is best known as a cause of pharyngitis, also known as strep throat to the general public, tonsillitis, and scarlet fever. Persistent throat infections may be because of the ability of the organism to hide from host defenses and form biofilms, as well as the presence of other colonizing, beta-lactamase-producing bacteria, which destroy penicillin used for therapy (Brook & Gober, 2008). In its capacity as the "flesh-eating" bacterium, it can cause severe damage associated with necrotizing fasciitis (Cunningham, 2000). Necrotizing fasciitis is legendary for its excruciating pain and gangrene, which can lead to death if not treated rapidly and aggressively with measures such as amputation. It can also be found as a mixed infection with *Staphylococcus aureus* in superficial skin infections such as boils and impetigo, as well as wound infections. ∞ Chapter 33, "Respiratory System," and ∞ Chapter 37, "The Integumentary System," describe diseases of these body systems and their laboratory diagnosis.

If left untreated a small percentage of group A streptococci cases go on to develop nonsuppurative or non-pus-forming sequelae such as reactive arthritis, rheumatic heart disease after rheumatic fever, or acute glomerulonephritis (AGN). Glomerulonephritis may be a result of immune complexes, made up of organisms coated with immunoglobulins, being deposited in the renal glomerulus, which affect the organ's function. AGN can occur after untreated pharyngitis and skin infections. Cross-reacting antibodies to streptococcal and renal antigens, complement activation, and damage because of streptokinase may also play a role. Nephrotoxins and cardiohepatic toxins are also produced by the organism and may directly damage the heart and kidney (Salyers & Whitt, 1994).

Rheumatic fever (RF) is considered an autoimmune disease. Antistreptococcal antibodies, against the organism's specific M protein, cross-react and attack receptors on the individual's heart muscle and valves. Each untreated infection with a new M protein serotype triggers a reoccurrence of the autoimmune process. This creates further heart valve damage. RF usually follows untreated pharyngitis but not skin infections.

REAL WORLD TIP

Mucoid strains of *S. pyogenes* have appeared in cultures prior to outbreaks of rheumatic fever. The increased capsule may protect the organism during phagocytosis, making it more virulent.

Streptococcal toxic shock syndrome (TSS) and other invasive diseases are associated with pyogenic exotoxin producing strains of group A *Streptococcus*. TSS involves bacteremia, intravascular coagulation, and rapid tissue destruction, which leads to multiple organ failure and shock. Death occurs in between 30% and 70% of infections (Bryant, 2003). There may be a connection between group A streptococcal infections and Tourette's syndrome and attention deficit disorders (Cunningham, 2000). Box 17-4 details the infectious diseases associated with *S. pyogenes*.

Serologic tests, such as the antistreptolysin O (ASO) and streptozyme test, may detect antibodies to streptolysin O, a hemolysin that is produced by this *Streptococcus*, and other extracellular products (anti-DNase B, antihyaluronidase,

✓ Checkpoint! 17–14 (Chapter Objective 7)

Two patients, with a history of pharyngitis, are examined by their physician. One individual has symptoms characteristic of arthritis and heart disease. The other has symptoms characteristic of renal disease. Both of their original throat cultures grew beta-hemolytic streptococci that were susceptible to bacitracin. The diseases these two individuals are experiencing are probably:

    A. *erysipelas and rheumatic fever.*
    B. *rheumatic fever and glomerulonephritis.*
    C. *scarlet fever and impetigo.*
    D. *scarlet fever and tonsillitis.*

REAL WORLD TIP

Direct detection methods for *S. pyogenes* are very specific for throat swabs, but false negative results can occur. The sensitivity of the kits is excellent if there are at least 10^5 organisms present on the swab. As the number of organisms decreases, so does the sensitivity of the test, so the laboratory must culture all negative screens for *S. pyogenes*.

✪ BOX 17-4

Infectious Diseases Associated with *S. pyogenes*

Pharyngitis/tonsillitis
Impetigo/pyoderma
Erysipelas
Cellulitis
Necrotizing fasciitis
Toxic shock syndrome
Scarlet fever
Septicemia
Pneumonia
Meningitis

antistreptokinase, or anti-NADase; Cunningham, 2000). A positive ASO or streptozyme result indicates prior infection with *S. pyogenes*. To review these immunologic tests, see ∞ Chapter 10, "Immunological Tests." Other beta-hemolytic streptococcus (groups C and G) may also produce a positive ASO result.

 REAL WORLD TIP

Other organisms can cause pharyngitis. Viruses, groups C and G beta *Streptococcus* and *Arcanobacterium haemolyticum* should be suspected if an individual exhibits signs and symptoms of pharyngitis but the group A *Streptococcus* screen is negative.

◆ Group B *Streptococcus* (*Streptococcus agalactiae*)

Identification

S. agalactiae is a particularly dangerous organism for newborns. When a suspicious colony is isolated from a baby, it is important to distinguish it from the other streptococci and *Listeria* spp. The physician should be notified immediately of its presence in a newborn.

 REAL WORLD TIP

A simple way to associate the significance of *S. agalactiae* is to remember group **B** is **b**ad for **b**abies.

Colony Morphology.   The group B streptococci are large, about 1 mm, translucent to opaque, flat, glossy, gray-white colonies, with a characteristic narrow zone of beta-hemolysis (Forbes et al., 1998). The beta-hemolysis can be very subtle or soft. It may require removal of a colony and viewing the area under it with light transmitted from behind the blood agar plate. Some strains are nonhemolytic and may be misidentified. *Listeria monocytogenes,* another significant organism for newborns, produces a colony that mimics that of *S. agalactiae. Listeria* spp. are ruled out by a Gram stain of small gram-positive rods and its positive catalase test reaction. ∞ Chapter 19, "Aerobic Gram-Positive Rods," provides more information on *Listeria* spp.

Key Biochemical Reactions.   Most laboratories test for streptococcal group antigens when catalase-negative, beta-hemolytic, gram-positive cocci are isolated. This provides a rapid result that is sensitive and specific. *Streptococcus agalactiae* agglutinates with the group B antiserum.

Another rapid test available is the hippurate test. Group B hydrolyzes sodium hippurate. Traditionally the CAMP test has been used for presumptive identification. Group B *Streptococcus* produces an enhanced arrowhead zone of complete hemoly-

sis, but the test requires overnight incubation. Group B is also pyrrolidonyl arylamidase (PYR) negative and bile esculin (BE) negative (Figure 17-14). Most strains are 6.5% NaCl negative (Figure 17-15), but a few strains as able to grow and produce turbidity.

Antibiogram Pattern.   Group B streptococci are sensitive to penicillin (Schuchat, 1998). No resistance to cephalosporins, such as ceftriaxone or cefotaxime, or vancomycin has been detected. Routine susceptibility testing on adults is not performed because of the predictable response to therapy (Forbes et al., 1998). Susceptibility testing is usually performed on isolates from babies.

Clinical Significance

Group B *Streptococcus* (GBS) is associated with stillbirth and life-threatening neonatal or infant infections such as meningitis, septicemia, and pneumonia. It can also cause postpartum (after childbirth) infections such as bacteremia and endometritis and nosocomial or community-acquired invasive disease in nonpregnant adults. GBS can be isolated from blood, spinal fluid, and urine specimens of newborns and when present often indicates a systemic infection such as septicemia or meningitis. Adults who are immunocompromised may present with this organism in the same specimen types. Other specimen types associated with this organism include skin and soft tissue, lower respiratory specimens, eye, ear, and sterile body fluids such as joint fluid, pleural fluid, or bone marrow. Vaginal and rectal swabs are collected specifically to screen pregnant women for the presence of GBS at 35 to 37 weeks gestation.

 REAL WORLD TIP

It is rare to isolate *S. agalactiae* causing an infection in a healthy adult. Its isolation suggests the presence of an underlying problem.

The organism colonizes mucous membranes, especially of the genitourinary and gastrointestinal systems, and can then spread to the bloodstream. GBS can also spread from localized infections such as cellulitis, foot ulcers, abscesses, and decubitus ulcers. Once in the bloodstream, it can reach the meninges, joints, or bone marrow to cause meningitis, arthritis, and osteomyelitis.

Virulence factors of GBS include a sialic acid capsule, β-hemolysin, group-specific polysaccharide, and peptoglycan. The sialic acid capsule inhibits activation of the alternate complement pathway and prevents phagocytosis (Koneman et al., 1997). The β-hemolysin is a pore-forming exotoxin whose interaction with epithelial and endothelial cells results in release of proinflammatory cytokines and production of nitric oxide in macrophages (Nizet, 2002). Release of proinflammatory cytokines is also induced by the group polysaccharide and peptoglycan (Mandell et al., 2000). The production of proinflammatory cytokines promotes inflammation.

Host factors play a significant role in the development of invasive disease. The very young, the elderly, and those with compromised immune systems are at greater risk (Schuchat, 1998). Refer to ∞ Chapters 4, 40, and 41 to review the host defenses and opportunistic and nosocomial infections.

Group B *Streptococcus* can colonize 15% to 35% of pregnant women in the vagina and rectum (Schuchat, 1998). The organism may ascend the vaginal canal to enter the uterus and spread into the amniotic fluid, where the fetus aspirates the organism. Transmission can also occur during birth by passing across prematurely ruptured membranes. It can also gain access through the newborn's nose, mouth, and ears as it moves through the birth canal. From these sites, the organism may enter the bloodstream, meninges, and other body sites. Neonatal sepsis, pneumonia, and meningitis are the most common acute infections. The baby appears well at birth but within hours become severely ill with fever, lethargy, hypotension, and poor feeding (Mandell et al., 2000). Prior to implementation of neonatal screening, the mortality rate was 55%, and now death occurs in 4% to 6% of the cases (Schuchat, 1998). If the baby survives infection, it may have permanent neurologic disability.

Neonatal group B invasive disease may present as early onset within the first 6 days of life, late onset within 7 days to 3 months of birth, or beyond early infancy at 3 to 18 months of age. Premature and low-birth-weight babies are at highest risk for this organism. Complications during delivery as well as heavy colonization of the mother by group B are also risk factors (CDC, 1996).

Physicians may request direct antigen testing on the blood and spinal fluid of the baby. Direct antigen testing on a urine specimen is no longer recommended because of false-positive results. A stained direct smear of the blood or spinal fluid has replaced this procedure in many labs.

CDC now recommends screening all expectant patients at 35 to 37 weeks gestation (Schrag, Gorwitz, Fultz-Butts, & Schuchat, 2002). The organism load can vary throughout the pregnancy, so screening just prior to delivery provides the most accurate picture. Rectal and vaginal specimens are collected on a swab and submitted to the laboratory for group B streptococcal culture. Selective liquid media enhances detection and isolation of the organism. It can be inoculated with the specimen and incubated overnight. Todd-Hewitt broth with colistin or gentamicin and nalidixic acid can be used. The antibiotics inhibit organisms other than *S. agalactiae*. Selective broth medium (SBM) or LIM broth media is available commercially (Schuchat, 1998).

After incubation, a portion of the selective broth is transferred to blood agar, and any colonies suspicious for *S. agalactiae* are tested. There have been cross-reactions reported between *S. porcinus,* a beta-hemolytic streptococcus usually associated with swine, and group B reagents in some streptococcal grouping kits. Performing a PYR test will help rule out this organism. *S. porcinus* is PYR positive, whereas GBS is negative (Thompson & Facklam 1997). *S. porcinus,* a rare human pathogen, can be recovered from the female genital tract and will grow in selective broth medium. The organism has been associated with stillbirth.

Selective broth media do have some issues in recovery of *S. agalactiae*. Overgrowth of group B streptococci by enterococci and other organisms can result in lower sensitivity and false negatives. Light colonization can also produce negative results. Several studies advocate the use of direct plating onto solid selective media, such as neomycin-nalidixic acid agar or Granada agar, in addition to the selective broth medium. This increases the chance of detecting group B streptococcal colonization and allows earlier identification (Dunne, 1999; Dunne & Holland-Staley, 1998; Gupta & Briski, 2004).

A selective, differential medium recently developed for primary isolation and detection of beta-hemolytic group B streptococci from clinical specimens is Granada medium. It contains antibiotics, methotrexate, and nutrients to select for group B. The methotrexate present enhances pigment production by this organism. The medium is incubated, under an aerobic or anaerobic environment, with a coverslip placed over the inoculated surface to detect colony pigmentation. Beta-hemolytic colonies of group B streptococci produce a red to orange pigment. Nonhemolytic strains are not detected because they do not produce pigment (Hardy Diagnostics, 2002).

Broth mediums based on the Granada medium method (GBS broth and StrepB Carrot Broth) are also available commercially. Observation of an orange to red color, similar to the color of a carrot, is positive for GBS. Figure 17-31 ■ displays positive and negative reactions for StrepB Carrot Broth. Only negative results require subculture resulting in faster turnaround time and cost savings. Performance of these broth mediums compare favorably to LIM broth according to recent studies (Church, Baxter, Lloyd, Miller, & Elsayed, 2008; Heelan, Struminshy, Lauro, & Sung, 2005).

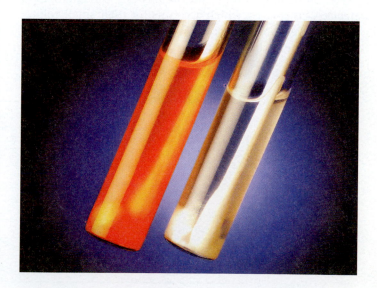

■ FIGURE 17-31 Positive (left) and negative (right) reactions for StrepB Carrot Broth.
Courtesy of Hardy Diagnostics.

Risk factors for the presence of *S. agalactiae* during labor and delivery include premature delivery at less than 37 weeks of gestation, rupture of placental membranes 18 hours or more before delivery, GBS bacteriuria, fever, or prior delivery of an infant with GBS disease. Antibiotics are administered during labor and delivery if risk factors are present or colonization is detected during screening (CDC, 1996).

Infections in adults occur primarily in those with underlying diseases such as diabetes mellitus, cancer, or cirrhosis. Nosocomial transmission may occur when central venous lines are placed. Underlying diseases such as congestive heart failure, diabetes, and seizure disorders are also associated with GBS nosocomial infections. The mortality rate in nonpregnant adults is 21% to 34% (Mandell et al., 2000). Recurrent infections occur in a small percentage of cases. Several cases presented initially as bacteremia then developed into focal infections of endocarditis or osteomyelitis (Mandell et al., 2000).

Checkpoint! 17–15 (Chapter Objective 9)

LIM media is used for selective isolation of:
   A. *Group B streptococci.*
   B. *salt-tolerant organisms such as Enterococcus spp.*
   C. *gram-positive organisms.*
   D. *pathogenic Staphylococcus spp.*

◆ Groups C, G, and F *Streptococcus*

Beta-hemolytic streptococci other than group A or B may be isolated from clinical specimens. These may be considered significant if isolated from normally sterile sites such as blood or in cases where the patient is displaying symptoms. *S. anginosus, S. constellatus,* and *S. intermedius* are microaerophilic *Streptococcus* species, which accounts for their small colony size. They were previously called the *Streptococcus milleri* group, but that term has been eliminated, and the individual species are now used for reporting. They are discussed in further detail in ∞ Chapter 24, "Anaerobic Bacteria."

Identification

The classification of groups C, G, and F *Streptococcus* can be confusing. Other organisms such as *S. dysgalactiae, S. anginosus, S. constellatus,* and *S. intermedius* can also possess group C, F, or G antigens. They can be distinguished by their small colony size and biochemical tests, as listed in Table 17-8. Many microbiology laboratories do not identify to species and just report group C, F, or G beta-hemolytic *Streptococcus* as present in a patient's specimen. The microaerophilic *S. anginosus, S. constellatus,* and *S. intermedius* usually possess the group F antigen.

Colony Morphology.   Groups C, G, and F streptococci are beta-hemolytic colonies of varying sizes. They can possess a wide-zone beta-hemolysis similar to *S. pyogenes*. Groups C and G may present as large colonies, greater than 0.5 mm or small colonies less than 0.5 mm in size. The large-colony type may be clinically significant, whereas the small colony type is usually considered normal flora. Group F grows as a small, pinpoint colony and possesses a sweet "caramel or butterscotch-like" odor (Mandell et al., 2000).

Key Biochemical Reactions.   The groups C, G, and F streptococci, isolated from humans, are pyrrolidonyl arylamidase (PYR), CAMP, and sodium hippurate hydrolysis negative. When tested with streptococcal grouping antisera, they can react with groups C, G, or F. To distinguish between the small and large-colony types that do not serotype, perform either the Voges-Proskauer (VP) test or β-glucuronidase (BGUR) test. The small-colony type, which is VP positive and BGUR negative, includes *S. anginosus, S. constellatus,* and *S. intermedius*. They are the only beta-hemolytic streptococci that are VP positive. This group of organisms is discussed later in this chapter and in ∞ Chapter 24, "Anaerobic Bacteria." The large-colony type, which is VP negative and BGUR positive, is *S. dysgalactiae*. Table 17-7✪ lists the test results for differentiation of the beta-hemolytic *Streptococcus*.

✪ TABLE 17-7

Differentiation of Beta-Hemolytic *Streptococcus* Species

Species	Colony size	Lancefield Group	PYR	Hippurate	CAMP	VP	BGUR
S. pyogenes	Large	A	+	−	−	−	v
S. anginosus	Small	A, C, F, or G	−	−	−	+	−
S. agalactiae	Large	B	−	+	+	−	v
S. dysgalactiae	Large	C	−	−	−	−	+
S. constellatus	Small	C or F	−	−	−	+	−
S. dysgalactiae	Large	G	−	−	−	−	+
S. intermedius	Small	Nongroupable	−	−	−	+	−

Large = >0.5 mm; Small = <0.5 mm; + = positive; − = negative; v = variable; PYR = pyrrolidonyl arylamidase; CAMP = Camp factor; VP = Voges-Proskauer; BGUR = β-glucuronidase.

Clinical Significance

Group C is normal flora in the nasopharynx, skin, and genital tracts. It is also found in many animals, and these animals can be the source for some human infections. Most infected individuals have underlying diseases such as diabetes melitis or malignancy. Group G colonizes the same sites as group C and is also found in the gastrointestinal tract. Sixty-five percent of individuals with a group G infection have a malignancy (Mandell et al., 2000). Other underlying conditions may also predispose an individual to a group G infection. Group F streptococci are considered commensals of the oral cavity and gastrointestinal tract. They may colonize the vagina (Mandell et al., 2000).

Large-colony types of groups C and G share some virulence factors of Group A *Streptococcus*. Both possess a similar M protein with the same functions described previously (Bisno, Collins, & Turner, 1996). Group C produces streptokinase and streptococcal streptolysin O. Group G may produce streptococcal streptolysin S and a streptolysin that is antigenically similar to streptolysin O (Humar et al., 2002; Mandell et al., 2000). Both organisms may stimulate the production of antibodies causing an increase in an ASO titer. They do not yet produce any streptococcal pyogenic exotoxins and are not usually responsible for nonsuppurative sequelae.

Group F possesses a capsule and a cell-surface protein that allows it to bind fibronectin, platelets-fibrin, clots, and fibrinogen. This adhesion is believed to play a role in the development of endocarditis in individuals infected with group F. It produces intermedilysin, which hemolyzes red blood cells and may also function as a superantigen. Many of the same enzymes already described, such as deoxyribonuclease and neuraminidase, are also manufactured to assist with its nutritional needs. IgG receptors are not apparent.

Large-colony types of group C and G infections may be pyrogenic, clinically significant, and resemble group A infections. Both are associated with pharyngitis, especially in college students and older adults (Dierksen, Ragland, & Tagg, 2000). Group C may spread into the bloodstream and is rarely associated with glomerulonephritis (Gerber & Shulman, 2004). Group G has been associated with sterile reactive arthritis. No cases of rheumatic fever have been reported yet. Some laboratories routinely report these organisms if isolated from throat specimens, whereas others do not consider it significant.

Groups C and G are also associated with skin and soft tissue infections, toxic shock-like syndrome, bacteremia, arthritis, osteomyelitis, respiratory infections, abscesses, endocarditis, and meningitis (Mandell et al., 2000; Murray et al., 1999). *S. anginosus, S. constellatus,* and *S. intermedius* include the small-colony types of group C and G as well as group F. These organisms are associated with bacteremia and abscess formation (Carmeli & Ruoff, 1995). Small-colony types can cause abscesses of the head, brain, neck, abdomen, and liver. They may also be considered commensal in the upper respiratory tract (Turner et al., 1993).

Other diseases include endocarditis, respiratory infections, osteomyelitis, and septic arthritis. Cellulitis also occurs, particularly in drug addicts (Mandell et al., 2000). Intravenous drug users may lick the needle to make insertion easier. This transfers the organism from the oral flora to the skin and blood.

Non-Beta-Hemolytic Streptococci

The appearance of alpha-hemolysis on sheep blood agar, produced by catalase-negative gram-positive cocci, is characteristic of *Streptococcus pneumoniae,* the group D *Streptococcus, Streptococcus gallolyticus* (previously known as *S. bovis*), and the viridans streptococci. Enterococci can also be alpha-hemolytic and may also need to be ruled out as a possibility. The non-hemolytic catalase-negative, gram-positive cocci include *Streptococcus gallolyticus* (previously known as *S. bovis*), viridans streptococci, or *Enterococcus* spp.

◆ *Streptococcus pneumoniae*

Identification

Streptococcus pneumoniae is a recognized pathogen when isolated from certain body sites such as the respiratory system. It also resides as normal flora in the same sites where disease may occur. Predominant numbers as well as the presence of white blood cells help to determine their significance. **Pneumococcus** is another name for *S. pneumoniae*. It is important to recognize the unique morphology characteristic of this potential pathogen so appropriate testing may be done.

Microscopic Morphology. *Streptococcus pneumoniae* has a characteristic microscopic morphology of gram-positive diplococci or cocci in pairs. The diplococci may appear lancet or football shaped, as seen in Figure 17-27. They may also appear in short chains similar to the other streptococci. On careful examination, a capsule may be visible as an unstained area or "halo" surrounding the cell. Older cells may over decolorize and appear gram-negative, but the lancet shape should be recognized.

Colony Morphology. *Streptococcus pneumoniae* produces alpha-hemolysis on sheep blood agar. ∞ Chapter 8 provides a photo of *S. pneumoniae* colonies. The colony itself is a small, about 0.5 mm, glistening, and gray. It may be mucoid, if encapsulated, or **umbilicated** and indented in the center (Forbes et al., 1998). The indentation is because of autolysis of the colony. The mucoid colonies can resemble green water droplets on the agar plate. Their appearance is because of excessive capsule production. The capsule can be serotyped. There are over 80 different serotypes, but most laboratories do not keep reagents to perform this testing. Without umbilication or encapsulation, its colony may be indistinguishable from the other alpha-hemolytic species. Figure 17-32a ■ provides a close-up view of the umbilicated or cratered colonies characteristic of *S. pneumoniae*. Figure 17-32b ■ provides a view of a mucoid colony of *S. pneumoniae*.

Growth may be better initially under anaerobic conditions. It is slightly fastidious because some strains require CO_2 for

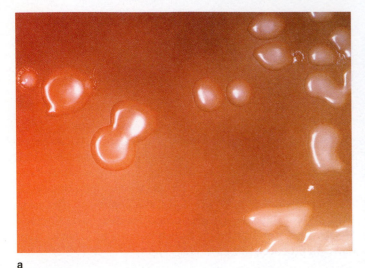

a

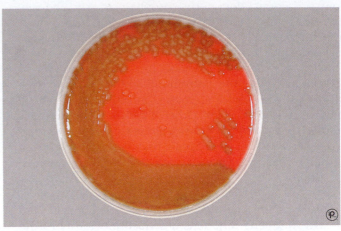

b

■ **FIGURE 17-32 a.** This close-up view of *S. pneumoniae* demonstrates its cratered or umbilicated colony. The colonies are initially domed, and this characteristic colony is created when the organism begins to autolyse. *From CDC and Dr. Richard Facklam. Website: http://phil.cdc.gov/phil/imageidsearch.asp.* **b.** This agar plate demonstrates the mucoid colony of *S. pneumoniae.* It appears as wet droplets because of the production of a large capsule. *From Marler LM, Siders JA, Kaufman CM, Owens EN, Korba GG and Allen SD, Bacteriology I Image Atlas CD-ROM, Indiana Pathology Images, 2005.*

growth. Some strains will completely autolyse without it. Liquid medium can also trigger autolysis. This makes the rapid detection and recovery of the organisms in blood cultures very important.

 ✓ **Checkpoint! 17–16 (Chapter Objective 5)**

Gram-positive lancet-shaped diplococci grow as an umbilicated, alpha-hemolytic colony. It is possibly:

   A. *Enterococcus spp.*
   B. *viridans streptococci.*
   C. *Streptococcus pneumoniae.*
   D. *Streptococcus gallolyticus (previously known as S. bovis).*

Key Biochemical Reactions.   Once a catalase-negative, alpha-hemolytic colony, which appears as gram-positive cocci on Gram stain, is isolated, there are two tests that help to identify the isolate as *S. pneumoniae.* Bile solubility is a rapid test that may provide identification within 30 minutes. *S. pneumoniae* lyses or solubilizes in the presence of bile salts. Some insoluble strains have been reported. The second test, optochin susceptibility, requires overnight incubation. *S. pneumoniae* is usually sensitive, whereas the viridans streptococci are usually resistant. There are reports of optochin resistant pneumococcus as well as optochin-sensitive viridans streptococci. *S. pneumoniae* does not possess a cell wall carbohydrate or "C" substance detected by the Lancefield serotyping. It can be divided into over 80 serotypes based on its capsular antigens.

 REAL WORLD TIP

Most laboratories do not maintain the antisera to test for the capsular antigen of *S. pneumoniae.* The most commonly encountered mucoid *S. pneumoniae* demonstrates a serotype III capsule. Most laboratories report a mucoid, alpha-hemolytic, optochin-susceptible colony as "*Streptococcus pneumoniae* presumptive type III" without performing the capsular serotype.

It is very important to correlate colony morphology with the test results. If an alpha-hemolytic colony is not mucoid, shiny, or indented in the middle, tests for both bile solubility and optochin susceptibility should be performed. Occasional isolates may require additional tests such as molecular or serologic assays (Kellogg, Bankert, Elder, Gibbs, & Smith, 2001). Figure 17-33 ■ provides an identification scheme designed for alpha-hemolytic *Streptococcus* spp.

 REAL WORLD TIP

S. pseudopneumoniae is an alpha-hemolytic colony that resembles that of *S. pneumoniae.* It is one of the viridans streptococci and has been isolated from lower respiratory cultures of individuals with cough and other symptoms. *S. pseudopneumoniae* is optochin resistant when incubated in CO_2 but susceptible when incubated in ambient air. It is also insoluble in bile.

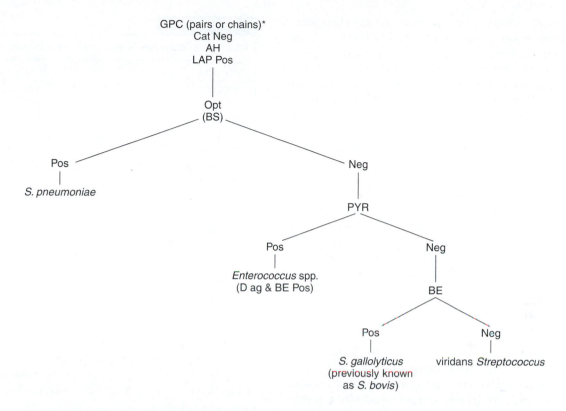

FIGURE 17-33 Identification of alpha-hemolytic *Streptococcus*.
GPC = gram-positive cocci; Cat = catalase; AH = alpha-hemolytic; LAP = leucine aminopeptidase;
Opt = optochin; BS = bile solubility; Pos = positive; Neg = negative; PYR = pyrrolidonase;
BE = bile esculin agar; ag = antigen; ( ) = alternate test.
Rule out Streptococcus-related cocci if the Gram stain shows clusters or tetrads, the LAP is negative, or it is resistant to vancomycin.

Antibiogram.   *Streptococcus pneumoniae* was historically a very sensitive organism. There is emerging resistance to penicillin and other β-lactam antibiotics, which is causing great concern. Pneumococci that are sensitive to penicillin are usually also sensitive to most other antibiotics. Tetracycline is one antibiotic where resistance is common. The early penicillin-resistant pneumococci were sensitive to the third-generation cephalosporins such as cefotaxime and ceftriaxone (Mandell et al., 2000). They are now becoming resistant to these antimicrobics. They remain sensitive to vancomycin, the drug of last resort for multiple-drug-resistant *S. pneumoniae* (Schrag, Beall, & Dowell, 2000). Any isolate that is resistant to fluoroquinolone or not sensitive to linezolid or vancomycin should be viewed as suspect. In some institutions resistance to penicillin or the third-generation cephalosporins would be unusual and also suspicious. Suspicious results should be checked for test organism purity, correct isolate identification and technical errors (NCCLS, 2003). Because *S. pneumoniae*'s response to antibiotic therapy is unpredictable, susceptibility testing should be performed. Testing with a method that reports a minimum inhibitory concentration (MIC) is preferred (Forbes et al., 1998). ∞ Chapter 11 reviews resistance mechanisms and susceptibility methods for *S. pneumoniae*.

Clinical Significance

Pathogenesis.   Colonization is necessary before disease can occur. Transmission is person to person via aerosolized droplets. Day-care and nursing home settings are especially prone to *S. pneumoniae* because of the close contact. The mechanism that determines when the organism becomes capable of causing disease in the host is not well understood. Certainly the organism's virulence factors play a role but it's not the full story. Underlying conditions such as viral infections, splenectomy, smoking, or cancer can affect the host's humoral and inflammatory response and play a role as well (Mandell et al., 2000; Spreer et al., 2004).

After colonization, local invasion may occur, resulting in access to the bloodstream or lymph system. From there the organism can gain entrance to sites that are normally free of microbes to cause meningitis, peritonitis, and septic arthritis. The organism may also be carried to a site whose clearance mechanism is not working effectively, such as the eustachian tubes or lungs. They can resist the host defenses to cause damage and inflammation characteristic of bronchitis, pneumonia, sinusitis, or otitis.

S. pneumoniae's capsule is the virulence factor that appears to help it most in resisting the host's defenses. Phagocytosis is less effective in allowing the organisms to survive their journey in the bloodstream. Components of its cell wall, such as peptidoglycan and polysaccharide, trigger inflammation resulting in damage to the areas cells and tissue (Sethi & Murphy, 2001). Few toxins are produced. Pneumolysin is a cytotoxin that harms respiratory epithelial cells and white blood cells. It also activates complement and causes the release of cytokines such as tissue necrosis factor and interleukin-1 (Mandell et al., 2000). An autolysin is produced prior to the organism reaching a stationary phase of growth releasing cell wall components. Complement is activated, and pneumolysin is released. Neuraminidase may enhance adherence to mucous membrane surfaces by cleaving sialic acid on the membranes exposing molecules for better adhesion. Pneumococcal surface protein A aids in resisting phagocytosis. *S. pneumoniae* also produces an IgA protease that may destroy IgA in the respiratory tract assisting in colonization (Sethi & Murphy, 2001).

Infectious Diseases.   *Streptococcus pneumoniae* is the most common cause of community-acquired pneumonia, especially in the elderly. It also causes invasive disease in newborns, infants, and adults. It can be isolated from respiratory, eye, ear, CSF, blood, and other sterile body fluid specimens. It is most frequently associated with otitis media, sinusitis, and meningitis. Occasionally it may cause endocarditis, septic arthritis, peritonitis, pericarditis, osteomyelitis, and soft tissue infections. It is a significant pathogen for individuals who do not possess a spleen. The spleen filters encapsulated organisms from the blood. Without vaccination against the most common capsular serotypes, individuals without a spleen, such as those with sickle cell anemia, would not survive each respiratory infection season. Box 17-5 ✪ lists the infectious diseases associated with *S. pneumoniae*.

✪ BOX 17-5

Infectious Diseases Associated with *S. pneumoniae*

Pneumonia
Meningitis
Sinusitis
Otitis media
Bacteremia
Endocarditis
Septic arthritis
Peritonitis
Pericarditis
Osteomyelitis
Soft tissue infections

✓ Checkpoint! 17–17 (Chapter Objective 8)

A physician has sent an expectorated sputum specimen, collected from an elderly female suspected of having pneumonia, to the laboratory. The Gram stain reveals many gram-positive diplococci and many white blood cells. The isolate grows as an alpha-hemolytic, mucoid, gray colony. It does not bubble with catalase reagent. The most appropriate action to take is:

   A. *report as "normal respiratory flora."*
   B. *repeat the catalase test.*
   C. *perform a PYR test.*
   D. *perform a bile solubility or optochin test.*

   REAL WORLD TIP

S. pneumoniae can be found as a colonizing organism in the throat. It is not a causative agent of pharyngitis and should not be identified and reported in this body site. Its presence in the throat is probably because of drainage from infected sinuses or transient colonization.

Streptococcus pneumoniae can be present in small numbers in the nasopharynx in 5% to 10% of adults and up to 40% of children, especially during the winter months of respiratory season. This makes processing of lower respiratory specimens such as sputum a challenge. When isolated as the predominant organism, along with the presence of white cells in the direct smear, it is assumed to be a pathogen. Processing of respiratory specimens is discussed in ∞ Chapter 33, "Respiratory System."

◆ *Streptococcus gallolyticus* (Previously known as *S. bovis*) or the Group D *Streptococcus*

Identification

The group D streptococci have gone through some taxonomic changes with the advent of DNA sequencing. They have been reclassified into new biotypes and subbiotypes based on genotypic and phenotypic testing. The most common human pathogen, *S. bovis*, has now been reclassified into two new biotypes, *S. gallolyticus* and *S. infantarius*. *S. gallolyticus* is found in humans with endocarditis, whereas *S. infantarius* is associated with neonatal meningitis. Because of the multitude of references to *S. bovis* in textbooks and journals, it will be used as the representative organism in this section for group D *Streptococcus*. The microbiologist must remain up to date on changes in nomenclature and educate physicians when these changes occur.

Streptococcus bovis shares the D antigen with *Enterococcus* spp. and some of the other related *Streptococcus*-like cocci. It is important to distinguish it from the others because it is not as commonly associated with disease and is more sensitive to antibiotics. Identification should correlate Gram stain results with the appropriate colony morphology and biochemical results.

Colony Morphology.   The colony of *S. bovis,* a group D *Streptococcus* now known as *S. gallolyticus,* is small at 0.5 mm, gray, and domed, exhibiting either alpha-hemolysis or gamma-hemolysis (Murray et al., 1999).

Key Biochemical Reactions.   Once an alpha-hemolytic, catalase-negative, gram-positive cocci in pairs and short chains is isolated, tests to rule out *Streptococcus pneumoniae, Enterococcus* spp., *S. bovis,* and the other related cocci are performed, as noted in Figure 17-33. *Streptococcus bovis* is insoluble in bile and optochin resistant, which distinguishes it from pneumococcus. Results for bile esculin (BE), esculin, and D antigen serotyping are positive, whereas pyrrolidonyl arylamidase (PYR) and growth in 6.5% NaCl is negative. This will differentiate it from alpha- and gamma-hemolytic *Enterococcus* and viridans streptococci. It is also leucine aminopeptidase (LAP) positive, whereas a negative result would be characteristic of some of the other related *Streptococcus*-like cocci. It is sensitive to vancomycin, whereas some *Enterococcus* spp. and some of the other related cocci are resistant.

Clinical Significance

Streptococcus bovis resides as normal flora in the gastrointestinal system. From this site, it can spread to the bloodstream or genitourinary system to cause infections. Infections include bacteremia and endocarditis. There is a strong correlation with its isolation from blood and the presence of an undetected colon cancer. The organism does not usually escape the gastrointestinal tract unless there are breaks in the mucosa because of malignant lesions.

Antibiogram.   *S. bovis* remains sensitive to penicillin. Any resistance should be investigated to ensure the identity of the organism or quality of the susceptibility testing procedure. Ceftriaxone is an alternative to penicillin for allergic patients. The aminoglycosides also remain an option for treatment.

◆ Viridans Streptococci

The viridans streptococci (a term which is not indicative of a particular genus or species) are a large number of alpha- and gamma-hemolytic streptococcal species that are PYR negative, and LAP positive. They are called viridans streptococci because many of the commonly isolated organisms display alpha-hemolysis. *Virde* is the Spanish word for *green.* Each species is placed into one of six groups based on phenotypic characteristics. The group D *Streptococcus, S. gallolyticus* (previously known as *S. bovis*) and *S. infantarius,* are actually members of the bovis group of the viridans streptococci. The bovis group is the only member of the viridans streptococci that possesses the group D cell wall antigen. This is why they are often not recognized as part of the viridans streptocci and have been separated from it.

Identification

Isolation of viridans streptococci is very common, as they are members of the normal flora in various body sites. They can cause infections in compromised individuals but are usually viewed as contaminants or normal flora isolates. The viridans streptococci may be isolated from the same types of specimens as those from which pathogens are isolated. This group of organisms may morphologically resemble *S. pneumoniae, Enterococcus* spp., *S. bovis* (now known as *S. gallolyticus*), and the other related *Streptococcus*-like cocci, so it is important to distinguish the viridans streptococci from these other known agents of disease.

Colony Morphology.   Colonies of the viridans streptococci are tiny, pinpoint to 0.5 mm in size, gray, domed, smooth, or matte (dull) (Forbes et al., 1998). They may be alpha-hemolytic or nonhemolytic on sheep blood agar. Their growth may be enhanced with incubation in CO_2.

Key Biochemical Reactions.   The viridans streptococci can be distinguished from *Enterococcus* spp. and *Streptococcus gallolyticus* (previously known as *S. bovis*) by the lack of the D antigen, negative reaction for bile esculin (BE), and no growth in 6.5% NaCl. Most do not possess a cell wall antigen that can be detected by the Lancefield grouping system. Some strains may possess the A, C, G, or F antigens. These were discussed earlier as the beta-hemolytic small-colony types. The small type colonies of microaerophilic *Streptococcus* can also be alpha- and gamma-hemolytic. They are also pyrrolidonyl arylamidase (PYR) negative. A positive leucine aminopeptidase (LAP) reaction will distinguish the group from some of the other related *Streptococcus*-like cocci. *Streptococcus pneumoniae* can be ruled out because the viridans streptococci present as optochin resistant and bile insoluble. Review Figure 17-33 for the identification of an alpha-hemolytic colony. Figure 17-34 ■ suggests a scheme for the identification of nonhemolytic *Streptococcus* spp.

Most laboratories report viridans streptococci without further identification to species. If further identification is necessary, as in the case of isolation from a significant specimen such as blood, additional tests must be performed. It is extremely difficult and cumbersome to identify the viridans streptococci to species. It may include checking enzyme activity using fluorogenic substrates, checking for production of extracellular polysaccharide using Mitis Salivarius Agar, and numerous biochemical tests. The viridans streptococci can be differentiated by their reactions for arginine hydrolysis, acetoin production, acid production from mannitol or sorbitol, and urease production. A table detailing their differentiation can be found on the Companion Website. Commercial systems for the identification of these organisms are available but vary greatly in their ability to identify the group to species.

Clinical Significance

The viridans streptococci are members of the resident flora of mucous membranes that line the oral cavity, gastrointestinal system, and female genital tract (Forbes et al., 1998). They may be isolated from respiratory specimens, urine, and genital cultures. Isolation from blood or CSF may indicate contamination or infectious disease. Their growth characteristics may

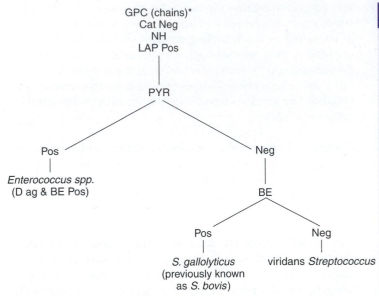

FIGURE 17-34 Identification of nonhemolytic *Streptococcus*. GPC = gram-positive cocci; Cat = catalase; Pos = positive; Neg = negative; NH = nonhemolytic; LAP = leucine aminopeptidase; PYR = pyrrolidonase; BE = bile esculin agar; ag = antigen; ( ) = alternate test.
Rule out Streptococcus-related cocci if the Gram stain shows clusters or tetrads, the LAP is negative, or it is resistant to vancomycin.

resemble that of potential pathogens, so adequate testing must be performed to rule out the potential pathogens that are associated with these specimens. Most laboratories do not continue with identification once the organism is known to be a member of the viridans streptococci. If isolated from sterile fluids, further identification may be necessary.

REAL WORLD TIP

Endocarditis, caused by the viridans streptococci, usually results in multiple positive blood cultures. If the organism is isolated from only one blood culture bottle when multiple sets are drawn, it is probably a contaminant.

Members of this group are also associated with endocarditis, bacteremia, and meningitis. Although they are not usually noted for their virulence, they do account for 50% to 60% of cases of subacute bacterial endocarditis. They are also responsible for gingivitis and dental caries. They produce "extra-cellular complex polysaccharides which can enhance attachment to and colonization of host cell surfaces" (Forbes et al., 1998). Most infections occur in compromised individuals who have had dental procedures, such as tooth extraction or cleaning, or other invasive medical procedures that may introduce the organism into the bloodstream (Forbes et al., 1998). Previously damaged or prosthetic heart valves may offer a new home to

REAL WORLD TIP

When catalase-negative gram-positive cocci are isolated, first note the colony hemolysis. Always rule out the most common isolates before considering more uncommon isolates such as the *Streptococcus*-like cocci.

- Alpha-hemolytic colonies could be:
  - *S. pneumoniae*
  - viridans streptococci
  - *Enterococcus* spp.
  - Group D *Streptococcus*
- Beta-hemolytic colonies could be:
  - *S. pyogenes*
  - *S. agalactiae*
  - Groups C, F, or G *Streptococcus*
  - rare *Enterococcus* spp.
- Gamma-hemolytic colonies may be:
  - *Enterococcus* spp.
  - Group D *Streptococcus*
  - viridans streptococci
  - rare *S. agalactiae*

The body site will also assist in narrowing down the potential isolates.

- Alpha-hemolytic streptococci in a respiratory site, ear, eye, CSF, or blood
  - Consider *S. pneumoniae* and viridans streptococci first
- Alpha-hemolytic streptococci in a genitourinary or gastrointestinal site or blood
  - Rule out possible Group D *Streptococcus*, *Enterococcus* spp., and viridans streptococci first
- Beta-hemolytic streptococci in a respiratory, wound, genital, CSF, or blood
  - Perform group serotyping first
  - If nontypable, consider the rare possibility of *Enterococcus* spp.
- Gamma-hemolytic streptococci in genitourinary, gastrointestinal, wound, CSF, or blood
  - Consider *Enterococcus* spp., Group D *Streptococcus*, and viridans streptococci first
  - There is also the possibility of rare nonhemolytic *S. agalactiae*, especially if it is found in a female genital body site or newborn

**Checkpoint! 17–18
(Chapter Objective 7)**

Microorganisms associated with bacterial endocarditis include:
1. *viridans streptococci.*
2. *S. gallolyticus.*
3. *Coagulase-negative Staphylococcus spp.*
   A. *1 & 2*
   B. *1 & 3*
   C. *2 & 3*
   D. *1, 2, & 3*

the blood-borne microbe. As the individual becomes more compromised, the organism may settle in other sites. Neutropenic patients are especially vulnerable (Murray et al., 1999).

STREPTOCOCCUS-LIKE COCCI

Some cocci resemble the streptococci and enterococci morphologically but are rarely isolated from clinical specimens. These organisms should be distinguished from potential pathogens as well as recognized as clinically significant in certain instances.

Growth Requirements

Most of the related *Streptococcus*-like cocci are facultative anaerobes. The two exceptions are *Aerococcus*, which is a microaerophile, and *Alloiococcus*, which is an obligate anaerobe (Murray et al., 1999).

Identification

This group of organisms can create problems for even the most experienced microbiologist. They are infrequently isolated and often do not identify accurately with most commercial kits available in the clinical laboratory. The microbiologist must remember this group of organisms when isolates do not fit the characteristics of a routinely encountered bacterium. Reference laboratories may need to be used for speciation.

Most of the time, identification will stop once a potential pathogen is ruled out. If the organism is repeatedly isolated in pure culture or from sterile body sites, further testing may be necessary (Murray et al., 1999). Consultation with the physician may be required to determine their clinical significance and the need for identification.

Microscopic Morphology.   The Gram stain is one of the most helpful clues as to the identity of this group of organisms. The best morphology is obtained by staining the growth of thioglycolate medium. Because these smears are prepared from growth in thioglycolate, fixation of these smears should be with methanol and not heat. Methanol fixation decreases distortion of cells and provides a cleaner background (Isenberg, 1998). The most common cellular morphology should be

noted, as there is usually a mixture of arrangements. If one observes gram-positive cocci in pairs or chains, *Globicatella, Lactococcus, Vagococcus, Dolosicoccus, Leuconostoc,* and nutritionally variant streptococci may be suspected. If clusters are observed, *Rothia* (previously known as *Stomatococcus*) is possible. If pairs or tetrads are observed, *Pediococcus, Aerococcus, Alloiococcus, Gemella, Tetragenococcus,* or *Helcococcus* are suspected (Facklam, 2001; Facklam & Elliott, 1995).

Colony Morphology.   These related *Streptococcus*-like cocci have similar colony morphology to staphylococci, streptococci, and enterococci (Murray et al., 1999). Many resemble the viridans streptococci and can be misidentified as such (Forbes et al., 1998). They may be alpha-hemolytic or nonhemolytic (Facklam, 2001). The nutritionally variant streptococci (NVS), *Abiotrophia* and *Granulicatella,* will not grow without the presence of pyridoxal (vitamin B_6). NVS may grow on chocolate agar.

 REAL WORLD TIP

If gram-positive cocci are observed in the Gram stain of liquid media, such as thioglycolate or blood culture bottles, but there is no growth on solid media, suspect a nutritionally variant streptococci. Test for satellitism using a *Staphylococcus aureus* streak or pyridoxal disk.

Key Biochemical Reactions.   Results from the catalase screening test are negative to weakly positive for the *Alloiococcus, Aerococcus,* and *Rothia.* The remainder are catalase negative.

Alloiococcus can be distinguished from the other catalase-positive cocci by its slower growth (Facklam & Elliott, 1995). It can take 2 to 3 days for detection of growth. *Aerococcus* can be distinguished from *Staphylococcus* by its sensitivity to bacitracin (Taxo A). *Aerococcus* is also distinguished from *Micrococcus* by its negative modified oxidase result. *Rothia* is also modified oxidase negative but can resemble *Staphylococcus.* It is unable to grow in a high concentration of salt, whereas most of the staphylococci can (Ruoff et al., 1999).

 REAL WORLD TIP

Think of *Rothia mucilaginosa* as a "sticky" *Staphylococcus.* The colony is white, nonhemolytic, and has gumlike consistency that likes to adhere to the agar. Because it can be weakly catalase positive, it is can be easily misidentified as *Staphylococcus* spp. The key to its accurate identification is the recognition of its unique sticky colony. Figure 17-35 ■ demonstrates the characteristic stickiness of its colony.

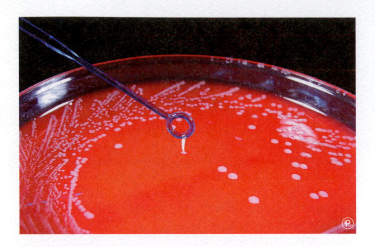

Tests useful in the identification of the catalase-negative cocci include the prolidonyl arylamidase or pyrrolidonase (PYR), leucine aminopeptidase (LAP), bile esculin (BE), 6.5% NaCl, β-glucuronidase (BGUR), and vancomycin susceptibility. Testing for growth at 10°C and 45°C are not as helpful as the other tests. Identification of most genera can be accomplished without testing for growth at 10°C and 45°C (Facklam, 2001). Table 17-8✪ presents test results for the differentiation of catalase-negative gram-positive cocci. Figures 17-36 ■ and 17-37 ■ provide a suggested scheme for identification.

The results listed in Table 17-8 are based on conventional test procedures. The results of these same tests performed by a rapid procedure may not correlate with conventional results. If using rapid test procedures, do not use this table, as it may result in misidentification (Facklam, 2001).

The nutritionally variant streptococci, *Abiotrophia* and *Granulicatella,* require pyridoxal or vitamin B₆ for growth. This growth enhancer must be added to the media to achieve the reactions listed in Table 17-8. Testing for satellitism best identifies NVS. A streak of *Staphylococcus aureus* is placed on to the surface of blood agar inoculated with the suspected NVS. If it is NVS, the organism will satellite or grow only around the *Staphylococcus* streak. Disks containing pyridoxal are commercially available.

✪ **TABLE 17-8**

Differentiation of Catalase-Negative Gram-Positive Cocci

Genus	GS	Van	PYR	LAP	BE	NaCl	Hem	Other Tests
Leuconostoc/Weisella	ch	R	−	V−	V	V	a/n	
Enterococcus group	ch	V	+	+	+	+	a/n	
viridans streptococci/*S. bovis*	ch	S	−	+	V	−	a/n	
NVS	ch	S	+	+	−	−	a/n	Satellites (SS)
Globicatella	ch	S	V+	−	+	+	a/n	
Dolosicoccus	ch	S	+	−	−	−	a	
Pediococcus	cl/t	R	−	+	V	V	a	
Tetragenococcus	cl/t	S	−	+	+	+	a	
Aerococcus	cl/t	S	V	V	V	+	a	Most Hipp +
Helcococcus	cl/t	S	+	−	−	+	n	Most Hipp −
Gemella	cl/t/ch	S	V+	V+	−	−	n	Porphyrin −
Salt-tolerant *Gemella*-like	cl/t/ch	S	+	+	−	+	n	
Rothia (previously *Stomatococcus*)	cl	S	V+	+	NT	−	n	Porphyrin +

GS = Gram stain morphology; Van = vancomycin; PYR = pyrrolidonyl arylamidase; LAP = leucine aminopeptidase; BE = bile esculin; NaCl = 6.5% NaCl; Hem = hemolysis; Hipp = Hippurate; ch = chains; cl/t = clusters and tetrads; cl/t/ch = clusters, tetrads, and chains; cl = clusters, R = resistant; S = sensitive; − = negative; + = positive; V = variable; V− = variable, but most are negative; V+ = variable, but most are positive; a = alpha-hemolytic; n = nonhemolytic, SS = staph. streak
Enterococcus group (*Enterococcus, Vagococcus, Lactococcus*)
NVS = nutritionally variant streptococci (*Abiotrophia, Granulicatella*)
Salt-tolerant *Gemella*-like (*Alloiococcus, Dolosigranulum, Facklamia, Ignavigranum*)

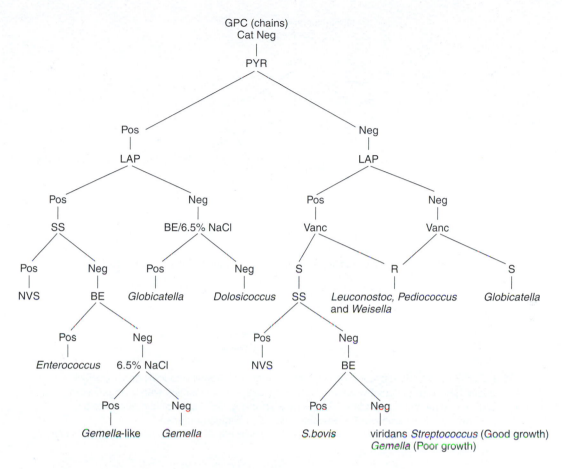

■ **FIGURE 17-36** Identification of non-beta-hemolytic "Streptococcal" gram-positive cocci.
GPC = gram-positive cocci; Cat = catalase; Pos = positive; Neg = negative; LAP = leucine amino-peptidase; PYR = pyrrolidonase; BE = bile esculin agar; SS = *Staphylococcus* streak (satellite test); Vanc = vancomycin; S = sensitive; R = resistant; NVS = nutritionally-variant *Streptococcus*.

The *Leuconostoc* group can be distinguished from the others by its intrinsic resistance to vancomycin and negative leucine aminopeptidase (LAP) and pyrrolidonyl arylamidase (PYR) reactions. *Pediococcus* is also intrinsically resistant to vancomycin, but it will appear as clusters and tetrads on Gram stain. It is usually LAP positive and PYR negative.

Gemella grows poorly in room or ambient air, so the vancomycin susceptibility test should be incubated in CO_2. Some strains are able to grow only anaerobically on initial isolation and become aerotolerant on transfer. They often resemble slow-growing viridans streptococci. Most testing can be incubated in air. Most *Gemella* are pyrrolidonyl arylamidase (PYR) and leucine aminopeptidase (LAP) positive. Most of the other related *Streptococcus*-like cocci that share the same microscopic morphology such as clusters, tetrads, or chains and sensitivity to vancomycin are either PYR and/or LAP negative. *Aerococcus*

 REAL WORLD TIP

Leuconostoc and *Pediococcus* can mimic vancomycin-resistant *Enterococcus* spp. Both can react with group D antiserum, hydrolyze esculin, and grow in 6.5% salt broth just like *Enterococcus* spp. A bile esculin slant and 6.5% salt broth should no longer be used to identify *Enterococcus* spp. because of the possibility of these other catalase-negative, vancomycin-resistant cocci. The LAP and PYR tests will differentiate the three organisms.

 Checkpoint! 17–19 (Chapter Objective 5)

You observe tiny colonies that satellite around a Staphylococcus aureus colony on sheep blood agar. The Gram stain reveals gram-positive cocci, which produce a red color when testing for PYR and LAP. This organism is most likely:

A. S. pyogenes.

B. Enterococcus spp.

C. Gemella spp.

D. nutritionally-variant streptococci.

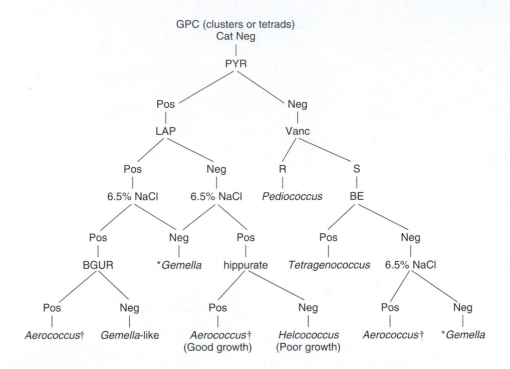

■ FIGURE 17-37 Identification of non-beta-hemolytic "Staphylococcal" gram-positive cocci. GPC = gram-positive cocci; Cat = catalase; Pos = positive; Neg = negative; LAP = leucine aminopeptidase; PYR = pyrrolidonase; BE = bile esculin agar; Vanc = vancomycin; S = sensitive; R = resistant; BGUR = B-glucuronidase.
*Catalase negative Rothia (previously known as Stomatococcus) are porphyrin positive; Gemella and the other related cocci are negative.
+PYR negative Aerococcus (A. urinae is LAP and BGUR positive; A. christensenii is LAP positive and BGUR negative; A. urinaehominis is LAP negative and BGUR positive); PYR positive Aerococcus (A. viridans is LAP negative; A. sanguinicola is LAP positive).*

sanguinicola is also PYR and LAP positive but is 6.5% NaCl and BE positive. *Gemella* is 6.5% NaCl and bile esculin (BE) negative (Facklam, 2001; Murray et al., 2007). The results for the other genera are presented in Table 17-8.

Clinical Significance

Many of these related *Streptococcus*-like cocci are found in the environment on plants, on vegetables, and in dairy products (Forbes et al., 1998). These organisms may also be members of the normal flora in the oral cavity, in respiratory and gastrointestinal systems, and on the skin (Murray et al., 1999). Infections are usually associated with compromised individuals (Forbes et al., 1998). They may be isolated from blood, CSF, urine, and wound specimens (Murray et al., 1999).

Gemella is associated with endocarditis, bacteremia, septic shock, and glomerulonephritis (Facklam 2001). *Gemella* has also been isolated from cultures of synovial fluid from a patient with septic arthritis and CSF from a patient with meningitis (Facklam & Elliott, 1995). *Pediococcus* have been isolated from blood cultures in individuals with bacteremia and abdominal abscesses. *Leuconostoc* are associated with meningitis, **odontogenic** infection, an infection of tissue involved in tooth

development, catheter-associated infection, and bacteremia or septicemia. Infections in compromised patients can be severe. Both *Pediococcus* and *Leuconostoc* have been isolated from infected patients after vancomycin therapy (Facklam & Elliott, 1995). *Aerococcus urinae* may cause urinary tract infections. Nutritionally variant streptococci are associated with endocarditis (Forbes et al. 1998) and ophthalmic infections (Murray et al., 1999). *Rothia* have been isolated in cases of meningitis and endocarditis.

SUMMARY

In this chapter the characteristics of gram-positive cocci isolates have been described. Figure 17-38 ■ visually demonstrates the characteristics that are shared among the gram-positive cocci and those that are different for each genus. The catalase test should be performed to distinguish a catalase-positive *Staphylococcus* or *Micrococcus* from the others. If the reaction is weak, suspect one of the related cocci. Staphylococci and micrococci can be differentiated with the modified oxidase and coagulase tests. The recognized pathogen among the catalase-positive cocci is *S. aureus,* which is also coagulase posi-

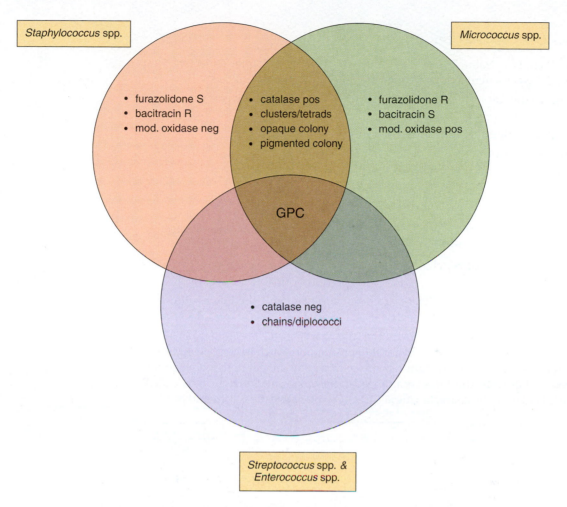

Staphylococcus spp.

Micrococcus spp.

- furazolidone S
- bacitracin R
- mod. oxidase neg

- catalase pos
- clusters/tetrads
- opaque colony
- pigmented colony

- furazolidone R
- bacitracin S
- mod. oxidase pos

GPC

- catalase neg
- chains/diplococci

Streptococcus spp. &
Enterococcus spp.

■ **FIGURE 17-38** GPC same-different. (Characteristics of GPC are the same where the circles overlap and different where they don't overlap.)
S = sensitive; R = resistant; pos = positive; neg = negative; GPC = gram-positive cocci; Pigmented colony = pink, yellow, white, tan, orange.

tive. The other catalase-positive cocci may cause infections in compromised patients.

If the gram-positive cocci are catalase negative, observe for hemolysis around the colonies growing on sheep blood agar. If beta-hemolytic, the PYR and antigen tests are helpful. *Streptococcus pyogenes* and *S. agalactiae* are recognized pathogens. Large-colony groups C and G and Group F are also associated with disease. If alpha-hemolytic, *S. pneumoniae* and *Enterococcus* spp. need to be ruled out as potential pathogens. Tests for optochin susceptibility, bile solubility, PYR, ability to grow in the presence of bile, and hydrolyze esculin (BE) are helpful. If suspect organisms are nonhemolytic, rule out *Enterococcus* spp. first as potential pathogens.

If a LAP result is negative or vancomycin resistance is observed, suspect one of the related *Streptococcus*-like cocci.

The Gram stain morphology in thioglycollate broth is most helpful with identification of these genera. Tests are selected after determination of "streptococcal" or "staphylococcal" cellular morphology. If gram-positive cocci are observed in Gram stains, but no growth occurs on solid media, suspect a nutritionally variant streptococci. Verify the suspect organism as a nutritionally-variant streptococci by testing for the requirement of pyridoxal (vitamin B_6) for growth.

Because both pathogenic and commensal gram-positive cocci may be isolated from the same specimens, it is important to perform sufficient biochemical tests to prevent misidentification.

LEARNING OPPORTUNITIES

1. On the Web: Play Name That Bug: Gram-Positive Cocci (Chapter Objective 5) at URL: http://www.karenkiser.com/Name.bug.html

2. You observe the following colony morphology on two specimens you are processing:

   Colony A = Umbilicate or mucoid, alpha-hemolytic colony, GPC

   Colony B = Translucent, 0.5 mm, beta-hemolytic colony, GPC

   Colony C = 2 to 3 mm, creamy, yellow, beta-hemolytic colony, GPC

   Which tests will you select for identification, and why?
   (Chapter Objectives 2, 5, and 8)

3. How does knowledge of the general characteristics of each genus assist in meeting growth requirements of these organisms? (Chapter Objectives 1 and 4)

4. How do cellular and colony characteristics help categorize the gram-positive cocci? (Chapter Objective 4)

5. Does the esculin test on the BactiCard Strep correlate with the bile esculin agar test? Why? (Chapter Objective 2)

6. Examine the figure below. Notice that some GPC characteristics are arranged in a hierarchal order on a ladder, with #1 being the most important characteristic and #3 of lesser importance. Can you determine why certain items are put in the same group? Can you establish why the items are arranged in the order which they are listed? Identify each ladder by the characteristics it lists. (Chapter Objectives 2, 4, and 8)

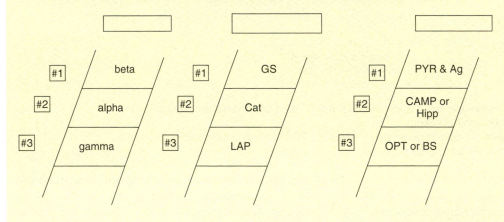

7. Name That Gram-Positive Cocci (Chapter Objective 5)

Name That Gram-Positive Cocci

Match each organism with the correct description (Number 1–11) by placing the number of the matching description with the correct name of bacteria.

Test	1	2	3	4	5	6	7	8	9	10	11
Catalase	−	−	+	−	−	+	−	+	−	+	−
Oxidase	−	−	−	−	−	−	−	−	−	−	−
Mod. Oxidase	−	−	−	−	−	−	−	+	−	−	−
α-hemolysis	−	+		+	+		+		+		−
β-hemolysis	+	−	+	+	−		−		−		+
Nonhemolytic	−	+		+	+	+	−	+	+	+	+
Antigen	A			D					D		B
Coagulase		+				−		−		−	
Novobiocin		S			S		S		R		
PYR	+	−		+	−		−		−		−
Optochin		R		R	R		S		R		
Bacitracin	S		R	R		R		S		R	R
Vancomycin	S	R		S	S		S		S		S
BE	−	+		+	−		−		+		−
6.5% NaCl	−	+/−		+	−		−		−		+
CAMP	−			−							+
Na Hippurate	−	−		−	−				−		+

Leuconostoc _____   S. gallolyticus (previously known as S. bovis) _____   S. agalactiae _____
Micrococcus spp. _____   Coagulase-negative Staphylococcus spp. _____   S. aureus _____
Enterococcus spp. _____   S. pneumoniae _____   S. saprophyticus _____
viridans streptococci _____   S. pyogenes _____

Use this address to access the interactive Companion Website created for this textbook. Simply select "Clinical Laboratory Science" from the choice of disciplines. Find this book and log in using your user name and password.

REFERENCES

Go to myhealthprofessionskit.com to view this chapter's references.

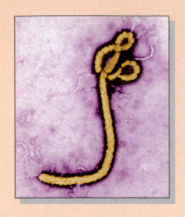

18

Aerobic Gram-Negative Cocci

Karen M. Kiser

■ LEARNING OBJECTIVES

Upon completion of this chapter, the learner should be able to:

1. Distinguish other organisms, such as *Staphylococcus,* from pigmented *Neisseria.*

2. Summarize the purpose, principle, interpretation, and sources of error of each differential test used in the identification of the gram-negative cocci.

3. Identify the purpose of the primary plating media used for isolation of *Neisseria.*

4. Relate key characteristics and natural habitat of *Neisseria* and *Moraxella.*

5. Relate the microscopic culture characteristics and environmental requirements for each gram-negative coccus.

6. Describe the virulence factors and clinical infections associated with gram-negative cocci.

   a. Correlate specific patient populations with potential pathogens.

7. Distinguish *N. gonorrhoeae* from *N. meningitidis.*

8. Differentiate pathogenic *Neisseria* from commensal *Neisseria.*

9. Distinguish *Neisseria* from *Moraxella catarrhalis, Acinetobacter, Capnocytophaga,* and *Kingella.*

10. Correlate patient history, body site or specimen type, colonial morphology, Gram stain reaction, identification test results, and /or susceptibility testing in order to identify the isolate and assess its clinical significance.

KEY TERMS

autolyze

carrier

commensal

exocytosis

fastidious

fulminant

gonococcus

    (pl. gonococci)

meningococcemia

meningococcus

    (pl. meningococci)

oligonucleotides

saprophytic

transcytosis

TAXONOMY

Family *Neisseriaceae* (nī-sé-rê-ā-sê-ê)
   Genus *Neisseria* (nī-sé-rē-a)
      N. gonorrhoeae (gon-or-rē-ā)
      N. meningitidis (me-niń-ji-ti-dis)
      N. polysaccharea (pol-ē-sak-ä-rē-ä)
      N. subflava (sŭb-flā-vä)
      N. flavescens (flā-ves-sins)
      N. cinerea (si-nē-rē-ä)
      N. elongata (ē-lon-gö-tä)
      N. lactamica (lak-tam-ĭ-cä)
   Genus *Kingella* (kĭng-ël-ŭh)
      K. denitrificans (dē-nī-tri-fi-kanz)

Family *Moraxellaceae* (mōŕ-ak-sel-ā-sē-ē)
   Genus *Moraxella* (mōŕ-ak-sel-a)
      M. catarrhalis (kā-tar-al-is)
   Genus *Acinetobacter* (AH-sin-ne-to-bac-ter)

This chapter focuses on the genera of *Neisseria* and the coccoid *Moraxella*. It includes a brief mention of *Kingella* and *Acinetobacter* because they may resemble *Neisseria* and the coccoid *Moraxella*. ∞ Chapter 22 provides more information on these nonfermentative bacilli.

▶ INTRODUCTION

These aerobic cocci are intriguing microorganisms. They share the common characteristic of presenting as gram-negative diplococci (GNDC) with flattened adjacent sides (like a pair of kidney or coffee beans) on gram-stained smears. They may resist decolorization and appear gram-positive, causing erroneous Gram stain reports and patient treatment (Das, Shah, & Levi, 1997). Some species reside as part of the normal flora of our body. Others are potential pathogens and one species is always a pathogen. Their growth requirements help distinguish them because two species are more **fastidious** or have complex nutritional requirements, and prefer enriched media, warmth, and CO_2 for growth. One of the fastidious species will **autolyze** or destroy the cell with its own digestive enzymes if its needs are neglected. The oxidase and catalase tests are useful screening tests for ruling out *Staphylococcus* spp. as well as other organisms that may resemble them. *Staphylococcus* spp. are oxidase negative whereas *Neisseria* and *Moraxella* are oxidase positive (Table 18-1✪). *Kingella* is catalase negative, differentiating it from the catalase-positive aerobic gram-negative cocci. Our job is to identify the presence of aerobic gram-negative cocci in clinical specimens and determine whether the isolate is a potential pathogen.

This chapter reviews the taxonomy of aerobic gram-negative cocci, describes useful biochemical tests, and concentrates on the genus *Neisseria* and *Moraxella catarrhalis*. The discussion of each organism includes the growth requirements, microscopic morphology, colony morphology, key presumptive and final identification tests, and clinical significance. The information for *N. gonorrhoeae* includes its antibiogram. Finally, the chapter covers other microorganisms that resemble gram-negative cocci and may cause confusion.

✔ Checkpoint! 18–1 (Chapter Objective 1)

Staphylococcus can be distinguished from Neisseria by performing a Gram stain and a/an:

   A. catalase test.
   B. oxidase test.
   C. DNase test.
   D. coagulase test.

✪ TABLE 18-1

Differentiation of *Neissera, Moraxella,* and Similar Organisms

Genus	Cell Morphology	Oxidase	Catalase
Neisseria	Diplococcus/Rod	+	+*
Moraxella catarrhalis	Diplococcus	+	+
Kingella	Coccobacillus	+	−
Moraxella spp. other than *M. catarrhalis*	Coccobacillus	+	+
Acinetobacter	Coccobacillus	−	+
Staphylococcus	Coccus	−	+
Streptococcus and *Enterococcus*	Coccus	−	−

+, positive; −, negative
N. elongata may be negative.

► USEFUL BIOCHEMICAL TESTS

Appropriate biochemical tests are selected after presumptive identification. Presumptive identification is based on Gram stain results, growth pattern on media incubated in various atmospheres, colony morphology, and oxidase and catalase test results. Final identification requires additional tests, which are described in the next section.

CARBOHYDRATE UTILIZATION

It is common to test isolates to determine whether they can produce acid from the oxidative metabolism of various carbohydrates. Glucose, maltose, lactose, and sucrose are routinely used. The pattern of utilization allows for differentiation among the various species. One must be cautious because without additional tests, **commensal** Neisseria or those that reside on the host, obtaining nutrients to sustain life without causing harm to the host, may be misidentified as a strict pathogen such as *N. gonorrhoeae* or a potential pathogen such as *N. meningitidis* or *M. catarrhalis*. Fructose may be helpful in the identification of commensal Neisseria.

Traditionally, cystine trypticase agar (CTA) medium with 1% carbohydrate was utilized for testing. This medium is no longer recommended because it is insensitive to acid produced by *Neisseria*. It is often a series of up to four tubes, including glucose (dextrose), maltose, lactose and sucrose, and a control tube with no carbohydrate. The oxidative process produces low concentrations of acid from metabolism of the sugar. Ammonia, produced as a byproduct of peptone metabolism, can neutralize the acid produced in the test medium. These problems can be avoided by using media with a low-protein-to-high-carbohydrate ratio and a sensitive pH indicator such

as phenol red. The medium is semisolid so any acids produced are concentrated. The tubes are incubated at 35°C, in ambient air, for up to four days. A change from red to yellow indicates the production of acid.

REAL WORLD TIP

CTA must be incubated in ambient air, rather than carbon dioxide, to prevent the formation of carbonic acid from CO_2. The presence of carbonic acid can cause a false-positive reaction with the pH indicator present. *Neisseria gonorrhoeae* requires CO_2 for growth so it does not survive well in this semisolid medium. The semisolid consistency and necessity for incubation for up to four days can promote the autolysis of *Neisseria gonorrhoeae*.

There is rapid testing available for the detection of acid from carbohydrates (Figure 18-1 ■). The carbohydrate suspensions are in smaller volumes so results usually only take 2 to 4 hours. One version is placed in microtiter wells and includes butyrate esterase and beta-lactamase in addition to the carbohydrates. The beta-lactamase results should be viewed with suspicion if the acidimetric method is used (Murray, Baron, Pfaller, Tenover, & Yolken, 1999).

REAL WORLD TIP

Neisseria cinerea can appear to be glucose positive in some rapid identification systems and be mistaken for *N. gonorrhoeae*. Both can be recovered from genital and rectal body sites. It is very important to differentiate the two organisms.

NITRATE TEST

The nitrate test is helpful in distinguishing *N. gonorrhoeae* (nitrate negative) from *K. denitrificans* and *M. catarrhalis* (both nitrate positive). It is also useful in identifying commensals when positive. See ∞ Chapter 9, "Final Identification," for a review of the nitrate test.

POLYSACCHARIDE SYNTHESIS FROM SUCROSE

This test determines an organism's ability to produce a starch-like polysaccharide from sucrose. This medium is not commercially available, but may be prepared if access to a media kitchen is available. It is useful for distinguishing *N. meningitidis* from *N. polysaccharea* and speciating the commensals.

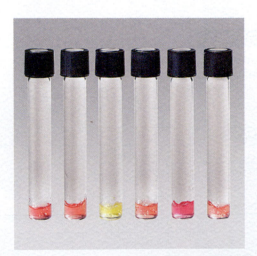

■ **FIGURE 18-1** Rapid fermentation agar: Control, sucrose, dextrose, fructose, maltose, and lactose showing positive (yellow) and negative (red) results for *N. gonorrhoeae*.
Photos courtesy of Remel, part of Thermo Fisher Scientific.

N. polysaccharea is positive whereas *N. meningitidis* is negative for polysaccharide synthesis from sucrose. Both organisms are able to ferment glucose and maltose so this test is important for their differentiation. Other commensal organisms are negative for the ability to produce polysaccharide from sucrose.

A starch-free medium with 1% sucrose is inoculated so that well-isolated colonies are obtained. After incubation for 24–48 hours, with or without CO_2, a drop of Gram's iodine (diluted 1:4) or Lugol's iodine is dropped onto the colonies. Observe for a dark blue–purple to black color in and around the colony (Hoke & Vedros, 1982). An alternative procedure is described by Koneman, Allen, Janda, Schreckenberger, and Winn (1997), which is performed using a rapid fermentation sucrose tube. One to two drops of regular Gram's iodine is added to the sucrose tube after 4 hours' incubation. A deep purple-to-blue color is positive (Figure 18-2). Iodine can be added to the maltose tube (a negative control) and will turn it into a tan color.

DNase

The DNase test evaluates an organism's ability to degrade DNA via the production of deoxyribonuclease. The organism is inoculated on DNase medium and incubated overnight. The growth is flooded with 1N HCL and observed for the formation of a clear zone around the inoculum. The appearance of a clear zone (Figure 18-3) is a positive reaction.

HCL will precipitate intact, polymerized DNA and cause the media to appear opaque. A clear zone (a positive result) will appear in the presence of **oligonucleotides**, a compound made up of a small number of nucleotides. The addition of dyes such as methyl green or toluidine blue enhances the visibility of the clear zone. *M. catarrhalis* and other coccoid *Moraxella* are the only aerobic gram-negative cocci that are DNase positive (Jannes et al., 1993).

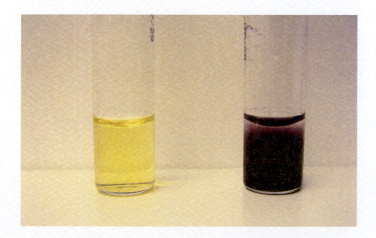

■ **FIGURE 18-2** Positive (right) polysaccharide synthesis from sucrose compared to a negative reaction on the left.

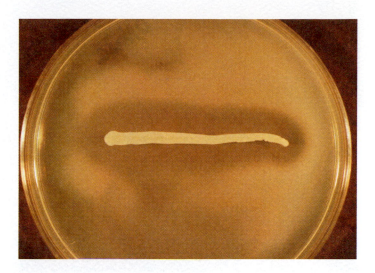

■ **FIGURE 18-3** Positive DNase test (clear zone) after flooding agar surface with hydrochloric acid.

> ✓ **Checkpoint! 18–2 (Chapter Objective 2)**
>
> *A positive DNase test would be indicated by:*
> A. *colonies becoming pink and finally black.*
> B. *clear zones around the growth.*
> C. *bubbling up from the colony.*
> D. *clotting of the plasma.*

SUPEROXOL TEST

The superoxol test is a catalase test that uses 30% hydrogen peroxide rather than the traditional 3% hydrogen peroxide concentration. It is useful for distinguishing *N. gonorrhoeae* from the other species. It is performed by dropping the reagent directly onto colonies growing on chocolate agar. Blood agar cannot be used for catalase testing because red blood cells may cause a false positive. One can also select a colony using a wooden stick, place it on a clean glass or plastic slide, and add a drop of 30% H_2O_2. A false positive may result if you reverse the order. The degree of bubbling is observed. *N. gonorrhoeae* gives an immediate explosive result (++++) (Figure 18-4 ■). Most other *Neisseria* species show weaker bubbling results (++). Some *N. meningitidis* and *M. catarrhalis* strains may also give a strong positive (++++) reaction if large amounts of organisms are used for testing.

> ℮ **REAL WORLD TIP**
>
> 30% H_2O_2 is extremely caustic and burns may occur if your skin comes into contact with the reagent. If this reagent is used, you should have 70% alcohol on hand to neutralize the reagent's action. Flood the exposed area with alcohol (not water) without delay in the event of skin exposure.

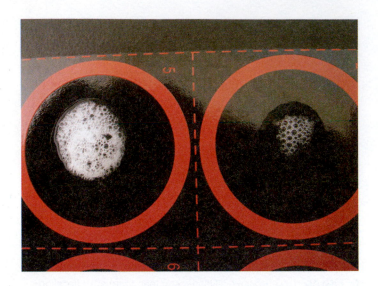

■ **FIGURE 18-4** The positive (left) superoxol reaction is suggestive of *Neisseria gonorrhoeae.* The weaker reaction on the right is seen with other *Neisseria* spp.

BUTYRATE ESTERASE

Organisms that produce butyrate esterase are able to act on indoxyl butyrate to produce indoxyl. The substrate can be placed on a paper disk or in suspension. The end-product, indoxyl, turns indigo or blue-green (Figure 18-5 ■). The disk test is rapid and only takes two minutes to results. *Moraxella catarrhalis* is positive for butyrate esterase while *Neisseria* spp. are negative.

MULTITEST IDENTIFICATION

There are commercially available test systems that include tests for sugar utilization and enzymes for substrates, such as phosphate, ortho-nitrophenyl-β-galactosidase (ONPG), proline aminopeptidase (PRO), γ-glutamylaminopeptidase (GGA),

resazurin, and urea. Testing also includes indole, ornithine decarboxylation, and nitrate reduction. These systems perform well to identify *N. gonorrhoeae, N. meningitidis,* and *M. catarrhalis.* Some systems also identify *N. cinerea, N. lactamica,* and other commensal *Neisseria.* PRO negative *N. gonorrhoeae* have been described so those test systems that include this reaction may result in misidentification. Additional tests may be required to accurately identify other species of *Neisseria* (Alexander & Ison, 2005). Figure 18-6 ■ shows a photo of the RapID™ Neisseria/Haemophilus (NH) identification panel from Remel Inc.

CHROMOGENIC ENZYME SUBSTRATE TESTS

Chromogenic enzyme substrate tests (Figure 18-7 ■) are used for rapid identification of 18- to 48-hour cultures of isolates that morphologically resemble the pathogens and grow on selective media. The substrate is impregnated on a paper disk rather than in a suspension. Substrates used include GGA, PRO, indoxyl butyrate (IB), and β-galactosidase (BGAL). These methods should be used to identify only *N. gonorrhoeae, N. meningitidis, N. lactamica,* and *M. catarrhalis* (Table 18-2✿). Only colonies from selective medium should be tested. *N. sicca, N. flavescens,* and *N. subflava* are able to produce GGA and PRO. These organisms can be misidentified as *N. meningitidis* because some strains may grow on selective media such as modified Thayer-Martin or Martin-Lewis medium.

Interpret results with caution as *N. gonorrhoeae* may be misidentified if these are the only tests used. Definitive identification of *N. meningitidis* should include additional tests (Dealler, Gough, Campbell, Turner, & Hawkey, 1991). PRO negative *N. gonorrhoeae* have been isolated.

It may be necessary to perform a test for butyrate esterase to identify *M. catarrhalis.* Rub disks containing indoxyl

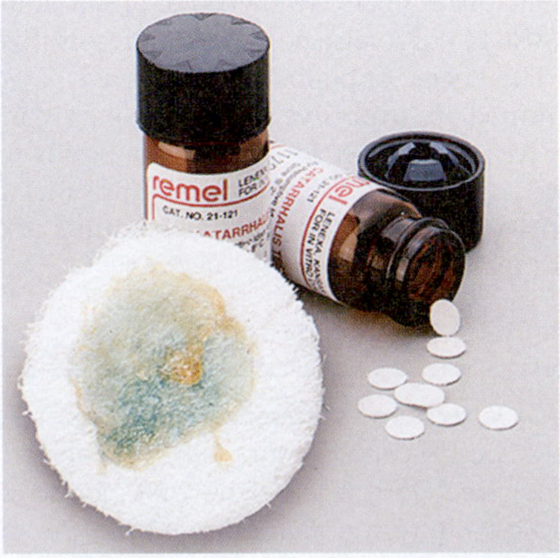

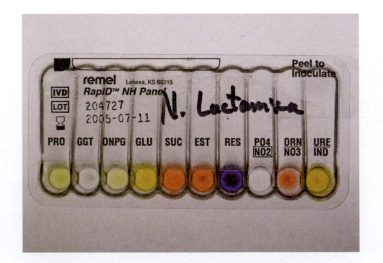

■ **FIGURE 18-5** Positive result for butyrate esterase.
Photo courtesy of Remel, part of Thermo Fisher Scientific.

■ **FIGURE 18-6** RapID™ NH panel from Remel.
Photo courtesy of Remel, part of Thermo Fisher Scientific.

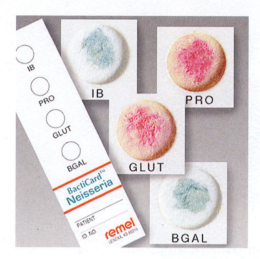

■ **FIGURE 18-7** Chromogenic enzyme test (BactiCard® Neisseria) from Remel (IB tests for Butyrate esterase; BGAL for beta-galactosidase; GLUT for gamma-glutamyl aminopeptidase; and PRO for prolyl aminopeptidase).
Photos courtesy of Remel, part of Thermo Fisher Scientific.

butyrate with colonies suspected of being *M. catarrhalis*. A blue reaction indicates the presence of the enzyme butyrate esterase (Dealler, Abbott, Croughan, & Hawkey, 1989). Other *Moraxella* species can be butyrate esterase and GGA positive.

 REAL WORLD TIP

It is important to correlate Gram stain, colony morphology, oxidase, and catalase results as well as perform sufficient testing to prevent misidentification of isolates.

▶ NEISSERIA

This genus contains two pathogenic species and many that are commensals. Let's look at the pathogenic *Neisseria* first, then consider the role of the **saprophytic** species or organisms able to live on the products of organic breakdown.

PATHOGENIC *NEISSERIA*

Neisseria gonorrhoeae is a strict pathogen and is always considered significant on isolation. *Neisseria meningitidis* is an opportunistic pathogen which can colonize the mucous membranes of humans and may cause significant infections.

General Characteristics

The pathogens share the Gram stain morphology of gram-negative cocci with the nonpathogenic *Neisseria*. Both of these pathogens may stimulate white blood cells, which results in their phagocytosis. A microbiologist is always interested in the bacteria that attract white blood cells. Their presence in a Gram stain, especially when observed inside white blood cells, indicates an inflammatory response. See ∞ Chapter 4 for a review of inflammation.

 REAL WORLD TIP

It's important to examine carefully any polymorphonuclear leukocytes (PMNs) in direct smears for the presence of intracellular and extracellular gram-negative diplococci.

The pathogens are more demanding in their growth requirements than the nonpathogens. They usually prefer enriched media, require a humid environment, a temperature of 35–37°C, and an atmosphere of CO_2 for growth.

Primary plating media designed to enhance the growth of these organisms is used routinely for those specimens that may contain these species as pathogens. Both chocolate and selective agars for *Neisseria* (Modified Thayer-Martin, Martin-Lewis, New York City, JEMBEC) are enriched with hemoglobin as well as other factors that enhance the growth of the pathogens. The selective agars for *Neisseria* also contain colistin and other antibiotics, which inhibit the growth of most commensals. Figure 18-8 ■ illustrates the necessity for the use of selective agar, such as Thayer-Martin, in the recovery of pathogenic *Neisseria* spp. from body sites with normal flora.

✪ TABLE 18-2

Expected Results for Chromogenic Enzyme Substrate Tests

	Indoxyl Butyrate Esterase (IB)	β-galactosidase (BGAL)	γ-glutamylaminopeptidase (GGA)	Proline-laminopeptidase (PRO)
Moraxella catarrhalis	+	−	−	−
Neisseria lactamica	−	+	−	+
N. gonorrhoeae	−	−	−	+
N. meningitidis	−	−	+	−/+

+, positive; −, negative; −/+, most negative with occasional positive.

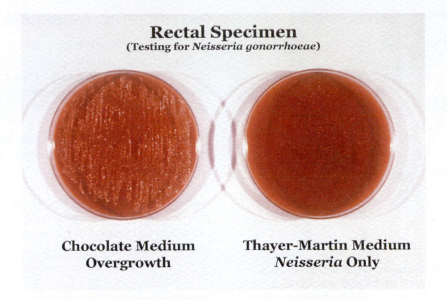

Rectal Specimen
(Testing for *Neisseria gonorrhoeae*)

Chocolate Medium
Overgrowth

Thayer-Martin Medium
Neisseria **Only**

■ **FIGURE 18-8** Body sites that contain normal flora, such as the rectum, require the use of selective agar to recover pathogenic *Neisseria* spp.
Public Health Image Library/CDC and Renelle Woodall

REAL WORLD TIP

Some strains of *Neisseria gonorrhoeae* are inhibited by the vancomycin present in Thayer-Martin agar. During specimen processing, always include a chocolate agar in addition to a Thayer-Martin agar to ensure the recovery of these vancomycin susceptible strains.

✓ Checkpoint! 18–3
(Chapter Objective 3)

A medium useful for the isolation of pathogenic Neisseria is:
  A. *sheep blood agar.*
  B. *MacConkey agar.*
  C. *Thayer-Martin agar.*
  D. *phenylethyl alcohol agar.*

NEISSERIA GONORRHOEAE

Identification

The identification of *N. gonorrhoeae* is based on microscopic morphology, colony morphology, and key biochemical reactions (Figure 18-9 ■). Nonculture tests such as nucleic acid probes and molecular amplification tests are used in most laboratories to identify the presence of *N. gonorrhoeae* in genital specimens. This approach is faster but can be costly and these results cannot be used in a court of law such as in cases of rape and sexual abuse. Cross reactions with commensal *Neisseria* and related organisms may also occur with nucleic acid amplification tests.

Molecular tests for the diagnosis of gonorrhea are more sensitive than culture and can detect *Chlamydia trachomatis*

in the same specimen (Centers for Disease Control and Prevention, 2002). Culture may be more appropriate for nongenital sites (unless approved by the Food and Drug Administration) and potential child abuse cases (Centers for Disease Control and Prevention, 2002; McNally et al., 2008; Schaechter, Moncada, Liska, Shayevich, & Klausner, 2008). False positives may occur in populations with low incidence of gonorrhea (Centers for Disease Control and Prevention, 2002). False positives can also occur for up to three weeks after treatment.

The Centers for Disease Control and Prevention (CDC) currently recommends confirmation of positive results, but a study by Moncada, Donegan, and Schacter (2008) shows that this confirmatory testing is "not warranted" for urethral swabs, cervical swabs, and first-catch urine because greater than 90% of all nucleic acid amplification tests were confirmed as positive. See ∞ Chapter 9, "Final Identification," and ∞ Chapter 36, "Genital System," to review the advantages and disadvantages of nucleic acid amplification testing and sexually transmitted diseases.

REAL WORLD TIP

The direct Gram stain of urethral specimens from symptomatic males is 95% sensitive and 100% specific for *N. gonorrhoeae.* Sensitivity drops to about 60% in asymptomatic males. Direct Gram stain is only presumptive for endocervical specimens. The sensitivity of a direct Gram stain is only about 70% for symptomatic females. Females possess normal genital flora, such as *Acinetobacter* and *Moraxella* spp., which can mimic *N. gonorrhoeae* on Gram stain.

Microscopic Morphology. Gram stain reveals gram-negative diplococci with flattened adjacent sides that resemble a pair of coffee or kidney beans (Figure 18-10 ■). It may be necessary to rule out gram-negative coccobacilli to ensure an accurate interpretation. This can be done by performing the cell elongation test or staining growth from liquid medium. The cell elongation test is performed by Gram staining or preparing a wet preparation from the growth at the edge of the zone of inhibition around a 10 international unit (IU) penicillin disk. Observation of long filaments (Figure 18-11 ■) or "snakes" is characteristic of coccobacilli. Observation of cocci is characteristic of most *Neisseria* and the coccoid *Moraxella* such as *M. catarrhalis* (Catlin, 1975).

Colony Morphology. *N. gonorrhoeae* is the most fragile and fastidious of the *Neisseria* spp. It requires enriched medium such as chocolate agar as well as CO_2 for growth. Growth on chocolate agar appears as 0.5–1 mm entire, gray, and sticky

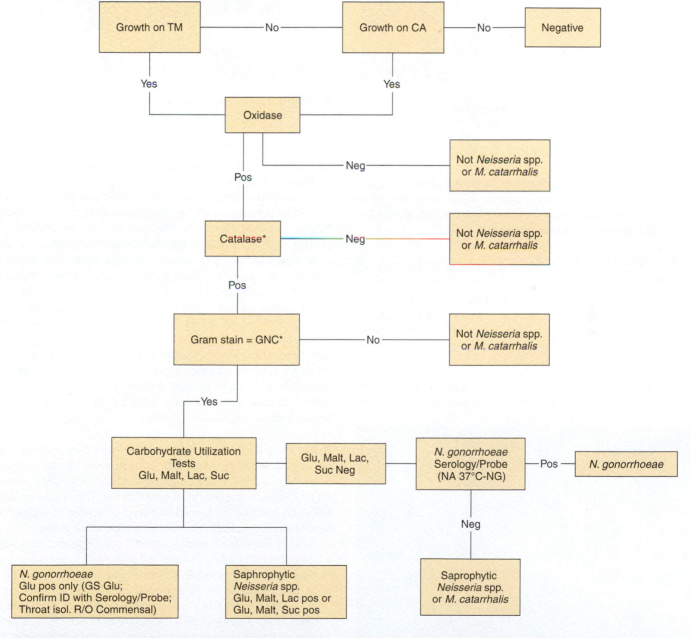

■ **FIGURE 18-9** Identification of *N. gonorrhoeae*.
TM = Thayer Martin; CA = Chocolate agar; GNC = Gram-negative cocci; GLU = Glucose; MALT = Maltose; LAC = Lactose; SUC = Sucrose; Neg = Negative; Pos = Positive; GS = Gram stain; NA = Nutrient agar; NG = No growth; ID = Identification; R/O = Rule out commensal *Neisseria* (colistin sensitivity, γ-glutamylaminopeptidase, Prolylaminopeptidase, pigment); CI = Colistin (10 μg); R = Resistant.
N. elongata is a gram-negative rod and may be catalase negative.

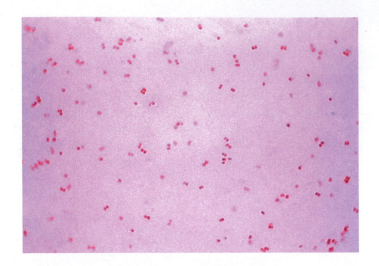

■ **FIGURE 18-10** Gram stain of *N. gonorrhoeae*.
From Public Health Image Library (PHIL), CDC/Joe Miller.

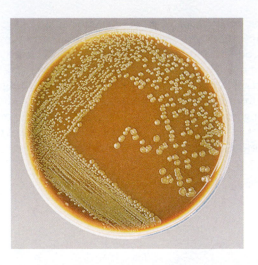

■ **FIGURE 18-12** Colonies of *N. gonorrhoeae* on chocolate agar.
Photo courtesy of Remel, part of Thermo Fisher Scientific.

colonies that may lift off the medium (Figure 18-12 ■). It may present with colonies demonstrating variations in size so that it gives a mixed culture appearance. Robust isolates can grow on blood agar but will only appear as discreet, pinpoint colonies. Most isolates grow on Thayer-Martin and other selective media used for *Neisseria* isolation.

> ℮ **REAL WORLD TIP**
>
> Because *Neisseria gonorrhoeae* may grow as pinpoint colonies on sheep blood agar, Gram stain any tiny colonies that appear on urine cultures in significant quantities.

Key Presumptive ID Tests. Colonies should be screened with the oxidase and catalase tests. ∞ Chapter 8 includes pho-

tos of positive results for these tests. *N. gonorrhoeae* is oxidase and catalase positive and ferments glucose but not lactose, maltose, or sucrose.

Presumptive identification can be made on the observation of oxidase positive, gram-negative diplococci, grown on selective agar such as Thayer-Martin. Most strains are positive for proline-aminopeptidase. PRO negative strains do exist and may cause a false-negative result for this enzyme and misidentification of the isolate. Additional tests must be performed to confirm identification. If isolated on nonselective medium or if test results do not correlate with growth characteristics or colony morphology, a test for resistance to colistin is recommended. Many commensal *Neisseria* are colistin sensitive. Resistance is usually demonstrated by the ability to grow on selective (Thayer-Martin, Martin-Lewis, New York City, or JEMBEC) medium, or no zone around a 10 μg colistin disk on chocolate agar. See ∞ Chapter 8 for a review of presumptive identification of bacterial colonies.

Key Final ID Tests. Additional tests may include biochemicals, serology, or nucleic acid probes. The isolation of *Neisseria gonorrhoeae* in a child, beyond the immediate neonatal period, indicates potential sexual abuse. The organism identification must be confirmed by two different methods such as biochemical, serologic, or non-amplified DNA probe.

Most *N. gonorrhoeae* strains produce acid in glucose only, and are negative for nitrate reduction. All positive glucose tests should be Gram stained, if possible, to ensure the reaction is due to carbohydrate oxidation by *N. gonorrhoeae* and no other microbe.

If isolated from the throat, a nutrient agar incubated at 35–37°C in CO_2, as well as a chocolate agar at room temperature, may help to rule out commensal *Neisseria*. *N. gonorrhoeae* and *N. meningitidis* will not grow but the commensal *Neisseria* do grow.

Maltose-negative *N. meningitidis*, weak glucose-positive *N. cinerea*, *M. catarrhalis*, and *K. denitrificans* could be misidentified as *N. gonorrhoeae*. *N. meningitidis* is positive for GGA

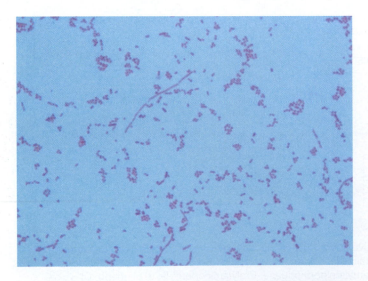

■ **FIGURE 18-11** Gram stain of *Acinetobacter* showing a positive cell elongation test.

✔ Checkpoint! 18–4 (Chapter Objectives 1 and 9)

A fastidious gram-negative cocci turns purplish-black with the oxidase reagent, bubbles with the catalase test, and produces acid in glucose only is potentially:

A. *Staphylococcus epidermidis.*
B. *Saprophytic Neisseria.*
C. *Neisseria meningitidis.*
D. *Neisseria gonorrhoeae.*

whereas *N. gonorrhoeae* is negative. *N. cinerea* should be sensitive to colistin, whereas *N. gonorrhoeae* is resistant. *M. catarrhalis* is DNase and butyrate esterase positive whereas *N. gonorrhoeae* is negative. *K. denitrificans* is nitrate positive whereas *N. gonorrhoeae* is negative (Knapp, 1988). See ∞ Chapter 9 for a review of final identification of bacterial isolates.

Serological confirmatory tests include a fluorescent antibody test as well as coagglutination tests. Some **gonococci**, the common name for *N. gonorrhoeae*, do not react with the fluorescent antibody test and false positives may occur with mixed cultures. See ∞ Chapter 10 for information on immunological tests.

Nucleic acid probes may also be used for confirmation. Their sensitivity and specificity can be good if appropriate specimens are used for testing. See ∞ Chapter 9 for information on molecular tests.

Antibiogram Pattern.   *Neisseria gonorrhoeae* has developed widespread resistance to agents used to treat gonorrhea. This resistance is both chromosomally mediated as well as plasmid mediated. Beta-lactamase testing is best conducted with the highly sensitive nitrocefin test method (Clinical and Laboratory Standards Institute, 2006). In the past penicillin, tetracycline, and spectinomycin were effective treatments. In 1993, the Centers for Disease Control and Prevention recommended that extended-spectrum cephalosporins or fluoroquinolones be used to treat uncomplicated infections. As a result of increasing resistance, only cephalosporins are currently recommended (Centers for Disease Control and Prevention, 2007). A single dose treatment of one of the quinolones and doxycylcine or azithromycin is often used for co-infections due to *N. gonorrhoeae* and *Chlamydia trachomatis*.

REAL WORLD TIP

Sensitivity testing is not routinely performed on *Neisseria gonorrhoeae* because it is fastidious and resistant strains are rare.

Culture and sensitivity testing should be performed in the event of treatment failure. Isolates resistant to third-generation cephalosporin or fluoroquinolone should be checked for purity and correct identification. Testing should be repeated, and results checked to ensure the absence of technical error and accurate test system function (Clinical and Laboratory Standards Institute, 2006). Confirmed resistant isolates should be reported to the public health department (Centers for Disease Control and Prevention, 2007). See ∞ Chapter 11 for a review of sensitivity testing.

Clinical Significance

Specimens of Choice for Isolation.   *Neisseria gonorrhoeae* is always considered a pathogen, even when isolated from anogenital and oropharyngeal specimens. Its only host is humans. *N. gonorrhoeae* can be isolated from endocervical, vaginal, urethra, rectum, pharynx, endometrium, fallopian tube, skin lesions, joint fluid, blood and conjunctiva specimens.

REAL WORLD TIP

Primary media should include chocolate and selective agars if normal flora is present in the body site or specimen type cultured. Cotton swabs should not be used to collect specimens for *N. gonorrhoeae*, unless their toxicity is neutralized by placing the swab in liquid media containing charcoal (Evangelista & Beilstein, 1993). Calcium alginate swabs may also be toxic for some strains (Lauer & Masters, 1988).

Sodium polyanethol sulfonate (SPS), the anticoagulant used in blood culture bottles, is toxic to *N. gonorrhoeae*. If the correct ratio of blood to broth is maintained at the time of collection, the lethal effects of SPS are diluted so the organism should grow. If the volume of blood drawn is less than recommended, 1% gelatin can be added. The Isolator system can also be used to collect blood when disseminated *N. gonorrhoeae* is suspected. See ∞ Chapters 6 and 7 for reviews of specimen collection and cultivation.

Host Encounter.   *N. gonorrhoeae* initiates infection by colonizing the host at the site of entry such as the columnar epithelial cells lining the mucosal surfaces of the genitourinary tract. Attachment to the host cell is facilitated by pili and cell wall lipoligosaccharide (LOS), which appears to be toxic to neighboring ciliated epithelial cells. Shortly after colonization, these neighboring cells stop beating and slough from the tissue. The organism appears to enter the cell and move across the cell via **transcytosis**, enclosed in a vesicle formed by enfolding of the cell membrane. It then exits via **exocytosis**, when a vesicle fuses with the cell membrane and ruptures, discharging its contents; and entering the subepithelial matrix. This ability to invade the epithelial cell appears to be related to a high level of opacity (Opc and/or Opa/class 5) proteins in their outer membrane. Bacteria that express these proteins on their surface have colonies that are visibly more opaque. These proteins allow the bacteria to become more tightly attached to the epithelial cells and contribute to cell invasion.

Receptors for iron binding compounds such as transferrin and lactoferrin are also present in their outer membrane (Nassif & So, 1995). See ∞ Chapter 3 for a review of cell wall structure.

Microbe Defense Strategies.   Ability to cause disease is also related to the organism's capacity to withstand the host defenses. *N. gonorrhoeae* hides from the immune system by changing the composition of its pili. This may also reduce the organism's adhesiveness. Sialic acid is a compound found on many of the host cells. By sialylating lipooligosaccharide (LOS), the organism is able to resist complement and avoids triggering the production of antibodies, so it is not perceived by the host as foreign (Nassif & So, 1995). It also produces an IgA protease, which provides some protection from antibody attack while attached to the mucosa. Outer membrane porins may impair a phagocyte's ability to kill by decreasing the oxidative burst or preventing phagolysosome fusion (Koneman et al., 1997). See ∞ Chapter 4 for a review of the host's encounter with microbes.

Pathogenic States.   Diseases caused by *N. gonorrhoeae* include gonorrhea, eye infections, disseminated gonococcal infections, and pelvic inflammatory disease (PID). A description of each follows.

Gonorrhea.   According to the CDC, gonorrhea (also known as the clap or GC) is one of the most common sexually transmitted diseases (STDs), second only to *Chlamydia trachomatis*. It is often found in co-infections with *C. trachomatis*. (See ∞ Chapter 31 for information on *Chlamydia*.) It is estimated that only half of the cases are reported to authorities. The incidence is highest among urban individuals under 24 years of age with multiple sex partners who practice unprotected sexual intercourse (Murray, Baron, Pfaller, Tenover, & Yolken, 1999). Females are often asymptomatic, which help contribute to its persistence as a cause of STD. Symptomatic males usually exhibit purulent penile discharge and dysuria.

REAL WORLD TIP

Neisseria gonorrhoeae infection is a reportable disease and confirmed cases must be reported to the state health department.

N. gonorrhoeae is very fastidious, and does not survive long outside of the host. Its survival is dependent upon direct contact transmission, most often of a sexual nature. Transmission to neonates can occur during birth. Isolation of this organism from older babies and children usually results in charges of sexual abuse.

Individuals practicing oral or anal intercourse risk exposure to this organism. Females who are not practicing anal intercourse may develop a rectal infection from autoinoculation with cervical secretions.

Eye infections occur most often in newborns and occasionally in adults. Neonates acquire the organism during birth while passing through an infected birth canal. The infection

is known as ophthalmia neonatorum. The infant exhibits a profuse, hyperpurulent discharge with eyelid edema and periorbital cellulitis. ∞ Chapter 38, "Central Nervous System," provides a discussion and figure of this condition. Adults can directly contaminate the eye by fingers or towels (Piehl, 1992). Blindness can occur if not treated promptly.

Disseminated Gonococcal Infection.   One to three percent of gonorrhea infections may become systemic (Murray, Baron, Pfaller, Tenover, & Yolken, 1999). In the past these infections were thought to be due to untreated asymptomatic infections but evidence seems to indicate that a deficiency in complement is more likely. This condition is discussed in depth in ∞ Chapter 40, "Opportunistic Infection." Patients may develop "dermatitis–arthritis" syndrome or septic arthritis. A few develop endocarditis or meningitis. Complications include pericarditis, pericardial effusions, and adult respiratory distress syndrome (Murray, Baron, Jorgensen, Landry, & Pfaller, 2007).

REAL WORLD TIP

Any gram-negative diplococci, resembling *N. gonorrhoeae*, recovered from blood, or cerebrospinal fluid should be differentiated from *N. meningitidis. Neisseria meningitidis* is the more common isolate from these sites and may be associated with a life-threatening community outbreak.

Pelvic Inflammatory Disease.   Ten to twenty percent of untreated *N. gonorrhoeae* infections in females, ascend or move upward from the endocervix to the uterus, fallopian tubes, ovaries, and peritoneal cavity. It causes endometritis, salpingitis, tubo-ovarian abscesses, and pelvic peritonitis. The inflammatory response may cause scarring and blockage of the fallopian tubes (Murray, Baron, Jorgensen, Landry, & Pfaller, 2007). The reproductive system may be permanently damaged, which can lead to infertility or ectopic pregnancies. The reader should review ∞ Chapter 36, "Genital System," for more information on STDs.

✓ Checkpoint! 18–5 (Chapter Objective 6)

The causative agent of gonorrhea is an oxidase positive GNDC that:
  A. *ferments glucose but not maltose, lactose, or sucrose.*
  B. *ferments glucose and maltose but not lactose or sucrose.*
  C. *is butyrate esterase positive.*
  D. *synthesizes polysaccharide from sucrose.*

NEISSERIA MENINGITIDIS

Identification

Identification of *N. meningitidis* is based on microscopic morphology, colony morphology, and key biochemical reactions (Figure 18-13). Microbiologists who work with

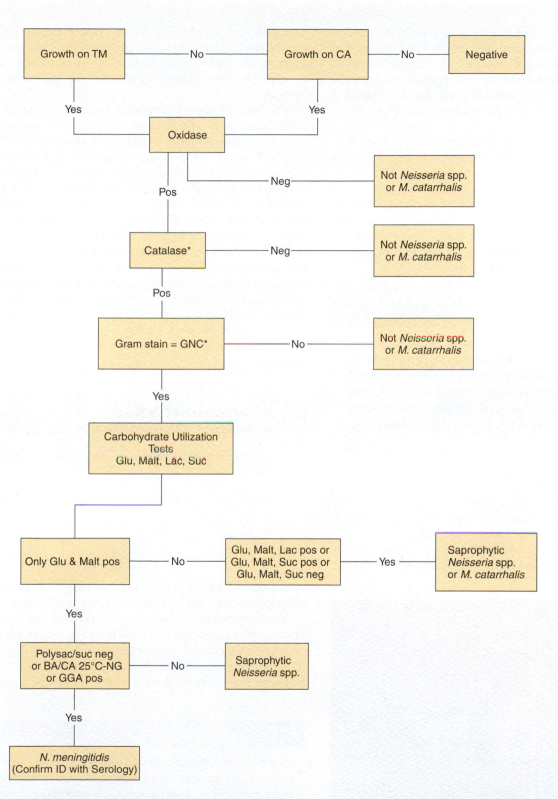

■ FIGURE 18-13 Identification of *N. meningitidis*.
TM = Thayer Martin; CA = Chocolate agar; GNC = Gram-negative cocci; GLU = Glucose; MALT = Maltose; LAC = Lactose; SUC = Sucrose; Neg = Negative; Pos = Positive; NA = Nutrient agar; NG = No growth; BA = Blood agar; Polysac/suc = Polysaccharide from sucrose; ID = Identification; GGA = Gamma-glutamylaminopeptidase.
N. elongata is a gram-negative rod and may be catalase negative.

N. meningitidis isolates are at increased risk of laboratory-acquired infections. Individuals who work with cultures that may contain the organism should perform all procedures in a Class II biosafety cabinet. Other barrier-type safety equipment does not appear to provide adequate protection from invasive disease when working with these isolates (Sejvar et al., 2005).

Microscopic Morphology. Gram stain reveals gram-negative diplococci with flattened adjacent sides that resemble coffee or kidney beans.

Colony Morphology. Growth can be observed on chocolate agar as 1–2 mm creamy and gray colonies. On blood agar they are blue-gray and may display alpha-hemolysis (Figure 18-14 ■). Most isolates will also grow on selective media used for isolation of pathogenic *Neisseria* spp.

Key Presumptive ID Tests. Colonies should be screened with the oxidase and catalase tests as described previously. *N. meningitidis* is oxidase and catalase positive and ferments glucose and maltose but not lactose and sucrose.

Presumptive identification of *Neisseria* spp. can be made on the observation of oxidase-positive, gram-negative diplococci.

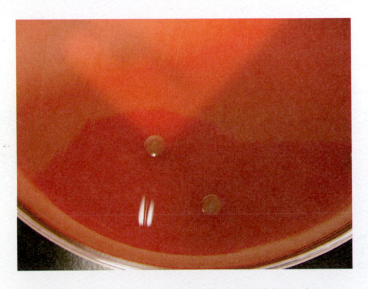

This pathogen is GGA positive and beta-galactosidase negative. *N. meningitidis* may be isolated from the same specimens as the commensal *Neisseria*. Additional tests must be performed to confirm identification and rule out the saprophytic *Neisseria*.

If isolated on nonselective medium, a test for colistin resistance based on its ability to grow on selective media or displaying no zone around a 10 µg colistin disk is helpful. It may help rule out *N. subflava* biovar *subflava* and biovar *flava*. Observation of *N. subflava*'s yellow pigment production will also aid in correct identification. Many commensal *Neisseriae* are colistin sensitive, unable to grow on selective media and may produce pigment. The production of polysaccharide from sucrose is an important test for ruling out *N. polysaccharea* and *N. subflava* biovar *perflava* isolates capable of growing on selective media with colistin. *N. polysaccharea* and *N. subflava* biovar *perflava* is positive for polysaccharide production, whereas *N. meningitidis* is negative. *N. polysaccharea* and *N. subflava* biovar *perflava* is also GGA and beta-galactosidase negative (Anand, Ashton, Shaw, & Gordon, 1991; Boquete, Marcos, & Sáez-Nieto, 1986; D'Amato, Eriquez, Tomfohrde, & Singerman, 1978).

Key Final ID Tests. Final identification of *N. meningitidis* relies on biochemical and serology tests (see Figure 18-13).

N. meningitidis produces acid in glucose and maltose, is negative for polysaccharide synthesis from sucrose, and is nitrate negative. An alternative test for lactose is the beta-galactosidase (ONPG) test. *N. lactamica* is positive whereas *N. meningitidis* is negative. See ∞ Chapter 9 for a review of the ONPG test.

The **meningococci**, the common name for *Neisseria meningitidis*, have 13 serotypes (A, B, C, D, 29E, H, I, K, L, X, Y, Z, W135) based on the specific polysaccharide capsule present (Murray, Baron, Jorgensen, Landry, & Pfaller, 2007). Serotypes A, B, C, Y, and W135 are the most frequent causes of systemic disease in the United States. Group B is most predominant followed by groups A and C. Groups A and C cause epidemic meningitis (Difco Laboratories, 1998). Groups B, W135, and other serotypes have been associated with outbreaks (Harrison, 2006). Serological tests can be used to test for the most common serotypes directly in body fluids such as cerebrospinal fluid, urine, or blood. They are no longer used in most laboratories because rapid bacterial antigen detection (BAD) lacks sensitivity and is not clinically useful (Perkins, Mirrett, & Reller, 1995; Tarafdar, Rao, Recco, & Zaman, 2001). ∞ Chapter 38, "Central Nervous System," provides a detailed discussion on BAD.

The meningococcal vaccine contains purified bacterial capsular polysaccharides of A, C, Y, and W-135 (Centers for Disease Control and Prevention, 2005). The Advisory Committee on Immunization Practices recommends that all persons with increased susceptibility or age 11–18; first-year college students living in dormitories; microbiologists that work with *N. meningitidis* routinely; military recruits; and persons traveling to countries with endemic meningococci be vaccinated. The vaccine may also be used to help control an outbreak of meningococcal disease (Centers for Disease Control and Prevention, 2005, 2007). Individuals with a history of Guillain-Barré syndrome should not receive the vaccine (Centers for Disease Control and Prevention, 2006). The vaccine may cause the production of auto-antibodies that attack the nervous system.

The group B serotype is not included in the vaccine because it is a poor immunogen and its capsular material resembles antigens found in human brain tissue. The body does not produce antibodies because it recognizes the organism capsule as "self." Any antibodies produced would attack the brain.

Clinical Significance

Specimens of Choice for Isolation.
N. meningitidis has been isolated from cerebrospinal fluid (CSF), blood, petechial aspirates, biopsy samples, joint fluid, conjunctiva, sputum, transtracheal aspirates, and nasopharyngeal specimens. Nasopharyngeal swabs, used to determine colonization, yield a greater number of isolates than throat swabs. This organism is more robust than *N. gonorrhoeae* but is still considered fastidious because it requires enriched media, such as sheep blood or chocolate agars, for growth. Humidity and CO_2 stimulate its growth but are not required. See ∞ Chapters 6 and 7 for specimen collection and cultivation information.

Host Encounter.
Like the gonococcus, *N. meningitidis* attaches to the epithelial cells that line the mucosa of the nasopharynx as well as other mucosal sites via their pili. Opacity proteins also play a role in adhesion and invasion. They appear to move through the epithelial cells as previously described, entering the subepithelial matrix and eventually the bloodstream. Tonsillar mucosal surface phagocytes (M cells) may also provide an additional route of invasion (Nassif & So, 1995). They multiply in the blood and disseminate. Strains isolated from blood and CSF usually possess a capsule. This capsule may play an important role in the later stages of infection once invasion has occurred by making the adhesions inaccessible. Non-encapsulated strains are rarely invasive.

Microbe Defense Strategies.
A capsule helps the meningococci resist phagocytosis and lysis by complement (van Deuren, Brandtzaeg, & van der Meer, 2000). A phenomenon called "capsular switching" allows the organism to change its capsule phenotype and may allow this pathogen to escape the patient's natural immunity (Harrison, 2006). Serotype B strains produce a capsule consisting of sialic acid that is not immunogenic. Therefore, antibodies for opsonization will not be produced (Salyers & Whitt, 1994). The same mechanisms used to resist host defenses by *N. gonorrhoeae* are utilized by the meningococcus. See ∞ Chapter 4 for a review of the host's encounter with microbes.

Carrier State.
Neisseria meningitidis may colonize the oro- and nasopharynx as a nonpathogen and result in a **carrier** state. A carrier is a person who possesses a specific infectious agent without signs or symptoms of disease, but is a potential source of infections for others. Up to 15% of the population may be carriers during the winter months. Meningococci may also colonize the anogenital mucous membranes. This carrier state may last for several weeks to months. When a certain population is confined, such as young adults in a college dorm or military base, up to 80% of the population may be carriers.

 REAL WORLD TIP

Neisseria meningitidis can be normal flora in upper respiratory sites. Family members or roommates of an individual with fulminant meningococcemia can carry the organism in their upper respiratory tract. If the organism is present, they have a higher risk of invasive infection. A full workup of *N. meningitidis* may be appropriate in these individuals but only at the request of the physician.

Pathogenic States.
Meningococcal disease occurs most often in infants under 6 months to 2 years of age, persons age 11–19, and young adults living in college campus dorms and military recruit bases. The mortality rate (10–14%) and morbidity rate (11–19%) is high. Since 1991, the frequency of localized outbreaks has increased (Centers for Disease Control and Prevention, 2005). College outbreaks have been linked to bar

patronage, cigarette smoke, and alcohol use (Centers for Disease Control and Prevention, 2005; Imrey et al., 1996).

This organism is spread by direct contact with respiratory secretions or aerosols. It colonizes the mucosa of the naso- and oropharynx. Infection occurs after exposure to a virulent strain in an individual who is lacking the antibody to the specific serotype. Most individuals have acquired antibodies through a carrier state and subclinical infections or have cross-reacting antibodies from other *Neisseria* spp.

Once an individual is colonized, if the organism becomes invasive, it may cause **meningococcemia**, the presence of *N. meningitidis* in the blood with or without meningitis. Shock and organ failure may occur with either invasive disease. This organism is the most common pathogen isolated from young adult cases of meningitis. Some cases produce a rapidly progressive disease that results in **fulminant** sepsis and the death of a previously healthy person within hours of displaying symptoms. Fulminant is the sudden occurrence of pathological processes with a rapid course and great severity or intensity. Death occurs in up to 50% of fulminant meningitis cases even with therapy (van Deuren et al., 2000). Those who have come into close contact with an infected individual are considered at risk and require prophylactic or preventative therapy. See ∞ Chapters 32 and 38 for reviews of the role that the cardiovascular system and central nervous system play in the development of meningitis.

Profound vascular effects may occur with meningococcemia. Seventy-five percent of patients may show a characteristic skin rash (Murray, Baron, Pfaller, Tenover, & Yolken, 1999). *N. meningitidis* possesses a higher concentration of lipopolysaccharide (LPS) in its cell wall compared to other gram negative organisms. The LPS triggers capillary bleeding under the skin called petechiae. As the skin hemorrhages enlarge and overlap, they become purpura and look like bruises.

Waterhouse-Friderichsen syndrome is characterized by fulminant sepsis and disseminated intravascular coagulation (DIC). DIC is triggered by the LPS of the organism. It results in widespread clot formation and rapid lysis within the bloodstream. Eventually the clotting factors are used up, leading to shock and death. Two thirds of patients die within 18 hours. Hemorrhaged adrenal glands are a classic marker of Waterhouse-Friderichsen syndrome (Murray, Baron, Jorgensen, Landry, & Pfaller, 2007).

A complication of blood infections is arthritis. Rarely *N. meningitidis* may cause endocarditis, primary pneumonia, sinusitis, and purulent conjunctivitis (van Deuren et al., 2000). Those individuals compromised by a deficiency in complement or without a functioning spleen are at increased risk for developing systemic infections and repeated infectious episodes. Survivors of invasive meningococcal disease may have sequelae that include hearing loss, loss of limbs due to vascular injury and tissue necrosis, or cognitive impairment (Centers for Disease Control and Prevention, 2005). See ∞ Chapter 40 for more information on opportunistic infections.

 Checkpoint! 18–7 (Chapter Objective 9)

A gram-negative coccobacillary organism isolated from CSF on chocolate agar resembles either a Kingella spp. or N. meningitidis. The single best test to distinguish between these two organisms is:

    A. *oxidase production.*
    B. *catalase production.*
    C. *beta-hemolysis.*
    D. *glucose utilization.*

COMMENSAL *NEISSERIA*

Commensal *Neisseria* reside on the mucous membranes of the upper respiratory system. They may resemble the pathogens or cause disease in compromised patients.

General Characteristics

The commensal *Neisseria* are similar to pathogenic *Neisseria* in that they grow best in warm (37°C), humid environments. Although they prefer CO_2, they do not require it. Many of these saprophytes will also grow in cooler temperatures (22°C or room temperature) and do not require enriched media for cultivation. Difficulty in differentiation occurs because some of the commensal species are resistance to colistin. This allows them to grow on *Neisseria* selective media and be easily confused with the pathogenic species.

The saprophytes resemble the pathogenic *Neisseria* microscopically as well. All but one species presents as gram-negative diplococci with flat adjacent sides that resemble kidney or coffee beans. *N. elongata* is the one exception. It occurs as a gram-negative rod (coccobacillary or diplobacillus).

Identification

Most of the time when a suspected saprophytic *Neisseria* is isolated, the objective is not speciation but ensuring that the pathogens can be ruled out.

Microscopic Morphology.   Microscopically, they resemble the pathogens as gram-negative diplococci. The exception is *N. elongata,* which resembles a gram-negative rod. The cell elongation test may be helpful in determining the true microscopic morphology.

 REAL WORLD TIP

Neisseria may underdecolorize with the Gram stain and resemble gram-positive cocci. One should be suspicious if no clusters or chains are observed. Take time to note whether the adjacent sides are flattened.

Colony Morphology.   Some of the commensal colony morphologies may resemble the pathogenic *Neisseria* in size and lack of pigmentation. Others vary in color and may be whitish, or produce a yellowish or yellow-green pigment. Some are beta hemolytic. The colonies may stick to the surface and be convex and glistening or wrinkled and flat after prolonged incubation. A few species may grow on MacConkey, but they don't grow very well and look very different from the colonies of *Enterobacteriaceae*.

Key Presumptive ID Tests.

As described before, presumptive identification of *Neisseria* spp. is made on the observation of oxidase-positive, gram-negative diplococci. The most helpful characteristics for ruling out the pathogens are pigment production and sensitivity to colistin as observed by a lack of growth on selective media for pathogenic *Neisseria*. Testing an isolate for the ability to grow on nutrient agar in ambient air at room temperature will assist in determining a possible pathogen. The pathogens are more fastidious in their growth requirements and do not grow at room temperature. (See Table 18-3.)

Key Final ID Tests.

The commensal *Neisseria* may be misidentified as either *N. gonorrhoeae* or *N. meningitidis* if sufficient testing is not performed. *N. cinerea* may be confused

REAL WORLD TIP

Growth on Thayer-Martin agar cannot be assumed to be *Neisseria gonorrhoeae* or *N. meningitidis*. *N. lactamica*, *N. cinerea*, and *Moraxella catarrhalis* can also grow on TM.

with *N. gonorrhoeae*; *N. lactamica* and *N. polysaccharea* with *N. meningitidis*; and *N. subflava* and *N. elongata* with both pathogens. Useful tests for distinguishing the pathogens from the saprophytic *Neisseria* include growth pattern, tests for chromogenic enzymes, lactose and sucrose utilization, the polysaccharide from sucrose test, and pigment production.

N. cinerea has been misidentified as a glucose-negative *N. gonorrhoeae*. It may grow on *Neisseria* selective agar. A colistin susceptibility test should be performed. *N. cinerea* should produce a zone size measuring equal to or greater than 10 mm. *N. gonorrhoeae* usually grows up to the edge of the disk (Murray, Baron, Jorgensen, Landry, & Pfaller, 2007).

✪ TABLE 18-3

Clinically Significant Aerobic Gram-Negative Cocci

Species	Growth on CA/BA (22°C)	NA (35°C)	Colistin Resistance (growth on ML, MTM, NYC)	G	M	L	Su	F	Polysaccharide from Sucrose	Nitrate	DNase	Pigment
Kingella denitrificans	–	–	R (+)	+	–	–	–	–	–	+	–	–
Neisseria gonorrhoeae	–	–	R (+)	+	–	–	–	–	–	–	–	–
N. meningitidis	–	–	R (+)	+	+	–	–	–	–	–	–	–
N. lactamica	[–]	V	R (+)	+	+	+	–	–	–	–	–	–†
N. polysaccharea	–	+	V	+	+	–	–	–	+	–	–	–
N. subflava												
biovar *subflava*	+	+	S (–)	+	+	–	–	–	–	–	–	+
biovar *flava*	+	+	S (–)	+	+	–	–	+	–	–	–	+
biovar *perflava*	+	+	[R] (+)	+	+	–	+	+	+	–	–	+
N. sicca	+	+	S (–)	+	+	–	+	+	+	–	–	V
N. mucosa	+	+	S (–)	+	+	–	+	+	+	+	–	–
N. cinerea	–	–	S (–)*	[–]	–	–	–	–	–	–	–	–†
N. flavescens	–	–	R (+)	–	–	–	–	–	+	–	–	+
N. elongata	+	+	S (–)	V	–	–	–	–	–	V	–	–
Moraxella catarrhalis	+	+	V	–	–	–	–	–	–	+	+	–

*Occasionally grows on *Neisseria* selective agar, no growth on subculture to *Neisseria* selective agar.
†Positive when swab is used for pigment observation rather than colony morphology.
G, glucose; M, maltose; L, lactose; Su, sucrose; F, fructose; S, sensitive; R, resistant (growth on *Neisseria* selective agar or no zone of inhibition around a 10 µg Colistin disk); V, variable; +, most positive; –, most negative; [ ], some weak positive reactions; CA, chocolate agar; BA, blood agar; NA, nutrient agar (with peptone); ML, Martin-Lewis agar; MTM, Modified Thayer-Martin agar; NYC, New York City agar.

N. lactamica and *N. polysaccharea* also grow on selective agar and can be confused with *N. meningitidis. N. lactamica* is lactose positive, beta-galactosidase positive, and GGA negative whereas meningococcus is lactose negative, beta-galactosidase negative, and GGA positive. *N. polysaccharea* produces polysaccharide from sucrose, whereas *N. meningitidis* does not. *N. polysaccharea* is beta-galactosidase and GGA negative.

N. subflava biovars and *N. elongata* are part of the normal flora in the oropharynx and nasopharynx and must be differentiated from the pathogens that may also be isolated from these sites. *N. subflava* should be checked for pigment production (Figure 18-15 ■) by sweeping the growth with a swab and observing for the yellowish color. The two biovars whose carbohydrate profile resembles *N. meningitidis* are sensitive to colistin and should not grow on selective agar used for *Neisseria.* The species that is resistant and grows on *Neisseria* selective agar will produce acid from sucrose and is positive for producing polysaccharides from sucrose. *N. elongata* is a gram-negative rod and will not grow on *Neisseria* selective agar.

Sterile body fluid isolates should be considered clinically significant and identified to species (see Table 18-3). Growth on enriched media at room temperature, the pattern of sugar utilization, pigment production, and positive results for poly-saccharide from sucrose and nitrate, is helpful for speciation. Add fructose to the carbohydrates tested to distinguish the *N. subflava* biovars.

Clinical Significance

The *Neisseria* species (other than *N. gonorrhoeae* or *N. meningitidis*) are considered part of the normal flora in the oro- and nasopharyngeal sites of healthy people. They are opportunistic and have been found to be the causative agents of bacteremia and endocarditis. They have also been associated with meningitis, septic arthritis, empyema, pericarditis, peritonitis, and pneumonia (Murray, Baron, Jorgensen, Landry, & Pfaller, 2007). When they are isolated from a normally sterile body site, they must be distinguished from pathogens. *N. cinerea* is associated with eye infections in young children (Dolter, Wong, & Janda, 1998). It has also been shown to be isolated from the rectum and is associated with proctitis.

℮ **REAL WORLD TIP**

Identify any *Neisseria* isolated from a normally sterile body site to species-level. Always ensure testing can rule out the pathogenic *Neisseria.*

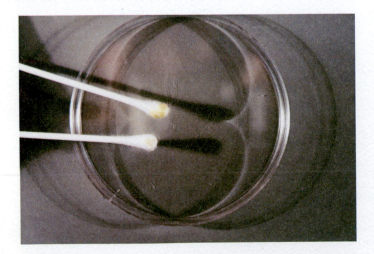

■ **FIGURE 18-15** Positive (bottom swab) and negative (top swab) results for the pigment.

▶ *MORAXELLA CATARRHALIS*

Moraxella catarrhalis colonizes the upper respiratory tract of children and older adults. It resembles *Neisseria* spp. in Gram stain and microscopic arrangement. It is the most common isolate of the genus *Moraxella.* The other species present as gram-negative rods and coccobacilli. They are discussed in ∞ Chapter 22, "Nonfermentative Bacilli."

General Characteristics

Moraxella catarrhalis is an aerobic microorganism that grows best at 35–37°C. It may also grow well at 28°C (Murray, Baron, Pfaller, Tenover, & Yolken, 1999). It does not have fastidious nutritional requirements. Colonies may be observed on chocolate agar, blood agar, and nutrient agar. Some strains may demonstrate colistin resistance by growing on Thayer-Martin and other similar selective media.

Identification

Identification of *Moraxella catarrhalis* is based on microscopic morphology, colony morphology, and key biochemical reactions (Figure 18-16 ■).

Microscopic Morphology.   Microscopically, the coccal *Moraxella* cannot be distinguished from the *Neisseria*. They are also gram-negative cocci with flattened adjacent sides that resemble kidney or coffee beans. *M. catarrhalis* can resist

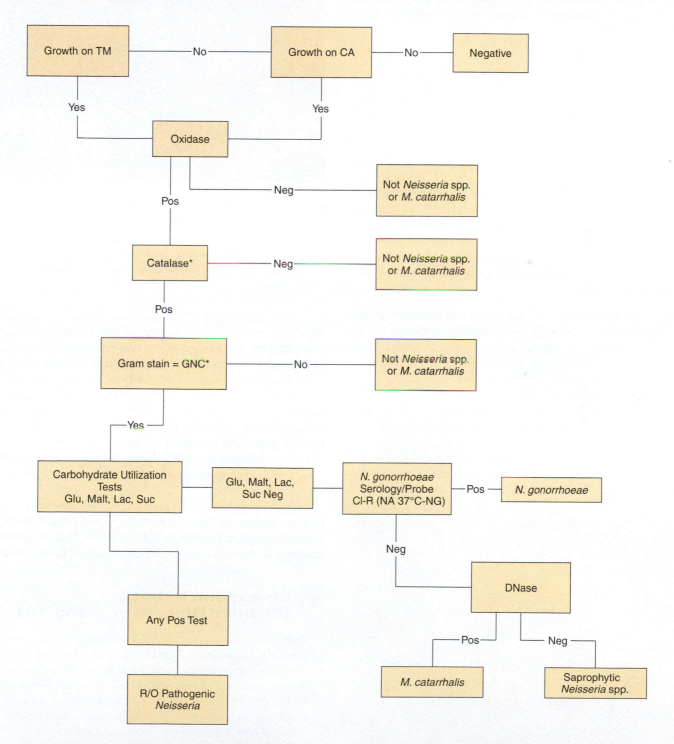

■ **FIGURE 18-16** Identification of *M. catarrhalis.*
TM = Thayer Martin; CA = Chocolate agar; GNC = Gram-negative cocci; GLU = Glucose; MALT = Maltose; LAC = Lactose; SUC = Sucrose; Neg = Negative; Pos = Positive; NA = Nutrient agar; NG = No growth; R/O = Rule out; CI = Colistin disk (10 μg) sensitivity; R = Resistant.
*N. elongata is a gram-negative rod and may be catalase negative.

decolorization and may appear as diplococci, tetrads, and small clusters (Ainsworth, Nagy, Morgan, Miller, & Perry, 1990; Das, Shah, & Levi, 1997).

Moraxella catarrhalis may be considered a potentially significant isolate when a direct Gram stain reveals gram-negative diplococci, accompanied by polymorphonuclear leukocytes (Figure 18-17 ■).

Colony Morphology.
Colonies are opaque, whitish to grayish-pink, 1 mm in size, and may be raised or dome-shaped (Figure 18-18 ■). Some have described the colonies as "hockey pucks" that move intact over the medium's surface. The colonies tend to grow slightly better on chocolate agar when compared to blood agar.

Key Presumptive ID Tests.
When screened with oxidase and catalase reagents, positive results are observed. *M. catarrhalis* is butyrate esterase positive. Other *Moraxella* species are also butyrate esterase positive. The colony of *M. canis,* another coccoid *Moraxella,* looks more like a gram-negative rod in colony morphology, grows on MacConkey, and usually produces a brown pigment on Mueller-Hinton agar. It is also GGA positive whereas *M. catarrhalis* is negative (Jannes et al., 1993).

Key Final ID Tests.
The pattern of carbohydrate utilization is helpful (see Figure 18-16). *Moraxella catarrhalis* is asaccharolytic, meaning sugars are not used. Asaccharolytic commensal *Neisseria* can be ruled out with the DNase test. They are DNase negative, whereas *M. catarrhalis* is DNase positive. Other *Moraxella* species are DNase negative except for *M. canis* (Jannes et al., 1993). As already described, colony morphology, brown pigment, and a positive reaction for GGA will rule out *M. canis.*

Clinical and Laboratory Standards Institute (CLSI) guidelines for rapid accurate identification of common isolates recommend the rapid identification of *M. catarrhalis* if (1) a

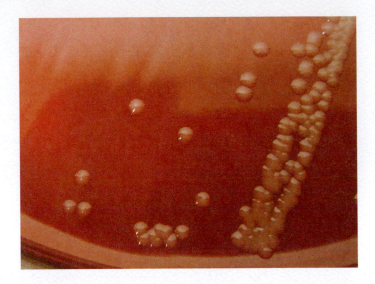

■ **FIGURE 18-18** Colonies of *Moraxella catarrhalis* on chocolate agar.

gram-negative diplococcus is isolated; (2) it grows at room temperature; and (3) it is oxidase and butyrate esterase positive (York, 1999).

Clinical Significance

Moraxella catarrhalis may be part of the normal flora in the nasopharynx, and carried in the oropharynx of children and older adults. It is associated with respiratory tract infections including bronchitis and pneumonia in older and immunocompromised adults, and otitis media and sinusitis in children. Most individuals infected have a predisposing pulmonary disease such as asthma. It is the third leading cause of chronic bronchitis behind *H. influenzae* and *S. pneumoniae.* It rarely disseminates to cause systemic infections. Specimens of choice include tympanocentesis fluid, sinus aspirate, and lower respiratory secretions.

Eighty-five percent of *Moraxella catarrhalis* isolates produce beta-lactamase, rendering it resistant to the penicillins (Murray, Baron, Pfaller, Tenover, & Yolken, 1999). Most laboratories assume a *M. catarrhalis* isolate is beta-lactamase positive and do

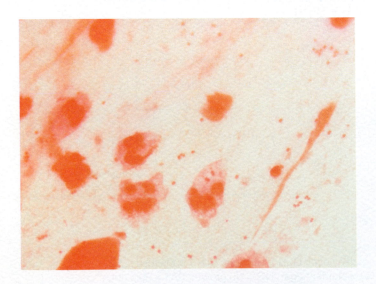

■ **FIGURE 18-17** Gram stain of sputum with *M. catarrhalis.*

 Checkpoint! 18–10 (Chapter Objectives 2 and 10)

A physician sent a sputum specimen collected from an older patient suspected of having pneumonia to the laboratory. The Gram stain reveals many gram-negative diplococci and white blood cells. The isolate grows better on chocolate agar, turns purplish-black with oxidase reagent and bubbles with 3% catalase reagent. Acid is not produced in glucose, lactose, maltose, and sucrose. The most appropriate action to take is:

    A. *identify as Neisseria spp. (saprophytic) and report it.*

    B. *repeat the rapid sugar tests.*

    C. *perform a DNase test.*

    D. *identify as N. gonorrhoeae and perform sensitivity tests.*

not test. *M. catarrhalis* have many of the outer membrane proteins described previously. These may help the organism establish itself at the site of infection, resist the killing power of serum, and retrieve iron from the host.

► MICROORGANISMS THAT RESEMBLE GRAM-NEGATIVE COCCI

Other organisms that may resemble the gram-negative cocci and possibly result in mistaken identification include *Kingella,* other *Moraxella* species, and other coccobacillary gram-negative organisms. Many can be ruled out using the oxidase test (see Table 18-1). *Neisseria* and *Moraxella catarrhalis* are oxidase positive. *Kingella* can be ruled out with the catalase test. It is negative whereas the *Neisseria* and *Moraxella catarrhalis* are positive. *Kingella* isolates have been misidentified as *N. gonorrhoeae* because it grows on selective media for *Neisseria* and utilizes glucose only (See Table 18-3). It also grows on nutrient agar and is nitrate pos-

itive. These characteristics should rule out *N. gonorrhoeae.* *Moraxella* has both coccoid and bacillary species. The cell elongation test may be helpful in determining the true microscopic morphology of *Moraxella* and other coccobacillary isolates. See ∞ Chapter 22, "Nonfermenting Gram-Negative Rods," to learn more about *Moraxella* and other coccobacillary bacteria.

SUMMARY

In this chapter the characteristics of gram-negative cocci isolates have been described (Figure 18-19 ■).

When a gram-negative diplococci grows, begin the identification by ruling out other coccobacillary organisms. The oxidase and catalase tests should be done first. If the isolate is oxidase positive and catalase negative, consider *Kingella.* If the isolate is oxidase positive and catalase positive, consider *Neisseria* and *Moraxella.* Demonstrating microscopic morphology of gram-negative rods would be typical of bacillary *Moraxella* and *N. elongata.*

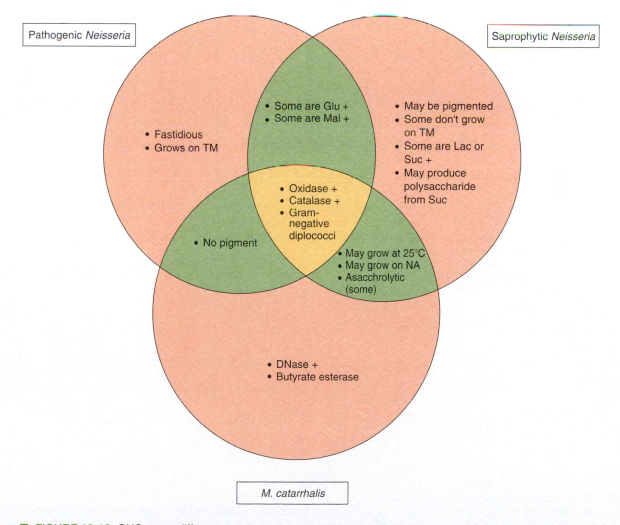

■ **FIGURE 18-19** GNC same-different.
TM = Thayer Martin; Glu = Glucose; Mal = Maltose; Lac = Lactose; Suc = Sucrose; NA = Nutrient agar; + = Positive; Yellow = Reaction shared by all three; Green = Reaction shared by two; Orange = Reactions that differentiate from other two.

Usually physicians are only interested in the two pathogens, *N. gonorrhoeae* and *N. meningitidis*. *M. catarrhalis* must be considered when isolated from sputum in older adults and ears and sinuses of children. Growth on *Neisseria* selective medium such as Thayer-Martin is helpful but not always reliable because commensals may also grow (Figure 18-20 ■). Testing for colistin resistance using a 10 μg colistin disk helps to rule out those strains of *N. cinerea* that may initially grow on *Neisseria* selective agar but are actually colistin sensitive. These strains do not grow on *Neisseria* selective agar on subculture.

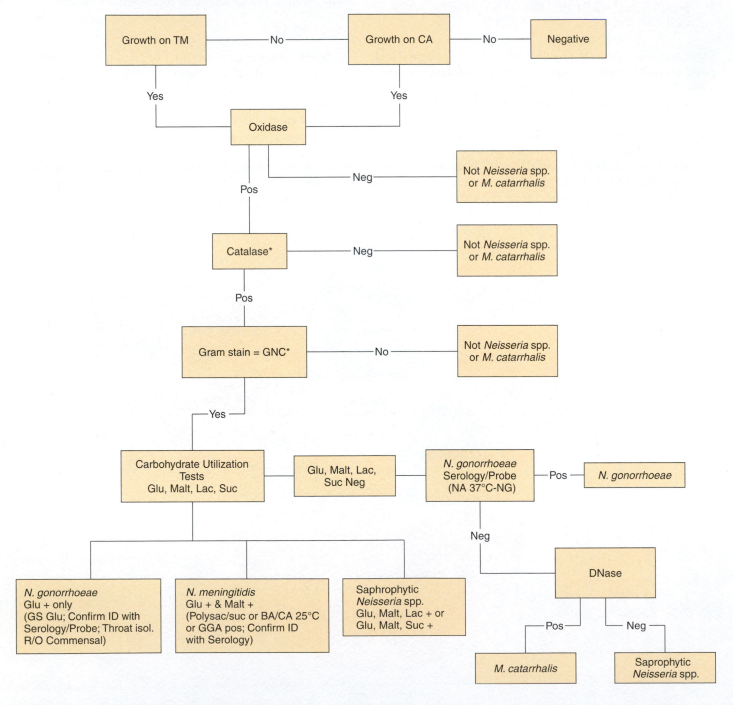

■ **FIGURE 18-20** Identification of gram-negative cocci.
TM = Thayer Martin; CA = Chocolate agar; GNC = Gram-negative cocci; GLU = Glucose; MALT = Maltose; LAC = Lactose; SUC = Sucrose; Neg = Negative; Pos = Positive; GS = Gram stain; NA = Nutrient agar; NG = No growth; ID = Identification; CL = Colistin (10 μg); R = Resistant; GGA = γ-glutamylaminopeptidase; R/O = Rule out commensal *Neisseria* (colistin sensitivity, pigment, γ-glutamylaminopeptidase, prolylaminopeptidase).
N. elongata is a gram-negative rod and may be catalase negative.

The pattern of sugar utilization is helpful. *N. gonorrhoeae* ferments glucose only and *N. meningitidis* ferments glucose and maltose. *M. catarrhalis* demonstrates negative results in all the sugars. The ability to grow on nutrient agar or at room temperature will also rule out the pathogenic *Neisseria*.

Observing pigmentation, a positive nitrate, polysaccharide production from sucrose, and positive DNase reactions are also helpful. The pathogenic *Neisseria* are negative for these characteristics. *M. catarrhalis* and the coccal *Moraxella* are the only gram-negative cocci that are DNase positive. Because both pathogenic gram-negative and commensal gram-negative cocci may be isolated from the same specimens, it's important to perform adequate biochemical tests to prevent misidentification.

LEARNING OPPORTUNITIES

1. On the Web (Chapter Objectives 1, 5, 7, 8, and 9):

    A. Take the cocci challenge at http://www.karenkiser.com/cocichal.html.

    B. Browse information related to the gram-negative cocci at http://www.karenkiser.com/Ilp.GNC.html.

2. Name That Bug

Name That Gram-Negative Cocci

Match each organism with the correct description (Number 1–11) by placing the number of the matching description with the correct name of bacteria.

Test	1	2	3	4	5	6	7	8	9	10	11
Cell morphology	Diplo	Diplo	Diplo	Diplo	Diplo	Diplo	Diplo	GNR	Diplo	Diplo	Diplo
Catalase	+	+	+	+	+	+	+	−	+	+	+
Oxidase	+	+	+	+	+	+	+	+	+	+	+
Glucose	−	+	+	+	+	+	+	+	+	−	−
Maltose	−	+	−	+	+	+	+	−	+	−	−
Lactose	−	−	−	−	+	−	−	−	−	−	−
Sucrose	−	−	−	−	+	−	−	−	+	−	−
Nitrate	+	−	−	−	−	+	−	+	−	−	−
Polysac. from suc	−	+	−	−	−	+	−	−	+	+	−
Grows TM	V	V	+	−	+	−	+	+	−	+	−
Grows NA/35°C	+	+	−	+	V	+	−	−	+	−	−
Grows 22°C	+	−	−	+	(−)	+	−	−	+	−	−
Pigment (colony)	−	−	−	+	−	−	−	−	V	+	−
DNase	+	−	−	−	−	−	−	−	−	−	−

N. gonorrhoeae _____   N. meningitidis _____   M catarrhalis _____   N. polysaccharea _____
K. denitrificans _____   N. subflava biovar subflava _____   N. sicca _____   N. flavescens _____
N. mucosa _____   N. lactamica _____   N. cinerea _____

3. How can knowledge of the characteristics of each genus be used in meeting growth requirements of these organisms (Chapter Objectives 1, 5, and 6)?

4. Which of the gram-negative cocci is clinically significant (Chapter Objective 6)?

5. How can you distinguish the pathogenic *Neisseria* from the nonpathogenic *Neisseria* (Chapter Objective 8)?

6. How can you distinguish the pigmented *Neisseria* from *Staphylococcus* (Chapter Objective 1)?

7. Situation: You isolate a *Neisseria* from a throat culture. Is it a potential pathogen or normal flora (Chapter Objective 10)?

8. Place the names of *N. meningitidis, N. gonorrhoeae, M. catarrhalis,* and commensal *Neisseria* at the head of the column that most matches their characteristics.

GNC Puzzle

1. Growth on selective agar medium	1. Growth on selective agar medium
2. Catalase positive	2. Catalase positive
3. Oxidase positive	3. Oxidase positive
4. Acid produced from glucose	4. Acid produced from glucose and maltose
5. No growth on BA or CA at 22°C	5. No growth on BA or CA at 22°C
6. No growth on NA at 35°C	6. No growth on NA at 35°C
7. DNase negative	7. DNase negative

1. Growth on selective agar medium (variable)	1. Growth on selective agar medium (variable)
2. Catalase positive (usually)	2. Catalase positive
3. Oxidase positive	3. Oxidase positive
4. Acid produced from sugars (variable)	4. No acid produced from sugars
5. Growth on BA or CA at 22°C (usually)	5. Growth on BA or CA at 22°C (variable)
6. Growth on NA at 35°C	6. Growth on NA at 35°C
7. DNase negative	7. DNase positive

PEARSON
myhealthprofessionskit™

Use this address to access the interactive Companion Website created for this textbook. Simply select "Clinical Laboratory Science" from the choice of disciplines. Find this book and log in using your user name and password.

REFERENCES

Go to myhealthprofessionskit.com to view this chapter's references.

19

Aerobic Gram-Positive Rods

Karen M. Kiser

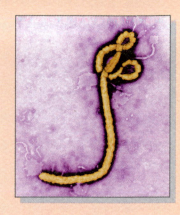

■ LEARNING OBJECTIVES

Upon completion of this chapter, the learner should be able to:

1. Categorize the aerobic gram-positive rods, using their general characteristics.
2. Describe specimen collection and transportation for aerobic gram-positive rods.
3. Determine appropriate media for selection and isolation of each gram-positive rod.
4. Summarize the principle and purpose of the following test procedures: CAMP inhibition or inverse CAMP, lysozyme resistance, and substrate decomposition of casein, xanthine, and tyrosine.
   a. Identify positive and negative reactions for each.
5. Relate the microscopic and culture characteristics for each aerobic gram-positive rod.
6. Identify clinically significant gram-positive rods using microscopic morphology, colony morphology, and biochemical results.
7. Distinguish *Listeria* spp. and *Arcanobacterium* spp. from beta-hemolytic streptococci.
8. Rule out *Bacillus anthracis* using appropriate biochemicals.
9. Correlate the natural habitat, virulence factors, and clinical significance associated with aerobic gram-positive rods.
   a. Associate patient populations at risk for disease.
10. Distinguish those aerobic gram-positive rods that are clinically relevant from those that are normal flora.
11. Summarize treatment strategies, antibiotic susceptibility results, and emerging resistance for aerobic gram-positive rods.
12. Correlate patient history, body site/specimen type, colonial morphology, Gram stain reaction, identification test results, and antibiotic susceptibility test results in order to identify an isolate and assess its clinical significance.

KEY TERMS

diphtheroids	heptamer	palisade
emetic	intracellular pathogen	protoplast
empyema	lipophilic	sporulation
erysipeloid	mediastinal	vegetative
eschar	metachromatic granules	vesicular
germination	necrotizing	zoonoses

TAXONOMY

Family *Bacillaceae* (băs-ĭ-lā′-sē-ē)
  Genus *Bacillus* (ba-sil′-ŭs)
    B. anthracis (an-THRĂ-sis)
    B. subtilis (SAb-til-us)
    B. cereus (SĒ-rē-us)
    B. thuringiensis (th-rin-gen-sis)
    B. mycoides (mî-koid-ēs)
Family *Corynebacteriaceae* (kŏ-rī′-nē-bak-tēr′-ē-ā-sē-ē)
  Genus *Corynebacterium* (kŏ-rī′-nē-bak-tēr′-ē-ŭm)
    C. diphtheriae (dif-thēr′-ēī)
    C. urealyticum (u-rē′-ah-lid-ik-cŭm)
    C. ulcerans (ul′-ser′-ranz)
    C. pseudotuberculosis (soo′-do-too-ber′-ku-lo′-sis)
    C. jeikeium (jei-kei-ŭm)
    C. resistens (rē-ziś-tens)
Family *Listeriaceae* (lis-tēr-ē-ā-sē-ē)
  Genus *Listeria* (lis-tēr-ē-ă)
    L. monocytogenes (mo-nō-sī-tŏ-jen-ēz)
Family *Lactobacillaceae* (lak-tō-bă-sil′ā-sē-ē)
  Genus *Lactobacillus* (lak-tō-bă-sil′-ŭs)
  Genus *Erysipelothrix* (er-i-sip′-ě-lō-thriks)
    E. rhusiopathiae (roo-ē-ō-PATH-ē-ī)
Family *Bifidobacteriaceae* (bī′-fī-dō-bak-ter′-ā-sē-ē)
  Genus *Gardnerella* (gard′-ner-el′-ă)
    G. vaginalis (va-ji-na′-lis)

Family *Actinomycetaceae* (ak′-ti-nō-mī-sē-tā-sē-ē)
  Genus *Actinomyces* (ak′-ti-nō-mī-sēz)
    A. israelii (is-Rā-lē-ā)
    A. naeslundii (nās-lun-dee-eye)
    A. turicensis (tû-rē-cen-sis)
  Genus *Arcanobacterium* (ar-kā′-nō-bac-tēr′-ē-ŭm)
    A. hemolyticum (he′-mo-lid-ĭ-cŭm)
    A. pyogenes (pie-ahj-e-neez)
    A. bernardiae (ber-nar-dē-eye)
Family *Norcardiaceae* (nō-kar′-dē-ā-sē-ē)
  Genus *Nocardia* (nō-kar′-dē-ă)
    N. asteroides (as-ter-oi-dēs)
    N. pseudobrasiliensis (soo′-do-bra′-zil-in-sis)
    N. brasiliensis (bra′-zil-in-sis)
    N. otitidiscaviarum (otī-ti-dis-ca-vi-a-rum)
    N. farcinica (far-ci-ni-ca)
    N. nova (nō-vă)
Family *Thermomonosporaceae* (ther-mō-mŏnō-spor-ā-sē-ē)
  Genus *Actinomadura* (ak′-ti-nō-mad′-yu-ră)
Family *Streptomycetaceae* (strep-tō-mī′-cēt-ā-sē-ē)
  Genus *Streptomyces* (strep-tō-mī′-sēz)
Family *Tsukamurellaceae* (tsoo-kă-mur-el-ā-sē-ē)
  Genus *Tsukamurella* (tsoo-kă-mur-ellă)

▶ INTRODUCTION

The aerobic gram-positive rods are a diverse group. Members differ in morphology, environment, and virulence. Most gram-positive rods isolated from clinical specimens are members of the genus *Bacillus, Corynebacterium,* or *Lactobacillus* (Koneman, Allen, Janda, Schreckenberger, & Winn, 1997). When isolated from clinical specimens, these genera may represent contamination or be clinically significant. Other less common isolates may be clinically significant in immunocompromised individuals.

Differences in microscopic morphology can be useful in the initial classification into possible genera. The spore-forming genera include *Bacillus.* Aerotolerant *Clostridium* may grow on medium incubated in CO_2 and need to be considered if large gram-positive rods with or without spores are observed. The non-spore-forming genera may be divided into those that are club shaped (the coryneforms), regular-shaped rods with two parallel sides, and irregular-shaped or branching rods.

Differences in pathogenicity or ability to cause infection exist. A few, such as *Bacillus anthracis,* are always considered pathogenic whereas others such as coryneform bacilli are often environmental or commensal organisms that are a danger to the immunocompromised but generally not for the healthy.

When gram-positive rods are isolated, the microbiologist must make a decision regarding clinical significance. This decision determines the extent of work-up performed on the isolate. A suggested guide for determining significance is outlined in Box 19-1 . In this chapter, the characteristic morphology and key biochemical reactions of the most clinically significant aerobic gram-positive bacilli are presented.

► SPORE-FORMING RODS

The first characteristic to note on a regular-shaped, gram-positive rod is the presence or absence of a spore. It appears as a nonstaining oval body inside the rod. It may also appear free of the cell in the background of the slide. Spores inside of the bacterial cell may be terminal, located at one end of the cell, or subterminal, or located off center of the rod, or central. The presence and location of a spore and whether it causes the cell body to appear swollen can be helpful in identification of a gram-positive rod. Spores may not be present in clinical specimens because higher CO_2 levels inside the body can prevent their production (Morse, 2002).

The two possible genera to consider when spores are observed in a gram-positive rod include *Bacillus* and *Clostridium*. *Bacillus* spp. are able to produce spores under aerobic conditions whereas *Clostridium* spp. produce spores under anaerobic conditions. Aerotolerant clostridia may show slight growth on medium incubated in CO_2 but better growth under anaerobic conditions.

BACILLUS

Bacillus species or their spores are present in the environment in thermal springs, fresh and salt water, soil, and on plant material. Some species may be found in the intestinal tract of humans and animals. They can be found in climates that vary from desert to subarctic. When isolated from clinical specimens they may be considered contaminants and ignored or clinically significant and identified. The culture work-up may only need to include enough tests to rule out *B. anthracis* or require complete identification and susceptibility.

General Characteristics

Bacillus spores are resistant to radiation, heat, desiccation, and disinfectants. Sterilization at 121°C with 15 pounds per square inch of pressure for 15 minutes kills spores. They are potential contaminants in the health care setting when spread by aerosol

or dust (Murray, Baron, Jorgensen, Pfaller, & Yolken, 2003). Once the spore finds favorable conditions, it germinates to create a vegetative cell.

Bacillus species do not have special requirements for growth. Most species are facultative anaerobes. Their optimum temperature is 35–37°C but they can grow in temperatures as low as 15°C and as high as 45°C (Murray et al., 2003). Some species are obligate aerobes.

They do not require special media for cultivation. They grow rapidly, sometimes within 6 to 8 hours, on sheep blood agar but not MacConkey agar. *Bacillus* species will usually not grow on CNA (colistin-nalidixic acid) agar due to sensitivity to nalidixic acid but will grow on PEA (phenylethyl alcohol) agar.

On Gram stain, *Bacillus* appear as large, straight-edged, gram-positive rods. Those species isolated from clinical specimens may appear gram-variable or gram-negative. Spores may not be visible on direct specimen smears but may appear on Gram stains from growth on media. ∞ Chapter 4, "The Host's Encounter with Microbes," shows a picture of gram-positive rods with spores (see Figure 4-3). Spore formation can be encouraged by inoculating the colony onto urea or bile esculin slants, or blood agar with vancomycin (Isenberg, 2004).

Bacillus anthracis appears encapsulated in cerebrospinal fluid (CSF) and blood smears. Other *Bacillus* species can also possess a capsule. India ink is one method used in many microbiology labs for visualizing capsules, as seen in Figure 19-1 . The capsule appears as a halo around the bacterial cell. Other methods to stain spores and capsules are available.

One spore stain can be carried out when the presence of spores is suspected on Gram stain. The immersion oil is stripped off the smear with acetone alcohol and the slide is restained with 10% malachite green. This stain is left on for up to 45 minutes if not heated and 3–5 minutes if heated. After washing the stain off, counterstain with 0.5% safranin for

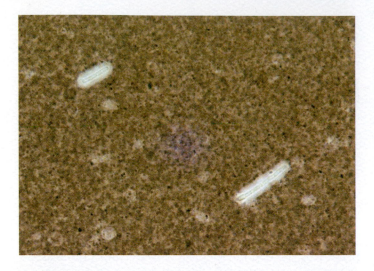

■ **FIGURE 19-1** Capsule of *Bacillus anthracis* using an India ink stain.
From Public Health Image Library (PHIL), CDC/Courtesy of Larry Stauffer, Oregon State Public Health Laboratory.

30 seconds. Spores will appear as green ovals within the pink rods (Murray et al., 2003). Methylene blue has also been recommended as a stain for observing spores (Burdon, 1956). It is important to note the location of the spore and whether it swells the bacterial cell.

A large, whitish-grayish, spreading colony with irregular edges is characteristic of *Bacillus* usually isolated from clinical specimens (Koneman et al., 1997). Colonies are usually nonpigmented, but may occasionally be green, pink, or blue-black in color (Bailey & Scott, 1998). Most species encountered in the clinical laboratory are strongly beta-hemolytic. *B. anthracis* colonies are nonhemolytic, an important characteristic for differentiation from other species.

As a group, *Bacillus* spp. are catalase positive. This characteristic will differentiate them from the anaerobic spore formers, *Clostridium* spp., which are catalase negative.

When a potential *Bacillus* spp. is isolated, most clinical laboratories usually only perform enough biochemical tests to rule out *Bacillus anthracis*. Species other than *B. anthracis* are usually viewed as environmental contaminants or considered to possess limited pathogenicity. Speciation of these other organisms may be important when evaluating cultures from compromised patients, those who abuse alcohol or drugs, or

suspected food-poisoning cases. The physician should be consulted to determine if speciation is needed. Table 19-1✪ contains key reactions for spore-forming, gram-positive rods frequently isolated in clinical laboratories.

Useful Biochemical Tests

Motility.   Motility can be tested by wet mount or motility medium (Morse, 2002). The wet mount is a rapid test whereas the motility medium requires overnight incubation. The motility medium may be difficult to interpret because many *Bacillus* spp. tend to grow on top of the media rather then along the stab line. The wet mount motility is therefore recommended (Bottone, Levine, Burton, & Namdari, 2003).

Some organisms may be immobilized when placed in distilled water. It is recommended suspected *Bacillus* spp. be suspended in trypticase soy broth rather then distilled water to avoid a false-negative wet mount motility result. Motility is enhanced by examining an organism suspension that has been agitated while incubating for 2–3 hours at 30°C (Cleary, Miller, & Martinez, 2002).

A motile or motility positive organism will show purposeful directional movement on a wet mount whereas a nonmotile or motility negative organism will stay in one place or show random Brownian movement. In motility medium a turbid cloud of growth diffusing out from the line of inoculum indicates a positive. No diffusion or growth other than that from the line of inoculum indicates a negative. *Bacillus anthracis* is nonmotile or negative whereas most other species of *Bacillus* are positive. Refer to Figure 9-12 in ∞ Chapter 9, "Final Identification," to review the motility test.

Phenylethyl Alcohol Agar (PEA).   Phenylethyl alcohol agar (PEA) is used to determine the ability of an organism to grow in the presence of phenylethyl alcohol. It can also be used to selectively isolate most of the *Bacillus* spp. If colonies are visible, the result is recorded as positive. If no colonies are visible, the result is recorded as negative. *B. anthracis* does not typically grow on PEA. Other *Bacillus* species usually do grow on PEA.

Lecithinase.   The lecithinase test is performed by inoculating the organism onto egg yolk agar. If the organism produces lecithinase it will break down lecithin in the egg yolk, producing a visible opaque zone around or underneath the colony, as seen in Figure 19-2 ■. *B. anthracis, B. cereus, B. thuringiensis,* and *B. mycoides* are positive, whereas the other species are negative. *B. anthracis* may be weakly positive with an opaque zone observed only beneath the colonies. The microbiologist should remove the colony to observe the reaction (MacFadden, 2000).

Mannitol Salt Agar (MSA).   Mannitol salt agar is most often used for the selection and differentiation of *Staphylococcus* spp., but it can be used to evaluate two growth characteristics of *Bacillus* spp. First, the ability of the *Bacillus* species

☣ TABLE 19-1

Key Reactions for Frequently Isolated, Spore-Forming, Gram-Positive Rods Encountered in the Clinical Laboratory

	Bacills subtilis	B. licheniformis	B. pumilus	B. cereus	B. anthracis	B. megaterium	B. circulans	B. sphaericus	Geobacillus stearothermophilus	Paenibacillus polymyxa	P. alvei	P. macerans	Brevibacillus brevis
Spore													
Shape	E	E (C)	C E	E (C)	E	E S	E	S (E)	E	E	E (C)	E	E
Position	S C	S C	S C	S C	S	S C	S T	S T	S T	S C	S C	S T	S C
Swollen	−	−	−	−	−	−	+	+	+	+	+	+	+
Motility	+	+	+	+	−	+	+	+	+	+	+	+	+
Lecithinase	−	−	−	+	+	−	−	−	−	−	−	−	−
Anaerobic growth	−	+	−	+	+	−	+	−	−	+	+	+	−
Starch hydrolysis	+	+	−	+	+	+	+	−	+	+	+	+	−
Gelatin hydrolysis	+	+	+	+	(+)	+	−	−	+	+	+	V	+
Nitrate reduction	+	+	−	(+)	+	−	V	−	V	V	−	−	+
Indole	−	−	−	−	−	−	−	−	−	−	+	−	−
VP	+	+	+	+	+	−	−	−	−	+	+	−	−
Citrate	+	+	+	+	V	+	−	−	−	−	−	−	V
Growth in 7.5% NaCl	+	+	+	+	+	+	V	V	−	−†	−†	−†	−†
Mannitol	+	+	+	−	−	+	+	−	−	+	−	+	(+)
Xylose	−	+	−	−	−	V	+	−	−	+	−	+	−
Arabinose	−	−	−	−	−	−	−	−	−	−	−	+	−

7.5%, growth on mannitol salt agar; VP, Voges-Proskauer (acetoin); +, positive; (+), weak positive; −, negative; V, variable reaction; E, ellipsoidal; S, spherical shape or subterminal position; C, cylindrical shape or central position; T, terminal position; (C) or (E), infrequent; †, growth in 7% NaCl.

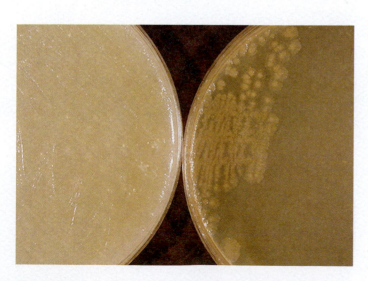

■ **FIGURE 19-2** Positive reaction (left) and negative reaction (right) for lecithinase agar.

to grow in the presence of 7.5% NaCl and, second, fermentation of mannitol. Fermentation of mannitol produces acid byproducts, which are observed as a yellow colony. Most *Bacillus* species that grow on MSA also ferment mannitol. *B. anthracis* and *B. cereus* will grow on MSA but are unable to ferment mannitol. ∞ Chapter 17, "Aerobic Gram-Positive Cocci," provides a photo of MSA and mannitol fermentation (see Figure 17-9).

Penicillin Susceptibility. This procedure determines the organism's ability to grow in the presence of 10 units of penicillin. A 15–20 mm zone of inhibition indicates a potential *B. anthracis*. Zones that measure less than 15 mm, as seen in Figure 19-3 ■, are typical of other *Bacillus* species (Gilchrist, McKinney, & Miller, 2000).

The tests discussed so far are used to presumptively identify *Bacillus anthracis* or speciate *Bacillus*. Clinically significant *Bacillus* species are described in depth in the following sections.

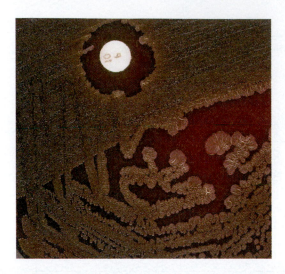

■ FIGURE 19-3 *Bacillus* species showing a zone of inhibition of less than 15 mm when tested against 10 units of penicillin.

B. anthracis

B. anthracis causes anthrax, primarily a disease of ruminants (cud-chewing animals). Humans become infected with the organism through accidental contact or a deliberate act of bioterrorism. Hospital laboratories are considered sentinel laboratories. They are the first line of detection and responsible for alerting public health authorities of the isolation of a potential *B. anthracis*. The laboratory must perform sufficient testing to rule in/rule out *B. anthracis*. Once the organism is identified as a potential *B. anthracis,* it is submitted to the nearest state public health laboratory for confirmatory testing.

Identification

One of the most important clues to the presence of *Bacillus anthracis* is its characteristic appearance on Gram-stained smears. Recognition of this organism is critical for positive patient outcomes and a quick response to a potential bioterrorism incident. Homeland security relies on the microbiologist's expertise as an important member of a sentinal laboratory. A sentinel laboratory is based in a hospital and is the first line of defense in the detection of potential bioterrorism organisms.

Microscopic Morphology. Microscopically *Bacillus anthracis* presents as large gram-positive rods that resemble bamboo plants, as noted in Figure 19-4 ■. The organisms are often rectangular with square ends and can appear in long chains. The rods may appear gram-negative if the cell is old, starving, or have been exposed to antibiotics (Mahon & Manuselis, 2000). Organisms may be absent in autopsy specimens due to destruction of the bacteria by decay after the host's death (Murray et al., 2003).

On smears of blood and cerebrospinal fluid, the microbiologist may observe short chains of two to four cells that are encapsulated. Nonencapsulated organisms usually do not pro-

duce toxin and are not associated with disease. These nonencapsulated isolates usually represent contamination from an environmental source (Murray et al., 2003). The Centers for Disease Control and Prevention (CDC) recommends the use of an India ink stain for capsule visualization.

Spores are only formed in the presence of atmospheric oxygen and may not be seen in direct patient smears (Klietmann & Ruoff, 2001). Smears made from growth on sheep blood, incubated in ambient air, reveal long chains of cells containing oval, central to subterminal spores. These spores do not cause the cell to appear swollen (Morse, 2002).

Ⓔ REAL WORLD TIP

It is important to remember the microscopic appearance of *B. anthracis* will be different in direct smears from patient specimens compared with colony smears. Spores may be observed in the colony smears but not in the direct patient smears. The presence of capsules surrounding large gram-positive rods is a key finding.

Colony Morphology.   On sheep blood agar, *B. anthracis* grows a large, tenaciously adherent, nonhemolytic colony. The 2–5 mm colonies are flat, slightly convex colonies with an irregular border and a ground glass appearance, as noted in Figure 19-5a ■. Finger-like or comma-shaped projections from the edge of the colony may produce a "Medusa-head" appearance. The colony stands up like a beaten egg white when teased with a loop, as seen in Figure 19-5b ■. Weak hemolysis under areas of heavy growth in older cultures should not be confused with true beta-hemolysis (Morse, 2002).

B. anthracis is susceptible to nalidixic acid, so it will not grow on CNA agar. *B. anthracis* will not grow on MacConkey agar, and most strains do not grow on PEA.

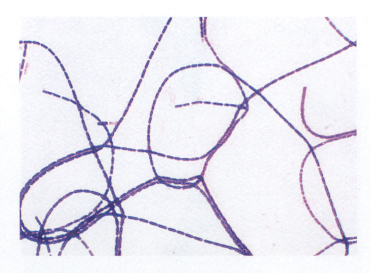

■ FIGURE 19-4 Gram stain of *B. anthracis.*
From Public Health Image Library (PHIL), CDC.

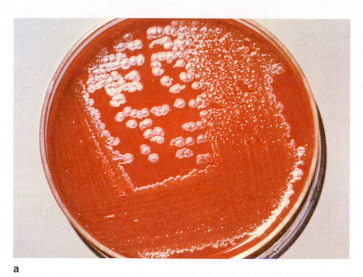

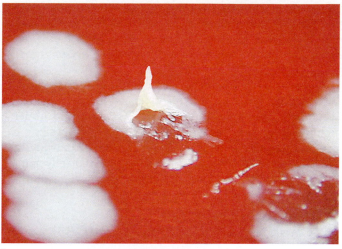

a

b

■ **FIGURE 19-5 a.** *B. anthracis* colonies. From Public Health Image Library (PHIL), CDC. **b.** "Beaten egg white" appearance of tenacious colony of *B. anthracis*.
From Public Health Image Library (PHIL), CDC/Courtesy of Larry Stauffer, Oregon State Public Health Laboratory.

Other species of *Bacillus* may also be nonhemolytic, so additional testing is required to rule out these species as well. The presence of beta-hemolysis automatically rules out *B. anthracis*.

 REAL WORLD TIP

If a colony is suspicious for *B. anthracis*, perform all examination of agar plates and testing within a class II biological safety cabinet. Gloves and gowns must be worn when handling the cultures (Morse, 2002).

 REAL WORLD TIP

Two selective media, polymyxin, lysozyme, ethylenediaminetetraacetic acid, thallium acetate (PLET) agar, and R&F Anthracis chromogenic agar (ChrA) are available for the isolation and selection of *Bacillus anthracis*. Due to the rarity of isolation and added expense, it is not practical for most clinical laboratories to keep such media in stock routinely.

Key Biochemical Reactions.   *Bacillus cereus* is probably the most common environmental isolate observed in the laboratory. Because *Bacillus anthracis* is closely related to *B. cereus*, it is important to perform key tests to ensure accurate differentiation of these two organisms. Initial screening tests on suspect *B. anthracis* colonies include catalase and motility. All *Bacillus* species are catalase positive. *B. anthracis* is nonmotile whereas most of the other *Bacillus* species are motile. It is important to quickly notify the physician and state reference

laboratory when a possible *B. anthracis* is isolated. Wet mount motility provides faster results than the use of semi-solid medium. Table 19-2✪ lists characteristics useful in distinguishing *B. anthracis* from other *Bacillus* species.

In 2001 the United States experienced an intentionally spread anthrax attack that used the postal system as a means to distribute *Bacillus anthracis* spores. This has resulted in increased surveillance for *Bacillus anthracis* from nasal, environmental, and clinical specimens. As a result, many species of *Bacillus* were isolated from these cultures.

Those gram-positive bacilli that met the initial screening criteria for *B. anthracis* were submitted to state reference laboratories. Reference laboratories subsequently identified many of these isolates as *Bacillus* spp. not *B. anthracis*. Recent articles recommend PEA or media testing for mannitol fermentation, such as MSA and lecithinase or egg yolk agar, be inoculated with potential *B. anthracis* colonies. During a bioterrorism alert, only colonies that are nonfermenting on MSA and lecithinase positive or do not grow on PEA should be submitted to the

✪ **TABLE 19-2**

Key Characteristics to Distinguish *B. anthracis* from Other *Bacillus* Species

Characteristic	*B. anthracis*	*B. cereus* group	Other *Bacillus*
Beta-hemolysis	–	+ or +^{w}	V
Growth on PEA	–	+	+
Motility	–	+	Most +
Lecithinase	+^{w}	+	–
Penicillin	S	R	V

+, positive; –, negative; w, weak; S, susceptible; R, resistant.

state reference laboratory (Bottone et al., 2003; Luna et al., 2005). The CDC has not made a recommendation for the addition of this media (Luna et al., 2005). Figure 19-6 provides the CDC recommendations for sentinel laboratory-presumptive identification of *B. anthracis*.

B. anthracis is lecithinase positive, nonmotile, and mannitol and xylose negative. *B. anthracis* will also grow in the presence of high concentrations of salt (7–7.5%), and under anaerobic conditions. Most of the other *Bacillus* species are lecithinase negative or motile. Those capable of growing in the presence of high concentrations of salt are typically mannitol or xylose positive. Another helpful test for differentiating *B. anthracis* from the other lecithinase-positive *Bacillus* is susceptibility to penicillin. *B. anthracis* is susceptible to penicillin, whereas the other species that are lecithinase positive are resistant to penicillin. Susceptibility to penicillin may change in the future if the organism acquires a penicillin-resistant gene through genetic engineering or via plasmids from other organisms.

Clinical Significance

Three forms of anthrax occur in humans. Cutaneous anthrax occurs as a result of handling products contaminated with the spores of *B. anthracis*. The spores are introduced into breaks in the skin. Black ulcers eventually form where the spores enter the skin. It is the most common type of anthrax. Inhalational anthrax can occur after handling animal products, such as goat hides or sheep wool, containing the spores, or after the intentional release of spores during a bioterrorism attack. Inhalation anthrax is almost always fatal. Gastrointestinal anthrax, the rarest form of the three, usually occurs after eating contaminated meat (Morse, 2002). The three forms of anthrax are discussed later in this chapter in the section "Infectious Diseases."

Specimens for Isolation.   *Bacillus anthracis* can be isolated from cutaneous **vesicular** fluid or fluid obtained from

---

> ✓ **Checkpoint! 19–2**
> **(Chapter Objectives 6 and 8)**
>
> *The best procedure(s) to differentiate Bacillus anthracis from other nonpathogenic Bacillus spp. include motility and hemolysis production because B. anthracis is:*
>
> A. *nonmotile and beta-hemolytic.*
> B. *motile and nonhemolytic.*
> C. *motile and beta-hemolytic.*
> D. *nonmotile and nonhemolytic.*

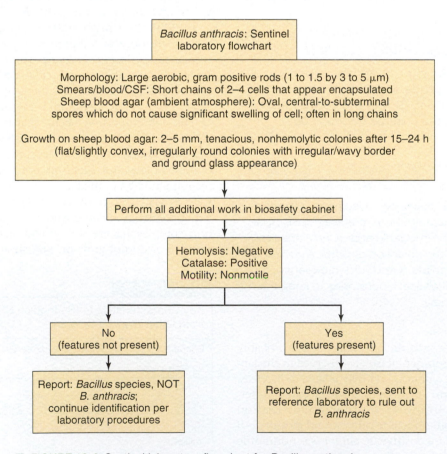

■ **FIGURE 19-6** Sentinal laboratory flowchart for *Bacillus anthracis.*
From American Society for Microbiology, http://asm.org/imags/pdf/bacillusanthracisprotocol.pdf.

blisters, lesion material, or blood cultures when cutaneous anthrax is suspected. Stool or rectal swabs and blood are appropriate specimens when gastrointestinal anthrax is suspected. Acceptable specimens for inhalational anthrax include blood and sputum (Morse, 2002). Blood cultures are often positive late in the course of disease. Cerebrospinal fluid (CSF) may be collected if meningitis is suspected. CSF cultures may be positive in late stages of disease (Snyder, 2006).

Pathogenesis.   The spores of *B. anthracis* enter the body through breaks in the skin, inhalation, or ingestion. Germination occurs at the entry site, producing vegetative cells that produce toxin. Toxin production results in necrosis and edema in the area. Macrophages may phagocytose the bacilli and carry them to the lymph nodes (Klietmann & Ruoff, 2001).

Inhaled spores are engulfed by alveolar macrophages where they germinate. The spores may also germinate in the **mediastinal** or thoracic lymph nodes. The bacteria multiply in the lymph nodes, resist phagocytosis, and produce a powerful exotoxin. Hemorrhagic mediastinitis, massive bacteremia, and secondary pneumonia are the results. Meningitis can also occur as a result of bacteremia (Klietmann & Ruoff, 2001). In

the lungs, the drainage of the pulmonary lymph may be blocked by peribronchial hemorrhagic lymphadenitis, causing pulmonary edema. Death occurs 1–7 days after exposure due to septicemia, toxemia, or pulmonary complications (Dixon, Meselson, Guillemin, & Hanna, 1999).

The exotoxin secreted by *B. anthracis* consists of two toxins: lethal toxin and edema toxin. Each consists of two proteins. One protein binds to a receptor on the cell's surface and ultimately aids in the movement of toxin across the cell membrane. The second protein has specific enzymatic activity. Protective antigen (PA) is the binding protein for both toxins. The enzymatic component of lethal toxin is lethal factor (LF). The enzymatic component of edema toxin is edema factor (EF). Intradermal injection of both PA and LF causes death. Intradermal injection of both PA and EF causes edema. None of the components have a lethal effect when injected alone (Koehler, 2000).

Toxin entry into host cells begins with the binding of the protective antigen to a receptor on the host cell, as seen in Figure 19-7 ■. A protease enzyme cleaves off a small fragment of the PA. The remaining fragment oligomerizes to form a seven-sided, ring-shaped **heptamer.** This heptamer competitively binds EF

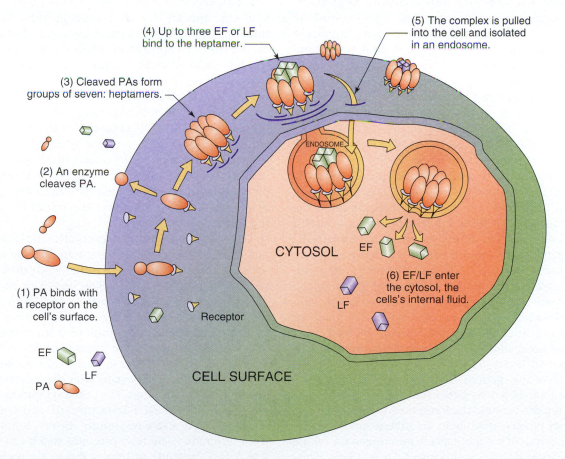

■ **FIGURE 19-7** Entry of anthrax toxin into the host cell.
Courtesy Los Alamos National Laboratory.

or LF and the entire complex is internalized via endocytosis. Once in the low pH environment of the endosome, the complex transforms into a pore. This creates an opening allowing the edema factor or lethal factor to move into the host cell (Koehler, 2000).

Microbe Defense Mechanisms.

B. anthracis has several defense mechanisms. Two virulence plasmids code for exotoxin and a capsule. "Both plasmids are required for full virulence; the loss of either one results in an attenuated strain" (Dixon et al., 1999). Anthrax is also capable of generating a spore when encountering adverse conditions.

The exotoxin assembly and actions on the host were described in the section on pathogenesis. It is believed that these toxins interfere with the immune response mounted by the host against the infection, causing inhibition of neutrophil function and the release of tumor necrosis factor and interleukin from macrophages (Dixon et al., 1999).

B. anthracis forms a capsule when grown in the right environment. This polypeptide capsule is strongly resistant to phagocytosis (Koehler, 2000). The protein capsule of *B. anthracis* is unique because most bacterial capsules are composed of polysaccharides.

B. subtilis studies reveal **sporulation**, the process of enclosing the genome in a spore coat; this occurs in stages and is completed in approximately 8 hours (Driks, 1999). A study by Liu et al. (2004) determined the pattern of gene expression during sporulation for *B. anthracis* is similar to *B. subtilis* and spores appear after 5 hours. Unknown environmental stimulation activates the gene expression of sporulation. Certain conditions, such as an intact tricarboxylic acid cycle and the presence of at least one external pheromone, must exist for sporulation to occur. These conditions are present during times of starvation and the cell responds by concentrating on spore formation rather than on growth (Driks, 1999).

Once the cell commits to sporulation, a septum divides the cell into a small forespore compartment and a larger mother cell compartment. The forespore will eventually become the endospore. The mother cell will nurture the forespore until it completes its development. Both compartments contain the sporulation gene expression program, resulting in the spore being built from both the inside and outside. After about 3 hours, the edge of the septum moves toward the forespore, engulfing and pinching the forespore off. This forms a cell without a rigid cell wall, a **protoplast**, which sits in the cytoplasm of the mother cell. After engulfment a cell wall–like layer is laid down between the double membranes of the protoplast. This cell wall has two layers. The inner layer will become the peptiglycan layer after germination. The outer layer helps to maintain the spore in a dehydrated state. At about 5 hours, a protein coat is placed around the forespore by the mother cell. The spore coat protects it while in an adverse environment. The final step is lysis of the mother cell, resulting in the release of the mature spore into the environment (Driks, 1999). Figure 19-8 ■ illustrates the stages of spore development.

Germination of a spore, which results in a cell capable of reproduction, occurs when it encounters suitable growth conditions. Specific amino acids and nucleosides are sensed by the spore and trigger the germination sequence. The interior of the spore rehydrates, the spore swells, and the coat cracks releasing the emerging cell. This results in a **vegetative** cell capable of growth and toxin production (Liu et al., 2004).

Infectious Diseases.

The primary disease associated with *B. anthracis* is anthrax. It is a worldwide disease with low incidence in the United States. The most affected parts of the world are central Asia and western Africa. An "anthrax belt" exists from Turkey to Pakistan as well as in Australia. Anthrax occurs in three forms: cutaneous, gastrointestinal, and inhalation. Cutaneous anthrax tends to remain localized while gastrointestinal and inhalation anthrax become systemic. Fatal septicemia can occur if cutaneous anthrax goes untreated (Koehler, 2000).

Cutaneous anthrax is also known as "woolsorters" or "ragpickers" disease. It is associated with those occupations that deal with animals and their hides. Farmers, large animal veterinarians, butchers, meat packers, sheep farmers, and weavers who work with animal hair or wool are susceptible. *B. anthrax* can infect all mammals, some birds, and possibly some reptiles (Koehler, 2000).

Cutaneous anthrax has two stages of infection. The vesicular stage appears first with a small pimple surrounded by fluid-filled vesicles that form at the point of entry. This fluid can be collected and submitted to the microbiology laboratory for examination. The **eschar** stage occurs when the lesion forms at the entry site, ulcerates, dries, and blackens, hence the name anthrax, which is Greek for coal. Figure 19-9 ■ demonstrates a characteristic black, crusty scab that covers the lesion formed at the infected site (Koehler, 2000). The lesion beneath the scab or eschar can be sampled by inserting a swab beneath the eschar and rotating to collect the lesion material. The organisms can be observed in both specimens but is best observed in the vesicular fluid (Snyder, 2006). The handlers of animals and their hides may also inhale the spores, resulting in inhalational anthrax.

Gastrointestinal anthrax occurs after the ingestion of contaminated or infected meat. Symptoms include anorexia, nausea, vomiting, and abdominal pain. Bloody diarrhea may also be present (Koehler, 2000). The organism can invade the bloodstream, resulting in death. Logan, Popovic, and Hoffmaster (2007) described it as cutaneous anthrax occurring on the intestinal mucosa. This form of anthrax occurs primarily in developing countries. An occurrence in the United States would be unusual and raise suspicions of a bioterrorism attack.

Inhalational anthrax occurs after the spores of *B. anthracis* are inhaled into the lungs. The initial symptoms are "flu-like," which consist of malaise, fever, myalgia, and a nonproductive cough. Sudden severe respiratory distress follows and death from respiratory failure, sepsis, and shock can occur within 2 to 3 days. Systemic anthrax is almost always fatal (Koehler, 2000).

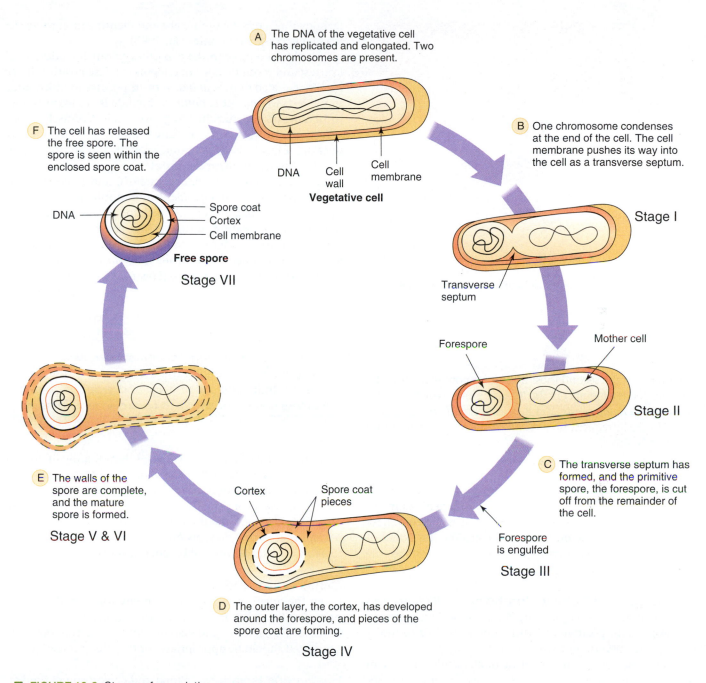

A The DNA of the vegetative cell has replicated and elongated. Two chromosomes are present.

DNA   Cell wall   Cell membrane
Vegetative cell

B One chromosome condenses at the end of the cell. The cell membrane pushes its way into the cell as a transverse septum.

Stage I

Transverse septum

Forespore   Mother cell

Stage II

C The transverse septum has formed, and the primitive spore, the forespore, is cut off from the remainder of the cell.

Forespore is engulfed

Stage III

F The cell has released the free spore. The spore is seen within the enclosed spore coat.

DNA   Spore coat
Cortex
Cell membrane
Free spore

Stage VII

Spore coat   Cortex   Cell membrane

E The walls of the spore are complete, and the mature spore is formed.

Stage V & VI

Cortex   Spore coat pieces

D The outer layer, the cortex, has developed around the forespore, and pieces of the spore coat are forming.

Stage IV

■ **FIGURE 19-8** Stages of sporulation.

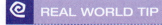

REAL WORLD TIP

Those laboratory professionals who work in agricultural states should be alert to the possibility of isolating *B. anthracis* as a potential pathogen in an infection not related to bioterrorism.

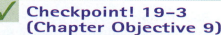

Checkpoint! 19–3 (Chapter Objective 9)

The etiological agent of anthrax is:
    A. *Bordetella pertussis.*
    B. *Corynebacterium diphtheriae.*
    C. *Staphylococcus aureus.*
    D. *Bacillus anthracis.*

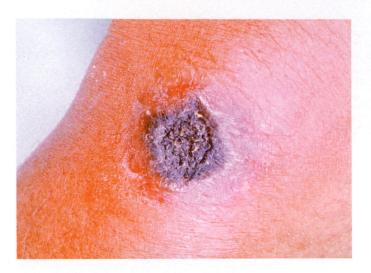

■ **FIGURE 19-9** Anthrax lesion or "eschar"on the skin of the forearm.
From Public Health Image Library (PHIL), CDC/James H. Steele.

B. cereus

Bacillus cereus is the second most important potential pathogen in the genus. It is a member of the *B. cereus* group, which includes *B. anthracis, B. thuringiensis,* and *B. mycoides. B. thuringiensis* and *B. mycoides* are infrequent isolates. All members of this group are lecithinase positive.

Identification

Isolation of *B. cereus* from an eye culture is a critical result and neonates may be especially vulnerable, so sufficient testing to identify to species should be performed on isolates from these specimens. Contact the physician to determine the extent of work-up for other specimen types. At minimum tests to rule out *B. anthracis* should be performed.

Microscopic and Colony Morphology. *Bacillus cereus* shares the same microscopic morphology as *Bacillus anthracis.* It is a large gram-positive rod with subterminal or centrally located spores that do not swell the cell.

It shares the colony characteristic of all *Bacillus* species, in that it is a large, uneven-edged, frosted-glass, greenish-appearing colony. Unlike *B. anthracis, B. cereus* is a hemolytic colony on blood agar. *B. cereus* can also grow on PEA, whereas *B. anthracis* cannot.

Key Biochemical Reactions. Most laboratories only perform enough testing to rule out anthrax. In cases of suspected food poisoning due to *Bacillus cereus,* most laboratories send feces or vomitus to the public health laboratory for isolation and identification of possible *B. cereus* and its toxin. *Bacillus cereus* may be isolated from feces of carriers so it is important to determine if the same strain is isolated from clinical specimens and food in significant numbers. This proves it is the cause of a food-associated outbreak. Isolates from ster-ile body fluids may be significant and identification to species may be necessary (Drobniewski, 1993).

Initial screening of the large *Bacillus* colony includes a catalase test and motility. *Bacillus cereus* is catalase positive. It can be differentiated from *B. anthracis* by its positive motility. Additional tests to rule out *B. anthracis* include *B. cereus'* resistance to 10 units/ml of penicillin and growth on PEA (Knisely, 1965). If further identification is required, useful tests include production of lecithinase, anaerobic growth, and ability to grow on MSA but not ferment mannitol.

B. cereus, B. anthracis, B. thuringiensis, and *B. mycoides* are lecithinase positive. *B. mycoides* is nonmotile. *B. thuringiensis* produces a "cuboid" or "diamond-shaped" crystal in addition to spores in sporulating cultures. These can be observed using a phase contrast microscope or by examining malachite green–stained smear. The other non–*Bacillus cereus* group species are lecithinase negative (Logan & Turnbull, 2003).

 REAL WORLD TIP

Bacillus thuringiensis produces an insecticidal toxin during spore formation. The insects ingest the toxin crystals that cause cell lysis and eventual death. Farmers spray it on crops to control insect damage.

Many of the other *Bacillus* species do not grow in anaerobic conditions, whereas *B. cereus* can. Those that do grow can be distinguished from *B. cereus* by their inability to grow on MSA (7.5% NaCl) or by mannitol fermentation. *B. cereus* grows on MSA (7.5% NaCl) but does not ferment mannitol. The other *Bacillus* species that do grow on MSA ferment mannitol. Refer to Table 19-1 for additional biochemical reactions.

Clinical Significance

Often the organism is considerd an environmental contaminant. *Bacillus cereus* is associated with gastrointestinal infections, local infections, and systemic infections. The specimens submitted should be appropriate for the site of infection.

Specimens Isolation. Blood and cerebrospinal fluid are the specimens submitted for systemic infections. *B. cereus* is a rare cause of pneumonia so sputum or pleural fluid may yield this organism. Local infections may result in wound, eye, bone marrow, and joint fluid being submitted for culture. Gastrointestinal infections are usually foodborne and feces or vomitus is submitted to the public health laboratory along with the suspected food source.

Pathogenesis. *Bacillus cereus* spores are present in the environment, including hospitals. Most infections are the result of trauma or contamination. Contamination of linens, dressings, catheters, indwelling lines or shunts, and solutions have been linked to cases of infection. Spores enter the host and germinate into a vegetative cell. The vegetative cell produces exotoxins including hemolysins, proteases, and phospholipases, which can contribute to successful local infection. **Necrotizing** infections are those that result in rapidly progressing death of the tissues. It may occur as a result of the effects of the necrotizing enterotoxin of the organism (Drobniewski, 1993).

Sporadic food poisoning outbreaks have recently been linked to fried rice, roasted chicken, baked beans, sliced turkey or ham, cheese, meat, vegetable pizza, and pasta (Centers for Disease Control, 2004). The vegetative cells or spores contaminate the food. When conditions are favorable, such as when food cools after heating, the spores germinate into vegetative cells that produce two types of toxins. The enterotoxins are cytotoxins that create pores or openings in the intestinal mucosa to produce diarrhea whereas the **emetic** toxin causes vomiting. The enterotoxins can also be produced in the small intestine after food is ingested (Amesen, Fagerlund, & Granum, 2008). The emetic toxin is resistant to heat and can cause illness even after the food has been heated (Maher, Pasi, Kramer, & Schulte, 1997). ∞ Chapter 35, "Gastrointestinal System," provides more information on other microbes associated with food poisoning.

Microbial Defense Mechanisms.   *Bacillus cereus* spores play the same protective role as already described for *Bacillus anthracis*. Phospholipase may aid the organism in resisting phagocytosis and hemolysins may cause lysis of leukocytes and macrophages (Drobniewski, 1993). The organism can also produce beta-lactamase, protease, and collagenase.

Infectious Diseases.   *Bacillus cereus* is a sporadic cause of food poisoning. Two syndromes may occur: diarrheal or emetic. The diarrheal syndrome occurs approximately 10 hours after eating the contaminated food. A patient's symptoms include profuse diarrhea, abdominal pain, and cramps; fever and vomiting may occur. The emetic syndrome resembles *Staphylococcus aureus* food poisoning. Symptoms occur approximately 5 hours after eating the contaminated food and include nausea, vomiting, abdominal cramps, and sometimes diarrhea. Both syndromes are self-limiting and rarely require supportive or antimicrobial therapy (Drobniewski, 1993). Liver failure has been associated with the emetic toxin and may be fatal without a transplant (Mahler et al., 1997).

B. cereus also causes local infections including postsurgical or traumatic wound, burn, and eye infections. Eye infections have increased especially in those who are immunocompromised and intravenous drug users. The organism is introduced into the eye via contaminated contact lens solution, trauma, or spread from the bloodstream as a result of contaminated drugs or drug paraphernalia, injection equipment, or a blood transfusion (Drobniewski, 1993). Isolation of *Bacillus cereus* from a specimen collected from the eye is a critical result and should be reported to the physician immediately. Loss of vision or the eye may occur if treatment is not begun in a timely manner (Murray et al., 2007).

 REAL WORLD TIP

Bacillus spp. are often isolated in initial burn wound cultures due to the "stop, drop, and roll" rule. Spores in the environment enter the burn wound then germinate.

Cases of meningitis, bacteremia, septicemia, endocarditis, and osteomyelitis have been described. The organism typically gains entrance into the site using intravenous lines or ventricular shunts. Most of these infections are in intravenous drug users or patients compromised due to malignancy, vascular disease, or indwelling lines. Rare pneumonia can also occur in this population and is life threatening (Drobniewski, 1993). Contamination of mechanical ventilators is associated with respiratory infections in newborns (Van Der Zwet et al., 2000).

Infections resembling anthrax and gas gangrene have been described (Cone, Dreisbach, Potts, Comess, & Burleigh, 2005; Darbar, Harris, & Gosbell, 2005). Reported cases of severe, life-threatening pneumonia resembling inhalation anthrax have occurred in previously healthy individuals. This is due to a new strain of *B. cereus* that is capable of producing a capsule and toxin similar to that produced by *B. anthracis* (Hoffmaster et al., 2004). The new strain has acquired a plasmid that codes for the anthrax toxin. Contact the patient's physician before calling the isolate a contaminant, especially if a capsule is observed (Hoffmaster et al., 2004).

 REAL WORLD TIP

Bacillus species are frequent contaminants of blood cultures but may also be isolated from septicemic patients. Before dismissing an isolate as a contaminant, consider the number of specimens or blood culture bottles from which the organism is isolated. If *Bacillus* is isolated from more than one blood culture bottle or multiple specimens, it may be a clinically significant isolate.

✓ **Checkpoint! 19–4 (Chapter Objective 9)**

Six fishermen on a camping trip ate reheated baked beans for supper. Later that evening they began vomiting. The most likely pathogen is:

    A. *Shigella.*
    B. *Bacillus cereus.*
    C. *Enterohemorrhagic E. coli.*
    D. *Vibrio parahaemolyticus.*

Other *Bacillus* species

Other species of *Bacillus* may be isolated as contaminants or cause infections in immunocompromised patients.

Identification

Initial dentification is based on Gram stain morphology and colony morphology. Most laboratories rule out *B. anthracis* but further testing may be performed if judged clinically significant.

Microscopic and Colony Morphology.

Gram stain morphology is the same as described for *B. anthracis* and *B. cereus*. They present as large gram-positive rods. If spores are observed they may be central, subterminal, or terminal. Some species produce spores that cause the cell to swell while others do not.

Other species of *Bacillus* often grow as large colonies. Their appearance may vary from moist to dry or wrinkled with even or uneven edges. They can even appear to spread. Their color ranges from buff, grayish white to orange colonies. They can demonstrate hemolysis or no hemolysis (Murray et al., 2003).

Key Biochemical Reactions.

Most clinical laboratories perform testing to rule out *B. anthracis*. Beta-hemolysis, growth on PEA, motility, and negative lecithinase will rule out *B. anthracis*. Lack of growth in the presence of 7.0–7.5% NaCl (no growth on MSA) and mannitol fermentation (acid in MSA) will also rule out *B. anthracis*. If isolated from sterile body sites or judged clinically significant, additional tests are needed to speciate. Refer to Table 19-1 for additional biochemical tests useful for identifying frequently isolated, spore-forming, gram-positive rods.

Clinical Significance

Other *Bacillus* species have been associated with rare systemic infections and food poisoning in the same patient population as has been described previously. The food-poisoning symptoms may resemble that of *Clostridium perfringens* or *Bacillus cereus*. The *B. subtilis* group is most often the villain in food-borne illness not caused by *B. cereus* (From, Pukall, Schumann, Hormazábal, & Granum, 2005). Refer to ∞ Chapter 24, "Anaerobic Bacteria," for more information about *C. perfringens*.

Cases of cutaneous lesions that resemble anthrax are rare but have been reported (Tena et al., 2007). Other *Bacillus* species may cause wound and eye infections (Callegan et al., 2005; Damgaard et al., 1997). When wound infections occur in immunocompetent individuals, the organisms may be self-injected with heroin or with material containing the spores such as septic tank contents or organic drain cleaner (Galanos et al., 2003; Hannah & Ener, 1999; McLauchlin et al., 2002).

Other *Bacillus* species are also linked to pseudoinfections. The spores are able to survive in many of the cleansing solutions used prior to venipuncture. Contamination of blood cultures may occur during collection. It is not necessary to swab the tops of blood culture bottles with alcohol because the rubber diaphragm covering the bottle is already sterile (Schreckenberger, 2003).

AEROTOLERANT *CLOSTRIDIUM*

Clostridium tertium and *Clostridium perfringens* are examples of an aerotolerant clostridia. They grow best without atmospheric oxygen, in an anaerobic environment, but may grow in an atmosphere with oxygen. An initial clue is the presence of sparse growth of tiny colonies on enriched medium incubated in CO_2 environments. Growth on media incubated in anaerobic conditions displays much more growth and larger colonies. Gram stain morphology is similar to *Bacillus* species in that *Clostridium* is a gram-positive rod with or without spores. *Bacillus* species will only form spores under aerobic conditions so the observation of spores in a smear of anaerobic growth would indicate *Clostridium*. *Clostridium* is usually catalase negative whereas *Bacillus* is catalase positive. For more information on aerotolerant *Clostridium*, refer to ∞ Chapter 24, "Anaerobic Bacteria."

▶ CORYNEFORM RODS

The coryneform bacilli share the common morphology of pleomorphic gram-positive rods with club-shaped ends but they do not form spores. They are often a member of the commensal or normal flora of the skin and mucous membranes. Improper specimen collection techniques result in their frequent isolation from contaminated specimens. There is one definitive pathogen, a toxigenic strain of *Corynebacterium diphtheriae*. The rest may cause infections in compromised individuals. This presents a dilemma to microbiologists and physicians in determining the clinical significance of coryneform isolates.

Isolation of coryneforms from multiple specimens, observation of polymorphonuclear leukocytes associated with coryneform bacteria on Gram stain, and the predominant growth of coryneforms among less pathogenic isolates in an individual with signs and symptoms of infection would be clues that organisms may be clinically significant (Murray et al., 2003).

Many clinical laboratories limit their identification to genus only after ruling out *Corynebacterium diphtheriae*. It may be important to identify to species if a coryneform is isolated from a sterile body site or if it is the predominant organism. Coryneform bacilli may be a significant isolate in a urine culture if it is the only isolate, the colony count is greater than 10,000 CFU/ml, or it is the predominant organism, among other organisms, and isolated with a colony count of greater than 10,0000 CFU/ml (Murray et al., 2003).

General Characteristics

The coryneform bacteria are irregular, slightly curved, gram-positive rods or **diphtheroids** with nonparallel sides and club-shaped or swollen ends, as seen in Figure 19-10 ■. They

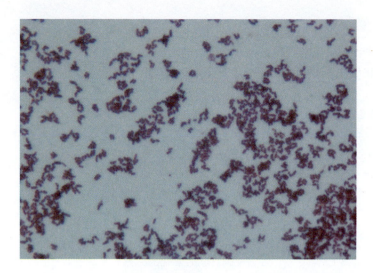

■ **FIGURE 19-10** Microscopic morphology of coryneform bacteria Gram stain of *C. urealyticum.*

are called diphtheroids because their Gram stain resembles that of the pathogen *C. diphtheriae.* They may **palisade** or form stacking patterns like a picket fence or log jam or appear as *V, L,* and *Y* shapes when grown in liquid medium (Bernard, 2005). Unless clinically significant, the microbiologist will call these coryneform bacteria "diphtheroids" based on the characteristic Gram stain and morphology.

Coccobacillary forms can be observed in older cultures. Coryneforms are facultative anaerobes that contain both fermenters and nonfermenters. *Corynebacterium* are catalase positive, oxidase negative, and the clinically significant species are nonmotile (Murray et al., 2003). *Arcanobacterium,* another gram-positive rod that can resemble diphtheroids on gram stain, is catalase negative.

Some species grow better in an atmosphere of carbon dioxide. Clinically relevant species prefer 35–37°C and may require 48 hours incubation for growth. Coryneforms will grow on blood and chocolate agars but not MacConkey agar. There may be sparse growth on phenylethyl alcohol (PEA) agar.

Useful Biochemical Tests. If a laboratory desires to speciate the coryneform, the following biochemicals are useful.

 Checkpoint! 19–5 (Chapter Objectives 1, 5, and 6)

An aerobic gram-positive rod with swollen, club-shaped ends is a suspected:
   A. *Corynebacterium species.*
   B. *Clostridium species.*
   C. *Bacillus species.*
   D. *Listeria species.*

Catalase. Colonies of *Listeria, Corynebacterium,* and other coryneforms will produce bubbles when exposed to hydrogen peroxide and so are considered catalase positive. Other gram-positive rods such as *Arcanobacterium, Actinomyces, Erysipelothrix, Gardnerella,* and *Lactobacillus* are catalase negative.

Motility. Demonstration of motility can be observed in a wet mount or semi-solid medium. The corynebacteria are nonmotile whereas *Listeria* is motile. Other less frequently isolated coryneforms may also be nonmotile. Refer to Table 19-3✪ for specific information.

Fermentation or Oxidation of Carbohydrates. Determining how a carbohydrate is metabolized by a coryneform is helpful information. Refer to Table 19-3 for details. Cystine trypticase agar (CTA) base medium is recommended for determining whether a sugar is metabolized fermentatively or oxidatively. If the organism is oxidative, acid is produced resulting in a yellow color, observed only on the surface, as seen in Figure 19-11 ■. If it is fermentative, acid is produced and a yellow color is observed throughout the tube (Murray et al., 2003).

Nitrate. Testing for nitrate reduction will help to distinguish nitrate negative *Arcanobacterium* from the *Corynebacterium* species that are able to reduce nitrates. Table 19-3 provides information on nitrate-negative *Corynebacterium* species. Refer to ∞ Chapter 9, "Final Identification," for more information on the nitrate test.

Urea. The urease enzyme is present in *C. urealyticum* so a positive or pink urea test result is a key finding, as noted in Figure 19-12 ■. *C. urealyticum* is also a lipid-requiring organism. Most of the other **lipophilic** or lipid-loving coryneforms are negative for this test. Nonlipophilic *Corynebacterium* may also be urease positive. Refer to Table 19-3 for more information. ∞ Chapter 9, "Final Identification," provides more information on the urease test.

Esculin. Most *Arcanobacterium* and *Corynebacterium* species are esculin negative so a positive test result will rule them out. ∞ Chapter 9, "Final Identification," describes the esculin test in detail.

CAMP Test and CAMP Inhibition (or Inverse CAMP) Test. The conventional CAMP test uses beta-hemolysin-producing *Staphylococcus aureus* to identify group B streptococci. ∞ Chapter 17, "Aerobic Gram-Positive Cocci," describes this test in detail. The CAMP test can also be used to help characterize the coryneforms.

A positive traditional CAMP test results in enhanced hemolysis at the intersection of the group B *Streptococcus* and *Staphylococcus aureus.* The enhanced hemolysis appears in the shape of an arrow.

A reverse version of the CAMP test is used for coryneform organisms. One observes a dark triangle, displaying a lack of

⊕ TABLE 19-3

Key Reactions for Selected Coryneforms Encountered in the Clinical Laboratory

	F/O	MOT	NIT	Urea	ESC	Reverse CAMP	Requirement for Lipids	Pyra	GLU	MAL	SUC	MAN	XYL
Corynebacterium													
C. diphtheriae	F	–	+/–	–	–	–	V	–	+	+	–	–	–
C. ulcerans	F	–	–	+	–	NHIB	–	–	+	+	–	–	–
C. pseudotuberculosis	F	–	V	+	–	NHIB	–	–	+	+	V	–	–
C. amycolatum	F	–	V	V	–	–	–	+	+	V	V	–	–
C. striatum	F	–	+	–	–	V	–	+	+	–	V	–	–
C. minutissimum	F	–	–	–	–/+	–	–	+	+	+	+	–/+	–
C. aurimucosum	F	–	–	–	–	NT	–	+	+	+	+^w	–	–
C. resistens	F	–	–	–	–	–	+	–	+	–	–	–	–
C. macgenleyi	F	–	+	–	–	–	+	–	+	–	+	V	–
C. jeikeium	O	–	–	–	–	–	+	+	+	V	–	–	–
C. urealyticum	O	–	–	+	–	–	+	+	–	–	–	–	–
C. pseudodiphtheriticum	O	–	+	+	–	–	–	+	–	–	–	–	–
Arcanobacterium													
A. haemolyticum	F	–	–	–	–	NHIB	NT	+	+	+	V	–	–
A. pyogenes	F	–	–	–	V	–	NT	NT	+	V	V	V	+
A. bernardiae	F	–	–	–	–	–	NT	NT	+	+	–	–	–

F, fermentative; O, oxidative; +, positive; –, negative; +/–, most positive, some negative; –/+, most negative, some positive; V, variable; +^w, weak positive; NHIB, inhibition of CAMP reaction or reverse CAMP positive; MOT, motility; NIT, nitrate reduction; ESC, esculin hydrolysis; Pyra, pyrazinamidase; NT, not tested.

inhibition of hemolysis, as seen in Figure 19-13 ■, at the intersection of *S. aureus* and the test coryneform organism. This is considered a positive CAMP inhibition or inverse CAMP test. This test is also referred to as a reverse CAMP test. The presence of phospholipase D in the coryneform organism inhibits the β-hemolysin produced by the *S. aureus,* resulting in a dark tri-angle (Murray, 1999). A positive inverse CAMP is characteristic of *Arcanobacterium hemolyticum, Corynebacterium ulcerans,* and *C. pseudotuberculosis.*

Requirement for Lipids. This test is used to identify lipid-loving corynforms and should only be performed on catalase-

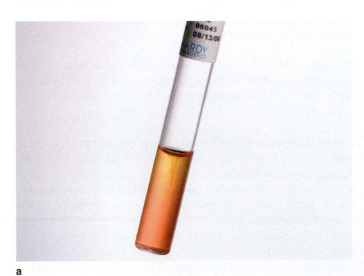

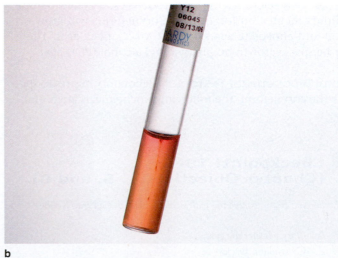

a   b

■ **FIGURE 19-11 a.** Positive reaction for oxidation of glucose in CTA medium. **b.** Negative reaction.
Photo courtesy of Hardy Diagnostics. www.HardyDiagnostics.com

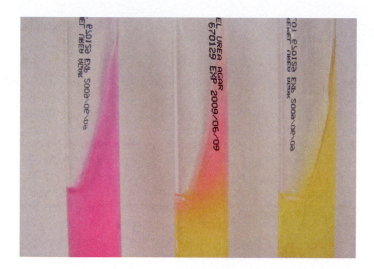

■ **FIGURE 19-12** Positive (left), weak positive (middle), and negative (right) reactions for urea agar.

Ⓔ **REAL WORLD TIP**

A positive inverse CAMP test or CAMP inhibition test result is opposite the expected result for a positive CAMP test in that it is an inhibition of hemolysis, rather than enhancement, which appears as a dark arrow or triangle.

Ⓔ **REAL WORLD TIP**

Another version of a reverse CAMP test may be performed using group B *Streptococcus* to identify *Clostridium perfringens*.

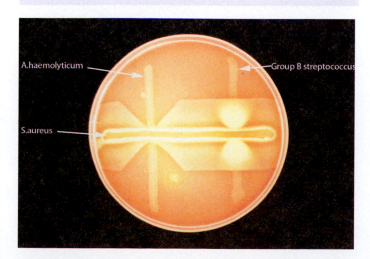

■ **FIGURE 19-13** Positive CAMP inhibition (or inverse or reverse) result (left) and positive CAMP test result (right).
Photo courtesy of Subhash Chandra Parija, Venkatesh Kaliaperumal, Saka Vinod Kumar, Sistla Sujatha, Venkateshwara Babu, and V Balu; BioMed Central Infectious Diseases.

✓ **Checkpoint! 19–6 (Chapter Objective 4)**

A CAMP inhibition test is positive when one observes:
 A. *no growth in the medium.*
 B. *inhibition of growth.*
 C. *a dark arrowhead or triangle.*
 D. *a beta-hemolytic arrowhead or triangle.*

positive colonies that are less than 0.5 mm in size. One half of a sheep blood agar plate is swabbed with a cotton swab dipped in 0.1–1% Tween 80. The test organism is struck so that it covers both sides of the plate, as seen in Figure 19-14 ■. The coryneform is lipophilic if the colony size increases after overnight incubation and is greater than 2 mm on the agar side struck with Tween 80 (Funke et al., 1999). *C. jeikeium, C. macgenleyi,* and *C. urealyticum* are lipophilic.

Ⓔ **REAL WORLD TIP**

Sterile olive oil can be swabbed onto the surface of an agar plate, prior to inoculation, to enchance the growth of lipophilic organisms such as *Corynebacterium urealyticum, C. jeikeium,* and the yeast *Malassezia furfur.*

Pyrazinamidase. Nontoxigenic strains of *Corynebacterium* spp. are able to hydrolyze pyrazinamide to pyrazinoic acid and ammonia. Pyrazinamidase activity is used in conjunction with colony morphology to presumptively identify *C. diphtheriae* and other potentially toxigenic species of *Corynebacterium* spp. A solution of pyrazinamide is heavily inoculated and incubated overnight. Two drops of ferrous sulphate reagent are

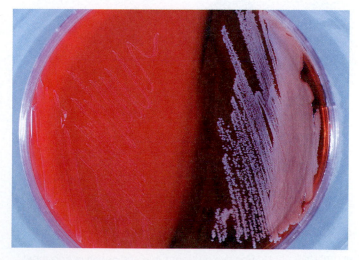

■ **FIGURE 19-14** Increased colony size on the side swabbed with Tween 80 (right) showing a requirement for lipid.

added and observed for an immediate color change. A positive result is an immediate color change to orange-red. If the test remains colorless it is a negative result. *C. diphtheriae, C. ulcerans,* and *C. pseudotuberculosis* are pyrazinamidase negative and potential toxin producers (Colman, Weaver, & Efstatiou, 1992).

REAL WORLD TIP

Pyrazinamide is an antibiotic used in combination with isoniazid and rifampicin for the treatment of *Mycobacterium tuberculosis.*

Gelatin Liquefaction.   The ability to dissolve gelatin into liquid is useful to distinguish *Arcanobacterium hemolyticum* from *A. pyogenes.* This test is illustrated in Figure 19-15 ■. The procedure for performing the tube gelatin liquefaction test is described later in this chapter with the *Nocardia* spp. An alternate procedure uses strips of exposed but undeveloped x-ray film. Sterile saline or distilled water, in the volume of 0.5 ml, is inoculated with a heavy suspension of test organism. The strip of x-ray film is inserted into the tube and incubated in a 37°C waterbath. The tube is observed every hour for 4 hours, after 24 hours of incubation, and again after 48 hours of incubation. A positive result is removal of the green gelatin emulsion from the immersed film, which leaves only the clear blue film strip. A negative result is an intact green emulsion on the immersed part of the film strip (MacFaddin, 2000). This method may no longer be a viable alternative because x-ray film may become a thing of the past with the use of digital imaging.

Arcanobacterium pyogenes is gelatin positive and shows liquefaction of the medium. *Arcanobacterium haemolyticum* is gelatin negative with no liquefaction. Gelatin reactions can

also be used to distinguish *Corynebacterium* spp. from other coryneform genera.

Rapid Sucrose Urea.   The rapid sucrose urea (RSU) test is a rapid screening test for the more common lipophilic species, *C. jeikeium* and *C. urealyticum. C. jeikeium* provides a negative result, which displays as no color change or yellowish-brown in color. Figure 19-16 ■ provides a view of a negative result. *C. urealyticum* produces a bright purple-violet color due to the hydrolysis of urea. Those coryneforms that ferment sucrose produce a bright yellow color. It is important to test isolates grown on nonglucose and nonselective medium such as sheep blood agar. Glucose present in the medium can interfere with sucrose utilization and cause a false positive. Most organisms prefer to utilize the simple sugar glucose before using the complex sugar sucrose. A false positive can also be caused by a heavy inoculum. Only two to three colonies are to be used for inoculation (Hardy Diagnostics, 2002).

Commercial Kits.   Several commercial kits are available to identify to species. These include conventional tests and chromogenic substrates. Many laboratories use rapid identification strips, such as API® Coryne, Remel™ CB Plus System, and BBL Crystal, as well as panels used in automated systems (Bernard, 2005).

Databases of these methods may not reflect recent changes to genera or contain the newer taxa. They also work best with the coryneforms that grow rapidly in air and actively utilize the substrates provided. Lipophilic, nonreactive, and slow-growing coryneforms may require additional tests. Identification of an isolate should be questioned if Gram stain morphology and colony morphology do not correlate.

***Corynebacterium diphtheriae* Group.**   *Corynebacterium diphtheriae* is the recognized pathogen in this group. Only tox-

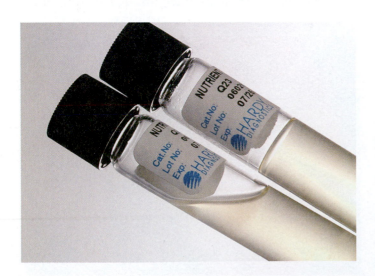

■ **FIGURE 19-15** Positive (bottom tube) and negative (top tube) results for nutrient gelatin liquefaction.
Photo courtesy of Hardy Diagnostics. www.HardyDiagnostics.com

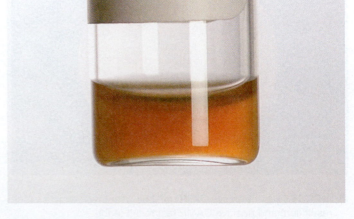

■ **FIGURE 19-16** Negative result for *C. jeikeium* in the rapid sucrose urea (RSU) test.
Photo courtesy of Hardy Diagnostics. www.HardyDiagnostics.com

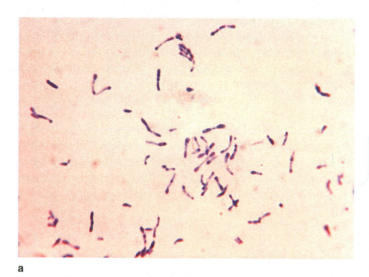

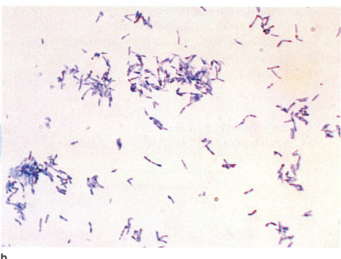

a   b

■ **FIGURE 19-17 a.** Gram stain of *Corynebacterium diphtheriae*. *From Public Health Image Library (PHIL), CDC.* **b.** *Corynebacterium diphtheriae* stained with methylene blue stain. *From Public Health Image Library (PHIL), CDC/Dr. P.B. Smith.*

igenic strains cause disease so testing for toxin expression is the key to determining its clinical significance. *C. diphtheriae* resides in the upper respiratory tract and must be distinguished from the commensal *Corynebacterium* species. It may also be found on the skin of individuals with poor hygiene (Murray et al., 2003).

Identification

Identification of *C. diphtheriae* is based on stain morphology, colony morphology on selective media, biochemical tests, and the presence of toxin.

Microscopic Morphology. *C. diphtheriae* are gram-positive rods that characteristically palisade, as noted in Figure 19-17a ■. **Metachromatic granules** appear as beaded areas within the cell. They can be observed best in growth from Loeffler's medium when stained with methylene blue, as noted in Figure 19-17b ■. These inclusion granules are thought to serve as energy reserves for the organism.

Colony Morphology. *C. diphtheriae* grows as a small whitish colony with variable beta-hemolysis, small gray, or transluscent colonies on sheep blood agar. Recovery of the organism requires the use of selective and nonselective culture media. Tellurite containing media such as Tinsdale, cystine tellurite, and potassium tellurite agars are selective and differential and designed to detect *C. diphtheriae*.

Media with tellurite inhibits the growth of most commensal flora. *C. diphtheriae*, some corynebacteria, staphylococci, and yeast are resistant to tellurite and will grow on this media (Efstratiou et al., 2000). *C. diphtheriae* appears as black colonies on cystine tellurite or potassium tellurite agar. Figure 19-18 ■ demonstrates the organism on cystine tellurite blood agar. Reduction of tellurite causes the blackening of the colonies.

Medium with cystine and sodium thiosulfate allows the detection of cystinase production by the isolate. Suspect colonies of *C. diphtheriae* will grow as gray-black colonies with brown halos on Tinsdale agar. The black color is due to tellurite reduction and the brown halo is due to the presence of cystinase.

REAL WORLD TIP

Tinsdale agar is probably the best medium for culturing *C. diphtheriae*. It is selective and differential but has a very short shelf life.

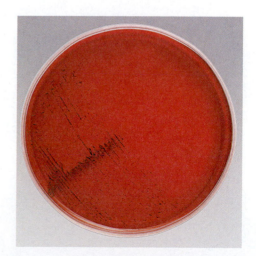

■ **FIGURE 19-18** Colonies of *C. diphtheriae* on cystine tellurite blood agar.
Photo courtesy of Remel, part of Thermo Fisher Scientific.

Loeffler's medium contains egg and serum for optimum growth of *C. diphtheriae* and is used for microscopic examination and biochemical testing. Loeffler's medium is nonselective but encourages the production of metachromatic granules, as noted in Figure 19-19 .

Checkpoint! 19–7 (Chapter Objectives 3 and 6)

Colonies suspicious for C. diphtheriae on Tinsdale agar:
   A. *are inhibited by the high cystine concentration.*
   B. *form blackish colonies with no change in the media.*
   C. *form whitish or translucent colonies.*
   D. *form gray-black colonies surrounded by a brown halo.*

Key Biochemical Reactions.   The *C. diphtheriae* group shares the catalase positive and nonmotile characteristics of the *Corynebacterium* genus. *C. diphtheriae* should be suspected if a urease-negative, cystinase-positive, and pyrazinamidase-negative colony is isolated (Colman et al., 1992; Efstratiou et al., 2000). Further testing is required to identify to species or biotype. *C. diphtheriae* metabolizes sugars fermentatively and may be lipophilic. Most strains are nitrate positive. *C. diphtheriae* is also negative for esculin hydrolysis and the inverse CAMP test. Refer to Table 19-3 for details of biochemical reactions that distinguish *C. diphtheriae* from other coryneforms.

There are four biotypes or subspecies of the organism: *C. diphtheriae* subspecies *gravis, mitis, belfanti,* and *intermedius*. *C. diphtheriae* subspecies *gravis* and *mitis* are the most common. The World Health Organization recommends that these biotypes be differentiated as part of the identification process (Murray et al., 2003).

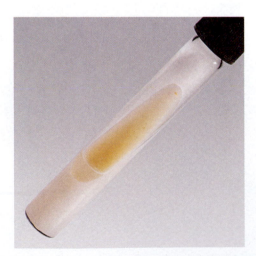

C. diphtheriae biotype *intermedius* is lipophilic and forms small gray or translucent colonies, whereas the other biotypes form larger, whiter, more opaque colonies. *C. diphtheriae* biotype *intermedius* can be distinguished from the others using microscopic morphology of methylene blue-stained smears of growth from Loeffler's media. The cells of biotype *intermedius* are long, barred, and clubbed whereas biotype *gravis* is short and stains uniformly and biotype *mitis* is long with metachromatic granules (Coyle, Nowowiejski, Russell, & Groman, 1993). *C. diphtheriae* biotype *gravis* is positive for fermentation of glycogen and starch whereas *C. diphtheriae* biotypes *mitis* and *intermedius* are negative (Coyle et al., 1993). *C. diphtheriae* biotype *belfanti* is nitrate negative while the other biotypes are nitrate positive (Funke, Stubbs, Pfyffer, Marchiani, & Collins, 1997).

Two other species, *C. pseudotuberculosis* and *C. ulcerans,* may produce brown halos on Tinsdale and are negative for pyrazinamidase. These two species may also produce diphtheria toxin if the *tox* gene is present. *C. pseudotuberculosis* and *C. ulcerans* are urea and CAMP inhibition positive whereas *C. diphtheriae* is urea and CAMP inhibition negative.

A diagnosis of diphtheria requires the identification of *C. diphtheriae* and confirmation of toxin production by the organism. There are non-toxin-producing strains of *C. diphtheriae* but they do not cause the disease. PCR can detect the *tox* gene but cannot determine if the protein is biologically active and producing toxin. A negative PCR result for the *tox* gene rules out a diagnosis of diphtheria and eliminates the need for special biosafety precautions (Efstratiou et al., 2000).

The modified Elek test is an immunoprecipitation test that determines if diphtheria toxin is present. A disk containing 10 International Units (IU) of diphtheria antitoxin is placed in the center of a petri dish containing Elek medium. A heavy inoculum of the suspected organism is placed 9 mm from the disk. Multiple organisms can be placed on the agar surface around the disk. The agar plate is examined after 24 hours incubation in ambient air. A positive result is indicated by a precipitin line in the agar between the antitoxin and organism (Engler, Glushkevich, Mazurova, George, & Efstratiou, 1997). Refer to Figure 19-20 ■ for a graphic representation of the modified Elek test.

Checkpoint! 19–8 (Chapter Objectives 6 and 9)

An organism resembling diphtheroids is isolated from a throat specimen. It grows as a black colony on cysteine tellurite agar and demonstrates a colorless reaction in the pyrazinamidase activity test. The next step is to:
   A. *confirm with catalase.*
   B. *confirm toxin production.*
   C. *confirm the serotype.*
   D. *check for a requirement for lipid.*

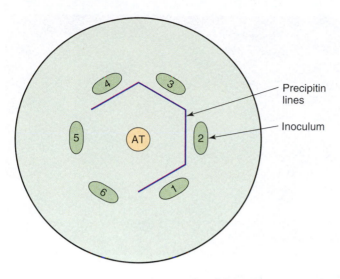

AT = Anti-toxin disk
1 = Test isolate (Toxigenic)
2 = Positive control
3 = Weak positive control
4 = Positive control
5 = Test isolate (Nontoxigenic)
6 = Negative control

■ FIGURE 19-20 Modified Elek test.

Clinical Significance

Specimens for Isolation. Specimens are usually received on a swab collected from the throat, nasopharynx, or cutaneous lesion. *C. diphtheriae* has also been isolated from lower respiratory tract specimens, blood, and prosthetic heart valves (Isenberg, 1998). Physicians should specify *C. diphtheriae* in the culture request, so Tinsdale agar and, if possible, Loeffler's media can be added to the primary culture media. CNA can also be used but the microbiologist will have to perform additional tests on suspect colonies to rule out *C. diphtheriae* (Murray et al., 2003).

Pathogenesis. Not all biotypes of *C. diphtheriae* cause the disease diphtheria. Pharyngeal diphtheria is only caused by toxigenic strains or those species infected by a bacteriophage or virus carrying the *tox* gene. The *tox* gene provides the blueprint for construction of the diphtheria toxin. The toxin blocks protein synthesis in eukaryotic cells. It is secreted by the bacteria and has no effect until exposed to proteases. Proteases cleave the toxin into fragments A and B. Fragment B binds to receptors on the cell membrane and forms endosomes that help fragment A enter the cytoplasm. Fragment A disrupts protein synthesis in the cell and is the toxic component of the toxin (Mims, Dimmock, Nash, & Stephen, 1995). Fragment A may also trigger cell lysis (Hadfield, McEvoy, Polotsky, Tzinserling, & Yakovlev, 2000)

C. diphtheriae reproduce in the infected site, usually the upper respiratory system, and secrete the toxin. Epithelial cells are damaged, inflammation is triggered, tissue necrosis results, and a tough, grayish-white pseudomembrane forms. Suffocation is a concern if the membrane blocks the airway. Prior to the discovery of antibiotics, ripping the membrane off was considered therapeutic. This action releases more toxin, which is absorbed into the bloodstream. The absorbed diphtheria toxin has systemic effects on the kidney, heart, and nervous system. Death can occur from cardiac failure. Paralysis can occur as a result of the diphtheria toxin demyelinating peripheral nerves (Mims et al., 1995). *C. diphtheriae* can also colonize surgical wounds, bites, and other skin lesions (Hadfield et al., 2000).

Infectious Diseases. Diphtheria is a communicable disease spread by aerosols due to coughing and sneezing and direct contact. Pharyngeal diphtheria results from infection with a toxigenic strain of *C. diphtheriae, C. ulcerans,* or *C. pseudotuberculosis.* Patients with pharyngeal diphtheria present with malaise, low-grade fever, and a sore throat. Because these symptoms are also associated with pharyngitis due to *Streptococcus pyogenes,* a blood agar plate is usually added to the primary media. Group A *Streptococcus* pharyngitis can also produce a white membrane in the back of the throat that can mimic that produced by *C. diphtheriae.*

Cutaneous diphtheria is a skin infection more commonly seen in tropical parts of the world. *C. ulcerans* and *C. pseudotuberculosis* infections are associated with contact with animals or unpasteurized dairy products (Mahon & Manuselis, 2000). Septic arthritis of the hip, splenic and hepatic abscesses, sepsis, and endocarditis have been associated with nontoxigenic *C. diphtheriae* strains (Hadfield et al., 2000).

Disease occurs in unvaccinated individuals or those who have not received booster immunizations. Diphtheria is a serious illness with a mortality of 5–10% in unvaccinated individuals (Centers for Disease Control, 1995). The disease is rare in the United States. There is concern diphtheria will reemerge due to the susceptibility of persons over the age of 30 because they have not received a 10-year booster vaccination.

Treatment is administration of an antitoxin, to bind the circulating toxin, and antibiotics to eradicate the bacteria. Penicillin and macrolides are recommended.

CORYNEBACTERIUM JEIKEIUM

One of the most frequently isolated *Corynebacterium* species, in blood and other sterile body fluids, is *C. jeikeium*. It is found on inanimate objects in hospitals. *C. jeikeium* is not usually part of the normal skin flora of healthy, nonhospitalized individuals. It is usually found in the inguinal, axillary, and rectal areas of hospitalized patients. The organism can be clinically significant especially as a nosocomial pathogen. It is highly antibiotic resistant and therefore difficult to treat without the appropriate antibiotics such as vancomycin.

Identification

Microscopic and Colony Morphology.
Corynebacterium jeikeium shares the microscopic morphology of the coryneforms, as seen in Figure 19-21 ■. It is a gram-positive small, pallisading coccobacillary or short rod (Cartwright, Stock, Kruczak-Filipov, & Gill, 1993).

The colony of *C. jeikeium* is similar to the other commensal coryneforms. This strict aerobe presents as a small, grayish-white, nonhemolytic colony, as seen in Figure 19-22 ■. It requires lipids for growth so the colonies can be pin-point on initial isolation.

Key Biochemical Reactions.
Initial screening includes a catalase test that is positive. Key biochemical results are nitrate negative and urea negative as most of the other lipophilic coryneforms encountered in the clinical laboratory are urea positive or nitrate positive. The remaining lipophilic *Corynebacterium* can be distinguished from *C. jeikeium* using glucose, fructose, and pyrazinamidase test results. *C. jeikeium* oxidatively uses glucose and is fructose negative and pyrazinamidase positive. Refer to Table 19-3 for additional biochemical reactions.

C. jeikeium is multiresistant. Resistance to most antibiotics can be used as an identification test rather than for susceptibility results. Because *C. jeikeium* is slow-growing, traditional antibiotic susceptibility methods do not provide valid results with this organism. Any results obtained can only be used as a part of the identification process. *C. jeikeium* will display resistance against most antibiotics other than vancomycin.

Many labs screen for *C. jeikeium* with rapid sucrose urea broth. Because it is urease and sucrose negative, no color change or a yellowish-brown color is observed. Cartwright and colleges (1993) recommend that any aerobic small gray colony that is a catalase positive, gram-positive bacilli or coccobacilli and RSU negative be presumptively identified as *C. jeikeium.* Another multidrug-resistant coryneform, *C. resistens,*

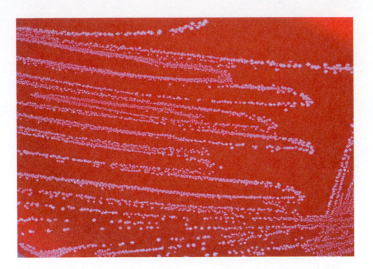

■ **FIGURE 19-22** Colonies of *C. jeikeium* on sheep blood agar.

is also RSU negative. *C. resistens* ferments glucose, is pyrazinamidase negative, and grows slowly anaerobically while *C. jeikeium* oxidizes glucose, is pyrazinamidase positive, and does not grow anaerobically (Otsuka et al., 2005).

Clinical Significance

C. jeikeium is the most common diphtheroid isolate. It is linked to infections associated with prosthetic devices or catheterization. Immunocompromised individuals with malignancies, those undergoing invasive procedures or prolonged hospital stays, and those receiving broad-spectrum antibiotic treatment are at highest risk of contracting this organism. Clinical infections include nosocomial septicemia, bacteremia, pneumonia, meningitis, and soft tissue infections (Funke et al., 1997). ∞ Chapter 40, "Opportunistic Infections," provides additional information on opportunistic infections.

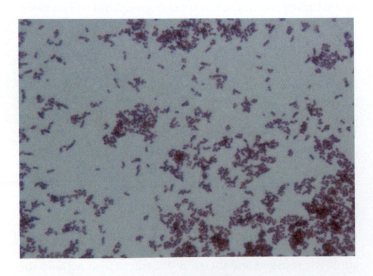

■ **FIGURE 19-21** Gram stain of *C. jeikeium.*

✓ **Checkpoint! 19–9**
(Chapter Objectives 5 and 6)

A gram-positive, non-spore-forming, diphtheroid rod is isolated from a blood culture. The following test results were observed:

    Catalase - bubbles
    Lipid Requirement - better growth with Tween 80
    Nitrate - colorless
    Urea - no change
    Sucrose - no change
    Pyrazinamidase - orange-red
This organism is most likely:
    A. *C. urealyticum.*
    B. *C. jeikeium.*
    C. *C. diphtheriae.*
    D. *C. amycolatum.*

Other Coryneform Bacilli.

Other coryneform bacilli that may be clinically significant include *C. urealyticum*, *C. resistans*, and *Arcanobacterium*. These rarely isolated species may cause infections in immunocompromised individuals or after invasive procedures. Infections include wound, bacteremia, endocarditis, urinary tract, eye, respiratory and genitourinary infections, and lymphadenitis.

C. urealyticum is a urinary tract pathogen that is lipophilic and may require 48 hours incubation to grow. Bacteruria occurs in long-term hospitalized, older individuals who are immunocompromised and catheterized (Funke et al., 1997). Individuals with hematological disorders may develop bacteremia due to this organism (Otsuka et al., 2005).

Its colony is pin-point to small, nonhemolytic, and whitish gray. Key biochemical reactions include a positive catalase and rapid urea. There are other urea-positive corynebacterium but they are not lipophilic. In addition, the other urea-positive *Corynebacterium* may be fermentative, glucose and maltose positive, or nitrate positive whereas *C. urealyticum* is oxidative, nitrate negative, and glucose and nitrate negative. Refer to Table 19-3 for details of differentiation of urea-positive *Corynebacterium*. *C. urealyticum* is usually multidrug resistant and only susceptible to vancomycin. Testing against antibiotics can be used as part of the identification process but not for reporting as susceptibility results.

The presence of alkaline urine and struvite crystals may be a clue for the presence of *C. urealyticum*. The organism splits urea to create crystals that deposit in the bladder wall, resulting in ulceration. Urine cultures must be held longer than 24 hours to isolate this slow-growing urinary tract pathogen (Murray et al., 2003).

Arcanobacterium haemolyticum is associated with pharyngitis in children and young adults ages 15–25, wound, and rare systemic infections (Parija et al., 2005). *Arcanobacterium pyogenes* is found in animals and most infections are acquired in rural settings. *A. pyogenes* has been isolated from blood cultures, abscesses, infected wounds, and respiratory specimens. *Arcanobacterium bernardiae* is a rare isolate from specimens of immunocompromised individuals including blood cultures and abscesses (Funke et al., 1997).

Any beta-hemolytic, catalase negative colony that does not serotype with streptococcal antisera may be an *Arcanobacterium*.

A. pyogenes can agglutinate with groups G and B streptococcus antisera, resulting in misidentification. A Gram stain must be performed to reveal short, sometimes pleomorphic gram-positive rods.

Both *A. haemolyticum* and *A. pyogenes* are beta-hemolytic, exhibiting narrow zone after 48 hours of incubation, and may be PYR positive like *Streptococcus pyogenes* (Coyle & Lipsky, 1990). Each of the two species can be distinguished with the reverse CAMP, xylose, and gelatin tests. *A. haemolyticum* is CAMP inhibition positive, as seen in Figure 19-13, xylose and gelatin negative. *A. pyogenes* is CAMP inhibition negative, xylose and gelatin positive. *A. bernardiae* grows as a nonhemolytic, small, glassy white colony. *A. bernardiae* is CAMP inhibition, xylose, and gelatin negative. Sarkonen, Kononen, Summanen, Kononen, and Jousimiies-Somer (2001) recommend the ONPG (β-galactosidase) test to distinguish *A. pyogenes* from *A. bernardiae*. *A. pyogenes* is ONPG positive and *A. bernardiae* is ONPG negative.

C. resistans is a multidrug resistant coryneform that causes rapidly fatal bacteremia in those that are immunocompromised. It is a lipophilic coryneform that forms a grayish-white, pearl colony. It is fermentative, nitrate, urea, pyrazinamidase, and reverse CAMP negative (Otsuka et al., 2005).

C. aurimucosum is associated with female genitourinary tract infections, pregnancy complications, and bone and joint infections (Shukla, Harney, Jhaveri, Andrews, & Reed, 2003; Roux et al., 2004). Colonies are sticky, charcoal black, pitting or slightly yellow. It is a nonlipophilic, fermentative coryneform.

▶ REGULAR RODS

Non-spore-forming, gram-positive rods that have two parallel sides with rounded ends include *Listeria*, *Lactobacillus*, and *Erysipelothrix*. Their colony morphology may be similar to other microorganisms so the Gram stain plays an important role in their identification.

USEFUL BIOCHEMICAL TESTS

Motility

L. monocytogenes exhibits an end-over-end tumbling motility that can be observed in a wet mount with nutrient broth. This motility also results in movement away from an inoculum stab in semisolid medium. The resulting growth occurs near the agar surface and looks similar to an open umbrella, as noted in Figure 19-23 ■. This unique result occurs only when

---

⊘ REAL WORLD TIP

A beta-hemolytic, gray, translucent colony isolated from an upper respiratory culture, such as the throat, requires a catalase test and Gram stain as part of the identification process. *Streptococcus pyogenes* is the most commonly isolated pathogen and is a gram-positive cocci that is catalase negative. The colonies of *Arcanobacterium haemolyticum* and *Actinomyces pyogenes* can mimic the colony of *S. pyogenes* but are catalase negative, gram-positive rods.

⊘ REAL WORLD TIP

The characteristic "umbrella" motility of *Listeria monocytogenes* is best observed in semisolid medium that contains 0.2–0.4% agar. An agar concentration greater than 0.4% will not allow the organism to spread away from the inoculum stab line.

incubated at room temperature (25°C). When incubated at 35–37°C, motility is negative or greatly reduced without the characteristic "umbrella" pattern.

Esculin

This test was discussed extensively in ∞ Chapter 17, "Aerobic Gram-Positive Cocci." It is a rapid test designed to detect the presence of esculinase. *L. monocytogenes* is positive.

@ **REAL WORLD TIP**

Listeria monocytogenes is bile esculin positive and grows in 6.5% NaCl broth. *Enterococcus* spp. produces the same reactions and can rarely be beta hemolytic. Both can be isolated from similar body sites and specimen types. To avoid misidentification of these organisms, a Gram stain and catalase test must be performed to differentiate the two. *L. monocytogenes* is a catalase-positive gram-positive rod whereas *Enterococcus* spp. is a catalase-negative gram-positive cocci.

CAMP TEST

The traditional CAMP test can be used to identify *L. monocytogenes*. It produces a shovel- or wedge-shaped area of enhanced hemolysis (Figure 19-24 ■) at the intersection of the beta-lysin-producing *Staphylococcus*.

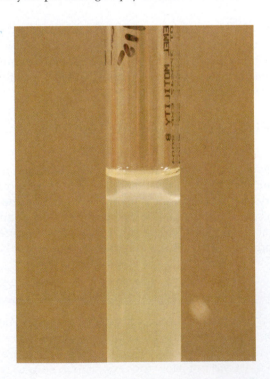

■ **FIGURE 19-23** Positive (umbrella) motility reaction characteristic of *L. monocytogenes*.

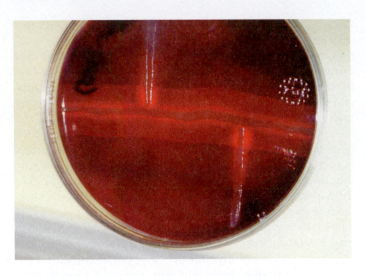

■ **FIGURE 19-24** Positive CAMP result for *L. monocytogenes*.

@ **REAL WORLD TIP**

The shovel-shaped CAMP reaction of *Listeria monocytogenes* is rarely used for identification in the clinical laboratory. It can be easily confused with the arrowhead CAMP reaction of group B *Streptococcus* (*Streptococcus agalactiae*). The CAMP test is only considered to be a presumptive test. It cannot be used as a single test to identify an organism.

Listeria monocytogenes

There are six species of *Listeria,* most of which are not associated with human disease. The human pathogen species is *L. monocytogenes*. Its environmental niche includes the soil, water, and decaying plant matter. Sheep, cattle, birds, fish, crustaceans, and insects such as flies and ticks may harbor this microbe. About 10% of the human population can carry this organism in their gastrointestinal tract. *Listeria monocytogenes* is an important foodborne pathogen. It has been isolated from lunch meat, hot dogs, soft cheeses, milk, butter, ice cream, raw vegetables, and unpasteurized apple cider (Wing & Gregory, 2002).

General Characteristics.   *Listeria* is a gram-positive, non-spore-forming, regular-shaped rod. They are facultative anaerobes that grow well on sheep blood and chocolate agars at routine incubation temperatures. A unique characteristic of *Listeria* is that it can grow in high concentrations of salt and cold environments. Cold enrichment at 4°C can be used to enhance the growth of *Listeria*. Growth as 4°C also allows it to continue to grow in contaminated food even when refrigerated. *Listeria monocytogenes* is catalase positive and oxidase negative.

Identification.   *Listeria monocytogenes* can be isolated from the same specimens as *Streptococcus agalactiae* (beta-hemolytic *Streptococcus* group B). These include blood, CSF, amniotic fluid, fetal and placental tissues, and stool. It is important to rule out group B streptococci during the identification process because they share similar biochemical reactions and colony morphologies. If this is not done, a clinically significant, erroneous report may be generated.

Microscopic Morphology.   *Listeria* are gram-positive, non-spore-forming, regular-shaped rods that may appear coccobacillary. They can be arranged in singles, chains, or palisading, as observed in Figure 19-25 ■. Because its Gram stain morphology can resemble streptococci or coryneforms, additional tests should be performed.

Colony Morphology.   The colony of *Listeria monocytogenes* closely resembles that of *Streptococcus agalactiae*. It is a small grayish-white colony with a narrow zone of beta-hemolysis. The catalase test, esculin test, and Gram stain will distinguish group B *Streptococcus* from *Listeria* because *L. monocytogenes* is a gram-positive rod that is catalase and esculin positive. Group B *Streptococcus* is gram-positive cocci that is catalase and esculin negative. If one relies on Gram stain alone, the result may be misleading as *Listeria* can appear coccobacillary. Both *L. monocytogenes* and group B streptococci are sodium hippurate hydrolysis positive. *Listeria monocytogenes* may react with groups B and G antisera when tested with streptococcal serotyping antigen kits.

 REAL WORLD TIP

The beta hemolysis of *Listeria monocytogenes* can be very subtle. The colony may have to be removed to see the weak beta hemolysis beneath it.

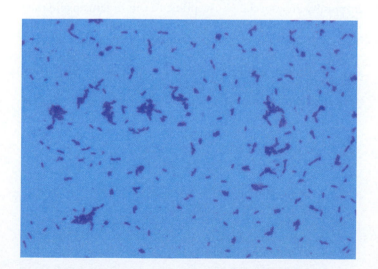
■ **FIGURE 19-25** Gram stain of *L. monocytogenes*.

 Checkpoint! 19–10 (Chapter Objective 7)

Listeria monocytogenes can be distinguished from Streptococcus agalactiae (group B Streptococcus) because it is:

1. *catalase positive.*
2. *gram positive.*
3. *sodium hippurate positive.*
    A. *1 only*
    B. *3 only*
    C. *1 and 3*
    D. *1 and 2*

Key Biochemical Reactions.   *Listeria* can be identified using Gram stain, motility, catalase, and esculin results. Acid from glucose and MRVP positive reactions confirm the identity (Murray et al., 2003). Tumbling or "end-over-end" motility is observed in a wet mount using nutrient broth. The semisolid motility test result is also helpful because of its unique appearance and temperature reactions. *L. monocytogenes* is nonmotile or displays reduced motility at 35–37°C and motile at 25°C. Its positive result is unique in that it resembles an open umbrella, as seen in Figure 19-23.

Listeria is catalase and esculin positive. *Corynebacterium* is esculin negative and nonmotile. Some of the coryneforms are also esculin positive and motile but do not demonstrate the tumbling motility feature. The motility test is not definitive and cannot be used to identify an organism without additional testing.

The traditional CAMP test may be used to presumptively identify *L. monocytogenes* because it is positive. It is important to remember group B *Streptococcus* is also positive. The area of enhanced hemolysis has a different appearance. *L. monocytogenes* looks like a shovel, as noted in Figure 19-24, whereas group B *Streptococcus* resembles an arrowhead.

Checkpoint! 19–11 (Chapter Objectives 5, 6, and 9)

The Gram stain of a newborn's CSF shows gram-positive, pallisading rods. Small, translucent colonies with narrow zones of beta-hemolysis appear on sheep blood agar after 24 hours in a carbon dioxide environment. Select the appropriate testing to presumptively identify this organism.

1. *wet mount motility*
2. *catalase*
3. *esculin hydrolysis*
4. *lipid requirement*
    A. *1, 2, and 3*
    B. *1 and 3*
    C. *4 only*
    D. *1, 2, 3, and 4*

Clinical Significance. Immunocompromised individuals, pregnant women, and infants are at higher risk of developing life-threatening infections from *L. monocytogenes*. *L. monocytogenes* can easily be mistaken for group B *Streptococcus* because of its similar colony morphology and it may be isolated from the same body sites and infect similar patient populations.

Specimens for Isolation. *Listeria monocytogenes* infection often begins as a foodborne illness. It can enter food during the manufacturing process and colonize the foodstuff. It has the unique ability to grow at refrigeration temperatures and be salt tolerant. Outbreaks in the food industry have been associated with soft cheeses, hot dogs, fish, shellfish, ice cream, and lunch meat (Koneman et al., 1997). Potentially contaminated food products and stool specimens are not routinely processed by clinical laboratories. These are usually submitted to public health reference laboratories.

> **⊘ REAL WORLD TIP**
>
> Immunocompromised individuals should avoid eating soft cheeses, such as feta, brie, camembert, and blue. They should also thoroughly heat cold cuts and hot dogs before eating.

Specimens submitted to clinical laboratories are those that reflect a systemic infection. Specimens include stool, cerebrospinal fluid, blood, amniotic fluid, and placental and fetal tissue (Isenberg, 1998). *Listeria* can cause sporadic infections in newborns, older adults, or immunocompromised patients. A pregnant woman's fetus is susceptible if exposed to this organism, so neonatal specimens may be submitted to the laboratory for analysis for this microbe.

> **⊘ REAL WORLD TIP**
>
> *Listeria meningitis* can imitate viral meningitis with lymphocytosis and tubercular or fungal meningitis due to the increased CSF protein, decreased CSF glucose, and increased white blood cell count. Listeriosis should be considered if organisms are not observed in the cerebrospinal fluid Gram stain of individuals considered at risk for this infection (Reynolds, 2006).

Pathogenesis. *Listeria monocytogenes* is ingested via contaminated food. Once ingested the microbe enters the bloodstream from the alimentary tract to cause a systemic illness. Depending on the immune response of the host, the bacteria are either eliminated in the liver or spread to the brain or placenta (Shechan et al., 1994). The susceptibility of an individual to this organism depends on gastric activity and host defenses. The bacterial inoculum amount is also an important factor.

Microbe Defense Mechanisms. *Listeria monocytogenes* is able to withstand the human defensive systems through a variety of mechanisms. These include enzymes that allow it to resist host defenses and become a pathogen within the cells. *Listeria* is able to infect hepatocytes, epithelial cells, and phagocytic cells (Reynolds, 2006).

Surface protein p60 triggers phagocytosis. Once inside the white cell, *Listeria* releases superoxide dismutase, which avoids the toxic effects of the oxidative products produced during the "respiratory burst." A pore-forming hemolysin, listeriolysin O, damages the phagosome membrane, releasing the organism to the cytoplasm. *Listeria* grows in the cytoplasm and rearranges the filaments, resulting in movement of the bacteria to the periphery of the cell. Pseudopod-like extrusions are extended until contact with an adjacent cell results in internalization of the microbe and a new cycle begins (Shechan et al., 1994).

This cell-to-cell spread enables the organism to become an **intracellular pathogen**, residing inside the cell, avoiding the host's circulating antibody and complement. Macrophages are unable to kill *Listeria* because they lack type 3 receptors for complement (Sheehan et al. 1994). Macrophages can serve as transport vehicles enabling the microbe to journey through the circulatory system unharmed. Refer to ∞ Chapter 4, "The Host's Encounter with Microbes," for more information on the host's defenses.

Infectious Diseases. Listeriosis is the infectious disease caused by *Listeria monocytogenes*. Food poisoning resulting in mild to severe gastroenteritis may occur (Wing & Gregory, 2002). Pregnant women exhibit "flu-like" symptoms. The symptoms include fever, headache, and muscle pain. The symptoms are usually not severe enough to warrant a visit to a physician. If the pregnant female becomes septic, the organism can cross the placenta, endangering the fetus. Infection may result in premature birth, spontaneous abortion, or stillbirth. The newborn may acquire this organism and develop sepsis and meningitis.

Older adults and those who have decreased cell-mediated immunity are especially susceptible to this organism and may develop life-threatening meningitis, encephalitis, and sepsis. There is a 20–50% mortality associated with central nervous system infections with *L. monocytogenes* (Murray et al., 2003). Eye infections, cellulitis, pneumonia, osteomyelitis, septic arthritis, and other systemic infections rarely occur (Reynolds, 2006). Refer to ∞ Chapter 36, "Genital System," and ∞ Chapter

> **Checkpoint! 19–12 (Chapter Objective 9)**
>
> *Spontaneous abortion or stillbirth during pregnancy may result from an infection with:*
>
> A. *E. coli.*
> B. *Staphylococcus aureus.*
> C. *Listeria monocytogenes.*
> D. *Gardnerella vaginalis.*

38, "Central Nervous System," to review infections associated with pregnancy and meningitis.

Lactobacillus

Lactobacilli may be isolated from specimens associated with mucous membranes. They play a significant role in defense against infection by being members of the commensal or normal flora.

General Characteristics.   *Lactobacillus* species can be obligate aerobes, facultative anaerobes, or obligate anaerobes. Under the microscope, they appear as gram-positive rods. They grow on sheep blood agar, chocolate agar, and gram-positive selective agars such as CNA and PEA.

Identification.   Suspect lactobacilli when a pinpoint alpha or gamma hemolytic colony appears after 48 hours of incubation. Colonies of *Corynebacterium* and streptococci may also be alpha or gamma hemolytic but can be ruled out using catalase test results and microscopic morphology.

Microscopic and Colony Morphology.   Lactobacilli are non-spore-forming gram-positive rods. They may appear different from the other regular gram-positive rods because they are long and filamentous, often appearing in chains as seen in Figure 19-26 ■. Other morphotypes may be present and include coccobacillary in chains and palisading, pleomorphic, gram-positive rods.

This chapter focuses on the aerobic lactobacilli. Their colony morphology varies from tiny, pin-point alpha-hemolytic colonies to large, rough, gray colonies. The colonies may require 48 hours of incubation for growth to be observed.

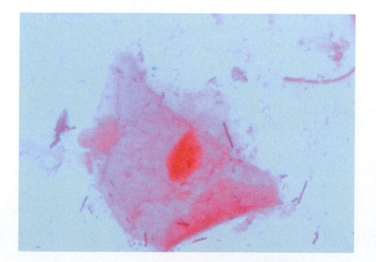

■ **FIGURE 19-26** Gram stain of vaginal direct smear showing *Lactobacillus* and vaginal squamous epithelial cells.

REAL WORLD TIP

The alpha-hemolytic colonies of *Lactobacillus* may resemble those of viridans streptococci. A Gram stain of the organism grown in thioglycolate growth will help rule out *Streptococcus* (Koneman et al., 1997). Growth in a liquid medium often provides the most accurate microscopic morphology.

REAL WORLD TIP

Small alpha hemolytic colonies isolated from the upper respiratory system are usually viridans streptococci. The same colonies isolated from the female genital tract are usually *Lactobacillus* spp.

Key Biochemical Reactions.   Most clinical laboratories only identify to genus based on the Gram stain. The biochemical test panel is designed to rule out other clinically significant gram-positive rods. *Lactobacillus* is biochemically inert, producing negative results in most tests. Useful tests include catalase, motility, esculin, glucose, hydrogen sulfide (H_2S) production, nitrate, and urease. Table 19-4✪ compares the biochemical reactions of *Lactobacillus* with the other aerobic gram-positive rods.

Lactobacillus is catalase negative, which differentiates it from *Listeria*, *Corynebacterium*, and *Bacillus*. *Erysipelothrix* is catalase negative but also produces H_2S in triple sugar iron agar (TSI) along the inoculum stab whereas lactobacilli do not. *Lactobacillus* is also nonmotile, esculin, glucose, nitrate, and urease negative.

Clinical Significance.   Lactobacilli are commensal or normal flora in the oral cavity, gastrointestinal tract, and female genital tract. Lactobacilli produce antimicrobial products such as bacteriocins and products of metabolism such as lactic acid or hydrogen peroxide, which prevents overgrowth of potential pathogens (Slover & Danziger, 2008). They play a significant role in maintaining the acidic environment needed for healthy vagina flora. Their absence is a key factor in the development of bacterial vaginosis. ∞ Chapter 36, "Genital System," provides more information on this disease. The presence of lactobacilli also contributes to the control of opportunistic pathogens that wait for the chance to cause disease.

REAL WORLD TIP

The loss of *Lactobacillus* spp., often due to antibiotic use, and subsequent growth of organisms such as *Gardnerella vaginalis*, *Mobiluncus* spp., and *Bacteroides* spp., leads to the development of bacterial vaginosis.

✪ TABLE 19-4

Key Reactions for Distinguishing Aerobic Gram-Positive Rods

Genus	Cat	Esc	H₂S (TSI)	Hemolysis	Motility	Other Characteristics
Bacillus	+	−	−	β, None	V	Spores in ambient air
Corynebacterium	+	−	−	β, None	−	Diphtheroid, palisades
Listeria	+	+	−	β	+ (25°C) −/+ (35°C)	May palisade; exhibits tumbling motility
Actinomyces	−/+	V	+/−	None, βʷ	−	Diphtheroid or branched rods; filaments
Arcanobacterium	−	V	−	β, None	−	Diphtheroid
Erysipelothrix	−	−	+	α, None	−	Bottle brush growth in gelatin; long filaments
Lactobacillus	−	−	−	α, None	−	Long filaments

Cat, catalase; Esc, Esculin; +, positive; −, negative; V, variable; −/+, most negative, some positive; α, alpha; β, beta; w, weak.

Immunocompromised individuals are susceptible to infection by lactobacilli. Endocarditis and bacteremia are the most commonly associated infections, with an overall mortality of 30% (Cannon, Lee, Bolaros, & Danziger, 2005). With bacteremia the source of the infecting lactobacillus is believed to be the gastrointestinal tract. A history of dental procedures or poor dental care has been associated with endocarditis. The ability of lactobacilli to aggregate platelets and cause fibrin to be produced is thought to contribute to their colonization of vegetative thrombi and the ability to escape the host defenses. Lactobacilli can also cause tooth cavities, abdominal abscesses, chorioamnionitis, pneumonia, and meningitis (Slover & Danziger, 2008).

 REAL WORLD TIP

Yogurt is created by the fermentation products of live *Lactobacillus*. Yogurt and *Lactobacillus* capsules can be used as a probiotic to reinstate normal vaginal flora.

 REAL WORLD TIP

Lactobacillus spp. is intrinsically resistant to vancomycin, which is unusual for most gram-positive organisms. Resistance to vancomycin can be used as part of the identification of the organism if needed.

Erysipelothrix

Erysipelothrix is a rare isolate and contains one clinically significant species. *E. rhusiopathiae* survives in water contaminated by a sick animal's feces or urine, soil, or plant material. Domestic swine are the main animal reservoir for this organism. Birds and fish may also carry this organism (Murray et al., 2003). It is highly resistant to food preservation practices including salting, smoking, and pickling.

General Characteristics. *Erysipelothrix* is a facultative anaerobe which appears microscopically as a gram-positive rod. It grows on most routinely used media and does not have any special growth requirements.

Identification. Use of certain biochemical tests and careful observation of microscopic morphology will distinguish *Erysipelothrix* from other microorganisms that can resemble it.

Microscopic and Colony Morphology. *Erysipelothrix* appears as long, filamentous gram-positive rods or short rods appearing singly, in pairs as a *V*, or in chains, as noted in Figure 19-27 ■. It decolorizes easily and may appear gram negative (Reboli & Farar, 1989).

Colonies appear after 1–3 days of incubation as pin-point alpha-hemolytic or nonhemolytic colonies on sheep blood agar. After 48 hours of incubation, as seen in Figure 19-28 ■, the colonies may appear small, smooth, and transparent with an entire edge or large, rough, and opaque with an irregular edge (Murray et al., 2003). Careful observation of a colony Gram stain should rule out a similar-looking organism, viridans streptococci.

 Checkpoint! 19–13 (Chapter Objectives 1 and 6)

A catalase negative, long, filamentous, gram-positive, non-spore-forming rod is most likely:

1. *Erysipelothrix.*
2. *Listeria.*
3. *Lactobacillus.*
   A. *1 and 2*
   B. *1 and 3*
   C. *2 and 3*
   D. *1, 2, and 3*

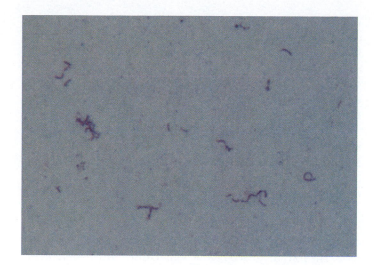

■ **FIGURE 19-27** Gram stain of *Erysipelothrix.*

Key Biochemical Reactions. *Erysipelothrix* can resemble lactobacilli in their microscopic morphology and negative test results for catalase, motility, nitrate, urease, and esculin. Lactobacilli are glucose negative whereas *Erysipelothrix* weakly ferments glucose. *Erysipelothrix* can also resemble *Listeria* because it is able to grow in cooler temperatures and withstand high salt concentrations. It cannot grow at 4°C and is catalase negative whereas *Listeria* grows at 4°C and is positive for motility and catalase.

Erysipelothrix is gelatin negative (at 22°C) but is unique in that is grows in gelatin with a "bottle brush" appearance. It is also a weak hydrogen sulfide (H_2S) producer, as seen in Figure 19-29 ■. It tends to produce H_2S only along the inoculum stab line. Most clinically significant gram-positive rods are H_2S negative. Review Table 19-4 for the biochemical reactions of the other aerobic gram-positive rods.

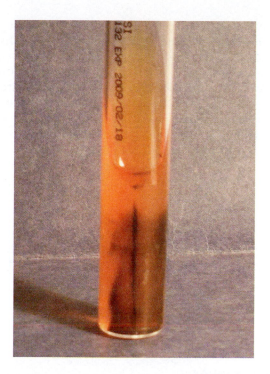

■ **FIGURE 19-29** Positive H_2S reaction in TSI characteristic of *Erysipelothrix.*

> **⊘ REAL WORLD TIP**
>
> *Erysipelothrix rhusiopathiae* is the most commonly isolated catalase negative gram-positive rod that produces H_2S in a KIA or TSI slant.

> **⊘ REAL WORLD TIP**
>
> *Erysipelothrix rhusiopathiae* is intrinsically resistant to vancomycin, which is unusual for gram-positive organisms. *Lactobacillus* spp. is also vancomycin resistant. A positive H_2S reaction will rule in *E. rhusiopathiae* and rule out *Lactobacillus* spp.

Clinical Significance. *Erysipelothrix* is found in soil and water. It is also carried in the digestive tract of many animals, especially turkey and swine. *E. rhusiopathiae* is known for causing **zoonoses**, or infections acquired from animals. It is usually associated with occupational exposure to animals. High-risk occupations include fishermen, butchers, veterinarians, and cooks. Specimens collected include blood and tissue.

The organism gains entry through a previous injury such as an abrasion or puncture wound. The typical infection begins with the formation of an **erysipeloid.** This is a local skin lesion with a reddish diamond-like pattern that usually occurs on the hands or fingers (Reboli & Farrar, 1989). The infected

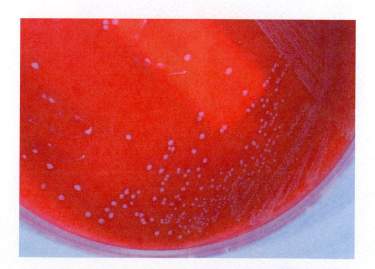

■ **FIGURE 19-28** Colonies of *Erysipelothrix* on sheep blood agar.

area is inflamed, swollen, and painful. Arthritis may be present and the regional lymph nodes may become swollen. The lesion appears 2–7 days after exposure to the bacteria. Usually the lesion heals within 2 to 4 weeks but may take months. The infection can become systemic in immunocompromised individuals, resulting in endocarditis or septicemia and a poor prognosis (Murray et al., 2003). Even with antibiotic therapy there is a 40% mortality rate with endocarditis.

The organism is located deep in the subcutaneous tissue so a swab of the skin surface will not be appropriate. A full thickness biopsy of the infected skin at the advancing margin of the lesion is required.

 Checkpoint! 19–14 (Chapter Objectives 6 and 9)

A gram-positive, non-spore-forming rod is isolated from a wound on a farmer's finger. The following test results were observed:

    Catalase - no change

    TSI - blackening along the stab line

    Bile esculin - no change

    Motility - no change

    Gelatin - no liquefaction and "bottle brush" growth

This organism can be identified as:

    A. *Erysipelothrix spp.*

    B. *Lactobacillus spp.*

    C. *Streptococcus agalactiae.*

    D. *Listeria monocytogenes.*

▶ IRREGULAR RODS

The genera discussed in this section are *Gardnerella, Actinomyces, Nocardia,* and *Streptomyces.* They are gram-positive rods that share a pleomorphic microscopic morphology. They may appear as branching rods or coccobacillary, with different sized cells.

GARDNERELLA

Gardnerella vaginalis has gone through several name changes since its discovery. It was first placed in the genus *Corynebacterium,* then *Haemophilus,* and now resides in the genus *Gardnerella.*

General Characteristics

G. vaginalis is a small, thin, gram-variable rod or coccobacilli. It grows as pinpoint non-hemolytic colonies on sheep blood agar. It grows a little better on chocolate agar. It also grows on PEA and CNA but not MAC. Human blood, incorporated into isolation medium, is used to demonstrate the organism's characteristic subtle beta-hemolysis. The best medium for growth is human blood bilayer-tween (HBT) agar. Its beta-hemolytic

reaction is more visible on HBT agar. This medium has a layer of Columbia agar base with antibiotics and Tween 80 and a layer of the same media with human blood. HBT agar is both selective and differential for *G. vaginalis* (Totten et al., 1982). V agar, with human blood, can be used to isolate and differentiate *G. vaginalis* from other vaginal flora (Greenwood & Pickett, 1979).

G. vaginalis is a capnophilic microbe requiring a CO_2-rich atmosphere for growth. It is inhibited by the anticoagulant SPS used in blood cultures so gelatin should be added to the blood culture broth if this organism is suspected (Forbes, Sahm, & Weissfeld, 2007).

Useful Biochemical Tests

Gardnerella isolates may resemble commensal coryneform bacteria. The tests discussed below help to differentiate *Gardnerella* from the other catalase-negative coryneforms. *Gardnerella* isolated from sites other than the vagina should be tested further to confirm the presumptive identification.

Starch Hydrolysis. Substrate containing starch is inoculated with the suspect organism. After overnight incubation in carbon dioxide, the growth is flooded with iodine. A clear zone around the inoculum indicates a positive result. Medium containing starch and a pH indicator can also be used to visualize a positive result, as seen in Figure 19-30 ■. *G. vaginalis* is able to ferment the starch, turning the medium from purple to yellow. This test alone is not sufficient to identify *Gardnerella* because other catalase-negative, gram-variable rods may also be positive.

Hippurate Hydrolysis. The sodium hippurate test has been discussed in this chapter previously for *Listeria. G. vaginalis* is able to hydrolyze sodium hippurate. Other coryneform bacteria may also be hippurate positive.

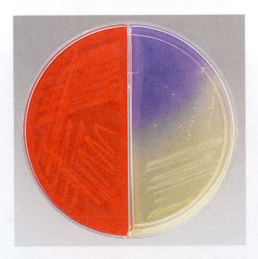

■ **FIGURE 19-30** Positive subtle beta hemolysis (left) and starch reaction (right) for *G. vaginalis* on V and starch agar with brom cresol purple.

Photo courtesy of Remel, part of Thermo Fisher Scientific.

Beta-Glucosidase and Alpha-Glucosidase. Substrate containing 4-nitrophenyl-α-D-glucopyranoside and 4-nitrophenyl-β-D-glucopyranoside are inoculated with the suspect organism and incubated at 37°C. A yellow color is considered positive (Piot, Van Dyck, Totten, & Holmes, 1982). *Gardnerella vaginalis* is alpha-glucosidase positive and beta-glucosidase negative

Rapid Identification Method. A rapid identification system using starch, raffinose fermentation, and hippurate hydrolysis may be helpful to identify *G. vaginalis* in those laboratories that do not keep human blood and starch agars available. Growth from chocolate agar can be used to prepare the inoculum (Lien & Hillier, 1989). A commercial version is available. Remel mini-ID™ *Gardnerella vaginalis* Rapid Tube Test (available from Fisher Scientific) consists of separate microtubes containing rapid carbohydrate degradation (RCD) starch and hippurate hydrolysis medium in a carrier tube containing RCD raffinose, as seen in Figure 19-31 ■. *G. vaginalis* can be identified within 4 hours if positive for hippurate (blue or purple) and starch (yellow), but negative (red) for raffinose. This test proves to provide a much quicker identification when compared to the traditional V and starch agars.

Identification. Most clinical laboratories presumptively identify *G. vaginalis* using the Gram stain, catalase, and colony morphology. If a more definitive identification is desired, additional tests selected from the above list may be performed. Table 19-5 ✪ provides selected reactions for *Gardnerella vaginalis*. The databases of rapid identification strips, such as API® Coryne and BBL Crystal, include this organism.

Microscopic and Colony Morphology. Analysis of the cell walls of *Gardnerella* reveals a composition characteristic of gram-positive bacteria. However, *Gardnerella* frequently stains gram negative. For this reason it is described as a gram-variable rod. Morphologically it is small and pleomorphic, appearing as short rods and coccobacilli.

Gardnerella colonies appear after 48–72 hours of incubation at 35–37°C with carbon dioxide. They are tiny white to gray colonies that are nonhemolytic on sheep blood agar but display a very subtle or soft beta-hemolytic on human blood or V agar, as seen in Figures 19-30 and 19-32 ■. There is no greening around colonies when grown on chocolate agar (Piot et al., 1982).

🔁 REAL WORLD TIP

It is easy to remember the Gram stain reaction of *Gardnerella vaginalis* by using the first letter of its genus and species. **G**ardnerella **v**aginalis is gram variable.

Key Biochemical Reactions. *Gardnerella vaginalis* can be presumptively identified when small, pleomorphic gram-

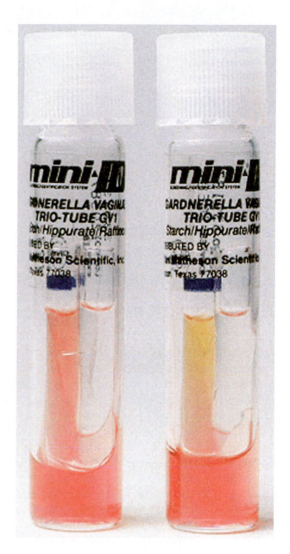

■ **FIGURE 19-31** Remel mini-ID™ *Gardnerella vaginalis* Rapid Tube Test.
Photo courtesy of Remel, part of Thermo Fisher Scientific.

✪ TABLE 19-5

Selected Reactions for *Gardnerella*	
Catalase	–
Oxidase	–
Hippurate hydrolysis	+
Alpha-glucosidase	+
Beta-glucosidase	–
Starch fermentation	+
Raffinose	–
Beta-hemolysis on human blood agar	+
Beta-hemolysis on sheep blood agar	–
Inhibition by SPS	+
Inhibition by viridans streptococci	+

+, positive; –, negative.

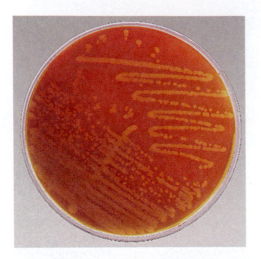

■ **FIGURE 19-32** *Gardnerella vaginalis* growing on HBT Bilayer medium.
Photo courtesy of Remel, part of Thermo Fisher Scientific.

variable rods are observed on Gram stain and the colonies are catalase negative and beta-hemolytic on HBT medium. Hippurate hydrolysis can also be performed and a positive result would be indicative of *G. vaginalis*. Nonvaginal isolates should be confirmed with additional tests. Additional tests include alpha-glucosidase, beta-glucosidase, and hydrolysis of hippurate and starch. *Gardnerella vaginalis* is alpha-glucosidase positive and beta-glucosidase negative, starch positive, and hippurate positive (Catlin, 1992).

Not all labs stock human blood agar routinely. Under these circumstances, a method such as Remel mini-ID™ *Gardnerella vaginalis* Rapid Tube Test (Fisher Scientific) may provide rapid identification of *G. vaginalis*. A hippurate- and starch-positive, raffinose-negative result would be characteristic of *G. vaginalis*.

Another identification scheme uses inhibition of growth by sodium polyanetholesulfonate (SPS) on V or HBT agar. *G. vaginalis* can also be inhibited on chocolate agar by the presence of alpha-hemolytic streptococci. Accurate results are method dependent and so are only considered presumptive. It requires use of a specific ATCC strain of *Streptococcus sanguis* (Reimer & Reller, 1985). Table 19-5 summarizes biochemical reactions for *Gardnerella*.

Clinical Significance.   *Gardnerella* can be isolated from genital, urine, and blood, as well as specimens from newborns. *Gardnerella* is a member of the normal flora in the female genital tract.

The loss of *Lactobacillus* spp. and the predominance of *Gardnerella vaginalis* and anaerobic gram-negative rods are associated with bacterial vaginosis, but a culture for the presence of *G. vaginalis* is not recommended. Its presence, along with anaerobic gram-negative rods, can be observed on the surface of squamous epithelial cells or "clue" cells on Gram stain of a vaginal specimen. Refer to ∞ Chapter 36, "Genital System," for information on the laboratory diagnosis of bacterial vaginosis.

G. vaginalis is also linked to maternal and neonatal infections. Bacteremia is more common in females than males. Successful isolation from blood is dependent on using SPS free growth medium or adding gelatin to the blood culture bottle broth to detoxify the SPS effect on *G. vaginalis* (Catlin, 1992). It is a rare cause of urinary tract infections in females and urogenital tract infections in males.

Isolation from nonvaginal specimens may be clinically significant if isolated in pure culture or if the patient is pregnant with a history of urinary tract infections or has had recent genital diagnostic procedures using instruments. Positive urine cultures in males are associated with prostatitis (Koneman et al., 1997). The physician should be able to provide guidance as to the isolates of potential significance.

Aerotolerant *Actinomyces*

Actinomyces species are non-spore-forming, non-acid-fast, pleomorphic, gram-positive rods. They are less frequent isolates than the other gram-positive rods previously discussed.

General Characteristics.   *Actinomyces* are facultative anaerobes that require carbon dioxide for optimum growth. Most species prefer an anaerobic environment but may grow aerobically on routine media incubated in CO_2.

Identification.   When a non-acid-fast, non-spore-forming, irregular, gram-positive rod is isolated, *Actinomyces* should be ruled out as part of the identification process. Identification to species can be difficult but identification to genus can be accomplished using Gram stain morphology, catalase result, and atmospheric preference. A branching gram-positive rod that is catalase negative and prefers an anaerobic environment over an aerobic environment can be presumptively identified as an *Actinomyces* species (Clarridge & Zhang, 2002). A slide culture is helpful in distinguishing *Actinomyces* from *Nocardia* and other *Actinomycetes*. It allows one to see aerial mycelium or conidia characteristic of *Actinomycetes*. Refer to ∞ Chapter 14, "Fungal Cultures," to review the slide culture procedure.

Microscopic and Colony Morphology.   Under the microscope, *Actinomyces* appear as irregularly staining, pleomorphic, gram-positive rods, as observed in Figure 19-33 ■.

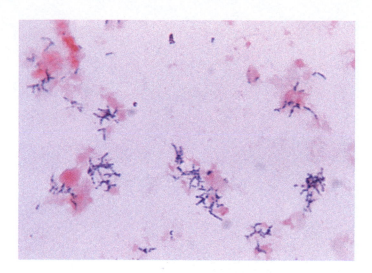

■ **FIGURE 19-33** Gram stain of pus revealing branched gram-positive rods characteristic of *Actinomyces*.
From Public Health Image Library (PHIL), CDC/Dr. Lucille Georg.

Filaments with branching may be observed in smears from microcolonies. Diphtheroidal and branching rods are commonly observed. Care must be taken to not misidentify the morphotypes as gram-positive cocci in short chains (Clarridge & Zhang, 2002). An acid-fast stain is helpful in ruling out *Nocardia; Actinomyces* is non-acid-fast whereas *Nocardia* is weakly acid-fast.

Actinomyces form microcolonies after 18 to 24 hours of incubation. A "spider" or granular-centered colony with peripheral branching filaments is highly suggestive of *Actinomyces*. Some *Actinomyces* species form smooth colonies without branching filaments, so further testing is needed. Mature colonies require 7 to 14 days to develop. They can form visible yellow to orange sulfur-like granular colonies in abscess drainage.

Key Biochemical Reactions. *Actinomyces* are catalase-negative, nonmotile fermenters. A few species may be catalase positive. Refer to Table 19-6✪ for more information on catalase-positive *Actinomyces*. *Actinomyces* can be distinguished from most of the other catalase-negative, gram-positive rods because most *Actinomyces* species produce H_2S. *Erysipelothrix* also produces H_2S but can be distinguished from *Actinomyces* using its growth pattern in gelatin. *Erysipelothrix* forms a bottle brush pattern in gelatin whereas *Actinomyces* grows in a straight line. Refer to Table 19-4 for more information on distinguishing *Actinomyces* from other gram-positive rods.

A. israelii is one of the most commonly isolated species and is discussed in ∞ Chapter 24, "Anaerobic Bacteria." *A. turicensis* and *A. naeslundii* are also common isolates (Clarridge & Zhang, 2002). The other species are less common isolates. *A. israelii* is catalase, traditional CAMP, and urea negative. It is also nitrate, esculin, ONPG, arabinose, sucrose, and trehalose positive. *A. turicensis* is catalase, CAMP, urea, esculin, nitrate, ONPG, and arabinose negative. It is also sucrose positive. *A. naeslundii* is catalase, CAMP, and arabinose negative. It is also urea, ONPG, sucrose, and trehalose positive (Sarkonen et al., 2001). Refer to Table 19-6 for test results that differentiate other selected *Actinomyces* species that may be isolated from clinical specimens.

Clinical Significance. *Actinomyces* are members of the commensal or normal flora in various body sites, especially the mouth. They are the causative agent of actinomycosis. Actinomycosis causes abscesses, often of the jaw, which drain

✪ **TABLE 19-6**

Key Reactions for Selected Aerotolerant *Actinomyces* Isolated in the Clinical Laboratory

Organism	Pigment	Cat	Traditional CAMP	Urea	Esc	Nit	ONPG	Ara	Suc	Tre
Actinomyces israelii	–	–	–	–	+	+	+	+	+	+
A. turicensis	–	–	–	–	–	–	–	–	+	V
A. europaeus	–	–	–	–	+	+	+	–	–	–
A. naeslundii	–	–	–	+	V	V	+	–	+	+
A. radingae	–	–	+	–	+	V	+	+	+	V
A. neuii ss neuii	–	+	+	–	–	+	+	+	+	–
A. neuii ss anitratus	–	+	+	–	+	–	+	–	+	+
A. odontolyticus	+	–	–	–	V^w	+	+	–	+	–
A. viscosus	–	+	=	V	V	+	+	–	+	V

+, positive; –, negative; V, variable; w, weak; Cat, catalase; Esc, esculin; Nit, nitrate; Ara, arabinose; Suc, sucrose; Tre, trehalose.

via sinus tracts to the skin surface. Small hard granules present in the abcess drainage are colonies of the organism. Refer to ∞ Chapter 24, "Anaerobic Bacteria," for more information on this disease. *Actinomyces* have also been isolated from human bite wounds, abscesses, blood, respiratory specimens, eye infections, skin, genital, intrauterine devices, and urinary tract infections (Sarkonen et al., 2001). The patient's physician should be consulted to assess clinical significance.

 **Checkpoint! 19–15
(Chapter Objective 9)**

The etiological agent of actinomycosis is:
 A. *Bacillus anthracis.*
 B. *Arcanobacterium.*
 C. *Actinomyces.*
 D. *Erysipelothrix.*

Aerobic *Actinomycetes*

The *Actinomycetes* consist of a group of gram-positive bacilli that form thin, beaded, branching filaments. Some species extend these filaments into the air, forming aerial mycelium similar to fungi. They also extend these filaments into the medium, forming substrate mycelium. Those that are weakly or partially acid-fast contain mycolic acids in their cell wall similar to *Mycobacterium* spp. These organisms can also form microcolonies in tissue (Forbes et al., 2002). The *Actinomycetes* grow on routine media but so slowly they can be hidden by overgrowth of commensal flora. An incubation time of 48 to 72 hours, at 30–36°C, is often required for colonies to become visible. Incubation of cultures up to 2 weeks may be necessary. They often have a tough, chalky, or waxy appearance with a damp soil or musty odor. They are infrequent isolates but do cause serious infectious diseases.

Useful Biochemical Tests

Lysozyme Resistance. Lysozyme resistance tests for the ability of the isolate to grow in the presence of lysozyme. Lysozyme is a muramidase that lyses gram-positive organisms. *Nocardia* are resistant to lysozyme. It is useful for distinguishing *Streptomyces* from *Nocardia*. The test organism is inoculated into one tube of glycerol broth, which contains 50µg/ml of lysozyme and one tube of glycerol broth without lysozyme and incubated for up to 7 days at 35°C. An organism that grows well in both tubes, in 5–20 days, is positive for lysozyme resistance, as noted in Figure 19-34 ■. An organism that does not grow in the tube with lysozyme but grows well in the tube without lysozyme is negative for lysozyme resistance (Kiska, Hick, & Pettit, 2002). *Nocardia* and *Tsukamurella* are positive or lysozyme resistant whereas *Streptomyces* is lysozyme susceptible and will not grow.

Substrate Decomposition of Casein, Xanthine, and Tyrosine. Substrate decomposition is useful in differenti-

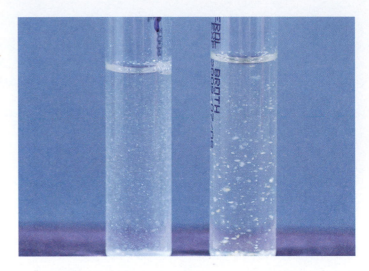

■ FIGURE 19-34 Positive reaction of *N. asteroides* for lysozyme resistance.

ating clinically significant *Nocardia* species. The organism is inoculated onto the surface of individual agar plates containing casein, xanthine, and tyrosine. The plates are incubated at room temperature. Casein is examined after 7 and 14 days of incubation. Xanthine and tyrosine is examined after 3–4 weeks of incubation. Any clearing or hydrolysis, as seen in Figure 19-35 ■, around or underneath the colonies is interpreted as positive (Berd, 1973). *N. brasiliensis* and *N. pseudobrasiliensis* decompose casein (positive) and tyrosine (positive) but not xanthine. *N. otitidiscaviarum* decomposes xanthine (positive) only. *N. asteroides*, *N. farcinia*, and *N. nova* do not decompose the substrates (negative).

Opacification of Middlebrook 7H10 Agar. Opacification, or clouding, of a Middlebrook 7H10 agar is useful in distinguishing *Nocardia farcinica* from other members of the

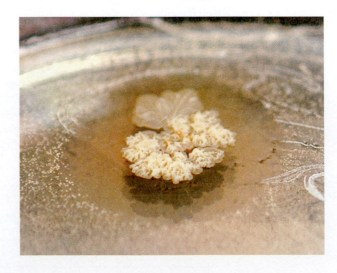

■ FIGURE 19-35 Hydrolysis of xanthine.
Photo courtesy of Hardy Diagnostics. www.HardyDiagnostics.com

Nocardia asteroides complex: *N. pseudobrasiliensis, N. asteroides,* and *N. nova.* The suspected *Nocardia* is inoculated onto Middlebrook agar and incubated at 28°C and 35°C. After 5–10 days of incubation the media is examined for a change in the media from clear to milky-white opacity. A positive result is characteristic of *N. farcinica* (Carson & Hellyar, 1994). Refer to ∞ Chapter 13, "Acid Fast Bacilli Cultures," for more information on Middlebrook 7H10 agar and its use in cultivating *Mycobacterium.*

Gelatin Liquefaction.   Gelatin liquefaction, as seen in Figure 19-15, differentiates *N. brasiliensis* and *N. pseudobrasiliensis* from the others in the genus. The test is performed by stabbing a loopful of growth into a tube of nutrient gelatin and incubating at 35°C for up to 7 days. The tube is then refrigerated (4°C) for 15 minutes. Observe for liquefaction by tilting the tube 45 degrees. Liquefaction of the medium is recorded as positive. If the medium remains solid, the result is recorded as negative (Kiska et al., 2002).

Acetamide.   Acetamide is useful for distinguishing *N. farcina* from the other clinically significant *Nocardia* species. The organism is inoculated onto the slant of acetamide agar and incubated at 35°C for up to 7 days. Observation of a pink color, as seen in Figure 19-36 ■, is positive. No color change is negative (Kiska et al., 2002). ∞ Chapter 22, "Nonfermenting Gram-Negative Rods," describes the use of acetamide to identify *Pseudomonas aeruginosa.*

Arylsulfatase.   Arylsulfatase production is used to differentiate *N. nova* from the other clinically significant *Nocardia* species. A tube of arylsulfatase broth is inoculated with the test organism. After 7 days of incubation at 35–37°C, six drops of 2N sodium carbonate is added to the tube. If the organism possesses the enzyme arysulfatase, development of a pink color, as seen in Figure 19-37 , is interpreted as positive (Kiska et al., 2002). ∞ Chapter 26, "*Mycobacterium* Species," provides information on using arylsulfatase reactions to speciate the *Mycobacterium.*

Citrate.   The use of citrate, as the sole source of carbon, can be used to separate *N. basiliensis* and *N. pseudobrasiliensis* from the other clinically significant *Nocardia* species. Simmon's citrate is inoculated with the test organism and incubated at 35°C for up to 7 days. A blue color is positive. Refer to Figure 9-11 to observe the citrate reaction. *N. brasiliensis* and *N. pseudobrasiliensis* are positive whereas the other *Nocardia* are negative (Kiska et al., 2002).

Commercial Kits.   Kiska et al. (2002) suggest the combination of susceptibility test results, colony pigment, citrate, and acetamide results as well as adonitol and inositol assimilation from API 20C can accurately identify *Nocardia* species in 4–7 days. MicroScan Rapid Anaerobe Identification panel and bioMerieux ID 32C yeast identification can also provide these additional tests. It is important only lysozyme-resistant isolates with aerial hyphae be identified with this scheme. This scheme does not include new species proposed since this paper was submitted.

✓ **Checkpoint! 19–16 (Chapter Objective 3)**

The medium that is most helpful in distinguishing Streptomyces from Nocardia is:

   A. *lysozyme.*
   B. *motility.*
   C. *arysulfatase.*
   D. *gelatin.*

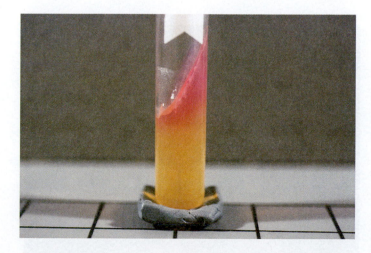

■ **FIGURE 19-36** Positive reaction for acetamide. This tube uses phenol red as the pH indicator rather than the traditional brom thymol blue.

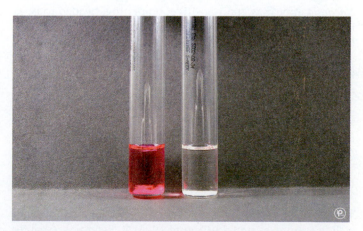

■ **FIGURE 19-37** Positive (left) and negative (right) reaction of arylsulfatase.
From Marler LM, Siders JA, Kaufman CM, Owens EN, Korba GG and Allen SD, *Bacteriology I Image Atlas* CD-ROM, Indiana Pathology Images, 2005.

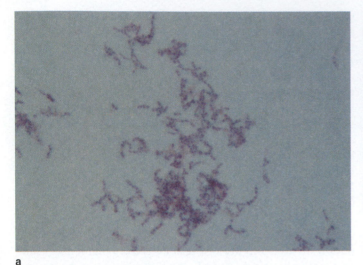

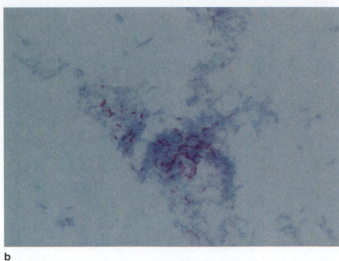

a

b

■ **FIGURE 19-38 a.** Gram stain of *N. asteroides*. **b.** Modified acid-fast stain of *N. asteroides*.

Nocardia

Nocardia are opportunistic pathogens and their infections occur worldwide. They exist in the environment in soil, water, and decaying plant matter. Isolation of the organism may indicate colonization, contamination, or infection.

General Characteristics. *Nocardia* are branching, beaded gram-positive rods. They grow at 35°C in ambient air. They do not grow anaerobically. Some species may require cooler temperatures, room temperature to 30°C, for optimum growth.

Identification. When a small colony resembling a "spider" is isolated after 48–72 hours of incubation, it is important to perform a Gram stain, an acid-fast stain, and look for aerial hyphae and conidia in a slide culture.

Microscopic and Colony Morphology. On Gram stain, *Nocardia* appear as gram-positive, branching, beaded rods, as noted in Figure 19-38a ■. It is important to determine the isolates acid-fast properties by using the modified Kinyoun stain, which uses 1% sulfuric acid to decolorize. *Nocardia* are partially or weakly acid-fast, as seen in Figure 19-38b ■, and appear as long, thin, beaded, branching rods.

 Nocardia colonies can be wrinkled, dry, chalky, adherent, white to yellow, orange, tan, or brown, and beta-hemolytic on sheep blood agar. The colony of *N. asteroides* is shown in Figure 19-39 ■. Selective media such as buffered charcoal yeast extract (BCYE) agar, used for *Legionella* spp., or Thayer-Martin agar, used for *Neisseria gonorrhoeae*, can be used to isolate *Nocardia* from specimens that contain commensal flora (Farrell, 2007). The presence of aerial mycelium and conida is best observed on a slide culture, as noted in Figure 19-40 ■. Refer to ∞ Chapter 14, "Fungal Cultures," to review the slide culture procedure.

Key Biochemical Reactions. *Nocardia* are very difficult to speciate without molecular testing. Conville and Witebsky

✓ **Checkpoint! 19–17
(Chapter Objective 5)**

An aerobic, partially acid-fast, branching, gram-positive rod is most likely:

  A. *Listeria*.

  B. *Corynebacterium*.

  C. *Actinomyces*.

  D. *Nocardia*.

(2004) recommend identification to a complex of organisms rather than species using biochemical tests and susceptibility results. A catalase-positive, partially acid-fast, branching gram-positive rod with aerial mycelium is suspicious for *Nocardia*. Lack of aerial hyphae and a lysozyme test will rule out the sec-

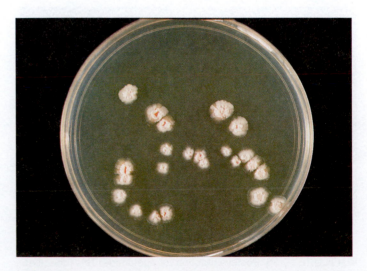

■ **FIGURE 19-39** Colony of *N. asteroides*.
From Public Health Image Library (PHIL), CDC/Dr. William Kaplan.

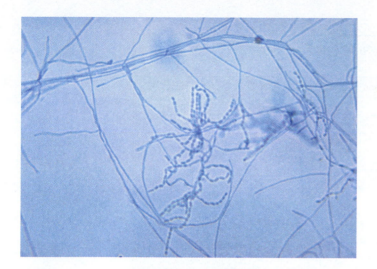

■ FIGURE 19-40 Slide culture showing aerial hyphae of *N. aster-oides.*
From Public Health Image Library (PHIL), CDC/Dr. Lucille K. Georg.

ond most commonly isolated *Actinomycetes* genus, *Streptomyces*. *Nocardia* is lysozyme positive while S*treptomyces* is lysozyme negative.

Nocardia are urease positive whereas the third most common *Actinomycetes* genus, *Actinomadura,* is urease negative. Table 19-7✪ provides information that can help separate *Nocardia* from other clinically significant aerobic actinomycetes. Presumptive identification to species requires additional tests. Refer to Table 19-8✪ for key reactions that can be used to presumptively identify medically relevant *Nocardia* species.

Clinical Significance. *Nocardia* can be isolated from sputum, abscess, skin lesions, eye specimens, tissue, blood, and cerebrospinal fluid.

An immunocompromised individual inhales the organism into their lungs and develops respiratory infections. From there it can disseminate to other parts of the body and isolated from blood and cerebrospinal fluid. Symptoms include fever, night sweats, and weight loss. Complications of the lung infections include pleural fluid build-up, pus formation or **empyema**, and mediastinitis. Disseminated nocardiosis has a poor prognosis.

Immunocompetent individuals usually develop skin infections. Invasive pulmonary infection is usually associated with a suppressed immune system. More than 80% of these lung infections are associated with *N. asteroides* (Forbes et al., 1998). *N. asteroides* is an intracellular pathogen that is able to evade the host defenses and grow in various human cells. *Nocardia* is able to inhibit phagosome fusion and produce increased amounts of catalase and hemolysins (Lerner, 1996).

N. brasiliensis causes 80% of the skin infections (Brown-Elliot, Brown, Conville, & Wallace, 2006). Skin infections are usually acquired as a result of traumatic injury. There are three types of cutaneous infections: mycetoma, lymphocutaneous, and superficial skin infections. Mycetoma is a chronic, local, painless, subcutaneous infection. The lower limbs swell, form nodules, and may discharge pus (Wallace et al., 1990). Granules resembling the yellow sulfur granules of *Actinomyces* spp. can be observed in the pus from the lesion. If a local cutaneous infection spreads to the lymph nodes, the disease is referred to as lymphocutaneous. Superficial skin infections include chronically draining ulcerative lesions, cellulitis, and abscesses (McNeil & Brown, 1994). Disseminated infections can spread from the blood to the brain, skin, eyes, kidney, joint, bones, and heart. Brain infections can be chronic, with the patient displaying strange behaviors and psychotic personalities along with tremors and seizures. Refer to ∞ Chapter 37, "Integumentary System," for more information on skin infections (Lerner, 1996).

Streptomyces

Streptomyces is the second most commonly isolated actinomycete and must be considered when a branching, gram-positive rod or "spider" microcolony is isolated.

General Characteristics. *Streptomyces* are catalase-positive, gram-positive rods exhibiting right-angle branching. These

✪ TABLE 19-7

Key Reactions for Presumptive Identification of Clinically Significant Aerobic *Actinomycetes*

Genus	Acid Fast	Aerial Mycelium	Conidia	Lysozyme	Motility	Nitrate Reduction	Urease
Nocardia	$+^w$	+	V	R	−	V	+
Gordonia	$+^w$	−	−	V	−	+	+
Rhodococcus	$+^w$	−	−	V	−	V	V
Tsukamurella	$+^w$	−	−	R	−	−	+
Nocardiopsis	−	+	+	−	−	+	+
Streptomyces	−	+	+	−	−	−	V
Actinomadura	−	V	+	S	−	+	−
Dermatophilus	−	+ (with increased CO_2)	−	S	+	−	+

$+^w$, weak positive; +, positive; −, negative; R, resistant; S, susceptible; V, variable; NT, not tested.

✪ TABLE 19-8

Key Reactions for Presumptive Identification of Common Human Pathogenic *Nocardia*

Organism*	Cas	Xan	Tyr	Opa	Urea	Ace	PYR	Gel	Ary	Esc	Cit
N. asteroides	−	−	−	−	+	V	−	−	−	−	−
N. farcinia	−	−	−	+	+	+	+	−	−	+	−
N. nova complex	−	−	−	+	−	+	−	−	+	−	−
N. cyriacigeorgica	−	−	−	−	−	+	−	−	NA	−	−
N. abscessus	−	−	−	−	+	−	−	−	−	−	+
N. transvalensis complex	−	−	−	+	−	+	−	−	−	+	+
N. brasiliensis	+	−	+	−	+	−	−	+	−	+	+
N. pseudobrasiliensis	+	−	+	−	+	+	−	+	−	+	+
N. otitidiscaviarum complex	−	+	−	−/+	+	−	−	−	−	+	

Cas, casein; Xan, xanthine; Tyr, tyrosine; Opa, opacity on Middlebrook agar; Ace, acetamide; PYR, pyrrolidonylamino-peptidase; Gel, gelatin; Ary, arysulfatase; Esc, esculin; Cit, citrate; +, positive; −, negative; −/+, most negative with some positive; V, variable; NA, not available.

N. abscessus was formerly known as *N. asteroides* Type I; *N. nova* complex was formerly known as *N. asteroides* Type III; *N. transvalensis* complex includes *N. asteroides* Type IV; *N. farcinica* was formerly known as *N. asteroides* Type V; *N. otitidiscaviarum* complex was formerly known as *N. caviae*.

organisms are commonly found in soil. They grow on the same nonselective media as bacteria, fungi, and mycobacterium. *Streptomyces* may require 2–3 weeks of incubation for growth to occur.

Identification.   *Streptomyces* should be ruled out when the Gram stain morphology or colony morphology suggests aerobic actinomycetes. Their colony can closely resemble that of *Nocardia*.

Microscopic and Colony Morphology.   The modified Kinyoun stain should be used to stain an organism that grows as a "spider-like" colony or appears as a gram-positive branching rod. *Streptomyces* is non-acid-fast. Branching at right angles is also characteristic of *Streptomyces*.

The *Streptomyces* colony can be glabrous, waxy, and heaped, as seen in Figure 19-41 ■. Most colonies are grayish-white. Aerial mycelium and conidia are best observed on slide cultures.

Key Biochemical Reactions.   Suspected aerobic actinomycetes should be tested for lysozyme resistance. *Streptomyces* is lysozyme negative and nitrate negative. The other non-acid-fast, aerobic actinomycetes that produce aerial mycelium and conidia are nitrate positive. *Streptomyces* will also decompose casein and tyrosine medium. Refer to Table 19-7 for additional tests to distinguish the clinically significant actinomycetes.

Clinical Significance.   *Streptomyces* are associated with head and neck mycetoma. They are also associated with penetrating wound and skin abrasions. *Streptomyces* can be isolated from sputum, wound, blood, and brain specimens.

SUMMARY

When aerobic gram-positive rods are isolated, a catalase test is a good starting point. Refer to Figure 19-42 ■ for information related to grouping of aerobic gram-positive rods.

If a catalase positive result is observed, the organism could be a coryneform, *Bacillus*, *Listeria*, *Actinomyces*, *Nocardia* or *Streptomyces*. Gram stain morphology provides clues to their identity. If spores are observed, it is a possible *Bacillus* species and *B. anthracis* should be ruled out. If palisading is observed, the organism is a possible *Listeria* or coryneform. A motility test will separate these two groups. *Listeria* is motile and coryne-

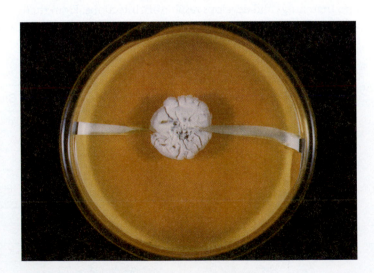

■ **FIGURE 19-41** Colony of *Streptomyces*.
From Public Health Image Library (PHIL), CDC/Dr. Ajello.

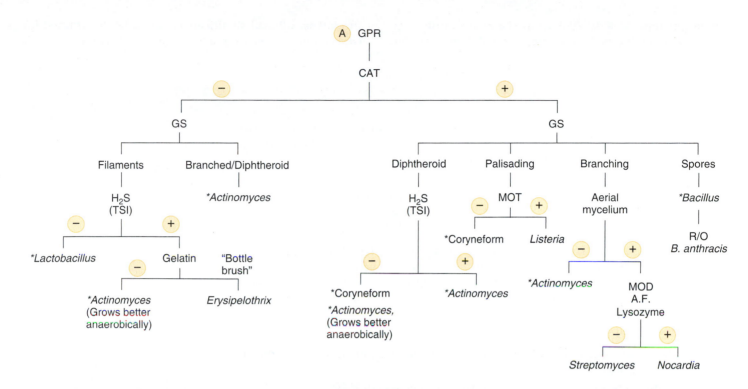

■ **FIGURE 19-42** Initial grouping of select aerobic gram-positive rods.
A = Aerobic; GPR = Gram-positive rod; CAT = catalase; GS = Gram stain; MOT = Motility; H_2S (TSI) = Hydrogen sulfide, triple sugar iron agar; MOD A.F. = Modified acid-fast stain; R/O = Rule out; + = positive; − = negative.
*Determine clinical significance.

forms are nonmotile. If diphtheroids are observed, the possibilities include coryneforms or occasional *Actinomyces* species. If H_2S is observed in TSI, it is *Actinomyces*. If H_2S negative, an esculin test may help. A positive esculin result is most likely *Actinomyces* because most coryneforms are esculin negative. If branching on Gram stain is observed, aerobic actinomycetes should be suspected. If aerial mycelium is present, a modified acid-fast stain and lysozyme tests should be performed. If acid-fast and lysozyme resistant (or positive), the isolate is most likely *Nocardia*. If non-acid-fast and lysozyme sensitive (or negative), the isolate is most likely *Streptomyces*. If aerial mycelium is absent and growth is better anaerobically then aerobically, the organism is probably *Actinomyces*.

If catalase is negative, the organism could be *Lactobacillus, Erysipelothrix,* or *Actinomyces*. Gram stain morphology will help

to group into possible genera. If filaments are observed, testing for H_2S is helpful. If H_2S negative, the isolate is most likely a *Lactobacillus*. If the H_2S result is positive, a gelatin test can distinguish *Erysipelothrix* from *Actinomyces*. Both genera are gelatin negative, but *Erysipelothrix* grows with the "bottle brush" appearance. Gelatin may not be available for use in all laboratories. If branching or diphtheroids are noted on Gram stain and the isolate grows better anaerobically then aerobically, the organism is most likely *Actinomyces*. An acid-fast stain and slide culture will rule out *Nocardia*. *Actinomyces* is non-acid-fast and lacks aerial hyphae.

The aerobic gram-positive bacilli are associated with diseases in immunocompetent and immunocompromised patients. There are specific diseases aligned with specific microbes. Refer to Table 19-9✪ for more information. The

✪ **TABLE 19-9**

Select Diseases Associated with Aerobic Gram-Positive Rods			
Anthrax	**Erysipeloid**	**Diphtheria**	**Listeriosis**
B. anthracis	*E. rhusiopathiae*	*C. diphtheriae*	*L. monocytogenes*
Actinomycosis	**Foodborne Illness**	**Diphtheria-like**	**Nocardiosis/Mycetoma**
A. israelii	*B. cereus*	*C. ulcerans*	*Nocardia*
A. naeslundii	*L. moncytogenes*	*Arcanobacterium haemolyticum*	*Streptomyces*

aerobic gram-positive bacilli may also be isolated from respiratory, wound, abscess, blood, cerebrospinal fluid, and other specimens. Clinical significance should be determined for *Lactobacillus*, *Actinomyces*, and coryneform isolates.

LEARNING OPPORTUNITIES

1. Sort the 12 items into three possible groups of gram-positive bacilli and name each with the possible genus. Use each item only once and each group should contain four items. (Chapter Objective 1)

Diphtheroids	Variable hemolysis	Filaments
Catalase positive	Umbrella	Nonhemolytic
Beta-hemolysis	H$_2$S positive	Esculin positive
Bottle brush	Nonmotile	Palisades

2. Situation: An arm wound culture inoculated on to sheep blood agar and chocolate agar grows a pure culture of an aerobic, gram-positive, palisading rod in all four quadrants. There is no growth on MacConkey agar. The organism is catalase positive. The direct Gram stain of the specimen reported white blood cells in addition to gram-positive rods. (Chapter Objectives 1, 6, and 10)

   a. What are the possible genera?

   b. What tests should be performed to assist in preliminary identification of the isolate to genus?

   c. Is this isolate clinically significant? What should you do?

3. The ideal specimen for the isolation of a catalase negative gram-positive rod displaying H$_2$S in TSI and test tube brush morphology in gelatin is:
   (Chapter Objective 2)

   a. Stool

   b. A swab of skin surface

   c. A full thickness skin biopsy of the advancing lesion

   d. Sulfur granules obtained from a mycetoma

4. Which of the following medium promotes the formation of metachromatic granules in *Corynebacterium diphtheriae*? (Chapter Objective 3)

   a. Loeffler's medium

   b. Tinsdale agar

   c. Potassium tellurite agar

   d. Cystine tellurite agar

5. If a branching gram-positive rod is plated to casein agar and turns positive after 14 days, it appears as: (Chapter Objective 4)

   a. Opacification of the agar under the colony

   b. Clearing of the agar under the colony

   c. Liquefaction of the agar

   d. A pink color after addition of 2N sodium carobonate

6. A small beta hemolytic gray colony was isolated as the predominant organism from a throat culture. The microbiologist should perform: (Chapter Objective 7)

   a. PYR hydrolysis

   b. streptococcal seroytping

   c. A catalase test

   d. A Gram stain

7. Select the organism that requires vancomycin for therapy: (Chapter Objective 11)

   a. *Lactobacillus* spp.

   b. *Erysipelothirx rhusiopathiae*

   c. *Corynebacterium jeikeium*

   d. *Bacillus anthracis*

8. A 35-year-old male presents to his physician with a sore throat, fever, and a white patch at the back of his throat. The group A *Streptococcus* rapid screen, performed in the office, was negative. A throat swab was sent to the microbiology laboratory for culture. At 24 hours, the sheep blood agar displays light growth of normal upper respiratory flora and heavy growth of a small gray-white nonhemolytic colony. Initial testing reveals:

   Gram stain – small, palisading gram-positive rods

   Catalase – bubbles

   The microbiologist should: (Chapter Objectives 5, 6, and 12)

   a. Report the organism as part of the normal upper respiratory flora

   b. Perform streptococcal serotyping

   c. Proceed with a full identification of the organism

   d. Perform a modified Elek test

   e. Both c and d

CASE STUDY 19-1   INHALATION ANTHRAX—PENNSYLVANIA AND NEW YORK CITY, 2006 (CHAPTER OBJECTIVES 1, 8, AND 9)

Patient: Charles, a drummer in a band

Admitting Diagnosis: Charles was admitted to the hospital in respiratory distress after collapsing after a performance. He had a 3-day history of shortness of breath, dry cough, and malaise. All four blood cultures grew gram-positive rods. The CDC confirmed the presence of *Bacillus anthracis* by PCR.

The patient made traditional African drums by using hard-dried animal skins. He had returned from Cote d'Ivoire with four hard-dried goat hides 2 months earlier. He soaked the hides and scraped the hair with a razor in order to make the drums (CDC, 2006).

1. Why were spores not observed on the smears of the blood cultures?

2. What is the probable source of this organism?

3. What is the probable route of infection?

4. What tests should be performed if *B. anthracis* is suspected?

CASE STUDY 19-2   CUTANEOUS NOCARDIOSIS—BAHAMAS (CHAPTER OBJECTIVES 1, 6, AND 10)

Patient: Roberta, a cancer patient

Admitting Diagnosis: Roberta, along with 15 other cancer patients, developed abscesses at multiple injection sites. *Nocardia asteroides* was isolated from the culture of the abscess specimen.

The patient had attended an immunotherapy clinic in the Bahamas. Human serum protein injections were prepared by the clinic and self-administered subcutaneously by the patient (Centers for Disease Control, 1984).

5. What is the typical microscopic morphology of *N. asteroides*? What additional procedures should be performed when this morphology is noted?

6. Which other microorganism(s) resemble *N. asteroides* microscopically and how are they differentiated?

7. Is *N. asteroides* part of the normal flora or a strict pathogen?

REFERENCES

Go to myhealthprofessionskit.com to view this chapter's references.

20

Fastidious Gram-Negative Rods

Daila S. Gridley

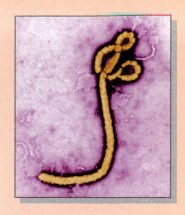

■ LEARNING OBJECTIVES

Upon completion of this chapter, the learner should be able to:

1. Differentiate fastidious bacteria from those that are not.
2. Identify the major characteristics that apply to the presented genera.
3. Correlate the major growth factor(s) required by each organism.
4. Choose the appropriate laboratory tests needed to support a diagnosis for each organism.
5. Relate the virulence factors produced by the organisms.
6. Correlate the major disease(s) associated with each organism.

KEY TERMS

bipolar staining	HACEK	subacute bacterial
Bordet-Gengou medium	Haverhill fever	endocarditis
brucellosis	Legionnaire's disease	tick fever
chancroid	L forms	tularemia
DTaP vaccine	pertussis toxin	V factor
fastidious	Pontiac fever	whooping cough
glandular fever	rat-bite fever	X factor

TAXONOMY

Family *Brucellaceae* (bru-sel-ay-see-ē)
   Genus *Brucella* (bru-sel-ah)
      B. abortus (a-bor-tus)
      B. canis (kay-nis)
      B. melitensis (mel-i-ten-sis)
      B. suis (su-is)
Family *Alcaligenaceae* (al-ka-lidg-en-ay-see-ē)
   Genus *Bordetella* (bor-de-tel-ah)
      B. pertussis (per-tus-is)
Family *Neisseriaceae* (nī-sé-rê-ā-sê-ê)
   Genus *Eikenella* (eye-ken-el-ah)
      E. corrodens (kor-rō-denz)
   Genus *Kingella* (king-el-ah)
      K. kingae (king-ee)
Family *Fusobacteriaceae* (fyou-zō-bak-ter-ee-ay-se-ē)
   Genus *Streptobacillus* (strep-toh-ba-sil-us)
      S. moniliformis (mo-nil-ee-form-is)
Family *Cardiobacteriaceae* (kar-dee-o-bak-ter-ee-ay-see-ē)
   Genus *Cardiobacterium* (kar-dee-o-bak-ter-ee-um)
      C. hominis (ha-min-is)
      C. valuarum (val-várum)

Family *Legionellaceae* (lee-jon-el-ay-see-ee)
   Genus *Legionella* (lee-jon-el-ah)
      L. pneumophila (new-mo-fil-ah)
Family *Pasteurellaceae* (pas-tur-el-ay-see-ee)
   Genus *Aggregatibacter* (ag-gri-gā-ti-bak-ter)
      A. actinomycetemcomitans (ak-ti-no-my-see-tem-ko-mi-tans) [formerly *Actinobacillus* (ak-tin-o-ba-sil-us) *actinomycetemcomitans*]
      A. aphrophilus (af-ro-fee-lus) [formerly *Haemophilus aphrophilus*]
   Genus *Haemophilus* (hee-mof-i-lus)
      H. ducreyi (du-kray-ee)
      H. influenzae (in-flu-en-zee)
      H. aegyptius (ee-gip-tee-us)
      H. parainfluenzae (para-in-flu-en-zee)
      H. pittmaniae (pitt-máni-ee)
Family *Francisellaceae* (fran-cis-el-ay-see-ē)
   Genus *Francisella* (fran-cis-el-ah)
      F. tularensis (too-lar-en-sis)

▶ INTRODUCTION

This chapter covers a broad range of gram-negative rods, all of which are **fastidious.** In other words, these are bacteria that have complex nutritional requirements and so do not grow readily on routinely used laboratory media. Nutritional growth factors are often added to culture media to make isolation and identification possible. Some of these organisms are facultative anaerobes, meaning they can grow in the presence or absence of air, whereas others are strictly aerobic or microaerophilic. They vary greatly in their natural habitats. Depending on the specific genus, they can be found in the environment, as part of the normal microbiota of humans, and in numerous animal populations. In most cases, human infection with these bacteria is relatively uncommon. In this chapter, emphasis is placed on *Haemophilus influenzae, Francisella tularensis* (a potential bioterror agent), *Legionella pneumophila,* and *Bordetella pertussis* because these are the organisms that cause the most serious disease and/or are the isolates most commonly recovered from infections, although a number of other organisms are also discussed (Brooks, Butel, & Morse, 2001a, 2001b, 2001c).

Among the other bacteria mentioned are the *Brucella,* the cause of **brucellosis** and a potential bioterror agent. This chapter also discusses, as a group, fastidious gram-negative bacteria that are implicated in **subacute bacterial endocarditis** (SBE). These organisms are known by the acronym **HACEK** and include *Haemophilus parainfluenzae* together with *Aggregatibacter, Cardiobacterium, Eikenella,* and *Kingella.* Finally, *Streptobacillus,* the slow-growing etiological agent of

rat-bite fever (also known as **Haverhill fever** and erythema arthriticum) is also briefly discussed.

▶ HAEMOPHILUS

GENERAL CHARACTERISTICS

Haemophilus species are facultative anaerobes (i.e., grow in the presence of air or without air) that generally require an enriched medium that contains fresh blood or some of its components (heme and/or NAD) for isolation and growth. The genus name is derived from "hemophilic," which means "blood loving," a reference to the fact that most of these bacteria need at least one of two factors: heme (**X factor**) and nicotinamide adenine dinucleotide (NAD) (**V factor**) that are present in fresh blood. They tend to multiply slowly in culture; some species require 5% to 10% carbon dioxide (CO_2).

In a Gram stained smear they are relatively short, pleomorphic (many forms), nonmotile gram-negative rods that sometimes assume coccobacillary morphology.

USEFUL TESTS

Useful laboratory tests include growth requirements for heme and NAD (originally known as factors X and V, respectively). The ability to synthesize heme and cause hemolysis on agar containing horse blood are also useful. Most species grow both aerobically and anaerobically. Growth is often stimulated in the presence of 5% to 10% CO_2. A polysaccharide capsule is frequently present on isolates from clinical specimens.

Colonies are usually visible after 24 hours of incubation, although in some cases incubation for up to 7 days may be required. In the case of *H. influenzae,* serotyping of capsular antigens is important because of the clinical significance of isolates with the type b capsule. Differentiation of the major species is presented in Table 20-1 ✪.

Aminolevulenic Acid (ALA) or Porphyrin Test

Some *Haemophilus* spp. are able to use delta-aminolevulenic acid (dALA) as a substrate to synthesize heme or factor X. In the process, porphyrins are created. Porphyrins produce a pink fluorescence under an ultraviolet light. ALA can be incorporated on a disk, in a liquid, or in an agar. In the disk method, the organism is rubbed onto a section and incubated for 4 to 24 hours. A pink fluorescence under ultraviolet light indicates synthesis of heme from ALA (positive), and so it is not required for growth. No color change indicates an inability to synthesize heme (negative), and the organism may require it for growth. In the tube method, 0.5 mL of Kovac's reagent is added to the broth and the appearance of red color indicates that ALA was used to create prophyrins (Figure 20-1 ■).

The ALA or porphyrin test is a much more accurate means of determining X factor requirement compared to using X and V factor disks. It is not possible to assume if an organism can make its own factor X then it must only require factor V. The ALA test provides no information on the V factor (NAD) requirement for the organism.

Horse Blood Agar (HBA)

Hemolysis of *Haemophilus* spp. is determined on horse blood agar. These organisms are not able to exhibit hemolysis on sheep blood agar. HBA contains both factors X and V to ensure growth. The hemolysis is subtle and best viewed with light originating from behind the agar plate. Stabbing the area of inoculation enhances the hemolytic reaction. The HBA reac-

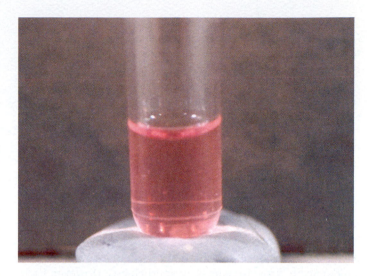

■ **FIGURE 20-1** Porphryn production test. A positive result (red) after addition of Kovac's reagent indicates an ability to produce heme precursors (porphyrins) from delta-aminolevulinic acid (ALA). This reaction correlates with a non-heme (X factor) requiring *Haemophilus* such as *H. parainfluenzae.* These organisms make their own factor X.

tion is used in combination with the ALA or factor requirement tests to identify *Haemophilus* spp.

X (Heme) and V (NAD) Factor Requirements

X factor is known as heme, hemin, or hematin. It is used in the synthesis of catalase, peroxidase, and in the cytochrome electron transport system. V factor is nicotinamide adenine dinucleotide (NAD). It is a coenzyme that transfers electrons from one reaction to another. Both are found inside red blood cells. Factor X can diffuse from intact red blood cells and is available in sheep blood agar. Factor V cannot diffuse from intact red blood cells and is only released due to hemolysis such as with *Staphylococcus aureus. S. aureus, Enterococcus* spp., and yeast can also produce NAD. Chocolate agar has high concentrations of both factors because sheep blood is added to the hot liquid agar, and the red cells are lysed releasing the factors.

Factor determination can be performed using paper disks impregnated with each factor alone on two different disks and one disk with both factors (XV) together. The factors can also be incorporated into an agar base eliminating the need for the disks. A lawn of organism growth is created on a non-nutrient agar such as Mueller-Hinton agar, and the disks are planted at equal distance from each other. The factors then diffuse into the agar. Growth appears around the disks that provide the factor(s) required by the organism (Figure 20-2a ■). It is important to make a broth suspension of the organism to be tested prior to inoculating the non-nutrient agar. This washes off excess X and V factors that can be carried over from the chocolate agar used for initial isolation of the organism. False-positive growth can occur if the organism is not washed prior to performing the test.

✪ **TABLE 20-1**

Growth Requirements and Hemolysis of Clinically Common *Haemophilus* Species

| Species | Factor Requirement | | | | Hemolysis on Horse Blood Agar |
	ALA	X	V	XV	
H. influenzae	–	+	+	+	–
H. aegyptius	–	+	+	+	–
H. parainfluenzae	+	–	+	+	–
H. ducreyi	–	+	–	+	–
H. haemolyticus	–	+	+	+	+
H. parahaemolyticus	+	–	+	+	+

ALA = delta-aminolevulinic acid or porphyrin test; X = heme; V = nicotinamide adenine dinucleotide (NAD)

Satellitism

Haemophilus spp. can grow on sheep blood agar if X and V factors are present in adequate concentrations. Hemolytic organisms release both factors from intact red blood cells. Factor X can also diffuse from intact red blood cells. *Staphylococcus* spp. and other organisms can produce NAD or factor V. Satelliting colonies appear as a pinpoint haze around other colonies on sheep blood agar where the amount of factor(s) present are optimal (Figure 20-2b ■). These satelliting colonies can be a clue to look for *Haemophilus* spp. on the chocolate agar.

◆ *H. influenzae* and *H. aegyptius*

Identification

Microscopic Morphology.   These are short, coccoidlike bacilli that measure approximately 1.5 µm in length and have a tendency to grow in pairs or in short chains. However, their morphology can vary, depending on the culture conditions and incubation time. They appear primarily as small coc-

  REAL WORLD TIP

- The ALA or factor requirements tests should always be used in combination with the horse blood agar test for hemolysis.

- The ALA test should only be used for respiratory specimen isolates. *Aggregatibacter aphrophilus* and *A. paraphrophilus* can cause endocarditis and be isolated from the blood. They are ALA positive and horse blood agar negative and would be misidentified as *H. parainfluenzae*.

cobacilli when incubated for a few hours in a rich medium; with extended incubation times, elongated, threadlike rods and high pleomorphism are evident. A capsule is frequently present on initial isolation, but can be rapidly lost on subculture.

Colony Morphology.   Colonial morphology depends on the type of culture medium. On brain–heart infusion agar containing blood, the colonies are small, round, and convex. An iridescent glow develops after approximately 1 day of incubation; there is no hemolysis. Growth on chocolate agar (heated blood agar) requires approximately 24 to 48 hours before small (~1 mm diameter), transparent, smooth, moist colonies appear. Addition of IsoVitaleX, an enrichment supplement, to media will enhance growth. Colonies of *H. influenzae* and *H. aegyptius* can form between two disks or strips containing heme (factor X) and NAD (factor V). The two factors diffuse and meet creating ideal concentrations of both for growth. In addition, small colonies may appear around colonies of hemolytic bacteria such as *Staphylococcus aureus*. *S. aureus* excretes factor V as well as releasing it from intact red blood cells with hemolysis. Other organisms such as *Enterococcus* spp. and yeast may also produce NAD. The satelliting is shown in Figure 20-2b.

Key Biochemical Reactions and Serotyping.   Typical specimens sent to the clinical laboratory are cerebrospinal fluid (CSF), blood, pleural fluid, joint fluid, and middle ear aspirates. After culture for 24 to 48 hours on chocolate agar enriched with IsoVitaleX, *H. influenzae* and *H. aegyptius* can be differentiated from other similar bacteria by their requirement for both heme (X factor) and NAD (V factor), and inability to lyse horse red blood cells or synthesize porphyrin (ALA negative). Heme is a heat-stable derivative of hemoglobin that is released by red blood cells into the medium, whereas NAD is a heat-labile factor that is bound to the cells and is not released until the

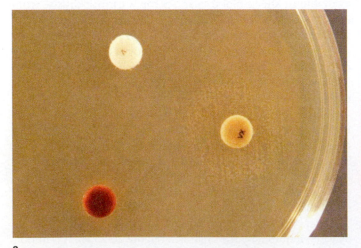

a

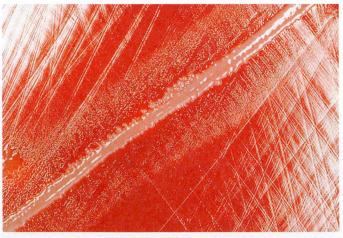

b

■ **FIGURE 20-2** *Haemophilus influenzae* colonies exhibiting the "satellite phenomenon." **a.** *H. influenzae* requires both heme (X factor) and NAD (V factor) for growth, and colonies can be seen around the disk on the right that supplies both of these factors. The growth occurs where the two factors have diffused outward into the medium compared to no growth around the V factor disk at the top left and the X factor disk at the bottom left. **b.** *H. influenzae* colonies can be seen growing around colonies of *Staphylococcus aureus*. It produces NAD as well as hemolyzes the red blood cells releasing the factor. Factor X can diffuse from intact red blood cells.
From Public Health Image Library (PHIL)/CDC/Dr. Mike Miller.

erythrocytes are lysed. Most isolates of *H. influenzae* produce acid (no gas) from glucose and xylose, but not lactose or sucrose; they are variable for urease and indole production. *H. aegyptius* can be distinguished from *H. influenzae* by a negative xylose reaction.

Most laboratories do not differentiate between the two organisms. Rather, they report them collectively as "*H. influenzae* or *H. aegyptius* biochemically similar." All *H. influenzae* from clinical cases should be serotyped, especially in patients under the age of 15 years. The organisms can produce six different antigenic types of capsule, designated as a, b, c, d, e, and f. Latex agglutination is a rapid and sensitive test for detection of these capsular antigens. Counterimmunoelectrophoresis is similar to the latex agglutination test, but is less sensitive and more difficult to perform. If large numbers of organisms are present, these tests can be performed directly on clinical specimens such as CSF, serum, and urine but is rarely performed due to cross reactions. Serotyping is usually done in state health departments or reference laboratories. Latex agglutination, counterimmunoelectrophoresis, serotyping, and other immunologic tests, are described in more detail in ∞ Chapter 10.

 REAL WORLD TIP

- Hemolytic reactions for *Haemophilus* can be observed on horse, bovine, and rabbit blood but not sheep blood.
- Sheep blood contains enzymes that inactivate V factor (NAD). The enzyme, NADase, is destroyed by heat and is not present in chocolate agar.

Clinical Significance

H. influenzae was first discovered by Richard Friedrich Johannes Pfeiffer during the great influenza pandemic of 1892 and is therefore also known as Pfeiffer's bacillus. It does not cause influenza ("the flu"), although it was originally believed to be the cause of the disease because it was present in most of the victims. It is often a secondary invader in individuals infected with influenza A, the true etiological agent. Adherence of the organisms to mammalian tissues is mediated by pili (fimbriae). *H. influenzae* with a type b capsule are the most notorious in causing disease. In the prevaccine era, approximately 95% of cases of invasive disease were caused by this serotype. Young children under the age of 5 years are especially susceptible to development of disease.

The organisms are transmitted person-to-person via respiratory droplets, frequently resulting in sinusitis and infection of the middle ear. Indeed, these bacteria, along with the pneumococci, are the most common causes of bacterial otitis media (inflammation of the middle ear) and acute sinusitis. Prior to 1989, *H. influenzae* type b was the most common cause of bacterial meningitis in the United States in children between the ages of 6 months and 5 years (Centers for Disease Control [CDC], 2002). Bacteremia and extension to the meninges of the brain can occur very rapidly (see Figure 38-9c). Prompt treatment is required to minimize the possibility of neurological and intellectual deficits that can result from localized accumulation of subdural fluid (Low, Pichichero, & Schaad, 2004). In untreated cases of meningitis, the mortality rate can be as high as 90%.

H. influenzae type b can also cause a variety of other illnesses such as pneumonia (especially in those with underlying lung problems), empyema, epiglottitis, cellulitis, and septic arthritis. In obstructive laryngotracheitis, an enlarged, cherry-red epiglottis in infants may require tracheostomy or intubation to prevent suffocation. The most common manifestations of illness in elderly or debilitated adults after *H. influenzae* type b infection are bronchitis and pneumonia. Treatment with β-lactam antibiotics (e.g., ampicillin) can be useful if the organism does not produce beta-lactamase. Other drugs such as ceftriaxone and the fluoroquinolones may be required because of increasing resistance (Anon 2005; Perez-Vasquez, Roman, Aracil, Canton, & Campos, 2004).

 REAL WORLD TIP

The organism's species name can help with remembering its factor requirement. Any *Haemophilus* spp. with the word "para" in its name will be ALA positive and require factor V only. Any species with "haemolyticus" in its name will be hemolytic on horse blood agar.

The original vaccine for *H. influenzae* type b consisted only of the type b polysaccharide. It was not very effective, although it was better than no vaccine at all. Today, four conjugated vaccines for type b *Haemophilus* are available that greatly reduce the risk for meningitis (the first one was approved in late 1987). In these vaccines, the type b polysaccharide (a poor antigen) is chemically bonded to a protein carrier, resulting in greatly enhanced immunogenicity and thus also much greater protection (Zhou et al., 2002). In children older than 2 months of age, type b polysaccharide conjugated either to a toxin protein from a mutant strain of *Corynebacterium diphtheriae* or an outer membrane protein of *Neisseria meningitidis* is effective. Children over 15 months of age can be immunized with a vaccine consisting of the type b polysaccharide conjugated to the diphtheria toxoid, which has low efficacy in younger children.

H. influenzae type b may be carried in the upper respiratory tract by approximately 2% to 4% of healthy individuals, although immunization has greatly reduced the incidence of carriage. The carrier rate is much higher (up to 80%) for nontypable forms of *H. influenzae* that do not have a capsule. The nonencapsulated strains are usually noninvasive. They tend to cause problems (e.g., tracheobronchitis and pneumonia) only in patients who already have chronic underlying conditions such as bronchitis, emphysema, or obstructive pulmonary disease.

Genetic analysis supports a separate species designation for *H. aegyptius*, a relatively common cause of conjunctivitis. *H. influenzae* biogroup *aegyptius* is implicated in Brazilian purpuric fever, which is characterized by fever, nausea, vomiting, hemorrhagic rash, and shock. *H. aegyptius* is often isolated from blood cultures, and many patients with the disease have a history of conjunctivitis caused by these organisms.

ANTIBIOGRAM PATTERN

Most strains of *H. influenzae* type b are susceptible to ampicillin, although 25% to 30% are resistant because they produce β-lactamase, an enzyme that breaks the β-lactam ring of the drug. Some medical centers have reported that 50% to 60% of their isolates are resistant to ampicillin. Children with serious *H. influenzae* type b infection should not receive ampicillin alone. Fortunately, strains are still susceptible to chloramphenicol, but resistance is possible due to chloramphenicol acetyltransferase. Most strains are susceptible to the newer cephalosporins such as cefotaximine and ceftriaxone (Arrieta & Singh, 2004).

◆ *H. parainfluenzae*

Identification

Microscopic and Colony Morphology. These bacteria resemble *H. influenzae* in both microscopic and colonial morphology. In blood cultures, the organisms may appear as large clumps of filamentous rods.

Key Biochemical Reactions. They differ from *H. influenzae* in that they are positive for ALA porphyrin synthesis and require only NAD (factor V) for growth; they are similar to *H. influenzae* in that they are nonhemolytic on horse blood agar. Most isolates produce acid and gas from glucose and sucrose, but not lactose or xylose. They are variable for urease and catalase and negative for indole.

Clinical Significance

H. parainfluenzae is part of the normal microbiota of the human respiratory tract. It has occasionally been identified as the etiologic agent in cases of endocarditis and urethritis and in infections of the respiratory tract. These organisms are also capable of colonizing the gastrointestinal tract and have been implicated in sporadic cases of peritonitis and cholecystitis (gallbladder infection; Frankard, Rodriguez-Villalobos, Struelens, & Jacobs, 2003).

◆ *H. ducreyi*

Identification

Microscopic Morphology. *H. ducreyi* are small gram-negative coccobacilli that tend to grow in short chains, clumps, or whorls within lesions. Occasionally they can be seen in "railroad track," school of fish, or fingerprint arrangements. Individual bacteria exhibit **bipolar staining** (the two ends of the bacteria stain more intensely than the central portion).

Colony Morphology. The organism is very difficult to culture. Isolation from scrapings of an ulcer is best accomplished on chocolate agar containing 1% IsoVitaleX and vancomycin and incubation at 33°C in 10% CO_2. Plates must be incubated for 10 days. The organisms will also grow on Mueller-Hinton agar with 5% sheep blood in a CO_2-containing atmosphere. The yellowish to gray colonies are variable in size, smooth, and dome-shaped; it is possible to push intact colonies across an agar surface.

Key Biochemical Reactions. *H. ducreyi* requires heme (factor X), but not NAD (factor V), for growth. It is similar to *H. influenzae* in that it is unable to synthesize porphyrin (ALA negative) and does not cause hemolysis on horse blood agar. Most strains are negative in the tests for catalase, urease, indole, and acid production from lactose, sucrose, and xylose; acid production from glucose is variable. Identification by rapid chromogenic enzyme substrate testing or PCR is recommended.

Clinical Significance

H. ducreyi is the cause of **chancroid**, a venereal disease that is found primarily in tropical countries. Chancroid is a chancre on the genitalia that typically is soft and swollen (Lewis, 2003). Considerable swelling of inguinal lymph nodes is also common. The bacteria are transmitted by direct sexual contact. In contrast to the chancre of syphilis, the lesion is painful. Several possible virulence factors have been identified, including a hemolytic cytotoxin, a cytolethal distending toxin, pili, a hemoglobin-binding protein, and lipooligosaccharide (LOS; Spinola et al., 2003; Sun et al., 2000). Immunity to the organisms does not develop after infection, possibly because its lipooligosaccharide resembles some blood group antigens found in human red blood cells. Treatment with ceftriaxone, trimethoprim-sulfamethoxazole, or erythromycin frequently results in healing of the ulcer within about 2 weeks. The use of condoms during sexual intercourse is usually effective in pre-

 REAL WORLD TIP

A new species of *Haemophilus, H. pittmaniae*, may be isolated from blood, bile, and specimens from the upper respiratory tract. It requires V factor for growth, can synthesize porphyrin and is beta-hemolytic. *H. pittmaniae* can be distinguished from *H. haemolyticus* and *H. parahaemolyticus* by its negative urease and positive ONPG reaction. *H. haemolyticus* and *H. parahaemolyticus* are urease positive and ONPG negative.

 ### Checkpoint! 20–1 (Chapter Objective 6)

Which of the following is most likely to cause meningitis in a child due to progression of a local infection?

    A. *H. ducreyi*
    B. *H. influenzae type b*
    C. *H. parainfluenzae*
    D. *H. influenzae biogroup aegyptius*
    E. *H. aphrophilus*

venting transmission. These organisms are found primarily in tropical countries.

► FRANCISELLA TULARENSIS

GENERAL CHARACTERISTICS

F. tularensis does not grow on most routinely used laboratory media. Very small, transparent colonies will generally appear on cysteine-supplemented agar when incubated for about 3 days at 37°C under aerobic conditions. Best growth is obtained on blood-cysteine-glucose agar, enriched chocolate agar, although they will also grow on Thayer-Martin agar, buffered charcoal yeast extract (used for isolation of *Legionella pneumophila*), or other similar media that contain the amino acid, cysteine. They will not grow on selective media such as MacConkey or eosin methylene blue (EMB) agar. The organisms are usually identified on the basis of their growth requirements, immunofluorescence staining, and agglutination with specific antisera. Because of its highly infectious nature, physicians should notify the laboratory if the organism is suspected. Presumptive identification of *F. tularensis* is done under Biological Safety Level 2 (BSL-2) conditions in clinical laboratories that have the appropriate facilities. Specimens are then forwarded to a BSL-3 laboratory (e.g., a state public health laboratory) for confirmation. All personnel handling clinical specimens suspected of having *F. tularensis* wear gloves and implement other safety precautions.

F. tularensis is an extremely small, intracellular gram-negative coccobacillus (0.2 × 0.5 μm) that stains poorly on Gram stain and is highly pleomorphic.

USEFUL BIOCHEMICAL TESTS

F. tularensis is relatively inert biochemically. Biochemical tests are not used for identification and not recommended, due to its infectious nature; a few biochemical characteristics are presented in the following sections.

IDENTIFICATION

Microscopic Morphology

Identification of these small coccobacilli is generally not done on the basis of microscopic morphology. The organisms are usually missed in smears from tissue specimens because of their small size, intracellular nature, high pleomorphism, and pale staining with Gram stain. The organisms have a thin capsule that consists of lipids, proteins, and carbohydrates.

Colony Morphology

Culture plates should be bagged and examined only under a laminar flow hood. Colonies on the appropriate media appear small and transparent after extended incubation. On supplemented chocolate agar, and often also on sheep blood agar, pinpoint colonies may appear after 24 hours of incubation; by 48 hours, colony size is approximately 1 to 2 mm.

Key Biochemical Reactions and Antibodies

These nonmotile organisms are oxidase, urease, indole, and ornithine negative; they test weakly positive for catalase and produce the β-lactamase enzyme. They are facultative anaerobes and thus can grow under aerobic or anaerobic conditions. Heme (X factor) and NAD (V factor) are not required for their growth, but the amino acid, cysteine, is required.

Direct fluorescence antibody techniques are available in specialized laboratories and are used for identification of the organisms in tissue and sputum specimens or after culture. Detection of serum antibodies by agglutination is a common method used to help make a diagnosis. An antibody titer of 160 in a single specimen is highly suggestive of *F. tularensis* infection, if the patient's history and clinical manifestations are compatible with a diagnosis of tularemia. A fourfold increase in antibody titer in paired serum samples taken 2 weeks apart is strongly indicative of active disease. In addition, all isolates can be tested for the presence of a polysaccharide antigen and at least one protein antigen.

CLINICAL SIGNIFICANCE

Francisella tularensis is the etiological agent of **tularemia**, a disease also known as **glandular fever**, **tick fever**, and occasionally as deer fly fever and rabbit fever. The genus name was given in honor of Edward Francis, who studied the organisms extensively, whereas the species name is based on the location where the organisms were discovered (Tulare County, CA). *F. tularensis* is present in a wide variety of wild animals, birds, and even some fish and amphibians. The most common animal reservoirs in the United States are wild rabbits, muskrats, and squirrels. Occasionally infection can occur by direct contact with a dog or cat that has had contact with an infected wild animal. Ticks and deerflies are the most common arthropod vectors. These highly infectious zoonotic organisms can be transmitted to humans via three different routes: (1) bite of an arthropod, (2) direct contact with an infected animal, and (3) ingestion of contaminated meat or water. Males and children under the age of 10 years have the highest incidence of tularemia, perhaps because of increased opportunity for exposure to the organisms. Individuals such as hunters, veterinarians, and taxidermists are at increased risk for infection.

There are two biotypes of *F. tularensis*. Biotype A is found primarily in the United States and other parts of North America. It is highly virulent. Transmission of biotype A to humans is primarily via the bite of a tick that has acquired the organism from infected wild rabbits. In contrast, biotype B is more widespread (found in both Western and Eastern Hemispheres of the world) and is associated mostly with water and rodents (water rats). Tularemia, a nationally reportable disease, declined dramatically in the United States during the second half of the 20th century, and the incidence today remains low.

As shown in Table 20-2✪, the manifestations of tularemia are highly dependent on the route of transmission. Fever,

⭐ TABLE 20-2

Routes of Transmission and Clinical Manifestations of *F. tularensis* Infection

Route	Disease	Description
Skin abrasions, direct contact	Ulceroglandular tularemia	As few as 10 organisms required to initiate skin infection
		Most common, occur in 50%–80% of cases
		Papule at entry site, painful, swollen
		Enlarged regional lymph nodes (necrotic)
		Fatality rate = 5%
Conjunctiva	Oculoglandular tularemia	Occurs in 3%–5% of cases
		Inoculation via infected finger or aerosol
		Inflamed conjunctiva, small ulcerations
		Enlarged cervical lymph nodes
		Photophobia, lacrimation, decreased visual acuity
		Fatality rate = 5%
Inhalation	Pneumonitis tularemia	Can be initiated by inhalation of as few as 25 organisms in aerosols
		Occurs most often because of dissemination from another site
		Pleural thickening, cough, may be tuberculosis-like
		Fatality rate = 30%
Ingestion of contaminated meat or water	Typhoidal tularemia	Most serious form (10%–30%)
		Acute, dehydration, vomiting, diarrhea
		No primary lesion, no lymph node swelling
		Fatality rate = 30%

malaise, headache, and pain in the involved region are noted in the great majority of cases, regardless of infection route. Infection occurs most often through minute abrasions in the skin, resulting in greatly enlarged regional lymph nodes that sometimes drain for weeks and become necrotic. This dramatic lymph node swelling is similar to what is seen in plague, a disease caused by *Yersinia pestis*. Streptomycin is the drug of choice, but administration of either streptomycin or gentamicin over a period of 10 days is a highly effective treatment. Individuals treated with tetracycline, also considered a relatively effective antibiotic, have a tendency to relapse; ceftriaxone is not effective. A live, attenuated vaccine has been available since 1959 from the U.S. Army Medical Research Institute of Infectious Diseases, Fort Detrick, Frederick, Maryland, for individuals at high risk for infection, such as laboratory personnel. However, the vaccine is not foolproof, as it provides only partial immunity.

Because of the increased possibility for bioterrorism, the awareness of clinical laboratory personnel for presence of *F. tularensis* in clinical specimens should be increased (Gallagher-Smith, Kim, Al-Bawardy, & Josko, 2004; Lamps, Havens, Sjostedt, Page, & Scott, 2004). *F. tularensis* is now classified as a Category A infectious agent. The criteria for Category A agents are as follows: (1) can be easily disseminated or transmitted by person-to-person contact, (2) causes high mortality and therefore has a major public health impact, (3) may cause public panic and social disruption, and (4) requires special action for public health preparedness. (See ∞ Chapter 42, "Global Threats." for more information.) Presumptive identification of *F. tularensis* requires notification of authorities to include the local FBI, state public health laboratory, and state public health department.

 Checkpoint! 20–2 (Chapter Objective 3)

Which of the following is the most important ingredient required for growth of F. tularensis?

    A. *protein*
    B. *lactose*
    C. *human serum*
    D. *lipid*
    E. *cysteine*

▶ **LEGIONELLA PNEUMOPHILA**

These bacteria were discovered after an outbreak of severe respiratory illness at an American Legion convention that took place in 1976 in Philadelphia. Hence, *Legionella* was selected as the genus name, and the disease itself became known as **Legionnaire's disease.** *L. pneumophila* can also cause **Pontiac fever**, an influenza-like illness that initially occurred during an outbreak in Michigan. Similar organisms have been identified as the etiologic agents of respiratory tract infections in retrospective studies of serum samples dating back to 1947. The legionellae are ubiquitous in the environment where warm and moist conditions prevail. They have been recovered from lakes, streams, mud, and soil in many parts of the world. There is no known animal reservoir. Of the more than 40 *Legionella* species that have now been identified, *L. pneumophila* is by far the most common cause of disease in humans (Brooks et al., 2001b). There are at least 10 serogroups of *L. pneumophila*, with serogroup 1 being the cause of the 1976 outbreak. The other species of *Legionella* are only rarely isolated from clinical specimens.

GENERAL CHARACTERISTICS

L. pneumophila is an aerobic gram-negative rod. The organisms can be isolated on buffered charcoal-yeast extract (BCYE) agar that is supplemented with 1% α-ketoglutarate. The organism requires iron salts, cysteine, and high humidity for growth. Best growth is obtained at a pH of 6.9, 37°C, and 90% humidity. Antibiotics are sometimes added to the medium to prevent overgrowth by other bacteria, such as the normal upper respiratory flora found in sputum. Growth in blood cultures usually requires at least 2 weeks of incubation. Culture and testing of these organisms is done in clinical laboratories that have a class II biological safety cabinet.

In a Gram stained smear the organisms are small, pleomorphic gram-negative rods. Silver or Giemsa stain is better for visualization in tissue.

USEFUL BIOCHEMICAL AND OTHER TESTS

L. pneumophila are usually detected in clinical specimens by direct fluorescence antibody testing. This species, and all other legionellae, are catalase positive; most also produce gelatinase and β-lactamase. Additional enzymes produced by *L. pneumophila* include metalloprotease, other proteases, lipase, DNase, RNase, and lipase. *L. pneumophila* can be distinguished from other members of the genus by its production of the oxidase enzyme and its ability to hydrolyze hippurate. Interestingly, metalloprotease, a major enzyme that is secreted and that has both hemolytic and cytotoxic properties, does not appear to be a required virulence factor.

IDENTIFICATION

Microscopic Morphology

On a Gram stain, the bacteria appear as relatively thin (0.5–1 μm width) rods, but can range from 2 to 50 μm in length. However, they do not stain well with the Gram stain. Basic fuchsin is often used as a counterstain, for up to 3 minutes, because uptake of safranin stains by the organism is poor. With the

Gimenez stain, small, coccobacillary and occasional filamentous forms are seen more readily, as shown in Figure 20-3 ■.

Colony Morphology

Visible colonies usually appear within about 3 to 4 days of incubation on an appropriate medium. There is considerable variation in their characteristics. The colonies may be round or flat with entire edges, glistening, and convex. They appear to have ground glass speckling like a shattered windshield. Pigmentation can vary from colorless, grayish, pale green, to iridescent pink or blue. In addition, the colonies may be translucent.

Key Biochemical and Other Reactions

Bronchial washings, lung biopsies, pleural fluid, and blood are typical specimens from which the organisms can be recovered. Sputum is not an optimal choice for culture, because of the abundance of other normal upper respiratory flora. If sputum is submitted, it tends to be very watery and not purulent as with most pneumonia specimens. The organisms are usually not seen during microscopic inspection of smears made directly from specimens. Direct staining with fluorescent antibody can be useful, but this test has low sensitivity compared to culture on BCYE agar containing antibiotics. A rapid differential screening test based on production of a pigment that fluoresces under long-wave fluorescent light (Wood's lamp) may be performed. In this test, *L. pneumophila* exhibits a pale yellow-green fluorescence. Immunologic methods are sometimes used to detect antigens of *L. pneumophila* in urine. Serum antibodies against the organisms rise slowly over the course of the illness and often do not reach peak levels until 4 to 8 weeks after infection. Tests for detecting these antibodies have a

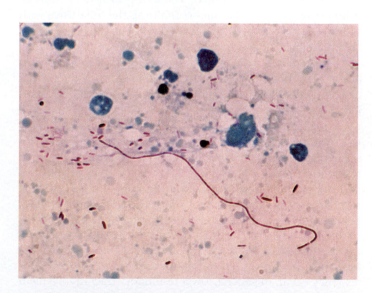

■ **FIGURE 20-3** Gimenez stain of *Legionella pneumophila*. Small red rods and long filamentous forms can be seen more readily using this stain because the organisms do not stain well with Gram stain.

From Public Health Image Library (PHIL)/CDC/Dr. Joseph McDade.

specificity of 95% to 99%, but a sensitivity of only 60% to 80%. Many patients are diagnosed retrospectively by an indirect fluorescent antibody test that detects antibodies. A four-fold rise in anti-*Legionella* antibody to a titer of 128 or greater is considered positive.

> **REAL WORLD TIP**
>
> ■ Growth on BCYE agar and yellow-green fluorescence of colonies supports a diagnosis of Legionnaire's disease because of *L. pneumophila*.
>
> ■ *Francisella tularensis* can also grow on BCYE and be found in the same respiratory specimens as *Legionella pneumophila*. Cultures for *L. pneumophila* should be examined under a laminar flow hood.

CLINICAL SIGNIFICANCE

L. pneumophila serogroup 1 is the major cause of Legionnaire's disease. The disease is most common in males over the age of 55 years who have risk factors such as smoking, emphysema, and other chronic respiratory tract conditions. Asymptomatic infection is possible among all age groups. The organisms are acquired through inhalation of aerosols created by contaminated air conditioners, showerheads, humidifiers, grocery store produce misters, and similar sources. The organisms infiltrate the lungs and survive in alveolar macrophages. They are also relatively resistant to destruction by polymorphonuclear white blood cells (i.e., neutrophils). The ability of the bacteria to inhibit fusion of phagosomes containing the organisms with lysosomes of phagocytic cells is thought to be the major mechanism accounting for virulence.

Disease ranges from a mild, short-term febrile illness to an acute purulent pneumonia with an intra-alveolar exudate that contains macrophages, neutrophils, erythrocytes, and proteinaceous material. High fever, chills, delirium, nonproductive cough, shortness of breath, and diarrhea occur frequently in severe cases. Additional manifestations include leukocytosis, hematuria, and abnormal liver function. Chest x-rays often reveal involvement of multiple lobes. There is usually little or no inflammation of the bronchioles and upper portions of the respiratory tract. The fatality rate can be as high as 10%. Legionellosis is a nationally reportable disease.

Pontiac fever is characterized by sore throat, cough, headache, fever, chills, malaise, and myalgia (muscle pain). Dizziness, confusion, photophobia, and stiffness of the neck also may occur. In general, lower respiratory tract involvement is much less likely than with Legionnaire's disease. Erythromycin is the drug of choice for infection because it can penetrate white blood cells to reach the intracellular organisms. Rifampin has been occasionally used when response to treat-

> **✓ Checkpoint! 20–3 (Chapter Objective 2)**
>
> Which of the following statements does **not** apply to L. pneumophila?
> A. Production of a fluorescent pigment can be useful in identification.
> B. The organisms are coccobacilli that sometimes produce filamentous forms.
> C. Resistance to erythromycin is common.
> D. Infection occurs after inhalation of contaminated aerosols produced by air conditioners.
> E. Males with predisposing factors are at greatest risk for disease after infection.

ment was delayed. Assistance with breathing and management of shock are frequently included in the treatment regimen.

▶ *BORDETELLA PERTUSSIS*

GENERAL CHARACTERISTICS

B. pertussis is a nonmotile, strictly aerobic bacterium that requires rich media for growth. The organisms are best cultured on a charcoal-containing medium to neutralize inhibitory substances. They can also be cultured on **Bordet-Gengou** (potato-sheep blood-glycerol) **medium** that includes penicillin G (Figure 20-4 ■). Regan-Lowe is often used as a transport medium. Incubation is for 3 to 7 days at 35°C to 37°C in a moist enclosure such as a sealed plastic bag.

The organisms are very small gram-negative coccobacilli that tend to grow singly or in pairs. Because staining is faint with

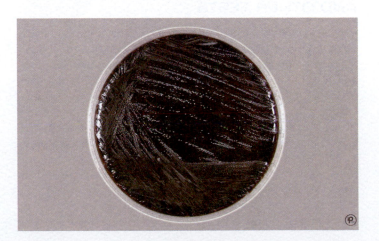

■ **FIGURE 20-4** Colonies of *Bordetella pertussis* growing on Bordet-Gengou (potato-blood-glycerol) medium. Small, glistening, mercury droplet colonies appear usually after 3 to 7 days of incubation under strict aerobic conditions in a moist atmosphere. *Photo courtesy of Indiana Pathology Images.*

the Gram stain, counterstaining with safranin O or aqueous basic fuchsin, for 3 minutes, is done to increase their visibility.

USEFUL BIOCHEMICAL TESTS

Although biochemical tests are usually not performed in clinical laboratories for identification of these bacteria, several observations can be made. *B. pertussis* forms acid, but not gas, from glucose and lactose. It does not require heme or NAD (V and X factors) when subcultured. Colonies of virulent strains will have a zone of hemolysis on blood-containing media.

IDENTIFICATION

Microscopic Morphology
The morphology of these small coccobacilli was described earlier.

Colony Morphology
Within 7 days on Bordet-Gengou agar that contains 20% blood, colonies will be surrounded by a diffuse zone of hemolysis. The colonial morphology is smooth, mucoid, and convex. The colonies are often described as having the appearance of shiny mercury drops with a pearly luster. On Regan-Lowe medium, the colonies are white with a mother-of-pearl opalescence.

Key Reactions
As mentioned earlier, biochemical reactions are generally not used for identification of these organisms. A saline nasal wash and nasopharyngeal swab are the most common specimens. Inoculation of an agar plate by droplets expelled during paroxysmal coughing ("cough plate"), a standard practice for many years, is no longer done. Direct fluorescent antibody (DFA) and slide agglutination tests are performed to detect the bacteria in nasopharyngeal aspirate specimens, as well as on colonies from culture. DFA must be used in tandem with culture, not in place of it, due to its low sensitivity of about 50%. Use of the polymerase chain reaction (PCR) provides the most sensitive method for identification of *B. pertussis* (Fry et al., 2004). It is recommended, however, that primers for both *B. pertussis* and *B. parapertussis* be included. Serologic tests for antibodies are not very useful for rapid diagnosis because those with agglutinating and precipitating properties do not appear until the third week of illness.

 REAL WORLD TIP

B. pertussis colonizes ciliated epithial cells. Specimens for culture or DFA must contain these cells.

CLINICAL SIGNIFICANCE

Humans are the only known source of *B. pertussis,* the etiologic agent of **whooping cough**, also known as pertussis (Latin: severe cough). Most cases occur in children under the age of 5 years, and most deaths occur in infants. Transmission occurs by inhalation of contaminated aerosols from individuals who have the early stage of the disease. Communicability rates ranging from 30% to 90% have been reported. After an incubation period of 2 weeks, the "catarrhal stage" is manifested by a mild cough and sneezing. During this time the patient is highly infectious, with large numbers of organisms in the respiratory droplets. The explosive "paroxysmal stage" that follows is characterized by a severe cough and a "whooping" sound during inhalation. Cyanosis, vomiting, and convulsions may also occur along with rapid exhaustion. The "whoop" and major complications occur primarily in infants, whereas the paroxysmal coughing is seen primarily in older children and adults. On rare occasions, encephalitis may develop. Recovery is slow and may take up to 6 months. There is marked lymphocytosis due to the organism's toxin.

Isolates obtained directly from patients exhibit hemolysis on blood-containing media and produce the **pertussis toxin**, the major virulence factor (Martin et al., 2004). The toxin paralyzes ciliated epithelial cells. Adherence to ciliated mucosal cells, a capsule, hemagglutinin, extracellular enzymes (adenylate cyclase), endotoxin, and other biologically active substances are among additional virulence factors produced by these bacteria.

Erythromycin is effective when administered during the catarrhal phase, but has little influence on the course of the disease when given after the onset of the paroxysmal phase. The antibiotic is also useful for prophylaxis, when given for 5 days to unimmunized infants or adults. Resistance to erythromycin has been reported. Immunity develops during the course of the disease, but second infections resulting in mild disease may occur. If infection occurs many years later in an adult, the disease may be severe. Several acellular vaccines, consisting of one to five antigens, are available and are usually administered together with the toxoids derived from *Corynebacterium diphtheriae* and *Clostridium tetani* (the **DTaP vaccine;** Purdy, Hay, Botteman, & Ward, 2004). These vaccines have lower risk for side effects compared to the previously used DPT vaccine that contained dead *B. pertussis* cells. Infants should receive three injections of a vaccine during the first year of life, followed by two booster injections. Adults who do not receive booster immunizations have decreased immunity. They are probably the primary reservoir for the organism. Pertussis is a nationally reportable disease.

 Checkpoint! 20–4 (Chapter Objective 4)

Which of the following is the most sensitive test for B. pertussis identification?

    A. *Polymerase chain reaction*
    B. *Direct fluorescent antibody test*
    C. *Growth on Bordet-Gengou agar*
    D. *Counterimmunoelectrophoresis*
    E. *Slide agglutination test*

▶ ADDITIONAL ISOLATES

◆ *Brucella*

The brucellae are intracellular bacteria that are usually found in animals, with humans being accidental hosts. These organisms were first isolated by Sir David Bruce on the island of Malta. Based on DNA analyses, it now appears that there is only one species, *B. melitensis,* with a number of biovars. However, these bacteria are often still referred to by their original "species" designations. The four that are known to infect humans, each having a typical animal reservoir, are *B. melitensis* (goats and sheep), *B. suis* (swine), *B. abortus* (cattle), and *B. canis* (dogs, especially beagles). Today, the disease in humans is most often referred to as brucellosis, but is also known as Malta fever and undulant fever.

General Characteristics

The brucellae are strictly aerobic, intracellular bacteria that have complex growth requirements. They will grow on well-defined media containing amino acids, vitamins, salts, and glucose. For isolation directly from patients, close contacts of patients, or animals, trypticase-soy agar or blood culture media are usually used (Almuneef et al., 2004). They tend to be slow growing on sheep blood or chocolate agars. Incubation is done in the presence of 5% to 10% CO_2, although only *B. abortus* has this requirement.

These organisms are nonmotile gram-negative rods that stain irregularly and pale with Gram stain.

Useful Biochemical Tests

The brucellae are relatively inactive metabolically. They are catalase and oxidase positive, use carbohydrates, but do not produce either acid or gas in significant amounts. All four biovars that infect humans produce catalase and oxidase. Many strains also produce H_2S and urease and reduce nitrates to nitrites.

Identification

Microscopic Morphology.   As shown in Figure 20-5 ■, short, coccobacillary forms dominate in early cultures, with rods being approximately 1.2 μm in length. Bipolar staining is sometimes evident.

Colony Morphology.   The colonies that appear after 3 to 5 days of incubation on enriched media are small, smooth, convex, transparent, and nonhemolytic. On subculture, the colonies tend to become rough because of loss of the capsule (avirulent form).

Key Biochemical and Other Reactions.   *Brucella* is a potential bioterror agent that can be presumptively identified using Gram stain morphology, oxidase, and urease tests. Tiny, faintly stained gram-negative coccobacilli that are oxidase and urease positive can be presumptively identified as *Brucella.*

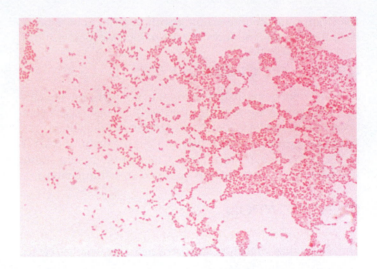

■ **FIGURE 20-5** Gram stain of *Brucella melitensis.* These are small gram-negative coccobacilli that stain irregularly and sometimes exhibit bipolar staining. This latter characteristic makes them appear like two cocci that are stuck together. *From Public Health Image Library (PHIL)/CDC.*

The different biovars express different amounts of lipopolysaccharide antigens, A and M. In addition, an L antigen that is similar to the Vi capsular antigen of *Salmonella typhi* may be present. As shown in Table 20-3 ✪, the biovars can be distinguished by differences in ability to produce H_2S, requirement for CO_2, and susceptibility to certain dyes. However, few clinical laboratories continue to perform these tests and thus do not identify the specific biovar that has been isolated. Biovar identification is available in some reference laboratories and is sometimes useful from the epidemiological viewpoint.

Blood and biopsy tissue from sites associated with the reticuloendothelial (RES) system such as lymph nodes and bone marrow are suitable for initial culture in trypticase soy broth and on thionine-tryptose agar. Incubation is in 10% CO_2 for at least 3 weeks, if the cultures remain negative. If bacteria resembling the brucellae are present, they are tested for H_2S production, dye sensitivity, and agglutination of absorbed sera.

Diagnosis may be based at least in part on serologic analyses. In the classical agglutination test, a standardized heat-killed, phenolized, smooth *Brucella* is used. An IgG titer of greater than 80 indicates active infection. In negative cases where the clinical presentation is strongly suggestive of brucellosis, additional tests may be done to determine presence of "blocking antibodies" of the IgA class. The IgA can interfere with agglutination by IgG and IgM, resulting in a false negative in low serum dilutions (i.e., prozone phenomenon; see ∞ Chapter 10). Addition of 2-mercaptoethanol to the patient's serum destroys IgM (which may remain at high titers for years after disease resolution) but leaves IgG intact for testing by agglutination. Although this test is not as sensitive as the classic agglutination test, the results correlate more accurately with chronic

⊗ TABLE 20-3

Selected Characteristics of the Brucellae

Biovar	CO$_2$ Requirement	H$_2$S Production	Growth in Presence of Dye*		Disease
			Thionine	Basic Fuchsin	
B. melitensis	–	–	+	+	Acute, severe
B. abortus	+	++	–	+	Mild, without suppurative complications, noncaseating
B. suis	–	V	+	V	Chronic, with suppurative lesions
B. canis	–	–	+	–	Mild, without suppurative complications, noncaseating

*Dye sensitivity test.

active disease. A skin test using a protein extract of brucella is available, but is rarely used because of its lack of reliability.

Clinical Significance

In animals, the brucellae localize in the pregnant uterus because of the presence of erythritol in allantoic and amniotic fluids. Erythritol is a four-carbon polyhydric alcohol that stimulates growth of the organisms. Abortion is a major manifestation of the disease in animals (humans do not have erythritol, and so there is no localization of the bacteria to the uterus of pregnant women). The disease in animals is sometimes referred to as "contagious abortion" because animals that eat or lick the aborted fetuses will frequently become infected because of the high invasiveness of the organisms. In addition, farmers who handle the aborted fetuses, have direct contact with infected animal feces or urine, or inhale airborne dust contaminated with the organisms can become infected. The bacteria remain viable in dry soil for up to 60 days. The brucellae localize in the mammary glands of animals and can be shed in milk for years. Ingestion of unpasteurized milk or cheeses and other products that contain unpasteurized milk is an important route of transmission. Farmers, veterinarians, and abattoir or slaughterhouse workers are at greatest risk for infection, but a number of laboratory-acquired cases have been reported (Robichard, Libman, Behr, & Rubin, 2004). It is the most common lab acquired infection.

The incubation period ranges from about 1 week to 6 weeks, and onset of illness is slow and insidious. The bacteria are disseminated via the lymphatics and bloodstream to many parts of the body. Granulomatous nodules, which may progress to abscesses, eventually form in sites that are especially rich in macrophages, such as the liver, spleen, and bone marrow of the RES system. Proliferation of mononuclear cells is a major histological finding. Fever, malaise, weakness, and nonspecific aches and pains are major manifestations of brucellosis. Gastrointestinal and nervous symptoms and lymph node and spleen enlargement are also frequently noted. The fever may have a daily periodicity, rising in the afternoon and falling at night, during which time the patient is drenched in sweat. Undulatant fever is seen primarily after infection with B. meliten-

sis. The generalized symptoms of brucellosis usually subside over a period of weeks to months, although localized symptoms may continue much longer, occasionally for years. The different biovars are associated with different degrees of disease severity (see Table 20-3).

Immunity is usually good after recovery, although reinfection is possible, resulting in a milder disease. The brucellae are usually susceptible to tetracycline, streptomycin, and ampicillin. However, because of their intracellular nature, the organisms are difficult to eradicate. Administration of streptomycin and a tetracycline for an extended period of time may be required. Rifampin prophylaxis is recommended for close contacts under 4 years of age.

Brucella is a potential bioterror agent and brucellosis is a nationally reportable disease. Appropriate authorities (local FBI, state public health laboratory, and state public health department) must be notified and the original specimen preserved (for a criminal investigation) if an isolate is presumptively identified as *Brucella*.

◆ HACEK

Most cases of subacute bacterial endocarditis (SBE) are caused by the viridans streptococci. Certain fastidious organisms, all of which are gram-negative coccobacilli, can also cause the disease. These bacteria have been given the acronym HACEK, based on the first letter of each genus involved: *Haemophilus parainfluenzae, Aggregatibacter, Cardiobacterium, Eikenella,* and *Kingella.* This group of bacteria is responsible for approximately 3% of endocarditis cases. They are occasionally implicated in infections other than SBE (Feder, Roberts, Salazar, Leopold, & Toro-Salazar, 2003) and may play a role in the formation of fatty plaques on the artery walls. Characteristics used to differentiate these bacteria (except *H. parainfluenzae*) are shown in Table 20-4⊗. The organisms are usually part of the normal oral flora and infections result because of poor oral hygiene or dental manipulations and damaged or diseased heart valves. As a group, they are often slow growing and require or are stimulated by carbon dioxide. Because of their slow growth, it may be necessary to hold blood cultures for up to 2 weeks to ensure their recovery.

✪ **TABLE 20-4**

Selected Characteristics of the HACEK Group

Bacteria	Oxidase	Catalase	Indole	Sugar Fermentation			
				Glucose	Lactose	Maltose	Sucrose
Aggregatibacter aphrophilus	weak +	−	−	+	+	+	+
A. actinomycetemcomitans	+	+	−	+	−	+	−
Cardiobacterium hominis	+	−	+	+	−	+	+
Eikenella corrodens	+	−	−	−	−	−	−
Kingella kingae	+	−	−	+	−	+	−

The "+" and "−" designations apply to the majority of isolates.

Organisms

H. parainfluenzae. The characteristics of this *Haemophilus* species were described earlier, along with the other members in the genus. The bacteria reside in the upper respiratory tract as part of the normal flora.

Aggregatibacter. *A. aphrophilus* (formerly known as *H. aphrophilus*) has variable morphology, although most strains have a coccobacillary shape. Colonies are round and convex and have a central opaque zone. It has an odor similar to grade school paste. *A. aphrophilus* requires 5% to 10% CO_2, but does not require either heme (factor X) or NAD (factor V) for growth; the requirement for heme is only on initial isolation. It can produce a weak positive ALA reaction even though it does not require heme for growth. This can result in its misidentification as *H. parainfluenzae*. Organisms isolated from blood cultures must be identified with a commercial system. The organisms do not cause hemolysis on horse blood agar and do not produce catalase, indole, and urease; they produce acid and gas from glucose and acid from lactose. It has occasionally been implicated in cases of endocarditis and pneumonia. These organisms have very low pathogenic potential and are considered to be opportunists.

A. actinomycetemcomitans is the most common of the HACEK group to be isolated from infective endocarditis (Brouqui & Raoult, 2001; Paturel, Casalta, Habib, Nezri, & Raoult, 2004). It is a small, nonmotile, slowly growing, capnophilic (requires an increased concentration of CO_2) coccobacillus. It will grow on trypticase soy blood agar supplemented with 0.5% yeast extract, hemin, and menadione (TSBY) at 37°C. After 48 to 96 hours, isolates form rough colonies and produce numerous peritrichous fimbriae that aggregate as bundles. On nutrient agar, colonies have a complex morphology characterized by irregular edges, a rough surface texture, a star-shaped internal structure, and pitting of the agar surface. In broth cultures, the liquid remains clear because the organisms adhere to plastic and glass surfaces. However, the expression of fimbriae and other adhesins is variable, depending on factors such as pH, temperature, oxygen, or iron concentration. On subculture, these organisms are irre-

versibly converted to a nonfimbriated phenotype, resulting in the appearance of smooth colonies.

The pattern of carbohydrate fermentation can be obtained within 4 hours using a medium that contains 20% carbohydrate, peptone, meat extract, and buffers. The organisms ferment glucose and maltose, but not lactose, sorbitol, and sucrose. They produce catalase. PCR may be useful for differentiating these organisms from certain *Haemophilus* species (Dogan, Asikainen, & Jousimies-Somer, 1999).

Many studies conducted in the United States, Europe, and Japan have reported that the organisms exhibit great genetic diversity that may be responsible for variations in virulence potential. Possible virulence factors include a secreted leukotoxin, a lipoprotein that kills human polymorphonuclear leukocytes and macrophages, and an immunosuppressive cytolethal-distending toxin that is similar to toxins produced by certain gram-negative bacteria.

In addition to SBE, these organisms have been recovered from abscesses, bacteremia, and cases of osteomyelitis. Overall, *A. actinomycetemcomitans* is most often associated with localized juvenile periodontitis, a severe and aggressive form of early onset infection that affects children 10 to 17 years of age; approximately 70,000 cases of this disease are reported each year in the United States. In adults, it has been associated with cases of refractory periodontitis. The organisms are susceptible to tetracycline and chloramphenicol. Treatment is also sometimes successful with penicillin G, ampicillin, and erythromycin.

🅔 **REAL WORLD TIP**

Comitans means *accompanying. Aggregatibacter actinomycetemcomitans* is frequently isolated with *Actinomyces israelii.*

Cardiobacterium. *C. hominis* is a facultative anaerobe that is part of the normal flora of the upper respiratory tract and bowel. The bacteria are pleomorphic, gram variable, and assume a rosette or flower-like arrangement on Gram stain.

Isolation is performed on samples of blood. After 48 hours of incubation in 5% to 10% CO_2 at 37°C, colonies will appear on blood agar and chocolate agar. A zone of α-hemolysis is seen around the colonies. Growth is very slow in routine blood culture media, and incubation for several weeks may be necessary before visible growth is evident. However, results for carbohydrate fermentation can be obtained within a few hours using a medium that contains 20% carbohydrate, peptone, meat extract, and buffers (as described above for *Aggregatibacter*). The organisms ferment glucose, maltose, fructose, mannitol, sucrose, and sorbitol, but not lactose. In addition, oxidase, indole, and nitrate reduction tests are positive, whereas the test for catalase is negative. Broad-base PCR amplification of ribosomal RNA, followed by single-strand sequencing, has been used occasionally to detect and identify these bacteria in arterio-embolic tissue (Mueller, Kaplan, Zbinden, & Altwegg, 1999). These organisms occasionally cause bacteremia and SBE, especially after dental work. However, the frequency of isolation from clinical specimens has been increasing in recent years. Penicillin is the drug of choice for treatment of *C. hominis* infection.

 REAL WORLD TIP

Cardiobacterium valvarum, a recently described cause of endocarditis, can be differentiated from *C. hominis* by its strongly positive spot indole reaction, and negative results for maltose, fructose, sucrose, and mannitol.

Eikenella.   *E. corrodens* is a small gram-negative bacillus that exists normally in the gingiva and bowel of 40% to 70% of humans. The organisms are facultative anaerobes that grow as small straight rods, although pleomorphism is sometimes observed. Several days of incubation on appropriate media are required for isolation. Growth on blood agar and chocolate agar is facilitated with 5% to 10% CO_2 and a high level of humidity. Typical colonies are small and grayish, produce a slight green discoloration on blood agar, and emit an odor resembling bleach. In some cases, the colonies may have a lemon yellow color when swiped up with a swab. Approximately one-half of the isolates form colonies that produce pits in or corrodes agar media. *Eikenella* does not ferment carbohydrates and is negative for catalase, urease, and indole. It produces oxidase and reduces nitrates to nitrites. Tests for lysine- and ornithine-decarboxylase are often positive. *E. corrodens* is most often associated with wounds inflicted by human bites or "fistfights," but has also been implicated in SBE. Infection has also been reported in addicts who lubricate needles with their saliva before injecting drugs (a practice known in the drug culture as "skin popping"). In addition, they are often found together with streptococci in a variety of mixed flora infections. In immunodeficient patients, endocarditis, meningitis, brain abscesses, and osteomyelitis may occur. *E. corrodens* is usually susceptible to ampicillin, the newer penicillins, and cephalosporins. Because they are invariably resis-

tant to clindamycin, incorporation of the antibiotic into media is useful for selective isolation of the eikanellae.

Kingella.   Within this genus, *K. kingae* is the most prominent cause of SBE. The nonmotile cells are short and plump with blunt ends; organisms may appear in pairs or chains. *K. kingae* will not grow on Thayer-Martin medium, in contrast to *K. denitrificans*. Incubation for several days in 5% to 10% CO_2 is often required for initial isolation on 5% sheep blood agar; a clear zone of β-hemolysis will eventually appear around the colonies. Colony morphology is variable. Some isolates form a "fried egg" structure with a thin haze surrounding the central growth and produce pits in the agar. The organisms are oxidase positive and most will reduce nitrates; they are negative for catalase. Carbohydrate fermentation results can be rapidly obtained using a special broth medium that contains 20% carbohydrate, as described earlier for *Actinobacillus* and *Cardiobacterium*. *K. kingae* ferments glucose and maltose, but not lactose, sucrose, and sorbitol. Although these bacteria are part of the normal oral microbiota, they can enter the blood circulation after trauma, even when it is a minor wound such as brushing the teeth. Poor dental hygiene is a predisposing factor, and children appear to be at greatest risk for infection. In addition to SBE, infection of bones, joints, and tendons have been reported. *K. kingae* appears to have a pronounced tropism or affinity for bones and the heart, although a few infections of skin have also occurred. Penicillin, ampicillin, and erythromycin are effective for treatment. The organisms are also susceptible to gentamicin and chloramphenicol.

Bacteria in the HACEK group should be suspected when a fastidious gram-negative coccobacillus is isolated from a case of SBE and fails to grow on MacConkey agar. In cases where a HACEK organism appears to be likely, a second-generation cephalosporin or ciprofloxacin is often administered until results of antibiotic susceptibility tests become available. Antibiotic therapy is usually continued for at least 6 weeks.

Clinical Significance

The clinical manifestations of SBE are quite variable. Fever (often intermittent), heart murmur, headache, cough, arthralgia, anemia, and hematuria occur in the majority of patients, whereas chills, anorexia, weight loss, skin lesions, and pain in the back, chest, and/or abdominal region are usually seen in 50% or less of patients. Some individuals may also exhibit neurologic signs or strokes. Because of the insidious nature of the disease, symptoms may evolve over a period of weeks to several months before a diagnosis is made. Many patients eventually develop congestive heart failure and need heart valve replacement. SBE is often associated with prosthetic heart valves or structural heart abnormalities. Dental caries and periodontal disease are among the most common predisposing factors. With the increasing popularity of body piercing in the United States and other countries, endocarditis because of members of the HACEK group has been occasionally reported after oral body piercing (e.g., *H. parainfluenzae*). As noted earlier, the HACEK bacteria can at times produce a number of other types of infections in addition to SBE. Overall, the mortality rate ranges from 10% to 20%.

◆ *Streptobacillus*

General Characteristics

S. moniliformis is a microaerophilic pleomorphic gram-negative rod that grows in media supplemented with serum protein, egg yolk, or starch. Best growth is obtained at 37°C, whereas at 22°C the organisms fail to grow.

These are highly pleomorphic bacteria that form long irregular chains containing fusiform enlargements and large round bodies that sometimes resemble a string of beads. **L forms** are readily observed in most cultures. These gram-negative bacteria have lost most of their cell wall but retained the outer membrane and entrapped peptidoglycan; if they are able to grow and divide, they are known as L forms. The typical morphology of streptobacilli reappears on culture of pure L forms in liquid media.

Useful Biochemical and Other Tests

S. moniliformis is a nonmotile bacteria that lacks a capsule. These organisms are negative for indole, oxidase, catalase, and reduction of nitrate. Mouse inoculation and serum agglutination tests can also be performed. Specific antibodies appear within 10 days after infection. However, serologic tests for serum antibodies are performed only in reference laboratories because disease caused by these organisms is rare.

Identification

Microscopic Morphology.   Bacteria that look like a string of beads or pearls on microscopic examination should alert the technologist that the organisms may very well be *S. moniliformis.*

Colony Morphology.   *S. moniliformis* may be isolated from blood, joint fluid, lymph nodes, or pus from lesions but are very difficult to culture. The organisms grow best when media contain blood, 10 to 20% serum, or ascitic fluid. On blood agar, the appearance of colonies is facilitated by incubation in a very moist atmosphere that contains 5% to 10% CO_2. After 48 hours of incubation at 37°C, colonies on brain–heart infusion agar that has been supplemented with 20% horse serum are small, colorless to grayish, smooth, and glistening; irregular edges may be apparent. Colonies in which the bacteria have undergone spontaneous transformation to L forms have a dark center with a flattened lacy edge that resembles fried eggs. On blood agar, cottonlike colonies appear after about 3 days of incubation. In a broth, the organisms will have the appearance of flocculent "fluff balls" or "bread crumbs" at the bottom of the tube or on top of sedimented red blood cells.

Clinical Significance

Streptobacillus is normally found in the throats of rats, mice, guinea pigs, and other rodents, although some carnivores (e.g., cats, ferrets, and dogs) that prey on these animals may also har-

bor the organisms. Human infection usually occurs following a rat bite, resulting in a disease known as rat-bite fever. The typical symptoms include fever and a petechial or blotchy rash that appears within the first 2 days after infection. The rash is present on the extremities, including the palms of the hands and soles of the feet. A very painful polyarthritis involving the knees, ankles, elbows, and other joints occurs in about 50% of patients (Wallet et al., 2003). Growth of bacteria in specimens from a patient with a history of a rat bite is useful in establishing a diagnosis because the other possible agent of rat-bite fever (*Spirillum minus*) does not grow in culture. When infection occurs by ingestion of contaminated milk, the disease is known as Haverhill fever. In this case, epidemics are possible. The clinical manifestations of Haverhill fever resemble those of rat-bite fever. Patients with *S. moniliformis* infection may cause a false positive in the VDRL (Venereal Disease Research Laboratories) screening test for syphilis. The organisms are susceptible to penicillin, although other antibiotics may also be effective. They are resistant to sulfonamides. L forms are resistant to penicillin because they lack a cell wall.

 Checkpoint! 20–5 (Chapter Objective 6)

Which of the HACEK organisms is most likely to cause subacute bacterial endocarditis (SBE)?

    A. *E. corrodens*
    B. *C. hominis*
    C. *A. actinomycetemcomitans*
    D. *K. kingae*
    E. *H. aphrophilus*

SUMMARY

The fastidious gram-negative rods encompass a wide range of natural habitats, characteristics, and diseases. A major unifying feature is that they require special nutrients and other additives for growth. Many of these organisms are transmitted to humans from animal sources, and some are part of the normal flora of humans, whereas others are found free-living in the environment. Insect vectors are occasionally involved. Most of these bacteria are facultative anaerobes, whereas a few are either strict aerobes or anaerobes. Microscopic morphology is generally coccobacillary, but long filamentous forms are common. Initial isolation is often accomplished after prolonged incubation in a CO_2-enriched atmosphere. Colony morphology is highly variable, ranging from white, smooth, glistening, round colonies to pigmentation, fried egg and irregular shapes, tuftlike growths, and pitting of agar. The diseases produced by these organisms involve numerous parts of the body, including the respiratory, genital, and urinary tracts, brain, heart, ears, bones, joints, spleen, liver, and skin,

The members of the *Haemophilus* genus require heme, NAD, or both for growth. *H. influenzae* requires both of these factors, forms "satellite" colonies on agar when both heme and NAD are supplied, and thus can be differentiated from most other *Haemophilus* species. *H. influenzae* type b is most likely to cause meningitis, otitis media, and other infections, especially in young children. Development of conjugated vaccines for *H. influenzae* type b has markedly decreased disease prevalence. *H aegyptius* is a common cause of conjunctivitis. *H. ducreyi* is the etiological agent of chancroid, a sexually transmitted disease found primarily in tropical regions. *H. parainfluenzae* is part of the normal flora of the human respiratory tract and causes infections infrequently.

F. tularensis, the cause of tularemia, is a highly invasive coccobacillus transmitted to humans during contact with wild animals or their carcasses and by bite of an arthropod vector. Wild rabbits are the most common cause of human infection in the United States. Laboratory diagnosis is based on culture and testing conducted in reference laboratories that use strict biosafety measures. These organisms have special significance in that they are in the most dangerous category (Category A) of potential bioterrorism agents.

L. pneumophila, the cause of Legionnaire's disease and Pontiac fever, is found worldwide in many lakes and streams. Humans become infected after inhalation of contaminated aerosols created by air conditioners, humidifiers, and other similar devices. Males with preexisting chronic respiratory tract conditions are especially susceptible. Isolation is done on BCYE agar supplemented with α-ketoglutarate under conditions that include 90% humidity. The organisms can be identified on the basis of direct fluorescent antibody staining, a fluorescent pigment, and production of many enzymes. Legionnaire's disease involves the lungs, with multiple lobes often being affected, whereas Pontiac fever is usually confined to the upper respiratory tract.

B. pertussis, found only in humans, causes an extremely contagious respiratory disease known as whooping cough in young children, although recently the incidence in older children and adults has been increasing. The catarrhal stage (mild coughing/sneezing) is followed by a paroxysmal stage that is characterized by a severe cough and a "whooping" sound during inhalation. The pertussis toxin is an important virulence factor. The organisms can be identified by the appearance of smooth, mucoid colonies that look like drops of mercury on Bordet-Gengou agar, by direct fluorescent antibody staining, and by PCR. An acellular vaccine, DTaP, which also contains toxoids derived from *C. diphtheriae* and *C. tetani*, has dramatically reduced disease prevalence.

The *Brucella* genus consists of four major biovars (*B. melitensis, B. suis, B. abortus,* and *B. canis*). These are tiny, intracellular, aerobic coccobacilli with occasional bipolar staining. They are transmitted to humans primarily from farm animals. Isolation is done in the presence of 5% to 10% CO_2. Differentiation of biovars is based on urease production, CO_2

requirement, H_2S formation, and growth in the presence of thionine and fuchsin dyes. BSL-3 conditions are necessary because of their highly invasive nature. Brucellosis is a disease that appears insidiously and has a long recovery time, even with treatment. Fever, which may or may not have a daily periodicity (i.e., undulation), and formation of granulomatous nodules are typical manifestations. The incidence of this disease has declined greatly in the United States since widespread pasteurization of milk and immunization of livestock were implemented. *Brucella* is a potential bioterrorism agent.

Members of the HACEK group (*H. parainfluenzae, A. aphrophilus* [formerly known as *H. aphrophilus*], *A. actinomycetemcomitans, C. hominis, E. corrodens,* and *K. kingae*) are normal oral microbiota, but can sometimes cause SBE and, less often, other infections. Most of them require extended incubation, 5% to 10% CO_2, and media such as TSBY. *A. aphrophilus* is a coccobacillus that forms round, convex colonies with a central opaque zone form on media typically used for *Haemophilus* species. It requires heme initially, but not NAD. The most common agent of SBE within the HACEK group is *A. actinomycetemcomitans.* These are small, capnophilic coccobacilli that form rough colonies, aggregate in bundles, and adhere to plastic and glass. Colonies may have a star-shaped internal structure with pitting of agar or a smooth surface. *C. hominis* is a facultative anaerobe that is sometimes recovered from SBE cases after dental procedures. These pleomorphic bacteria form rosettes and produce α-hemolysis on blood agar. *E. corrodens* is a small, pleomorphic, facultative anaerobe that produces small, gray colonies with a bleachlike odor on blood agar in the presence of CO_2 and high humidity. Infection is associated primarily with wounds inflicted by human bites and intravenous drug use by addicts. *K. kingae* is a short, plump, nonmotile rod that grows in pairs or chains and forms colonies with a zone of β-hemolysis; some isolates form "fried egg" colonies. The pattern of carbohydrate fermentation for at least some of the HACEK bacteria (*K. kingae, A. actinomycetemcomitans,* and *C. hominis*) can be determined within a few hours after inoculating a special medium that contains 20% carbohydrates.

S. moniliformis is a highly pleomorphic, microaerophilic organism that grows on media supplemented with serum protein, egg yolk, or starch. The organisms often have branching filaments and beadlike chains. Colonies on supplemented blood agar and in liquid media look like balls of fluff. Spontaneous transformation to L forms is common, resulting in fried egg colony morphology. Humans are infected primarily by the bite of a rat and may develop rat-bite fever. When transmission occurs by less-common routes such as food, milk, and water, the disease is called Haverhill fever. Symptoms are similar in both cases (i.e., acute onset of fever, headache, severe joint pain).

LEARNING OPPORTUNITIES

1. What characteristics do the bacteria presented in this chapter have in common? (Chapter Objective 1)

2. How can these bacteria be differentiated in the clinical laboratory? (Chapter Objectives 2, 3, and 4)

3. What are the circumstances under which these bacteria cause disease, and are there any specific factors associated with disease production? (Chapter Objective 5)

4. What are the major types of diseases associated with the presented bacteria? (Chapter Objective 6)

CASE STUDY 20-1   OTITIS MEDIA BECAUSE OF *HAEMOPHILUS INFLUENZAE*

Patient: 4-year-old female

Admitting Diagnosis: A lethargic 4-year-old girl with a high fever, headache, vomiting, and other signs of acute meningitis is admitted to the hospital. The mother states that several days earlier, her daughter had an extremely painful ear. Blood cultures are initially negative, but microscopic examination of cerebrospinal fluid (CSF) reveals the presence of many polymorphonuclear cells. Colonies with typical *H. influenzae* morphology appear within 24 hours after culture of the CSF on enriched chocolate agar. A positive serotyping result for *H. influenzae* type b antigen is also obtained with the CSF.

Background: Questioning of the mother reveals that the child has not received any of the routinely administered immunizations. Although appropriate antibiotic therapy is initiated rapidly, the child's condition worsens and ends in death.

1. Is there a vaccine that could have prevented infection with *H. influenzae* type b?

2. What are the growth requirements for these bacteria?

3. What other types of infections can *H. influenzae* type b cause in addition to meningitis?

CASE STUDY 20-2   SUBACUTE BACTERIAL ENDOCARDITIS AFTER A VISIT TO THE DENTIST

Patient: 40-year-old male

Admitting Diagnosis: A 40-year-old man arrived in the emergency room because of fever, chills, and severe shortness of breath. After admission to the hospital, it was learned that the fever and chills had begun several weeks earlier, but were becoming progressively more severe. The patient complained of persistent chest and back pain and stated that he had lost a considerable amount of weight because he "did not feeling like eating" (anorexia).

Background: After further questioning, it was learned that the patient had a root canal procedure performed several months earlier. Physical examination revealed an enlarged spleen. His heart size appeared normal based on percussion and chest x-ray films, but a diastolic murmur consistent with mitral valve stenosis was heard on auscultation. Echocardiography revealed an enlarged left atrium and thickened mitral valve leaflets, one of which had a vegetation. Two blood cultures, obtained on the day of admission, were positive for gram-negative rods that required enriched media for growth. A diagnosis of subacute bacterial endocarditis because of *Eikenella corrodens* was eventually made.

1. What are the morphological properties of this bacterium?

2. What is the normal habitat of these organisms?

3. Does this bacterium have any unusual characteristics that may be helpful in diagnosis?

4. What are the most common bacteria that cause subacute bacterial endocarditis?

PEARSON
myhealthprofessionskit™

Use this address to access the interactive Companion Website created for this textbook. Simply select "Clinical Laboratory Science" from the choice of disciplines. Find this book and log in using your user name and password.

REFERENCES

Go to myhealthprofessionskit.com to view this chapter's references.

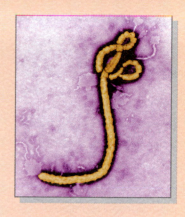

21

Enterobacteriaceae

Daila S. Gridley

■ LEARNING OBJECTIVES

Upon completion of this chapter, the learner should be able to:

1. Relate the general characteristics and the antigenic properties of the *Enterobacteriaceae*.

    a. Differentiate from nonfermenters and other organisms.

2. Describe major distinguishing features of the presented genera and name the species of greatest importance in human infections.

    a. Determine appropriate specimen for isolation.

    b. Determine appropriate media for selection and differentiation of these organisms.

    c. Describe any growth and environmental requirements for each organism.

3. Correlate the various organisms with the major type(s) of infection(s) they cause.

    a. Associate patient populations at risk for disease.

    b. Identify organisms that have the potential to be used as bioterrorism agents.

4. Describe the significance of lipopolysaccharide (LPS) and other major virulence factors that are associated with these organisms.

5. Select the major types of tests that are useful in isolation and identification of the most common *Enterobacteriaceae*.

    a. Predict limitations and potential sources of errors.

    b. Differentiate one organism from another.

6. Summarize treatment strategies, expected antibiotic susceptibility results, and emerging resistance for the *Enterobacteriaceae*.

7. Correlate patient history, body site or specimen type, colonial morphology, Gram stain results, identification test results, and antibiogram results in order to identify an isolate and assess its clinical significance.

KEY TERMS

coliform

disseminated intravascu-
  lar coagulation (DIC)

dysentery

endotoxin

granuloma inguinale

heat-labile toxin (LT)

heat-stable toxin (ST)

hemolytic uremic
  syndrome (HUS)

hemorrhagic colitis

K antigens

Kligler's iron agar (KIA)

lipid A

lipopolysaccharide (LPS)

O antigen

P pilus

plague

salmonellosis

shiga toxin

shigellosis

Triple sugar iron agar
  (TSI)

typhoid fever

verotoxin

Vi antigen

TAXONOMY

Family *Enterobacteriaceae* (en-te-ro-bak-te-ree-a-ce-ee)
  Genus *Citrobacter* (sit-ro-bak-ter)
    C. koseri (ko-ser-i)
    C. freundii (froyn-dee-i)
  Genus *Edwardsiella* (ed-ward-see-el-ah)
    E. tarda (tar-dah)
  Genus *Enterobacter* (en-te-ro-bak-ter)
    E. aerogenes (air-ah-dgen-ees)
    E. cloacae (clo-a-cae)
  Genus *Escherichia* (esh-er-eesh-ah)
    E. coli (kol-i)
  Genus *Hafnia* (haf-nee-ah)
    H. alvei (al-vee-eye)
  Genus *Klebsiella* (kleb-see-el-ah)
    K. granulomatis (gran-you-lo-ma-tis)
    K. oxytoca (oxee-to-ka)
    K. pneumoniae (new-mo-nee-ee)
  Genus *Morganella* (mor-ga-nel-la)
    M. morganii (mor-ga-nee-eye)
  Genus *Pantoea* (pan-toe-a)
    P. agglomerans (ag-glo-mer-ans)
  Genus *Plesiomonas* (ple-see-o-mo-nas)
    P. shigelloides (shi-gel-loi-des)
  Genus *Proteus* (pro-tee-us)
    P. mirabilis (mi-ra bi-lis)
    P. vulgaris (vul-ga-ris)

Genus *Providencia* (pro-vi-den-see-ah)
    P. alcalifaciens (al-cal-ee-fac-i-ens)
    P. rettgeri (ret-ger-ee)
    P. stuarti (stu-ar-tee-i)
  Genus *Salmonella* (sal-mon-el-ah)
    S. serotype Cholerae-suis (kol-er-ah-su-is)
    S. serotype Enteritidis (en-te-ri-ti-dis)
    S. serotype Newport (new-port)
    S. serotype Paratyphi (pa-ra-ty-fee)
    S. serotype Typhi (ty-fee)
    S. serotype Typhimurium (ty-fee-mur-ee-um)
  Genus *Serratia* (ser-ra-tea-a)
    S. marcescens (mar-ses-cens)
  Genus *Shigella* (shi-gel-la)
    S. boydii (boy-d-eye)
    S. dysenteriae (dis-en-ter-ee-ee)
    S. flexneri (flex-ner-ee)
    S. sonnei (son-ne-i)
  Genus *Yersinia* (yer-si-nee-a)
    Y. enterocolitica (en-ter-o-co-li-ti-ca)
    Y. pestis (pes-tis)
    Y. pseudotuberculosis (pseu-do-tu-ber-q-lo-sis)

▶ INTRODUCTION

The *Enterobacteriaceae* family is very large, consisting of more than 25 genera and 110 species or groups. Many of the members reside within the intestinal tracts of both humans and animals, and so they are often referred to as "the enterics."

They can also be found in food and water contaminated with feces. Classification of these gram-negative rods has always been difficult because of their numerous shared and overlapping properties. Changes in taxonomy have become even more common place since the introduction of DNA and RNA analyses. Classification is based at least partly on the presence of characteristic antigens, some of which are associated with pathogenicity and virulence. Biochemical reactions, of course, also play a major role in classification. A broad range of selective and differential media are used to assist in identification of isolates.

Most of the enterics are part of the normal flora and do not produce disease unless they reach parts of the body that they do not usually inhabit. However, some may be pathogenic under certain conditions in certain individuals, and some are always considered to be pathogenic. Clinically, these organisms are extremely important. Together with the staphylococci and streptococci, they are among the most common causes of bacterial disease in humans. The bacteria in the *Enterobacteriaceae* family are responsible for a high percentage of the estimated 76 million cases of food-borne illnesses that occur in the United States each year. Contamination with *E. coli* O157:H7 is responsible for the biggest food recalls that have ever been imposed by the Food and Drug Administration (FDA). The *Enterobacteriaceae* are implicated in a large percentage of the more than 7 million episodes of diarrhea that occur each year and are the leading cause of urinary tract infections and bacteremia in the United States (Centers for Disease Control [CDC], 2003a; Clarke, 2001; Mead et al., 1999). Overall, these organisms account for approximately 80% of clinically significant gram-negative isolates and approximately 50% of all clinically significant isolates. Unfortunately, many of the enterics are now resistant to virtually all of the older antibiotics, and many are becoming resistant to the newest and best drugs available (Ryan, 2004). Some of these bacteria also produce exotoxins and a variety of other factors that play significant roles in pathogenesis and virulence. Infections, as well as deaths, because of these bacteria are increasing in the United States. In recent years, there has been a great increase in nosocomial infections (hospital-acquired infections) because of many of the *Enterobacteriaceae*, as well as multidrug resistance. Therapy is often initiated on the basis of susceptibility patterns. However, there is no guarantee that a particular isolate will respond as expected. Therefore, it is important for statistics on drug susceptibility patterns to be updated frequently and laboratory personnel, as well as clinicians, are well informed.

The clinically most important genera within the *Enterobacteriaceae* family discussed in this chapter are *Salmonella, Shigella, Edwardsiella, Escherichia coli, Klebsiella, Enterobacter, Serratia, Proteus-Providencia-Morganella* group, *Citrobacter,* and *Yersinia*. Brief descriptions of less-common enteric organisms such as *Ewingella, Hafnia, Kluyvera, Cedecea, Moellerella,* and *Plesiomonas* are also presented on the Companion Website. General and distinguishing characteristics (microscopic and colonial morphology), key biochemical reactions, and serologic procedures useful for isolation and identification are presented. Brief discussions of the clinical importance of the various organisms are also included. Additional information can be obtained from other sources (Abbot, 2003; Bopp, Brener, Fields, Wells, & Strockbine, 2003; Brooks, Butel, & Morse, 2001a; Gridley, 1998).

► GENERAL CHARACTERISTICS OF ENTERIC GRAM-NEGATIVE RODS

The *Enterobacteriaceae* are gram-negative rods or coccobacilli that grow well as facultative anaerobes. Their dimensions usually range from 0.3 to 1.0 μm in width and 0.6 to 6 μm in length. Most genera are motile because they possess peritrichous flagella that are scattered all over the body of the organism (peritrichous). However, at least two genera are consistently nonmotile. Presence of a capsule is also a variable feature. The organisms produce pili, also known as fimbrae, that stick outward from the wall and are used for conjugation and adherence. In some cases, the type of pili produced can increase the virulence of the organisms. As is the case with all gram-negative bacteria, the *Enterobacteriaceae* have **lipopolysaccharide (LPS)**, also known as **endotoxin** because it is part of the organism's structure. The LPS is an important structural feature that also plays a major role in pathogenesis, although the degree of toxicity varies considerably from one genus to the next, as well as among members within the same genus. The morbidity and mortality caused by enteric infections are often associated with the pathophysiological properties of LPS.

The organisms are nonfastidious, meaning that they do not have any special nutrient requirements and will grow readily on many routinely used laboratory media. Colonies appear wet, gray, circular, convex, and smooth with definite edges. Colony diameter on many different types of media is usually within the range of 2 to 4 mm after a 24-hour incubation period. Most *Enterobacteriaceae* are nonhemolytic. Growth and colony characteristics on selective, as well as differential media, are frequently used to narrow down the large number of possibilities when an enteric bacteria is suspected as the cause of disease. The *Enterobacteriaceae* tend to be very active metabolically. They ferment many different carbohydrates, resulting in a variety of end products. They also exhibit great antigenic variation, in part because of free exchange of genetic material via transfer of small pieces of circular DNA known as plasmids. This genetic exchange from one bacterium to another, processes known as transduction or conjugation, can occur even among members belonging to different genera. Furthermore, certain antigens may be lost completely or partially, depending on the microenvironment and/or innate properties of the bacteria. Thus, resistance to multiple antibiotics, as well as loss of protective immunity, may occur as a result of this genetic and antigenic variation. In addition to high antigenic variability, virulence factors associated with members of this family include LPS (endotoxin), presence of a capsule, expression of certain types of colonization factors (pili), resistance to killing by humoral factors present in serum, and sequestration of growth factors. According to the official definition, three characteristics that are common to all *Enterobacteriaceae* are: (1) they ferment glucose with the production of acid, (2) they reduce nitrates to nitrites, and (3) they do not produce oxidase (except for the recently added genus *Plesiomonas*). Efforts are being made to develop computer programs that can be used to expedite the identification of both common and uncommon isolates that belong in this very large family.

▶ BIOCHEMICAL IDENTIFICATION

Identification of an enteric gram-negative rod begins with the examination of differential media, Colonies are tested biochemically to confirm the characteristics of the *Enterobacteriaceae* and determine the species. Gram stain and colony morphology should always be correlated to biochemical reactions, antibiogram, and the organism's identification prior to reporting the laboratory result. If the identity does not correlate, then purity of the test organism should be checked and tests repeated to ensure accurate laboratory reports.

SELECTIVE AND DIFFERENTIAL MEDIA

In addition to the routinely inoculated agar plates, many different types of media have been developed to assist in identification of the enteric bacteria. Selective media contain ingredients that allow the growth of the bacteria of interest, but inhibit the growth of other bacteria that may also be present in the specimen. Some selective media contain dyes that allow growth of the enterics in general or a specific type of bacteria, but suppress the growth of other organisms; some also contain specific carbohydrates. Examples include eosin-methylene blue (EMB) agar; eosin Y, a dye, is bacteriostatic for gram-positive bacteria. Salmonella-Shigella (SS) agar selects for the growth of the salmonellae and shigellae, but inhibits gram-positive bacteria because of the presence of bile salts. Bismuth sulfite (BIS) medium (Figure 21-1 ■) is highly selective for the salmonellae. Differential media contain ingredients that may or may not be used by a given organism, and the subsequent appearance of colonies is helpful in identification. One very frequently used differential medium is MacConkey agar that contains lactose, as well as crystal violet and bile salts. Enterics that ferment lactose form pink colonies on MacConkey agar, whereas colorless colonies are formed by those that do not ferment the sugar. Sorbitol-MacConkey (SMAC) agar is used to screen for a specific strain of *E. coli* that secretes **verotoxin** or shiga-like toxin. *Salmonella* species are easily identified on xylose-lysine-deoxycholate (XLD), hektoen enteric (HE), Salmonella-Shigella (SS), and bismuth sulfite (BIS) (Figure 21-1) medium by the production of colonies with black centers because of the formation of H_2S. In many cases, a particular type of medium can have both selective and differential properties. Photos of many of these media can be viewed in ∞ Chapter 35, "Gastrointestinal System." Examples of some of the most commonly used selective and differential media are presented in Table 21-1✪.

USEFUL BIOCHEMICAL TESTS

Initial identification is often based on the oxidase test (with one exception, the *Enterobacteriaceae* are oxidase negative) and reactions seen after inoculation of either **Kligler's iron agar (KIA)** or **triple sugar iron (TSI) agar.** Both KIA and TSI have a small amount of glucose (0.1% w/v), a 10-fold amount of lactose (and sucrose in the case of TSI agar; 1% w/v), and phenol red as an indicator of pH (phenol red turns yellow if acid is produced). These media are used to demonstrate whether the isolate ferments lactose (KIA) or lactose and sucrose (TSI), produces gas during sugar fermentation, and has the ability to produce H_2S from an inorganic source of sulfur (i.e., ferrous sulfate). In preparation of these media, the agar is poured into a test tube that is then tilted at an angle before the agar hardens so that a slant with a deep butt is created. The agar is inoculated by stabbing a wire "needle" with the isolated organisms deep into the butt, carefully withdrawing the wire, and then streaking the slant. After a short incubation, the slant and butt will initially turn yellow if the bacteria produce a small amount of acid by fermenting glucose; however, the slant will eventually become red (alkaline) because of oxidation of the fermentation products to CO_2 and H_2O and formation of amines because of oxidative decarboxylation of proteins (alkaline/acid reaction). If the organisms ferment either sucrose or lactose, a large amount of acid will be produced so that both the butt and slant remain yellow (acid/acid reaction). Formation of "bubbles" in the medium is indicative of gas production. Some of the enterics, such as the great majority of the salmonellae, will use ferrous sulfate to produce H_2S gas that is manifested as a black iron-containing precipitate. Further tests are then selected on the basis of these reactions ∞ Chapter 9 provides further information on KIA and TSI testing.

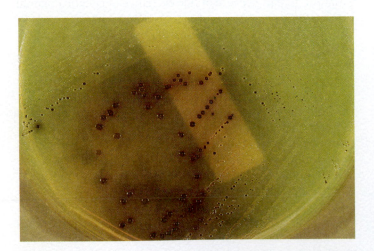

■ **FIGURE 21-1** *Salmonella* ser. Typhimurium growing on bismuth sulfite agar. The black colonies indicate hydrogen sulfide production.

> ℮ **REAL WORLD TIP**
>
> Black colonies on differential media should correlate with positive reactions for H_2S in the TSI/KIA and other test panels.

✪ TABLE 21-1

Examples of Commonly Used Selective and Differential Media

Medium	Carbohydrate	Color of Colonies	
		Fermenter	Nonfermenter
MacConkey	lactose	red or pink	colorless
Eosin methylene blue (EMB)	lactose	red or black with sheen	colorless
Salmonella-Shigella (SS)	lactose	red	colorless
Xylose-lysine-deoxycholate (XLD)	lactose, xylose	yellow	red (colorless)
Hektoen enteric (HE)	lactose, sucrose, salicin	yellow-orange	green, blue-green (colorless)
Thiosulfate citrate bile salts sucrose (TCBS)	sucrose	yellow	colorless

Source: Adapted from Reisner, B. S., & Woods, G. L. (2001). Medical bacteriology. In J. B. Henry (Ed.), Clinical diagnosis and management by laboratory methods (20th ed., pp. 1088–1118). Philadelphia: Saunders.

Tests that detect fermentation of specific carbohydrates, activities of enzymes, and ability to generate certain end products from substrates are extensively used for identification of specific isolates. Among the most often included tests are the following: oxidase, indole, methyl red, Voges-Proskauer (VP), citrate, motility, phenylalanine (or tryptophan) deaminase, ornithine decarboxylase, lysine decarboxylase, arginine dihydrolase, gelatin hydrolysis, growth in KCN, urease, H_2S, and fermentation of glucose (with or without the production of gas), lactose, and other carbohydrates. Lactose fermentation (as discussed earlier with KIA and TSI media) is an especially important test in that it distinguishes the major pathogens (*Salmonella* and *Shigella*) that are lactose negative from the **coliform** or enteric bacteria such as *E. coli, Enterobacter,* and *Klebsiella* that are lactose positive. Clinical laboratories vary to some extent in the series of biochemical tests that they use. Numerous commercially available kits consist of a panel of miniaturized and well-standardized tests. The basic principle in the reactions is the same as for conventional tube tests. The advantages of using kits include savings in turnaround-time and increased number of tests that can be rapidly set up with a minimum amount of inoculum. Kits usually contain anywhere from 12 to 50 different tests. In some cases, the reading of results and interpretation can be carried out by an instru-

ment. A disadvantage of automation is that some of the newer or less-common species may not be included in the database. For members of the *Enterobacteriaceae,* the API 20E (bio-Mérieux), Enterotube II (Becton Dickinson), and Fox Extra Gram Negative MIC/ID (MicroMedia) systems are available, among others. A photo of one example of these miniaturized tests, the API 20E strip, can be found in ∞ Chapter 9. Typical reaction patterns for some of the more commonly isolated and/or clinically most important isolates are shown in Table 21-2✪.

▶ SEROLOGIC IDENTIFICATION

The antigenic structure of the *Enterobacteriaceae* is very complex. More than 150 O antigens (somatic), more than 100 K antigens (capsular), and more than 50 H antigens (flagellar) have now been identified with the use of highly specific monoclonal antibodies. The identified **O antigens** are predominantly located in the LPS portion. The antigens found on a particular isolate constitute what is often referred to as the serotype of the organism. By convention, the antigenic formulas that are generated always list the antigens in the same sequence (O, K, and H). For example, *Salmonella typhi* (also known as *Salmonella* serotype Typhi) with O antigens 9 and 12, the **Vi antigen** (virulent capsular), phase 1 flagellar antigen d, and no phase 2 flagellar antigen, would have the following antigenic formula: 9,12(Vi):d:–. *Salmonella* serotype Typhimurium that has O antigens 1, 4, 5, and 12, no capsule, phase 1 flagellar antigen i, and phase 2 flagellar antigens 1 and 2 would have the following antigenic formula: 1,4,5,12:i:1,2. Identification of the O, K, and H antigens can be very useful because they may reveal serotypes that are associated with pathogenicity and provide epidemiologic information below the species level. The locations of the O, K, and H antigens are shown in Figure 21-2 ■. Serotyping of the *Enterobacteriaceae* is usually performed only in state health department or other reference laboratories. Although the organisms also have pili that

℮ REAL WORLD TIP

Remember that the IMViC (indole, methyl-red, Voges-Proskauer, citrate) reactions can be used to place an isolate into a possible genus. Refer to ∞ Chapter 9 to review Figure 9-14, "Presumptive Identification of Clinically Significant *Enterobacteriaceae* to Genus." This is useful when correlating test results to the identity of the isolate prior to reporting the laboratory result. If the presumptive genus and isolate identity do not match, do not report the results without investigating the cause of the discrepancy. *E. coli*, the most common isolate, is IMViC ++––.

✪ TABLE 21-2

Typical Biochemical Reactions of Selected *Enterobacteriaceae*

Organism	I	MR	VP	Cit	H₂S	U	PAD/TDA	Lys	Orn	MOT	Glu A	Glu G	Lac
Pathogens: *Salmonella typhi*	−	+	−	−	+	−	−	+	−	+	+	−	−
Salmonella, other	−	+	−	+	+	−	−	+	+	+	+	+	−
Shigella sonnei	−	+	−	−	−	−	−	−	+	−	+	−	−
Shigella, other	+/−	+	−	−	−	−	−	−	−	−	+	−	−
Edwardsiella tarda	+	+	−	−	+	−	−	+	+	+	+	+	−
Yersinia enterocolitica	+/−	+	−	−	−	+	−	−	+	+(22°C) −(35°C)	+	−	−
Yersinia pestis	−	+	−	−	−	−	−	−	−	−	+	−	−
Opportunists: *Escherichia coli*	+	+	−	−	−	−	−	+	+	+	+	+	+
Citrobacter koseri	+	+	−	+	−	+	−	−	+	+	+	+	+/−
Citrobacter freundii	−	+	−	+	+	+/−	−	−	−	+	+	+	+
Enterobacter aerogenes	−	−	+	+	−	−	−	+	+	+	+	+	+
Enterobacter cloacae	−	−	+	+	−	+	−	−	+	+	+	+	+
Pantoea agglomerans	−	+/−	+	+	−	−	−	−	−	+	+	−	−
Klebsiella pneumoniae	−	+	+	+	−	+	−	+	−	−	+	+	+
Klebsiella oxytoca	+	−	+	+	−	+	−	+	−	−	+	+	+
Serratia marcescens	−	−	+	+	−	−	−	+	+	+	+	+/−	−
Hafnia alvei	−	−	+	−	−	−	−	+	+	+	+	+	−
Proteus mirabilis	−	+	+/−	+	+	++	+	−	+	+	+	+	+
Proteus vulgaris	+	+	−	−	+	++	+	−	−	+	+	+	−
Morganella morganii	+	+	−	−	−	+	+	−	+	+	+	+	−
Providencia rettgeri	+	+	−	+	−	+	+	−	−	+	+	−	−
Providencia stuartii	+	+	−	+	−	−	+	−	−	+	+	−	−
Providencia alcalifaciens	+	+	−	+	−	−	+	−	−	+	+	+	−

I = indole production; MR = methyl red; VP = Voges-Proskauer; Cit = citrate; H₂S = production of hydrogen sulfide; U = urea hydrolysis; PAD/TDA = phenylalanine deaminase/tryptophan deaminase; Lys = lysine decarboxylase; Orn = ornithine decarboxylase; Mot = motility; Glu = glucose fermentation with production of acid (A) and gas (G); Lac = lactose fermentation. + = >50% of isolates; +/− = ~50% of isolates; − = <50% of isolates; ++ = rapid positive (within 4 hours).

are protein antigens, they are currently not included in any formal classification scheme.

O ANTIGENS

The letter *O* designation is derived from the German words "**O**hne hauch," meaning "without film." These antigens extend outward from the body of the bacteria, consist of complex hydrophilic polysaccharide, and exhibit great variation. They confer a high degree of immunologic specificity to a particular isolate. In most enterics, they consist of a basic trisaccharide unit (e.g., galactose-mannose-rhamnose) that is repeated many times. Basic units consisting of tetra- and pentasaccharides are also possible.

H ANTIGENS

The letter *H* stands for hauch, which means "film" in German. These antigens are found on the flagella. They are very fragile and can be easily denatured by heat, alcohol, and other treatments. They can also be mechanically knocked off by agitation of liquid media, although in this case they regenerate within about 3 to 6 minutes. They consist of several thousand molecules of a protein known as flagellin that contains a novel amino acid (ε-*N*-methyl lysine). The protein aggregates to form tubular structures that confer motility to the organism. Some of the *Salmonella* can express two different sets or phases of H antigens. A given cell produces H antigens in either phase 1 or phase 2, but not both. However, a single cell can "flip-flop" from one phase to another, and thus may evade immune destruction.

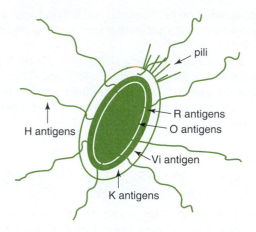

■ **FIGURE 21-2** Location of *Enterobacteriaceae* antigens. O antigens (somatic) are present on the body of the bacteria; H antigens are found on the flagella; K antigens are on the capsule; the Vi antigen is a capsular antigen that is produced primarily by *Salmonella typhi.*

K ANTIGENS

The **K antigens** are found on the capsule (kapsel in Danish). These are densely packed polysaccharides that closely surround the bacteria. Presence of a capsule allows the organism to evade phagocytosis and is indicative of increased virulence. The Vi antigen is a special type of K antigen that is produced primarily by *Salmonella typhi.* It consists of a simple carbohydrate (*N*-acetyl galactosaminouronic acid). *S. typhi* strains that produce Vi are more virulent than their counterparts that have lost the ability to produce it.

LPS

LPS consists of **lipid A**, the core or R antigens, and O antigens all in one long continuous piece that sticks outward from the outer membrane of the cell wall (Figure 21-3 ■). If LPS is still attached to the bacteria, it has no pathological effects. However, when the organisms are disrupted or lysed because of immune attack or when the correct antibiotic is administered, the lipid A portion can mediate numerous toxic effects. Pathophysiological consequences include fever, transient leukopenia, hypotension that may lead to shock, impaired oxygen perfusion into tissues resulting in acidosis, activation of the alternative complement cascade, and **disseminated intravascular coagulation (DIC)**. Death can occur as a result of massive organ dysfunction, shock, DIC, or a combination thereof. A photo showing the pooling of blood under the skin of a patient with endotoxemia is shown in ∞ Chapter 38, "Central Nervous System." Many of the effects of LPS effects are thought to be mediated by tumor necrosis factor-α (TNF-α) and possibly also by interleukin-1 (IL-1), both of which are major cytokines secreted by activated macrophages (see ∞ Chapter 10). Indeed, LPS is among the most potent, if not the most potent, activator of macrophages.

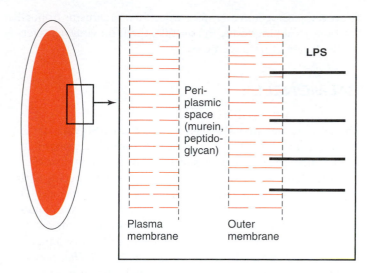

■ **FIGURE 21-3** Lipopolysaccharide (LPS) in cell wall. The diagram shows that the LPS of *Enterobacteriaceae,* as well as other gram-negative bacteria, protrudes outward from the outer membrane of the cell wall. LPS is the major factor associated with morbidity and mortality in patients infected with *Enterobacteriaceae.*

 Checkpoint! 21–1 (Chapter Objectives 1 and 5)

Which of the following characteristics apply to the Enterobacteriaceae family?

   A. *Glucose fermentation*
   B. *Lack of oxidase*
   C. *Nitrate reduction*
   D. *A and C are correct*
   E. *A, B, and C are correct*

 Checkpoint! 21–2 (Chapter Objective 4)

Fever, leucopenia, disseminated intravascular coagulation, and shock caused by infection with the Enterobacteriaceae are most strongly associated with which of the following?

   A. *Flagella*
   B. *LPS*
   C. *Exotoxin*
   D. *Capsule*
   E. *Pili*

▶ ENTERIC PATHOGENS

A pathogen is a biological agent that causes disease or illness to its host. The term is most often used for agents that disrupt the normal physiology of a multicellular animal or plant.

However, pathogens can infect unicellular organisms from all the biological kingdoms. In contrast, the term *virulence* refers to the degree of pathogenicity.

SALMONELLA

General Characteristics

The salmonellae, first discovered more than 100 years ago by an American scientist by the name of Salmon, were originally given names as if they were species. However, it is now clear that they represent a long continuum of a single species, with more than 2,400 different serologic types based on the O, H, and Vi antigens. In light of this information, some recent publications have opted to not italicize the serotype name and to begin it with a capital letter. In addition, at least two names have been proposed for the one species (i.e., *S. choleraesuis, S. enterica*). In this chapter, the nomenclature in use by the CDC is used, except for *S. typhi* (Brenner et al., 2000). Based on DNA-DNA hybridization studies, there are seven groups. Human infections are caused almost exclusively to group I, which contains more than 1,400 serotypes; in rare cases, isolates belonging to groups IIIa and IIIb have been reported.

Useful Cultural, Biochemical, and Other Characteristics

In general, these motile bacteria do not ferment either lactose or sucrose and produce H_2S (see Table 21-2). They tend to be resistant to chemicals such as sodium deoxycholate, brilliant green, and sodium tetrathionate that inhibit the growth of other enteric organisms. These compounds are often incorporated into media that are used for isolation of the salmonellae. The great majority can be found in the intestinal tracts of both humans and animals (e.g., poultry, pigs, cattle, rodents, parrots, pet turtles, and pet iguanas). Infection is the result of ingestion of food and water that has been contaminated with either human or animal feces. A large number of the organisms (in the range of 10^5 to 10^8) must be ingested for infection to occur because these organisms are susceptible to the acidity of the stomach.

Stool, blood, urine, and bone marrow are the usual types of specimens used for culture. Duodenal drainage may be obtained in the case of carriers with gallbladder problems. Media such as EMB, MacConkey, or deoxycholate are frequently used to demonstrate lack of lactose fermentation. Bismuth sulfite (Figure 21-1) medium is used to rapidly detect H_2S production of *S. typhi* and other *Salmonella* that results in formation of black colonies. Salmonella-Shigella (SS) agar, hektoen enteric agar, XLD, or deoxycholate-citrate agar select for growth of the *Salmonella* and *Shigella* and prevent or minimize the growth of other enteric bacteria. H_2S production can also be detected on SS, HE, and XLD. Stool specimens may be incubated in enrichment media such as gram-negative, selenite F or tetrathionate broth which facilitate growth of the salmonellae and inhibit other enterics, prior to inoculation of selective and differential media. Final identification of isolated

organisms is based on biochemical reaction patterns and slide agglutination tests with antibodies specific for antigens of the salmonellae.

Other genera may produce H_2S (Table 21-2). A positive lysine decarboxylase and negative indole and ONPG is characteristic of *Salmonella*. *S. typhi* can be differentiated from other *Salmonella* species by its negative citrate and ornithine decarboxylase test results.

 REAL WORLD TIP

The PYR test can be used to quickly separate *Salmonella* and *E. coli* from *Citrobacter* species. *Salmonella* and *E. coli* are negative while *Citrobacter* species are positive (Inoue et al., 1996; York et al., 2000).

The agglutination test is usually performed using commercially available kits that detect O antigens so that the isolate can be placed into one of the A, B, C_1, C_2, D, or E serogroups. The Widal test is a tube agglutination assay that detects serum antibodies against specific O and H antigens, as well as the Vi antigen. Agglutinating antibodies increase dramatically during the second and third weeks after infection. Twofold dilutions of two serum samples, taken 1 to 2 weeks apart, are tested against representative salmonellae. A high or rising titer ($\geq$160) of antibodies against O antigens indicates active infection; a high titer ($\geq$160) of anti-H antibody suggests past infection or immunization; a high titer against the Vi capsular antigen occurs in some carriers. Potential cross-reactivity with other *Enterobacteriaceae*, however, limits the usefulness of this test.

 REAL WORLD TIP

Appearance of a black color in KIA, TSI, and bismuth sulfite media is strongly suggestive of *Salmonella*.

Clinical Significance

Pathogenesis and Infectious Diseases. The salmonellae are considered to be overt pathogens because they frequently cause disease in humans. Every year approximately 40,000 cases of **salmonellosis** are reported in the United States, although the true number of infections is thought to be 30-fold (or more) higher; approximately 600 deaths/year are attributed to these bacteria. The salmonellae are often implicated as the cause of severe infections in patients with AIDS. Typhoid fever ("enteric fever"), bacteremia, and enterocolitis are the three major types of diseases produced (Table 21-3✿).

✪ TABLE 21-3

Clinically Distinguishable Infections Caused by *Salmonella* and *Shigella*

Serotype/Species	Disease	Comments

Salmonella
  Salmonella ser. Typhi
  Salmonella ser. Paratyphi A/B
	Typhoid fever	High fever, constipation followed by bloody diarrhea, weakness, stomach pain, headache; rash (rose spots) may be present; carriers possible

Salmonella ser. Cholerae-suis
  Salmonella ser. Enteritidis
  Salmonella ser. Dublin, etc.
	Bacteremia	Early invasion of blood, fever, focal lesions in lungs, bones, meninges; diarrhea often absent; seen primarily in elderly, debilitated persons

Salmonella ser. Typhimurium
  Salmonella ser. Potsdam
  Salmonella ser. Loma linda, etc.
	Enterocolitis	Diarrhea, low-grade fever, nausea, vomiting, headache; illness usually resolves within a week without treatment

Shigella
  S. dysenteriae
  S. flexneri
  S. boydii
  S. sonnei
	Dysentery	Abrupt onset of fever, abdominal pain, watery diarrhea followed by bloody diarrhea (blood, mucus, pus in stools); meningismus (meningeal irritation) possible

The incidence of typhoid fever has decreased dramatically in the United States, whereas the incidence of the latter two continues to steadily increase (Crum, 2003).

S. typhi or *Salmonella* ser. Typhi, is the major cause of **typhoid fever.** Each year approximately 400 cases are reported in the United States, with 70% having been acquired while traveling outside the country (www.cdc.gov/travel/diseases/typhoid.htm). In developing countries, the disease occurs in an estimated 12.5 million persons. Unlike the vast majority of the other salmonellae, *S. typhi* is found exclusively in humans. The course of infection follows a typical pattern, as summarized in Figure 21-4 ■. A large number of these organisms must be ingested, as they are susceptible to the acidity of the stomach, which at times reaches a pH as low as 2. However, if viable bacteria reach the small intestine, they proliferate in the Peyer's patches (small collections of lymphoid tissue). The Peyer's patches become infiltrated with inflammatory cells, resulting in enlargement, hyperplasia, and necrosis at the site. From there the organisms travel through the lymphatic and blood circulatory systems and become disseminated to many parts of the body, including gallbladder, liver, spleen, and kidneys. After an incubation period of approximately 2 weeks, fever rises to a high plateau (up to 104°F or 40°C) and may stay high for 4 to 8 weeks in untreated cases.

Early in the disease (first week after infection) there is constipation; bloody diarrhea appears thereafter. Weakness, stomach pains, headache, loss of appetite, hepatomegaly, and splenomegaly are often noted. Necrotic lesions appear in the liver, and there is inflammation of the gallbladder, lungs, periosteum, and other organs. A pale, pinkish skin rash (referred to as "rose spots" because the lesions resemble a

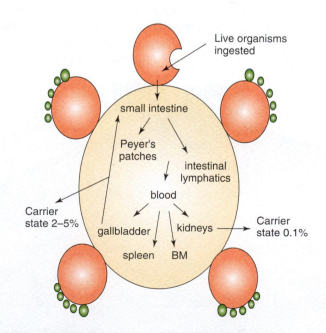

■ **FIGURE 21-4** Overview of *Salmonella typhi* infection.
Diagram was originally conceived by Leonard Bullas, Ph.D., Emeritus Professor at Loma Linda University, Loma Linda, CA. Reproduced with permission.

rosebud) may be visible on the abdomen or chest (Figure 21-5 ■) in some cases while the bacteria are in the blood. The white blood cell (WBC) count is either normal or low. Blood cultures are positive during the first and second weeks after infection; stool cultures are positive from the second week on. Mortality is approximately 10% to 15%, and intestinal hemorrhage and perforation are relatively common without treatment. With appropriate antibiotic treatment, mortality is less than 1%, and complications are rare. A carrier state is established in approximately 2% to 5% of individuals after resolution of the disease. The major reservoir in these cases is the gallbladder because bile is a good culture medium for these bacteria. The gallbladder dispenses bile into the small intestine and also the organisms if they are present. Carriers usually shed the bacteria in the stool, although shedding in urine is also possible. Infection with either *S. typhi* or *Salmonella* ser. Paratyphi usually results in some degree of immunity after recovery. IgA at the intestinal mucosa may prevent attachment of the organisms. Serum antibodies against the O and Vi antigens are generally associated with resistance. However, reinfection followed by mild disease is possible as early as a few weeks after recovery, despite the presence of antibodies.

 REAL WORLD TIP

A person who has recovered from typhoid fever may continue to shed *S. typhi* for a long time. Thus, family members and other close contacts of the recovered individuals may become infected.

Bacteremia with focal lesions is most often seen after infection with *Salmonella* ser. Choleraesuis, but can occur following infection with virtually any serotype. Elderly, debilitated individuals with chronic underlying diseases and children with

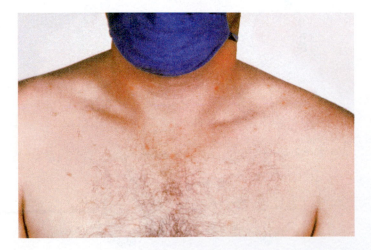

■ **FIGURE 21-5** Rose spots on the chest of a patient with typhoid fever.
Photo courtesy of CDC, Armed Forces Institute of Pathology, Charles N. Farmer.

enterocolitis are the most susceptible. Persons who are homozygous for sickle cell anemia are especially prone to infections with *Salmonella*. The incubation period is variable, and onset of illness is abrupt. There is early invasion of the blood, a rapidly rising fever that spikes, and development of lesions in the lungs, bones, meninges, and other organs. Thus, patients exhibit symptoms of pneumonia, osteomyelitis, and meningitis. Blood cultures are positive during high fever. Diarrhea usually does not occur, and the organisms are only rarely isolated from stool specimens.

Enterocolitis (old name: gastroenteritis) is by far the most common manifestation of infection with the salmonellae. *Salmonella* ser.Typhimurium and *Salmonella* ser. Enteritidis are the most commonly isolated from these cases, but the condition can be caused by any of the group I serotypes (Bender et al., 2001; CDC, 2003a). A substantial increase in *Salmonella* ser. Newport has been observed in the United States since the mid-1990s. It appears that the large outbreak of multi-drug-resistant *Salmonella* ser. Newport in 2002 may be linked to the emergence of this strain in cattle and the consumption of ground beef (CDC, 2002). The disease of enterocolitis is manifested as diarrhea (with few, if any, leukocytes in stool), fever, nausea, vomiting, and headache that occur 8 to 48 hours after ingestion of the organisms. Fever is low-grade and common; inflammation of the small and large intestine occurs frequently. The illness usually resolves on its own within about 4 to 7 days. Stool cultures, however, may remain positive for several weeks after recovery. According to FoodNet, *Salmonella* together with *Shigella* and *Campylobacter* are responsible for the highest incidence of bacterial food-borne illness in the United States (CDC, 2003b; www.cdc.gov/foodnet/surveillance.htm). Infants, the elderly, and those with immunodeficiency (e.g., AIDS patients) are more likely to have severe illness.

Treatment and Prevention.   The great majority of individuals with enterocolitis do not require treatment, although it is strongly recommended that neonates be treated. Treatment can cause the organism to retreat to the gallbladder and create a carrier state. In contrast, typhoid fever and bacteremia must be treated with an appropriate antibiotic. Unfortunately, multidrug resistance has increased dramatically over the years, worldwide in the case of *S. typhi*. A fluoroquinolone drug is the empiric drug of choice for typhoid fever. Ampicillin, trimethoprim-sulfamethoxazole, and third-generation cephalosporins such as ciprofloxacin may be effective. Patients usually feel much better within just 2 to 3 days. Cases of untreated typhoid fever may continue to have fever for weeks to months, and up to 20% may die from complications. Because multidrug resistance is a problem with the salmonellae, at least partly because of the use of antibiotics as growth promoters in food animals, antibiotic susceptibility testing should be performed. Eradication of the organisms in chronic carriers frequently requires long-term ampicillin together with cholecystectomy (i.e., surgical removal of the gallbladder). Although there are usually no long-term consequences of infection, a small percentage of individuals develop joint pains, eye irritation, and other symptoms typical of Reiter's syndrome (a reactive, inflammatory arthritis) that can lead to chronic arthritis. Antibiotic treatment does not appear to be a determining factor as to whether or not the person will later develop arthritis.

There are now two different vaccines available for immunization. A third heat-phenol-inactivated vaccine manufactured by Wyeth-Ayerst that was previously approved for use has now been discontinued. The live attenuated vaccine consisting of rough strains of *S. typhi* is taken orally in capsular form four times with a 2-day interval between doses and is considered to be protective for 5 years. The other vaccine consists of purified Vi polysaccharide, is given in a single injection, and provides protection for about 2 years. However, immunity is not absolute with either vaccine (60% to 80% efficacy), and disease may develop if a large enough number of organisms are ingested. These vaccines are used primarily during outbreaks of salmonellosis, although travelers to countries where typhoid fever is common are often encouraged to receive immunization. Prevention of infection with the salmonellae relies on proper methods of sewage disposal, maintenance of unpolluted water supplies, proper handling of food supplies of animal origin, proper cooking of foods immediately prior to eating, proper health control of public eating places, and identification and treatment of carriers in the case of *S. typhi*.

 Checkpoint! 21–3 (Chapter Objective 3)

In carriers of Salmonella typhi, the organisms are most likely to reside in which of the following sites?

    A. *Liver*
    B. *Gallbladder*
    C. *Lungs*
    D. *Kidneys*
    E. *Spleen*

SHIGELLA

General Characteristics

New isolates of *Shigella*, like *Salmonella*, were originally given species names. However, because of great similarity, these organisms have now been classified into four serogroups: serogroup A (*S. dysenteriae*, 12 serotypes), serogroup B (*S. flexneri*, 6 serotypes), serogroup C (*S. boydii*, 23 serotypes), and serogroup D (*S. sonnei*, 1 serotype). In this chapter, the traditional nomenclature is used. Historically, **shigellosis** was always thought of as a "disease of armies." Whenever two armies fought, both would invariably develop severe diarrhea, but the losing army would be the one that always developed the disease first. Interestingly, it did not seem to matter which army had more soldiers, horses, cannons, or other weapons of war. Thus, it appears that these bacteria may have changed the course of history a number of times. Today, shigellosis is

primarily thought of as a "disease of institutions," especially where there is crowding and substandard conditions. Day-care centers, jails, prisons, mental institutions, and inner-city apartments are common sites of outbreaks. Children below the age of 10 years who regularly attend day-care centers account for approximately 50% of cases in the United States. Well-publicized outbreaks have also occurred on luxury cruise ships. In some cases, the ships have had to return to port because so many of the passengers and crew were seriously ill. Transmission occurs person-to-person via the five "Fs" (friends, flies, fingers, feces, and food), as well as contaminated water. The shigellae are naturally found only in the intestinal tracts of humans and some nonhuman primates. Recent DNA analyses have indicated that they are virtually identical to *E. coli* (Lan & Reeves, 2002).

 REAL WORLD TIP

Remember *Shigella* spp. as the "do nothing" organism. Most of the biochemical reactions, including motility, are negative for this genus.

Useful Cultural, Biochemical, and Other Characteristics

The shigellae are slender gram-negative rods, although coccobacillary forms are often seen in early cultures. They are consistently nonmotile because they lack flagella. They are facultative anaerobes, but tend to grow better in the presence of oxygen. The organisms do not ferment lactose, but do ferment glucose and other carbohydrates with the production of acid and no gas (see Table 21-2). The round colonies that appear on blood agar are convex, and transparent. Properties often used to distinguish *Shigella* from *Salmonella* include lack of motility, citrate utilization, lysine decarboxylation, and no production of H_2S.

Figure 21-6 ■ demonstrates that the four serogroups can be differentiated on the basis of relatively few biochemical tests: mannitol, lactose, and indole. More than 40 serotypes, based on the O antigens, have been identified so far. There is considerable overlap, however, in the O antigens among the different serogroups, as well as with other enteric bacilli. Overall, the biochemical tests and antigenic serotyping after isolation on selective and differential media are as described for the salmonellae.

Clinical Significance

Pathogenesis and Infectious Disease. The organisms are responsible for **dysentery**, a diarrheal disease also known as bacillary dysentery or shigellosis when *Shigella* is isolated (see Table 21-3). Although dysentery can be caused by a variety of other agents such as some amoeba, parasitic worms, and caustic chemicals, these bacteria are the leading cause in the United States.

Dysentery is characterized by an intense inflammatory response against the organisms, resulting in the hallmark

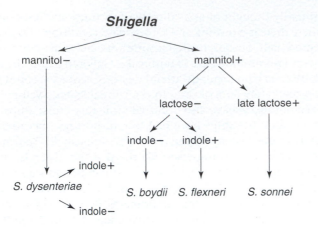

FIGURE 21-6 Scheme for identification of pathogenic *Shigella*. The species of *Shigella* can be differentiated on the basis of relatively few biochemical tests, as shown in this diagram.

presentation of blood and pus in the stool (Figure 21-7 ■). Disease severity is somewhat dependent on the serogroup causing the infection, with *S. dysenteriae* causing the most severe, *S. flexneri* and *S. boydii* causing moderately severe, and *S. sonnei* causing relatively mild disease. Protracted epidemics and pandemics and complications such as leukemoid reaction and hemolytic uremic syndrome have been linked to *S. dysenteriae*. In the United States and other industrialized countries, *S. sonnei* is the most common isolate. The disease is caused by the endotoxin (LPS) and also an exotoxin (**shiga toxin**) that is produced primarily by *S. dysenteriae*. The heat-labile exotoxin is somewhat similar to one of the toxins produced by *E. coli,* but is more versatile. It can act as an enterotoxin in producing diarrhea and also as a neurotoxin, potentially resulting in meningismus (intense pain and hyperactivity of the meningocortical area of the brain), coma, and death.

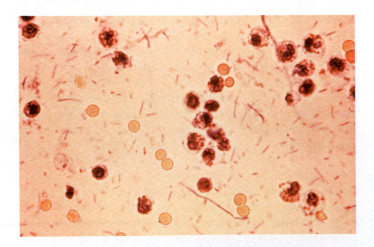

FIGURE 21-7 Stool from patient with shigellosis. *Shigella* cause bacillary dysentery that is characterized by the appearance of blood and pus in the stool. Note the presence of both red and white blood cells.
Photo courtesy of the Centers for Disease Control (CDC).

In contrast to the salmonellae, the shigellae are highly infectious; ingestion of less than 1,000 organisms can result in disease. Once the organisms reach the intestinal tract, they invade mucosal epithelial cells (i.e., M cells) by induced phagocytosis, exit from the phagocytic vacuole, multiply in the epithelial cell cytoplasm, and spread to other cells in the vicinity. After an incubation period of only 1 to 2 days, there is abrupt onset of fever, abdominal pain, and watery diarrhea (attributed to the action of the exotoxin). These very early manifestations are followed approximately 1 day later by increasing passage of stools that are less liquid, but contain blood, mucus, and dead cells sloughed from the intestinal wall. Bowel movements are accompanied by intense pain in the lower abdomen and rectal spasms (tenesmus). Meningismus, facial contortions, and vomiting may occur in some individuals. More than 50% of cases in the United States are mild and subside spontaneously in about 2 to 5 days. Bacteremia, in contrast to the salmonellae, is very rare. Children and the elderly are most likely to develop dehydration and acidosis, which can lead to death. After recovery, most individuals shed the organisms in the stool for only a short period of time, although a few may become chronic carriers and have recurrent disease episodes. Serum antibodies do develop, but these are not protective against reinfection.

Treatment and Prevention.   If treatment is necessary, ciprofloxacin, ampicillin, trimethoprim-sulfamethoxazole, tetracycline, and chloramphenicol can be effective. However, multiple-drug resistance is very common among the shigellae and can be transmitted by plasmids. Chemoprophylaxis has been attempted in military personnel for brief periods of time, but resistant strains have emerged rapidly. Prevention is dependent on sanitary food and water supplies, appropriate sewage disposal, disinfection of feces, fly control, and isolation of patients. In addition, subclinical cases and carriers should be identified and treated.

EDWARDSIELLA TARDA

General Characteristics
E. tarda is primarily found in freshwater fish, both feral and farmed. They cause hemorrhagic septicemia in several commercially important fish species. However, the organism has a very broad host range and has been isolated from turtles, lizards, snakes, alligators, crayfish, birds, and mammals, as well as directly from lakes, rivers, and sewage water.

Useful Cultural, Biochemical, and Other Characteristics
These bacteria are motile, gram-negative rods that produce H_2S and ferment glucose with the production of gas, but do not ferment lactose, sucrose, or most other sugars. The great majority of isolates are positive in the tests for indole, methyl red, and lysine and ornithine decarboxylases. Results from the Voges-Proskauer, citrate, urease, phenylalanine deaminase,

gelatin hydrolysis, and arginine dihydrolase assays are negative. The organisms resemble the salmonellae morphologically and in colony appearance on standard enteric plating media. The positive indole reaction and negative results in agglutination tests using antisera specific for *Salmonella* are useful in distinguishing *E. tarda* from *Salmonella*.

 REAL WORLD TIP

E. tarda is intrinsically resistant to colistin, so a sensitive susceptibility result should be investigated as a potential identification error.

Clinical Significance

Pathogenesis and Infectious Diseases. In humans, the most likely site for localization is the intestinal tract. Indeed the great majority (>80%) of human cases are associated with gastrointestinal disease. It appears likely that their prevalence is under reported because they are often found together with other potential pathogens and because many clinical laboratories do not identify all gram-negative isolates from the intestinal tract. *E. tarda* is also known to cause wound infections such as fish hook injuries, osteomyelitis, peritonitis, myonecrosis, cholecystitis, and sepsis (Slaven, Lopez, Hart, & Sanders, 2001; Wang et al., 2005). One report describes a case of neonatal sepsis caused by the same strain of *E. tarda* that was acquired by the infant's mother at 6 months of gestation while swimming in lake water (Mowbray, Buck, Humbaugh, & Marshall, 2003). Although these organisms are only occasionally isolated from human infections, they have been found in stool, blood, urine, CSF, peritoneal fluid, bile, and wound specimens.

The organisms are similar to the salmonellae in at least some pathogenic mechanisms. Invasion through epithelial cells in the intestinal lumen, resulting in systemic disease, has been reported. *E. tarda* can apparently evade host immune defenses and proliferate rapidly in a seemingly uncontrolled manner. Survival and replication, even in macrophages, has been reported. Recent studies in which genes involved in iron transport, survival in serum, motility, and catalase production were disrupted suggest that there is a correlation with these factors and virulence. Using proteomic analysis, flagellin and SseB have been identified as virulent strain-specific proteins (Tan et al., 2002), whereas a functional genomics approach has been used to identify 14 virulence genes (Srinivasa Rao, Lim, & Leung, 2003).

Treatment and Prevention. The bacteria are almost always susceptible to antibiotics that are commonly used for gram-negative bacteria (e.g., aminoglycosides, cephalosporins, imipenem, and ciprofloxacin). However, in extraintestinal cases, which are usually seen only in patients with hepatobiliary disease, hemoglobinopathies, or other significant underlying medical condition, the fatality rate is nearly 50%.

Suitable immunodiagnostic tests have been difficult to develop because of high cross-reactivity among antigens of *E. tarda* with those of certain *Aeromonas* and *Pseudomonas* species. There is currently no vaccine available to prevent infection.

Other species of *Edwardsiella* that are rarely isolated from human infections include *E. hoshinae* and *E. ictaluri,* both of which have been associated with diarrhea, wound infections, and sepsis.

 Checkpoint! 21–4 (Chapter Objective 7)

One day after a picnic featuring potato salad and chicken, 10 of the attendees developed diarrhea. Two of them became sick enough to be hospitalized. A motile gram-negative rod that was negative for lactose fermentation but positive for H₂S production, was isolated from stool samples of both patients. Given this scenario, which of the following is most likely to be the cause of the diarrhea?

A. Escherichia coli
B. Salmonella ser. Typhimurium
C. Enterobacter aerogenes
D. Shigella flexneri
E. Klebsiella pneumoniae

YERSINIA SPECIES

General Characteristics

The *Yersinia* are facultatively anaerobic or microaerophilic short, ovoid to rod-shaped gram-negative bacilli. The organisms are nonmotile at 37°C, although some species become motile at temperatures below 30°C. *Y. pestis,* the cause of **plague** ("Black Death" and pestilence), is by far the most notorious species in this genus, having killed many millions of people over the course of centuries. Although it is not found in the intestinal tracts of humans or animals, it is a member of the *Enterobacteriaceae* family. These bacteria have a long and infamous history as the cause of plague in humans, rodents, and many other mammals. In addition, this species is classified by the Centers for Disease Control and Prevention (CDC) in Category A, which contains the most dangerous of all potential bioterrorism agents (see ∞ Chapter 42 for further information). *Y. pestis* exhibits a striking bipolar ("safety pin") appearance, especially with Wayson's stain, and to a lesser extent also with Wright's stain and Giemsa; it does not have bipolar morphology on a Gram stain. The other two species of concern to humans are *Y. enterocolitica* and *Y. pseudotuberculosis,* both of which can cause enterocolitis and mesenteric adenitis. *Y. pseudotuberculosis* causes pseudotuberculosis in birds, a variety of other animals, and, on rare occasions, humans. The *Yersinia* species produce a large number of virulence factors, some of which are antigens that induce a potent inflammatory response.

Useful Cultural, Biochemical, and Other Characteristics

Yersinia species ferment mannitol, but not lactose, and they are PYR, methyl red, and catalase positive. They do not use citrate as a sole source of carbon. Blood, aspirates of enlarged lymph nodes, sputum, and cerebrospinal fluid (CSF) are typical specimens taken from patients suspected of being infected with *Y. pestis*. Isolation and culture is done in laboratories with biosafety level 3 facilities. Growth of *Y. pestis* is relatively slow on blood and MacConkey agar and in infusion broth. Best growth is obtained at ~25°C to 28°C. Colonies on blood agar resemble fried eggs. The peripheral growth around the central portion contains capsular material that forms strings when scooped up with a loop. The layer of polysaccharide that forms around *Y. pestis* is less densely packed compared to the capsules of most other bacteria and hence is sometimes referred to as a "slime layer." The organisms are relatively inert biochemically, although they ferment both glucose and mannitol. *Y. pestis* is negative for urease.

Molecular techniques for *Y. pestis* identification are available at the CDC. *Y. pestis* produces at least 19 different antigens, 15 of which are shared by closely related *Y. pseudotuberculosis*. The most important ones associated with virulence are (1) LPS, similar to the LPS of enteric bacteria, but is 50 to 100 times more potent; (2) fraction I (FI), a heat-labile envelope protein that is the main antigen responsible for both virulence (it is antiphagocytic) and immunity and is produced mainly at 37°C; (3) the V-W antigen system (V antigen is a cell-bound protein, W antigen is an excreted lipoprotein); (4) an exotoxin that appears to act on the peripheral vascular system of humans, leading to hemoconcentration and shock; (5) coagulase that is produced at 28°C; and (6) bacteriocin that kills some bacteria, including *Yersinia* species other than *Y. pestis*. For lethal infection to occur, *Y. pestis* must produce at least the first four factors. Serum samples may be tested for specific antibodies. A convalescent serum antibody titer of 16 or greater is presumptive evidence for *Y. pestis* infection. A twofold rise in the titer in acute, and convalescent serum samples confirm the diagnosis of plague. Additional information on *Yersinia* species is readily available (Bockemuhl & Wong, 2003; Brooks et al., 2001b).

 REAL WORLD TIP

Wild and commensal animals (e.g., ground squirrels, rats, feral cats) that are sick should not be handled because they may have plague.

For *Y. enterocolitica* and *Y. pseudotuberculosis,* stool samples and rectal swabs are collected. Types of media inoculated include blood agar, MacConkey agar, Hektoen enteric agar, XLD agar, and gram-negative enrichment broth. Colonies on blood and MacConkey agar are smooth, colorless, and <1 mm in diameter. The celfsulodin-irgasan-novobiocin (CIN) medium is designed specifically for *Y. enterocolitica* and is commercially available. It contains a peptone agar base with mannitol, neutral red, and crystal violet, as well as cefsulodin, irgasan (3,3',4',5-tetra-chlorosalicylanilide), and novobiocin that have antibacterial properties. Fecal specimens are streaked onto the agar and incubated at room temperature for 48 hours. *Y. enterocolitica* colonies look like a target with a red center and a clear edge. *Aeromonas* species may grow on CIN agar, but most other bacteria will not. "Cold enrichment" is another procedure that is sometimes used to increase its isolation. A small fecal sample or rectal swab is placed into buffered saline with a 7.6 pH and incubated at 4°C for 2 to 4 weeks. Because *Y. enterocolitica* and *Y. pseudotuberculosis* survive this process well, whereas most other enterics do not, the preparation becomes "enriched" with *Yersinia*. In addition, both species usually produce urease and most other bacteria in stool samples do not, the rapid urea test is useful in facilitating identification. Motility is another useful characteristic; both species are motile at room temperature (~25°C), but not at 37°C, which is unique among the *Enterobacteriaceae*. In some cases, serotyping may be performed. *Y. enterocolitica* has more than 50 serotypes, with 03, 08, and 09 being the most common isolates from humans. *Y. pseudotuberculosis* has at least 6 serotypes, with 01 being the most often isolated from humans. The two species can be differentiated on the basis of two tests: *Y. enterocolitica* is positive for ornithine decarboxylase and ferments sucrose, whereas *Y. pseudotuberculosis* is negative for both.

Clinical Significance

Pathogenesis and Infectious Disease.
Y. pestis, as mentioned earlier, is not found in the intestinal tracts of either humans or animals. Humans develop plague after the bite of an infected flea, direct contact with an infected animal such as a rat or ground squirrel, or via inhalation of contaminated aerosols. Shortly after entry, the organisms are phagocytized by neutrophils and macrophages, but can multiply both intra- and extracellularly. Robust production of a capsule (the "slime layer" that includes FI) at 37°C, allows many of the organisms to escape destruction and travel via the lymphatics to the lymph nodes. The lymph nodes swell to large proportions, sometimes up to 4 cm in diameter, because of a strong inflammatory response and form what are known as "buboes." At this point, the patient has bubonic plague, which represents about 95% of human plague cases in the United States. Following an incubation period of 1 to 7 days, the onset of symptoms is abrupt. The large buboes are very painful, and there is high fever, delirium, vomiting, diarrhea, edema, and disseminated intravascular coagulation. Fatality rate is ~50% within about 3 to 5 days in untreated individuals. Pneumonic plague (~5% of human plague cases in the United States) occurs when the buboes burst, releasing the organisms into the blood circulation or via inhalation of contaminated aerosols. The lungs become filled with fluid, the sputum is bloody and frothy, and the patient has great difficulty breathing. In cases of untreated pneumonic plague, the fatality rate approaches 100% within 3 days. Isolation of patients suspected of having plague, either

bubonic or pneumonic, is mandatory. Patients with bubonic plague have a high incidence of pulmonary involvement, and the organisms can be easily spread by aerosols. *Y. pestis* is frequently referred to as the "ultimate pathogen" because it is a highly virulent infectious agent that can rapidly kill even the healthiest of individuals within a very short time. Streptomycin is the drug of choice, although chloramphenicol and tetracycline are also effective. Sometimes streptomycin is used in combination with one of the two alternative drugs. Unfortunately, high-level multi-drug-resistant *Y. pestis* strains have been reported to the World Health Organization. In some cases, the resistance has been linked to transmissible plasmids. The incidence of human plague in the United States remains low, with an annual average of about 13 cases.

Y. enterocolita and *Y. pseudotuberculosis* are found in the feces and lymph nodes of both healthy and sick animals, in materials contaminated with feces, and in cadavers of decaying domestic, farm, and wild animals. The most likely route of transmission to humans is by ingestion of food or water contaminated with animal feces; person-to-person transmission is thought to be rare. Fever, abdominal pain, and occasional bloody diarrhea are typical symptoms that appear in about 5 to 10 days after ingesting a large number of the organisms ($10^8 - 10^9$). Multiplication in the gut (especially ileum) leads to inflammation, ulceration, and the appearance of blood in the stool, although diarrhea can range from watery to bloody. Sometimes the infection progresses to the mesenteric lymph nodes (mesenteric adenitis), resulting in severe pain. In some patients, the pain occurs in the right lower quadrant of the abdomen, mimicking appendicitis. Laparotomy (exploratory surgery) is then often performed to determine the etiology. After the acute phase, the development of arthritis, arthralgia, and erythema nodosum in some individuals suggests an aberrant immunological reaction to the bacteria.

A cluster of *Y. enterocolitica* infections in 2002 involved nine Chicago infants under the age of 1 year (CDC, 2003c). All the infants had either eaten contaminated chitterlings (pork intestines) or had been in a household in which they were prepared. Clinical illness was limited to gastroenteritis, which in six cases was very severe and required hospitalization. All the infants eventually recovered. In the early 1990s, several episodes of bacteremia and shock, followed in some cases by death, were linked to transfusion of contaminated packed red blood cells. These *Yersinia* species can multiply to high numbers in erythrocytes, even when refrigerated, with no visible evidence of growth. Invasiveness into eukaryotic cells is thought to contribute to the pathogenicity of these bacteria. On rare occasions, the organisms have been isolated from cases of conjunctivitis, meningitis, and pneumonia. Overall, the incidence of yersiniosis has been decreasing for a number of years, although the reasons for the decline remain unclear. Most *Yersinia* infections causing diarrhea are self-limiting; deaths usually occur only in immunocompromised patients because of meningitis or sepsis. Some strains of *Y. enterocolitica* produce a heat-

stable enterotoxin, although its significance in diarrheal disease is not clear.

Treatment and Prevention. If treatment is required, aminoglycosides, chloramphenicol, trimethoprim-sulfamethoxazole, tetracycline, piperacillin, fluoroquinolones, and third-generation cephalosporins are usually effective. Resistance to ampicillin and first-generation cephalosporins is common.

Checkpoint! 21–5 (Chapter Objective 3)

Infection with which of the following organisms is most likely to lead to a condition simulating acute appendicitis?
  A. *Klebsiella pneumoniae*
  B. *Yersinia pestis*
  C. *Salmonella typhi*
  D. *Brucella melitensis*
  E. *Yersinia enterocolitica*

▶ ENTERIC OPPORTUNISTS

Opportunists are organisms that usually do not cause harm to a person with a healthy immune system, but can affect people with poorly functioning or suppressed immune defenses. The immune system consists of soluble substances, cells, tissues, and organs that work in concert to protect against infectious agents, as well as inanimate materials that may enter the body (see ∞ Chapters 4 and 10 for further information). Depression or dysfunction of this interactive and highly complex system increases the risk for infection and subsequent development of clinically relevant disease. Numerous factors can lead to immune depression, including malnutrition, certain infectious and other diseases (e.g., AIDS, diabetes mellitus), genetic predisposition, chemotherapy for cancer, and other medical procedures. There are literally many millions of people that are immunocompromised at least to some extent.

Many of the *Enterobacteriaceae* have developed antibiotic resistance mechanisms. Additional testing such as the Hodge test or ESBL screen may need to be performed in order to detect antibiotic resistance mechanisms. Go to ∞ Chapter 11, "Susceptibility Testing," to review ESBL producing gram-negative rods.

E. COLI

General Characteristics

E. coli are small, straight, usually motile gram-negative rods that can grow with or without oxygen. They tend to occur singly, rather than in pairs or chains and can be easily dispersed into a single-celled suspension by swirling a scooped up colony in a liquid medium (Figure 21-8 ■). They are a part of

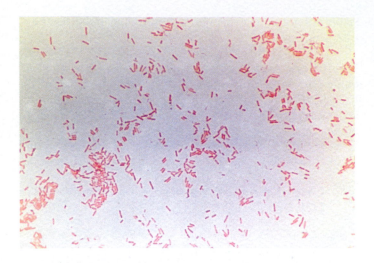

■ FIGURE 21-8 *E. coli* in a liquid medium. These bacteria are straight rods that tend to grow singly or in pairs. They can be easily dispersed into a single-celled suspension when swirled in a liquid medium, as shown here.

the normal flora in the intestinal tracts of humans and many animals. Although these bacteria are generally considered to be nonpathogenic, under certain conditions they can cause urinary tract infections, gastrointestinal disease, and meningitis. *E. coli* is a serious cause of nosocomial (hospital-acquired) infections. Some *E. coli* have specialized pili with colonization factor antigens (CFA) or bundle-forming pili (BFP) in addition to the usual type 1. Use of pulsed-field gel electrophoresis and comparison of patterns by PulseNet has increased the speed and accuracy in identifying outbreaks caused by certain serotypes such as O157:H7 that are linked with serious illness.

Useful Cultural, Biochemical, and Other Characteristics

Common specimens collected for laboratory diagnosis are urine, stool, and CSF. The flat, wet, gray colonies of *E. coli* exhibit β-hemolysis on blood agar. Beta hemolysis is rare for most genera of the *Enterobacteriaceae*. They ferment lactose and glucose with the production of acid and gas. Because they are lactose positive, they form rose-pink colonies, sometimes

REAL WORLD TIP

E. coli can be rapidly identified using colony characteristics and spot or rapid tests. A large, gray, non-spreading colony on blood agar that is oxidase negative and spot indole positive can be identified as *E. coli* if it is hemolytic or PYR negative and lactose-fermenting on MAC/EMB or MUG positive. Lactose negative colonies from abdominal sites should not be tested with MUG because of the possibility of misidentifying *M. morganii* and *P. vulgaris* as *E. coli*. Both of these organisms are indole positive.

surrounded by precipitated bile, on MacConkey agar (go to ∞ Chapter 8 to view a photo); on EMB agar, the colonies have an iridescent, almost metallic, sheen (Figure 21-9 ■). Sorbitol MacConkey agar (SMAC) can be used to isolate shiga toxin producing *E. coli* O157:H7. This specific serotype is unable to ferment sorbitol while most *E. coli* strains can ferment it. The medium has fallen out of use because there are serotypes other than O157:H7 that can also produce shiga toxin. *E. coli* can grow at 42°C, whereas the great majority of other enteric bacteria cannot. There are several hundred serotypes based on O, K, and H antigens.

Clinical Significance
Pathogenesis and Infectious Diseases.
Overall, *E. coli* is most notorious for causing urinary tract infections, especially community acquired. Indeed, these bacteria are the leading cause of urinary tract infections in the United States. However, a broad range of other types of infections are also possible. Table 21-4✪ shows the six groups that are considered as pathogenic. The nephropathogenic *E. coli* (NPEC) can infect any part of the urinary tract, resulting in uretitis (ureter), cystitis (bladder), and pyelonephritis (kidney). Common signs and symptoms include urinary frequency, dysuria, hematuria, pyuria, and flank pain when the upper urinary tract is involved. Urinary tract infections caused by *E. coli* are very common in young women, toddlers in diapers, and patients with indwelling catheters. Many strains carry plasmids with a gene that encodes a hemolysin. Pyelonephritis is associated with the presence of capsule and type **P pilus,** a structure that helps with adhesion. In severe cases, bacteremia and sepsis can occur. It has been reported that the organisms can form biofilm-like communities inside bladder cells in infected mice. If this phenomenon is shown to be true in humans, it may explain why these uropathogenic *E. coli* are able to persist despite aggressive antibiotic therapy and intact host immune responses.

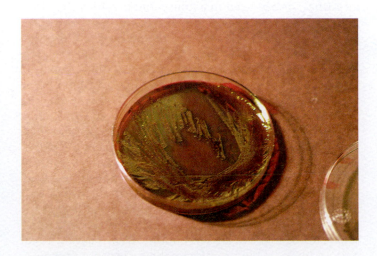

■ FIGURE 21-9 EMB medium showing the dark colonies and metallic sheen produced by *E. coli.*

⭐ TABLE 21-4

Classification of the Pathogenic *E. coli*

Name	Disease	Virulence Factor
Nephropathogenic *E. coli* (NPEC)	Urinary tract infection	P pilus, capsule, hemolysin
Enterotoxigenic *E. coli* (ETEC)	Traveler's diarrhea; may be severe if toxins are produced	Heat labile and heat stable toxins Colonization factors
Enteropathogenic *E. coli* (EPEC)	Infantile diarrhea	(certain serotypes)
Enterohemorrhagic *E. coli* (EHEC)	Hemorrhagic colitis, hemolytic uremic syndrome	Verotoxin (Shiga-like toxin)
Enteroinvasive *E. coli* (ETEC)	Diarrhea	—
Enteroaggregative *E. coli* (EAEC)	Diarrhea	—
(Unclassified)	Neonatal meningitis	K1 capsule

LT = heat-labile toxin; ST = heat-stable toxin

The diarrhea associated with out-of-country travel by Americans ("traveler's diarrhea") is often because of infection with serotypes of *E. coli* that are uncommon in the United States. The hypermobility of the gut generally lasts for only a few days and is self-limiting. However, cases caused by enterotoxigenic *E. coli* (ETEC) may be relatively severe because of the production of enterotoxins. Genes for two different enterotoxins are carried in plasmids that may also contain genes for colonization factors that facilitate attachment to the intestinal epithelium. The **heat-labile toxin (LT)** activates adenylate cyclase, resulting in increased cAMP and intense and prolonged hypersecretion of fluid (Figure 21-10 ■). This mechanism of action is similar to that of toxins produced by *Vibrio cholerae* and *Bacillus cereus*. The **heat-stable toxin (ST)** activates guanylate cyclase, resulting in increased cGMP and increased fluid secretion

The enteropathogenic *E. coli* (EPEC) are responsible for outbreaks of infantile diarrhea in nurseries with newborn infants. The watery diarrhea is generally self-limiting, but relapses and chronic infections are relatively common. The isolates often express certain O antigens (e.g., O55, O111, O125), and chromosomal genes code for adherence factors that allow the organisms to bind tightly to mucosal cells of the small intestine. Adults do not have a problem with these *E. coli* strains, but medical personnel can be carriers and transmit them to newborns.

The enterohemorrhagic *E. coli* (EHEC) cause a very severe form of bloody diarrhea known as **hemorrhagic colitis.** Approximately 2,100 patients are hospitalized annually in the United States because of this disease. In about 10% of cases, most of which are in children under the age of 5 years, progression to **hemolytic uremic syndrome (HUS)** occurs. HUS is characterized by microangiopathic anemia and thrombocytopenia. There is a very real danger for acute renal failure in these cases. The fatality rate is relatively low (3% to 5%), but prolonged hospitalization, massive blood transfusions, multiple bouts of hemodialysis, and long-term follow-up are frequently required. Survivors often have extensive urinary tract damage, and some require surgery to remove part of the bowel. Neurologic impairment such as seizures and stroke are also possible. Serotype O157:H7 is the most common EHEC in the United States, but other serotypes have been associated with disease. The organisms exist in the intestinal tracts of apparently healthy cattle, as well as other ruminants. Transmission to humans occurs primarily by consumption of undercooked ground beef, although cases have also been linked to unpasteurized milk, fresh apple cider, salami, lettuce, sprouts, and even contaminated water. Waterborne transmission may also occur by swimming in contaminated lakes and inadequately chlorinated pools. Person-to-person transmission in day-care centers has also been reported. In contrast to many other *Enterobacteriaceae,* the CDC's Emerging Infections Program Foodborne Diseases Active Surveillance Network (FoodNet) has determined that food-borne illness caused by this serotype

Enterocyte

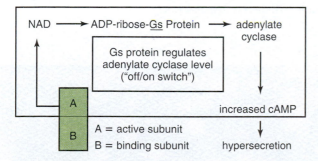

FIGURE 21-10 Mechanism of action of the LT toxin. Some *E. coli* secrete the LT toxin (heat-labile toxin) that activates adenylate cyclase, resulting in increased cAMP and hypersecretion of fluid by enterocytes into the intestinal lumen. The toxin consists of two subunits; the B subunit binds to the enterocyte so that the A subunit can enter and cleave NAD, thereby releasing ADP-ribose that then forms a complex with Gs protein. Gs is part of a family of proteins that function in numerous signal transduction pathways. In this case, the ADP-ribose-Gs protein complex turns on the "switch" for increased activity of the adenylate cyclase enzyme. *Vibrio cholerae* and *Bacillus cereus* produce toxins with a similar mechanism of action.

has not declined since 1996. Currently, an estimated 73,000 cases occur annually, with approximately 60 of these being fatal. *E. coli* O157:H7 secretes verotoxin (given this name because it kills Vero cells, a kidney cell line derived from the African Green monkey). The toxin is similar to the shiga toxin produced by *Shigella dysenteriae*. In 2002 there were 647 cases of shiga toxin–producing *E. coli* O157 identified by FoodNet. In addition, some non-O157 serotypes of *E. coli*, such as O26 and O111, can also produce this same toxin. Stool specimens can be tested directly or after enrichment (for example, using gram-negative broth) by immunoassay to detect the shiga toxin antigen. All O157 positive and shiga toxin positive specimens should be submitted to local public health laboratories for verification and further testing (CDC, 2009). A Vero cell assay is used for virulence testing of verotoxigenic *E. coli*. The test requires a 48- to 96-hour incubation period before microscopic examination for cytotoxicity.

The remaining two categories of pathogenic *E. coli* are found primarily in developing countries. Enteroinvasive *E. coli* (EIEC) produce a diarrhea in young children that is similar to shigellosis (dysentery), but milder. They can be invasive, resulting in inflammation and ulcers. Transmission is primarily by the fecal–oral route. Enteroaggregative *E. coli* (EAEC) cause acute and chronic diarrhea with mucoid, watery stools. The organisms produce an adherent biofilm.

The *E. coli* strain that causes neonatal meningitis are as yet unclassified. They account for 40% of neonatal meningitis cases. Infants are exposed to the organisms during birth. Infection has a very high mortality rate (40% to 80%). Most strains (75%) have a capsule with the K1 antigen. Interestingly, the K1 antigen is similar to an antigen found on the capsule of group B *Neisseria meningitidis* and may account for cross-reacting antibodies.

Treatment and Prevention.   There is no single specific therapy that is effective for all isolates. Great variation in antibiotic susceptibility exists, and multiple-drug resistance, often under the control of transmissible plasmids, is common. Thus, antibiotic susceptibility testing is essential. Sulfonamides, trimethoprim-sulfamethoxazole, ampicillin, cephalosporins, chloramphenicol, tetracyclines, and aminoglycosides are useful. The organisms are usually resistant to the penicillins (including penicillinase-resistant penicillins), erythromycin, clindamycin, vancomycin, and ampicillin. In the case of urinary tract infection, a catheter or other urinary obstruction usually must be removed for best results. Bismuth subsalicylate and tetracyclines have been sometimes prescribed for persons traveling outside the United States. However, because this practice is not foolproof and may select for resistant variants, it is generally no longer recommended. In severe cases of bacteremia or septic shock, restoration of fluid and electrolyte balance are important.

KLEBSIELLA

General Characteristics

The *Klebsiella* are facultatively anaerobic gram-negative bacilli that produce a large capsule and lack motility. They occur singly, in pairs, and in short chains. These bacteria cause a substantial proportion of nosocomial, as well as community-acquired, infections involving the respiratory tract, urinary tract, and wounds. *K. pneumoniae* (also known as Friedländer's bacillus) is relatively common in the intestinal tracts of humans and animals, but can also be found in water, in soil, and on grain. *K. pneumoniae* is most often implicated in clinically relevant disease, but infections caused by *K. oxytoca* also occur.

Useful Cultural, Biochemical, and Other Characteristics

Identification of *K. pneumoniae* is relatively easy on the basis of their glistening, highly mucoid colonies on agar (Figure 21-11 ■), positive lactose fermentation, and lack of motility. Additional useful reactions include fermentation of glucose with the production of acid and gas and positive citrate and lysine decarboxylase tests. They usually do not liquefy gelatin. *K. pneumoniae* is intrinsically resistant to ampicillin and carbenicillin. The two major species can be differentiated on the outcome of the indole test: *K. pneumoniae* does not produce indole, whereas *K. oxytoca* does.

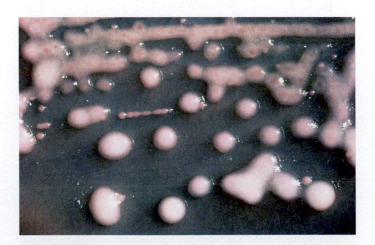

■ **FIGURE 21-11** *Klebsiella pneumoniae* colonies on MacConkey agar. These bacteria form large, mucoid, glistening colonies.
Photo courtesy of Centers for Disease Control (CDC).

✓ **Checkpoint! 21–6 (Chapter Objective 2)**

Which of the following represents the main reservoir for E. coli O157:H7?

   A. *Cattle*
   B. *Rodents*
   C. *Poultry*
   D. *Pigs*
   E. *Sheep*

Clinical Significance

Pathogenesis and Infectious Disease. The *Klebsiella* are well known for their unusually large, gelatinous capsule that is composed of polysaccharide. The capsule provides the organisms with a virulence mechanism by preventing engulfment by phagocytic cells such as neutrophils and macrophages. It also covers somatic antigens so that antibodies cannot readily bind them and, if released, soluble polysaccharide antigens can intercept antibodies. Hence the possibility for opsonization is greatly minimized (see ∞ Chapter 10 for further explanation). Specific serotypes can be identified through the use of antisera directed against the more than 70 capsular antigens that have been characterized to date. This information can be especially useful when tracking outbreaks of infection in the hospital setting. Some of these antigens are similar to those found on other encapsulated bacteria such as *Haemophilus influenzae* and *Streptococcus pneumoniae*. The *Klebsiella* also have several types of pili on their surface, some which may increase their adherence to epithelial cells in the respiratory and urinary tracts.

K. pneumoniae can be found in the respiratory tracts, as well as in the intestinal tracts, of ~5% of healthy humans. Hospitalized patients are often colonized with this organism. It then goes on to cause respiratory tract infections primarily in elderly and debilitated individuals. It is responsible for approximately 1% of acute bacterial pneumonias. Infection has also been reported in alcoholics and persons with compromised pulmonary function, diabetes mellitus, and other medical conditions. Many isolates from these cases have a capsule with K1 and K2 antigens. There is hemorrhagic necrotizing consolidation of the lungs that may resemble lobar pneumonia, the classical etiological agent of which is *Streptococcus pneumoniae*. The sputum is thick and reddish, resembling currant jelly. Many rod-shaped bacilli with a large capsule that looks like a surrounding halo are evident (go to ∞ Chapter 33, "Respiratory System," to view a photo). Infection is often severe, resulting in destruction of alveolar spaces, cavity formation, and empyema. If septicemia occurs, the fatality rate is high. *K. pneumoniae* can also cause urinary tract infections and bacteremia in debilitated individuals. Isolates from the urinary tract frequently have a capsule that expresses the K1, K8, K9, K10, and K24 antigens.

 REAL WORLD TIP

Presence of gram-negative rods with an unusually large capsule in a sputum specimen should alert the laboratory technologist that the bacteria may be *K. pneumoniae*.

Other species of *Klebsiella* have been implicated in chronic inflammatory diseases of the upper respiratory tract. *K. ozaenae* causes a progressive, foul smelling atrophy of the nasal mucosa, and *K. rhinoscleromatis* causes a destructive granuloma of the nose and pharynx. Both species are biochemically much less active than *K. pneumoniae*. Infection with these two species is rare in the United States.

K. granulomatis (formerly known as *Calymmatobacterium granulomatis*) has been recently transferred into the *Klebsiella* genus, based on genetic analysis and similarity with the clinical and pathological manifestations induced by *K. ozaenae* and *K. rhinoscleromatis*. *K. granulomatis* is the etiologic agent of **granuloma inguinale**, a granulomatous disease affecting the genital and inguinal areas. The disease is seen primarily in tropical parts of the world such as New Guinea and the Caribbean; it is rare in the United States. The bacteria are relatively small, having dimensions of only 0.5 to 1.0 × 1.5 μm. A typical course after infection is the appearance of subcutaneous nodules within weeks to months and subsequent breakdown of the nodules, resulting in granulomatous lesions that may coalesce. Scrapings of infected tissues stained with Wright's or Giemsa reveal bacilli with a large capsule in the cytoplasm of polymorphonuclear cells, plasmacytes, and histiocytes (visit ∞ Chapter 36, "Genital System," to see a photo). Transmission is by sexual contact or trauma to the genital or inguinal areas.

Treatment and Prevention. The *Klebsiella* are among the most antibiotic-resistant organisms in the *Enterobacteriaceae* family. Currently, a third-generation cephalosporin (e.g., cefotaxime or cefuroxime) is the drug of choice; alternative drugs include trimethoprim-sulfamethoxazole, an aminoglycoside; imipenem or meropenem, a fluoroquinolone; piperacillin; mezlocillin; and aztreonam. Trimethoprim-sulfamethoxazole, tetracycline, and erythromycin are usually effective for treatment of granuloma inguinale. Review ∞ Chapter 11 for potential resistance mechanisms and detection methods.

 Checkpoint! 21–7 (Chapter Objective 6)

An organism identified as K. pneumoniae is ampicillin sensitive. You should:

    A. *report the identity and susceptibility result.*
    B. *check isolate for purity and repeat all tests.*
    C. *investigate the atypical antibiogram pattern.*
    D. *report the identity and repeat the susceptibility test.*

ENTEROBACTER

General Characteristics

Enterobacter aerogenes (proposed new name: *Klebsiella mobilis*) is a facultative anaerobe that closely resembles *E. coli* in morphology and habitat and also usually does not cause disease. It is a very common part of the normal flora of the intestinal tract, but may also be found free-living in the environment.

Useful Cultural, Biochemical, and Other Characteristics

These motile bacteria are consistently different from *E. coli* in certain biochemical tests such as the Voges-Proskauer and indole. *E. aerogenes* is Vogues-Proskauer positive (acetylmethylcarbinol is produced) and indole negative, whereas the reactions for *E. coli* are opposite. It also differs from *E. coli* in that colonies on EMB agar do not have a metallic sheen and appear more viscous, somewhat reminiscent of *Klebsiella*. The organisms produce smooth, raised colonies on blood agar and slightly mucoid, pink colonies on MacConkey agar (Figure 21-12 ■) because of lactose fermentation. The organisms have many different antigenic types, and a small capsule is usually present. *Enterobacter aerogenes* is intrinsically resistant to cephalothin.

Clinical Significance

Pathogenesis and Infectious Disease.
Enterobacter species cause urinary tract infections and sepsis, primarily in those who are immunocompromised, and only rarely in immunocompetent individuals. Several outbreaks of infection in hospitals have been linked to parenteral fluids contaminated with these organisms. Most often, however, they are found as part of a mixed flora in clinical specimens. It can be a nosocomial pathogen in the intensive care unit (ICU).

Treatment and Prevention.
These organisms are frequently multidrug resistant. Trimethoprim-sulfamethoxazole and imipenem are among the most effective drugs. Production of β-lactamase occurs frequently, thus rendering the organisms resistant to many β-lactam antibiotics, including cephalosporins.

SERRATIA

General Characteristics

Serratia is a small, gram-negative rod that can grow in oxygen or without it. The organisms are ubiquitous in the environment (water, soil, vegetation) and can also be found in food and milk. They are occasional inhabitants in the colons of healthy humans, and hence qualify as being included among the enterics. Some strains produce a capsule.

Useful Cultural, Biochemical, and Other Characteristics

Although these organisms are usually lactose negative, some strains ferment lactose very slowly, and a positive result may be obtained after 3 to 4 days of incubation. These bacteria ferment glucose with the production of acid, but not gas. Positive results are usually obtained in VP, citrate, lysine, and ornithine decarboxylase tests. Some organisms produce a bright red pigment, a property that has been exploited in studies of bacterial dispersal in the atmosphere (biological warfare) and air currents in hospitals. Needless to say, once it was discovered that *Serratia* is a serious cause of nosocomial infections, the air current studies in hospitals were terminated. The red pigmented strain is more often an environmental organism and may be a contaminant rather than the infecting organism. On solid media, the red colonies have a tendency to look like drops of blood (Figure 21-13 ■). However, clinical isolates are usually achromogenic. Another rather unusual feature for an *Enterobacteriaceae* is that these bacteria produce an extracellular DNase. It is unclear whether or not this enzyme plays a role in pathogenesis. *S. marcescens* is intrinsically resistant to cephalothin, polymyxins, and nitrofurantoin.

Clinical Significance

Pathogenesis and Infectious Disease.
In general, disease occurs only in individuals who are already debilitated or who are addicted to drugs, with *S. marcescens* being

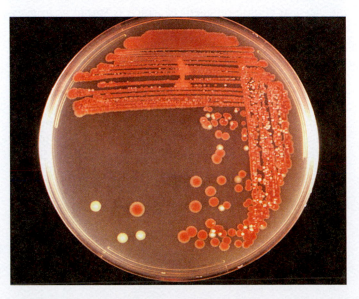

■ **FIGURE 21-13** Colonies of *Serratia marcescens* on blood agar. *S. marcescens* isolated from the environment, or that may be present as a contaminant, often produces a bright red pigment that makes the colonies look like drops of blood. However, most isolates from clinical specimens are achromogenic.
Photo courtesy of Centers for Disease Control (CDC), Dr. Negut.

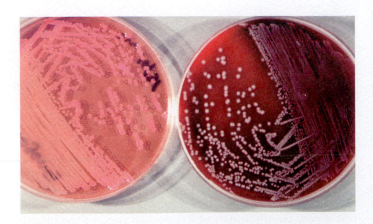

■ **FIGURE 21-12** *Enterobacter aerogenes* growing on MacConkey (left) and blood agar (right).

the species most often isolated. Indeed, the frequency of *S. marcescens* isolation in the hospital setting has been steadily increasing over the past two decades. Manifestations of infection are typical of an opportunist and include pneumonia, bacteremia, septicemia, endocarditis, localized cellulitis, burn infections, and urinary tract infections developing from indwelling catheters.

Treatment and Prevention.   As is the case with many other opportunists, *S. marcescens* is highly drug resistant and multidrug resistance has been often linked with plasmid-encoded resistance factors. Treatment with the newer cephalosporins (e.g., cefatoximine, cefoperazone, cefuroxime), gentamicin, tobramicin, and trimethoprim-sulfamethoxazole has been successful. The organisms are consistently resistant to ampicillin and cephalothin; resistance to tetracycline is common. A very recent study of footbaths at several dairy factories found that *S. marcescens* was resistant to amphoteric and alkyl amino acetate-based disinfectants. It was concluded that disinfecting footbaths may serve as a source of contamination in food factories and that careful monitoring should continue to be implemented.

 REAL WORLD TIP

Remember *Serratia marcescens* by its ability to possess "ases"—lipase, gelatinase, and DNase.

PROTEUS-PROVIDENCIA-MORGANELLA GROUP

General Characteristics

This is a group of closely related gram-negative rods. There are two major species of *Proteus* (*P. mirabilis* and *P. vulgaris*), *Providencia* has at least three species (*P. rettgeri*—most common, *P. alcalifaciens,* and *P. stuartii*), and only one species of *Morganella* (*M. morganii*). The genus *Proteus* was named after a sea god who was able to change his form, a characteristic strongly associated with these bacteria. Although these bacteria are ubiquitous in the environment, they can be found as normal colon flora and in both normal and diarrheal stools. Overall, *P. mirabilis* is the species most frequently isolated from urine and other clinical specimens.

Useful Cultural, Biochemical, and Other Characteristics

The members of this group can assume coccoid and large irregular and filamentous forms under certain conditions. The members of this group grow well on many types of routinely used laboratory media. The organisms are motile and lactose negative, but ferment xylose and glucose; fermentation of the latter sugar is accompanied by the production of acid or acid and gas. They produce phenylalanine deaminase and are able

to grow on potassium cyanide (KCN) medium. An interesting sidelight is that certain strains of *P. vulgaris* (e.g., X-19) have the same polysaccharides as some of the *Rickettsia,* gram-negative bacteria that cause typhus. Because *Rickettsia* are strictly intracellular organisms and difficult to culture, this antigenic cross-reactivity has been used in the past in the Weil-Felix test (now obsolete) to help make the diagnosis of typhus. Antibodies against the *Rickettsia* in a patient's serum would agglutinate the bacteria because of the strongly cross-reactive antigens.

P. mirabilis and *P. vulgaris* are very highly motile, exhibiting what is often referred to as "swarming motility" (Figure 21-14 ■). They move rapidly over the surface of agar plates, forming a thin film of growth that covers other bacteria that may also be present. Sometimes the swarming has a periodicity, resulting in a series of ripples similar to what is seen when a pebble is tossed into a quiet pool of water. The swarming is inhibited when the organisms are streaked onto MacConkey, CLED (cystine-lactose-electrolyte-deficient) medium or exposed to chemicals such as phenylethyl alcohol. *Proteus* spp. can produce a unique odor that has been described as burnt chocolate.

P. mirabilis and *P. vulgaris* produce H_2S. *Proteus* species, and *Providencia rettgeri* produce a urease enzyme that rapidly breaks down urea, giving off an odor of ammonia, whereas the other *Providencia* species are usually urease negative. *M. morganii* is weakly urease positive. The major species can be, at least partly, differentiated on the basis of the reactions shown in Table 21-2. Spreading colonies that are oxidase negative, gram-negative rods can be rapidly identified using the spot indole test. An indole-positive result is reported as *P. vulgaris*. An indole-

■ **FIGURE 21-14** *Proteus* swarming. *Proteus* species produce many more flagella than other *Enterobacteriaceae* and hence exhibit a high degree of motility. Sometimes the motility has a periodicity, resulting in successive waves of growth that extend outward from the site of inoculation, as shown here. The organisms can also form a thin, continuous, and barely visible film over the entire surface of the agar. In this latter case, it is virtually impossible to collect a pure colony of any other bacteria that may also be present because of overgrowth by *Proteus.*

negative result is reported as *P. mirabilis* as long as the isolate is ampicillin sensitive. *P. penneri* has a spreading colony and is indole negative, but it is ampicillin resistant. *M. morganii* is citrate negative but ornithine decarboxylase positive. *P. alcalifaciens* ferments adonitol and produces gas from glucose fermentation, while *P. stuartii* does not ferment adonitol or produce gas from glucose fermentation

P. mirabilis, P. vulgaris, M. morganni, and *Providencia rettgeri* are intrinsically resistant to polymyxins, tetracycline, and nitrofurantoin. *P. vulgaris* is also intrinsically resistant to ampicillin; *M. morganni* and *Providencia rettgeri* are also intrinsically resistant to cephalothin. Other *Providencia* species are intrinsically resistant to polymyxins and nitrofurantoin.

 REAL WORLD TIP

Be careful when performing a spot indole test on *Proteus* spp. As it swarms, it can carry the indole produced by other organisms and may give a false positive reaction. The spot indole can only be reliably performed on a pure isolation of *Proteus* spp.

Clinical Significance

Pathogenesis and Infectious Disease.
In the case of *Proteus,* especially *P. mirabilis,* urinary tract infections are common (Mobley & Belas, 1995). Production of a very potent urease by the organisms results in the breakdown of urea and formation of CO_2 and ammonia. This raises the pH of the urine (i.e., it becomes alkaline), resulting in damage to the uroepithelium. In addition, the alkalinity of the urine causes the precipitation of calcium and magnesium salts that, in turn, facilitate the formation of kidney stones (calculi). Acidification of the urine to solubilize the kidney stones is virtually impossible with concurrent *Proteus* infection. Wound infections, pneumonia, and septicemia caused by members of this group have also been reported.

Some of these organisms, especially *M. morganii,* produce high levels of histamine by decarboxylating histidine (an amino acid present in many proteins). This can result in histamine poisoning after consumption of contaminated foods (Church, Norn, Pao, & Holgate, 1987; Lehane & Olley, 2000; Taylor, Stratton, & Nordlee, 1989). Spoiled fish (tuna, mackerel, bonito, mahi-mahi, bluefish, and sardines) have been especially implicated. This form of histamine poisoning is also known as scombroid fish poisoning because many of the fish belong in the *Scombridae* and *Scomberesocidae* families. The disease has also been linked to consumption of spoiled cheeses, especially Swiss cheese. Foods containing high levels of histamine may not outwardly appear to be spoiled and therefore are freely consumed. The clinical presentation is very similar to what is seen in IgE-mediated allergies. Symptoms (nausea, vomiting, diarrhea, hives, and itching) appear within minutes

after ingesting the food and usually resolve on their own within a time interval of 24 hours or less. In addition, *P. vulgaris,* as well as several other members of the *Enterobacteriaceae* (e.g., *E. coli, Enterobacter cloacae,* and *Klebsiella pneumoniae*), can induce the release of histamine from human lung and tonsillar mast cells. Antihistamines are used to effectively treat these conditions.

Treatment and Prevention.
The bacteria in this group are often antibiotic resistant. Ampicillin, newer cephalosporins (e.g., cefotaxime, cefuroxime), aminoglycosides, and trimethoprim-sulfamethoxazole have been successfully used. *P. mirabilis* tends to be the most susceptible to antibiotics, including penicillin, compared to the others in this group.

 Checkpoint! 21–8 (Chapter Objective 5)

The development of kidney stones in patients with urinary tract infections caused by Proteus species is strongly associated with which of the following factors?
   A. *Phenylalanine deaminase*
   B. *Swarming motility*
   C. *Histamine*
   D. *Urease*
   E. *Acid*

CITROBACTER SPECIES

General Characteristics

Citrobacter (previously called the Bethesda-Ballerup group) is a gram-negative rod found in the intestinal tracts of humans and animals as part of the normal flora, as well as in the environment.

Useful Cultural, Biochemical, and Other Characteristics

These motile organisms grow well on routine laboratory media used for other *Enterobacteriaceae.* They use citrate as the sole source of carbon, grow on potassium cyanide (KCN) medium, produce trimethylene glycol from glycerol, and are PYR positive. Overall, the members in this genus have strong biochemical and serologic similarities with *Salmonella.* They ferment lactose very slowly or not at all; some strains produce a Vi positive capsule like *S. typhi.* Differentiation from the salmonellae is relatively easy because they do not decarboxylate lysine and are ONPG positive. *C. freundii* and *C. koseri* are the two major species isolated from patients. Differentiation between these two is possible because *C. freundii* usually produces H_2S, does not ferment adonitol, and does not produce ornithine decarboxylase, whereas *C. koseri* is negative for H_2S, decarboxylates ornithine, and ferments adonitol. *C. koseri* is indole positive, while *C. freundii* is indole negative.

C. freundii is intrinsically resistant to cephalothin, and *C. koseri* is intrinsically resistant to cephalothin and carbenicillin.

Clinical Significance

Pathogenesis and Infectious Disease.   These organisms rarely cause infection in healthy persons; nosocomial infections account for the majority of relevant cases. The two major species, and to a lesser extent others such as *C. amalonaticus,* have been isolated from urinary tract infections, the most common health problem associated with *Citrobacter.* However, wound infections, cellulitis, and sepsis are also possible. In the literature, both *C. freundii* and *C. koseri* have been reported to have a high tendency to cause meningitis and brain abscesses in young infants, but the incidence is low. It appears that the organisms may evade host immune defense mechanisms because of their ability to survive and multiply within macrophages. Several relatively new species that have been isolated from clinical specimens include *C. gillenii* (old name: *Citrobacter* species 10) and *C. murliniae* (old name: *Citrobacter* species 11). Overall, these organisms are uncommon opportunists in immunodeficient and otherwise seriously debilitated persons. In one report, most cases of *Citrobacter* infection were found in patients with underlying hepatic, biliary, or pancreatic disease.

Treatment and Prevention.   Aminoglycosides, tetracycline, and chloramphenicol are usually effective for treatment. However, resistant strains are common in long-term hospitalized patients, especially those who have received prior antibiotic therapy. Significant risk factors for ceftriaxone resistance include peripheral vascular disease, AIDS, cerebrovascular disease, and length of time in an intensive care unit. Antibiotic resistance is most prevalent in *C. freundii,* the species that has also been associated with the highest fatality rate.

▶ OTHER ENTERICS

HAFNIA

General Characteristics

Hafnia was originally called *Enterobacter hafnia* because of the close similarity of these organisms to *Enterobacter* species. *H. alvei* is the only species in this genus. These motile organisms have been isolated from drinking water, water at fish farms, intestines of fish and rabbits, and a variety of wild rodents. Although they appear to be quite ubiquitous in the environment, no known environmental source is specific for these bacteria.

Useful Cultural, Biochemical, and Other Characteristics

Biochemical analyses have shown that they are usually indole and urease negative, are Voges-Proskauer reaction positive, and produce decarboxylase enzymes for lysine and ornithine (but not arginine), *o*-nitrophenyl-D-galactopyranoside (ONPG),

and acid and gas from glucose fermentation. They are metabolically more active at 25°C than at 37°C. *Hafnia alvei* is intrinsically resistant to cephalothin. Its colony gives off a characteristic odor of human feces.

Clinical Significance

Pathogenesis and Infectious Disease.   *H. alvei* has been linked most often to pediatric cases of gastroenteritis. On rare occasions, it has been isolated from patients with respiratory tract infections, urinary tract infections, liver abscesses, appendicitis, and postoperative endophthalmitis (Ramos & Damaso, 2000). In some cases, blood cultures have been positive. Extraintestinal infection, although very unusual, has been reported in both immunocompromised and immunocompetent adults, with more cases being found in the former than in the latter. In addition, the organisms appear to have a tendency to localize in the gallbladder and produce biliary abscesses. The antibiotic susceptibility profile is somewhat similar to that of *Enterobacter.*

Treatment and Prevention.   Susceptibility to aminoglycosides, imipenem, cotrimoxazole, ciprofloxacin, piperacillin, and cefotaxime is usually noted; most strains are resistant to cephalothin.

PLESIOMONAS

General Characteristics

At various times, *Plesiomonas shigelloides* has been thought to belong to the *Pseudomonas, Aeromonas,* and *Vibrio* genera. The recent inclusion of these organisms in the *Enterobacteriaceae* family is based on ribosomal RNA sequencing studies that have demonstrated very close similarity to *Proteus,* especially *P. vulgaris.*

Useful Cultural, Biochemical, and Other Characteristics

P. shigelloides is a glucose but not lactose and sucrose fermenting gram-negative rod that possesses the common enterobacterial antigens. It grows well on blood agar, forming opaque, convex colonies. It also grows well on CIN medium on which colonies are opaque; there is no pink center because the organisms do not ferment mannitol. Other oxidase positive bacteria such as *Aeromonas* will produce colonies with a pink center and an opaque periphery. Positive results for inositol fermentation, and the tests for lysine, arginine, and ornithine, are also helpful in identification. Interestingly, because these bacteria are oxidase positive and the formal definition of *Enterobacteriaceae* states that the members do not produce oxidase, the definition for this family will undoubtedly be rewritten in the near future.

Clinical Significance

P. shigelloides is best known for causing self-limiting diarrhea in persons consuming seafood and living in or traveling to tropical countries. Severe cases of diarrhea may also occur, especially in individuals with debilitating underlying conditions. The nature of the diarrhea is variable, ranging from watery to bloody. Dehydration, severe abdominal pain, and fever are relatively common. In some cases, the diarrhea can persist for up to 2 weeks. The organisms are capable of invading and multiplying in human gastrointestinal cells. Although no specific virulence factors have yet been clearly identified, a β-hemolysin may be important in pathogenesis because it releases the organisms from vacuoles within colon cells. Production of cholera-like toxins from some isolates has also been recently described. There is, unfortunately, no good animal model for study of these organisms that would facilitate identification of virulence factors expressed in vivo. ∞ Chapter 23 provides details on distinguishing *Plesiomonas* from other oxidase positive, glucose fermenting gram-negative rods. Information on less commonly isolated enterics, such as *Cedecea* and *Kluyvera* can be found on the Companion Website.

clinical significance. They are among the most common infectious agents isolated in the clinical laboratory and are also among the most common in causing disease (Box 21-1 ✪). Diarrhea, urinary tract infections, and bacteremia are frequent clinical manifestations. LPS, the endotoxin present in the wall, is a major cause of morbidity and mortality. Its effects can rapidly lead to DIC, shock, and organ dysfunction. However, a variety of other factors may contribute to pathogenicity and virulence.

The organisms grow rapidly and well on many laboratory media. Because they are often part of a mixed flora (especially in the case of stool specimens and rectal swabs), many variations in selective and differential media have been developed to speed up the process of isolation and identification (e.g., MacConkey, EMB, SS, HE, XLD, BS, and TCBS media). Formation of large, circular, smooth, convex colonies on blood agar

---

Checkpoint! 21–9 (Chapter Objective 5)

The biochemical and serological characteristics of which of the following organisms most closely resemble Salmonella?

  A. *Hafnia*
  B. *Citrobacter*
  C. *Ewingella*
  D. *Moellerella*
  E. *Cedecea*

SUMMARY

Members of the *Enterobacteriaceae* family are facultatively anaerobic, non-spore-forming gram-negative rods that grow singly, in pairs, or in short chains and that sometimes exhibit considerable pleomorphism. The family consists of many genera, species, groups, and literally thousands of serological types based on O, H, and K antigens. Classification of these bacteria has always been a difficult and never-ending process because of the many overlapping and shared characteristics that these organisms possess. The ability to pass genetic material from one species to another within a genus, as well as between different genera, contributes to taxonomic complexity. Advances in molecular biology such as nucleic acid hybridization and sequencing, computer technologies, and automation continue to provide new information that is used to help clarify classification schemes.

Many of the *Enterobacteriaceae* are natural inhabitants of the intestinal tracts of humans and animals, although some are primarily found in the environment. Some, like *Salmonella* and *Shigella*, are overt pathogens, whereas many others are merely opportunists. Although not found in the intestinal tract, the family also includes *Y. pestis*, the cause of bubonic and pneumonic plague. This bacteria is in class A in the list of bioterrorism agents. Overall, the *Enterobacteriaceae* have great

---

✪ BOX 21-1

Selected Diseases Associated with *Enterobacteriaceae*

Bacteremia/Septicemia	Enterocolitis/Diarrhea
E. coli	*E. coli*
Edwardsiella	*Edwardsiella*
Salmonella	*Salmonella*
Klebsiella	*Shigella*
Enterobacter	*Yersinia enterocolitica*
Serratia	*Y. pseudotuberculosis*
Proteus	*Hafnia alvei* (pediatric)
Providencia	*Proteus* (histamine food poisoning)
Citrobacter	

Nosocomial/Opportunistic

Citrobacter
Enterobacter
Serratia
Providencia
Morganella

Wound

Edwardsiella
Citrobacter
Enterobacter
Serratia
Providencia
Proteus

Bacteriuria

E. coli (community acquired)
Klebsiella
Enterobacter
Serratia
Proteus
Providencia
Citrobacter

Meningitis

E. coli
Edwardsiella

Neonatal Sepsis

E. coli

Pneumoniae

Klebsiella
Serratia marscens

Plague

Yersinia pestis

Mesenteric Adenitis

Y. pseudotuberculosis
Y. enterocolitica

Enteric Fever

Salmonella
Edwardsiella

Dysentery

Shigella

Hemolytic Uremic Syndrome

E. coli

and MacConkey agar within 24 hours of inoculation is typical for many isolates. Some strains of *E. coli* produce β-hemolysis on blood agar; *Klebsiella* produces very large mucoid colonies; spreading or swarming colonies are typical of the proteae. Most of the enterics are motile via peritrichous flagella, the major exceptions being *Shigella* and *Klebsiella*. Overall, these bacteria are metabolically very active. They ferment many different sugars, resulting in many different end products. Major features that are common to the family include reduction of nitrates to nitrites, glucose fermentation with the production of acid or acid and gas, and lack of the oxidase enzyme (except for *Plesiomonas*).

Community- and hospital-acquired infections caused by the *Enterobacteriaceae* are becoming increasingly common, as is multidrug resistance. Especially troublesome are the noso-comially acquired cases, many of which involve the bloodstream and lungs. Surveillance data indicate that 5% to 10% of patients admitted to hospitals in the United States become infected during hospitalization. This translates into approximately 1.75 to 3.5 million cases per year that are difficult to manage because of drug resistance and an already debilitated population. Although treatment is usually begun empirically, based on generally accepted drug susceptibility patterns, it is no longer possible to predict with certainty that a particular isolate in the *Enterobacteriaceae* family will be susceptible to any one given antibiotic. Hence, drug susceptibility testing of these infectious agents is a critical service performed by personnel in clinical laboratories. The accuracy and care with which all these tests are done have a direct impact on the health and well-being of many patients.

LEARNING OPPORTUNITIES

1. What are the major unifying characteristics of the *Enterobacteriaceae* family? (Chapter Objective 1)

2. What are some of the distinguishing features of the major genera that are useful in identification? (Chapter Objective 2)

3. What types of diseases do the presented organisms cause? (Chapter Objective 3)

4. What role does LPS play in diseases associated with the *Enterobacteriaceae*? (Chapter Objective 4)

5. Construct a flowchart to identify the major species of *Enterobacteriaceae* (listed in taxonomy section) using no more than four biochemical reactions for each species. (Chapter Objective 5)

6. The following reactions are obtained on four isolates (Chapter Objectives 5 and 7):

    Isolate A (NLF colony): Ind +, MR +, VP −, Cit −, TSI K/AG + H_2S, Lys +

    Isolate B (NLF colony): Ind −, MR +, VP −, Cit −, TSI K/A, Lys −, Orn +, MOT −

    Isolate C (LF colony): Ind −, MR −, VP +, Cit +, TSI A/AG, Lys +, Orn −, MOT −

    Isolate D (LF colony): Ind +, MR +, VP +, Cit +, TSI A/AG + H_2S, Lys +, Orn +, PAD +

    a. Do these results correlate with colony morphology?

    b. If yes, what is the identity of each isolate?

    c. If no, what are the possible causes of the discrepancy?

CASE STUDY 21-1.   LONG-TERM SHEDDING OF *S. TYPHI*

Patient: Female (nickname: "Typhoid Mary")

Background: In 1904, when an epidemic of typhoid fever broke out in Oyster Bay, New York, the pattern of contamination put health officials on the trail of Mary Mallon, who had been employed in the area as a cook. Nicknamed "Typhoid Mary," she managed to elude authorities until 1907, when she was discovered working as a cook in a Park Avenue home. Overtaken with considerable difficulty, she was taken to Willard Parker hospital, where she was found to be so loaded with typhoid bacilli that some officials referred to her as a human culture tube! Mary, the first typhoid carrier identified in America, was committed that year to North Brother Island in New York harbor. Despite a Supreme Court appeal, she remained there until 1911, when health officials released her on her promise not to accept food-handling employment. However, 4 years later, when an epidemic of typhoid broke out in a New Jersey sanitarium and the Sloane Maternity Hospital, authorities feared that she had broken her promise. Investigations revealed that she had been employed in the kitchens of both institutions. She managed to escape before investigators arrived. She was finally "captured" in a suburban New York home. Attributed with 51 original cases of typhoid and 3 deaths, "Typhoid Mary" was sent back to North Brother Island, where

she remained in isolation until 1938, when she died after a stroke—still excreting *S. typhi*.

1. What laboratory tests would distinguish between *Salmonella* and *Shigella?*
2. What was the most likely route of transmission of the *S. typhi?*
3. If current antibiotics had been available during "Typhoid Mary's" lifetime, which one(s) might have been useful for treatment?

CASE STUDY 21-2.   OUTBREAK OF DIARRHEA AFTER A PICNIC

Patients: Children

Background: Thirty children were hospitalized with bloody diarrhea, diffuse abdominal pain, and severe hematological abnormalities during a 1-week period of time. A 4-year-old girl died of kidney failure shortly after admittance. Laboratory testing revealed a heavy growth of a gram-negative rods with the O157:H7 serotype in all examined stool specimens. Epidemiologic investigation established that all the children

developed symptoms soon after consuming hamburgers from the same fast-food restaurant chain.

1. Which bacteria is most likely to be the etiological agent?
2. What types of laboratory tests should be performed to distinguish the bacteria from other well-known enteric pathogens?
3. Does the bacteria produce a virulence factor that likely contributes to the disease?

CASE STUDY 21-3.   NOSOCOMIAL URINARY TRACT INFECTION

Patient: 65-year-old male

Background: A 65-year-old patient with an episode of acute urinary retention was catheterized. Three days later, he developed fever and suprapubic pain. Culture of the urine revealed a thin film of bacterial growth over the entire blood agar plate, and the urease test was positive.

1. Which organism is the most likely cause of this infection?
2. Why would antibiotic susceptibility testing be especially important in this case?
3. What are the long-term implications for the patient, if the infection is not cured?

PEARSON
myhealthprofessionskit™

Use this address to access the interactive Companion Website created for this textbook. Simply select "Clinical Laboratory Science" from the choice of disciplines. Find this book and log in using your user name and password.

REFERENCES

Go to myhealthprofessionskit.com to view this chapter's references.

22

Nonfermenting Gram-Negative Rods

Joy T. Henderson

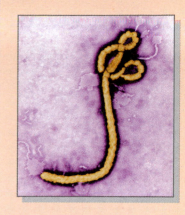

■ LEARNING OBJECTIVES

After completion of this chapter, the learner should be able to:

1. Categorize the nonfermenters using general characteristics.

   a. Differentiate from the family *Enterobacteriaceae* and other organisms.

2. Recognize clues that indicate the presence of nonfermenters.

3. Determine appropriate media for selection and differentiation of these organisms.

   a. Determine appropriate specimens for isolation.

   b. Describe growth and environmental requirements for each organism.

   c. Correlate its presence in culture with specific diseases.

4. Summarize the purpose and principle of identification methods discussed.

   a. Recognize limitations and potential sources of errors.

5. Relate the microscopic and colony morphologies and key identification results for each organism.

   a. Differentiate one organism from another.

6. Summarize natural habitats and virulence factors for each organism.

   a. Associate patient populations at risk for disease.

   b. Identify organisms that have the potential to be used as bioterrorism agents.

7. Summarize treatment strategies, expected antibiotic susceptibility results, and emerging resistance for the nonfermenters.

8. Correlate patient history, body site or specimen type, colonial morphology, Gram stain reaction, identification test results, and antibiotic susceptibility results in order to identify an isolate and assess its clinical significance.

KEY TERMS

alginate slime	denitrifier	pyocyanin
asaccharolytic	melioidosis	pyoverdin
cystic fibrosis	nonfermenter	siderophore

TAXONOMY

Family *Pseudomonadaceae* (sü-də-'mōn-a-dāsē-ē)
  Genus *Pseudomonas* (sü-'də-mōn-əs)
    P. aerugionosa ('ar-ə-jə'-nō-sə)
    P. stutzeri (stüt'-zeri)
    P. fluorescens/putida (flu-oh-res-cens/pu-ti-da)
Family *Moraxellaceae* (mor'-ak-sel'-a-s-ē'-ē)
  Genus *Acinetobacter* (AH-sin-neto-bacter)
    A. baumannii (buh-ma'-ne-i)
  Genus *Moraxella* (mor'-ak-sel'-a)
Family *Xanthomonadaceae* (zan'-thō-mŏ'-na-dās-ē'-ē)
  Genus *Stenotrophomonas* (ste-no-tro-fo-mo'-nas)
    S. maltophilia (mal-to-fĭl'-e-a)

Family *Burkholderiaceae* (burk-hold-er'-ē-ā-sē-'ē)
  Genus *Burkholderia* (burk-hold-er'-e-a)
    B. cepacia (se-pa'-se-a) complex
    B. pseudomallei (su-do-mal'-e-i)
Family *Flavobacteriaceae* (flā'-vō-bak-tēr-'ē-ā-sē-'ē)
  Genus *Elizabethkingia* (ee-liz-uh-beth-kin'-gē-a)
    E. meningoseptica (mě-nin-jo-sěp'-te-kah)
Family *Alcaligenaceae* (ăl-kă-lĭj-ă-nā-s-ē'-ē)
  Genus *Alcaligenes* (al-ka-lij-a-nēz)
    A. faecalis (fee-kay-lis)
  Genus *Achromobacter* (ā-krō-mo-bak-tər)
    A. xylosoxidans (zy-los-ox'-idans)

▶ INTRODUCTION

In this chapter, nonfermentative bacilli are discussed and distinguished based on their general characteristics and microscopic and macroscopic morphology as well as conventional identification systems. Their role as opportunistic pathogens and their presence in the environment are also described.

These organisms share similar properties such as their inability to ferment carbohydrates. If these organisms are able to utilize carbohydrates, they are oxidized rather than fermented. Some do not utilize carbohydrates at all for energy

▶ GENERAL CHARACTERISTICS

Nonfermentative bacilli tend to prefer wet environments such as sinks, respiratory equipment, flower vases, even ice from ice machines. They are usually not part of the healthy human normal flora. They are considered opportunistic and can colonize and infect immunocompromised individuals when the opportunity arises. In addition, they are often found as transient or colonizing flora of hospitalized individuals and can become nosocomial pathogens.

As a group, these aerobic gram-negative rods either do not use carbohydrates as a source of energy or degrade them through metabolic pathways other than fermentation. Most are obligate aerobes and grow poorly, if at all, under anaerobic conditions. They are oxidizers, or **nonfermenters**, compared to the *Enterobacteriaceae*, which are fermenters. Those that do not degrade carbohydrates at all are described as **asaccharolytic.**

These organisms usually display abundant growth on sheep blood agar and chocolate agar within 24 to 48 hours. Most

grow on MacConkey media with the exception of *Moraxella* species. Those that do grow on MacConkey media are not able to ferment lactose and so usually appear as nonlactose fermenters (NLF) after 18 to 24 hours of incubation. Table 22-1 compiles the key biochemical reactions for the organisms discussed in this chapter.

✔ **Checkpoint! 22–1 (Chapter Objective 1)**

By which process do nonfermentative rods utilize carbohydrates?
  A. *oxidation*
  B. *fermentation*
  C. *reduction*
  D. *denitrification*

▶ CLUES THAT SUGGEST THE ISOLATION OF A NONFERMENTER

There are several clues that should lead the microbiologist to consider the presence of nonfermenting gram-negative rods. These include:

- The organism does not ferment carbohydrates and creates an alkaline (K) slant and no change (NC) deep butt reaction in triple sugar iron agar (TSI) and Kligler's iron agar (KIA) slants.
  - These organisms require oxygen for the metabolism of carbohydrates if they are able to use them at all. A triple

TABLE 22-1

Key Biochemical Reactions and Other Characteristics of the Common Nonfermenting Gram-Negative Rods

Organism	Oxidase	Motility	Pyocyanin	Pyoverdin	Growth on MacConkey	Acetamide	Growth at 42°C	Oxidation of Carbohydrates — Glucose	Lactose	Maltose	Sucrose	Xylose	Decarboxylases — Arginine	Lysine	Ornithine	Gelatin Hydrolysis	Nitrate Reduction	Other
Pseudomonas aeruginosa	+	+	+	+	+NLF	+	+	+	–	–	–	+	+	–	–	+	+	• Can be beta-hemolytic • Grape-like odor
P. fluorescens	+	+	–	+	+NLF	–	–	+	–	–	+/–	+	+	–	–	+	–	• Can grow at 4°C
P. putida	+	+	–	+	+NLF	–	–	+	–	–	–	+	+	–	–	–	–	
P. stutzeri	+	+	–	–	+NLF	–	+/–	+	–	+	–	+	–	–	–	–	+	• Wrinkled colony • Starch hydrolysis +
Acinetobacter baumannii	–	–	–	–	+NLF	–	–	+	+/–	–	–	+	–	–	–	–	–	• NLF but can appear pink-blue due to oxidation of lactose
Stenotrophomonas maltophilia	–	+	–	–	+NLF	–	+/–	+	+/–	++	+	–	–	+	–	+	V	• DNase + • Polymyxin B susceptible • Ammonia-like odor
Burkholderia cepacia complex	+	+	–	–	+NLF	+	=	+	+	+/–	+	+	–	+	–	+	–	• Dirt-like odor • Polymyxin B resistant • Yellow pigment
B. pseudomallei	+	+	–	–	+NLF	–	+	+	+	+	+	+	+	–	–	V	+	• Wrinkled colony • NLF but can appear pink due to oxidation of lactose • Musty or earth-like odor
Elizabethkingia meningoseptica	+	–	–	–	+NLF	–	–/+	+	–	+	–	–	–	–	–	+	–	• Indole positive • Yellow pigment
Alcaligenes faecalis	+	+	–	–	+NLF	+	–	–	–	–	–	–	–	–	–	–/+	–	• Green apple odor • Alkaline reaction in OF medium • Reduces nitrites but not nitrates
Achromobacter xylosoxidans	+	+	–	–	+NLF	+	+/–	+	–	–	–	+	–	–	–	–	+	
Moraxella spp. (other than *M. catarrhalis*)	+	–	–	–	–	–	–/+	–	–	–	–	–	NA	NA	NA	–	+/–	• Asaccharolytic

+, positive; ++, strong positive; –, negative; +/–, more are positive then negative; –/+, more are negative than positive; V, variable; NA, not available or not applicable; NLF, nonlactose fermenter; NG, no growth; unshaded boxes are important differentiating reactions.

sugar iron or Kligler's iron agar slants provide the first big clue. They fail to ferment carbohydrates. Nonfermenters produce weak acids, if any at all. The pH indicators present in the TSI and KIA slant cannot detect these weak acids. During incubation, the nonfermenter uses the proteins aerobically as an energy source. When proteins are degraded on the surface of the agar slant, alkaline byproducts are created that turn the phenol red pH indicator from red/orange to pink. This produces an alkaline slant (K) and no reaction changes in the deep butt (NC) of the tube and so the name nonfermenter (NF). Figure 22-1 ■ displays the typical K/NC nonfermenter reaction on a TSI slant. ∞ Chapters 8 and 9 discuss the principle of the TSI slant.

■ Nonfermenters can be oxidase positive.

• Most *Enterobacteriaceae* are oxidase negative. The one exception is *Pleisiomonas,* which was recently named a member of the *Enterobacteriaceae.* Some of the more commonly isolated non-fementers are oxidase positive. While a positive oxidase reaction is not exclusive for

nonfermenters, it is a valuable clue. An oxidase-positive gram-negative rod must still be screened with a TSI or KIA to determine how it uses carbohydrates.

■ Nonfermenting gram-negative rods may fail to grow or show poor growth on MacConkey agar.

• While the inability to grow on MacConkey agar is not an absolute guideline, it does indicate a possible NF. If a NF does grow on MacConkey agar it appears as a NLF after 24 hours incubation.

■ Some of the nonfermenters have sweet, fruity, or unique odors. They also may display unique colony morphologies and pigmentation.

■ Many of the more common nonfermenters, such as *Pseudomonas aeruginosa* and *Acinetobacter* spp., are often multidrug resistant.

■ The organisms display limited biochemical reactivity in commercial identification systems used for the *Enterobacteriaceae.*

Nonfermenting gram-negative rods have proven to be a frustrating group of organisms that are difficult to identify. Other than *Pseudomonas aeruginosa, Stenotrophomonas maltophilia,* and *Acinetobacter* spp., these organisms are not frequently isolated. Most microbiologists do not have adequate experience with the uncommon organisms. Conventional medium is often not suitable for identification of these organisms. Some of the nonfermenters are slow growers and their biochemical reactions tend to be weak, which extends the time required for their detection and identification. Media used for isolation and identification is expensive and tends to outdate due to infrequent use. Commercial identification systems have

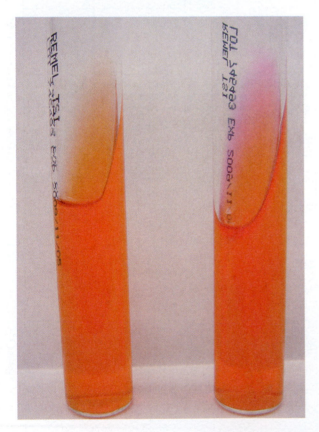

■ **FIGURE 22-1** Nonfermenters produce weak acids from oxidation of the sugars present. These weak acids cannot be detected on TSI agar so there is no color change on the slant or in the deep butt. The subtle pink color on the TSI slant on the right is due to deamination of the proteins present by the organism. This is a typical reaction for nonfermenters. Compare it to the uninoculated TSI slant on the left.

⊘ REAL WORLD TIP

Realize there are other organisms that are unable to ferment carbohydrates. Some can also share other characteristics of the nonfermenting gram-negative rods such as being oxidase positive or unable to grow on MacConkey agar. These organisms can include *Francisella tularensis, Eikenella corrodens, Pasteurella multocida, Bordetella* spp., and others.

✓ Checkpoint! 22–2 (Chapter Objective 2)

Which of the following biochemical tests or physical characteristics can definitely determine if a gram-negative rod is a member of the Enterobacteriaceae or a true nonfermenter?

A. Oxidase
B. Growth on MacConkey agar
C. TSI slant
D. Pigmentation

a lower rate of accuracy. They also often require additional testing, which adds to the expense.

▶ BIOCHEMICAL TESTS FOR IDENTIFICATION

HUGH-LEIFSON OXIDATION-FERMENTATION (OF) MEDIUM

Hugh-Leifson OF medium determines how NF utilize glucose and other carbohydrates more effectively than the media used for the *Enterobacteriaceae*. Testing usually requires two tubes of each carbohydrate in a base medium for testing and a control tube with no carbohydrate present in the base medium. A series of duplicate tubes are usually set up using glucose, lactose, maltose, and other carbohydrates. The base medium is semisolid, to contain the weak acids produced, and uses a brom thymol blue pH indicator. The pH indicator turns yellow with acid by-products and blue with alkaline by-products.

The tube is inoculated by stabbing the organism down the center of the tube to within ¼ inch of the bottom. One of the two specific carbohydrate tubes is overlaid with about 1 to 2 mL of sterile mineral oil or paraffin to create an anaerobic environment to detect fermentation. This is called the closed tube. The other tube remains open to the air, with a loosened lid, to detect oxidation. This is called the open tube.

The tubes are incubated in ambient air at 35–37°C for up to 4 days. Remember, these organisms can grow slowly and are weak acid producers so they need more time for positive reactions. A control tube is required to ensure the organism does not react with anything other than the carbohydrate present. It should remain its original color after incubation.

REAL WORLD TIP

- Only one series of carbohydrate tubes (open) need be used if the isolate is known to be a nonfermenter or if either a TSI or KIA is inoculated at the same time.
- If the OF medium is incubated in a carbon dioxide atmosphere, there is the potential for a false-positive reaction. Incubation in carbon dioxide creates carbonic acid in the medium, which converts the brom thymol blue pH indicator from green to yellow.

An organism that is unable to use the specific carbohydrate displays no reaction in either the open or closed tube, as seen in Figure 9-2. Figure 9-2 demonstrates an organism that is an oxidizer. The open tube (tube C) is positive while the closed tube (tube D) is negative, meaning the organism requires oxygen to metabolize the carbohydrate present. Figure 9-2 also presents the reactions of an organism that ferments the carbohydrate present. Fermenting gram-negative rods will display a positive reaction in both the open (tube A) and closed tubes (tube B).

OF medium is best for NF because it contains a greater concentration of carbohydrates compared to other media. The more carbohydrates present, the more weak acids produced. There is less protein present so less amines are produced, which can raise the medium pH. Amines can neutralize the weak acids produced. The brom thymol blue indicator is more sensitive than other pH indicators and detects the weak acids better. The semisolid medium concentrates the weak acids produced so the pH change is easier to detect.

✓ Checkpoint! 22–3 (Chapter Objective 4)

A microbiologist inoculates two duplicate sets of OF media (control, glucose, lactose, and fructose). One set is left open to the atmosphere and the other set is overlaid with sterile mineral oil. Both sets are placed in the CO_2 incubator. After 24 hours all four of the open tubes are yellow. The closed tubes remained green. Which of the following statements explains these results?

A. *The organism is a fermenting gram-negative rod rather than one that is nonfermenting.*

B. *The open tubes are false-positive reactions.*

C. *The tubes are acceptable because the organism in a nonfermenter.*

D. *The tubes should be incubated for 3 more days before interpretation.*

OXIDASE

The oxidase test is used to differentiate the oxidase-positive pseudomonads from the oxidase-negative *Enterobacteriaceae*. Cytochrome c oxidase is the last enzyme in the electron transport chain of some organisms. The enzyme converts molecular oxygen into water. In the process, ATP is synthesized for energy.

In the oxidase test the reagent, para-phenylenediamine dihydrochloride, substitutes for oxygen in the reaction. The reagent is initially colorless and turns purple when oxidized by the organism. The most common reagent used is 0.5–1.0% tetramethyl-*p*-phenylenediamine dihydrochloride. A drop of the liquid is placed onto a filter paper. A wooden stick is used to rub a colony of the organism into the moistened area. An oxidase-positive organism turns the inoculated area purple within 10–30 seconds. ∞ Chapter 8 provides more discussion on the oxidase reaction.

REAL WORLD TIP

Place the oxidase filter paper in the lid of a clean petri dish prior to use. If the moistened filter paper is placed on the counter surface, the oxidase reagent can react with the bleach used to clean the bench counter and cause a false-positive reaction.

DECARBOXYLATION OF AMINO ACIDS

The traditional decarboxylase procedure relies on the development of decarboxylase enzymes after the organism ferments glucose. The low pH triggers the enzymes to form and break down the amino acids to form alkaline amines, which cause the pH indicator to turn purple. It is a series of four tubes: one tube for each amino acid, arginine, lysine, and ornithine, and a base medium control tube with no amino acid present. Nonfermenters may not demonstrate decarboxylation by this method. They are also unable to ferment the glucose present and must be tested in a different manner. ∞ Chapter 9 discusses the traditional use of decarboxylase to identify the *Enterobacteriaceae*.

Nonfermenters display weak decarboxylase activity. This can be overcome by using only 1–2 mL of the amino acid broth and inoculating with a heavy inoculum of pregrown organisms. Pregrown organisms ensure the highest concentration of enzymes. The tubes are overlaid with only about 4 mm of sterile mineral oil. The tubes are incubated up to 5 days before reporting as negative.

NF are not able to ferment the glucose present so the control base medium will not turn yellow as with the *Enterobacteriaceae*. It remains a dirty gray color. Examine the tubes for a purple color stronger than the control tube. It will not be the vivid purple as seen with the *Enterobacteriaceae*. Figure 22-2 ■ demonstrates the appearance of a decarboxylase control tube and lysine tube with *Burkholderia cepacia*.

MOTILITY

Due to the limited biochemical reactions of the NF, motility may be needed for differentiation. Use of a semisolid medium such as SIM or motility with TTC may not work well to demonstrate motility. These organisms may only grow on the surface of the agar because of their need for oxygen. It may be possible to observe motility in these tubes if the stab line is only about 4 mm into the semisolid medium. The tube is incubated at room temperature because the flagellar proteins are produced better. Figure 22-3 ■ demonstrates a motile nonfermenter in medium with a red dye, TTC.

A hanging drop is more accurate but cumbersome. A loopful of a 6- to 24-hour broth culture is placed in the center of a coverslip. The coverslip is then suspended over the concave surface of a depression slide. Motile organisms display directional movement. Nonmotile organisms remain in place. Any shaking seen is due to Brownian movement.

Another option is to melt a tube of motility B medium and pour it into a small petri dish, 60×15 mm, to harden. Stab the agar down the center about 4 mm and incubate at room temperature overnight. Observe for motility by reading from the side of the agar plate. Motility appears as haziness away from

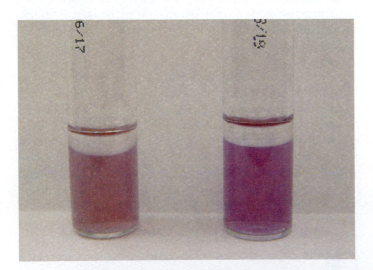

■ **FIGURE 22-2** The decarboxylase reaction of the non-fementers is read slightly differently than that of the *Enterobacteriaceae*. Note the decarboxylase control tube on the left does not turn yellow, as with *Enterobacteriaceae*, because the nonfermenters are unable to ferment the glucose present. A positive reaction is a deeper purple color, as noted in the tube on the right, when compared to the gray-purple control tube.

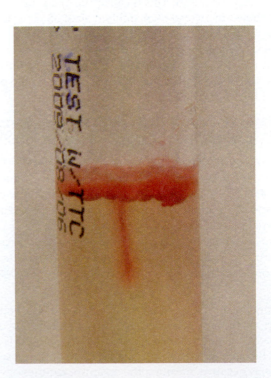

■ **FIGURE 22-3** Nonfermenters are obligate aerobes and require oxygen to grow. This motility medium tube with a red dye, TTC, demonstrates motility. The red hazy growth away from the stab line can be observed. Semisolid medium can be used to demonstrate motility for NF, provided the organism is not stabbed too deeply into the agar.

the stab line. Ignore any growth across the surface of the agar. While more difficult to read, this method allows the organisms the oxygen they need for growth.

Flagellar stains can be used to determine the placement and amplitude of flagella. These stains are very difficult to perform and are not routinely done in most clinical laboratories. A wet-mount technique using RYU flagella stain is a simple way to observe flagella on organisms grown on blood agar for 16 to 24 hours. A small drop of water is placed on a microscope slide. A sterile inoculating loop is dipped into sterile water. The loopful of water is touched to a colony edge, allowing motile cells to swim into the water. The loop droplet containing the motile cells is gently touched to the drop of water on the slide, then covered with a cover slip. The turbid wet-preparation is examined for motile cells. If motile cells are seen, the slide is left at room temperature for 5 to 10 minutes then 2 drops of RSU stain is added to the edge of the coverslip. The slide is left at room temperature for 5 to 10 minutes more, then examined for flagella under oil immersion (Forbes et al., 2007, p. 227). Figure 22-4 ■ demonstrates *Pseudomonas aeruginosa* stained with the RYU flagella stain. It shows a monotrichous, or single, flagellum at one end.

NITRATE REDUCTION

Nitrate reduction is discussed in detail in ∞ Chapter 9. Some of the NF are able to reduce nitrate beyond nitrite to nitrogen gas and other byproducts. Testing may require the use of zinc dust for detection of nitrogen gas and other byproducts.

ACETAMIDE

Acetamide broth or slant determines if the organism is able to use acetamide as the sole source of carbon. When acetamide is deaminated, the brom thymol blue pH indicator turns blue due to an alkaline pH, as seen in Figure 22-5 ■. Yellow or no change in the original green indicates assimilation and a negative reaction. If a phenol red indicator is used instead of brom thymol blue, a pink reaction is positive.

GROWTH AT 42°C

Some nonfermenters demonstrate the unique ability to grow at 42°C. A non-nutrient broth or slant such as brain heart infusion (BHI) can be used. The organism is lightly inoculated onto the slant or into the broth. After 24 hours' incubation, the tube is inspected for growth.

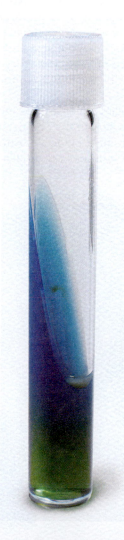

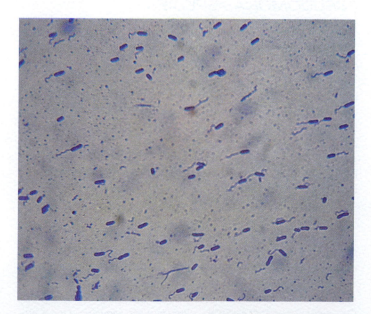

■ **FIGURE 22-4** The flagella stain may be used as part of the identification process of nonfermenters. This illustrates a bacterium, *Pseudomonas aeruginosa* (stained with RYU flagella stain), with a single flagellum at one end of the cell.

■ **FIGURE 22-5** The deamination of acetamide provides the organism a source of carbon. A positive reaction is seen as a blue color change in the green agar slant.
Photo courtesy of Remel, part of Thermo Fisher Scientific.

PIGMENTS, COLONY MORPHOLOGIES, AND DISTINCT ODORS

The nonfermenting gram-negative rods may produce colorful colony pigments, unique colony morphologies, and distinct odors that are helpful in identification. Colonies can appear yellow-orange, violet, red, maroon, brown, and coral. The pigments may also diffuse into the agar beyond the boundaries of the colony. Pigments play a protective role by absorbing ultraviolet rays and resisting antibiotics.

Pyocyanin is a distinctive blue, water soluble, pigment. This pigment acts as a **siderophore**, which helps in the acquisition and metabolism of iron by *Pseudomonas aeruginosa*. While often easily recognized, special isolation and identification media can be used to enhance its detection. Figure 22-6 ■ demonstrates the production of the blue pigment, pyocyanin.

Pyoverdin or fluorescein is a water-soluble, yellow fluorescent pigment produced by *Pseudomonas aeruginosa* and other fluorescent pseudomonads. It is important in helping the organisms acquire iron when grown in an environment low in iron. Figure 22-7 ■ illustrates the pigment's ability to fluoresce under UV light. The combination of pyocyanin and pyoverdin create the blue-green pigment so commonly associated with *P. aeruginosa*.

Colony morphologies can be unique and are discussed with individual organisms later in this chapter. Organisms can create odors due to byproducts of metabolism. While it is not recommended to sniff colonies on an agar plate, often it is

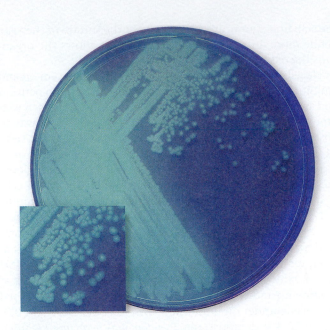

■ **FIGURE 22-7** *Pseudomonas* F agar allows for the detection of pyoverdin or fluorescein under ultraviolet light.
Photo courtesy of Remel, part of Thermo Fisher Scientific.

possible to detect an odor when the agar plate is initially opened. Distinct odors are discussed with individual organisms later in the chapter.

▶ COMMON NONFERMENTERS

PSEUDOMONAS SPECIES

Pseudomonas spp. can be found in many different environments such as soil, water, plant, and animal tissue but rarely inhabits the skin or mucosal surfaces of healthy individuals. Many different species of this genus are opportunistic pathogens that can colonize and infect humans, animals, and plants. *Pseudomonas aeruginosa*, the most common opportunistic pathogen of the genus, usually does not infect uncompromised, intact tissues, however, it can infect once they are compromised (Todar, 2004). Because of its invasive nature and frequency in the environment and nature, transmission to humans can occur in a variety of ways.

Pseudomonas fluorescens, *Pseudomonas putida,* and *Pseudomonas stutzeri* are also environmental inhabitants, but they are much less often encountered in clinical specimens than *Pseudomonas aeruginosa*. Because of their rarity in clinical specimens, the mode of transmission to humans remains uncertain.

Pseudomonas aeruginosa
General Characteristics. *Pseudomonas aeruginosa* is a gram-negative, aerobic rod that may be encapsulated. Most strains are motile by means of a single polar flagellum. This organism is a common inhabitant of the environment such as soil, water, and plants. It survives well in wet environments, such as hot tubs,

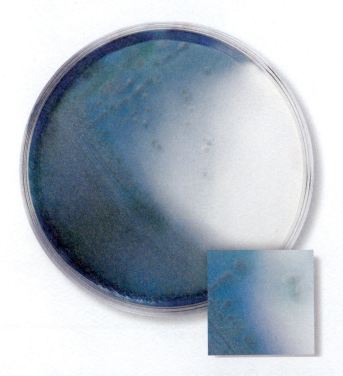

■ **FIGURE 22-6** The blue pigment, pyocyanin, of *Pseudomonas aeruginosa* is enhanced on this *Pseudomonas* isolation agar. The water-soluble pigment diffuses into the medium.
Photo courtesy of Remel, part of Thermo Fisher Scientific.

whirlpools, and contact lens solutions. It can be found in hospitals in sinks, showers, and respiratory equipment.

REAL WORLD TIP

- *Pseudomonas aeruginosa* tends to be a longer, thinner, pale staining gram-negative rod (Figure 22-8 ■) with slightly pointed or rounded ends on Gram stain. While it is not possible to identify *Pseudomonas aeruginosa* based on its Gram stain alone, an experienced microbiologist may be able to differentiate it from *Enterobacteriaceae*, which appear as shorter, fatter gram-negative rods with rounded or squared ends. (Go to ∞ Chapter 21 to see a photo of *E. coli* stained with Gram stain.)
- On a direct specimen Gram stain, mucoid *Pseudomonas aeruginosa* are encapsulated and tend to clump together.

Its metabolism is oxidative and requires the presence of oxygen. It is not able to ferment like the *Enterobacteriaceae*. Its optimum temperature for growth is 35–37°C but is able to grow at temperatures as high as 42°C. It is very tolerant to a wide variety of environmental conditions and resistant to high

REAL WORLD TIP

Pseudomonas aeruginosa will grow in the absence of oxygen if nitrate is available as a respiratory electron acceptor. This means it is possible to see this organism growing on media under anaerobic conditions even though it is considered an obligate aerobe.

concentrations of salts and dyes, weak antiseptics, and many commonly used antibiotics.

Pseudomonas aeruginosa is rarely part of human flora in healthy individuals. Even though this organism is an environmental inhabitant, it rarely causes community-acquired infections even in immunocompromised individuals (Van Delden et al., 1998). As a result, this organism is considered an opportunistic pathogen.

Colonial Appearance. *Pseudomonas aeruginosa* isolates are often beta-hemolytic with rough, spreading, flat colonies with a ground glass consistency and serrated or jagged edges. The colonies often display an aluminum foil or metallic sheen and blue-green pigment that diffuses into the agar. Figure 22-9 ■ demonstrates the typical, slightly irregular, spreading colonies of *P. aeruginosa*. Pigmentation can also be red or brown. The colonies are often beta-hemolytic with a sweet, fruity odor described as grape-like or corn taco shell–like. The odor is due to the production of 2-aminoacetophenone.

REAL WORLD TIP

While *Pseudomonas aeruginosa* is best known for its grape-like odor, there are strains that have a rotten potato odor. The odor is so strong it can permeate throughout the incubator and work area and linger for days.

Culture can also yield one of two smooth colony types. One type is large and smooth with flat edges and an elevated appearance in the center. Another type displays a mucoid appearance. It is frequently obtained from respiratory specimens

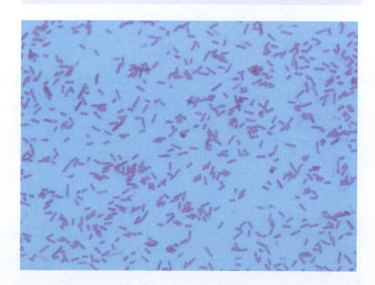

■ **FIGURE 22-8** This Gram stain of *Pseudomonas aeruginosa* shows the long, thin, gram-negative rod that is characteristic of most nonfermenters.

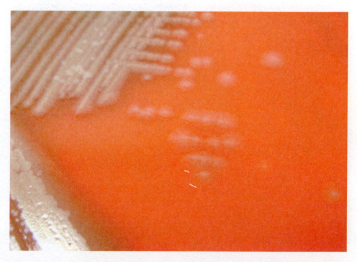

■ **FIGURE 22-9** This colony is typical for *Pseudomonas aeruginosa*. It is often flat and spreading. While it is not visible in this photograph, it is often beta hemolytic. Note the aluminum foil sheen present on the lower left. It often appears where colonies overgrow one another.

of individuals with **cystic fibrosis** (CF). CF is an inherited chronic disease that affects the lungs and digestive system. A defective gene causes the body to produce unusually thick mucus that clogs the lungs and leads to life-threatening lung infections and obstructs the pancreas and prevents enzymes from helping the body break down and absorb food.

The mucoid colony consistency is attributed to the production of **alginate slime**, an exopolysaccharide made up of mannurionic and glucoronic acid (Todar, 2004). The presence of the slime plays a role in prevention of phagocytosis. Both the smooth and mucoid colonies play a role in its ability to colonize and cause disease. Figure 22-10 ■ displays the mucoid colony often associated with infection in individuals with cystic fibrosis.

On a MacConkey agar, *Pseudomonas aeruginosa* is usually described as a nonlactose fermenter. It produces two types of water-soluble pigments. The first is a fluorescent pigment pyoverdin or fluorescein that is yellow and seen only as fluorescence under a UV light. The second is the blue pigment pyocyanin. The latter is produced abundantly in media of low-iron content and functions in iron metabolism in the bacterium. Blue pus is frequently seen in wound infections caused by this organism (Todar, 2004). When combined, the two pigments produce the characteristic blue-green pigment often seen in cultures with *Pseudomonas aeruginosa*.

Key Biochemical Reactions. *Pseudomonas aeruginosa* grows well on most routine laboratory media such as 5% sheep blood, chocolate, and MacConkey agars. It is so common an isolate in the laboratory that it can be rapidly identified, on the same day as isolation, with only a few characteristics. It can be identified as *Pseudomonas aeruginosa* based on being an oxidase-positive NLF that produces a blue-green pigment and possesses a grape-like odor, as noted in Box 22-1.

If the isolate does not meet the rapid identification criteria then conventional testing must be performed. It is identified on the basis of its Gram stain morphology and a positive oxidase reaction, its ability to oxidize glucose, fructose, and xylose but not lactose or sucrose, and its ability to deaminate acetamide and growth at 42°C as well as on the basis of nitrate reduction, positive motility, and arginine decarboxylation. Fluorescence, under ultraviolet light, of the culture plates suggests the presence of the organism. Other *Pseudomonas* spp. can be fluorescent as well so it is not considered a definitive test. Due to its common isolation, most commercial identification systems can be used to identify *P. aeruginosa* accurately.

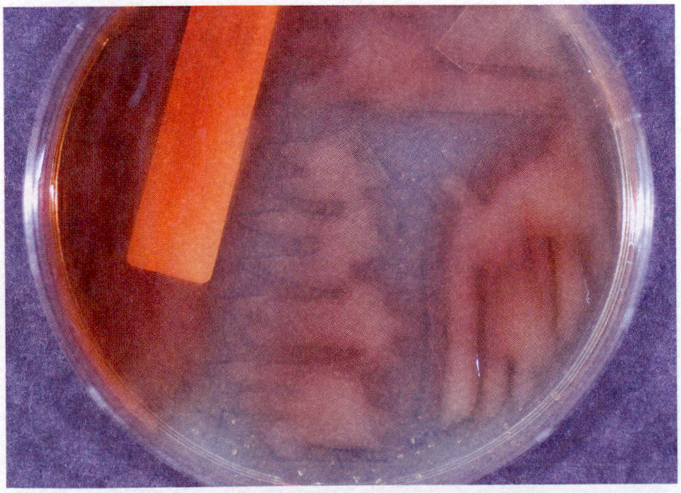

✓ Checkpoint! 22–4 (Chapter Objective 5)

An oxidase-positive, gram-negative rod demonstrates a flat colony with aluminum sheen on the surface of the colonies. It is a nonlactose fermenter but demonstrates a green pigment that extends beyond the colonies on MacConkey. What additional characteristic is necessary to identify the organism as Pseudomonas aeruginosa *using rapid identification criteria?*

A. *The presence of a diffusible yellow pigment*
B. *Beta-hemolysis*
C. *A mucoid colony*
D. *A grape-like odor*

Clinical Significance. *Pseudomonas aeruginosa* requires a break in the body's defenses for an infection to begin. Specimens for cultures include blood, urine, sputum, and other lower respiratory specimens, skin and wound samples, and bone and cartilage.

Microbe Defense Mechanisms. Because *Pseudomonas aeruginosa* is a normal soil and water organism, it has a natural resistance to many antibiotics produced by bacteria and fungi in the environment. *Pseudomonas aeruginosa* possesses a wide array of virulence factors that result in a wide range of diseases, which include septicemia, urinary tract infections, pneumonia, chronic lung infections, endocarditis, skin and wound

■ **FIGURE 22-10** Some strains of *Pseudomonas aeruginosa* can produce alginate slime and appear very mucoid. The mucoid colony is often associated with individuals who have cystic fibrosis. Note the red-brown pigment, pyorubin, produced by this strain rather than the more common blue-green pigment, pyocyanin.

✪ BOX 22-1

Rapid Identification Criteria for *Pseudomonas aeruginosa*

- Nonlactose fermenter
- Oxidase positive
- Presence of a blue-green diffusible pigment
- Grape-like odor

infections, and bone and cartilage infections. It is invasive and toxinogenic. Infections consist of three stages: (1) bacterial attachment and colonization, (2) local invasion, and (3) dissemination, by means of the blood, and systemic disease (Todar, 2004; Qarah & Cunha, 2005).

As with most opportunistic organisms, colonization usually precedes infection. *Pseudomonas* spp. are found everywhere in nature so its exact source and mode of transmission may be difficult to determine. While it may present as part of normal flora, it is not often associated with individuals in the community. It is most often found in hospitalized individuals. Colonization of the respiratory tract by *Pseudomonas* requires adherence to human cells by means of fimbriae. Protease enzymes, released by the organism, break down protein to expose the fimbrial receptors on the surface of epithelial cells. This contributes to tissue injury of the respiratory tract and so plays a large role in colonization.

Pili or filamentous appendages on *P. aeruginosa* are attracted to receptors on epithelial cells. Mucoid strains are able to overproduce exopolysaccharide to form alginate slime. Alginate slime creates the matrix of the *Pseudomonas* biofilm, which anchors it to mucous membranes and prevents its clearance by the ciliated epithelial cells of the respiratory system. It also protects the bacteria from the host defenses by inhibiting phagocytosis and opsonic killing. It is a significant contributor to infections in individuals with cystic fibrosis. *Pseudomonas aeruginosa* growing in an alginate "slime matrix" are resistant to antibiotics and disinfectants. The exact nature of resistance is unclear but has been attributed to slower growth of the organism, protection due to a physical barrier, beta-lactamase production, and other factors (Van Delden & Iglewski, 1998).

The ability of *Pseudomonas aeruginosa* to invade tissues is usually due to toxins and enzymes that break down physical barriers, damage host cells, and help the organism evade host immune defenses. Two known extracellular proteases have been associated with virulence due to their invasive properties: elastase and alkaline protease. Elastase enzymes cleave elastin, protein, collagen, IgG, IgA, and complement. It also lyses fibronectin, a protein, to expose receptors so the organism can attach to the respiratory mucosal lining. This disrupts the lung epithelium and interferes with ciliary function.

Alkaline protease contributes by interfering with fibrin formation and causes tissue destruction. Together these two enzymes can destroy corneal substance and other supporting structures composed of fibrin and elastin (Todar, 2004; Van Delden & Iglewski, 1998). Both enzymes have been reported to cause inactivation of cytokines such as gamma interferon and tumor necrosis factor. This results in the inability to activate the immune cells.

Pseudomonas aeruginosa produces cytotoxins that are toxic for most human cells, including neutrophils. Hemolysins, such as phospholipase and lecithinase, act together to break down lipids and lecithin. The cytotoxins and hemolysins together allow the organism to invade cells (Todar, 2004; Van Delden & Iglewski, 1998; Allewelt, Coleman, Grout, Priebe, & Pier, 2000).

The blue pigment, pyocyanin, appears to impair the ability of the upper respiratory cilia to sweep out mucous and debris such as bacteria. It also kills cells of the lung epithelium by preventing catalase activity within the cell. In addition, it causes apoptosis or death of white blood cells.

Other virulence factors include lipopolysaccharide or endotoxin that causes the signs and symptoms associated with gram-negative septicemia such as fever, hypotension, and disseminated intravascular coagulation. Exoenzyme S is an exotoxin produced by *P. aeruginosa* growing in tissue that has been damaged due to burns. It may be detected in the blood before the bacteria disseminate. This enzyme has a cytotoxic effect on cells in the lung and may be necessary for bacterial dissemination (Van Delden & Iglewski, 1998). It impairs phagocytic cells making invasion by *Pseudomonas aeruginosa* easier (Todar, 2004).

Exotoxin A has exactly the same mechanism of action as the toxin produced by *Corynebacterium diphtheriae*. Both toxins inhibit protein synthesis in eukaryotic cells. It also has a necrotizing effect at the site of bacterial colonization and is responsible for tissue damage, bacterial invasion, and possible immunosuppression due to the ability to kill phagocytes. Purified exotoxin A is highly lethal for human cells (Todar, 2004; Van Delden & Iglewski, 1998).

Pathogenesis and Infectious Diseases.   *Pseudomonas aeruginosa* causes a variety of diseases. It is involved in respiratory infections, which usually occur in individuals with either a compromised lower respiratory tract, such as chronic lung disease, or immunosupression. It is especially prevalent in intensive care unit patients on a ventilator and receiving long-term therapy with broad-spectrum antibiotics. Long-term antibiotic use wipes out the normal upper respiratory flora, making it easier for the resistant *P. aeruginosa* to colonize. Bacteremia associated with pneumonia is commonly seen in individuals undergoing chemotherapy. They are unable to fight infection due to neutropenia (Qarah & Cunha, 2005).

REAL WORLD TIP

Neutropenic individuals should avoid raw vegetables, live plants, flowers in vases, and ice from an ice machine. All of these are potential sources of bacteria, such as *Pseudomonas aeruginosa*, which can cause infection in these compromised individuals.

Individuals with cystic fibrosis (CF) are often colonized by a unique mucoid strain of the bacterium that is very difficult to eradicate. This particular organism has been the leading pathogen associated with cystic fibrosis. Review Figure 22-10 to see this characteristic mucoid colony. The organism is probably acquired from the environment and is probably not passed person to person.

Once colonized, infection leads to the destruction of lung tissue and significant reduction of lung function, both of which often result in early death. In 1996, the U.S. Cystic Fibrosis Foundation database reported the median survival of CF individuals who were colonized with *Pseudomonas aeruginosa* was 28 years old while the median survival for non-colonized individuals was 39 years old. The presence of a mucoid colony in CF individuals predicts a more unfavorable patient outcome than the presence of nonmucoid *Pseudomonas aeruginosa*. The presence of nonmucoid strains of the organism can serve as the reservoir for the development of mucoid strain bacterial biofilms and colonization (Van daele et al., 2005; O'Carroll et al., 2004). Cystic fibrosis and associated infections are discussed in detail in ∞ Chapter 33, "Respiratory System."

 REAL WORLD TIP

- The presence of a mucoid strain of *Pseudomonas aeruginosa* in culture should be reported. Its presence is most often associated with cystic fibrosis but it can also be found in the lungs of adults with chronic obstructive pulmonary disease (COPD).
- A healthy individual is rarely colonized by *Pseudomonas aeruginosa*. If it is isolated from a body site such as the throat, the physician should investigate to determine why the organism is present.

Pseudomonas aeruginosa is associated with bacteremia and septicemia in individuals with immunosuppression, underlying diseases such as diabetes, and severe burns.. It can account for about 25% of all hospital-acquired gram-negative bacteremias, which makes it an important nosocomial organism. In addition, it causes endocarditis in intravenous drug users and those with prosthetic heart valves (Qarah & Cunha, 2005). The organism invades the bloodstream to reach the damaged or artificial heart valves (Todar, 2004).

P. aeruginosa is well known as the cause of "swimmer's ear." Because the organism likes water, the wet environment of the external auditory canal of a swimmer's ear is the perfect place for the organism. Those afflicted often complain of pain, itching, and discharge (Qarah & Cunha, 2005).

The organism is a major cause of bacterial keratitis. It most often occurs after trauma to the cornea such as extended contact wear or poor contact lens hygiene. Individuals who have been

REAL WORLD TIP

Individuals can purchase colored and novelty contacts over the Internet without a prescription from an eye doctor. Often contact lens hygiene is nonexistent because these individuals have not been properly instructed and they may share the lenses with others. *Pseudomonas aeruginosa* and other organisms can be isolated from these lenses.

admitted to the intensive care unit are at risk also. It can cause a rapid destructive infection, which may lead to the loss of the entire eye (Todar, 2004; Qarah & Cunha, 2005; Zhu et al., 2004).

Bones and joints may be sites for potential infection. The organism can be directly inoculated into these sites or spread from other sites of infection via the bloodstream. *Pseudomonas aeruginosa* seems to prefer the cartilage joints of the bones of the skull and trunk. It can cause chronic osteomyelitis due to direct inoculation of the bone. This can occur after a puncture wound to the foot.

 REAL WORLD TIP

Kids like to jump and play in mud puddles while wearing their sneakers. The sneaker liners often stay wet for days. *Pseudomonas aeruginosa* likes to grow in this moist lining. When a child steps on a nail or other sharp object, it can push the organism into the bone of the heel, leading to osteomyelitis.

Urinary tract catheterization, instrumentation, or surgery can lead to urinary tract infections in hospitalized individuals due to its status as a nosocomial pathogen. While not known as a common cause of diarrhea, *Pseudomonas aeruginosa* can produce disease in the gastrointestinal tract, especially in immunocompromised patients. It has been associated with necrotizing enterocolitis in infants. Even though *Clostridium difficile, Staphylococcus aureus,* drug-resistant *Salmonella* species, and *Candida* species have been reported to cause most of antibiotic-associated diarrhea or colitis, there have been reports that suggest *Pseudomonas aeruginosa* could be a potential cause of antibiotic-associated diarrhea (Woo Kim et al., 2001). Colonization of the gastrointestinal tract of a hospitalized patient can be the source of the organism if the individual develops bacteremia.

Pseudomonas aeruginosa is well known for skin and soft tissue infections, including burn wound infections, pyoderma with large sores, and dermatitis. Predisposing factors include the breakdown of the natural barrier of the skin and high moisture conditions. Individuals with AIDs and underlying diseases such as diabetes are easily infected. The organism is a common pathogen in burn wound patients. The loss of the protective skin barrier, leaking capillaries, loss of blood flow, and subsequent inability of white blood cells to reach the area and the presence of necrotic tissue promote the colonization of a burn wound by *Pseudomonas aeruginosa*.

 REAL WORLD TIP

Fresh flowers are not allowed to be sent to patients in the burn unit. They can be a source of *Pseudomonas aeruginosa*.

Pseudomonas has been shown to cause folliculitis or infection of the hair follicles. It is due to bacterial colonization of hair follicles after exposure to contaminated wet environments such as whirlpools, hot tubs, and swimming pools (Krivda & Toner, 2006). Body parts covered by the wet swimming suit, such as the buttocks, are most often infected. The organism can flourish when adequate chlorine levels are not maintained.

 Checkpoint! 22–5 (Chapter Objective 6)

*Which of the following individuals is **least** likely to be colonized or infected with Pseudomonas aeruginosa?*

  A. *14-year-old female with cystic fibrosis*
  B. *24-year-old male firefighter with third-degree burns*
  C. *20-year-old male who teaches swimming classes*
  D. *17-year-old female student with a urinary tract infection*

Prevention and Treatment. *Pseudomonas aeruginosa* is a common environmental inhabitant. Within the hospital, the bacterium finds many places to flourish ranging from disinfectants, respiratory equipment, food, sinks, taps, and mops. It is constantly reintroduced to the hospital environment on raw fruits and vegetables, flowers, plants, and even ice as well as visitors and patients transferred from other facilities. Spread occurs from patient to patient on the hands of hospital personnel, by direct patient contact with contaminated reservoirs and by the ingestion of contaminated foods and water. The spread of the organism can be controlled by observing proper isolation procedures, aseptic techniques, and careful cleaning and monitoring of respirators, catheters, and other instruments.

The emergence of bacterial strains resistant to antimicrobial agents is a major challenge today. *Pseudomonas aeruginosa* is now a major problem pathogen showing intrinsic resistance to many antibiotics. This is partly due to its low outer membrane permeability and secondary resistance mechanisms such as beta-lactamases and multidrug active efflux pumps (Van Delden et al., 1998; Ochs, McCusker, Bains, & Hancock, 1999). It also has the ability to acquire resistance mechanisms from other organisms.

Antimicrobial agents effective against the organism include the antipseudomonal beta-lactams, fluoroquinolones, and aminoglycosides (Hsu, Okamoto, Murthy, & Wong-Beringer, 2005). The fluoroquinolones are an oral treatment option but resistance among *Pseudomonas aeruginosa* strains has increased. Ciprofloxacin and levofloxacin may someday no longer be options for empirical antipseudomonal therapy (Hsu et al., 2005).

The current standard for treatment is an antipseudomonal beta-lactam agent combined with an aminoglycoside (Infections in Medicine, 2007). Although many strains are susceptible to gentamicin, tobramycin, colistin, and amikacin, resistant forms have now developed. In addition, imipenem,

a carbapenem, is useful in treatment because of its high potency, broad spectrum, and general lack of microbial resistance (Ochs et al., 1999). The combination of gentamicin and carbenicillin is frequently used to treat severe *Pseudomonas* infections.

Treatment of infection in individuals with cystic fibrosis often requires the use of an aerosolized aminoglycoside such as tobramycin and oral azithromycin. The aerosol can reach the organism deep in the lungs. Burn wounds are often treated with topical cream containing antibacterial agents coupled with surgical debridement and intravenous antibiotics. This type of therapy dramatically reduces the prevalence of *Pseudomonas* sepsis in burn patients (Todar, 2004).

 REAL WORLD TIP

Cystic fibrosis individuals require high doses of nebulized or aerosolized tobramycin to penetrate the thick respiratory secretions present. They must be monitored for tobramycin levels to prevent neurotoxicity and nephrotoxicity.

Other *Pseudomonas* species

Pseudomonas fluorescens and *P. putida* (Fluorescent Group).

Pseudomonas fluorescens and *P. putida* are closely related and often described together. Both are motile, aerobic, oxidase-positive, gram-negative bacilli that resemble *Pseudomonas aeruginosa* because they produce pyoverdin or fluorescein but not pyocyanin. *P. aeruginosa*, *P. fluorescens*, and *P. putida* are considered the fluorescent pseudomonad group.

 REAL WORLD TIP

Pyoverdin is a siderophore that functions to bind iron for essential metabolic processes. It is produced when the iron content of the environment is low. Its production may be linked to virulence (Cox & Adams, 1985).

Pseudomonas fluorescens is an environmental organism found in soil, water, plants, and contaminated food such as milk. It is rarely isolated from clinical specimens because the majority of isolates grow poorly at 35°C, which is the temperature of clinical laboratory incubators. Its optimal growth temperature is 25–30°C. Its colony, on sheep blood agar, is the same typical wet and gray associated with most gram-negative rods. It appears as a nonlactose fermenter on MacConkey agar.

Pseudomonas putida is also an environmental organism found in soil and water. It is known for its ability for bioremediation such as the breakdown of oil and toluene. It has been isolated from lizards, insects, and mammals. Its optimal temperature for growth is 25°C or room temperature. Growth on MacConkey is as a nonlactose fermenter.

Pseudomonas fluorescens and *P. putida* are both motile and oxidase positive. Often the two species are not differentiated and reported as a group name. They can be distinguished from the most common fluorescent nonfermenter, *Pseudomonas aeruginosa*, by their inability to grow at 42°C and failure to deaminate acetamide. *P. aeruginosa* is positive for both reactions.

Pseudomonas fluorescens can be distinguished from *Pseudomonas putida* by the latter's ability to grow at 4°C and hydrolyze gelatin. These characteristics explain *P. fluorescens'* frequent involvement in the spoilage of refrigerated food, especially chicken and processed meats. Its love for cooler temperatures also explains it implication in transfusion-related septicemia. Table 22-2✪ differentiates the biochemical reactions for the most common fluorescent pseudomonads.

Both organisms that have been isolated include respiratory tract specimens, pleural fluid, urine, cerebrospinal fluid, feces, blood, and a variety of other materials. The clinical importance of *Pseudomonas fluorescens* and *Pseudomonas putida* is debatable. Their love for cooler temperatures may explain why they are rarely pathogenic for humans even though they have been found associated with abscesses, urinary tract infections, septicemia, and septic arthritis. They have been implicated as nosocomial pathogens in immunosuppressed individuals.

⊚ REAL WORLD TIP

Special medium that enhances the production of pyoverdin is available. There is also medium that enhances the production of pyocyanin. The use of the two may assist in the presumptive identification of some *Pseudomonas* spp.

P. fluorescens can be treated with aminoglucosides, fluoroquinolones and trimethoprim-sulfamethoxazole. Imipenem and ceftazadime are effective against *P. putida*.

Pseudomonas stutzeri. *Pseudomonas stutzeri* is a non-fluorescent gram-negative rod that is widely distributed in the environment. It has been isolated as a rare opportunistic pathogen in humans. It is best known as a soil **denitrifier** in which nitrogen is reduced in the soil and returned to the atmosphere.

Pseudomonas stutzeri is often recognized by its unusual colony. On blood agar the colonies are adherent, wrinkled or leathery, hard and dry with either a yellow or brown pigment. It tends to be difficult to mix into suspension, making its identification and susceptibility testing complicated. The colony can resemble that of *Burkholderia pseudomallei*, a potential bioterrorism organism, so accurate identification is necessary. Figure 22-18, later in this chapter, displays the wrinkled colony of *B. pseudomallei*. The organism appears as a nonlactose fermenter on MacConkey media.

Growth temperatures ranging from 4°C to 45°C have been noted. Most strains can grow at 40–43°C. The optimum temperature for growth is approximately 35°C (Lalucat, Bennasar, Bosch, Garcia Valde, & Pallero, 2006).

P. stutzeri is a motile, gram-negative rod that is oxidase positive. It is a denitrifier, which means that it has a respiratory metabolism and oxygen is the main terminal electron acceptor but it can also use nitrate as an alternative electron acceptor for cellular processes (Lalucat et al., 2006). No fluorescent pigment is produced, which differentiates it from the fluorescent group of *Pseudomonas* species. It is arginine decarboxylase negative while most of the common pseudomonad isolates are positive. This reaction can also differentiate it from *Burkholderia pseudomallei*, which it can physically resemble. *Bukholderia pseudomallei* is arginine positive. It is also able to oxidize maltose and hydrolyze starch while most of the other *Pseudomonas* spp. cannot.

While a rare source of infection, *Pseudomonas stutzeri* has been associated with bacteremia and septicemia, bone infection, endocarditis, eye infection, meningitis, skin infections, and urinary tract infections in those with underlying conditions and immunosupression.

The tough wrinkled colony of *P. stutzeri* makes it difficult to suspend in liquid. It is challenging to achieve a 0.5 McFarland suspension for susceptibility testing. *Pseudomonas stutzeri* demonstrates at least two antibiotic resistance mechanisms. They include an alteration in outer membrane proteins and lipopolysaccharide profiles and the presence of beta-lactamases that hydrolyze natural and semi-synthetic penicillins, broad-

---

⊚ REAL WORLD TIP

An outbreak of pseudobacteremia due to *Ralstonia pickettii* has been reported (Verschraegen et al., 1985). This organism contaminated the chlorhexidine solution used to disinfect the skin prior to venipuncture. When multiple blood cultures drawn from multiple patients become positive with rarely isolated organisms such as nonfermenters, investigate the possibility of pseudobactermia due to contamination.

✪ TABLE 22-2

Biochemical Differentiation of *Pseudomonas aeruginosa*, *P. fluorescens*, and *P. putida*

Test	P. aeruginosa	P. fluorescens	P. putida
Pyocyanin production	+	–	–
Pyoverdin production	+	+	+
Growth at 42°C	+	–	–
Acetamide deamination	+	–	–
Gelatin hydrolysis	+	+	–
Nitrate reduction	+	–	–

+, positive; –, negative.

spectrum cephalosporins, and monobactams (Lalucat et al., 2006). Treatment may include the use of aminoglycosides, trimethoprim-sulfamethoxazole, tetracycline, fluoroquinolones, and the third-generation cephalosporins.

ACINETOBACTER SPECIES

Acinetobacter spp. are gram-negative coccobacilli that normally thrive in water and soil. It may be found on the skin and in the upper respiratory tract of healthy individuals. There are at least 25 different species of *Acinetobacter*. A few species, especially *Acinetobacter baumannii*, can cause infections in hospitalized individuals. The hospital-acquired strains are the second most commonly isolated nonfermenters after *Pseudomonas aeruginosa*. *Acinetobacter baumannii* tends to be very resistant to many antibiotics and the infections they cause can be difficult to treat.

Acinetobacter baumannii

General Characteristics. *Acinetobacter baumannii* is a pleomorphic aerobic gram-negative rod that tends to appear as a coccobacillus in singles, pairs, and short chains. Figure 22-11 ■ demonstrates its typical Gram stain. It can be confused with the gram-negative diplococci of the *Neisseria gonorrhoeae* and *Moraxella* spp. The organism has a tendency to retain crystal violet when grown in a liquid medium such as blood culture broth or stained from the direct specimen. The microbiologist must be aware that they can resemble gram-positive cocci in positive blood cultures.

It has gained recognition in the past 15 years as a significant nosocomial pathogen. In the environment it is a soil and water organism. They have become a significant nosocomial

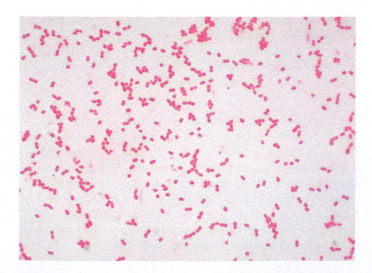

■ **FIGURE 22-11** This Gram stain of *Acinetobacter baumannii* shows its characteristic gram-negative coccobacilli morphology. It can be confused with the gram-negative diplococci of *Neisseria* and *Moraxella* spp. or overdecolorized gram-positive cocci.

From Public Health Image Library (PHIL), CDC/Dr. W. A. Clark.

pathogen and can be found in moist environments in the hospital such as ventilation equipment, waterbaths, and humidifiers. As with other nosocomial pathogens, the organism must first colonize those with underlying diseases or immunosuppression then it can go on to cause infection. It tends to colonize the skin, oral cavity, respiratory tract, and intestine of hospitalized patients.

Colonial Appearance. In general, the macroscopic morphology of *Acinetobacter baumannii* is a nonhemolytic smooth, opaque, raised, wet-looking, gray-white colony on sheep blood agar after overnight incubation. These organisms are able to grow well on most routine media. On MacConkey agar, they are considered nonlactose fermenters but can exhibit a slightly bluish-pink tint, which may cause the organism to be mistaken for a late lactose-fermenter. The organism is able to oxidize lactose over time, which can drop the pH of the agar and change the pH indicator to slightly pink. Figure 22-12 ■ demonstrates the colonies of *A. baumannii* on sheep blood and MacConkey agars.

ⓔ REAL WORLD TIP

The Gram stain of *Acinetobacter baumannii* can falsely appear as gram-positive coccobacilli when grown in blood culture broth medium. Its colony can appear nonhemolytic and white on sheep blood agar and it is catalase positive. Microbiologists have been fooled into thinking it is a *Staphylococcus* spp. The susceptibility will offer a clue. *A. baumannii* is always vancomycin resistant. Vancomycin-resistant *Staphylococcus* spp. are rare to date and should trigger an investigation of the organism's identification.

Key Biochemical Reactions. *A. baumannii* is a nonmotile nonlactose fermenter. It can be easily confused with members of the *Enterobacteriaceae* because it is oxidase negative. The TSI slant reaction will differentiate them. *A. baumannii* produces a K/NC reaction compared to that of the *Enterobacteriaceae* that demonstrate at least an acid-deep butt.

The genus is divided into two groups: one that contains the saccharolytic or glucose-oxidizing species and the other contains the assacharolytic or noncarbohydrate-utilizing species. Most glucose-oxidizing, nonhemolytic strains are designated *Acinetobacter baumannii*, while the nonglucose-using, nonhemolytic strains are identified as *Acinetobacter lwoffi*. The majority of beta-hemolytic organisms are called *Acinetobacter haemolyticus* (Forbes, Sahm, & Weissfeld, 2007).

Its negative-oxidase reaction differentiates it from organisms with a similar Gram stain such as *Neisseria* and *Moraxella* spp. Because it is nonmotile, it may be necessary to differentiate it from other nonmotile nonfermenters such as *Moraxella* spp., *Chryseobacterum* spp., and *Elizabethkingia* spp. An oxidase

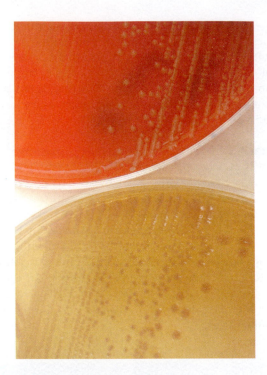

■ **FIGURE 22-12** The colonies of *Acinetobacter baumannii* can resemble those of other gram-negative rods. Microbiologists may misinterpret its slightly blue-pink colonies on MacConkey agar as lactose fermentation.

negative result will point to *Acinetobacter* spp. whereas the others are oxidase positive.

Stenotrophomonas maltophilia is oxidase negative, similar to *A. baumannii*. *S. maltophilia*'s ability to hydrolyze gelatin, decarboxylate lysine, and motility will differentiate the two organisms.

Clinical Significance

Microbe Defense Mechanisms. *A. baumannii* is able to form biofilms on inanimate objects, which explains its current success as a nosocomial pathogen. The presence of pili allows the organism to adhere to epithelial cells. Once it adheres, it is able to create proteins that can cause cell death. As a gram-negative organism, it possesses lipopolysaccharide as part of its cell wall. It tends to be resistant to disinfectants and can survive on moist and dry surfaces. It is best known now for its multidrug resistance.

Pathogenesis and Infectious Diseases. Because *Acinetobacter baumannii* is a common colonizer of hospitalized patients, its clinical significance may be difficult to determine. The organism seems now to be most widespread in burn units and intensive care units (ICUs). This is probably related to the frequent use of antibiotics in these areas.

In addition to intrinsic resistance, *Acinetobacter baumannii* has the ability to acquire resistance to many major classes of antibiotics, including newer beta-lactams. The presence of

resistance plasmids is a significant virulence feature of this organism (Joshi, Litake, Geetanjali, Ghoe, & Niphadkar, 2003; Villers et al., 1998). *Acinetobacter baumannii* has been nicknamed the "gram-negative MRSA," and measures directed at controlling it are similar to those used to control MRSA even though their reservoirs and mode of transmission vary dramatically (Rello, 1999).

The digestive tract, skin surface, and mucous membranes of patients in the ICU environment may be the reservoir sites for the organism. Transmission occurs due to contact from the hands of health care workers or from environmental reservoirs such as humidifiers, ventilators, and other medical equipment. It is essential to maintain good infection control measures to prevent its transmission.

Acinetobacter baumannii infections outside the hospital are very rare. In hospitalized patients, it may be difficult to determine if it is a colonizer or a true pathogen when isolated in the respiratory tract. As a nosocomial pathogen, it most often causes pneumonia in individuals admitted to the ICU and on a ventilator or with an endotracheal tube or tracheostomy. It is also associated with bacteremia in ICU patients. It can cause catheter-related urinary tract infections. *A. baumannii* is also nicknamed "Iraqibacter" because it is the most common isolate from soldiers injured in Afghanistan and Iraq (Peleg, Seifert, & Paterson, 2008). Hosptialized burn patients are extremely susceptible to colonization and infection.

 Checkpoint! 22–6 (Chapter Objective 7)

Which of the following organisms has been nicknamed the "gram-negative MRSA"?
A. *Pseudomonas aeruginosa*
B. *Acinetobacter baumannii*
C. *Stenotrophomonas maltophilia*
D. *Pseudomonas stutzeri*

Prevention and Treatment. An outbreak due to *Acinetobacter baumannii* can close entire floors of hospitals, take many lives, and cost facilities a lot of money. Hand hygiene, either traditional hand washing or with the use of alcohol-based hand sanitizer, remains effective. Microbiology cultures performed allow the infection control team to perform surveillance and place infected individuals on isolation. Standard and contact precautions can decrease the reservoir of organisms and control its dissemination. Careful use of antibiotics decreases antibiotic selective pressures (Rello, 1999).

Acinetobacter baumannii is a multiresistant gram-negative bacillus susceptible to very few antibiotics. In one report, *Acinetobacter baumanii* is defined as multidrug resistant when the organism is resistant to piperacillin/tazobactam, cefepime, ceftazidime, aztreonam, ciprofloxacin, gentamicin, and tobramycin, but susceptible to amikacin, ampicillin-sulbactam, imipenem, meropenem, and minocycline (Abbo et al., 2005). Multidrug-resistant *Acinetobacter baumannii* is probably not a new or emerging phenomenon but has always been an organism inherently resistant to multiple antibiotics (Cunha, 2007; Appleman et al., 2000).

Treatment should be based on susceptibility test results. Most *Acinetobacter baumannii* are susceptible to the carbapenems, imipenem and meropenem. However, reports of carbapenem resistance among *Acinetobacter* species are now being reported (Yu et al., 2004; Afzal-Shah, Villar, & Livermore, 1999). Other treatment options include piperacillin/tazobactam, most third-generation cephalosporins, and aminoglycosides. Quinolones once had good activity but resistance has now emerged in clinical isolates.

Multiple-resistant *Acinetobacter baumannii* infections are usually treated with imipenem or sulbactam but resistance has been reported. Colistin is among one of the few antimicrobial agents that can still be used to treat infections caused by multiresistant strains (Li et al., 2006). The downside of colistin is its potential for nephrotoxicity, neuromuscular block leading to respiratory distress, and neurotoxicity (Vila et al., 2002). A new fluoroquinolone, clinafloxacin, is being studied as a therapeutic option in the treatment of severe infections caused by multidrug-resistant *Acinetobacter baumannii* (Vila et al., 2002).

A beta-lactam agent combined with an aminoglycoside is often used to treat serious infections, such as pneumonia or bacteremia. A new potent tetracycline agent, tigecyline, has shown promise against *A. baumannii*. Because this organism is able to acquire multidrug resistance, susceptibility testing is recommended for clinically relevant isolates.

STENOTROPHOMONAS MALTOPHILIA

General Characteristics

Stenotrophomonas maltophilia is a motile, oxidative, gram-negative rod found in a wide variety of environments including soil, plants, and water as well as a nosocomial pathogen. It likes a moist environment similar to *Pseudomonas aeruginosa*. Originally it was included in the genus *Pseudomonas* then moved to the genus *Xanthomonas*. It is now the only species in the genus *Stenotrophomonas*.

Colonial Appearance

Stenotrophomonas maltophilia appears as nondistinct, straight or slightly curved gram-negative rods in singles or pairs. On a blood agar medium, the colonies are nonhemolytic, large, smooth, and shiny. They can be gray-white but may have a slight yellow pigment with a distinctive ammonia-like odor when the agar lid is initially removed. The colonies may exhibit a lavender-green discoloration of the agar in areas of heavy growth on blood agar medium. It is a nonlactose fermenter and may exhibit a brownish discoloration of MacConkey agar. Figure 22-13 ■ demonstrates the colonies of *S. maltophilia* on sheep blood and MacConkey agars. *Stenotrophomonas maltophilia* is an obligate aerobe. Its optimal growth is at 35°C.

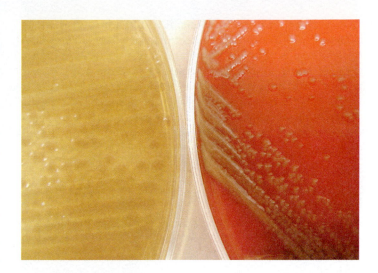

■ **FIGURE 22-13** The colonies of *Stenotrophomonas maltophilia* can possess a light yellow pigment, as seen here on the sheep blood agar. While its colonies on MacConkey agar are considered non-lactose-fermenting, they also may have a slight yellow pigment.

Key Biochemical Reactions

The key biochemical reactions of *Stenotrophomonas maltophilia* include negative-oxidase reaction, rapid and strong oxidation of maltose (therefore the species name *maltophilia,* or "maltose loving"), weaker oxidation of glucose, ability to decarboxylate lysine, and positive reaction for DNase enzyme.

Its negative-oxidase reaction and NLF colony can be confused with members of the *Enterobacteriaceae*. Its TSI reaction, K/NC, will differentiate it from the acid-deep butt of the *Enterobacteriaceae*. *Acinetobacter* spp. is also an oxidase-negative NLF. Motility and decarboxylation of lysine will differentiate *S. maltophilia* from the nonmotile and lysine-negative *Acinetobacter* spp.

There are two clinically significant lysine-positive nonfermenters, *S. maltophilia* and *Burkholderia cepacia*. The two organisms may be differentiated by the oxidase reaction. *B. cepacia* is usually oxidase positive but may be such as weak reaction that it can be read as negative. A positive DNase reaction will identify the organism as *S. maltophilia*.

Clinical Significance

Microbe Defense Mechanisms. Over the last decade, *Stenotrophomonas maltophilia* has gained recognition as an important nosocomial pathogen in debilitated and immunosuppressed individuals (Denton & Kell, 1998; Gasparetto, Bertholdo, Davaus, Marchiori, & Escuissato, 2007; Tatman-Otkun, Gurcan, Ozer, Aydoslu, & Bukavaz, 2005). Little is known about the virulence factors associated with this organism. It does produce proteases and elastases similar to those of *Pseudomonas aeruginosa*. As a gram-negative rod, it possesses lipopolysaccharide (LPS) as part of its cell wall.

As with other nonfermenters, it is difficult to distinguish between colonization and infection. *Stenotrophomonas maltophilia* may actually be an organism of very limited pathogenicity. Some studies were unable to attribute death of any patient directly to the presence of the organism (Denton & Kerr, 1998; Nseir et al., 2006). It has been suggested that the presence of *Stenotrophomonas maltophilia* is only significant when it acts in combination with other pathogens present (Denton & Kerr, 1998).

> ### ⊚ REAL WORLD TIP
>
> *S. maltophilia* can survive in disinfectants and antiseptic soaps, which can lead to outbreaks of pseudobacteremia.

Pathogenesis and Infectious Diseases. *Stenotrophomonas maltophilia* is a very common colonizer of immunosuppressed individuals, those with cystic fibrosis, and hospitalized patients. Its presence does not mean an infection is present. There is an increased risk of death if *S. maltophilia* is isolated from a respiratory source in a patient over the age of 40 who is admitted to the intensive care unit and receives broad-spectrum antibiotics. While it may not cause the infection that leads to death, its presence is a marker that the patient is deteriorating. It presence is most common when medical devices such as intravenous, central venous, and urinary catheters are present.

Pneumonia, due to *S. maltophilia,* is the most common infection and is usually associated with the use of mechanical respiratory ventilators and endotracheal tubes. Individuals with lung problems are also at risk for pneumonia with this organism. Cystic fibrosis patients can be colonized with *S. maltophilia* in addition to other nonfermenters. It is probably not a true pathogen for this patient population and should not be treated.

Individuals with intravascular devices, such as catheters and arterial monitoring equipment, are at increased risk for bacteremia with *S. maltophilia*. Its presence in urine is usually due to colonization of the urinary catheter or manipulation of the urinary tract due to surgery or other invasive procedures. Urinary tract infections are not a common occurrence. *S. maltophilia* can be isolated from wounds. Unless there is the presence of white blood cells in the form of pus, it may be only a colonizer.

Prevention and Treatment. Because *Stenotrophomonas maltophilia* is a nosocomial organism, hand hygiene and infection control measures are important in preventing the spread of the organism from patient to patient. The physician must be careful not to attempt therapy to eradicate the organism when it is present as a colonizer and not a true pathogen. Unnecessary treatment can predispose the individual to infections due to other nosocomial pathogens.

S. maltophilia is intrinsically resistant to many antibiotics due to production of beta-lactamases and carbapenemases, plasmids, alteration of outer membrane proteins, and an efflux mechanism. It is well known for developing resistance to new antibiotics quickly. Surprisingly it is susceptible to trimethoprim-sulfamethoxazole, which is unusual for the nonfermenters, but resistance is now being reported (Al-Jasser, 2006). It is also susceptible to colistin and polymyxin B, which are antibiotics not used frequently today. Treatment options are limited. The newer fluorquinolones may be effective. It is somewhat susceptible to cephalosporins and penicillins. Therapy usually requires rifampin plus a fluoroquinolone or a beta-lactam.

Susceptibility testing can be an issue with *S. maltophilia*. The disk diffusion method can produce inaccurate and nonreproducible zone sizes, leading to the potential for false susceptibility or resistance. Broth dilution is the method recommended by the Clinical and Laboratory Standards Institute (CLSI). Susceptibility testing is discussed in detail in ∞ Chapter 11.

Burkholderia cepacia Complex

General Characteristics. *Burkholderia cepacia* is a very significant motile gram-negative rod that is most often associated with a specific patient population: individuals with cystic fibrosis. This previous member of the *Pseudomonas* genus inhabits the environment in soil and water and is not considered part of normal human flora. It is well known as a plant pathogen but not as a nosocomial pathogen and does not cause harm to healthy individuals. It can be found in the hospital environment in tap water, disinfectants, soaps, and lotions. *B. cepacia* is actually a complex of nine subspecies. They are usually not differentiated but can be based on biochemicals or molecular genetics. It is often reported as *B. cepacia* complex.

Colonial Appearance. *B. cepacia* is able to grow on sheep blood, chocolate, and MacConkey agars. On sheep blood agar, colonies appear smooth and slightly raised with a dirt-like odor. Some strains can possess a yellow or green pigment. On MacConkey agar, they are NLF but after 4–7 days they may become dark pink or red due to oxidation of lactose. Figure 22-14 ■ demonstrates *B. cepacia* colonies on sheep blood and MacConkey agars.

Because of their significance, it is very important to isolate *B. cepacia* from among the numerous organisms, especially mucoid strains of *Pseudomonas aeruginosa*, potentially present in the respiratory secretions of those with cystic fibrosis. Selective medium has been developed to ensure its recovery. Recovery may require up to 3 days. *Burkholderia cepacia* selective agar (BCSA) selects and differentiates the organism based on the presence of crystal violet, polymyxin B, gentamicin, and vancomycin. Figure 22-15 ■ demonstrates its colonies on BCSA.

Another selective and differential agar for *B. cepacia* is OFPBL agar. Its initials stand for oxidative, fermentative,

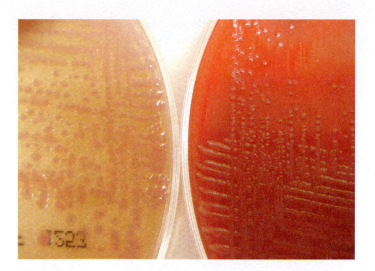

■ **FIGURE 22-14** While the colonies of *Burkholderia cepacia* can possess a slight yellow pigment on sheep blood agar, the colonies shown here do not exhibit the pigment. Its colonies on MacConkey agar may appear light pink due to its ability to oxidize lactose rather than ferment it.

polymyxin B, bacitracin, and lactose. Colonies of *B. cepacia* are yellow due to oxidation of lactose. Figure 22-16 ■ demonstrates its colonies on OFPBL agar. Both agars are incubated in ambient air rather than carbon dioxide.

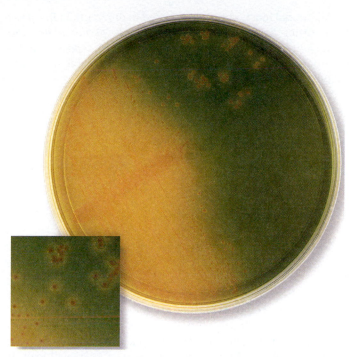

■ **FIGURE 22-16** *Burkholderia cepacia* creates yellow colonies on OFPBL agar. The addition of polymyxin B and bacitracin inhibit other organisms that may be present.
Photo courtesy of Remel, part of Thermo Fisher Scientific.

REAL WORLD TIP

Other nonfermenters such as *Burkholderia gladioli* and *Ralstonia* spp. can also grow on BCSA and OFPBL agars. Growth on these agars is not definitive for the presence of *B. cepacia*. The organism must still be identified.

Key Biochemical Reactions. Because there are nine subspecies within the *B. cepacia* complex, identification can prove to be difficult. It is extremely important to correctly identify this organism in cystic fibrosis patients. It is recommended two different identification methods be used to ensure its accurate identification. Commercial identification systems may have difficulty in the identification of *B. cepacia*. Molecular methods are now recommended.

The *B. cepacia* complex is oxidase positive but the reaction may be weak and misinterpreted as negative. If read as oxidase negative, it may be confused with the NLF members of the *Enterobacteriaceae*. Its K/NC TSI reaction will differentiate it from the *Enterobacteriaceae*.

B. cepacia is able to decarboxylate lysine. Only it and *Stenotrophomonas maltophilia* possess this characteristic among the nonfermenters. Both are also able to oxidize glucose, maltose, and lactose. To differentiate them, *B. cepacia* is able to oxidize mannitol while *S. maltophilia* is DNase positive.

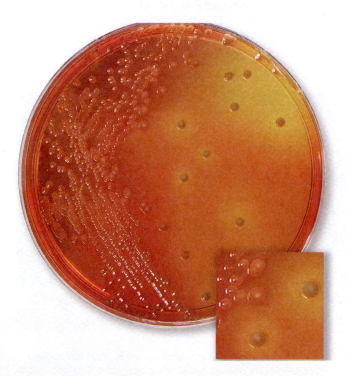

■ **FIGURE 22-15** BCSA is a selective and differential agar for the isolation of *B. cepacia.* Its colonies are variable in size and demonstrate a pink to yellow zone around each.
Photo courtesy of Remel, part of Thermo Fisher Scientific.

Additional biochemicals are needed to differentiate *B. cepacia* from other *Burkholderia* spp. such as *B. pseudomallei* and *B. gladioli*. The negative arginine reaction of *B. cepacia* will differentiate it from *B. pseudomallei*. *B. gladioli* is unable to oxidize maltose and lactose.

Checkpoint! 22–7
(Chapter Objective 5)

Which other nonfermenter shares a positive lysine decarboxylase result with Burkholderia cepacia?

    A. *Pseudomonas aeruginosa*
    B. *Stenotrophomonas maltophilia*
    C. *Acinetobacter baumannii*
    D. *Pseudomonas stutzeri*

Clinical Significance

Microbe Defense Mechanisms. While *B. cepacia* is extremely pathogenic for those with cystic fibrosis, it seems to possess very few virulence factors. As a gram-negative rod, it does have lipopolysaccharide (LPS) as part of its cell wall. It has the ability to adhere to mucin, a tracheobronchial protein, produced by CF patients. One of its most important virulence factors is it resistance to multiple antibiotics and the ability to develop resistance to others rapidly.

Pathogenesis and Infectious Diseases. Individuals with cystic fibrosis initially become colonized with *Pseudomonas aeruginosa*. Later in their disease process they may become colonized with *B. cepacia*. Once established there is a rapid decline in lung function and frequent bacteremia. There is a higher mortality rate in the year following colonization. Death often occurs due to lung failure.

The presence of *B. cepacia* in the respiratory secretions is often considered a death sentence for the CF patient. They are no longer able to associate with other CF patients to prevent its spread to others. The CF community is a close-knit community and the inability to interact with other CF individuals is devastating. Even worse, they are no longer eligible for a lung transplant once colonized. Studies show the presence of *B. cepacia* prior to transplant often results in death after transplantation. These consequences indicate why it is so important to ensure recovery and accurate identification of *B. cepacia*.

Prevention and Treatment. The presence of *B. cepacia* in CF patients requires isolation of the patient when hospitalized. This prevents its transmission to other CF individuals. Antibiotic therapy rarely eradicates the organism from the CF respiratory tract.

B. cepacia is resistant to aminoglycosides, which is unusual for most nonfermenters. This characteristic can be used as a clue to its identity. Often multiple antibiotics are necessary for treatment. Antibiotics used include minocycline,

meropenem, ceftazidime, fluoroquinolones, and chloramphenicol. It is susceptible to trimethoprim-sulfamethoxazole, similar to *S. maltophilia*.

Checkpoint! 22–8
(Chapter Objectives 3, 5, and 6)

A sputum culture from a 10-year-old cystic fibrosis patient is received in the laboratory. The sheep blood and chocolate agars grew heavy growth of a mucoid, oxidase-positive gram-negative rod with a blue-green pigment and a grape-like odor. The MacConkey agar shows heavy growth of a mucoid NLF.

The culture also included an OFPBL agar, which grew light growth of a yellow colony. This organism will probably be:

    A. Oxidase positive, acetamide positive, and display growth at 42°C
    B. Oxidase negative, lysine positive, and maltose positive
    C. Oxidase positive, lysine positive, and mannitol positive
    D. Oxidase negative, nonmotile, and glucose positive

Burkholderia pseudomallei

Burkholderia pseudomallei is an oxidase-positive, motile, aerobic gram-negative bacillus that is straight or slightly curved. It grows on most standard laboratory media such as sheep blood, chocolate, and MacConkey agars at 35–37°C in a CO_2 atmosphere. It has a smooth and mucoid colony or a dry and wrinkled colony similar to *Pseudomonas stutzeri* when grown on sheep blood agar. Figure 22-17 ■ demonstrates the smooth colony of *B. pseudomallei*. Figure 22-18 ■ demonstrates the

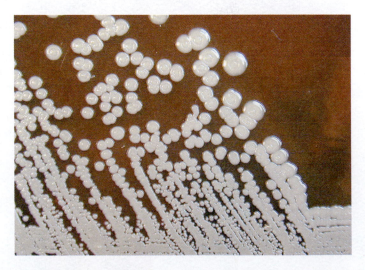

■ **FIGURE 22-17** While the wrinkled colony is often associated with *Burkholderia pseudomallei*, the colony can also be smooth, as seen here. With further incubation the colony can become wrinkled.
From Public Health Image Library (PHIL), CDC/Larry Stauffer, Oregon State Public Health Laboratory.

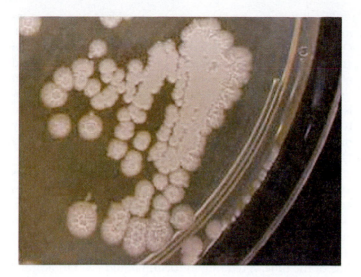

■ **FIGURE 22-18** *Burkholderia pseudomallei* is most often recognized by its wrinkled colony after 3 days of incubation. This same colony morphology can also be seen with *Pseudomonas stutzeri*. It is very important to accurately identify *B. pseudomallei*.
From Perumal, S., et al. (2006). BMC Infectious Diseases, 6, 100, http://www.biomedcentral.com/1471-2334/6/100

wrinkled *B. pseudomallei* colonies on tryptic soy agar after 3 days of incubation.

When the lid of the agar plate is opened, a characteristic musty or earthy odor is noted. On MacConkey agar, it is a NLF but after 4 to 7 days the colony can appear pink due to its oxidation of lactose. Figure 22-19 ■ demonstrates the rough, wrinkled pink colony of *B. pseudomallei* on MacConkey agar.

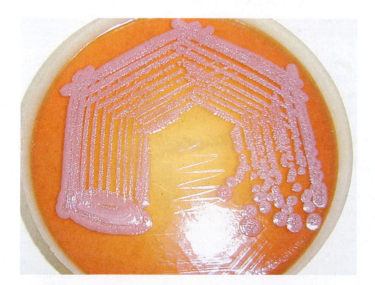

■ **FIGURE 22-19** While *Burkholderia pseudomallei* does not ferment the lactose present in MacConkey agar, it can oxidize it and create enough acids to turn the pH indicator pink as demonstrated here.
From Dhodapkar et al. (2008). Cases Journal, 1, 224, http://www.casesjeditorial.com/content/1/1/224

 REAL WORLD TIP

Some nonfermenters can oxidize the lactose present in MacConkey agar. This may give them the appearance of a light or late lactose fermenter. They are actually oxidizing the carbohydrate, which in turn creates weak acids that are able to change the pH indicator pink. Traditionally microbiologists assume a lactose fermenter or late lactose fermenter on MacConkey agar is a member of the *Enterobacteriaceae*. An oxidase test may not be performed because the *Enterobacteriaceae* are oxidase negative. If the organism does not identify with the commercial system used for *Enterobacteriaceae*, perform an oxidase on a colony from sheep blood agar. If positive, then the organism may be a nonfermenter. If negative, it may still be a nonfermenter and screening with a TSI or KIA slant may be necessary.

A biochemical screening test should be performed if the isolate is suspected to be *Burkholderia pseudomallei*. Because its colony can resemble that of *Pseudomonas stutzeri*, key biochemical reactions needed to differentiate include oxidation of lactose and decarboxylation of arginine. *B. pseudomallei* is positive for both reactions whereas *P. stutzeri* is negative. The organism is resistant to colistin and polymyxin B, which can help differentiate it from *Pseudomonas* spp. and *Stenotrophomonas maltophilia,* which are susceptible (Gales, Jones, Andrade, & Sader, 2005). Within the common *Burkholderia* genus members, it is able to decarboxylate arginine whereas *B. cepacia* and *B. gladioli* cannot.

Burkholderia pseudomallei is a motile, gram-negative rod found in soil and water of southeast Asia and northern Australia. It is associated with rice paddy surface waters and most likely obtained naturally by direct contact with soil and water or associated aerosols. It can also be transmitted person to person through aerosols.

B. pseudomallei causes **melioidosis**, an infectious disease, which exhibits as either a local infection, a pulmonary infection such as pneumonia, or a rapid, fatal septicemia in individuals with underlying diseases or immunosuppression. It is important for the microbiologist to be aware of this organism. It is known as the Vietnamese time bomb. During the Vietnam War in the late 1960s and early 1970s soldiers inhaled the organism as they marched through swamps and rice paddies in Southeast Asia. They also inhaled dust stirred up by helicopters. The organism survives in phagocytes and can reactivate decades after the initial infection. This organism can be cultured today due to Vietnam veterans becoming compromised by cancer, diabetes, and other underlying conditions. The disease reactivates when the individual's immune system is compromised. Reactivation often appears as multiple abscesses throughout the body and skin. It is important to quickly identify this organism in order to reduce mortality due to septicemia.

REAL WORLD TIP

- *Burkholderia mallei* is the causative agent of glanders. It causes the same type of infections as *B. pseudomallei* but the infections occur in animals such as horses. It can be transmitted to humans via aerosols and is seen in those with occupations that require exposure to horses, donkeys, and mules. It is considered a zoonotic disease

- *Burkholderia pseudomallei* and *Burkholderia mallei* have the potential to used as bioterrorism agents. Both have the ability to be spread by aerosols and are resistant to routinely used antibiotics. Both are considered category B bioterrorism agents by the Centers for Disease Control and Prevention (CDC). They are moderately easy to disseminate in an aerosolized version, display moderate morbidity and low mortality, and are not routinely isolated in most laboratories so it would probably require more time and resources to identify than more common organisms. Once isolated, both are reportable organisms to the public health department.

The organism is resistant to routinely used antibiotics. Treatment includes trimethoprim-sulfamethoxazole, ceftazidime, meropenem, and tetracycline. Because the organism hides within white blood cells, long-term therapy for up to 6 months is necessary.

✓ Checkpoint! 22–9 (Chapter Objective 6)

How can an organism such as Burkholderia pseudomallei be used as a bioterrorism agent?

A. *It is easily spread by aerosolization*
B. *It displays moderate morbidity and low mortality*
C. *It is not easily recognized in most clinical laboratories*
D. *All of the above*

ELIZABETHKINGIA MENINGOSEPTICA (PREVIOUSLY *CHRYSEOBACTERIUM MENINGOSEPTICUM*)

Elizabethkingia meningoseptica has gone through several name changes. Previously it was known as *Chryseobacterium meningosepticum*, and prior to that it was *Flavobacterium meningosepticum*. As an environmental organism, it may be found in soil, plants, water, food, and hospital water sources including incubators, sinks, faucets, saline solutions, and respiratory equipment (Kambal, Arora, AlZeer, & Babay, 1997). It is not considered part of normal human flora and individuals are probably exposed via contaminated medical devices or solutions. Its ability to survive in chlorinated water makes it difficult to eradicate from hospital water.

Elizabethkingia meningoseptica is an oxidase-positive, nonmotile, slightly filamentous or thread-like gram-negative rod. On routine laboratory media such as 5% sheep blood agar and chocolate agar, it is described as being circular, smooth, and glistening with a light yellow pigment. It may not grow well on MacConkey, if at all. If it does grow it is a NLF. The organism will produce adequate growth after 24 hours when incubated at 35°C in either carbon dioxide or ambient air. Its key biochemical reaction is a positive indole result using the Ehrlich method rather than the traditional Kovac's reagent.

The Ehrlich method, recommended for nonfermenters, uses xylene to extract and concentrate indole. One mL of xylene is added to the broth tube (tryptophan, peptone, or heart infusion broth) after 24 or 48 hours incubation at 35°C. Shake well and wait for the xylene to rise to the surface of the broth. Tilt the tube and add 0.5 mL Ehrlich's reagent so it runs down the side of the tube. A red ring in the top liquid layer indicates a positive result, no color is a negative result, and an orange color may indicate a possible precursor to indole and is considered a variable result.

Elizabethkingia meningoseptica is often associated with meningitis and bacteremia in premature infants. They become colonized via a nosocomial source. There can be outbreaks of infection in neonatal units. This particular organism has also been associated with fatal infections, such as pneumonia, cellulitis, and abscesses in immunocompromised patients (Kambal et al., 1997; Holmes, 1987).

REAL WORLD TIP

*Elizabethkingia **mening**o**septic**a's* name tells one its clinical significance. It causes meningitis and septicemia.

Antibiotics suitable for therapy include ciprofloxacin, rifampin, clindamycin, trimethroprim-sulfamethoxazole, vancomycin, and the newer fluoroquinolones. Most produce beta-lactamases so the beta-lactams are not suitable.

ALCALIGENES FAECALIS

Alcaligenes faecalis, the most common species of the genus, inhabits the environment and is not part of normal human flora. It can be found in moist hospital environments such as respiratory equipment and disinfectants. This oxidase-positive, motile gram-negative rod produces a thin, spreading colony with irregular edges on sheep blood agar. It can produce a green discoloration of the agar. Its species name does not tell its true odor. Surprisingly it smells of green apples. It appears as a NLF on MacConkey agar.

Alcaligenes faecalis is asaccharolytic, meaning it does not oxidize the carbohydrates present in OF medium. It tends to create a strong alkaline reaction in OF medium, which appears as a blue color. A key biochemical reaction is its ability to reduce nitrite but not nitrate.

While rarely pathogenic, it can cause opportunistic infections in immunocompromised individuals and those with underlying disease. Often they are exposed through medical devices requiring water such as humidifiers. It has the ability to colonize cystic fibrosis patients who are intubated.

ACHROMOBACTER XYLOSOXIDANS

Achromobacter xylosoxidans is the most common species within the genus and is an aerobic, motile, oxidase-positive, non-lactose-fermenting gram-negative rod. It is found in moist environments and has been isolated from a wide range of clinical samples (Clermont, Harmant, & Bizet, 2001; Liu et al., 2002). Based on its species name, it can oxidize glucose and xylose. It is an opportunistic pathogen capable of causing a variety of infections, including bacteremia, meningitis, pneumonia, and peritonitis. Similar to *Alcaligenes faecalis*, it is capable of colonizing the respiratory tract of persons with cystic fibrosis. Medical equipment and solutions have been found to be contaminated with this organism, thus nosocomial outbreaks have been attributed (Liu et al., 2002).

 REAL WORLD TIP

Shewenella putrifaciens and *S. algae* are motile, oxidase-positive nonfermenters that can produce an orange-tan pigment. They are often found in water sources and can cause wound infections or bacteremia. They are unique among the nonfermenters because of the production of hydrogen sulfide in a TSI or KIA slant. *S. putrifaciens* is usually an environmental organism whereas *S. algae* has been isolated in immunocompromised individuals.

MORAXELLA SPECIES

While *Moraxella catarrhalis* is discussed in ∞ Chapter 18, "Aerobic Gram-Negative Cocci," there are other species of the genus that can be encountered in the clinical laboratory. As a genus, *Moraxella* are nonmotile, oxidase-positive, aerobic, asaccharolytic gram-negative diplococci. The species, other than *M. catarrhalis,* can appear more like rods when exposed to antibiotics. They are often normal flora of the upper respiratory and genital tracts and rarely cause infection. They can be confused with *Neisseria* spp. based on the positive-oxidase and gram-negative diplococcus morphology.

Moraxella spp. routinely do not grow on MacConkey agar. The most commonly isolated species, *M. nonliquefaciens,* may grow on MacConkey but rarely. Other more commonly isolated species include *M. osloensis,* which can grow on MacConkey agar, and *M. lacunata,* which does not grow on MacConkey. Colonies are often pin-point on sheep blood and chocolate agars. The colonies of *M. nonliquefaciens* and *M. lacunata* may pit these agars.

Other than *M. catarrhalis,* the other species are not routinely identified unless isolated from a significant body site or specimen type. *M. catarrhalis* is the only species to produce DNase. Differentiation of the other species can prove to be difficult due to their variable or negative reactions. Most laboratories choose to report the organisms other than *M. catarrhalis* as *Moraxella* spp.

M. nonliquefaciens is a known causative agent of bacteremia as well as respiratory tract infections. *M. lacunata* is well known for conjunctivitis as well as eye and upper respiratory infections. *M. osloensis* has been isolated in cases of bacteremia, other systemic infections, and upper respiratory infections.

Only *M. catarrhalis* typically produces beta-lactamase. This means beta-lactams are appropriate for treatment of the other species. To ensure beta-lactams can be used, each species should be tested for beta-lactamase. Quinolones and aminoglycosides are also therapeutic agents.

 REAL WORLD TIP

Methylobacterium spp. and *Roseomonas* spp. are pink-pigmented nonfermenters. Both organisms are oxidase-positive gram-negative rods.

 Checkpoint! 22–10 (Chapter Objective 5)

Which of the following organisms is an asaccharolytic gram negative that characteristically produces a strong alkaline reaction in OF medium?

A. *Alcaligenes faecalis*
B. *Chromobacterium violaceum*
C. *Achromobacter xylosoxidans*
D. *Moraxella lacunata*

 REAL WORLD TIP

Most organisms are not always 100% positive or negative for all biochemical reactions. This is especially true for the nonfermenters. Often their reactions are variable, making their identification even more difficult. It may require multiple biochemical reactions to rule in or rule out a nonfermenting organism's identification.

SUMMARY

Nonfermenting gram-negative rods can prove to be a challenge for most microbiologists. *Pseudomonas aeruginosa, Acinetobacter baumannii,* and *Stenotrophomonas maltophilia* are the most commonly isolated infectious agents and are recognized and identified more easily than other nonfermenters.

There are clues that can lead the microbiologist to suspect an organism is a nonfermenter. These include a K/NC TSI or KIA; positive oxidase reaction; no growth on MAC; a sweet, fruity, or unique odor; multidrug resistance; and limited biochemical reactions in commercial systems used to identify *Enterobacteriaceae*.

The identification of nonfermenters can be difficult due to need for conventional biochemical testing. Commercial identification systems may not be accurate and reliable for the less commonly isolated organisms. Table 22-1 summarizes the key biochemical reactions and other characteristics of the more commonly isolated nonfermenting gram-negative rods.

Most nonfermenters are found naturally in soil and water and so can also be found as contaminating organisms in the hospital setting. Several are associated with outbreaks of pseudobacteremia due to contamination of disinfectants.

They are also opportunistic pathogens able to cause disease in those who are immunocompromised or have underlying conditions such as cancer or diabetes. The organisms must first colonize the host in order to eventually cause infection. Individuals with cystic fibrosis are extremely vulnerable to colonization and infection with nonfermenters. The presence of *Burkholderia cepacia* in respiratory secretions can be a death sentence for the CF patient.

Because the nonfermenters are environmental organisms, they tend to be antibiotic resistant and can be a challenge for susceptibility testing. Antibiotics available for treatment may be limited.

Nonfermenters have proven to be a source of emerging pathogens and potential bioterrorism agents. This chapter has only touched on some of the more common nonfermenters encountered in the laboratory or those that are very clinically significant. A detailed reference book should always be available for information on nonfermenters that are not frequently isolated. Microbiologists must continue to update their knowledge base to ensure they are able to recognize and identify nonfermenters.

LEARNING OPPORTUNITIES

1. A 50-year-old male drunk driver was rushed to the emergency department severely burned and badly bruised. The man had a long-standing history of alcoholism. He was intubated, given intravenous fluids, and transfused with packed red blood cells in the intensive care unit. He remained intubated and ventilator dependent for several weeks. He developed fevers and was treated with broad-spectrum antibiotics. Culture of his tracheal aspirate initially grew *Staphylococcus aureus*. After further antibiotic therapy, Gram stain of his tracheal aspirate showed many white blood cells and many gram-negative rods. A culture of a second tracheal aspirate grew an oxidase-positive gram-negative rod that was a nonlactose fermenter on MacConkey agar and showed a bluish green sheen on 5% sheep blood agar with a grape-like odor.

   a. Which is the identification of the gram-negative rod?
   (Chapter Objectives 5, 6, and 8)

   b. The organism produces an exotoxin that is similar to the exotoxin of which other bacteria? How do they act on the host cells? (Chapter Objective 6)

   c. What factors put the patient at risk for developing infection with this organism? (Chapter Objective 6)

   d. This organism was isolated after the patient received a prolonged course of broad-spectrum antibiotics. How did this therapy predispose the patient to infection with this organism? Why is this organism able to survive in the presence of antimicrobial agents? (Chapter Objective 6)

   e. Neutropenic patients are at increased risk for bacteremia with this organism. What steps can be taken to reduce this risk? (Chapter Objective 6)

   f. Patients with cystic fibrosis are frequently chronically infected with this organism. What unique feature does this organism usually possess when it chronically colonizes and infects this patient population? (Chapter Objective 6)

2. Hugh-Leifson OF medium is used to determine the ability of nonfermenting gram-negative rods because: (Chapter Objective 4)

   a. It contains more carbohydrates than most media so more weak acids are produced

   b. It contains less protein so less amines are produced, which can neutralize weak acids produced

   c. It is semi-solid to concentrate the weak acids produced

   d. All of the above

3. *Burkholderia cepacia* and *Stenotrophomonas maltophilia* share the following characteristics: (Chapter Objectives 5 and 7)

   a. Lysine decarboxylase

   b. Susceptible to trimethoprim-sulfamethoxazole

   c. Oxidase positive

   d. a and b

4. A 67-year-old male enters the hospital due to congestive heart failure. He recently retired from a lifelong career in the military where he fought in several wars and participated in other military actions throughout the world over the past four decades. While in the hospital, he develops multiple abscesses on his skin and over his lymph nodes. The organism isolated from one of the ulcers has a colony that is dry, wrinkled, and leathery on sheep blood agar. MacConkey agar demonstrates what appears to be a very faint lactose fermenter. You would expect this organism to be: (Chapter Objectives 5, 6, and 8)

   a. Oxidase positive, arginine decarboxylase positive, and able to oxidize lactose

   b. Oxidase positive, arginine decarboxylase negative, and able to hydrolyze starch

   c. Oxidase negative, lysine decarboxylase positive, and able to oxidize maltose

   d. Oxidase negative, nonmotile, and able to oxidize glucose

5. A gram-negative coccobacilli is isolated from the endotracheal tube of a 54-year-old female hospitalized in the intensive care unit after surgery for removal of an aneurysm. The organism provides the following results:

Sheep blood agar = white, wet, nonhemolytic colony

MacConkey agar = clear colony with a trace of faint pink

Oxidase = no color change

Motility = negative

TSI slant = pink/red-orange

OF carbohydrates	Open tube	Closed tube
Glucose	yellow	no color change
Lactose	yellow	no color change
Maltose	no color change	no color change

Decarboxylase

    Arginine = no color change

    Lysine = no color change

This organism can be identified as: (Chapter Objectives 5, 6, and 8)

a. *Stenotrophomonas maltophilia*

b. *Pseudomonas aeruginosa*

c. *Acinetobacter baumannii*

d. *Acinetobacter lwoffi*

6. Which of the following organisms can potentially be used as a bioterrorism agent? (Chapter Objective 6)

a. *Pseudomonas stutzeri*

b. *Burkholderia pseudomallei*

c. *Burkholderia cepacia*

d. All of the above

PEARSON myhealthprofessionskit™

Use this address to access the interactive Companion Website created for this textbook. Simply select "Clinical Laboratory Science" from the choice of disciplines. Find this book and log in using your user name and password.

REFERENCES

Go to myhealthprofessionskit.com to view this chapter's references.

23

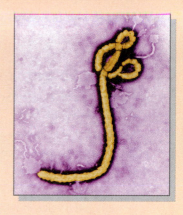

Vibrio, Aeromonas, Plesiomonas, Campylobacter, Helicobacter, and Chromobacterium

Teresa A. Taff

■ LEARNING OBJECTIVES

Upon completion of this chapter, the learner should be able to:

1. Describe specimen collection and transportation requirements for each organism.
   a. Evaluate specimen acceptability of patient specimens.
   b. Determine the specimen of choice for isolation.
2. For each organism discussed:
   a. Describe enzymes, toxins, and antigens produced.
   b. Discuss environmental requirements (atmosphere, temperature, etc.) for isolation.
   c. Describe the Gram stain reaction and microscopic morphology.
   d. Select media for isolation and/or differentiation and describe the expected results.
   e. Establish key identification characteristics.
   f. Determine the source or origin and potential transmission mechanisms.
   i. Determine the potential to cause an epidemic.
   g. Correlate with specific diseases or syndromes.
   h. Describe mechanisms of pathogenicity.
   i. Define patient populations prone to disease.
   j. Differentiate from other organisms based on objectives 2a–i.
3. Correlate patient history, body site or specimen type, colonial morphology, Gram stain reaction, identification test results and/or susceptibility results to identify an organism, assess its clinical significance, and recognize problems or discrepancies.
4. Propose a cost-effective and timely identification scheme.
   a. Determine alternative or additional testing required.

■ **LEARNING OBJECTIVES (*continued*)**

5. For each medium, identification, or test procedure discussed:

   a. Explain the principle.

   b. Recognize potential sources of errors and limitations.

   c. Discuss incubation requirements.

   d. Interpret the results.

   e. Evaluate the sensitivity and specificity.

   f. Judge the value in relation to ease of use, turnaround time, cost, results provided, and other factors.

6. Summarize treatment strategies and potential patient outcomes.

KEY TERMS

bullae	epidemic	radioisotope
classic biotype	Guillain-Barré syndrome	vibriostatic
debridement	halophilic	violacein
El Tor biotype	necrosis	zoonotic
endemic	pandemic	

TAXONOMY

Family *Vibrionaceae* (vĭb′-rē-ōn-ā′-sē′-ē)
   Genus *Vibrio* (vib-rē-ō)
      V. cholerae (käl-ə-ra)
      V. parahaemolyticus (pär′-ə-hē′-mə-lĭt′-ĭ-kus)
      V. vulnificus (vŭl-nĭf′-i-kus)
      V. alginolyticus (al-gi-no-lyt-i-kus)
   Family *Aeromonadaceae* (ār-ō-mō′-nad-ē′-ā′-sē′-ē)
      Genus *Aeromonas* (ar-ō-mō-nəs)
      A. hydrophila (hī-drō-fīl-ŭh)
Family *Enterobacteriaceae* (ĕn′-tēr′-ô′-băk′-tēr′-ē′-ā′-sē′-ē)
   Genus *Pleisiomonas* (plē′-sē-ō-mō′-năs)
      P. shigelloides (shi-gel-ó-id-ēz)

Family *Campylobacteraceae* (kam-pə-lō-bak-tər-ā′-sē′-ē)
   Genus *Campylobacter* (kam-pə-lō-bak-tər)
      C. jejuni (ji-jū-nē)
      C. coli (kō-lī)
      C. fetus (fēt-us)
   Family *Helicobacteraceae* (hel-i-kō-bak-tər-ā′-sē′-ē)
      Genus *Helicobacter* (hel-i-kō-bak-tər)
      H. pylori (pī-lōr-ē)
   Family *Neisseriaceae* (nī-sir-ē-ā-sē-ē)
      Genus *Chromobacterium* (krō-mō-bak-tir-ē-um)
      C. violaceum (vī-o-lāce-ē-um)

▶ INTRODUCTION

The organisms discussed in this chapter consist of the *Vibrio* species, which includes *V. cholerae, Aeromonas hydrophila, Plesiomonas shigelloides, Campylobacter* species, *Helicobacter pylori,* and *Chromobacterium violaceum*. These organisms are usually not considered part of the normal flora of humans. Most are able to cause disease in the gastrointestinal tract. Infections can range from self-limiting gastroenteritis to massive diarrhea, which can lead to death. Although diarrhea may not be a thrilling subject to most individuals, a microbiologist is always interested in determining the causative agents in a culture.

Some of the organisms discussed in this chapter are also able to cause skin and tissue infections and septicemia after exposure. The *Campylobacter* species are probably the most easily recognizable of the group and the most commonly isolated enteric pathogen in most laboratories. The other organisms may not be routinely seen in most laboratories and may prove to be a challenge for microbiologists.

▶ VIBRIONACEAE

VIBRIO CHOLERAE

V. cholerae is the causative agent of cholera. The disease probably originated in Asia, specifically India. The Ganges River may serve as a reservoir source for the organism. Although cholera is always present today throughout southern Asia, it can only be sporadically found in the United States.

In 1853, John Snow made the connection between drinking contaminated water and acquiring cholera during a London outbreak (Uthman, 1998). Robert Koch discovered the organism in 1883. Since its discovery, the organism has caused at least seven **pandemics** (a wave of infection that spreads across the world in a large-scale epidemic). The pandemics have stretched across Asia, Europe, Africa, and South America (Todar, 2005).

General Characteristics

Vibrio species are gram-negative rods known for their characteristic comma-shaped morphology and motility through the means of a single polar flagellum (Figure 23-1 ■). The translation of "vibrio" means to vibrate. As a group, they possess a somatic or cell wall (O) antigen and flagellar (H) antigen similar to the *Enterobacteriaceae* family. Their somatic antigen is used to differentiate between pathogenic and nonpathogenic strains of the organisms. Currently, 139 serotypes, based on the somatic antigen, have been identified (Mégraud & Thijsen, 2004).

V. cholerae serotypes O1 and O139 are known to cause **epidemic** (a disease that affects many people in a period of time) cholera. Serotype O1 can be further differentiated into the **El Tor** (a subtype of *Vibrio cholerae* O1 serotype) and **classic** (a subtype of *Vibrio cholerae* O1 serotype) **biotypes** (subtype within a species that can be differentiated by biochemical or serologic properties). The El Tor biotype is responsible for most cases of cholera in the world.

Environment.   *Vibrio cholerae* is an aquatic microorganism with humans as its only known host. It prefers salt water but can be found in freshwater contaminated with human feces. *V. cholerae* can remain as a free-living organism among plankton, algae, crustaceans, and fish, provided the temperature, saline level, and nutrients remain adequate (Seas & Gotuzzo, 2000). It has the ability to tolerate an alkaline (pH of 9.0) environment that kills most organisms. This characteristic is used to design media for its transportation and isolation.

Outbreaks have been associated with the warm seasons and poor sanitation. Contaminated food and water serve to transmit the organism to humans. Undercooked seafood and fish are the most common food sources. While cholera is primarily linked with developing countries, it can be found in the United States because of the ability of individuals to travel virtually anywhere in the world in a short time frame. Exposure to ocean waters along the coastal states is another factor involved in its transmission.

Microscopic Morphology.   While other organisms can be comma shaped, gram-negative rods, the small curved rods are characteristically associated with *Vibrio species* (Figure 23-2 ■). Only an experienced microbiologist working in a coastal state may be able to presumptively diagnose cholera from just observing the Gram stain of a loose, watery stool specimen. A culture is still required to recover the organism and provide a definitive diagnosis.

During cholera epidemics, darkfield microscopy can be used to rapidly diagnose infections. Fresh stool is examined for the organism's characteristic motility described as a shooting star (Mégraud & Thijsen, 2004). Antiserum against the cholera O1 and O139 serotypes can then be added to the darkfield exam. The loss of motility confirms the diagnosis of cholera (Finkelstein, 1996). Diagnosis outside an epidemic situation requires culture and identification.

Biochemical Characteristics.   *Vibrio cholerae* can be identified using biochemical testing or serology. It is a gram-

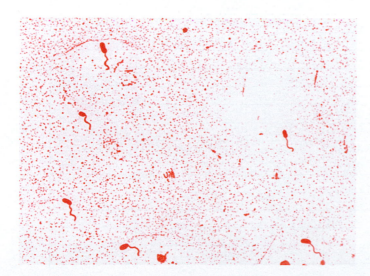

■ **FIGURE 23-1** The prominent single polar flagellum of *Vibrio cholerae* is easily observed on this Leifson flagella stain of the organism.
From CDC PHIL/Dr. William Clark.

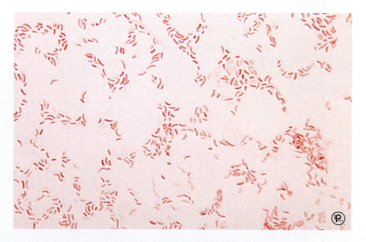

■ **FIGURE 23-2** Note the curved appearance of the gram-negative rods of *Vibrio* spp. Although characteristic for *Vibrio*, definitive identification of the organism is still necessary.
From Marler LM, Siders JA, Kaufman CM, Owens EN, Korba GG and Allen SD, *Bacteriology I Image Atlas* CD-ROM, Indiana Pathology Images, 2005.

negative rod that does not require NaCl for growth on medium or in biochemical tests even though it is predominantly associated with a marine environment. Table 23-1✪ compiles the identification tests and their reactions for *V. cholerae*. It is characterized by a positive oxidase reaction (purple), which separates it from members of the family *Enterobacteriaceae,* which are also present in stool specimens. *Vibrio* species as a group are able to ferment carbohydrates to produce acid by-products. *V. cholerae* is able to ferment glucose and sucrose but not lactose. On a triple sugar iron (TSI) slant, it produces an acid (yellow) slant and acid (yellow) butt because of the fermentation of both the glucose and sucrose present. On a Kligler iron agar (KIA) slant, the reaction is alkaline (pink) slant and acid (yellow) butt because of the fermentation of only the glucose present. *V. cholerae* is able to decarboxylate the amino acids, lysine, and ornithine but not arginine. It is also able to break down tryptophan to produce indole. Refer to ∞ Chapter 9 for details of the principle, performance, and interpretation of the oxidase, TSI, KIA, decarboxylase, and indole tests.

ⓔ REAL WORLD TIP

The oxidase test must be performed from a sheep blood agar. A false-negative reaction may occur if colonies grown on a medium with a fermentable carbohydrate are used. The fermentation of carbohydrates produces acid by-products, which may inhibit the oxidase reaction at a pH of less than 5.1. MacConkey, hektoen enteric, and thiosulfate citrate bile salts sucrose agars all contain fermentable carbohydrates. Colonies from these media should not be used to perform the oxidase test.

Within the O1 serogroup, the El Tor and classic biotypes can be differentiated based on β (beta) hemolysis on sheep blood agar and in the presence of red blood cells in a tube and the production of acetoin from pyruvate, as seen in the Voges-Proskauer test. The El Tor biotype is characteristically

---

✪ TABLE 23-1

Differentiation of *Vibrio* species, *Aeromonas hydrophila*, *Chromobacterium violaceum*, and *Plesiomonas shigelloides*

	Vibrio cholerae	*Vibrio parahaemolyticus*	*Vibrio vulnificus*	*Aeromonas hydrophila*	*Chromobacterium violaceum*	*Plesiomonas shigelloides*
Oxidase	+	+	+	+	V	+
Growth in:						
0% NaCl	Growth	No growth	No growth	Growth	Growth	Growth
1% NaCl	Growth	Growth	Growth	No growth	No growth	No growth
6% NaCl	No growth	Growth	Growth	No growth	No growth	No growth
TSI	A/A	K/A	A/A	A/A	K or A/A	K or A/A
KIA	K/A	K/A	K/A	K or A/A	K/A	K/A
TCBS growth	Yellow	Blue-green	Blue-green	No growth	Not Done	No growth
MacConkey	NLF	NLF	LF	NLF>LF	NLF	NLF>LF
Indole	+	+	+	+	−	+
Decarboxylase						
Arginine	−	−	−	+	+	+
Lysine	+	+	+	+	−	+
Ornithine	+	+	V	−	−	+
String test (within 60 seconds)	+ 7 mm or greater	− ≤3 mm	− 4–6 mm	− no string	− no string	− no string
O/129						
10 µg	S	R	S	R	R	S
150 µg	S	S	S	R	R	S
Salicin	−	−	+	V	−	V
Gelatinase	+	+	+	+	V	−
DNase	+	+	+/−	+	+	−

+ = positive, − = negative, +/− = more positive reactions than negative, A = acid, K = alkaline, NLF = nonlactose fermenter, LF = lactose fermenter, V = variable, mm = millimeters, > = greater than, ≤ = less than or equal to, S = susceptible (zone of inhibition), R = resistant (no zone of inhibition)
Note: Biochemical reactions for *V. parahaemolyticus* and *V. vulnificus* are based on the addition of 1% NaCl to each test medium.

hemolytic (Figure 23-3 ■) and Voges-Proskauer (VP) positive, whereas the classic biotype is nonhemolytic and VP negative. During the last pandemic, a mutated strain of the El Tor biotype was observed, and most of the isolates had lost the ability to produce a hemolytic reaction (Finkelstein, 1996). Although it is possible to differentiate the biotypes with biochemicals, it may only be necessary for epidemiology studies because both biotypes cause the same disease because of the enterotoxin produced. Refer to ∞ Chapter 9 for details on the principle, performance, and interpretation of the Voges-Proskauer test.

Halotolerance. Most species of *Vibrio* are naturally **halophilic** (salt-loving) and able to tolerate a wide range of salt concentrations. Salts make up about 3.5% of ocean water. Most of the salt present in the ocean is in the form of NaCl (sodium chloride). Nutrient broth tubes with various concentrations ranging from 1.0 to 12.0% NaCl can be used to establish an organism's ability to grow in salt. The growth pattern may be helpful in the identification of specific *Vibrio* species. Most genus members other than *V. cholerae* will grow in 6.0% NaCl. This is a key reaction for differentiating other *Vibrio* species from *V. cholerae* and *Aeromonas* species, *Plesiomonas shigelloides,* and *Chromobacterium violaceum,* which are other organisms associated with water exposure.

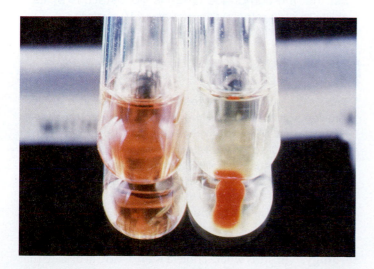

■ **FIGURE 23-3** The *Vibrio cholerae* serogroup O1 El Tor biotype characteristically hemolyzes red blood cells, as observed in the test on the left.
From CDC.

Because of their close relationship with the ocean, the growth and biochemical reactions of the majority of the *Vibrio* species are enhanced by the addition of at least 0.5% sodium chloride (NaCl or saline). Surprisingly, *V. cholerae* is one of only two species that do not require saline for growth despite its close relationship with ocean water. It can, however, grow in the presence of 1.0% NaCl.

Most routine media such as sheep blood agar and MacConkey agar contain at least 0.5% sodium chloride and will support the growth of most *Vibrio* species. Commercial identification systems are available and have shown an overall accuracy rate of approximately 72.0% when attempting to identify *Vibrio* species. If 0.85% saline is used as the inoculum fluid, the results tend to be slightly better. Care must be taken when evaluating the results of these systems when used to identify *Vibrio* species (O'Hara, Sowers, Bopp, Duda, & Strockbine, 2003).

String Test. The string test may be useful for differentiating *V. cholerae* from *Aeromonas* species, another oxidase-positive gram-negative rod associated with water exposure. A loop full of 18- to 24-hour growth from a noninhibitory medium is mixed with a drop or two of 0.5% sodium deoxycholate solution on a glass slide. In the string test, the sodium deoxycholate lyses the *Vibrio* bacterial cells, and the organism's viscous DNA is released. A long string forms as the inoculating loop is pulled away from the mixture (Figure 23-4 ■). The

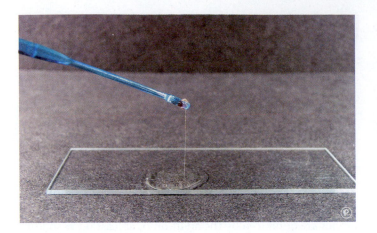

DNA string of *V. cholerae* forms within 60 seconds and can be pulled up to about 7 millimeters from the slide (Keast et al., 1997). *V. cholerae* O1 and O139 serotypes produce a DNA string, whereas *Aeromonas* species cells are not lysed. Other *Vibrio* species may give what appears to be a weak positive reaction, but their DNA string cannot be pulled as high as that of *V. cholerae*. Their string lengths usually run from 1 to 6 millimeters (Keast & Riley, 1997).

The string test is very subjective depending on the medium used for growth of the organism as well as the fine motor and interpretive skills of the microbiologist performing the test. This test should not be considered a definitive or confirmatory test for *V. cholerae*. Its sensitivity and specificity average about 86.0% and 70.0%, respectively, and therefore make it a test with very limited value in today's clinical microbiology laboratory setting (Keast & Riley, 1997). A positive test can

REAL WORLD TIP

The *V. cholerae* string test should not be confused with the potassium hydroxide (KOH) solubility test. The KOH solubility test is used to determine the true Gram stain reaction of organisms that produce variable or weak reactions. A loopful of the suspect organism is stirred into a few drops of 3.0% KOH on a glass slide. Most gram-negative organisms will become sticky within 60 seconds. A string is created when the loop is pulled about 1 centimeter away from the suspension. Gram-negative organisms lyse in the alkaline solution. Cellular DNA is released, and the suspension becomes viscous.

only lead the microbiologist to suspect a potential *Vibrio* species. Further testing is necessary to confirm the organism's definitive identification. A negative test should probably be confirmed by identification methods as well because of its low specificity.

Susceptibility to O/129. O/129 (2, 4-diamino-6, 7-diisopropylpteridine phosphate) is a **vibriostatic** compound that inhibits the growth of *Vibrio* species but not *Aeromonas hydrophila*. It has been an important test because of the limited number of biochemical tests that can accurately differentiate *V. cholerae* and *Aeromonas* species (Abbott, Cheung, Portoni, & Janda, 1992). *Aeromonas hydrophila* is an oxidase-positive glucose-fermenting gram-negative rod that can be found in the same types of environments as *V. cholerae*.

The O/129 test is run on heart infusion agar with disks of two different concentrations of the disk. One disk contains 10 µg, whereas the other contains 150 µg. Two different concentrations are used because *Vibrio* species can vary in their results between the two disks. *V. cholerae* is sensitive (susceptible) to both concentrations. Other *Vibrio* species are usually sensitive to only the higher concentration. Sensitivity is defined as any size zone of inhibition around the disk. Resistance is defined as no zone of inhibition. It is disturbing that O/129 resistant *V. cholerae* strains are now being reported (Abbott et al., 1992). *Aeromonas hydrophila* is resistant to both concentrations of O/129.

REAL WORLD TIP

O/129 is not used in treatment of *Vibrio* infections. It is only used to screen for *Vibrio* species that are usually susceptible to the compound. An easy way to remember that the compound O/129 is vibriostatic is by its ability to stop (stasis) the growth of *V. cholerae*.

REAL WORLD TIP

The O/129 susceptibility test is performed on a heart infusion agar rather than the traditionally used Mueller-Hinton agar. Most *Vibrio* species require a minimum of 0.5% NaCl to grow. Mueller-Hinton agar, used for Kirby-Bauer susceptibility testing, does not provide adequate salt for the growth of *Vibrio* species. Heart infusion agar provides 0.5% NaCl and so allows the growth of most *Vibrio* species.

Serology. In areas where cholera is **endemic** (a disease that is continually present in a location or group), screening with biochemicals may not be necessary provided *V. cholerae* O1 and O139 antisera are available. Growth from a nonselective medium must be used for serologic testing. Colonies from thiosulfate-citrate-bile salts-sucrose agar (TCBS) agar can result in false-negative reactions in both biochemical and serologic tests (Centers for Disease Control [CDC], 1999). A polyvalent antisera containing antibodies to both O1 and O139 serogroups is mixed with the test organism and observed for agglutination. If agglutination is observed, then the organism can be reported as presumptive *V. cholerae* O1 or O139 serogroup. The use of antisera is probably not a cost-effective option for most laboratories in the United States. It is usually performed only by state, federal, or reference laboratories.

Organisms that identify as *V. cholerae* but do not agglutinate with O1 or O139 antisera are called noncholera *Vibrio* or *V. cholerae* non-O1, non-O139 (Figure 23-5 ■). They do not produce cholera toxin but can still cause mild to severe diarrhea. They have been recently added to the CDC's list of nationally notifiable infectious diseases.

Special Considerations

Specimen Collection.
Obtaining an adequate amount of specimen is not an issue for someone experiencing cholera. Because *V. cholerae* is not common in the United States, the physician must notify the laboratory if cholera is suspected. Most laboratories do not routinely culture stool for *Vibrio* species. Ideally, a stool specimen or rectal swab should be collected prior to administration of antibiotics. If a rectal swab is used, it should be transported in Cary-Blair medium but not in buffered glycerol saline (Reller et al., 2003).

Alkaline peptone water (APW) can be used as a transport medium as well as to enhance the recovery of suspected *V. cholerae*. APW provides the alkaline environment (pH 8.6–9.0) in which *V. cholerae* is able to grow, but normal flora organisms are inhibited. After 6 to 8 hours of incubation, the trans-

port medium can be subcultured to a selective and differential medium for *Vibrio* species.

Media for Isolation.
V. cholerae is able to grow on 5% sheep blood and MacConkey agars. Both media contain at least 0.5% NaCl, which is the minimum concentration of salt required by most *Vibrio* species for growth. Most species of *Vibrio* are nonhemolytic on sheep blood agar, but the El Tor biotype is usually beta hemolytic. All laboratories can theoretically screen for *V. cholerae* because they can search for oxidase-positive colonies on sheep blood agar or oxidase-positive nonlactose fermenters on MacConkey agar if isolation is requested on a stool culture. The use of selective and differential agar can make the process easier.

> ## REAL WORLD TIP
>
> To easily screen for *Vibrio* species on a stool culture, perform a swipe or sweep oxidase test from the original sheep blood agar. Using a wooden stick, swipe up representative growth from the primary area of growth on the sheep blood agar. Perform an oxidase test using the swipe of growth. If the test shows a positive reaction, then the microbiologist can begin the detailed search for the specific colony causing the positive oxidase reaction.

TCBS is a selective and differential medium that selects for *Vibrio* species and differentiates them based on their ability to ferment the carbohydrate sucrose. The agar provides 1% NaCl, which allows halophilic *Vibrio* species to grow. *V. cholerae* is able to ferment sucrose, the acid by-products produced that change the pH indicator (brom thymol blue) from its original blue-green to yellow. A few other *Vibrio* species, such *V. aginolyticus,* can also ferment sucrose so yellow colonies are not definitive for the presence of *V. cholerae*. *Vibrio* species that do not use sucrose as a carbohydrate source remain as blue-green colonies (Figure 23-6 ■). It may not be cost effective for most laboratories to keep this medium on hand because the organism is

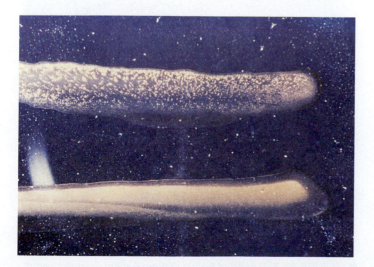

■ **FIGURE 23-5** The use of O1 or O139 *V. cholerae* antiserum can presumptively identify the organism. The suspicious organism is mixed with antiserum and observed for agglutination as seen in the top half of this slide.
From the CDC.

> ✓ ## Checkpoint! 23–1
> ## (Chapter Objective 1)
>
> *A 42-year-old male, recently returned from a business trip to India, has developed severe watery diarrhea. His physician suspects the gastroenteritis is caused by Vibrio cholerae. Select the most useful medium for isolation and differentiation of this organism from stool.*
> A. *MacConkey agar*
> B. *5% sheep blood agar*
> C. *Thiosulfate citrate-bile salts agar*
> D. *Hektoen enteric agar*

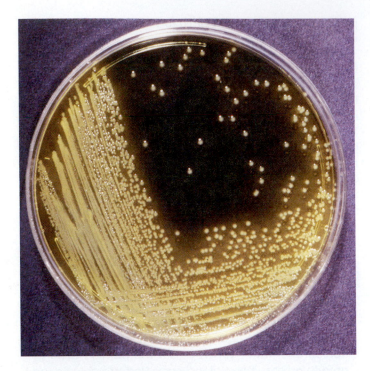

■ **FIGURE 23-6** This TCBS demonstrates *V. cholerae*'s ability to ferment the sucrose present as seen by the yellow colonies on the blue-green agar.
From the CDC.

so uncommon in most of the United States. Coastal laboratories may choose to add this medium routinely to stool cultures because the organism is much more likely to be present with exposure to ocean water. Surprisingly, a survey of Gulf Coast laboratories revealed that although almost 85% kept TCBS agar in stock, the agar was only added to about one of every four stool cultures performed (Marano et al., 2000).

Clinical Significance

V. cholerae enters the body in contaminated water or food, especially raw or undercooked shellfish. The organism cannot survive the acid environment of the stomach, so a high infectious dose of 10^3 to 10^6 organisms is required (Handa, 2003). Water or food may further serve to dilute the acid produced in the stomach. Individuals who use antacids or acid reduction medications have an increased risk for infection when exposed to the organism (Handa, 2003). Interestingly, blood group O individuals are at increased risk for cholera caused by the El Tor biotype (Handa, 2003). The reason for this increased risk remains unknown.

Once in the small bowel, the organism adheres to the intestinal epithelial cells. As they grow, they produce an enterotoxin. The cholera toxin is very similar in structure and function to that produced by enterotoxigenic *Escherichia coli,* which causes traveler's diarrhea. The enterotoxin initiates a cascade of events within the intestinal cells that can eventually lead to massive diarrhea. Non-O1 and non-O139 strains of *V. cholerae* do not produce the characteristic enterotoxin and are not

responsible for epidemics of severe disease. They typically produce a self-limiting gastroenteritis, wound infections, or septicemia.

The cholera enterotoxin binds to the intestinal epithelial cells. The toxin stimulates the cells to hyperproduce adenylate cyclase from ATP. This in turn causes the hyperproduction of cyclic AMP (cAMP). The high levels of cAMP produced trigger chloride, sodium, potassium, and bicarbonate ions to be pumped out of the cell and into the intestinal lumen. Water passively follows the electrolytes into the intestinal lumen by osmosis. As the old saying goes, where sodium goes, so goes water. The cells immediately replace the water and electrolytes lost from their nearby blood supply only to quickly lose it again because of the nonstop hyperproduction of cAMP. The bowel cannot absorb the steady and excessive release of water, and massive diarrhea results. There are no fecal red blood cells or leukocytes present because the organisms do not invade and damage the intestinal mucosa. They only alter the intestinal cells' ability to retain electrolytes and water. Vomiting can also occur early in the disease process.

The diarrhea produced can lead to dehydration because of the massive loss of fluids. An untreated individual can lose several gallons of fluid over a few hours. The loss of so much fluid and electrolytes can lead to metabolic acidosis, cardiac complications, shock, and circulatory failure (Todar, 2005). The stool contains very little fecal material. It is described as rice water stool, which is a colorless liquid, resembling the water left after boiling rice, with flecks of mucus (Figure 23-7 ■). Untreated cholera can lead to fluid depletion within 12 hours and death within 1 to 2 days (Reller & Tauxe, 2003).

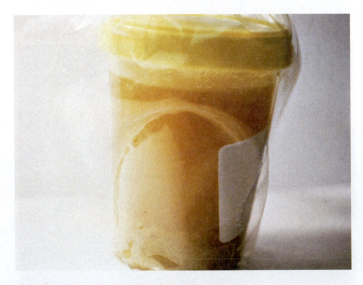

■ **FIGURE 23-7** This stool from a cholera patient is comprised of mostly liquid with flecks of mucus, as seen on the bottom of this collection container. As the diarrhea progresses, the liquid stool becomes clear and contains small white flecks. It resembles the water left over after boiling rice.
From CDC.

✓ Checkpoint! 23–2 (Chapter Objective 2)

The pathogenic enteric organism that characteristically produces rice water stools causes disease because of

- A. *an enterotoxin.*
- B. *a cytotoxin.*
- C. *invasion of the intestinal cells.*
- D. *adherence to the intestinal cells.*

In endemic areas, special cots can be used for the cholera patient (Thaker, 2003). The cot contains a hole cut out for the patient's buttocks and a bucket placed under the hole to catch the liquid stool. The volume of fluid lost can be easily assessed and treated accordingly.

Although cholera is not a major concern in the United States, it is a potential threat wherever sanitation systems are inadequate, such as seen in the aftermath of Hurricanes Katrina and Rita. Two cholera cases were attributed directly to flooded living conditions and improperly cooked shellfish after Hurricanes Katrina and Rita (CDC, 2006). Increases in other *Vibrio* species infections were also reported after the 2005 hurricanes and are discussed later in this chapter.

Travelers to developing countries must be aware of the potential for cholera and how to prevent its transmission. They should avoid high-risk behaviors such as drinking water that is not boiled or treated or eating raw or uncooked foods, especially fish or shellfish.

The most important step in the treatment of cholera is the rapid replacement of fluid and electrolytes lost because of vomiting and diarrhea. Patients who receive adequate fluid replacement are more likely to survive, even without antimicrobial agents. The World Health Organization (WHO) oral rehydration solution (ORS), consisting of sugars, salts, and water, is used in developing countries because of its ease of preparation and delivery. The sugar present aids in the absorption of the electrolytes by the bowel. The water follows the electrolytes as they are taken in by the intestinal cells (Mégraud & Thijsen, 2004).

Once fluids have been replaced, antibiotics can be administered to shorten the length of illness and excretion of the organism. Tetracycline, doxycycline, erythromycin, and ciprofloxacin are the drugs of choice. They are usually given as a single dose. Resistant strains have been observed and are a growing concern.

Once an individual recovers from cholera, immunity can last as long as 3 years (Seas & Gotuzzo, 2000). This observation has led researchers to investigate the development of a vaccine against cholera. Although past vaccines have proven they are good at stimulating an immune response in individuals who had previously experienced cholera, they are not good for immunization of individuals who have never had the disease (Seas & Gotuzzo, 2000). Cholera vaccines are no longer available in the United States because of the low risk of contracting the disease and the incomplete immunity offered.

The recent development of an oral vaccine, outside the United States, has shown promise. It has been reported to also provide protection against enterotoxigenic *Escherichia coli,* the causative agent of traveler's diarrhea (Seas & Gotuzzo, 2000). Even with the ideal cholera vaccine available, vaccination in developing countries with epidemic cholera would prove to be challenging and problematic. Improvements to sanitation systems would provide a more logical solution to the prevention of the spread of cholera.

 REAL WORLD TIP

The isolation of *Vibrio cholerae* is considered a reportable disease. It should be reported to public health officials and submitted for further epidemiologic testing.

VIBRIO PARAHAEMOLYTICUS

General Characteristics

Vibrio parahaemolyticus is a halophilic (salt-loving) gram-negative rod that is a member of the noncholera *Vibrio* species. Although it can cause gastroenteritis, it is not associated with epidemic outbreaks like *V. cholerae*. Its disease state is less severe in a healthy individual but can be deadly in a compromised individual. It is one of the most frequently encountered *Vibrio* species in the United States. There are as many as 3,000 cases per year (CDC, 2005b). It is also known to cause skin infections and septicemia.

Environment. *V. parahaemolyticus* can be found as a free-living microorganism in ocean waters. It can be present in brackish lakes and streams but does not indicate fecal contamination (Beatty & Tuxe, 2003). The organism is most prevalent during the summer months and is naturally found in seafood such as oysters, clams, mussels, shrimp, or crabs. It is easy to see why the old adage of not eating oysters in any month without an *R* in its spelling should be followed. During those months, the organism proliferates in the warm ocean water. Raw or undercooked seafood and exposure to ocean water are the primary modes of transmission.

Microscopic Morphology. *V. parahaemolyticus* can appear as a straight or curved gram-negative rod. Its Gram stain and microscopic morphology are not characteristic enough to be able to presumptively identify it directly from a patient specimen. The organism is motile with a single polar flagellum similar to the other members of the genus.

Biochemical Characteristics. This gram-negative rod is oxidase positive similar to the majority of the genus. Its decarboxylase and indole reactions are similar to those of *V. cholerae* (arginine negative, lysine and ornithine positive, and indole positive). The TSI and KIA reactions appear as an alkaline (pink) slant over and acid (yellow) butt or deep because of the organism's ability to ferment only the glucose present in both tubes. Its inability to ferment sucrose on TCBS agar will help differentiate it easily from *V. cholerae*. The blue-green colony it produces on TCBS is easily distinguished from the characteristic yellow colony of *V. cholerae*.

Halotolerance.   *V. parahaemolyticus* requires 1.0% NaCl for growth. Some strains will grow in NaCl concentrations as high as 8.0%. It will grow on 5.0% sheep blood, MacConkey, and TCBS agars because of the presence of an adequate amount of NaCl. It is important to remember that biochemical test results will provide false-negative results for *V. parahaemolyticus* if 1.0% NaCl is not added prior to incubation.

String Test.   *V. parahaemolyticus* can produce what appears to be a positive string test when tested with 0.5% sodium deoxycholate. The key difference is that the string produced by *V. parahaemolyticus* is usually shorter than 3 millimeters versus the 7 millimeters produced by *V. cholerae*. The string test is not considered confirmatory for *Vibrio* species. This test is very subjective in its performance and interpretation, and results should be used with caution. It must always be followed up with additional biochemical testing.

Susceptibility to O/129.   *V. parahaemolyticus* is usually sensitive to O/129 at a concentration of 150 µg. It is usually resistant at a concentration of 10 µg, but results can be variable. The 150 µg concentration will differentiate *Aeromonas* species (resistant) from most *Vibrio* species, which are susceptible.

Special Considerations

Specimen Collection.
V. parahaemolyticus infection can be diagnosed by culture of stool, wound site, or blood, depending on the disease presentation. Cary-Blair medium can be used if a delay in transportation is anticipated. The physician should notify the laboratory if *V. parahaemolyticus* is suspected. A history of exposure to ocean water or ingestion of seafood can assist the clinical microbiologist.

Special Media.
V. parahaemolyticus will grow on routine sheep blood agar. To select and differentiate *V. parahaemolyti-*

cus from stool specimens, TCBS can be used. It does not ferment the sucrose present and produces a clear colony, which takes on the blue-green coloration of the agar (Figure 23-8 ■). It appears as a nonlactose fermenter on MacConkey agar.

Clinical Significance

The virulence factors of *V. parahaemolyticus* include cytotoxin, hemolysin, and enterotoxin. The cytotoxin and its ability to damage intestinal cells accounts for the blood that can accompany the watery diarrhea because of the enterotoxin. The hemolysin present has been associated with pathogenicity, but its exact mechanism is unknown (Finkelstein, 1996). Dehydration is not a common complication as with cholera. Fecal leukocytes are often present because of the intestinal cell damage. Abdominal cramps, nausea, and vomiting can accompany the diarrhea. The gastroenteritis is usually self-limiting and often resolves in 2 to 3 days.

Wound infections are associated with open wound exposure to contaminated water or seafood. Although the organism can invade the bloodstream, it is rare except in the case of immunocompromised patients. Following Hurricane Katrina there was an increase in *Vibrio parahaemolyticus* wound infections (CDC, 2005b).

Diarrhea caused by *V. parahaemolyticus* does not require any treatment other than fluid replacement in healthy individuals. Antibiotics do not usually have any effect on the gastrointestinal symptoms produced. Wound infections and septicemia require antibiotics such as doxycycline, cefotaxime, ciprofloxacin, and the beta-lactam/beta-lactamase inhibitor combinations.

Avoiding raw or undercooked seafood, especially oysters, prevents infection. Although probably not realistic, individuals should avoid exposure to ocean water during the warm months, especially if open wounds or an immunocompromised state exists.

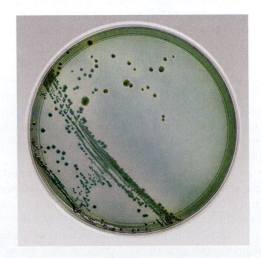

■ **FIGURE 23-8** *Vibrio parahaemolyticus* is unable to ferment the sucrose present in TCBS and presents as a clear colony against a blue-green background.
Photo courtesy of Remel, part of Thermo Fisher Scientific.

 Checkpoint! 23–3 (Chapter Objective 4)

A 38-year-old HIV-positive male is hospitalized with diarrhea and septicemia. He admitted a recent visit to New Orleans, where he indulged in eating raw oysters. The stool culture grew a non-lactose-fermenting, oxidase-positive gram-negative rod. The biochemicals were set up, but after 24 hours of incubation, they showed little to no growth. What should you do next?

A. Add more organism to the biochemicals and reincubate.

B. Reincubate the biochemicals for up to 48 hours.

C. Repeat the organism identification using another methodology.

D. Repeat the identification using 1% NaCl as the inoculum.

VIBRIO VULNIFICUS

Vibrio vulnificus has become the most common noncholera *Vibrio* species isolated after Hurricane Katrina (CDC, 2005b). This halophilic gram-negative rod is known for its virulence. It produces aggressive tissue infections and septicemia similar to that of the flesh-eating *Streptococcus pyogenes*. It is found in ocean water, with its highest concentrations during the warm months of the year. Ocean water and raw or undercooked seafood such as oysters, clams, mussels, shrimp, and crabs are known sources of the organism.

Healthy individuals can exhibit gastrointestinal symptoms, including vomiting and diarrhea if infected with the organism. Immunocompromised individuals, especially those with liver disease, are more prone to tissue infection and septicemia (Figure 23-9 ■). About half the patients with septicemia die because of septic shock (Mégraud & Thijsen, 2004).

V. vulnificus requires iron as a growth factor. Compromised patients with high serum iron levels are especially prone to infection (Mégraud & Thijsen, 2004). Serum iron levels can be elevated in individuals with hemolytic anemia, hemochromatosis, lead poisoning, or liver problems such as hepatitis and cirrhosis. Additional virulence factors include a polysaccharide capsule and cell wall lipopolysaccharide (LPS). Both virulence factors explain the dramatic invasive properties of this organism.

The organism is usually acquired by eating raw oysters or contamination of an open wound by ocean water. The symptoms appear rapidly with the possibility of death within 48 hours. Tissue infections present initially with fever, swelling, and intense pain at the site. Wounds are usually located on the extremities such as the hands and arms or feet and legs. Within hours, hemorrhagic **bullae** (blood-filled black blisters) and tissue **necrosis** (death) appear. The necrotic tissue can develop into necrotizing fasciitis and rapidly lead to secondary septicemia.

The organism can enter the bloodstream without ever causing gastrointestinal tract symptoms, especially in the compromised host (Neill & Carpenter, 2000). It invades the intestinal mucosa to reach the bloodstream. Septicemia presents rapidly with fever, chills, and pain and edema of the lower extremities (Ho, 2002). Multiple hemorrhagic bullae eventually form on the extremities.

Cultures of the wound, blood, and stool can provide the definitive diagnosis. See ∞ Chapters 32, 35, and 37 for more information on blood, stool, and wound cultures. *V. vulnificus* is able to grow on MacConkey agar. Unlike other *Vibrio* species, it is a lactose fermenter. The microbiologist may overlook the organism on culture if there are other gram-negative rods such as *Enterobacteriaceae* present in the body site, such as in stool. Ideally the physician can provide the laboratory with the necessary patient history to ensure its recovery. On TCBS agar, most strains appear as nonsucrose fermenters, which present as clear, blue-green colonies. A small percentage may ferment sucrose and develop yellow colonies on TCBS agar just like *V. cholerae.*

V. vulnificus is a halophilic *Vibrio* species. It will grow in NaCl concentrations of up to 1.0%. It produces what appears to be a positive string test, but it can only be held at lengths of 3 to 6 millimeters. The organism is also susceptible to both concentrations of O/129. This oxidase-positive, lysine decarboxylase, and arginine dihydrolase-negative and indole-positive organism is unique among the *Vibrio* species because of its ability to ferment lactose. The ability to produce acid from salicin will also help differentiate it from *V. parahaemolyticus.* Table 23-1 compiles the biochemical reactions for *V. vulnificus* and differentiates it from other *Vibrio* species.

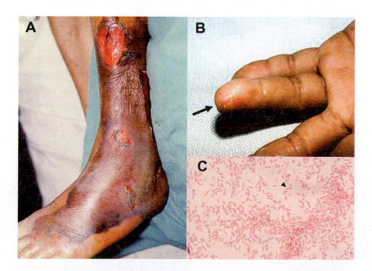

■ **FIGURE 23-9** *Vibrio vulnificus* is known for its aggressive tissue infections and ability to invade the bloodstream. Picture A shows a patient's leg with the typical hemorrhagic bullae and tissue necrosis associated with the organism. Picture B displays its ability to rapidly infect a fish bone puncture injury. This patient developed bacteremia within 1 day of the injury. Picture C demonstrates the characteristic curved gram-negative rods (noted at the arrowhead) of *V. vulnificus* isolated from a blood culture.

From CDC, Emerging Infectious Diseases, Volume 10, Number 8, August 2004.

℮ REAL WORLD TIP

Because *V. vulnificus* is a lactose fermenter on MacConkey and spot indole positive, it could be misidentified unless an oxidase test is performed. *E. coli* can be presumptively identified by its beta hemolysis, positive spot indole test, and dark lactose-fermenting colony. It could be easy to overlook *V. vulnificus'* lack of beta hemolysis and presumptively classify its colony as an *E. coli* from the stool or wound without the oxidase reaction.

Healthy individuals with gastroenteritis usually do not require treatment with antibiotics. Fluid replacement may be the only intervention required. Immunocompromised patients require early and aggressive treatment because of the organism's rapid ability to cause infection. Wound infections require **debridement** (removal of dead tissue to reinstate blood flow to a body site) of the necrotic tissue. If the infection is advanced, amputation of the extremity may be necessary. Early antibiotic therapy has been shown to have a positive impact on patient survival. As with any organism, necrotizing fasciitis and septicemia require aggressive therapy. Antimicrobial agents for treatment include tetracycline, cefotaxime, and ciprofloxacin. One-third of septic patients perish even if antibiotics are initiated within 24 hours of the start of the infection (Neill & Carpenter, 2000).

 Checkpoint! 23–4 (Chapter Objective 5)

You have isolated an oxidase-positive gram-negative rod from a blood culture. It is a lactose fermenter on MacConkey agar. You believe one potential pathogen is Vibrio vulnificus. Select the patient history that led you to suspect this organism.

　A. *16-year-old male from Los Angeles who went deep sea fishing*
　B. *56-year-old male from New Orleans who is waiting for a liver transplant*
　C. *38-year-old female from St. Louis who has recently traveled to India*
　D. *29-year-old female from Rhode Island who has ingested raw seafood*

▶ AEROMONAS HYDROPHILA

GENERAL CHARACTERISTICS

The genus *Aeromonas* was originally considered a member of the family *Vibrionaceae*. It is now included in the family *Aeromonadaceae*. The genus proves to be a confusing group of organisms for the inexperienced clinical microbiologist. Although *Aeromonas hydrophila* is the most common isolate and probably the easiest to identify, other *Aeromonas species* have proven to be a challenge for current identification systems.

Environment

Aeromonas hydrophila is the most common human isolate of the genus. Based on its species name, this organism loves water. It can be found in fresh- and salt water. Because it is found in water, it can also be present as normal flora in leeches, oysters, fish, frogs, and other water reptiles such as alligators. It is known to cause disease in cold-blooded animals such as frogs and fishes and so may be present in freshwater aquariums.

Because it can be found in freshwater, household fixtures such as faucets, showerheads, and sink traps can harbor the organism. Its presence in these devices can place it in the hospital environment, where it has the potential to become a nosocomial pathogen.

Microscopic Morphology

The human pathogens of the *Aeromonas* genus are motile. It appears as a straight or curved gram-negative rod on Gram stain. Its Gram stain is not unique, and the microbiologist will not be able to differentiate it readily from other gram-negative rods.

Biochemical Characteristics

A. hydrophila is a gram-negative rod that is oxidase positive. This reaction will differentiate it from the *Enterobacteriaceae*, even if it appears as a lactose fermenter on MacConkey agar. An easy screen, which can be used to detect *Aeromonas* species in stool culture, is the swipe or sweep oxidase. Growth on a 5% sheep blood agar can be swiped up and tested for oxidase. Once a positive reaction is observed, the microbiologist can test individual colonies to find the specific organism providing the positive result.

Vibrio species can be confused with *Aeromonas hydrophila* because of several characteristics they have in common. Both are found in water sources, able to cause diarrhea and wound infections related to water exposure and produce positive oxidase reactions. Both are also motile, lysine decarboxylase positive, indole positive, DNase positive and gelatinase positive. Commercial identification systems have experienced difficulty in differentiating *Vibrio* species from *Aeromonas* species (Abbott, Sell, Catino, Hartley, & Janda, 1998). Care should be taken when interpreting the results of these commercial identification systems.

 REAL WORLD TIP

Aeromonas hydrophila can appear as beta-hemolytic, lactose-fermenting gram-negative rods that are oxidase and indole positive. *E. coli* is presumptively identified based on its beta-hemolytic colony, lactose fermentation on MacConkey agar and positive spot indole. Without the oxidase reaction, *A. hydrophila* can be easily mistaken for *E. coli* and missed in a stool or misidentified in a wound culture.

　Aeromonas hydrophila can be differentiated from *Vibrio* species by its negative ornithine decarboxylase reaction, an inability to grow in the presence of 6.0% NaCl, its failure to grow on TCBS agar, and its resistance to the vibriostatic agent O/129 at concentrations of both 10 μg and 150 μg. The string test is negative for *A. hydrophila*. Sodium deoxycholate does not lyse the organism, so its DNA is not available to form a string when pulled away from the glass slide with a loop. Table 23-1 lists the most common identification reactions for *Aeromonas hydrophila* and differentiates it from *Vibrio* species and *Plesiomonas shigelloides*.

Triple Sugar Iron (TSI) Agar and Kligler Iron Agar (KIA) Slants.　*Aeromonas hydrophila* is able to ferment glu-

cose and sucrose consistently. Some strains can ferment lactose also. On TSI, the organism produces a yellow (acid) slant and yellow (acid) butt. It ferments the glucose and sucrose present and possibly the lactose present, depending on the strain present. On KIA, the slant is may be pink (alkaline) if lactose is not utilized and yellow (acid) if it is used. The butt is yellow because of the fermentation of glucose. The TSI and KIA slant reactions of *Aeromonas hydrophila* can mimic those of *V. cholerae.* Additional testing is required to differentiate them.

Gelatin Hydrolysis. *Aeromonas hydrophila* produces protein degrading enzymes. Proteinases are often associated with virulence. Gelatin is made up of amino acids and acts as the substrate for the protein-degrading enzymes. *V. cholerae, V. parahaemolyticus,* and *V. vulnificus* produce gelatinase provided 1.0% saline is used as the test medium to ensure the halophilic organisms will grow. *Aeromonas* species also produce gelatinase. The test is useful for differentiating these organisms from *Plesiomonas shigelloides,* which does not produce gelatinase.

DNase. Organisms that produce gelatinase usually also produce other "ases" or enzymes. DNase is another enzyme produced by *V. cholerae, V. parahaemolyticus, V. vulnificus,* and *Aeromonas* species but not by *Plesiomonas shigelloides.* DNase is an enzyme that breaks down deoxyribonuclease acid (DNA). The presence of DNase is usually associated with virulence.

In one method, DNA is incorporated into an agar plate. The use of toluidine blue as an indicator eliminates the use of reagents to detect DNA degradation. Toluidine blue is an indicator dye that is blue when bound to intact DNA. As the DNA is degraded, oligonucleotides and mononucleotides are created. The dye turns from blue to pink with the presence of nucleotides (Figure 23-10).

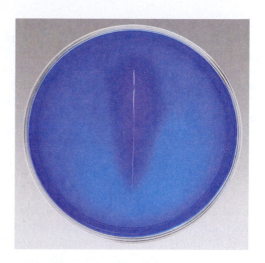

FIGURE 23-10 DNase test agar with toluidine blue can be used to determine the ability of an organism to produce deoxyribonuclease and break down intact DNA. A pink halo around the organism is because of the presence of nucleotides after degradation of the DNA. The toluidine blue dye turns pink in the presence of nucleotides.
Photo courtesy of Remel, part of Thermo Fisher Scientific.

The agar is inoculated with organism and incubated at 35°C to 37°C for 18 to 24 hours. A positive DNase reaction demonstrates a pink coloration around the organism's inoculation site. A negative DNase reaction remains blue.

✓ **Checkpoint! 23–5 (Chapter Objective 6)**

A gram-negative rod isolated from a fishhook injury in the right thumb of a 15-year-old healthy male produced the following reactions:

> *Sheep blood agar—large gray colony with beta hemolysis*
> *MacConkey—pink colony*
> *Oxidase test—purple*
> *Spot indole—pink*
> *TSI slant—yellow slant over a yellow butt*
> *Arginine dihydrolase—yellow*

The organism will also be
>   A.   *DNase negative.*
>   B.. *lysine decarboxylase positive.*
>   C.   *ornithine decarboxylase positive.*
>   D.   *gelatinase negative.*

SPECIAL CONSIDERATIONS

Specimen Collection

There are no special requirements for the collection, transportation, or isolation of *Aeromonas hydrophila.* Appropriate specimens should be collected to ensure the organism will be recovered. Stool specimens are preferred to a rectal swab for gastrointestinal infections.

Special Media

Most *A. hydrophila* isolates are beta-hemolytic on 5.0% sheep blood agar. It is able to grow on routine media used for the isolation of stool pathogens. Although the majority of strains are nonlactose fermenters on MacConkey agar, up to 15% of *A. hydrophila* isolates may be overlooked because of their ability to ferment lactose. This characteristic can prompt even an experienced microbiologist to mistake it for a member of the *Enterobacteriaceae* in a stool culture. On hektoen enteric agar, it appears as a sucrose fermenter (yellow colony) and will again be mistaken for normal stool flora. It will not grow on TCBS agar.

Because the organism may be overlooked in the vast number of normal enteric bacteria that can be present in stool, selective and differential media for *Aeromonas* species have been developed. Cefsulodin-irgasan-novobiocin (CIN) is an agar that was developed for the isolation of *Yersinia enterocolitica,* another enteric pathogen. *A. hydrophila* can be selectively isolated on this agar. Its colony can mimic the typical bull's-eye colony (red center with transparent edges) produced by *Yersinia enterocolitica.* Most laboratories that perform stool cultures probably have this medium available. A full identification must be performed on any characteristic colony found on a CIN agar. Blood agar incorporated with 10 μg/mL of ampicillin (Figure 23-11 ■) can also be used to select the organism from normal enteric flora in a stool specimen.

Alkaline peptone water (APW) was developed for the isolation of *Vibrio* species. Its alkaline environment (pH 8.6 to 9.0) is ideal for *V. cholerae.* APW can also be used to selectively isolate *Aeromonas* species as well in stool. The broth is inoculated and incubated overnight and then subcultured to sheep blood and MacConkey agars. The agars are then screened for colonies typical of *A. hydrophila.*

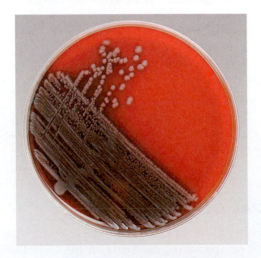

■ **FIGURE 23-11** The use of selective media such as blood agar with ampicillin can be used to selectively isolate *Aeromonas hydrophila* from normal enteric flora in stool cultures.
Photo courtesy of Remel, part of Thermo Fisher Scientific.

CLINICAL SIGNIFICANCE

Humans are at an increased risk of infection during the summer months, which coincides with the increased recreational use of water sources. Contact with contaminated food, water, or cold-blooded animals provides the more common modes of transmission. Occupations associated with increased risk of infection include veterinarians, fish and reptile handlers, and fishermen. Even seemingly harmless hobbies such as keeping a fish aquarium may put its owner at risk for infection.

The use of leeches after reattachment of amputated appendages, such as a finger, is a common practice in most hospitals today. The anticoagulation effect of the leech's saliva maintains blood flow to the reattached appendage so it remains viable. The leech carries *Aeromonas* species as part of its normal gut flora. The organism helps the leech break down the blood in its digestive tract and use it for nutrition. The presence of this organism provides a potential source of infection. Infections associated with the use of leeches include soft tissue infections, myonecrosis, and septicemia.

ⓔ REAL WORLD TIP

In 2004, the U.S. Food and Drug Administration (FDA) approved the use of leeches as a medical device. Leeches produce anticlotting agents and a natural anesthetic in their saliva, which keep the blood flowing in regrafted amputated appendages without causing patient discomfort because of the their presence. The leeches used are raised under very controlled conditions by FDA-approved companies. It is impossible to raise leeches that do not contain *Aeromonas* species because of their interdependent relationship. Infections caused by the medicinal use of leeches have been reported. About 40 minutes after attachment, the leech finishes feeding, drops off the patient, and is then discarded as biohazardous waste.

This gram-negative rod can be the causative agent of gastroenteritis, skin and tissue infections, and septicemia. Gastroenteritis is probably caused by enterotoxin production, which leads to a self-limiting watery diarrhea (Winn et al., 2006). Although much is written about *A. hydrophila* as a potential enteric pathogen, it has not been proven. Volunteers fed up to 10^{10} organisms did not develop gastroenteritis (Atkins & Cleary, 2003a). Skin infections are often associated with lacerations that are exposed to contaminated water. A classic case study would involve the formation of an abscess after a fisherman removes an impaled fishhook from his thumb. Septicemia is a serious complication of *Aeromonas hydrophila* infection in individuals with an impaired immune system (Winn et al., 2006).

Prevention of infection requires avoiding potentially contaminated food and water. An open wound should never be washed with lake or river water. The use of leeches, although necessary to save an amputated appendage, may introduce a potential infection. The administration of antibiotics prior to the use of leeches may be necessary.

Diarrhea is usually self-limiting with only fluid replacement required. *Aeromonas* species can produce several beta-lactamases. They are resistant to penicillin, ampicillin, vancomycin, and carbenicillin. Fluoroquinolones, tetracycline, and trimethoprim-sulfamethoxazole have proven to be effective for treatment of gastroenteritis if needed. More serious infections such as skin and tissue infections and septicemia can be treated with a third-generation cephalosporin in combination with an aminoglycoside. Tissue infections may require tissue debridement.

▶ PLESIOMONAS SHIGELLOIDES

Plesiomonas shigelloides is an oxidase-positive gram-negative rod that is now included in the family *Enterobacteriaceae* (Murray, Baron, Jorgenson, Pfaller, & Yolken, 2003). The family *Enterobacteriaceae* has always been defined as oxidase-negative gram-negative rods that ferment glucose and reduce nitrates to nitrites. With the addition of *Plesiomonas shigelloides,* the family definition now needs to be revised.

This gram-negative rod is another in a long line of organisms that can be transmitted by contact with freshwater and cold-blooded animals. Human infections are rare but can take the form of gastroenteritis or tissue infections. Like *Aeromonas* species, the incidence of infection rises with the warm summer months.

P. shigelloides has always been linked with self-limiting gastroenteritis but it has not been proven to date (Atkins & Cleary, 2003b). Studies have been done in which volunteers were fed the organism but none developed diarrhea (Atkins & Cleary, 2003b). The CDC reported a case in which a child developed watery diarrhea and fever after bathing in a bathtub in which a fish aquarium had been emptied earlier (CDC, 1989).

P. shigelloides grows easily on routine media used for isolation of stool pathogens. Although most isolates of this gram-negative rod appear as a nonlactose fermenter on MacConkey agar, approximately one-third of strains may ferment lactose. This can hinder its detection on initial observation in a stool culture because lactose fermenters are usually disregarded as normal enteric flora. *P. shigelloides* is a gray, nonhemolytic colony on sheep blood agar. On hektoen enteric agar, the organism appears as green (nonsucrose fermenter) colonies, which should be screened as a potential stool pathogen. The organism will not grow on TCBS agar, which can help differentiate it from *Vibrio* species.

The oxidase test is valuable in the detection of *P. shigelloides* in a stool culture. An oxidase swipe or sweep screen performed on growth on a 5% sheep blood agar will detect this oxidase-positive organism. If a positive oxidase reaction is detected, then the microbiologist can search for individual oxidase-pos-

itive colonies. This screen will aid in detection of the organism, especially if its MacConkey agar isolates are lactose fermenters. Lactose-fermenting gram-negative rods on a MacConkey agar from a stool specimen are routinely ignored as normal flora in most clinical laboratories.

Identification requires differentiation of *P. shigelloides* from *Aeromonas* species. The organism proves to be gelatin hydrolysis and DNase negative and ornithine decarboxylase positive. These reactions are opposite those observed in its close cousin, *Aeromonas hydrophila.* On TSI and KIA agar slants, most strains of *P. shigelloides* produce an alkaline (pink) slant over a yellow (acid) butt. The organism ferments glucose. If lactose is fermented, then the TSI slant reaction is acid (yellow) slant over a yellow (acid) butt. It can be differentiated from other *Aeromonas* species and *Vibrio* species by its fermentation of inositol (Winn et al., 2006). It does not require NaCl for growth. It is susceptible to both concentrations of the vibriostatic agent O/129. This test is not useful in differentiating it from the *Vibrio* species. Table 23-1 compiles biochemical reactions for *P. shigelloides* and its differentiation from *Aeromonas hydrophila* and the more commonly isolated *Vibrio* species.

Because most individuals are exposed to this organism through contaminated food or water, hand washing and adequate cooking of food items is essential for prevention of disease. Treatment of gastroenteritis is usually not required because the infection is often self-limiting. Trimethoprim-sulfamethoxazole and the fluoroquinolones may be used to as treatment options. *Plesiomonas shigelloides* has the ability to produce beta-lactamases just like *Aeromonas* species.

> ✓ **Checkpoint! 23–6 (Chapter Objective 7)**
>
> *Which of the following tests can easily differentiate Plesiomonas shigelloides from the other members of the family Enterobacteriaceae?*
>   A. *Catalase*
>   B. *Fermentation of lactose*
>   C. *Oxidase*
>   D. *Beta hemolysis*

▶ CAMPYLOBACTERACEAE

As a group, the *Campylobacter* species are well known for their association with diarrhea and systemic infections. They are **zoonotic** organisms that are usually found in animals but able to cause disease in humans. With the Gram stain, these small, curved gram-negative rods can appear as loose spirals (squiggles) or *S* shapes (Figure 23-12). They can characteristically resemble the gull-winged birds that children make in grade school drawings. A "darting" motility can be observed in a wet preparation made with trypticase soy broth (TSB). Saline and water may inhibit their motility. Most of the

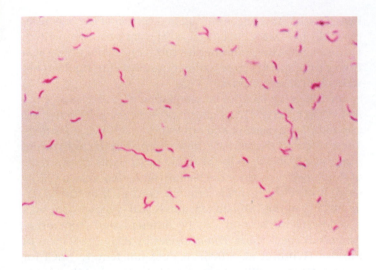

Campylobacter species that cause human disease are microaerophilic (love decreased levels of O_2) and capnophilic (love increased levels of CO_2). Most of these slow-growing organisms only thrive in an atmosphere that provides 5 to 10% oxygen and 3 to 10% carbon dioxide. Special isolation media, unique temperatures, and 2 to 3 days of incubation are usually required to ensure in their isolation.

 REAL WORLD TIP

Campylobacter is the only enteric pathogen that can be presumptively identified from a direct Gram stain of stool. The unique Gram stain morphology can be observed along with the presence of fecal red blood cells and polymorphonuclear leukocytes. *Campylobacter* species do not take up safranin well in the Gram stain procedure. Either the safranin stain must be left on longer than usual (2 to 3 minutes) or alternate counterstains such as carbol fuchsin or aqueous basic fuchsin can be substituted.

CAMPYLOBACTER JEJUNI

General Characteristics

Campylobacter jejuni is the most common of all of the *Campylobacter* species isolated. It is the leading causative agent of diarrhea worldwide. In the United States, approximately 2.5 million cases occur each year (Ruiz-Palacios, 2003). There are more reported cases of diarrhea because of *Campylobacter* species than *Salmonella* or *Shigella* species combined. Animals, such as cattle, domesticated pets, and poultry, serve as the reservoir for the organism. It lives in their digestive tracts.

Chickens may account for 50 to 70% of infections (Javid et al., 2005). The organism can be found in about 50% of the poultry sold in the United States (Perez-Perez & Blaser, 1996). Humans become infected through contaminated food, such as raw milk, and water or contact with infected animals or carcasses. The juice of raw chicken is often contaminated with the organism. The typical case study involves an individual developing diarrhea after ingesting improperly cooked chicken or playing with a puppy that has diarrhea.

Environment.   An environment of 5 to 10% oxygen (microaerophilic) and 3 to 10% carbon dioxide (capnophilic) is perfect for the isolation and growth of *C. jejuni*. The ideal atmosphere can be purchased as a tank of gas (5% O_2, 10% CO_2, and 85% N_2) or created chemically with an atmosphere-generating packet.

REAL WORLD TIP

In an emergency, a microaerophilic and capnophilic atmosphere can be created without the need for a special gas tank or chemical generating packs. The culture plates can be placed in a glass jar with a culture plate of *E. coli* and a burning nonscented tea candle. After the jar is closed, the candle will extinguish when it has used up most oxygen present and create carbon dioxide. *E. coli* uses more oxygen as it grows and creates carbon dioxide also. The action of both creates a microaerophilic, capnophilic environment, which will grow *Campylobacter* species in an emergency situation. An agar plate with a known *Campylobacter* species should be included as a quality control measure. The microbiologist must ensure the environment generated will support the growth of the organism when using this method.

Special Media.   Isolation media have been developed to select for the organism from the vast numbers of normal flora present in stool. The addition of antibiotics such as vancomycin, cephalothin, and trimethoprim to sheep blood agar can inhibit the growth of most of the normal fecal flora. Although *C. jejuni* is able to grow at 37°C, it can also grow at 4°C and 42°C. The use of a higher temperature plus the selective medium plus the unique atmosphere provides for the optimum recovery of the organism (Figure 23-13 ■). Medium must be held at least 3 days because of the slow growth of the organism.

Enrichment broths, such as Campy broth, can enhance the recovery of the organism from a stool specimen. After overnight incubation at 4°C, the broth is subcultured to a Campy selective agar. Because *C. jejuni* is microaerophilic, the broth should be inoculated with stool about 1 inch below the surface. After incubation, the same region of the broth is removed with a pipette for culture to a selective medium.

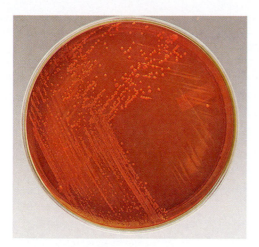

■ **FIGURE 23-13** The use of selective *Campylobacter* medium, in a microaerophilic, capnophilic atmosphere at 42°C, can inhibit the normal enteric flora found in stool while allowing *Campylobacter jejuni* to proliferate.
Photo courtesy of Remel, part of Thermo Fisher Scientific.

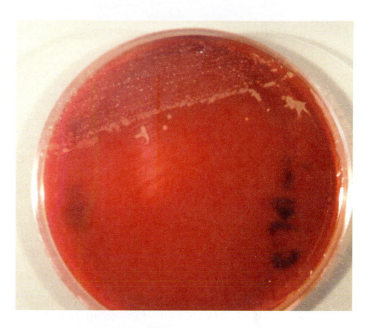

■ **FIGURE 23-14** *C. jejuni* colonies growing on sheep blood agar. Notice some of the colonies are following the agar streak lines rather then forming individual colonies.

Many laboratories have eliminated the use of Campy enrichment broth as a cost-saving strategy. They have chosen to inoculate the selective agar directly with the specimen. Each laboratory must assess the value of the use of an enrichment broth versus direct inoculation for their patient population.

Filtration of stool through a membrane can selectively allow *Campylobacter* species to pass through while holding back the normal enteric flora present. The key is the pore size of the membrane. They must be within the range of 0.45 to 0.65 μm to ensure only *Campylobacter* species can pass through (Murray et al., 2003). The membrane is inoculated with several drops of a mixture of sterile saline and stool and placed onto a sheep blood agar or selective Campy agar. After 30 to 60 minutes, the filter is removed, and the culture plate is incubated at the appropriate temperature and atmosphere.

 Checkpoint! 23–7 (Chapter Objective 5)

A 28-year-old female developed bloody diarrhea after a picnic lunch of fried chicken. The enteric pathogen isolated Gram stained as small loosely spiraled gram-negative rods. From what atmosphere and temperature did you take the culture medium to make this Gram stain?

	Atmosphere	Temperature
A.	5% oxygen, 10% CO_2, 85% nitrogen	42°C
B.	10% oxygen, 5% CO_2, 85% nitrogen	42°C
C.	5% oxygen, 10% CO_2, 85% nitrogen	35°C
D.	10% oxygen, 10% CO_2, 80% nitrogen	25°C

Biochemical Characteristics. *C. jejuni* appears as gray to pink-tan, flat colonies that may have a tendency to follow the agar streak lines (Figure 23-14 ■), rather than form individual colonies on fresh medium with high moisture content. As an agar plate loses moisture with storage, there is a tendency for the organism to form distinct colonies. This gram-negative rod is catalase and oxidase positive. Refer to ∞ Chapter 9 for details on the principle of these two biochemical reactions and their interpretation. The positive oxidase and catalase reactions plus the characteristic Gram stain of the organism isolated from the appropriate selective medium incubated in a microaerophilic, capnophilic atmosphere can be used to presumptively identify *Campylobacter jejuni*. Because it is such a commonly encountered enteric pathogen, the use of presumptive identification criteria can provide cost savings for the laboratory and rapid diagnosis for the patient. Traditional biochemical testing can be used to differentiate *Campylobacter* species other than *C. jejuni*. Table 23-2✪ lists the biochemical reactions for the three most common *Campylobacter* species isolated from humans.

Hippurate Hydrolysis. Hydrolysis of hippurate can be used to differentiate *C. jejuni* from other species if necessary. This test determines the organism's ability to hydrolyze sodium hippurate. It is a critical test for differentiating *C. jejuni*, which is positive, from its closest cousin, *C. coli*, which is negative. *C. jejuni* is the only *Campylobacter* species that can hydrolyze sodium hippurate.

The test can be performed using two different methods. One uses ferric chloride as the detection reagent and can take 24 to 48 hours for results. The rapid test is only incubated for 2.5 hours. For all organism identifications, rapid results are critical to the clinical microbiologists. They provide the fastest turnaround time, which in turn improves patient outcomes, as well as decreasing length of stay and costs.

The rapid hippurate hydrolysis test begins with a suspension of 1% sodium hippurate solution. A heavy inoculum of

TABLE 23-2

Differentiation of *Campylobacter* Species and *Helicobacter pylori*

	Campylobacter jejuni	*Campylobacter coli*	*Campylobacter fetus*	*Helicobacter pylori*
Oxidase	+	+	+	+
Catalase	+	+	+	+
Hippurate hydrolysis	+	–	–	–
Indoxyl acetate	+	+	–	–
Urease production	–	–	–	+ (rapid)
Growth at:				
25°C	–	–	+	–
37°C	+	+	+	+
42°C	+	+	–	V

+ = positive, – = negative, V = variable

fresh organism is created in 0.4 mL of the solution and incubated for 2 hours at 35°C to 37°C. After incubation, 0.2 mL of ninhydrin detection reagent is overlaid onto the inoculum. The tube is incubated for an additional 10 minutes. Glycine is one of end products produced from the hydrolysis of sodium hippurate. The ninhydrin reagent reacts with glycine to create a deep blue-purple color. A negative test must be incubated for 30 minutes and shows no color change. Refer to ∞ Chapter 17, "Gram-Positive Cocci," to view a photo of a positive and negative hippurate reaction. ∞ Chapters 17 and 19 describe how hippurate hydrolysis is used to identify gram-positive cocci and gram-positive rods.

Indoxyl Acetate.   *Campylobacter jejuni* and *C. coli* are both able to hydrolyze indoxyl acetate, whereas most other *Campylobacter* species are not (Figure 23-15 ■). A commercial disk impregnated with indoxyl acetate is available. Suspected organisms are rubbed onto the moistened disk. Hydrolysis of the substrate is detected by the presence of a blue color within 10 minutes. There is no color change with a negative reaction.

Other.   Polymerase chain reaction (PCR) methods are available for detection of *Campylobacter* species directly in stool specimens. This method allows for rapid speciation of organisms and epidemiological studies. Immunologic tests (INDX Campy-JCL, Hardy Diagnostics, and Fisher Scientific or Dry Spot Campylobacter Test Kit, Remel) and a molecular probe (Gen-Probe) are available to identify an isolate as a *Campylobacter* species.

Specimen Collection.   No special handling of fecal specimens is required unless there is a delay of 2 hours or more. If a transportation delay is possible, the specimen can be placed in Cary-Blair transport medium or Campy enrichment thioglycolate broth.

Although the organism will grow in the blood culture medium of automated detection systems, its slow growth may require incubating the bottles for up to 2 weeks for detection

(Forbes, Sahm, & Weissfeld, 2002). Subcultures should be incubated in the microaerophilic, capnophilic atmosphere and held for at least 3 days.

Clinical Significance

As few as 500 organisms can initiate enteric disease, especially if taken in with water or milk (Ruiz-Palacios, 2003). *C. jejuni* has the ability to penetrate the intestinal epithelium of the jejunum, ileum, and colon. They multiply and destroy cells to cause bloody diarrhea. Invasion of the intestinal cells also leads to the presence of fecal white blood cells in stool. White and red blood cells are the classic indicator cell on Gram stain for invasive enteric pathogens. Patients often complain of fever and abdominal cramps. Culture is required because the gas-

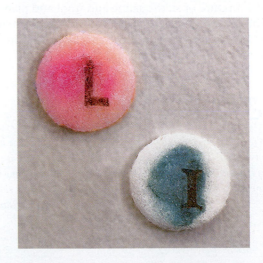

■ **FIGURE 23-15** Indoxyl acetate (lower right disk) is a rapid test that can be used to identify and differentiate *Campylobacter jejuni* and *C. coli* from other *Campylobacter* species. The development of a blue color indicates a positive reaction. (LAP [upper left disk] is used for rapid differentiation of the *Streptococcus* and is discussed in ∞ Chapter 17.)
Photo courtesy of Remel, part of Thermo Fisher Scientific.

trointestinal signs and symptoms reported are very similar to those of other enteric pathogens.

The organism may also create a cholera-like enterotoxin that causes fluid to accumulate in the intestine leading to a watery diarrhea. The production of several cytotoxins has also been reported in some isolates (Ruiz-Palacios, 2003). The organism rarely causes disease beyond the gastrointestinal tract, such as septicemia, except in those who are immunocompromised or have underlying conditions.

A unique potential complication of *Campylobacter* infection is **Guillain-Barré syndrome** (GBS; a potentially paralytic disease; Perez-Perez & Blaser, 1996). GBS is caused by an autoimmune response that may occur about once every 1,000 infections (CDC, 2005a). As soon as two weeks after infection, the antibodies produced against *C. jejuni* may cross react with the myelin of the peripheral nerves (Ruiz-Palacios, 2003). Symptoms can range from weakness of the limbs to complete paralysis and respiratory failure requiring airway ventilation. Most cases reverse and resolve after a few weeks or months. About 20% of patients can be left with some type of neurological deficit such as an unsteady gait (Nachamkin, Allos, & Ho, 1998). GBS has also developed after infections with organisms other than *Campylobacter* species.

Treatment and Prevention

Because most enteric infections are self-limiting, replacement of fluids and electrolytes are usually all that are necessary for most patients. Antibiotics should be considered for compromised individuals or those with extraintestinal infections. Erythromycin is usually the antibiotic of choice. Ciprofloxacin may be used, but resistance is on the increase in the United States (Mégraud & Thijsen, 2004). Tetracycline may be an alternate choice.

Transmission of the organism can be interrupted by properly cooking food, avoiding contaminated water and unpasteurized milk, or washing hands after contact with animals. Washing hands, utensils, and surfaces such as cutting boards after contact with raw poultry can dramatically break the transmission cycle within the home.

Other *Campylobacter* species

C. jejuni and *C. coli* are the most common species isolated in humans. Both require the same media, atmosphere, and temperature for isolation. *C. coli* is usually food borne and produces infections very similar to *C. jejuni* but usually follow a less severe course (Mégraud & Thijsen, 2004). *C. coli* has been isolated more frequently in individuals with close contact with hogs (Ruiz-Palacios & Pickering, 2003).

The two organisms are rarely differentiated in most laboratories. Treatment is similar, so differentiation may only be necessary for epidemiological studies. If identification is required, *C. coli* is oxidase and catalase positive but unable to hydrolyze hippurate.

Campylobacter fetus is an animal pathogen that may cause infections in compromised patients. It is the third-most-isolated

species, but only accounts for about 0.3% of all *Campylobacter* species isolated (Ruiz-Palacios & Pickering, 2003). Although it may cause gastroenteritis, it is primarily known for leaving the intestine to cause bacteremia and other extraintestinal infections. It has a fondness for vascular sites such the placenta and the brain (Javid, 2005). This organism is sensitive to the antibiotics present in the selective media used to isolate *C. jejuni* from stool cultures. Filtering the stool through a selective membrane can hold back most of the normal flora organisms present while allowing the small *Campylobacter* rods to move through it. The filtrate is then cultured on noninhibitory blood media. Blood cultures should be held at least 2 weeks to ensure detection of this slow-growing organism.

C. fetus does grow at 25°C and 37°C but not 42°C. It is unique among *Campylobacter* species in its growth at 25°C. *C. jejuni* and *C. coli* will grow at 37°C and 42°C but not at 25°C. *C. fetus* requires the same atmosphere as *C. jejuni* for growth. The laboratory must be informed if the physician suspects this organism. This vital information can ensure the laboratory uses the proper temperature and media for its isolation.

▶ *HELICOBACTER PYLORI*

In 2005, two scientists received the Nobel Prize in medicine for culturing *Helicobacter pylori* for the first time and determining its role in gastritis, duodenal, and peptic ulcer disease (Watts, 2005). They used unusual methods to prove Koch's postulates. One of the scientists swallowed the organism to prove its ability to cause gastritis. He developed the disease and proved the correlation between the presence of the organism and the occurrence of disease. Their discovery squashed the myth that stress causes stomach ulcers.

CULTURAL CHARACTERISTICS

A gastric biopsy collected by means of an endoscope provides the specimen of choice for culture of *H. pylori*. This small, curved gram-negative rod will grow under the same microaerophilic atmosphere used to isolate *C. jejuni*. The biopsy should not be delayed in transport. If a delay is anticipated, a commercial transport medium can be used. A physician may also choose to inoculate a commercial rapid urease test, such as the CLOtest (Figure 23-16 ■) at the patient's bedside. The specimen can be ground prior to plating.

A nonselective agar such as brain heart infusion, tryptic soy, or brucella with at least 5% blood provides the best growth (Winn et al., 2006). Thayer-Martin may be used as a selective agar if mixed cultures are expected. The agar should be incubated in a humidified, microaerophilic atmosphere at 37°C for up to 10 days. Small, round, translucent colonies usually appear within 3 to 4 days.

A Gram stain of a touch preparation of the gastric biopsy can be prepared. Because the organisms do not take up the safranin counterstain well, carbol fuchsin can be substituted.

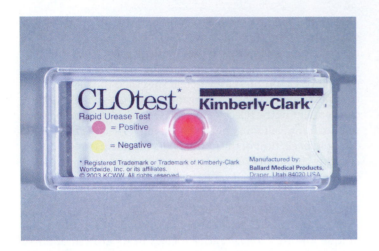

■ **FIGURE 23-16** Positive reaction (pink) for the CLOtest.

Ideally the counterstain should be allowed to sit for 2 to 3 minutes. Histologic stains such as hematoxylin and eosin, Giemsa, or Warthin-Starry silver may also be used to observe and identify the organism in gastric biopsy tissue sections.

⟳ REAL WORLD TIP

H. pylori is rarely diagnosed by culture methods in the clinical laboratory. It is usually detected by serology, direct histologic examination of gastric tissue, or urease production tests.

✓ Checkpoint! 23–8 (Chapter Objectives 3, 5, and 6)

A patient complains of stomach pain after eating. The physician suspects peptic ulcers. What specimen will the laboratory probably receive to confirm the diagnosis?

   A. *Gastric biopsy*
   B. *Stool*
   C. *Blood*
   D. *Stomach contents*

IDENTIFICATION INCLUDING RAPID TESTS

H. pylori colonies require limited testing for identification. The unique Gram stain along with the positive catalase, oxidase, and urease reactions confirm the identification. *H. pylori* is very similar to *C. jejuni* in its Gram stain and environmental requirements. *H. pylori* is unable to hydrolyze sodium hippurate and indoxyl acetate and usually will not grow at 42°C.

   H. pylori possesses the enzyme, urease, which allows it break down urea to ammonia. This characteristic provides an alkaline cloud around the organism, which allows it to survive in the highly acidic environment of the stomach. The urea sub-

strate can be prepared as an agar slant or a solution. The test can be inoculated with organism from culture or directly with a gastric biopsy. After incubation, the phenol red indicator turns pink (positive) with the presence of alkaline by-products caused by the breakdown of urea. No color change indicates a negative result. *H. pylori* produces a bright pink or magenta color, sometimes within minutes to hours of inoculation. The characteristic intense, rapid positive urease result observed is similar to that seen with *Proteus* species.

   Culture requires several days for isolation and may not be practical for all laboratories. Other methods, both invasive and noninvasive, are available, for diagnosis of *H. pylori*.

   Because the stomach rarely contains organisms other than *H. pylori,* the laboratory can use its unique intense, rapid urease reaction for its detection from a gastric biopsy specimen. After removal, the tissue is placed in urea incorporated into a semisolid agar or solution, incubated at 37°C, and read at intervals for urease production. A positive urease reaction produces a bright pink or magenta color (Figure 23-17 ■). The test should be incubated a full 24 hours before calling negative.

✓ Checkpoint! 23–9 (Chapter Objective 6)

Which of the following characteristics differentiate Helicobacter pylori from Campylobacter species?

   A. *Oxidase*
   B. *Catalase*
   C. *Urease*
   D. *Gram stain*

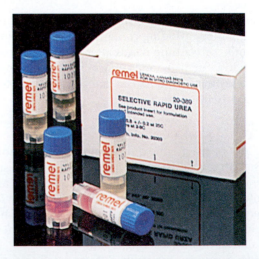

■ **FIGURE 23-17** A gastric biopsy is usually collected via an endoscope. The biopsy is placed in a urea broth, incubated, and observed. A positive reaction is noted by the development of a bright pink or magenta color as noted in the picture. The color is because of the alkaline by-products from the breakdown of urea by *H. pylori*.
Photo courtesy of Remel, part of Thermo Fisher Scientific.

Although urease is specific for *H. pylori,* other transitory urease-positive organisms may present with a false-positive reaction.

The urea breath test provides an alternate patient procedure that is rapid and noninvasive. The patient drinks a urea solution labeled with a carbon isotope (^{13}C or ^{14}C). *H. pylori* breaks down the urea, and the patient releases the carbon isotope as labeled CO_2. The patient breathes into a collection tube 30 minutes after drinking the solution. The concentration of ^{13}C or ^{14}C released is measured. The expense of this procedure and the use of **radioisotopes** (an atom of a chemical element that emits radiation as it breaks down) have limited its use in most facilities (Blaser, 2005). It can be used to monitor therapy because the level of labeled CO_2 should correlate with the number of *H. pylori* organisms present.

Serology can provide a rapid, inexpensive diagnosis with only a blood sample. The presence of antibodies against *H. pylori* is detected using an enzyme-linked immunosorbent assay (ELISA). The test has a high sensitivity and specificity for detection of new cases of infection (Santacroce & Miragliotta, 2005). Because antibodies remain elevated for a long time after infection, the test cannot be used to monitor treatment.

Clinical Significance

This small curved gram-negative rod is found in the human stomach. It is able to survive a highly acid environment that kills most organisms. Humans appear to be the only reservoir. It is probably passed via mouth-to-mouth transmission or with fecal-to-oral contact. Initial contact with the organism probably begins in childhood. The organism may stay with the individual for life. Individuals raised in a low socioeconomic level are at an increased risk for development of disease (Mégraud & Thijsen, 2004). Crowded conditions, large families and poor sanitation add to an increased risk for infection (Blaser, 2005).

Once ingested, *H. pylori* is able to move rapidly into the jellylike layer of mucus covering the gastric mucosa. In this layer, it is better protected from the acid environment and can be free-living or adhere to the mucus-producing cells (Blaser, 2005). It produces urease, which in turn breaks down urea present to produce ammonia as a by-product. An alkaline ammonia cloud is created around the organism to further buffer its exposure to the acid environment.

Gastric or duodenal lesions form not because of invasion by the organism but rather because of contact with the organism, its by-products, and other host factors (Blaser, 2005). The ammonia produced by the organisms, because of urease activity, damages the stomach cells to expose the underlying tissue (Perez-Perez & Blaser, 1996). Once the damaged tissue is exposed to stomach acid, it leads to gastritis and duodenal and peptic ulcers. Continuous cell damage over decades can eventually lead to the development of gastric carcinoma.

The organism needs to be eliminated to avoid potential complications such as gastric carcinoma. A combination of antibiotics is used to ensure elimination of the organism. Clarithromycin in combination with amoxicillin or metronidazole is used (Mégraud & Thijsen, 2004). The addition of a bismuth salt (such as Pepto-Bismol) results in eradication of the organism in up to 90% of cases (Blaser, 2005). One month after treatment, the patient should be retested using a biopsy or urea breath test to ensure the organism has been eliminated (Blaser, 2005). Serology can be used if 6 months have elapsed since treatment (Blaser, 2005). Relapses can occur because of antibiotic resistance.

> ✓ **Checkpoint! 23–10 (Chapter Objective 5)**
>
> *A patient has been on treatment for gastric ulcers caused by H. pylori for the past 4 months. Which of the following tests should **not** be used to determine the effectiveness of this patient's treatment schedule?*
>
> A. *Serology*
> B. *Biopsy*
> C. *Urea breath test*
> D. *B and C*

► *CHROMOBACTERIUM VIOLACEUM*

Chromobacterium violaceum is an oxidase-positive, glucose-fermenting, motile, facultative anaerobic, slightly curved gram-negative rod that grows on MacConkey agar. Even though it is a glucose fermenter rather than glucose oxidizer, it is oxidase positive and may be confused with the oxidase-positive nonfermenters. Its primary habitat is fresh water and soil in the tropics and subtropics. It can be found in the southeastern United States so it is possible for microbiologists to see it in culture. It is not considered part of normal human flora and transmission to humans usually occurs by ingestion of contaminated water (Bilton & Johnson, 2000) or by exposure of broken skin and mucosal surfaces to contaminated water.

This organism grows on 5% sheep blood and chocolate agars after 24 hours at 35°C. It is easily recognized by the production of a characteristic violet pigment, **violacein**, especially when incubated on sheep blood and MacConkey agars at room temperature (Bilton & Johnson, 2000). Figure 23-18 demonstrates the distinctive pigment of *C. violaceum.* The colonies smell of ammonium cyanide, which is similar to almonds. Pigmented strains of *Chromobacterium violaceum* are so distinctive a presumptive identification can be made based on pigment production and positive oxidase reaction. The violet pigment can interfere with the positive purple reaction of the oxidase test. The organism can be grown under anaerobic conditions where it cannot produce pigment and then retested. Table 23-1 details laboratory tests that differentiate *C. violaceum* from other oxidase-positive glucose fermenters.

While wound infections are more common, extraintestinal infections, such as septicemia, due to this organism can be

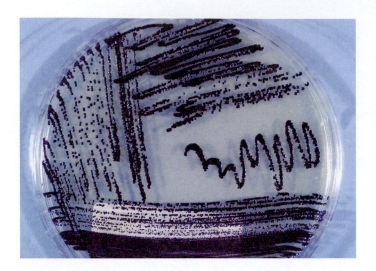

■ **FIGURE 23-18** The characteristic violet color produced by *Chromobacterium violaceum.*

SUMMARY

With the exception of *C. violaceum,* the organisms discussed in this chapter are oxidase-positive gram-negative rods that are able to attack the gastrointestinal system. The diseases they cause can range from stomach ulcers to death because of massive diarrhea. Although most are known for their ability to cause diarrhea, some are known for their role in skin and tissue infections as well as septicemia. The physician must notify the laboratory to ensure the appropriate media and atmosphere are used to isolate the organisms because they can easily be overlooked due to the predominance of normal flora in specimens such as stool. Identification can be easily accomplished for most. Tables 23-1 and 23-2 provide a summary of differentiating biochemical reactions for the organisms discussed in this chapter. The *Vibrio* species may require the addition of saline to biochemicals to ensure accurate results. Treatment depends on the infecting organism and the extent of the infection.

A clinical microbiologist must be well educated on these organisms because of their potential for isolation. The ability of people to travel to anywhere in the world and return in a time period as short as 24 hours can provide organisms a free ride to geographic locations where they may never have been cultured before.

life-threatening in compromised individuals. Potential active agents for treatments include cefotaxime, ceftazidime, imipenem, and aminoglycosides. The activity of the penicillins is variable and the activity of first- and second-generation cephalosporins is poor (Chang, Lee, Liu, Wang, & Tsao, 2007).

LEARNING OPPORTUNITIES

1. A gram-negative rod, isolated from a stool culture, produces a yellow colony on TCBS agar. It provides the following reactions: (Chapter Objectives 2d, 2e, and 2j)

   TSI—yellow slant/yellow butt

   Oxidase—purple

   Decarboxylase

   - Lysine—purple
   - Ornithine—purple

   This organism would also be:

   a. able to grow in a 6% saline solution

   b. a lactose fermenter on MacConkey agar

   c. string test negative

   d. susceptible to O/129 at 10 μg and 150 μg

2. A gram-negative rod that produces a yellow colony on TCBS agar, a yellow slant/yellow butt on TSI, and a pink slant/yellow butt on KIA is able to ferment: (Chapter Objectives 5a and 5d)

   a. lactose only

   b. sucrose only

   c. glucose and sucrose

   d. glucose and lactose

3. An oxidase-positive gram-negative rod, isolated from the hand wound of a hurricane victim, was found to produce a clear colony on MacConkey agar and a clear colony on TCBS agar. This organism is also known to commonly cause: (Chapter Objective 2g)

   a. self-limiting gastroenteritis

   b. septicemia

   c. rice water stools

   d. necrotizing fasciitis

4. A 65-year-old male went to the beach to vacation after his long-awaited retirement. He cut his right foot on a seashell and proceeded to wash it off in the ocean water. He went on with his vacation but later that night he developed pain, swelling, and reddening in his right calf with the cut. He also noticed large blisters filled with serous fluid and immediately went to the emergency room. Blood cultures were taken, and he was started on IV antibiotics. His right leg had to be amputated below the knee to halt the aggressive infection.

   Blood cultures grew an oxidase-positive gram-negative rod, which produced pink colonies on MacConkey agar. Initial identification methods did not produce any positive reactions. The identification methods were repeated using 2% saline as the inoculum. Testing revealed: (Chapter Objectives 2e, 2f, 2g, 2h, 2i, 2j, 3, and 6)

   TSI slant—yellow slant/yellow butt

   Decarboxylase

   - Arginine—yellow
   - Lysine—purple
   - Ornithine—purple

   O/129 at 10 µg—a zone of inhibition of 15 mm

   O/129 at 150 µg—a zone of inhibition of 17 mm

   DNase agar with toluidine blue—pink halo around the organism

   Which underlying disease state could have led to this patient's outcome with this organism?

   a. Diarrhea

   b. Gastroenteritis

   c. Cirrhosis

   d. Gastric ulcer

5. A beta-hemolytic gram-negative rod from a stool culture provides the following reactions: (Chapter Objectives 2e, 2g, and 2j)

   MacConkey agar—pink colonies

   TCBS agar—no growth

   Oxidase—purple

   Spot indole—pink

   O/129 at 10 µg—no zone of inhibition

   O/129 at 150 µg—no zone of inhibition

   DNase on toluidine blue agar—pink halo around the colony

You suspect the organism to be:

a. *Vibrio* species

b. *Aeromonas hydrophila*

c. *Plesiomonas shigelloides*

d. *Campylobacter* species

6. *Plesiomonas shigelloides* is easily differentiated from *Aeromonas hydrophila* by its: (Chapter Objectives 2e and 2j)

a. oxidase reaction

b. colony on MacConkey agar

c. negative DNase reaction

d. negative ornithine reaction

7. The most commonly isolated 42°C stool pathogen is an oxidase-positive gram-negative rod that will also be: (Chapter Objectives 2e and 2j)

a. hippurate positive

b. urea positive

c. indoxyl acetate negative

d. catalase negative

8. Which of the following organisms is prone to causing intravascular infections (septicemia or bacteremia)? (Chapter Objective 2g)

a. *Vibrio cholerae*

b. *V. vulnificus*

c. *Campylobacter fetus*

d. b and c

9. *H. pylori* is able to survive living in the stomach because of its ability to produce: (Chapter Objectives 2a and 2e)

a. oxidase

b. catalase

c. urease

d. hippuricase

10. Treatment of *H. pylori* infection requires: (Chapter Objective 6)

a. clarithromycin

b. a plus metronidazole

c. b plus a bismuth salt

d. surgery

PEARSON
myhealthprofessionskit™

Use this address to access the interactive Companion Website created for this textbook. Simply select "Clinical Laboratory Science" from the choice of disciplines. Find this book and log in using your user name and password.

REFERENCES

Go to myhealthprofessionskit.com to view this chapter's references.

24

Anaerobic Bacteria

Teresa A. Taff

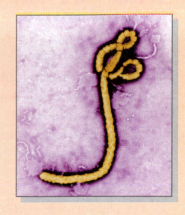

■ LEARNING OBJECTIVES

Upon completion of this chapter, the learner should be able to:

1. Define the normal anaerobic flora for each body site or specimen type and patient population.
   a. Discuss the factors that promote anaerobic infections.
2. Describe proper specimen selection, preparation, collection, and transportation requirements for anaerobes.
   a. Evaluate specimen acceptability.
   b. Describe clues that indicate the presence of anaerobes and correlate each with specific organisms, if possible.
   c. Differentiate suitable and unsuitable specimens for anaerobic culture.
3. Summarize the atmosphere, incubation, and culture plate examination requirements for anaerobes.
   a. Categorize organisms based on their ability to tolerate oxygen.
   b. Describe reasons for the varying levels of oxygen sensitivity/tolerance among anaerobes.
   c. Evaluate methods used to achieve anaerobic conditions.
      i. Explain the principle.
      ii. Recognize and resolve potential errors.
   d. Describe methods used to ensure the anaerobic atmosphere is maintained appropriately.
   e. Discuss the use of aerotolerance testing and its interpretation.
4. Select media for selection and differentiation of organisms.
   a. Describe the principle, incubation, and interpretation.
   b. Describe growth factors required and correlate with specific organisms.
5. Outline the process of anaerobic culture workup.

■ LEARNING OBJECTIVES (*continued*)

6. For each identification or test procedure:

   a. Explain the principle.

   b. Recognize potential sources of errors.

   c. Recognize incubation requirements.

   d. Interpret results.

   e. Evaluate sensitivity and specificity.

   f. Judge its value in relation to ease of use, turnaround time, cost, and other factors.

7. For each organism:

   a. Describe enzymes, toxins, and antigens produced.

   b. Describe the Gram stain reaction and microscopic morphology.

   c. Describe macroscopic colony morphology.

   d. Establish key identification characteristics.

   e. Determine additional or alternative testing required

   f. Determine the source or origin and potential transmission mechanism(s).

   g. Correlate with specific diseases or syndromes.

   h. Define patient populations affected.

   i. Differentiate from other organisms.

8. Discuss susceptibility testing for anaerobes.

   a. Determine appropriate treatment options based on the disease state or organism iso-lated.

9. Correlate patient history, body site/specimen type, colonial morphology, Gram stain results, identification test results, and susceptibility results in order to identify an organism, assess its clinical significance, recognize discrepancies, and resolve problems.

KEY TERMS

actinomycosis

aerotolerance

anaerobe

endogenous

facultative anaerobe/
   aerobe

fusiform

gingiva

Lemierre's disease

microaerophilic
   organism

microaerotolerant
   anaerobe

myonecrosis

obligate or strict aerobe

obligate or strict
   anaerobe

oxygen reduction (redox)
   potential (E_h)

periodontitis

tetanospasim

Vincent's angina

TAXONOMY

Family *Clostridiaceae* (kläs-'trid-ē-ās-ē'-ē)
    Genus *Clostridium* (kläs-'trid-ē-əm)
        C. perfringens (pĕr-frin'-jenz)
        C. tetani (tĕt'-a-ne)
        C. botulinum (bot-chu'-li-num)
        C. difficile (dif-e-sēl)
        C. septicum (sep'-ti-kum)
Family *Actinomycetaceae* (ak'-ti-no-mi'-sə-ta-se-ē)
    Genus *Actinomyces* (ak'-ti-no-mi'-sez)
        A. israelii (iz-ra'-le-i)
Family *Propionibacteraceae* (pro'-pe-on-i-bak-ter'-ās-ē'-ē)
    Genus *Propionibacterium* (pro'-pe-on-i-bak-ter'-e-um)
        P. acnes (äk'-nēz)
Family *Lactobacillaceae* (lak'-to-ba-sil'-ās-ē'-ē)
    Genus *Lactobacillus* (lak'-to-ba-sil'-us)
Family *Bifidobacteriaceae* (bi'-fi-do-bak-ter'-e-ās-ē'-ē)
    Genus *Bifidobacterium* (bi'-fi-do-bak-ter'-e-um)
Family *Eubacteriaceae* (yu'-bak-ter'-e-ās-ē'-ē)
    Genus *Eubacterium* (yu'-bak-ter'-e-um)
    Genus *Eggerella* (ĕgg-ĕr-ĕl-lŭ)
        E. lenta (lĭn-tŭ)
Family *Bacteroidaceae* (bak-ter-oy'-d-ās-ē'-ē)
    Genus *Bacteroides* (bak-ter-oy'-dez)
        B. fragilis group
        B. fragilis (fraj'-i-lis)
        B. distasonis (dis-ta-so'-nis)
        B. thetaiotaomicron (thā'-tŭ-ī-ō-tā-ō-mī'-krŏn)
        B. vulgatus (vul-gat'-ŭs)

Family *Fusobacteriaceae* (fu'-zo-bak-ter'-e-ās-ē'-ē)
    Genus *Fusobacterium* (fu'-zo-bak-ter'-e-um)
        F. nucleatum (nu-kle-a'-tum)
        F. necrophorum (nĕ-krō'-fôr-ŭm)
Family *Prevotellaceae* (prev'-ō-tel-ās-ē'-ē)
    Genus *Prevotella* (prev'-ō-tel'-ä)
        P. melaninogenica (mel'-a-nin-o'-jen'-ĭ-k-a)
        P. intermedia (in-tĕr'-me'-de-a)
Family *Porphyromonadaceae* (pōr'-fir-om'-ō-näd-ās-ē'-ē)
    Genus *Porphyromonas* (pōr'-fir-om'-ō-näs)
        P. asaccharolytica (a-sak'-a-ro-lĭ'-tĭk-a)
        P. gingivalis (jĭn'-jĭ-väl'-ĭs)
Family *Peptostreptococcaceae* (pĕp''-tō-strĕp''-tō-kŏk-ās-ē'-ē)
    Genus *Finegoldia* (fīn'-gohld-ē'-a)
        F. magna (mäg'-na)
    Genus *Peptoniphilus* (pĕp'-tŏn-ĭ-fī-lŭs)
        P. asaccharolyticus (a-sak'-a-ro-lĭ-tĭk-ŭs)
    Genus *Peptostreptococcus* (pĕp''-tō-strĕp''-tō-kŏk'ŭs)
        P. anaerobius (än'-ĕr-ō'-bē-ŭs)
Family *Streptococcaceae* (strep-to-kok'-ā-sē'-ē)
    Genus *Streptococcus* (strĕp''-tō-kŏk'-ŭs)
        S. anginosus (än'-jĭ-nō'-sŭs)
        S. constellatus (kŏn'-stŭ-lŏt-ŭs)
        S. intermedius (ĭn'-tĕr-mē'-dē-us)
Family *Veillonellaceae* ('vāl-yō-nə'-lās-ē'-ē)
    Genus *Veillonella* ('vāl-yō'-nel-ə)

▶ INTRODUCTION

Anaerobes, organisms that can live without oxygen, populate almost every niche of the human body and surprisingly even those regularly exposed to oxygen. As a bacterial group, they vary in their ability to tolerate exposure to oxygen. Some can live and grow in up to 10% oxygen whereas others cannot tolerate the presence of any oxygen. Anaerobes vary in their frequency of isolation depending on the body site and specimen type. Two thirds of anaerobic infections involve mixed infections with aerobic organisms (Chow, 2005). Infections can range from minor such as chronic sinus infections to deadly such as botulism or tetanus.

Because anaerobes are unique in their environmental requirements, care must be taken to ensure a quality specimen. Microbiologists must be knowledgeable of proper specimen collection, transportation procedures, appropriate media, and a suitable incubation environment to ensure their recovery. A poorly collected specimen will provide poor and possibly even deadly results for the patient depending on the treatment selected by the physician.

The identification of anaerobes has proven to be a challenge for most microbiologists. There are clues that can help narrow down the possibilities. Once isolated, the microbiologist must employ traditional identification procedures or commercial identification systems to identify significant organisms. Once identified, susceptibility testing proves to be another challenge in the clinical laboratory.

▶ CLASSIFICATION

ENVIRONMENTAL REQUIREMENTS

Anaerobes were probably one of the first organisms to appear on the face of the earth. Prior to the appearance of oxygen, organisms probably used sulfur to live and reproduce. Early anaerobes were probably the source of oxygen in the earth's atmosphere. Once there was sufficient atmospheric oxygen, most organisms began to use it to live and grow. Oxygen metabolism produces energy more efficiently than other processes.

Anaerobes adapted to live without oxygen but some can survive with up to 10% oxygen for a limited amount of time as part of their environment. Most organisms have enzymes that allow them to react with oxygen. When they react with oxygen, superoxide is produced, which can cause cell damage.

Superoxide must be eliminated or they will die. Aerobic organisms produce an enzyme, superoxide dismutase (SOD), which converts superoxide to hydrogen peroxide, another toxic substance. Aerobic organisms then produce catalase and/or peroxidase, which break down hydrogen peroxide, rendering it harmless. Obligate anaerobes do not usually possess SOD or catalase or peroxidase. Any exposure to oxygen kills them because of the accumulation of toxic products, which they cannot eliminate. Some anaerobes, such as *Clostridium perfringens,* possess SOD and can survive after limited exposure to oxygen. Oxygen has a bacteriostatic effect on it rather than bactericidal, which is why it can be called a microaerotolerant anaerobe. Possessing any one of the enzymes—SOD, catalase, and peroxidase—possibly explains the varying sensitivity of anaerobes to oxygen.

The **oxygen reduction (redox) potential (E_h)** of an environment is a measurement of its ability to lose (a reduced environment) or gain (an oxidized environment) electrons. Aerobes like to live in an environment that is oxidized and so has a high oxygen reduction potential. They use oxygen to make their energy via aerobic respiration. As the oxygen is used up, the surrounding tissues become reduced with a low oxygen reduction potential. With blood flow, oxygen is returned to the environment and the tissues become oxidized again. Anaerobes need reduced conditions with a low oxygen reduction potential to grow and metabolize. Whenever there is necrotic tissue or a lack of blood flow, oxygen cannot reach the tissue and any aerobes present use up the remaining oxygen. The tissue becomes reduced and anaerobes flourish. They produce their energy via fermentation or anaerobic respiration, which does not require oxygen.

A reduced environment allows the metabolic enzymes of anaerobic organisms to function properly. With oxygen, these essential enzymes become inactive and the anaerobe can die if not returned to an anaerobic environment quickly. If returned to an anaerobic environment before too much damage is done, then they may survive and begin to grow again. This may partially explain why some anaerobes are able to survive even after exposure to oxygen.

 Checkpoint! 24–1 (Chapter Objective 1a)

*A ruptured appendix can predispose an individual to an anaerobic infection. Select **all** possible explanations that support this statement.*

A. *Release of normal gastrointestinal flora*
B. *Loss of blood flow to the tissue*
C. *Tissue necrosis*
D. *Reduced oxygen present due to metabolism by aerobic organisms*

One method used to classify organisms is based on their level of oxygen requirements. Room air contains about 21% oxygen, 78% nitrogen, and trace amounts of carbon dioxide, hydrogen, and eight other gases. Environments with varying levels of oxygen can be produced in the clinical laboratory. Knowing an organism's ideal growth environment can be useful in its cultivation and identification. Table 24-1 differentiates organisms based on their ideal environment requirements for growth, metabolism and the effect of toxic oxygen byproducts (superoxide and hydrogen peroxide) on each.

 Checkpoint! 24–2 (Chapter Objectives 3a, 3b)

An organism displays the following growth pattern:

　Ambient room air – no growth
　Microaerophilic atmosphere – no growth
　Anaerobic environment – growth

This organism probably possesses the following enzyme(s):

A. *Superoxide dismutase (SOD)*
B. *Catalase/peroxidase*
C. *SOD and catalase/peroxidase*
D. *Neither SOD nor catalase/peroxidase*

❷ REAL WORLD TIP

Pseudomonas aeruginosa is considered an obligate aerobe but it may grow on anaerobic medium if there is a nitrate source present. Nitrate can act as a substitute for oxygen for this organism.

CLUES TO THE PRESENCE OF ANAEROBES

The process of diagnosing anaerobic infections begins with the physician examining the patient. There are often physical signs that lead the physician to suspect an anaerobic infection. Early diagnosis of anaerobic infections is important because of the seriousness of some infections such as gas gangrene. Anaerobic cultures are time consuming and the physician must often act quickly before culture results are even available. Just as the physician uses physical signs and symptoms to help diagnose potential anaerobic infections, the microbiologist employs bacteriological clues that may suggest the presence of anaerobes. Table 24-2 explains some of the common clinical and bacteriological clues of anaerobic infections.

 Checkpoint! 24–3 (Chapter Objective 2b)

A purulent aspirate obtained from the jaw is received in the laboratory. The physician suspects actinomycosis. What clue(s) should the microbiologist look for when processing the specimen for culture?

A. *Squamous epithelial cells*
B. *Sulfur granules*
C. *Gas in the specimen*
D. *Black discoloration of the specimen*

✪ TABLE 24-1

Differentiation of Organisms Based on Environmental Requirements, Energy Metabolism, and Effect of Toxic Oxygen Byproducts

Term	Environmental Requirements	Energy Metabolism	Effect of Toxic O_2 Byproducts	Representative Organism
Obligate or strict anaerobe	Will not grow in the presence of any oxygen	Fermentation or anaerobic respiration	Unable to protect themselves due to the lack of superoxide dismutase (SOD) and catalase/peroxidase	*Clostridium botulinum*
Micro-aerophilic organism	■ Can grow scantily in the presence of oxygen ■ A microaerophilic environment with 5–10% oxygen and 10–15% carbon dioxide is ideal for these organisms.	Fermentation or aerobic respiration	Limited ability to protect themselves in only low levels of oxygen due to the presence of SOD but not catalase/peroxidase	Microaerophilic *Streptococcus* species
Facultative aerobe/ anaerobe	■ Able to grow either in the absence or presence of room air oxygen ■ They have the faculty or ability to switch back and forth in their energy metabolism depending on the environment.	■ Fermentation or anaerobic respiration without O_2 ■ Aerobic respiration with O_2	Able to protect themselves due to the presence of SOD and catalase/peroxidase	*Escherichia coli*
Microaero-tolerant anaerobe	Does not require oxygen for growth but also not killed by *limited* exposure to room air	Fermentation with or without O_2	Able to partially protect themselves due to the presence of SOD and/or catalase/peroxidase	*Clostridium perfringens*
Obligate or strict aerobe	Requires oxygen (room air) for growth	Aerobic respiration	Able to protect themselves due to the presence of SOD and catalase/peroxidase	*Pseudomonas aeruginosa*

SPORE FORMATION, GRAM STAIN, AND MICROSCOPIC MORPHOLOGY

Anaerobes are often classified initially based on their ability to form spores and then based on the Gram stain and morphology. A spore is a survival structure formed by the organism when the environment does not meet its basic needs to survive and grow. It provides the organism a dormant state, and, once conditions are ideal again, it germinates and the organism is revived. The anaerobic genus *Clostridium* is well known for its ability to produce spores. Go to ∞ Chapter 19, "Aerobic Gram-Positive Rods," for a review of the process of spore formation.

Spores appear as clear zones within the organism cell on Gram stain. The Gram stain reagents cannot penetrate the thick wall of the spore. Malachite green, applied with heat, can penetrate the spore wall. Safranin is used as a counterstain for the organism's cell wall. Figure 24-1 ■ demonstrates the presence of subterminal spores, stained with malachite green, within the rods of *Clostridium* spp.

Spore-Formers

***Clostridium* species.** The genus *Clostridium* includes gram-positive rods that characteristically produce spores. The presence of a spore may make the cell appear swollen. The location of the spore can be useful in the identification of certain species. A spore located at one end of the rod is called terminal. A subterminal spore is located between the rod's center and one end. Figure 24-1 shows a *Clostridium* spp. exhibiting subterminal spores. Spores located in the center of the rod are called central. While the presence of spores is characteristic for the genus *Clostridium*, some only produce them under strongly reduced conditions. Their absence does not eliminate *Clostridium* spp. as a possible identification.

The gram-positive rods of *Clostridium* can be pleomorphic because they vary in shape. Their microscopic morphology ranges from large, straight-edged rods to thin, curved rods. They may even stain gram variable in both direct patient cultures as well as in culture. Gram-negative *Clostridium* may be seen with age or with the production of spores. The presence of large rectangular gram-negative rods should still suggest a potential *Clostridium* spp. infection.

Nonspore Formers

Gram-Positive Rods. The most common anaerobic nonspore-forming gram-positive rods include the genera *Actinomyces, Bifidobacterium, Eubacterium, Lactobacillus,* and *Propionibacterium.* They can be highly pleomorphic ranging from short, fat rods to long, branching twig-like structures.

⭐ **TABLE 24-2**

Clinical and Bacteriological Clues Suggestive of Anaerobic Infection

Clue	Explanation
Infection close to a mucosal surface	The mucous membranes are colonized with aerobic and anaerobic normal flora. If a break occurs in the skin, mouth, upper respiratory, gastrointestinal, or genitourinary tracts, the organisms can escape to cause infections.
Poor blood flow and presence of necrotic tissue	The loss of blood flow causes tissue to die due to the lack of oxygen. The lack of oxygen and dead tissue creates a reduced environment that favors the growth of anaerobes. Surgery or trauma can reduce blood flow to a body site.
Foul odor	Some anaerobes create putrid-smelling metabolic byproducts.
Gas in tissues	*Clostridium perfringens* is known for its ability to form gas under anaerobic conditions. While the production of gas is not limited to *C. perfringens,* it is characteristic.
Presence of sulfur granules in drainage	The colonies of *Actinomyces* species can appear as hard yellow particles in specimens.
Black discoloration of specimen/colonies	Some *Prevotella* species and *Porphyromonas* species can create a dark pigment due to their ability to break down hemoglobin to create heme.
Fluorescence of specimen/colonies	In the process of producing heme, some *Prevotella* species and *Porphyromonas* species produce red fluorescing porphyrins. Other anaerobes also have the ability to produce fluorescence of various colors.
Inability to grow organisms seen on Gram stain	Aerobic cultures that do not grow but demonstrate organisms on Gram stain could be due to anaerobes. A properly collected and transported specimen is necessary to insure the isolation of anaerobes.
Infection that continues despite anti-microbial therapy	Most anaerobes are resistant to aminoglycosides and quinolones. *Bacteroides* species are usually resistant to tetracycline and the beta-lactams.
Specific infections	Brain abscesses, gas gangrene, oral and dental infections, human bites, peritonitis, aspiration pneumonia, and Vincent's angina are usually associated specifically with anaerobes.
Unique microscopic morphologies on the direct Gram stain	*Fusobacterium nucleatum* appears as fusiform (long, thin, with pointed ends) gram-negative rods, *Clostridium perfringens* appears as large gram-positive rods in long chains, most *Clostridium* species produce spores, and branching gram-positive rods may suggest *Actinomyces* species.

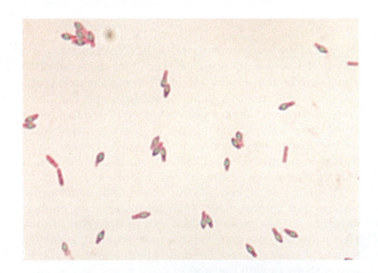

■ **FIGURE 24-1** Spores do not stain with routine Gram stain reagents. The application of heat while staining with malachite green will force the stain into the spore. Safranin is then used as a counterstain to stain the organism's cell wall. *Clostridium* spp. vary in the placement of the spore within the cell and it can be used for identification of some species. This photo depicts sub-terminal spores located between the rod's center and one end of the cell.
From CDC and Larry Stauffer, Oregon State Public Health Laboratory.

Gram-Positive Cocci.   The anaerobic gram-positive cocci include the most common genera *Finegoldia, Peptoniphilus,* and *Peptostreptococccus.* These organisms commonly appear as cocci in pairs, chains, or clusters.

Gram-Negative Rods.   The commonly isolated anaerobic gram-negative rods consist of the genera *Bacteroides, Fusobacterium, Porphyromonas,* and *Prevotella.* They range from gram-negative coccobacilli to long, thin, toothpick-like rods.

Gram-Negative Cocci.   The anaerobic gram-negative cocci include only one genus, *Veillonella.* These organisms appear as tiny gram-negative diplococci in pairs, chains, and clusters. They can mimic *Neisseria* spp. on Gram stain.

▶ **SPECIMEN COLLECTION AND TRANSPORT**

It is critical that specimens for anaerobic culture be properly collected and transported. The clinical microbiologist must educate physicians and nurses to ensure appropriate clinical specimens are selected for culture and sent to the laboratory in proper transport systems. Remember the adage "garbage in, garbage out." A poorly collected and transported specimen will only provide poor results for the patient.

Anaerobic infections are frequently **endogenous** because they originate from within the body as part of the normal flora. The skin and mucous membranes of the upper respiratory, genitourinary, and gastrointestinal systems harbor normal aerobic and anaerobic flora. Infections begin when organisms are able to leave their normal surroundings and enter a sterile area through trauma, surgery, or disease such as cancer. The first goal of collecting specimens for anaerobic culture is avoiding contamination with normal aerobic and anaerobic flora while still selecting for the potential pathogen present. ∞ Chapter 4, "The Host's Encounter with Microbes," summarizes the commensal or normal flora related to each specimen type. It is critical the laboratory creates standard operating procedures and criteria for specimen rejection to ensure anaerobic specimens of the highest quality. Poorly collected specimens provide poor results and potentially poor outcomes for the patient. Table 24-3 describes the clinical specimens that are considered acceptable and unacceptable for anaerobic cultures.

The ideal specimen for anaerobic culture is whole tissue or aspiration via needle and syringe. If a needle and syringe is used, it is essential for the safety of all health care workers that the needle is removed after aspiration. Excess air must be expelled and the syringe end sealed prior to transportation. Room air can permeate through the plastic syringe so the spec-

imen must be processed within 30 minutes of retrieval (Brook, 2003a).

A swab is the least favorable method for collection but is probably the most common type submitted by physicians and nurses because it is the easiest to obtain. Specimens on swabs are often minimal, can easily dry out during transportation, and expose anaerobes to room air. They should not be accepted for anaerobic culture unless transported in a proper anaerobic environment.

Whole tissue can be transported in a sterile container with a small amount of sterile saline to prevent drying, if necessary. Intact tissue can protect anaerobes from exposure to room

---

✓ **Checkpoint! 24–4
(Chapter Objectives 2a and 2c)**

A physician suspects anaerobic pneumonia in a 57-year-old male. He has a history of alcoholism with frequent blackouts and vomiting spells. She calls the laboratory to discuss how to collect sputum for anaerobic culture. Which of the following specimens would be acceptable for anaerobic culture?

    A. *Expectorated sputum*
    B. *Sputum collected via suction*
    C. *Transtracheal aspirate*
    D. *Bronchial washings via nonprotected endoscope*

✪ TABLE 24-3

Acceptable and Unacceptable Clinical Specimens for Culture of Anaerobes

Body Site/ Specimen Type	Acceptable	Unacceptable	Notes on Collection
Aspirate	Majority are acceptable if collected and transported properly	Drainage collected from skin surface	Surface must be decontaminated prior to aspiration. Ideally the aspirate is collected with a needle and syringe.
Body fluids	Normally sterile fluids from an enclosed body space such as blood, CSF, peritoneal, joint, pericardial, pleural, etc.	Fluids that come in direct contact with mucous membranes such as urine	Skin surface must be decontaminated prior to collection
Genitourinary	Suprapubic urine, *intrauterine	Voided or catheterized urine, cervical, urethral, or vaginal discharge	Skin surface must be decontaminated prior to collection
Intestinal	Feces for *Clostridium difficile* toxin detection or culture for *C. perfringens* and *C. botulinum* only	Intestinal contents, ileostomy and colostomy drainage	Feces may be collected for detection of toxin produced by certain *Clostridium* spp.
Respiratory	Transtracheal aspirate, †bronchial washing	Expectorated or suctioned sputum, oral or throat swab, nasopharyngeal swab, or secretions	Skin surface must be decontaminated prior to collection
Tissue, biopsy, or bone	Majority are acceptable if collected and transported properly	Swab of infected tissue	Surface must be decontaminated prior to biopsy.
Wound	Decubitus (bed sore) and diabetic ulcers	Swab of superficial wounds and lesions	Biopsy or aspiration after surface cleansing and debridement

*Must be collected via a protected catheter to avoid contamination with normal genitourinary flora
†Must be collected via a protected catheter to avoid contamination with normal upper respiratory flora

air. It should be sent to the laboratory within 30 minutes for processing (Isenberg, 2004).

To minimize the lethal effect of oxygen, anaerobic transport systems are available. Currently there are three options for anaerobic specimen transportation: (1) a tube containing oxygen-reduced semi-solid agar transport medium, (2) a tube containing an enclosed anaerobic gas environment, and (3) a gas-impermeable bag with its own gas-generating environment. Each minimizes the lethal effect of oxygen on obligate anaerobes. Anaerobes have been shown to survive 24–72 hours in these systems (Brook, 1987). The only organisms that may not survive prolonged transposition in anaerobic transport systems are obligate aerobes such as *Pseudomonas aeruginosa*. Figures 24-2 ■ and 24-3 ■ provide two examples of anaerobic specimen transportation systems.

Most anaerobic transportation systems contain an indicator, resazurin, which is colorless when reduced but turns pink when exposed to oxygen. It serves as a visual security system to alert the microbiologist to potential problems during specimen transportation. If the indicator displays signs of oxygen exposure, the specimen should be rejected if recollectable. If the specimen is not recollectable, such as tissue obtained in surgery, then a disclaimer should be added to the culture results indicating that the specimen may be suboptimal, which could hinder the recovery of anaerobes. Additional information on specimen collection is available in ∞ Chapter 6.

▶ SPECIMEN PROCESSING

Whole tissue or bone must be ground to ensure a homogenous specimen. A small amount of anaerobic thioglycolate broth can be added prior to grinding. Fluids should be cen-

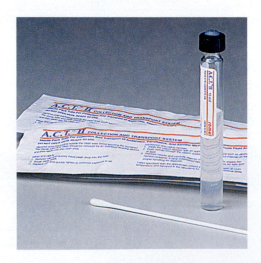

■ FIGURE 24-2 This anaerobic transportation system uses a semi-solid, nonnutritive medium to maintain aerobic, facultative, and anaerobic organisms. It can be used with a swab or fluid specimens.
Photo courtesy of Remel, part of Thermo Fisher Scientific.

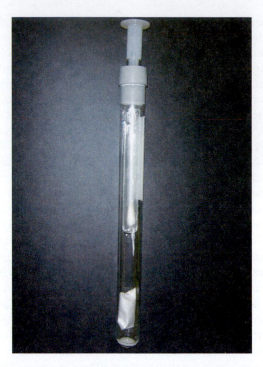

■ FIGURE 24-3 This enclosed anaerobic environment tube is used for collection and transportation of anaerobic specimens. The swab is used to collect the appropriate specimen. After collection the swab plunger is pushed into the gray rubber top. This forces the inner glass tube to drop and exposes the swab to the anaerobic environment inside of the large glass tube. Any oxygen that enters with the swab combines with hydrogen, present in the anaerobic environment, to create water that collects on the desiccant pack at the bottom of the tube. The white indicator disk will turn pink if exposed to excessive amounts of oxygen.

trifuged to create sediment, which is used for media inoculation and Gram stain. Swabs, while least favorable, can be used to directly inoculate media or washed in a small amount of anaerobic thioglycolate broth. The broth washings are then used to inoculate media and make the Gram stain.

DIRECT EXAMINATION

The appearance and odor of the specimen may provide valuable clues for the presence of anaerobes. Anaerobic infections typically produce foul odors due to their metabolic end-products. The presence of small, hard yellow granules in the specimen is distinctive for an infection with *Actinomyces israelii*. The yellow granules are actually the colonies of the organism. A black discoloration of the specimen may suggest the presence of pigmented *Prevotella* and *Porphyromonas* spp.

Some anaerobic Gram stains and microscopic morphologies are so characteristic that the direct specimen may provide a presumptive identification of the offending anaerobe. Presumptive identification may assist the physician in beginning appropriate therapy as early as possible. *Clostridium perfringens* appears as large gram-positive straight-edged rods that line up like a chain of box cars being pulled by a train engine. The presence of gram-negative **fusiform** or toothpick-shaped rods suggests the presence of *Fusobacterium nucleatum*. *Actinomyces* spp. display branching non-spore-forming gram-positive rods. *Veillonella* spp. appear as gram-negative cocci in clusters. Pale staining gram-negative coccbacilli suggests *Bacteroides* spp., *Prevotella* spp., or *Porphyromonas* spp. Visual examples of the Gram stain reaction and microscopic morphology of individual organisms will be provided later in this chapter.

Anaerobic infections often produce purulent material. White blood cells are usually found in abundance on the direct Gram stain. Specimens containing *Clostridium perfringens* often do not exhibit white blood cells. The organism produces powerful toxins that destroy any white bloods cells produced by the body. The absence of white blood cells in a clinical specimen should not rule out a potential anaerobic infection.

℮ REAL WORLD TIP

The skin is covered by dead stratified keratinized squamous epithelial cells. Mucous membranes are lined by nonkeratinized stratified squamous epithelial cells or simple columnar epithelial cells. All of these surfaces are populated by normal aerobic and anaerobic flora that serve a protective function by preventing potential pathogens from finding a place to colonize and flourish.

The presence of squamous epithelial cells is a good indication of the quality of anaerobic specimens. There should not be any squamous epithelial cells present in the Gram stain. If they are present then there is potential for the presence of normal aerobic and anaerobic flora. It can be difficult to determine the significant pathogens in the midst of normal flora present. The specimen should not be processed for anaerobic culture.

The direct specimen Gram stain also provides a means to ensure the quality of the results being reported. There should be close correlation between the quantity and microscopic Gram stain and morphology of organisms seen on the Gram stain and the organisms reported on final culture plate results. Daily supervision of the accuracy of the Gram stain results can help monitor both the preanalytical and postanalytical stages of the testing process. A significant variance between the original specimen direct Gram stain and the reported results could be due to an error in the Gram stain technique, misinterpretation of the Gram stain, a mislabeled specimen,

a break in processing policies and procedures, or a failure to grow fastidious organisms such as anaerobes. Discrepancies should be investigated, corrections made, and reeducation of microbiologists and other health care personnel initiated as needed.

GROWTH FACTORS

Vitamin K and hemin are routinely added to anaerobic media to enhance the recovery and growth of some anaerobes. *Prevotella melaninogenica,* an obligate anaerobic gram-negative rod, has been proven to require both compounds in order to fuel several of its critical metabolic processes and reach maximum growth (Gibbons & Macdonald, 1960). Hemin enhances the growth of most anaerobes. Vitamin K seems to be more critical to the growth of this obligate anaerobic gram-negative rod than hemin (Robins, Yee, & Bentley, 1973). Other organisms that may be present in mixed infections, such as *Staphylococcus aureus,* are able to synthesize vitamin K and may promote the growth of *Prevotella melaninogenica* when grown on media without the compound (Gibbons & Macdonald, 1960). *P. melaninogenica* can produce satelliting colonies around *S. aureus* on blood containing media deficient in vitamin K, similar to that seen with *Haemophilus influenzae*. Figure 24-9, later in this chapter, demonstrates the satelliting phenomenon exhibited by *P. melaninogenica.*

MEDIA FOR ANAEROBES

Because of the fastidious nature of anaerobes, media selection is an important decision for any microbiology laboratory. Freshly prepared, enriched media appears to provide the best possible growth of anaerobes but often proves to be too costly and time consuming for most clinical laboratories (Hanson & Martin, 1976). When stored in room air, anaerobic media absorbs oxygen, which causes the production of toxic byproducts. Their presence prevents the growth of anaerobes. The only way to prevent their production is to maintain the media under reduced or anaerobic conditions as all times, which is usually impractical for most clinical laboratories.

The incorporation of palladium chloride, L-cysteine HCl, and dithiothreitol into anaerobic media allows it to reach a low oxidation-reduction potential fairly quickly so it can support the growth of anaerobes. Prepared media with reducing agents must be stored in an anaerobic environment for a minimum of 24 hours prior to use. The reducing agents drive off any oxygen that may be present in the media. The use of commercially prepared, reducible media is a viable option that just takes a little planning and organization on the part of the clinical laboratory to ensure it is always available for use.

Another option for the clinical laboratory is to purchase prereduced media. This media is prepared, packaged, and sold under anaerobic conditions so it guarantees that oxygen is not an issue. It is often much more expensive than reducible media, which can be a decision breaker for most clinical laboratories.

A combination of enriched nonselective and selective and differential media should be used for isolation and presumptive identification for anaerobes (Isenberg, 2004). All must contain nutrients and growth factors required by clinically significant anaerobes. Because aerobic organisms may be involved in anaerobic infections, appropriate aerobic media must be inoculated at the same time as anaerobic media. The aerobic media used is determined by the body site or specimen type and the potential pathogens that may be encountered.

Nonselective Media

A nonselective blood agar will support the growth of most obligate and facultative (can grow in the presence or absence of oxygen) anaerobic organisms. Agar bases used include brucella, brain heart infusion, Columbia, CDC, or Schaedler. The addition of 5% sheep blood provides nutrients as well as allows for detection of hemolysis. Nonselective media must also be supplemented with vitamin K and hemin to insure the recovery of *Prevotella melaninogenica*.

Anaerobic thioglycolate broth is available as a backup to culture plates, if needed. It must contain the supplements vitamin K and hemin. The tubes can be reduced by placing in a boiling water bath for 10 minutes with the lids loose and then recapping tightly. The oxygen is driven off as it is boiled. The tubes can be stored in an anaerobic environment to maintain the reduced state.

One disadvantage of the use of a broth is the strong possibility of overgrowth of slow-growing anaerobes by the facultative anaerobic organisms that may be present. It should only be subbed if original culture plates do not grow and the broth displays turbidity or if an organism is observed on Gram stain but not found on culture. It should not be used to recover anaerobes when the original specimen was not collected properly for the transport of anaerobes. It is not possible to determine the true significance of any anaerobes isolated in this instance. Many laboratories have discontinued the use of thioglycolate broth because it does not provide valued-added information for the patient.

 Checkpoint! 24–5 (Chapter Objectives 5 and 9)

A physician used a swab to collect drainage from the left leg wound of a 28-year-old male involved in a motorcycle accident. The swab was processed for aerobic culture in the laboratory. The direct Gram stain revealed:

> *Many pleomorphic gram-negative rods*
> *Few gram-positive cocci in clusters*
> *Moderate white blood cells*

At 24 hours, the culture results revealed:

> *Blood agar plate = 10 colonies of Staphylococcus not S. aureus*
> *MacConkey agar = no growth*
> *Phenylethyl alcohol agar = 12 colonies of Staphylococcus not S. aureus*
> *Thioglycolate broth Gram stain = gram-negative rods and gram-positive cocci in clusters*

The next step in the work-up of this culture is:

> *A. Report Staphylococcus not S. aureus but ignore the gram-negative rods since they did not grow*
> *B. Report Staphylococcus not S. aureus and gram-negative rods—unable to grow*
> *C. Sub the thioglycolate broth to a reducible blood agar plate to try to recover the gram-negative rods*
> *D. Request a recollect specimen for anaerobic culture*

Selective Media

The most commonly used selective medium for isolation of anaerobes is laked blood–kanamycin–vancomycin (LKV) agar. It selects for most anaerobic gram-negative rods, especially *Bacteroides* and *Prevotella* species. The presence of hematin, from the laked blood, promotes the development of black pigment by some *Prevotella* spp. Kanamycin inhibits most facultative anaerobic gram-negative rods whereas vancomycin inhibits most gram-positive organisms. It almost resembles a MacConkey agar for anaerobic gram-negative rods but without the ability to differentiate them. Some facultative anaerobes have the ability to grow on LKV so one cannot assume a colony on LKV is automatically an anaerobe. One disadvantage of LKV is the inability to isolate the anaerobic gram-negative rod, *Porphyromonas* spp. This organism is sensitive to the vancomycin present and will not grow. Its inability to grow on this medium may be useful in its presumptive identification. *Fusobacterium* spp. may be inhibited or not grow at all on LKV due to their sensitivity to kanamycin.

 REAL WORLD TIP

An anaerobic thioglycolate broth can be used to selectively recover *Clostridium* spp., spore-forming gram-positive rods, when culture plates are overgrown with a swarming organism such as *Proteus* spp. The broth is heated to 80°C for 10 minutes. The clostridial spores survive heating but all other organisms are killed. The broth is subbed to an anaerobic blood agar and the spores will germinate under anaerobic conditions. Another option to recover *Clostridium* spores is with the use of 95–100% ethanol. Ethanol is added in equal volumes to the thioglycolate broth and allowed to sit. After one hour the broth is subbed to anaerobic media and under anaerobic condition the spores germinate.

Vancomycin-resistant *Enterococcus* (VRE) can grow on LKV agar. LKV agar contains 7.5 µg/mL of vancomycin and the agar screen used to routinely detect VRE contains 6 µg/mL of vancomycin. If *Enterococcus* spp. is identified on the aerobic portion of the culture, a quick review of the LKV agar plate may indicate if it is a possible VRE.

Bacteroides bile esculin (BBE) agar is used to select for the anaerobic gram-negative rod, *Bacteroides fragilis* group. The bile and gentamicin present inhibit most other organisms. The organism is stimulated to grow in the presence of bile. The esculin present is hydrolyzed by the *Bacteroides fragilis* group, which turns the colonies black. The black, esculin-hydrolyzing colonies of *Bacteroides fragilis* (Figure 24-4 ■) are easily recognizable on BBE agar.

An anaerobic phenylethyl alcohol (PEA) agar or colistin-naladixic acid (CNA) agar can be added if swarming *Proteus* spp. is a possibility in a clinical specimen or as a semi-selective medium for the isolation of *Clostridium* spp. and other anaerobic gram-positive organisms. PEA inhibits facultative anaerobic gram-negative rods due to the alcohol present. CNA employs antibiotics to inhibit most gram-negative rods. Both will allow most facultative gram-positive organisms to grow on these agars as well as the obligate and microaerotolerant anaerobic gram-positive organisms.

Other selective and differential anaerobic media are available for specific organisms. They are discussed in detail with the organisms throughout the chapter.

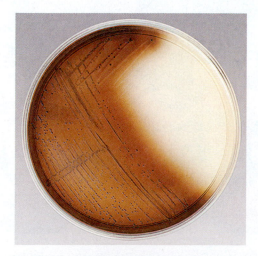

■ **FIGURE 24-4** BBE (*Bacteroides* bile esculin) agar can be used to selectively isolate and presumptively identify *Bacteroides fragilis*. This organism has the ability to grow in the presence of bile and hydrolyze the esculin present to create black colonies. *Photo courtesy of Remel, part of Thermo Fisher Scientific.*

▶ **ANAEROBIC INCUBATION ENVIRONMENT**

Once the clinical specimen is inoculated onto appropriate medium, the agar plates must be incubated at 35°C under anaerobic conditions as quickly as possible. The ideal anaerobic environment is composed of 80–90% nitrogen, 5% hydrogen, and 5–10% carbon dioxide. There are several ways to generate this environment. The decision on which anaerobic generation and incubation system to use may depend on the initial and maintenance costs, amount of space required, training involved, number of cultures processed daily, and ease of daily inspection of agar plates.

Any anaerobic incubation system used must incorporate a method to monitor maintenance of an anaerobic environment. A methylene blue strip can be used to monitor an anaerobic environment. Its indicator is blue when oxidized and white or colorless when reduced. Figure 24-5 ■ demonstrates a sealed anaerobic jar with a gas-generating envelope and methylene blue indicator. Another indicator used is resazurin, which is colorless in the appropriate anaerobic environment but turns pink with the presence of oxygen. Both provide semi-real-time monitoring results but can dry out and lose their ability to detect oxygen. Color change is not an instant reaction but rather a gradual process. Once a color change is noted there should not be a delay in finding the source of the oxygen present in the environment and correcting the issue. Both indicators must be replaced daily to ensure accurate and continuous quality control of the anaerobic environment.

An alternate method to monitor the anaerobic incubation system is to inoculate an anaerobic agar plate with an

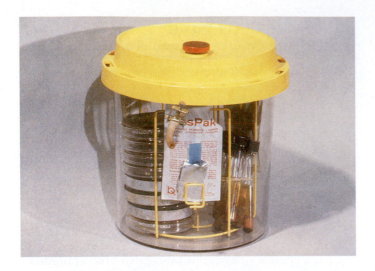

■ FIGURE 24-5 This sealed anaerobic jar employed a gas-generating envelope to create an anaerobic environment. The methylene blue indicator strip is indicative of the presence of oxygen. If the jar has only recently been closed, it may take up to 30 minutes to remove the oxygen initially present and the strip will then revert to white. If the jar has been closed for over 30 minutes, a blue strip indicates the environment is not appropriate for the recovery of anaerobes. The jar should be reopened, examined for cracks and leaks, and a new gas-generating envelope employed.
From Public Health Image Library (PHIL)/CDC.

obligate anaerobe every 48 hours, incubate it in the anaerobic environment, and monitor for growth. Most obligate anaerobes take 48 hours to display good growth. Poor growth at 48 hours means the environment has been breached by oxygen. The delay in quality control results means all cultures incubated in the anaerobic environment have been compromised in the past 48 hours. While extremely cost effective, the lack of real-time quality control results is a major disadvantage for this oxygen monitoring method.

SELF-CONTAINED ANAEROBIC AGAR

A unique approach to an anaerobic incubation system is a self-contained anaerobic culture medium. The brucella-based blood and LKV agars contain an enzyme that reduces oxygen in the culture medium. The unique agar plate lid sits very close to the surface of the agar to create an air-tight seal. A methylene blue indicator in the plate lid monitors the anaerobic environment. The enzyme remains active during the life of the agar plate and continues to reduce oxygen after each opening.

The self-contained anaerobic agar provides a viable method for performing anaerobic cultures when there are a small number of anaerobic cultures and space for equipment is limited. The self-contained system has proven to grow most but not all clinically significant anaerobes (Wiggs, Cavallaro, & Miller, 2000). Growth of *Clostridium* spp. can be a challenge for this unique system (Wiggs et al., 2000).

ANAEROBIC GENERATING SYSTEMS

The smaller anaerobic generating systems use a gas-impermeable bag, container, or jar to incubate agar plates in the anaerobic environment, as seen in Figures 24-5 and 24-6 ■. The bag holds one to two plates while the container and jar can hold up to 10–12 plates. The advantage of using a gas-impermeable bag versus a closed container or a jar is the ability to view the agar plates without having to expose them to oxygen. Another advantage to the bag is the ability to process specimens as soon as they arrive in the clinical laboratory. With a container or jar, the anaerobic environment must be regenerated each time the container or jar is opened to add culture plates, unless a holding system is used. Each system must employ either a methylene blue or resazurin indicator to ensure an anaerobic environment.

The anaerobic atmosphere is usually generated by a chemical reaction. In one method an ampule of weak hydrochloric acid is broken prior to sealing the container. The acid reacts with a tablet of potassium borohydride and sodium bicarbonate. Carbon dioxide and hydrogen are generated. Hydrogen combines with the oxygen present to form water in the presence of the palladium catalyst. A desiccant absorbs excess water produced.

A second anaerobic atmosphere generation system uses a packet that absorbs oxygen and in turn generates carbon dioxide without a palladium catalyst. A third system consists of a hydrogen- and carbon dioxide–generating envelope. Water is added to the envelope and the hydrogen produced reacts with oxygen to form water in the presence of the palladium catalyst. A desiccant absorbs excess water produced.

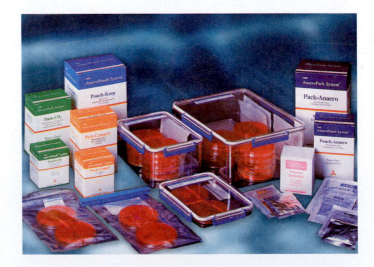

■ FIGURE 24-6 The use of gas impermeable bags allows ease of examination of the anaerobic agar plates without opening the bag. The plastic containers, while holding more agar plates, do require opening them to exam the agar plates individually. This requires the anaerobic atmosphere to be regenerated after each opening, adding to the cost of an anaerobic culture.
Photo courtesy of Remel, part of Thermo Fisher Scientific.

The anaerobic generating systems have proven to be a good alternative for small clinical laboratories where space is limited and there are a small number of anaerobic cultures processed. One downfall and ongoing expense is the need to use a new generating envelope each time the bag, container, or jar is opened. Figures 24-5 and 24-6 provide some examples of gas-generating envelopes.

While good growth is usually seen with most clinically significant anaerobes, there were some organisms such as *Fusobacterium* species and *Peptostreptococcus anaerobius* that had poor recovery in these systems (Downes, Mangels, Holden, Ferraro, & Baron, 1990). The poor recovery is probably due to the time delay in reaching an anaerobic environment after closure (Downes et al., 1990).

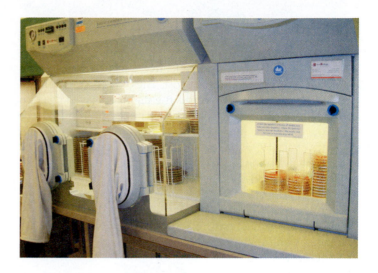

■ **FIGURE 24-7** This gloveless anaerobic chamber provides an anaerobic environment for incubation of cultures. The port allows specimens to be transported in and out of the chamber. All work can be done inside the chamber with minimal exposure of the anaerobic culture plates to oxygen.

 REAL WORLD TIP

The removal of oxygen from an anaerobic environment is accomplished by the addition of hydrogen in the presence of a catalyst. The palladium catalyst accelerates the chemical reaction without being consumed in the process. The chemical reaction looks like this: $2H_2 + O_2 \xrightarrow{\text{Catalyst}} 2H_2O$ The catalyst can be rejuvenated by heating.

ANAEROBIC CHAMBER

The anaerobic chamber is a self-contained system that acts like a workbench enclosed within a gas-tight cabinet that is continuously bathed in an anaerobic environment. It allows for processing of specimens, incubation, and workup of culture plates without having to expose them to oxygen. The atmosphere is provided by a gas tank that contains a tri-gas mixture of 80–90% nitrogen, 5% hydrogen, and 5–10% carbon dioxide. The anaerobic chamber is considered the "gold standard" for anaerobic cultures. Figure 24-7 ■ provides an example of a working anaerobic chamber.

 REAL WORLD TIP

Hydrogen explosion is a potential hazard in an anaerobic chamber. Hydrogen and oxygen mixed in just the right proportions can ignite in the presence of the palladium catalyst or heat from a sterilizing coil. The combination of 10% hydrogen and 6–12% oxygen is flammable (Cox, 1997). Oxygen can enter the chamber during transition from aerobic to anaerobic conditions in the entry port. The use of 5% hydrogen in purchased gas mixtures is adequate to maintain anaerobic conditions and does not present the potential for explosion.

Work is done through gloved or gloveless openings in the front of the cabinet. The common name for an anaerobic chamber is a glove box. A vacuum pump and entry/exit port provides a means to transition specimens and culture plates to and from the cabinet. The cabinet can be equipped with a heating coil for sterilizing needles and loops or plastic disposable loops can be used. An incubator and an optional microscope port for viewing culture plates complete the package. Foot pedals allow the operator to control the vacuum pump and sterilizer. All work can be done inside the cabinet without ever having to expose the cultures to oxygen.

The anaerobic atmosphere is maintained with palladium catalysts and dessicants. Hydrogen from the tri-gas mixture combines with oxygen to form water vapor in the presence of the palladium catalyst. The dessicant absorbs the water formed. Both are regenerated by heating at 160°C for 2 hours on a daily schedule. Depending on the volume of cultures, the palladium chloride and dessicants may need complete replacement every 6–12 months. A charcoal filter is used to capture hydrogen sulfide and other metabolic byproducts produced by organisms. Hydrogen sulfide and other metabolic byproducts can break down the palladium catalyst and inactivate it.

Holding systems can be used to provide reduced conditions while processing and working up specimens if an anaerobic chamber is not practical. Anaerobic jars with vented lids can be hooked up with a rubber hose to a nitrogen-containing gas tank. Inoculated plates can be stored in the jars until a sufficient number of plates accumulate to "fill" a jar or the workup of the culture is complete. Ideally, a holding system would be placed at the specimen processing "bench" and another at each culture workup site. One must be careful to minimize the introduction of atmospheric oxygen when placing plates into the jar, not open the jar too often, or leave the cultures in the holding jar for more than an hour.

Anaerobic conditions must be monitored continuously. While an indicator strip is cost effective, there are oxygen analyzers available for a significant cost. The oxygen analyzer provides real-time monitoring versus the slightly delayed reaction of the indicator strip. The anaerobic chamber has proven to be superior to other methods for cultivation of anaerobes (Downes et al., 1990). It requires a large amount of space and initial capital of about $15,000 for start-up. Once in place it can be less expensive to operate than other methods. At one large facility, the cost of reaching anaerobic conditions for a plate was shown to be $0.09 for the anaerobic chamber versus $0.96 for the anaerobic generating systems (Downes et al., 1990). The cost of one self-contained anaerobic agar plate is about $2.50 (Oxyrase, 2007).

Checkpoint! 24–7 (Chapter Objectives 3c and 3d)

Oxygen has accidentally entered the laboratory's anaerobic chamber. Which component of the chamber will transform it into water in the presence of hydrogen from the anaerobic atmosphere?

    A. *Methylene blue indicator*
    B. *Palladium chloride catalyst*
    C. *Dessicant*
    D. *Charcoal filter*

▶ ANAEROBIC CULTURE WORKUP

A microbiologist cannot differentiate anaerobes from facultative anaerobes by simply looking at them. Just as with any microorganism encountered in the clinical laboratory, there should be a workflow that determines the level and extent of workup.

Organism workup begins with examination of the Gram stain of the specimen. Anaerobes can present with unique Gram stain reaction as described in the "Spore Formation, Gram Stain, and Microscopic Morphology" section of this chapter. The physician may be able to initiate therapy based on the direct Gram stain results.

Once the specimen is plated and incubated, a decision must be made on when to first visually examine the anaerobic culture plates. It is well known that the sooner the patient results are available, the sooner appropriate treatment can be started and the sooner the patient is able to show improvement and leave the hospital. Slow-growing anaerobes may take up to 48 hours before they appear. The challenge to the clinical microbiologist is whether to examine plates at 24 hours and possibly lose some organisms due to oxygen sensitivity or wait until 48 hours and delay results for the patient. The anaerobic incubation system used may determine how to approach this problem.

REAL WORLD TIP

Anaerobic culture plates must be exposed to minimal amounts of oxygen during work-up. Obligate anaerobes can be killed with less than 15 minutes of exposure to oxygen.

The use of self-contained anaerobic agar allows organism workup at 24 hours without the possibility of losing organisms. The enzymes in the medium continue to maintain a reduced environment after each opening. The use of anaerobic generating systems in bags allows the plates to be viewed at 24 hours. The bag must be opened to work with the plates so organisms are exposed to potentially toxic oxygen. Anaerobic generating systems that use containers or jars must be opened just to be able to examine plates. The anaerobic chamber allows examination of plates and workup at 24 hours without having to expose the organisms to oxygen. It may prove to be the gold standard for anaerobic workup but may not be a viable option for smaller laboratories. Most laboratories elect to examine incubated plates at 48 hours to ensure the viability and detection of most anaerobes. Anaerobic plates are usually reexamined at 3, 4, and 5 days to ensure the detection of any additional slow-growing anaerobes.

Just as with aerobic organism workup, colonies must be examined visually and by Gram stain. Unique colony morphologies characteristic for specific anaerobic organisms are discussed later in this chapter. The colonies on the agar plates are quantified, differentiated, and described based on macroscopic morphology and hemolysis.

Because facultative anaerobes can grow on anaerobic media, the clinical microbiologist must test each potentially significant colony type for **aerotolerance** to determine its oxygen requirements before identification. After differentiation, each unique colony is quantified, Gram stained, and subcultured to a quarter section of a chocolate agar and an entire anaerobic blood agar. Ideally, one colony is used to perform all three functions. This ensures a pure isolation plate of the organism. Up to four organisms can be placed on the aerotolerance chocolate isolation plate to save costs. The use of a stereomicroscope or dissecting microscope allows for much better colony differentiation than with the naked eye. Both scopes allow the microbiologist to magnify and view 3D objects such as colonies on the agar plates. With experience the microbiologist can learn to manipulate colonies under the dissecting scope easily.

After review of the Gram stain, screening disks useful for presumptive identification of some organisms can be placed on the primary area of the aerotolerance anaerobic blood agar isolation plate. This saves time since it takes most anaerobes at least 48 hours to grow. A sodium polyanethol sulfonate (SPS) disk can be used to differentiate the anaerobic gram-positive cocci, *Peptostreptococcus anaerobius*, which is uniquely sensitive to this substance. Differentiation of the anaerobic gram-negative and -positive organisms is made easier with several special potency disks such as 1000 µg (1 mg) kanamycin, 5 µg vancomycin, and 10 µg colisitin. The patterns of susceptibility or resistance can assist in the presumptive differentiation of organisms. The use of the special potency disks is discussed in greater detail later in this chapter.

The aerotolerance chocolate isolation agar is placed in a 35°C CO_2 incubator for 48 hours and the anaerobic blood isolation agar plate is incubated in an anaerobic environment for 48 hours. A facultative anaerobe shows growth on both agars. The microbiologist must then determine if this organism correlates with a previously identified aerobic isolate or is a new potentially significant isolate that requires workup. An obligate or strict anaerobe will not grow on the chocolate agar but does grow on the anaerobic blood agar. Some microaerophilic organisms may display inhibited, pinpoint growth on the chocolate agar but shows much better growth on the anaerobic blood agar. Rarely, microaerotolerant anaerobes may show inhibited growth on the chocolate agar and better growth on the reducible blood agar, similar to that of a microaerophilic organism. A microaerotolerant anaerobe can overcome the oxygen's lethal effect for only a limited amount of time and will eventually stop growing aerobically. If an aerobic subculture was performed with this organism, it would not grow. Figure 24-8 ■ visually illustrates the aerotolerance testing results of a facultative anaerobe (a), either a microaerophilic organism or an aerotolerant anaerobe (b), and an obligate anaerobe (c). Visit ∞ Chapter 7 to review the cultivation of microorganisms.

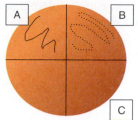
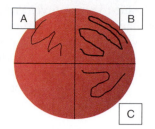

Chocolate agar at 35°C CO_2 Reducible blood agar at 35°C trigas

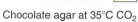

■ **FIGURE 24-8** Organism A displays equal growth in both environments, indicating a facultative anaerobe. Organism B demonstrates the growth pattern of either a microaerophilic organism or aertolerant anaerobe. It grows sparsely in the 2–8% CO_2 aerobic environment but shows much better growth in the 10% CO_2 enriched anaerobic environment. This organism requires further testing to determine its true oxygen requirements. Organism C indicates the results of an obligate anaerobe. It displays no growth in an aerobic environment and enhanced growth in the anaerobic environment.

REAL WORLD TIP

Chocolate agar is used as the aerobic aerotolerance screen plate because *Haemophilus* spp. are facultative anaerobes. If a sheep blood agar plate is used, they appear as an obligate anaerobe on aerotolerance testing and would be misidentified as an anaerobic gram-negative rod.

Isolation and identification of anaerobic organisms can be very time consuming and use up valuable technologist time and supplies if the results obtained are not relevant to the patient's current health state. Once a pure isolation plate of an anaerobe is available, the microbiologist must determine the level of workup required such as (1) should any workup be done, (2) is presumptive identification adequate, or (3) is definitive identification workup necessary. The final decision must be a cooperative effort that serves the needs of the laboratory, physician, and patient. The majority of anaerobic isolates will be a mixture of organisms and may require only identification to genus and/or species with the use of limited testing and will probably not require susceptibility testing.

A pure culture of an anaerobe from any site or those from sterile or clinically significant sites, such as a prosthetic joint infection or blood culture, should be identified to species level with a reliable identification system and tested for antimicrobial resistance. Literature recommends limiting complete iden-

tification to those specimens that grow less than three anaerobes (Engelkirk & Duben-Engelkirk, 1992). Isolation of more than three anaerobes suggests potential contamination with normal flora and should be limited to reporting based on Gram stain results or presumptive identification criteria. Significant anaerobic organisms with variable antibiotic susceptibility patterns should also be identified. *Fustobacterium* spp. can be

REAL WORLD TIP

If you report an organism by genus and species, you make it important in the mind of the physician. When a specimen is contaminated with commensal or normal flora, each normal flora organism present should not be reported individually due to the possibility of unnecessary treatment. The normal flora should be grouped together and reported based on the body site or specimen type of isolation.

For example, an aerobic/anaerobic foot wound culture of a diabetic patient demonstrates the presence of *Staphylococcus aureus*, *Staphylococcus not S. aureus*, diphtheroids, viridans streptococci, and *Bacteroides fragilis* group. The microbiologist should quantitate, identify, and report the presence of *Staphylococcus aureus* and *Bacteroides fragilis* group. *Staphylococcus not S. aureus*, diphtheroids, and viridans streptococci represent normal skin flora and should not be identified. These three organisms should be quantified and reported collectively as "normal skin flora." The use of this type of reporting procedure prevents the unnecessary treatment of contaminating organisms and focuses the physician on the true potential pathogens.

resistant to clindamycin and penicillin, certain *Clostridium* spp. can prove to be resistant, and the *Bacteroides fragilis* group can vary greatly in their resistance to many antimicrobial agents (Citron & Appelbaum, 1993). Ultimately it is a team effort between the physician and the microbiologist to determine the extent of anaerobic workup. There should be close communication to ensure the best outcome for the patient.

▶ ANAEROBES AS NORMAL FLORA

Before a microbiologist begins the task of isolating and identifying anaerobes, a working knowledge of endogenous anaerobes for each body site and specimen type is essential.

✓ Checkpoint! 24–8 (Chapter Objectives 3e, 5, and 7d)

A peritoneal fluid is processed for aerobic and anaerobic culture. The direct Gram stain demonstrated:

> *Few gram-negative rods*
> *Few large gram-positive rods*
> *Many white blood cells*

After 48 hours of incubation, the culture of peritoneal fluid reveals:

> *Blood agar plate, MacConkey agar, and phenylethyl alcohol agar = no growth*
> *RBAP = 6 colonies of a gray gamma colony and 10 colonies of a large gray colony with double beta hemolysis*
> *LKV = 5 colonies of a gray colony*

The next step in the work-up of this culture is:

> A. *perform aerotolerance testing.*
> B. *perform presumptive anaerobic identification testing.*
> C. *to turn out the final report as anaerobic GPR and anaerobic GNR isolated.*
> D. *A and then B*

Knowledge of normal anaerobic organisms can save the microbiologist time, energy, and supplies in the workup of potential contaminants. Anaerobes colonize all of the mucous membranes and skin surface of the human body. On the skin and in the mouth, upper respiratory tract, and genitourinary and intestinal tracts, anaerobes can outnumber aerobes by a factor of up to 1000:1 (Chow, 2005). Table 24-4 lists the concentration of anaerobic normal flora based on body site.

Knowing the origin of an anaerobic isolate may help determine the level of identification required. Based on Table 24-3, one can see that certain anaerobes are associated with body sites above or below the waist and may indicate to the physician the source of infection. There is a clinical correlation between isolation of *Clostridium septicum* from the blood and the presence of malignancy of the colon. This organism should be identified to species level. The isolation of *Porphyomonas* spp. usually indicates an oral or upper respiratory source whereas *Bacteroides fragilis* group indicates an intestinal source. The isolation of a non-spore-forming gram-positive diphtheroid-like rod from a single blood culture probably indicates *Propionibacterium acnes*. It usually does not require full identification because its presence indicates possible skin contamination.

▶ RAPID AND TRADITIONAL METHODS FOR IDENTIFICATION OF ANAEROBES

Anaerobic identification can prove to be difficult for microbiologists. Most do not have a lot of experience with these organisms because of their infrequent isolation. There are commercial identification systems available but traditional and rapid biochemicals and other criteria may provide enough information for presumptive identification. Presumptive identification can be cost effective and may prove to be adequate

---

✪ TABLE 24-4

Concentration and Predominance of Anaerobic Normal Flora by Body Site

Body Site	Concentration of Anaerobes (Organisms/cm^2)	Predominant Anaerobic Organisms
Skin	10^4–10^5	*Propionibacterium* spp. (primarily *P. acnes*), *Peptostreptococcus* spp., other anaerobic gram-positive cocci
Mouth and upper respiratory tract	10^6–10^{11}	*Bacteroides* spp. (but rarely *B. fragilis* group), *Prevotella* spp., *Porphyromonas* spp., *Fusobacterium* spp., *Veillonella* spp., *Actinomyces*, spp., *Peptostreptococcus* spp., *Propionibacterium* spp., microaerophilic *Streptococcus*
Intestinal tract	10^{11}–10^{12}	*Bacteroides* spp. (primarily *B. fragilis* group), *Bifidobacterium* spp., *Clostridium* spp., *Eubacterium* spp., *Peptostreptococcus* spp., *Lactobacillus* spp.
Female urethra and vagina	10^8–10^{10}	*Lactobacillus* spp. (primarily in the vaginal tract), *Bacteroides* spp., *Prevotella* spp., *Porphyromonas* spp., *Fusobacterium* spp., *Propionoibacterium* spp., *Peptostreptococcus* spp.

depending on the source of the isolate, its significance, and the physician's needs. Table 24-5✪ lists cost-effective identification criteria in order to presumptively identify some anaerobic organisms. Descriptions and the suggested use of traditional and rapid testing methods follow.

PIGMENT PRODUCTION

The pigmented *Prevotella* and *Porphyromonas* spp. are known for their ability to produce tan to black pigmentation with time on blood containing media. The pigment is due to the breakdown of the hemoglobin in red blood cells to produce heme. The pigment has a catalase-like effect to protect the organisms from the toxic effect of hydrogen peroxide and acts as a barrier against oxygen (Smalley, Silver, Birss, Withnall, & Titler, 2003).

Media with laked blood, such as laked kanamycin–vancomycin agar, accelerates their pigment production. It can take 4–6 days for most colonies to display pigment. If pigment production is delayed beyond 6 days, then fluorescence under ultraviolet light may be helpful for presumptive identification. While pigment production is not a rapid test it is distinctive for the pigmented *Prevotella* and *Porphyromonas* spp. if present. Figure 24-9 ■ demonstrates the characteristic black pigment produced by *Prevotella melaninogenica*.

FLUORESCENCE

The colonies of some anaerobes produce distinctive colors under a Wood's lamp with ultraviolet light at 366 nm (long wavelength). In the process of producing heme, red fluorescing porphyrins are created. Fluorescence is best viewed on culture plates containing blood that is 48–72 hours old.

The original culture plate is held under the UV light in a darkened room for 15–30 seconds. The pigmented *Prevotella* and *Porphyromonas* spp. fluoresce brick-red to orange when exposed to UV light. In Figure 24-10 ■, this reducible blood agar plate, under ultraviolet light, demonstrates the pink-red colonies characteristic of *Prevotella* and *Porphyromonas* spp. *Fusobacterium* spp. and some *Clostridium* spp. such as *C. difficile* display a chartreuse (yellow-green) color, as seen in Figure 24-10. *Veillonella* spp. can display a red fluorescence but it is not due to heme production as seen in *Prevotella* and *Porphyromonas* spp. A Gram stain will easily differentiate this

---

✪ TABLE 24-5

Presumptive Identification of Anaerobes	
Cost-Effective Identification Criteria for Anaerobes	**Presumptive Identification**
A large, box car–shaped gram-positive rod exhibiting double-zoned beta hemolysis	*Clostridium perfringens*
A swarming gram-positive rod with prominent terminal spores	*Clostridium tetani*
A non-spore-forming gram-positive rod resembling "diphtheroids" that is catalase and indole positive	*Propionibacterium acnes*
A non-spore-forming gram-positive rod that reduces nitrate and whose colony fluoresces red	*Eggerthella lenta* (previously known as *Eubacterium lentum*)
A gram-negative rod or coccobacilli that is resistant to kanamycin, vancomycin, and colistin as well as stimulated by bile	*Bacteroides fragilis* group
A gram-negative rod or coccobacilli that is resistant to kanamycin, vancomycin, and colistin, stimulated by bile, catalase positive, indole negative, and esculin negative	*Bacteroides vulgatus*
A gram-negative rod or coccobacilli that is resistant to kanamycin, vancomycin, and colistin, stimulated by bile, catalase positive, and indole positive	*Bacteroides thetaiotaomicron*
A gram-negative rod that is resistant to vancomycin, sensitive to kanamycin and colistin, as well as indole and lipase positive	*Fusobacterium necrophorum*
A fusiform gram-negative rod that is resistant to vancomycin, sensitive to kanamycin and colistin, as well as indole positive and lipase negative	*Fusobacterium nucleatum*
A pigmented gram-negative rod or coccobacilli which is sensitive to vancomycin and indole positive	*Porphyromonas* spp.
A pigmented gram-negative rod or coccobacilli that is resistant to vancomycin and indole and lipase positive	*Prevotella intermedia*
A gram-positive cocci that is sensitive to SPS	*Peptostreptococcus anaerobius*
A gram-positive cocci that is resistant to SPS and indole positive	*Peptoniphilus asaccharolyticus* (previously known as *Peptostreptococcus asaccharolyticus*)
A gram-negative cocci that reduces nitrate	*Veillonella* species
A gram-positive cocci displaying a tiny colony with beta-hemolysis and PYR negative and Voges-Proskauer (VP) positive	Microaerophilic *Streptococcus* spp. (*S. anginosis*, *S. constellatus*, and *S. intermedius*)

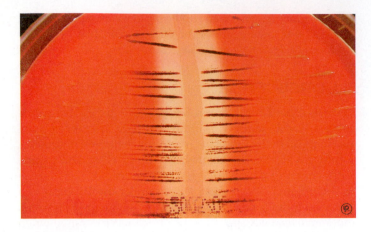

■ **FIGURE 24-9** The pigmented *Prevotella* spp. and *Poryphyro-monas* spp. are easily recognizable by the production of black pigment after 4–6 days. This photograph also demonstrates the ability of *P. melaninogenica* to satellite. If the media does not provide the vitamin K the organism requires for growth, it can satellite around other organisms, such as *S. aureus*, which can synthesize the compound.

From Marler LM, Siders JA, Kaufman CM, Owens EN, Korba GG and Allen SD, *Bacteriology I Image Atlas* CD-ROM, Indiana Pathology Images, 2005.

anaerobic gram-negative cocci from gram-negative rods. Care must be taken with the original plate. Overexposure to UV light can kill the organisms present as well as be potentially damaging to human skin. UV safety glasses should be worn to protect the microbiologist's eyes.

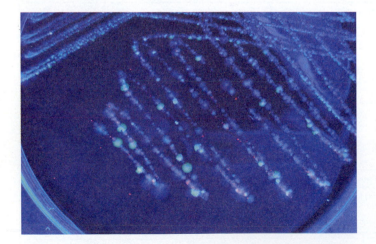

■ **FIGURE 24-10** This reducible blood agar plate of a mandible culture has been incubated for 5 days in an anaerobic environment. Under ultraviolet light, the red-pink colonies of *Prevotella* and *Porphyromonas* spp. are easily recognizable among the many other isolates present. The chartreuse (green-yellow) colonies represent *Fusobacterium* spp.

SPOT INDOLE

Anaerobic media enriched with blood contains tryptophan, which makes them appropriate for performing a rapid spot indole test. At 24–48 hours, a colony is rubbed into a drop of the indole reagent, p-dimethyl-aminocinnamaldehyde, placed on a piece of filter paper. This method is recommended over Kovac's for anaerobes. A blue-green color indicates the organism is able to break down tryptophan into indole, which reacts with the reagent to form the color change. A positive spot indole is helpful in the identification of *Propionibacterium acnes* and *Peptoniphilus asaccharolyticus,* differentiating *Fusobacterium nucleatum* and *F. necrophorum* from other *Fusobacterium* spp. and differentiating within the *Bacteroides fragilis* group. Indole can diffuse into the agar and be carried with swarming organisms such as *Proteus* spp. Only isolation plates with pure colonies should be used for testing. The presence of a positive nitrate disk can cause a possible false-negative indole reaction (Isenberg, 2004).

SPECIAL POTENCY DISKS

Three disks, 1000 µg (1 mg) kanamycin, 5 µg vancomycin, and 10 µg colisitin, can be used to initially categorize and differentiate anaerobes. The disks are placed on a pure isolation plate, such as the anaerobic aerotolerance agar plate, at equal intervals in the primary area. A zone of inhibition of >10 millimeters (mm) is considered susceptible. gram-positive organisms are usually sensitive to vancomycin and resistant to colistin whereas gram-negative organisms are usually resistant to vancomycin. These disks do not predict the use of these antimicrobial agents as therapy. They are only meant to screen organisms for categorization and presumptive identification.

The most common isolate, the *Bacteroides fragilis* group, is resistant to all three agents. *Fusobacterium* spp. are resistant to vancomycin but susceptible to kanamycin and colistin. *Porphyromonas* spp. are susceptible to vancomycin but resistant to kanamycin and colistin. *Clostridium perfringens* is susceptible to vancomycin and kanamycin yet resistant to colistin. The disks can be especially useful with *Clostridium*

 Checkpoint! 24–9 (Chapter Objectives 3e and 7d)

Interpret the following results to provide the most likely identification of the organism:

■ *No growth on chocolate agar at 35°C CO_2*
■ *Growth on reduced blood agar plate (RBAP) at 35°C, anaerobic (tri-gas)*
■ *A gram-negative coccobacillus that displays resistance to vancomycin, kanamycin, and colistin*

A. *Bacteroides fragilis* group
B. *Fusobacterium nucleatum*
C. *Porphyromonas spp.*
D. *Prevotella intermedia*

spp. isolates, which have a tendency to overdecolorize easily. Use of the three disks will ensure it is not misidentified as a gram-negative rod.

SODIUM POLYANETHOL SULFONATE (SPS) DISK

Most microbiologists recognize sodium polyanethol sulfonate (SPS) as the anticoagulant used in blood culture medium. It can also be used to identify the anaerobic gram-positive cocci, *Peptostreptococcus anaerobius*. The 5% concentration disk is placed on the primary area of a pure isolation culture plate. A zone of inhibition of >12 millimeters (mm) is considered presumptive for *P. anaerobius*.

 REAL WORLD TIP

Commercial blood culture media contains 0.25–0.5% sodium polyanethol sulfonate (SPS) as an anticoagulant. *Peptostreptococcus anaerobius* is sensitive to 0.1% SPS and can be inhibited in blood culture medium. Most commercial blood culture broths also contain gelatin at a concentration that is four times that of SPS (Wilkins & West, 1976). The gelatin neutralizes the effect of SPS on *P. anaerobius* by an unknown mechanism so the organism is able to grow.

NITRATE

Some organisms have the ability to reduce nitrates to nitrites and other nitrogen byproducts. Nitrate, applied to a paper disk, is placed in the primary area of a pure isolation plate of an anaerobic organism and allowed to incubate. After addition of reagent A (alpha-naphthylamine) and reagent B (sulfanilic acid), if the organism is able to reduce nitrates to nitrites, the disk will turn red. The lack of a color change does not automatically mean the test is negative. The two reagents used are only able to detect nitrites and not the other nitrogen byproducts if the organism is able to reduce nitrate beyond nitrite. If there is a lack of color change after 5 minutes, then a sprinkle of zinc dust is added to the disk. Zinc is able to reduce nitrates to nitrites. After the addition of zinc, a lack of a color change means that no nitrates were present so the organism was able to reduce nitrates to other nitrogen byproducts besides nitrites. A red color after the addition of zinc means nitrate was present and the organism did not reduce it. Zinc reduced the nitrate present to nitrite, which then reacted with the two reagents. Review the conventional nitrate test in ∞ Chapter 9, "Final Identification."

CATALASE

The catalase test is performed in the same manner as for aerobic organisms except a 15% concentration of hydrogen peroxide is used rather than a 3% solution. The higher concentration is more sensitive for anaerobes (Jousimies-Somer, 2002). Care must be taken to avoid picking up media containing blood which can cause a false-positive reaction. Sustained, effervescent bubbles, similar to the bubbles in carbonated soda, indicate a positive reaction. No bubbles or delayed or weak trails of bubbles should be interpreted as a negative reaction.

LIPASE

Egg yolk agar (EYA) is used to demonstrate an organism's ability to break down fat with the enzyme lipase. The resulting glycerol and fatty acids causes an iridescent or oil-on-water effect with a multicolored shine on the colony surface. The agar plate may have to be examined in natural light while being tilted back and forth to best see the rainbow of colors effect. Figure 24-11 ■ shows lipase production of *Clostridium* spp. on egg yolk agar. Lipase production is associated with several *Clostridium* spp. as well as *Fusobacterium necrophorum*. EYA can be included with routine anaerobic media on initial specimen processing if *Clostridium* spp. are suspected.

LECITHINASE

EYA also demonstrates lecithinase production by some *Clostridium* spp. Lecithin is a lipid present in egg yolk. Lecithinase is an enzyme that splits lecithin into diglycerides. The diglycerides appear as an opaque white halo in the agar around the colony. Figures 24-11 and 24-12 ■ demonstrate the ability of a *Clostridium* spp. to produce lecithinase.

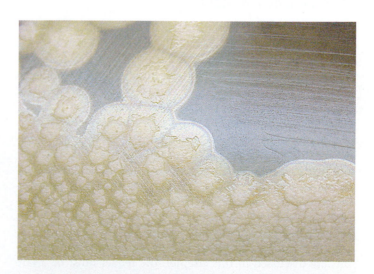

■ **FIGURE 24-11** On egg yolk agar, organisms that produce lipase can break down the fat present. This creates a rainbow-like sheen on the agar surface due to glycerol and fatty acids present as by-products of fat degradation.
From CDC and Larry Stauffer, Oregon State Public Health Laboratory.

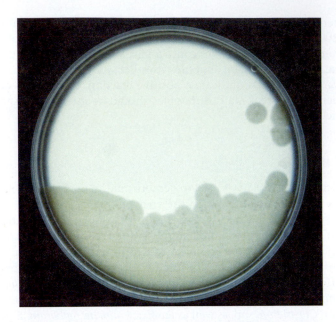

■ **FIGURE 24-12** On egg yolk agar, an organism that produces lecithinase is able to break down the lecithin present to produce diglycerides. An opaque, white halo around the colony indicates the presence of diglycerides.
From Public Health Image Library (PHIL)/CDC.

 REAL WORLD TIP

Protease-producing clostridia (e.g., *C. sporogenes*) may produce a clear zone around the colony on EYA. This reaction is recorded as proteolysis positive.

BILE STIMULATION

Bacteroides fragilis group and *Fusobacterium mortiferum* are stimulated to grow in the presence of 20% bile. A bile disk is placed in the primary area of a pure culture plate of the unknown isolate and incubated. Any zone of inhibition is considered a negative reaction whereas growth up to the disk is a positive reaction for bile stimulation.

Bacteroides bile esculin (BBE) agar can be included with routine anaerobic media on initial specmen processing if members of the *Bacteroides fragilis* group are suspected. The agar contains 20% bile, which inhibits the growth of most anaerobes other than *Bacteroides fragilis* group. The *Bacteroides fragilis* group is also able to break down the esculin present to produce a black discoloration around the colony. Refer to Figure 24-4 for a review of BBE agar.

As the identification results of individual anaerobic organisms are discussed in this chapter, the reader must be aware that only the more commonly recognized anaerobic isolates are discussed. The microbiologist is encouraged to utilize additional resources when determining the definitive identification and significance of anaerobes isolated from clinical specimens.

 Checkpoint! 24–10 (Chapter Objectives 4, 6a, + 6f)

A microbiologist observes large box car–shaped gram-positive rods in the direct Gram stain of purulent material from an abdominal abscess after surgery for a bowel obstruction. To hasten the identification of this organism, which medium should be added at processing?

  A. *Anaerobic Thioglycolate broth*
  B. *BBE*
  C. *LKV*
  D. *EYA*

► COMMERCIAL IDENTIFICATION SYSTEMS

Definitive identification should be performed on isolates that grow in pure culture, are from sterile body sites such as blood, require susceptibility testing due to potential resistance, and are associated with specific infections such as *Clostridium perfringens* and gas gangrene. Many commercial identification systems are able to identify most common isolates accurately and may provide same-day results. The microbiologist must weigh the value of same-day results with the higher cost of most commercial identification systems against the need for definitive identification.

Most commercial biochemical systems require turbid suspensions for inoculation. Most call for a suspension of organisms greater than or equal to a 3.0 McFarland standard. It is essential a pure isolation plate is used for suspension inoculation to ensure accurate results.

 REAL WORLD TIP

A 3.0 McFarland standard equals 9×10^8 organisms per milliliter.

Biochemicals can be miniaturized and lined up on a strip or in micro-titer wells. They are usually inoculated outside an anaerobic environment due to the fine manipulations necessary. They must be returned to an anaerobic environment to be incubated for up to 48 hours before interpretation. Most require the addition of regents prior to interpretation of some biochemical reactions.

The biochemicals are number coded and a multidigit code is created based on the interpreted reactions. A code book or online database interprets the number to provide the organism identification. Additional testing may be required when the database does not provide a clear-cut answer.

A rapid miniaturized identification system has evolved based on detection of preformed enzymes. As anaerobes grow they produce enzymes that are used for metabolism. The enzymes are able to hydrolyze chromogenic substrates to create a color change. The advantage of this system is the ability to incubate the substrate strip in an aerobic environment. Once the enzymes are formed, they function regardless of whether the organism is alive or dead and in any environment.

The rapid enzyme-based identification systems require a heavy inoculum of at least 3.0 McFarland or greater. The biggest advantage is the 4-hour incubation at 35°C in ambient air. After the addition of reagents, a multidigit code is generated and compared to a database for interpretation. Supplemental tests may be required. Interpretation of the colors can prove to be subjective. A color comparison chart is usually provided to ensure accurate interpretation and results.

► GAS LIQUID CHROMATOGRAPHY

Prior to commercial identification systems, gas liquid chromatography (GLC) and traditional biochemical testing were used to identify anaerobic isolates. GLC detects the metabolic end-products of glucose fermentation by anaerobes. The volatile fatty acids, alcohols, and nonvolatile organic acids produced are unique and can be used for presumptive and definitive identification.

The anaerobe to be identified is grown in peptone yeast glucose broth for 48 hours. A portion of the broth is treated with ether to solubilize the short-chained volatile fatty acids, which include acetic, propionic, isobutyric, butyric, isovaleric, valeric, isocaproic, and caproic. The detection of the nonvolatile fatty acids: pyruvic, lactic, and succinic, requires treatment of a second sample with methanol and chloroform prior to testing.

After treatment the sample is injected into the heated chromatograph column. The sample is initially vaporized and carried along the column by a carrier gas such as helium or nitrogen through the liquid phase of the column. Compounds that are less soluble move quickly through the column whereas those that are more soluble are held longer and detected much later. The compounds are measured when they reach a detector. A recorder draws a peak on paper that corresponds to each compound and its concentration as it is detected. GLC peak patterns for specific organisms are discussed with individual organisms later in this chapter.

A standard known solution is used to ensure that both the sample preparation and instrument are functioning properly. The organism sample peaks are compared to the standard solution peaks. If the sample peak is larger than the corresponding standard peak, the metabolic end-product is considered a major metabolic end-product and reported with a capital letter. For example, if the organism produces acetic acid (A/a) at a quantity greater than the standard, it is reported as a capital letter *A* when listing the GLC products pattern. If the sample peak is smaller than the corresponding standard, then the compound is considered a minor metabolic end-product and reported as a lowercase letter *a*. All of the letters of the compounds produced by an organism provide the GLC pattern for the organism. Some patterns are very recognizable for certain organisms. Figure 24-13 ■ demonstrates an example of the detection of major and minor metabolic end-products.

The GLC procedure is complicated, time consuming, and many instrument and technologist variables can affect the results. The use of chloroform and ether in the laboratory should be avoided due to their potential health and safety hazards. Many clinical laboratories have given up the procedure for the convenience and ease of commercial identification systems.

COMMON ANAEROBES INVOLVED IN INFECTIONS

Two-thirds of anaerobic infections are due to a combination of aerobic as well as anaerobic organisms (Chow, 2005). Both make up the normal flora of the skin and mucous membranes. Any trauma, surgery, or disease to these surfaces releases aerobic and anaerobic organisms that can colonize and eventually infect previously sterile sites. In addition, trauma, surgery, and disease can disturb blood flow to body sites. The loss of blood flow prevents oxygen from reaching tissues and eventually the tissues can begin to die. The presence of facultative anaerobes also promotes anaerobic infections by using up the oxygen present for their aerobic respiration. All of these processes lower the oxidation reduction potential of the environment, making it more hospitable for the growth of anaerobes.

► SPORE-FORMING GRAM-POSITIVE RODS

Clostridium spp. make up about 10% of all anaerobic infections (Brook, 2003c). The diseases produced by these spore-formers are usually due to powerful exotoxins. They are found in the

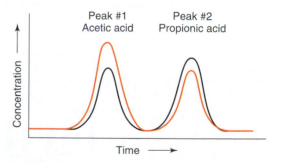

Red line = Organism metabolic end-products
Black line = Known standard end-products

■ **FIGURE 24-13** The black line represents two end-product peaks (acetic acid and propionic acid) produced by a standard known solution on the gas-liquid chromatograph. The red line demonstrates an unknown organism that produces major acetic acid and minor propionic acid as metabolic end-products when compared to the standard. The organism's production of acetic acid is considered major because it creates more than the known standard while its propionic acid production is minor because the peak is smaller than the standard. This organism's GLC pattern would be reported as A, p.

soil as well as part of human and animal intestinal tract flora. While most *Clostridium* spp. produce endospores, *C. perfringens* is known for producing them under only the harshest conditions so they are rarely seen in patient specimens or in culture. A few of the *Clostridium* spp., such as *C. perfringens,* have proven to be microaerotolerant. While they do not grow on media in room air oxygen, they can endure limited exposure to oxygen and survive once returned to an anaerobic environment.

Clostridium spp. can prove to be difficult to Gram stain because of their tendency to lose the ability to retain the crystal violet-alkaline iodine complex after decolorization. The use of special potency disks assist in determining their true Gram stain reaction. Gram-positive organisms are usually sensitive to 5 µg of vancomycin and resistant to 10 µg of colistin whereas gram-negative organisms are usually resistant to van-

comycin. Table 24-6 lists the more commonly recognized *Clostridium* spp. and their differentiation based on biochemical and other results.

CLOSTRIDIUM PERFRINGENS

Clostridium perfringens is the most common *Clostridium* spp. isolated from tissue infections and bacteremia (Lorber, 2005b). The Gram stain of *C. perfringens* demonstrates the typical large, straight-edged positive rods in chains that resemble train box cars in a line. Figure 24-14 ■ demonstrates the Gram stain of *C. perfringens.* The organism is usually unwilling to produce its central to subterminal spores in a patient sample or culture isolates. On direct Gram stain there is an unusual absence of

✪ TABLE 24-6

Biochemical and Other Characteristics of the More Recognized Isolated *Clostridium* Species

Organism	Vancymycin (5 µg)	Kanamycin (1000 µg)	Colistin (10 µg)	Lipase	Lecithinase	Swarming Colony	Spore Location	Fluorescence	Indole	Oxygen Tolerance	Other
Clostridium perfringens	S	S	R	–	+	–	C or ST*	None	–	MA	Distinct double beta hemolysis
C. tetani[†]	S	S	R	–	–	+	T	None	+	OA	Tennis racket–shaped cells
C. botulinum	S	S	R	+	–	–	ST	None	–	OA	Not considered normal flora in humans
C. difficile	S	S	R	–	–	–	ST	Chartreuse	–	OA	Yellow on CCFA agar
C. septicum	S	S	R	–	–	+	ST	None	–	OA	Isolation may correlate with gastrointestinal malignancy

C, central; MA, microaerotolerant (can grow in presence of up to 10% oxygen); OA, obligate anaerobe; S, susceptible; ST, subterminal; T, terminal; R, resistant; unshaded areas indicate presumptive identification reactions.

*Spores are rarely detected

[†]Rarely isolated

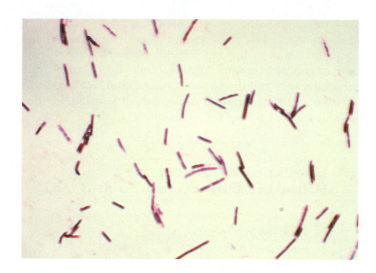

■ **FIGURE 24-14** The typical Gram stain of *C. perfringens* shows large, rectangular gram-positive rods with the absence of spores. The only other genus that can possess this same Gram stain reaction and microscopic morphology is *Bacillis* spp. The two can be differentiated by the catalase reaction. *Clostridium* spp. are catalase negative while *Bacillus* spp. are positive. *From Public Health Image Library (PHIL)/CDC.*

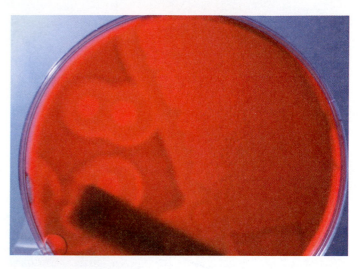

■ **FIGURE 24-15** Note the two zones of beta hemolysis around the colonies of *C. perfringens*. This colony morphology is so unique to this organism that it can be presumptively identified on its presence and Gram stain results.

white blood cells. Numerous enzymes and toxins produced by the organism are able to lyse neutrophils and destroy platelets (Lorber, 2005b). Several of its histotoxic toxins are responsible for the hemolysis, extensive tissue necrosis, and muscle damage associated with infection with the organism. It also produces collagenase, which allows the organism to rapidly spread through tissues.

On blood containing medium, *C. perfringens* produces a medium- to large-sized colony with a characteristic double zone of beta hemolysis. The inner complete beta zone is due to theta (θ) toxin whereas the outer subtle beta zone is due to alpha (α) toxin (Lorber, 2005b). Theta toxin is responsible for destruction of endothelial cells and white and red blood cells. Its alpha toxin hydrolyzes lecithin and sphingomyelin in the cell membranes of red blood cells, platelets, white blood cells, and endothelial and muscle cells. Both are responsible for massive hemolysis and necrotic tissue associated with infection.

The double zone of beta hemolysis is unique to *C. perfringens* and can be used along with its characteristic Gram stain in its presumptive identification. Figure 24-15 ■ demonstrates the unique double beta hemolysis of this organism.

Egg yolk agar can be used to detect lecithinase and lipase production of some *Clostridium* spp. While it can be set up on initial specimen processing, organisms other than *Clostridium* spp. can produce lipase and its results must be interpreted carefully. *C. perfringens* is unable to produce lipase but does produce lecithinase. Lecithinase splits lecithin into water-insoluble diglycerides (Isenberg, 2004). A positive result appears as a distinct opaque zone in the medium around the colony, as seen in Figure 24-12.

C. perfringens is best known as the most common causative agent of **myonecrosis** or gas gangrene, a rapid and widespread necrotic infection of the muscle with distinctive gas formation in the tissues. *C. perfringens* causes up to 90% of cases of gas gangrene (Revis, 2006). The other 10% of cases are caused by other *Clostridium* spp. *Clostridium perfringens* is also able to cause less virulent infections without progressing to myonecrosis.

℮ REAL WORLD TIP

Other *Clostridium* spp., such as *C. septicum*, *C. novyi*, *C. histolyticum*, *C. bifermentans*, and *C. sordelli*, can also be rare causes of gas gangrene.

The organism is introduced through deep penetrating trauma or surgery, especially if associated with the gastrointestinal tract. Compromised or loss of blood supply, tissue necrosis, and a low oxidation-reduction potential are essential for initiation of infection. The organism requires many amino acids and growth factors, which are only available in necrotic tissue (Kasper et al., 2007). Gas gangrene progresses rapidly and appears within 1 to 3 days. The infected area is very painful and the skin turns bronze or purple red and develops large, fluid-filled blisters, as demonstrated in Figure 24-16 ■. Hydrogen and nitrogen gases are produced by the organism in the tissues (Lorber, 2005b). The skin crackles when manipulated due to the presence of gases in the tissue. Muscle and other tissues liquefy due to histotoxic toxins produced. In addition, the patient can experience septicemia. A hematocrit of 0% is possible, but not compatible with life, due to

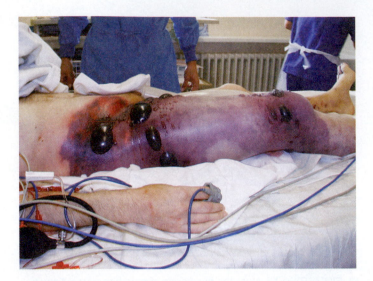

■ **FIGURE 24-16** This graphic picture demonstrates gas gangrene due to *Clostridium perfringens.* The discolored skin and large fluid filled blisters are prominent. Gas, produced by the organism, can be felt beneath the skin.
Source: Schröpfer, Rauthe, and Meyer. (2008). Diagnosis and misdiagnosis of necrotizing soft tissue infections: Three case reports. Cases Journal, 1, 252, http://www.casesjournal.com/content/1/1/252.

intravascular hemolysis as a result of toxins and hemolysins produced (Stevens, 2004). Without intervention shock and organ failure develop.

C. perfringens is also associated with perirectal and diabetic foot ulcers. It has been isolated as the causative agent of infections of the uterus such as endometritis, which can occur after an incomplete abortion and premature rupture of the placental membrane.

Treatment of gas gangrene involves antibiotics, aggressive necrotic tissue debridement, including amputation, and the possible use of a hyperbaric oxygen chamber. Antibiotics such as penicillin, vancomycin, clindamycin, and chloramphenicol are effective. Most anaerobes, including *C. perfringens,* are susceptible to metronidazole because this antibiotic must be reduced to become effective. It works best in an anaerobic environment. Surprisingly, with all of the enzymes produced by *C. perfringens,* beta-lactamase is not one of them so penicillin remains an effective option.

Tissue debridement is necessary to restore the blood supply to the area, promote healing, and reduce the number of bacteria present. Amputation may be necessary if the infection does not respond to antibiotics. A rapidly advancing infection may benefit from use of hyperbaric oxygen therapy (Bowler, Duerden, & Armstrong, 2001). Raising the oxygen level of tissues can inactivate some of the powerful toxins produced by *C. perfringens* (Bowler et al., 2001).

The histotoxic toxins of *C. perfringens* can cause gastrointestinal diseases such as food poisoning. Spores and toxin are ingested in food such as meat and meat byproducts (Lorber, 2005b). The spores germinate in the small intestine and pro-

duce an enterotoxin. The enterotoxin produces watery diarrhea due to the loss of water and electrolytes, nausea, and abdominal pain. Symptoms usually resolve with time. Diagnosis can only be confirmed by isolation of the organism from the food source and the patient's stool (Brook, 2003c). Looking for *C. perfringens* in stool is one of the few instances when feces should be cultured for anaerobic organisms.

> ✓ **Checkpoint! 24–11**
> **(Chapter Objectives 7c and 7d)**
>
> *A key identification characteristic of Clostridium perfringens is its:*
> A. *double beta hemolysis.*
> B. *production of central spores.*
> C. *positive lipase reaction.*
> D. *ability to produce beta-lactamase.*

CLOSTRIDIUM TETANI

On Gram stain, *Clostridium tetani* is easily recognized by its characteristic gram-positive rod with terminal spores. The spore causes the cell to swell so it looks like a tennis racket, lollipop, or chicken drumstick. Figure 24-17 ■ demonstrates the characteristic terminal spores of *Clostridium tetani.*

The organism is the causative agent of tetanus and is rarely isolated from clinical specimens in patients with the disease (Jousimies-Somer, 2002). Diagnosis is usually made by the physician at the bedside based on signs and symptoms. On isolation, the organism produces a slightly beta hemolytic, swarming colony. The extent of swarming can match that of *Proteus* spp. and cover the entire plate. Few *Clostridium* spp.

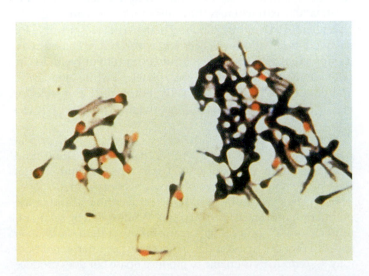

■ **FIGURE 24-17** This spore stain of *Clostridium tetani* reveals the prominent terminal spores associated with the organism. The swollen cells resemble a tennis racket or chicken drumstick.
Source: CDC.

swarm. The characteristic Gram stain with the presence of the unique terminal spores and a swarming colony are adequate for presumptive identification of the organism. Due to the severity of the disease *C. tetani* causes, a commercial system should be used for definitive identification if isolated. The organism is lecithinase negative and usually lipase negative.

Tetanus is rare in the United States due to the widespread use of the diphtheria–pertussis–tetanus (DPT) vaccine. Most cases occur in unvaccinated individuals or those who do not receive booster vaccinations. The organism is usually introduced through traumatic injury or open wound contaminated with soil, dust, or animal dung.

Once in the wound, the spores are able to germinate under a reduced oxidation-reduction potential. Powerful toxins produced cause the signs and symptoms seen with the disease. **Tetanospasim** is a neurotoxin that moves through the bloodstream to affect nerves throughout the body. The toxin causes almost constant muscle contraction. The first muscles affected are usually the jaw because they have the shortest nerves. Lockjaw, the inability to open the mouth completely, is usually the first complaint. As the disease progresses, the back muscles eventually are affected and can contract all at once so only the head and feet touch the bed. Figure 24-18 ■ shows a patient displaying severe hyperextension of the spinal column due to the neurotoxin. The patient may require airway ventilation if the respiratory system nerves are affected.

Patients can survive tetanus with early detection and treatment but it carries about a 20–25% mortality rate even with treatment (Bartlett, 2004). Treatment requires supportive care such as ventilation, control of muscle spasms, immunization to promote antibody production, antitoxin to neutralize unbound toxin, and antibiotics such as penicillin, metronidazole, clindamycin, or erythromycin to eliminate the organism. Recovery can be complete but may take months (Kasper et al., 2007).

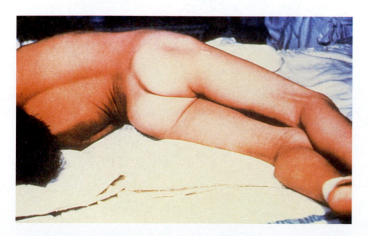

■ **FIGURE 24-18** This patient is exhibiting the severe muscle spasms associated with tetanus. The powerful neurotoxin causes the body's muscles to continually contract.
From Public Health Image Library (PHIL)/CDC.

CLOSTRIDIUM BOTULINUM

Clostridium botulinum is a soil and water organism best known for its lethal toxin associated with consumption of contaminated food. This gram-positive rod is the causative agent of botulism. The organism produces subterminal spores. Egg yolk agar can be used for initial isolation of the organism. All strains of *C. botulinum* produce lipase but not lecithinase on egg yolk agar. The inability to produce lecithinase differentiates it from other lipase-producing *Clostridium* spp. Identification among the strains can be accomplished by carbohydrate fermentation and gas liquid chromatography.

The signs and symptoms of botulism are due to the powerful exotoxin released by the organism. There are at least eight different strains of the organism. All strains produce the lethal toxin but each differs slightly in their toxin's serologic properties (Shapiro, 1998). It is a neurotoxin that binds to and blocks the body's peripheral neurons to produce paralysis and loss of muscle tone. Foodborne botulism occurs after consumption of food containing the preformed toxin. Inadequate cooking and improper home canning techniques do not kill the spores present. The spores germinate under the anaerobic conditions created by canning and the organisms produce toxin.

Infant botulism occurs after the ingestion of spores of *C. botulinum*. The spores germinate in the intestine and form toxin. Raw honey and common house dust have been implicated as sources of *C. botulinum* spores (Nevas et al., 2005). Wound botulism is rare but is being seen more in injection drug users, especially those who use black tar heroin (Chan-Tack & Bartlett, 2006). The organism can also be introduced by trauma associated with soil contamination.

@ REAL WORLD TIP

Clostridium botulinum toxin, which is one of the most poisonous substances on earth, can be used medically to treat muscle spasms, wrinkles, and excessive sweating. In November 2004, four individuals received 2,857 times the lethal dose due to the use of an unlicensed preparation of botulinum toxin. All four individuals received the toxin for cosmetic purposes. The toxin used was highly potent and labeled for research purposes only. Remarkably, all four patients survived after long hospital stays (Chertow, Tan, & Maslanka, 2006).

The gastrointestinal version of botulism may present with constipation, due to paralysis of the intestinal muscles, 18–36 hours after ingestion. As the toxin spreads through the body, there is descending paralysis. The muscles of the head are affected first, then the upper extremities, followed by the respiratory system, and finally the lower extremities. Wound botulism has an incubation period of approximately 7 days.

Rapid diagnosis of botulism is essential for positive patient outcomes. Detection of toxin in serum, stool, and food source aids the physician in establishing the diagnosis. Cultures can support the detection of toxin. The presence of *C. botulinum* in a stool culture may be adequate for diagnosis because the organism is not considered normal flora for humans. Most clinical laboratories are not equipped to detect botulism toxin. State public health laboratories usually perform the laboratory testing required for confirmation of the diagnosis of botulism.

Botulism is a rapidly lethal disease that must be recognized quickly, especially if there is the potential for a major outbreak due to contaminated commercial foods. Supportive care and airway ventilation are essential. Antitoxin is the only treatment available and must be released by epidemiologists at the Centers for Disease Control and Prevention (CDC). Botulism is a reportable disease that must be communicated to public health as soon as suspected.

 Checkpoint! 24–12 (Chapter Objective 7a)

The pathogenicity of Clostridium tetani and C. botulinum is due to their ability to:

    A. *produce neurotoxin.*
    B. *produce spores.*
    C. *resist the stomach acids.*
    D. *resist antitoxin.*

CLOSTRIDIUM DIFFICILE

Clostridium difficile is best known as the most common causative agent of antibiotic associated diarrhea and pseudomembranous colitis (PMC) during or after treatment with antibiotics. PMC can occur in both hospitalized individuals and outpatients. The organism is an anaerobic gram-positive rod that produces subterminal spores on Gram stain. Its colony on blood containing media is not unique among the *Clostridium* spp. but it does produce a characteristic horse manure or barnyard odor. Surprisingly, even though it is relatively easy to grow, culture for the organism is not recommended.

The organism is known to live in the intestine of healthy infants and young children (Gronczewski & Katz, 2006). Spores enter the environment and individuals can become colonized with antibiotic use. Some go on to become asymptomatic carriers while others go on to develop serious diarrhea. Colonized individuals are the major source of spores in the hospital environment. The spores can live in the environment for up to 6 months and contaminate inanimate objects such as blood pressure cuffs, bed railings, and sinks (Martitrosian, 2006). Hospital personnel can provide the major means of transmission from patient to patient.

The presence of *C. difficile* in stool does not automatically correlate with disease. The organism is only considered sig-nificant when it produces toxins that ultimately cause colitis. This means a routine stool culture is no longer considered useful for diagnosis of PMC. It is possible to isolate *C. difficile* from stool using cycloserine–cefoxitin–fructose and egg yolk (CCFA) agar. The agar is selective and differential for the organism. Initially the agar is pink and the organism produces a large, yellow colony with a yellow ring, due to fermentation of fructose, that extends into the area around the colony, as observed in Figure 24-19 . The colony also produces characteristic chartreuse (yellow-green) fluorescence under long-wave ultraviolet light. Remember, culture cannot determine if an isolated colony is a toxin producer and results will be delayed for the patient while further testing is done. Detection of toxin is much more reliable for diagnosis of *C. difficile*-associated PMC.

C. difficile is an important nosocomial pathogen. The patient becomes colonized via spores in the hospital environment. With antibiotic use, normal stool flora is inhibited and the spores germinate and proliferate to produce toxin. The organism produces two types of toxins, A and B, which cause the clinical signs of disease. Toxin A is an enterotoxin that causes the loss of fluids and electrolytes from intestinal cells while toxin B is a cytotoxin that damages the cells and promotes the formation of the characteristic plaque-like pseudomembrane that coats the intestinal wall.

REAL WORLD TIP

There have been recent reported outbreaks of severe *Clostridium difficile*–associated disease due to a strain that produces 16 times more toxin A and 23 times more toxin B than other toxigenic strains. The increased toxin production is probably due to a mutation that caused the deletion of a regulatory gene (Sunenshine & McDonald, 2006).

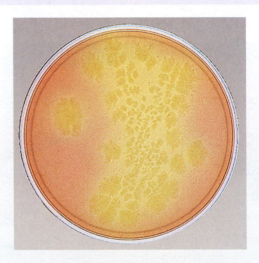

■ **FIGURE 24-19** While culture for *Clostridium difficile* is not recommended, selective agar is available. It will also differentiate the organism based on fermentation of fructose.
Photo courtesy of Remel, part of Thermo Fisher Scientific.

Watery diarrhea, fever, abdominal cramps, and leukocytosis can appear after 5–10 days of antibiotic therapy (Knoop, 1993). Lesions form in the intestine that can eventually be covered by a pseudomembrane made up of leukocytes, fibrin, mucous, and cellular debris. The pseudomembrane can be viewed using a gastrointestinal endoscope and is considered diagnostic but the procedure is not practical for some hospitalized patients.

REAL WORLD TIP

The key indicator of *Clostridium difficile*–associated disease is diarrhea. A formed stool should not be accepted for detection of the presence of *C. difficile* or its toxins (Gerding, Johnson, Peterson, Mulligan, & Silva, 1995). Asymptomatic carriers harbor the organism but they do not display the classic diarrhea associated with true disease. While identifying asymptomatic carriers may be important from an infection control standpoint, using formed stools only serves to dilute the sensitivity and specificity of the disease detection tests used in the clinical laboratory.

Diagnosis of antibiotic-associated *C. difficile* disease can be made by detection of toxin in the stool by enzyme immunoassay or cytopathic effect on cell line culture or culture for the organism with subsequent toxin detection. Enzyme immunoassay (EIA) has proven to be rapid, with results often available in 2–4 hours. The test is less sensitive then cell culture assay. It is important for the microbiologist to recognize that some EIA test kits detect only toxin A whereas others detect both toxins. There have been reported cases of *C. difficile*, which produce only toxin B so the diagnosis of PMC would be missed using an EIA kit, which detects only toxin A. ∞ Chapters 9 and 10 have information related to EIA methods.

The cytotoxic effect of filtered stool on cell lines has proven to be the most specific and sensitive test available (Schroeder, 2005). It is considered the "gold standard" for detection of *C. difficile* toxin because of its ability to accurately correlate with disease. The specimen is processed, added to fibroblast cells, incubated, and read for cytopathic changes in the cells. Once cell changes are detected, antiserum is added to the cell line. After reincubation, the cell line is examined for neutralization of the cytopathic effect. Neutralization of the toxin ensures the cytopathic effect is due to *C. difficile* toxin only. Results can take up to 3 days and requires an experienced microbiologist to read tissue culture assays. Culture for *C. difficile*, while the most sensitive, requires up to 5 days for recovery of the organism. Further testing must be done to test for toxin-producing strains, which can take up to 3 additional days.

REAL WORLD TIP

Repeat testing for *C. difficile* is discouraged. One or two specimens are all that is needed. If the first test result is negative, then a second more specific test, such as PCR or tissue culture cytotoxin assay, can be performed if the patient is symptomatic. Alternatively, if the first EIA result is negative, then a second EIA test can be performed approximately 48 hours later. If the first test result is positive, a repeat test should not be performed within 7 days. "Test of cure" toxin assays should not be performed on any patients (Welch, 2006; Borek, Aird, & Carroll, 2005; Cardona & Rand, 2008).

To prevent PMC in hospitalized patients, physicians should use antibiotics wisely in the treatment of any infection. Rapid diagnosis and early treatment can reduce the effect of diarrhea and the spread of spores in the environment. Adherence to infection control measures assist in the prevention of outbreaks. Once in the hospital environment, the spores are difficult to eradicate. Bleach is one of the few disinfectants that is recommended for the inactivation of *C. difficile* spores. The use of penicillins, cephalosporins, and clindamycin as well as the second and third cephalosporins such as cefotaxime, ceftriaxone, cefuroxime, and ceftazadime are associated with the development of PMC (Steiner, 2004). Treatment includes supportive care and discontinuation of the offending antibiotic(s). Metronidazole or vancomycin can be used to relieve symptoms. Relapses can occur after therapy has been stopped.

OTHER *CLOSTRIDIUM* SPECIES

Clostridium septicum is an aerotolerant gram-positive rod with subterminal spores. It is the second most common *Clostridium* spp. isolated after *C. perfringens*. This organism is recognized by its swarming colony, similar to that of *Proteus* spp. On reducible blood agar, it initially produces a "Medusa head" colony, which continues to grow to create a barely visible film across the agar surface after 24 hours, much like *Proteus* spp. It is called a "Medusa head" colony because of the snake-like projections around the edge of the colony. The other swarming *Clostridium* spp. is *C. tetani*. The two can be differentiated by *C. septicum*'s subterminal spores versus the terminal spores of *C. tetani*. Another differentiating test is the production of indole. *C. tetani* is indole positive whereas *C. septicum* does not produce indole. Figure 24-20 ■ demonstrates the unique irregular edges of a young colony of *C. septicum*.

The organism can be part of the normal gastrointestinal flora but is rarely found outside the intestine. Isolation of the organism from blood cultures should alert the physician to examine the patient for malignancies such as leukemia or colon cancer. Cancer is found in 70–80% of cases of *C. septicum* bacteremia (Lorber, 2005b). The organism escapes due to malignant lesions in the intestine.

■ **FIGURE 24-20** The colony of *C. septicum* begins as an irregular colony with finger-like tentacles originating from its edges. Within 24 hours, the colonies swarm to cover the entire agar plate, very much like *Proteus* spp.
From Public Health Image Library (PHIL)/CDC.

> ✓ **Checkpoint! 24–13 (Chapter Objective 1)**
>
> *Which of the following Clostridium spp. can be normal enteric flora but is not considered pathogenic until it produces toxin?*
>
> A. *C. tetani*
> B. *C. difficile*
> C. *C. septicum*
> D. *C. botulinum*

▶ NON-SPORE-FORMING GRAM-POSITIVE RODS

Most of the anaerobic non-spore-forming gram-positive rods are considered normal flora. Some, especially *Lactobacillus* spp., are an important first line of defense against colonization by potential pathogens. They vary in their tolerance to oxygen. Some are able to grow in the presence of oxygen and can produce tiny colonies in room air. While commonly isolated, *Propionibacterium* spp., *Bifidobacterium* spp., *Eubacterium* spp., and *Lactobacillus* spp. are usually considered to be of low virulence. *Actinomyces* spp. can be a significant pathogen of the head and neck, brain, and pulmonary and female genital systems. Most of the anaerobic non-spore-forming gram-positive rods, except for *Eubacterium* spp., are resistant to metronidazole, which is a common antibiotic used specifically in the treatment of anaerobic infections. Table 24-7✪ distinguishes the more commonly recognized anaerobic non-spore-forming gram-positive rods based on biochemical reactions and other characteristics.

ACTINOMYCES SPECIES

Actinomyces species are long, thin gram-positive rods that tend to branch like a tree and grow in a mass. The long rods can break into short club-shaped rods similar to those of "diphtheroids." They can exhibit a beaded or banded look due to irregular staining. Figure 24-21 ■ is a Gram stain of an aspirate of a brain abscess due to *Actinomyces* spp.

Actinomyces spp. are able to demonstrate aerotolerance and produce tiny colonies on enriched aerobic media in CO_2. Growth is much better under anaerobic conditions. Colonies are slow growing and may take 1–2 weeks to be visible. The

✪ TABLE 24-7

Biochemical and Other Characteristics of the More Commonly Recognized Anaerobic Non-Spore-Forming Gram-Positive Rods

Organism	Vancomycin (5 µg)	Kanamycin (1000 µg)	Colistin (10 µg)	Catalase	Indole	Nitrate Reduction	Metabolic End-Products	Oxygen Tolerance	Other
Actinomyces israelii	S	S	R	–	–	+	A, L, Su	MA	Molar tooth colony
Propionibacterium acnes	S	S	R	+	+	+	A, P	MA	Anaerobic diphtheroid
Bifidobacterium species	S	S	R	–	–	–	A > L	OA	Dog bone Gram stain morphology
Eubacterium species	S	S	R	–	–	–	A, B	OA	Sensitive to metronidazole
Eggerthella lenta	S	S	R	–	–	+	A	OA	Red fluorescence
Lactobacillus species	R	V	R	–	–	–	L	MA	Colony can resemble viridans *Streptococcus*

A, acetic acid; B, butyric acid; L, lactic acid; MA, microaerotolerant (can grow in presence of up to 10% oxygen); OA, obligate anaerobe; P, propionic acid; R, resistant; S, susceptible; Su, succinic acid; >, greater than; unshaded areas indicate presumptive identification reactions.

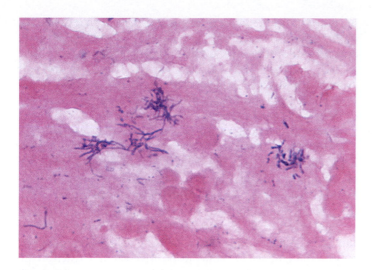

■ **FIGURE 24-21** The thin, branching gram-positive rods of *Actinomyces* spp. tend to grow in a mass and can mimic the hyphae of fungi on Gram stain. The long branches tend to break into short rods, as shown in this Gram stain of a brain abscess aspirate.
From Public Health Image Library (PHIL)/CDC.

organism may be missed when isolated with other organisms because they grow so slow. *Actinomyces israelii* is the most common pathogen of the genus and produces a characteristic white molar tooth colony. Figure 24-22 ■ demonstrates a young colony of *Actinomyces* spp. ∞ Chapter 19, "Aerobic Gram-Positive Rods," contains additional information on *Actinomyces*.

Actinomyces israelii is catalase negative, indole negative, and able to reduce nitrates. Fermentation of glucose, lactose, mannitol, and rhamnose differentiate it from other *Actinomyces*

spp. Biochemical testing and gas liquid chromatography are necessary to differentiate it from other non-spore-forming gram-positive rods. *A. israelii* produces succinic acid as one of its major metabolic products.

A. israelii is normal flora on the mucous membranes of the upper respiratory, gastrointestinal, and female genital tracts. Most infections are associated with individuals with a compromised immune system, especially those with acquired immunodeficiency syndrome (AIDS). Once the mucous membrane has been breached such as with surgery or trauma, the organism enters the soft tissues and causes **actinomycosis.** It involves the formation of purulent masses with the eventual development of sinus tracts to the body surface so the pus can escape. *A. israelii* is the most common cause of actinomycosis.

The purulent masses can be found anywhere in the body but especially in the jaw, chest, abdomen, and pelvic region. Foreign devices such as an intrauterine device (IUD) can also trigger infection. Most infections are chronic and occur in the jaw region due to poor oral hygiene, after dental surgery, or having a tooth pulled. Actinomycosis of the jaw is called lumpy jaw due to the prominent tissue swelling. Figure 24-23 ■

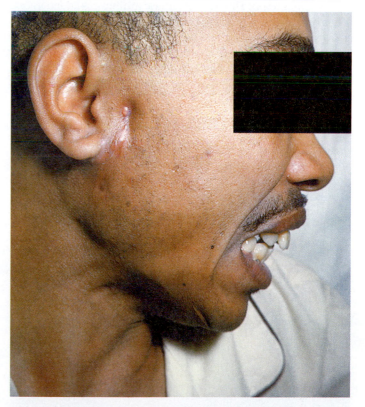

■ **FIGURE 24-23** An infection due to *Actinomyces* spp. in the soft tissue surrounding the jaw is present in this individual. A purulent discharge has worked its way to the skin surface through a sinus tract. While there is not significant swelling, this individual has actinomycosis of the jaw, which is also known as lumpy jaw.
From Public Health Image Library (PHIL)/CDC/Dr. Thomas F. Sellers/Emory University.

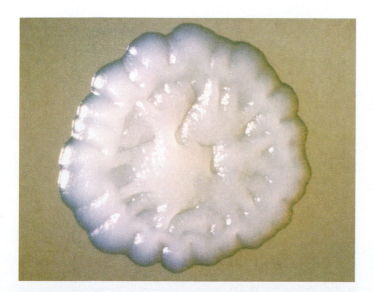

■ **FIGURE 24-22** This colony of *Actinomyces* spp. is 3 days old. The colony will continue to grow and heap upon itself until it looks similar to a molar tooth.
From Public Health Image Library (PHIL)/CDC/Dr. George.

demonstrates the purulent discharge draining from a sinus tract that has developed along the jawline.

The purulent discharge often contains characteristic sulfur granules. The small, yellow, hardened granules are actually colonies of the organism. The granules can be crushed and Gram stained to view the characteristic Gram reaction and microscopic morphology. The presence of sulfur granules in a purulent discharge is highly suspicious for actinomyosis. Figure 24-24 ■ illustrates a yellow colony of *Actinomyces* spp., which can mimic a sulfur granule in a purulent discharge.

  REAL WORLD TIP

Bifidobacterium spp., *Eubacterium* spp., and *Propionibacterium* spp. can also cause actinomycosis. All three genera are branching, non-spore-forming gram-positive rods similar to *Actinomyces* spp.

High doses of intravenous penicillin and a beta-lactamase inhibitor for 4–6 weeks are required for treatment of infections by *Actinomyces* spp. The beta-lactamase inhibitor is added in case other organisms, which are beta-lactamase producers, are present. This is followed by oral penicillin for 6–12 months (Chow, 2005). Abscesses must be drained and infected tissue debrided. Tetracycline, erythromycin, and clindamycin are viable options for penicillin-allergic patients but are not quite as effective.

PROPIONIBACTERIUM SPECIES

Propionibacterium spp. is the most common isolate of the anaerobic non-spore-forming gram-positive rods. They appear as clubbed, pleomorphic gram-positive rods in pallisades. Their log jam or Chinese letter arrangement mimics that of aerobic diphtheroids so much so that it should probably be called an anaerobic diphtheroid. Colonies are small and gray to white. It can be microaerotolerant in the presence of CO_2 so it can be confused with facultative diphtheroids but it grows better under anaerobic conditions. Figure 24-25 ■ demonstrates the diphtheroid-like appearance of *P. acnes* on Gram stain. Figure 24-26 ■ shows its colony on reducible blood agar.

Propionibacterium acnes is the most common isolate of the genus. It is normal skin flora and often isolated as a blood culture contaminant. It is best known as the causative agent of acne in adolescents. The organism can be presumptively identified based on its diphtheroid-appearing Gram stain, positive catalase reaction, production of indole, and ability to reduce nitrate. It produces propionic acid as one of its major metabolic end-product, hence its name. Its positive-catalase reaction differentiates it from other non-spore-forming gram-positive rods such as *Actinomyces israelii*, *Bifidobacterium*, *Eubacterium*, and *Lactobacillus* spp.

P. acnes has an affinity for artificial medical devices, just like another common normal skin flora organism, *Staphylococcus not S. aureus*. It can cause infections associated with artificial joints, intravenous catheters, central nervous system shunts, and prosthetic heart valves. It is also associated with keratitis when the cornea has been cut or punctured, such as in cataract surgery. Bacteremia can lead to endocarditis. Care must be taken in determining the significance of blood and other sterile body fluid isolates since they are common skin contaminants but also able to cause significant infections. Repeated isolation from sterile body sites probably indicates a true infection.

■ FIGURE 24-24 This yellow colony mimics a granule of sulfur. It may be present in the purulent discharge associated with actinomycosis. If present, it should be processed for culture.
From Public Health Image Library (PHIL)/CDC/Dr. George.

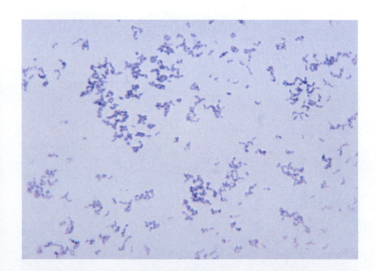

■ FIGURE 24-25 The Gram stain of *Propionibacterium acnes* can mimic that of the *Corynebacterium* spp. known as diphtheroids. These pleomorphic gram-positive rods can be clubbed and appear to palisade.
From Public Health Image Library (PHIL)/CDC/Bobby Strong.

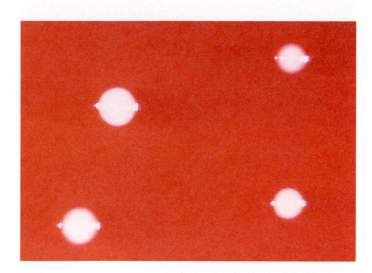

 FIGURE 24-26 The photograph demonstrates colonies of *P. acnes* on reducible blood agar after 3 days of incubation. While the organism may demonstrate pin-point colonies on the aerobic agar plate used for aerotolerance testing, due to microaerotolerance with CO_2, it will produce better growth on the anaerobic agar plate. This will help differentiate it from facultative diphtheroids.
From Public Health Image Library (PHIL)/CDC/Bobby Strong.

@ ■ **REAL WORLD TIP**

Each facility must monitor its blood culture contamination rate in order to ensure the quality of specimen collection and transportation, which is part of the pre-analytical phase of the clinical diagnosis process. A contamination rate of 2–3% is usually used to determine the quality of blood culture specimens received. The isolation of skin flora such as *Staphylococcus not S. aureus* and *Propionibacterium acnes* can be monitored to determine the blood culture contamination rate. If the established contamination rate is exceeded, an improvement plan must be implemented.

Propionibacterium acnes is usually susceptible to most antimicrobial agents including penicillin, carabapenems, and clindamycin (Midura, 1996). Effective treatment requires the removal of infected medical devices and the use of appropriate antimicrobial agents.

@ ■ **REAL WORLD TIP**

Acne is caused by the body's response to the metabolism of lipids by *Propionibacterium acnes* in the skin follicles and sebaceous glands. Topical erythromycin and clindamycin are commonly used as treatment options. *P. acnes* can develop resistance to both during treatment for acne (Mascini & Verhoff, 2005).

LACTOBACILLUS SPECIES

Lactobacillus spp. are long, thin, non-spore-forming gram-positive rods that may form long chains. They can also appear as coccobacilli. Figure 24-27 ■ demonstrates the characteristic Gram stain of these organisms. As a group, they are microaerotolerant and may appear as pin-point colonies when incubated in CO_2. Colonies may display alpha or gamma hemolysis. The organism produces lactic acid as one of their major metabolic product, hence its name.

Lactobacillus spp. can resemble the viridians streptococci with their colony morphology and negative catalase, indole, and nitrate reduction. *Lactobacillus* spp. will produce long, thin gram-positive rods when grown in a thioglycolate broth while the viridians streptococci form gram-positive cocci in chains. It is difficult to differentiate to species level even with commercial identification systems.

@ ■ **REAL WORLD TIP**

Small alpha-hemolytic colonies in the upper respiratory tract are usually viridians streptococci whereas the same colony type in a female genital tract are usually *Lactobacillus* spp.

Lactobacillus spp. are best known as the predominant normal flora organism of the female genital tract. It can also be a member of the normal flora of the intestine and oral cavity. Its major metabolic byproduct, lactic acid, maintains the acidic

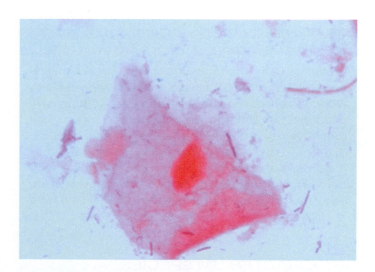

 FIGURE 24-27 This Gram stain of a female genital tract demonstrates the characteristic long, thin, non-spore-forming gram-positive rods of *Lactobacillus* spp. These organisms maintain the normally acidic pH of the female vaginal tract by their production of lactic acid. They are shown here adhering to a squamous epithelial cell. These cells line the wall of the vaginal tract.

pH of the vagina, which prevents colonization by potential pathogens. The loss of *Lactobacillus* spp., often due to antibiotic use, allows other organisms to overgrow and cause disorders such as bacterial vaginosis and yeast infections. ∞ Chapter 36, "Genital System," provides information on the laboratory diagnosis of bacterial vaginosis.

 REAL WORLD TIP

Lactobacillus spp. produce hydrogen peroxide, which is bactericidal to *Prevotella bivia* and *Gardnerella vaginalis*. With antibiotic use, there is a potential for the loss of vaginal *Lactobacillus* spp. *P. bivia*, *G. vaginalis*, and other anaerobic gram-negative rods can then overgrow and cause the signs and symptoms of bacterial vaginosis.

Infections are rare. Even though the organism is fairly innocent and usually considered beneficial, it can cause endocarditis and septicemia in immunocompromised patients or those with severe underlying disease. It is associated with a high mortality rate in cases of subacute endocarditis (Mascini & Verhoff, 2005). Organisms that cause disease are usually endogenous. Care must be taken in determining the significance of isolation of *Lactobacillus* spp. Repeated isolation from sterile body sites may assist in the decision. *Lactobacillus* spp. are intrinsically resistant to vancomycin and display variable resistance to the cephalosporins. Pencillin and an aminoglycoside provide the best synergistic therapy for *Lactobacillus* endocarditis (Mascini & Verhoff, 2005).

 REAL WORLD TIP

Probiotics allow live organisms to be taken internally in order to benefit the host. *Lactobacillus* species and *Bifidobacterium* species have been shown to survive passage through the gastrointestinal tract. They reestablish the intestinal flora, especially after antibiotic use. The Federal Drug Administration (FDA) has determined it is safe to take these organisms internally because they are already part of normal human flora. The organisms are available commercially in the form of cheese, yogurt, dairy drinks, and capsules.

BIFIDOBACTERIUM SPECIES

Bifidobacterium spp. appear as gram-positive, highly pleomorphic rods with branching or bifurcated ends. They can resemble bone-shaped dog biscuits due to their splint ends. Figure 24-28 ■ demonstrates the typical gram stain of *Bifidobacterium* spp. The obligate anaerobic colonies are usually small and

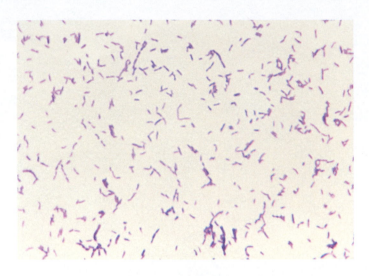

■ **FIGURE 24-28** This Gram stain of *Bifidobacterium* spp. reveals its pleomorphic nature. The gram positive rods can appear branching due to their bifurcated or "Y"-shaped ends.
From Public Health Image Library (PHIL)/CDC/Bobby Strong.

white, as seen in Figure 24-29 ■. The organism is considered normal flora in the mouth and intestine. As a group, the genus is catalase, indole, and nitrate reduction negative. It produces more acetic acid than lactic acid as its major metabolic endproducts. The organism is rarely isolated but may be a major pathogen for dental caries (Becker et al., 2002). It has been associated with infections such as peritonitis, brain abscesses, decubitus ulcers, and wound infections of the genitourinary tract. If infection of a sterile body site occurs, penicillin or amoxicillin, vancomycin, carabapenems, cefoxitin, and clindamycin are considered effective. *Bifidobacterium* species are

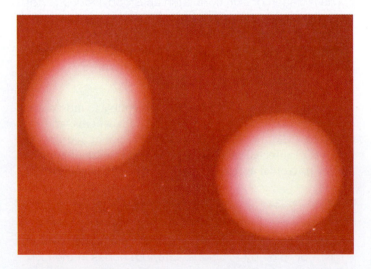

■ **FIGURE 24-29** *Bifidobacterium* spp., at 3 days incubation, displays smooth, white colonies on reducible blood agar. It is rarely isolated as a significant pathogen.
From Public Health Image Library (PHIL)/CDC/Bobby Strong.

intrinsically resistant to aminoglycosides (Moubareck, Gavini, Vaugien, Butel, & Doucet-Populaire, 2005).

 REAL WORLD TIP

An easy way to remember the Gram stain morphology of *Bifidobacterium* spp. is to think of a bone-shaped dog biscuit. The ends of these gram-positive rods often split like that in the fork of a tree or the end of a bone. Just remember the "fido" in *Bi**fido**bacterium* in order to remember the dog bone morphology.

 REAL WORLD TIP

On initial Gram stain, *Bifidobacterium* spp. can resemble *Actinomyces* spp. Both are very similar in their biochemical reactions. To differentiate, place the organism in a thioglycolate broth and incubate overnight. *Actinomyces* spp. will retain their characteristic branching morphology but *Bifidobacterium* spp. will produce pleomorphic, diphtheroid-like rods with little or no branching.

EUBACTERIUM SPECIES

Eubacterium spp. is a very pleomorphic rod or coccobacilli in pairs and chains. Its colony is small and gray. One species' colony can resemble the molar tooth morphology of *Actinomyces israelii*. It is found as normal flora in the mouth and intestine.

As a group, *Eubacterium* spp. are catalase negative, indole variable, and nitrate negative. Its major metabolic end-product is butyric acid. One organism, *Eggerthella lenta,* previously known as *Eubacterium lentum,* can be presumptively identified based on its ability to reduce nitrate and fluoresce red under an ultraviolet light (Isenberg, 2004).

These organisms have been found in infections of the female genital tract associated with the use of an intrauterine device (Mascini & Verhoff, 2005). Most infections are associated with the oral cavity or colon as a source for the organism. It can cause bacteremia in individuals with malignancy of the gastrointestinal tract. Treatment can include penicillin, most

 Checkpoint! 24–14 (Chapter Objective 7b)

Which of the anaerobic non-spore-forming gram-positive rods is considered the "anaerobic diphtheroids"?

A. *Actinomyces species*
B. *Biofidobacterium species*
C. *Eubacterium species*
D. *Propionibacterium species*

cephalosporins, and clindamycin. It is susceptible to metronidazole, unlike other anaerobic gram-positive non-spore-forming rods (Mascini & Verhoff, 2005).

▶ GRAM-NEGATIVE RODS

The anaerobic gram-negative rods are the most commonly isolated anaerobes associated with infection (Tzianabos & Kasper, 2005). They can also be some of the most antibiotic-resistant anaerobes isolated. Most infections are usually related to surgery, trauma, or disease of the mucous membranes where they reside. *Bacteroides* spp. are found primarily in the colon and female genital tract whereas *Prevotella* spp., *Porphyromonas* spp., and *Fusobacterium* spp. are usually considered residents of the upper respiratory tract and vaginal canal. Table 24-8✿ differentiates the more commonly recognized anaerobic gram-negative rods based on biochemical reactions and other important characteristics.

The pathogenicity of the anaerobic gram-negative rods relates to several factors they possess. The presence of histolytic enzymes allows them to destroy tissue and spread throughout the body. Because they are gram-negative organisms, their outer cell membrane contains lipopolysaccharide (LPS). The LPS of some anaerobic gram-negative rods seems to be less toxic than that of aerobes. The decreased pathogenic effect may be due to a slight change in the chemical structure of the LPS molecule (Chow, 2004). *B. fragilis* group is known for its capsule production, which promotes abscess formation. This group of organisms also possesses structures (pili or fimbriae) that allow them to adhere to the epithelium.

Most of the anaerobic gram-negative rods, especially the *B. fragilis* group, are able to produce beta-lactamase. This enzyme destroys the beta-lactam ring of penicillins and other related antibiotics. The ability to destroy penicillin not only benefits the anaerobic gram-negative rods but also other facultative organisms that are usually present in an infection.

BACTEROIDES FRAGILIS GROUP

The *Bacteroides fragilis* group appears as gram-negative coccibacilli or rods that may stain irregularly so they appear to have vacuoles or clear areas within the cell. They may even appear to have swellings within the cells but they do not produce spores. The group consists of about 10 different species, with *B. fragilis* as the most common isolate. *B. distasonis, B. thetaiotaomicron,* and *B. vulgatus* are occasional isolates. Figures 24-30a–30d ■ illustrate the pleomorphic nature of the *Bacteroides fragilis* group on Gram stain.

The *Bacteroides fragilis* group makes up the largest portion of the normal flora in the gastrointestinal tract. Surprisingly, *B. fragilis,* one member of the group, comprises only 0.5% of the GI flora but accounts for most human anaerobic infections (Lorber, 2005a). They typically appear as large, wet, gray colonies on reducible blood agar and laked kanamycin–

⭐ TABLE 24-8

Differentiation of the More Commonly Isolated Anaerobic Gram-Negative Rods

Organism	Vancomycin (5 µg)	Kanamycin (1000 µg)	Colistin (10 µg)	Catalase	Lipase	Indole	Stimulated by Bile	Esculin	Salicin	Trehalose	Pigmentation	Fluorescence	Oxygen Tolerance	Other
Bacteroides fragilis group	R	R	R	+	–	–	+	+	V	V	–	–	OA	
B. distasonis	R	R	R	+	–	–	+	+	+	+	–	–	OA	Member of *B. fragilis* group
B. fragilis	R	R	R	+	–	–	+	+	–	–	–	–	OA	Member of *B. fragilis* group
B. thetaiotaomicron	R	R	R	+	–	+	+	+	–	+	–	–	OA	Member of *B. fragilis* group
B. vulgatus	R	R	R	+	–	–	+	–	–	–	–	–	OA	Member of *B. fragilis* group
Fusobacterium necrophorum	R	S	S	–	+	+	–	–	–	–	–	Chartreuse	OA	
F. nucleatum	R	S	S	–	–	+	–	–	–	–	–	Chartreuse	OA	Long, thin, fusiform gram-negative rods
Prevotella melaninogenica	R	R	V	–	–	–	–	–	–	–	Tan to black	Red	OA	
P. intermedia	R	R	S	–	+	+	–	–	–	–	Tan to black	Red	OA	
Porphyromonas asaccharolytica	S	R	R	–	–	+	–	U	U	U	Tan to black	Red	OA	
P. gingivalis	S	R	R	–	–	–	–	U	U	U	Tan to black	–	OA	

OA, obligate anaerobe; R, resistant; S, susceptible; U, unknown; V, variable; unshaded areas indicate presumptive identification reactions.

vancomycin agar after 48 hours of incubation. Figure 24-31 demonstrates the typical colony of *Bacteroides fragilis*.

 REAL WORLD TIP

There are about 10^{11}–10^{12} organisms per gram of stool. Anaerobes make up about 99.9% of these organisms and are represented by 300–400 different species (Brook, 2004).

REAL WORLD TIP

Bile acids are produced by the liver to aid in the digestion and adsorption of fats in the intestine. *Bacteroides* spp. are stimulated by the presence of bile and have the ability to deconjugate the unused bile acids. The deconjugated bile salts are returned to the liver and reconjugated for use again. This prevents the loss of bile acids in the feces.

The *B. fragilis* group is resistant to all three special potency disks: kanamycin, vancomycin, and colistin. They are further grouped based on their ability to grow in the presence of 20% bile. *Bacteroides* bile esculin (BBE) agar can be used to selectively isolate these organisms based on their ability to grow in high concentrations of bile. It further differentiates this group from other gram-negative rods based on their ability to hydrolyze esculin. Most of the *B. fragilis* group appear as large black colonies with dark halos on BBE agar due to esculin hydrolysis. Refer to Figure 24-4 to view *B. fragilis* group colonies on BBE agar.

Resistance to all three potency disks and ability to grow in the presence of 20% bile can presumptively identify an anaerobic gram-negative rod as a member of the *B. fragilis* group. All four of the most common species isolated are usually catalase positive. *B. vulgatus* is the only member of the *B. fragilis* group that does not hydrolyze esculin. *B. thetaiotaomicron* can be differentiated from the other three species by its ability to produce indole. *B. distasonis* is able to ferment salicin whereas the others cannot. *B. fragilis* produces biochemical reactions very similar to *B. distasonis* but *B. fragilis* is unable to ferment salicin and trehalose.

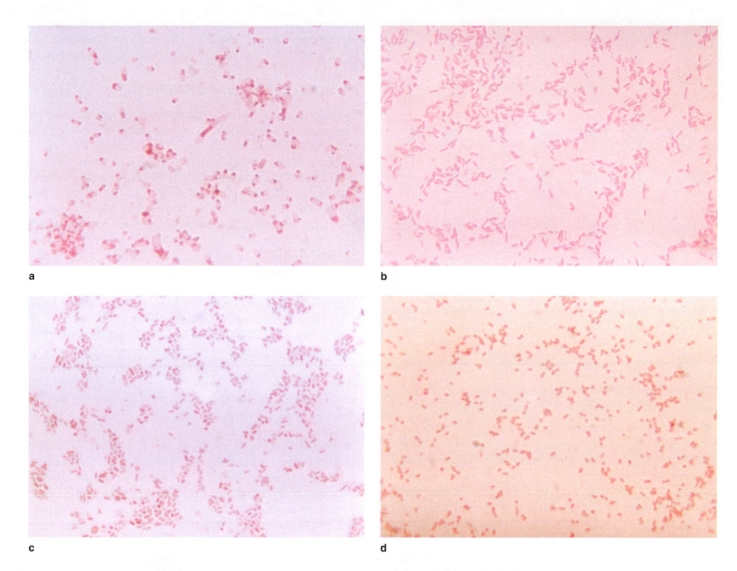

a

b

c

d

■ **FIGURE 24-30** These four Gram stains of the *Bacteroides fragilis* group illustrates the variability in the size, shape, and staining of this collection of anaerobic gram-negative rods. **a.** Demonstrates vacuoles in *B. thetaiotaomicron*. **b.** Shows the typical gram-negative rod in the Gram stain of *B. fragilis*. **c.** Displays the faint staining gram-negative rods and coccobacilli of *B. vulgatus*. **d.** Shows *B. distasonis* exhibiting gram-negative coccobacilli morphology.
From Public Health Image Library (PHIL)/CDC/Dr. V. R. Dowell, Jr.

For an infection to become established there is usually some type of traumatic event in the gastrointestinal or female genital tracts. The aerobic and anaerobic organisms escape to enter the surrounding tissues. As the facultative anaerobes begin to grow, they reduce the redox potential of the tissue to create an anaerobic environment. The obligate anaerobes begin to grow and flourish. Once established, the anaerobes can gain access to the bloodstream and spread throughout the body.

The *B. fragilis* group is known for infections in the peritoneal area. A ruptured appendix or abdominal surgery provides the classic patient history for infection with these anaerobic gram-negative rods. Intra-abdominal infections are usually polymicrobic, consisting of up to three anaerobes, espe-

cially *B. fragilis,* and at least two facultative aerobes such as *E. coli* and *Enterococcus* spp. (Lorber, 2005a).

Decubitus ulcers or bed sores can develop on the bony portions of the body such as at the base of the tailbone and hips due to constant pressure from lying in bed. The loss of blood flow, presence of necrotic tissue, and potential for fecal contamination set up an environment ideal for the *B. fragilis* group.

About 10% of cases of bacteremia are due to anaerobic gram-negative rods (Brook, 2004). *B. fragilis* is isolated about 70% of the time (Lorber, 2005a). Bacteremia with *B. fragilis* group is usually due to infection somewhere in the body that seeds to the bloodstream.

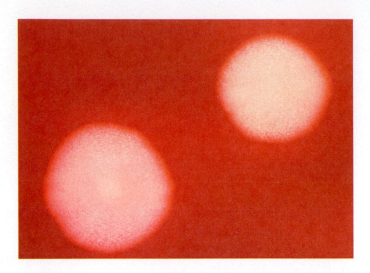

■ **FIGURE 24-31** These colonies of *B. fragilis*, on reducible blood agar after 48 hours of incubation, demonstrate the typical large, gray, shiny, slightly speckled appearance associated with this group of organisms.
From Public Health Image Library (PHIL)/CDC/Dr. V. R. Dowell, Jr.

 REAL WORLD TIP

Blood cultures commonly involve the use of both aerobic and anaerobic media for the recovery of organisms. The incidence of anaerobic bacteremia is decreasing. One study showed that anaerobic bloodstream infections occurred in only 0.14% of their facility's high-risk patient population (Chandler, Morton, Byrd, Fields, & Roy, 2000). It has been proposed that anaerobic blood cultures be used selectively rather than routinely. A cost savings could be realized if a policy establishing criteria for the selective use of anaerobic blood culture was in place. A second study revealed that when the entire volume of blood collected was used for two aerobic blood culture bottles rather than the traditional aerobic and anaerobic blood culture bottles, the yield of clinically significant aerobic isolates rose by about 6% (Morris, Wilson, Mirrett, & Reller, 1993).

Treatment of anaerobic gram-negative rod infections often requires surgical intervention in combination with antimicrobial therapy. Surgery is necessary to drain purulent material, remove necrotic tissue, improve tissue oxygenation, and repair mucous membrane trauma, if possible. Because the *B. fragilis* group can vary in their resistance to antimicrobial agents, susceptibility testing should be performed when isolated as a significant pathogen.

The antimicrobial agents most active against the *B. fragilis* group include a beta-lactam plus a beta-lactamase inhibitor, the carbapenems, cefoxitin, chloramphenicol, clindamycin, and metronidazole. Penicillin, used alone, is ineffective due to the ability of these organisms to produce beta-lactamase.

FUSOBACTERIUM SPECIES

These long, thin, fusiform, and sometimes very pleomorphic anaerobic gram-negative rods are resistant to vancomycin but sensitive to kanamycin and colistin. Based on their special potency disk pattern they may not grow or grow poorly on laked kanamycin–vancomycin agar. *Fusobacterium* spp. are considered normal flora of the oral cavity, upper respiratory tract, and female genital tract. Infections are usually found in the head and neck area and respiratory tract due to a break in the mucous membranes.

They produce enzymes that help them penetrate tissues and their cell membrane lipopolysaccharide (LPS) has the ability to initiate disseminated intravascular coagulation as seen with some facultative anaerobic gram-negative rods. The two most common isolates, *Fusobacterium nucleatum* and *F. necrophorum*, are catalase negative, produce indole, and are not stimulated to grow in 20% bile. Their colonies display a chartreuse (yellow-green) color under long-wave ultraviolet light, as seen in Figure 24-10. They typically produce a rancid butter odor due to the production of butyric acid from glucose.

Fusobacterium nucleatum

Fusobacterium nucleatum appears as a long, slender, fusiform gram-negative rod, as seen in Figure 24-32 ■. The organism has three different colony morphologies that can be observed: (1) irregular and resemble kosher salt grains or bread crumbs; (2) large, smooth with a speckled or ground-glass appearance, as noted in Figure 24-33 ■; and (3) small, smooth, gray-white.

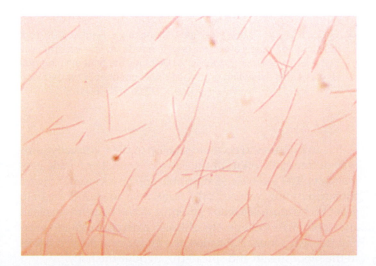

■ **FIGURE 24-32** *Fusobacterium nucleatum*, an anaerobic gram-negative rod, possesses a characteristic microscopic morphology that mimics toothpicks. These long, thin, tapered rods are easily recognizable.
From Public Health Image Library (PHIL)/CDC/Dr. V. R. Dowell, Jr.

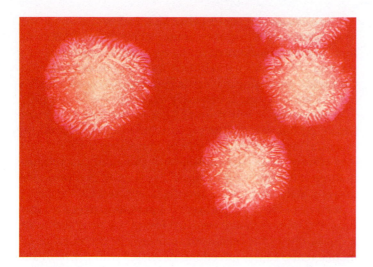

■ **FIGURE 24-33** One of the three colony morphologies of *F. nucleatum* is shown here. It is described as a large, white-gray, and translucent colony with a speckled or crystal-like appearance.
From Public Health Image Library (PHIL)/CDC/Dr. V. R. Dowell, Jr.

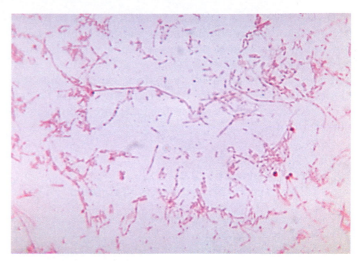

■ **FIGURE 24-34** *Fusobacterium necrophorum* is an extremely pleomorphic organism ranging from coccobacilli to very long, filamentous gram-negative rods. Note the bulbous (swollen), dark staining ends of some of the rods.
From Public Health Image Library (PHIL)/CDC/Dr. V. R. Dowell, Jr.

This catalase-negative and indole-positive species can be differentiated from *F. necrophorum* by its negative lipase.

F. nucleatum is one of the predominant anaerobes in the oral cavity, especially in dental plaque and the upper respiratory tract. It usually causes infections in the same areas. It is often one of the multiple aerobes and anaerobes found in cases of aspiration pneumonia (Lorber, 2005a). With complications of oral and respiratory infections, *F. nucleatum* can escape to cause bacteremia and infections in other body sites such as the brain and bone.

F. nucleatum is able to produce beta-lactamase so the use of penicillin is not advised. If a beta-lactam antibiotic is used it must be combined with a beta-lacatamse inhibitor such as clavulinic acid, sulbactam or tazobactam. Metronidazole, cefoxitin, chloramphenicol, and piperacillin are usually effective.

Fusobacterium necrophorum

F. necrophorum is the most commonly isolated species (Brook, 2003b). It appears as extremely pleomorphic gram-negative rods or coccobacilli. It may display swollen, rounded ends. Figure 24-34 ■ demonstrates the pleomorphic morphology associated with the organism. Its colony on reducible blood agar appears as a dull gray-yellow colony with a nipple-like projection in its center. It may display beta hemolysis but there is usually a greening effect around the colonies on blood containing media when exposed to oxygen.

F. necrophorum is the only *Fusobacterium* spp. that produces lipase on egg yolk agar. The rainbow sheen is characteristic for this organism. An indole-positive, lipase-positive, anaerobic gram-negative rod that is resistant to vancomycin and sensitive to kanamycin and colistin can be presumptively identified as *Fusobacterium necrophorum*.

Because of *F. necrophorum*'s close association with upper respiratory mucosal membranes, it can be recovered from cases of otitis media, tonsillar and pharyngeal abscesses, sinusitis, and deep neck abscesses after head and neck surgery. It is a key pathogen in a synergistic infection called **Vincent's angina**, an acute necrotizing infection of the pharynx occurring in children. Spirochetes play a synergistic role and escalate the infectious process. There appears to be shift toward a predominance of anaerobes in the makeup of the flora in the mouth similar to the process of bacterial vaginosis. The patient complains of a bad taste in the mouth and foul-smelling breath. Physical examination shows a purulent discharge that coats the throat and tonsils in addition to bleeding ulcers. Because of its resemblance to the pseudomembrane of diphtheria, the two must be differentiated. Necrotizing ulcerative gingivitis or "trench mouth" can be a complication of Vincent's angina. This was a common condition in World War I troops due to the terrible conditions of trench warfare. Trench mouth is associated with painful, bleeding gums that are covered with a grayish membrane. A Gram stain or methylene blue stain of the exudate of Vincent's angina will display a predominance of rods and spiral organisms. A culture should not be performed. The infection can spread to reach the blood and eventually other sterile body sites. The infection can result from poor oral hygiene and immunodeficiency.

F. necrophorum is also associated with **Lemierre's disease** in adolescents. After bacterial pharyngitis, this organism can cause deep peritonsillar abscesses. The abscesses penetrate into the neck tissue to eventually reach the jugular vein. The organism then penetrates the large neck vein to cause emboli or clots. Pieces of the infected clots break off and spread to the lungs, liver, and other organs of the body. There is a high mortality rate with this disease even with treatment.

Depending on the extent of infection, surgery to remove necrotic tissue and antibiotics may be necessary. *Fusobacterium* spp. can produce beta-lactamase so if pencillin is used it must be accompanied by a beta-lactamase inhibitor as well. Clindamycin, chloramphenicol, cefoxitin, carbapenems, and metronidazole are also effective. Erythromycin and tetracycline are not effective as well as the first- and second-generation quinilones.

 Checkpoint! 24–15 (Chapter Objectives 7d and 7i)

The Bacteroides fragilis group can easily be differentiated from Fusobacterium necrophorum by its:

A. *ability to grow in bile.*

B. *level of oxygen tolerance.*

C. *pigmentation.*

D. *ability to produce beta-lactamase.*

BILE-SENSITIVE, PIGMENTED GRAM-NEGATIVE RODS

The *Prevotella* spp. and *Porphyromonas* spp. are known for their ability to produce tan to black pigmented colonies after growing about 1–3 weeks on medium containing laked red blood cells. Prior to pigment production, they can be recognized by their brick red fluorescence under ultraviolet light.

As a group, they appear as pleomorphic gram-negative rods or coccobacilli. They are not able to grow in the presence of bile. *Prevotella* spp. are resistant to kanamycin and vancomycin and display variable reactions against colistin. *Porphyromonas* spp. are sensitive to vancomycin but resistant to kanamycin and colistin. These special potency disk patterns can assist in the differentiation of the two. Most *Porphyromonas* spp. capable of causing disease in humans are indole positive. An indole positive, pigmented gram-negative rod that is sensitive to vancomycin can be presumptively identified as a member of the genus *Porphyromonas*.

Both genera are considered normal flora of the mucous membranes of the mouth and upper respiratory tract while *Prevotella* spp. is usually found more often than *Porphyromonas* spp. in the female genital tract. They are able to produce enzymes that break down tissue allowing them to move from breaks in the mucosal membranes to deep in the body. They also have the ability to produce beta-lactamase.

Prevotella melaninogenica

Prevotella melaninogenica, a pale-staining gram-negative coccobacilli, is one of the most commonly isolated organisms of the genus. On reducible blood agar, the colony presents as medium gray and slightly wet. Its species name comes from its ability to eventually produce a brown or black (melanin) pigmented colony on laked kanamycin–vancomycin agar. The colonies produce a typical brick-red fluorescence.

P. melaninogenica requires vitamin K and hemin for growth so all media used for isolation must include these compounds. In its natural environment in the body, other organisms may produce the vitamin K required by *P. melaninogenica*. Biochemically, the organism is catalase, indole, and lipase negative but additional testing is necessary to definitively identify it.

P. melaninogenica is normal flora in the oral cavity and female genital system. The presence of a capsule around the organism increases its virulence by promoting abscess formation (Chow, 2005). Its capsule and the ability to produce numerous enzymes aid in tissue destruction and promotes invasion into other tissues and the bloodstream.

It is one of the causative agents of **periodontitis** with gum tissue inflammation and eventual loss of the bone and teeth. It can be one of the organisms recovered in aspiration pneumonia. It also causes infections associated with the head and neck area such as tonsillar abscesses. Because of its ability to cause oral infections and the close proximity to the brain, the organism can invade and spread to cause brain abscesses. In the female genital tract, it is found in mixed aerobic and anaerobic infections both postsurgery and postpartum (Chow, 2005).

P. melaninogenica produces beta-lactamase so they automatically display resistance to penicillin. Metronidazole, imipenem (a penicillin and beta-lactamase inhibitor), and clindamycin are considered firstline-use antibiotics. Cefoxitin, chloramphenical, and piperacillin may be used as second line use antibiotics.

Prevotella intermedia

This gram-negative coccobacilli produces a black pigmented colony on blood containing agar. Its pigment production is usually much darker on laked kanamycin–vancomycin agar than on reducible blood agar. It is considered normal oral and vaginal flora. A pigmented, indole, and lipase-positive gram-negative rod can be presumptively identified as *P. intermedia*. It has the ability to produce enzymes that allow the organism to invade epithelial cells and it is associated with oropharyngeal and pulmonary infections. It can produce beta-lactamase so the use of penicillin is not advised. Metronidazole, a penicillin in combination with a β-lactamase inhibitor, chloramphenicaol, and imipenem are recommended for treatment.

Porphyromonas asaccharolytica

Porphyromonas asaccharolytica is a pleomorphic gram-negative rod that grows as a gray colony, eventually producing brown to black pigment with time. Because it is sensitive to vancomycin, it will not grow on laked kanamycin–vancomycin agar. It produces the typical red fluorescence seen with other pigmented gram-negative rods. Biochemically *P. asaccharolytica* is indole positive. Its special potency disk pattern will differentiate it from another indole-positive pigmented gram-negative rod, *Prevotella intermedia*. Additional biochemical testing is necessary to differentiate it from other pigmented *Porphyromonas* spp.

It is primarily an oropharyngeal organism known for infections of the oral cavity such as periodontal disease. It can be part of the normal vaginal flora. Once infection is established, a local infection can become systemic. It has the ability to produce beta-lactamase so penicillin is not advised unless used in tandem with a beta-lactamase inhibitor.

Porphyromonas gingivalis

Porphyromonas gingivalis is a pleomorphic gram-negative rod that grows as a black-pigmented colony within 7–10 days. It is unique because it does not display red fluorescence like the other pigmented *Prevotella* and *Porphyromonas* spp. It is indole positive like most others in the genus. Additional biochemical testing is required to differentiate it from others in the genus.

As its species name implies, it is found primarily in the mouth, especially in the **gingiva** or gum tissue. The organism is able to bind to gingival epithelial cells, invading them using enzymes. Once it has invaded the tissue, the organism causes inflammation of the gingiva, destruction of the periodontal tissues and the bone that holds the teeth in place, and eventually tooth loss. As the infection progresses, the organism can enter the bone of the jaw and eventually become systemic.

 REAL WORLD TIP

The identification of some anaerobes can provide the physician with an indication to the original source of the organism. Certain anaerobes are known to reside "above the waist/diaphragm" or "below the waist/diaphragm." Regardless of the site of infection, the isolation of *Porphyromonas gingivalis* should guide the physician to look for an oral source while the isolation of *B. fragilis* group indicates an intestinal origin.

Because of potential resistance due to beta-lactamase production, the beta-lactam antibiotics such as penicillin should not be used unless accompanied by a beta-lactamase inhibitor. Imipenem, metronidazole, and chloramphenicol are usually considered effective.

 ### Checkpoint! 24–16 (Chapter Objectives 7d and 7i)

A key characteristic that will easily differentiate Prevotella spp. and Porphyromonas spp. is:

  A. *pigmentation.*
  B. *fluorescence.*
  C. *ability to grow on LKV.*
  D. *Gram stain.*

BILE-SENSITIVE, NONPIGMENTED GRAM-NEGATIVE RODS

There are many other clinically significant *Bacteroides, Prevotella,* and *Porphyromonas* spp. that are gram-negative rods, do not grow in the presence of bile, and are not able to produce pigment. The colony of *Bacteroides ureolyticus,* a member of the normal flora of the upper respiratory tract and intestine, has a unique colony that is able to pit the agar. It is also able to hydrolyze urea. *Prevotella oralis* and *P. oris-buccae* are normal mouth flora known to cause infection of the orofacial area. *Prevotella bivia* and *P. disiens* are members of the normal vaginal flora and important in obstetric and gynecological infections. They are known for causing endometritis, amnionitis, and septic abortion as well as pelvic inflammatory disease (PID) and abscesses of the fallopian tubes and ovaries. Both are able to fluoresce light orange to pink rather than the traditional brick-red color.

▶ GRAM-POSITIVE COCCI

The anaerobic gram-positive cocci include the most commonly isolated genera *Peptostreptococcus, Peptococcus, Peptoniphilus,* and *Finegoldia.* This group is the second most commonly isolated anaerobes after gram-negative rods (Isenberg, 2004). They are most often isolated in mixed cultures but can occur in pure culture in up to 10% of cases (Brook, 2003b). They can be found on the skin, upper respiratory tract, intestine, and genitourinary tract. Infections can occur in all body sites. The anaerobic gram-positive cocci are sensitive to vancomycin and variable in their reaction with kanamycin and resistant to colistin. Table 24-9✿ differentiates the more commonly recognized anaerobic gram-positive cocci, gram-negative cocci, and microaerophilic *Streptococcus* based on biochemical and other characteristics.

There have been recent updates to the classifications of some of the more commonly isolated organisms. Most organisms were previously included in the genus *Peptostreptococcus.* Two new genera have been proposed, *Finegoldia* and *Peptoniphilus.*

The microaerophilic *Streptococcus* are gram-positive cocci that appear as obligate anaerobes on initial isolation but display microaerophilic growth on subculture. They have been removed from the anaerobic gram-positive cocci and placed with the viridians streptococci. It is important to be able to differentiate them from the anaerobic gram-positive cocci because each requires different antibiotics treatment.

FINEGOLDIA MAGNA

Finegoldia magna (previously known as *Peptostreptococcus magnus*) is the most pathogenic of the anaerobic gram-positive cocci as well as the most commonly isolated (Murdoch, 1998). It is a gram-positive cocci that appears as singles, pairs, tetrads, and clusters. Its cells are larger than other anaerobic gram-positive

⊘ TABLE 24-9

Differentiation of the More Commonly Recognized Anaerobic Gram-Positive Cocci, Gram-Negative Cocci, and Microaerophilic *Streptococcus*

Organism	Vancomycin (5 µg)	Kanamycin (1000 µg)	Colistin (10 µg)	Catalase	Susceptible to SPS	Indole	Fluorescence	Nitrate Reduction	Esculin	PYR	Oxygen Tolerance	Other
Finegoldia magna	S	V	R	–	–	–	–	–	–	U	OA	
Peptostreptococcus anaerobius	S	R	R	–	+	–	–	–	–	U	MA	Sickening sweet odor
Peptoniphilus asaccharolyticus	S	S	R	–	–	+	–	–	–	U	OA	Musty odor
Veillonella species	R	S	S	V	–	–	Red	+	–	U	MA	
Microaerophilic *Streptococcus*	S	V	R	–	–	–	–	–	+	–	MA	Tiny aerobic colony, butterscotch odor, beta hemolysis, VP positive

MA, microaerotolerant (can grow in presence of up to 10% oxygen); OA, obligate anaerobe; R, resistant; S, susceptible; U, unknown; V, variable; unshaded areas are presumptive identification reactions.

cocci but this characteristic may not be easily recognized by most microbiologists. Its Gram stain morphology and arrangement may be confused with *Staphylococcus* species. If the direct Gram stain reveals gram-positive cocci in clusters and *Staphylococcus* species is not recovered, the microbiologist should suspect *Finegoldia magna*. Figure 24-35 ■ illustrates the Gram stain of *F. magna*.

The gray to white colonies of *F. magna* are small and can take more than 48 hours to appear. They can be easily lost in a mixed culture. Figure 24-36 ■ demonstrates the small

colonies associated with *F. magna*. Biochemically, *F. magna* is catalase negative, resistant to sodium polyanethol sulfonate (SPS), and indole negative.

F. magna can be normal flora on the skin, in the oral cavity, intestine, and female genital tract. It is associated with skin and soft tissue infections such as diabetic foot ulcers, human bites, and decubitus ulcers. Gynecological and obstetric infections often include a mixture of aerobes and anaerobes that include *F. magna*. Oral and female genital tract infections can lead to bacteremia. Because of its presence as

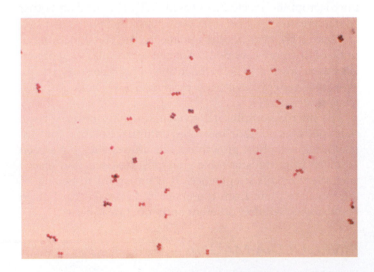

■ **FIGURE 24-35** The morphology of the gram positive cocci of *Finegoldia magna* can resemble those of *Staphylococcus* spp. *F. magna* is an obligate anaerobe whereas most *Staphylococcus* spp. are facultative anaerobes.
From Public Health Image Library (PHIL)/CDC/Dr. V. R. Dowell, Jr.

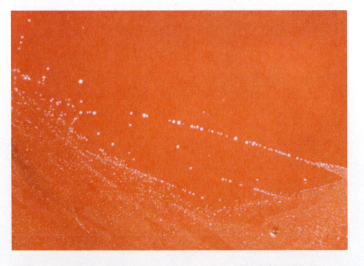

■ **FIGURE 24-36** *Finegoldia magna* appears as small, white colonies on reducible blood agar. It may take up to 48 hours to observe its colonies. In culture, they can be easily overgrown by other organisms present.
From Public Health Image Library (PHIL)/CDC/Dr. Gilda Jones.

normal skin flora, it has been recovered in cases of septic arthritis and bone infection associated with orthopedic surgery. The presence of a prosthetic device such as an artificial joint enhances infection.

Penicillin is the drug of choice for anaerobic gram-positive cocci. Clindamycin and metronidazole are also effective. Treatment must include necrotic tissue debridement and removal of any foreign device present.

PEPTOSTREPTOCOCCUS ANAEROBIUS

Peptostreptococcus anaerobius appears as gram-positive cocci in pairs and chains. Its cells are often more elongated like those of *Streptococcus* spp. compared to the round cocci of *Staphylococcus* spp. Figure 24-37 ■ demonstrates the Gram stain of *P. anaerobius*.

P. anaerobius is sensitive to SPS. An anaerobic gram-positive cocci that is sensitive to SPS can be presumptively identified as *P. anaerobius*. The organism is also catalase negative and indole negative.

It appears as a small gray-white colony within 24–48 hours. It gives off a unique odor that is described as sickeningly sweet, like that of overripe cantaloupe (Isenberg, 2004). The odor is due to the volatile fatty acids produced by the organism.

P. anaerobius is found as normal flora on the skin, in the mouth, intestine, vagina and urethra. Most isolates are found in oral, skin and soft tissue, gastrointestinal, female genitourinary, and bone and joint infections. It can be involved in infections of the head and neck, lungs, brain, skin, and soft tissue. Treatment includes penicillin, cephalosporins, chloramphenicol, clindamycin, and vancomycin. Because anaerobic gram-positive cocci are usually isolated in mixed cultures, treatment may require use of broad-spectrum antibiotics or multiple antibiotics to ensure adequate coverage for all organisms present.

PEPTONIPHILUS ASACCHAROLYTICUS

Peptoniphilus asaccharolyticus (previously known as *Peptostreptococcus asaccharolyticus*) appear as gram-positive cocci in pairs, short chains, tetrads, and small clusters. As the organism ages, it loses its ability to retain crystal violet and may appear gram negative. Its colonies are often small to medium with a distinctive yellow color. They have a musty odor due to indole production.

P. asaccharolyticus is resistant to SPS, catalase negative, and indole positive. An anaerobic gram-positive cocci that is SPS resistant and indole positive can be presumptively identified as *P. asaccharolyticus*.

It can be found as normal flora of the skin and intestinal and genitourinary tracts and is associated with obstetric and gynecological infections. It has been isolated in cases of endometritis, pelvic infections, and Bartholin gland abscesses (Brook, 2003a). Treatment includes most antibiotics usually used to treat other anaerobic infections.

MICROAEROPHILIC *STREPTOCOCCUS* SPECIES

The microaerophilic *Streptococcus* spp. are discussed in this chapter because of their unusual growth pattern. They are also discussed in ∞ Chapter 17, "Aerobic Gram-Positive Cocci," in relation to the *Streptococcus* spp. As a group they require up to 10% of carbon dioxide for growth and will not grow in room air without it. Most aerobic incubators are only able to achieve a level of 2–8% carbon dioxide. Even with increased carbon dioxide they produce very tiny colonies. They appear to grow better under anaerobic conditions, due to the presence of 5–10% carbon dioxide, but the colonies are still small compared to other *Streptococcus* spp. A microbiologist can be confused and call them anaerobic gram-positive cocci if the aerobic culture grows poorly or not at all.

The microaerophilic *Streptococcus* spp. were previously known as the *Streptococcus milleri* group. The use of the group name has been eliminated. Three distinct species names, *S. anginosus*, *S. constellatus*, and *S. intermedius*, are now used for reporting. They are each considered a member of the viridans group of the genus *Streptococcus*. Most are found as normal flora of the mouth and gastrointestinal and genitourinary tracts.

On Gram stain they cannot be distinguished from other *Streptococcus* spp. They present as gram-positive cocci in pairs and chains. The colonies can be alpha, beta, or gamma hemolytic but are usually beta hemolytic. They are characteristically very small, often one-half the size of other *Streptococcus* spp. Figure 24-38 ■ demonstrates the small beta-hemolytic colony morphology characteristic of the microaerophilic *Streptococcus* spp. As a group they are most often discovered due to their characteristic butterscotch or caramel odor. The

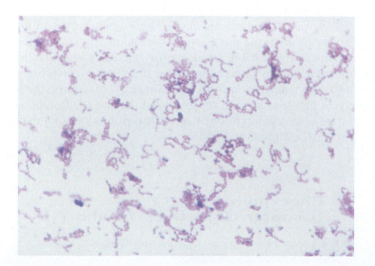

■ **FIGURE 24-37** The gram-positive cocci in pairs and chains of *Peptostreptococcus anaerobius* resembles those of the facultative anaerobic *Streptococcus* spp. It grows quicker than other anaerobic gram-positive cocci.
From Public Health Image Library (PHIL)/CDC/Dr. Gilda Jones.

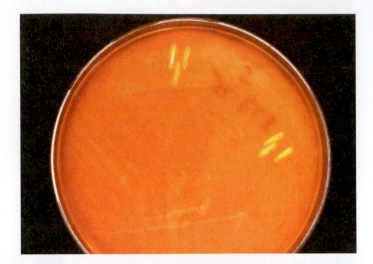

■ **FIGURE 24-38** The colonies of microaerophilic *Streptococcus* spp. grow poorly in an aerobic environment, as observed in this figure. Better growth in an anaerobic environment should alert the microbiologist to their presence.
From Public Health Image Library (PHIL)/CDC/Richard R. Facklam, PhD.

odor is due to the production of the metabolite, diacetyl (Chew & Smith, 1992). Its presence can help the microbiologist recognize the organism as a possible member of the microaerophilic *Streptococcus* spp.

Each species can exhibit multiple Lancefield groups such as A, C, F, or G. This makes Lancefield grouping of little value in their identification. The presence of the A antigen can misidentify them as *S. pyogenes* (group A beta *Streptococcus*) if they present as beta hemolytic. The very small colonies, better growth in an anaerobic environment, and characteristic butterscotch odor should warn the microbiologist that the identification does not correlate. With Lancefield grouping, the presence of the F antigen indicates the organism is probably a microaerophilic *Streptococcus* spp.

Biochemical testing can identify the microaerophilic *Streptococcus*. They are catalase negative and rapidly hydrolyze esculin but not L-pyrronlidonyl-α-naphthylamide (PYR). Review ∞ Chapter 17, "Aerobic Gram-Positive Cocci," for the principle and interpretation of the esculin and PYR hydrolysis tests. The microaerophilic *Streptococcus* spp. can be misidentified as group D *Streptococcus* based on their positive esculin and negative PYR reactions. The presence of small beta-hemolytic colonies with a butterscotch odor should alert the microbiologist to question the identification. Group D *Streptococcus* are commonly alpha or gamma hemolytic.

A gram-positive cocci displaying a tiny colony with beta-hemolysis and testing as PYR negative and Voges-Proskauer (VP) positive can be presumptively identified as a member of the microaerophilic *Streptococcus* spp. Extensive testing is required to differentiate among the three species. Commercial systems have proven to have difficulty in the identification of the species within this group of organisms (Mirzanejad & Stratton, 2005).

The microaerophilic *Streptococcus* spp. produce enzymes that allow them to dissolve tissue and move to other body sites to cause infections. Infections typically produce thick pus and abscesses. The organisms are usually introduced into the tissue through trauma or surgery. The most common sites for infection are the abdomen, head, and neck. *S. anginosus* and *S. constellatus* are most commonly isolated from infections in the abdomen such as liver abscess, peritonitis, and appendicitis. *S. intermedius* is primarily associated with brain abscesses. It has been isolated in 50–80% of brain infections (Mirzanejad & Stratton, 2005). If they are isolated and identified from blood cultures, it should direct the physician to look for an abscess somewhere in the body as the original source of the organism.

Treatment of infections due to these organisms requires surgery to drain the pus as well as antibiotic therapy. These organisms are showing an increasing resistance to penicillin but most remain susceptible at this time (Han & Kerschner, 2001). Vancomycin, cefotaxime, clindamycin, and erythromycin may also be used for treatment. Due to the fastidious nature of this group of organisms, susceptibility testing may prove to be difficult to perform.

 Checkpoint! 24–17 (Chapter Objectives 7d and 7i)

Which anaerobic gram-positive cocci are easily differentiated from the others with the use of an SPS disk?

    A. *Finegoldia magna*
    B. *Peptoniphilus asaccharolyticus*
    C. *Microaerophlic Streptococcus*
    D. *Peptostreptococcus anaerobius*

► GRAM-NEGATIVE COCCI

Veillonella is the only significant genus in this organism group. On Gram stain, *Veillonella* spp. appear as small gram-negative cocci in clusters. They may display a diplococci arrangement and mimic that of *Neisseria* spp. Figure 24-39 ■ displays the characteristic cluster of gram-negative cocci associated with the genus. *Veillonella*'s small gray-white colonies can display red fluorescence on blood containing agar under a long-wave ultraviolet light. The fluorescence is weaker when compared to other organisms and rapidly fades with exposure to oxygen and may be overlooked (Brazier & Riley, 1988).

Using special potency disks, *Veillonella* spp. are vancomycin resistant and kanamycin and colistin sensitive. They will not grow on laked vancomycin–kanamycin agar. Biochemically, *Veillonella* spp. are usually able to reduce nitrates and this result can be used to presumptively identify the genus.

Veillonella spp. can be found as normal flora in the upper respiratory system, intestine, and genitourinary system. *V. parvula* is the most commonly encountered anaerobic gram-negative cocci. It is usually isolated in mixed culture with other organisms. This makes it difficult to determine when *V. parvula* is significant or should be considered a contaminant. When isolated in pure culture, the organism can be significant in cases of aspiration pneumonia, chronic sinusitis, bite wound infections, osteomyelitis, and bacteremia after gastrointestinal endoscopy, especially in immunocompromised patients such as those with leukemia or other underlying diseases (Brook, 1996). *Veillonella* spp. are usually sensitive to most antibiotics used to treat anaerobic infections but resistant to vancomycin and tetracycline. They display variable susceptibility to erythromycin (Brook, 1996).

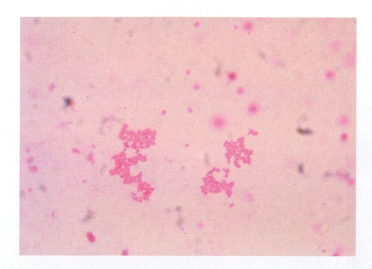

■ **FIGURE 24-39** *Veillonella* spp. is the only significant anaerobic gram-negative cocci. It characteristically appears in clusters. It could be misinterpreted on Gram stain as a member of the genus *Neisseria*.
From Public Health Image Library (PHIL)/CDC/Dr. Gilda Jones.

 Checkpoint! 24–18
(Chapter Objectives 7d and 71)

The fluorescence of Veillonella species can resemble that of:
   A. *Prevotella melaninogenica*
   B. *Fusobacerium nucleatum*
   C. *Clostridium difficile*
   D. *Porphyromonas gingivalis*

► SUSCEPTIBILITY TESTING

Susceptibility testing of anaerobes has proven to be a source of frustration for many clinical laboratories. Due to the increased time required for isolation and identification of anaerobes, susceptibility testing results are often reported long after treatment has been initiated. Results may not be available until 6 to 7 days after submission of the original specimen.

Susceptibility testing is not required for every anaerobic isolate. Many are predictably susceptible to antimicrobial agents such as metronidazole, chloramphenicol, and the cephalosporins. Anaerobes, such as *Bacteroides fragilis* group, *Prevotella* spp., *Fusobacterium nucleatum*, *F. mortiferum*, and *Clostridium perfringens*, can be resistant to numerous antimicrobial agents and should be routinely tested (Jousimies-Somer et al., 2002). Anaerobes isolated in pure culture as well as those isolated from significant body sites/specimen types such as central nervous system, bone, joint, endocarditis, and bacteremia should be routinely tested.

Beta-lactamase testing, using the chromogenic cephalosporin method, can provide the physician useful information before susceptibility testing results are available. Anaerobic gram-negative rods should be routinely tested using this method. If the organism is beta-lactamase positive then the beta-lactam antimicrobial agents should not be used unless accompanied by a beta-lactamase inhibitor such as clavulinic acid. If the result is negative, it cannot be assumed that beta-lactams antibiotics will be effective because the organism may be resistant by another mechanism.

The antimicrobial agents selected for testing should be a combined decision of the microbiology department, infectious disease specialists, and the pharmacy department. The method used for susceptibility testing should follow the protocols provided by the Clinical and Laboratory Standards Institute (CLSI)

 Checkpoint! 24–19
(Chapter Objective 8a)

The treatment of most anaerobic infections requires:
   A. *no intervention.*
   B. *antibiotics and tissue debridement.*
   C. *susceptibility testing.*
   D. *use of a hyperbaric chamber.*

to ensure accurate and reliable results. Review ∞ Chapter 11, "Susceptibility Testing," for details on testing anaerobes.

SUMMARY

Anaerobes remain a challenge for most microbiologists. Their isolation requires very specific collection and transport methods, incubation systems that provide an oxygen-free environment as well as specialized media. This often proves to be costly for smaller laboratories. If a laboratory has the resources to perform anaerobic cultures, they must decide the level of workup. Anaerobes are not isolated as frequently as aerobes and require at least 48 hours incubation before subcultures can be performed. Most microbiologists are not as experienced in the workup of anaerobes as they are for most aerobic organisms. These factors only add to their complexity.

Anaerobes are found as part of the normal flora present on the skin and mucous membranes. Anaerobic infections can affect most body systems. Most infections are endogenous but there are some that can originate from an exogenous source. Endogenous anaerobes often cause infection due to a break in the natural protective barrier of the skin and mucous membranes. Breaks can occur with trauma, surgery, or disease. Knowledge of the normal flora of specific body sites is essential when determining the significance of organisms isolated.

This is especially important because most anaerobic infections are actually mixed infections that include aerobes as well. This makes determining the significance of isolated organisms even more challenging.

Some of the most frequently isolated anaerobes include the *Bacteroides fragilis* group, *Porphyromonas* spp., *Prevotella* spp., *Fusobacterium nucleatum,* and *F. necrophorum,* the anaerobic gram-positive cocci and *Clostridium* spp. They often provide valuable clues to their presence that can guide the physician and microbiologist in their recovery and identification. Presumptive identification of organisms can save valuable resources while providing the physician accurate results to guide treatment. It is important to recognize that not all anaerobes can be presumptively identified and may require additional testing.

Treatment of anaerobic infections usually involves drainage of abscesses, debridement of necrotic tissue to improve blood circulation, and oxygenation of the tissue and the use of antibiotics. Routine susceptibility testing of anaerobes is usually not required. Certain agents such as metronidazole are effective against almost all anaerobes, except the non-spore-forming gram-positive rods, because it works best in a reduced state. Penicillin is also very effective unless the organism is able to produce beta-lactamase. Important beta-lactamase producers include many of the anaerobic gram-negative rods such as the *Bacteroides fragilis* group.

LEARNING OPPORTUNITIES

Interpret the following data in order to presumptively identify each organism.

1. An anaerobic gram-positive cocci was isolated in pure culture from the blood of a 19-year-old motorcycle accident victim. The gray-white colony grew on RBAP but not LKV. Biochemically it produced the following reactions:
(Chapter Objectives 7 and 9)

    Catalase = no bubbles
    SPS disk = 14 millimeters zone—see the image below
    Spot indole = no color change
    Nitrate = red after the addition of zinc dust

Name that organism _____

2. A large anaerobic gram-positive rod was isolated from a necrotic leg wound of a 64-year-old farmer who was injured in a tractor accident. The gray colony produced a zone of double beta hemolysis on RBAP. There was no growth on LKV. It produced the following reactions: (Chapter Objectives 7 and 9)

   Catalase = no bubbles
   Spot indole = no color change
   EYA = opaque zone around the colony without a rainbow sheen

   Name that organism _____

3. A very pleomorphic anaerobic gram-negative rod was isolated from a deep neck abscess of a 27-year-old male after oral surgery. The gray colony produced a green haze around each colony on RBAP. The LKV did not grow. Testing performed in the microbiology department revealed the following reactions: (Chapter Objectives 7 and 9)

   5 µg Vancomycin disk = 0 millimeters
   1 mg Kanamycin disk = 12 millimeters
   10 µg Colistin disk = 13 millimeters
   Bile stimulation disk = 15 millimeters
   Spot indole = blue-green
   Lipase = rainbow sheen

   Name that organism _____

4. An anaerobic clubbed, non-spore-forming gram-positive rod has been isolated from multiple blood cultures of a 46-year-old female suspected of having bacterial endocarditis. The small white colony grew on RBAP but not on LKV. Biochemical testing provided the following results:

   Catalase = effervescent bubbles
   Spot indole = blue-green
   Nitrate = red after addition of reagents A and B

   Name that organism _____

5. A pleomorphic anaerobic gram-negative coccobacilli was isolated from an abdominal abscess in a 77-year-old female. The abscess developed after gastrointestinal surgery for an obstruction. The large gray colony grew on both the RBAP and LKV. The following results were obtained:

   Bile stimulation disk = 0 millimeters
   Special potency disks (vancomycin, kanamycin, and colistin)—see the image
      below = 0 millimeters
   Esculin = black colony
   Fluorescence = None
   Pigmentation = None
   Spot indole = no color change

   Name that organism _____

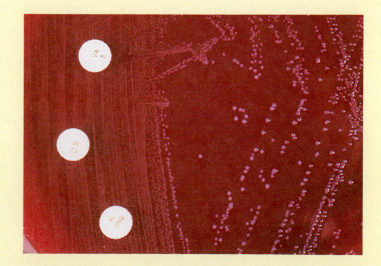

6. An anaerobic gram-positive cocci in short chains was isolated from the endometrium of a 28-year-old female after childbirth. The small yellow colony grew on RBAP but not LKV. The laboratory performed the following tests:

  Catalase = no bubbles
  SPS disk = 0 millimeters
  Spot indole = blue-green
  Fluorescence = none

  Name that organism _____

7. A physician submits a formed stool from a 79-year-old female patient who has been hospitalized for the past 2 weeks with bacterial pneumonia. He writes an order for a stool culture and includes a special request for isolation of *Clostridium difficile*. The microbiologist working at specimen processing should: (Chapter Objectives 2 and 6)

   a. Add a CCFA agar plate to the stool culture

   b. Test the specimen for *C. difficile* toxins A and B by an EIA method

   c. Test the specimen for *C. difficile* toxins A and B using a cell line culture

   d. Reject the specimen

8. Which of the following disease state/causative organism combinations is **correct?** (Chapter Objective 7)

   a. Periodontitis/*Bacteroides fragilis* group

   b. Tonsillar abscess/*Fusobacterium necrophorum*

   c. Peritonitis/*Prevotella melaninogenica*

   d. Lumpy jaw/*Bifidobacterium* spp.

9. Due to the low numbers of anaerobic cultures processed, a laboratory uses an anaerobic jar and a gas-generating pack for incubation of inoculated agar plates. After 48 hours of incubation, the microbiologist notices the anaerobic stock organisms, kept in the same jar as the culture plates, are not growing. Which of the following reasons does **not** explain the lack of growth for the anaerobic stock organisms? (Chapter Objective 3)

   a. The jar was opened too early and the organisms were exposed to oxygen.

   b. There was a crack in the jar lid seal, which allowed oxygen to enter.

   c. The palladium catalyst was not reheated prior to use.

   d. The gas-generating pack failed to create the appropriate environment.

10. Determine a method in which the microbiologist, in learning opportunity 9, could have ensured the jar's anaerobic environment was appropriate. (Chapter Objective 3)

11. Vitamin K and hemin enhances the growth of which of the following anaerobes? (Chapter Objective 4)

   a. A large box car–shaped gram-positive rod exhibiting double beta hemolysis

   b. A gram-negative rod that is resistant to kanamycin, vancomycin, and colisitin and stimulated by bile

   c. A red fluorescing gram-negative rod that is resistant to kanamycin and vancomycin, lipase negative, and indole negative

   d. A gram-positive cocci that is sensitive to SPS

12. Two sets of blood cultures, collected from a 28-year-old male with peritonitis, grow a gram-negative rod on reducible blood agar and laked kanamycin–vancomycin agar and displays black colonies on BBE agar. Aerotolerance testing proves the organism is an obligate anaerobe. In the workup for this organism, the microbiologist should perform: (Chapter Objectives 4, 5, and 8)

   a. A presumptive identification
   b. A full identification
   c. Susceptibility testing
   d. Both a and c
   e. Both b and c

PEARSON myhealthprofessionskit™

Use this address to access the interactive Companion Website created for this textbook. Simply select "Clinical Laboratory Science" from the choice of disciplines. Find this book and log in using your user name and password.

REFERENCES

Go to myhealthprofessionskit.com to view this chapter's references.

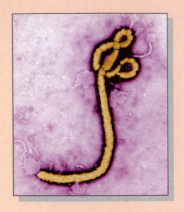

25

Spirochetes

Lisa A. Morici

■ LEARNING OBJECTIVES

Upon completion of this chapter, the learner should be able to:

1. Identify the pathogenic spirochetes.
   a. Correlate each with their respective diseases.
2. Discuss the general characteristics of spirochetes.
3. Identify the stage-specific diseases of spirochetes and their relevance in the diagnosis of spirochete infection.
4. Differentiate treponemal and nontreponemal tests.
   a. Determine potential sources of errors for each.
5. Differentiate venereal and nonvenereal treponemal disease.
6. Discuss the need for species-specific diagnostic tests for spirochetes.

KEY TERMS

adhesins	Lyme disease	spirochete
antigenic variation	nontreponemal tests	syphilis
chancre	pinta	treponemal tests
endemic syphilis	prozone phenomenon	Venereal Disease
endemic	Rapid Plasma Reagin	Research Laboratory
treponematoses	(RPR)	(VDRL)
erythema migrans	relapsing fever	Weil's disease
gumma	serofast state	yaws
leptospirosis		

► INTRODUCTION

The **spirochetes** are highly motile, corkscrew-shaped bacteria. Their cell wall is composed of a cytoplasmic membrane surrounded by peptidoglycan and axial fibrils as well as a loosely associated outer membrane. In fixed, Wright-stained differential smears, spirochetes appear as loose coils. They tend to stain poorly on Gram stain. The pathogenic spirochetes known to cause human disease are summarized in Table 25-1 ✪. This chapter will examine the general characteristics of spirochetes, their respective diseases, and the diagnostic tests used to discriminate spirochetal infection.

► *LEPTOSPIRA* SPECIES

GENERAL CHARACTERISTICS

Leptospires are coiled, motile spirochetes with bent or hooked ends (Figure 25-1 ■). They measure 6 to 25 microns in length and 0.25 microns in width. They are obligate aerobes that share features of both gram-negative and gram-positive bacteria. Leptospires are oxidase and catalase positive. The genus *Leptospira* is classified into 17 species based on DNA relatedness. The pathogenic leptospires are grouped in the *interrogans* complex, whereas the saprophytic strains are placed in the *biflexa* complex. Leptospiral strains are most commonly referred to by serovar. Both the *interrogans* and *biflexa* complex have been divided into several serovars based on the cross-agglutinin adsorption test (CAAT). In the *interrogans* complex, more than 200 pathogenic serovars are recognized. The genome of *Leptospira* is much larger than the genomes of *Borrelia* and *Treponema* spp. The possession of additional genes that are expressed under specific environmental conditions likely enables leptospires to survive in the environment as well as in mammalian hosts. Potential virulence factors include proteins involved in attachment and invasion of host tissues and hemolytic, phospholipase, and sphingomyelinase activities (Bharti et al., 2003).

✪ TABLE 25-1

Pathogenic Spirochetes

Pathogenic Spirochete	Human Disease	Vector or Source
Borrelia		
B. burgdorferi	Lyme disease	Ixodid (hard bodied) ticks
B. recurrentis	Epidemic relapsing fever	Body louse
B. turicatae	Endemic relapsing fever	Ornithodoros (soft bodied) ticks
Leptospira		
L. interrogans	Leptospirosis	Animal urine
Treponema		
T. pallidum		
subspecies *pallidum*	Syphilis	Human
ssp. *endemicum*	Endemic syphilis	Fomites
ssp. *pertenue*	Yaws	Human skin lesions
T. carateum	Pinta	Human skin lesions

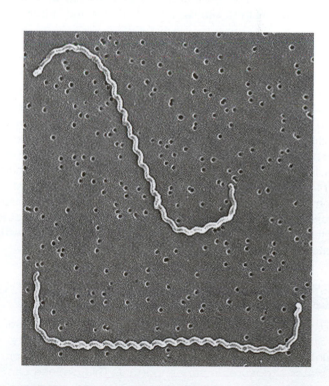

■ **FIGURE 25-1** The hooked ends of this spirochete are characteristic for *Leptospira* spp.
From Centers for Disease Control and Prevention.

SPECIMEN COLLECTION AND PROCESSING

Specimens for culture of *Leptospira* spp. should be collected during the first 10 days of illness. Those taken during episodes of fever are optimum. Leptospires appear first in the blood and cerebrospinal fluid (CSF) during the first week of illness. At 1–3 weeks, they appear in the urine. Urine may be the best specimen because the organisms remain in the kidneys longer than other body sites. Clinical specimens should be transported within one hour of collection to prevent loss of organisms. Blood and CSF can be collected in sodium oxalate or heparin if there is delay in transportation. Citrate anticoagulant is inhibitory and should not be used, and specimens should not be frozen.

Specimens can be cultured in artificial semisolid media containing 10% rabbit serum or 1% bovine serum albumin plus long-chain fatty acids (i.e., Tween 80) at pH 6.8 to 7.4. Commercial formulations are available, such as Fletcher's and Stuart's media. Media are made selective by the addition of 5-flurorouracil and neomycin sulphate. Other antibiotics can also be used, such as polymyxin B, rifampicin, and vancomycin. They grow optimally at 28°C to 30°C in the dark. Cultures should be checked for bacterial contamination after 3 to 4 days of growth and then subcultured after 1 to 3 weeks. *Leptospira* can survive in liquid media for months to years. *Leptospira* stain poorly on Gram stain so darkfield or phase-contrast microscopy of wet preparations is required for direct visualization. Cell debris and artifacts can easily be confused with the spirochetes. Histological or immunofluorescence stains can be used to observe the organisms in tissues such as liver and kidney.

CLINICAL SIGNIFICANCE

Leptospirosis is a zoonotic disease, due to *Leptospira interrogans,* that can be passed to humans via the urine of infected animals. It is an emerging infectious disease with a worldwide distribution. Although rats are the primary reservoir, other animals, including mice, skunks, opossums, wildcats, foxes, raccoons, shrews, dogs, cattle, and swine, can be infected and transmit the leptospires in urine. Those who work with animals and have prolonged exposure to water are at an increased risk for infection. Indirect contact, through abraded skin, mucous membranes, conjunctiva, or inhalation, is the more common route of transmission to humans and usually occurs from contact with water or soil contaminated with infected urine.

> **REAL WORLD TIP**
>
> The highest incidence of leptospirosis in the United States occurs in Hawaii. A thorough patient history, including geographic locations visited and animal or water exposure, is very important. This disease can mimic others such as hantavirus and rickettsial disease.

The disease manifests with highly variable clinical symptoms, ranging from asymptomatic to febrile illness and jaundice to life-threatening renal failure and pulmonary hemorrhage. The clinical syndrome is divided into a biphasic illness and fulminant disease. In the biphasic illness, bacteremia causes a febrile illness of sudden onset. The organism spreads throughout the body and enters the tissues, including the central nervous system and aqueous fluid of the eye. Fever, chills, severe headache, myalgias (especially in the legs and lower back), nausea, vomiting, and conjunctival redness are common during this acute stage of disease. The organism appears to cause damage to the blood vessel endothelium.

Resolution of symptoms coincides with IgM antibody production, but fever reoccurs after 3 to 4 days. The acute phase can be followed by either a lessening of symptoms or progression to a delayed secondary phase of severe disease possibly due to the inflammation produced. Aseptic meningitis, in which leptospires cannot be cultured from the CSF, can occur in a majority of cases. Possibly the organisms are cleared quickly from the body but subsequent inflammation accounts for the signs and symptoms of meningitis.

Weil's disease represents the most severe form of leptospirosis. It is characterized by jaundice, acute renal failure, and hemorrhage. There can be multi-organ failure. Case fatality rates range from 5 to 15% (Bharti et al., 2003).

Diagnosis of Leptospirosis

Diagnosis of leptospirosis is made by clinical suspicion, knowledge of the epidemiology of the disease, and diagnostic tests. General laboratory findings may include the following:

1. Increases in transaminases, alkaline phosphatase, bilirubin, CSF protein, plasma creatinine, serum creatine phosphokinase, and serum amylase

2. Abnormal urinalysis with proteinuria, pyuria, and microscopic hematuria

3. Peripheral leukocytosis with a shift to immature neutrophil band forms and anemia

Microbiologic diagnosis of leptospirosis can be made by culture of the spirochete or by serology. *Leptospira* can be cultured from the blood or CSF during the first week of illness and from urine for up to a month. Fletcher's medium is semisolid and a drop or two of the clinical specimen is dispersed throughout the agar. Growth appears as turbidity below the surface. Culture of leptospira is slow, insensitive, and requires appropriate media. If performed, cultures should be kept for a minimum of 6 weeks.

Serologic tests are most often used to diagnose leptospirosis and include microscopic agglutination using live antigen, enzyme linked immunosorbent assay (ELISA) to detect leptospiral IgM antibodies, and microagglutination tests (MAT). The MAT is the reference standard test for serologic diagnosis (Bharti et al., 2003). It is highly sensitive and specific, but requires considerable user expertise. A positive MAT is defined by a fourfold increase in antibody titer or a conversion from seronegative to a titer of 1:100 or greater. Several assays for determination of IgM antibodies against crude whole-cell lysate or cell-surface antigens are commercially available.

Molecular tests, such as real-time quantitative polymerase chain reaction (PCR), are sensitive and can differentiate between pathogenic and nonpathogenic species.

 REAL WORLD TIP

Most laboratories do not keep Fletcher's medium in stock. They usually cannot perform the serology testing necessary for diagnosis of leptospirosis. It is often too expensive to maintain the necessary reagents for a test that is infrequently ordered. A reputable reference laboratory is necessary for esoteric testing.

TREATMENT

Antibiotics are effective against *Leptospira* spp. Oral doxycycline is recommended for those with less severe disease. Intravenous penicillin G is effective with severe disease. Erythromycin and the third-generation cephalosporins are also effective. In severely ill individuals, supportive therapy is essential due to potential kidney failure. Upon recovery, the kidneys regain full function. A vaccine is available but has not been shown to be very successful in humans. Currently the vaccine is used primarily for animals to prevent the organism's transmission to others.

 Checkpoint! 25–1 (Chapter Objective 2)

To culture Leptospira, one should:
  A. *maintain cultures for at least 6 weeks.*
  B. *incubate the cultures at 28°C to 30°C in the dark.*
  C. *avoid the use of citrate during sample collection.*
  D. *All of the above*

▶ *TREPONEMA* SPECIES

GENERAL CHARACTERISTICS

The treponemes are spirochetes that are helical and tightly coiled. The organism is encased in a sheath that tends to hide its surface antigens from the host's immune system. Treponemes cause both venereal and nonvenereal disease. The treponemal diseases of humans comprise **syphilis**, a sexually transmitted disease, and the **endemic treponematoses:** yaws, pinta, and endemic syphilis. Regardless of the treponeme causing infection, clinical manifestations of treponemal disease occur in stages.

The inability to readily grow treponemes in vitro has hindered the determination of virulence factors and therapeutic targets. However, the sequencing of the genome of *T. pallidum* subspecies *pallidum* may aid in the development of appropriate culture mediums as well as more specific diagnostic tests. In particular, the development of a molecular or serologic test that can distinguish between pathogenic subspecies of *T. pallidum* is urgently needed.

At present, it is impossible to differentiate the human pathogenic treponemes either morphologically, biochemically, or serologically. Clinically important features of all treponemes are that they are intrinsically susceptible to penicillin, and they have a relatively slow generation time of 30 to 33 hours.

SPECIMEN COLLECTION AND PROCESSING

Treponema pallidum subspecies *pallidum,* the etiologic agent of venereal syphilis, cannot be grown in culture. Darkfield microscopic examination in the hands of a well-trained microbiologist is the only test that provides a correct diagnosis of syphilis in 100% of cases during primary- and secondary-stage syphilis. With the exception of the macular rash lesions, all cutaneous and mucous membrane lesions contain *T. pallidum* (Baughn & Musher, 2005). Thus, spirochetes can be obtained in the serous exudate of a gently abraded lesion and examined under a microscope equipped with a darkfield condenser. Issues with direct examination of lesions by darkfield microscopy include: (1) it does not differentiate virulent treponemes from those that are avirulent and (2) many laboratories no longer perform darkfield microscopy for syphilis.

Clinical diagnosis now relies largely on serologic confirmation. Serum serology, such as nontreponemal tests used for screening and treponemal tests used for confirmation, can be used for diagnosis of syphilis and endemic treponematoses. The use of serology tests is discussed in later in this chapter.

CLINICAL SIGNIFICANCE

◆ **Venereal Syphilis**

Syphilis is a sexually transmitted disease caused by the spirochete, *Treponema pallidum* subspecies *pallidum* (Salyers & Whitt, 2002). The discovery of penicillin in the 1940s and its effectiveness in treating syphilis decreased the prevalence of this disease for many decades. Unfortunately, the United States experienced a dramatic increase in syphilis cases in the 1980s and 1990s, partially as a result of the AIDS epidemic.

Like most spirochetal diseases, syphilis occurs in stages. The organism enters through breaks in the mucous membranes or skin. After infection with *T. pallidum*, a primary lesion forms at the site of inoculation approximately 2 to 3 weeks after infection. Typically, like many STDs, the primary syphilitic **chancre** or ulceration occurs in the genital, anal, perineal, or oral areas of the body (review Figure 36-5 in ∞ Chapter 36, "Genital System"). The organism can be visualized, using darkfield microscopy or immunofluorescence, from the scrapings of the surface of the lesion as seen in Figure 36-17 in ∞ Chapter 36, "Genital System." A remarkable feature of the syphilitic chancre is that the ulcer is painless and heals spontaneously after 3 to 8 weeks so an individual may not be aware of its presence. In addition to the chancre, the primary stage of disease may include modest inguinal lymph node enlargement.

Ⓔ REAL WORLD TIP

Darkfield examination of oral syphilitic lesions should not be performed. The mouth contains many commensal nonpathogenic spirochetes which cannot be differentiated from those of *T. pallidum*.

In untreated individuals, the spirochete disseminates via the lymphatics to the bloodstream and other parts of the body, resulting in secondary syphilis. A characteristic finding is the appearance of a rash and secondary lesions 4 to 10 weeks after the initial primary chancre. Both involve the entire trunk of the body and the extremities, including the palms of the hands and soles of the feet. ∞ Chapter 36, "Genital System," provides a view of a syphilis rash in Figure 36-6.

In addition, numerous clinical manifestations are associated with this stage of the disease, including secondary lesions on the mucous membranes; condyloma lata (broad, flat, wart-like growths in moist creased areas of the body); lymphadenopathy; systemic symptoms such as fever, weight loss, and malaise; hepatitis; uveitis, arthritis; and neurologic complications such as headache, meningitis, cranial nerve disorders, and cerebrovascular accidents (Baughn & Musher, 2005). Loss of hair, including the eyebrows, is not uncommon. Interestingly, although infection with *T. pallidum* results in the production of antibodies and a cellular response, it is not sufficient to eradicate the organism and does not provide long-lasting immunity. Reinfection with *T. pallidum* can occur.

In addition to primary and secondary disease, the spirochete can form a latent infection. Latent infection is characterized by seroreactivity with no clinical manifestations. During latent infection, vertical transmission can occur from mother to infant, resulting in congenital syphilis. Congenital syphilis is usually severe, resulting in deformities, interstitial keratitis, and death.

Tertiary or late syphilis develops one or more years after the initial infection and can manifest in almost any organ system. Typically, the lesions of tertiary syphilis involve the cardiovascular, central nervous, and musculoskeletal systems. The spirochetes can scar and weaken the aorta leading to aneurysm. In addition, **gummas** or large granulomas with extensive necrosis can develop in the bones, CNS, spleen, and on the skin. Neurosyphilis is especially problematic in individuals coinfected with HIV. It results in the loss of mental and physical abilities.

Diagnosis of Syphilis

Serological testing remains the most widely used means for diagnosis of syphilis. Of the various stages of disease, secondary syphilis is the least difficult to diagnose clinically (Table 25-2 Ⓒ). Serologic tests for *T. pallidum* include both treponemal and nontreponemal tests.

Nontreponemal tests are considered screening tests because they are not specific for *T. pallidum* antigens, and they are inexpensive and can be done easily to test large numbers of serum samples. IgG and IgM anti-lipid antibodies are formed in response to material released because of the organism's reaction with the tissues and lipid from the surface of the organism itself. Antibodies produced against *T. pallidum* cross react with lipoidal antigens (cardiolipin cholesterol lechithin). These antigens, also known as Wassermann antigens, are found in the mitochondrial membranes of mammalian tissues.

The two nontreponemal tests are the **Venereal Disease Research Laboratory test (VDRL)** and the **Rapid Plasma Reagin test (RPR).** Nontreponemal tests are less sensitive in patients with primary-stage disease. Titers are low (less than 1:8) and are only positive in 80 to 86% of patients with primary syphilis. However, the tests are positive in greater than 98% of patients with secondary and latent syphilis at high dilutions (>1:32) (Brown & Frank, 2003). Dilutions are usually requested by the physician when syphilis is suspected because of the **prozone phenomenon**, in which high concentrations of antibody overwhelm the antigens present and may not be detected in undiluted serum and thus yield a false negative. Therefore, a negative nontreponemal test in a patient

Ⓒ TABLE 25-2

Stage-Specific Diagnosis of Syphilis

Stage	Clinical Manifestations	Diagnostic Test(s)[a]	Sensitivity
Primary	Painless chancre	Darkfield microscopy	100%
	Lymphadenopathy	Nontreponemal test	80–86%
Secondary	Secondary skin or genital lesions	Darkfield microscopy	100%
		Nontreponemal test	>98%
	Systemic symptoms	Treponemal test	>98%
	CNS involvement		
	Arthritis		
	Hepatitis		
	Glomerulonephritis		
	Condyloma latum		
Latent	None	Nontreponemal test	>98%
		Treponemal test	>98%
Tertiary	Neurosyphilis	Treponemal test	>98%
	Cardiovascular disease		
	Gumma		

[a]Note: The inability to grow treponemes in vitro excludes "culturing" the organism for diagnosis.

with a disseminated rash cannot exclude syphilis (Baughn & Musher, 2005).

A positive VDRL in CSF is specific for neurosyphilis, but a negative result cannot rule it out. False-positive results may occur with autoimmune disorders or pregnancy. After adequate treatment of syphilis, the nontreponemal tests eventually become nonreactive and can be used to assess treatment efficacy. Titers typically drop fourfold within 6 months of therapy. A small percentage of syphilis patients retain low-grade VDRL positivity throughout their life (known as the **serofast state**). A positive VDRL or RPR test must be confirmed with a treponemal test due to the potential for false positive results.

Treponemal tests measure antibody to antigens of *T. pallidum* and are used to confirm the diagnosis of syphilis in a patient with a positive nontreponemal test result. Treponemal tests include the *T. pallidum* hemagglutination assay (TPHA), the microhemagglutination test with *T. pallidum* antigen, fluorescent treponemal antibody-adsorption test (FTA-ABS), and ELISA.

These tests are positive in nearly 95% of primary-stage patients, yet a negative test result cannot exclude a diagnosis of syphilis. Treponemal tests are highly specific (>98%) and sensitive in secondary-stage patients, and a negative test result can exclude secondary or late-stage syphilis and neurosyphilis. High titers (>1:16) in the treponemal test indicates active infection (Brown & Frank, 2003).

Positive treponemal tests will likely remain positive for an individual's lifetime, whereas seropositivity in the nontreponemal tests will wane over time. This is an important feature because reinfection with *T. pallidum* can occur. Furthermore, treponemal specific tests will remain positive after treatment and are not used to assess treatment efficacy as are the nontreponemal tests. False-positive results in the treponemal tests can occur in patients with systemic lupus erythematosus or Lyme disease, another spirochete disease that is discussed later in this chapter.

 Checkpoint! 25–2 (Chapter Objective 3)

During the latent stage of venereal syphilis, which of the following diagnostic tests is most reliable for detecting T. pallidum?

   A. Culture of the spirochete from a skin lesion
   B. Culture of the spirochete from the CSF
   C. A nontreponemal test on diluted serum
   D. A nontreponemal test on undiluted serum

◆ Yaws

Yaws is an infectious, relapsing nonvenereal skin disease caused by *Treponema pallidum* subspecies *pertenue*. It is highly endemic in rural tropical areas with heavy rainfall such as Africa and South America. Yaws typically affects the poorest areas of the world and predominantly infects children. Approximately 75% of new cases occur in individuals less than 15 years of age (Koff & Rosen, 1993).

The clinical manifestations of yaws occur in two stages: early and late. Similar to primary syphilis, infection with *T. pallidum* subspecies *pertenue* results in a primary lesion at the site of infection. It begins as a small papule that enlarges and then ulcerates. This initial "mother" yaw usually appears 2 weeks to 6 months after infection and can persist for up to 6 months before spontaneously resolving. It is full of spirochetes and can be passed person to person by contact.

The onset of "daughter" yaws (Figure 25-2 ■), which are smaller, widespread, cutaneous lesions, follows the development of the mother yaw. Other features can include systemic symptoms, lymphadenopathy, and inflammation of bone and joints. The late stage of yaws follows a variable period of latency in approximately 10% of untreated individuals. Manifestations of late-stage yaws include painful thickening of the skin on the palms and soles of the feet, ulceration of the skin, gumma formation, and bone and cartilage destruction causing disability and deformity (Walker & Hay, 2000).

Diagnosis

Diagnosis of yaws is similar to that for syphilis. The disease is suspected based on clinical manifestation and supported by serology. It is important to remember that serologic tests for the treponemes, such as *T. pallidum* hemagglutination assay,

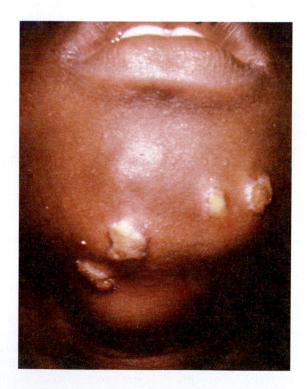

■ **FIGURE 25-2** These lesions are characteristic for yaws.
From Centers for Disease Control and Prevention.

cannot distinguish between subspecies. This can make a definitive diagnosis difficult, especially in those areas where both venereal syphilis and the endemic treponematoses are prevalent.

◆ Pinta

The causative organism of **pinta** is *Treponema carateum*. Pinta was likely the first treponematosis to occur in humans and is considered to be the most benign of the treponemal diseases (Engelkens, Niemel, van der Sluis, Meheus, & Stolz, 1991). Most infections with pinta are acquired by young adults in Central and South America. Transmission occurs through contact with infected skin or mucous membranes. Both early and late stages of disease are recognized. The initial stage of pinta is characterized by the appearance of a papule or plaquelike lesion several weeks to months after infection. The lesions can become pigmented, thickened, and scaly and then disappear spontaneously. Months to years later, smaller more extensive lesions called "pintids" appear and may remain for years or recur. The pintids lead to extensive changes in skin pigmentation, causing disfiguring appearance, lack of pigmentation, skin atrophy, and hyperkeratosis. However, the skin appears to be the only organ affected. Severe mutilations do not occur, and cardiologic and neurologic complications have not been observed (Engelkens et al., 1991).

Diagnosis

Diagnosis of pinta depends largely on clinical suspicion, epidemiological association, and geographic location. Silver and immunofluorescent stains and darkfield microscopy have aided in the visualization of *T. carateum* in the epidermis and early lesions. Late pigmented skin lesions are often colored copper, grey, or blue and contain treponemes and an inflammatory infiltrate composed of lymphocytes, whereas late nonpigmented skin lesions do not contain either. No specific serologic test for *T. carateum* is available. The same nontreponemal and treponemal tests used for venereal syphilis are used for diagnosis of yaws, pinta, and endemic syphilis as well.

◆ Endemic Syphilis

Endemic syphilis is caused by a nonvenereal skin infection with *T. pallidum* subspecies *endemicum* and is typically found in dry, hot climatic zones such as the Middle East and Sahara Desert (Engelkens et al., 1991). The main reservoir of infected individuals is children from 2 to 15 years of age. Unlike venereal syphilis, endemic syphilis is not transmitted sexually, but rather through direct contact with infectious lesions on the skin or mouth. The disease manifests in early and late stages. The early stage is unique among the treponematoses in that a primary lesion frequently does not occur. Instead, primary manifestations include the ulcers of the oropharyngeal mucosa, skin eruptions, lymphadenopathy, and painful

inflammation of bone and its periosteum. After a period of clinical latency, a late stage occurs that can affect the skin, bones, and cartilage and lead to severe deformity, especially of the nose and palate. Neurologic and cardiologic complications are rare (Engelkens et al., 1991).

Diagnosis

The diagnosis of endemic syphilis is dependent on clinical, epidemiologic, and geographic factors. Darkfield examination of early lesions demonstrates the spirochete. Like the other treponematoses, positive serologic tests can help confirm the diagnosis. A positive treponemal test result in a person from a region where the nonvenereal treponematoses are endemic should caution a hasty diagnosis of venereal syphilis.

Treatment

Treponemes are highly sensitive to penicillin, and it is the drug of choice for both venereal and nonvenereal diseases. Tetracycline, erythromycin, and chloramphenical may be alternatives for pinta, yaws, and endemic syphilis.

Checkpoint! 25–3 (Chapter Objective 5)

The venereal and nonvenereal treponematoses share all the following features except

    A. *involvement of the skin.*
    B. *sexual transmission.*
    C. *early and late stages of disease.*
    D. *periods of clinical latency.*

▶ *BORRELIA* SPECIES

GENERAL CHARACTERISTICS

Borrelia species vary in length, diameter, number of flagella, and tightness of the spiral coils (Figure 25-3 ■). They can range from 3 to 30 microns in length and 0.2 to 0.5 microns in width. *Borrelia* flagella are characteristically unsheathed, as opposed to treponemal flagella that are enclosed within a sheath. They grow optimally at 30°C to 40°C under microaerophilic conditions and have a generation time of 7 to 20 hours. *Borrelia* are very adaptable and survive in both cold and warm-blooded hosts.

The genome of *B. burgdorferi*, the sole causative agent of **Lyme disease** or borreliosis, has been completely sequenced. It has a linear chromosome as well as linear and circular plasmids. The plasmids encode special outer-surface proteins (Osp). Different surface proteins are expressed depending on whether the organism is in the tick vector or mammal host (Salyers & Whitt, 2002). Furthermore, other outer surface proteins of *Borrelia* spp. allow it to exhibit **antigenic variation.** It can

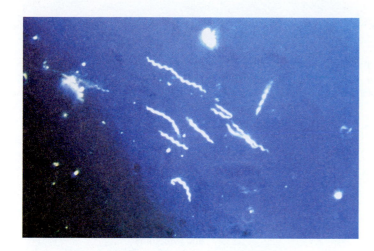

■ **FIGURE 25-3** This darkfield examination demonstrates the spirochete *Borrelia burgdorferi.*
From Centers for Disease Control and Prevention.

change its surface proteins to avoid detection by the host immune system. One other recognized virulence factor is the presence of **adhesins** that allow the spirochete to adhere to various host tissues and enhance dissemination.

SPECIMEN COLLECTION AND PROCESSING

Borrelia spp. are known for two diseases, Lyme disease and relapsing fever. The specimen used for diagnosis depends on the disease suspected. In cases of suspected Lyme disease, the organisms may be found in the skin and tissues and detected by silver stains, immunofluorescence, and molecular methods. Culture is possible early in the disease, using a skin biopsy of the characteristic lesion or citrated blood. CSF can also be cultured if there are signs of meningitis. Liquid Barbour-Stoenner-Kelly (BSK) medium is available. It is incubated at 30–34°C, in the dark and under microaerophilic conditions, for up to 12 weeks. The medium is examined for the presence of spirochetes by darkfield examination. Culture is usually too cumbersome and not productive. It is also not available in most laboratories. Serology is currently the best tool for diagnosis.

@ **REAL WORLD TIP**

It is possible to culture the tick if the patient has saved it after removal. The midgut of the tick should be removed and used for culture.

For diagnosis of relapsing disease, a Wright- or Giemsa-stained peripheral blood smear, taken during an episode of fever, will demonstrate the spirochete among the red blood cells. A buffy coat smear can also be stained. It is possible to see the organism swimming and pushing red bloods cells around in a wet preparation of peripheral blood. Culture is also available.

@ **REAL WORLD TIP**

Often relapsing fever is detected in the hematology department upon seeing the spirochete during the review of the stained differential smear.

CLINICAL SIGNIFICANCE

◆ Lyme Disease

Lyme disease, also known as Lyme borreliosis, is an inflammatory disease caused by the spirochete, *B. burgdorferi.* The disease can affect multiple organ systems, including the nervous system, cardiovascular system, joints, and muscles (Singh & Girschick, 2004). Infection occurs when the soft bodied tick vector, mainly of the genus *Ixodes*, transmits the spirochete during a blood meal.

Lyme disease is now the most commonly reported arthropod-borne disease in the United States and Europe. According to the Centers for Disease Control and Prevention (CDC), more than 100,000 cases of Lyme disease were reported in the United States from 1990 to 2000, and the highest incidence occurred in Connecticut. The peak seasonality is during the months of May through August, when both the tick activity and human outdoor activity are also at their peak. Fortunately, even in endemic areas where a large number of ticks can be infected, the chance of acquiring the disease from tick exposure is not great. The spirochete appears to disseminate from the tick to the human host after at least 48 hours of attachment. Thus, ticks removed before this period of time are unlikely to transmit the spirochete (Steere, Coburn, & Glickstein, 2004).

@ **REAL WORLD TIP**

Lyme disease has been reported in every state except Hawaii. The northeastern coastal states still maintain the highest incidence of infection. Certain regions of Minnesota and Michigan also have a high risk for contracting Lyme disease.

The clinical findings of Lyme disease manifest in three stages (Stanek & Strie, 2003; Figure 25-4 ■). Stage 1, primarily localized to the skin, lasts a median of 4 weeks, but can vary from person to person. In this stage of the disease, the only sign that provides a reliable diagnosis is the appearance of a characteristic lesion at the site of the tick bite. **Erythema migrans** (EM) is a small, red, pigmented spot on the skin that slowly enlarges, resulting in a ringlike or target lesion (Figure 25-5). It is often accompanied by flulike symptoms, such as fatigue, headache, joint and muscle pain, and fever. The characteristic lesion may only appear in about two-thirds of those infected.

Stage 2 occurs within days or weeks and results from hematogenous dissemination. During this stage, the spirochete

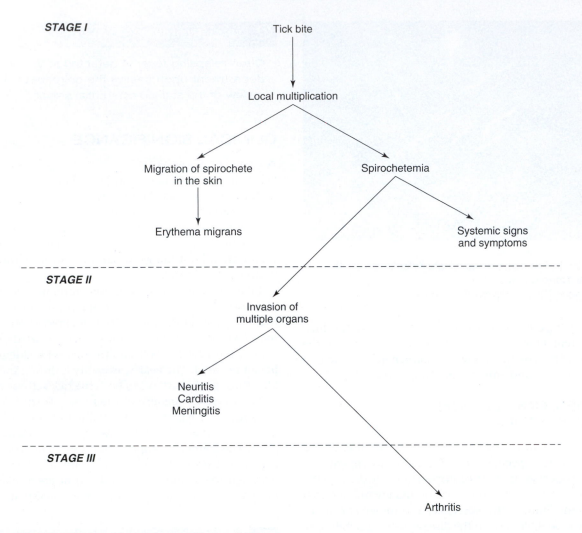

FIGURE 25-4 Clinical stages of Lyme disease.

can be recovered from blood and CSF. Symptoms can include smaller secondary skin lesions similar to the original EM, meningitis, acute muscle and joint pain, conjunctivitis, and neuropathy.

Stage 3 disease occurs months to years later and is characterized as a persistent infection. In untreated patients, most will experience intermittent bouts of arthritis, especially in the large joints. Despite antibiotic treatment, a small percentage of patients may develop severe fatigue, musculoskeletal pain, or neurocognitive disorders. The symptoms of *B. burgdorferi* infection may be the result of the formation of antigen-specific immune complexes that result in autoimmune-mediated injury (Singh & Girschick, 2004).

Diagnosis of Lyme Disease

The diagnostic criteria for Lyme disease have been established by the CDC. A clinical case is defined by the presence of erythema migrans approximately 5 cm in diameter or at least one late manifestation, such as musculoskeletal, nervous, or cardiac involvement, and laboratory confirmation of infection. The laboratory criteria for diagnosis are:

1. Isolation of *B. burgdorferi* from clinical specimens
2. Demonstration of diagnostic levels of IgM or IgG to the spirochete in serum or CSF
3. Significant change in IgM or IgG in paired acute and convalescent serum samples

Among the laboratory criteria for diagnosis, culture of *B. burgdorferi* from clinical specimens in Barbour-Stoenner-Kelly medium may provide a definitive diagnosis. However, although the spirochete grows well in vitro, it is infrequently recovered from human specimens. This is likely because of the short-lived spirochetemia and the low density of organisms in the tissue. Positive cultures are usually only obtained early in the course of disease, primarily from biopsies of the erythema migrans lesions and occasionally from plasma and CSF samples. Visualization of the organism in the tissue is also rare because of the small numbers of spirochetes.

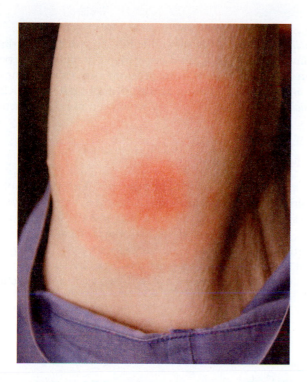

■ **FIGURE 25-5** Erythema migrans is the target-like skin lesion associated with Lyme disease.
From Centers for Disease Control and Prevention.

Serology provides the best means of diagnosis if no EM is present. Current serologic tests include indirect immunofluorescence assay (IFA), ELISA, hemagglutination, and Western blotting. A two-step detection of antibody response to *B. burgdorferi*, determined by first ELISA and then confirmed with Western blot, provides a positive diagnosis.

In most cases of stage 1 disease, the sensitivity of serology is low. In the early stages of disease, less than half of patients have detectable IgM antibodies. In the late stage of disease, a majority of patients are seropositive and display a shift from IgM to IgG antibodies. IgM peaks 3 to 6 weeks after onset, and IgG peaks in 2 to 3 months. Individuals in stage 1 or stage 2 disease may take as long as 3 to 6 months after exposure to become seropositive. Usually, patients with stage 3 disease have seropositive results. Serological testing is full of cross reactions and nonspecific results when used for the diagnosis of Lyme disease. Serology results and the presence of the characteristic skin lesion often make diagnosis easier. The physician must understand the limitations of each test used for diagnosis. Even molecular testing has limitations due to the scarcity of the organism in specimens.

◆ **Relapsing Fever**

Relapsing fever is a disease characterized by recurrent bouts of fever and nonspecific symptoms such as headache, myalgia, arthralgia, and abdominal pain. It is caused by infection with *Borrelia* spirochetes through the bite of an infected tick or contact with the body fluid of an infected louse. Tick-borne relapsing fever (TBRF) is caused by *Borrelia hermsii*, *B. parkeri*, *B. duttoni*, and *B. turicatae*, whereas louse-borne relapsing fever (LBRF) is caused by *Borrelia recurrentis*. TBRF is found throughout most parts of the world and is endemic in the western United States. Cases rarely occur east of Texas in the United States (Dworkin, Schwan, & Anderson, 2002). LBRF is often associated with war, overcrowding, homelessness, and poor personal hygiene. Humans are the only reservoir for LBRF while animals, such as squirrels and rabbits, serve as reservoir hosts for TBRF.

Unlike the ticks that transmit Lyme disease, the ticks that transmit relapsing fever may need only 30 seconds of attachment to the skin to transmit the spirochetes. In the case of louse-borne disease, the organism can be transmitted through breaks in the skin or via the mucous membranes. The incubation period ranges from 4 to 18 days. The episode of the first set of symptoms usually lasts around 3 to 5 days, and a week usually passes before relapse. Symptoms include high fever, headache, muscle and joint pain, and fatigue.

During fever the organisms are numerous in the blood. Once recognized by the host immune system, the organisms hide in the internal organs where they modify the composition of their surface proteins. When they remerge into the blood stream, fever returns. This happens multiple times with TBRF but often only once with LBRF. Complications of relapsing fever can include involvement of the hepatic, renal, cardiovascular, gastrointestinal, and central nervous systems.

Diagnosis of Relapsing Fever

Observation of routine differential, fixed blood smears during the acute stage of disease may reveal as many as five spirochetes per 100× oil immersion field (Dworkin et al., 2002). However, spirochetes in infected patients may be missed by microscopy if they are below a density of 10^4/mL. Spirochetes may also be visualized by direct or indirect immunofluorescent staining and fluorescence or darkfield microscopy. A wet mount of a blood specimen can be examined with a brightfield microscope. During urologic involvement, dysuria, proteinuria, and microhematuria may be observed, and spirochetes may be observed in the urine during acute disease. However, during asymptomatic infection, spirochetes are undetectable by microscopy.

Serologic diagnosis of relapsing fever is determined by a fourfold increase in antibody titer between paired acute and convalescent sera or sera that is reactive. ELISA is the most frequently performed test. Indirect immunofluorescent antibody test (IFA) and Western blot are also performed. The phenomenon of antigenic variation may contribute to false-negative test results. Serologic tests, particularly ELISA and IFA, may yield false-positives if patients have been previously infected with other species of spirochetes due to cross reaction with flagellin proteins.

Many *Borrelia* species can be distinguished by PCR amplification and analysis of specific genomic DNA markers. Due to its complexity, molecular testing for *Borrelia* is not routinely performed in most laboratories.

Checkpoint! 25–4 (Chapter Objective 7)

A reliable and specific serologic test to distinguish between pathogenic Borrelia species would likely target which of the following bacterial components?

    A. *Flagellin*
    B. *Osp*
    C. *Constitutively expressed proteins*
    D. *Surface proteins that undergo antigenic variationt*

Treatment

Borrelia spp. are sensitive to antibiotics. Amoxicillin and doxycycline are often used. Third-generation cephalosporins, penicillin G, and erythromycin are other options. Doxycycline has the advantage of working against other organisms, such as *Ehrlichia* and *Rickettsia* species, which can also be carried by ticks.

SUMMARY

The spirochetes are a fascinating group of bacteria, capable of causing a wide spectrum of human disorders. Fortunately, standard serologic tests are available to diagnose the spirochetal diseases. However, a major obstacle in the medical laboratory is the inability to discriminate between species. The development of molecular or serologic tests that are species specific remains a significant challenge in the diagnosis of spirochetal infections.

LEARNING OPPORTUNITIES

1. A patient with a disseminated rash tests positive with both the nontreponemal and treponemal tests. What do these observations most likely indicate and why? (Chapter Objectives 1, 3, and 4)

2. A patient presents to the clinic with clinical signs and symptoms of Lyme disease. Describe three laboratory findings that would confirm the diagnosis. (Chapter Objectives 1, 3, and 6)

3. How is *Treponema pallidum,* the agent of syphilis, distinct from the nonvenereal treponemes? (Chapter Objectives 1 and 5)

4. What distinguishes the spirochete from other bacterial organisms? (Chapter Objective 2)

Further Reading: *Bad Blood: The Tuskegee Syphilis Experiment* by James Jones (New York Free Press, 1981).

PEARSON
myhealthprofessionskit™

Use this address to access the interactive Companion Website created for this textbook. Simply select "Clinical Laboratory Science" from the choice of disciplines. Find this book and log in using your user name and password.

REFERENCES

Go to myhealthprofessionskit.com to view this chapter's references.

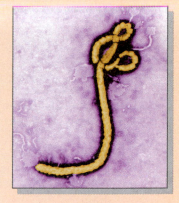

26

Mycobacterium Species

Jaya Prakash

■ LEARNING OBJECTIVES

Upon completion of this chapter, the learner should be able to:

1. List the major medically important *Mycobacterium* species.
2. Relate the epidemiology of the medically important *Mycobacterium* species.
3. Classify mycobacteria on the basis of pathogenicity, pigment production, and growth rate.
4. Differentiate the most commonly isolated *Mycobacterium* species on the basis of:
   a. microscopic morphology
   b. colony morphology
   c. key biochemical reactions
   d. molecular methods
5. Relate the clinical significance of various species of mycobacteria.
6. Select the appropriate form of treatment for mycobacterial infections.

KEY TERMS

acid-fast bacilli

atypical mycobacteria

leprosy

Mantoux test

TAXONOMY

Family *Mycobacteriaceae* (my-kō-bak-tēr'-e-a-sē'-ē)
  Genus *Mycobacterium* (my-kō-bak-tēr'-ee-uhm)
    Mycobacterium tuberculosis complex (the tubercle bacilli)
      M. tuberculosis (too-bûr'-kyə-lŏ'-sis)
      M. bovis (bŏ'-vis) and a related organism the Bacille Calmette Guérin (bă-seel' kăl-mĕt' gă-răn') or BCG strain
      M. africanum (af'-ree-kah-num)
      M. microti (my-krŏ'-tee)
      M. canetti (kah'-net-ee)

Mycobacterium avium complex
    M. avium (ā-vee-uhm)
    M. intracellulare (in'-trə-sel-yoo'-lâr)
  M. kansasii (kan-zəs-ee-eye)
  M. marinum (mə-reen-uhm)
  M. ulcerans (ul-sə-rans)
  M. fortuitum (fôr-too-i-tuhm)
  M. chelonae (che-lŏ'-nee)
  M. malmoense (mal-mŏ'-en-see)
  M. xenopi (zə-nŏ'-pee)
  M. gordonae (gôr'-dŏn-ee)
  M. haemophilum (hee-mof-i-lum)

▶ INTRODUCTION

The term **acid-fast bacilli** refers to a number of aerobic, non-spore-forming, rod-shaped bacteria that resist decolorization with acid-alcohol decolorizing reagents. While acid-fast bacilli is the term frequently used to describe these bacteria, these microorganisms may appear as coccoid and filamentous forms, as well as bacillary forms. Most species of mycobacteria will grow on media containing simple substrates. Only a few are fastidious, such as *M. haemophilum,* which requires hemin, or *M. leprae,* an organism that cannot be cultivated *in vitro.* The genus *Mycobacterium* includes a number of species, most of which are harmless saprobes that can be isolated from soil and water. There are species that are native to animals other than humans (but which may infect humans, such as *M. bovis, M. avium,* and *M. microti*), and pathogenic species that primarily infect humans, such as *Mycobacterium tuberculosis, M. africanum,* and *M. leprae.* Mycobacteria are responsible for many cases of human illness and death throughout the world.

Mycobacteria have very complex cell walls with high lipid content, including mycolic acids (long chain, branched fatty acids: up to 90 carbons) and waxy substances, and, as a consequence, are relatively resistant to unfavorable environments. They are quite capable of surviving arid, acid, or alkaline conditions that destroy or inhibit the growth of most other organisms. The unique nature of the cell wall constituents also makes mycobacteria microorganisms able to evade the immune system. Defense mechanisms, including antibody production, complement lysis, and phagocytosis, are basically ineffective in dealing with invasion by organisms such as *M. tuberculosis,* the most common cause of tuberculosis. Mycobacteria not only survive phagocytosis, but they are capable of multiplying within the cytoplasm of macrophages.

Another consequence of the cell wall complexity is the relatively long generation time, which is close to 20 hours. In contrast, the generation time of *E. coli* is about 20 minutes. Because of the long generation time, and exceedingly slow growth rate of mycobacteria, isolation from clinical specimens may take as long as 6–8 weeks. For this reason identification by conventional means and susceptibility testing can be a lengthy process, requiring up to 12 weeks before a final report can be rendered.

According to the latest estimates by the World Health Organization, nearly one-third of the world's population is infected with *Mycobacterium tuberculosis.* Nine million new cases of tuberculosis occur each year, with nearly 2 million deaths attributed annually to this disease (a case fatality rate of 23%). The greatest numbers of cases per capita occur in Africa where factors such as population growth, migration from rural settings to urban centers, poverty and poor living conditions, and the spread of HIV contribute greatly to the spread of tuberculosis.

Only a small number of active cases of tuberculosis are seen in industrialized countries but infections caused by acid-fast bacteria are increasing as the population of immunocompromised individuals increases. Leukemia and lymphoma patients, transplant patients, AIDS patients, cancer patients, patients on corticosteroid therapy, and patients subjected to irradiation and chemotherapy are particularly vulnerable to infection with *Mycobacteria* species.

▶ CLASSIFICATION OF THE MYCOBACTERIA

Over the years different classification schemes have been devised to categorize the many different *Mycobacterium* species. The criteria that have been used to classify these organisms include biochemical tests, serological tests, physiological characteristics (particularly colony morphology), and pathogenicity.

CLASSIFICATION BASED ON PATHOGENICITY

The simplest classification scheme is to use pathogenicity as a distinguishing characteristic. Two groups can be established in this manner. The first group is the *Mycobacterium tuberculosis* complex, also referred to as the "tubercle bacilli." The

Mycobacterium tuberculosis complex includes those mycobacteria that are primary agents of human tuberculosis (Table 26-1 ✪). Tuberculosis is a disease that is characterized by the formation of spherical granulomatous lesions, called tubercles, and caseous (cheese like) necrosis. The tubercle bacilli include *M. tuberculosis, M. bovis, M. africanum, M. microti,* and *M. canetti.*

- *M. tuberculosis* is the most common cause of pulmonary tuberculosis or "consumption," a slowly progressive, respiratory illness that is very contagious.

- *M. bovis,* an organism with a wide host range, is associated with tuberculosis in humans, other primates, goats, cats, dogs, deer, buffalo, and bison, as well as cattle. Presently, the number of human infections caused by *M. bovis* is quite low, but prior to the introduction of pasteurization and other public health measures it was spread to humans through the consumption of milk from infected cows. Interestingly, individuals who work with infected cattle are more likely to develop pulmonary disease than alimentary disease (O'Reilley & Daborn, 1995).

- *M. africanum* is an organism that occasionally causes pulmonary tuberculosis in Africa.

- *M. microti* is an organism that causes tuberculosis primarily in small wild rodents such as voles (vole tuberculosis). There have been reported cases of this organism causing severe pulmonary tuberculosis in immunocompetent individuals (Van Soolingen et al., 1998). *M. microti* is a very slow growing organism that is very difficult to isolate and differentiate because of its extended incubation period, which may be as long as 9 weeks for visible growth. Because of this, molecular methods (∞ Chapter 8, "Final Identification") are often the means sought to characterize isolates as *M. microti.*

- *M. canetti:* Tuberculosis caused by this organism is an emerging disease found in northwest Africa (the Horn of Africa). Unlike *M. tuberculosis,* which grows slowly and produces rough, thick, dry, light buff-colored colonies on Lowenstein-Jensen medium, *M. canetti* grows much quicker and produces smooth, white, glossy colonies (Miltgen et al., 2002).

In contrast, **atypical mycobacteria** species, those that are not in the *M. tuberculosis* complex, are referred to as nontuberculous mycobacteria (NTM), or mycobacteria other than tubercle (MOTT) bacilli. This group includes such organisms as *M. avium, M. intracellulare, M. kansasii, M. malmoense, M. chelonae, M. xenopi,* and *M. gordonae.* Some of these organisms are capable of producing a pulmonary disease identical to that produced by the tubercle bacilli and have been recovered from the respiratory samples of patients with a high index of clinical suspicion of tuberculosis. Unlike the tubercle bacilli, however, there is no evidence of person-to-person transmission. The population at risk is immunocompromised individuals and the route of transmission is more than likely direct contact with these organisms, many of which are found in environmental reservoirs such as fresh water (*M. gordonae*) or soil.

CLASSIFICATION BASED ON PHYSIOLOGY

In 1959, E. H. Runyon classified the nontuberculous mycobacteria into four groups on the basis of pigment production and their rate of growth (Table 26-1). Formerly called Runyon groups I, II, III, and IV, these groups are presently designated as follows:

- Photochromogens (Runyon group I)—slow-growing *Mycobacterium* species (requiring 2–6 weeks of incubation in order for mature colonies to form), which are nonpigmented when they are grown in the absence of light (Figure 26-1 ■). They, however, are able to produce yellow or orange carotenoid pigments when they are subsequently exposed to light and reincubated, a phenomenon known as photoactivation. The activity of the enzyme responsible for the production of the soluble beta carotene pigments is not only light-dependent but also oxygen-dependent.

- Scotochromogens (Runyon group II)—slow-growing species that produce yellow to orange pigment whether they are grown in the dark or in the light. The pigment produced in the absence of light deepens to orange or dark red when the organisms are exposed to light (Figure 26-2 ■).

- Nonphotochromogens (Runyon group III)—slow-growing organisms that may be lightly pigmented (buff, tan, or

---

✪ TABLE 26-1				
Medically Important *Mycobacterium* Species				
***M. tuberculosis* Complex**	**Photochromogens**	**Scotochromogens**	**Nonphotochromogens**	**Rapid Growers**
M. tuberculosis	*M. kansasii*	*M. scrofulaceum*	*M. avium* complex (MAC) [*M. avium* and *M. intracellulare*]	*M. fortuitum*
M. bovis and BCG	*M. marinum*	*M. szulgai*	*M. xenopi*	*M. chelonae*
M. africanum	*M. simiae*	*M. gordonae*	*M. malmoense*	*M. abscessus*
M. microti			*M. paratuberculosis*	
M. canetti				

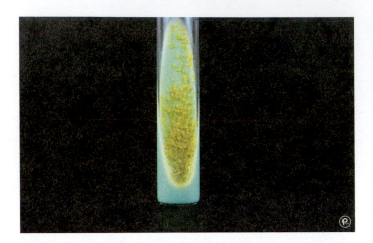

pale yellow). The pigment does not intensify when they are exposed to light (Figure 26-3 ■).

■ Rapid-growers (Runyon group IV)—organisms that form mature colonies that are readily visible to the naked eye within 7 days of incubation (Figure 26-4 ■).

Differentiation to the genus-species level is dependent on further testing. Biochemical tests, such as nitrate and tellurite reduction, Tween 80 hydrolysis, urease and catalase production, and the niacin test are frequently employed. Fatty acid analysis, mycolic acid analysis, and DNA hybridization tech-

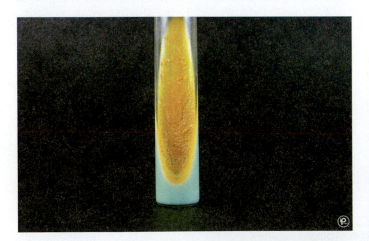

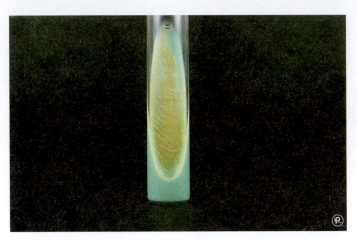

niques such as the polymerase chain reaction are more recent procedures that can be used to identify mycobacteria. Refer to ∞ Chapter 13, "Acid-Fast Bacilli Cultures," to review specimen processing and presumptive identification of acid-fast bacilli.

CLASSIFICATION INTO COMPLEXES

Mycobacteria have also been grouped into complexes. Certain species share similar biochemical, serological, and pathogenic characteristics, allowing them to be grouped into complexes. The *M. tuberculosis* complex (the tubercle bacilli) has previously been mentioned. Complexes such as the *M. avium* complex (MAC), which includes *M. avium* and *M. intracellulare*

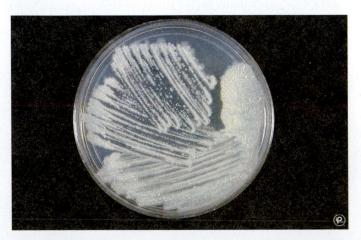

biovariants, and the *M. fortuitum* complex, which includes bio-variants of *M. fortuitum* and *M. chelonae,* have become well recognized as groups of closely related organisms.

 **Checkpoint! 26–1
(Chapter Objectives 1 and 2)**

Mycobacterium bovis is classified as a member of:
  A. *Nontuberculous mycobacteria (NTM).*
  B. *M. tuberculosis complex.*
  C. *M. avium complex (MAC).*
  D. *M. fortuitum complex.*

 **Checkpoint! 26–2
(Chapter Objective 2)**

_____ *are slow growing mycobacteria which may be lightly pigmented when grown in the dark and, when exposed to light and re-incubated, the pigment does not intensify.*
  A. *Photochromogens*
  B. *Scotochromogens*
  C. *Nonphotochromogens*
  D. *Rapid growers*

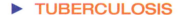

▶ TUBERCULOSIS

There are certain populations that are at a higher risk of acquiring mycobacterial infections, such as immunosuppressed patients, those living in close quarters (such as prison inmates), those with a low socioeconomic status (homeless persons and recent immigrants from underdeveloped countries), and health care workers.

Tuberculosis, a disease that may be asymptomatic, might be suspected based on the appropriate clinical history (contact with infected individuals shedding the organism), results of the **Mantoux** or tuberculin skin test, or examination of chest radiographs for evidence of granulomatous lesions within lung tissue. Tuberculosis is often associated with the production of very viscous sputum. Mycobacteria, which may be seen within the mucous threads on sputum smears, do not stain well, if at all, with Gram stain reagents, and may appear as "ghost cells" (unstained bacteria) or they may exhibit a beaded appearance when examined microscopically. With acid-fast stains, such as the Ziehl-Neelsen or Kinyoun carbol fuchsin-based stains or auramine-rhodamine fluorescent stains, mycobacteria are typically slightly curved or straight rods about 0.2–0.6 microns in diameter and 1–10 microns in length. *M. tuberculosis* can exhibit serpentine cording on smear from liquid and solid media. The rope-like strands of organisms are often presumptive for *M. tuberculosis.* ∞ Chapter 8, "Presump-

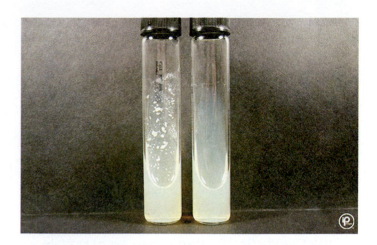

■ **FIGURE 26-5** TCH medium inoculated with mycobacteria showing growth or resistance (left) and no growth or susceptibility (right).
From Marler LM, Siders JA, Kaufman CM, Owens EN, Korba GG and Allen SD, *Bacteriology I Image Atlas* CD-ROM, Indiana Pathology Images, 2005.

tive Identification," and ∞ Chapter 13, "Acid-Fast Bacilli Cultures," have photos of acid-fast bacilli stained with carbol fuchsin and fluorescent stains.

Mycobacterium tuberculosis will not grow on routine media, whereas most other bacterial pathogens grow well on blood or chocolate agars within 24 to 72 hours. On suitable growth media, including egg-based media such as Lowenstein-Jensen slants, or chemically defined media, such as Middlebrook 7H10 and 7H11, 4–8 weeks are required for visible growth to appear. *M. tuberculosis* will appear as dry, granular, buff-colored colonies. ∞ Chapter 13 has photos of the buff and rough *M. tuberculosis* colonies. This organism is niacin production and nitrate reduction positive, 68° C catalase test negative, and not inhibited (Figure 26-5 ■) by thiopene-2-carboxylic acid hydrazide (TCH). These biochemicals are discussed in more detail later in this chapter.

FDA-approved tests based on the polymerase chain reaction (PCR) can be used in the identification of members of the *M. tuberculosis* complex. In addition, nucleic acid probes are available to test clinical samples, as well as to identify organisms that have been cultivated.

▶ CLINICAL SIGNIFICANCE OF THE *MYCOBACTERIUM TUBERCULOSIS* COMPLEX

As mentioned earlier, the *M. tuberculosis* complex is comprised of those *Mycobacterium* species that are strict pathogens and the primary agents of tuberculosis, a highly contagious disease spread by the airborne route. It is estimated that as many as 3 million people are killed annually by tuberculosis. The body's primary immune defense against TB is through cell-mediated immunity. A finding supported by the fact a positive tuberculin skin test, a procedure in which a small amount of purified protein derivative is injected just under the top layer of skin on the forearm, is a reaction associated with delayed-type hypersensitivity. Radiographic evidence from Egyptian mummies has shown that members of the *M. tuberculosis* complex have been associated with human infection since antiquity.

℮ REAL WORLD TIP

- Criteria for a positive tuberculin test (also known as the purified protein derivative or PPD test) vary. For example, a raised hardened area around the injection site of greater than 15 mm is positive in those being tested prior to entering the work site if they have no risk factors. Greater than 10 mm would indicate a positive reaction in recent immigrants including those that have been vaccinated with BCG. Greater than 5 mm would indicate a positive result in HIV-positive individuals (Centers for Disease Control, 2000).

- A new test (QuantiFERON TB Gold, Cellestis, Valencia, CA), for detection of latent tuberculosis infection and tuberculosis disease, measures the release of interferon-gamma by lymphocytes, in whole blood, in response to PPD. Results are not affected by the BCG vaccine, but the test takes 12 hours for completion.

MYCOBACTERIUM TUBERCULOSIS

Mycobacterium tuberculosis, the primary agent of human tuberculosis, most commonly enters the host through the respiratory tract, although the gastrointestinal tract or skin may also serve as portals of entry. Transmission occurs through inhalation of respiratory droplets expelled from infected persons as they talk, sneeze, or cough.

Organisms entering the upper respiratory tract through the oropharynx and nasopharynx are drawn into the lower respiratory tract where they eventually settle into the air sacs or alveoli of the lungs. Alveolar macrophages (dust cells), whose job it is to remove dust, microbes, and other particulate matter from the lungs, phagocytize the acid-fast bacteria. Most other types of bacteria are destroyed by the processes involved in phagocytosis, but mycobacteria, having cell walls that are resistant to harsh chemicals, continue to survive. These organisms, which are able to multiply intracellularly as well as extracellularly, may be disseminated through the lymphatics and bloodstream by hitching a ride in the cytoplasm of phagocytic cells.

As mentioned earlier, organisms that have invaded host tissues induce a type IV or delayed-type hypersensitivity reaction, eventually becoming surrounded by mononuclear inflammatory cells that have entered the infected area. Macrophages are also recruited into the area, eventually maturing into elongated epithelioid cells, which, along with Langhans giant cells, are arranged in concentric circles to form granulomatous tubercles. Lymphocytes, plasma cells, immature macrophages, and fibroblasts then form an outer cellular

zone. The center of the tubercle disintegrates to form a homogenous, cheese-like mass in a process called caseation.

In immunocompetent individuals mycobacteria stimulate a strong cell–mediated immune response whereupon multiplication and dissemination ceases. In the last stage, lesions in the middle and lower lobes of the lungs undergo fibrosis and calcification, a process that makes them readily visible on radiographs (X-rays) of the chest (Figure 26-6 ■).

If the immune system of the infected person is insufficient to contain the organisms, the caseous mass in the lungs is liquefied by the hydrolytic enzymes of the macrophages. Within the lesions bacteria multiply in large numbers and, when the lesion ruptures, organisms are released into the environment. They are expelled from the respiratory tract when these infected individuals talk, sneeze or cough. This large outpouring of mycobacteria is responsible for the highly contagious nature of tuberculosis.

If the lesion ruptures into a pulmonary blood vessel, organisms can be spread to other parts of the body through the bloodstream, producing a condition known as miliary tuberculosis. Miliary tuberculosis is a severe disease and has a high mortality rate. Small nodular lesions, 1–3 mm in size (and thought to resemble millet seeds), appear in organs throughout the body. Organisms that have spread to the kidneys may multiply and subsequently be expelled in the urine.

Even in individuals with a strong immune response, conditions such as old age, diabetes, immunosuppression, or lung disease may lead to a weakening of the host's cellular immune system. In these cases tuberculous lesions may become necrotic, undergo liquefaction, and infectious bacteria may be released. This phenomenon is known as secondary tuberculosis.

Cord factor, a cell surface glycolipid that serves as a virulence factor for *M. tuberculosis,* plays a major role in the development of the granulomatous lesions of the tubercle bacilli.

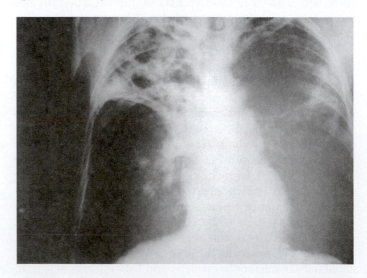

■ **FIGURE 26-6** A radiograph of the chest of a patient diagnosed with advanced bilateral pulmonary tuberculosis. The white cloudy areas represent where the organism has infiltrated.
From Public Health Image Library (PHIL), CDC.

MYCOBACTERIUM BOVIS

Mycobacterium bovis is another member of the *M. tuberculosis* complex or tubercle bacilli. Although this organism is an animal pathogen, it can also infect humans. It is mainly transmitted by the consumption of unpasteurized milk and diary products, whereupon it can cause gastrointestinal infection. *M. bovis* is rarely seen in the United States.

Bacille Calmette Guérin (BCG) is an attenuated strain of *M. bovis* that is used for vaccination against tuberculosis. It is rarely used in the United States because individuals who receive the vaccine become PPD positive. This leads to the loss of a valuable screening test. In rare cases this organism may cause infection in individuals who have been vaccinated (vaccinosis), especially those who are immunocompromised.

M. bovis is morphologically similar to *M. tuberculosis* when observed on acid-fast smears but can be differentiated from *M. tuberculosis* using biochemical tests. The organism grows poorly on traditional Lowenstein-Jensen slants but grows better when pyruvate is incorporated into the medium. Colonies are typically flat, round, thin, transparent, and have irregular edges. *M. bovis* is niacin, nitrate reduction, and pyrazinamidase negative and does not grow (Figure 26-6) on TCH medium (TCH susceptible).

MYCOBACTERIUM AFRICANUM

Mycobacterium africanum, another species in the *M. tuberculosis* complex that is morphologically similar in appearance to *M. tuberculosis,* also produces a disease similar to that associated with *M. tuberculosis.* It may produce disseminated disease in immunocompromised individuals. The organism, which is likely spread by inhalation of infectious respiratory droplets, is endemic to equatorial Africa. It has been reported in Europe and on rare occasion in the United States (CDC, 2004).

M. africanum is niacin, nitrate reduction, pyrazinamide, and tellurite reduction negative. Variable results are seen with TCH susceptibility. Differentiation from *M. tuberculosis* may require genotyping.

▶ DISEASES ASSOCIATED WITH NONTUBERCULOUS MYCOBACTERIA (NTM)

Diseases associated with nontuberculous mycobacteria occur primarily in individuals who are immunocompromised. As mentioned previously, these organisms are common environmental saprophytes and occur in fresh water and soil, the likely point of contact. NTM may colonize the respiratory, gastrointestinal, and urinary tract (*M. smegmatis*) without causing disease. Underlying conditions that lower host resistance contribute to the propensity of these organisms to cause significant morbidity and death. Because a host's defense against mycobacteria is largely dependent upon cell-mediated immunity, individuals with AIDS, leukemia, lymphoma, and other immunosuppressed states are very susceptible to these diseases. In industrialized countries, where tuberculosis is uncommon, infections due to NTM are predominant. AIDS patients, in particular, succumb to massive infections caused by members of the *M. avium* complex (MAC), which can be isolated from blood and stool specimens.

NTM have been associated with a number of different diseases, such as:

- Chronic pulmonary diseases, which closely resemble tuberculosis and are caused by the MAC and *M. kansasii.*

- Colonization and severe lung disease caused by *M. abscessus* (formerly known as *M. chelonae,* subspecies *abscessus*) in cystic fibrosis patients. Risk factors seem to be systemic steroids and allergic bronchopulmonary aspergillosis (Mussaffi, Rivlin, Shalit, Eprhos, & Bau, 2005). The organism is apparently picked up from the environment and is not nosocomially acquired or transmitted (Jönsson et al., 2007; Gaillard, 2003).

- Chronic lymphadenitis in young children caused by the MAC and *M. scrofulaceum*

- Skin infections characterized by ulcerative lesions and localized cutaneous granulomas are often caused by organisms such as *M. ulcerans* and *M. marinum.* These cases usually begin as injuries associated with watery environments, such as aquariums and swimming pools. Injuries to the knees and elbows from swimming pools and injuries to the fingers and hands of individuals who own or work with aquariums produce breaks in previously intact skin and then environmental organisms invade the subcutaneous tissues. *M. ulcerans* and *M. marinum* grow optimally at 30°C, a temperature close to that of the skin surface.

Checkpoint! 26–3 (Chapter Objective 4)

_____ *tuberculosis is a severe disease in which the TB organisms have disseminated to other parts of the body, producing nodular lesions.*
A. *Miliary*
B. *Nontubercular*
C. *Gastrointestinal*
D. *Subcutaneous*

Checkpoint! 26–4 (Chapter Objective 4)

Bacille Calmette Guérin is an attenuated mycobacterial strain that is used to immunize individuals in order to build resistance to tuberculosis. Which Mycobacterium species is used to create the BCG vaccine?
A. *M. tuberculosis*
B. *M. bovis*
C. *M. africanum*
D. *M. microti*

These organisms often do not grow well, if at all, at internal body temperatures (37°C).

■ Regional ileitis (also known as Crohn's disease) may be associated with *Mycobacterium avium* subspecies *paratuberculosis* (MAP). It is believed that MAP triggers a massive immune reaction against the body's own tissues. In this case the immune system reacts to an individual's own intestinal tissues, leading to ulcerative lesions that give the intestinal mucosa a "cobblestone" appearance. Individuals with Crohn's disease may suffer debilitating bouts of diarrhea, nausea, vomiting, and fever. In severe cases, repeated surgical resection of the colon may be the only treatment that promises relief from this painful condition (Greger, 2001).

Useful biochemical tests to identify acid-fast bacilli, which are discussed in detail later in this chapter, include photoreactivity, niacin production, nitrate reduction, catalase at 68°C, pyrazinamidase production, iron uptake, arylsulfatase production, and thiophene-2-carboxylic acid hydrazide (TCH) inhibition.

PHOTOCHROMOGENS

Photochromogens are nontuberculous mycobacteria that form pigment when exposed to light but that do not produce a pigment when the organism is grown and kept in the dark. Discussed below are photochromogens that are associated with human infection.

Mycobacterium kansasii

M. kansasii is second only to the MAC in causing NTM pulmonary infections in the United States. Classic lung infection is the most common manifestation. This organism can also produce cutaneous infections, lymphadenitis, and other soft tissue infections. It only causes disseminated disease in severely immunocompromised patients.

M. kansasii forms smooth, raised, buff-colored colonies in the absence of light and yellow colonies after exposure to light. Some colonies may be rough and wrinkled. Microscopically the acid-fast bacilli have a beaded appearance. *M. kansasii* is nitrate positive, hydrolyzes Tween 80 (Figure 26-7 ■), strongly catalase positive, and pyrazinamide negative. A 16sRNA nucleic acid probe is a molecular method that is currently available for identification purposes.

Mycobacterium marinum

M. marinum grows best at 30°C with little or no growth at 37°C similar to *M. ulcerans* and *M. haemophilum*. This organism, which is found in water, soil, and many other habitats, causes chronic skin infections associated with swimming pools and aquariums. A papule or nodule usually develops at the site of inoculation (often through breaks in the skin such as cuts or abrasions) and may ulcerate later on.

Buff-colored, smooth to slightly rough colonies are produced when grown in the dark. Following exposure to light

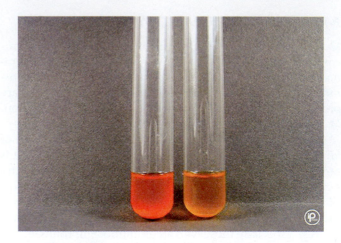

■ **FIGURE 26-7** Tween 80 test results showing hydrolysis or positive pink-to-red color (left) and negative amber color (right) results.
From Marler LM, Siders JA, Kaufman CM, Owens EN, Korba GG and Allen SD, *Bacteriology I Image Atlas* CD-ROM, Indiana Pathology Images, 2005.

and reincubation, a yellow pigment is produced. The organism is nitrate reduction positive, pyrazinamide positive, and hydrolyzes Tween 80. Microscopically, long rods with cross bands are observed.

Other photochromogens have recently emerged as opportunistic pathogens. *M. abscessus* causes disseminated infections in immunocompromised patients. *M. chelonae, M. mucogenicum,* and *M. smegmatis* are known to cause skin and soft tissue infections.

SCOTOCHROMOGENS

Scotochromogens produce a deep yellow to orange pigment whether they are grown in the dark or in the light. The pigment produced in the absence of light deepens to orange or dark red when the organisms are exposed to light. Scotochromogens of medical importance include the following.

Mycobacterium scrofulaceum

M. scrofulaceum was a common cause of cervical lymphadenitis, especially in children, and is still common in Africa. In fact, its scientific name is associated with the characteristic swollen, glandular swellings, which at one time were called "scrofulae."

Smooth colonies that are deep yellow to orange pigmented in the dark, and that may or may not deepen after exposure to light, can be seen on the proper growth media. Microscopically the organisms are similar to *M. tuberculosis* in appearance. Identification can be accomplished with the aid of biochemical reactions such as niacin production and Tween 80 hydrolysis (Figure 26-7), which are both negative. *M. scrofulaceum* is catalase positive (both semi-quantitative and 68°C).

Mycobacterium gordonae

M. gordonae, also known as the tap water bacillus, is a non-pathogen that is occasionally seen as a laboratory contaminant because it can be found in tap water. Until identified, it may be considered to be the cause of an infection or "pseudo" outbreaks when it is isolated on media or observed on smears.

Colony morphology consists of smooth, yellow- to orange-colored colonies in conditions of light and dark. Colonies may be raised or dome-shaped with regular or irregular edges. The organism is nitrate reduction and urea negative, Tween 80 hydrolysis, and catalase positive. The polymerase chain reaction (PCR) and nucleic acid probes are also available. Microscopically *M. gordonae* is similar in appearance to *M. tuberculosis,* but it does not show cording.

NONPHOTOCHROMOGENS

Nonphotochromogens do not produce pigment in the dark or after exposure to light. The *M. avium* complex consists of two organisms, *M. avium* and *M. intracellulare,* that are often difficult to differentiate. They are opportunistic pathogens and are able to cause a variety of diseases.

Mycobacterium avium and Mycobacterium intracellulare

Both organisms produce a colony morphology exhibiting considerable variation, most commonly appearing as small, smooth, thin colonies. Some colonies are rough and wrinkled. Microscopically they are similar to *M. tuberculosis* in acid fastness. These organisms are nitrate reduction, niacin, and Tween 80 negative. In addition, they reduce tellurite and are pyrazinamide positive (4 days). Nucleic acid probes and 16sRNA genotyping are needed to distinguish between *M. avium* and *M. intracellulare.*

Members of the MAC are widely distributed in nature. They are important pathogens of poultry and swine. Occasionally they are isolated from disease and symptom-free individuals. In AIDS patients they are major pathogens and may cause disseminated disease. In heavy smokers, alcoholics, and those with preexisting disease, members of the MAC can cause pulmonary infections. These organisms are an important cause of cervical lymphadenitis in children 1–5 years of age.

Mycobacterium ulcerans

M. ulcerans is the etiological agent of a chronic ulcerative disease affecting the skin and subcutaneous tissues. The highest incidence occurs in children and is endemic in the tropical areas of Africa, Central and South America, Asia, and Australia. In Africa the disease is known as Buruli ulcer while in Australia it is known as Bairnsdale ulcer. Buruli ulcer is the third most common mycobacterial disease in humans following tuberculosis and leprosy (Centers for Disease Control and Prevention, 2004).

The initial lesion, which appears 7–14 days after the initial skin trauma, is seen most often on the lower leg or arm and usually begins as a small papule resembling an insect bite. As the disease slowly progresses, the lesion becomes a nodule that can be felt under the skin. Eventually the skin over the nodular lesion erodes, producing a shallow ulcer. The ulcerative lesions are typically painless with surrounding induration and extensive subcutaneous necrosis. Histologically, numerous extracellular acid-fast bacilli are seen. Systemic symptoms such as fever are usually absent.

Treatment consists of complete surgical removal of all necrotic tissue, often extending well beyond the visible margins of the ulcer and skin grafting of large lesions. Antimycobacterial therapy without prior surgical intervention appears to be ineffective. *M. ulcerans* is sensitive, in vitro, to streptomycin, clofazimine, and ethambutol (Jenkin, Smith, Fairley, & Robinson, 2002).

This slow-growing nonphotochromogen grows best at temperatures approximating 30°C (32–33°C is recommended) and produces rough colonies. The organism is nitrate reduction, Tween hydrolysis, and arylsulfatase negative. A positive reaction is seen with the 68°C catalase test.

Other nonphotochromogens causing pulmonary infections and disseminated disease include the following species: *M. xenopi, M. malmoense, M. shimoidei,* and *M. simiae.* Disseminated infections have been caused by *M. haemophilum* and *M. genavense.*

RAPID GROWERS

Organisms classified as rapid growers are nontuberculous mycobacteria that grow readily on blood or chocolate agar in 3–5 days and take less than 7 days to grow on Lowenstein-Jensen medium. This group of organisms may not stain with auramine O fluorescent stain but do stain with the carbolfuschin stains. Most laboratories prefer the ease of use of the fluorescent stain so these organisms could be missed on smear.

Mycobacterium fortuitum Complex

Members of the *M. fortuitum* complex are weakly gram positive and resemble diphtheroids. These bacilli are weakly acid fast and form round, convex, rough, wrinkled, multilobulate

---

 Checkpoint! 26–5 (Chapter Objective 4)

Mycobacterium marinum is one of two medically important organisms that grow optimally at temperatures close to _____. This is consistent with the fact these organisms are associated with lesions affecting the skin and subcutaneous tissues.

    A. *25°C*
    B. *30°C*
    C. *37°C*
    D. *42°C*

colonies, which sometimes have filamentous extensions, on Lowenstein-Jensen medium. These organisms grow on Mac-Conkey agar without crystal violet, tolerate 5% sodium chloride, and are niacin negative. In addition, they are arylsulfatase and iron uptake positive.

Members of the *M. fortuitum* complex have been isolated from soil and water. They are responsible for a variety of diseases including surgical and traumatic wound infections, osteomyelitis, as well as skin and other soft tissue infections.

 Checkpoint! 26–6
(Chapter Objective 4)

Which of the nontuberculous mycobacteria is a photochromogen that is associated with pulmonary infections but may also cause cutaneous lesions, lymphadenitis, and other soft tissue infections?

A. *M. tuberculosis*
B. *M. fortuitum*
C. *M. kansasii*
D. *M. intracellulare*

► BIOCHEMICAL TESTS FOR THE DIFFERENTIATION OF MYCOBACTERIA

While physiological criteria are used to assign isolates to a particular subgroup such as photochromogen, scotochromogen, nonphotochromogen, or rapid grower, identification to the genus species or complex level requires a more sophisticated approach. A number of biochemical tests may be used to differentiate mycobacteria. This section of the chapter is devoted to a brief description of some of the commonly used biochemical tests (in alphabetical order).

ARYLSULFATASE

Arylsulfatase is an enzyme that catalyzes the breakdown of trispotassium phenolphthalein disulfate producing free phenolthalein, which can be detected by the addition of a solution that creates alkaline conditions.

To perform the test, arylsulfatase medium is inoculated with a loopful of freshly grown test organism or 0.1 mL from a 1-week broth culture. After an incubation period of 3 days for rapid growers or 14 days for slow growers, 1 ml of 1M sodium carbonate solution is added. A pink color (Figure 26-8 ■) is indicative of a positive reaction and no color change is considered to be a negative reaction.

CATALASE

The catalase enzyme causes the breakdown of hydrogen peroxide (H_2O_2) into water and oxygen, which produces effervescence (bubbles). There are two types of catalase tests, one that tests for a form of catalase that is stable at 68°C. The other test is a semiquantitative catalase test.

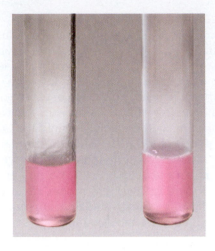

■ **FIGURE 26-8** A positive arylsulfatase reaction for *Mycobacterium fortuitum*.
Photo courtesy of Remel, part of Thermo Fisher Scientific.

To test for the heat stable catalase (Figure 26-9 ■), a heavy suspension of the organism in 0.5 ml of phosphate buffer is made. The suspension is heated to 68°C in a heating block or water bath for 20 minutes. The tube is cooled to room temperature and 0.5 ml of a 10% Tween 80 and 30% hydrogen peroxide solution (1:1 mixture) is then added. The tube is recapped loosely and, after 5 minutes, examined for the presence of a column of bubbles (a positive reaction). Tubes in which there is no effervescence must be observed after a period of 20 minutes before recording as negative and discarding.

To perform the semi-quantitative catalase test, inoculate the flat (not slanted) surface of Lowenstein-Jensen deep tubes with 0.1 mL of a week-old broth culture or loopful of a colony. Incubate at 37°C for 2 weeks. Place the tube in an upright position and add 1.0 mL of a Tween 80 and 30% hydrogen peroxide solution (1:1 mixture) to the inoculum and observe for

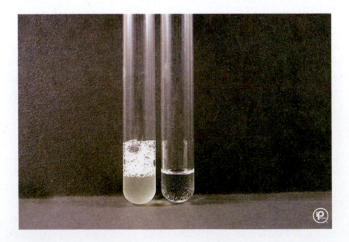

■ **FIGURE 26-9** 68°C catalase test showing positive (left) and negative (right) results.
From Marler LM, Siders JA, Kaufman CM, Owens EN, Korba GG and Allen SD, Bacteriology I Image Atlas CD-ROM, Indiana Pathology Images, 2005.

5 minutes. Measure the column of bubbles in millimeters (mm). Greater than 45 mm is considered positive.

IRON UPTAKE TEST

The iron uptake test is used to demonstrate the ability of an isolate to convert ferric ammonium citrate (FAC), which is incorporated into the growth medium, to iron oxide, a substance more commonly known as rust. This occurrence is indicated by the presence of rust-colored colonies on the surface of the growth medium and a tan discoloration of the medium in the vicinity of the growth itself.

To perform the test, an L-J slant is inoculated. When visible growth is obtained, sterile FAC (1 drop for each milliliter of medium), is added to the slant and the tube is reincubated for up to 3 weeks. The color of the colonies is then evaluated. The presence of rust-colored colonies constitutes a positive test result (Figure 26-10 ■) and no color change is negative.

NIACIN ACCUMULATION TEST

All mycobacteria are capable of synthesizing niacin but most species then degrade it to nicotinamide. A few *Mycobacterium* species, and in particular, *M. tuberculosis,* are capable of producing a sufficient amount of niacin to accumulate in the growth medium in demonstrable quantities.

To demonstrate the presence of niacin, 1.5 ml of sterile distilled water or saline is instilled onto the surface of a 4-week-old L-J slant inoculated with the test organism. Using a sterile inoculating loop or needle, the surface of the slant is stabbed several times. The tube of growth is then positioned so liquid covers the surface of the growth medium and is allowed to remain in this position for a minimum of 30 minutes up to 2 hours. Using a sterile Pasteur pipette, 0.6 ml of extract is transferred to a sterile test tube. Forceps are then used to place

a niacin reagent strip into the extract at the bottom of the test tube. (Note: The reagent, cyanogen bromide, is highly toxic and could produce cyanide gas.) The tube should be tightly sealed and allowed to remain at room temperature for 15–20 minutes. After the appropriate time period the liquid at the bottom of the test tube is examined for the development of a yellow color, a positive reaction (Figure 26-11 ■). If the solution is turbid or colorless, then the test is negative for the presence of niacin. At the conclusion of the test procedure the used reagent test strips should be discarded into a 10% NaOH solution to neutralize the cyanogen bromide.

NITRATE REDUCTION TEST

The nitrate reduction test is used to demonstrate the presence of the enzyme nitrate reductase, which allows a microorganism to reduce nitrate to nitrite. Some organisms can reduce the substrate even further to nitrogen gas (N_2). Negative test results are confirmed by the addition of zinc dust. (With a true negative, the nitrate is reduced to nitrite by the zinc, resulting in the formation of a red color after the zinc is added.)

To demonstrate the presence of nitrate reductase, nitrate broth is inoculated with a sufficient quantity of the test organism (4-week-old growth) to make a heavy suspension. The mixture is shaken gently and incubated at 35–37°C for 2 hours. At the end of the incubation period, a small amount of a crystalline reagent, comprised of a mixture of sulfanilic acid, N-(1-naphthyl) ethylenediamine dihydrochloride, and tartaric acid (the exact amount is not critical), is added. The suspension is examined immediately for the development of a pink to red color, a positive reaction (Figure 26-12 ■). If there is no color change a small amount of powdered zinc should be added for confirmation. If there is still no color development, the organism has reduced the nitrate to nitrite and even further to nitrogen gas. If there is a red color after the addition of

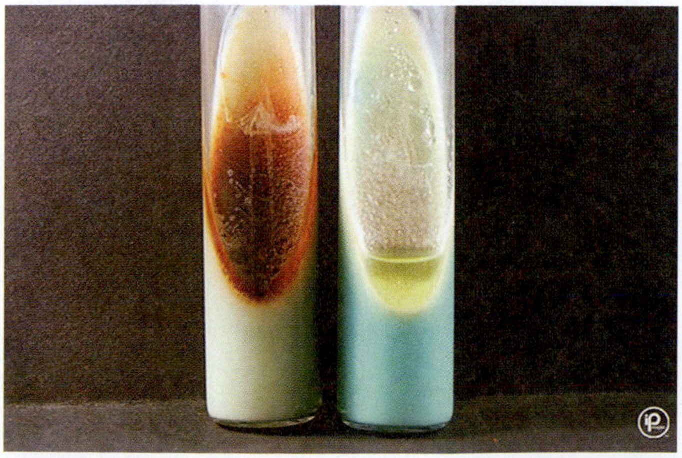

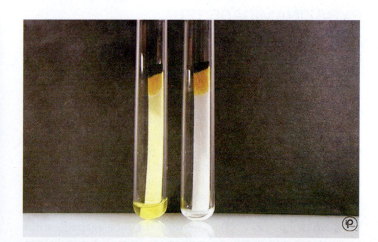

■ **FIGURE 26-10** Iron uptake test showing positive (left) and negative (right) results.
From Marler LM, Siders JA, Kaufman CM, Owens EN, Korba GG and Allen SD, *Bacteriology I Image Atlas* CD-ROM, Indiana Pathology Images, 2005.

■ **FIGURE 26-11** Niacin test showing positive (left) and negative (right) results.
From Marler LM, Siders JA, Kaufman CM, Owens EN, Korba GG and Allen SD, *Bacteriology I Image Atlas* CD-ROM, Indiana Pathology Images, 2005.

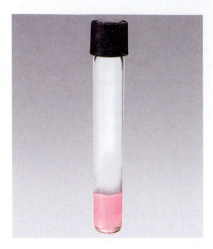

■ **FIGURE 26-12** A positive nitrate substrate broth result for *Mycobacterium tuberculosis*.
Photo courtesy of Remel, part of Thermo Fisher Scientific.

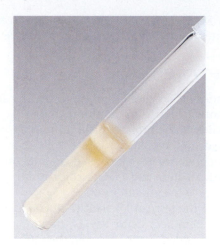

■ **FIGURE 26-13** Pyrazinamidase agar inoculated with *Mycobacterium intracellulare* showing a positive result.
Photo courtesy of Remel, part of Thermo Fisher Scientific.

the zinc, unreduced nitrate was present and the organism is nitrate reductase negative.

PYRAZINAMIDASE TEST

The enzyme pyrazinamidase hydrolyzes pyrazinamide (PZA) to pyrazinoic acid and ammonia. The presence of the pyrazinoic acid can be detected by the addition of a 1% ferrous ammonium sulfate reagent.

To perform the test, two PZA slants are inoculated heavily with the test organism. An uninoculated slant can be used as a control. The tubes are incubated at 35–37°C in a non-CO_2 atmosphere. After 4 days, one tube is removed and 1 ml of freshly prepared 1% ferrous ammonium sulfate solution is added to the slant. The slant is kept at room temperature for 30 minutes, then refrigerated at 2–8°C for 4 hours. The slant is then examined for the presence of a pink band in the medium (Figure 26-13 ■) by holding the tube against a white background and using incident room light. If this tube produces a negative result, the second tube is held for an additional 3-day incubation period (a total of 7 days). Ferrous ammonium sulfate is then added to the second tube and the procedure repeated.

TELLURITE REDUCTION

This test evaluates the ability of an organism to reduce potassium tellurite to metallic tellurium within 3 days.

To perform the test, Middlebrook 7H9 broth is inoculated heavily and incubated at 37°C for 7 days. Two drops of sterile potassium tellurite solution are added and the mixture is reincubated for 3 days undisturbed. The tube is examined for the presence of a black precipitate, a positive reaction. The absence of a black precipitate is a negative reaction (Figure 26-14 ■).

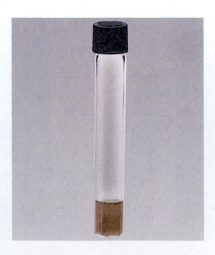

■ **FIGURE 26-14** Middlebrook 7H9 broth with Tween 80 (tellurite reduction medium) inoculated with *Mycobacterium tuberculosis* showing a negative result.
Photo courtesy of Remel, part of Thermo Fisher Scientific.

✪ TABLE 26-2

Biochemical Tests for Mycobacteria

Name of Test	Test Results	Control Organisms
Arylsulfatase	Positive: production of a pink color	Positive: *M. fortuitum* ATCC 6841
	Negative: no color change	Negative: *M. intracellulare* ATCC 13950
68°C Catalase	Positive: effervescence	Positive: *M. fortuitum* ATCC 6841
	Negative: no bubbles	Negative: *M. tuberculosis* ATCC 25177
Semi-quantitative catalase	Weak positive: column of bubbles less than 45 mm	Weak positive: *M. tuberculosis* ATCC 25177
	Strong positive: column of bubbles ≥45 mm	Strong positive: *M. fortuitum* ATCC 6841
	Negative: no bubbles	Negative: uninoculated medium and reagent
Iron uptake test	Positive: rust-colored colonies	Positive: *M. fortuitum* ATCC 6841
	Negative: no color change	Negative: *M. chelonae* ATCC 35751
Niacin accumulation test	Positive: yellow color	Positive: *M. tuberculosis* ATCC 25177
	Negative: no color change	Negative: *M. intracellulare* ATCC 13950
Nitrate reduction	Positive: pink to deep red color	Positive: *M. tuberculosis* ATCC 25177
	Negative: no color change	Negative: *M. intracellulare* ATCC 13950
Pyrazinamidase	Positive: pink color	Positive: *M. intracellulare* ATCC 13950
	Negative: no color change	Negative: *M. kansasii* ATCC 12478
Tellurite reduction	Positive: black precipitate	Positive: *M. intracellulare* ATCC 13950
	Negative: no black precipitate	Negative: *M. tuberculosis* ATCC 25177
Urease	Positive: red color	Positive: *M. fortuitum* ATCC 6841
	Negative: yellow color	Negative: *M. gordonae* ATCC 44470

UREASE PRODUCTION

Mycobacteria that produce urease can hydrolyze urea to ammonia and carbon dioxide. This test is useful in differentiating members of the *Mycobacterium avium* complex from other nonphotochromogens.

Urea broth is inoculated heavily with an actively growing mycobacterial culture and incubated at 35–37°C in ambient air up to 7 days. Mycobacteria that produce urease will hydrolyze urea to ammonia, creating alkaline conditions. At an alkaline pH, the phenol red pH indicator will be pink to red, a positive reaction. No color change is a negative reaction.

Table 26-2✪ lists helpful biochemical tests used in the identification of mycobacteria, their test results, and quality control organisms. Table 26-3✪ summarizes the biochemical reactions of selected mycobacteria.

✪ TABLE 26-3

Identification of Selected *Mycobacterium* Species

Organism	PIG	ROG	NCN	NIT	s-CAT	68-CAT	T80	ARY	URE	TEL	IRON	PYZ
M. tuberculosis	Non	S	+	+	−	−	−	−	+	−	−	+
M. avium complex	Non	S	−	−	−	+	−	−	−	+	−	+
M. kansasii	Photo	S	−	+	+	+	+	−	+	−	−	−
M. marinum	Photo	S	−	−	−	−	+	−[d]	+	−	−	+
M. szulgai	Scoto	S	−	+	+	+	−	V	+	+	−	+
M. scrofulaceum	Scoto	S	−	−	+	+	−	V	V	V	−	+
M. fortuitum	Non	R	−	+	+	+	V	+	+	+	+	+

+, most strains are positive; −, most strains are negative; ARY, arylsulfatase test (3 days); 68-CAT, 68°C catalase test; d, delayed (positive at 14 days); IRON, iron uptake; NCN, niacin accumulation; NIT, nitrate reduction; Non, nonphotochromogen; Photo, photochromogen; PIG, pigmentation; PYZ, pyrazinamidase (4 days); R, rapid grower; ROG, rate of growth; S, slow grower; s-CAT, semiquantitative catalase; Scoto, scotochromogen; T80, Tween 80 hydrolysis (5 days); TEL, tellurite reduction; URE, urease production; V, variable (positive or negative).

Checkpoint! 26–7 (Chapter Objective 3)

Which biochemical test used in the identification of mycobacteria requires heavy growth of the test organism, extraction of the metabolite, and the generation of a yellow color as a positive reaction?

A. *Tellurite reduction*

B. *Nitrate reduction*

C. *Urease production*

D. *Niacin accumulation*

 ## Checkpoint! 26–8 (Chapter Objective 3)

Which methodology is more accurate at identifying mycobacterial isolates?

A. *Acid-fast staining*

B. *Photoreactivity*

C. *Molecular testing*

D. *Biochemical tests*

 ## ▶ LEPROSY

M. leprae is the etiological agent of Hansen's disease or **leprosy**, a disease that affects the skin and nerves. The leprosy bacillus was first identified in 1873 by Gerhard Hansen, a Norwegian physician. At the age of 32, Hansen, a tireless researcher and physician who was trained in histology in Vienna, was able to find rod-shaped bodies in cells taken from leprous nodules.

While leprosy has been virtually eradicated from Western countries, it is still endemic to nations of the Southern hemisphere, such as India, South America, Africa, and Southeast Asia. The World Health Organization (WHO) estimates the prevalence of leprosy worldwide to be about 11 million cases. While the number of cases of leprosy in the United States is extremely low, there are areas where endemic foci exist, including Texas, California, Louisiana, Puerto Rico, and Hawaii (Figures 26-15 ■ and 26-16 ■). Many of the cases of leprosy seen in the United States are believed to be "imported" cases, seen in recent immigrants from areas of high prevalence. In areas where leprosy is endemic, many people may be exposed to the bacillus, but the number of people who contract the disease is very small. With available treatment regimens the numbers of infected individuals has dropped drastically over the last 20 years with more than 14 million patients being cured.

It is believed armadillos may serve as a reservoir for the bacillus. The organism can be grown in the footpads of mice or nine-banded armadillos, a procedure that is performed for research purposes and is not useful in the clinical laboratory. The organism is less acid fast than *M. tuberculosis*.

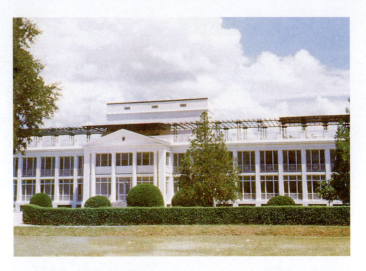

■ **FIGURE 26-15** Historic photograph of the front of the Carville, Louisiana, Leprosarium's infirmary. This health care facility, built in 1894, was used to house leprosy patients.
From Public Health Image Library (PHIL), CDC.

MYCOBACTERIUM LEPRAE

As with other *Mycobacterium* species, *M. leprae* exhibits a very slow growth rate. The incubation period of leprosy may be as long as 5 years, with symptoms taking as long as 20 years to appear (World Health Organization, 2009). The leprosy bacillus has a predilection for skin, mucous membranes, and peripheral nerves, leading to three clinical manifestations of leprosy.

The majority of individuals who come in contact with the leprosy bacillus and become infected remain asymptomatic (no clinical symptoms). In these cases, it is believed, infected

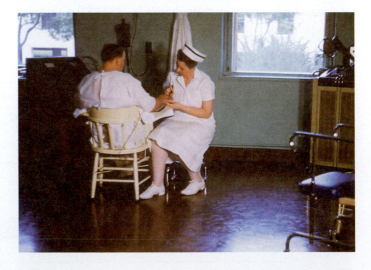

■ **FIGURE 26-16** A patient receiving therapy to prevent the crippling effects of leprosy on the hands and feet. This public health nurse is performing her duties in the Physical Therapy Room at the Carville, Louisiana, Leprosarium.
From Public Health Image Library (PHIL), CDC.

persons possess an adequate immune defense to prevent clinical disease.

Tuberculoid (also called paucibacillary, or PB) leprosy is seen in individuals who exhibit some resistance to infection but the immune response appears to be inadequate. There is usually a single or just a few erythematous or hyperpigmented plaques with raised outer edges and a flattened, clearing center. Peripheral nerves, as well as skin, where the temperature is lower than that of the core body temperature are invaded, leading to a complete sensory loss. Histologically, lesions resemble a tubercle but acid-fast bacilli are few in number and may be difficult to find. In individuals with strong resistance to infection, spontaneous recovery may occur.

Lepromatous (also known as multibacillary, or MB) leprosy is seen in patients whose resistance is low. If untreated the disease is progressive. There is extensive skin involvement with numerous, small, poorly defined lesions. In severe cases, macules (spots or blotches on the skin) may be seen over the entire body surface but the effect on peripheral nerves is less severe than that of tuberculoid leprosy. Large numbers of organisms are found in the nasal mucous membranes, which serve as a source for the shedding of large numbers of organisms. Transmission of leprosy is most likely respiratory in nature, through nasal discharges rather than skin-to-skin contact.

Collections of acid-fast bacilli in macrophages with a honeycomb-like cytoplasm (leprae cells) may be seen in stained tissue sections made from skin biopsies (Figure 26-17). The earliest skin lesion is usually a hypopigmented, erythematous macule that usually heals.

Leprosy bacilli, which invade peripheral nerves, may affect sensory, sensorimotor, or both types of nerves, leading to anesthesia of the affected area. Paralysis and deformity follow sensory loss. One common manifestation of leprosy is seen as the claw hand, a deformity that follows paralysis of the muscles of the hand. With flexor muscles dominating the hand, the fingers are curled into a claw-like position. Sensory loss often leads to destruction of the fingers and toes as a consequence of trauma and infection. Because infected individuals experience no pain sensations, burns from handling objects heated to high temperatures and other injuries to the extremities may be ignored. Further assault may occur from rats, who may take advantage of the opportunity to gnaw on fingers and toes during the night as individuals sleep.

DIAGNOSIS OF LEPROSY

Because of the inability to cultivate the leprosy bacillus in an artificial medium, the diagnosis of Hansen's disease is often made on the basis of demonstrating acid-fast organisms in tissues obtained by a skin biopsy. Determination of the type of leprosy may be achieved with a delayed type hypersensitivity skin test using a suspension of the organism as the antigen. The test determines the level of an individual's immune response.

> ✓ **Checkpoint! 26–9**
> **(Chapter Objective 4)**
>
> *Which of the following statements aptly describes lepromatous leprosy?*
> A. *The organism responsible has a predilection for the central nervous system leading to sensory loss.*
> B. *There is usually a single or just a few erythematous or hyperpigmented plaques with raised outer edges and a flattened, clearing center.*
> C. *Lesions resemble a tubercle but organisms are few in number.*
> D. *Large numbers of organisms are found in the nasal mucous membranes, which serve as a source for the shedding of large numbers of organisms.*

► SUSCEPTIBILITY TESTING FOR *MYCOBACTERIUM* SPECIES

During the Industrial Revolution, tuberculosis devastated Europe and the United States, becoming the leading cause of death a century ago. Inferior living and working conditions, poor nutrition, and poverty spawned its rapid spread during the nineteenth century, particularly in lower socioeconomic circles of society. Today, with the deterioration of the public health infrastructure in large metropolitan areas, the influx of infected immigrants, increased poverty, homelessness, and substance abuse, the inner cities are a breeding ground for new and dangerous strains of multidrug-resistant *M. tuberculosis* (Brown & Body, 1993). The recent emergence of these multidrug-resistant strains of *Mycobacterium tuberculosis* (MDR TB) has made susceptibility testing a necessity for public health labs. There are three factors that may have led to the emergence of drug resistance: inadequate treatment regimens, patient noncompliance (patients must take the drugs from

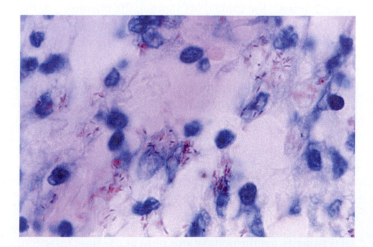

■ **FIGURE 26-17** A photomicrograph depicting leprosy bacilli in material taken from a skin lesion.
From Public Health Image Library (PHIL), CDC.

6 months to a year in some cases), and spontaneous mutations within the organism that render the drug ineffective.

The conventional diffusion techniques, such as the disc agar diffusion technique, where filter paper impregnated discs are placed on the surface of a suitable solid growth medium, is not the method used to determine which drug of choice should be prescribed. These methods are used for rapidly growing organisms, primarily aerobic and facultatively anaerobic organisms such as streptococci, staphylococci, and members of the family *Enterobacteriaceae*. In order to test the susceptibility of *Mycobacterium* species to antimicrobial agents, the antibiotics are incorporated into the growth medium itself. Visit ∞ Chapter 13, "Acid-Fast Bacilli Cultures," to see a photo of this method of susceptibility testing.

The drugs commonly administered to treat mycobacterial diseases include isoniazid (INH), streptomycin, rifampin, ethambutol, p-aminosalicylic acid, and pyrazinamide. The current recommendation for drug therapy is to prescribe a regimen consisting of combinations of multiple drugs. This strategy appears to prevent the development of drug resistance by attacking the organism through different modes of action. Secondary drugs, which can be used to treat resistant strains, include antimicrobial agents such as ethionamide, capreomycin, ciprofloxacin, ofloxacin, kanamycin, cycloserine, and the latest addition, rifabutin. Patient-centered case management includes directly observed therapy (DOT) by a health care worker or another designated person. Anyone taking drugs fewer than 7 days per week must be watched while swallowing each dose of anti-TB drugs (Centers for Disease Control, 2003).

Some of the nontuberculous mycobacteria, such as those in the *M. avium* complex, have shown high resistance to the effect of drug therapy (especially to INH). Organisms in the *M. fortuitum-chelonae* complex are usually resistant to antituberculosis drugs but may be susceptible to conventional drugs, such as aminoglycosides, cephalosporins, and sulfonamides (Howard, 1994).

Proper nutrition, availability of clean water, improved housing, and better hygiene practices has contributed to a decline in the number of cases of leprosy worldwide. Diagnosis and treatment with multidrug therapy are key elements in the fight to eliminate leprosy as a major health threat. The drugs used in the treatment of leprosy include a combination of rifampicin, clofazimine, and dapsone for the treatment of MB leprosy patients. Rifampicin and dapsone are used to treat patients suffering from PB leprosy. The combination of dapsone, rifampicin, and clofazimine is used in the treatment of both forms of leprosy (World Health Organization, 2009).

SUMMARY

Mycobacterial diseases have been known to man since antiquity. *M. tuberculosis* is the etiological agent of tuberculosis, a slowly progressive respiratory illness that is very contagious and once known as "consumption" in medieval Europe. Tuberculosis is a worldwide disease, which has declined significantly in industrialized countries during the twentieth century. With the emergence of drug-resistant strains of *M. tuberculosis*, epidemiologists fear tuberculosis will once again become the scourge it once was when it devastated Europe and the United States during the Industrial Revolution.

Diseases associated with organisms in the genus *Mycobacterium* have resurged. This increase in the number of infections has been associated with the increased population of immunocompromised individuals, and in particular, among AIDS patients.

Tuberculosis is acquired by the respiratory route via droplet nuclei and on occasion through the gastrointestinal tract. Mycobacteria settle in the peripheral alveoli in the lungs. They are then carried by macrophages and lymph fluids to the hilar lymph nodes. Depending on a person's immune status, clinical disease will differ from individual to individual. In those with good immunity, the lymphadenopathy will resolve but bacteria may persist in the lesion and the tuberculin test will be positive. In a person with poor immunity, mycobacteria may spread by the hematogenous route to the rest of the body, causing disseminated or "miliary" tuberculosis. *M. tuberculosis* can infect any tissue in the body. Sites other than the lungs can be involved, such as the skin, the gastrointestinal tract, the urogenital tract, the spine (Pott's spine), the meninges, or the brain. Secondary tuberculosis results from reactivation or reinfection with the tubercle bacilli.

M. bovis is an animal pathogen rarely seen in the United States. It is mainly transmitted by consumption of unpasteurized milk and diary products. Ingestion of the organism may lead to gastrointestinal infection. Bacille Calmette Guérin (BCG) is an attenuate strain of *M. bovis* that can be used for vaccination and on rare occasions has caused BCG vaccinosis.

While *Mycobacterium tuberculosis* is the main pathogen, many other species, often referred to as nontuberculous mycobacteria (NTM), can cause disease in humans (Table 26-4 ✪). These organisms may cause a pulmonary disease very similar to that of *M. tuberculosis* and infections of the skin and soft tissues as well. Immunocompromised patients, such as AIDS patients, are the populations most at risk from infection. NTM include organisms such as the *M. avium* complex (MAC), the *M. fortuitum* complex, *M. kansasii*, *M. malmoense*, *M. xenopi*, *M. ulcerans*, and *M. marinum*.

> ✓ **Checkpoint! 26–10**
> **(Chapter Objective 5)**
>
> *The most effective therapy to treat tuberculosis and prevent the emergence of resistant strains is the administration of:*
>
>   A. *aminoglycosides.*
>   B. *cephalosporins.*
>   C. *sulfones such as dapsone.*
>   D. *sulfonamides.*
>   E. *multidrug therapy.*

⭐ **TABLE 26-4**

Important Characteristics of Mycobacteria

Species	Epidemiology	Clinical Significance	Important Characteristics
M. tuberculosis	Worldwide distribution Transmitted by droplet nuclei Highly infectious	Causes tuberculosis and pulmonary, cutaneous, spinal, genitourinary, and disseminated infections	AFB with serpentine cording on smear from culture, slow growth with rough, dry, buff-colored colonies, niacin and nitrate positive, 68°C catalase negative
M. bovis	Rare in the United States Transmitted primarily through unpasteurized dairy products	Gastrointestinal tuberculosis, rarely pulmonary infection	Tiny, translucent, smooth colonies TCH susceptible, niacin, pyrazinimidase, and nitrate negative
M. africanum	Seen mostly in Africa	Similar to *M. tuberculosis*	Colonies resemble *M. tuberculosis* Biochemically inactive but urease positive
M. kansasii	Widely distributed in nature	Lung disease: second most common NTM infection in the United States Disseminated disease in immunocompromised patients	Photochromogen, usually smooth colonies, pigment in light Niacin negative, nitrate, catalase, pyrazinimidase, and urease positive
M. marinum	Fresh water as well as salt water and soil habitat	Cutaneous infection Swimming pool/fish tank granuloma	Photochromogen Grows at 30°C Tween 80 hydrolysis, urease, and pyrazinimidase positive Nitrate and catalase negative
M. gordonae	Tap water, frequent laboratory contaminant	Nonpathogenic	Scotochromogen Nitrate and urea negative Tween 80 hydrolysis and catalase positive
MAC complex— *M. avium* and *M. intracellulare*	Widely distributed in nature, major pathogen of poultry and swine	Most common cause of disseminated disease in immunocompromised patients (AIDS, leukemia, lymphoma, and transplant patients) Occasional respiratory colonization without disease	Nonphotochromogen, variable colony morphology, for the most part, biochemically inactive, tellurite and pyrazinimidase positive
M. scrofulaceum	Common in Africa	Cervical lymphadenitis in children—scrofula	Scotochromogen Nitrate and Tween 80 hydrolysis negative Catalase and urease positive
M. fortuitum	Mainly skin flora, water	Postop infections on the chest and other soft tissue infections	Rapid grower (3–5 days) Growth on MacConkey without crystal violet Nitrate, arylsulfatase, and iron uptake positive
M. chelonae	Skin flora and water	Skin, soft tissue, and bone infections	Rapid grower (2–4 days), nonphotochromogen, growth on MacConkey without crystal violet, arysulfatase positive, nitrate and iron uptake negative
M. leprae	Worldwide but most cases now in South and Southeast Asia	Leprosy—lepromatous and tuberculoid (Hanson's disease)	Noncultivable
M. haemophilum	Unknown	Ulcers and abscesses in individuals with AIDS and transplant recipients	Nonphotochromogen, pyrazinimidase positive, most biochemicals negative, requires hemin for growth so should be suspected when seen on stain but unable to grow organism, grows at 30°C

Leprosy, a disease known since ancient times, is another important mycobacterial disease that causes significant morbidity and mortality. *Mycobacterium leprae,* the etiological agent of leprosy, is endemic to tropical countries such as India, South America, Africa, and Southeast Asia. In the United States there are a few isolated areas where the organism is endemic. Cases of leprosy occur sporadically in Texas, California, Louisiana, Puerto Rico, and Hawaii.

Leprosy occurs in two clinical forms. In lepromatous leprosy many AFB may be seen in smears made from skin biopsies. In tuberculoid leprosy, a few isolated AFB will be seen. Because the leprosy bacillus prefers skin and nerve tissue it may cause sensory loss, skin lesions, and deformity. The organism cannot be cultured in artificial media, making inoculation into the footpads of mice or armadillos the means of cultivating the organism. For this reason, the primary means of diagnosing leprosy is based on clinical signs and symptoms and identification of acid-fast organisms in stained material obtained by skin biopsy.

The overwhelming majority of the mycobacterial infections do not respond to the use of conventional antibiotics. When left untreated, tuberculosis kills more than half of its victims. There are several drugs that are approved for the treatment of diseases caused by *Mycobacterium* species, including isoniazid (INH), streptomycin, rifampin, ethambutol, p-aminosalicylic acid, and pyrazinamide. The current recommendation for drug therapy is to prescribe a regimen consisting of combinations of multiple drugs. This strategy appears to prevent the development of drug resistance by attacking the organism through different modes of action.

Improved living conditions have led to a decrease in the number of new leprosy cases. Treatment regimens for curing individuals infected with the leprosy bacillus, like those recommended for the treatment of tuberculosis, depend on the administration of multiple drugs to ensure success. The drugs used in the treatment of leprosy include a combination of rifampicin, clofazimine, and dapsone.

LEARNING OPPORTUNITIES

1. Which *Mycobacterium* species is the most common cause of human tuberculosis worldwide? (Chapter Objectives 1 and 4)

2. Describe the typical appearance of *Mycobacterium tuberculosis* on a slant composed of an egg-based medium such as Lowenstein-Jensen. (Chapter Objective 3)

3. What useful purpose does Bacille Calmette Guérin (BCG) an attenuated strain of *M. bovis,* serve? (Chapter Objective 4)

4. What is the primary means of transmission for *M. tuberculosis?* (Chapter Objective 2)

5. What is the main source of infection for the nontuberculous mycobacteria (NTM)? (Chapter Objective 2)

6. Which *Mycobacterium* species is the most common cause of disseminated disease in immunocompromised patients, such as individuals with AIDS? (Chapter Objectives 1 and 4)

7. Which *Mycobacterium* species are associated with skin and subcutaneous tissue infections? These infections are usually associated with breaks in the skin and exposure to watery environments where the organisms are thought to thrive. Optimal growth is obtained at temperatures approximating 30°C. (Chapter Objectives 1 and 5)

PEARSON myhealthprofessionskit™

Use this address to access the interactive Companion Website created for this textbook. Simply select "Clinical Laboratory Science" from the choice of disciplines. Find this book and log in using your user name and password.

REFERENCES

Go to myhealthprofessionskit.com to view this chapter's references.

27

Miscellaneous Microorganisms

Lisa A. Morici

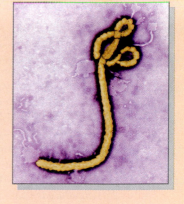

■ LEARNING OBJECTIVES

Upon completion of this chapter, the learner should be able to:

1. Differentiate the miscellaneous microorganisms associated with bite wounds, chronic bacteremia, and endocarditis.
   a. Select major types of tests that are useful in identification of *Bartonella, Pasteurella,* and *Capnocytophaga.*
   b. Separate one organism from another
2. Relate the general characteristics of *Bartonella.*
3. Correlate various organisms with the major type(s) of infectious diseases they cause.
   a. Identify species-specific diseases of *Bartonella.*
   b. Associate patient populations at risk for disease.
4. Distinguish between human oral and cat and dog oral *Capnocytophaga* organisms.
5. Predict the growth requirements of *Bartonella, Pasteurella,* and *Capnocytophaga*
   a. Determine appropriate specimen for isolation.
   b. Choose appropriate media for selection and identification of these organisms.
   c. Describe any growth and environmental requirements for each organism.
6. Correlate patient history, body site or specimen type, colonial morphology, Gram stain results, and identification test results in order to identify an isolate and assess its clinical significance.

KEY TERMS

bacillary angiomatosis	Carrión's disease	trench fever
bacillary peliosis	cat scratch disease	verruga peruana
bartonellosis	endocarditis	

TAXONOMY

Family *Bartonellaceae* (bar-to-nel-la'-ce-ee)
  Genus *Bartonella* (bar-to-nel'-la)
    B. bacilliformis (ba-cil-li-for'-mis)
    B. clarridgeiae (clar-ridge'-i-a-e)
    B. elizabethae (e-liz'-a-beth-a-e)
    B. henselae (hen'-sel-a-e)
    B. quintana (quin-ta'-na)
Family *Pasteurellaceae* (pas-teu-rel-la'-see-ee)
  Genus *Pasteurella* (pas-teu-rel'-la)
    P. multocida (mul-to-ci'-da)
    P. canis (ca'-nis)
    P. dagmatis (dag-ma'-tis)
    P. stomatic (sto-ma'-tis)

Family *Flavobacteriaceae* (fla-vo-bac-ter-eay'-see'-ee)
  Genus *Capnocytophaga* (cap-no-cyto-pha-ga)
    C. canimorsus (ca-ni-mor'-sus)
    C. cynodegmi (sy-no-deg'-mi)
Family *Bradyrhizobiaceae* (bra-dy-rhi-zo-bee-a'-ce-ee)
  Genus *Afipia* (a-fip'-i-a)
    A. felis (fe'-lis)

▶ INTRODUCTION

The spectrum of miscellaneous microorganisms associated with human disease is too numerous to include in this chapter. Therefore, this chapter will discuss those organisms commonly associated with bite wounds and other diseases such as chronic bacteremia and endocarditis. In most circumstances, these organisms cause higher morbidity and mortality in individuals with compromised immune systems. This chapter will discuss the general characteristics of *Bartonella*, *Pasteurella*, and *Capnocytophaga*, their respective diseases, and the diagnostic tests used to discriminate infection with these miscellaneous microorganisms.

▶ *BARTONELLA*

GENERAL CHARACTERISTICS

The *Bartonella* species are emerging infectious agents with a worldwide distribution. The genus *Bartonella* includes 19 identified species, although only 6 of them are responsible for human disease (Greub & Raoult, 2002). *Bartonella* species are facultative, intracellular, gram-negative coccobacilli. The name *Bartonella* was derived from the Peruvian physician, Alberto Barton, who discovered *Bartonella bacilliformis* as the etiologic agent of Carrión's disease. The term "bartonellosis" is now used to describe a group of diverse clinical disorders caused by the major *Bartonella* species (Massei, Gori, Macchia, & Maggiore, 2005).

CLINICAL SIGNIFICANCE

Specimens for Analysis

Blood and tissue specimens should be collected prior to antibiotic treatment. Laboratory diagnosis in most clinical laboratories usually uses molecular or serological analysis. Laboratory diagnosis of bartonellosis is discussed later in this chapter.

Virulence Factors and Pathogenesis

The major virulence factors of bartonellae enable them to infect red blood cells and vascular endothelial cells, resulting in persistent circulatory system infections. Type IV secretory systems inject molecules into host cells that 1) rearrange the endothelial cytoskeleton, internalizing bacterial cells by creating an invasome within the cell, 2) activate proinflammatory factors that cause angiogenesis (proliferation of vessel endothelial cells that lead to the abnormal creation of blood vessels) as well as expression of cell adhesions, and 3) inhibit apotosis.

The bartonellae are transmitted by direct contact or blood-sucking arthropods. They colonize the vascular endothelium and possibly the cells of the reticuloendothelial system (RES). The microbes spread into the bloodstream after approximately 5 days and adhere to erythrocytes and reinfect the endothelial cells and RES. This cycle repeats until the immune response produces an antibody that kills the microbe and ends the cycle of reinfection. The red cell internalizes the adhered bacteria where they multiply and remain for the life of the erythrocyte, except for *B. bacilliformis* that causes lysis of the RBC (Dehio, 2008).

Clinical Manifestations

Cat Scratch Disease (CSD). Cat scratch disease is
caused by infection with *Bartonella henselae* and consists of a subacute, solitary, or regional lymphadenopathy that occurs 1 to 3 weeks after a scratch, bite, or other contact with an infected cat or kitten. Most cases appear in children and young adults. Clinical signs and symptoms include 3 to 5 mm papules at the site of inoculation, as well as minor symptoms such as anorexia, malaise, arthralgia, fever, and headache. The affected lymph nodes draining the site of the infection will gradually

---

 REAL WORLD TIP

Afipia felis, the organism originally thought to be the cat scratch bacillus, can be differentiated from *Bartonella* by its positive hemolysis, nitrate, and urease. *Bartonella* is negative for these reactions.

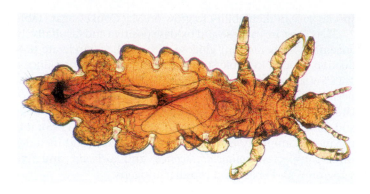

■ **FIGURE 27-1** Body louse, *Pediculus humanus var. capitis*, the vector for *B. recurrentis* and *B. quintana*.
Source: Centers for Disease Control, Dr. Dennis and D. Juranik.

enlarge and then resolve within 9 weeks. Because the disease is self-limiting, antibiotic treatment is only recommended for unresolved lymphadenopathy or when there is significant morbidity or systemic involvement. In most cases of CSD, treatment is based on the symptoms presented.

Carrión's Disease. **Carrión's disease** is caused by *B. bacilliformis* and is endemic in South America. It is transmitted by the sand fly, *Lutzomyia verrucosum*, which inhabits altitudes of 500 to 3200 meters above sea level. Therefore, Carrión's disease is geographically distinct and is also characterized by two clinically and chronologically distinct features. The first overt sign of disease is Oroya fever—an acute fever and anemia that can be fatal. Several months after infection, an eruption of cutaneous red-purple hemangiomatous lesions called **verruga peruana**, or verrucae, can follow. These eruptions are pathognomonic or characteristic for Carrión's disease.

Trench Fever. *B. quintana* causes a persistent or relapsing fever known as **trench fever** and is transmitted by the body louse *Pediculus humanus corporis* (Figure 27-1 ■). This disease is usually characterized by myalgia, arthralgia, bone pain, particularly in the shins, and splenomegaly. Today the disease primarily affects the poor, homeless, and alcoholics living in urban areas.

Bacillary Angiomatosis. Immunocompromised hosts, particularly AIDS patients, may develop disseminated disease from *Bartonella* infection that may involve the brain, liver, spleen, bone marrow, or lungs. **Bacillary angiomatosis** is characterized by systemic symptoms such as fever, chills, night sweats, anorexia, and weight loss. It may or may not present with characteristic skin lesions. Fortunately, the incidence of bacillary angiomatosis has declined significantly following the introduction of antiviral triple therapy and antibiotic prophylaxis.

Bacillary Peliosis. Similar to bacillary angiomatosis, **bacillary peliosis** occurs in terminally ill AIDS patients and affects the parenchymal organs with reticuloendothelial elements. Thus it primarily affects the liver and can lead to hepatitis, but can also involve the spleen, bone marrow, and abdominal lymph nodes.

Endocarditis. Several *Bartonella* species (Table 27-1 ✪) can cause a subacute, insidious (silent but deadly) **endocarditis** that often presents with acute cardiac failure (Brouqui & Raoult, 2001). Laboratory findings are not specific and include a normal white blood cell count, thrombocytopenia, and elevated blood creatinine levels. Echocardiographic vegetations are evident in most patients, but blood cultures are usually negative.

Treatment of *Bartonella* infections may include erythromycin or doxycycline or azithromycin. Clarithromycin or ciprofloxacin may also be prescribed (Miller, 2007).

LABORATORY DIAGNOSIS OF *BARTONELLA*

Diagnosis of *B. henselae* infection is made by serologic testing and often aided by a history of contact with a cat or kitten. Indirect fluorescent antibody (IFA) test and enzyme immunoassay (EIA) are the most common tests used for the detection of specific serum antibody to *B. henselae*. There are often fluctuations in the IgM and IgG responses in patients; however, IFA is 88% sensitive and 97% specific for both IgM and IgG antibodies. A titer of >1:256 is currently used to indicate infection (Massei et

✪ **TABLE 27-1**

Diseases Caused by *Bartonella*

Disease	Clinical Manifestation	*Bartonella* species
Cat scratch disease	Lymphadenopathy, mild fever, myalgia, arthralgia	*B. henselae*
Carrion's disease		
Oroya fever	Acute febrile fever, hemolytic anemia	*B. bacilliformis*
Verruga peruana	Skin eruptions	*B. bacilliformis*
Trench fever	Relapsing fever, myalgia, arthralgia	*B. quintana*
Bacillary angiomatosis	Red popular cutaneous lesions, lymphadenopathy, fever, weight loss	*B. quintana, B. henselae*
Bacillary peliosis	Abdominal pain, hepatosplenomegaly, fever, hepatitis	*B. henselae*
Endocarditis	Fever, cardiac murmur, emboli and vegetations	*B. quintana, B. henselae, B. vinsonii, B. elizabethae*
Chronic bacteremia	Fever, myalgia, leg pain, thrombocytopenia	*B. quintana*

al., 2005). Serologic tests cannot reliably distinguish between *Bartonella* species because of cross-reactivity of bacterial antigens. Therefore, polymerase chain reaction can be used to differentiate the *Bartonella* species. Although *Bartonella* can be cultured from various tissues, it is not practical in the clinical microbiology laboratory. *Bartonella* grows slowly (9 to 40 days) on chocolate agar at 35°C with carbon dioxide and humidity. The colonies are small, dry, and embedded in the agar. It has an incubation period of 6 weeks, and live organisms are rarely isolated from blood or tissues of infected patients. Biopsy of infected tissue may demonstrate the presence of bacilli within granulomatous lesions by the Warthin-Starry stain reaction or by PCR.

 Checkpoint! 27–1 (Chapter Objective 3)

Bartonella henselae can cause which of the following diseases?
A. *Cat scratch disease*
B. *Endocarditis*
C. *Bacillary angiomatosis*
D. *All of the above*

▶ *PASTEURELLA*

GENERAL CHARACTERISTICS

Pasteurella species are gram-negative, nonmotile, coccobacilli with a worldwide distribution. There are currently more than 17 species of *Pasteurella*. These bacteria are part of the normal flora of the gastrointestinal tract and nasopharynx in dogs, cats, and wild animals, but they are rare in the respiratory tract of healthy individuals. Microscopically, they are pleomorphic organisms (Figure 27-2 ■) appearing as ovoid to short rods to filamentous forms, and bipolar staining is common. All *Pasteurella* grow as flat, gray, wet colonies on blood agar and chocolate agar, but

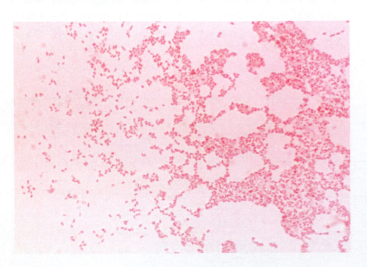

■ **FIGURE 27-2** Gram stain of *Pasteurella multocida*.
Source: Centers for Disease Control and Dr. R. Weaver.

species vary in their ability to grow on MacConkey agar (Table 27-2✿). They are catalase and oxidase positive and facultatively anaerobic. They ferment glucose with weak to moderate production of acid. In triple sugar iron (TSI) agar, they produce a "sick" weak acid that helps distinguish them from other gram-negative rods. *Pasteurella multocida* is the major pathogen isolated from cat bites and is also associated with bites from dogs and other animals (Griego, Rosen, Orengo, & Wolf, 1995). It is the most commonly isolated *Pasteurella* species and includes three subspecies: *multocida*, *septica*, and *gallicida*, and five serogroups (A–F) based on capsular antigens.

CLINICAL SIGNIFICANCE

Specimens for Analysis

Purulent material or tissue from a bite wound can be collected and submitted for culture. Care should be taken to collect the specimen without contamination with skin flora. Other specimens may include joint fluid, sputum, and systemic specimens such as CSF and blood.

Virulence Factors and Pathogenesis

Possible pasteurellae virulence factors include endotoxin, a capsule, hemagglutins, a cytotoxin and iron-acquiring proteins (Harper et al., 2003). Transmission occurs by bites, scratches, and licking of skin lesions by dogs, cats, pigs, hamsters, horses, and other animals. The organism is most often associated with a cat bite due to the animal's needle-like teeth, which can inject the organism deep into tissue and joints. Dog bites tend to crush bones and tissue.

Clinical Manifestations

Clinical infection with *P. multocida* is characterized by the development of a rapid inflammatory response at the site of a bite. Pain and swelling occurs within 24 to 48 hours (Griego et al., 1995). *P. multocida* has also been associated with meningitis, sepsis, pneumonia, osteomyelitis, endocarditis, septic arthritis, and abscess formation especially in immunocompromised patients and those with underlying disease such as liver cirrhosis (Brouqui & Raoult, 2001; Kirby, 2007).

Treatment includes antibiotic therapy such as penicillin, ampicillin, or amoxicillin; doxycycline, ampicillin-clavulanic acid, trimethoprim-sulfamethoxazole, or extended spectrum cephalosporins and tissue debridement.

LABORATORY DIAGNOSIS OF *PASTEURELLA*

The diagnosis of *Pasteurella* is usually suspected for animal bite or scratch wounds. In such cases, *Pasteurella* can usually be cultured from wound scrapings or aspirates. Identification of the *Pasteurella* species is based on the phenotypic and biochemical characteristics presented in Table 27-2. One caveat to the culture of bite wounds is that specimens cultured both aerobically and anaerobically will typically yield approximately

⚙ **TABLE 27-2**

Differentiation of *Pasteurella* Species and Related Organisms

Species	Cat	Ox	ODC	Ind	Ur	Man	Growth on Mac	Hemolysis
P. multocida	+	+	+	+	−	+	−	−
P. pneumotropica	+	+	+	+	+	−	+/−	−
Mannheimia haemolytica	+	+	−	−	−	+	+	+
P. trehalosi	V	+	−	−	−	+	+	+
P. aerogenes	+	+	+/−	−	+	−	+	−
P. dagmatis	+	+	−	+	+	−	−	−
P. canis	+	+	+	+/−	−	−	−	−
P. bettyae	+/−	+/−	−	+	−	−	+/−	−
P. caballi	−	+	+/−	−	−	+	−	−

Cat = catalase; Ox = oxidase; ODC = ornithine decarboxylase; Ind = indole; Ur = urease; Man = mannitol fermentation; + = positive; − = negative; V = variable; +/− = more strains are positive then negative.

five different species of bacterial isolates per culture. Common aerobes identified in bite wounds include streptococci, staphylococci, *Moraxella*, and *Neisseria*. Typical anaerobes observed in bite wound isolates include *Fusobacterium*, *Bacteroides*, *Porphyromonas*, and *Prevotella*. However, *Pasteurella* is the most frequent bacteria isolated from dog bites (50%) as well as cat bites (75%; Talan, Citron, Abrahamian, Moran, & Goldstein, 1999). CLSI document M45 provides guidance for standardized susceptibility testing of this microbe.

 REAL WORLD TIP

The spot indole test can be used to presumptively identify *P. multocida*. The test should be performed on oxidase and catalase positive colonies grown for 24 hours on blood agar. A positive result is typical for *P. multocida* (Oberhofer, 1981). Organisms that produce indole tend to have a musty odor.

✓ **Checkpoint! 27–2 (Chapter Objective 6)**

Carole was bitten by a dog. Several days later, a culture of the bite site grew an oxidase- and catalase-positive, gram-negative coccobacillus on blood agar. The MacConkey agar showed no growth. A spot indole test yielded a positive result. The organism's probable identity is:

A. *Pseudomonas aeruginosa.*

B. *Pasturella multocida.*

C. *Bartonella spp.*

D. *Neisseria spp.*

▶ *CAPNOCYTOPHAGA*

GENERAL CHARACTERISTICS

The *Capnocytophaga* species are normal flora of the mouth and oral cavities. They are gram-negative, fastidious bacilli with a fusiform or pointed appearance microscopically (Figure 27-3 ■). On agar, the colonies exhibit a characteristic gliding motility with spreading edges similar to swarming but not as extensive as *Proteus* spp. (Figure 27-4 ■). *Capnocytophaga* may require an increased CO_2 concentration for growth. They are nonhemolytic and produce a yellow-orange pigment. These bacteria can ferment sucrose, glucose, maltose, and lactose. They are usually negative in most biochemical reactions, although they may hydrolyze esculin and reduce nitrate. The genus *Capnocytophaga* includes seven species: *C. gingivalis* (human oral), *C. canimorsus* (dog and cat oral), *C. ochracea*

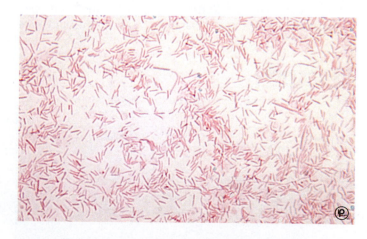

■ **FIGURE 27-3** Gram stain of *Capnocytophaga.*
Source: Indiana Pathology Images.

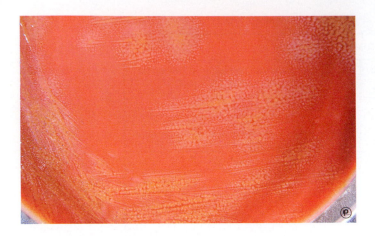

■ **FIGURE 27-4** Colonies of *Capnocytophaga*. The spreading colony is the result of the organism's gliding motility.
Source: Indiana Pathology Images.

(human oral), *C. haemolytica* (human oral), *C. sputigena* (human oral), *C. granulosa* (human oral), and *C. cynodegmi* (dog and cat oral). Those species normally found in the human oral cavity were previously known as dysgonic fermenters (DF-1) because they are difficult to grow on artificial media. They are distinguishable from the dog and cat oral organisms, previously known as DF-2, by the absence of oxidase and catalase production. Table 27-3 ✪ lists reactions that differentiate the human oral *Capnocytophaga* from those of the oral cavities of dogs and cats. The sodium polyanetholesulfonate disk can be used to distinguish *C. ochracea* and *C. canimorsus* (both SPS susceptible) from *Haemophilus* species (other then *H. ducreyi*), *Cardiobacterium hominis*, *Eikenella corrodens*, *P. multocida*, and *Moraxella* species, which are SPS resistant (Shawar, Sepulveda, & Clarridge, 1990).

CLINICAL MANIFESTATIONS

Capnocytophaga species may produce an immunosuppressive factor (Ochiai, Senpuku, Kurita-Ochiai, 1998), and *C. canimorsus* may produce a cytotoxin that destroys phagocytes and other immune cells (Fischer et al., 1995). The most commonly isolated *Capnocytophaga* species is *C. ochracea*. Common sites of infection include juvenile periodontal disease, endocarditis (Sandoe, 2004), and oral ulcers in the granulocytopenic patients. *C. canimorsus* (DF) can cause fulminant septicemia following a dog or cat bite (Griego et al., 1995). Clinical infection with *C. canimorsus* can present with sepsis, fever, leukocytosis, petechiae, rash, disseminated intravascular coagulation, cellulitis, hypotension, renal failure, meningitis, or pneumonia (Le Moal, Landron, Grollier, Robert, & Burucoa, 2003; Lion, Escande, & Burdin, 1996). The case fatality rate is 25% and occurs mostly in immunocompromised individuals, alcoholics, or those without a spleen; although deaths have occurred in immunocompetent individuals. In addition to *C. canimorsus*, other *Capnocytophaga* species can cause bacteremia and sepsis in immunocompromised patients (Dudley, Czarnecki, & Wells, 2006; Mantadakis, Danilatou, Christidou, Stiakaki, & Kalmanti, 2003; Mirza et al., 2000).

Treatment of *C. canimorsus* infections includes amoxicillin-clavulanate, ciprofloxacin, or penicillin G. *C. ochracea* is treated with clindamycin, amoxicillin-clavulanate, ciprofloxacin, or penicillin G (Miller, 2007).

LABORATORY DIAGNOSIS OF *CAPNOCYTOPHAGA*

The organism grows slowly on blood agar, chocolate agar, or heart infusion agar with 5% rabbit blood in the presence of 5 to 10% CO_2 at 37°C. Blood cultures may at first appear negative, and subcultures may take up to 7 days of incubation before growth is visible. Gram staining of peripheral blood smears and cerebrospinal fluid is also helpful in diagnosing bacteremia and meningitis (Mirza et al., 2000). Because *Capnocytophaga* grows slowly (2 to 7 days) and will not grow on MacConkey agar, it is advisable to inform the laboratory that it is being considered in the diagnosis. Selective media have been developed, and fastidious anaerobe agar supports the growth of all *Capnocytophaga* strains.

A yellow-pigmented colony that Gram stains as a thin, fusiform, gram-negative rod, that demonstrates gliding motility (wet mount motility) or spreading colony and does not grow in ambient air can be presumptively identified as *Capnocytophaga* species.

✪ TABLE 27-3

Selected Tests That Differentiate the Human Isolates from the Animal Isolates of *Capnocytophaga*

Organism	Oxidase	Catalase	Sucrose
C. canimorsus (dog and cat oral flora)	+	+	–
C. cynodegmi (dog and cat oral flora)	+	+	+
Capnocytophaga (Human oral isolates)	–	–	+

+ = positive; – = negative

✓ **Checkpoint! 27–3 (Chapter Objective 5)**

Capnocytophaga will not grow on which of the following?
    A. *Chocolate agar*
    B. *Blood agar*
    C. *MacConkey agar*
    D. *Brain heart infusion agar with blood*

✪ TABLE 27-4

Differentiation of *Bartonella*, *Pasteurella*, and *Capnocytophaga*

Organism	Indole	Catalase	Oxidase	Glucose	Urease	Motility on Wet Mount
Pasteurella	+	+	+	A	V	–
Capnocytophaga	–	V	+	A	–	+
Bartonella	–	–	–	–	–	V

A = acid; + = positive; – = negative; V = variable reactions

SUMMARY

These miscellaneous microorganisms are a fascinating group of bacteria, associated with animal bites and capable of causing a wide spectrum of human disorders. Fortunately, standard serologic or microbiologic tests are available to diagnose infections caused by *Bartonella*, *Pasteurella*, and *Capnocytophaga*. They can be differentiated from each other using the tests listed in Table 27-4✪ as well as Gram stain, colony morphology, and growth pattern. However, a major obstacle in the medical laboratory is the inability to culture these organisms rapidly during early infection. The development of molecular or serologic tests that are rapid and species specific remains a significant challenge in the diagnosis of these organisms.

LEARNING OPPORTUNITIES

1. A patient presents to the clinic with a suspected case of cat scratch disease. Explain why you would or would not culture for the presence of *Bartonella* to confirm the diagnosis. (Chapter Objectives 1, 2, 3, and 5)

2. A culture specimen obtained from a bite wound yields bacterial growth on blood agar, but fails to produce bacterial colonies when cultured on MacConkey agar. Explain why this observation cannot rule out infection with the gram-negative bacteria *Pasteurella* or *Capnocytophaga*. (Chapter Objectives 1, 4, and 5)

PEARSON
myhealthprofessionskit™

Use this address to access the interactive Companion Website created for this textbook. Simply select "Clinical Laboratory Science" from the choice of disciplines. Find this book and log in using your user name and password.

REFERENCES

Go to myhealthprofessionskit.com to view this chapter's references.

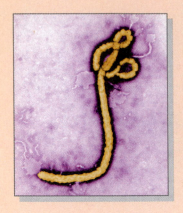

OUTLINE

28

Mycoplasma and *Ureaplasma*

Ken Baker Waites

■ LEARNING OBJECTIVES

Upon completion of this chapter, the learner should be able to:

1. Relate the characteristics of the *Mollicutes* that make them unique among prokaryotic organisms.
2. Describe the epidemiology and virulence factors of *M. pneumoniae*.
3. Recognize the four major human pathogens, *Mycoplasma pneumoniae, M. genitalium, M. hominis,* and *Ureaplasma* species and the diseases they cause.
4. Describe the requirements for cultivation of human mycoplasmas and ureaplasmas and the limitations of culture as a means for diagnosis.
5. Determine key features that allow the pathogenic mycoplasmas to be identified and distinguished from one another.
6. Identify and describe the methods of antimicrobial susceptibility testing of mycoplasmas and ureaplasmas and the drugs used for the treatment of infections because of them.
7. Summarize the current and future potential for use of molecular diagnostics tests such as nucleic acid amplification in detection of mycoplasmas and ureaplasmas.
8. Discuss the role of serology and types of serologic tests available for diagnosis of *M. pneumoniae* infections.
9. Correlate the impact of cold agglutinins produced by *M. pneumoniae* and urinary stones associated with *Ureaplasma* infections on results produced by nonmicrobiology laboratory departments.

KEY TERMS

cold agglutinins	*Mollicutes*	primary atypical
cranial nerve palsy	nongonococcal urethritis	pneumonia
enzyme immunoassay	polymerase chain	sterol
hypogammaglobulinemia	reaction	transverse myelitis

TAXONOMY	
Family *Mycoplasmataceae* (mi-ko-plaz-me-ta-se-e)	*M. pneumoniae* (new-mo-ne-i)
Genus *Mycoplasma* (mi-ko-plaz-ma)	*M. primatum* (pri-ma-tum)
M. amphoriforme (am-pho'-ri-for'-me)	*M. salivarium* (sal-i-var-i-um)
M. buccale (boo-kal-e)	*M. spermatophilum* (sper-ma-to-fil-um)
M. fermentans (fer-men-tans)	Genus *Ureaplasma* (u-rea-plaz-ma)
M. genitalium (gen-i-ta-li-um)	*U. urealyticum* (u-re-a-li-ti-cum)
M. hominis (hom-i-nis)	*U. parvum* (par-vum)
M. orale (o-ral-e)	Family *Acholeplasmataceae* (a-ko-le-plaz-ma-ta-se-e)
M. penetrans (pen-e-tranz)	Genus *Acholeplasma* (a-ko-le-plaz-ma)
M. pirum (peer-um)	*A. laidlawii* (laid-law-ee)

▶ INTRODUCTION

Mycoplasmas are the smallest free-living organisms and are unique among bacteria in many ways. *Mycoplasma* (Greek, fungus form) describes the growth pattern of one species, *M. mycoides*. In the 1950s these organisms were known as pleuropneumonia-like organisms (PPLO; Waites, Katz, & Schelonka, 2005). Although numerous species are known to produce diseases in humans, animals, and plants, their small size, often slow growth, and diverse and demanding nutritional requirements have hindered development of diagnostic testing methods and led to a widespread lack of appreciation of their pathologic significance. Improved methods for laboratory testing have enabled a greater understanding of the role of mycoplasmas as agents of human disease. This chapter reviews the taxonomy, biological characteristics, clinical importance, methods for detection by culture, nucleic acid amplification, and serologic means, and the antimicrobial susceptibilities of mycoplasmas that infect humans.

▶ BIOLOGICAL CHARACTERISTICS

Bacteria commonly referred to as mycoplasmas are eubacteria that have evolved from clostridial-like gram-positive cells by gene deletion. They are included within the Class **Mollicutes** (soft skin), which now includes 4 orders, 5 families, 8 genera, and approximately 200 known species (Waites & Taylor-Robinson, 2007). Mycoplasmas are common in practically all mammals, as well as many other vertebrates in which they have been sought. The mycoplasmal species for which humans are the primary host are shown in Table 28-1⬦. Among these, the most important human pathogens are *Mycoplasma pneumoniae*, *Mycoplasma hominis*, *Mycoplasma genitalium* and *Ureaplasma* species. Members of the *Mycoplasmataceae* require **sterols** (steroids with at least one alcoholic hydroxyl group such as cholesterol for growth). The *Acholeplasmataceae* do not require sterols and are found in soil, plants, animals, and occasionally as commensal organisms in humans. They are also notorious for causing contamination of tissue culture cell lines.

Mycoplasmas associated with humans range from coccoid cells of about 0.2 to 0.3 μm diameter for *Ureaplasma* spp. to tapered rods 1 to 2 μm in length for *Mycoplasma hominis*. Mycoplasmal cells are contained by a trilayered membrane (Waites & Taylor-Robinson, 2007). The permanent lack of a cell wall barrier in all members of Class *Mollicutes* makes these organisms unique among prokaryotes and differentiates them from bacterial L forms, which lack the cell wall only as a temporary situation because of the environmental conditions such as exposure to antibiotics (Waites & Taylor-Robinson, 2007). Lack of a rigid cell wall also renders mycoplasmas insensitive to the activity of beta-lactam antimicrobials, such as penicillin, prevents them from staining by Gram stain, and is largely responsible for their pleomorphic form. *M. pneumoniae* is often even smaller, existing as rod-like forms that cannot be classified as cocci or rods as other bacteria are. The extremely small genome size, approximately 580 kilobase pairs for *M. genitalium*, and limited abilities for biosynthesis explain the parasitic or saprophytic nature of these organisms, their sensitivity to adverse environmental conditions, and fastidious growth requirements for cultivation in vitro. Species infecting humans are facultative anaerobes (see ∞ Chapter 7, "Cultivation of Microorganisms") and produce colonies better when grown in an atmosphere supplemented with CO_2 or anaerobically. Both *Mycoplasma* and *Ureaplasma* spp. require sterols in growth media, supplied by the addition of serum to synthesize their cell membranes. *Mycoplasma* spp. isolated from humans hydrolyze glucose, arginine, or both to generate ATP, whereas *Ureaplasma* spp. hydrolyze only urea as a metabolic substrate (Waites & Taylor-Robinson, 2007). Growth rates in culture medium vary among individual species, with generation times of approximately 1 hour for *Ureaplasma* spp., 6 hours for *M. pneumoniae,* and 16 hours for *M. genitalium* (Waites, Bebear, Robertson, Talkington, & Kenny, 2001).

Mycoplasmas and ureaplasmas are primarily mucosal pathogens of the respiratory and urogenital tracts. They rarely invade systemically, except in cases of immunosuppression or instrumentation. Several mycoplasmal species occur as commensals in the oropharynx, with *M. salivarium* and *M. orale* being the most common.

⊕ TABLE 28-1

Mycoplasmas and Ureaplasmas of Humans[a]

Species	Primary Site(s) of Isolation	Metabolic Substrate		Associated Diseases
		Glucose	Arginine	
Acholeplasma laidlawii	Oropharynx; skin	+	−	None
Mycoplasma amphoriforme	Respiratory tract	+	−	Possible association with chronic bronchitis in antibody-deficient persons
M. buccale	Oropharynx	−	+	None
M. faucium	Oropharynx	−	+	None
M. fermentans	Oropharnyx; GU tract	+	+	Pneumonia; possibly nephropathy and disseminated disease in HIV-infected persons, arthritis
M. genitalium	GU tract	+	−	Urethritis, pelvic inflammatory disease, cervicitis
M. hominis	GU tract; blood; wounds	−	+	Pelvic inflammatory disease; amnionitis and postpartum sepsis; cervicitis; pyelonephritis; pneumonia, meningitis, bacteremia in neonates; wound infections; abscesses; and arthritis in immunosuppressed persons
M. lipophilum	Oropharynx	−	+	None
M. orale	Oropharynx	−	+	None
M. penetrans	GU tract in HIV-infected persons	+	+	Unknown
M. pirum	Blood in HIV-infected persons	+	+	Unknown
M. pneumoniae	Respiratory tract	+	−	Pneumonia; bronchitis; extrapulmonary complications
M. primatum	Respiratory tract; GU tract	−	+	None
M. salivarium	Oropharynx	−	+	None
M. spermatophilum	GU tract	−	+	Unknown
Ureaplasma urealyticum/ parvum[b]	GU tract; respiratory tract in neonates	−	−	Urethritis; urinary calculi; chorioamnionitis; pneumonia, meningitis, bacteremia in neonates; arthritis in antibody-deficient persons, wound infections

+ = positive; − = negative; GU = Genitourinary tract

[a]Some of the commensal mycoplasmas that typically reside in the oropharynx have occasionally been recovered from normally sterile sites in association with disease, usually in hosts with an impaired immune system, but such isolations are extremely rare, and these organisms are more appropriately considered nonpathogenic for most humans

[b]Metabolizes urea.

✓ Checkpoint! 28–1 (Chapter Objective 1)

Mycoplasmas can be differentiated from other prokaryotes in that they do not possess:

    A. *a membrane-bound nucleus.*
    B. *a rigid cell wall.*
    C. *ribosomes.*
    D. *DNA.*

VIRULENCE FACTORS AND TRANSMISSION

The ability to be intracellular, by some mycoplasmas such as *M. genitalium,* may be responsible for protecting them from antibodies and antibiotics, as well as contributing to disease chronicity and difficulty in cultivation. The ability of *M. hominis* and *Ureaplasma* spp. to vary surface antigens may be related to persistence of these organisms at invasive sites (Waites & Taylor-Robinson, 2007). Other virulence factors that have been suggested for the genital mycoplasmas include the phospholipases and immunoglobulin A protease of *Ureaplasma* spp. and arginine depletion, ammonia production, phospholipase, and aminopeptidase production in *M. hominis* (Blanchard & Bebear, 2002)

M. pneumoniae has a specialized tip structure, the P1 and P30 adhesins that facilitate attachment to the respiratory epithelium (Balish & Krause, 2002). The close interaction between the mycoplasma and host cells protects it from removal by the mucociliary clearance mechanism. The tip structure is actually a network of interactive proteins and adherence accessory proteins that cooperate structurally and functionally to mobilize and concentrate adhesins at the tip of the organism and permit mycoplasmal colonization of mucous membranes and eukaryotic cell surfaces. A similar type of attachment structure has also been described in *M. genitalium* (Hu et al., 1987). *Ureaplasma* adhesins stick to red blood cells, sperm, and urethral epithelial cells. They also attach to neutrophils and activate complement (Waites et al., 2005).

It is not known precisely how *M. pneumoniae* injures the respiratory epithelial cell after attachment, but a number of biochemical and immunologic properties of the organism have been described that are likely to be involved. Close approximation of the organism to the host cells facilitated by the adhesin proteins appears to be important to facilitate localized tissue disruption and cytotoxicity. The P1 protein also serves as a primary antigen against which a vigorous antibody response is elicited during acute *M. pneumoniae* infections and is the antigenic component in some of the serologic tests used for diagnostic purposes (Waites et al., 2001). Hydrogen peroxide and superoxide radicals synthesized by *M. pneumoniae* act in concert with endogenous toxic oxygen molecules generated by host cells to induce oxidative stress in the respiratory epithelium. *M. pneumoniae* apparently lacks superoxide dismutase and catalase, as well as iron-containing cytochromes and has minimal abilities to produce other enzymes for biochemical reactions that are common in many conventional bacteria. Hydrogen peroxide is known to be important as a virulence factor in *M. pneumoniae* and is the molecule that confers hemolytic activity (Pollack, Williams, & McElhaney, 1997). Recently, an ADP-ribosylating protein that causes vacuolation and ciliostasis (lack of cilia movement) in cultured host cells was identified in *M. pneumoniae*, suggesting it functions as an exotoxin (Kannan et al., 2005).

Autoimmune response is also a very important component of many *M. pneumoniae* infections. This may be manifested by development of **cold agglutinins**, IgM antibodies that react with the red blood cell I antigen and cause agglutination of erythrocytes at 4°C (and sometimes 25°C to 31°C), and a wide array of other autoantibodies against other tissues that may be a factor in the extrapulmonary complications that are sometimes associated with *M. pneumoniae* infections (Clyde, 1979; Harmening, Steffey, Prihoda, & Green, 2005). These cold agglutinins may also interfere with cell counts performed in the hematology laboratory and blood bank procedures such as blood typing and compatibility testing. Mycoplasma species are also known to act as immunomodulators by their direct interactions with lymphocytes that may result in stimulation of T cell mitosis, activation of cytotoxic T cells in vitro, and induction of polyclonal B cell activation (Waites & Taylor-Robinson 2007).

In humans, mycoplasmas and ureaplasmas may be transmitted by direct contact between hosts (i.e., venereally through genital–genital or oral–genital contact), vertically from mother to offspring either at birth or in utero, by respiratory aerosols or fomites in the case of *M. pneumoniae,* or even by nosocomial acquisition through transplanted tissues (Sanchez, 1993).

► CLINICAL SIGNIFICANCE

Mycoplasma and *Ureaplasma* can cause respiratory disease, urogenital infections, and invasive disease.

RESPIRATORY SYSTEM INFECTIONS

M. pneumoniae was first identified as a bacterium and not a virus and described in the early 1960s although it had already been implicated as the etiologic agent of **primary atypical pneumonia**, also known as "walking pneumonia" because it is usually of less severity than typical bacterial pneumonias caused by organisms such as *Streptococcus pneumoniae*. *M. pneumoniae* causes approximately 20% of all community-acquired pneumonias and infects persons in all age groups, although school-aged children and young adults have historically been the patient populations most likely to have clinically significant infections because of this organism. Closed populations such as prisoners, college students, and military personnel have experienced several well-documented outbreaks during recent years (Talkington, Waites, Schwartz, & Besser, 2001).

The most common clinical syndrome is tracheobronchitis, often accompanied by upper respiratory tract manifestations. Pneumonia develops in about one-third of persons who are infected. The incubation period is generally 2 to 3 weeks, and spread throughout households is common. Though not considered to be normal flora, *M. pneumoniae* may persist in the respiratory tract for several months after initial infection, possibly because it attaches strongly to and invades epithelial cells. Disease tends not to be seasonal, subclinical infections are common, and the disease is ordinarily mild. However, in a minority of cases, severe infection requiring hospitalization and resulting in death sometimes occur, especially in the middle-aged and elderly.

Usual manifestations include persistent hacking cough, low-grade fever, headache, sore throat, earache, and coryza (runny nose). Extrapulmonary complications include meningoencephalitis, ascending paralysis (Guillain-Barré Syndrome), **transverse myelitis**, or acute inflammation of the spinal cord that may progress to loss of sensation and paralysis below the lesion; **cranial nerve palsy**, or paralysis of cranial nerves that affects vision, hearing, facial expression, and balance; pericarditis; autoimmune hemolytic anemia; arthritis; and mucocutaneous lesions in some cases (Waites & Taylor-Robinson 2007; Waites & Talkington, 2004). An autoimmune response is thought to play a role in some extrapulmonary complications. However, *M. pneumoniae* has been isolated directly from cerebrospinal (CSF), pericardial, and synovial fluids, as well as other extrapulmonary sites (Talkington et al., 2001). Protective immunity does not usually occur following *M. pneumoniae* respiratory infections, so reinfections are common.

✓ ### Checkpoint! 28–2
(Chapter Objective 2)

Which of the following is a major virulence factor of M. pneumoniae *that is believed to be important for its ability to cause disease in the lower respiratory tract?*

  A. *Production of urease*
  B. *Lipopolysaccharide*
  C. *A proteinaceous attachment organelle*
  D. *An impermeable cell wall surrounded by a capsule*

M. fermentans has been recovered from the throats of children with pneumonia, adults with an acute influenza-like illness, and bronchoalveolar lavages, peripheral blood lymphocytes, and bone marrow from patients with the acquired immunodeficiency syndrome (AIDS) and respiratory disease (Waites & Taylor-Robinson 2007). ∞ Chapter 33 provides more information on respiratory system infections.

UROGENITAL TRACT INFECTIONS

Following puberty, *Ureaplasma* spp. and *M. hominis* can be isolated from the lower genital tract in many sexually active adults, with ureaplasmas being the more common organisms detected. Both *Ureaplasma* spp. and *M. genitalium* may cause non-chlamydial, **nongonococcal urethritis** (NGU), an acute inflammatory condition of the urethra in sexually active men, and rarely conjunctivitis (Björnelius, Jensen, & Likbrink, 2004; Taylor-Robinson & Furr, 1998). *Ureaplasma* spp. also produce urease and induce crystallization of struvite and calcium phosphates in urine and have been found in urinary calculi of patients with infection-type stones more frequently than those with metabolic-type stones.

 REAL WORLD TIP

Urinary calculi or stones, due to *Ureaplasma* spp., may correlate with urinalysis results of hematuria or blood in the urine, crystals (calcium phosphate), white blood cells, and an alkaline pH.

M. hominis has been isolated from the upper urinary tract only in patients with concurrent symptoms of acute pyelonephritis. *M. hominis* and *M. genitalium* may play a role in endometritis and female pelvic inflammatory disease. *M. hominis* and possibly *Ureaplasma* spp. may also be associated with bacterial vaginosis, although the mechanism of their contribution in this disease is not known (Taylor-Robinson & Furr, 1998). Ureaplasmas can invade the amniotic sac early in pregnancy in the presence of intact fetal membranes, causing persistent infection, chorioamnionitis, and adverse pregnancy outcome (Cassell et al., 1983). Isolation of *M. hominis* from the blood of about 10% of women with postpartum fever and endometritis, but not from afebrile women who have had abortions or from healthy pregnant women suggests a possible role for this organism in this condition. Clinical and animal studies have shown that ureaplasmas alone may play a role in spontaneous abortion and premature birth (Waites, Katz, & Schelonka, 2005; Novy et al., 2009).

An infant may be colonized by the mother's genital mycoplasmas in utero or via vertical transmission during delivery. The organisms may be transient with no sequelae for the newborn. *M. hominis* and *Ureaplasma* spp. from cord blood and the blood of newborns indicate a hematogenous route of transmission. The CSF of neonates may be invaded by both organisms. Colonization of healthy full-term infants declines after 3 months of age, and fewer than 10% of older children and sexually inexperienced adults are colonized with genital mycoplasmas (Waites, Katz, & Schelonka, 2005).

INVASIVE DISEASE

There is considerable evidence that *Mollicutes* can cause invasive disease of the joints and respiratory tract with bacteremic dissemination in immunosuppressed persons, especially individuals with **hypogammaglobulinemia** (a deficiency of all immunoglobulins). Mycoplasmas are probably the most common etiologic agents of septic arthritis in individuals with antibody deficiency (Furr, Taylor-Robinson, & Webster, 1994). *M. hominis* bacteremia has been demonstrated after renal transplantation, trauma, and genitourinary manipulations. *M. hominis* has also been found in wound infections, brain abscesses, peritonitis, endocarditis, and osteomyelitis lesions (Taylor-Robinson & Furr, 1998). Numerous mycoplasmal species, including *M. fermentans, U. urealyticum*, and *M. salivarium,* have been detected in the synovial fluid of persons with rheumatoid arthritis, although the precise contribution of these organisms to this disease condition is still uncertain (Schaeverbeke et al., 1999). It may be because of an autoimmune process related to the deposition of antigen-antibody complexes in synovial and cartilage tissues. The significance of *M. fermentans, M. penetrans*, and other mycoplasmas in progression of disease in persons infected with HIV has received a great deal of attention for several years. However, there is no conclusive evidence to date that indicates a role of these organisms other than that of opportunistic pathogens. Refer to ∞ Chapter 36 for more information on genital system infections.

 Checkpoint! 28–3 (Chapter Objective 3)

Which of these mycoplasmas is known to cause pelvic inflammatory disease, meningitis, postpartum sepsis, and pyelonephritis?

A. *M. pneumoniae*
B. *M. hominis*
C. *M. genitalium*
D. *M. fermentans*

▶ DIAGNOSIS BY CULTURE

Diagnostic evaluations for mycoplasmas should be performed only for a patient suspected of having a type of infection with which mycoplasmas have been associated. Routine screening of respiratory tracts for *M. pneumoniae* is not indicated, nor is screening of the lower urogenital tracts of adults for genital mycoplasmas. Neonates with clinical, radiographic, or laboratory evidence of pneumonia or central nervous system infection without a proven bacterial etiology should have specific cultures obtained for genital mycoplasmas because these organisms would not be recovered in routine bacterial cultures. Because culture is rather insensitive and very time consuming for detection of *M. pneumoniae*, alternative procedures such as serology and/or the **polymerase chain reaction** (PCR) assay, a procedure that amplifies and detects the presence of minute amounts of microbial DNA, are preferred and culture is rarely performed (Waites & Taylor-Robinson, 2007). Slower-growing, fastidious organisms such as *M. genitalium* and *M. fermentans* may sometimes be of diagnostic interest. However, culture techniques are less well established for these organisms and are not undertaken routinely. Therefore, information provided in subsequent sections on culture techniques apply only to *M. pneumoniae, M. hominis,* and *Ureaplasma* spp.

SPECIMEN TYPES

Specimens suitable for mycoplasmal culture and PCR include blood, synovial fluid, amniotic fluid, CSF, urine, prostatic secretions, semen, wound aspirates, sputum, pleural fluid, bronchoalveolar lavage, or other tracheobronchial secretions. Urine from women should only be cultured for genital mycoplasmas if the specimen is collected by catheterization or suprapubic aspiration. Other suitable specimens include swabs from the nasopharynx, throat, cervix/vagina, wounds, and urethra. Biopsy or autopsy tissue, including placenta, endometrium, bone chips, and urinary calculi, can also be cultured. Care must be taken to roll the swab across the desired site vigorously to obtain as many cells as possible because mycoplasmas adhere closely to cells. Avoid collection of specimens that are contaminated by lubricants or antiseptics commonly used in gynecologic practice since they may be inhibitory to mycoplasmas and ureaplasmas. Preferred swabs include calcium alginate, Dacron, or polyester swabs with aluminum or plastic shafts. Avoid wooden shaft cotton swabs because of potential inhibitory effects.

SPECIMEN TRANSPORT AND STORAGE

Mycoplasmas lack a protective cell wall and are extremely sensitive to adverse environmental conditions, especially drying and heat. Specimens should be inoculated at bedside whenever possible. Commercial mycoplasma media such as SP4 or 10B broths or sucrose phosphate (2 SP) are acceptable transport media. Other media suitable for transport and storage of specimens are Stuart's medium and trypticase soy broth with 0.5% bovine serum albumin. Liquid specimens do not require special transport media if protected from evaporation and inoculated into culture medium within 1 hour. Tissues can be placed in a tightly closed, sterile container and delivered to the laboratory immediately. Tissue specimens should be placed in transport media if culture inoculation is delayed. Refrigerate specimens that cannot be immediately transported to the lab-

oratory. Mycoplasmas can be isolated from anticoagulant-free blood by inoculating into liquid mycoplasmal growth media at the bedside in a 1:10 ratio, using as much blood as possible. Use of commercial blood culture media with or without automated blood culture instruments is not recommended for detection of mycoplasmas because mycoplasmas are inhibited by sodium polyanethol sulfonate, the anticoagulant used in most commercial blood culture media. If specimens must be shipped and/or if the storage time is likely to exceed 24 hours prior to processing, the specimen in transport medium should be frozen at –70°C to prevent loss of viability and to minimize bacterial overgrowth if the specimen is from a non-sterile site. Mycoplasmas can be stored for long periods in appropriate growth or transport media at –70°C or in liquid nitrogen. Dry ice can be used to ship frozen specimens to a reference laboratory if necessary.

 REAL WORLD TIP

Mycoplasmal or ureaplasmal infections will not normally be detected in diagnostic specimens using procedures designed to detect conventional bacteria. Specialized growth media and conditions must be provided. Laboratories that cannot provide these requirements must ship specimens to a reference laboratory for diagnosis, paying careful condition to the appropriate environmental conditions necessary to prevent loss of viability of these fastidious microbes.

DIRECT EXAMINATION

Gram Stain

Because of their cellular dimensions, mycoplasmas cannot be seen using routine brightfield microscopy. Mycoplasmas do not stain with the Gram stain. This procedure may prove useful to rule out contaminating bacteria. *M. hominis* may occasionally appear as pinpoint colonies on bacteriologic media, and the lack of a Gram reaction by these colonies gives a clue as to their possible mycoplasmal identity, warranting further investigation and subculture to mycoplasmal media.

Giemsa Stain

Giemsa stains may be used to examine clinical specimens for mycoplasmas, but the results can be difficult to interpret because of debris and artifacts in clinical specimens, which can be confused with mycoplasmas because of their small size.

DNA Fluorochrome Stain

Hoechst DNA fluorochrome stain 33258 or Acridine orange has sometimes been used to detect the presence of mycoplasmas in a sterile body fluid or contaminated cell culture. The fluid of interest is fixed in glacial acetic acid, stained with the fluorochrome, and examined under a fluorescent microscope. Mycoplasmas appear as small fluorescing oval bodies. It is important to always examine a positive and negative control slide to aid in the interpretation of DNA fluorochrome preparations. ∞ Chapter 8, "Presumptive Identification," has a photo of acridine orange and provides information on fluorescent microscopy.

Dienes' Stain

The Dienes' methylene blue stain (Figure 28-1 ■) is a nonspecific stain that imparts a contrasting appearance to mycoplasmal colonies on agar, thereby allowing improved visualization of the colonial morphology and characteristics.

CULTURE PROCESSING AND INOCULATION

To maximize potential yield, both broth and agar should be inoculated for detection of mycoplasmas and/or ureaplasmas and processed as described in Figures 28-7 and 28-8. Specimens should always be mixed well before inoculating media, and fluids should be centrifuged (600 g × 15 min) and the pellet inoculated. Urine can be filtered through a 0.45 μm filter if bacterial contamination is suspected. Furthermore, it is wise to mince, not grind, tissues in broth prior to diluting. Serial dilution of specimens in broth to at least 10^{-3} with subculture of each dilution onto agar is an extremely important step in the cultivation process because it will help overcome possible interference by antibiotics, antibodies, and other inhibitors, including bacteria, that may be present in clinical specimens. Omission of this critical dilution step can be one reason why some laboratories have difficulty recovering the organisms. Dilution also helps to overcome the problem of rapid decline in culture viability, which is particularly common with ureaplasmas.

GROWTH MEDIA

In addition to providing serum as a cholesterol source needed for development of cell membranes, growth factors such as yeast extract, and a metabolic substrate such as glucose, arginine, or urea, depending on the species sought are required for successful in vitro cultivation. Addition of a pH indicator, such as phenol red, is important for detection of growth because mycoplasmas do not produce turbidity in broth culture because of their small cell size. Addition of penicillin is helpful to minimize bacterial overgrowth, especially for specimens from nonsterile sites. No single medium formulation is ideal for all pertinent species because of different properties, optimum pH, and substrate requirements. SP4 broth and agar (pH 7.5) can be used for both *M. pneumoniae* and *M. hominis*, provided arginine is added for the latter. Shepard's 10B broth (pH 6.0) can be used for *M. hominis* and *Ureaplasma* spp. with A8 agar as the corresponding solid medium (Figure 28-2 ■).

> ### @ REAL WORLD TIP
>
> Remel Laboratories (Lenexa, KS) manufactures and sells 10 B (Figure 28-2) and SP4 broths (Figure 28-3 ■), as well as SP4 and A8 agar, commercially in the United States.

Biphasic media have been used successfully for many years for cultivation of *M. pneumoniae*. An agar slant is prepared in a small screw-capped bottle to which broth is added to fill half to two-thirds the height of the agar. The rationale for this approach is that it supplies a wide range of atmospheric conditions, and inhibitor metabolites present in the specimen may be absorbed by the agar, further promoting the possibility of growth. Biphasic media have been sold commercially in

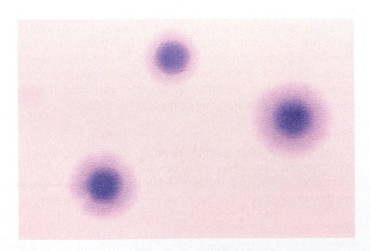

■ **FIGURE 28-1** PPLO agar with *M. hominis* with Dienes' stain.
Photo courtesy of Remel, part of Thermo Fisher Scientific.

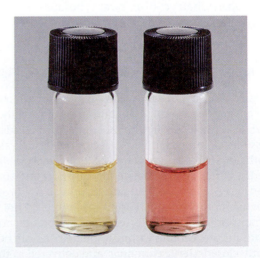

■ **FIGURE 28-2** Uninoculated (left) and positive (right) reaction for 10B Arginine broth.
Photo courtesy of Remel, part of Thermo Fisher Scientific.

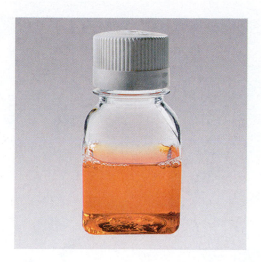

■ **FIGURE 28-3** SP4 Glucose broth.
Photo courtesy of Remel, part of Thermo Fisher Scientific.

the United States for several years (Mycotrim; Irvine Scientific, Irvine, CA) for *M. pneumoniae* as well as the genital mycoplasmas. A number of other commercial kits and media, most of which have been designed primarily for detection of *M. hominis* and *Ureaplasma* spp., are sold in Europe, and some are now beginning to be distributed in the United States. There have not been extensive comparative evaluations made of many of the various commercial media with the original formulations developed by mycoplasma researchers, so it is not possible to recommend any specific product. Commercial media are certainly more convenient to use than the nonproprietary broths and agars because of the labor-intensive preparation and quality control time for the latter, and some types can be purchased in a lyophilized form to prolong shelf life. However, the commercial products are substantially more expensive to purchase.

 Checkpoint! 28–4 (Chapter Objective 4)

An essential component of Mycoplasma pneumoniae growth media that must be included to enable the organisms to synthesize cell membranes is:

A. *penicillin.*
B. *arginine.*
C. *urea.*
D. *serum.*

INCUBATION CONDITIONS AND SUBCULTURES

Broth cultures are incubated at 37°C in ambient air. Agar plates yield the best growth if they are incubated in an atmosphere of room air supplemented with 5 to 10% CO_2 or in an anaerobic environment of 95% N_2 plus 5% CO_2. A candle jar or anaerobe jar with GasPak catalyst is adequate if dedicated incubators are not available. The relatively rapid growth rates of *M. hominis* and *Ureaplasma* spp. make identification of most positive cultures possible within 2 to 4 days, and cultures can be reported as negative if no growth is evident by 7 days. *M. pneumoniae* typically requires 21 days or longer and this is the reason that most laboratories recommend PCR-based detection rather than culture. Cultures must be held a minimum of 4 weeks before being designated as negative. Several mycoplasmal species of human origin can produce similar biochemical reactions, and identification can only be accomplished by immunologic or molecular-based tests on organisms once isolated. All broths that have changed color, because of a pH change, should be subcultured into a fresh tube of the corresponding broth (0.1 mL into 0.9 mL) and onto agar (0.02 mL) since the primary culture may not always grow on solid media. Subcultures must be performed soon after the color change occurs, particularly if the organism belongs to *Ureaplasma* spp. because the culture can lose viability within a few hours. This means that broth cultures must be examined at least twice daily if ureaplasmas are suspected. Subculture of apparently negative broths, a blind subculture, periodically during incubation may improve the yield of *M. pneumoniae* and other mycoplasmas because a color change may not always be evident, even if growth occurs.

COLONIAL APPEARANCE

Due to their small size, mycoplasmal and ureaplasmal colonies require a stereomicroscope for visualization and identification. Mycoplasmal colonies must be distinguished from artifacts such as air bubbles, water or lipid droplets, or other debris, which can be confusing. Application of the Dienes' methylene stain directly to the agar plate (Figure 28-1) containing mycoplasma colonies can sometimes help in distinguishing them from artifacts. If there is any doubt about whether mycoplasmal colonies are present, a plug of agar can be removed and subcultured to fresh broth, which should eventually show color change if viable organisms are present to metabolize the substrate. *Ureaplasma* colonies can be identified on A8 agar by urease production in the presence of $CaCl_2$ indicator contained in the medium (Figure 28-4 ■). Incorporation of the $CaCl_2$ directly into A8 medium eliminates the need for adding an indicator for urease activity such as $MnCl_2$. The typical colony is described as being granular and having a bird's nest appearance. The larger *M. hominis* colonies are urease negative and often have the typical fried egg appearance (Figure 28-5 ■). *M. pneumoniae* will produce much smaller spherical colonies, which may or may not demonstrate the fried egg appearance (Figure 28-6 ■). *M. hominis* is the only pathogenic mycoplasma of humans cultivable on bacteriological media such as chocolate agar or Columbia agar, but the pinpoint translucent colonies are easily overlooked, and routine bacterial cultures may be discarded sooner than the time needed for *M. hominis* colonies to develop, which may require 4 days or more in some cases. Occurrence of suspicious colonies warrants subculture to appropriate mycoplasma media.

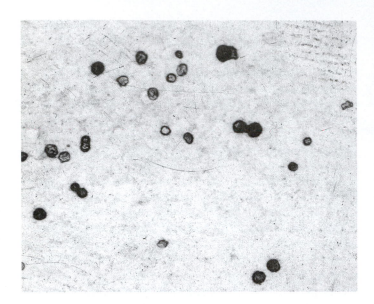

■ **FIGURE 28-4** Granular colonies of *Ureaplasma* species on A8 agar viewed under a stereomicroscope.

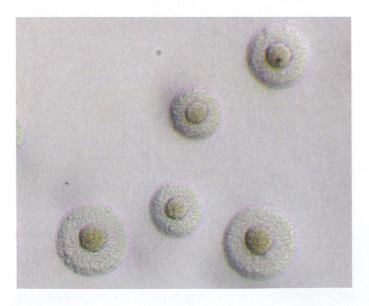

■ **FIGURE 28-5** Fried egg colonies of *M. hominis* on A8 agar viewed under a stereomicroscope.

![Spherical colonies of M. pneumoniae on SP4 agar]

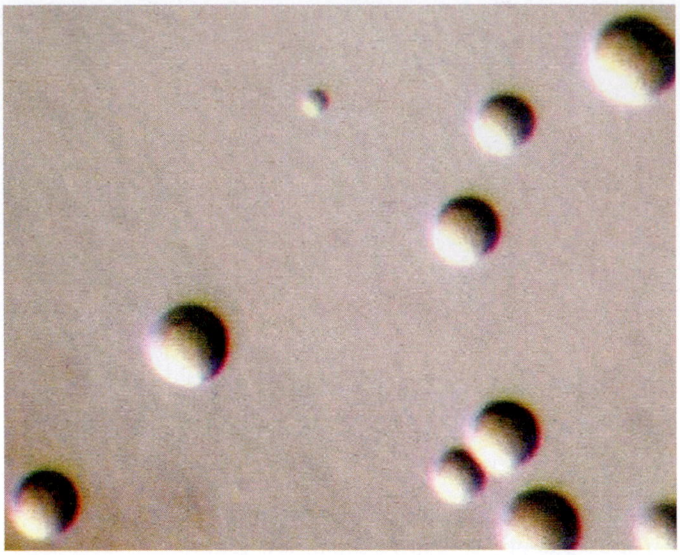

■ **FIGURE 28-6** Spherical colonies of *M. pneumoniae* on SP4 agar viewed under a stereomicroscope.

SPECIES IDENTIFICATION

Utilization of glucose by a mycoplasma in SP4 broth (Figure 28-3) will produce an acidic pH indicator shift (red to yellow), whereas use of arginine will produce a red to deeper red color change in this broth. Urea or arginine hydrolysis in 10B broth (Figure 28-2) causes an alkaline pH shift of orange to deep red. Thus, a slow-growing glycolytic organism grown from the respiratory tract that produces spherical colonies on SP4 agar after approximately 5 to 20 days of incubation is likely to be *M. pneumoniae* (Figure 28-7 ■). An alkaline color change that occurs after overnight incubation without turbidity in 10B broth containing urea is almost certain to contain *Ureaplasma* spp., whereas a urogenital specimen that produces an alkaline reaction within 24 to 72 hours in broth supplemented with arginine is likely to contain *M. hominis* (Figure 28-8 ■). Examination of colonial morphology is sufficient to identify *Ureaplasma* spp. (granular or bird's nest-like), and it is important to keep in mind that these organisms often coexist with *M. hominis* in urogenital specimens.

The genus *Ureaplasma* is now separated into two species, *U. urealyticum* and *U. parvum* (Robertson et al., 2002). This separation was based on evaluation of the DNA homologies of the two clusters within the 14 recognized serovars of *U. urealyticum*. Formerly *U. parvum* was referred to as *U. urealyticum* biovar 1 and consisted of serovars 1, 3, 6, and 14. *U. urealyticum* biovar 2, the T960 biovar, was comprised of serovars 2, 4, 5, and 7 to 13. It is not practical or necessary for diagnostic purposes to separate the species.

ⓔ REAL WORLD TIP

Ureaplasma colonies can be easily identified to genus level by their characteristic granular brown appearance on A8 agar, and it is not necessary to identify them to species level for clinical purposes. In contrast, large-colony mycoplasmas require additional procedures to characterize them to the species level, and this may be needed to differentiate pathogens such as *M. pneumoniae* from oral commensal species that can sometimes cause diagnostic confusion.

To identify a large-colony mycoplasma completely to species level, a number of different techniques are available. Numerous

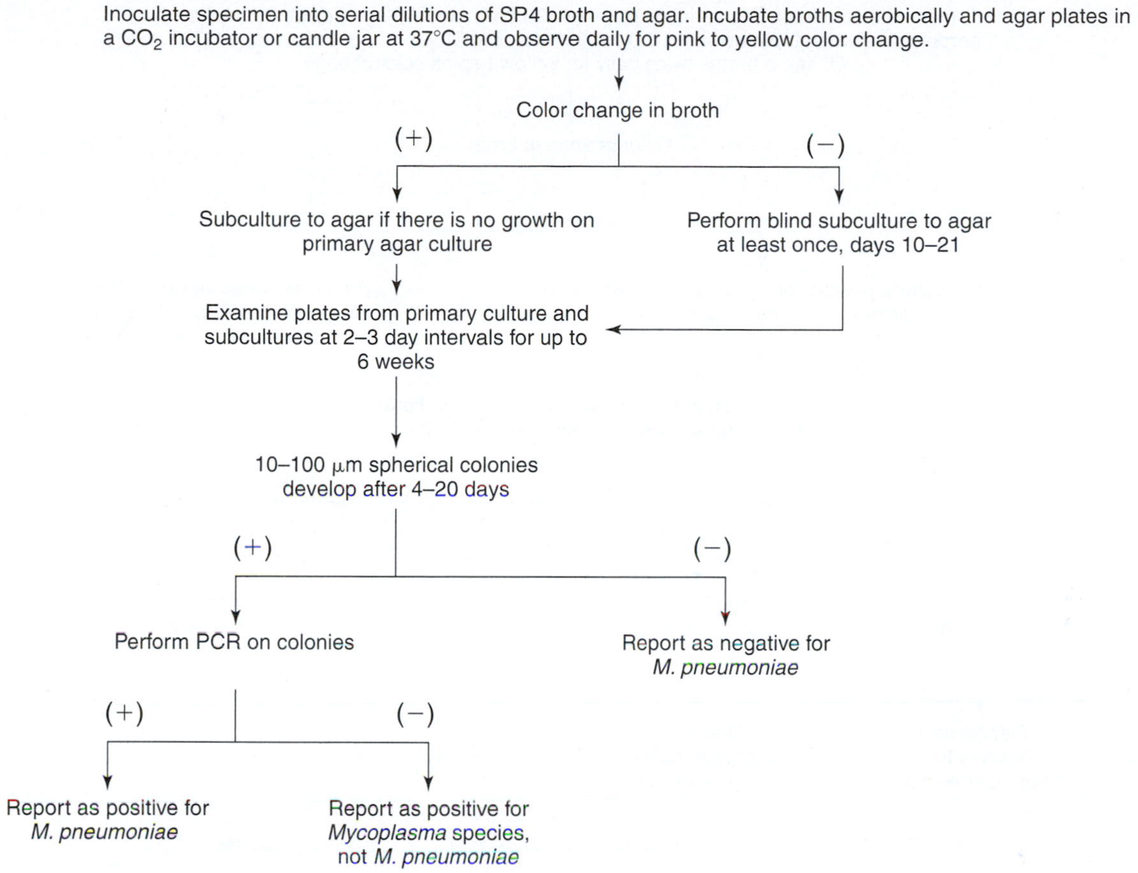

Inoculate specimen into serial dilutions of SP4 broth and agar. Incubate broths aerobically and agar plates in a CO_2 incubator or candle jar at 37°C and observe daily for pink to yellow color change.

Color change in broth

(+)   (−)

Subculture to agar if there is no growth on primary agar culture   Perform blind subculture to agar at least once, days 10–21

Examine plates from primary culture and subcultures at 2–3 day intervals for up to 6 weeks

10–100 μm spherical colonies develop after 4–20 days

(+)   (−)

Perform PCR on colonies   Report as negative for *M. pneumoniae*

(+)   (−)

Report as positive for *M. pneumoniae*   Report as positive for *Mycoplasma* species, not *M. pneumoniae*

■ **FIGURE 28-7** Detection of *Mycoplasma pneumoniae* by culture.

biochemical and immunological phenotypic tests have been developed to identify large-colony mycoplasmas to species level, but from a practical standpoint, they have now been replaced by PCR-based technology, which is available from specialized reference laboratories. Identification of mycoplasmas to the species level is most important for respiratory tract specimens due to the possibility of confusion of *M. pneumoniae* with various oral commensal species. Since PCR is needed to positively identify mycoplasmas isolated from respiratory tract specimens, it is most logical, time saving, and cost-effective in most clinical settings to obtain PCR assays directly on respiratory specimens at the outset rather than processing a culture.

 Checkpoint! 28–5 (Chapter Objective 5)

M. hominis can be differentiated from M. pneumoniae biochemically in that it hydrolyzes which of the following metabolic substrates to generate energy?

    A. *Arginine*
    B. *Urea*
    C. *Glucose*
    D. *Maltose*

INTERPRETATION OF CULTURE RESULTS

Isolation of *M. pneumoniae* from respiratory tract specimens is clinically significant in most instances, although it may occasionally be carried asymptomatically for variable periods and may be shed for some time after clinical resolution of a symptomatic infection. *M. pneumoniae* will sometimes disseminate and infect normally sterile sites such as CSF, synovial fluid, or pericardial fluid. Isolation of *Ureaplasma* spp. or *M. hominis* in any quantity from normally sterile body fluids or tissues is significantly associated with disease. The presence of *M. hominis* or *Ureaplasma* spp. in a nonsterile site such as urethra or cervix is somewhat more problematic in its interpretation, and laboratory data should be correlated with the patients' overall condition. Fewer than 10^4 ureaplasmas in the male urethra is unlikely to be significant.

▶ ANTIMICROBIAL SUSCEPTIBILITIES

Because of lack of a cell wall, mycoplasmas and ureaplasmas are intrinsically resistant to beta-lactams. Sulfonamides, trimethoprim, and rifampicin are also inactive. Resistance to macrolides and lincosamides is variable according to species,

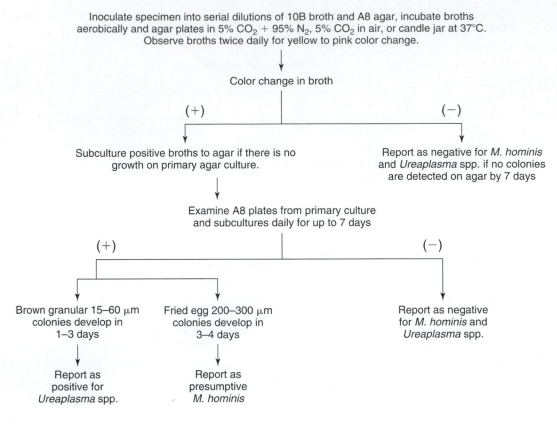

Inoculate specimen into serial dilutions of 10B broth and A8 agar, incubate broths aerobically and agar plates in 5% CO_2 + 95% N_2, 5% CO_2 in air, or candle jar at 37°C. Observe broths twice daily for yellow to pink color change.

Color change in broth

(+)

(−)

Subculture positive broths to agar if there is no growth on primary agar culture.

Report as negative for *M. hominis* and *Ureaplasma* spp. if no colonies are detected on agar by 7 days

Examine A8 plates from primary culture and subcultures daily for up to 7 days

(+)

(−)

Brown granular 15–60 μm colonies develop in 1–3 days

Fried egg 200–300 μm colonies develop in 3–4 days

Report as negative for *M. hominis* and *Ureaplasma* spp.

Report as positive for *Ureaplasma* spp.

Report as presumptive *M. hominis*

■ **FIGURE 28-8** Detection of *Mycoplasma hominis* and *Ureaplasma* species by culture.

with *M. hominis* being resistant to erythromycin but susceptible to clindamycin. For *Ureaplasma* spp. the reverse is true. New macrolides have activity comparable to erythromycin for *M. pneumoniae* and *Ureaplasma* spp. (Waites & Taylor-Robinson, 2007).

M. pneumoniae has remained predictably susceptible to newer fluoroquinolones and tetracyclines. Macrolides have been considered to be the treatment of choice, but recent data from Asian countries indicate a strikingly high rate of high-level macrolide resistance that is also being documented in the United States (Xiao et al., 2009). Tetracycline resistance has been well documented in recent years in both *M. hominis* and *Ureaplasma* spp. and may occur in up to 50% in isolates, depending on the patient population (Waites, Katz, & Schelonka, 2005). Other agents such as streptogramins, ketolides, fluoroquinolones, and chloramphenicol usually show in vitro inhibitory activity against genital mycoplasmas. Susceptibility profiles for *M. fermentans* are generally similar to those of *M. hominis,* whereas susceptibilities of *M. genitalium* are similar to those of *M. pneumoniae.* Eradication of extragenital infections, especially if they occur in immunocompromised hosts, can be quite difficult, requiring prolonged therapy, even when organisms are susceptible to expected agents.

Agar dilution is a useful reference method for susceptibility testing, but this technique is not practical for testing small numbers of strains or occasional isolates of mycoplasmas or

ureaplasmas that may be encountered. Agar disk diffusion is not useful for mycoplasmas because there has been no correlation between inhibitory zones and MICs, and the relatively slow growth of some of these organisms further limits this technology. Microbroth dilution is the most practical and widely used method. The agar gradient diffusion (Etest) technique has been used for determination of in vitro susceptibilities of *M. hominis* and *Ureaplasma* spp. to various antimicrobials and has yielded results comparable to both agar dilution and broth

REAL WORLD TIP

Antimicrobial susceptibility procedures adapting both the agar dilution and microbroth dilution methods to determine antimicrobial susceptibilities of human mycoplasmas and ureaplasmas are available through reference laboratories. The main value for performing antimicrobial susceptibility testing for mycoplasmas and ureaplasmas for clinical purposes is for a patient with a systemic infection, especially if he or she is an abnormal host because of a congenital or acquired immunocompromised condition, or because of a prior treatment failure.

dilution. Visit ∞ Chapter 11 to review susceptibility methods. Susceptibility testing methods for human mycoplasmas has been the subject of a multicenter international collaboration that has taken place over several years organized by the Clinical and Laboratory Standards Institute, and a publication detailing these methods will be forthcoming.

 **Checkpoint! 28–6
(Chapter Objective 6)**

Which one of the following antimicrobial groups would usually be appropriate for treatment of an infection caused by Mycoplasma pneumoniae?

    A. Penicillin

    B. Cephalosporin

    C. Macrolide

    D. Carbapenem

▶ NONCULTURE METHODS FOR DIAGNOSIS

NONAMPLIFIED ANTIGEN DETECTION AND NUCLEIC ACID PROBES

Although culture is well adapted to species that can be isolated easily and rapidly from clinical specimens such as *M. hominis* and *Ureaplasma* spp., it is not ideal for detection of fastidious and/or extremely slow-growing organisms such as *M. genitalium* and *M. pneumoniae*. Therefore, alternate means of detection should be used for these organisms.

Antigen detection systems for diagnosis of *M. pneumoniae* respiratory infections have been hampered by low sensitivity and cross-reactivity with other mycoplasmas found in the respiratory tract. DNA hybridization techniques were studied for several years, but like nonamplified antigen detection techniques, they have not been developed commercially because of the attractiveness of more sensitive techniques such as the PCR assay.

POLYMERASE CHAIN REACTION (PCR) ASSAY

PCR assays have been developed for all the clinically important mycoplasma species that infect humans. Several PCR assays are commercially available in various European countries, but none are yet approved in the United States. While PCR is the only practical means for direct detection of *M. pneumoniae* and *M. genitalium* in clinical specimens, it is less valuable for routine diagnostic purposes in the case of the more rapidly growing and easily cultivable organisms, such as *M. hominis* and *Ureaplasma* spp. The PCR assay is also a very good tool for identification of an unknown mycoplasma previously obtained by culture. It can be used for characterization of strains within a species and for detection of a specific feature, such as the presence of an antibiotic resistance determinant. Currently, PCR detection of human mycoplasmas and ureaplasmas is available only in specialized reference laboratories. Use of the real-time PCR assay technique theoretically enables results to be available on the same day the specimen is collected, providing the assay is done on-site and also enables quantitative determination of the numbers of organisms present in a clinical specimen. Even if overnight shipment to a reference laboratory is necessary, PCR still provides the best turnaround time for any diagnostic technique used for human mycoplasmas and ureaplasmas. Over the past several years, as more comparisons of PCR assays with traditional methods for diagnosis including both culture and serology have been made, PCR appears to be the test of choice for both *M. pneumoniae* and *M. genitalium*, even though serology is still widely used for indirect detection of *M. pneumoniae* infection. Concern still remains regarding how to interpret results of an extremely sensitive PCR assay that detects *M. pneumoniae* in someone without apparent respiratory illness or if corresponding serology is negative, a situation that sometimes occurs. It is anticipated that once PCR assays become commercially available on a more widespread basis and are sold in the United States, more clinical laboratories will adopt this method for diagnosis of mycoplasmal infections.

 **Checkpoint! 28–7
(Chapter Objective 7)**

Which of the following are theoretical advantages of the PCR assay to detect infections with Mycoplasma pneumoniae?

    A. The PCR assay does not require viable mycoplasmas to detect their presence in a clinical specimen.

    B. The PCR assay can detect much smaller numbers of mycoplasmas that may be present in a clinical specimen than would be detected using culture.

    C. The PCR assay can detect acute infection in a single clinical specimen within a few hours after collection.

    D. All of the above choices are correct.

▶ SEROLOGIC METHODS

Detection of an antibody response has long been the primary means for diagnosis of infections with *M. pneumoniae*, despite a number of limitations inherent in the methods that are currently available. Antibody responses in clinical infections caused by *M. pneumoniae* can be detected after about 1 week of illness, peaking at 3 to 6 weeks, followed by a gradual decline. Complement fixation (CF) was the first method developed for serological testing for *M. pneumoniae*, but it has a number of limitations, including false-positive results because of cross-reactive autoantibodies induced by acute inflammation from other unrelated causes. In most clinical laboratories CF has been replaced by alternative techniques such as **enzyme**

immunoassays (EIAs; Waites et al., 2001). EIA technology is based on the absorption of an immunogenic antigen of the organism of interest to a solid phase (e.g., a plastic microtiter plate). Serum dilutions are added, then incubated, washed, and reincubated with anti-immunoglobulin labeled with an enzyme. Enzyme activity is measured by adding the specific substrate and estimating a color reaction which is a direct function of the amount of antibody bound. EIA is widely available, less labor intensive than CF, more sensitive than culture, and may be comparable in sensitivity to PCR for detection of acute *M. pneumoniae* infection, provided a sufficient time has elapsed for the host to mount an immune response. Several EIA test formats are marketed commercially by various companies in the United States. Acute and convalescent sera, collected 2 to 4 weeks apart and tested simultaneously for both IgG and IgM, are necessary to accurately detect acute *M. pneumoniae* infection. A membrane-based EIA specific for IgM, called the Meridian ImmunoCard (Meridian Diagnostics, Cincinnati, OH), has been developed for rapidly detecting an acute *M. pneumoniae* infection using a single serum specimen. The ImmunoCard (Figure 28-9) has the advantages of being technically much simpler and quicker (10 minutes) to perform than other types of assays. Its potential disadvantages are lack of sensitivity for detection of *M. pneumoniae* infections in some adults in whom the IgM response may be minimal and the fact that IgM, when present, may persist for up to several months after a single infection. The Remel EIA is another rapid point-of care qualitative serologic assay that detects both IgM and IgG simultaneously. This test has shown reasonably good sensitivity and specificity when compared to other EIAs and CF tests. Among several EIA-based tests sold commercially to measure the immune response to *M. pneumoniae*, some direct comparisons among them have been reported (Talkington et al., 2004). Despite some claims that diagnosis of an acute *M. pneumoniae* infection can be made by testing a single serum sample, the available data suggest that optimum detection still requires paired sera, meaning two clinical visits and a retrospective disgnosis. Cold agglutinins, detected by agglutination of type O Rh-negative erythrocytes at 4°C, sometimes occur in association with *M. pneumoniae* infection. Titers of 64 to 128, or a fourfold or greater rise in titer, suggest a recent *M. pneumoniae* infection, but the test is nonspecific, and cold agglutinins may be induced by a wide variety of viral infections as well as noninfectious conditions. Because of these limitations, detection of cold agglutinins is not recommended for serologic diagnosis of *M. pneumoniae* infection. No serologic tests for genital mycoplasmas have been standardized and made commercially available in the United States, and they cannot be recommended for routine diagnostic purposes at present. Visit ∞ Chapter 10, "Immunological Tests," to review the use of EIA for diagnosis of infectious disease.

REAL WORLD TIP

Though it suffers from some limitations, measurement of IgM and IgG antibodies remains the most widely used method to diagnose respiratory infections with *M. pneumoniae*.

✓ Checkpoint! 28–8 (Chapter Objective 8)

The most widely used method for diagnosis of respiratory infections because of Mycoplasma pneumoniae *is:*

    A. *culture in fibroblast monolayers.*
    B. *culture on A8 agar.*
    C. *detection of antibody in serum.*
    D. *detection of antigen in sputum by immunofluorescence.*

SUMMARY

Commonly encountered organisms such as *Mycoplasma* and *Ureaplasma* spp. are no more difficult to detect and identify than other fastidious bacteria, provided appropriate attention to their specific cultivation requirements is given. Still, these organisms are often ignored by clinical laboratories because of the perception that they cannot be readily recovered from clinical specimens. Given the potentially serious infections that can potentially occur because of these organisms, clinical laboratories should have appropriate procedures in place to collect and transport specimens for their detection by cultural or noncultural methods, even if the diagnostic procedures are not performed on site. The future of mycoplasma diagnostics should ideally include development and refinement of commercial

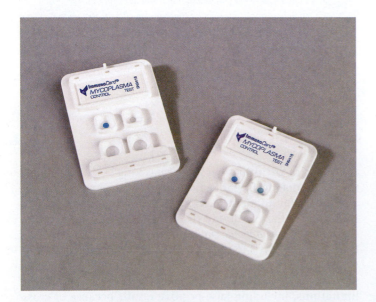

■ **FIGURE 28-9** Negative result (left) and positive result (right) for the ImmunoCard Mycoplasma.
Photo courtesy of Meridian Bioscience.

PCR kits for detection of *M. pneumoniae* that could be used as a screening device for the presence of respiratory infection for this organism, other mycoplasmas, and perhaps even unrelated bacteria that cause pneumonias simultaneously. Use of the PCR assay to detect and identify unknown or uncommon mycoplasmas is also likely to become important, but the use of such technology would be limited primarily to mycoplasma research or reference laboratories. Further improvements and simplification of commercial serologic tests that can accurately and rapidly measure IgM, IgA, and IgG antibodies against *M. pneu-*

moniae, ideally in an acute care clinic setting, will also be important goals to achieve. Given that culture is likely to remain the preferred diagnostic method for detection of *M. hominis* and *Ureaplasma* spp. for some time to come, the most obvious need is for reliable commercial products to be sold more widely and that media capable of detecting these organisms in all types of clinical specimens be validated. Widespread availability of complete diagnostic kits may further increase the likelihood that hospital-based microbiology laboratories will begin offering diagnostic services for mycoplasmas.

LEARNING OPPORTUNITIES

1. Which mycoplasmal species pathogenic for humans has the slowest growth rate (Chapter Objective 5)?

2. Which mycoplasma that infects humans is sometimes discovered accidentally because of the ability of some strains to grow on chocolate or Columbia agar (Chapter Objective 5)?

3. Discuss the implications of having such a small genome on the biological characteristics of mycoplasmas and ureaplasmas that infect humans (Chapter Objective 1).

4. What laboratory departments other then microbiology may have patient results affected by *Mycoplasma* or *Ureaplasma* infections (Chapter Objective 9)?

PEARSON myhealthprofessionskit™

Use this address to access the interactive Companion Website created for this textbook. Simply select "Clinical Laboratory Science" from the choice of disciplines. Find this book and log in using your user name and password.

REFERENCES

Go to myhealthprofessionskit.com to view this chapter's references.

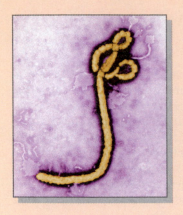

29

Medical Mycology

William C. Payne

■ LEARNING OBJECTIVES

Upon completion of this chapter, the learner should be able to:

1. Describe the physiological characteristics and cellular structures that differentiate fungi from prokaryotic cells (bacteria) and eukaryotic organisms such as plants and animals.
2. Discuss aspects of nonspecific immunity that work to protect humans from fungal diseases.
3. Explain the importance of fungi as causes of human disease, including risk factors that predispose individuals to fungal infections.
4. Describe microscopic and macroscopic structures that allow identification of yeasts and moulds.
5. State the role of asexual and sexual reproduction in the propagation of fungi.
6. Define the role of saprophytic fungi in the environment (soil, plants, and decaying vegetation) and human disease.
7. Explain the importance of histological stains in the diagnosis of fungal diseases.
8. Correlate the etiology, epidemiology, clinical manifestations, and laboratory diagnosis of the following fungal diseases:
   a. Opportunistic mycoses
   b. Superficial mycoses
   c. Dermatophytosis
   d. Subcutaneous mycoses
   e. Systemic mycoses
9. Differentiate filamentous fungi (moulds) and yeasts based on macroscopic and microscopic morphologies and biochemical tests.
   a. Select key identification characteristics and biochemical testing required to identify organisms.

■ LEARNING OBJECTIVES (continued)

10. Formulate a probable diagnosis given the following information:

    a. Signs and symptoms of the disease

    b. Patient history (geographic location, history of exposure, travel history, etc.)

    c. Specimen type

    d. Pathogenesis

    e. Results of laboratory tests (stain results, histology, serology, cultures, biochemical testing, etc.)

11. Discuss the treatment of infections due to yeast and moulds.

KEY TERMS

Note: Additional key terms can be reviewed in ∞ Chapter 14, "Fungal Cultures."

anamorph (or asexual form)	mould	stolon
biseriate	mycelium (pl., mycelia)	synamorph
chlamydoconidia	mycology	teleomorph (or sexual form)
columella	mycosis (pl., mycoses)	uniseriate
dematiaceous	rhizoids	vesicle
metulae	sclerotic bodies	yeast
	septate	

TAXONOMY

The classification of fungal species into phyla, classes, orders, and families has undergone a number of changes in recent years and changes will continue to occur as more information is uncovered using molecular methods. The sexual stage is used in classification but in some cases beginning mycologists will be more familiar with the name given to the asexual stage. It should be noted that some sexual names are used for more than one asexual stage and genera may be included in more than one family. To simplify the information for the learner, in this chapter, the fungi are classified by genus and species based on the type of clinical disease they cause rather than the traditional taxonomy headings such as phylum, class, and family. Realize some organisms may cross classifications and appear under multiple headings.

CLASSIFICATION OF MEDICALLY IMPORTANT FUNGI:

Opportunistic
Genus *Aspergillus* (as-per-jil′-lus)
   A. fumigatus (fume-uh-got′-us)
   A. flavus (flay-vus)
   A. niger (nī-jur)
Genus *Penicillium* (pen-uh-sil′-ee-um)
Genus *Acremonium* (ak′-ruh-moan′-ee-um)

Genus *Rhizopus* (rye′-zō-pus)
Genus *Mucor* (myoo′-kor)
Genus *Rhizomucor* (rye′-zō-myoo′-kor)
Genus *Absidia* (ab-sid′-ee-ah)
Genus *Fusarium* (fyoo-sar′-ee-um)
   F. solani (sō′-lan-ē)
Genus *Paecilomyces* (pay-sil′-ō-my′-seez)
   P. lilacinus (lī-lăk-ĭn-ŭs)
Genus *Scopulariopsis* (skop′-yoo-lar-ee-op′-sis)
   S. brevicaulis (brēv-ĭ-call-ŭs)
Genus *Cryptococcus* (krip′-tō-kok′-kus)
   C. neoformans (nē-ō-for′-munz)
Genus *Candida* (kan-dee′-dah)
   C. albicans (al′-buh-cans)
   C. tropicalis (trop-uh-cal-lous)
   C. parapsilosis (pŭ-răp-sĭ-lō-sĭs)
   C. stellatoideae (stĕl-lŭ-tōy-dē-ā)
   C. glabrata (glŭ-bra-tŭ)
   C. dubliniensis (dŭb-lĭ-nĭn-sĭs)
   C. krusei (crew-sē-ī)
   C. lusitaniae (loo-sĭ-tā-nē-ā)
Genus *Geotrichum* (jee′-ah-tree-kum)
   G. candidum (can-deed′-um)
Genus *Trichosporon* (try-kuh-spôr′-on)
   T. beigeli (bay-juh-lee)

(continued)

TAXONOMY (*continued*)

Superficial

Genus *Malassezia* (mal-uh-see'-zee-ah)
  M. furfur (fur-fur)
Genus *Hortaea* (previously *Phaeonellomyces*) (hoor-tē-ā)
  (fay"-oh-nell-oh-my'-seez)
  H. werneckii (wur-neck-ee)
Genus *Trichosporon* (try-kuh-spôr'-on)
  T. beigeli (bay-juh-lee)
Genus *Piedraia* (pee-eh'-dree-uh)
  P. hortae (hoar-tay)

Dermatophytes

Genus *Microsporum* (my-krō-spôr'-um)
  M. audouini (aw-dough'-een-ee)
  M. canis (kane'-us)
  M. gypseum (jip'-see-um)
Genus *Trichophyton* (try-kō'-fyt-on) or (trick-ō-fyt'-en)
  T. mentagrophytes (men-tah"-grow-fyt'-eez)
  T. rubrum (roob'-rum)
  T. schoenleinii (show-en-leen-ee)
  T. verrucosum (věr-rû-kō-sǔm)
  T. tonsurans (tǒn-sir-ǎns)
  T. violaceum (vī-ō-lā-sē-ǔm)
Genus *Epidermophyton* (ep-i'-dur'-mof-uh-ton)
  E. floccosum (flock-oh-sum)

Subcutaneous

Genus *Fonsecaea* (fahn-seek'-uh)
  F. pedrosoi (puh-drow-so-ee)
Genus *Phialophora* (fy'-uh-loff'-ôr-uh)
  P. verrucosa (ver-uh-kō-suh)
Genus *Cladosporium* (klad-ō-spôr'-ee-um)
  C. carrioni (care-ee-own'-ee)

Genus *Alternaria* (âl'-ter-nar'-ee-uh)
Genus *Curvularia* (kurv'-yoo-lar'-ee-uh)
Genus *Bipolaris* (by'-pō-lar'-us)
Genus *Exophiala* (ěk-sō-fī-ǎl-ǔ)
  E. jeanselmei (jēn-sěl-mē-ī)
Genus *Wangiella* (wān-gē-ěl-ǔ)
  W. dermatitidis (derm-uh-tit-uh-dis)
Genus *Pseudallescheria* (sood-uh-lesh-er-ē-uh)
  P. boydii (boy-dē)
    ■ Asexual forms
      Genus *Scedosporium* (skē'-dō-spore'-ee-um)
        S. apiospermum (ape-ee-oh-sperm-um)
      Genus *Graphium* (grǎf-ē-ǔm)
Genus *Sporothrix* (spôr-oh-thriks)
  S. schenckii (schenk-ee)

Systemic

Genus *Blastomyces* (blast-ō-my'-seez)
  B. dermatitidis (derm-uh-tit-uh-dis)
Genus *Histoplasma* (hist-ō-plas'-mah)
  H. capsulatum (kap-suh-lot-um)
Genus *Paracoccidioides* (par'-e-kok-sid'-ee-oy'-deez)
  P. brasiliensis (bruh-zill-ee-en-sis)
Genus *Coccidioides* (kok-sid'-ee-oy'-deez)
  C. immitis (imm-uh-tis)
Genus *Penicillium* (pen-uh-sil'-ee-um)
  P. marneffei (mǎr-něf-fē-ī)

Other

Genus *Pneumocystis* (new-mō-sis-tiss)
  P. jiroveci (yee–row–vet-zee)

► INTRODUCTION

The study of fungi is called **mycology.** This group of organisms includes **yeasts** that are unicellular organisms and **moulds** that are multicellular filamentous organisms. Moulds frequently tend to be a source of annoyance when they contaminate laboratory media, spoil foodstuffs, or destroy items made of wood and other fibrous materials. Yeasts have been employed for centuries in the production of food and beverages. Yeast, such as *Saccharomyces cerevisiae* (baker's yeast), is used to raise bread dough through the fermentation of carbohydrates and the production of carbon dioxide. Fermentation also results in the generation of by-products such as alcohol, a property exploited by brewers, winemakers, and distillers in the making of alcoholic beverages. Fungi are also used in the production of soy sauces and cheeses.

 REAL WORLD TIP

Textbooks may use different spellings of the word "mould." Some may use the spelling "mold." *Mould* is probably the more accurate spelling. It originated in the Old English language. *Mold* is used to describe a hollow container used to cast or shape mediums such as clay, wax, or metal.

Fungi are ubiquitous and many thrive in moist environments where they play an important role in returning nutrients to the soil by contributing to the decomposition of animal and vegetable matter. As a means of propagation fungi produce spores. The inhalation of fungal spores has brought misery to individuals who are prone to allergies and asthma.

It is estimated that anywhere from 50,000 to 100,000 species of fungi have been identified and within that number approximately 150 species are known to cause human disease. The importance of bacteria as etiological agents of human illness is well known, but most individuals are much less familiar with the role of fungi as the cause of significant morbidity and mortality. Fortunately, most humans have an innate resistance to fungal infection. This can be reviewed in ∞ Chapter 4. Most fungi have only a transient existence on body surfaces but a few species cause disease as a result of inhalation, invasion of mucous membranes, or implantation into the tissues by trauma.

In this chapter taxonomy, terminology, and the etiological (causative) agents of fungal diseases are discussed. **Mycoses**, or fungal infections, will be presented according to the tissue levels affected, beginning with superficial infections and progressing to systemic infections. Saprophytic or nonpathogenic fungi and yeast can cause superficial and systemic infections depending on the immune status of the individual and are discussed under their respective headings. As each fungal disease is presented, pathophysiology, symptoms, etiological agents, treatment regimens, diagnosis by direct examination of clinical specimens, diagnosis by examination of fungal cultures, and serological tests, where appropriate, are discussed. The routes of transmission and the recommended specimen types are discussed within the narrative and are summarized in tables. As an aid in identifying fungal species, both macroscopic (colony growth on fungal media) and microscopic characteristics are provided. For detailed discussions describing the handling, processing, staining, culturing, and microscopic morphology of fungi, see ∞ Chapter 14, "Fungal Cultures."

► GENERAL CHARACTERISTICS OF FUNGI

Observing the microscopic morphology of fungal species gives the impression these organisms are simply incredibly small plants. Earlier scientists considered fungi to be simple forms belonging to the plant kingdom, but more recently it is has been accepted that fungi are neither plants nor animals and a separate kingdom was designated for these organisms. Despite the unicellular nature of yeast, fungi are not related to other unicellular organisms such as bacteria and protozoans.

Bacteria are prokaryotes, and while they have a nuclear region, their DNA is not enclosed by a nuclear membrane. Prokaryotic cells lack other membrane-bound organelles such as mitochondria and possess a 70S ribosome. The cell wall of bacteria is composed primarily of peptidoglycan or lipid components and the cytoplasmic membrane lacks sterols. Mycoplasmas are an exception to this rule. Bacteria reproduce through binary fission and are incapable of sexual reproduction through meiosis.

In contrast, fungi are eukaryotic organisms. Eukaryotes have a true nucleus bound by a nuclear membrane, mitochondria,

endoplasmic reticulum, and 80S ribosomes. The differentiation of fungi and plants can be made on the basis of cell structures and physiology. Plants, which are autotrophic, possess chlorophyll and obtain nutrition by absorption of inorganic compounds and through photosynthesis. Fungi, which lack chlorophyll, are heterotrophic and as such, require preformed organic compounds. They secrete extracellular enzymes into the environment to break macromolecules into their subunits, which are then absorbed. The cell walls of plants are composed of cellulose whereas those of fungi contain chitin.

The major sterol in the cytoplasmic membrane of fungi is ergosterol as opposed to animals, which have cholesterol in their cell membranes. Amphotericin B, which is an effective antifungal drug, binds very strongly to ergosterol, causing potassium to leak from the cell interfering with respiration and glycolysis. Fortunately, amphotericin B has a greater affinity for ergosterol than cholesterol, providing a selective advantage in which the antifungal agent has a more pronounced effect on the cytoplasmic membrane of fungal cells than that of mammalian cells. Azole derivatives, which are also antifungal drugs, are effective because they inhibit the synthesis of ergosterol.

Fungi, which are primarily aerobic organisms, grow well in room air. Yeast and some mould forms are facultative anaerobes and therefore are able to grow under anaerobic conditions. They do not require increased levels of CO_2, as some bacteria do, but tend to prefer a moist environment. Both yeast and mould forms tolerate a wide range of acidic or alkaline conditions, and while they can grow in environments with pH values from 2 to 10, a neutral pH tends to encourage their best growth. Since fungi are environmental organisms they also grow over a wide range of temperatures, typically growing under refrigeration (0–8°C) to temperatures as high as 45°C. Optimal growth occurs at 25–37°C depending on the species involved. Many clinical laboratories use a 30°C incubator for fungal cultures since all fungi can grow well at this temperature.

Checkpoint! 29–1 (Chapter Objective 1)

The cytoplasmic membrane of fungi:
  A. *lacks sterols.*
  B. *is composed primarily of chitin.*
  C. *is composed of lipopolysaccharides.*
  D. *contains cholesterol.*
  E. *contains ergosterol.*

THE MEDICAL IMPORTANCE OF FUNGI

Even with the large number of fungal species known, only a small percentage cause disease in humans. The fungal infections that occur most frequently are vaginal yeast infections, diaper rash, and athlete's foot. Virtually all fungal infections are of an exogenous origin (the source of infection is outside the body of the host). Because of the ubiquitous nature of fungi and the ability of spores to become airborne, mould colonies growing on media were often considered to be "contaminants." Contributing to this attitude is the fact that, unlike viruses, protozoan parasites, and some bacteria, fungi do not need to colonize or infect tissues to survive. With the increasing population of immunocompromised individuals, that assumption is no longer acceptable. Fungal species that were considered to be saprophytic can cause life-threatening illnesses. Factors that predispose individuals to infection with organisms of low pathogenic potential include:

- debilitation through metabolic imbalance such as diabetes, pregnancy, or menstruation
- debilitating infectious diseases such as human immunodeficiency virus infection
- neoplastic diseases such as leukemias, lymphomas, or sarcomas
- immunosuppression through the administration of corticosteroids or cytotoxic drugs
- therapeutic measures such as radiation therapy
- administration of long-term broad-spectrum antibiotics that disrupt the balance of microbial flora of mucous membranes

In addition, there must be factors inherent to fungal species that influence the pathogenic potential of microorganisms. Fungi must be able to evade host defenses, grow at 35–37°C, and grow under conditions where oxygen is at a partial pressure lower than that of air. See Table 29-1 ✪ for clinical classifications of human mycoses.

FUNGAL STRUCTURES OF MOULDS

Mycologists rely heavily on recognition of the macroscopic and microscopic morphology and arrangement of vegetative and reproductive structures in the identification of moulds. Budding mycologists (pun intended) must therefore become well versed in the terminology employed in this discipline to describe fungal structures. The next four sections present terminology that should become part of the vocabulary of individuals working in the mycology section of the laboratory. Review ∞ Chapter 14, "Fungal Cultures," for terms and figures that have been previously discussed.

Moulds are a multicellular, filamentous form of fungi that are often described as "fluffy" or "fuzzy." The body of moulds, referred to as a thallus, is composed of long, cylindrical, or tube-like structures called hyphae. Depending on the species in question, the diameter of hyphae ranges from 3 to 20 microns (or micrometer; a unit of measure equal to one millionth of a meter). **Septate** hyphae contain crosswalls at regular intervals which separate it into sections within the tubular growth as seen in *Aspergillus fumigatus*. See Figure 14-17 to view septate hyphae. Because septae contain pores, cytoplasm within the

hyphae is actually continuous. In aseptate or nonseptate hyphae, the septae are very sparse or absent rather than being regularly spaced. Aseptate hyphae are associated with the Zygomycetes such as *Mucor* species. Review Figure 29-4 to observe aseptate hyphae. With the lack of septae, the nuclei and cytoplasm are essentially continuous throughout the hyphae. Both types of hyphae elongate by growth from the tip or apical zone. **Mycelium** is the term applied to the mass that develops as hyphae grow, branch, and intertwine. Hyphae penetrate the surface of a growth medium in order to absorb nutrients forming the vegetative mycelium. The vegetative mycelium gives a mould colony a very tenacious hold onto the growth medium and contributes to the topography or surface contour of moulds. Fortunately removal of even a small portion of the mycelium is sufficient to transfer a mould to a fresh growth medium. Other hyphae grow above the surface of the growth medium to support reproductive structures forming the aerial mycelium. Aerial hyphae are responsible for the textural appearance of mould colonies. Review Figure 14-12 to observe aerial and vegetative mycelium. **Dematiaceous** moulds have darkly pigmented hyphae due to the presence of a melanin-like pigment. An example of a dematiaceous mould is *Bipolaris* species. The dark pigmentation is evident when the mould colony is examined macroscopically or microscopically as seen in Figures 14-8 and 14-17. Moulds that are nonpigmented are referred to as hyaline moulds. Hyaline mould colonies begin as white colonies that may produce color as reproductive structures mature as seen with *Aspergillus fumigatus* (Figure 29-1 ■). Other fungal elements include **rhizoids** and **stolons**, structures found in the Zygomycetes such as *Rhizopus* species as seen in Figure 29-4. Rhizoids are root-like structures that are part of the vegetative mycelium. Stolons are structures that are homologous to the runners of strawberry plants.

THE FUNGAL STRUCTURES OF YEAST

Yeasts are a form of fungus that is unicellular in nature. As they grow on a solid growth medium they form discrete, round, smooth, moist, or mucoid colonies similar to those of bacteria. These colonies are composed of spherical to ellipsoid cells that range in diameter from 3 to 15 microns. Yeasts reproduce asexually by budding or fission. During the budding process a swelling appears along the cell wall of the mother cell as a result of a weakening of a small portion of the cell wall. The nucleus of the mother cell divides by mitosis and as a result the cell now contains two nuclei. As the swelling continues to enlarge, cytoplasm and one of the nuclei flows into the daughter cell. Eventually a septum forms between the mother or parent cell and the daughter cell. Eventually separation of the two cells occurs, leaving a bud scar that is clearly visible in an electron micrograph. The end-product of this asexual reproduction or budding process is a blastoconidium or bud. *Candida glabrata* is known for its production of these structures.

On some occasions the two cells elongate but remain connected, continuing to divide until a chain of blastoconidia is

Classification of Human Mycoses

Mycosis	Route of Transmission	Etiological Agents (Representative Species)
Opportunistic Infections		
Aspergillosis	Inhalation	*Aspergillus fumigatus*
Zygomycosis		*A. flavus*
		A. niger
		A. terreus
Mucoromycosis	Inhalation	*Rhizopus arrhizus*
		Mucor spp.
		Rhizomucor spp.
		Absidia spp.
Mycotic keratitis	Accidental or surgical trauma and ocular topical corticosteroids or antibiotics	*Fusarium solani*
		Aspergillus spp.
		Acremonium spp.
		Pseudallescheria boydii
		Bipolaris spp.
		Curvularia spp.
Mycotic otitis	Colonization of ear canal	*Aspergillus niger*
		A. fumigatus
		Candida spp.
		Penicillium spp.
Superficial mycoses		
Pityriasis (tinea) versicolor	May be part of normal skin flora. Predisposing factors are uncertain but may include excess sweating, corticosteroid therapy, malnutrition, and poor health	*Malassezia furfur*
Superficial phaeohyphomyco-sis or tinea nigra	Route of transmission and predisposing factors are unknown	*Hortaea* (previously *Phaeoannello-myces*) *werneckii*
White peidra	Route of transmission is unclear. The etiological agent is occasionally isolated from the skin of healthy individuals	*Trichosporon beigelii*
Black peidra	Route of transmission is uncertain	*Piedra hortae*
Dermatophytosis		
Anthropophilic dermatophytes	Spread by combs, brushes, clothing, furniture, and bathing facilities	*Microsporum audouinii*
		Trichopyton rubrum
		T. shoenleinii
		Epidermophyton flocossum
Zoophilic dermatophytes	Direct contact with infected animals	*Microsporum canis*
		T. mentagrophytes
		T. verrucosum
Geophilic species	Direct contact with soil or infected animals	*Microsporum gypseum*
Subcutaneous mycoses		
Chromoblastomycosis	Traumatic implantation	*Fonseceae pedrosoi*
		Phialophora verrucosa
		Cladophialophora carrionii
Phaeohyphomycosis	Traumatic implantation	*Alternaria, Bipolaris, Curvularia, Exophiala,* and *Phialophora* spp.
Eumycotic mycetoma	Traumatic implantation	*Pseudallescheria boydii*
		Exophiala jeanselmei
Sporotrichosis	Traumatic implantation or inhalation	*Sporothrix schenckii*

(continued)

TABLE 29-1

Classification of Human Mycoses (continued)

Mycosis	Route of Transmission	Etiological Agents (Representative Species)
Systemic mycoses		
Histoplasmosis	Inhalation of conidia	*Histoplasma capsulatum*
Blastomycosis		*Blastomyces dermatitidis*
Coccidioidomycosis		*Coccidioides immitis*
Paracoccidioidomycosis		*Paracoccidioides brasiliensis*
Penicilliosis		*Penicillium marneffei*
Opportunistic yeast infections		
Cryptococcosis	Inhalation	*Cryptococcus neoformans*
Candidiasis	*Candida* species are often part of an individual's resident microflora	*Candida albicans* and other species
Geotrichosis	Etiological agent may be part of the normal microflora of the skin and gastrointestinal tract	*Geotrichum candidums*
Other infections		
Interstitial plasma cell pneumonia	Inhalation	*Pneumocystis jiroveci*

produced, forming a filamentous structure referred to as pseudohyphae as seen in *Candida tropicalis*. Pseudohyphae differ from true hyphae as a constriction is apparent at the common septum between the parent or mother cell and the daughter cell (blastoconidium or bud). There is no constriction or pinching at the point of septation in true hyphae. In other words, the walls of true hyphae are parallel and lack indentations where the septae (crosswalls) are found. Blastoconidia and pseudohyphae can be observed in Figure 29-40.

Yeast cells may also produce a filament by apical growth (growth at the tip) in which there is no constriction at the origin from the parent cell. This is a germ tube, as seen in Figure 14-6, and it can be useful in the identification of *Candida* species especially *C. albicans*. Germ tubes eventually become true hyphae as septae develop along the length of the filament. Identification of yeast species is usually accomplished through a combination of biochemical testing and observation of microscopic morphology to determine which fungal elements are present as growth occurs on cornmeal agar with Tween 80.

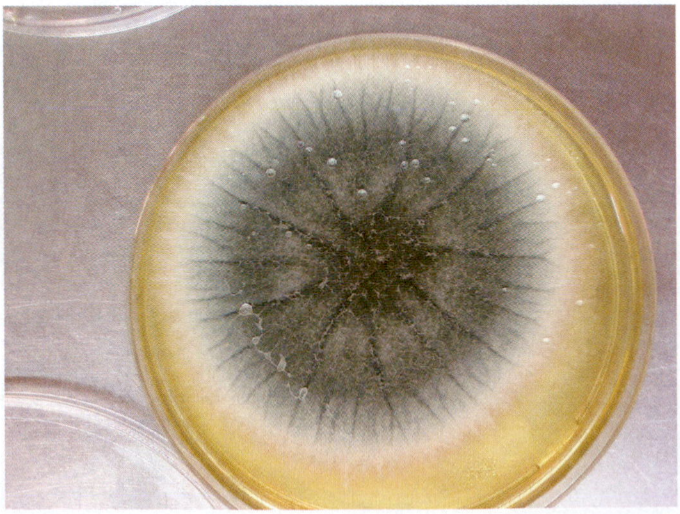

Some fungal species are able to grow in two different forms, exibiting both yeast and filamentous mould phases. They are known as dimorphic fungi. The determining factor as to which form predominates is usually temperature and therefore this condition is referred to as being temperature dependent. If the microorganism is growing within host tissue or on an enriched medium a yeast form can be seen. The enriched medium recommended to induce the yeast phase is brain heart infusion agar with sheep blood incubated at a temperature of 35–37°C. The same organism will be seen in a mould form when grown on a non-nutritive type medium (a medium containing minimal nutrients). To demonstrate the mould form, subculturing the test organism onto sabouraud's dextrose or potato dextrose agar incubated at room temperature or 22–25°C is recommended.

■ **FIGURE 29-1** The characteristic colony of *Aspergillus fumigatus* is dark green with a velvet-like appearance.

✓ Checkpoint! 29-2 (Chapter Objective 4)

Hyphae in which the septae are very sparse rather than being regularly spaced are called:

A. *aseptate or nonseptate.*

B. *septate.*

C. *hyaline.*

D. *dematiaceous.*

ASEXUAL REPRODUCTION IN FUNGI

Asexual reproduction in yeast results in the formation of blastoconidia, and in the filamentous moulds results in the formation of some type of conidium (Latin, *dust;* pl. conidia) or spore. Conidia, which can survive harsh environmental conditions such as a dry atmosphere, are produced as the result of mitosis. These asexual spores are usually produced on the tips of specialized aerial hyphae called conidiophores as seen with *Aspergillus* spp. in Figure 29-2 ■. Conidia, which may be formed in long chains, are easily airborne and allow moulds to spread a great distance from the parent mould. The fungal structure that produces conidia is called a phialide as seen with *Penicillium* species in Figure 29-10. In some species having septate hyphae, terminal segments become slightly enlarged. These segments have thickened cell walls and are called arthroconidia. They separate from each other and may become airborne. Arthroconidia are prevalent in *Geotrichum* species and can be observed in Figure 29-42. In some species, round, thick-walled conidia called **chlamydoconidia** are produced as noted in Figure 14-22. These spores, which represent a resting stage, may be located at the tips of hyphae (terminal) or inserted along the hyphae (intercalary). Chlamydoconidia are known to be produced by *Candida albicans* and *C. dublinensis.*

In the Zygomycetes, asexual spores are formed within a sac-like structure called a sporangium. *Mucor* species are known for their production of sporangium. Specialized aerial hyphae, called sporangiophores, bear the sporangium containing sporangiospores, and may be branched or unbranched. A rounded, sterile, supporting structure called a **columella** is formed at the tip of the sporangiophore. It extends into the sporangium and serves to separate the sporulating and nonsporulating areas. All three of these structures can be observed in Figure 14-16.

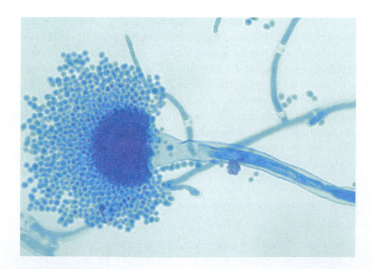

■ **FIGURE 29-2** *Aspergillus glaucus.* Note the slightly oval vesicle, on top of the stalk-like conidiophore, with its bottle-shaped phialides. The numerous round conidia, resting on top of the phialides, are slightly rough.

SEXUAL REPRODUCTION IN FUNGI

Sexual reproduction involves the union of two haploid (n) nuclei, each possessing a single set of chromosomes, to form a zygote having a diploid (2n) nucleus with 2 sets of matched chromosomes. Meiosis or reductive division then follows producing four haploid (n) nuclei. To avoid confusion it should be noted that the sexual form, called a **teleomorph**, and asexual form, called an **anamorph**, are given different genus-species names. For example: *Pseudoallescheria boydii* (sexual stage) and *Scedosporium apiospermum* (asexual stage) refer to the same organism but represent two different microscopic morphologies. It is important to note that sexual reproduction has not been demonstrated in all fungal species. Those species that do not undergo sexual reproduction as well as those species for which the sexual stage has not been demonstrated are classified as Fungi Imperfecti. The majority of human pathogens belong to this group. Demonstration of a sexual stage allow other species to be placed into the classes Ascomycetes, Basidiomycetes, or Zygomycetes, based on the morphological characteristics of the sexual stage. The sexual stage of fungi is rarely demonstrated in the clinical laboratory setting because two compatible isolates are required and infections usually involve only one mating type. There are, however, some clinically important species that are sexually self-fertile and no discussion of sexual reproduction would be complete without a description of the structures involved in the process of sexual reproduction found in these three classes. In such cases morphology could play an important role in identifying the sexual stage of a particular isolate.

The Ascomycetes include fungi whose sexual spores are encased in a sac-like structure called an ascus. The spores are called ascospores (Figure 14-20) and can be seen with *Saccharomyces* species. The Basidiomycetes include fungi whose sexual spores, basidiospores, are borne on minute stalk-like structures called sterigmata. Mushrooms are known for the presence of this structure. Basidiospores are produced on the tip of a small, swollen, club-shaped, terminal hyphal element called the basidium. This group also includes smuts and rusts, which are important causes of agricultural losses but will not be discussed in this textbook. The Zygomycetes includes fungi whose sexual spores are produced when fusion of the cytoplasm of two gametangia (organs which form gametes) form a multilayered, thick-walled, reproductive structure called a zygosporium containing a single zygospore. *Rhizopus, Mucor,* and *Absidia* species are representatives of this group. See Table 29-2 .

> ✓ **Checkpoint! 29–3 (Chapter Objective 5)**
>
> *The sexual state of a fungus is called a/an:*
> A. synamorph.
> B. teleomorph.
> C. anamorph.
> D. holomorph.

TABLE 29-2

Propagation of Fungi

Category	Reproductive Structures	Representative Genera	
		Teleomorph (Sexual Form)	Anamorph (Asexual Form)
Ascomycetes	Ascospore (sexual) Conidia (asexual) Blastoconidia (asexual)	Ajellomyces Arthroderma Pseudallescheria	Blastomyces Histoplasma Trichophyton Microsporum Scedosporium
Basidiomycetes	Basidiospore (sexual) Blastoconidia (asexual)	Filobasidiella	Cryptococcus
Zygomycetes	Aygospore (sexual) Sporangiospores (asexual)	Absidia Mucor Rhizopus	
Fungi Imperfecti	(asexual stages only) Conidia Blastoconidia Arthroconidia		Aspergillus Phialophora Cladosporium Geotrichum

SAFETY MEASURES IN HANDLING FUNGUS CULTURES

In order to determine the identity of fungi, the microscopic morphology of the organism must be examined. The presence and arrangement of fungal elements may be observed by examining preparations made from fungus cultures. Experienced mycologists know fungal cultures must be handled very carefully because fungal infections may be acquired by inhalation of conidia. It is critically important that individuals who work with these organisms use a biological safety cabinet because these devices control the flow of air and prevent exposure to aerosols. Laboratory safety in mycology can be reviewed in ∞ Chapter 14, "Fungal Cultures."

REAL WORLD TIP

Microbiologists may encounter moulds growing on routine agar plates. Practice scanning through the closed lids to look for the presence of moulds before opening the routine agar plates. Never open an agar plate that contains a mould colony. Tape it shut and open it only in a biological safety cabinet.

▶ SAPROPHYTIC FUNGI

When "fuzz" appears on food stored under refrigerated conditions after long-term storage the reaction is more one of dismay than surprise since this occurrence is not infrequent. Fungal conidia and spores are ever present in the air unless stringent measures are taken to prevent their dispersal. Even at temperatures of 0–8°C saprophytic fungi are able to thrive and reproduce. Some fungi are capable of thriving at elevated temperatures such as in decaying vegetation. Under extenuating circumstances, some fungi are capable of abandoning their saprophytic existence in favor of growth within a host species. Because these species can initiate an infection only when the host is immunocompromised, they are referred to as opportunists and the diseases they cause are called opportunistic infections. Patients suffering from human immunodeficiency virus infection, leukemia, and lymphomas, transplant patients, diabetics, cancer patients, pregnant women, and individuals with other debilitating conditions constitute the population most at risk. *Aspergillus* species and *Candida* species are two of the most common fungi capable of evading weakened host defenses, growing at body temperature, and existing in the low partial pressure of oxygen occuring in host tissues.

OPPORTUNISTIC INFECTIONS CAUSED BY SAPROPHYTES

Most species of fungi are found primarily in soil, decaying vegetation, and other warm, moist environments where they contribute to the return of important nutrients to the nitrogen and carbon cycles in nature. In most cases these organisms of low pathogenicity pose little, if any, threat to the health of immunocompetent individuals who are capable of mounting a normal response to an antigenic stimulus. The population most at risk for succumbing to diseases caused by these organisms is immunocompromised individuals whose immune systems have been weakened by disease or immunosuppressive agents. See ∞ Chapter 4, "The Host's Encounter with Microbes," ∞ Chapter 40, "Opportunistic Infections," and ∞ Chapter 41, "Nosocomial Infections," for a review. A discussion of different types of opportunistic infections, etiological agents, methods for diagnosis, and treatment regimens is presented in the following sections. As with other mycology texts, these sections are organized according to the type of infection, rather

REAL WORLD TIP

An opportunistic fungus may be a pathogen if: (1) it is repeatedly isolated from an individual's clinical specimens, (2) it has been demonstrated in clinical material, and (3) it is the only or predominant organism isolated.

than discussing each fungal species, since different species, even different genera, can cause the same disease syndromes.

Aspergillosis

Diseases caused by species in the genus *Aspergillus* are collectively referred to as aspergillosis. *Aspergillus fumigatus, A. flavus, A. niger,* and *A. terreus* are the species that are responsible for most cases of human illness. Four major syndromes are caused by members of this group, as noted in Table 29-3 ✪. Details of these syndromes can be found on the Companion Website. In addition to the four major syndromes, *Aspergillus* species may occasionally cause otomycosis (saprophytic colonization of the ear canal), keratomycosis (invasion of the cornea), pneumonia, sinusitis, cutaneous ulcers, or the organism may invade the internal organs following invasion of the blood.

A. fumigatus is one of the most commonly isolated species of fungi in the clinical laboratory and subsequently is considered to be the most common cause of aspergillosis. Other *Aspergillus* species appear to be less pathogenic but can occasionally cause human illness, most often in immunocompromised individuals. *Aspergillus flavus* is not a frequent cause of aspergillosis but is medically important because of its production of powerful carcinogens called aflatoxins. These mycotoxins are produced as the organism grows in foods such as peanuts and grains. Evidence points to an association between ingestion of foods contaminated with *A. flavus* and hepatocarcinoma. For this reason the consumption of bread or other foods with spots of mould is not considered to be a safe practice.

Diagnosis of Aspergillosis by Direct Examination.

Potassium hydroxide (KOH), a cellular clearing agent, and the Gram stain can reveal the presence of fungal elements associated with aspergilli. When the KOH preparation is examined, the organic material, in clinical specimens, clears to reveal the refractile cell wall of the fungal elements. When a properly performed Gram-stained preparation of respiratory secretions is examined the fungal elements will be seen to be gram positive whereas mucus and host tissues appear pink. Tissue sections can be sent for cytological examination, where various stains such as the periodic acid-Schiff (PAS), Gomori methenamine silver (GMS), hematoxylin and eosin (H & E) stains, and calcofluor white can demonstrate the presence of fungal elements in the tissues. Septate hyphae, 2.5–8.0 µm in diameter, with parallel walls and exhibiting dichotomous branching at 45° angles are characteristic of mycelial elements of aspergilli in tissue. Dichotomous branches are those that divide into two branches from the main branch. See Table 29-4 ✪ for a brief summary of the diagnosis of opportunistic fungal infections.

Diagnosis of Aspergillosis Using Fungus Cultures.

There are many different types of media that have been formulated to grow fungi. When cultured on a medium such as sabouraud dextrose or potato dextrose agar, aspergilli grow rapidly, requiring 2–6 days to form mature colonies. At first the surface color of the colony is white and as colonies mature the color may be yellowish green, dark green, greenish blue, blue-gray, tan, or brown to black depending on the species. Surface texture is usually velvety or cottony. The reverse (underside of the colony) usually remains white or lightly colored. Figure 29-1 demonstrates the typical colony of *Aspergillus fumigatus*.

Microscopic examination of material from a slide culture will allow one to observe the arrangement of specific fungal elements. Slide cultures of aspergilli should reveal the presence of hyaline, septate hyphae, with conidiophores that may be smooth or rough, arising from the base, which is called a "foot cell." The conidiophore terminates in a swollen round or vase-shaped structure referred to as a **vesicle.** Flask- or bottle-shaped phialides may attach directly to the vesicle. This is known as **uniserate.** The phialides may be supported by a secondary structure called the **metulae** to become the **biserate** form. It is called biserate because there are two structures supporting the conidia rather than one in the uniserate. Compare it to the structure of the bones of the fingers; the proximal phalanx, closest to the hand, would be the metulae and the middle phalanx above it would be the phialide. The phialides and/or metulae may cover the entire vesicle or varying degrees of it. Phialides produce chains of round conidia, 2–6 µm in diameter, which may be smooth or rough depending on the species (Figure 29-2). The terms "rough" or "echinulate" refer to fungal structures that are covered with tiny pointed spines.

✪ TABLE 29-3

The Four Major Syndromes of Aspergillosis

Syndrome	Underlying Cause
Allergic bronchopulmonary aspergillosis	Asthma accompanied by an allergic reaction to inhaled conidia
Saprophytic bronchopulmonary aspergillosis	Pre-existing damage to lung architecture through conditions such as recurrent bacterial infections, silicosis, carcinoma, sarcoidosis, and tuberculosis
Aspergillomas or fungal balls (a type of saprophytic bronchopulmonary aspergillosis)	Preexisting cavitary lesions as seen in tuberculosis or healed abscesses
Invasive pulmonary aspergillosis	Often associated with immunocompromised individuals (AIDS, cancer, and transplant patients)

 REAL WORLD TIP

Aspergillus fumigatus can be distinguished from the other *Aspergillus* spp. by its bluish-green colony and single row of phialides (uniserate) that cover the upper two-thirds of the vesicle.

⊛ TABLE 29-4

Diagnosis of Opportunistic Fungal Infections

Common Etiological Agents	Specimen Types	Microscopic Examination	
		Cytological Examination	Slide Cultures
Aspergillosis: *Aspergillus fumigatus* *A. flavus* *A. niger*	Sputum, tracheal aspirates, bronchial brushing, tissue, biopsy material, pus	Hyaline, septate hyphae, 2.5–8.0 µm in diameter, with parallel walls and dichotomous branching	Hyaline, septate hyphae with smooth or rough conidiophores, foot cells, vesicles, phialides produce chains of round conidia, 2–6 µm in diameter
Mucormycosis: *Absidia* species *Mucor* species *Rhizopus* species	Respiratory secretions, necrotic tissue, biopsy materials, skin scrapings, drainage from lesions	Broad (6–25 µm in diameter), hyaline, aseptate hyphae, branching is rarely seen	Long sporangiphores connected by stolons, columella, large, round sporangia with sporangiospores, rhizoids dependent upon species
Mycotic keratitis: *Fusarium* species *Aspergillus* species *Acremonium* species *Paecilomyces* species *Scopulariopsis* species *Bipolaris* species *Curvularia* species	Corneal scrapings or biopsy, exudates and swabs are not adequate because fungi are located within the tissue	Hyaline, septate hyphae if agent is a hyaline mould or darkly pigmented, septate hyphae if agent is a dematiaceous (black) mould	Depends on the etiological agent
Mycotic otitis: *A. niger* *A. fumigatus* *Penicillium* species *Scopulariopsis* species *Candida* species	Ear swab to collect discharge	Hyaline fungal elements if agent is a filamentous mould or blastoconidia and pseudohyphae in cases of candidiasis	Depends on the etiological agent

 REAL WORLD TIP

Aspergillus niger produces a colony that changes from white to yellow and eventually turns a salt and pepper black. The entire vesicle is covered by metulae and phialides (biserate) in a sunburst effect.

 Checkpoint! 29–4 (Chapter Objectives 4 and 9)

Which characteristic microscopic morphotype is seen in the tissues of individuals suffering from invasive aspergillosis?

A. *Dichotomous branching*
B. *Branching sporangiophores*
C. *Aseptate hyphae*
D. *Darkly pigmented hyphae*

Zygomycosis

Fungi in the class Zygomycetes have also been implicated as etiological agents of human disease. This includes the genera: *Rhizopus, Mucor, Rhizomucor,* and *Absidia.* The term zygomycosis includes the clinical condition known as mucormycosis. Predisposing factors include immunosuppression, lymphoma, leukemia, malnourishment, metabolic disorders, and trauma.

Mucormycosis

Mucormycosis refers to any disease caused by *Rhizopus, Mucor,* and rarely *Absidia* species. The normal habitat for these fungal species is soil and decaying matter. In the human host they are capable of causing several disease states including rhinocerebral, pulmonary, gastrointestinal, subcutaneous, and disseminated disease. Most infections follow inhalation of spores and as a consequence nasal sinuses and the lungs are the most common sites of initial infection.

Rhinocerebral mucormycosis is the clinical form most frequently encountered and *Rhizopus arrhizus,* an opportunist, is the major etiological agent. Predisposing or risk factors that enhance susceptibility to disease include uncontrolled acute diabetes mellitus, hyperglycemia, metabolic ketoacidosis (as a result of untreated diabetes), and leukopenia. The infection begins in the turbinates and nasal sinuses and has a tendency to spread into the orbit of the eye (Figure 29-3), the palate, and eventually into the brain where cranial nerves are destroyed. If left untreated this disease is rapidly progressive and may end with coma and death occurring in less than one week's time.

The fungus exhibits a preference for blood vessels. Vascular invasion leads to thrombosis (blood clots), infarction (occlusion of the blood vessel), and tissue necrosis. Early symptoms include headache, nasal congestion and pain, and a serous, black, or blood-tinged nasal discharge. As the infection progresses, deeper tissues are invaded. Periorbital swelling and pain with erosion and perforation of the nasal septum and palate then follow. Successful treatment involves correction of the ketoacidosis induced by uncontrolled diabetes, surgical removal of infected tissue, and administration of amphotericin B.

Diagnosis of Mucormycosis by Direct Examination.

The examination of sputum, excised necrotic tissue, biopsy material, and skin scrapings, which reveals the presence of fungal elements in clinical specimens, provides important additional evidence to support the diagnosis of mucormycosis. KOH and calcofluor white preparations, PAS, H & E, and methenamine silver stains can be used to demonstrate aseptate hyphal elements. Characteristically the hyphae are broad (6–25 μm), hyaline, and irregular in shape and diameter with right-angled branching (see Table 29-4). They may appear as wide ribbons and tend to fold onto themselves or break easily as seen in Figures 14-7 and 14-16.

> **REAL WORLD TIP**
>
> Because the organisms that cause mucormycosis are invasive, often tissue is submitted for culture. The tissue should not be homogenized using a tissue grinder because it destroys the hyphae. The tissue should be minced and plated.

Diagnosis of Mucormycosis Using Fungal Cultures.

Refrigeration of clinical specimens and maceration of tissues (cutting and grinding in preparation for plating) may decrease viability of the organism. Inoculation of fungal media that does not contain cyclohexamide is recommended for culturing the Zygomycetes. These organisms grow rapidly; mature colonies develop within 1 to 4 days when media is incubated at 30°C.

Observation of colonial morphology reveals white, cottony colonies that turn gray as the colony matures. Differentiation of *Rhizopus*, *Absidia*, and *Mucor* species is accomplished by microscopic examination of a tease mount or slide culture stained with lactophenol cotton blue. *Rhizopus* species typically have unbranched sporangiophores, similar to a flower stem and occurring singly or in clusters, with rhizoids at the base. The sporangium, similar to a balloon, is round and darkly pigmented, containing numerous lemon-shaped sporangiospores (Figure 29-4 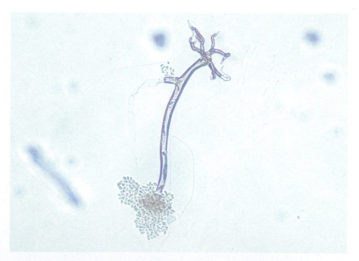). *Absidia* species typically have branching sporangiophores arising from stolons and are located between the rhizoids rather than directly on them. The

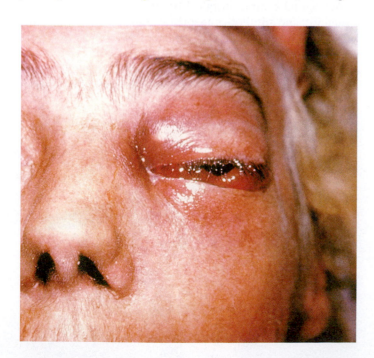

FIGURE 29-3 Mucormycosis typically involves the nasal sinuses and eyes. The fungi can invade tissues to reach the brain. *Public Health Image Library (PHIL)/CDC/Dr. Thomas F. Sellers and Emory University*

FIGURE 29-4 *Rhizopus* species. The root-like rhizoids as well as the aseptate hyphae are easily seen. The sporangium has released the sporagiospores.

sporangium is usually pear-shaped and contains numerous round to oval sporangiospores. *Mucor* species typically have branching sporangiophores and lack rhizoids. The sporangium is round and filled with round to oval sporangiospores as seen in Figure 14-16.

 REAL WORLD TIP

The rhizoids of *Absidia* spp. are difficult to see microscopically. A dissecting microscope may be required to see them on organisms growing on agar (Larone, 1995).

MYCOTIC KERATITIS

Many different species of fungus have been associated with mycotic keratitis (fungal invasion of the corneal epithelium) but in the United States the most common cause appears to be *Fusarium solani* (Figure 29-5 ■). *Fusarium* species are often noted for pink or lilac colonies as seen in Figure 14-12. The color varies with the species. *Fusarium* produces hyaline, septate hyphae with large curved canoe- or banana-shaped multicellular macroconidia at the end of right angle phialides. The organism can also produce clusters of single-celled microconidia on short phialides.

 REAL WORLD TIP

Acremonium species can resemble *Fusarium* species macroscopically. The key to differentiation is the presence of the large curved macroconidia, microscopically, in *Fusarium* species. *Acremonium* species produces septate hyphae with fine and narrow phialides which form at 90-degree angles. Oval conidia form in clusters at the tip of the phialide.

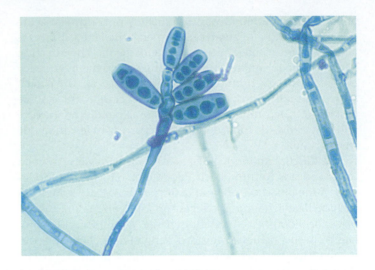

■ **FIGURE 29-6** *Bipolaris* species. The macroconidia are large, thick-walled and multicellular. They create slight bends in the conidiophore where they attach.

Other genera include hyaline saprobes, organisms that derive their nutrition from non-living materials, such as *Aspergillus*, *Acremonium*, *Pseudallescheria boydii* (Figure 14-14), *Candida albicans*, and dematiaceous fungi such as *Bipolaris* (Figure 29-6 ■), *Curvularia* (Figure 29-7 ■), and *Cladosporium* species. *Blastomyces dermatitidis* and *Cryptococcus neoformans* have been isolated from eye cultures but their presence more likely occurs by dissemination through hematogenous spread.

Accidental trauma, surgical trauma, ocular topical corticosteroids, and antibiotics are predisposing factors for mycotic keratitis. Farmers, fruit pickers, gardeners, and others who work outside are at greatest risk of minor injury to the eye through airborne debris, stalks, and sticks. Saprophytic fungi that normally inhabit soil, plants, and decaying organic matter con-

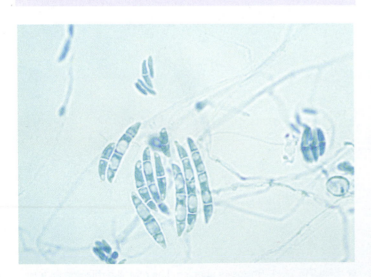

■ **FIGURE 29-5** *Fusarium solani.* Note the long, curved multicellular macroconidia. They resemble canoes.

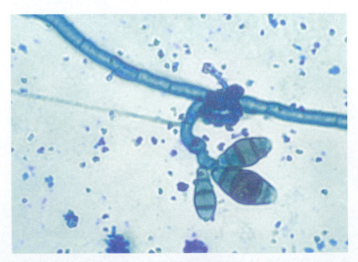

■ **FIGURE 29-7** *Curvularia* species. The macroconidia are multicelluar and thick-walled. Note the center cell is larger than the others.

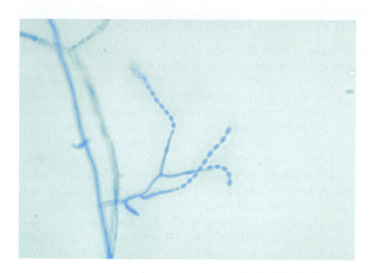

■ FIGURE 29-8 *Paecilomyces* species. The phialides are long and slender and create chains of oval conidia.

taminate the site of the ocular abrasion and invade the corneal stroma.

Paecilomyces lilacinus (Figure 29-8 ■) has been reported to cause keratitis, corneal ulcers, and endophthalmitis. This pink to lilac colony produces septate, hyaline hyphae with branching conidiophores possessing long, slender, tapering phialides. The conidia are often oval shaped and arranged in chains.

There are reports that *Scopulariopsis brevicaulis* (Figure 29-9 ■), another soil saprophyte, has been an agent of onychomycosis (infection of the nail), otomycosis, and keratitis. The colony can be tan with a brown center on its underside or reverse. The septate, hyaline hyphae produce a structure very similar to *Pencillium* species. The structure resembles a hand with the

fingers spread apart. The conidiophores are often spiked, like a cockle burr, and arranged in a single row.

The initial discomfort associated with a foreign object on the surface of the eye is followed by pain that intensifies over the next several days. Redness of the eye is readily apparent and examination by the clinician will reveal the corneal ulcer surrounded by a white, gray, or yellowish corneal infiltrate. Satellite lesions and hypopyon (a collection of pus in the anterior chamber of the eye) will be evident as the infection progresses. Without treatment, loss of the eye is inevitable.

It is important that histological evidence (the presence of fungal elements, such as hyphae, in corneal tissue) support cultural evidence of fungal invasion. A KOH preparation, Giemsa stain, or Gram stain of a portion of the corneal scrapings should be examined to demonstrate the presence of pseudohyphae (*Candida albicans*) or hyphal elements. The remaining portion should be cultured on blood agar medium and fungal media containing chloramphenicol, to inhibit bacterial growth, but should not contain cyclohexamide, which can inhibit the growth of some saprophytic fungi.

MYCOTIC OTITIS

Saprophytic fungi may invade the outer ear, leading to another opportunistic infection, mycotic otitis. *Aspergillus niger*, *Aspergillus fumigatus*, *Candida* species, and *Penicillium* species (Figure 29-10 ■) are the fungi that are most commonly associated with this condition. Symptoms such as hearing loss, itching, pain, and discharge from the external ear canal are common manifestations. Fungal growth may even be observed within the ear canal (see Table 29-4). Cleaning the ears and application of topical ointments can lead to resolution of the infection.

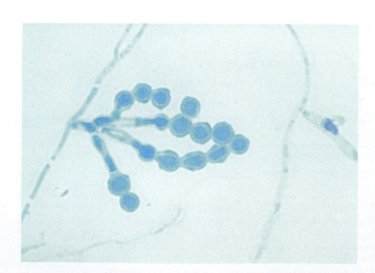

■ FIGURE 29-9 *Scopulariopsis* species. The large lemon-shaped conidia have a rough outer wall.

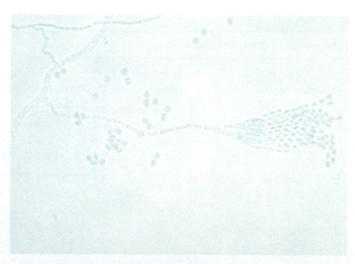

■ FIGURE 29-10 *Penicillium* species. The brush-like appearance is characteristic. The metulae extend from the conidiophore. Next are the phialides that contain chains of conidia.

Checkpoint! 29–5
(Chapter Objectives 5, 7, and 9)

Which of the following circumstances provides substantial support for a diagnosis of mycotic keratitis caused by the saprophytic fungus, Fusarium solani?

A. *Presence of pus and other signs of inflammation around the affected eye*

B. *Presence of septate, hyaline hyphae within tissues obtained from corneal scrapings*

C. *Presence of a velvety, bluish-green-colored mould colony growing on the blood agar plate only*

D. *Numerous pus cells with intracellular gram-negative diplococci on the Gram stain of inflammatory material*

▶ SUPERFICIAL MYCOSES

Superficial mycoses involve the outermost layers of skin and hair, which are composed of a protein called keratin. These infections of the skin are confined to the outermost layer, the stratum corneum, sparing the deeper layers of tissue such as the dermis and subcutaneous tissues. Infections involving the hair are characterized by masses of hyphae surrounding the hair shaft. The hair follicles are usually not invaded. The overwhelming majority of infections are not serious but skin infections may lead to discoloration, so treatment is primarily for cosmetic purposes. In the following sections the different superficial mycoses are discussed, including predisposing factors, signs and symptoms, treatment, etiological agents, and methods employed in diagnosis of these infections. Table 29-5✪ summarizes diagnosis of the superficial fungi.

PITYRIASIS (TINEA) VERSICOLOR

Pityriasis or tinea versicolor is a superficial skin infection that is chronic in nature. The highest incidence of infection occurs in young adults and most often in tropical countries. High ambient temperatures, hyperhidrosis (excessive sweating), high humidity, corticosteroid therapy, and malnutrition are thought to be contributing factors to the disease process. The upper back, shoulders, upper arms, chest, and abdomen are the areas most commonly infected. The lesions are described as hyperpigmented or hypopigmented, scaly, macular lesions with a mild itching in approximately one-third of affected individuals. In light-skinned individuals the hyperpigmented lesions have a reddish or brownish discoloration while dark-skinned individuals have hypopigmented lesions that may be confused with vitiligo, a benign skin disease of unknown origin characterized by areas of depigmented skin. Treatment of pityriasis versicolor includes topical therapy with selenium sulfide, tolnaftate, or imidazole (ketaconazole) creams.

The etiological agent of pityriasis versicolor is *Malassezia furfur*. Unlike many other fungi, *M. furfur* has not been recovered as a saprophyte in nature nor from animal species. This organism is part of the normal flora of skin in healthy individuals and has been recovered from the scalp and trunk of more than 90% of individuals in one study, who showed no evidence of disease. Because of this organism's association with epithelial surfaces, additional ailments may be caused by *M. furfur,* including folliculitis and sepsis associated with the use of intravascular catheters to deliver lipids to premature infants, neonates, and adults. In cases of *Malassezia furfur* sepsis, removal of the catheter results in resolution of the illness.

✪ TABLE 29-5

Diagnosis of Superficial Infections

Etiological Agents	Specimen Types	Microscopic Examination	
		Cytological Examination	Slide Cultures
Pityriasis versicolor: *Malassezia furfur*	Skin scrapings	"Spaghetti and meatballs": round or oval yeast-like cells with elongate hyphal elements among epithelial cells	Round to oval yeast-like cells with small collarettes and single buds; hyphal elements are usually absent
Superficial phaeohyphomycosis: *Hortaea* (previously known as *Phaeoannellomyces*) *werneckii*	Skin scrapings	Brown, closely septate, branching hyphae up to 5 μm in diameter and elongated budding cells	Brown, septate, branching hyphae and one- or two-celled, dark, elongated, budding yeast-like cells with a double septum (annellides)
White piedra: *Trichosporon beigelii* (also known as *T. cutaneum*)	Infected hairs	Light-colored, segmented hyphae, 2–4 μm in diameter with round to rectangular arthroconidia and blastoconidia	Septate hyphae and arthroconidia, predominate but blastoconidia and psuedohyphae may also be seen
Black piedra: *Piedraia hortae*	Infected hairs	Dark brown, septate hyphae, arthroconidia, and numerous asci containing two to eight spindle-shaped ascospores within cavities	Darkly pigmented, thick-walled, septate hyphae and intercalary chlamydoconidia

Diagnosis of Pityriasis Versicolor by Direct Examination

Diagnosis can be accomplished through the use of KOH as a clearing agent, PAS, and GMS stains of skin scrapings. The microscopic morphology seen in stained skin scrapings has been described as "spaghetti and meatballs." Clusters of single budding, round to bottle-shaped yeast cells (3–7 µm in diameter), and short, unbranched, hyaline hyphal elements are characteristic of infected areas of skin (Figures 14-3 and 29-11 ■).

Diagnosis of Pityriasis Versicolor by Fungus Cultures

Skin scrapings should be plated on sabouraud agar with or without antibiotics. *M. furfur* is lipophilic, requiring a source of lipid for growth. Long-chain fatty acids, essential for growth of the organism, must be provided as part of the growth medium. Successful culturing can be accomplished by the addition of a drop of sterile mineral or olive oil to the skin scrapings and spreading the mixture over the surface of the solid medium. Smooth, cream-colored yeast-like colonies can be observed in a matter of days when incubated at 30–37°C. Little or no growth occurs at 25°C. With age the colonies become dull in appearance and develop a tan to brownish color. Microscopic examination reveals round-to-oval yeastlike cells with small, broad, and square collarettes, where the single buds form. Hyphal elements are usually absent in culture.

SUPERFICIAL PHAEOHYPHOMYCOSIS OR TINEA NIGRA

Superficial phaeohyphomycosis means a brown hyphae fungal infection. It is a chronic superficial skin infection that is more prevalent in young people (less than 20 years of age) and occurs primarily in tropical countries including Africa, Asia, and Central and South America. It is occasionally seen in the United States and Europe. A single, brown to black, irregularly shaped spot with a sharply distinct border is typically seen. Occasionally infected persons may experience slight itching. The lesion is rarely scaly. Most lesions occur on the palmar surface of the hands or the plantar surface of the feet and occasionally on the neck or chest. Factors that predispose individuals to tinea nigra have not been clearly defined and the route of transmission is unknown, although similar fungi are found in soil and decaying vegetation. The etiological agent of superficial phaeohyphomycosis is *Hortaea* (previously known as *Phaeoannellomyces*) *werneckii,* one of the dematiaceous or black fungi.

Effective treatment involves the administration of oral griseofulvin or topical application of amphotericin B, tolnaftate, or azoles such as miconazole and ketaconazole.

Diagnosis of Superficial Phaeohyphomycosis by Direct Examination

Examination of skin scrapings using 10–20% KOH and gentle heat will differentiate the lesions from melanoma. The presence of brown, septate, branching hyphae up to 5 µm in diameter and elongated budding cells among the epithelial cells are characteristic of the infection.

Diagnosis of Superficial Phaeohyphomycosis by Fungus Culture

On sabouraud dextrose agar, gray-colored, shiny, moist, yeastlike colonies are seen within 1 week. As the colony of *H. wernickii* ages it quickly becomes olive black to black. Microscopic examination of growth reveals the presence of brown, septate, branching hyphae and one- or two-celled, dark, elongated, budding yeast-like conidia with a distinct division within the cell (Figure 29-12 ■).

WHITE PIEDRA

White piedra is a fungal infection that is uncommon in temperate regions and occurs primarily in the tropics. The nature of the route of transmission and predisposing factors is still in question. This condition involves the hair shaft only so neither hair follicles nor skin are affected. The axilla, beard, mustache, scalp, and genital area are the areas most commonly infected. Examination of infected hairs reveals the presence of white to tan nodules that adhere loosely to the hair shaft and are easily stripped off. Mycelia grow inward, penetrating beneath the hair cuticle, and may weaken the cuticle to the point hair shafts may break off above the nodule. This superficial infection, which is caused by *Trichosporon beigelii* (also known as *Trichosporon cutaneum*), a yeast-like organism, must be differentiated from the nits (eggs) of lice. White piedra may be treated by cutting or shaving infected hair close to the scalp and observing practices of good hygiene.

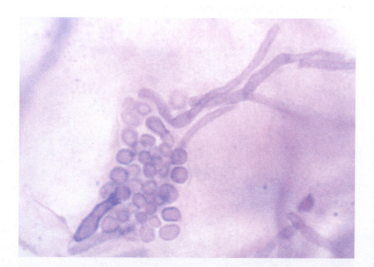

■ **FIGURE 29-11** *Malassezia furfur,* the etiological agent of pityriasis versicolor, seen in a skin scraping stained with the periodic acid-Schiff (PAS) stain. Note the hyphae and budding yeasts, resulting in the characteristic spaghetti and meatballs appearance.

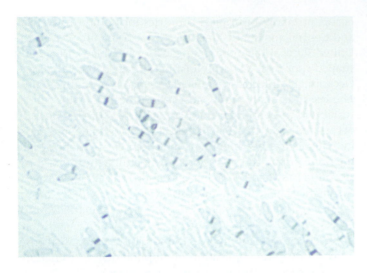

■ FIGURE 29-12 *Hortaea* (previously known as *Phaeoannello-myces*) *werneckii*, the etiological agent of superficial phaeohy-phomycosis or tinea nigra, from a fungus culture grown on potato dextrose agar. The long yeast cells have a distinct division within each.

 REAL WORLD TIP

The taxonomy of *Trichosporin* spp. has been revised based on molecular methods. What was thought to be *T. beigelii* is now *T. cutaneum*. Other new species include *T. asteroides*, *T. ovoides*, *T. ashaii*, *T. inkin*, and *T. mucoides*. *T. ovoides*, rather than *T. beigelii*, affects the scalp while *T. inkin* affects the genital area. It will take time for textbooks to adopt this new classification. Because it is still not fully accepted across the mycology community, this textbook has chosen to use the traditional taxonomy (Patterson and McGinnis, 2009).

Diagnosis of White Piedra by Direct Examination

Examination of infected hairs reveals the presence of white to tan nodules that adhere loosely to the hair shaft. A KOH preparation of the hair or lactophenol cotton blue solution will reveal the nodule is composed of light colored, segmented hyphae, 2–4 μm in diameter. The crushed nodules show round to rectangular arthroconidia and blastoconidia surrounding the hair shaft (Table 29-5).

Diagnosis of White Piedra by Fungus Culture

When cultured on sabouraud dextrose agar with chloramphenicol but without cycloheximide or cornmeal agar with Tween 80 agar incubated at 25°C, moist, white, yeast-like colonies with a butyrous (creamy) consistency are seen with *T. beigelii*. As the colonies mature they darken to a yellowish, gray color and tend to be heaped, wrinkled, and appear to be

drier. Microscopic examination through the bottom of the agar plate reveals the presence of septate hyphae, which are easily fragmented into arthroconidia. Hyphae and rectangular arthroconidia predominate, but single or short-chained blastoconidia and psuedohyphae may also be seen.

 REAL WORLD TIP

Geotrichum spp. is also recognized by its production of arthroconidia. *T. beigelii* can be differentiated by its production of blastoconidia and hyphae in addition to arthroconidia.

BLACK PIEDRA

Black piedra, an infection of the hair shaft, occurs primarily in tropical countries such as Africa, eastern Asia, and South America. The causative agent is a dematiaceous (black) fungus, *Piedraia hortae*, which usually infects only the hairs of the scalp. Exposure to stagnant and river water and frequent wetting of the hair may be risk factors associated with black piedra. Hard, black nodules that adhere tightly to the hair shaft and are not easily dislodged are characteristic for black piedra (Figure 29-13 ■). The infected hair may become fragile and break.

Diagnosis of Black Piedra by Direct Examination

The hard, black nodule of *P. hortae* is composed of a cemented mass of fungal cells including dark brown hyphae and arthroconidia. Because the sexual state of the fungus is involved in the infection, numerous asci, sac-like structures, containing two to eight spindle-shaped or fusiform ascospores, 5–8 μm

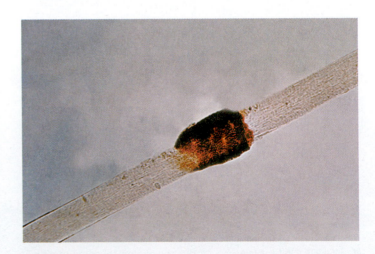

■ FIGURE 29-13 The hard, black nodule of *P. hortae* is composed of a cemented mass of dark brown hyphae and arthroconidia.
Public Health Image Library (PHIL)/CDC and Dr. Lucille K. George

by 35–55 μm, are seen within cavities when a KOH preparation of infected hair is made. The presence of these structures is diagnostic but cultures may also be attempted.

Diagnosis of Black Piedra by Fungus Culture

On Sabouraud dextrose agar with chloramphenicol the asexual stage is most commonly seen. Examination of the slowly growing, dark greenish, brown to black, velvety colonies reveal dark pigmentation. *P. hortae* displays thick-walled, septate hyphae with intercalary chlamydoconidia located within the hyphae rather than at the end (Figure 29-14 ■). Treatment is through cutting or shaving the infected hairs and proper hygiene is required to avoid reinfection.

▶ DERMATOPHYTOSIS

The term "dermatophytosis" describes mild to severe diseases of the keratinized layers of the skin, hair, and nails, but spares the subcutaneous tissues. Infection is not confined to the stratum corneum and as a result the deeper vascularized layers of skin, such as the dermis, are involved. Invasion of tissue with a blood supply allows the presence of the invading organisms to be recognized by the immune system, and a cellular immune response is elicited. Pain and itching are often symptoms of dermatophytosis.

Over the years dermatophytosis has also been known as ringworm or tinea (Latin, *worm*) because of the characteristic appearance of the skin lesions, which are ring-like and look like a worm burrowing under the skin (Figure 29-15 ■). The outermost margins, where the infection is active and spreading, are typically red, scaly, raised, and distinct. As the infection spreads across the skin a central area of healing is observed.

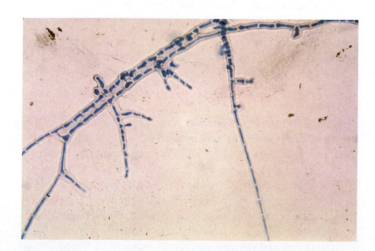

■ **FIGURE 29-14** The hyphae of *Piedra hortae* are septate, dark, and thick-walled. There can be intercalary chlamydoconidia-like cells present.
Public Health Image Library (PHIL)/CDC and Dr. Lucille K. George

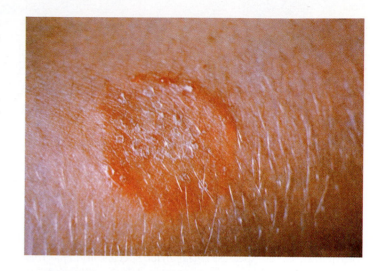

■ **FIGURE 29-15** Ringworm on the arm, or tinea corporis, due to *Trichophyton mentagrophytes*.
Public Health Image Library (PHIL)/CDC and Dr. Lucille K. George

Clinical manifestations are commonly named according to the body site affected:

- tinea barbae refers to infection of the beard and moustache
  - most commonly caused by *Trichophyton verrucosum*, *T. mentagrophytes*, and *Microsporum canis*
- tinea capitis is infection of the scalp, eyebrows, and eyelashes. Lesions may be confined to discrete areas but with time may involve the entire scalp. Infected hairs may break off, creating areas of hair loss characterized by black dots, which are the remnants of the hair shafts.
  - most commonly caused by *T. tonsurans*, *T. mentagrophytes*, *M. audouinii*, and *M. canis*
- tinea coporis refers to infection of areas of the body, such as the trunk, where body hair is more sparse
  - usually caused by *T. rubrum*, *T. mentagrophytes*, *T. tonsurans*, *M. canis*, and *Epidermophyton floccosum*
- tinea cruris is commonly referred to as "jock itch," and involves infection of the groin or perineal region
  - most frequently caused by *T. rubrum*, *T. mentagrophytes*, and *E. floccosum*
- tinea manuum involves infection of the palms of the hands and between the fingers
  - associated with *T. rubrum*
- tinea pedis, or athlete's foot refers to infection of the plantar surfaces of the feet and the toe webs
  - commonly caused by *T. mentagrophytes*, *T. rubrum*, and *E. floccosum*
- tinea unguium refers to onychomycosis or infection of the nails
  - usually caused by *T. rubrum*, *T. interdigitale*, and *E. floccosum*

■ tinea favosa or favus refers to infected hair that has hyphal elements surrounding the base of the hair follicle at the scalp line with hyphal elements penetrating the hair shaft

• caused by *T. schoenleinii*

■ tinea imbricate is an unusual form of tinea corporis characterized by concentric rings of scaling spreading out in a centrifugal pattern (somewhat like a bull's-eye)

• caused by *T. concentricum*

ETIOLOGICAL AGENTS OF DERMATOPHYTOSIS

Approximately 20 species of dermatophytes are responsible for human disease. Three genera are known by their asexual forms: *Microsporum* species, *Trichophyton* species, and *Epidermophyton* species. *Microsporum* species attack the skin and hair but not the nails. *Epidermophyton floccosum* attacks the skin and nails but not the hair. *Trichophyton* species attack the skin, hair, and nails.

Dermatophytes are also classified according to their natural habitat and host preferences. Humans are the primary or only reservoirs for the anthropophilic (Greek, *anthropos,* human + *philein,* to love) dermatophytes and are spread by combs, brushes, hats, clothing, furniture, locker rooms, and bathing facilities. Anthropophilic species include:

Microsporum audouinii
Trichophyton concentricum
T. rubrum
T. interdigitale
T. tonsurans
T. violaceum
T. shoenleinii
Epidermophyton floccosum

Domestic and wild animals are the primary reservoirs for the zoophilic (Greek, *zoon,* animal + *philein,* to love) dermatophytes. Transmission occurs through direct contact with infected animals or from troughs and stalls used by infected animals. Zoophilic species include:

Microsporum canis (cats and dogs)
T. mentagrophytes (rodents, cats, dogs, cattle, and sheep)
T. verrucosum (cattle and horses)

Geophilic (Greek, *ge,* earth + *philein,* to love) dermatophytes are species that are native to the soil and while direct contact with the soil can result in transmission, human infection more likely orginates from infected animals. Geophilic species, which are isolated from the soil, include:

Microsporum gypseum
M. nanum (isolated from soil in pig yards and in rare cases transmitted to humans from pigs)
M. fulvum
T. ajelloi
T. terrestre

Anthropophilic dermatophytes, which have adapted to parasitizing humans, cause chronic infections that range from mild to severe and are often difficult to treat. Zoophilic and geophilic species, which are not native to humans, cause acute diseases with pain and itching and are usually self-limiting.

Topical therapy, using azole antifungals, is often applied to the affected areas to treat many cases of ringworm. Griseofulvin taken orally is safe and effective in treating ringworm systemically.

Diagnosis of Dermatophytosis by Direct Examination

To collect skin and nail specimens the area should first be cleansed with 70% alcohol. Material may then be collected using a sterile scalpel to gently and carefully scrape the leading edge of the skin lesion or the nail. Scrapings may be collected in a sterile petri dish and transported to the laboratory. In the laboratory skin scrapings may be used to inoculate fungal media and a portion placed on a slide to which 10–20% KOH is added and gently heated. When the host cells have been cleared, the presence of dermatophytic invasion is seen as long, branching, thick-walled, hyphal elements. Older hyphae may produce arthroconidia.

Some dermatophytic infections of the hair can be identified using a Wood's lamp. Species such as *M. audouinii, M. canis,* and *T. schoenleinii* fluoresce blue-green or green-yellow under ultraviolet light and this method has been used in the past to screen large numbers of individuals for signs of infection.

ⓔ REAL WORLD TIP

■ *T. tonsurans* is the most frequent causative agent of tinea capitis, but it does not fluoresce under a Wood's lamp.

■ *Malassezia furfur,* the causative agent of tinea (pityriasis) versicolor can also fluoresce. It will appear yellow to white but is found in skin and not hair.

Some hair infections produce characteristic patterns of hair invasion. These patterns may be beneficial in narrowing down the etiological agents. One pattern is referred to as ectothrix hair invasion and is characterized by a sheath of hyphae and arthroconidia surrounding the hair shaft. Hyphae penetrate the hair shaft destroying the cuticle. As the hyphae age, they are converted into arthroconidia 2–8 µm in diameter. Although fungal invasion begins inside the shaft, arthroconidia occur as masses located on the surface or outside of the shafts of infected hairs. Species that produce ectothrix hair invasion include *M. audouinii, M. canis, M. gypseum* (sparse chains inside and outside of the hair shaft), *T. mentagrophytes,* and *T. verrucosum.*

Endothrix hair invasion is characterized by hyphae that grow down along the hair shaft and penetrate the inside of the hair. Arthroconidia, 5–8 μm in diameter, accumulate within the hair shaft. Species capable of endothrix hair invasion include *T. tonsurans*, the most common cause of tinea capitis in the United States, *T. violaceum*, and, in rare cases, *T. rubrum*.

In favic hair invasion, which is caused by *T. schoenleinii*, hyphae surround the hair shaft near the opening of the hair follicle and penetrate the hair shaft, creating tunnels within the strands. These tunnels run parallel to the long axis of the hair. Fat droplets may be seen within the tunnels but arthroconidia are not produced.

Diagnosis of Dermatophytosis Using Fungus Cultures

Because many different dermatophyte species produce a similar appearance in clinical specimens such as skin and hair, identification using fungal cultures is required. Hair, skin, and nail scrapings should be cultured on media such as sabouraud with chloramphenicol and cycloheximide to inhibit normal bacterial flora, which could overgrow dermatophytes, making recovery very difficult. Inoculated media should be incubated at 25–30°C for a minimum of 4 weeks. Dermatophyte test medium (DTM) is also used to isolate dermatophytes. They turn the medium red because of production of alkaline by-products. Growth from these media can be removed and placed on a slide containing a drop of lactophenol cotton blue (LPCB), which kills and stains the organism. The mycelium may be teased apart using teasing needles. A coverslip is then placed on top of the growth and the eraser of a pencil can be used to apply gentle pressure before examining with a bright-field microscope. Scan using the low power objective, then use the high power objective to obtain greater detail.

Dermatophytes are capable of producing macroconidia and microconidia. The macroconidia may be smooth or rough (echinulate), multiseptate, and thick or thin walled. They may be clavate (club-shaped), fusiform (spindle-shaped), or cylindrical. Microconidia can be globose (round), clavate, or pyriform (pear-shaped), 2–4 μm in diameter, and attached directly to the hyphae or on short conidiophores.

Identification of Dermatophytes Using Physiological and Biochemical Tests

In addition to macroscopic or colony morphology, physiological and biochemical tests can be used to identify the species in question.

Nutritional tests determine which vitamins and amino acids are required for the different species to grow. Inositol, histidine, and vitamins, such as thiamine (B1) and nicotinic acid or niacin (B3) are added to a basal medium. The amount of growth is graded from 0 (none) to 4+ (excellent). The tube that shows maximum growth is recorded as 4+ and the other tubes are read by comparison. Identifying the vitamins and amino acids that are required as growth factors aids in differentiating

the different dermatophytes, which can produce similar conidia. Basal medium without vitamins or amino acids is used as a control. See Table 29-6✪ for reactions of common dermatophytes on trichophyton agars.

As with other filamentous fungi, microscopic morphology is very important in differentiating the different etiological agents. *T. mentagrophytes* and *T. rubrum*, however, are two species that are morphologically similar, produce similar reactions on Trichophyton nutritional agars, and may be difficult to distinguish based on microscopic examination alone. This is especially true when macroconidia are not produced. For this reason additional biochemical tests such as pigment production, urease production, sorbitol assimilation, and hair perforation (*in vitro*) testing can be used to assist in the differentiation of these two species.

Pigment production is determined by subculturing the test organism to cornmeal agar with 1% dextrose. *T. rubrum* produces a blood red pigment whereas *T. mentagropytes* does not. The urease hydrolysis test is designed to detect the production of urease production. Christensen's urea agar or broth is inoculated with the test organism and incubated at 25–30°C for up to 7 days. *T. rubrum* is negative for urease activity while *T. mentagrophytes* produces urease that leads to the development of a bright pink to purple-red color (positive).

Carbohydrate assimilation tests are designed to demonstrate the ability of an organism to utilize a particular carbohydrate as the sole carbon source under aerobic conditions. *T. rubrum* is able to use sorbitol as the sole source of carbon in a growth medium (positive) whereas *T. mentagrophytes* does not assimilate sorbitol and therefore is unable to grow (no growth = negative).

The *in vitro* hair perforation test demonstrates the ability of an organism to penetrate hair. Hair cultures are set up by adding approximately 20 ml of sterile distilled water to several strands of sterile hair in a petri dish. Three drops of a 10% yeast extract solution are added aseptically and then each culture is inoculated with a test organism. This test system is incubated up to 4 weeks and periodically a strand of hair is extracted aseptically and examined using lactophenol cotton blue. The production of conical or wedge-shaped perforations perpendicular to the long axis of the hair constitutes a positive reaction. *T. rubrum* is negative (no wedge-shaped perforations) whereas *T. mentagrophytes* is positive (Figure 29-16 ■).

℮ REAL WORLD TIP

The blonde hair of a prepubescent child provides the best results for a hair perforation test. The hair should not have any hairspray or coloring on it. It is easier to view the wedge-shaped perforations using light colored hair.

Rice cultures can be used to differentiate isolates of *M. audouinii* and *M. canis* that do not produce macroconidia. To prepare this medium, distilled water is added to polished,

⭐ **TABLE 29-6**

Reactions of Common Dermatophytes on Trichophyton Agars

Species	Casein Basal Agar					NH$_4$NO$_3$ Basal Media	
	#1 Casamino Acids Base Agar (no vitamins)	#2 Inositol	#3 Inositol and Thiamine	#4 Thiamine	#5 Nicotinic Acid (Niacin)	#6 Ammonium Nitrate Base Agar (no vitamins)	#7 Histidine
Trichophyton verrucosum							
84% of strains	0	1+	4+	0	0		
16% of strains	0	0	4+	4+	0		
T. shoenleinii	4+	4+	4+	4+	4+		
T. concentricum							
50% of strains	4+	4+	4+	4+	4+		
50% of strains	2+	2+	4+	4+	2+		
T. tonsurans	1+	1+	4+	4+	1+		
T. mentagrophytes	4+	4+	4+	4+	4+		
T. rubrum	4+	4+	4+	4+	4+	2+	
T. violaceum	1+	1+	4+	4+	1+		
T. equinum	0	0	0	0	4+		
T. magninii	2+					0	4+
Microsporum gallinae	3+					4+	4+

4+, rich abundant growth; 3+, good growth; 2+, fair growth; 1+, poor growth; 0, no growth.

non-fortified rice. The rice should have no added ingredients such as calcium. The mixture, one part rice to three parts water, is sterilized using an autoclave. The rice culture is inoculated with the test organism, incubated at 25–30°C for 2 weeks and examined periodically. *M. audouinii* grows very poorly, pro-ducing a salmon- or peach-colored reverse (underside of the colony) whereas *M. canis* grows well on polished rice and produces a yellow to yellow-brown color (Figure 29-17 ■).

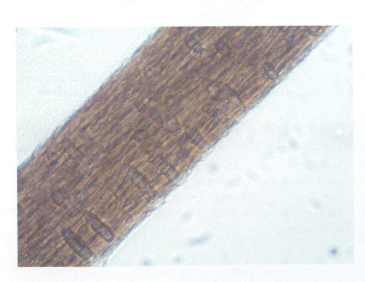

■ **FIGURE 29-16** Positive hair perforation (invasion) test (*T. mentagrophytes*).

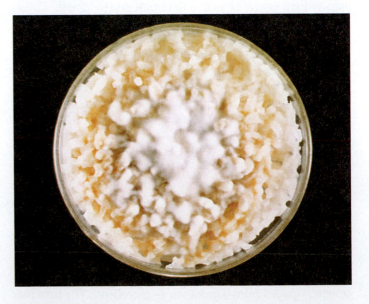

■ **FIGURE 29-17** *Microsporum canis* is able to grow on boiled polished rice grains.
Public Health Image Library (PHIL)/CDC and Dr. Lucille K. George

Microsporum canis grows on polished rice. An easy way to remember this is **cani**ne**s** or dogs will eat anything including rice.

Key identification characteristics for *M. audouinii* include absent or rare conidia, poor growth on rice, and negative in-vitro hair perforation test.

Macroscopic or Colonial Morphology of the Dermatophytes

The dermatophytes require 6 days to as long as 2–3 weeks to produce mature colonies. Their surfaces are usually flat and most produce white to tan colonies, but occasionally pinkish colonies are seen. Textures range from fluffy or velvety to powdery as the colony ages. On some occasions red or yellow pigments, which diffuse into the surrounding medium, are produced. The reverse varies according to species and may be colorless, yellow, red, purplish, or brown.

Microscopic and Macroscopic Morphology of the Dermatophytes

Microsporum audouinii usually does not produce conidia but terminal chlamydoconidia with nipple-like or beak-like projections may be seen. Septate hyphae with pectinate (narrow and slender) structures, similar to the teeth on a hair comb, are characteristic of this species. Occasionally clavate or clubbed microconidia are produced. Macroconidia, while rarely seen, are spiny or rough, long, thick-walled, fusiform, and contain few or no septa (Figure 29-18 ■). They may resemble the macroconidia of *M. canis* but are usually narrower. Its colony is usually beige with a consistency similar to suede. The colony reverse is a light pink-orange with the possibility of a red-brown to red-orange center.

Microsporum canis usually produces numerous rough, thick-walled, spindle-shaped macroconidia, which vary in length from 60 to 125 μm. These macroconidia are multiseptate, containing 3–15 compartments, and taper to a curved knobby end where the spines are more prominent (Figure 29-19 ■). Microconidia, which are usually less abundant, may be clavate or pyriform shaped. Its colony is fluffy and white to cream with a light yellow pigment at the edge. The reverse is often bright yellow.

- To remember the microscopic morphology of *M. canis*, the macroconidia taper like a big (macro) dog's or canine's snout and has whiskers (spines).

- There are two varieties of *M. canis: canis* and *distortum*. *M canis var. distortum* has very distorted macroconidia.

- Key identification characteristics for *M. canis* include spiny, dog-snout macroconidia, good growth on rice, and ability to perforate hair in the in-vitro test.

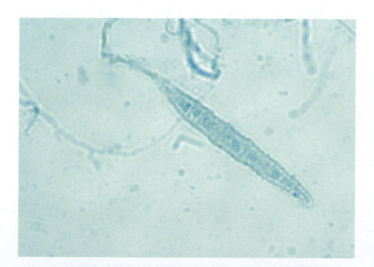

■ **FIGURE 29-18** *Microsporum audouinii.* The often rare macroconidia are long, thick-walled, and spiny or rough.

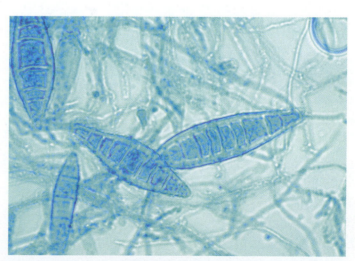

■ **FIGURE 29-19** *Microsporum canis.* The macroconidia are multicelled and thick-walled with a tapered tip.

Microsporum gypseum produces large numbers of macroconidia that are broadly spindle shaped and vary in length from 25 to 60 μm in length. Macroconidia are numerous and may be smooth or rough and contain four to six septa (Figure 29-20 ■). Microconidia are clubbed-shaped and form along the hyphae. Thickness of the conidial walls helps to differentiate *M. gypseum* from *M. canis,* as those of *M. gypseum* tend to be much thinner. Microconidia are sparse and clavate in shape. The colony begins white and turns cinnamon. The colony reverse is beige to red-brown.

Trichophyton mentagrophytes may produce either few (anthropophilic strains) or numerous macroconidia (zoophilic strains). Macroconidia are typically smooth, thin walled, cigar or club shaped, contain three or four septa, and measure 20–50 μm in length (Figure 29-21 ■). Microconidia are tear shaped and tend to occur in grape-like clusters. There may be only a few, or they are produced in large numbers. When grown on sabouraud's agar, the colony is variable but is most often white to cream. A brown, yellow, or dark red color, resembling that of *T. rubrum* may appear on the reverse. This dark red pigment is not produced by *T. mentagrophytes* on potato dextrose agar (PDA) or cornmeal agar (CMA) with 1% dextrose as occurs with *T. rubrum.*

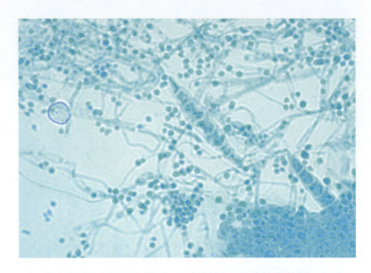

■ **FIGURE 29-21** *Trichophyton mentagrophytes.* The macroconidia are multicelluar and thin-walled. They resemble cigars or clubs. The smaller microconidia often occur in clusters.

Isolates of *Trichophyton rubrum* produce slow-growing colonies, which mature in 14 days. On sabouraud's agar the surface is typically white to buff in color, with a downy to

 REAL WORLD TIP

T. mentagrophytes may develop spiral hyphae shaped like a "corkscrew" that can be observed on slide culture.

Trichophyton rubrum typically produces small tear-shaped microconidia on septate hyphae but rarely macroconidia (Figure 29-22 ■). Macroconidia are produced in strains that are highly sporulating and are long, narrow, thin walled and contain two to eight compartments. They are often described as pencil or cigar shaped. Microconidia may form on the macroconidia.

REAL WORLD TIP

■ To remember the microscopic morphology of *T. rubrum,* the microconidia often form on the hyphae and macroconidia (if present) like small cardinal (rubrum means red) birds sitting on a picket fence (septate hyphae).

■ The in-vitro hair perforation test will differentiate *T. mentagrophytes* and *T. rubrum. T. menta**gro**phytes* tells one its ability to grow into hair.

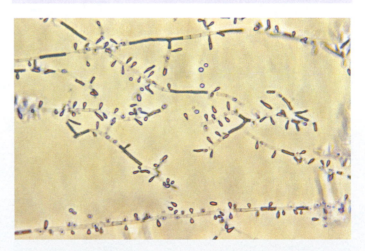

■ **FIGURE 29-22** *Trichophyton rubrum* typically produces small tear-shaped microconidia on septate hyphae but rarely macroconidia.
Public Health Image Library (PHIL)/CDC and Dr. Libero Ajello

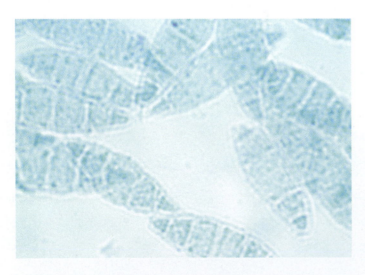

■ **FIGURE 29-20** *Microsporum gypseum.* The macroconidia are multicellular and thin-walled with a rounded tip.

fluffy or granular texture. The reverse is deep red or purplish in color, but may be brown, yellow-orange, or even colorless. Pigment production is enhanced by growing the organism on cornmeal agar with 1% dextrose so the typical deep red pigment is observed.

Trichophyton tonsurans rarely produces macroconidia, but when present they are irregular in form. Microconidia are usually abundant and club to tear shaped. One distinguishing characteristic of *T. tonsurans* is the tendency of some microconidia to enlarge, producing "balloon" forms. Intercalary and terminal chlamydoconidia may form as the colony ages. The colony can be white to light yellow to bright yellow. The reverse is yellow to dark brown.

 REAL WORLD TIP

*T. **tons**urans* has **tons** of microconidia and prefers **th**iamine over the other vitamins.

Epidermophyton floccosum typically produces large (8–15 μm in length), smooth, club-shaped macroconidia with two to six septa. The base where macroconidia are attached to the hyphae is broad (Figure 29-23 ■). The macroconidia can be in characteristic clusters, but they can also appear solitary. Microconidia are not produced. As the organism ages, the macroconidia can transform into chlamydoconidia. Its colony is often olive or khaki colored with a brown reverse. Table 29-7✿ summarizes the identification of the more common dermatophytes.

 REAL WORLD TIP

*E. **floc**cosum* produces only **flock**s or clusters of macroconidia.

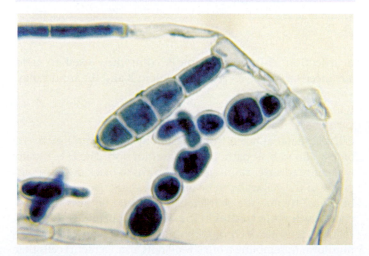

■ **FIGURE 29-23** *Epidermophyton floccosum* typically produces macroconidia in characteristic clusters. Microconidia are not produced.
Public Health Image Library (PHIL)/CDC and Dr. Libero Ajello

 Checkpoint! 29–6 (Chapter Objectives 8 and 11)

Skin scrapings are submitted from a patient suffering from a severe case of tinea pedis. The skin scrapings were plated to fungal media and after 14 days, mature white, powdery colonies grew on the sabouraud agar with chloramphenicol and cycloheximide. A lactophenol cotton blue preparation revealed the presence of septate, hyaline hyphae with numerous, round microconidia in clusters. No macroconidia were seen but spiral hyphae were noted. Because the microscopic morphology from the fungus cultures was not sufficient to identify the organism, biochemical tests were performed. The organism was urease positive, and after 4 weeks incubation at room temperature in a hair culture, wedge-shaped perforations were noted on the in vitro hair perforation test. The test organism was nonpigmented on cornmeal agar supplemented with 1% dextrose. What is the most probable identification of this isolate?

    A. *T. mentagrophytes*
    B. *T. tonsurans*
    C. *T. rubrum*
    D. *Epidermophyton floccosum*

► SUBCUTANEOUS MYCOSES

Subcutaneous mycoses are fungal infections involving the deep layers of skin and subcutaneous tissues resulting in a cellular mediated immune response involving lymphocytes, plasma cells, eosinophils, macrophages, and neutrophils. Numerous species of fungi serve as etiological agents of subcutaneous mycoses but all are primarily plant pathogens or soil saprobes. Because these fungi are not able to penetrate intact skin, they must gain access to host tissues through some type of traumatic inoculation such as a penetrating wound made by a thorn or splinter. Fungal elements within the tissue produce subcutaneous infections that may disseminate to multiple organ systems. Chromoblastomycosis, phaeohyphomycosis, mycetoma, and sporotrichosis are included in the subcutaneous mycoses. Table 29-8✿ summarizes the diagnosis of subcutaneous mycoses.

CHROMOBLASTOMYCOSIS

Chromoblastomycosis follows traumatic implantation of dematiaceous fungi through minor trauma such as small cuts or puncture wounds. This chronic infection develops over many months with slowly progressive lesions that occur primarily on the lower extremities such as the legs and feet. The characteristic lesion begins as a small, scaly papule that gradually increases in size. If untreated, large, raised, verrucous (cauliflower or wart-like) lesions and satellite lesions will develop since spontaneous remission usually does not occur. Hematogenous spread is rare and, unlike mycetoma, there is

✪ TABLE 29-7

Identification of Common Dermatophytes

Organism	Colony	Macroconidia	Microconidia	In-vitro Hair Perforation	Urea Hydrolysis	Other
Microsporum audouinii	Top – beige; Reverse – pink-orange	Rare fusiform, thick walled and spiny (may resemble those of *M. canis*)	Rare and clubbed	Negative	Negative	■ Terminal chlamydoconidia with a nipple or beak ■ Poor or absent growth on rice
M. canis	Top – white to cream with yellow edge; Reverse – bright yellow	Numerous spindle, thick walled and spiny with a knobby curved end	Less abundant and clubbed	Positive	Positive	■ Good growth on rice with a bright yellow pigment
M. gypseum	Top – cinnamon; Reverse – red-brown	Large numbers of broad, spindle shaped with thin walls	Sparse and clubbed	Positive	Positive	■ Poor or absent growth on rice
Trichophyton mentagrophytes	Top – white to cream; Reverse – brown	Thin walled, cigar or club shaped when present	Numerous grape-like clusters	Positive	Positive	■ Spiral hyphae ■ No red pigment on PDA or CMA with 1% dextrose
T. rubrum	Top – white to buff; Reverse – red	Rare long, narrow, thin walled like a pencil or cigar	Clubbed or tear shaped along the hyphae and macroconidia	Negative	Positive	■ Deep red pigment on PDA or CMA with 1% dextrose
T. tonsurans	Top – white to yellow; Reverse – yellow to dark brown	Rare wavy or irregular	Abundant clubbed or tear shaped	Usually negative	Positive	■ Microconidia may balloon ■ Intercalary and terminal chlamydoconidia with age ■ Prefers thiamine
Epidermophyton floccosum	Top – olive or khaki; Reverse – brown	Club shaped and in clusters	None	Negative	Positive	■ Macroconidia can transform into chlamydoconidia with age

no invasion of bone. Although the lesions are disfiguring and may itch, there is little pain unless secondary bacterial infection occurs. The etiological agents of chromoblastomycosis include *Fonsecaea pedrosoi,* the most common cause worldwide, *Fonsecaea compacta, Philophora verrucosa,* and *Cladophialophora carrionii. Exophilia jeanselmei* has recently been implicated in chromoblastomycosis but is usually associated with mycetoma and phaeohyphomycosis. All of these organisms are dematiaceous fungi that produce dark colonies.

Most cases occur in tropical and subtropical areas of South America and Africa but cases have been reported in Asia, Europe, and the United States. The disease is often an occupational hazard for agricultural workers because these organisms live in the spoil and vegetation. Puncture wounds and cuts provide a means of entry for the organism into the tissues.

Treatment of chromoblastomycosis requires surgical excision and is often successful if performed during the early stages

of infection. 5-fluorocytosine is commonly used to treat advanced cases as well as amphotericin B and the imidazoles.

Diagnosis of Chromoblastomycosis by Direct Examination

Clinical material taken from a lesion by a procedure such as a biopsy allows histopathological examination. The H & E stain is superior to silver staining as the brown to black melanin pigments of the cell wall can be observed. Dematiaceous, septate, branched hyphae are characteristically seen but it is the presence of **sclerotic bodies** in the skin and subcutaneous tissues that is diagnostic of chromoblastomycosis. Sclerotic bodies are muriform (resembling a brick wall in its arrangement) cells that reproduce by septal division rather than budding. As these cells enlarge they are divided by septae which grow along two intersecting planes, resulting in a cluster of three to four cells. Sclerotic bodies are described as thick walled, chestnut brown or

✪ TABLE 29-8

Diagnosis of Subcutaneous Mycoses

Etiological Agents	Specimen Types	Microscopic Examination	
		Cytological Examination	Slide Cultures
Chromoblastomycosis Genera include: *Fonsecaea* *Phialophora* *Cladophialophora* *Rhinocladiella* *Exophiala*	Subcutaneous tissues and skin biopsies	Dematiaceous, septate, branched hyphae but sclerotic bodies are diagnostic of chromoblastomycosis Sclerotic bodies are divided by septae along two intersecting planes and are described as thick walled, chestnut brown or copper colored, spherical to ovoid in shape, and ranging in size from 4 to 12 μm in diameter	Depends on species involved
Phaeohyphomycosis Genera include: *Alternaria* *Bipolaris* *Curvularia* *Exophiala* *Phialophora*	Subcutaneous tissues and skin biopsies	Yellowish-brown hyphal elements with or without budding cells Pigmentation of the fungal elements may be too faint to be detected in some cases	Depends on species involved
Eumycotic mycetoma *Pseudallescheria boydii*	Draining pus, aspirate from abscesses, biopsy of subcutaneous tissues, and granules	Intertwined masses of septate hyphae 2–5 μm in diameter	Septate hyphae and one-celled, egg-shaped conidia that are produced singly or in small groups at the tips or conidiogenous hyphae that may be short or long
Sporotrichosis *Sporothrix schenckii*	Draining pus, aspirate from abscesses, lymph node aspirate, tissue biopsies, and respiratory secretions	Oval or spindle- to cigar-shaped forms called "cigar bodies"	37°C: multiple budding round, oval, or cigar-shaped forms (cigar bodies) 22–25°C: septate hyphae, conidia are oval, elliptical to pyriform, and are connected by threadlike denticles forming a "rosette"-like cluster

copper colored, spherical to ovoid in shape, and ranging in size from 4 to 12 μm in diameter (Figure 29-24 ■).

REAL WORLD TIP

Remember the sclerotic bodies as copper pennies for the organisms which cause chromoblastomycosis. These structures will differentiate the lesions, which can resemble those of leishmaniasis, leprosy, and other fungi.

Diagnosis of Chromoblastomycosis Using Fungus Cultures

Differentiation of the agents of chromoblastomycosis requires fungus cultures since all of these fungal species produce dematiaceous hyphae with sclerotic bodies within the tissues. As a group these soil saprobes grow slowly on fungal media, often requiring 7–10 days to produce mature colonies. Macroscopically the colonies are heaped, slightly folded, with a gray, dark olive color, similar to the color of army fatigues, or black with

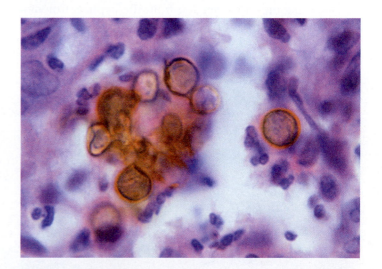

■ **FIGURE 29-24** Sclerotic bodies seen in hemotoxylin and eosin stained section of a tissue sample. Note the presence of the thick-walled, yeast-like sclerotic bodies that are chestnut brown in color. These histological changes are associated with chromoblastomycosis.
From Public Health Image Library (PHIL), CDC/Dr. Libero Ajello.

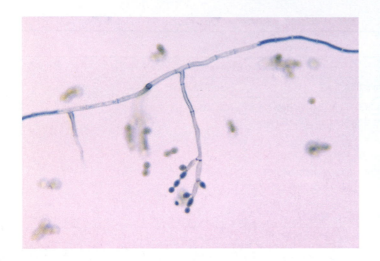

■ FIGURE 29-25 *Cladosporium* species. Note the long chains of oval conidia.
Public Health Image Library (PHIL)/CDC and Dr. Leanor Haley

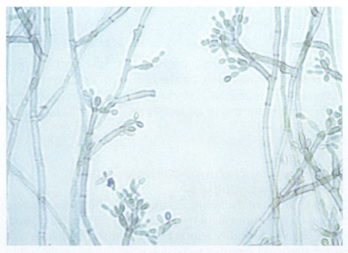

■ FIGURE 29-27 *Phialophora* species. There are clusters of conidia at the end of vase-like phialides.

a velvety surface and a jet black reverse. Microscopic examination using a slide culture technique allows differentiation based on the different morphotypes exhibited.

Cladosporium (Figure 29-25 ■) and *Cladophialophora* species (Figure 29-26 ■) typically have long, sparsely branching chains of elliptical or lemon-shaped blastoconidia from erect conidiophores. *Cladosporium* spp. is very tree-like with short chains of oval blastoconidia on large thick branches (conidiophores) often called shields. *Cladosporium* spp. is considered non-pathogenic but must be differentiated from *Cladophialiphora carronii*. Its colony is deep olive to black with a black reverse.

C. carronii consists of long delicate chains of blastoconidia that look like they are emerging from the hyphae. Conidiophores present are not easily recognizable. At first glance its structure resembles a blade of grass ready to seed. To differen-

tiate the two, *C. carronii* has long chains of blastoconidia, indistinct conidiophores and no shields. Its colony is gray-green to black with a black reverse.

Phialophora species (Figures 29-27 ■ and 14-15) produce short, flask or vase shaped to tubular phialides with well-defined cup-shaped collarettes. Clusters of conidia accumulate in the opening of the phialides in a gelatinous mass. It looks like a vase of flowers. Its colony is green-brown to black with a black reverse.

Fonsecaea pedrosoi (Figure 29-28 ■), the most common causative agent of chromoblastomycosis, produces a polymorphic or mixed type of sporulation characteristic of the *Cladosporium, Phialophora,* and *Rhinocladiella* species. The fonsecaea type is the most common. The conidiophores develop denticles, or small projections, which bear the single conidia.

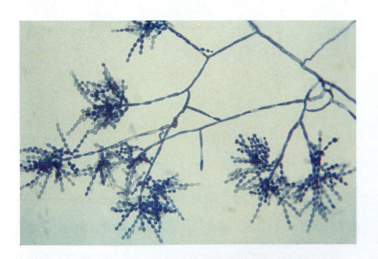

■ FIGURE 29-26 *Cladophialiphora carronii* has long chains of blastoconidia, indistinct conidiophores and no shields.
Public Health Image Library (PHIL)/CDC and Dr. Lucille K. George

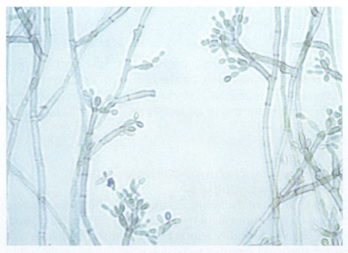

■ FIGURE 29-28 *Fonsecaea* species. The single conidia are produced at the end of denticles, which are located on end of the conidiophores.

Rarely do the conidiophores branch more than three times. The cladosporium type of sporulation consists of very short spore chains formed by successive budding. The phialophora type of sporulation consists of flask-shaped phialides with distinctive collarettes and clusters of conidia. Phialides, which are typically few in number and may be lost on subsequent cultures, are sometimes produced on the same conidiophore, which produces the cladosporium type of spores. The rhinocladiella type of sporulation consists of one-celled primary conidia on denticles and is seen on either side of sympodial conidiophores. In sympodial conidiophores, each time a conidium forms, another conidiophore forms at its base leading to a new conidium. Its colony is dark brown to black with a black reverse.

PHAEOHYPHOMYCOSIS

Phaeohyphomycosis refers to fungus infections that are also caused by dematiaceous fungi but is distinctly different from chromoblastomycosis. Extensive epithelial hyperplasia and the presence of sclerotic bodies are not found in phaeohyphomycosis. Clinical conditions range from cutaneous to systemic infections including keratomycosis, subcutaneous abscesses, sinusitis, pulmonary infection, and fatal cerebral infections seen as brain abscesses. The route of transmission is through traumatic implantation or inhalation. A large number of fungal species have been implicated but the most common include soil saprophytes such as *Alternaria* (Figure 29-29 ■), *Bipolaris*, *Curvularia*, *Exophilia*, *Phialophora*, and *Wangiella* species.

Diagnosis of Phaeohyphomycosis by Direct Examination

Clinical specimens, such as pus aspirated from cysts, biopsy materials, or skin scrapings, contain yellowish-brown hyphal elements with or without budding cells. In some cases pig-

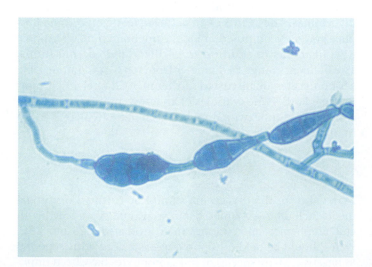

■ **FIGURE 29-29** *Alternaria* species (lactophenol cotton blue stain) from a slide culture. The macroconidia are broad and multicellular. Note the long slender end, which connects it to the rounded end of the next.

mentation of the fungal elements may be too faint to be detected. Regardless of the etiological agent the forms found within the tissues are identical so fungus cultures are required to establish the identity of the invading fungus.

Diagnosis of Phaeohyphomycosis by Fungus Cultures

The fungi that cause phaeohyphomycosis are commonly encountered as airborne contaminants. Observation of fungal elements in clinical specimens and isolation on plated media ensure the organism is a true pathogen. Colonial morphology of the phaeohyphomycotic agents varies from smooth, moist, yeast-like colonies to velvety or woolly colonies. The surface is darkly pigmented, ranging in color from gray to olive to dark brown to black (Figure 14-8) while the reverse is dark brown to black. These organisms may initially present with budding conidia and resemble yeast. They are commonly known as the black (dematiaceous) yeasts.

> **@ REAL WORLD TIP**
>
> The black yeasts eventually develop into the typical mould colony. This is different than the dimorphic fungi. The dimorphic fungi develop into yeast or mould depending on the temperature. Their yeast phase is seen at 35 to 37°C while the mould phase is present at 25 to 30°C. The black yeasts are not temperature dependent and eventually grow to form the familiar fuzzy mould.

Alternaria spp. possesses conidiophores which may zig-zag. The conidia are large and may resemble the spindle macroconidia of the dermatophytes. They may even have a snout or beak like that of *Microsporum canis*. The conidia of *Alterneria* spp. have horizontal and vertical septations which make them look like they contain layers of bricks (Figure 29-29).

The conidiophores of *Bipolaris* spp. bend at the formation of each conidium, giving them a knobby appearance. The conidia are oval, thick walled, and contain four or five septations (Figure 29-6). The dark hyphae will differentiate this organism from the dermatophytes.

Curvularia spp. produce knobby conidiophores with boomerang-shaped conidia that contain four cells (Figure 29-7). The conidia appear to curve (thus the genus name) due to the enlargement of one of the central cells.

Exophiala jeanselmei is the most common isolate of the genus. The slender conidiophores are called annellides and extrude the conidia into the environment. The annellide tends to taper to point with a cluster of oval conidia. The conidia may also be seen in clusters along the sides of the conidiophores and hyphae (Figure 29-30 ■). Early in growth the organism may appear as darkly pigmented conidia only.

The colony of *Wangiella dermatitidis* can appear creamy like that of yeast, but it is pigmented black. With time it develops

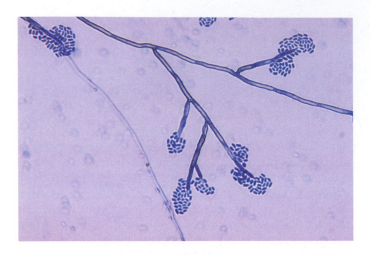

■ **FIGURE 29-30** *Exophiala jeanselmei* produces septate hyphae with slender conidiophores and clusters of oval conidia.
Public Health Image Library (PHIL)/CDC and Dr. Libero Ajello

the fuzziness associated with moulds. The phialide is slightly vase shaped and oval conidia collect at the top. The conidia may also appear along the side of the phialides.

 **Checkpoint! 29–7
(Chapter Objectives 7 and 8)**

What fungal structure, seen in host tissues and detected by direct histological examination, is unique for chromoblastomycosis?

  A. *Sclerotic bodies*
  B. *Darkly pigmented, septate hyphal elements*
  C. *Asci with four ascospores*
  D. *Aseptate hyphae*

MYCETOMA

The term *mycetoma* refers to a chronic fungal infection characterized by localized, swollen yet painless, granulomatous lesions that occur primarily on the feet and lower legs but may also affect the hands and arms. Suppurative abscesses and draining sinuses are found within the subcutaneous tissues and multiple sinus tracks discharge serosanguinous pus (thin, red-tinged discharge composed of serum and blood) to the surface of the skin. This discharge often contains colony granules, which may be white, yellow, red, or black.

Mycetomata involve cutaneous and subcutaneous tissues but may also spread into the fascia and bone and occasionally disseminate to other organs including the brain. If not treated, amputation may be required to resolve the infection. Most cases occur in the tropics and subtropics among those who work outdoors without protective clothing. Many cases involve immigrant workers from Mexico.

Approximately 50% of the cases of mycetoma are caused by the aerobic actinomycetes *Nocardia*, *Actinomadura*, and *Streptomyces* and are therefore bacterial infections. This is

referred to as an actinomycotic mycetoma. The remaining cases are caused by fungi and are referred to as a eumycotic mycetoma. The etiological agents include a heterogenous group of fungi possessing septate hyphae and include *Pseudallescheria boydii*, *Exophiala jeanselmei*, *Acremonium* species, and *Curvularia* species, as well as others.

The teleomorph or sexual state, *Pseudallescheria boydii*, is the most common cause of mycetoma in the United States. *P. boydii* is an unusual fungus because it has two anamorphs or asexual states. In other words, the conidial states are found in two forms, *Scedosporium* and *Graphium*. The predominant asexual form is *Scedosporium* and, in fact, some isolates may lack the *Graphium* form. *P. boydii*, like other saprophytic fungi, is an environmental organism and has been recovered from soil, water, manure, and sewage. From such sources the portal of entry into the host is through traumatic implantation of the etiological agent into the tissues.

It is important to determine the etiological agent of mycetoma because successful treatment relies on the administration of the appropriate chemotherapy. Antibacterials are appropriate to treat actinomycotic mycetoma but will be ineffective for the agents of eumycotic mycetoma. The administration of antifungal agents work against the agent of eumycotic mycetoma. In cases of eumycotic mycetoma, surgical intervention is usually required in addition to the use of antifungal drugs such as ketaconazole, which must be administered on a long-term basis, even as long as 12 months.

Diagnosis of Mycetomata by Direct Examination

Pus or biopsy material should be examined for the presence of granules. Each granule is a mass of organisms. The granules range in size from 0.2 to 5.0 μm or more and may be visible to the unaided eye. Gram staining crushed granules will allow differentiation of actinomycotic and eumycotic mycetomas. The agents of an actinomycotic mycetoma produce granules composed of long, thin, branching, gram-positive filaments in addition to bacillary and coccoid forms. The filaments range in diameter from 0.5 to 1.0 μm. Aerobic actinomycetes are discussed further in ∞ Chapter 19, "Gram-Positive Rods." The granules of an eumycotic mycetoma are composed of intertwined masses of septate hyphae 2–5 μm in diameter.

Diagnosis of Mycetomata Using Fungus Cultures

Material from the mycetoma should be cultured on fungal media including sabouraud dextrose agar (SDA) and SDA with chloramphenicol and cycloheximide incubated at 25 and 37°C. Plates should be held for up to 6 weeks before being reported as negative. Many species of soil saprophytes have been implicated as etiological agents of mycetoma but only the morphological characteristics of *Pseudallescheria boydii*, the most common cause of mycetoma in the United States, are discussed here. The others are discussed in other sections of this chapter.

Colonial Morphology of *Pseudallescheria boydii* (Anamorph, *Scedosporium aspiospermum*, and Synamorph, *Graphium* spp.). *Pseudallescheria boydii* is a moderately rapid-growing fungus producing mature colonies within 7 days. The colonies are initially white with a cottony texture and with age the surface darkens to a grayish brown color. The reverse is initially white but eventually becomes gray or black.

 REAL WORLD TIP

P. boydii is inhibited by cyclohexamide while *S. aspiospermum* may or may not be inhibited.

Microscopic Morphology of *Pseudallescheria boydii* (Anamorph, *Scedosporium apiospermum*, and Synamorph, *Graphium* spp.). The anamorph, *Scedosporium apiospermum,* produces septate hyphae. One-celled, egg-shaped conidia are produced singly or in small groups at the tips of conidia-producing hyphae, which may be short or long (Figures 29-31 ■ and 14-14). There is a **synamorph** (an additional anamorphic or asexual state) that occasionally occurs on fungal media. The *Graphium* spp. synamorph consists of rope-like bundles of hyphae fused to form long stalks (synnemata). Clusters of one-celled conidia, which are cylindrical to clavate (club-shaped), are produced. These conidia are somewhat smaller than those of the *Scedosporium* type.

In the sexual state of this fungus, cleistothecia (multicellular structures in which asci and ascospores are formed and held) are found below the surface of the agar. These sac-like structures are darkly pigmented, spherical in shape, and range in size from 140 to 200 µm in diameter. When mature, the cleistothecia rupture releasing asci containing eight one-celled, oval to ellipsoidal, pale brown to copper ascospores. The cleistothecia may be better seen on CMA or PDA.

SPOROTRICHOSIS

Sporotrichosis, also called "rose gardener's disease," is a fungal disease of worldwide distribution, with most cases occurring in temperate and tropical countries. The disease ranges from a localized cutaneous infection to a disseminated or systemic infection. The etiological agent is *Sporothrix schenckii*, a dimorphic fungus whose normal habitat is plants and soil.

Sporotrichosis is an occupational hazard, affecting persons who spend time working with plants and soil, such as gardeners, plant nursery workers, florists, and foresters. The mode of entry into host tissues is through thorns and splinters, which drive the organism into the skin and subcutaneous tissues. However, outbreaks have been recorded in miners who acquired the disease through abrasions caused by contact with supporting timbers.

The most common form of sporotrichosis is the lymphocutaneous form. In these cases the initial lesion is a small, erythematous, relatively painless nodule that forms at the point of entry, usually the hand or forearm but occasionally the feet and legs. The local lymph drainage channels and nodes are invaded and the organism multiplies. A sinus tract may lead to the surface of the skin, which erodes to form an ulcerative lesion (Figure 29-32 ■). Chronic cases can occur on the face, neck, trunk, or arm. On rare occasions the organism disseminates to mucocutaneous areas, the skeletal system, and other organ systems. This hematogenous spread is secondary to cutaneous sporotrichosis and is termed mucocutaneous sporotrichosis. Pulmonary sporotrichosis can develop following inhalation of the organism.

Immunological Tests for Sporotrichosis
In most cases sporotrichosis is diagnosed on the basis of clinical symptoms and cultural findings. Immunological tests are available but are usually performed in reference laboratories.

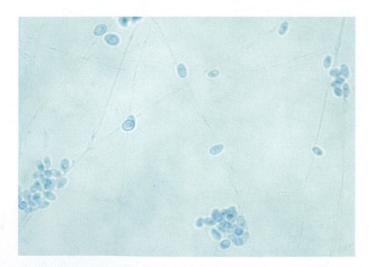

■ FIGURE 29-31 *Scedosporium apiospermum.* The thin delicate conidiophores end with a large single conidium.

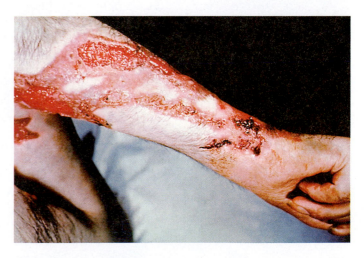

■ FIGURE 29-32 Sporothrichosis occurs after spores of *Sporothrix schenckii* are implanted by a thorn or splinter.
Public Health Image Library (PHIL)/CDC and Dr. Lucille K. George

The best known immuological test is the delayed-type hypersensitivity test in which sporotrichin, a protein extracted from the organism, is injected just under the skin. A positive reaction resembles that of the tuberculin skin test. Latex agglutination and tube agglutination tests are also available to detect antibody to the fungus.

Diagnosis of Sporotrichosis by Direct Examination

Sporothrix schenckii is one of the dimorphic fungi. Dimorphic means it can exist in one of two states depending on the temperature: yeast at 35 to 37°C or mould at 25 to 30°C. The yeast form is exhibited in the tissues while the mould form can be found in cultures incubated at room temperature. The yeast form may be seen in a Gram-stained smear made from a sputum specimen, in a KOH preparation of pus, and in a PAS- or GMS-stained section from a tissue biopsy. Unfortunately, direct examination of clinical specimens may not be productive since the number of yeast cells is usually low and multiple slides may have to be examined to demonstrate the presence of the yeast cells. Fluorescent antibodies may be applied to tissue sections in an attempt to demonstrate the yeast form. Typically oval and fusiform budding yeast forms are diagnostic. The spindle or cigar-shaped forms have been referred to as "cigar bodies" (Figure 29-33 ■).

Diagnosis of Sporotrichosis by Fungus Cultures

Biopsy material may be ground aseptically using sterile broth and a mortar and pestle designed for grinding tissue. The liquid can then be used to inoculate fungal media including SDA and SDA with chloramphenicol and cycloheximide, or enriched media such as blood, chocolate, or brain heart infusion supplemented with blood. Pus, blood, and bone marrow can be used to inoculate the media also. The SDA and SDA with antibiotics should be incubated at 25–30°C in order to isolate the mould form. The enriched media should be incubated at 35–37°C under increased CO_2 in order to demonstrate the yeast or tissue form. All media should be held for up to 4 weeks.

Colonial Morphology of *Sporothrix schenckii* (Mould Form).   Initially the color of the colony is white to cream colored but with age becomes dark gray, brown, or nearly black. The colonies are typically smooth, moist, and yeast-like in appearance with flat or finely wrinkled surfaces. Later colonies often become leathery or velvety, especially after several subcultures.

Microscopic Morphology of *Sporothrix schenckii* (Mould Form).   The hyphae are thin (usually less than 3 µm in diameter), septate, branching, and hyaline (colorless). Conidia may be hyaline and thin walled or dark brown and thick walled. They are oval, elliptical to pyriform, and are produced in a bouquet at the swollen tip of the conidiophore connected by small, threadlike denticles forming a "rosette" or flower-like cluster (Figure 29-34 ■). Later the thick- and thin-walled conidia can form along the conidiophores and hyphae.

Colonial Morphology of *Sporothrix schenckii* (Yeast Form).   Conversion of the mycelial mould form to the yeast-like form is essential for identification. The colonies are cream or tan colored, smooth, and yeast-like.

Microscopic Morphology of *Sporothrix schenckii* (Yeast Form).   Microscopically, the yeast forms produced *in vitro* are oval, globose (spherical), or fusiform (the "cigar bodies") and may produce multiple buds. This form is most often visualized in the tissues.

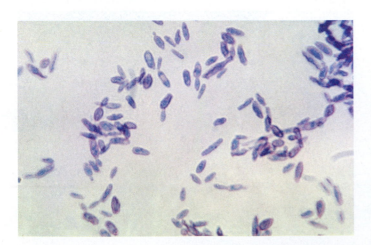

■ **FIGURE 29-33** The yeast form of *Sporothrix schenckii* reveals elongated budding cells that are described as "cigar bodies." *Public Health Image Library (PHIL)/CDC and Dr. Lucille K. George*

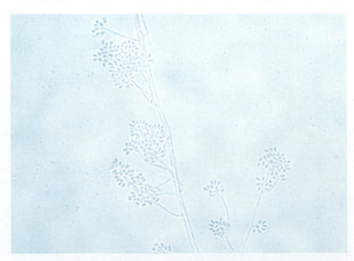

■ **FIGURE 29-34** Mould form of *Sporothrix schenckii* from a slide culture. Conidia are produced in a bouquet at the swollen tip of the small, threadlike denticles forming a "rosette," or flower-like cluster.

REAL WORLD TIP

To perform a mould-to-yeast conversion, brain heart infusion (BHI) agar plus 20% blood is used. Two agars are inoculated within a biological safety cabinet. One is incubated at 25°C (for the mould phase) and the other at 35–37°C (for the yeast phase). It may take several weeks for the conversion to occur.

► SYSTEMIC MYCOSES

Some species of fungi have the ability to disseminate or spread from the portal of entry to infect multiple organ systems. For example, a fungus may gain entry into the host by inhalation of conidia, then multiply within the host and spread to other tissues, such as the skin or central nervous system, through the bloodstream. Even organisms of low pathogenicity, such as *Aspergillus fumigatus,* may cause a life-threatening illness in immunocompromised hosts. In other cases, organisms such as *Sporothrix schenckii,* a fungus that usually causes a localized infection following traumatic implantation, may disseminate to internal organs such as the bone or central nervous system. *Candida albicans,* a yeast that is often found as part of the normal flora of mucous membranes, may also spread to cause multiorgan infections. In contrast, the four classic agents of systemic mycoses are strict pathogens rather than opportunists. These organisms include *Histoplasma capsulatum, Blastomyces dermatitidis, Coccidioides immitis,* and *Paracoccidioides brasiliensis.* They share some common characteristics that justify studying these organisms as a group:

- these organisms are able to cause disease in otherwise healthy individuals
- they tend to be endemic to particular geographic regions
- they exhibit a dimorphism that is temperature dependent
- their primary target organ is the lungs from which they may spread to secondary organ systems.

In the following sections the systemic fungal diseases, the etiological agents, and the microscopic and macroscopic or colonial morphology of the etiological agents are presented. The route of transmission, which is through inhalation of conidia, is the same for all of the systemic fungi. From the lungs these organisms may spread to other organ systems such as the skin and mucous membranes. The greatest risk of significant morbidity and mortality occurs when fungal agents spread throughout the body and involve multiple organ systems.

The fungi included in this section are dimorphic and exist in two forms. The yeast or parasitic form is found within host tissues and is seen when the organism is grown *in vitro* at 37°C on media enriched with sheep blood. The mould or saprophytic form occurs in soil and decaying vegetation and can be grown on a peptone medium at room temperature. When identifying the systemic fungi on fungal cultures, it is necessary to demonstrate the mould phase can be converted to the yeast phase.

HISTOPLASMOSIS

Histoplasmosis, also called Darling's disease, cave disease, spelunker's disease, and reticuloendothelial cytomycosis, is a disease of worldwide distribution (Deepe, 1997). It is found in temperate, subtropical, and tropical regions of the world. In the United States, histoplasmosis is endemic to the Mississippi, Missouri, Ohio, and St. Lawrence River valley regions.

The etiological agent is *Histoplasma capsulatum.* It grows best in soil enriched with the feces of birds (especially chickens and starlings) and bats. Birds are not infected possibly due to body temperatures that are higher than that of humans and other mammals. Bats are naturally infected and often have intestinal lesions containing the yeast form. Human infections may occur when individuals engage in activities such as cleaning chicken coops, attics, barns, and other roosting areas, demolishing old abandoned buildings, and exploring caves (spelunking). These activities create infective aerosols leading to inhalation of conidia produced by the organism.

An estimated half million persons are exposed to *H. capsulatum* each year in the United States. Conidia or hyphal elements that are inhaled are phagocytized predominantly by macrophages, convert to the yeast phase, and are able to replicate within the cytoplasm of the macrophage. In immunocompetent individuals the immune system is able to contain the mould. About 95% of infections are asymptomatic, self-limiting infections in immunocompetent hosts and are likely due to a light exposure to the fungus. Heavy exposure in uncompromised individuals will usually result in an illness that resembles influenza. Necrotic lesions in the lungs become encapsulated by a fibrous material and eventually become calcified and may be visible on radiographs. Cavitary lesions develop due to destruction and necrosis of lung tissue.

Immunocompromised individuals are at high risk of developing disseminated histoplasmosis as a result of primary exposure to *H. capsulatum* or reactivation of dormant histoplasmosis. Individuals with serious invasive infections usually complain of fever, night sweats, and weight loss. Examination of the peripheral blood smear may reveal the presence of small intracellular yeast in the cytoplasm of polymorphonuclear leukocytes. Specimens for examination and culture include blood, bone marrow, urine, sputum, cerebrospinal fluid, and tissue.

Serological Tests for the Diagnosis of Histoplasmosis

The complement fixation test, which measures antibodies directed against *H. capsulatum,* is the standard serological test to diagnose histoplasmosis. Histoplasmin (a sterile culture filtrate of *H. capsulatum* that has been grown in broth for 2–3 months) and intact formalin-treated yeast can be used as the antigen source. Titers >1:32 or a fourfold rise in titer between acute and convalescent titers indicates active infection. The major drawback is the problem of cross-reactivity with other fungal infections such as coccidioidomycosis and blastomycosis.

Immunodiffusion tests, using precipitating antibodies, have also been employed. They are less sensitive but more specific for a diagnosis of histoplasmosis. In this test histoplasmin is tested against sera containing reactive antibody leading to the formation of precipitin bands where antigen and antibody combine in optimal proportions. The exoantigen test, which employs the use of antigen extracts from an agar growth medium, can be used in culture confirmation. Anti-histoplasma antibody is used in an immunodiffusion test where precipitin lines of identity that form with control histoplasmin antigens are interpreted as a positive identification. Commercially available nucleic acid probes are also available to confirm the identification.

Diagnosis of Histoplasmosis by Direct Examination

Small intracellular yeasts can be seen by histopathological examination of infected tissue. Bone marrow and peripheral blood smears can be stained with the Giemsa or Wright stain. The small intracellular yeasts are usually seen within the cytoplasm of phagocytes and occasionally extracellularly (Figure 29-35 ■).

REAL WORLD TIP

The phagocytized yeast cells of *Histoplasma capsulatum* can resemble the amastigotes of *Leishmania* spp. Both are the same size and are engulfed by white blood cells. The amastigote of *Leishmania* spp. contains a nucleus and kinetoplast often referred to as a dot (nucleus) and dash (kinetoplast).

Spleen, liver, lymph nodes, and lung tissues stained with H & E, PAS, GMS, calcofluor white, and fluorescent antibody stains can also be used to demonstrate the presence of yeast in the tissues in cases of disseminated histoplasmosis.

Diagnosis of Histoplasmosis by Fungus Cultures

In diagnosing histoplasmosis, specimens such as sputum, blood, bone marrow, and ground tissues can be used to inoculate fungal media. Sabouraud's dextrose agar and SDA with chloramphenicol and cycloheximide are recommended to isolate the fungus from body sites that contain normal bacterial flora. It must be remembered that high concentrations of chloramphenicol and gentamycin may inhibit the growth of *H. capsulatum*. Fungal media should be incubated at 30°C, inspected every 2–4 days for growth, and held for at least 4 weeks before reporting as negative for fungal growth.

Colonial or Macroscopic Morphology of *Histoplasma capsulatum*.

Histoplasma capsulatum is a slow-growing fungus and usually requires a minimum of 2 weeks to produce mature colonies, and in some cases up to 8 weeks. At 25–30°C on sabouraud agar the colony is white to brown with a fine, dense, cottony texture. The reverse is usually white but may be yellowish.

Microscopic Morphology of *Histoplasma capsulatum*.

At 25–30°C septate hyphae are present in the mould phase. Smooth or spiny, round to pear-shaped microconidia (2–5 μm in diameter) are produced on short conidiophores or directly on the sides of the hyphae. Large, thick-walled, round, tuberculate (knobby) macroconidia (7–15 μm in diameter) are formed as the colony ages (Figure 29-36 ■). The macroconidia can resemble the spiky fruit of the sweetgum or

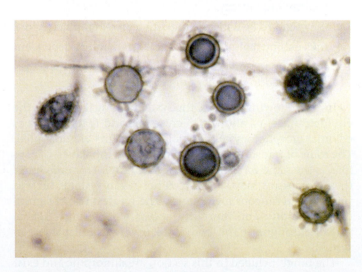

■ FIGURE 29-36 Mould form of *Histoplasma capsulatum*. Note the presence of the large, thick-walled, tuberculate or spiked macroconidia.
Public Health Image Library (PHIL)/CDC

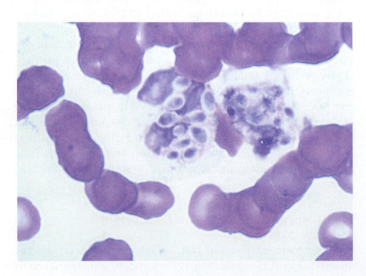

■ FIGURE 29-35 *Histoplasma capsulatum* intracellular yeast on a Wright-stained peripheral blood smear of an AIDS patient.

gumball tree. These structures resemble the macroconidia of *Sepedonium* species, a nonpathogenic mould species, but it is not dimorphic. This differentiates it from *H. capsulatum*, which is dimorphic.

Demonstration of dimorphism, by conversion of the mould phase to the yeast phase, is required to identify the organism if cultures are used for definitive identification. At 35–37°C on an enriched medium, small, round to oval budding cells are seen. A medium such as brain heart infusion agar enriched with sheep blood is recommended for this purpose. Sabouraud brain heart infusion (Sabhi) agar should not be used for the conversion of the mould to yeast phases of dimorphic fungi. Repeated subculture may be required to demonstrate the yeast form.

BLASTOMYCOSIS

Blastomycosis, also called Chicago disease, Gilchrist's disease, and North American blastomycosis, is a disease of worldwide distribution, although the majority of cases occur in the North American continent. The disease is primarily endemic to the Ohio and Mississippi River valley regions, with the St. Lawrence and Arkansas River valleys, Minnesota, and southern Canada to a lesser extent. Dogs and horses serve as additional hosts for the organism in endemic areas. *Blastomyces dermatitidis*, the etiological agent of blastomycosis, has been isolated from riverbank soil and beaver dams, however, the natural reservoir and ecological niche of the organism is not known for certain.

Blastomycosis is acquired by inhalation of conidia resulting in a primary pulmonary infection of the host. Similar to histoplasmosis, the majority of infections are asymptomatic and self-limiting. A chronically progressive blastomycosis may involve one or more organs including the lungs, followed by skin and bone infection. Osteomyelitis develops in nearly one-third of patients with disseminated blastomycosis. The genitourinary tract, especially the prostate and epididymis, is another organ system targeted by *B. dermatitidis*. Following inhalation of the organism, the yeast form emerges and is phagocytized by macrophages. The yeast cells within the cytoplasm of the macrophage are not killed so viable organisms are carried to other sites and are released when the host cell dies. It is well known that skin lesions result from hematogenous (bloodborne) dissemination of the organism from the lungs to other tissues. Skin lesions are ulcerated, verrucous, granulomatous processes that may become extensive. Patients with diabetes are at increased risk of contracting blastomycosis.

Diagnosis of Blastomycosis Using Serological Tests

Serological and immunological tests for blastomycosis are less diagnostic because of a high degree of cross-reactivity with other mycoses, especially histoplasmosis and coccidioidomycosis.

Diagnosis of Blastomycosis by Direct Examination

Microscopic examination of KOH preparations of sputum, purulent fluid from abscesses, and tissue sections may reveal the presence of yeast forms as well as histopathological examination of infected tissues (Figure 29-37 ∎) using fungal stains such as direct fluorescent antibody (DFA), H & E, PAS, GMS, or calcofluor white.

Colonial Morphology of *Blastomyces dermatitidis*.

Blastomyces dermatitidis is another slow-growing fungus producing mature colonies within 2 weeks. Cultures should be kept for up to 8 weeks before reporting as negative for fungal growth. At 25–30°C on sabouraud agar, young colonies may be thin and membranous, eventually acquiring a spiky or prickly appearance, and finally a white cottony aerial mycelium. Color varies from dirty white to tan or brown with age. The reverse is often tan. At 35–37°C on enriched media, the yeast-like colonies are cream to tan in color and waxy in appearance.

> ## ℮ REAL WORLD TIP
>
> The yeast phase of *Blastomyces dermatitidis* will not grow on media with cyclohexamide while its mould phase is resistant to cyclohexamide and will grow.

Microscopic Morphology of *Blastomyces dermatitidis*.

At 25–30°C the mould phase of *B. dermatitidis* forms septate hyphae bearing small, round to oval, smooth-walled conidia borne on short, lateral, hypha-like conidiophores of

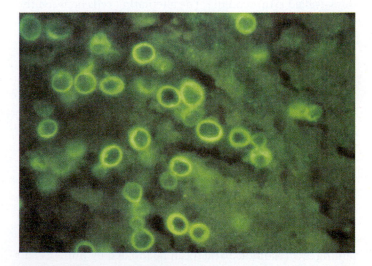

∎ **FIGURE 29-37** Yeast form of *Blastomyces dermatitidis* revealed by direct fluorescent antibody (DFA) staining of lung tissue. Note the presence of the mother cell with a single blastoconidium attached by a broad-based septum.
From Public Health Image Library (PHIL), CDC/Dr. William Kaplan.

varying lengths or directly on the hyphae. With time, chlamydoconidia may be present. This organism may resemble *Scedosporium apiospermum* or *Chrysosporium* species, both non-pathogen moulds that are not dimorphic. Demonstrating the dimorphic nature of *B. dermatitidis* allows these species to be differentiated.

Conversion to the yeast phase requires growth on an enriched medium and incubation at 35–37°C. If accomplished, large, spherical, thick and double-walled yeast cells (8–15 μm in diameter) with a single blastoconidium attached to the parent cell by a broad-based septum can be seen. The mother and daughter cell are usually very nearly the same size, a characteristic seen with *B. dermatitidis* and much less likely to occur in the yeast phase of the other dimorphic fungi.

 REAL WORLD TIP

Remember the unique **b**road **b**ase yeast morphology of ***B**lastomyces dermatitidis* by using the letter "b" in its genus name.

COCCIDIOIDOMYCOSIS

Coccidioidomycosis, also known as San Joaquin Valley fever, desert fever, desert rheumatism, and Posada's disease, is endemic to the southwestern United States, especially Arizona and California, northwestern Mexico, and Central and South America. The etiological agent is *Coccidioides immitis,* an organism that thrives in a semiarid climate where rainfall is low, summer temperatures are high, winters are moderate, and growth is supported by an alkaline, sandy soil. As the fertile, septate hyphae grow in the soil, alternating cells form into thick-walled arthroconidia. The alternating cells between the arthroconidia undergo autolysis, becoming hollow, thin-walled cells called disjunctor cells (Figure 14-19). Disjunctor cells readily fragment, allowing the arthroconidia to become easily airborne. Once inhaled, the infectious arthroconidia develop into the parasitic tissue stage, the spherule. The spherule is filled with endospores.

The organism can soon overwhelm the immune system, leading to disseminated infection, especially if the spherule should rupture adjacent to a blood vessel. Sputum, urine, feces, purulent material, and the carcasses of animals are probably the mechanism by which the pathogen is returned to the soil. Spherules that seed the environment convert to the mycelial form in the soil.

Activities such as farming, construction work, archeological digs, and wind storms produce infectious aerosols containing arthroconidia, which can be inhaled by humans and inhalation of as few as 10 arthrospores can result in disease. Coccidioidomycosis is usually an asymptomatic disease (60% of cases) or a mildly symptomatic, self-limited disease of the lungs (40% of cases). Symptomatic cases often present as a severe, acute, upper respiratory tract infection with nonspe-cific, influenza-like symptoms such as fever, malaise, headache, anorexia, and myalgia. This leads to pleuritic or dull, aching chest pain and a dry or productive cough. This productive cough may be characterized by white, purulent, or blood-streaked sputum. Less than 1% of cases may progress to serious or fatal cases of disseminated coccidioidomycosis.

Serological Diagnosis of Coccidioidomycosis

Tube precipitin and complement fixation tests are serological tests that have been widely accepted as reliable methods in the diagnosis of coccidioidomycosis. A high titer exceeding 1:16 and persistent or rising titers are indicative of disseminated disease. In addition, skin reactivity to coccidioidin or spherulin (cell-free filtrates from fungus cultures) appears 2–4 weeks following infection. Other tests such as latex particle agglutination and agar immunodiffusion have largely replaced the tube precipitin and complement fixation tests.

Diagnosis of Coccidioidomycosis by Direct Examination

Direct microscopic examination of clinical specimens, such as a KOH preparation of sputum or abscess material and histopathological sections of infected tissues, is especially useful in the diagnosis of coccidioidomycosis. The parasitic form consists of spherules or sporangia (singular, sporangium), which are usually 10–80 μm in diameter and contain granular material or endospores (sporangiospores), which are 2–5 μm in diameter. These spherules with endospores are characteristic enough to be diagnostic. The usual fungal stains, such as the H & E, PAS, or Gridley fungus stains, are suitable for staining tissue sections, however, the GMS stain with a bright-green counterstain is far more sensitive.

Diagnosis of Coccidioidomycosis by Fungus Culture

Of the four dimorphic fungi discussed under the topic systemic mycoses (*Histoplasma capsulatum, Blastomyces dermatitidis, Coccidioides immitis,* and *Paracoccidioides brasiliensis*), *C. immitis* is the most rapidly growing, requiring only 3–5 days for growth to appear. Cultures of *C. immitis* require practices consistent with that of a biosafety level 3 containment facility because of the hazard of inhaling arthroconidia of the mycelial phase. Slide cultures should not be made to study the microscopic structures of *C. immitis*. After wetting down the tubed growth with sterile, distilled water, a tease mount using a drop of lactophenol cotton blue, which kills in addition to staining the hyphal elements, should be prepared using a biological safety cabinet. After the mount is covered with a coverslip the preparation may be examined microscopically.

The Parasitic Phase of *Coccidioides immitis.* When *Coccidioides immitis* is cultured it does not behave in the same manner as the other dimorphic fungi. Growth on enriched media at 37°C does not induce conversion to the parasitic form found in host tissues. Unlike the other systemic fungi, the form found within the tissues is not yeast-like but is the spherule with endospores (Figure 14-11). Conversion to the spherule phase requires animal inoculation or use of a special, synthesized, liquid medium called Converse medium. The medium must be incubated under an atmosphere of increased CO_2 at a temperature of 40°C.

Colonial (or Macroscopic) and Microscopic Morphology of the Mycelial Phase.

Inoculation of SDA with or without antibiotics and subsequent incubation at 25–30°C or even inoculation of a medium enriched with sheep blood incubated at 35–37°C results in production of the mycelial phase of growth. Incubation at 37°C on an enriched medium does not induce conversion, so the organism remains filamentous and does not form a yeast phase. Mould colonies are initially moist, grayish in color, and membranous. As the culture ages the texture becomes white and cottony and the color may progress to a tan to brown color. The reverse is often white to gray.

Microscopic examination of material from colonies at least 1–2 weeks of age should reveal the presence of arthroconidia. The arthroconidia are characteristically thick walled, barrel shaped, and measure approximately 3×6 μm in size. Arthroconidia alternate with hollow, thin-walled disjunctor cells (Figure 14-19). Branching of septate, hyaline hyphae usually occurs at approximately 90° angles. An immunodiffusion test for exoantigen and nucleic acid probes are also available to confirm the identification of *C. immitis*.

Microscopic Morphology of the Parasitic Phase of *C. immitis*.

When *C. immitis* grows within host tissues or on special media, the arthroconidia of the mycelial phase become spherical, enlarge, and develop into spherules containing endospores. To demonstrate the dimorphic nature of this fungus in the laboratory, the organism must be subcultured to Converse medium and incubated at 40°C under increased CO_2.

PARACOCCIDIOIDOMYCOSIS

Paracoccidioidomycosis is also called South American blastomycosis because distribution is restricted geographically to Central and South America. The etiological agent *Paracoccidioides brasiliensis* thrives in areas that have hot, humid summers and dry, mild winters, as evidenced by areas of high incidence within the countries of Brazil, Venezuela, and Colombia. Typically, paracoccidioidomycosis involves adult males because estrogen has an inhibitory effect on the transformation of the saprophytic to parasitic forms of the fungus.

Pulmonary infection follows inhalation of fungal elements and is most often asymptomatic but can develop into a progressive pulmonary disease that can be either an acute or chronic pneumonia. Symptomatic infection may be associated with a primary infection or reactivation of a dormant infection. Symptoms associated with pneumonia or disseminated paracoccidioidomycosis include fever, cough, sputum production, chest pain, dyspnea or difficulty in breathing, hemoptysis, malaise, and weight loss.

Oral and nasal lesions are prominent and represent hematogenous spread from a pulmonary infection to the mucous membranes of the oral cavity. Other sites of dissemination include lymph nodes, spleen, liver, gastrointestinal tract, bone, the central nervous system, and adrenal glands.

Diagnosis of Paracoccidioidomycosis by Direct Examination

Histopathological examination of biopsy materials or crusts and granulomatous bases of ulcers or KOH preparations of sputum or pus from draining lymph nodes may reveal the presence of yeast-like cells of *P. brasiliensis*. The fungal cells may be demonstrated within H & E stained sections or by the use of other fungal stains. These yeast-like cells often exhibit the typical peripheral budding in which the parent cell is a large, spherical, double-walled blastoconidium that measures 10–30 μm in diameter surrounded by globose, oval, or pear-shaped buds measuring 2–10 μm in diameter and attached to the mother cell by very narrow denticles (small, tooth-like projection on which spores are produced). This morphology is said to resemble a ship's steering wheel or "pilot's wheel."

Diagnosis of Paracoccidioidomycosis by Fungal Cultures

SDA with or without antibiotics may be used in isolation of *P. brasiliensis*. When incubated at 25–30°C the filamentous or mould form will be seen. On an enriched medium incubated at 35–37°C, the yeast form is displayed.

The Filamentous (Mould) Form and Yeast Forms.

When incubated at room temperature on nutritive media, colonies grow very slowly and may require as long as 21 days to mature. The mould is typically white with a short, white aerial mycelium that turns brown with age. The typical microscopic morphology includes septate, branched, hyaline hyphae with intercalary and terminal chlamydoconidia. A few microconidia may be observed along the hyphae.

Incubation at 37°C leads to the growth of yeast colonies that are cream to tan, moist, and yeast-like. Microscopically, large, round, thick-walled cells with single and multiple buds are seen. The buds are attached by narrow connections and nearly surround the parent cell, providing the typical "pilot's wheel" appearance. Conversion to the yeast form is required for identification as *P. brasiliensis* (Figure 29-38 ■). The diagnosis of systemic mycoses is summarized in Table 29-9✪.

SYSTEMIC PENICILLIOSIS DUE TO *PENCILLIUM MARNEFFEI*

One form of systemic mycosis is caused by a unique dimorphic fungus belonging to the genus *Pencillium*. The organism is endemic to southern China and Southeast Asia where it is the

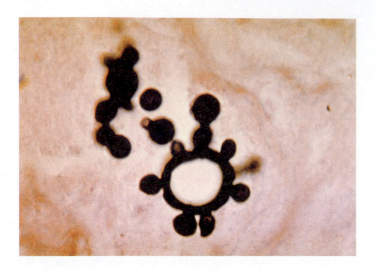

■ **FIGURE 29-38** Yeast form of *Paracoccidioides brasiliensis.*
Note the buds formed around the edge of the central yeast.
Public Health Image Library (PHIL)/CDC and Dr. Lucille K. George

third most common cause of disseminated opportunistic infection in AIDS patients living in the region. The etiological agent is *Penicillium marneffei* and it displays a typical *Penicillium* mould morphology at room temperature but a yeast morphology in tissue. The primary source in the environment has not been determined.

Because members of this genus are among the most common of all laboratory contaminants, the recovery of *Penicillium* species from patient specimens does not necessarily implicate these fungi as pathogens unless the typical fungal elements are demonstrated in tissue sections or smears from exudates.

Penicillinosis is seen most frequently in immunocompromised individuals but has also been diagnosed in immunocompetent individuals. The organism has been isolated from blood, bone marrow, skin lesions, lung tissues, mucosa, lymph nodes, urine, stool, spinal fluid, and other internal organs.

At body temperature *Penicillium marneffei* forms small, round to oval yeast cells within the cytoplasm of phagocytes and may be identical to the yeast phase of *Histoplasma capsulatum.* Unlike *H. capsulatum,* which multiplies by budding, *P. marneffei* divides by fission.

At 25–30°C *Penicillium marneffei* grows rapidly, producing mature colonies in 3–5 days. Colonies are flat, powdery to velvety, and may be bluish-green to reddish yellow with a yellow or white periphery. A unique soluble red to maroon pigment diffuses into the agar and the reverse is brownish red. Microscopically, hyaline, septate hyphae are seen. There are smooth conidiophores with four to five metulae that support four to six phialides, which produce chains of smooth or slightly rough oval conidia (Figure 29-39 ■). At 35–37°C on enriched media oval, yeast-like forms develop. The organism measures 2–6 μm in size and cross-walls or internal septae in the absence of budding may be seen with careful examination.

@ **REAL WORLD TIP**

For the dimorphic fungi, remember that the mould phase is present at 25–30°C while the yeast phase is present at 35–37°C. The letter "m" comes before "y" and 25°C comes before 35°C.

✪ **TABLE 29-9**

Diagnosis of Systemic Mycoses

Etiological Agents	Specimen Types	Microscopic Examination	
		Cytological Examination	Slide Cultures
Histoplasmosis: *Histoplasma capsulatum*	Sputum, blood, bone marrow, spleen, liver, lymph nodes, lungs	Examination of bone marrow or peripheral blood smears may reveal small intracellular yeasts within the cytoplasm of phagocytes	Septate, hyaline hyphae with round to pear-shaped microconidia (2–5 μm in diameter) and large, round, thick-walled tuberculate macroconidia (7–15 μm in diameter)
Blastomycosis: *Blastomyces dermatitidis*	Sputum, skin and tissue biopsy, purulent material from abscesses	Large, spherical, thick-walled yeast (8–15 μm in diameter) with a single bud attached by a broad-based septum; mother and daughter cell nearly the same size	Septate hyphae with small, round to oval conidia on short conidiophores
Coccidioidomycosis: *Coccidioides immitis*	Sputum, purulent material from abscesses, infected tissue	Large, round, thick-walled spherule (10–80 μm in diameter) containing endospores (2–5 μm in diameter); spherules may be ruptured, releasing endospores	Hyaline, septate hyphae with thick-walled, barrel-shaped arthroconidia (3 × 6 μm) alternating with hollow disjunctor cells
Paracoccidioidomycosis: *Paracoccidioides brasiliensis*	Sputum, purulent material, infected tissue, biopsy of material at base of ulcerative lesions	Large, spherical, thick-walled parent cell (10–30 μm in diameter) with multiple oval to pear-shaped buds attached to parent cell by narrow denticles	Septate, branched, hyaline hyphae with intercalary and terminal chlamydoconidia; a few microconidia may be observed

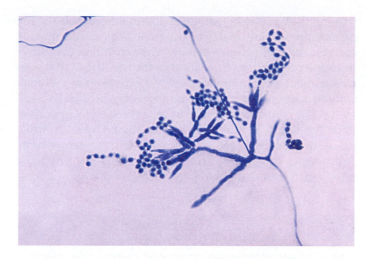

■ FIGURE 29-39 *Penicillium marneffei* produces hyaline, septate hyphae with smooth conidiophores possessing four to five metulae. The metulae support four to six phialides that produce chains of smooth or slightly rough oval conidia.
Public Health Image Library (PHIL)/CDC and Dr. Libero Ajello

 ## Checkpoint! 29–8 (Chapter Objective 8)

Biopsy material from a well-demarcated granulomatous skin lesion with crusted central ulceration is sent to the histopathology section for H & E and PAS stains. Microscopic examination revealed the presence of large, spherical to oval, thick-walled yeast cells averaging 10–12 μm in diameter. A single bud approximately of equal size to the parent cell is attached to the parent cell by a broad-based septum. What is the most likely etiological agent fitting this description?

A. Paracoccidioides brasiliensis
B. Coccidioides immitis
C. Histoplasma capsulatum
D. Blastomyces dermatitidis

▶ OPPORTUNISTIC YEASTS

Yeast are the most common fungi isolated from human patients, with two species, *Candida albicans* and *Cryptococcus neoformans*, being the major yeast pathogens. Other species are becoming an increasing problem, particularly for immunocompromised patients with cellular and humoral immunodeficiencies. Many factors may contribute to this immunosuppression, including the use of cytotoxic drugs, radiation therapy and corticosteroids, cancer, leukemia and lymphomas, HIV infection, transplanted organs, hormonal imbalances, and antibiotics that disrupt the host's normal microbiota.

There are several characteristics that serve to distinguish yeasts from the filamentous moulds. Yeasts are round to oval, unicellular organisms that reproduce by budding and that usually produce smooth, moist colonies that may be membra-nous or butyrous (creamy or butter-like in consistency). Yeasts may produce white to tan, brightly colored, or dematiaceous (black) colonies (*Exophiala* and *Wangiella* species). With few exceptions, yeast do not produce aerial hyphae but may produce many other fungal structures including blastoconidia, arthroconidia, phialides, capsules, chlamydoconidia, germ tubes, pseudohyphae, and true hyphae.

For yeast that have a sexual state, ascospores may be stained with an acid-fast stain or the spore stain. Hyphae, pseudohyphae, or both can be produced under conditions of reduced oxygen tension, as exists in host tissues. To achieve a reduced oxygen tension, yeasts can be submerged below the surface of agar, or when sedimented at the bottom of tubes of liquid media. Identification of yeasts usually involves a combination of morphological characteristics and biochemical characteristics such as urease production, nitrate and carbohydrate assimilation, and carbohydrate fermentation.

Yeasts may be part of the normal microbiota of the mucous membranes of human hosts where they compete with bacteria for space and nutrients, helping to maintain a healthy balance that prevents pathogenic organisms from becoming established and causing disease. This makes it difficult to determine the significance of yeast being isolated from clinical specimens obtained from areas containing resident microbes. Yeast is commonly found in the mucous membranes of the upper respiratory tract, gastrointestinal tract, and urogenital tract. As a general rule, the recovery of small numbers of yeast from nonsterile sites and in mixed cultures is usually not a concern. In direct contrast, the recovery of pure cultures of yeast in large numbers, or even just one or two colonies of the yeast form of systemic fungi from any sterile body site, should be considered significant. The recovery of yeast on several successive specimens should also be suspect.

The following sections cover the species of yeast that are a major cause of human disease, including cryptococcosis, candidiasis, and disseminated infection caused by *Trichosporon beigelii* (an organism previously discussed in the section covering superficial mycoses). *Candida dubliniensis, Pneumocystis jiroveci,* and *Geotrichum* spp. cause infections that are usually encountered only in severely immunocompromised patients (AIDS, leukemia, lymphoma, and transplant patients).

CRYPTOCOCCOSIS

Cryptococcosis is a fungal infection that may cause acute or chronic infection in humans. Like other sytemic fungal infections, the primary infection is acquired by inhalation of the etiological agent *Cryptococcus neoformans,* leading to a pulmonary infection that may spread to other body sites. *C. neoformans* is known to have a preference for the central nervous system and is spread via the bloodstream. It is the leading cause of fungal meningitis and brain abscesses. Dissemination to other areas of the body, such as the skin, bones, and joints, also occurs.

C. neoformans is able to produce systemic disease in individuals who have no apparent underlying immune or metabolic defects, but is more often associated with predisposing conditions such as human immunodeficiency virus (HIV) infection, leukemia, lymphomas, Cushing's syndrome, and systemic lupus erythematosus. Signs and symptoms of cryptococcal meningitis may include fever, headache, nausea, dizziness, irritability, impaired memory, and eventually gait ataxia (a staggering gait due to a loss of coordination).

The presence of a mucopolysaccharide capsule serves as a virulence factor for the organism because the capsule is antiphagocytic. The capsule may be very prominent, appearing as a wide halo in stained specimens, or may be a lighter zone surrounding the organism that is nearly undetectable. India ink stain may be helpful in demonstrating the presence of encapsulated yeasts in body fluids such as cerebrospinal fluid (Figure 14-2). Because of the presence of capsular material, *C. neoformans* usually forms large, mucoid colonies with colors ranging from cream or tan to yellow or pink (Figure 14-9). The yeast cells vary greatly in size, with a size range from 3.5 to 8 µm in diameter, and in most cases there is only a single bud attached to the parent cell by a thin connection.

C. neoformans appears to survive well in alkaline, nitrogen-rich, hypertonic environments and has been most frequently associated with the feces of pigeons and other birds, or soil contaminated with bird droppings (Garcia-Hermoso et al., 1997). A bird is not naturally infected with *C. neoformans* nor is the organism found in their fresh droppings; instead, it is the accumulation of droppings near roosting sites that serves as a reservoir for human infection.

Diagnosis of Cryptococcosis Using Serological Tests

The fact that cryptococcosis is such an important cause of morbidity and mortality in AIDS patients has led to the presence of the organism as being one of the markers of progression to AIDS in HIV-positive individuals. While many other fungal diseases can be diagnosed by demostrating the presence of detectable levels of antibody to the etiological agents, diagnosis of cryptococcosis is frequently made by demonstrating the presence of detectable capsular antigen in body fluids such as spinal fluid, serum, and urine. Latex agglutination methods employ antibody-coated latex particles, which react with polysaccharide capsular antigen producing agglutination of the particles. This method is very popular because it is sensitive, specific, rapid, and simple to perform.

A serum titer of 1:4 or higher often indicates cryptococcal infection. Titers of 1:8 or greater suggest active infection due to *C. neoformans*. Physicians may use the titer to monitor effective therapy, which is indicated by a falling titer level. Individuals with AIDS may possess very high titers.

Diagnosis of Cryptococcosis by Direct Examination

India ink, which is a colloidal suspension of carbon particles, can be used to demonstrate the hyaline capsule of *C. neoformans* in body fluids. Under conditions of reduced lighting

(closing the iris diaphragm of the light microscope), the ink particles, which are unable to penetrate the capsule, provide contrast and highlight the capsule. The percentage of positive India ink preparations in relation to the number of true positives is about 50%, so negative preparations must be cultured. Only in AIDS patients where numbers of yeast can be quite high is this method considered to be very reliable. Other specimen types such as sputum can be examined by KOH, while tissues may be examined using fungal stains to demonstrate the presence of spherical, single, or multiple budding yeast cells, which may be 4–8 µm in diameter.

REAL WORLD TIP

Most yeast stain gram positive in clinical specimens and from cultures. The blastoconidia are much larger than the gram-positive cocci of organisms such as *Staphylococcus* spp. Look for the presence of budding if yeast is suspected. *Cryptococcus neoformans* and other yeasts can exhibit a gram-variable or speckled effect. They may also appear gram negative and be easily overlooked.

REAL WORLD TIP

The CSF india ink stain is only effective about two-thirds of the time for individuals with AIDS and only about half the time in non-AIDS individuals with meningitis due to *Cryptococcus neoformans*. If capsules are not present, the organism can be grown in a 1% peptone solution to promote its formation.

Diagnosis of Cryptococcosis by Fungus Cultures

Diagnosis can be made by culturing clinical specimens such as cerebrospinal fluid and blood but urine cultures should not be overlooked as a valuable source of the organism, since *C. neoformans* is often cultured from the urine of patients with disseminated infection. *C. neoformans* is easily cultured on most fungal media. Media containing cycloheximide may inhibit growth of the yeast.

Macroscopic (Colonial) Morphology of *Cryptococcus neoformans*.
Colonies are usually large, tan, and mucoid because of the presence of the polysaccharide capsule but may become drier and darker with age. Niger seed (birdseed) or caffeic acid agar is often employed in differentiating *C. neoformans* from other yeasts because of the organism's ability to produce phenol oxidase, an enzyme that converts phenolic compounds to melanin, resulting in the production of dark brown to black colonies. Figure 14-25 demonstrates a rapid caffeic acid test for

the detection of phenol oxidase. Other biochemical tests include the rapid production of urease, nitrate (KNO_3) utilization, carbohydrate utilization, and fermentation of carbohydrates. *Cryptococcus* species are nonfermentative aerobes.

 REAL WORLD TIP

The rapid presumptive identification of *Cryptococcus neoformans* can be accomplished by: (1) gram-positive spherical budding yeast, (2) +/− presence of capsule on India ink stain, (3) production of caffeic acid using a disk test, and (4) positive rapid urea hydrolysis using a broth test.

Microscopic Morphology of *Cryptococcus neoformans*.   When *C. neoformans* is subcultured to cornmeal with polysorbate (Tween) 80, large, round to oval budding yeast are seen. Rarely rudimentary pseudohyphae may be noted.

CANDIDIASIS

Candidiasis refers to any infection caused by a member of the genus *Candida*. *Candida* species, such as *C. albicans, C. tropicalis,* and *C. parapsilosis,* are responsible for a wide variety of illnesses from chronic cutaneous and mucocutaneous infection to fatal disseminated disease. Onychomycosis (infection of the nails), *Candida* diaper rash, infection of the perineum and skin folds under the breasts and in the groin area, infection between the toes, and athlete's foot are examples of cutaneous infections which can be treated with topical ointments.

Hormonal influences may also trigger candidiasis, as evidenced by the increased risk posed to individuals such as diabetics or women using oral contraceptives or during menstruation and pregnancy. Antibiotic use can eliminate normal flora leaving only yeast, which then proliferate. Deficiencies in phagocytosis also predispose individuals to *C. albicans* infection, as is seen in chronic granulomatous disease (a congenital abnormality affecting neutrophils).

Colonization of mucosal surfaces by yeast species is not uncommon; however, a disseminated yeast infection can be life threatening if prompt treatment is not administered. In severely immunocompromised patients, these same yeast species, which may reside in the mucous membranes of healthy individuals without harm, may invade the mucosa, enter the bloodstream, and disseminate to other organs and organ systems.

Treatment of Candidiasis

Superficial infections of the skin and mucous membranes (such as vulvovaginitis) may be successfully treated with nystatin, a polyene antifungal agent that may be administered in a powdered form for moist intertriginous areas (such as the groin, armpit, and beneath pendulous breasts), given as oral tablets to treat intestinal candidiasis, or as a vaginal suppository. However, this antifungal agent cannot be used parenterally (intravenously) because of its toxicity. In the treatment of vulvovaginitis, azole creams and suppositories are more convenient and effective than nystatin suppositories. Oral systemic therapy such as ketoconazole or fluconazole may be preferred by some patients as a matter of convenience. The drug of choice to treat systemic candidiasis is amphotericin B administered intravenously but toxicity can be a problem with this antifungal agent. As an alternative, the azoles, in particular fluconazole, one of the newer imidazole antifungal agents licensed for the treatment of candidiasis and cryptococcosis, may be prescribed. Both the azoles and amphotericin B target ergosterol, a sterol found in the cell membrane of fungal cells. Unfortunately the development of resistance to the azoles has been documented.

Diagnosis of Candidiasis by Direct Examination

The presence of blastoconidia in a specimen from a nonsterile body site, such as the mucous membranes, may or may not be significant because yeast, especially *Candida albicans*, may colonize many body sites including the skin and mucous membranes. Without information on the clinical symptoms of the patient it would not be clear whether the organism had simply colonized the patient or is involved in an invasive process. The presence of yeast in a normally sterile body site, however, is a significant finding. In either case, the wisest course of action is to report the presence of yeast and allow the clinician to decide the relative importance of the organism's presence.

Yeast may produce blastoconidia (Figure 29-40 ■), pseudohyphae (Figure 29-40) that appear pinched rather than

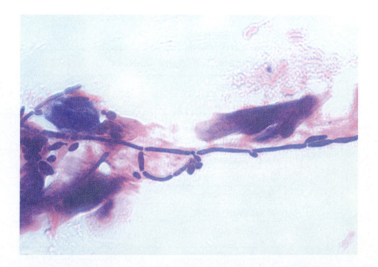

■ **FIGURE 29-40** The small oval budding blastoconidia and the long pseudohyphae can be seen on this Gram-stained smear of vaginal secretions. Note the presence of numerous epithelial cells. The etiological agent is most likely *Candida albicans*, the most common cause of candidiasis. In this case candidiasis may be a sexually transmitted disease.

possessing septates, arthroconidia, or true hyphae with septates, depending on the species involved. Gram staining is an excellent method to demonstrate the presence of yeast in clinical specimens.

For skin specimens fungal elements may be seen following the use of potassium hydroxide (KOH) to clear the specimen, allowing visualization of the fungal elements. Calcofluor white, PAS, GMS, and the H & E stain may be used to detect yeast in tissue sections and exudates. The Giemsa or Wright stain may be used to identify yeast on peripheral blood smears or bone marrow smears.

Diagnosis of Candidiasis Using Fungus Cultures

Candida species grow very well on enriched media such as brain heart infusion, blood, and chocolate agars. It is not unusual to see yeast growing on eosin methylene blue agar, which typically inhibits the growth of gram-positive organisms. Most *Candida* species should grow well on SDA with and without antibiotics including cycloheximide. SDA with antibiotics is recommended for specimens from nonsterile sites to suppress the growth of resident microbiota, which helps the yeast to proliferate.

Diagnosis of Candidiasis Using Biochemicals

∞ Chapter 14, "Fungal Cultures," presents information on the presumptive identification of *Candida*. Definitive identification requires assimilation studies and the evaluation of the yeast's ability to ferment carbohydrates and produce urease. Table 29-10✪ provides specific information on the biochemical identification of yeast.

REAL WORLD TIP

Assimilation and fermentation of carbohydrates is often used to differentiate within the *Candida* spp. Assimilation determines if the organism is able to use carbohydrates aerobically as the sole source of carbon. Turbidity is considered a positive reaction. Fermentation of carbohydrates determines if the organism is able to use carbohydrates to form energy with the production of carbon dioxide gas, ethyl alcohol, and acid by-products. A positive reaction is often determined by an acid change in the pH indicator as well as accumulation of gas in a Durham tube. Some yeast are able to assimilate carbohydrates but not ferment them.

CANDIDA ALBICANS

Candida albicans has frequently been isolated from the mucous membranes of the upper respiratory tract, the gastrointestinal tract, and the urogenital tract in asymptomatic individuals. Problems can arise, however, following the adminstration of broad-spectrum antibiotics on a long-term basis. In these cases the antibiotic disturbs the normal balance of bacteria that inhabit these nonsterile sites. Without the normal competition for attachment sites and nutrients provided by different species of bacteria, *C. albicans* is able to proliferate, becoming the predominant organism.

C. albicans frequently causes an infection of the mucosa of the oral cavity called thrush. The mouth, tongue, and throat are coated with a film of yeast (Figure 29-41 ■). It is not

✪ TABLE 29-10

Identification of Yeast Species

Yeast species	GLU	LAC	CEL	SUC	XYL	URE	GT	BLC	PSH	TRH	ARC	CMC
Candida albicans	+	−	−	+	+	−	+	+	+	+	−	+
Candida tropicalis	+	−	+	+	+	−	−	+	+	+	−	−
Candida parapsilosis	+	−	−	+	+	−	−	+	+	−	−	−
Candida glabrata	+	−	−	−	−	−	−	+	−	−	−	−
Cryptococcus neoformans	+	−	+	+	+	+	−	+	−	−	−	−
Trichosporon species	+	+	+	+	+	+	−	+	+	+	+	−
Rhodotorula species	+	−	+	+	+	+	−	+	−	−	−	−
Saccharomyces species	+	−	−	+	−	−	−	+	−	−	−	−

GLU, glucose assimilation; GT, germ tube production; LAC, lactose assimilation; BLC, blastoconidia; CEL, cellibiose assimilation; PSH, pseudohyphae; SUC, sucrose assimilation; TRH, true hyphae; XYL, xylose assimilation; ARC, arthroconidia; URE, urease production; CMC, chlamydoconidia

The germ tubes of *Candida albicans* are produced within 2–3 hours; urease production may vary according to strain; *Cryptococcus*, *Rhodotorula*, and *Saccharomyces cerevisiae* may occasionally produce short hyphae; assimilation of the various carbohydrates are subject to strain variation; (+), positive or (−), negative denotes the reaction of the majority of strains.

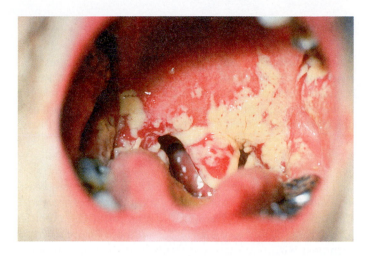

■ **FIGURE 29-41** *Candida albicans* is well known as the causative agent of thrush.

Public Health Image Library (PHIL)/CDC

uncommon to find this condition in newborns because the normal microbiota of the oral cavity is not yet well established. Thrush is also a major problem for AIDS patients, where, in conjuction with esophageal candidiasis, it may lead to dysphagia (difficulty in swallowing) because of the pain associated with these conditions. The administration of antibiotics may lead to the isolation of *C. albicans* from the stool. The gastrointestinal flora is reduced, and the yeast, which is resistant to such antibiotics, invades the mucosa, causing diarrhea. Studies have shown that the carrier rate of *C. albicans* in the GI tract may be as high as 80%.

Approximately one-fifth of urinary tract infections are caused by *C. albicans*. In such cases the organism should be quantitated in the same manner as that established for bacterial UTIs. Care should be taken to note the collection time since urine is an excellent growth medium, and specimens maintained at room temperature for extended periods of time may have falsely elevated colony counts. Balanitis (inflammation of the glans penis) and vulvovaginitis (inflammation of the female urogenital tract) can be caused by *C. albicans* and are considered to be sexually transmitted diseases. It has been postulated that recurrent vulvovaginitis may be due to an intestinal reservoir, a sexual partner with candidal balanitis, or from organisms that persist in the vagina.

Immunocompromised individuals with an intravenous catheter are at risk for candidemia. Colonization of the catheter site can occur due to a lengthy hospital stay and antibiotic use. Catheters can prove to be the portal of entry for the organism to the bloodstream. Treatment includes antifungal therapy and the removal of the colonized medical device. A peptide nucleic acid probe (PNA) fluorescent in-situ hybridization (FISH) is available to rapidly detect the presence of *C. albicans* directly from blood culture bottles (Figure 14-21).

Colonial (Macroscopic) Morphology of *Candida albicans*

Colonies grown on SDA are white to cream colored, smooth, and glistening. In many cases colonies of *C. albicans* have extensions growing from the periphery of the colonies, giving what has been termed a "spider-like," feet or fringe appearance. Growth occurs rapidly, with mature colonies within 3 days.

REAL WORLD TIP

Yeast may be able to grow on MacConkey agar. They can appear as pinpoint colonies that may be pink due to the ability to use lactose.

Microscopic Morphology of *Candida albicans*

In thrush, vaginitis, and from blood culture bottles, it is quite common to see blastoconidia, pseudohyphae, and true hyphae of *Candida albicans* that are typically 3–5 μm in diameter. In the filamentous form the hyphae are able to skewer and infiltrate host cells. These fungal elements, which are gram positive (purple colored), can readily be seen in sputum, vaginal, and stool specimens when the Gram stain is employed. They can also be seen when a KOH preparation is used to examine skin, sputum, and vaginal specimens.

When *Candida albicans* is grown on cornmeal agar with polysorbate (Tween) 80 at 22–25°C for 72 hours and examined microscopically, blastoconidia, pseudohyphae, true hyphae, and chlamydoconidia can be seen using the low power objective. By placing a light inoculum in tryptic soy broth or beef serum and incubating at 37°C for 2 hours, germ tubes (Figure 14-6) can be produced. The formation of germ tubes along with the assimilation of sucrose is sufficient to identify test organisms such as *Candida albicans*. *Candida stellatoideae* (which some consider to be a subspecies of *C. albicans*) is also germ tube positive but usually requires more than 3 or 4 hours of incubation for germ tube formation. The fact that *C. stellatoideae* fails to assimilate sucrose serves to separate the two species.

REAL WORLD TIP

Rapid identification of *Candida albicans* can be accomplished by: (1) the presence of oval budding yeast, (2) colony with fringe-like extensions, (3) production of L-prolineaminopeptidase, and (4) production of β-galactosaminidase.

REAL WORLD TIP

A RIOT (rice infusion, oxgall, and Tween 80) agar can be used to identify *C. albicans*. A small area of the agar surface is inoculated with the suspect yeast. The area is overlaid with a glass cover slip. After 3 hours incubation at 35°C, examine the cover-slipped area of the agar, using the 45× objective of the microscope, for the presence of germ tubes. The agar is held at room temperature for an additional 24 hours and examined for the presence of chlamydoconidia. *C. albicans* is germ tube positive and chlamydoconidia positive.

REAL WORLD TIP

Candida tropicalis and *C. krusei* can also produce colonies with feet or fringe.

CANDIDA GLABRATA

This organism is an opportunistic organism, causing infection in immunocompromised individuals primarily. This organism may be part of the normal microflora of the GI tract, the upper respiratory tract, and the skin of healthy individuals but has been isolated in cases of fungemia and occasionally is seen in urinary tract infections. The organism has been found to disseminate to tissues such as the lungs, kidneys, heart, and central nervous system, where it may be confused with *Histoplasma capsulatum*. Fluorescent antibody techniques and additional tests can be used to differentiate the two organisms.

Colonial (Macroscopic) and Microscopic Morphology of Candida glabrata

Candida glabrata usually forms small (pin-point), smooth, white- to cream-colored yeast colonies that require 72 hours to form mature colonies. When grown on cornmeal with polysorbate 80, the organism is seen as small blastoconidia with single buds that do not form pseudohyphae or true hyphae.

REAL WORLD TIP

Hold the sheep blood agar plate of urine cultures an additional 24 hours after reporting "no growth at 24 hours." After 48 hours of incubation, pinpoint colonies that stain as gram-positive oval budding yeast and exhibit blastoconidia after incubation on RIOT agar can be presumptively identified as *Candida glabrata.*

TRICHOSPORON BEIGELII

Trichosporon beigelii (*T. cutaneum*), the etiological agent of white piedra, was discussed previously under superficial mycoses. This organism is opportunistic. It may cause disseminated disease in immunocompromised individuals with neutropenia. Even though this organism is known to cause disease in humans it has also been recovered from the skin of healthy individuals.

Colonial (Macroscopic) and Microscopic Morphology of Trichosporon beigelii

On SDA *T. beigelii* forms smooth, moist, cream-colored yeast-like colonies. With age the colonies take on a drier appearance and have a folded topography. At this point the colonies adhere more firmly to the growth medium. When grown on cornmeal with polysorbate 80, this organism may produce blastoconidia, pseudohyphae, true hyphae, and arthroconidia. The presence of blastoconidia serves to differentiate *Trichosporon* species from *Geotrichum* species, another organism that produces arthroconidia.

CANDIDA DUBLINIENSIS

Oral candidiasis is an infection frequently seen in humans infected with the human immunodeficiency virus (HIV). In immunocompromised individuals, *Candida albicans* is the major cause of candidiasis, with other *Candida* species such as *C. tropicalis*, *C. krusei*, and *C. glabrata* playing an increasing role in the number of cases of candidiasis. In 1995 a new species of *Candida* was described based on electrophoretic karyotyping methods such as restriction fragment length polymorphism or DNA fingerprinting and pulsed field gel electrophoresis (Jabra-Risk et al., 1999). This new species, named *Candida dubliniensis,* is primarily associated with HIV-seropositive individuals, particularly those suffering from recurrent episodes of oral candidiasis, but has also been recovered from other body sites including the lungs and vagina. This organism is phenotypically similar to *Candida albicans* in its ability to form germ tubes and chlamydoconidia, colonial coloration on differential media such as CHROMagar Candida and methyl blue-sabouraud agar, and carbohydrate assimilation. It is believed that many cases of candidiasis caused by *C. dubliniensis* have falsely been attributed to *C. albicans* because germ tube and chlamydoconidia formation is the standard clinical laboratory procedure to identify *C. albicans.*

Concern over the clinical significance of *C. dubliniensis* is due to a study that indicates this organism may be more virulent than *C. albicans* because of higher levels of proteinase activity and stronger adherence to buccal epithelial cells. In addition, *C. dubliniensis* is capable of developing fluconazole resistance *in vitro* at a high frequency and therefore this organism may emerge as a resistant organism when *C. albicans* infection is successfully treated with fluconazole or some other antifungal drug.

In order to afford better treatment of immunocompromised patients suffering from recurrent bouts of candidiasis following the initially successful use of flunconazole, it may be important to distinguish between infections caused by *C. albicans* and those due to *C. dubliniensis*. Studies have shown that a combination of routine tests, including carbohydrate assimilation tests, the germ tube test, and microscopic morphology seen on cornmeal with polysorbate 80, can accomplish this (Salkin et al., 1998). *C. dubliniensis* fails to assimilate xylose and α-methyl-D-glucoside, will not grow at 45°C, produces germ tubes and abundant chlamydoconidia, and forms a dark green color on CHROMagar Candida medium.

Chlamydoconidia of *C. dubliniensis* are often attached at the end of short, hyperbranching pseudohyphae and in a characteristic triplet or pair arrangement. *C. albicans* also produces germ tubes but typically produces fewer chlamydoconidia on longer hyphae. The test that will likely appeal to mycologists in the clinical laboratory will be testing for growth at 45°C for which *C. dubliniensis* gives a negative result (growth at 42°C is not as reliable since some strains of *C. dubliniensis* grow weakly at that temperature). *C. albicans* is able to grow at 45°C, although weak or negative growth has been observed in some strains.

OTHER *CANDIDA* SPECIES

Other *Candida* species that are isolated in the clinical laboratory include: *C. tropicalis, C. parapsilosis, C. krusei,* and *C. lusitaniae*. All are known to cause infections in immunocompromised individuals. They cannot be differentiated by colony morphology. Chromogenic agar (Figure 14-10) is available, which can presumptively identify *C. albicans, C. tropicalis, C. dubliniensis,* and *C. krusei*.

C. tropicalis produces long pseudohyphae with blastoconidia along its surface. *C. parapsilosis* demonstrates blastoconidia along its long, slightly curved pseudohyphae. *C. krusei* produces long blastoconidia on the rare branches of tree-like pseudohyphae. *C. lusitaniae* demonstrates curved, branched pseudohyphae with chains of blastoconidia along its surface. It is necessary to employ additional testing, such as assimilation and fermentation of carbohydrates, to differentiate the clinically important species of *Candida*.

 REAL WORLD TIP

It is important to differentiate *C. lusitaniae* and *C. krusei* from other *Candida* spp. due to their intrinsic resistance to antifungal agents often used for treatment. *C. lustitaniae* is resistant to amphotericin B. *C. krusei* is resistant to fluconazole.

PNEUMOCYSTIS JIROVECI INFECTION (INTERSTITIAL PLASMA CELL PNEUMONIA)

Pneumocystis jiroveci, previously known as *P. carinii,* is an organism that was considered to be a sporozoan for many years until DNA relatedness studies showed this organism to be more closely related to fungi than protozoan parasites (Forbes, Sahm, & Weissfeld, 2007). This organism can be visualized using fungal stains such as methenamine silver (Figure 14-4), toluidine blue, or Giemsa stain (Figure 14-5). The cyst wall of *P. jiroveci* and the cell wall of fungi have similar ultrastructures and the intracystic structures found in the cysts of *P. jiroveci* are similar to the ascospores of ascomycetes. The 16S rRNA subunit of *P. jiroveci* is structurally similar to that of the ascomycetes and the 5S rRNA subunit to that of zygomycetes.

Pneumocystis jiroveci is the etiological agent of interstitial plasma cell pneumonia and is a particularly important pathogen of premature or malnourished infants and older adults. Other high-risk groups are immunocompromised individuals such as AIDS patients, those receiving cytotoxic or immunosuppressive drugs, and leukemia, lymphoma, and transplant patients. Although the infectious form of the organism has not been explained, inhalation is thought to be the mode of transmission. In addition to primary infection, reactivation of a latent childhood infection in immunosuppressed patients is believed to occur. Symptoms of severe *P. jiroveci* infection include rapid onset of fever, nonproductive cough, tachypnea, tachycardia, and cyanosis. Radiological examination may demonstrate a bilateral diffuse infiltrate, consolidation, and pneumothorax as terminal sequelae. Histopathological examination of lung tissue often reveals alveoli filled by a gelatinous exudate. Interstitial plasma cell pneumonia is associated with a mortality rate approaching 100%, due to acute respiratory distress and asphyxiation, if untreated. Cases in which the organism has disseminated to the spleen, lymph nodes, and bone marrow have been documented.

Treatment of *Pneumocystis jiroveci* Infection
Treatment options for *P. jiroveci* are not the same as those of other fungal infections because of the different nature of *P. jiroveci* from other fungal species, warranting their special consideration here. The treatment of choice for patients with severe *P. jiroveci* infection is trimethoprim-sulfamethoxazole given intravenously. Pentamidine isethionate administered as an inhalant spray is also available. Both medications are toxic and may produce serious side effects, necessitating careful monitoring of patients.

Diagnosis of *Pneumocystis jiroveci* Infection by Direct Examination
Because the organism cannot be cultured on artificial media, detection by histopathological staining is the primary method to diagnose infection. Many different clinical specimens can be sent to the microbiology section of the clinical laboratory, including sputum, induced sputum, tracheal aspirates, bronchoalveolar lavage, transbronchial biopsy, bronchial brushings, and tissue obtained by open thorax lung biopsy. The specimen recommended for immunocompromised patients is a lung biopsy or bronchial lavage specimen. Sputum is not recommended because the number of organisms is usually low and the organism is firmly attached to host cells. However,

AIDS patients are the exception because diagnosis can usually be accomplished by processing sputum specimens. AIDS patients exhibit numbers of organisms that are substantially higher than those seen in other patients.

The same stains used for other fungal pathogens, GMS, PAS, and calcofluor white, work well in staining cyst forms of *P. jiroveci*. The Gram-Weigert and toluidine blue stains also are used to demonstrate the presence of cyst forms. The cyst forms are spherical in shape, 4–12 µm in diameter, and contain eight intracystic forms. Fungal stains reveal the outer wall of the cyst form and two comma-shaped cyst wall thickenings but fail to stain the trophic forms (2–4 µm in diameter) or intracystic bodies. The Giemsa, Wright, and Romanowsky stains readily stain the trophic and intracystic bodies but not the cyst wall (Figure 14-5). The nuclei stain a violet color while the cytoplasm stains blue. Low cost, speed, reliability, and simplicity are advantages of using these staining methods. Immunofluorescent stains work well because both trophic and cyst forms can be demonstrated.

GEOTRICHOSIS

Geotrichosis is an infection caused by *Geotrichum candidum*, a yeast-like organism that has been found on a variety of fruits and vegetables. It also may be part of the normal microbiota of the skin and gastrointestinal tract of healthy individuals. *G. candidum* is an opportunistic pathogen that rarely causes infection except in individuals who are extremely debilitated. The organism has been implicated in wound infections and oral thrush and has been isolated from skin lesions and infected nails. It has been seen in sputum specimens as gram-positive arthroconidia and has also been isolated from urine, skin, stool, vaginal secretions, and the conjunctiva.

Colonial (Macroscopic) and Microscopic Morphology of *Geotrichum* species

G. candidum is a rapidly growing organism and produces smooth, moist, white- to cream-colored, yeast-like colonies. Microscopically, septate, hyaline hyphae that fragment into one-celled, rectangular arthroconidia (Figure 29-42 ■) that vary in length from 4 to 10 µm are seen when the organism is grown on cornmeal agar with polysorbate 80. No blastoconidia, pseudohyphae, or chlamydoconidia are produced. Diagnosis of geotrichosis and other yeast infections is summarized in Table 29-11 ✪.

REAL WORLD TIP

The pink mucoid colony of *Rhodotorula* spp. is easily recognizable. It is often found in areas with high moisture such as the bathroom. It produces oval blastoconidia but no pseudohyphae. It is usually considered an environmental contaminant.

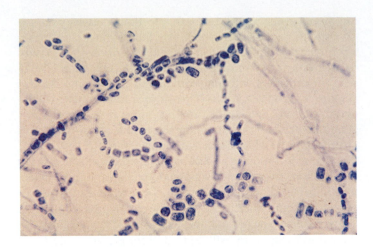
■ **FIGURE 29-42** *Geotrichum* spp. produces septate, hyaline hyphae that fragment into one-celled, rectangular arthroconidia. *Public Health Image Library (PHIL)/CDC and Dr. Lucille K. George*

✓ **Checkpoint! 29–9 (Chapter Objective 8)**

Which yeast species, although it is transmitted by inhalation and initially invades lung tissue, has a predilection for the central nervous system leading to meningitis and brain abscesses?

   A. *Candida albicans*
   B. *Candida glabrata*
   C. *Cryptococcus neoformans*
   D. *Pneumocystis jiroveci*

SUMMARY

Fungi are an integral part of the human environment, being associated primarily with soil, water, plants, and decaying vegetation. These organisms serve an important role in the decomposition of organic matter, returning valuable nutrients to the soil. When examined microscopically fungi resemble small plants but unlike plants, fungi do not possess chlorophyl and therefore require preformed organic compounds since they cannot undergo photosynthesis. Fungi have an absorptive type of nutrition whereby they secrete enzymes into the environment in order to catabolize macromolecules into their subunits, which are then absorbed. In addition, fungi have cell walls composed of chitin instead of cellulose, which makes up the cell wall of plants. Fungi reproduce asexually and also have sexual stages of reproduction. Those species in which no sexual form has been demonstrated are classified as Fungi Imperfecti. Asexual reproduction results in the formation of cells with haploid nuclei such as conidia, blastoconidia, arthroconidia, chlamydoconidia and sporangiospores. Fungi can be divided into three other phyla based on the type of sexual spore produced. The mating of two individual fungi results in spores having diploid nuclei. Ascomycetes have septate hyphae and produce sexual spores called ascospores within a sac-like

⊕ TABLE 29-11

Diagnosis of Yeast Infections

Etiological Agents	Specimen Types	Microscopic Examination	
		Cytological Examination	Slide Cultures
Cryptococcosis: *Cryptococcus neoformans*	Spinal fluid, brain abscesses, sputum, infected tissue	Spherical, single, or multiple budding yeast cells (4–8 µm in diameter)	Spherical, single, or multiple budding yeast cells (4–8 µm in diameter)
Candidiasis: *Candida albicans* (major cause of candidiasis)	Skin, respiratory secretions, feces, urine, blood, vaginal secretions, tissues	Blastoconidia with or without pseudohyphae	Blastoconidia, true hyphae, pseudohyphae, and terminal chlamydoconidia may be seen
White piedra and (rarely) disseminated infections: *Trichosporon beigelii*	Hair, infected tissues	Light-colored, segmented hyphae, 2–4 µm in diameter with round to rectangular arthroconidia and blastoconidia	Septate hyphae and arthroconidia predominate but blastoconidia and pseudohyphae may also be seen
Interstitial plasma cell pneumonia: *Pneumocystis jiroveci*	Bronchial secretions, lung tissue	Cyst forms: spherical (4–12 µm in diameter) containing eight intracystic forms Fungal stains reveal the outer wall of cyst form and two comma-shaped cyst wall thickenings Giemsa stains trophic and intracystic bodies but not the cyst wall Nuclei stain violet while cytoplasm stains blue Slide cultures are not feasible as this organism cannot be cultured on artificial media	

structure called an ascus. Basidiomycetes, which include mushrooms, produce sexual spores called basidiospores. They are formed at the tip of a pedestal called a basidium. Zygomycetes have aseptate hyphae and have sexual spores, called zygospores, which are produced from the fusion of the nuclei of two cells, resulting in the formation of a large spore enclosed in a thick wall.

Yeasts are round to oval, unicellular organisms that form smooth, creamy, discrete colonies when grown *in vitro* on a solid medium. They reproduce by budding where a swelling appears on the parent cell and enlarges by a blowing-out process. As the blastoconidium elongates, the parent cell's nucleus divides with one nucleus migrating into the daughter cell and one nucleus remaining in the parent cell. A cell wall eventually divides the two cells and in some cases the blastoconidium separates from the parent cell. At other times the blastoconidium remains attached and elongates to produce pseudohyphae. Fungi may metabolize carbohydrates in the presence of oxygen in a process called assimilation or may metabolize carbohydrates anaerobically in a process called fermentation. These and other biochemical processes along with microscopic morphology allow yeasts to be identified in the clinical laboratory.

Moulds are filamentous, multicellular organisms that grow by extension at the apical end of tubelike structures called hyphae. Masses of hyphae make up the mycelium, which spreads across the surface of a growth medium. The mycelium is responsible for the color, texture, tenacity, and topography of a mould colony. Using slide cultures the microscopic morphology of a mould may be examined, noting the fungal elements present, especially the reproductive structures that may allow the mould to be identified. Dimorphic fungi are capable of existing in two forms. They are able to grow as either moulds or yeast in a process that is temperature dependent. In the laboratory the mould form may be induced to grow by culturing on a nutrient medium at room temperature (22–25°C) while the yeast form is induced by culturing on an enriched medium such as a brain heart infusion medium supplemented with sheep blood and incubated at 35–37°C.

Of the 100,000 or so fungi that have been classified, only about 150 are associated with human illness. Some species are strict pathogens and are able to cause disease in previously healthy individuals who are immunocompetent, while others are opportunistic pathogens that normally exist on plants and in soil. Opportunistic pathogens usually pose the greatest danger to immunocompromised individuals such as AIDS patients, patients undergoing chemotherapy or radiation therapy, or leukemia, lymphoma, and transplant patients. These are individuals whose cell-mediated immunity has been compromised by conditions that affect a patient's white blood cell population.

Mycoses, or fungal infections, can range from asymptomatic infections to life-threatening infections, which, if untreated, will eventually result in the death of the patient. Some fungi, such as *Candida albicans,* can affect multiple body systems with symptoms depending on the body systems affected. Because of the ubiquitous nature of fungi, direct examination of clinical specimens may provide important clues as to the significance of isolating different fungal species on laboratory media. Many procedures are available to identify the presence of fungal elements in clinical specimens, including potassium hydroxide preparations and fungal stains, such as hemotoxylin and eosin (H & E), periodic acid-Schiff (PAS), Gomori methenamine silver (GMS), calcofluor white, and Giemsa and Gridley fungal stains. Then again, because many fungi may have similar morphological features in host tissues, it is important to recover and identify the etiological agent.

Based on the tissues affected, mycoses have been classified as superficial, cutaneous, subcutaneous, and systemic. Superficial mycoses involve the outermost layers of skin and the hair shafts. Most cases are seen in the tropics and since the tissues involved are nonvascularized there is little or no inflammation and treatment is usually for cosmetic reasons. Superficial mycoses include pityriasis or tinea versicolor, tinea nigra, white piedra, and black piedra.

Cutaneous mycoses or dermatomycoses affect keratinized tissues such as the skin, nails, and hair. Infections may be acute and self-limiting if geophilic or zoophilic species are involved or may be chronic and difficult to treat when anthropophilic species are the etiological agents. Transmission is from human to human or animal to human by direct contact with infected hairs or epidermal cells. Symptoms include itching, burning sensations, erythema (redness), scaling lesions, and brittle and broken hairs. Older lesions are ring-like in shape with a well-defined advancing margin, leaving a central area with some clearing. Clinical manifestations depend on the tissues affected and are named based on the body area affected: tinea capitis, tinea barbae, tinea corporis, tinea cruris, tinea pedis, and tinea unguium. Etiological agents include *Epidermophyton floccosum*, *Microsporum*, and *Trichophyton* species.

As the name implies, subcutaneous mycoses are fungal infections in which subcutaneous tissues are invaded. The route of transmission is through traumatic implantation in which fungal elements gain entrance through some type of puncture wound usually involving thorns, splinters, or other sharp objects that push the fungus or soil and plant material containing the fungus into the tissues. Many of the etiological agents are dematiaceous fungi, which have melanin within the cell wall so the hyphal elements are darkly pigmented. The fungi involved with subcutaneous mycoses are normally soil saprobes such as *Cladosporium*, *Phialophora*, and *Fonsecaea* species, *Scedosporium apiospermum*, and *Sporothrix schenckii*, which can cause diseases such as eumycotic mycetoma, chro-

moblastomycosis, and sporotrichosis when introduced into host tissues. Direct examination and fungus cultures are important in the diagnosis and treatment of subcutaneous mycoses.

The systemic mycoses are fungal infections of the deep tissues and may affect many different tissues and body systems. The etiological agents are fungi that are normally found in soil but may gain entrance into humans through inhalation of spores. Most infections are either asymptomatic infections or pulmonary infections, which produce influenza-like symptoms. These infections primarily involve the lungs but in some cases the organism may disseminate to other organ systems such as the skin and bones, producing granulomatous lesions. Histoplasmosis, blastomycosis, and coccidioidomycosis are the systemic fungal diseases encountered most often in the United States but immunocompromised patients are at high risk of developing aspergillosis and mucormycosis, rare diseases caused by saprophytic fungi. Because the agents of the systemic mycoses have characteristic morphotypes in host tissues, direct examination of clinical specimens can be very beneficial in beginning antifungal therapy as soon as possible. When fungal cultures are attempted it is important to remember that these diseases are transmitted by inhalation and safety precautions to prevent conidia from becoming airborne must be followed.

Pathogenic yeasts such as *Candida albicans* and *Cryptococcus neoformans* are a major source of morbidity and mortality in humans. *C. albicans* is commonly seen as a cause of thrush, diaper rash, and vulvovaginitis but is also known to colonize moist areas of skin and the mucous membranes where the organism may be a part of an individual's normal microbiota. Cases of disseminated candidiasis and fungemia are serious infections attributed to *C. albicans* and other members of the genus *Candida*. *Cryptococcus neoformans* can be found in a saprophytic existence in soil enriched with excreta of birds and bats. Humans are infected following inhalation of the organism where an asymptomatic or pulmonary infection may result. Because the *C. neoformans* has a predilection for the central nervous system it may be seen in cases of meningitis and brain abscesses where procedures such as an India ink preparation may be employed to demonstrate the presence of encapsulated yeast or demonstration of the polysaccharide capsular antigen in spinal fluid may be used in the diagnosis of cryptococcosis. Table 29-12✪ summarizes some of the unique macroscopic and microscopic characterisitics that may help in the initial workup of fungi.

Unique Macroscopic and Microscopic Characteristics Associated with Some Fungi

If You See:	Consider:	Other Possibilities:
Chlamydoconidia	Candida albicans	C. dubliniensis C. stellatoidea
Arthroconidia	Geotrichum spp.	Trichosporon beigelii Coccidioides immitis
Pinpoint yeast colonies	Candida glabrata	Malassezia furfur
Pink mucoid yeast colonies	Rhodotorula spp.	
Mucoid white yeast colonies	Cryptococcus neoformans	
Cream or white yeast colony with feet or fringe	Candida albicans	C. tropicalis C. krusei
Black yeast	Exophiala jeanselmei Wangiella dermatitidis Hortaea wernickii	
Yeast within white blood cells	Histoplasma capsulatum	
Broad base budding yeast	Blastomyces dermatitidis	
Yeast with buds around its periphery like a ship's steering wheel	Paracoccidioides brasiliensis	
Cigar-shaped yeast cells	Sporothrix schenckii	
White mould at 25°C and yeast at 35°C	Dimorphic fungi ■ Sporothrix schenckii ■ Histoplasma capsulatum ■ Blastomyces dermatitidis ■ Paracoccidioides brasiliensis	
Spherules	Coccidioides immitis	
Lavender or purple mould	Fusarium spp.	
Black mould	Dematiaceous fungi ■ Bipolaris spp. ■ Exophiala spp. ■ Scedosporium spp. ■ Curvularia spp. ■ Fonsecaea spp. ■ Cladosporium spp. ■ Alternaria spp. ■ Wangiella spp. ■ Hortaea werneckii	Other moulds
Red mould	Penicillium marneffei	
Broad, ribbon-like, aspetate hyphae which tends to fold onto itself or break	Zygomycetes ■ Mucor spp. ■ Rhizopus spp. ■ Absidia spp.	Rhizomucor spp.
Septate hyphae with 45° branching	Aspergillus spp.	
Granules in pus	Pseudallescheria boydii Exophiala jeanselmei Acremonium spp. Curvularia spp. Madurella spp.	Other moulds Nocardia spp. Actinomadura spp. Streptomyces spp.
Sclerotic bodies	Cladosporium spp. Fonsecaea spp. Phialophora spp.	

LEARNING OPPORTUNITIES

1. What important role in nature do saprophytic fungi serve? (Chapter Objective 6)

2. List five aspects of nonspecific immunity that contribute to host resistance to fungal infection. (Chapter Objective 2)

3. Why would a patient who has undergone an organ transplant be at greater risk of developing a fungal infection than a person in the general population? (Chapter Objective 3)

4. Matching: (Chapter Objective 9)

   Match the fungal disease with the clinical presentation.

   Superficial Mycosis

   _____ Pityriasis versicolor

   _____ Superficial phaeohyphomycosis

   _____ White piedra

   _____ Black piedra

   Characteristic Features

   a. White to tan nodules

   b. Brown to black macules

   c. Brown to black macules

   d. "Spaghetti and meatballs"

5. Why is it important to distinguish between cases of actinomycotic mycetoma and cases of eumycotic mycetoma? (Chapter Objective 11)

CASE STUDY 29-1   (CHAPTER OBJECTIVES 8, 9, AND 10)

A 55-year-old male living in Ohio who enjoys horticulture as a hobby and a source of fresh vegetables embedded a splinter into the palmar surface of his right hand near the base of the thumb while handling the wooden poles he used to stake his tomato plants. The splinter was at such a depth he was unable to pull it out easily and the splinter remained embedded until the soreness disappeared in a few days. At this point he was able to remove the splinter using a straight pin sterilized over a flame. The injured area healed without incident and the initial wounding remained largely forgotten until weeks later when a small subcutaneous swelling, which was firm to the touch but painless, developed on his right hand. A few more weeks passed in which the swollen area enlarged very gradually but very little pain was experienced. Eventually a blister appeared at the base of the thumb, which soon opened to discharge a serosanguinous exudate. This development alarmed the man to the point he sought medical attention. His clinician expressed more fluid from the tumorlike lesion, noticing the presence of yellowish, firm granules, ranging in size from 1 to 2 mm. Abscess drainage, which was collected using a needle and syringe after careful cleansing of the overlying skin, was submitted to the microbiology section for routine, anaerobic, and fungus cultures. In the laboratory a KOH preparation was made revealing the presence of hyaline hyphae, 2–5 μm in diameter, in the central part of the granule. At the periphery of the granule, the hyphae were swollen, producing oval cells of 10–20 μm.

For fungus cultures, the exudate was subcultured to sabouraud dextrose agar, sabouraud's 2% dextrose agar with chloramphenicol, and a tryptose agar base supplemented with 10% sheep blood. The sheep blood agar medium was incubated at 37°C and the sabouraud's agar media were incubated at 30°C. After 3 days, sabouraud's culture yielded white, cottony, spreading colonies that later turned gray. The reverse was at first white but became gray with age. Microscopic examination showed septate hyaline hyphae, which were 2–4 μm in diameter, with unicellular conidia 9 × 5 μm in diameter borne terminally, singly, or in small groups on elongated, narrow, erect, simple, or branched conidiophores. The conidia were ovoid, with the larger end toward the apex, appeared to be cut off at the base, and had a distinct brown wall. This organism did not exhibit dimorphism.

1. What is the identity of the etiological agent recovered from the sabouraud agars? Give the name of the anamorph. (Chapter Objectives 5 and 8)

2. What clinical entity (type of mycosis) is represented in this case study? (Chapter Objective 10)

3. What is the sexual state of this fungus? (Chapter Objective 5)

CASE STUDY 29-2   (CHAPTER OBJECTIVES 8, 9, AND 10)

A 24-year-old female who is diabetic and sexually active is seen by her gynecologist with complaints of itching and burning in the vagina. She tells the clinician that symptoms are exacerbated just prior to menstruation. Pelvic examination revealed vulvar erythema and the vaginal mucosa is reddened with whitish patches that can be removed by gentle scraping. The vaginal discharge is white and curd-like. Three swabs are sent to the laboratory with a request for a Gram stain, vaginal culture, and fungus cultures.

The Gram stain revealed the presence of numerous pus cells, epithelial cells, long, slender, gram-positive rods in short chains and singly, and a few gram-negative rods. Most notable was the presence of oval blastoconidia and pseudohyphae that measure 3–5 μm in diameter. The pseudohyphae exhibit branching, oval budding yeast, and constriction at the septae.

On the blood and chocolate agar plates and on the sabouraud agar plates, white- to cream-colored, yeast-like colonies with "spider-like" extensions from the periphery appear after 24–48 hours. The colonies are smooth and glistening and have a butyrous consistency. A Gram stain reveals the organisms are oval-shaped blastoconidia.

1. What is the diagnosis for this patient? (Chapter Objective 10)

2. What is the most likely etiological agent in this case? (Chapter Objectives 8, 9, and 10)

3. What biochemical and physiological tests are commonly used to identify this agent and what are the anticipated results? (Chapter Objective 9)

4. What fungal elements are typically seen when this organism is subcultured to cornmeal with polysorbate (Tween) 80? (Chapter Objective 9)

5. What antifungal therapy is likely to be prescribed to control this infection of the mucous membranes? (Chapter Objective 11)

PEARSON
myhealthprofessionskit™

Use this address to access the interactive Companion Website created for this textbook. Simply select "Clinical Laboratory Science" from the choice of disciplines. Find this book and log in using your user name and password.

REFERENCES

Go to myhealthprofessionskit.com to view this chapter's references.

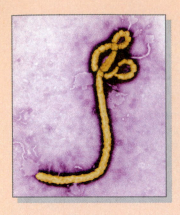

30

Parasitology

William C. Payne

■ LEARNING OBJECTIVES

Upon completion of this chapter, the learner should be able to:

1. Discuss factors that promote or prevent the transmission of parasites.
2. List the common and scientific names of each parasite.
3. Describe the general morphological characteristics of each parasite.
   a. Differentiate parasites among and within classes based on morphological characteristics.
   b. Differentiate parasites from common fecal artifacts.
4. Diagram the life cycle of each parasite.
   a. Identify the diagnostic stage to include the specimen of choice and optimal conditions for recovery.
   b. Associate intermediate, defininitve, reservoir hosts and/or vectors involved in transmission and the parasite form found in each.
   c. Relate the geographic distribution of each.
   d. Determine laboratory procedures for detection and diagnosis.
5. Associate the disease state(s) for each parasite.
   a. Summarize the major symptoms and pathology of infection.
   b. Relate parasites more common in immunosuppressed individuals.
6. Correlate patient history, specimen type/body site, laboratory test results, clinical signs and symptoms, and other data to predict potential parasites.
   a. Select the most probable parasite.
   b. Assess the clinical significance of each.
   c. Determine if additional testing is necessary for confirmation.
7. Recognize critical results.
8. Discuss methods to control, prevent, and treat parasitic infections.

KEY TERMS

definitive host	periodicity	sporogony
ectoparasite	pseudoparasite	steatorrhoea
endoparasite	reservoir host	vector
enzootic	schizogony	xenodiagnosis
intermediate host		

TAXONOMY

Kingdom: Protoctista
  Subkingdom: Protozoa
    Phylum: Sarcomastigophora
      Class Lobosea
        Order Amoebida
          Acanthamoeba (ay-kanth′-uh-mee-buh)
          Endolimax nana (en-doe-lī-maks)
            (nay′-nuh)
          Entamoeba coli (en′-tuh-mee′-buh) (kō′-lye)
          E. dispar (dis′-par)
          E. hartmanni (hart-man′-nee)
          E. histolytica (his-toe-lit′-ee-kuh)
          E. polecki (pō-lek′-ee)
          Iodamoeba bütschlii (eye-oh′-dah-mee′-bah)
            (boot-shlee′-eye)
        Order Schizopyrenida
          Naegleria fowleri (nah′-glâr-ee′-uh)
            (fow-ler′-eye)
      Class Zoomastigophorea
        Order Retortamonadida
          Chilomastix mesnili (kī″-lō-mast′-iks)
            (mes′-nil′-eye)
        Order Trichomonadida
          Dientamoeba fragilis (dye-en′-tuh-mee′-buh)
            (fradj″-i-lis)
          Trichomonas hominis (trik″-oh-mō′-nas)
            (hom′-i-nis)
          T vaginalis (vaj-i-nal′-is)
        Order Diplomonadida
          Giardia lamblia (jee′-are-dee′-uh)
            (lam-blee′-uh)
        Order Kinetoplastida
          Leishmania donovani (līsh-may′-nee-uh)
            (don″-ō-vah′-nigh)
          L. braziliensis (bra-zil″-ē-en′-sis)
          L. tropica complex (trop′-i-kuh)
          Trypanosoma brucei gambiense (trip-an″-ō-
            sō′-muh) (brew′-see-eye) (gam-bee-en′-see)

          T. brucei rhodesiense (brew′-see-eye)
            (rō-dee″-zee-en′-see)
          T. cruzi (kroo′-zye)
          T. rangeli (ran-jel′-ee)
    Phylum: Ciliophora
      Class Litostomatea
        Order Vestibuliferida
          Balantidium coli (bal′-an-tid′-ee-um)
            (kō′-lee)
    Phylum: Apicomplexa
      Class Sporozoasida
        Order Eucoccidiorida
          Babesia microti (bab-ee″-zee′-uh)
            (mī-krot′-ee)
          Cryptosporidium parvum (krip″-toe-spor-i′-
            dee-um) (par′-voom)
          Cyclospora species (sī′-klō-spor-uh)
          Isospora belli (eye″-sos′-por-uh) (bell′-eye)
          Plasmodium falciparum (plaz-mō′-dee-um)
            (fal-sip′-uh-rum)
          P. malariae (ma-lair′-ee-ee)
          P. ovale (ovay′-lee)
          P. vivax (vī′-vaks)
          Sarcocystis (sahr″-kō-sis′-tis)
          Toxoplasma gondii (tok″-sō-plaz′-muh)
            (gon′-dee-eye)
  *Uncertain phylogenetic affinity:
          Blastocystis hominis (blast′-oh-sis-tis)
            (hom-in′-is)
    Phylum: Microspora
      Class Microsporididea
        Order Pleistophoridida
          Encephalitozoon (ën-sëf-ŭ-līt-ë-zō-än)
          Pleistophora (plēs-tä-fō-rŭ)
        Order Nosematidida
          Nosema (nō-sē-më)

(continued)

TAXONOMY (*continued*)

Phylum: Nematoda
  Class Enoplea
    Order Trichurida
      Trichinella spiralis (trik″-i-nel′-uh) (spi′-rä′-lis)
      Trichuris trichiura (trik-yoo′-ris)
        (trik″-ee-yoo′-ruh)
    Order Rhabditida
      Strongyloides stercoralis (stron″-jee-loy′-deez)
        (stir″-kor-rä′-lis)
    Order Strongylida
      Ancylostoma braziliensis (an″-si′-lō-stō′-muh)
        (bra-zil″-ē-ën′-sis)
      A. caninum (kay′-nī-num)
      A. duodenale (dew″-ŏ-dë-nä′-lee)
      Necator americanus (ne-kay′-tur)
        (ah′-mer″-i-kä′-nus)
    Order Ascaridida
      Anisakis species (an″-i-sō′-kis)
      Ascaris lumbricoides (as′-kâr-is) (lum-bri-koy′-deez)
      Toxocara canis (tok″-sō-kah′-rah) (kay′-nis)
      T. cati (ca′-tī)
    Order Oxyurida
      Enterobius vermicularis (en″-tur-ō′-bee-us)
        (vur-mik-yoo-lair′-us)
  Family Dracunculidea
    Dracunculus medinensis (drah-kun″-ku-lus)
      (med″-in-nen′-sis)
  Family Onchocercidae
    Brugia malayi (broo′-jee-ah) (mah-lay-eye)
    Dirofilaria immitis (dye″-rō-fil-air-ee-ah)
      (im′-mi-tis)
    Loa loa (lō′-uh) (lō′-uh)
    Mansonella ozzardi (man″-so-nel′-ah)
      (o-zar′-dee)
    M. perstans (per′-stans)
    M. streptocerca (strep′-to-sir′-cuh)

    Onchocerca volvulus (on′-kō-sir′-kuh)
      (vol-vyoo-lus)
    Wuchereria bancrofti (wooch-ur-rare′-ee-uh)
      (ban-krof′-tĭ)
Phylum: Platyhelminthes
  Class Cercomeridea
    Subclass Trematoda
    Infraclass Digenea
      Clonorchis sinensis (klo-nor′-kis) (si-nen′-sis)
      Fasciola hepatica (fä-see′-oh-luh) (he-pat′-i-kuh)
      Fasciolopsis buski (fä-see′-oh-lop′-sis) (bus′-kī)
      Heterophyes heterophyes (het-ur-off′-ee-eez)
        (het-ur-off′-ee-eez)
      Metagonimus yokogawai (met′-uh-gon-i-mus)
        (yō-kō-gah-wah′-eye)
      Paragonimus westermani (par″-i-gon′-i-mus)
        (wes-tur-man′-eye)
      Schistosoma haematobium (shis′-toe-sō′-muh)
        (hee-muh′-toe-bee-um)
      S. japonicum (ja-pon′-i-kum)
      S. mansoni (man-so′-nī)
  Infraclass Cestodaria
    Cohort Cestoidea
      Order Pseudophyllidea
        Diphyllobothrium latum (dye-fil″-o-both′-ree-um) (lay′-tum)
      Order Cyclophillidea
        Dipylidium caninum (dip″-i-lid′-ee-um)
          (kay-nī′-num)
        Echinococcus granulosus (eh-kī″-nō-kok′-us)
          (gran-yoo-lō′-sus)
        Hymenolepis diminuta (high″-men-ō-lep′-is)
          (dim-in-oo′-tuh)
        H. nana (nay′-nuh)
        Taenia saginata (tee′-nee-uh) (sa-ji-nät′-uh)
        T. solium (sō-li-um)

▶ INTRODUCTION

Parasitology is the field of study that deals with organisms (parasites) that live within or upon another organism for the purpose of obtaining nourishment. Parasites have interacted with humans and other animals for millennia and only within recent history have medical practitioners been able to effectively deal with many parasitic diseases.

Several conditions have contributed to the fact that parasitic diseases are not prevalent in the United States and other industrialized countries. Advances in sanitation and proper disposal of human waste and practicing good hygiene are important in preventing the spread of parasites. In addition, the dormant stages of parasites, which allow survival in a less than ideal environment, cannot thrive in the cold weather conditions experienced in countries with a temperate climate. Finally, most of these countries lack suitable **vectors** (the organism that transmits the parasite), **intermediate hosts** (where the parasite must develop for a short time), and **reservoir hosts** (harbor the parasite indefinitely with no ill effects), which the parasites need to continue their life cycles.

Unfortunately, in recent years parasitic diseases have again become a medical and public health problem, even in industrialized countries where parasites had ceased to become a major source of human morbidity and mortality. A number of factors have contributed to an increase in the number and variety of parasitic infections occurring worldwide. Jet travel and international wars have exposed uninfected individuals to parasitic diseases that are not found in their country of origin. War refugees who flee from areas of conflict to other countries may present a clinician with parasitic diseases that are not normally found in their adopted countries.

Another factor contributing to an increase in parasitic diseases is the emergence of strains of mosquitoes that are resistant to pesticides. In addition, some parasitic species have become resistant to drugs used in the prevention and treatment of parasitic diseases. For example, strains of *Plasmodium falciparum,* which are resistant to chloroquine (a synthetic antimalarial drug), have emerged.

Our use of technology has been both beneficial and detrimental. By improving sanitation in underdeveloped countries we have decreased certain parasitic diseases, but in turn, building projects have changed the environment and taken construction workers into areas where they are exposed to **enzootic** parasites (those capable of infecting man and animals). These parasites are endemic to the area and to animals that serve as vectors and hosts.

The increased population of immunosuppressed individuals has led to an increase in the number of parasitic diseases seen in industrialized countries. The immune system can be damaged by underlying illnesses or our attempt to treat serious illnesses. Such individuals are now more susceptible to uncomon parasitic infections.

Newer diagnostic techniques that are more sensitive, and more specific, such as the polymerase chain reaction (PCR) coupled with an increased awareness that parasitic infections can be a likely source of human illness, should lead to a realization of the importance of parasitology in medical curricula.

 **Checkpoint! 30–1
(Chapter Objective 1)**

Which of the following are factors that have contributed to the increase in the number and variety of parasitic infections?

A. *Environmental changes*
B. *Emergence of resistance to antimicrobials and insecticides*
C. *Faster modes of transportation*
D. *An increase in the number of susceptible hosts*
E. *All of the above*

▶ MEDICAL PARASITOLOGY

Symbiosis, a permanent association of two organisms that cannot exist independent of one another, may be epitomized by the old proverb, "Adversity makes strange bedfellows." This relationship gives one or both organisms an advantage in the competition for space and nutrients that exists between all living organisms. In mutualism both organisms are benefitted. In other symbiotic relationships one organism (the host) provides shelter and nutrients to the benefit of another organism (the parasite). The parasitic organism obtains part or all of its nourishment from the host and derives all the benefit from the association. The host may show no detrimental or harmful effects or may suffer various diseases or disorders.

An important concept in this relationship is that a successful parasite does not kill the host. In most cases, the death of the host would lead to the death of the parasite and this, in turn, would interrupt further propagation of the parasite by terminating the life cycle. Humans, other animals, and even plants may serve as hosts for parasitic organisms. The subject matter in this chapter centers on human parasites and enzootic parasites (those that may infect man and other animals).

CLASSIFICATION OF PARASITES

The host–parasite relationship is seen in many variations. If the parasite lives outside the host's body it is referred to as an **ectoparasite** and results in an infestation of the host. If the parasite lives within the body of the host it is called an **endoparasite** and the result is an infection of the host. Some parasites are capable of leading both a free existence (apart from the host) and parasitic existence depending on the stage of the life cycle and the availability of a suitable host. In such cases the term "facultative parasite" is used. In other cases the organism establishes a permanent residence in the host and may not be capable of existing apart from the host. The appropriate term in this case is obligate parasite. In this situation the parasite is completely dependent upon the host for its existence. An incidental parasite is one that establishes itself in a host in which it does not ordinarily live. If the parasitic organism causes injury to the host in procuring nourishment, by its migration through the tissues of the host, or by the production of toxins it is a pathogenic parasite.

For an inexperienced laboratory worker an artifact may be easily mistaken for a parasite. Objects such as yeast, pollen, WBCs, organic debris, and undigested vegetable matter may appear to be parasitic forms but are, in truth, **pseudoparasites** or artifacts. A spurious parasite is a foreign species that has passed through the gastrointestinal tract without causing an infection. It is a true parasite, but its native host is another species. Some parasites can only infect a specific host or a closely related host species and residence in any other species does not result in a parasitic relationship. For example, it is possible to find the eggs of a plant nematode in the feces of humans who have eaten root vegetables but this does not represent a true infection.

LIFE CYCLES

In studying parasites, especially parasitic helminths, it is evident that these organisms have developed rather complicated life cycles. Some spend their entire lives within the host, one generation after another. *Trichomonas vaginalis,* a protozoan parasite, is transmitted by direct contact between an infected and uninfected host. No cyst stage (an environmentally resistant form) has yet been demonstrated so exposure to the environment would have to be brief. Other parasites are capable of leaving the host's body as environmentally resistant forms such as cysts, eggs, or larvae. At these stages in the life cycle the parasite remains in a quiescent or dormant stage until they are introduced into the body of another host to begin a new cycle of growth and propagation. *Entamoeba histolytica* and *Enterobius vermicularis* (the pinworm) are good examples.

Some parasites undergo a period in which they can exist in a free state. This free-living stage may still undergo growth and development while in the external environment as they await the opportunity to infect a new host. *Necator americanus* and *Ancylostoma duodenale* (human hookworms) are prime examples of this. In a more complex life cyle the parasite may have developmental stages that must occur in another host before infecting the final host. *Plasmodium* species, which cause malaria, and *Clonorchis sinensis,* the Chinese liver fluke, provide excellent examples of this. When more than one host species is involved different terms are used to denote the role the host plays in the life cycle of the parasite in question. The **definitive host** harbors the adult (sexually mature) parasite or the sexual stage of the parasite. The intermediate host is any species in which part or all of the developmental stages may be passed. If there is more than one intermediate host it is so designated by number (i.e., the first intermediate host or the second intermediate host). In addition, there may be animals that harbor the same species as man and that may serve as additional sources of infection. In other words, a parasite may be transmitted from man to man or from another animal to man. This animal species is referred to as the reservoir host. While medicines are available to treat humans, it may not be feasible to treat all susceptible animal species, making control of parasitic infections involving intermediate hosts more difficult.

Whenever the existence of a parasite is discovered, knowledge of the life cycle is important because it allows treatment to be applied at stages where preventative measures are the most effective. It also enables the technologist to possess greater insight as to the best means to isolate and identify the diagnostic stage of the parasite. In addition, knowing where an organism is endemic may be important in the identification of the parasite (i.e., differentiation of West African sleeping sickness versus East African sleeping sickness is usually accomplished on the basis of geographic distribution because the two strains are morphologically indistinguishable).

PREDISPOSING FACTORS

Simply harboring a parasite does not guarantee the host will suffer clinically apparent infection. Certain factors seem to be associated with symptomatic infection. Hosts infected with low numbers of hookworms will likely be asymptomatic but if large numbers of hookworms are involved the loss of blood may be greater than the capacity of the host to replenish the blood loss and an anemia may result. *Ascaris* in low numbers may not cause apparent injury to the host but in large numbers this parasitic roundworm may cause intestinal obstruction. *Entamoeba histolytica,* a protozoan parasite, elaborates proteolytic enzymes that erode the intestinal wall, resulting in ulceration, bleeding, and diarrhea. Parasites of sufficiently large size may traumatize host tissues through their physical activities. *Fasciolopsis buski,* a large intestinal fluke, may damage the intestinal mucosa because of its powerful suckers. *Ascaris* may perforate the bowel wall in response to drugs and other noxious stimuli in an effort to escape the gastrointestinal tract.

ARTIFACTS AND PSEUDOPARASITES

The most impressive characteristic that is noted upon examining fecal material is the large amount of debris present. For the novice parasitologist it may at first be difficult to decipher what is "organic and inorganic debris" and artifacts from that which is truly a parasite. It is equally important to distinguish body cells of the host from parasitic forms. Those who are very proficient at this task have acquired this capability through experience and careful observation. In this section the most commonly encountered pseudoparasites and artifacts are discussed along with morphological characteristics that serve to distinguish them from true parasitic forms such as cysts, eggs, and larvae.

The most common artifacts that are confused with true parasites are leukocytes or white blood cells. Neutrophils may appear to have two to four nuclei, which very closely resemble the nuclei of certain amoeba species (Figure 30-1 ■). Compare Figure 30-1 (neutrophil) to Figure 30-18 (*E. coli* cyst) to see the resemblence. When stained, white blood cells appear to have peripheral chromatin around the edge of the nuclear membrane and a karyosome in the center of the nucleus, which leads them to be confused with the cysts of *Entamoeba* species. Distinguishing characteristics that allow the differentiation of amoebic cysts from body cells of the host include the lack of cyst walls, chromatoidal bars, or glycogen vacuoles in human body cells. In addition, human cells have a higher nuclear material to cytoplasm (N/C) ratio (the amount of nuclear material relative to the amount of cytoplasm).

Macrophages possess a single nucleus and sometimes ingest red blood cells and for this reason may be mistakenly identified as *Entamoeba histolytica* trophozoites. Again, the nuclear to cytoplasmic ratio is higher than that of amoebae. Sometimes degenerate macrophages are seen. They can be identified

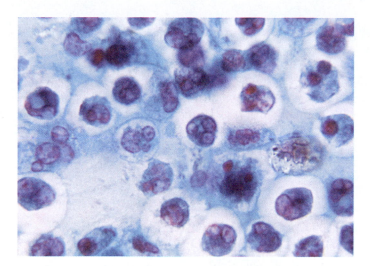

■ FIGURE 30-1 Fecal leukocytes (Trichome stain). Many appear to have two to four nuclei with peripheral chromatin and a karyosome. Fecal leukocytes may be confused with the cysts of *Entamoeba* species.
From Public Image Library (PHIL), CDC.

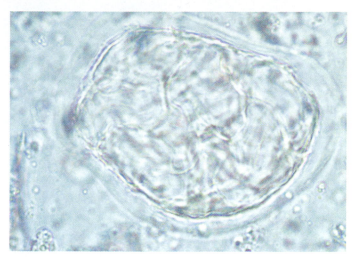

■ FIGURE 30-2 Plant parenchymal cells (direct wet mount preparation 400× magnification). Note the presence of the highly refractile cell wall and irregular cell interior.

by the presence of darkly staining inclusions and the lack of a visible nucleus.

Yeasts are commonly found in stool specimens and their presence is not considered to be significant when fecal material is examined for the presence of parasites. Yeast cells are frequently confused with protozoan cysts, especially those of *Chilomastix mesnili* because of their small size and oval shape. Morphological characteristics that distinguish yeast cells from cyst forms include their variation in size, budding, and the presence of multiple, solid nuclei of differing size that are scattered throughout the cytoplasm.

Parenchyma cells of plants are about the same size and shape as helminth eggs. Parenchymal cells containing starch granules may resemble eggs in packets or the early cleavage stage of hookworm eggs. Because humans cannot digest cellulose, the building block of plant cell walls, whole cells or empty cell walls may be found in feces. Plant cells characteristically have thick, smooth cell walls and are frequently irregular in shape and size (Figure 30-2 ■). Starch granules stain blue to black when an iodine solution is used as an aid in the microscopic examination of stool specimens for eggs and protozoan parasites. These characteristics are helpful in distinguishing plant parenchymal cells from true parasites.

Plant root hairs are commonly confused with hookworm larvae because of their size and shape. Differential characteristics include thick refractile cell walls, a hollow central canal extending throughout their length, and the lack of distinct internal structures such as the digestive tract of free-living larval forms of hookworms and *Strongyloides*. The posterior (or caudal) (tail) end of free-living larval forms is tapered while the anterior (head) end contains the buccal cavity.

Oil droplets, pollen grains, and diatoms may resemble cyst forms because they are small and uniform in size but they lack

internal structures. A fat stain such as Oil Red O or Sudan black can be used to verify the presence of oil droplets. They are removed by concentration procedures when a solvent such as ethyl acetate is used.

Pollen grains (Figure 30-3 ■) and diatoms (Figure 30-4 ■) are very regular in shape and size and may be present in large numbers depending on the host's dietary habits. Both diatoms and pollen grains can be ingested in food and water sources. While pollen grains are of plant origin, diatoms are a type of algae that can be found in fresh water, marine water, and moist soil. Diatoms are single celled and encased within a silicon-based cell wall. Consistency in shape and size is a characteristic of parasitic forms and therefore a novice may be tempted to regard pollen grains or diatoms as a parasite egg. The lack

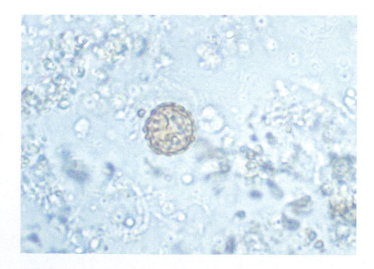

■ FIGURE 30-3 Pollen grain (direct wet mount preparation 400× magnification).

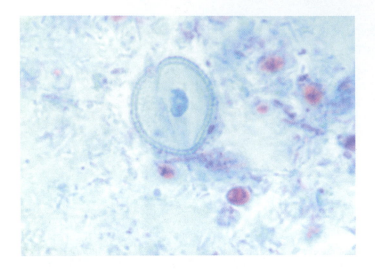

■ FIGURE 30-4 Diatom (direct wet mount preparation 400× magnification).

of internal structures is a good clue that the object in question is probably not a parasite.

Vegetable fibers, which are part of the supportive structures of plants, exhibit a spiral structure and are not likely to be confused with parasitic forms. Mention is made here simply to satisfy the curiosity of those wishing to identify these interesting, large structures, which are readily apparent even when the low power or scanning objective is employed (Figure 30-5 ■).

Muscle fibers may also be found when the direct wet mount or the sediment from a concentration procedure is examined. These objects may appear when intestinal mobility is so great food cannot be completely digested (as seen in cases of severe diarrhea). In other illnesses, such as pancreatic insufficiency, the enzymes that degrade protein are not produced in sufficient quantity to digest flesh foods and therefore undigested

muscle fibers may be found. Undigested muscle fibers can be distinguished by the striations that can be seen even when the low power objective is employed.

Charcot-Leyden crystals are frequently seen in smears made from stool specimens. They stain red on the trichrome stain and are seen as highly refractile, fusiform-shaped (long, thin, with pointed ends) crystals in wet mounts (Figure 30-6 ■). These crystals are thought to be the by-product of eosinophil degradation. Eosinophils may be associated with allergic reactions and parasitic infections.

INTESTINAL AND UROGENITAL PROTOZOAN PARASITES (AMOEBAE, FLAGELLATES, AND CILIATES)

Protozoa, single-celled eukaryotes that infect humans, may be classified as *amoebae* (singular, *amoeba*), flagellates, or ciliates. Amoebae have a naked protoplast during their trophozoite stage and move in a manner that is termed "amoeboid motion." When observing motile amoebae the protoplasm seems to glide forward in the direction of locomotor organelles called *pseudopodia* (singular, *pseudopodium*), which begin as a bulge on the surface of the organism and elongate into blunt or fingerlike projections of the protoplasm.

Flagellates are unicellular organisms that possess one to several long, delicate, thread-like extensions of the cytoplasm, termed *flagella* (singular, *flagellum*), which serve as locomotor organelles. Most species of flagellate protozoa possess a rudimentary oral depression, called a cytostome.

Ciliates are unicellular organisms that possess short, thread-like projections from the cytoplasmic membrane called cilia. The cilia beat in a coordinated rhythm, producing wave-like movements along the surface of the organism, moving the organism forward or backward. Many ciliates also possess a distinct cytostome that functions as a feeding organelle.

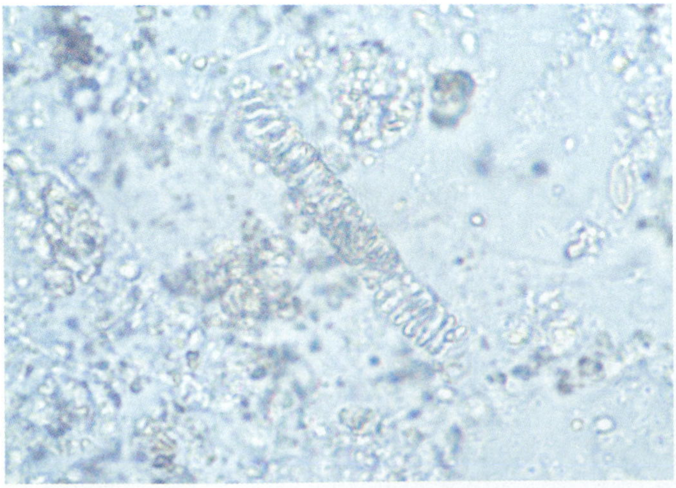

■ FIGURE 30-5 Plant spiral, a type of vegetable fiber (direct wet mount preparation 400× magnification).

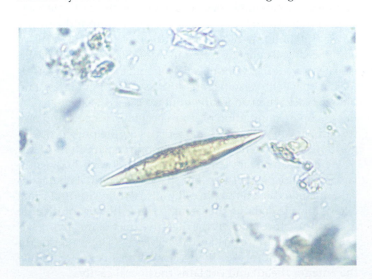

■ FIGURE 30-6 Charcot-Leyden crystals (direct wet mount preparation 400× magnification).

While many parasites are confined to the tropics and sub-tropics, protozoan parasites may be found throughout the world, even in temperate climates where temperatures fall below the freezing point of water. The incidence of protozoan parasitic infections is, however, generally higher in the tropics and subtropics than in temperate climates. Outbreaks of intestinal protozoan infection have occurred when public water supplies have been contaminated with sewage or in crowded conditions such as prisons or day care facilities.

The life cycle of intestinal protozoans is far simpler than that of many helminth parasites because intermediate hosts are not required. There are two stages in the life of these organisms: the trophozoite stage and the cyst stage. Trophozoites are the form that is motile, feeding, metabolically active, capable of undergoing cell division, but very susceptible to a hostile environment. They are able to survive outside the body for only a very brief period of time. On the other hand, cysts are the stage that is more resistant to the environment and are the dormant stage, which allows survival outside of the body. Cyst forms are able to gain entrance into a new host by ingestion of food or water that has been contaminated with fecal material and are therefore considered to be the infective stage of intestinal protozoans. Trophozoites are most often found in loose, watery stools while cysts are often seen in formed stools.

The best specimen to demonstrate the presence of intestinal parasites is a properly collected and properly preserved stool specimen (∞ Chapter 15, "Ova and Parasites"). Trophozoites, cysts, and in some cases both cysts and trophozoites may be present in the stool of infected individuals. For this reason either trophozoites or cysts can be considered the diagnostic stage of intestinal protozoa. ∞ Chapter 15, "Ova and Parasites," discusses the laboratory procedures used to recover, detect, and identify parasites.

 REAL WORLD TIP

Concentrated fecal wet mounts are used to detect and differentiate the large ova of parasites and ciliates whereas a stained fecal smear is used to detect small amoeba and flagellates. The two methods must be performed on all fecal specimens suspected of harboring parasites.

When fecal specimens are sent for examination, identification of intestinal protozoans requires consideration of several differential characteristics of trophozoites:

1. The number of nuclei. Trophozoites may be either mononucleate or binucleate.
2. The presence and pattern of peripheral chromatin. (Is it present or absent? Is it uniformly or unevenly distributed around the nuclear membrane?)
3. The appearance of the karyosome. (Is it large, small, round, or irregular in shape? Is it in the center of the nucleus or eccentric [off-center]?)
4. The appearance of the cytoplasm. (Is it smooth or coarsely granular?)
5. The presence of inclusions in the cytoplasm. (Is there bacteria, yeast, red blood cells, or other organic debris present?)
6. The size of the parasite. Because parasites tend to be uniform in size and shape there is usually a characteristic size range for each species.
7. The type of motility may be characteristic in some species (e.g., the "falling leaf" motility of *Giardia lamblia*).

Much the same can be said of the cyst stage of an individual parasitic species. The number of nuclei varies with each species and the presence of cytoplasmic inclusions, such as chromatoidal bars (crystalline or condensed RNA) and glycogen vacuoles, is often characteristic for some species. As with trophozoites, the shape and size varies with each species, but may be very important in the identification of a few species. This will become clearer as the different protozoan parasites are discussed below.

 Checkpoint! 30–2 (Chapter Objective 3)

Long, delicate, thread-like extensions of the cytoplasm that serve as locomotor organelles for protozoans are known as:
   A. *cilia.*
   B. *flagella.*
   C. *pseudopodia.*
   D. *cytostomal fibrils.*

Checkpoint! 30–3 (Chapter Objective 4)

Cyst forms that are commonly passed in formed stools of infected individuals possess readily identifiable morphological characteristics, are resistant to environmental conditions, and can be found in food or water sources contaminated with feces. For these reasons cysts, when present, constitute the
   A. *active, motile, feeding stage.*
   B. *diagnostic and infective stage.*
   C. *intermediate stage.*
   D. *transition stage.*

PATHOGENIC PROTOZOANS

Entamoeba histolytica

Entamoeba histolytica is the etiological or causative agent of amoebic dysentery. Approximately 1% of the world's population is colonized with *E. histolytica*. Of those individuals, only 1 in 10 is symptomatic, so it seems the overwhelming majority of infections are asymptomatic. The trophozoite is capable of invading the bowel wall, causing deep flask-shaped ulcers, where it feeds on blood and tissue, leading to the passage of stools that contain blood and mucus. Acute, symptomatic infection is characterized by diarrhea or dysentery, abdominal pain, cramping, flatulence, anorexia, weight loss, and chronic fatigue. Asymptomatic carriers of the organism harbor the infective stage (cysts) and are the individuals responsible for spreading the infection. Cysts are more resistant to the environment but are killed by drying, temperatures above 55°C, chlorine, and iodine. They are found in formed stools. A diagram of the life cycle of *E. histolytica* is available on the Companion Website.

E. histolytica may spread from the intestine to the liver through the bloodstream, producing symptoms such as liver tenderness and enlargement (hepatomegaly), fever, and weight loss. Radiography may reveal single or multiple liver abscesses. The trophozoite can be recovered from biopsy material obtained from the wall of the abscess. Once in the bloodstream, the organism can spread to the brain to cause secondary amebic meningoencephalitis. Liver abscesses can rupture in the pleural cavity to reach the lungs. Trophozoites can be recovered in sputum.

 REAL WORLD TIP

The bloody, thick purulent material aspirated from the liver is often referred to as "anchovy paste" due to its consistency and color.

 REAL WORLD TIP

The meningitis caused by *E. histolytica* is called secondary amebic meningoencephalitis. It is called secondary because it enters the brain as a result of seeding from another body site rather than directly infecting the CSF and brain.

 REAL WORLD TIP

E. histolytica can be released into the pleural and peritoneal cavities upon rupture of a liver abscess. The organisms can enter the lung and be found in the sputum and upper respiratory tract. Another amoeba that can be found in the upper respiratory tract is *Entamoeba gingivalis.* It lives in the gumline. The single nucleus of *E. gingivalis* trophozoite can have peripheral chromatin and a karysome similar to that of *E. histolytica. E. gingivalis* ingests white blood cells and this unique characteristic can be used in its identification and differentiation from *E. histolytica.*

E. histolytica may also be responsible for a sexually transmitted disease, which may be spread among the homosexual population following anal intercourse with an infected individual. It is also possible for amebiasis of the penis to occur as a result of intercourse with a female suffering from vaginal amebiasis.

 REAL WORLD TIP

As each parasite is covered in this chapter, characteristics of the microscopic morphology of the organism and its characteristic motility (if noteworthy) are described in detail. This is important because visual recognition of the parasite is the primary means of identifying many of the parasites responsible for a patient's illness. Eventually molecular diagnostics may come to play a significant role in diagnosis but, at the present time, microscopic examination remains the mainstay of the investigative methods employed in parasitology.

Diagnosis of Amebic Dysentery.   The specimen of choice to diagnose amebic dysentery is stool. Any areas with blood or mucus should be sampled as this is where the organism is most likely to be found.

Concentration procedures are used to increase the number of organisms and reduce fecal debris. Stained wet mounts and fecal smears are used to detect and identify *E. histolytica* trophozoites and cysts. Due to the pathogenic nature of this organism, enzyme immunoassays are recommended for antigen detection. Molecular testing is also available.

Distinguishing Characteristics of *Entamoeba histolytica* Trophozoites.   When the nucleus is examined in stained preparations, the nuclear membrane appears to be a distinct, very thin line. Typically the peripheral chromatin granules, which lie just underneath the nuclear membrane, are small, evenly distributed, and uniform in size. The karyosome is usually small, round, compact, and centrally located. There is only one nucleus in the trophozoite (Figure 30-7 ■).

The cytoplasm reveals the endoplasm has a fine granular appearance with a clear, clean ectoplasm. Cytoplasmic inclusions can consist of one or more ingested red blood cells (RBCs). The presence of RBCs is considered diagnostic for *E. histolytica*. The size range of this protozoan is between 12 and 60 microns (μm), with an average size of approximately 20 μm. The typical motility of *E. histolytica* is described as progressive and directional as though the microorganism were moving with purpose. As the amoeba moves, long, finger-like pseudopodia are protruded forcefully and in rapid succession (John & Petri, 2006).

Distinguishing Characteristics of *Entamoeba histolytica* Cysts.   Cyst stages are recognized by the presence

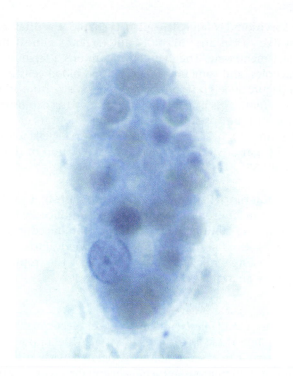

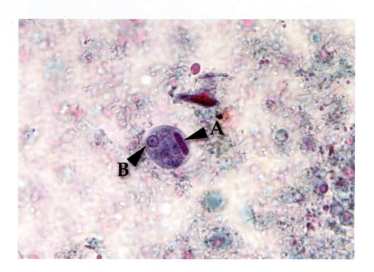

■ FIGURE 30-8 An immature *Entamoeba histolytica/E. dispar* cyst stained with the trichrome stain. Note the typical morphology of the nucleus (B), which is similar to that of the troph and the presence of a chromatoidal bar within the cytoplasm (A). *From Public Health Image Library (PHIL), CDC/DPDx—Melanie Moser.*

■ FIGURE 30-7 *Entamoeba histolytica* trophozoite with ingested red blood cells within the cytoplasm (trichrome stain, 1000× magnification). Note the typical morphology of the single nucleus: small, round, compact, centrally located karyosome with evenly distributed peripheral chromatin.

of a hyaline cyst wall that is highly refractive in unstained preparations. During the trichrome staining process, the cytoplasm may shrink away from the cyst wall, giving the appearance of a halo or clear space around the cytoplasm. Cysts of *E. histolytica* are usually spherical. They typically contain one to four nuclei, which may not be visible in a direct wet mount preparation. The nuclear peripheral chromatin is similar to that of troph, with a layer of peripheral chromatin granules that are evenly distributed. The karyosome is centrally located.

The cytoplasm of the cyst has a clean, fine granular appearance. Before trophozoites encyst they extrude all ingested material and assume a rounded form. Other cytoplasmic inclusions such as chromatoidal bars may be found. In *E. histolytica*, *E. dispar*, and *E. hartmanni*, they appear red on the trichrome stain. The elongated bars with rounded ends can look like a cigar (Figure 30-8 ■). A large, round glycogen vac-

uole, which pushes the nucleus to one side, is often found in immature cysts. On iodine wet preparations, the glycogen mass stains dark brown due to the presence of starch. Cysts range in size from 10 to 20 μm.

ⓔ REAL WORLD TIP

The trophozoite and cyst stage of *Entamoeba dispar* look exactly like those of *E. histolytica*. *E. dispar* is considered nonpathogenic. The presence of red blood cells in the trophozoite indicates the pathogen, *E. histolytica*. Without the presence of red blood cells, only immunoassays or molecular methods can differentiate the two organisms.

ⓔ REAL WORLD TIP

It is often necessary to review many organisms before making a definitive identification. There is variation in the placement of the karysome and appearance of the peripheral chromatin in both trophozoites and cysts. It is also possible to have multiple parasites causing infection.

Naegleria fowleri

Naegleria fowleri is a free living amoebae normally found in fresh or brackish water, moist soil, and decaying vegetation. This opportunistic pathogen occurs in two trophozoite phases, an amoeboid phase (seen in humans) and a pear-shaped biflagellate phase (seen in culture and water), depending on the environmental conditions. The cyst stage can be found in nature and in culture. *N. fowleri* is the etiological agent of primary amoebic meningoencephalitis (PAM), which is a fatal intracerebral infection of brain tissue of previously healthy children and young adults.

Most cases occur during the summer months in association with exposure to fresh or brackish water. The organism likely enters through the nasal passages in aerosols associated with diving, swimming, and water-skiing. After invasion of the nasal mucosa, the organism migrates from the cribiform plate and sinuses to the olfactory bulb. From the olfactory bulb, the amoeba migrates across the olfactory nerve into the tissues of the brain. Symptoms begin as a sore throat, stuffy nose, and headache, which progress to severe headache, fever, nausea, vomiting, and other signs of meningitis such as stiff neck and photophobia occur after an incubation period of 1–3 days. Coma and death occur within a period of 3–10 days after the onset of symptoms. With rare exception, this disease is invariably fatal, with death occuring early, usually within a matter of 3 days. Diagnosis is often made on autopsy unless the physician has a high index of suspicion early in the infectious process. A flowchart of the life cycle of *Naegleria fowleri* can be found on the Companion Website.

Diagnosis of Primary Amoebic Meningoencephalitis.

The specimen of choice is cerebrospinal fluid (CSF) or brain tissue. The presence of a high number of white blood cells, some red blood cells, and motile trophozoites in centrifuged CSF is diagnostic. Stained smears of CSF can be prepared from the sediment. Brain tissue may be stained with the hematoxylin and eosin stain.

 REAL WORLD TIP

Meningitis due to *N. fowleri* yields CSF that resembles that of bacterial meningitis. The CSF glucose is decreased, protein is increased, and the WBC count is greater than 20,000/μL consisting of neutrophils. When no bacteria are seen on a Gram-stained smear of purulent CSF, consider the possibility of meningitis due to *N. fowleri*.

 REAL WORLD TIP

On culture, a drop of the CSF is placed on medium seeded with a lawn of the bacterium, *E. coli*. The amoeba eats the bacteria, creating tracks in the bacterial growth, and, using a dissecting microscope, can be found at the end of one of the tracks.

 REAL WORLD TIP

In hematology, the trophozoites of *N. fowleri* can mimic white blood cells in a counting chamber used for body fluids. The amoeba are better visualized with a wet prep using a slide and coverslip.

Distinguishing Characteristics of Trophozoites.

The trophozoite of *N. fowleri* possesses a single nucleus. Careful evaluation of the nucleus will reveal the absence of peripheral chromatin so there appears to be a halo around the karyosome.

The karyosome is large, irregular in shape. It is often called "blot-like" as in an "ink blot" and extends almost to the nuclear membrane. The cytoplasm contains a large number of vacuoles, and sometimes ingested red blood cells may be seen (Figure 30-9 ■). Trophozoites range in size from 10 to 20 μm and motility is usually characterized by the explosive formation of blunt pseudopodia. The amoeboid form may be transformed to the elongated form with two flagella following the addition of sterile distilled water to a drop of the sedimented CSF.

Distinguishing Characteristics of Cysts.

Cyst forms exist in the environment and may be produced when the organisms are cultured but they are not produced when the parasite is found in tissues of the host. Spherical to oval cysts contain a single nucleus similar to that of the trophozoite. They have an average size of 10 μm.

Acanthamoeba species

The genus *Acanthamoeba* includes several species of free-living amoeba but these organisms may also be opportunistic pathogens. The disease states associated with this genus include granulomatous amoebic encephalitis (GAE), progressive corneal ulceration that may lead to blindness, and chronic granulomatous infections of the skin. The progression of these diseases is chronic and prolonged, with an incubation period of at least 10 days or more. The route of transmission leading to GAE may involve inhalation of cysts leading to infection of the lower respiratory tract and subsequent spread, via the blood, to the central nervous system (CNS). Trauma to the skin and contamination of the affected area with soil, water, or decaying vegetation containing the organism may lead to

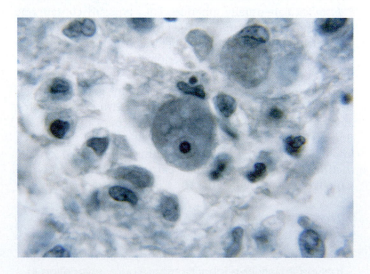

■ **FIGURE 30-9** The trophozoite of a free-living amoeba (*Naegleria fowleri* or *Acanthamoeba* species). *Naegleria fowleri* is the etiological agent of primary amoebic meningoencephalitis (PAM). This photomicrograph shows a trophozoite within the brain tissues of an infected individual.
From Public Health Image Library (PHIL), CDC/Dr. Martin D. Hicklin.

granulomatous skin infections and possible hematogenous spread from these sites to the CNS. Corneal ulceration has been associated with the use of "homemade" saline solutions for storing and washing contact lenses, which has been prepared with tap water.

While *Naeglaria fowleri* infections usually occur in previously healthy individuals with intact immune systems, *Acanthamoeba* infection usually requires some underlying medical condition that predisposes the host to infection. For this reason, such infections occur, in most cases, in immuocompromised or debilitated hosts, such as alcoholics.

REAL WORLD TIP

The keratitis caused by *Acanthamoeba* spp. can resemble that of herpes simplex virus. Viral therapies used are ineffective against *Acanthamoeba* spp.

Distinguishing Characteristics of Trophozoites. The trophozoites of *Acanthamoeba* species are very similar to those of *Naeglaria* but no flagellate stage has been demonstrated (Figure 30-10). Examination of stained preparations should reveal the presence of a single nucleus with a karyosome that is very large and darkly stained and no peripheral chromatin. The cytoplasm contains numerous vacuoles and spine-like or thorny projections extend off of the surface of the pseudopodia, creating what are known as acanthopodia. The size range is from 20 to 50 μm in length and descriptions of the

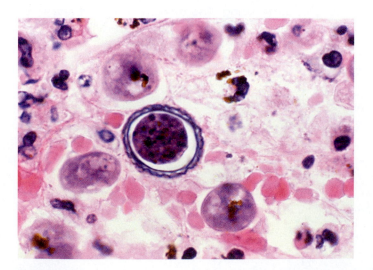

■ **FIGURE 30-10** The trophozoite and cyst stages of an *Acanthamoeba* species within the brain tissue of an infected patient. The cyst stage is located off-center and to the left. Note the presence of the double cyst wall; the outer cyst wall has an irregular shape. There are at least five trophozoites within the field.

From Public Health Image Library (PHIL), CDC.

characteristic motility simply state the organism is a slow-moving trophozoite. In contrast to infection caused by *Naeglaria fowleri*, both trophozoites and cysts may be found in host tissues infected with *Acanthamoeba* species.

Distinguishing Characteristics of Cysts. Cysts contain a single nucleus that closely resembles that seen in the trophozoite. A morphological characteristic that differentiates the cysts of *Acanthamoeba* from those of *Naeglaria fowleri* is the cyst wall. The cysts of *Acanthamoeba* species possess a cyst wall that is double layered with an uneven, wrinkled outer cyst wall. The average size of these cysts is 10–25 μm in diameter (Figure 30-14).

Checkpoint! 30–4 (Chapter Objective 4)

The specimen of choice to diagnose primary amoebic meningoencephalitis is

   A. *a fresh stool specimen paying particular attention to areas containing blood and mucus.*

   B. *serum to demonstrate a significant rise in titer between acute and convalescent specimens.*

   C. *cerebrospinal fluid concentrated by centrifugation, sampling the sediment.*

   D. *a thick and thin blood smear stained with the Giemsa or Wright's stain.*

Giardia lamblia

Giardiasis or "beaver fever" is acquired through the ingestion of contaminated food and water. As with many gastrointestinal parasitic infections, infection can be through hand-to-mouth transmission. Backpackers and mountain climbers are at increased risk because aquatic mammals such as beavers, muskrats, or water rats are carriers of *Giardia lamblia* (also known as *G. intestinalis*), a flagellate, and may pass the cysts into water. Humans who use streams, lakes, or ponds as sources of drinking water without using some means of water purification (such as boiling, filtering, or halide tablets) may ingest the cysts and acquire the infection. Another source of infection is through contamination of a community's water supply with raw sewage. Sewer workers are at high risk. Outbreaks in nursery school settings can occur. A visual representation of the life cycle can be found on the Companion Website.

Trophozoites of *G. lamblia* are most likely to be found in the duodenum of the small intestine. Infection is often characterized by **steatorrhoea**, or the production of loose, pale-yellow, fatty, foul-smelling stools. This is a direct result of mechanical damage to the villi of the small intestine. The organisms coat the intestine surface and lead to a malabsorption syndrome. Individuals often complain of flatulence and explosive diarrhea.

Diagnosis of Giardiasis.   The specimen of choice is a stool specimen or duodenal aspirate. The procedures employed in preparing material to be examined is the same as those used in the diagnosis of amoebic dysentery, including direct wet mounts, concentration procedures, and permanent stains. In addition, duodenal biopsies may be examined by the pathologist. Enzyme immunoassay procedures are employed by many laboratories because it is a very common pathogenic parasite.

Distinguishing Characteristics of the Trophozoite. The trophozoite of *Giardia lamblia* is binucleate. The two nuclei give the organism the appearance of having eyes. Examination of the nucleus should reveal that there is no peripheral chromatin and the karyosome is usually centrally located. Trophozoites of this organism are among the easiest of the protozoan parasites to recognize because of its "pear" or teardrop shape, the presence of two distinct nuclei, and other structures that are somewhat unique to this organism. Cytoplasmic structures include the presence of four pair of flagella, which are readily apparent on motile organisms in saline wet mounts made from freshly passed stools. The flagella are not apparent when the trichrome or iron hematoxylin stains are used.

In addition to the eight flagella there are two axonemes, which are the intracytoplasmic portion of the pair of caudal (tail) flagella. Think of the axoneme like a backbone for the organism. It divides the organism in half so it exhibits bilateral symmetry if you were to fold the organism in half lengthwise.

There is a prominent sucking disk, shaped like the bowl of a spoon, that comprises nearly all of the anterior portion of the organism. There are also two median bodies, curved, rod-shaped organelles located posterior to the sucking disk, giving the organism the appearance of a grin (Figure 30-11 ■). The sucking disk, which may be difficult to observe, provides a means of attachment to the intestinal mucosa and may be the cause of damage to the villi, which interferes with the proper absorption of nutrients.

The average size of *G. lamblia* trophozoites is 9–21 μm in length and 5–15 μm in width. Living, actively motile trophozoites can be observed to move with a slow, erratic, oscillatory type of motility referred to as "falling leaf" motility. When caught in mucus, the organisms appear to flutter.

Distinguishing Morphological Characteristics of Cysts.   The shape of the cysts of *G. lamblia* has been described as elliptical, ovoid, or "football shaped." One to four nuclei may be seen within the cytoplasm. Basically, the number of cytoplasmic structures is double that seen within the trophozoite (Figure 30-12 ■). The axonemes are usually visible. The organism may appear to pull away from the cyst wall, especially in formalinized specimens. On iodine stained concentrated wet preparations, they appear as golden footballs. The average size of *G. lamblia* cysts is 8–14 μm in length and 7–10 μm in width, which is two to three time larger than a yeast cell (4 μm).

> **ⓔ   REAL WORLD TIP**
>
> *Giardia lamblia* trophozoites can be securely attached to the intestinal mucosa and may not appear in stool samples readily. A noninvasive specimen from the duodenum may provide the diagnosis. A gelatin capsule containing a coiled string is swallowed by the patient. One end of the string is taped to the patient's face so the string can be recovered. After 4 hours the string reaches the duodenum. *Giardia* trophozoites will adhere to the string. The string is removed and the mucus is stripped and examined for parasites.

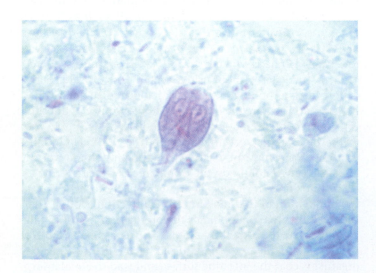

■ FIGURE 30-11 *Giardia lamblia* trophozoite (Trichrome stain, 1000× magnification).

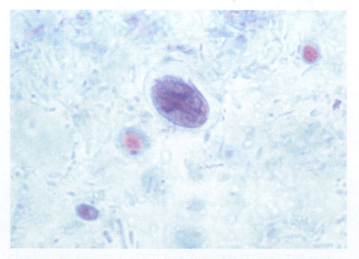

■ FIGURE 30-12 *Giardia lamblia* cyst (Trichrome stain, 1000× magnification).

Dientamoeba fragilis

Because of the genus name of this organism one might be led to believe that this discussion centers on an amoeba, and, indeed, at one time *D. fragilis* was classified as such. Examination of the organism in a stained fecal specimen using conventional microscopy would also give the impression that the microorganism in question is an amoeba, but, despite the lack of any apparent flagella, electron microscopy has revealed this parasite to be a flagellate (Windsor, 1999).

This organism is transmitted by the fecal-oral route. Because no cyst stage has been demonstrated, it is unknown how the trophozoite is able to survive passage through the acid environment of the stomach. There is evidence that transmission may be associated with the acquisition of pinworm or other helminth eggs (www.cdc.gov, 2008). A flowchart of the life cycle can be found on the Companion Website.

The pathogenicity of *D. fragilis* has been in question because it rarely invades tissue. It may be considered a pathogen when an individual exhibits symptoms in the absence of any other intestinal parasites (Spencer & Garcia, 1979). Typical symptoms include diarrhea, abdominal pain, anorexia, weight loss, and the presence of blood and mucus in the stools. The presence of the parasite should be reported and left to the discretion of the clinician to decide if treatment is warranted.

Diagnosis of *Dientamoeba fragilis* Infection.
If the fecal specimen has not been mixed with a preservative solution, the trophozoites are likely to have been lysed in the wash steps of concentration techniques when distilled water is used. For this reason concentration procedures are not usually productive. On a stained fecal smear the diagnosis of *D. fragilis* infection may be made if characteristic trophozoites are noted.

Distinguishing Characteristics of Trophozoites.
Trophozoites of *D. fragilis* may be either mononucleate or binucleate. On average 80% of the organisms will be binucleate and 20% will be mononucleate. The character of the nucleus in both forms is identical: no peripheral chromatin and the karyosome can appear to be fragmented and composed of three-to-five chromatin granules (Figure 30-13). Obviously, the genus-species name *Dientamoeba fragilis* (*di*, two, and *fragilis*, fragile or fragmented) reflects the character of the nucleus of this organism. The size range is typically between 7 and 12 μm and one should be cautioned that mononucleate forms may be confused with the trophozoites of other intestinal protozoans, *Endolimax nana* and *Iodamoeba bütschlii*, which share the same size range. The presence of binucleate forms or a characteristic broken karysome should clear up any confusion. As previously mentioned, no cyst stage has been demonstrated.

 REAL WORLD TIP

The broken pieces of karyosome of *Dientamoeba fragilis* often resemble a "Maltese" cross pattern.

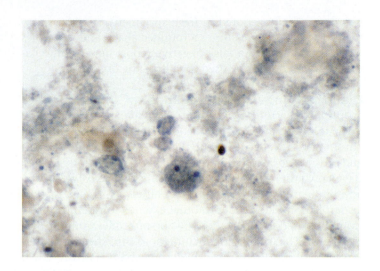

■ **FIGURE 30-13** *Dientamoeba fragilis* trophozoite. While the karyosomes are not fragmented, the presence of two nuclei is a feature characteristic of this protozoan parasite. *From Public Health Image Library (PHIL), CDC/Dr. Mae Melvin.*

REAL WORLD TIP

If *Dientamoeba fragilis* only possesses one nucleus, then it can be confused with *Entamoeba nana* and *Iodamoeba butschlii*. To differentiate, review several organisms and look for the broken karyosome of *Dientamoeba fragilis*. *E. nana* and *I. butschlii* have a blot-like karyosome that remains intact.

Trichomonas vaginalis

Trichomonas vaginalis, a flagellated urogenital parasite, is passed from host to host as a sexually transmitted disease. Typically the organism is found in the vaginal tract or urethra, but in a small percentage of females may be a cause of cystitis (bladder infection). Symptoms include itching, burning, and a frothy, yellow or greenish, foul-smelling vaginal discharge. Trophozoites may be found in vaginal or urethral discharge and are frequently seen in the urine of infected females. Cystitis is characterized by dysuria (painful urination) and polyuria (an increased frequency of urination). In many cases males are asymptomatic carriers and act as a source of infection for uninfected females. The organism may be found in the prostate, seminal vesicles, and the epididymis. The prostate may be enlarged and tender and a urethral discharge present. Neonates can acquire the organism from an infected mother at birth, causing neonatal pneumonia. A flowchart of the life cycle can be found on the Companion Website.

Diagnosis of *Trichomonas vaginalis* Infection.
Wet preparations of vaginal or urethral discharge, prostatic secretions, and centrifuged urine may be used for diagnosis. The whipping action of the flagella and rippling of the undulating

membrane is often noted in fresh specimens. In older specimens, the organism assumes a rounded shape and resembles white blood cells so a false-negative report may result. Diamond's medium can be used to culture the organism.

Distinguishing Characteristics of Trophozoites.

Trophozoites of *T. vaginalis* are pear shaped with a single nucleus located at the anterior end of the body. The peripheral chromatin is evenly distributed and the karyosome is small and centrally located. This organism has four anteriorly located flagella. Cytoplasmic structures such as the axostyle, costa, and undulating membrane may be observed. The axostyle is a sharply pointed, slender rod that extends through the body from the anterior to posterior end and protrudes from the posterior end. The undulating membrane, a thin sheet of fluttering protoplasm, is short and extends about halfway down the body of the organism toward the posterior end (Figure 30-14 ■). The size range is generally from 5 to 15 μm but some trophozoites may be up to 30 μm in length. The characteristic motility is described as jerky and nondirectional. No cyst stage has been demonstrated.

Checkpoint! 30–5 (Chapter Objective 3)

Which of the following flagellates is a gastrointestinal parasite whose trophozoite form may be mononucleate or binucleate? The nuclei lack peripheral chromatin and the karyosome is fragmented.

A. *Entamoeba histolytica*
B. *Giardia lamblia*
C. *Dientamoeba fragilis*
D. *Trichomonas vaginalis*

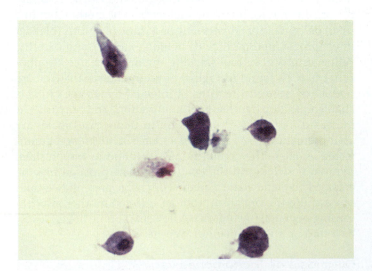

■ **FIGURE 30-14** Photomicrograph of *Trichomonas vaginalis* trophozoites from a laboratory culture (Giemsa stain). *From Public Health Image Library (PHIL), CDC.*

REAL WORLD TIP

Infection with *Trichomonas vaginalis* is often diagnosed on the urinalysis microscopic examination. The organism can be detected when it exhibits an undulating membrane or jerky motility.

Balantidium coli

B. coli, the only ciliate that parasitizes humans, inhabits the large intestine where it feeds on bacteria. The organism thrives on starch, so when an individual's diet is low in starch, it can invade the intestinal mucosa. This organism has been known to produce ulcerative lesions that can become infected. It rarely escapes the intestine like *E. histolytica*. A visual representation of its life cycle can be found on the Companion Website.

Diagnosis of *B. coli* Infection.

Concentration techniques such as formalin-ethyl acetate are instrumental in the diagnosis of *B. coli* infection. The organism is so large it is often overlooked on a stained fecal smear.

Distinguishing Characteristics of the Trophozoite.

Trophozoites are egg-shaped with one end slightly flattened. There are two nuclei, a small, round micronucleus that may not be readily apparent even in stained specimens, and a large, kidney bean–shaped macronucleus which is very conspicuous especially. Cytoplasmic structures include cilia that cover the surface of the body and the cytostome (feeding organelle), which is a funnel-shaped opening at the slightly pointed end of the body (Figure 30-15 ■). *B. coli* trophozoites may attain a length 50 to 100 μm and a width of 40 to 70 μm. Motility is directional with a rotary or boring action.

Distinguishing Characteristics of the Cyst.

Like the trophozoites, the cysts of *B. coli* are binucleate but only the

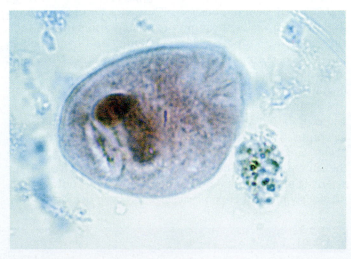

■ **FIGURE 30-15** *Balantidium coli* trophozoite. Note the presence of the anteriorly located cytostome and the kidney bean–shaped macronucleus (400× magnification).

macronucleaus is easily seen. The distinguishing characteristic of the cyst stage is the presence of a round cyst wall. The size range for cysts is typically 50–75 μm in length and width. Refer to Tables 30-1 ✪ and 30-2 ✪ for a summary of the distinguishing morphological characteristics of pathogenic protozoans previously discussed.

▶ COMMENSAL PROTOZOANS

It is important to be able to identify the commensal or non-pathogenic protozoan because: (1) the route of transmission is the same as the pathogens; (2) the presence of commensal parasites increases the likelihood of pathogenic parasites being present; and (3) misidentification as a pathogen initiates unecessary treatment. Demonstration and identification of commensal protozoans is accomplished in the same manner as the pathogenic species (i.e. using saline and iodine direct wet mounts, concentration techniques, and permanent stains).

COMMENSAL AMOEBAE

Entamoeba dispar

Only recently has the name *Entamoeba dispar* (Latin, *dispar*, unequal or different) been adopted as the name of organisms that were formerly considered to be a noninvasive strain of *E. histolytica*. The trophozoites and cysts (refer to Figure 30-8) of this organism are morphologically indistinguishable from *E. histolytica* and but can be differentiated using genetic, biochemical, or immunological tests (Hamzah, Petmitr, Mungthin, Leelayoova, & Chavalishewinkoon-Petmitr, 2006).

Because *E. dispar* does not invade the tissues, the cytoplasmic inclusions found in the trophozoite include organic debris, bacteria, and yeast. Red blood cells are rarely ingested. The average size of the trophic forms is 14 μm with a size range of

✪ TABLE 30-1

Distinguishing Morphological Characteristics of Pathogenic Protozoan Trophozoites

Parasite	Size (microns)	No. of Nuclei	Character of Nucleus	Cytoplasmic Inclusions	Other Characteristics
Entamoeba histolytica	12–60	1	Small, round, centrally located karyosome Evenly distributed peripheral chromatin	Ingested red blood cells (RBCs)	Progressive and directional motility with long, finger-like pseudopodia, finely granular endoplasm, clear ectoplasm
Naegleria fowleri	10–20	1	Thin, delicate nuclear membrane No peripheral chromatin Karyosome is large and irregular in shape (blot-like)	Numerous vacuoles Sometimes ingested RBCs	Explosive formation of blunt pseudopodia
Acanthamoeba species	20–50	1	Thin, delicate nuclear membrane No peripheral chromatin Karyosome is large and irregular in shape (blot-like)	Numerous vacuoles	Sluggish motility Hyaline projections (acanthopodia)
Giardia lamblia	9–21 in length	2	Thin, delicate nuclear membrane No peripheral chromatin Karyosome is centrally located	Eight flagella, two axonemes, two median bodies	Large sucking disk
Dientamoeba fragilis	7–12	1 or 2	Thin, delicate nuclear membrane No peripheral chromatin Karyosome appears to be fragmented (Maltese cross pattern)	Numerous vacuoles with ingested bacteria, yeast, or organic debris	Binucleate and mononucleate forms
Trichomonas vaginalis	5–15	1	Small, centrally located karyosome Evenly distributed peripheral chromatin	Four flagella, undulating membrane ½ the length of the body axostyle	Jerky, nondirectional motility
Balantidium coli	50–100	2	Small, round micronucleus, large kidney bean– or horseshoe-shaped macronucleus	Large cytostome Numerous cilia	Directional motility

✪ TABLE 30-2

Distinguishing Morphological Characteristics of Pathogenic Protozoan Cysts

Parasite	Size (microns)	No. of Nuclei	Character of Nucleus	Cytoplasmic Inclusions	Other Characteristics
Entamoeba histolytica	10–20	1–4	Small, round, centrally located karyosome Evenly distributed peripheral chromatin	Immature cysts: glycogen vacuole, elongated chromatin bars with rounded ends	Spherical or oval shape Finely granular cytoplasm
Naegleria fowleri	7–15	1	Thin, delicate nuclear membrane No peripheral chromatin Karyosome is large and irregular in shape (blot-like)	None	Spherical or oval shape Smooth cyst wall
Acanthamoeba species	10–25	1	Thin, delicate nuclear membrane No peripheral chromatin Karyosome is large and irregular in shape (blot-like)	None	Double cyst wall with wrinkled outer wall
Giardia lamblia	8–14 in length	1–4	Karysome is centrally located No peripheral chromatin	Four axonemes, four median bodies	Elliptical or ovoid shape (football-shaped) May pull away from cyst wall
Dientamoeba fragilis	Cyst stage has not been demonstrated				
Trichomonas vaginalis	Cyst stage has not been demonstrated				
Balantidium coli	50–75	2	Small, round macronucleus and kidney bean– or horseshoe-shaped macronucleus	Cilia in early cyst stage	Round shape

12–40 μm. Motility is directional and purposeful as opposed to random or multidirectional.

E. dispar does not cause symptomatic disease and does not elicit the production of serum antibodies. Because *E. histolytica* and *E. dispar* are morphologically indistinguishable, one can no longer rely on microscopy alone for the definitive detection of *E. histolytica* infection. *E. histolytica* does not always invade the intestinal mucosa in asymptomatic individuals. The key to differentiation of the two is the presence of ingested erythrocytes within the cytoplasm of the trophozoites. It is diagnostic for *E. histolytica* but not *E. dispar*.

If *E. histolytica*-like organisms are found in the stool and there are no ingested red blood cells, then a positive serological response, antigen detection methods (such as enzyme immunoassay), or genetic techniques support the diagnosis of an *E. histolytica* infection. If additional testing is not performed, suspicious organisms should be reported out as *E. histolytica/E. dispar*. The clinician must determine if therapy is necessary based on the clinical symptoms.

Entamoeba hartmanni

Entamoeba hartmanni is an amoeba that is morphologically identical to *E. histolytica/E. dispar* except for differences in size. As a matter of fact, the organism now known as *E. hartmanni* was formerly designated as the "small race" of *E. histolytica*. The presence of trophozoites that are morphologically consistent with descriptions of *E. histolytica/E. dispar* (Figure 30-16) but less than 12 μm in size should be identified as *E. hartmanni*. Cysts that are morphologically consistent with those of *E. histolytica/E. dispar* but are less than 10 μm in size and possess chromatoidal material identical to that of *E. histolytica* should be identified as the cysts of *E. hartmanni*. Measurement with a calibrated ocular micrometer is essential.

℮ REAL WORLD TIP

If the patient is asymptomatic, it is not possible to differentiate *E. histolytica* and *E. dispar* trophozoites unless there are ingested red blood cells present. If there are no ingested red blood cells, identify the organism as *E. histolytica/E. dispar*.

℮ REAL WORLD TIP

It is important to use a calibrated ocular micrometer on the microscope for the accurate measurement of parasites. It must be calibrated for each objective and done annually to verify the accuracy.

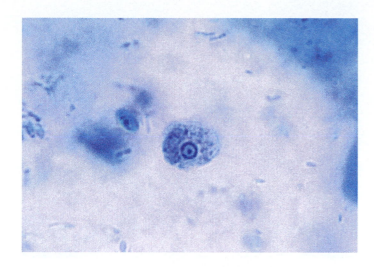

■ FIGURE 30-16 *Entamoeba hartmanni* trophozoite (Trichrome stain).
CDC/Dr. L.L.A. Moore, Jr.

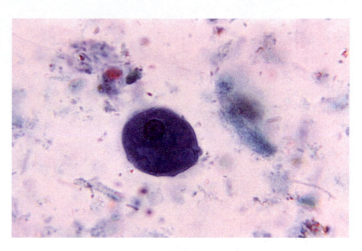

■ FIGURE 30-17 *Entamoeba coli* trophozoite (Trichrome stain, 1000× magnification). Note the presence of the eccentric karyosome and numerous food vacuoles. The organism tends to take up the trichrome stain very well.
CDC

 REAL WORLD TIP

If an amoebic trophozoite or cyst resembling *E. histolytica/E. dispar* is less than 10 µm in size, then it is probably *E. hartmanni*. If it is greater than 10 µm, then it is more likely to be *E. histolytica/E. dispar*.

Entamoeba coli

Entamoeba coli is another nonpathogenic amoeba that can be confused with *E. histolytica*.

Distinguishing Characteristics of Trophozoites.
E. coli trophozoites possess a layer of peripheral chromation that lies against the nuclear membrane. The chromatin granules are coarse, irregular in size, unevenly distributed, and more abundant than that of *E. histolytica*. The karyosome is often large, irregularly shaped, and eccentrically located. The cytoplasm is coarsely granular and contains numerous vacuoles (Figure 30-17 ■). Inclusions found within the cytoplasm include ingested bacteria, yeast, and organic debris. The cytoplasm is often called "dirty" due to the presence of a lot of debris. Because this organism is commensal, host tissues are not invaded and ingested red blood cells are usually not observed. Motility has been described as slow, progressive, and characterized by the formation of short blunt pseudopodia. The size range is from 15 to 50 µm.

 REAL WORLD TIP

The trophozoite and cyst of *E. coli* tends to take up the trichrome stain very well. On stained smear, *E. coli* may appear very dark.

Differential Characteristics of the Cyst Stage.
In *E. coli* cysts the number of nuclei may range from one to eight depending on the stage of maturity (Figure 30-18 ■). The character of these nuclei is essentially the same as those of the trophozoite just smaller in size. The cytoplasm is coarsely granular and inclusions that may be present in immature cysts include chromatoidal bars with splintered ends (compared to the rounded ends seen within the cysts of *E. histolytica*) and a glycogen vacuole. The glycogen vacuole, if present, can be so large that it pushes the nucleus to the periphery of the cytoplasm. The size of an *E. coli* cyst is 10–35 µm.

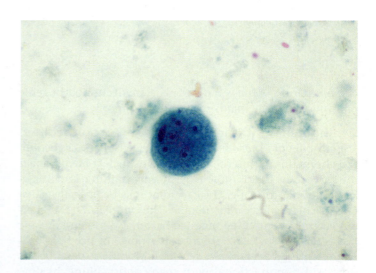

■ FIGURE 30-18 *Entamoeba coli* cyst. Note the presence of multiple nuclei within the coarsely granular cytoplasm. A chromatin bar is also present in this immature cyst.
From Public Health Image Library (PHIL), CDC/Dr. Mae Melvin.

REAL WORLD TIP

Entamoeba coli has one of the few amoeba cysts that can be identified on iodine wet prep. If there are greater than four nuclei present then the cyst must be *E. coli*. Remember cysts are three-dimensional so you must focus up and down in order to see all of the nuclei present.

 ## Checkpoint! 30–6 (Chapter Objective 3)

What cytoplasmic inclusions often used differentiates E. histolytica trophozoites from those of the other Entamoeba species?

A. *Ingested red blood cells*
B. *Chromatoidal bars with rounded ends*
C. *Bacteria, yeast, and organic debris*
D. *Axonemes*

 ## Checkpoint! 30–7 (Chapter Objectives 3 and 6)

A smear made from a stool specimen preserved in polyvinyl alcohol (PVA), a fixative and preservative solution, is dried, stained, mounted, and examined using the oil immersion lens. Many spherical-shaped cysts that range in size from 5 to 9 μm in diameter are clearly seen. These cysts have one to four nuclei with small, round, centrally located karyosomes and evenly distributed peripheral chromatin. The cytoplasm is finely granular and some cysts have large empty glycogen vacuoles and elongated chromatoidal bars with rounded ends. This microscopic morphology is consistent with

A. *Entamoeba histolytica*
B. *E. dispar*
C. *E. hartmanni*
D. *E. coli*

Endolimax nana

E. nana (Greek, *nannos* = dwarf) is a small, nonpathogenic intestinal amoebae that is seen quite commonly.

Distinguishing Characteristics of Trophozoites. Trophozoites of *E. nana* have a single nucleus that lacks peripheral chomatin. Within the thin, delicate nuclear membrane is the karyosome that is quite large, deeply staining, and irregular or blot-like in shape. The karysome may be pushed against one side of the nuclear membrane. The cytoplasm has numerous vacuoles containing ingested bacteria, yeast, and organic debris (Figure 30-19 ■). Trophozoites range in size from 5 to 12 μm with an average size of 7 μm. Motility is described as slow and nondirectional with many short, blunt, hyaline pseudopodia being formed.

Distinguishing Characteristics of Cysts. Cysts of *E. nana* may be spherical or ovoid in shape. Typically four

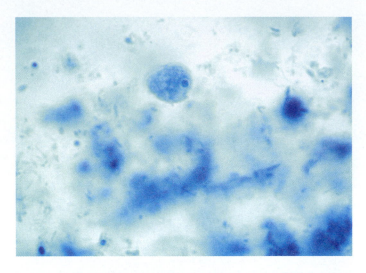

■ **FIGURE 30-19** *Endolimax nana* trophozoite (Iron hematoxylin stain, 1000× magnification).

nuclei are present, but the number of nuclei can vary from one to four. The karyosomes are large and may be eccentric or centrally located. The lack of peripheral chromatin may create the appearance of a halo around the karyosome. The cytoplasm is coarsely granular and chromatin granules may occasionally be seen within the cytoplasm (Figure 30-20 ■). Cysts range in size from 5 to 12 μm.

 REAL WORLD TIP

Amoeba with the genus name *Entamoeba* possess peripheral chromatin. Those with the genera names *Endolimax* or *Iodoamoeba* do not have peripheral chromatin.

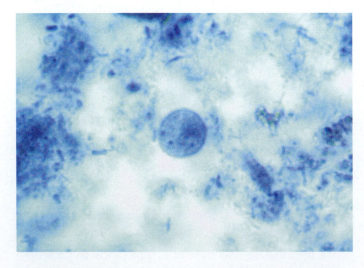

■ **FIGURE 30-20** *Endolimax nana* cyst (Iron hematoxylin stain, 1000× magnification). Note the presence of four pin-point nuclei within the cytoplasm.

Iodamoeba bütschlii

I. bütschlii is another nonpathogenic amoeba known to inhabit the lumen of the intestine. This organism is very similar in appearance to *E. nana*, but tends to be somewhat larger in size.

Distinguishing Characteristics of Trophozoites.

Trophozoites of *I. bütschlii* have a single nucleus bound by a thin, delicate nuclear membrane. The lack of peripheral chromatin gives it the appearance of a halo around the karyosome. The karyosome is large, irregularly shaped. While difficult to see, the karysome may be surrounded by small chromatin granules, giving it the appearance of a basket with a handle. Numerous vacuoles containing ingested bacteria, yeast, or organic debris are found within the cytoplasm (Figure 30-21 ■). Motility is often described as being slowly progressive accompanied by the formation of hyaline pseudopodia. The size range of *I. bütschlii* trophozoites overlaps that of *E. nana*, being from 4 to 20 μm with an average size of 9–14 μm. The key to differentiation is often based on its unique cyst stage.

Distinguishing Characteristics of Cysts.

Cysts of *I. bütschlii* possess a single nucleus with a karyosome that is large, irregularly shaped, and eccentric. They are spherical, ovoid, or elliptical. The cytoplasm is coarsely granular and characteristically contains a large glycogen vacuole. This glycogen vacuole stains dark brown on iodine stained wet preparations. During the fecal smear staining process, the glycogen is dissolved and the vacuole appears as an empty space within the cytoplasm (Figure 30-22 ■). Cysts range in size from 9 to 11 μm.

  REAL WORLD TIP

The trophozoites of *Iodamoeba butschlii* and *Endolimax nana* are difficult to differentiate. The cysts help because those of *E. nana* have up to four nuclei but those of *I. butschlii* have only one nucleus and often possess a glycogen vacuole. *E. nana* is more frequently isolated.

Trichomonas hominis

T. hominis (also known as *Pentatrichomonas hominis*) is a nonpathogenic flagellate transmitted through fecal contamination. This organism also inhabits the lumen of the intestine and, although related to *T. vaginalis*, it does not colonize the urogenital tract. These two organisms have adapted to survival in specific areas of the host's body.

Distinguishing Characteristics of Trophozoites.

Trophozoites of *T. hominis* are teardrop shaped. They have a single nucleus located in the anterior of the organism, close to the point of origin of the flagella. The karyosome is small and centrally located with evenly distributed peripheral chromatin. This organism possesses four anterior and one recurrent flagellum that form the border of the undulating membrane and extends out of the posterior end. Other cytoplasmic inclusions include an axostyle that runs the entire length of the organism's body and protrudes posteriorly. The undulating membrane

REAL WORLD TIP

Most amoeba cysts can possess glycogen vacuoles. The cysts of *Iodamoeba butschlii* consistently possess glycogen vacuoles. Think of the cysts as having the appearance of a Greek mythology cyclops (one nucleus with a blot like karyosome) with a large open mouth (glycogen vacuole).

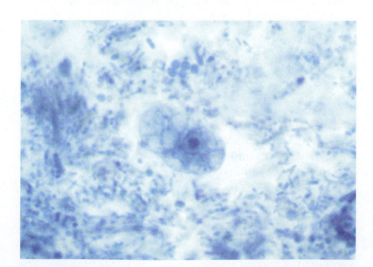

■ **FIGURE 30-21** *Iodamoeba butschlii* trophozoite (Iron hematoxylin stain, 1000× magnification).

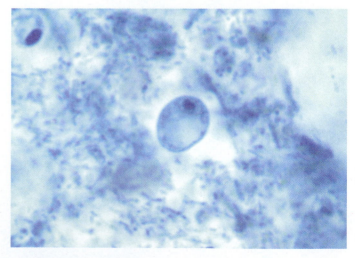

■ **FIGURE 30-22** *Iodamoeba butschlii* cyst (Iron hematoxylin stain, 1000× magnification).

extends the length of the body, as opposed to that of *T. vaginalis,* which runs only half the length of the body. Trophozoites range in size from 7 to 15 µm and exhibit jerky, nondirectional motility. No cyst stage has been demonstrated so it is unknown how the organism survives the stomach acid when passed through the fecal-oral route.

Chilomastix mesnili

This nonpathogenic flagellate has the same route of transmission as other intestinal protozoans, the fecal–oral route. It is important to recognize *C. mesnili* so it is not confused with other flagellates, particularly *Giardia lamblia,* which is the etiological agent of giardiasis, a significant cause of gastrointestinal distress.

Distinguishing Characteristics of Trophozoites. The pear-shaped trophozoites of *C. mesnili* have a single nucleus that is anteriorly located. The nucleus has peripheral chromatin, and a karyosome may be eccentric or centrally located. This organism possesses three anteriorly located flagella and a cytostome, or oral depression, that is bordered by cytostomal fibrils that are said to resemble a "shepherd's crook" (Figure 30-23 ■). Motility is directional and this may be due to the presence of a groove running in a spiral manner along the length of the body. In profile this spiral groove may be seen as an indentation of the cytoplasm. The size range of *C. mesnili* trophozoites is 10–20 µm.

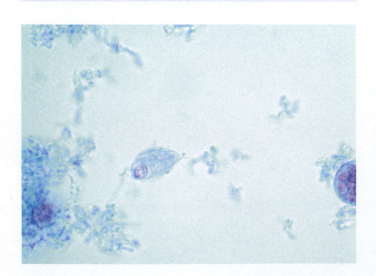

ⓔ **REAL WORLD TIP**

Often *Chilomastix mesnili*'s "shepherd's crook" and spiral groove are very difficult to see. The organism usually appears as a teardrop with a nucleus located at the fat end of the drop on stained fecal smears.

■ **FIGURE 30-23** *Chilomastix mesnili* trophozoite (Trichrome stain, 1000× magnification).

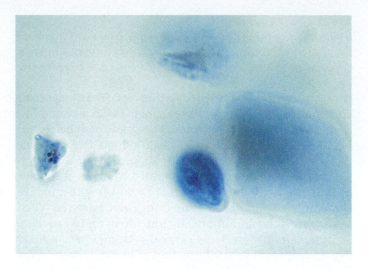

■ **FIGURE 30-24** *Chilomastix mesnili* cyst (Trichrome stain, 1000× magnification).

Distinguishing Characteristics of Cysts. Cysts have a single nucleus similar to that seen in the trophozoite. Cytoplasmic structures include the curved cytostomal fibrils in the shape of a "shepherd's crook." There is a nipple-like protuberance that makes the cyst appear to be "lemon shaped" (Figure 30-24 ■). Cysts range in size from 6 to 10 µm.

✓ **Checkpoint! 30–8 (Chapter Objectives 3 and 6)**

Numerous oval structures that range in size from 9 to 11 microns are seen in an iodine direct wet mount preparation. These objects have a clearly visible cyst wall and a large glycogen vacuole that stains a deep brown color. It is very difficult to see morphological characteristics of the single nucleus found within the cysts, but there appear to be no other cytoplasmic structures other than the glycogen vacuoles. This organism is most likely

    A. *Iodamoeba butschlii*
    B. *Entamoeba hartmanni*
    C. *Endolimax nana*
    D. *Trichomonas hominis*

Entamoeba polecki

E. polecki is an intestinal parasite of pigs and monkeys that is only rarely seen in humans. It is, however, the most common intestinal amoeba of man in parts of New Guinea.

Distinguishing Characteristics of Trophozoites. *E. polecki* shares morphological characteristics of the nucleus and cytoplasm with both *E. histolytica* and *E. coli.* Peripheral chromatin may appear as fine granules that may be evenly distributed or massed at one or both poles of the nucleus. The karyosome is typically small, compact, and centrally located. The cytoplasm is coarsely granular and contains numerous

Checkpoint! 30–9
(Chapter Objectives 3 and 6)

A stool specimen is sent to the lab for routine culture and susceptibility testing and ova and parasite examination. The patient has been diagnosed with episodes of severe diarrhea. Occasional teardrop-shaped trophozoites are detected on the permanent smear. These forms have a single, anteriorly located nucleus with eccentric karyosomes and unevenly distributed peripheral chromatin. A cytostome is present and cytostomal fibrils in the shape of a "shepherd's crook" are distinctly visible. This protozoan parasite is most likely

- *A. Trichomonas vaginalis*
- *B. T. hominis*
- *C. Chilomastix mesnili*
- *D. Giardia lamblia*

vacuoles. Inclusions include ingested bacteria, yeast, and organic debris and give the cytoplasm a "dirty" appearance. Motility is typically sluggish with pseudopodia formed slowly but occasionally the pseudopodia are extended in an explosive manner similar to that of *E. histolytica*. The size range is from 15 to 20 μm.

Differential Characteristics of Cysts.   As opposed to the multinucleate mature cysts of *E. histolytica* and *E. coli,* those of *E. polecki* are mononucleate. The nucleus is similar to that of the trophozoite. The cytoplasm is coarsely granular and inclusions may include abundant, pointed, thread-like chromatin bars with angular ends. Quite unique is the presence of an inclusion mass that stains lightly and uniformly and is of unknown composition. The size range of these cysts is 11–15 μm (John & Petri, 2006). Refer to Tables 30-3✪ and 30-4✪ for specific information on the distinguishing morphological characteristics of commensal protozoan trophozoites and cysts. Tables 30-3 and 30-4 summarize the morphological characteristics of the nonpathogenic protozoans.

✪ TABLE 30-3

Distinguishing Morphological Characteristics of Commensal Protozoan Trophozoites

Parasite	Size (microns)	No. of Nuclei	Character of Nucleus	Cytoplasmic Inclusions	Other Characteristics
Entamoeba dispar	12–40	1	Indistinguishable from that of *Entamoeba histolytica*	Ingested bacteria, yeast, organic debris	Indistinguishable from *Entamoeba histolytica*
Entamoeba hartmanni	Less than 12	1	Indistinguishable from that of *Entamoeba histolytica*	Ingested bacteria, yeast, and organic debris	Indistiguishable from *E. histolytica/dispar* except for size
Entamoeba coli	15–50	1	Large, irregularly shaped karyosome that is eccentrically located, peripheral chromatin abundant and not evenly distributed	Ingested bacteria, yeast, and organic debris	Coarsely granular cytoplasm Slow, progressive motility Blunt pseudopodia
Entamoeba polecki	15–20	1	Small, centrally located karyosome, peripheral chromatin evenly distributed or massed at one or both poles	Ingested bacteria, yeast, and organic debris	Coarsely granular cytoplasm Sluggish motility
Endolimax nana	5–12	1	Thin, delicate nuclear membrane No peripheral chromatin Karyosome is large and irregular in shape (blot-like)	Ingested bacteria, yeast, and organic debris	Slow, nondirectional motility Blunt pseudopodia
Iodamoeba bütschlii	4–20	1	Thin, delicate nuclear membrane No peripheral chromatin Karyosome is large and irregular in shape (blot-like)	Ingested bacteria, yeast, and organic debris	Slowly progressive motility, hyaline pseudopodia
Trichomonas hominis	7–15	1	Small, centrally located karyosome Evenly distributed peripheral chromatin	Four anterior flagella Undulating membrane Axostyle	Jerky, nondirectional motility
Chilomastix mesnili	10–20	1	Eccentric or centrally located karyosome Peripheral chromatin present	Three anterior flagella, cytostome with fibrils in shape of "shepherd's crook"	Spiral groove Directional motility

✪ TABLE 30-4

Distinguishing Morphological Characteristics of Commensal Protozoan Cysts

Parasite	Size (microns)	No. of Nuclei	Character of Nucleus	Cytoplasmic Inclusions	Other Characteristics
Entamoeba dispar	12–40	1–4	Indistinguishable from that of *E. histolytica*		
Entamoeba hartmanni	Less than 10	1–4	Indistinguishable from that of *E. histolytica/dispar*		
Entamoeba coli	10–35	1–8	Large, irregularly shaped karyosome that is eccentrically located, peripheral chromatin abundant, and not evenly distributed	Immature cysts: large glycogen vacuole, chromatoidal bars with splintered ends	Round to oval shape, coarsely granular cytoplasm
Entamoeba polecki	11–15	1	Small, centrally located karyosome, peripheral chromatin evenly distributed or massed at one or both poles	Angular chromatoidal bars with pointed ends, lightly staining inclusion mass	Coarsely granular cytoplasm
Endolimax nana	5–12	1–4	Thin, delicate nuclear membrane No peripheral chromatin Karyosome is large and irregular in shape (blot-like)	Chromatin granules	Ovoid shape, coarsely granular cytoplasm
Iodamoeba bütschlii	9–11	1	Thin, delicate nuclear membrane No peripheral chromatin "Basket of flowers" appearance	Large glycogen vacuole	Coarsely granular cytoplasm
Trichomonas hominis	Cyst stage has not been demonstrated				
Chilomastix mesnili	6–10	1	Eccentric or centrally located karyosome Peripheral chromatin present	Fibril in the shape of a "shepherd's crook"	Nipple-like protuberance produces a "lemon-shaped" cyst

---

℮ REAL WORLD TIP

Care must be taken not to misidentify *E. polecki* as *E. histolytica*. If the organism is misidentified, then unnecessary treatment will be prescribed.

▶ COCCIDIA AND SPOROZOA

THE COCCIDIAN/ SPOROZOAN PARASITES

This class of parasitic organisms includes intestinal protozoans such as *Isospora belli*, *Sarcocystis* species, *Cryptosporidium parvum,* and *Cyclospora cayetanensis* as well as blood and tissue parasites such as the *Plasmodium* species, *Babesia microti*, and *Toxoplasma gondii*. Many of these parasites (coccidia) are acquired by the fecal–oral route through the ingestion of contaminated food and water or through the ingestion of animal tissues containing the organism. *Plasmodium* and *Babesia* species are spread through arthropod (insect) vectors that inject the infective stage into the host when they obtain a blood meal. All of these parasites share one thing in common: life cycles that include asexual and sexual reproduction. In asexual reproduction, propagation is accomplished through division within a host cell (hepatocytes, erythrocytes, or cells of the intestinal epithelium), whereas sexual reproduction involves the production of male and female gametes that unite to form a zygotic cell.

During asexual reproduction, or **schizogony**, trophozoites within infected host cells increase in size until they nearly fill the cell. The nucleus undergoes multiple divisions followed by division of the body of the parasite (segmentation) to produce merozoites, which are released when the cytoplasmic membrane of the host cell is ruptured. Merozoites are now free to infect other host tissues where the cycle of reproduction may occur for a number of generations. Host cells containing maturing merozoites are referred to as schizonts.

During sexual reproduction, or **sporogony**, maturing trophozoites within infected host cells increase in size but cell division fails to occur, leading to the development of immature sexual forms called gametocytes. The male form of the sexual cell is referred to as a microgametocyte, while the female form is referred to as a macrogametocyte. As the microgametocyte matures, the nucleus divides and a number of microgametes are produced. The macrogametocyte matures into a single macrogamete that is fertilized by one of the microgametes, forming a zygote. In time the zygote secretes a cyst wall and this new form is called an oöcyst.

Isospora belli Infection

Isospora belli is a parasite that is distributed worldwide, infecting both immunocompetent and immunosuppressed individuals. It is different from the other coccidian because both the sexual and asexual forms can inhabit the human intestine. A second host is not required. The asexual reproductive cycle occurs within cells of the intestinal epithelium, allowing the infection to spread throughout the tissues of the bowel. Sexual reproduction also occurs within the tissues of the intestinal tract producing oöcysts, which undergo development in the stool. These eliptical or spindle-shaped oöcysts make their way into the environment when the infected host passes feces. Maturation of the oöcyst occurs in the soil.

Immature oöcysts contain a single spherical mass of protoplasm that eventually divides into two spherical sporoblasts. As the oöcyst continues to mature each sporoblast undergoes further cell division to produce four sausage-shaped sporozoites. The end-product, the mature oöcyst, now contains two sporocysts each containing four sporozoites. Immature or, less frequently, mature oöcysts may be found in the stool of infected individuals and are considered to be the diagnostic stage. Mature oöcysts containing sporozoites require 4–5 days of development and are considered to be the infective stage. The sporozoites go on to infect mucosal cells. The mode of transmission is ingestion of food or water contaminated with fecal material. An illustrated version of the life cycle is available on the Companion Website.

Symptoms of *I. belli* infection include anorexia, nausea, abdominal pain, and diarrhea. Spread of the infection throughout the intestine leads to destruction of the surface layer of the intestinal epithelium (villous atrophy), which is associated with a malabsorption syndrome characterized by the presence of increased fecal fat, diarrhea, and cramps. The infection can go on for months to years and lead to massive weight loss in immunocompromised individuals. Death can occur due to water loss and electrolyte imbalance. Stools passed by infected individuals are typically loose, pale yellow in color, and particularly foul-smelling; however, asymptomatic cases of *I. belli* are not uncommon.

Diagnosis of *Isospora belli* Infection. A direct wet mount using saline or a concentration procedure such as Sheather's sugar flotation can be used as the recommended method. Other methods such as zinc-sulfate flotation, or formalin-ethyl acetate sedimentation can be employed to evaluate stool specimens. Because oöcysts are very pale and transparent, careful examination of the area directly beneath the coverslip with reduced illumination is strongly advised. Oöcysts are 30 by 12 microns in size, transparent, and appear as a long oval with tapered ends.

Examination of a stool smear stained with the modified acid-fast or auramine-rhodamine fluorescent stain allows the mature or immature oöcysts to be seen more easily. While the oöcyst wall does not take up the stain, the sporocysts stain a deep red color.

Sarcocystis Infection

Sarcocystis species exist as parasites of both humans and animals such as mice, dogs, cats, cattle, pigs, and sheep. Man can be the definitive host for two species, *Sarcocystis hominis* and *S. suihominis*. After ingestion of infective oöcysts (usually in undercooked beef or pork), male and female gametes develop in the small intestine and unite to produce oöcysts, which are passed in the feces and may be ingested by another definitive host to perpetuate the cyle.

For those *Sarcocystis* species for which animals are the definitive host, humans may act as intermediate hosts. Under these circumstances humans accidentally ingest the oöcysts (usually in contaminated food or water containing oöcysts) of *Sarcocystis* species other than *S. hominis* and *S. suihominis*. In the intestine, the oöcysts release two sporocysts. A sporocyst then releases four infective sporozoites. The sporozoites penetrate the intestine and migrate, via the bloodstream, and develop in muscle, via schizgony, into a mass called a sarcocyst. Most infections are asymptomatic but myositis may be seen in symptomatic cases. Severe diarrhea and weight loss can occur in immunocompromised individuals.

Diagnosis of *Sarcocystis* Infection. Diagnosis of intestinal infection relies upon demonstration of sporocysts in fecal specimens. Because the oöcysts have very thin oöcyst walls, sporocysts frequently rupture out of the oöcyst and are found singly or in pairs. Examination of saline direct wet mounts or concentrates of fresh stool specimens can reveal the presence of ovoid sporocysts that measure from 11 to 17 microns in length and 7.7 to 11 microns in width.

When extra-intestinal infection occurs sarcocysts may be found in a muscle biopsy using histological methods. These sarcocysts vary in length and may be less than 100 microns and invisible to the unaided eye or as large as 5 centimeters. Macroscopically these bodies appear as minute white streaks within the muscle fibers whereas microscopically they typically appear as elongated cylindrical bodies enclosed within a limiting membrane containing radial striations. Sarcocysts may contain many thousands of trophozoites (4–8 microns in diameter) and may be divided into compartments by septa.

Toxoplasma gondii Infection (Toxoplasmosis)

T. gondii is another parasite that is found worldwide and is able to infect a wide variety of animals both carnivorous and herbivorous. The majority of infections are most likely asymptomatic or mild. Even in asymptomatic disease, serological tests can show evidence of past infection.

Members of the cat family (felines) act as the definitive host where both schizogony and sporogony occur in the small intestine. Mature oöcysts contain two sporocysts, which in turn contain four sporozoites. These oöcysts are passed out in the feces and may accidentally be ingested by other animals that are not members of the cat family. These animals then serve as intermediate hosts.

In the intermediate host the sporozoites invade the intestinal mucosa, gain access to the bloodstream, and spread to other tissues, especially the lungs, heart, lymphoid tissues, and the central nervous system. The crescent-shaped tachyzoite (Figure 30-25 ■) is metabolically active and rapidly dividing. It spreads throughout the body destroying host tissues. The bradyzoite develops slowly and, with time, enters a dormant state to become a mass of organisms encysted in host tissues. If the infected host's tissues are ingested by a feline, the organisms are released in the cat's intestines to begin the cycle over again. An illustrated version of the life cycle of *T. gondii* is available on the Companion Website.

The majority of infections are usually asymptomatic. Symptomatic infection is characterized by chills, fever, headache, myalgia, lymphadenitis, prostration, and may be confused with infectious mononucleosis, a viral disease. Immunocompromised individuals, such as individuals with AIDS, transplant patients, those with leukemia and lymphoma or treated with corticosteroids, radiation, or chemotherapy, are subject to acute or severe infection. Severe infection involves invasion of internal organs and is characterized by hepatitis, myocarditis, encephalomyelitis, retinochoroiditis, and possibly blindness. These infections may be the result of primary infection with *T. gondii* or reactivation of cysts of dormant bradyzoites.

Intratuterine infection during the first and second trimesters of pregnancy, can have catastrophic consequences. Severe injury to the fetal central nervous system could result in hydrocephalus, mental retardation, blindness, and possibly death. Pneumonitis, fever, and convulsions may also be associated with neonatal infection. Because an infected cat can pass the organisms in its feces, pregnant females should not clean or change the litter box.

Diagnosis of Toxoplasmosis. Because humans are not the definitive host of *T. gondii,* examination of stool specimens would not yield the infective form, the oöcyst. Biopsies of a patient's tissues might be attempted but histopathological evaluation might be confusing since the encysted organisms very closely resemble the sarcocysts seen with *Sarcocystis* infection. Another issue is that many individuals have been exposed to this parasite during their lifetime and cysts may not represent a current infection. Serology is traditionally used to diagnose toxoplasmosis. Procedures such as indirect fluorescent antibody testing or ELISA can be used to demonstrate the presence of a significant rise in titer of IgG antibodies to *T. gondii.*

@ **REAL WORLD TIP**

Serology testing for *T. gondii* is riddled with problems in interpretation. PCR testing has now proven much more reliable in detecting acute infections.

Cryptosporidum parvum Infection

C. parvum is another coccidian parasite that is found worldwide and infects a wide variety of animal species. Until recently it was seen primarily in other mammals such as calves, pigs and chickens. With the increased population of immunosuppressed individuals, the incidence of *C. parvum* infection has increased correspondingly. Another species, *C. hominis,* is primarily a human pathogen.

The organism is resistant to disinfectants and may be found in drinking water when chlorine levels are diluted. The presence of the organism in drinking water could potentially paralyze an entire city, as it did in 1993 in Milwaukee, WI. An outbreak cost the city almost a million dollars due to medical costs and loss of productivity for 300,000 infected individuals.

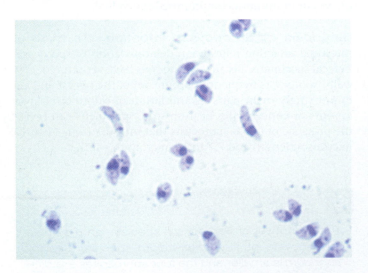

■ **FIGURE 30-25** Tachyzoite of *Toxoplasma gondii* (Giemsa stain, 1000× magnification).

Cryptosporidium spp. infections are acquired through the ingestion of contaminated food and water or contact with infected animals. Mature oöcysts contain four sporozoites, which are released within the intestine to enter epithelial cells where they undergo asexual reproduction and eventually sexual reproduction. As with other coccidia, sexual reproduction results in the production of gametes and spherical oöcysts but in contrast to other coccidian species, the oöcysts of *C. parvum* contain sporozoites that are not contained within sporocysts. Oöcysts shed in the feces are the infective and diagnostic stages. They can contaminate water and ground vegetation where they may be ingested by a new host to complete the cycle. The Companion Website provides a visual illustration of the life cycle of *Cryptosporidium* spp.

Symptoms of cryptosporidiosis include a profuse, cholera-like, watery diarrhea, cramping, nausea, and anorexia. The more liquid the fecal specimen, the more oöcysts present. In immunocompetent hosts the disease is self-limiting, but in immunocompromised patients the severe diarrhea may last for weeks or months. Fluid losses can reach up to 17 to 20 liters per day, which leads to electrolyte imbalance.

Diagnosis of Cryptosporidiosis.   The modified acid-fast procedure (Figure 30-26 ■) or auramine-rhodamine fluorescent dyes may be used to stain direct smears, revealing the

℮ REAL WORLD TIP

The *Cryptosporidium* spp. oöcyst is 5–6 μm, which is about the size of a yeast cell. An experienced parasitologist can recognize this highly-refractile parasite on a concentrated wet prep or trichrome stained smear of a fecal sample.

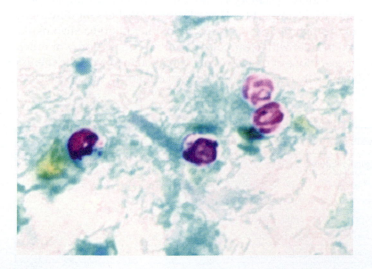

■ **FIGURE 30-26** *Cryptosporidium parvum* oöcysts. The acid-fast (red) parasites are easily recognized against the blue-green background.
From Public Health Image Library (PHIL), CDC/DPDx.

presence of the small oöcysts. Concentration procedures such as formalin-ether and Sheather's sugar flotation may also be employed but requires an experienced parasitologist to detect the small organism. The use of enzyme immunoassays has proven to be effective and easily incorporates into the workflow of most laboratories.

Cyclospora cayetanensis Infection

Cyclospora cayetanensis has recently been identified as the cause of several outbreaks of diarrheal illness associated with contaminated water and foods such as raspberries and lettuce. The life cycle appears to be quite similar to that of *Isospora* species, with oöcysts being produced within cells of the small intestine and maturation occuring outside the host's body over a period of a week or more. *C. cayetanensis* infection is associated with prolonged watery diarrhea (3 or more weeks) accompanied by nausea, vomiting, anorexia, low-grade fever, fatigue, weight loss, and cramps.

Diagnosis of *Cyclospora cayetanensis* Infection. Oöcysts of *C. cayetanensis* may be observed in direct wet mounts as spherical oöcysts, 8–10 microns in diameter. Immature oöcysts are unsporulated and contain six to nine refractile globules whereas mature oöcysts contain two sporocysts each containing two cresent-shaped sporozoites. Staining is variable when the modified acid-fast stain is used, with some appearing pink and others dark red. The modified safranin technique is superior for staining *C. cayetanensis* because the organisms stain more uniformly (www.dpd.cdc.gov). If a microscope equipped with an ultraviolet light source is used, oöcysts autofluoresce, appearing as bluish-green objects.

℮ REAL WORLD TIP

Cyclospora cayetanensis is acid fast just like *Cryptosporidium parvum*. To differentiate, a measurement of the oocyst is necessary. *C. cayetanensis* is 8–10 μm whereas *C. parvum* is 5–6 μm.

Blastocystis hominis

The taxonomic status of *B. hominis* has been in question for years. This organism has been classified as a yeast-like organism, a coccidian parasite, and recently a more amoeboid form seen in cases of diarrhea has been described. The pathogenicity of *B. hominis* has come into question because the organism has been recovered in patients with no symptoms of disease whereas in other instances it has been recovered from symptomatic patients (diarrhea, abdominal pain, pruritis ani, flatulence, and weight loss) in the absence of any other parasites. The best course of action to follow is to report the organism when seen in a clinical specimen, allowing the clinician to make the decision for or against treatment.

Diagnosis of *Blastocystis hominis* Infection. *B. hominis* cysts are spherical in shape and range in size from

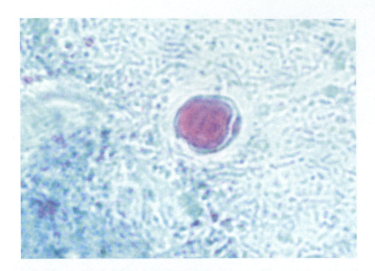

■ **FIGURE 30-27** *Blastocystis hominis* in a trichrome-stained fecal smear (1000× magnification). Note the presence of the large fluid-filled vacuole surrounded by a thin strip of cytoplasm in which multiple nuclei are embedded.

5 to 30 microns. In a direct wet mount made with saline or stained with iodine the organism may be identified by the thin strip of cytoplasm surrounding a large, centrally located, fluid-filled vacuole. On trichrome stain, the multiple red nuclei look like they are pushed to the outer wall leaving a large vacuole in the center (Figure 30-27 ■). Concentration procedures are not productive because the cyst forms are lysed by the use of distilled water. Table 30-5 ✪ summarizes the morphological characteristics of oöcysts, sporocysts, and cysts of intestinal coccidian/sporozoans.

REAL WORLD TIP

Blastocystis hominis is one of the few intestinal protozoan that should be quantitated. It is a potential pathogen in symptomatic individuals if there are no other infectious agents present.

Microsporidial Infection

The microsporidia are obligate intracellular parasites that infect a wide variety of animals (including invertebrates) and humans. There are more than 100 genera that have been described with *Enterocytozoon* and *Encephalitozoon* as the most common infective agents.

Microsporidial infections are found worldwide. Most infections are likely transmitted by the fecal–oral route or airborne transmission. The population most commonly infected has been AIDS patients but increasing numbers of infections have been seen in other types of immunocompromised states as well as immunocompetent individuals. Enteric infections are more common but disseminated infections can be seen in immunocompromised individuals.

The spore is the infective stage. They range in diameter from 1 to 2.5 microns and possess polar tubules or filaments that are unique to the microsporidia. The tubule extends from the spore and injects its contents into the host cell where more spores are formed.

In AIDS patients the disease is typically associated with prolonged diarrhea but other symptoms may include fever, malaise, weight loss, nausea, and anorexia. Four to eight episodes of watery diarrhea may occur, resulting in the passage of one to several liters of liquid feces in a single day. Dehydration and electrolyte imbalance are not uncommon.

Diagnosis of Microsporidial Infection. Because microspordia species are able to cause disseminated infections, any number of specimens may be processed in order to diagnose infection. Enteric infections are diagnosed primarily through the examination of stool specimens, but systemic infections may be best detected with urine sediments, biopsy specimens, or other body fluids such as respiratory secretions.

A variety of stains have been used to demonstrate the presence of microsporidia. Using Ryan's or Weber's modifications of the trichrome stain, the spores of microsporidia are pinkish-red in color with clear polar or central zones. Biopsy or touch preparations of tissue sections can be stained with the Giemsa stain. Other stains that have been employed in the detection

✪ **TABLE 30-5**

Morphological Characteristics of Oöcysts, Sporocysts, and Cysts of Intestinal Coccidian/Sporozoans

Parasite	Size (microns)	Shape	Morphological Features
Isospora belli oöcysts	30 × 12	Ellipsoidal	Immature oöcyst: single, large, spherical mass of protoplasm
			Mature oöcyst: two sporocysts, each containing four sporozoites
Sarcocystis species sporocysts	11–17 × 7.7–11	Ovoidal	Mature oöcyst: two sporocysts, each containing four sporozoites
			Oöcysts often rupture so sporocysts may be found singly or in pairs
Cryptosporidium parvum oöcysts	4–5 (diameter)	Spherical	Oöcysts contain one to six dark granules
Cyclospora cayetanensis oöcysts	8–10 (diameter)	Spherical	Immature oöcyst: contains six to nine refractile granules
			Mature oöcyst: two sporocysts, each containing two cresent-shaped sporozoites
Blastocystis hominis cysts	8–30 (diameter)	Spherical	Thin strip of cytoplasm, with nuclei, surrounds a large, centrally located, fluid-filled vacuole

of microsporidia include the Gram stain (gram positive), acid-fast, and periodic acid-Schiff stains.

MALARIA

Four species in the genus *Plasmodium* are the major etiological agents of malaria in humans (*P. falciparum, P. malariae, P. ovale,* and *P. vivax*). Malaria species native to monkeys, such as *P. knowlesi, P. cynomolgi,* and *P. anui,* have been known to infect humans and may represent emerging health problems as human populations seek to convert forest lands to farmland. As much as 70% of malarial infections diagnosed in regional hospitals in Borneo and other areas of the Far East are the result of *P. knowlesi* infection (McCutchan, Piper, & Makler, 2008).

Female *Anopheles* mosquitos are the definitive host as well as the arthropod vector (route of transmission) of malaria. Their presence in the environment is a crucial factor in the spread of malaria.

INVERTEBRATE PHASE IN THE LIFE CYCLE OF MALARIA PARASITES

Sexual reproduction or sporogony occurs within the female mosquito tissues. Macrogametocytes and microgametocytes are ingested along with human blood. The gametocytes quickly mature into macrogametes and microgametes within the gut of the mosquito. Maturation of the microgametocyte involves a phenomenon called exflagellation in which thin, delicate, spider-like microgametes are extruded from the body of the microgametocyte. Fertilization occurs when the microgamete penetrates the macrogamete and the resulting zygote enlongates to form the next developmental stage, the oökinete, an actively motile form. The oökinete penetrates one of the epithelial cells of the gut wall and migrates to the opposite side of the cell where it matures into an oöcyst about 50 microns or more in size. Cell division takes place within the oöcyst, producing thousands of sporozoites that eventually rupture the oöcyst wall, releasing fusiform-shaped organisms into the body cavity of the mosquito. These sporozoites migrate to the salivary glands of the mosquito and are injected, along with the saliva, into a new host. Injection of saliva, which contains an anticoagulant to facilitate the flow of blood into the gut of the mosquito, acts as the transfer mechanism of the infective stage (the sporozoite) into humans, the intermediate host of the parasite.

VERTEBRATE PHASE OF THE LIFE CYCLE

Once the malarial parasite has entered the bloodstream of the human host it travels to the liver where hepatocytes are invaded. Within the hepatic parenchymal cells the pre-erythrocytic (outside the red blood cell) stage of asexual multiplication, referred to as exoerythrocytic schizogony, occurs.

After the malarial parasite has entered the liver cell, a period of cell division occurs. This asexual reproduction results in the production of merozoites, which eventually rupture the host cell and invade the bloodstream. The merozoites invade red blood cells to begin the erythrocytic stage of asexual reproduction.

In *P. vivax* and *P. ovale* there is a unique resting stage that occurs with a number of the sporozoites. These quiescent or dormant parasitic forms are referred to as hypnozoites and they are believed to be responsible for the relapses characteristic of cases of malaria caused by these two species of malarial parasite. These recurrences of malaria may occur weeks, months, or even years after the initial clearing of the malarial parasites from the bloodstream. Eradication of the parasite from the peripheral blood results in a remission of the symptoms of malaria. Reactivation of hypnozoites and reinvasion of the bloodstream results in a sudden reappearance of the symptoms of malaria.

ERYTHROCYTIC SCHIZOGONY

Merozoites from the liver travel through the blood and invade red blood cells to begin the erythrocytic stage. This is the diagnostic stage for malaria. When a peripheral smear is examined they can appear to be attached to the outer margin of the red blood cell and are known as accolé or applique forms. After penetrating the red blood cells the malarial parasites grow and develop into trophozoites. The earliest trophic form is called the "ring," which consists of a small amount of chromatin material and a thin ring of cytoplasm surrounding a vacuole. These early forms are not distinctive for any of the four species infecting man.

As the trophozoite continues to grow within the red blood cell, it may appear as irregular ameboid shapes. In some cases the trophozoite assumes an elongated form in which it stretches across the red blood cell, often referred to as "band" forms. The parasite feeds on hemoglobin, producing a waste product that shows up as brown-colored malarial pigment when a stained peripheral smear is examined.

After the trophozoite has matured the nucleus begins to undergo mitosis. As soon as cell division or schizogony begins to occur the parasitic form is referred to as a schizont, which is made up of a mass of merozoites. When cell division is completed the newly formed merozoites rupture the red blood cell and are free to invade other red blood cells and repeat the erythrocytic cycle again. The term "merozoites" refers to parasitic forms that result from both exo-erythrocytic and erythrocytic schizogony.

After several erythrocytic cycles, some merozoites grow until they nearly fill the red blood cell and then develop into microgametocytes (female) and macrogametocytes (male) in a process referred to as gametogony. The male and female gametocytes circulate in the bloodstream and may then be ingested by an *Anopheles* mosquito to complete the life cycle. The Companion Website offers a visual representation of the life cycle of *Plasmodium* spp.

If red blood cell destruction exceeds the capacity of the bone marrow to replenish the supply, the end result is anemia and this may be accompanied by hepatosplenomegaly. Other symptoms of malaria include headache, photophobia, muscle pain, nausea, malaise, and anorexia. When the red blood cells rupture to release the merozoites, the toxic metabolic by-products lead to the paroxysms (fever, chills, sweats) that are the hallmark of malaria. The chills and fever of malaria may become cyclical in nature with the appearance of febrile periods occuring at regular intervals. These 48- or 72-hour cycles of fever may be characteristic of infection with the different species of malarial parasites. Symptoms appearing every 48 hours are described as tertian, while those occurring every 72 hours are known as quartan.

Checkpoint! 30–10 (Chapter Objective 4)

In malarial infections, asexual reproduction in liver and red blood cells results in the production of parasitic forms called

   A. *hypnozoites.*
   B. *merozoites.*
   C. *sporozoites.*
   D. *gametocytes.*

Plasmodium vivax

The most prevalent form of malaria is *Plasmodium vivax,* an organism found in tropical, subtropical, and even temperate climates around the world. *P. vivax* is the cause of "vivax malaria" or "benign tertian malaria." Its **periodicity**, or ability to appear at regular intervals of the fever cycle, is 48 hours. *P. falciparum* and *P. vivax* account for up to 95% of all malarial infections. *P. vivax* accounts for 80% of those cases.

P. vivax likes to invade reticulocytes or young red blood cells. Reticulocytes account for 2–5% of the red blood cells present. Stained infected cells contain a number of fine red granules called "Schüffner's dots" or "Schüffner's stippling."

Using the Giemsa stain, the developing trophozoite appears first as a minute blue disc with a vacuole and a single red chromatin dot, the ring stage. In most cases only one parasite is found within the cytoplasm of the red blood cell. As the trophozoite matures, it assumes irregular and somewhat bizarre shapes (Figure 30-28). The malarial pigment appears as granules of brownish pigment. When the trophozoite is mature it nearly fills the infected red blood cell. Trophozoites become somewhat more compact in size just before cell division begins. Twelve to 24 merozoites, with an average count of 16, can be found in mature schizonts (Figure 30-29 ■).

P. vivax produces gametocytes that are very similar to those of *P. malariae* and *P. ovale,* therefore it is better to rely on the asexual stages to distinguish the different species. Microgametocytes and macrogametocytes are round to oval in shape and often fill the entire red blood cell prior to rupture. Gametocytes may be differentiated by examining the nucleus closely.

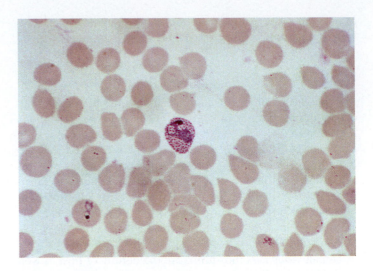

■ **FIGURE 30-28** *Plasmodium vivax* trophozoite within a red blood cell.
CDC/Dr. Mae Melvin

Microgametocytes have a nucleus with a pale, loose network of chromatin whereas macrogametocytes have a denser, more compact nucleus.

It is common for individuals to relapse with malaria due to *P. vivax.* It can have a dormant phase in the liver. Up to 50% of individuals can relapse as late as 5 years after the initial infection.

REAL WORLD TIP

The macrogametocytes of *Plasmodium vivax, P. ovale,* and *P. malariae* are the female gametocytes. There is often condensed, eccentric, compact chromatin present in the macrogametocyte. The microgametocyte often has dispersed chromatin. It is easier to differentiate the two by remembering the female has her act together when it comes to her chromatin.

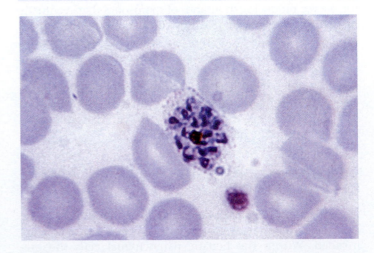

■ **FIGURE 30-29** *Plasmodium vivax* schizont with 15 merozoites and a mass of malarial pigment in the center.

Plasmodium ovale

Plasmodium ovale, the least common species of malaria infecting humans, is found in tropical Africa, primarily along the west coast, but may also be found in South America, the South Pacific islands, and Asia. *P. ovale* is the cause of "ovale malaria," which has a fever cycle with a periodicity of 48 hours.

P. ovale invades reticulocytes or young red blood cells and, as a result, infected red blood cells appear to be larger than normal and pale. Schüffner's dots are present but are fewer in number and more prominent than those of *P. vivax.* In stained blood smears *P. ovale*-infected red cells can be elongated or oval shaped with ragged or jagged cell margins (fimbriated) and typically there is a single parasite in each cell (Figure 30-30 ■). The ring form is indistinguishable from that of *P. vivax* but the developing trophozoite is more compact, less amoeboid, and malarial pigment occurs in smaller amounts. Schizonts contain 4–12 merozoites, with an average of 8. Gametocytes closely resemble those of *P. vivax.*

With their life cycles are similar, *P. ovale* has a less severe course than *P. vivax.* Relapses are possible. Infected individuals usually have a spontaneous recovery.

Plasmodium malariae

Plasmodium malariae is common in tropical and subtropical areas of the world. It is found in tropical Africa, certain parts of Malaysia and Indonesia, and areas in India. *P. malariae* is the cause of "quartan malaria," so named because the periodicity of the fever cycle is 72 hours instead of the typical 48-hour period of other species.

Merozoites tend to infect older red blood cells so fewer cells are available for infection. Schüffner's dots or stippling is not present. While the ring forms resemble those of *P. vivax,* maturing forms are more distinctive. The trophozoites become elongated and often appear to stretch across the body of the red blood cell, forming what is often called "band" forms. In addition, malarial pigment is usually abundant (Figure 30-31 ■). At the completion of schizogony, a total of 6–12 merozoites can be found in the schizont. Most often there is an average of eight merozoites almost entirely filling the red blood cell and surrounding a moderate amount of dark malarial pigment. This morphological characteristic is said to resemble "rosettes" or a flower. The gametocytes closely resemble those of *P. vivax* and *P. ovale.* Untreated infections can last up to 20 years.

Plasmodium falciparum

Plasmodium falciparum is common in tropical and subtropical areas of Africa and Asia. Before the advent of malaria eradication programs it was fairly common in the southern United States and around the Mediterranean. This organism is the etiological agent of "falciparum malaria" or as it was commonly referred to in the past, "malignant tertian malaria." The periodicity of the fever cycle is a 36- to 48-hour period, similar to that of *P. vivax* and *P. malariae.* The term "malignant" carried with it the understanding this form of malaria could be a significant cause of mortality in areas where it was endemic. High fever, up to 107°C, cerebral malaria, and blackwater fever are complications that contribute to a high mortality rate.

Cerebral malaria results from the invasion of the central nervous system where small blood vessels in the brain are clogged by masses of parasitized red blood cells. This may cause sudden attacks of severe headaches, and if untreated, may progress to coma and eventually death. Blackwater fever is associated with massive intravascular hemolysis and the resulting hemoglobinuria as the kidneys attempt to clear hemoglobin from the blood. This condition is associated with repeated attacks of malaria, and, while hemoglobin is undoubtably

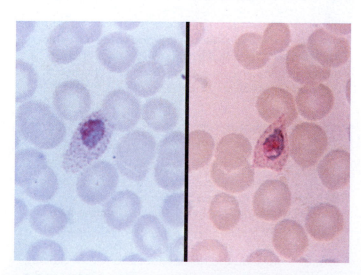

■ **FIGURE 30-30** *Plasmodium ovale* trophozoite within a red blood cell displaying a fimbriated edge. The cell on the left also demonstrates Schüffner's dots.
From Public Health Image Library (PHIL), CDC/Steven Glenn, Laboratory and Consultation Division.

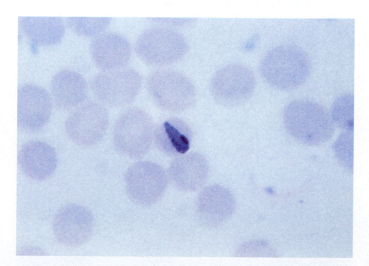

■ **FIGURE 30-31** *Plasmodium malariae* trophozoite within a red blood cell.
From Public Health Image Library (PHIL), CDC/Steven Glenn, Laboratory and Consultation Division.

released when merozoites rupture red blood cells, there is also the possibility that hemolysis may involve some type of an autoimmune reaction.

P. falciparum merozoites show no age preference when invading red blood cells and as a result a large number of red blood cells may be parasitized. The asexual stages of this species of malaria remain largely confined to the deep vessels of vital organs such as the brain, lungs, heart, and intestine so ring forms and gametocytes are the stages that are prevalent in peripheral blood smears. Many of the ring forms have two small chromatin dots rather than having a single chromatin dot. In addition, multiple infections of parasitized red cells is quite common, with two- or three-ring forms found in one red blood cell. Malarial pigment is rarely seen in parasitized red blood cells recovered from peripheral blood.

Gametocytes of *P. falciparum* are easily distinguished from those of *P. vivax*, *P. ovale,* and *P. malariae* by their large size and distinctive shape. They have been described by such various terms as "crescent"-, "banana"-, or "sausage"-shaped gametocytes (Figure 30-32 ■). In some cases the remnants of the red blood cell membrane are intact and are seen as a thin, pink line connecting the poles of the crescent.

Although schizonts are rarely seen on a peripheral blood smear it is important they are recognized when seen. The number of merozoites ranges from 8 to 36, with an average of 24, another distinguishing feature of *P. falciparum.*

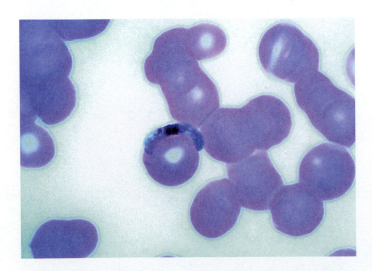

■ **FIGURE 30-32** Gametocyte of *Plasmodium falciparum* (Giemsa-stained blood smear, 1000× magnification).

Diagnosis of Malaria

The method that is most often used to diagnose malaria is examination of thick and thin blood smears made from peripheral (the preferred specimen) or venous blood. ∞ Chapter 15, "Ova and Parasite," describes the procedure. Smears should be made at 6- to 12-hour intervals in order to find the different stages of the parasite. Very early in the infection, ring forms tend to predominate and identification of *Plasmodium* species is difficult without other more mature forms. However, the presence of multiple parasites and double chromatin dots may be indicative of *P. falciparum* infection.

Morphological characteristics of mature forms, schizonts, and gametocytes are used to identify the malarial parasite to the genus-species level. Thick smears can be used to screen individuals rapidly for the presence of malarial parasites, which may be few in number. The parasites may be distorted when the red blood cells are hemolyzed in the preparation process. Thin smear preparations should be used for definitive identification because trophozoites can be found within intact red blood cells. Table 30-6✪ lists the distinguishing characteristics of malarial parasites.

Molecular methods such as the use of the polymerase chain reaction and DNA fingerprinting (restriction fragment length polymorphism) may become important in the diagnosis of malaria as the sequence of the parasites genome become

⭐ **TABLE 30-6**

Distinguishing Characteristics of Malarial Parasites

| Malarial Parasite | Infected Red Blood Cells (RBCs) | | Schüffner's Stipppling | Periodicity (hours) | No. of Merozoites in Schizonts | Other Characteristics |
	Size	Shape				
Plasmodium vivax	Reticulocytes–enlarged and pale	Normal	Present	48	12–24 (average 16)	Single chromatin dot in ring forms Singular infections of red blood cells Very amoeboid trophozoites with bizarre, irregular shapes
P. ovale	Reticulocytes–enlarged and pale	Oval	Present	48	4–12 (average = 8)	Single chromatin dot in ring forms Singular infections of red blood cells Red blood cells exhibit ragged or jagged margins
P. malariae	Older cells–smaller than normal	Normal	Absent	72	6–12 (average = 8)	Single chromatin dot in ring forms Singular infections of red blood cells Abundant malarial pigment Mature troph often assumes "band" form "Rosette"-shaped arrangement of merozoites in schizont
P. falciparum	Normal	Normal	Absent	36–48	8–36 (average = 24)	Ring forms often have double chromatin dots Multiple infections of red blood cells Mature troph and schizont seldom seen in peripheral blood smear Crescent- or banana-shaped gametocytes

 REAL WORLD TIP

Mosquitos can survive the nonpressurized cargo cabins of airplanes. If an individual lives near or works at an international airport, malaria is possible. It is very important for a physician to take a detailed patient history.

 REAL WORLD TIP

Some degree of resistance to *Plasmodium falciparum* infection is conferred on individuals with red blood cell anomalies such as hemoglobin S, C, and E and thalassemia. Additionally, an individual possessing red blood cells lacking Duffy antigen (Fy negative) possesses some degree of resistance to infection with *P. vivax*.

known. The use of monoclonal antibodies may also prove to be an important advance in the identification process, especially in differentiating closely related animal species that may infect humans (McCutchan et al., 2008).

 Checkpoint! 30–11 (Chapter Objective 7)

The observation of which of the following organisms is considered a medical emergency and should be reported to the physician immediately?

    A. *Plasmodium malariae*
    B. *P. ovale*
    C. *P. vivax*
    D. *P. falciparum*

Babesia species

Babesia microti. Babesiosis is a febrile illness of several weeks duration and in most cases a self-limited disease. Symptoms include fever, chills, headache, myalgia, arthralgia, and general malaise. It is found across the United States with outbreaks associated with states along the northeast coast. This disease can be carried by wild animals where it may spread to domestic animals. *Babesia microti* is the species that appears to be native to humans. The arthropod vector for the *Babesia* species are hard-bodied ticks in the genus *Ixodes*. Ixodid ticks serve as the definitive host where sexual reproduction occurs.

Diagnosis of Babesiosis. *Babesia* parasites, like the *Plasmodium* species, target red blood cells, although there is no exoerythrocytic stage as is seen with malarial parasites. The specimen of choice is thick and thin peripheral blood smears where the trophozoite's appearance very closely resembles the ring forms seen in malaria. This could make it difficult to differentiate these parasites from those of *Plasmodium falciparum* where ring forms predominate in the peripheral blood. Like *P. falciparum,* it is not unusual for the red blood cells to have multiple parasites with more than one chromatin dot. To differentiate babesiosis from malaria, review the stained blood smear for extracellular parasites, a greater variation in size (size range = 1–5 microns), the lack of malarial pigment within the red cell, and the absence of schizonts. A "Maltese cross" form is considered diagnostic, but the cross-like arrangement of four rings may not be commonly seen.

REAL WORLD TIP

Babesia microti can be transmitted via blood transfusions. It can be fatal in immunocompromised individuals.

REAL WORLD TIP

Asplenic individuals can have very high levels of parasitemia with *Babesia* and *Plasmodium* species. Both organisms can be rapidly fatal in those without a spleen.

✓ Checkpoint! 30–12 (Chapter Objective 3)

A peripheral blood smear stained with Giemsa stain was examined for the presence of malarial parasites. Several infected host cells, which tend to be smaller than normal, were found to be infected with a single ring form having a bright red chromatin dot, a large vacuole, and a thin blue strip of cytoplasm. Smears made over the next 48 hours revealed mature trophozoites, many of which extend from one side of the cell to the other. Occasionally schizonts, with an average of eight or nine merozoites in the form of a rosette, are found. Although malarial pigment is plentiful, Schüffner's stippling is not present. Which parasite is most likely the cause of this patient's illness?

A. Plasmodium vivax

B. P. malariae

C. P. ovale

D. P. falciparum

E. Babesia microti

► HEMOFLAGELLATES

Members of the family *Trypanosomatideae* include parasites that have both invertebrate and vertebrate hosts (*Leishmania* and *Trypanosoma* species). All of these species are transmitted by insects and must pass through developmental stages in the insect host. Review the life cycles of *T. brucei* and *Leishmania donovani,* on the Companion Website, for a visual representation of each of the four stages present in hosts:

- Trypomastigotes (Figure 30-33 ■) are long, slender, spindle- or fusiform-shaped parasites with pointed ends. They possess a centrally located nucleus and a kinetoplast (DNA containing organelle) that is located in the posterior portion of the organism. The flagellum also originates in the posterior portion of the organism but passes forward across the body to the anterior portion, forming the outer edge of the undulating membrane (similar to a fish dorsal fin). The flagellum may project free of the undulating membrane to provide motility through a whipping motion. In fresh blood the trypanosomes may be seen as colorless spindle-shaped forms that move rapidly between red blood cells, imparting a spinning motion.

- Epimastigotes (Figure 30-34 ■) are long, slender, fusiform parasites that closely resemble the trypomastigotes. They are differentiated by the location of the kinetoplast and flagellum, which are just anterior to the centrally located nucleus. The flagellum originates at the kinetoplast and forms the outer border of the undulating membrane on one-half of the organism's body. The membrane ends in a flagellum.

- Promastigotes (Figure 30-35 ■) are also long, slender, and fusiform in shape. The flagellum originates from the kinetoplast, which is located in the far anterior portion of the

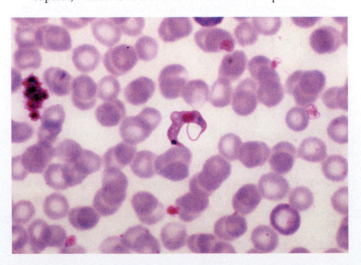

■ **FIGURE 30-33** Trypomastigote form of *Trypanosoma cruzi* in a blood smear stained with the Giemsa stain (1000× magnification).
Public Health Image Library (PHIL)/CDC/Dr. Mae Melvin

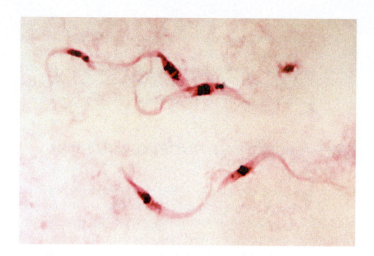

■ **FIGURE 30-34** Epimastigote form of *Trypanosoma cruzi*.
Public Health Image Library (PHIL)/CDC

organism. The nucleus is centrally located and there is no undulating membrane.

■ Amastigotes (refer to Figure 30-37) are ovoid in shape and lack an undulating membrane and flagellum. The kinetoplast and a short intracytoplasmic flagellum are situated anterior to the nucleus.

The genus *Trypanosoma* contains three species that infect humans.

TRYPANSOMA CRUZI

American Trypanosomiasis or Chagas Disease

Trypanosoma cruzi is the etiological agent of Chagas disease. This organism is endemic to South and Central America and southern United States.

The insect vector is the reduviid or kissing bug. Kissing bugs are most likely to be found in rural settings in countries

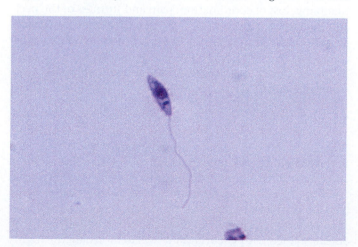

■ **FIGURE 30-35** Promatigote form of *Leishmania* spp.
Public Health Image Library (PHIL)/CDC/Dr. Mae Melvin

with warm climates where houses are constructed of adobe, wooden poles, or thatch. The insects hide within cracks and holes during the day and come out at night to feed while its victims are asleep. The bite is usually painless and the insect often feeds on the face at junctions of cutaneous and mucous surfaces such as the eyes or mouth, hence the name "kissing bug."

T. cruzi has two phases in its life cycle: one that occurs in the blood and tissues of infected humans and animals, which serve as reservoir hosts, and another phase that occurs in the intestinal tract of the insect. Humans are infected with the bite of the reduviid bug. A small trypomastigote, called the metacyclic trypomastigote, is found in the rectum of the insect and is passed out in the feces when it feeds. This infective stage gains entry into the body of the host when it is rubbed into the puncture wound made by the bite of the insect, or it may gain entrance through a break in the skin such as an abrasion.

Having gained access to the host's body the parasite is carried to other tissues through the peripheral blood. When tissue cells have been invaded, the trypomastigote loses its flagellum and undulating membrane, and is transformed into the amastigote stage, which undergoes binary fission. When the host cell is filled with amastigotes it ruptures, releasing the parasite.

Nests of amastigote may be found in the myocardium, in macrophages in the liver, spleen, lungs, bone marrow, and in glial cells of the brain. They develop into trypomastigotes, which are ingested by reduviid bugs. In the insect the trypomastigote becomes an epimastigote that multiplies in the posterior portion of the midgut. Eventually the epimastigote develops into the metacyclic trypomastigote form, which moves into the hindgut and rectum to be passed in the feces where they can infect a new host and complete the cycle. A visual representation of the life cycle of *T. cruzi* is available on the Companion Website.

Chagas disease is seen most often in children who are less than 5 years of age. In the acute form, a high fever correlates with the appearance of trypomastigotes in the blood. The liver and spleen can be enlarged (hepatosplenomegaly). Encephalomyelitis or meningoencephalitis are possible. If untreated, death may occur within 2–4 weeks. Swelling of the face with marked edema of the eyelids of one or both eyes is a called a chagoma. It is associated with Chagas disease and is referred to as Romaña's sign. It is a reaction to the bite of the insect and, early in infection, may yield amastigotes and trypomastigotes.

In older children and adults, the chronic form is most likely to occur. Myocarditis is common and damage to heart tissue causes it to enlarge and results in congestive heart failure. Invasion of the central nervous system may be accompanied by neurological disorders that follow destruction of motor centers. Nerves that control peristalsis of the gastrointestinal tract may also be destroyed. This leads to dialation and edema of the digestive tract, which, in turn, is seen as conditions known as megaesophagus and megacolon.

In the chronic form, trypomastigotes are fewer in number and more difficult to demonstrate on a peripheral blood smear. A special technique has been devised to diagnose Chagas disease under such circumstances. **Xenodiagnosis** is a process in which trypanosome-free, laboratory-bred reduviid bugs in specially constructed boxes are attached to the arm of patients suspected of having trypanosomiasis. The insects are allowed to feed and if the patient harbors the parasite they will multiply within the hindgut of the insect. The intestinal contents of the insects are examined microscopically after a period of 10–30 days. Metacyclic trypomatigotes will be present if the patient has trypanosomiasis.

Diagnosis of Chagas Disease

A Giemsa-stained peripheral blood smear is employed to diagnose trypanosomiasis. Trypanomastigotes appear, among the red blood cells, as long, slender, fusiform shapes that have an average size of about 20 microns (refer to Figure 30-33). They can assume a "C" or "U" shape, but this is not diagnostic for a species identification. The cytoplasm stains blue whereas the centrally located nucleus and the posteriorly located kinetoplast stain a deep red to violet color.

The amastigotes, usually appear in clusters in monocytes and the tissues of the heart, lymph nodes, and other organs. An amastigote is round to oval in shape and measures 1.5–4 microns in diameter. The nucleus is large, round, and dot like and stains a deep violet. Sometimes the short intracytoplasmic flagellum can appear as a small dash next to the nucleus within the organism.

> **Checkpoint! 30–13 (Chapter Objective 4)**
>
> *Which parasitic form does T. cruzi assume when it has been ingested by macrophages in organs such as the spleen or when it has invaded cardiac tissues?*
>
>   A. *Amastigote*
>   B. *Promastigote*
>   C. *Epimastigote*
>   D. *Trypomastigote*

TRYPANOSOMA RANGELI

Trypanosoma rangeli Infection

Trypanosoma rangeli is a nonpathogenic hemoflagellate with a wide range of host species, including domestic animals, wild animals, and humans. Most human infections occur in children with no apparent symptoms even when the parasite is seen in blood smears. The vector is the same reduviid bug as for *T. cruzi*. It is clinically important to be able to recognize the diagnostic stage of this commensal parasite in order to avoid confusion with *T. cruzi*.

Diagnosis of *Trypanosoma rangeli* Infection

When trypomastigotes of *T. rangeli* are seen on a blood smear the average size is 31 microns. The body of the parasite is in the typical long, slender, fusiform or spindle shape of a typical trypomastigote. This organism possesses a relatively broad, undulating membrane and a free anterior flagellum that is less than half the length of the body. The kinetoplast is minute, round, and located in the posterior end of the parasite. The nucleus is somewhat anterior to the actual center of the body. No intracellular form has been reported.

TRYPANOSOMA BRUCEI GAMBIENSE

West African Sleeping Sickness

Trypanosoma brucei gambiense is the etiological agent of West African sleeping sickness and is endemic to the equatorial region of west and central Africa. Tsetse flies (*Glossina* species), both males and females, feed on infected persons and, in doing so, ingest trypomastigotes in the blood meal. The parasite migrates to the salivary glands to become epimastigotes. The epimastigotes develop into the metacyclic trypomastigotes that infect a new host following the bite of the tsetse fly. A visual representation of the life cycle is available on the Companion Website. While the organism can be transmitted to animals, there are no known animal reservoirs for *T. gambiense*.

Initially the parasite resides in the tissues surrounding the bite site forming a nodule. The organism appears in the peripheral blood and invasion of the lymph nodes occurs. The swollen lymph nodes on the neck are called Winterbottom's sign. This chronic stage can last for months. In the acute phase, the organism invades the central nervous system leading to coma. *T. gambiense* usually causes a mild, chronic disease that, if untreated, debilitates the host over a period of several years before producing a fatal outcome.

During the chronic stage, the infected individual may experience a number of other symptoms including headache, anorexia, nausea, vomiting, and night sweats. Invasion of the central nervous system produces symptoms such as severe headache, increasing apathy and confusion, muscle spasms, trembling, loss of coordination, pain and stiffness of the neck, and increasing periods of somnolence (sleepiness). Individuals suffering from sleeping sickness are often extremely emaciated but in contrast, the face is edematous (John & Petri, 2006). As the disease progresses the individual lapses into a coma and shortly thereafter dies.

Diagnosis of West African Trypanosomiasis

Blood, lymph node fluid, and cerebrospinal fluid may be sent to the laboratory for study. Organisms are present in the lymph fluid during febrile periods but they may also be recovered from the blood in large numbers at the same time. During afebrile periods the numbers of trypanosomes in the blood may be few and difficult to demonstrate. A peripheral blood smear, stained with Giemsa stain, will demonstate the highly pleomorphic trypomastigotes (Figure 30-36 ■). The organism measures 33 microns in length and 1.5–3.5 microns in width and resembles that of other Trypanosoma species.

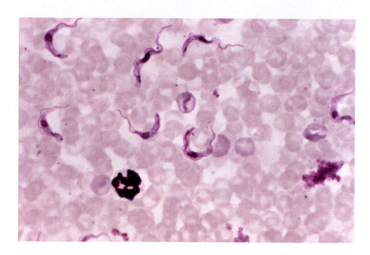

■ **FIGURE 30-36** Trypomastigote forms of *Trypanosoma brucei* in a blood smear stained with the Giemsa stain (1000× magnification). *CDC/Dr. Mae Melvin*

 REAL WORLD TIP

During the chronic stage of West African sleeping sickness, trypomastigotes are found in nodules and lymph nodes. The organisms are also in the blood but in low numbers. The concentration in the blood is highest during a fever. In the acute stage of the disease, the trypomastigotes are found in the CSF.

TRYPANOSOMA BRUCEI RHODESIENSE

East African Sleeping Sickness

Trypanosoma brucei rhodesiense is the etiological agent of East African sleeping sickness. This organism is endemic to Eastern and Central African countries. The life cycle is the same as that of *T. gambiense* and trypomastigote forms of *T. rhodesiense* are morphologically indistinguishable from those of *T. gambiense* when stained peripheral blood smears are examined. A differential diagnosis is based on the particular geographic areas where the patient lives or has traveled. Difficulties arise in individuals who have been in areas, such as Uganda, where tsetse flies and both *Trypanosoma* species can be found.

T. rhodesiense produces a disease very similar to that of gambian form except it is of a more virulent nature. The rhodesian form has a shorter incubation period so the trypomastigotes appear earlier. In addition, they are found in greater numbers in the blood. The disease progresses more rapidly, with the central nervous system being invaded early on. Winterbottom's sign often is not manifested in the rhodesian form because there is little glandular involvement and patients frequently die within 9 months to a year after the onset of symptoms.

Control of this disease is difficult because, unlike *T. gambiense,* which has humans as the only host species, there are a number of animal reservoirs, including domestic animals, such as cattle, and game animals.

Diagnosis of East African Trypanosomiasis

Diagnosis employs the same methods as those used in the diagnosis of West African trypanosomiasis. Because of the greater number of parasites in the peripheral blood of patients suffering from East African trypanosomiasis, the infection is more readily diagnosed. Table 30-7✪ lists the distinguishing characteristics of *Trypanosoma* species.

✓ **Checkpoint! 30–14 (Chapter Objective 4)**

Which of the following does not include reservoir hosts in its life cycle?
 A. *Trypanosoma cruzi*
 B. *T. rangeli*
 C. *T. brucei gambiense*
 D. *T. brucei rhodesiense*

LEISHMANIASIS

The hemoflagellates responsible for leishmaniasis occur in only two stages: promastigotes and amastigotes. The life cycle requires an insect vector, sandflies, and may involve a number of vertebrate hosts including humans.

The promastigote is the infective stage, which is introduced into the human host when the sandfly feeds. The stage seen in blood and tissues of man is the amastigote, which has been engulfed by phagocytic cells. Amastigotes, the diagnostic stage, proliferate within the cytoplasm of macrophages until the cell is destroyed and they are released to infect other macrophages in the skin, mucous membranes, and reticuloendothelial (RES) system (organs such as the liver, spleen, and bone marrow that are rich in macrophages). As these phagocytic cells circulate in the peripheral bloodstream they may be ingested by a sandfly when it obtains its blood meal. Within the midgut of the insect the amastigotes are transformed into the promastigote form. These promastigote forms migrate forward from the midgut into the salivary glands where they can be introduced into a new host when the sandfly feeds again. A flow chart depicting the life cycle is available on the Companion Website.

Cutaneous Leishmaniasis

Cutaneous leishmaniasis is transmitted by sandflies of the genus *Phlebotomus* (Old World forms) and *Lutzomyia* (American forms). The Old World forms are endemic to Asia, India and Pakistan, Russia, the Middle East, North and Central Africa, and European countries surrounding the Mediterranean Sea. The American forms are found in Central and South America.

Old World Cutaneous Leishmaniasis (Oriental Sore).

Following the bite of the sandfly there is an incubation period, which may be just a few days in length or as much as several months duration. The *Leishmania tropica* complex, which contains a number of subspecies, produces a chronic skin disease that lasts a year or more. The Old World form of cutaneous

❂ TABLE 30-7

Distinguishing Characteristics of *Trypanosoma* Species

Parasite	Vector	Disease	Key Facts
Trypanosoma cruzi	Reduviid or kissing bugs	American trypanosomiasis or Chagas disease	Trypomastigotes approximately 20 microns in length Large, oval, posteriorly located kinetoplast "C"-shaped trypomastigotes on stained peripheral blood smears Wide range of reservoirs
T. rangeli	Reduviid or kissing bugs	Nonpathogenic parasite	Average size of trypomastigotes is 31 microns Small, round, posteriorly located kinetoplast Nucleus located somewhat anterior to the center Wide range of animal reservoirs
T. brucei gambiense	Tsetse flies of the *Glossina* species	West African sleeping sickness or West African trypanosomiasis	Highly pleomorphic trypomastigotes 15–33 microns Small, round, posteriorly located kinetoplast No known animal reservoirs
T. brucei rhodesiense	Tsetse flies	East African sleeping sickness or East African trypanosomiasis	Trypomastigote morphologically indistinguishable from *T. brucei gambiensi* More virulent form of West African sleeping sickness Winterbottom's sign frequently not manifested Wide range of reservoirs

leshmaniasis is characterized by a lesion that eventually erodes into a shallow ulcer with a raised, indurated edge. In the majority of cases there is a single lesion, and it is not uncommon for secondary bacterial infections of the sore to occur. *L. tropica* occurs primarily in urban areas where it is transmitted from human to human through its insect vector. There is evidence that dogs may be infected but they are not considered to be an important reservoir for human infection.

REAL WORLD TIP

Cutaneous leishmaniasis has been seen in military personnel who have served in Afghanistan, Iraq, and Iran.

Diagnosis of Cutaneous Leishmaniasis.   It is very difficult to demonstrate the organism if the specimen is taken from the surface of the ulcer as bacteria may destroy the parasite when the lesion is secondarily infected. Cutaneous leishmaniasis is diagnosed most easily by aspirating fluid from beneath the ulcer bed and tissue scrapings or biopsies from the margin or base. Amastigote forms, which are identical in all of the *Leishmania* species, may be seen within the cytoplasm of large monocytic cells. With the Giemsa or Wright's stain, the amastigote forms will appear as ovoid-shaped organisms 4.5×3.3 microns in size. The nucleus is large and stains red or purple whereas the cytoplasm is a pale blue color. A short intracytoplasmic flagellum may be seen as a dash within the cytoplasm and close to the nucleus. Think of the organism as having a large dot (nucleus) and small dash (intracytoplasmic flagellum).

Mucocutaneous Leishmaniasis (Espundia)

Mucocutaneous leishmaniasis is endemic to Central America, from southern Mexico to Paraguay, and South America in northern Argentina and Brazil. It has also been seen in Texas and Arizona. *Leishmania braziliensis* is the etiological agent that affects not only the skin but the mucous membranes as well. The initial cutaneous lesion very closely resembles that of oriental sore but the organism spreads to the mucocutaneous areas, which may involve the nasal septum, buccal mucosa, nasopharynx, larynx, and ears. Without effective treatment the disease can produce very destructive lesions that destroy the soft tissues. This includes cartilage, and can lead to the loss of the soft parts of the nose, lips, and the soft palate. Secondary bacterial infections are very serious and can result in septicemia and death. Rodents are an important reservoir host.

Diagnosis of Mucocutaneous Leishmaniasis.   The

specimen of choice to diagnose mucocutaneous leishmaniasis is a biopsy of the initial cutaneous lesion or material from ulcerations in the mucous membranes. Examination of material from lymph nodes in the vicinity is also an option. Examination of this material should reveal the presence of amastigotes identical to those seen in cutaneous leishmaniasis.

Visceral Leishmaniasis

Visceral leishmaniasis is widely known by its East Indian name "kala-azar," which means "black fever," a name derived from one of the symptoms associated with the illness, a darkening of the skin. It is found in North and Central Africa, India, Asia, the Middle East, and Central and South America where various sandflies are responsible for its spread. This disease is found in both urban and rural areas and a number of animals may serve as reservoirs for human infection, principally rodents and canines.

Leishmania donovani is the etiological agent of this disease. Following an incubation period of 2 weeks to 18 months, the organism infects not only subcutaneous tissues and mucous membranes, but other areas of the body including the viscera or internal organs. Tissues that comprise the reticuloendothelial system, such as liver, spleen, bone marrow, and mesenteric lymph nodes, are the target organs of this parasite and infection leads to hyperplasia of the tissues. It results in hepatosplenomegaly and swelling of the abdomen. Infected persons may experience anemia, weight loss, and intermittent fevers, as well as dysentery or diarrhea.

Although skin lesions like those of cutaneous leishmaniasis do not commonly occur, a condition known as post-kala-azar dermal leishmanoid may arise after treatment. In this case, measle-like lesions can spread throughout the body followed by swollen, nodular lesions that may arise over a period of months. These signs and symptoms tend to mimic leprosy. Untreated visceral leishmaniasis has a mortality rate of 75–95%, with death occurring in as little as 2 weeks. Some patients may survive for 2 or 3 years before succumbing to infection in chronic cases.

Diagnosis of Visceral Leishmaniasis.   Because visceral leishmaniasis can mimic other diseases, diagnosis cannot be made on the basis of signs and symptoms alone but relies upon demonstration of amastigotes in a clinical specimen from the patient (Figure 30-37 ■). For decades the specimen of choice has been biopsy material obtained by splenic puncture because of its high rate of success in demonstrating the presence of amastigote forms, but this procedure carries the risk of hemorrhage and acute blood loss due to spleen enlargement. Liver biopsy, while not as successful in demonstrating the parasite,

is considered to be much safer but still carries an element of risk. From the standpoint of safety, bone marrow from a sternal or iliac puncture may be the specimen of choice over other biopsy procedures and can effectively be used to demonstrate the presence of the parasite. Table 30-8 provides information on the vector, disease, and key facts pertinent to leishmaniasis.

> ✓ **Checkpoint! 30–15 (Chapter Objective 4)**
>
> The infective stage of the Leishmania species is
>   A. amastigotes.
>   B. promastigotes.
>   C. epimastigotes.
>   D. metacyclic trypomastigotes.

> ✓ **Checkpoint! 30–16 (Chapter Objective 4)**
>
> What is the diagnostic stage of Leishmania donovani in the human host?
>   A. Amastigotes
>   B. Promastigotes
>   C. Epimastigotes
>   D. Metacyclic trypomastigotes

▶ HELMINTHS

Parasitology involves not only unicellular parasites, or protozoa but also multicellular parasitic organisms. Because many of these organisms are worm-like in nature they are referred to as helminths ("helmins," Greek, worm). Unlike protozoan parasites, which are microscopic, the adult stages of the helminths are visible to the unaided eye as they range in size from a few millimeters to a meter or more in length. In fact, some helminths may damage host tissues simply by virtue of their size. Some are free-living, while others are exclusively parasitic, and some may even lead both forms of existence depending on the stage of their life cycle.

Their interaction with the host species may be simple, involving a single host species, but in some cases the routes of transmission are quite complex and involve one or more intermediate hosts in which multiplication and development of larval stages must take place before invasion of the definitive host, which contains the adult stage. In most cases the eggs of the parasite exit the host and develop in the environment and for this reason, warm, humid climates favor their survival. It is not surprising, therefore, that the highest infection rates are seen in tropical and subtropical countries where the mean temperature year round is never lower than 20°C. Not only is the environment more conducive to their existence but levels

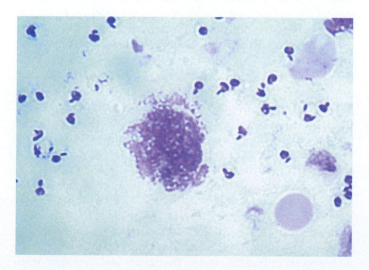

■ **FIGURE 30-37** *Leishmania donovani* amastigotes in a Giemsa-stained preparation from splenic tissue.

✪ TABLE 30-8

Leishmaniasis

Parasite	Vector	Disease	Key Facts
Leishmania tropica	*Plebotomus* species (sandflies)	Cutaneous leishmaniasis (Old World form)	Chronic skin disease of long duration Single lesion usually Typically seen as dry ulcerative lesions Transmission primarily human to human
L. major	*Phlebotomus* species	Cutaneous leishmaniasis (Old World form)	Acute skin disease of short duration Lesions are moist and primarily on lower limbs Secondary or satellite lesions are common Rodents are important reservoir hosts
L. mexicana	*Lutzomyia* species (sandflies)	American cutaneous leishmaniasis (chiclero ulcer or bay sore)	Single lesion, most often found on the ear Extensive destruction of cartilage possible
L. pifanoi	*Lutzomyia* species (sandflies)	American cutaneous leishmaniasis (chiclero ulcer or bay sore)	Diffuse, nodular lesions that resemble those of leprosy Rodents are important reservoir hosts
L. braziliensis	*Lutzomyia* species *Psychodopygus* species (sandflies)	Mucocutaneous leishmaniasis	Affects skin and mucous membranes Destructive lesions affect soft tissue including nasal cartilage Secondary bacterial infections can be fatal Rodents are important reservoir hosts
L. donovani	*Phlebotomus* and *Lutzomyia* species (sandflies)	Visceral leishmaniasis	Affects mucous membranes, subcutaneous tissues, and viscera In untreated patients mortality rates can be as high as 75–95%

of sanitation and hygiene in these countries are poor and this facilitates transmission via the fecal–oral route.

Eggs and larval forms that are ingested must have a shell (eggs), integument (larvae), or, in the case of adults, a cuticle that is tough enough to resist digestion. Adults and larval forms may also have secretory glands that can produce enzymes that digest skin and other body tissues, allowing entrance through the skin and migration through host tissues. Although the immune system does react to the presence of helminth parasites, especially those that enter the circulation or traverse internal organs, there is no lasting immunity to reinfection.

Within the different classes of these parasites there may be partial or complete loss of the digestive tract, either of which would necessitate a parasitic existence. Peristalsis, the muscular action of the gastrointestinal tract that propels its contents downward, would eventually expel intestinal parasites from the body of the host. Trematodes (flukes) and cestodes (tapeworms) possess muscular attachment organs with suckers and hooks that allow the organism to maintain a stationary position within the host. Hookworms have a buccal cavity with teeth or cutting plates for attachment.

Although helminths differ in how well developed their digestive tracts are, all species have very well-developed reproductive systems. Enough eggs must survive conditions outside the host's body, and a sufficient number of larvae must survive the search for a suitable host, to propagate the species. In their favor most trematodes and all cestodes are hermaphroditic,

having both male and female reproductive systems. In contrast, nematodes exist as separate sexes, with females typically much larger than males. Helminths as a group are very prolific, with females being able to produce as many as 200,000 eggs in a 24-hour period. Females have specialized organs that produce yolk material, to be used as food during development into larval stages, and a protective shell that protects the egg against dessication, temperature variation, and bacterial or fungal attack. The size, shape, shell thickness, and developmental stage of the egg when passed in the feces are all important characteristics that aid in the identification of the parasite.

Examination of a direct wet mount and a concentrated wet mount for eggs, larvae, and adults are useful methods employed in the diagnosis of helminth infections. In some cases stained tissue sections allow detection of larval or adult forms that migrate through host tissues. Examination of a fecal smear that has been fixed and stained with the iron hematoxylin or Gomori's trichrome stain is indispensable in diagnosing protozoan infections, but in most cases is not productive in the diagnosis of helminth infections. The dehydration steps required in the preparation of fecal smears that are fixed and stained often distort eggs and larval forms.

Classification schemes for metazoan parasites may differ slightly but in this text the following phyla are considered to be medically important: Nematoda; Platyhelminthes (which includes two important classes, Trematoda and Cestoda); Acanthocephala, the thorny-headed worms; Pentastomida, the tongue worms; and Arthropoda, segmented organisms with chitinous exoskeletons and jointed appendages. In the following discussions of the major pathogens, modes of transmission or host entry, target sites, pathogenicity, symptoms, and methods of diagnosis are covered.

INTESTINAL NEMATODES

Nematodes or roundworms are long, cylindrical in shape, tapered anteriorly and posteriorly, and in some cases resemble the common earthworm. Nematodes are widespread in nature and may be recovered from fresh and marine water environments, decaying vegetation, and moist soil. The nematodes can be free-living, saprophytic organisms as well as obligate plant, animal, and human parasites. The eggs of free-living and plant nematodes, which pass through the gastrointestinal tract of humans following their ingestion in food and water, may be a source of confusion to novice clinical parasitologists. They are referred to as spurious parasites.

Eggs of parasitic nematodes that pass out of the host's body may be undeveloped, unembryonated (containing only an undifferentiated egg mass), at an early cleavage stage containing a few cluster of cells, or may contain a well-differentiated larval stage. For some nematode species the female is viviparous, implying the discharge of live larvae instead of eggs.

As they mature, some nematodes demonstrate two stages: rhabditiform larvae, which are free-living, and the filariform larvae, which is the infective stage. The infective stage can be introduced into a new host by ingestion, skin penetration, or through an insect vector. Once ingested, the larvae may develop into the adult stage within the intestinal tract or there may be a migratory period where the larvae undergo development in organs other the digestive tract.

Adult forms are found primarily in the intestines where they may attach to the mucosa by their anterior end, which may have spines or hooks, or there may be a well-developed buccal cavity containing teeth or cutting plates. Nematodes exist as separate sexes that may easily be differentiated on the basis of size. Males may possess copulatory spicules or bursae which are thought to aid the mating process.

Checkpoint! 30–17 (Chapter Objective 4)

In most cases the infective stage for nematodes are
  A. *filariform larvae.*
  B. *rhabditiform larvae.*
  C. *cysticercoid larvae.*
  D. *hydatidiform larvae.*

Ascaris lumbricoides

Ascaris lumbricoides Infection. *Ascaris lumbricoides*, commonly referred to as human roundworm, infects more humans than any other intestinal parasite. This organism is found in both tropical and subtropical countries and is even endemic to more temperate climates such as the southeastern area of the United States. Infection is transmitted through the ingestion of plant foods or water contaminated with human fecal material containing embryonated eggs, the infective stage. Underdeveloped countries use human waste, referred to as "night soil," as fertilizer, which aids transmission.

When eggs reach the duodenum the larval form hatches, penetrates the intestinal mucosa, and, via the bloodstream, travels to various organs including the liver, heart, and eventually the lungs. Once in the lung, they migrate from the capillaries into the alveoli. In the alveoli the larvae grow and molt over a period of approximately 3 weeks before migrating up the trachea where they are swallowed to enter the small intestine. In the small intestine the larvae mature into adults, mating occurs, and females begin producing eggs, as many as 200,000 a day. With such prolific breeding it is not surprising that *A. lumbricoides* infects as much as one-fourth of the world's population. A visual representation of the life cycle is available on the Companion Website.

Because the female discharges her eggs into the lumen of the intestine they are passed out with the feces. In freshly passed stool, *A. lumbricoides* eggs will be unembryonated and are usually surrounded by an albuminous coating, giving them a bumpy or wavy appearance. The term "mammillated" is used to describe eggs with this outer protein coating. The eggs are bile colored (brown), round to oval in shape, have a very thick shell, and range in size from 45 to 75 microns (Figure 30-38 ■). Unfertilized eggs can be differentiated from fertile eggs in that they are longer and narrower, ranging in size from 88 to 94 microns, and the albuminoid coating and egg shell may be thinner. In some cases *A. lumbricoides* eggs lack the wavy albuminoid coating and are called "decorticated" eggs. Decorticated fertile eggs may be misidentified as hookworm eggs if the thickness of the shell is not taken into consideration. Hookworm eggs have a very thin shell in comparison to the thick-shelled

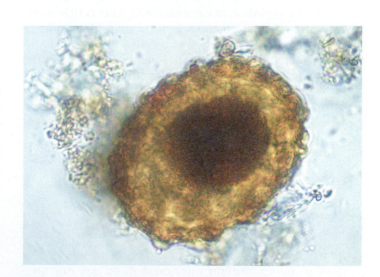

■ **FIGURE 30-38** Fertilized mammillated *Ascaris lumbricoides* egg in a direct wet mount (400× magnification).

A. lumbricoides eggs. Another problem encountered by novices is misidentifying decorticated, infertile eggs as the eggs of *Trichostrongylus* species, which are in the same size range but also have a very thin shell like the eggs of human hookworms. *Trichostrongylus* species usually infects herbivores. Information on *Trichostrongylus* spp. can be found on the Companion Website.

A. lumbricoides eggs require 2–3 weeks of development in warm, moist soil before they reach the infective stage. Unless they are killed by excessive heat or dessication these eggs may remain viable for months even though they are outside the body of the host. Ingestion of just a few embryonated eggs will result in a light infection, which may be asymptomatic. Ingestion of a large number of eggs will likely result in a heavy infection and patients may develop pneumonitis due to the large numbers of larvae migrating into lung tissue.

Large numbers of adult *A. lumbricoides* may form into large masses, called a bolus, and can lead to bowel obstruction especially in young children because their intestinal lumen tends to be small in diameter. Serious sequelae to intestinal obstruction include gangrene of the bowel and death, unless surgical intervention is employed. Another danger is posed by the large size of adult roundworms and the fact that they are covered by a tough outer cuticle. Fever, drugs, and anesthesia may irritate the roundworms and cause them to perforate the bowel in an attempt to escape noxious stimuli. This can result in peritonitis as bowel contents leak into the peritoneal cavity.

Diagnosis of *Ascaris lumbricoides* Infection.

A freshly passed or properly preserved stool is the specimen of choice in the diagnosis of *A. lumbricoides* infection. The procedures recommended include examination of both saline and iodine-stained direct wet mounts and concentrated wet mount preparations. Using a concentration procedure increases the likelihood eggs will be detected when they are few in number. The diagnostic stages include adults or eggs, fertile, unfertile, mammillated, or decorticated. *A. lumbricoides* adults are creamy white to pinkish in color and their outer cuticle is covered with fine circular striations. Females range in size from 20 to 35 centimeters (8–14 inches) in length and 3 to 6 millimeters in diameter. Males are slightly smaller than females and range in size from 15 to 30 cm in length and 2 to 4 mm in diameter. One distinguishing characteristic that allows males to be differentiated from females is the male's incurved tail, which is likely an aid in copulation.

Trichuris trichiura

Trichiuriasis. *Trichuris trichiura*, often referred to as the human whipworm, is another roundworm that is prevalent in tropical, subtropical, and temperate areas of the globe. *T. trichiura* is the etiological agent of the second most common nematode infection in the United States. It is seen primarily in the South where infections are usually light.

The whipworm gains entry to the host through the ingestion of embryonated eggs in contaminated food and water in much the same manner as *Ascaris lumbricoides*. In the small intestine the egg shell is digested and the larval forms grow and molt for a short period of time before eventually moving to the cecum or large intestine where they attach themselves and begin to reproduce. A visual representation of the life cycle is available on the Companion Website.

As with *A. lumbricoides*, light infections are asymptomatic whereas heavy infections may be accompanied by abdominal pain and bloody or mucoid diarrhea. Anemia, eosinophilia, and edema of the rectum may also occur with heavy infections. Small children with heavy infections may suffer from a prolapsed rectum with adult worms being clearly visible. The thin anterior portion of adult whipworms is firmly embedded in the intestinal mucosa while the posterior end remains in the lumen of the intestine so that eggs produced by the female are discharged into the feces and are then passed to the outside with the stool. Freshly passed eggs are unembryonated and require an incubation period of 10–14 days in warm, moist soil for the embryo to develop.

Diagnosis of Trichuriasis.

Examination of saline and iodine-stained direct and concentrate wet mounts of freshly passed stool is the recommended procedure to diagnose trichuriasis. The spindle-shaped eggs of *T. trichiura* are often described as "barrel or football shaped." It has also been described as a "tea tray" morphology. The eggs are bile colored with the exception of the unstained, highly refractile, bipolar plugs or prominences, which are a distinguishing characteristic. When passed in feces eggs are unembryonated, 50–54 microns in length, 22–23 microns in diameter, and have a moderately thick shell (Figure 30-39 ■).

Adult worms are 3–5 cm in length with the anterior three-fifths of the body being much thinner than the posterior end of the organism. Males are slightly smaller than females and examination of the thickened, curled posterior end may reveal

---

✪ REAL WORLD TIP

Seeing only unfertilized eggs in a concentrated fecal sample may indicate infection with all female *Ascaris* adults.

✪ REAL WORLD TIP

Unfertilized *Ascaris* ova will not float with the zinc-flotation concentration method and so will not be recovered.

✪ REAL WORLD TIP

The quantitiation of *Trichuris* eggs in the stool may indicate the level of treatment needed. Light infestations usually do not require treatment.

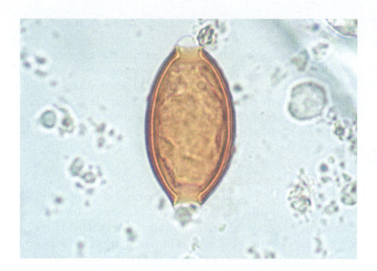

FIGURE 30-39 *Trichuris trichiura* egg in a direct wet mount from a stool specimen (400× magnification).

the presence of a retractable copulatory spicule. Because the anterior end of whipworms is so firmly embedded in the mucosa, adults are not frequently recovered from the stool.

Hookworm

Hookworm Infection.
Hookworms are found in tropical, subtropical, and temperate areas of the world. There are two species for which man is the definitive host, *Ancylostoma duodenale,* known as the Old World hookworm, and *Necator americanus,* referred to as the New World hookworm. *A. duodenale* is the only human hookworm found in southern Europe, countries bordering the Mediterranean Sea, and the west coast of South America. *N. americanus* is the predominant human hookworm found in the southern United States, Central America, Cuba, much of South America and Africa, and Australia. In India, China, Southeast Asia, and islands of the South Pacific, both species may be found in the same geographic area. Hookworms, human roundworms, and whipworms are found in very much the same areas of the globe and some parasitologists have referred to *A. lumbricoides, T. trichiura,* and hookworms as "the big three" because patients are often infected with all three parasites in areas where these organisms are endemic.

The life cycle of both species of hookworm is essentially the same, with the filariform larva being the infective stage. The preferred environment for filariform larvae is the uppermost layer of warm, moist soil containing decaying vegetation where they wave about in a nearly vertical position, waiting for a chance to make contact with the exposed skin of a suitable host. Although the larvae may penetrate any area of skin, entrance is most likely to be gained in the feet as individuals walk barefoot across the soil. Larvae then migrate through the subcutaneous tissues where they enter venules and are carried in the bloodstream to the heart and from there to the lungs. In the lungs they break out of the capillaries and

into the air sacs and migrate up the trachea to be swallowed. The larvae reach the jejunum and attach to the intestinal mucosa with their buccal capsule. Growth and maturation occurs in the small intestine where adults ingest blood and tissue fluids of the host. Symptoms of hookworm infection may include diarrhea, abdominal pain, and nausea. With heavy infestations, sufficient blood loss can lead to anemia.

REAL WORLD TIP

After the hookworm filariform larvae invade the skin, their tunneling causes severe allergic itching. This is known as "ground itch." The tunnels can become secondarily infected with bacteria.

REAL WORLD TIP

With a heavy hookworm burden, an individual can lose 100 milliliters per day. The anemia caused by hookworm is an iron-deficient anemia. Red bloods cells appear microcytic and hypochromic.

Shortly after mating, the production of eggs begins and since the body of the female is in the intestinal lumen, the unembryonated eggs she deposits are passed out with the feces. Eggs found in freshly passed stool are either unembryonated or at the two- to eight-cell stage of cleavage. Eggs passed onto warm, moist soil continue to develop and in 24–48 hours will contain well-developed larval forms. Because such a short time is required for development of the first larval stage, it is possible to find embryonated eggs and occasionally actively motile rhabditiform larvae in the stools of patients who are constipated or in unpreserved stool specimens. In such cases it will be necessary to differentiate these free-living hookworm larvae from those of *Strongyloides stercoralis*.

Rhabditiform larvae, which develop within the egg in the soil, hatch and for about 3 days feed on bacteria and organic debris before molting to become the non-feeding, infective filariform larvae. Filariform larvae are unable to subsist in the soil and therefore must find a suitable host and penetrate the skin to continue the life cycle. A flow chart of the life cycle can be found on the Companion Website.

Diagnosis of Hookworm Infection.
Examination of saline or iodine-stained direct or concentration wet mounts can reveal the presence of either hookworm adults or eggs. The eggs of *A. duodenale* and *N. americanus* are identical and differentiation of the etiological agent requires the adult stage. For this reason one cannot assign a genus-species name to the hookworm infection. If neither adults nor rhabditiform larvae are observed the cause of the infection is reported as "hookworms."

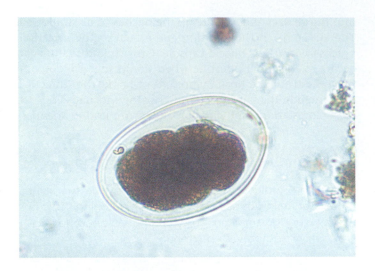

■ FIGURE 30-40 Human hookworm egg in a direct wet mount preparation (400× magnification).

Hookworm eggs are broadly oval, with a size range of 55–75 microns. The egg shell is very thin (a distinguishing feature) and hyaline or colorless. Freshly passed eggs are either unembryonated or in the early cleavage stage, with two to eight cell clusters (Figure 30-40 ■). In cases of intestinal stasis or constipation, rhabditiform larvae may be seen in the stool. Hookworm rhabditiform larvae must be differentiated from those of *S. stercoralis* and this is possible with careful examination using the high power objective. Hookworm rhabditiform larvae have a long, narrow buccal cavity (Figure 30-41 ■), a flask-shaped, muscular esophagus in the anterior third of the digestive tract, and an inconspicuous genital primordium (a cluster of cells about two-thirds of the way down the body). *Strongyloides stercoralis* rhabditiform larvae have a short buccal cavity and a large genital primordium. The hookworm filariform larvae dis-

play a pointed tail, whereas *Strongyloides stercoralis* has a notched tail (Figure 30-42 ■).

The name "hookworm" is derived from the appearance of the adult stage. The anterior-most portion of the adult is sharply bent in relation to the body. Male hookworms are 5 to 10 mm in length and have a prominent copulatory bursa in the posterior end of the body. Females are longer, attaining lengths of 10–13 mm. Both males and females are grayish-white or pinkish in color.

Cutaneous Larval Migrans

Cutaneous larval migrans is a disease caused by nonhuman roundworms. In this case the infective larvae of *Ancylostoma braziliensis*, the dog and cat hookworm, or *A. caninum*, the dog hookworm, penetrate the skin of humans. Infection is a result of exposure to warm, moist soil in which dogs and cats have defecated. Because man is an accidental host of these animal hookworms, the larvae are not able to complete development into the adult stage to establish an intestinal infection. As a

> ✓ **Checkpoint! 30–18 (Chapter Objectives 3 and 6)**
>
> *Examination of a saline direct wet mount preparation revealed the presence of a few spindle-shaped, bile-colored, unembryonated eggs with the following characteristics: size range = 50–54 μm, shell thickness is moderate, and highly refractile bipolar plugs or prominences were noted. This parasite is most likely*
>
> A. *Ascaris lumbricoides.*
> B. *Trichuris trichiura.*
> C. *Necator americanus.*
> D. *Ancylostoma duodenale.*
> E. *A. braziliensis.*

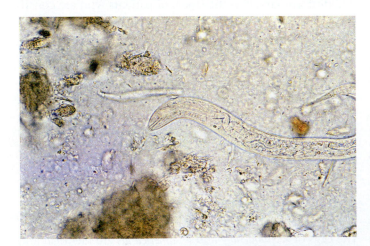

■ FIGURE 30-41 The buccal cavity of the rhabditiform larvae of *Hookworm* spp. is considered long when compared to that of *Strongyloides stercoralis.* It is equal in length to the width of the larvae.

Public Health Image Library (PHIL)/CDC/Dr. Mae Melvin

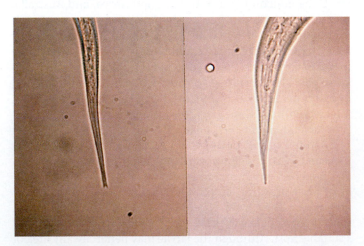

■ FIGURE 30-42 The tail of filariform larvae must be used to differentiate *Hookworm* spp. from *Strongyloides stercoralis.* The tail of *S. stercoralis* is notched (left) while that of *Hookworm* spp is pointed (right).

Public Health Image Library (PHIL)/CDC

result, the larvae continue to migrate through the subcutaneous tissue until they die and are absorbed. The immune response to the presence of the larval forms is a severe allergic reaction characterized by intense itching. Lesions are seen as tunnels in the tissue. These symptoms are the reason cutaneous larval migrans is also known as "creeping eruption." The tunnels often become secondarily infected with bacteria.

Checkpoint! 30–19 (Chapter Objectives 4 and 8)

To prevent the transmission of hookworm infection, one should:
A. wash hands after cleaning the cat litter box.
B. avoid eating sushi.
C. wear shoes outdoors.
D. throughly cook pork prior to eating.

Anisakiasis

Anisakiasis is a roundworm infection caused by nematodes in the genus *Anisakis*. *Anisakis* species are native to marine mammals such as seals, whales, and dolphins. Marine mammals acquire the infective larvae through eating infected fish or squid. The adult stage develops, in their intestinal tract, to produce eggs. Human infection is acquired by the ingestion of raw or undercooked fish, which harbor the larval form in their tissues. The life cycle is visually represented on the Companion Website.

Infection is often characterized by nausea, vomiting, and abdominal pain. In some cases, adult worms or larval forms may be expelled in vomitus or with coughing. Following ingestion, larval forms penetrate the mucosa where they form eosinophilic granulomas in the stomach or intestines. Surgical excision and histologic examination of tissue sections is a means of demonstrating the presence of the roundworms.

REAL WORLD TIP

After capture, if fish are not gutted properly or kept frozen, the *Anisakis* spp. larvae can leave the fish intestine and enter the flesh. There is an increased incidence of this parasite due to the popularity of sushi and sashimi bars.

REAL WORLD TIP

Often there is only one *Anisakis* nematode present in an individual. It must be physicaly removed using a fiber optic device and forceps.

Strongyloides stercoralis

Strongyloidiasis. *Strongyloides stercoralis*, the human threadworm, has a life cycle very similar to that of hookworms, with filariform larvae penetrating the skin of humans to initiate infection. The larvae reach the lungs via the bloodstream, where they

undergo a series of molts before migrating up the trachea to be swallowed. Adult females burrow into the intestinal mucosa and deposit their eggs. Adult females, in the intestine, are parthenogenic so the eggs develop into larvae without male fertilization. The eggs hatch while they are still in the mucosal layer, and the rhabditiform larvae migrate into the lumen of the intestine where they can be passed with the stool. A flow chart of the life cycle is available on the Companion Website.

On occasion rhabditiform larvae become filariform larvae while they are still within the intestine and these larvae may reinfect the host by penetrating the intestinal mucosa and gaining access to the bloodstream. This is known as autoinfection and usually occurs in immunocompromised individuals. The rhabditiform larvae, passed in the feces, develop in the soil and may become filariform larvae able to infect a new host or they may develop into free-living male and female adults and produce eggs that hatch in the soil, releasing free-living rhabditiform larvae.

Light *S. stercoralis* infections may be asymptomatic whereas heavy infections may be characterized by pneumonitis, dyspnea, wheezing, fever, and gastrointestinal symptoms including sloughing of the intestinal mucosa leading to ulcerations and fibrosis. Disseminated strongyloidiasis may occur in immunocompromised hosts such as transplant patients and those on steroids. Disseminated strongyloidiasis is characterized by large numbers of migrating larvae, which leads to major damage of organs such as the liver, heart, pancreas, kidneys, and brain.

Diagnosis of Strongyloidiasis. *S. stercoralis* infection may be diagnosed in the same manner as hookworm infection. Examination of a wet mount preparation can reveal the presence of actively motile rhabditiform larvae approximately 275 μm in length and 16 μm diameter. These larval forms have a short buccal cavity of small diameter (Figure 30-43 ■), a muscular, hourglass-shaped esophagus (diagnostic for the genus),

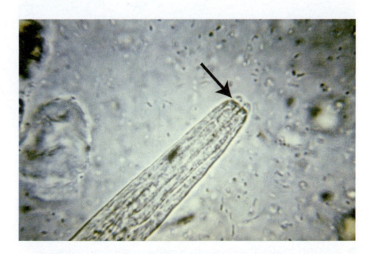

■ **FIGURE 30-43** The buccal cavity of the rhabitiform larvae of *Strongyloides stercoralis* is considered short when compared to that of *Hookworm* spp. (Figure 30-41).
Public Health Image Library (PHIL)/CDC

and a relatively conspicuous genital primordium (a packet of cells that will develop into the genitalia) that is located ventrally, halfway down the midgut region (Figure 30-44 ■). The filariform larvae may be seen in the stool with autoinfection. It is about 600 μm in length and 20 μm in width and recognized by its notched tail (refer to Figure 30-42).

In cases of disseminated strongyloidiasis, filariform larvae may be found in the sputum. In bacterial sputum cultures, they leave tracks in the organism colonies as they travel across the agar plate. Because adult females are within the intestinal mucosa they are not usually recovered in feces but in patients with severe diarrhea, embryonated eggs, 50–58 microns in length and 30–34 microns in diameter, may be seen in the stool. They are similar to those of hookworm but smaller in size.

 REAL WORLD TIP

Differentiation of the rhabditiform larvae of *Strongyloides stercoralis* is made by its short buccal cavity and large, prominent genital primordium. Just remember it is "short" and "sexy."

 REAL WORLD TIP

Prior to transplantation, patients must be screened for *Strongyloides stercoralis*. With immunosuppression, the organism can cause hyperinfections and disseminate throughout the body.

Enterobius vermicularis

Pinworm Infection.   *Enterobius vermicularis,* also known as the pinworm or seatworm, is the most common helminth in countries with temperate climates. Infection is acquired by inges-

tion of embryonated eggs that hatch in the duodenum, freeing the larvae. Once mature they become attached to the mucosa where they establish an infection in the large intestine. After mating, the adult female pinworm migrates out of the anus into the perianal region. As she moves around the perianal region she discharges her eggs onto the perineal skin rather than the lumen of the intestine. Occasionally she migrates back into the anus and large intestine but in most cases she usually dies, whereupon her body may dry out, rupture, and release more eggs. Those eggs that are deposited in the perianal region are fully embryonated and infective within a few hours. The life cycle is visually represented on the Companion Website.

The clothing and bedding of infected individuals becomes contaminated with eggs and can be the source of infection for others. Eggs can remain viable for up to 2 weeks outside the body under moist or humid conditions. Pinworm infection, which results from a hand-to-mouth transfer of embryonated eggs, is easily transmitted to all members of the family, especially under crowded conditions. Symptoms of intense itching in the perianal region, referred to as "pruritis ani," may occur in individuals who have a hypersensitive reaction to secretions of the worm. The adults can migrate into the female genital tract and eventually the uterus and fallopian tubes.

Diagnosis of Pinworm Infection.   Light, yellowish-white adult females and occasionally males may be seen in the perianal region and it is not at all uncommon to find females on the surface of the stool. Females are 8–13 mm (about one half inch) in length and about 0.5 mm in diameter while males range in length from 2–5 mm and about 0.2 mm in diameter. Females have a long, thin, sharply pointed tail that gives this nematode their common name, "pinworm." Both sexes lack a buccal capsule but the oral end does have a characteristically dorso-ventrally flattened cuticle (like a fish fin), creating what are called "cephalic alae."

E. vermicularis eggs are oval or spindle shaped and flattened on one side and look like an Italian loaf of bread. The length

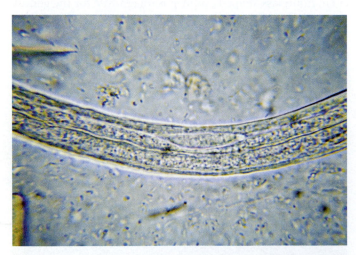

■ **FIGURE 30-44** The *Strongyloides stercoralis* rhabditiform is recognized by its genital primordium about two-thirds of the way down the organism. It is a packet of cells that will become genitalia when the organism matures.
Public Health Image Library (PHIL)/CDC/Dr. Mae Melvin

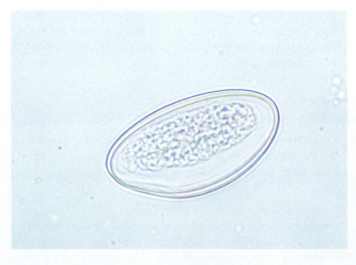

■ **FIGURE 30-45** *Enterobius vermicularis* egg.

of the egg may be from 50 to 60 microns, and the shell is of moderate thickness and translucent (Figure 30-45 ■). The eggs are seldom found in large numbers in the stool. Therefore a stool specimen is not recommended for diagnosis of pinworm infection. Instead, an attempt should be made to recover eggs from the perianal region using a pinworm paddle or scotch tape preparation. Table 30-9 ✪ lists the distinguishing characteristics of nematode eggs.

Checkpoint! 30–20 (Chapter Objective 4)

The adult stage of _____ is normally found in the intestines of marine animals such as seals, dolphins, and whales. Occasionally larval forms infect humans through the ingestion of raw or poorly cooked fish.

    A. *Trichuris trichiura*
    B. *Strongyloides stercoralis*
    C. *Anisakis* species
    D. *Enterobius vermicularis*

Checkpoint! 30–21 (Chapter Objective 4)

Transmission of Strongyloides stercoralis infection is through

    A. *ingestion of contaminated food and water.*
    B. *skin penetration by rhabditiform larvae.*
    C. *skin pentration by filariform larvae.*
    D. *ingestion of embryonated eggs.*

BLOOD AND TISSUE NEMATODES

Nematodes are responsible for extra-intestinal infections as well as intestinal infections. As a general rule invasion of blood and tissues is more serious than establishment of an infection within the lumen of the intestinal tract. Transmission of blood and tissue nematodes may occur through ingestion of embryonated eggs, ingestion of infective larval forms, or through the bite and feeding of an insect vector.

Microfilarial Infections

The filariae are threadlike worms that inhabit the vessels of blood and lymph as well as the subcutaneous and deeper tissues. All are introduced into the definitive host through insect vectors, which act as intermediate hosts. The infective larval forms are transmitted when the biting insect obtains its blood meal. Infective larvae mature into male and female adults, which mate and produce larval forms called microfilariae. In some cases the microfilariae may be encased in a thin, transparent sheath. They may be found in the peripheral blood or the subcutaneous tissues where they may be ingested when another biting insect feeds, thus completing the life cycle.

Wuchereria bancrofti

Bancroftian Filariasis. *Wuchereria bancrofti* is endemic to tropical countries of Asia, the Far East, the Pacific islands, India, and central and northern Africa. The infective filariform larvae enters the bite wound of female *Culex, Anopheles,* and *Aedes* mosquitos. After gaining entrance into the host, larvae migrate into the peripheral lymphatics to the regional lymph nodes and larger lymph vessels where they mature into adults, where

✪ TABLE 30-9

Distinguishing Characteristics of Nematode Eggs

Parasite	Shape	Size (microns)	Color	State of Development (when passed)	Key Characteristics
Ancylostoma duodenale	Ovoid	55–75 × 35–45	Colorless	Unembryonated or early cleavage stage	Size, shape, very thin shell, and early stage of development
Ascaris lumbricoides (fertile)	Round to oval	45–75 × 35–50	Brown (bile-colored)	Unembryonated	Very thick shell and mammilated outer albuminoid coating May lack the mammilated coating (decorticated)
Ascaris lumbricoides (unfertile)	Elongated	85–95 × 35–45	Brown (bile-colored)	Unembryonated	Very thick shell and mammilated outer albuminoid coating
Enterobius vermicularis	Elongate with one side flattened	50–60 × 20–30	Colorless	Embryonated	Moderately thick shell with flattened side Found on perianal skin not in stool
Necator americanus	Morphologically indistinguishable from those of *Ancylostoma duodenale*				
Trichostrongylus species	Ovoid with somewhat pointed ends	75–95 × 40–50	Colorless	Unembryonated or early cleavage stage	Size, shape, very thin shell, and early stage of development
Trichuris trichiura	Barrel or tea tray shaped	50–54 × 20–29	Brown (bile-colored)	Unembryonated	Thick shell with highly refractile bipolar prominences (plugs)

they mate and produce microfilariae that circulate in the peripheral blood. The greatest number of larvae occurs during the hours of 10:00 P.M. and 4:00 A.M., a phenomenon referred to as nocturnal periodicity. This ensures the microfilariae are in the peripheral blood during the time the intermediate host, the mosquito, takes its blood meal. A visual representation of the life cycle is available on the Companion Website.

Ingested microfilariae bore through the stomach of the mosquito, enter the body cavity, and eventually migrate to the thoracic muscles where they grow and molt. The resulting larval form is the infective stage, which migrates from the thorax into the proboscis of the mosquito where it is able to infect a new host to complete the life cycle. Man is the only definitive host for *W. bancrofti*. No reservoir hosts serve as additional sources of infection.

During the early stage of the illness, symptoms include fever, lymphangitis, and lymphadenitis. As the disease progresses the lymphatic vessels of affected limbs become dilated and the walls of the vessels thicken. Proliferation of connective tissues or fibrosis, edema, and thickening of the epidermis leads to enlargement of the lower extremity limbs, a condition known as "elephantiasis." With some infections the breasts or vulva of women and the scrotum of males may also be affected and greatly enlarged. Not only can elephantiasis be terribly disfiguring, but this condition may be life threatening due to impairment of circulation to the affected body part and possible secondary invasion by bacteria or fungi. Involvement of the lymphatics of the kidney or bladder may result in rupture of the distended lymph vessels, resulting in chyluria. Adult worms that die may become calcified, providing radiographic evidence of the disease.

Diagnosis of *Wuchereria bancrofti* Infection.   Examination of thick and thin smears of peripheral blood is the method recommended for diagnosis of bancroftian filariasis. In cases where only small numbers of microfilaria are present concentration procedures and filters can be employed. Examination of Giemsa-stained smears can reveal the presence of the diagnostic stage, the microfilariae. *Wuchereria bancrofti* microfilariae are long and thin, with a blunt, rounded anterior end, tapered tail, and range in size from 245 to 300 microns. The organisms are surrounded by a thin, delicate shell; they are said to be "sheathed." The body of the embryo contains numerous nuclei but the posterior portion of the tail is free of nuclei (Figure 30-46 ■). Adults are rarely seen but may be found in the lymph nodes and larger vessels. Males are 2.5–4 centimeters in length while females are 5–10 centimeters in length.

Brugia malayi

***Brugia malayi* Infection.**   *Brugia malayi* infection is endemic, as its name applies, to Malaysia but is also found in other Far Eastern countries, New Guinea, and the subcontinent of India and Sri Lanka. The life cycle of *B. malayi* is very similar to that of *W. bancrofti* except the insect vectors include

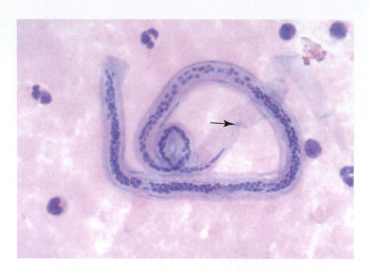

■ **FIGURE 30-46** Sheathed microfilaria of *Wuchereria bancrofti* in a Giemsa-stained blood smear (400× magnification). Note the nuclei stop before the end of the tail as noted by the arrow.

Mansonia, Anopheles, and *Aedes* mosquitos. While *W. bancrofti* does not have reservoir hosts, monkeys, dogs, and cats can serve as definitive hosts and additional sources of infection with Malayan filariasis. A flow chart of the life cycle can be found on the Companion Website. The disease caused by *B. malayi* is very similar to that of *W. bancrofti* except the genitalia are rarely involved and chyluria is usually not present.

Diagnosis of *Brugia malayi* Infection.   Thick and thin smears are commonly used in the diagnosis of Malayan filariasis. Like *W. bancrofti*, *B. malayi* also exhibits nocturnal periodicity. The microfilariae are sheathed, range in size from 175 to 230 microns in length, and nuclei do extend into the tip of the tail. Careful examination will reveal the two terminal nuclei are distinctly separate from the other caudal nuclei (Figure 30-47 ■).

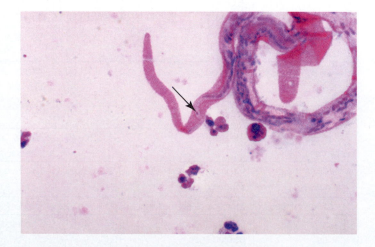

■ **FIGURE 30-47** Sheathed microfilaria of *Brugia malayi*. One of the two distinct terminal nuclei is easily observed.
Public Health Image Library (PHIL)/CDC/Dr. Mae Melvin

Loa loa

Loa loa Infection. *Loa loa,* a filarial parasite that is also known by its common name, the African eye worm, is endemic to the Congo, the Sudan, and the rain forests of West Africa. The infective filariform larva gains entrance into a new host through the bite wound left by its insect vector, *Chrysops,* the mango fly. Adults migrate through the subcutaneous and deeper tissues and have been known to enter the viscera. A visual representation of the life cycle is available on the Companion Website.

Localized, edematous, inflammatory reactions to the metabolic by-products of adult worms, called "Calabar swellings," may develop as a result of the wanderings of adult worms. While little or no pain may be associated with the migration of the adults, feeling and observing worms traveling beneath the conjunctiva is especially irritating and unnerving.

Adult worms may be present a year or more before microfilariae are produced. While adults are found in the tissues, the microfilariae are found in the blood and appear in greatest concentration during daylight hours, a phenomenon referred to as diurnal periodicity. Microfilariae in the peripheral circulation may be ingested by another mango fly. Once the infective stage is reached the infected mango fly may transmit the disease to other humans through its painful bite.

Diagnosis of Loa loa Infection. Adult worms have been surgically removed from different areas of the body including the conjunctiva, eyelids, scalp, back, breasts, groin, and penis. Adult males are 2–3.5 centimeters in length while females range in size from 5–7 centimeters.

Examination of Giemsa-stained thick and thin blood smears may reveal the presence of microfilariae of *Loa loa.* They range in size from 250 to 300 microns in length, are sheathed, and possess caudal nuclei that are continuous to the tip of the tail (Figure 30-48 ■).

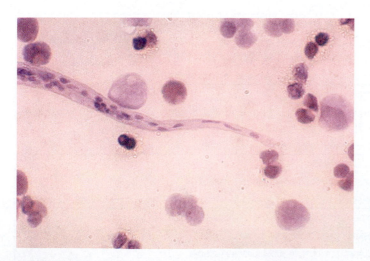

■ **FIGURE 30-48** Sheathed microfilaria of *Loa loa.* Giemsa-stained blood smear (400× magnification). While the sheath is difficult to see, the nuclei go to the end of the tail.

 REAL WORLD TIP

The morphology of the *Loa loa* microfilariae is easy to remember because the nuclei go low (to the end) in the tail.

Onchocerca volvulus

River Blindness. *Onchocerca volvulus* is the cause of river blindness and is also known as the "blinding worm." This filarial parasite is endemic to central Africa, the Middle East, and Central and South America. It is transmitted through the bite of *Simulium* species, insects that are also known as black flies or buffalo gnats, which breed along fast flowing rivers. In areas where *O. volvulus* is endemic, blindness is found to be six times more common than in areas where the parasite is not found, earning its common name.

As with the other microfilariae, the infective larvae enter the host through the bite wound left by the feeding insect. The larval filarial worms migrate through the subcutaneous tissues as they mature, finally gathering in groups of two or more. Adult worms soon become encased in a fibrous capsule, producing tumor-like masses that come in varying sizes. After mating the adult parasites produce microfilariae that migrate out of the nodule into the subcutaneous tissue and the dermis. The life cycle is visually represented on the Companion Website.

The subcutaneous nodules, which may be numerous, appear most often in the pelvic region, at the junction of the long bones, and in the temporal or occipital regions of the scalp. While the nodules may be disfiguring they usually are not painful. Some individuals experience acute inflammatory reactions in which the skin overlying the nodules thickens, loses elasticity, and becomes tender and edematous. Often the individual experiences severe itching. The host immune response attacks the microfilariae in the eyes, which leads to blindness.

When the host goes to fast-flowing streams to obtain drinking water, bathe, wash clothes, or fish, they may be bitten by blackflies. If the insect bites an infected host they will ingest microfilariae along with its meal of blood and tissue fluids. Within the fly the microfilariae migrate from the stomach to the thoracic muscles producing the infective stage filariform larvae.

Diagnosis of River Blindness. Surgery can be employed to remove the subcutaneous nodules. Adults that lie coiled within the fibrous tissue capsules are whitish in color and wire-like in appearance. Males may attain a length of 5 centimeters but females may reach lengths of 50 centimeters.

Because the microfilariae are found in the subcutaneous tissues and dermis, examination of peripheral blood smears is not helpful in diagnosing *Onchocercus volvulus* infection. Instead, the specimen of choice is a skin snip. This specimen is procured by raising a small cone of skin using a needle and cutting

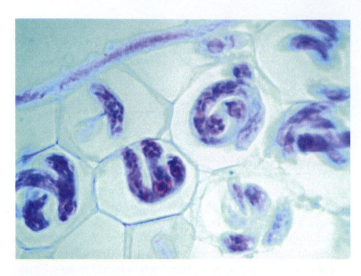

FIGURE 30-49 Tissue cross section containing microfilaria of *Onchocerca volvulus* (400× magnification).

the tissue with scissors or a razor blade. Alternately the skin may be folded upward and a razor can be used to excise material from the raised area. Skin biopsies have also proven effective in demonstrating the presence of microfilariae.

The excised tissue must be teased apart after placing it in a small amount of saline on a slide. This will allow the embryos to be examined microscopically. Employing Wright's or Giemsa stain will facilitate identification of the species of filarial parasite.

O. volvulus microfilariae range in length from 150 to 370 microns, lack the sheath seen around those found in the peripheral blood, and the tip of the tail is free of nuclei (Figure 30-49).

> ✓ **Checkpoint! 30–22 (Chapter Objectives 2 and 5)**
>
> *The microfilarial species known as the "blinding worm" is*
> A. Dirofilaria immitis.
> B. Brugia malayi.
> C. Loa loa.
> D. Wuchereria bancrofti.
> E. Onchocerca volvulus.

Nonpathogenic Microfilariae

There are microfilariae species that can be found in the blood and tissues but that are not known to cause disease. The importance of being familiar with the nonpathogenic species is in recognizing them as such so they are not reported as pathogens. *Mansonella ozzardi*, a nonpathogenic species that might possibly be recovered in a skin biopsy, should not be mistaken for *Onchocerca volvulus*, the pathogen that is often diagnosed using skin biopsies.

The nonpathogenic species are found in the same areas of the tropics where pathogens are seen and are also transmitted by insect vectors in which essential developmental stages must take place. They gain entrance through the bite left by the

⊘ TABLE 30-10

Differential Characteristics of Microfilariae

Parasite	Vector	Size	Sheath	Key Facts
Wuchereria bancrofti	*Anopheles, Aedes, Culex* (mosquitos)	245–300 µm	Present	Nocturnal periodicity Posterior portion of the tail is free of nuclei No reservoir hosts
Brugia malayi	*Anopheles, Aedes, Mansonia* (mosquitos)	175–230 µm	Present	Nocturnal periodicity Nuclei extend into the tip of the tail with the two terminal nuclei distinctly separate from the other caudal nuclei Monkeys, dogs, and cats serve as reservoir hosts
Brugia timori	*Anopheles*	310 µm (avg.)	Present	Nocturnal periodicity The cephalic space of *B. timori* is significantly longer than that of *B. malayi* and the sheath stains more lightly than that of *B. malayi* No reservoir hosts
Loa loa	*Chrysops* species (mango flies or deerflies)	250–300 µm	Present	Diurnal periodicity Nuclei are continuous into the tip of the tail "Calabar swellings" may develop as a result of the wanderings of the adult worms
Onchocerca volvulus	*Simulium* species (black flies or buffalo gnats)	150–370 µm	Absent	No periodicity, skin snip is the specimen of choice (not blood smear) Posterior portion of the tail is free of nuclei Adult worms found in subcutaneous nodules
Dirofilaria immitis	Many species of mosquito	307–322 µm	Absent	Natural infections found in dogs and cats, occasionally seen in humans

✪ TABLE 30-11

Differential Characteristics of Nonpathogenic Microfilariae

Parasite	Vector	Size	Sheath	Key Facts
Mansonella ozzardi	*Culicoides* species (midges) *Simulium* species (blackflies)	About 88 µm	Absent	Nuclei do not extend into the posterior portion of the tail
Mansonella perstans	*Culicoides* species	About 93 µm	Absent	Nuclei extend into the tip of the tail where the terminal pair of nuclei are separated slightly from the other caudal nuclei
Mansonella streptocerca	*Culicoides* species	180–240 µm	Absent	The tail is bent in the shape of a shepherd's crook with nuclei extending into the tip

feeding insects. In contrast to the pathogenic species they do not exhibit diurnal or nocturnal periodicity. Morphological characteristics and insect vectors are presented in Tables 30-10✪ and 30-11✪.

OTHER BLOOD AND TISSUE NEMATODES

Visceral Larval Migrans

Toxocara canis and *Toxocara cati* are the roundworms of dogs and cats, respectively, which inhabit the small intestines of their host species. These organisms have life cycles that are very similar to that of the human roundworm, *Ascaris lumbricoides*. The unembryonated eggs, which are passed out with the feces, develop outside the host into the infective embryonated eggs, which must then be ingested by a new host. In their native host the larvae burrow into the intestinal mucosa and migrate through the tissue, developing into second-stage larvae. In *T. canis* the complete life cycle—maturation to adults, mating, and egg production—only occurs in puppies less than 5 weeks old that ingest embryonated eggs. Infection may also occur *in utero* in pregnant females who harbor the second-stage larvae, which cross the placenta to infect the unborn puppies.

If embryonated eggs are ingested by older puppies, adult dogs, or humans they are unable to develop beyond second-stage larvae and continue to migrate until they eventually encyst in the tissues. This wandering of the larval form through the tissues of humans is accompanied by hemorrhage, necrosis, and infiltration by lymphocytes and eosinophils. Invasion of the viscera can be associated with a number of symptoms, depending on the organs involved, and can include epilepsy, myocarditis, hepatosplenomegaly, chronic pulmonary inflammation, visual impairment, and possibly death.

Trichinella spiralis

Trichinosis. *Trichinella spiralis* is a parasite that is not confined to the tropics and subtropics but is found worldwide. This organism is able to infect a wide range of carnivorous and omnivorous hosts including humans. In the wild, rats are commonly infected and perpetuate the infection through canni-

balism. Bears, cats, dogs, and wild boars, which consume the flesh of infected animals, can also acquire the infection.

Human infection occurs primarily through ingestion of raw, poorly processed, or poorly cooked pork, especially homemade sausages. This is most likely to occur when the flesh of pigs, which are fed household garbage and slaughterhouse scraps, is eaten. The infective larval forms are encysted in the meat and, unless the meat is thoroughly cooked, the larvae contained within cysts are not killed. The cysts are freed in the stomach and excyst in the duodenum. The larvae penetrate the mucosa of the duodenum and the jejunum where they mature into thread-like adult worms within 2 days.

After fertilization, females produce larvae, which migrate into the lymph vessels and veins that drain the intestinal tract. Once in the circulatory system the larvae are carried to tissues throughout the body but the target organs of the immature parasite is the striated muscle. The larval forms leave the capillaries, which supply the muscles, and penetrate the sheath of the muscle fibers.

Muscles that are constantly active and well vasculated, such as the diaphragm, abdomen, pectorals, and those of the arms and legs, are most heavily infected. Larvae, coiled into a spiral within a sheath, produce degeneration and inflammation of the muscles and within a year may become calcified and visible on radiographs. A visual representation of the life cycle is available on the Companion Website.

Symptoms of trichinosis depend on the severity of the infection and include fever, eosinophilia, and myositis accompanied by severe pain. Infection of the central nervous system may be accompanied by meningitis, encephalitis, cerebral vascular accident, acute psychosis, ocular disturbances, deafness, and diplegia. Fatal cases have been reported. Encysted larvae may remain viable for years awaiting ingestion by a new host and completion of the life cycle.

Diagnosis of Trichinosis. Diagnosis of *Trichinella spiralis* infection is rarely accomplished through the examination of stool for the presence of adults or larval forms as adults are located within the intestinal mucosa and not the lumen of the intestine. Diagnosis can be made through muscle biopsy and histological stains in which encysted larval forms may be found (Figure 30-50 ■). Intradermal injection of trichina antigen has been

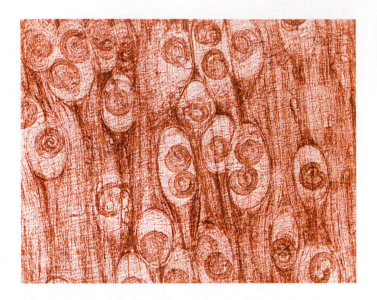

■ FIGURE 30-50 *Trichinella spiralis* cysts in a muscle biopsy.
Public Health Image Library (PHIL)/CDC

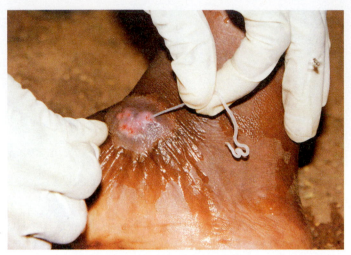

■ FIGURE 30-51 Adult female Guinea worm, *Dracunculus medinensis*. The worm emerges from a blister-like lesion when the affected body part (usually the legs or feet) is immersed in water. Larval forms are then released.
From Public Health Image Library (PHIL), CDC/The Carter Center.

successful in demonstrating an immune response to infection and would be considered evidence of *T. spiralis* infection. A positive response is the development of a small, white swelling surrounded by an unraised wheal or welt about 5 cm in diameter.

Dracunculus medinensis

Dracunculus medinensis Infection.
Dracunculus medinensis, also known as the guinea worm, is a parasite of carnivores and omnivores that is found in central equatorial Africa, the west coast of Africa, the Nile Valley, central India, and the Middle East.

The parasite is transmitted in humans through the ingestion of water containing aquatic arthropods, called copepods or water fleas in the genus *Cyclops*. The copepods themselves are not parasitic but they are infected with the larval stage of the parasitic roundworm and therefore act as an intermediate host. The infective larval stage is liberated within the duodenum of the human host, penetrates the intestinal mucosa, and travels through the circulation to the deep connective tissues where they mature into adults without causing overt symptoms to the host.

Gravid females, which may attain a length just under a meter, migrate through the subcutaneous tissues and eventually locate themselves just under the skin in the distal portion of the limbs, particularly the lower legs, ankles, and feet (Figure 30-51 ■). The dermis, overlying the female, progresses from a reddish papule to a blister-like lesion. The blister ruptures on contact with water, to form a small ulcerative lesion. The female lies in the ulcer opening, and first-stage rhabditiform larvae are discharged. This process is repeated until the uterus is emptied, a process that may take up to 3 weeks to accomplish. The larval forms must be ingested by copepods where they mature into infective forms that are accidentally ingested by a suitable intermediate host. A flow chart of the life cycle is available on the Companion Website.

Symptoms such as erythema, intense itching, nausea, vomiting, diarrhea, and severe dyspnea develop a few hours before eruption of the cutaneous lesion. These symptoms are thought to be associated with the buildup of toxic by-products produced by the gravid female. The ulcerative lesions may heal without further complications once discharge of larvae is completed and the female withdraws back into the subcutaneous tissues, dies, and is resorbed.

In some cases the female may be expelled from the cutaneous lesion. With the appearance of this large roundworm erupting from an extremity, some individuals attempt to remove the female by winding her onto a stick a few centimeters per day. If the female is removed successfully (more often by modern surgical means) the lesion heals promptly. In some cases the ulcerative lesion becomes secondarily infected with bacteria, especially if attempted removal of the worm is unsuccessful and the worm is pulled apart in the process. If the worm is broken during removal, there is an intense inflammatory reaction

Diagnosis of Dracunculus medinensis Infection.
Diagnosis of *D. medinensis* infection is made based on the appearance of systemic symptoms and the presence of cutaneous lesions. Larvae can be seen in ulcer washings. Past infection may be diagnosed if calcified worms are identified on radiographs.

 REAL WORLD TIP

Dracunculus medinensis is not a true filarial worm. It does not produce microfilariae in the blood or tissues.

CESTODES

Cestodes, or tapeworms, are hermaphroditic and therefore each adult contains both male and female reproductive organs and is capable of self-fertilization. Adult cestodes are white or yellowish in color, flat, and ribbon-like. They may be composed of just a few or hundreds of reproductive units and measure several meters in length. Adult worms, which are attached to the intestinal mucosa, are found in the small intestines and have no well-developed digestive tract and therefore must depend on predigested food supplied by the host species. The nervous system is rudimentary at best but the reproductive organs are well developed with the shape, size, and pattern of the gravid (pregnant) uterus being diagnostic in many species.

The life cycles of cestodes are complex and involve passage through one or more intermediate hosts in which development into another larval stage occurs. In some cases humans may serve as either the definitive host or an intermediate host, as is the case for *Taenia solium* and *Hymenolepis nana*. Man can only act as the definitive host for several species of cestodes such as *Diphyllobothrium latum, Taenia saginata,* and *Hymenolepis diminuta*. For other tapeworms, humans can only serve as an incidental intermediate host because larval forms, which are found in the tissues, cannot develop into the adult form. In such cases, as occurs with *Echinococcus granulosus,* man is never the definitive host. As a general rule the presence of larval stages in the tissues is much more serious than infection involving adult cestodes in the intestinal tract.

Transmission of the infection usually involves ingestion of the infective stage, which may either be the embryonated egg or an infective larval stage. There are three different infective larval stages. The cysticercus or bladder worm is the infective larval stage for the *Taenia* species and consists of a scolex (head with hooks or suckers) that is invaginated (pushed into) the proximal portion of a bladder-like covering. The cysticercoid larva is the infective larval form for *Dipylidium caninum* and the *Hymenolepis* species. The cysticercoid larva consists of a small anteriorly located bladder into which only the head may be invaginated. The elongated caudal portion is solid tissue. The plerocercoid larva is the infective stage for *Diphyllobothrium latum,* the broad fish tapeworm. The plerocercoid larva has no bladder-like portion but is instead an elongated organism with a scolex that may be invaginated into the neck.

Adult tapeworms are composed of different sections, and diagnosis of tapeworm infection can be made by finding any of the following forms:

- the scolex, an anteriorly located attachment organ, which is equivalent to the head
- a proglottid, the segments that follow the scolex and make up most of the body; on some occasions terminal proglottids break off and may be recovered in the feces
- larvae, which may be found in the tissues in an extra-intestinal infection
- eggs, which may be recovered in the feces or seen enclosed within the uterus of a gravid or pregnant proglottid

To avoid being evacuated with the stool through peristalsis, the tapeworm must be firmly attached to the intestinal mucosa. To accomplish this, the scolex may possess four muscular, cup-shaped suckers. In most species the scolex also has a rostellum, a centrally located, elongated structure that may be protruded or retracted. The rostellum may also be supplied with spines or hooks to provide additional stability. If the rostellum possesses hooks it is said to be "armed." If hooks are lacking it is referred to as an "unarmed" rostellum. The scolex of the broad fish tapeworm is an exception to this because it has neither suckers nor a rostellum and is discussed later in this chapter. The scolex must be removed to halt the infection.

The portion of the scolex below the suckers is often referred to as the "neck." Extending from the neck are the progottids, the segments that make up the body of the tapeworm. The most anterior proglottids are the newly formed segments that do not contain any internal structures. These are referred to as immature proglottids. Larger segments, which contain one full set of male and female reproductive organs, are found near the middle of the body. These are mature proglottids. Mature segments that are filled with eggs are referred to as gravid proglottids. The entire chain of proglottids that grows by proliferation of immature proglottids is called the strobila.

The first larval form, which is contained within the egg, is called an oncosphere or hexacanth larva because of the presence of six hooklets. In the broad fish tapeworm the onchosphere is ciliated and is referred to as a coracidium.

Diphyllobothrium latum

Broad Fish Tapeworm Infection. *Diphyllobothrium latum,* the broad fish tapeworm, is a common parasite of man and is found worldwide, especially countries where freshwater fish forms a major part of the diet. Places with temperate climates, such as Finland, Sweden, Canada, and Alaska, are areas where a high incidence of disease occurs. It can be found in the Great Lakes in the continental United States.

D. latum passes through two intermediate hosts before infecting the definitive host, man. Eggs that are passed in the feces must be deposited in a fresh water source in order for the first larval form, the coracidium, to be ingested by an aquatic crustacean, a copepod or water flea (*Diaptomus* or *Cyclops* species). Within the body cavity of the copepod the coracidium is transformed into a procercoid larva, the second larval form. When the infected copepod is ingested by a fish, the second intermediate host, the procercoid larva, develops into the plerocercoid larva, the third larval form. The plerocercoid larva, the infective stage that is found in the tissues of the fish, can then infect humans if a person eats raw, inadequately cooked, or pickled fish. When the plerocercoid larva reaches the intestines it develops into the adult form. A visual representation of the life cycle can be found on the Companion Website.

The strobila of the broad fish tapeworm may be several meters in length, running throughout the small intestines.

The scolex lacks suckers and a rostellum, and is instead elongated, spoon shaped, and possesses two lateral or longitudinally situated grooves. Mature and gravid proglottids are described as being wider than long (hence the name "broad" fish tapeworm) and there is a centrally located, unique, rosette- or flower-shaped uterus.

The presence of the adult tapeworm in the intestine usually causes minimal damage, if any, to the host and in such cases the patient is asymptomatic. If the parasite is attached at the level of the jejunum it may lead to pernicious anemia because the worm selectively absorbs vitamin B_{12}, preventing it from combining with intrinsic factor and being absorbed into the intestinal lining. This condition, also called "bothriocepahalus anemia," is most likely to occur in individuals who are already genetically predisposed to pernicious anemia.

Diagnosis of Broad Fish Tapeworm Infection. Both eggs and proglottids may be recovered in the stool. *Diphyllobothrium latum* eggs are a light yellowish-brown color, ovoid in shape, measuring 58–76 microns by 40–51 microns, have a moderately thick shell and are unembryonated when passed (Figure 30-52 ■). The fish tapeworm is the only trematode of man that produces eggs that are operculated or possess a lid. There is a small knob on the end opposite of the egg's lid.

Hymenolepis nana
Hymenolepis nana Infection.
Hymenolepis nana, the dwarf tapeworm, is found throughout the world but the highest incidence occurs in countries with warm climates. The infection may be transmitted through ingestion of the egg or the infective larval stage (the cysticercoid larva) by the definitive host, which may be humans, mice, or rats. It is the only tapeworm that does not require an intermediate host.

In areas where hygiene is poorly practiced, embryonated eggs, which are passed in the feces, may be transmitted by hand to the mouth. Following ingestion and arrival in the small intestines, the onchosphere hatches from the egg, penetrates the intestinal wall, and is transformed into the cysticercoid larva. The cysticercoid larva emerges from the intestinal wall and matures into the adult form, which begins to produce eggs that are passed in the feces. In this instance humans may act as both intermediate and definitive hosts. A flow chart of the life cycle is available on the Companion Website.

Alternatively the eggs passed in the feces may contaminate grain products, which serve not only as a food for humans and rodents but also grain beetles. The grain beetle may ingest the embryonated egg and the onchosphere may be transformed into the cysticercoid larva in the beetle. When the beetle, acting as an intermediate host, is ingested by a definitive host, the infective larva arrives in the intestines where it attaches, matures to the adult stage, and begins to produce eggs that will be passed in the feces. Eggs shed in the intestine are immediately infective so autoinfection is possible.

Hymenolepis nana adults attain a length of just a few centimeters. The scolex possesses four suckers and an armed rostellum. Proglottids are wider than long.

Diagnosis of Hymenolepis nana Infection.
The eggs of *Hymenolepis nana* are hyaline, broadly spherical, and measure 30–47 microns in diameter. They are nonoperculated, fully embryonated, and contain an onchosphere with three pairs of hooklets. The eggs are surrounded by a thick shell. One unique characteristic of *H. nana* eggs is the presence of a thin inner envelop that surrounds the onchosphere. This inner membrane possesses bipolar knobs or thickenings, and from each, four to eight filaments arise (Figure 30-53 ■).

Hymenolepis diminuta
Hymenolopis diminuta Infection.
Hymenolepis diminuta, the rat tapeworm, is found throughout much of the world, including the United States. It is primarily a parasite of rats but cases of human infection are not uncommon. Eggs are passed in the feces, which may in turn contaminate grain on which the rat feeds. Various insects, such as grain beetles, feed on the contaminated grain and ingest the eggs, and the larvae contained within hatch in the intestines. Eventually the ingested larvae are transformed into cysticercoid larva. If

---

✔ ## Checkpoint! 30–23 (Chapter Objective 4)

In human infection the infective stage of Diphyllobothrium latum is the

A. *cysticercus.*
B. *cysticercoid larva.*
C. *plerocercus larva.*
D. *plerocercoid larva.*
E. *procercoid larva.*

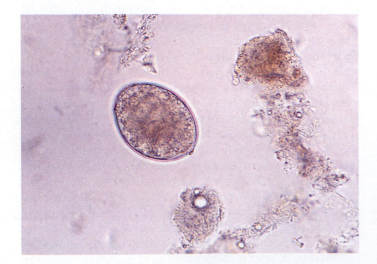

■ **FIGURE 30-52** Egg of *Diphyllobothrium latum* in a direct wet mount (400× magnification). Note the presence of a characteristic small knob on one end of the egg.
From Public Health Image Library (PHIL), CDC/Dr. Mae Melvin.

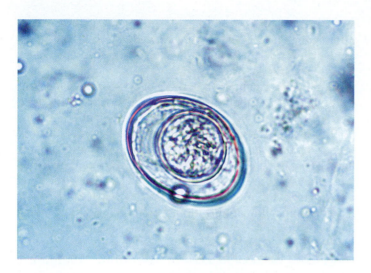

■ **FIGURE 30-53** Direct wet mount preparation containing a *Hymenolepis nana* egg (400× magnification).

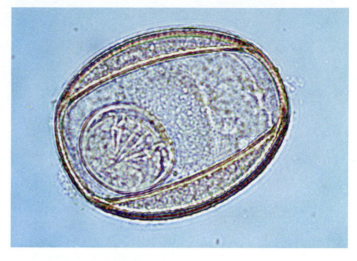

■ **FIGURE 30-54** Direct wet mount preparation containing a *Hymenolepis diminuta* egg (400× magnification).

the insect vector is accidentally eaten along with the grain, the cysticercoid larvae, which is the infective stage for both humans and rats, ends up in the small intestines. They then attach to the intestinal mucosa and mature into the adult form, which begins to produce eggs and complete the life cycle. In this case, the insect serves as the intermediate host and is required for the life cycle to be complete. The life cycle is visually represented on the Companion Website.

Despite its name, *H. diminuta* adults are much larger than those of *H. nana*. The rat tapeworm adult may attain a length of 50–60 cm. The scolex, which is small and rounded, possesses four deeply cupped suckers and an unarmed rostellum. Gravid proglottids, which eventually become detached, disintegrate in the lumen of the intestine, allowing the eggs to be released and passed in the feces.

Diagnosis of *Hymenolepis diminuta* Infection.

Diagnosis of *H. diminuta* relies upon recovery of eggs in the feces. They are broadly oval, brown in color, and have a relatively thick shell. The eggs range in size from 60 to 79 microns by 72 to 86 microns, are fully embryonated when passed, and, although the onchosphere is covered by two membranes, there are no polar filaments (Figure 30-54 ■). The larger size and lack of polar filaments clearly distinguishes the eggs of *H. diminuta* from those of *H. nana*.

Taenia saginata

Taenia saginata Infection. *Taenia saginata*, the beef or unarmed tapeworm, is found throughout the world. The infection is transmitted to humans through the ingestion of poorly cooked beef containing the infective stage, the cysticercus larva. After passing unharmed through the stomach, the scolex of the cysticercus larva evaginates (pops out) and attaches to the intestinal mucosa. The worm matures into the adult stage and begins to produce eggs, which are passed out in the feces.

Eggs remain viable in the soil for 8 weeks or more. Cattle graze and accidentally ingest the eggs. Once the egg is in the duodenum, the onchosphere hatches, penetrates the intestinal wall, and is carried to the striated muscle through the blood and lymphatics. In the muscles of the intermediate host the onchosphere is transformed into the cysticercus larvae, a fluid-filled sac with an invaginated scolex. This completes the life cycle if ingested by man. A visual representation of the life cycle is available on the Companion Website.

Adult beef tapeworms may attain a length of several meters, up to as much as 25 meters. The scolex possesses four muscular suckers but lacks a rostellum and therefore has no hooklets. This accounts for its name as the unarmed tapeworm.

Diagnosis of *Taenia saginata* Infection.

Gravid proglottids may detach from the stobila and pass in the feces. They look like cooked macaroni. Careful examination of a stool specimen may reveal their presence and with the aid of a microscope they may easily be identified. These gravid proglottids are longer than wide, measuring 5–7 mm by 20 mm. The uterus contains 15–20 lateral uterine branches, which is diagnostic for the species (Figure 30-55 ■). India ink can be injected into the genital pore of the proglottid to visualize the uterine branches.

T. saginata eggs are spherical, have a very thick shell, lack an operculum, and are fully embryonated when passed. Six hooklets can be distiguished in the onchosphere. Typically the

 REAL WORLD TIP

The eggs of *Taenia saginata* and *T. solium* cannot be differentiated and are identified as *Taenia* spp. when observed.

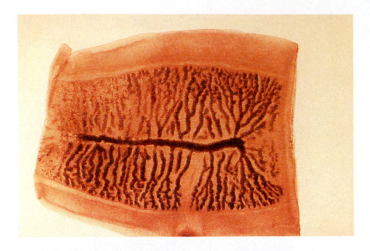

■ FIGURE 30-55 A proglottid of *Taenia saginata* injected with India ink to show the uterine branches. Count the branches on one side of the central stem. *T. saginata* averages about 18 uterine branches.
Public Health Image Library (PHIL)/CDC

℮ REAL WORLD TIP

Taenia saginata has more letters in its species name and so one can remember it also has more uterine branches in its proglottid than *T. solium*.

eggs range in diameter from 31 to 43 microns, are brown or bile-colored, and by carefully focusing up and down, radial or sunburst striations can clearly be seen in the thick shell surrounding the larva (Figure 30-56 ■).

Taenia solium

Taenia solium Infection.   The life cycle of *T. solium*, the pork or armed tapeworm, is essentially the same as that of *T. saginata*. The two main differences include: the intermedi-

ate host is the pig instead of cattle and man may serve as the intermediate host as well as the definitive host. The eggs are immediately infective so autoinfection is possible if they hatch prior to leaving the intestine.

If humans accidentally ingest the eggs of *Taenia solium*, the eggs hatch in the small intestine and the onchosphere penetrates the bowel wall, gaining access to the blood and lymphatics. The onchosphere is carried by the blood to tissue as well as the brain and eyes. Invasion of the brain and development into the cysticercus larva leads to the symptoms of meningitis but may also result in seizures and death. The presence of cysticercus larvae in the eyes can lead to visual impairment. Extra-intestinal human infection, which involves the presence of cysticercus larvae in host tissue, is called cysticercosis.

Diagnosis of Taenia solium Infection.   Diagnosis is usually accomplished through recovery of eggs in the feces. The eggs of *T. solium* and *T. saginata* are identical and a differential diagnosis must rely on recovery of the scolex or gravid proglottids. The scolex of *T. solium* is small, possesses four muscular suckers, and a rounded, armed rostellum containing a double row of hooks. The gravid proglottids are longer than wide, are usually much smaller than those of *T. saginata*, and contain 7–13 lateral uterine branches (Figure 30-57 ■). Diagnosis of cysticercosis may be made on the basis of radiographic evidence as the encysted cysticercus larvae often become calcified after 2 months.

℮ REAL WORLD TIP

The presentation of epilepsy in an individual with no family or previous history of seizures should cause the physician to consider *Taenia solium* cysticercosis in the differential diagnosis.

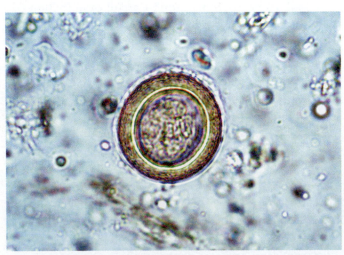

■ FIGURE 30-56 *Taenia* species egg in a direct wet mount preparation (400× magnification).

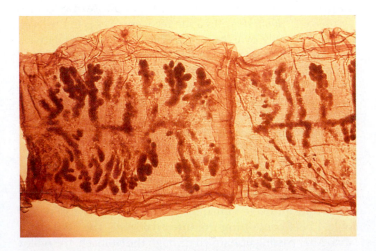

■ FIGURE 30-57 A proglottid of *Taenia solium*. *T. solium* averages about 9 uterine branches on one side of the central stem.
CDC

REAL WORLD TIP

The eggs of *Taenia* spp. stains very dark due to bile and on iodine wet prep of the stool it may be overlooked. Look for its regular and round shape.

Checkpoint! 30–24
(Chapter Objectives 3 and 6)

Hyaline eggs, which average 39 microns in diameter, are seen in the direct wet mount made from a freshly passed stool specimen. They are nonoperculated but an onchosphere can easily be seen with the confines of the thick shell. By focusing up and down carefully the parasitologist is able to discern bipolar knobs from which four to eight filaments project. Identify the parasite that produces eggs fitting this description.

A. *Hymenolepis nana*
B. *H. diminuta*
C. *Taenia solium*
D. *T. saginata*
E. *Diphyllobothrium latum*

Checkpoint! 30–25
(Chapter Objectives 3 and 4)

Recovery of gravid proglottids, which are longer than wide and contain 15–20 lateral uterine branches, is diagnostic for which cestode?

A. *Hymenolepis nana*
B. *H. diminuta*
C. *Taenia solium*
D. *T. saginata*
E. *Diphyllobothrium latum*

Dipylidium caninum
Dipylidium caninum Infection. *Dipylidium caninum,* the double-pored dog tapeworm, is in actuality a parasite that is common in both cats and dogs worldwide. On occasion humans may be accidental definitive hosts and acquire the infection if the infective larval stage, the cysticercoid larva, is ingested.

The eggs of *D. caninum,* which are deposited on the ground and in the perianal region, are ingested by larval cat (*Ctenocephalides cati*) and dog (*C. canis*) fleas as they feed on organic debris. The onchosphere hatches in the intestine of the insect and migrates into the hemacoel where it develops into a cysticercoid larva. This larval form of the parasite is maintained in the flea as it matures to the adult stage. When the host animal nips and licks itself, it accidentally ingests the adult flea infected with the cysticercoid larva. Children who kiss the animal or allow their pet to lick their face can also accidentally ingest the adult fleas or their internal contents.

When the cysticercoid larva finds itself in the intestine of the definitive host, including humans, it attaches to the intestinal mucosa, matures to the adult stage, and begins to grow a chain of proglottids. Gravid proglottids detach from the strobila and may be passed out with the feces. In some cases, because they are actively motile, the proglottids may actually migrate outside the anus where they contract, forcefully releasing eggs. Proglottids that are passed in the feces will eventually disintegrate, releasing the eggs into the environment where they may be ingested by larval fleas. A flow chart of the life cycle can be found on the Companion Website.

REAL WORLD TIP

In the home environment, such as on the carpet, the proglottid of *Dipylidium caninum* looks like a cucumber seed when moist or fresh and like a grain of rice once it dries.

D. caninum adult tapeworms are relatively small and attain a length between 10 and 70 cm. The scolex possesses four, muscular, oval-shaped suckers, and an armed rostellum with one to seven rows of hooks.

Diagnosis of *Dipylidium caninum* Infection. Diagnosis can be made on finding either the proglottids or eggs of *D. caninum* in the feces of infected animals or humans. In most cases it is the proglottid that is found in the stool. Mature and gravid proglottids are said to be shaped like a pumpkin or cucumber seed, with mature proglottids having two sets of male and female reproductive organs and a genital pore located on both sides. Gravid proglottids are considerably longer than wide and full of eggs.

The eggs of *D. caninum* are spherical or ovoid in shape, 30–40 microns in diameter, nonoperculated, and fully embryonated. The shell is moderately thick, the eggs are colorless, and in packets. Eggs that are released will be found packets of seven to as many as 30 eggs and are enclosed in an embryonic membrane (Figure 30-58 ■).

Echinococcus granulosus
Hydatid Cyst Disease. *Echinococcus granulosus,* the hydatid worm, is a tissue cestode and is found in greatest abundance in countries that raise sheep, cattle, and other herbivores. This parasite is endemic to many South American countries, Australia, New Zealand, Europe, Siberia, China, Japan, Israel, and Arabia. Cases do occur in the southwestern United States.

Eggs, found in the soil, are ingested by intermediate hosts such as herbivores, pigs, or humans, and the onchosphere hatches in the duodenum. This larval form penetrates the intestinal wall and escapes to the mesenteric venules where it is carried by the circulation to various organs such as the liver, lungs, and brain. The parasite forms cysts that continue to enlarge over time. In less than 6 months the hydatid cyst reaches a diameter of 1 cm and is characterized by an outer limiting membrane and an inner germinal layer. As the cyst

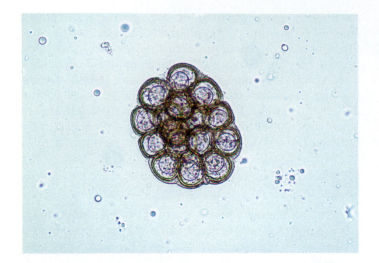

■ **FIGURE 30-58** Egg packet of *Dipylidium caninum* (100× magnification).

continues to develop, vacuolated, stalked masses of cells, called brood capsules, bud off the germinal epithelium. The brood capsules themselves are lined with a germinal layer that develops protoscolices resembling the scolex of the adult tapeworm. Trauma may rupture the mother cyst and daughter cysts may be produced, which, in turn, also produce brood capsules and protoscolices. In older cysts the brood capsules may break down, releasing the protoscolices. This material, composed of daughter cysts, free protoscolices, free hooklets, and amorphous material that remains contained within the cysts, is often referred to as hydatid sand and may be aspirated for diagnostic purposes. It is called hydatid sand because the hooklets crunch under the glass coverslip used for microscopic examination of the fluid.

To complete the cycle, the definitive host, which is a dog, wolf, or other canine species, must ingest the larval form, the protoscolices, which are encysted within the viscera of infected intermediate hosts (herbivores, cats, rodents, rabbits, and kangaroos). Once the protoscolex is in the intestine of the dog, it attaches to the intestinal mucosa and matures to the adult tapeworm. Adult dog tapeworms are very small and consist of the scolex and three proglottids, an immature, mature, and gravid proglottid. The scolex is small, possessing four suckers and an armed rostellum. Eggs released from the gravid proglottid are passed with the feces onto the soil where they may be ingested. The eggs are not found in human feces because humans can only act as intermediate hosts. They are indistinguishable from those of the *Taenia* species.

Symptomatic infection depends on the size and location of the hydatid cyst. In the liver, the most common body site, the cyst may put pressure upon the bile duct if it reaches sufficient size. Cysts located in the lungs may produce coughing, dyspnea, and pain in the chest. Cysts in the central nervous system may be devastating if growth occurs in the spinal column or within

the skull. Anaphylactic shock is a possible consequence if hydatid fluid should leak into the tissues as a result of surgical intervention or trauma.

Diagnosis of Hydatic Cyst Disease.   As stated previously, the eggs of *E. granulosus* are only found in the feces of the definitive host, canines. Because man can only serve as the intermediate host, diagnosis depends on demonstration of the presence of a hydatid cyst. Fluid-filled cysts of sufficient size can readily be demonstrated on a radiograph of the infected area. Serological methods are also available. The specimen of choice to diagnose hydatid cyst disease is an aspirate of cyst contents examined using a direct wet mount (Figure 30-59 ■). Table 30-12✪ reviews the distinguishing characteristics of cestode eggs.

✔ **Checkpoint! 30–26 (Chapter Objective 5)**

Hydatic cysts occur most often in the _____ .
  A. *liver*
  B. *central nervous system*
  C. *lungs*
  D. *subcutaneous tissues*

TREMATODES

Most trematodes, or flukes, are hermaphroditic or monoecious (Greek for "one house"). These terms refer to organisms that possess both male and female reproductive organs and therefore capable of self-fertilization. In the trematodes the one exception to this rule is the blood flukes or schistosomes, which are diecious (Greek for "two houses"). These trematodes are separated into the two sexes, males and females.

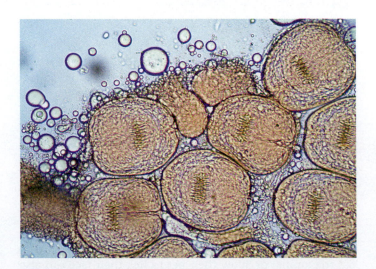

■ **FIGURE 30-59** *Echinococcus granulosus* protoscolices from hydatid sand (direct wet mount preparation 100× magnification).

TABLE 30-12

Distinguishing Characteristics of Cestode Eggs

Parasite	Shape	Size (microns)	Color	State of Development (when passed)	Key Characteristics
Diphyllobothrium latum	Ovoid	58–76 × 40–51	Yellowish-brown	Unembryonated	Moderate shell thickness with operculum and abopercular knob
Dipylidium caninum	Spherical or ovoid	30–40 × 27–48	Colorless	Embryonated (onchosphere)	Moderate shell thickness Eggs in packets of 5–30 eggs
Hymenolepis diminuta	Ovoid	70–86 × 60–80	Brown	Embryonated (onchosphere)	Size, color, and lack of polar filaments
Hymenolepis nana	Broadly oval	30–47 × 30–50	Colorless	Embryonated (onchosphere)	Two polar knobs or thickenings with four to eight polar filaments
Taenia species	Spherical	31–43	Brown (bile-colored)	Embryonated (onchosphere)	Thick shell with radial striations

Eggs, which are produced by adult trematodes located within organs or tissues of the vertebrate host, are expelled to the outside in feces, urine, or sputum. Some eggs are embryonated when passed and others develop outside the host depending on the parasitic species. In either case the larval form that hatches from the egg, called a miracidium, swims off to find the first intermediate host. The first intermediate host is a mollusk, usually a snail or clam, in which multiplication and development into a second larval form occurs. The second larval form, the cercaria, must find a second intermediate host, which may be a fish, crustacean, or even an aquatic plant. Another developmental stage takes place in the second intermediate host, resulting in a third larval form, the metacercaria. The metacercaria is ingested by the vertebrate host and is therefore the infective stage larval form. Once again the schistosomes are an exception to this general rule because they do not require a second intermediate host. Because there is no second intermediate host, cercariae are the infective stage of the schistosomes instead of metacercariae. The diagnostic stage for trematodes may be eggs or adults.

The Blood Flukes

Schistosoma species. The genus *Schistosoma* contains a number of different species. Three species are of major importance to humans, *Schistosoma mansoni, S. haematobium,* and *S. japonicum. S. intercalatum* and *S. mekongi* are blood flukes that are able to infect humans but are of lesser significance and will not be discussed here.

S. japonicum, as its name implies, is found in the Far East, particularly Japan, China, the Philippines, Thailand, Laos, and Cambodia. *S. haematobium* is endemic to most of Africa, Asia Minor, and India. *S. mansoni* is found throughout much of Africa, with high numbers of people infected in the delta region of the Nile River. As a result of the slave trade this parasite is found in South America and the West Indies as well as Puerto Rico.

Schistosomiasis is acquired through exposure to water containing the appropriate intermediate host, usually fresh water snails. Cercariae are released from the snails and swim about until they encounter the skin of a suitable host. On contact with the skin of human hosts the cercariae lose their tails, penetrate the skin, and migrate into the cutaneous capillary beds using proteolytic enzymes to move through the tissues. The parasites then enter the venous circulation where they are carried to the heart, the lungs, back to the heart, and from there to the liver sinusoids. Adult schistosomes must then migrate against the backflow of the portal venous system, into the veins draining the intestines (*S. japonicum* and *S. mansoni*) and bladder (*S. haematobium*). The female leaves the male and deposits her eggs in the veins, which drain the submucosal tissues surrounding the lumen of the target organ. Eggs lie wedged in the venules until the miracidium matures and secretes an enzyme that facilitates destruction of the tissues, a process that eventually allows the eggs to be released into the lumen of the intestine or bladder depending on the species of schistosome. Eggs are passed out of the definitive host in the feces or urine and, if deposited in water, the miracidium ruptures the egg and swims off to find the first intermediate host, the snail. In the tissues of the snail the parasite multiplies and develops into cercariae, the infective stage for man. It is the cercariae that escape the snail's body and must then seek a suitable human host to complete the cycle. Humans are infected following exposure to water sources containing cercariae liberated from the tissues of suitable snail species. This often occurs during activities such as bathing or immersion of the feet when obtaining water for drinking and washing. A visual representation of the life cycle is available on the Companion Website.

The symptoms associated with schistosomiasis are dependent upon how heavily the host is infected, with light infections causing few, if any, symptoms. In heavier infections, skin penetration may be associated with dermatitis, and localized hemorrhaging and eosinophilic accumulations in the lungs due to migration of larvae. The most profound effect is on the liver and intestinal tract.

Hepatitis may result from the growth of larval forms to adults in the hepatic portal veins. Inflammatory reactions to the eggs result in the formation of pseudoabscesses, fibrosis, portal cirrhosis of the liver, and eventually the accumulation of ascites fluid and in some cases esophageal varices. Patients with severe cases of schistosomiasis have greatly distended abdomens, due to splenomegaly and ascites, emaciated upper limbs, and edema of the lower limbs.

Hyperemia of the wall of the small intestine follows the arrival of adult worms in the mesenteric venules and in time pseudoabscesses, fibrosis, papilloma formation, and hypertrophy of the affected sections of the bowel impairs the normal functioning of the intestines and results in poor digestion. Eggs that are deposited in mesenteric veins are carried to venules in the mucosa and submucosa and as the larvae mature they produce highly irritating secretions that destroy host tissues, allowing the eggs to escape and fall into the lumen of the target organ. The period of egg extrusion is associated with profuse dysentery, allowing the eggs to be expelled from the body in the feces with *S. mansoni* and *S. japonicum* infections. In *S. haematobium* infections the female discharges her eggs in the venules supplying the bladder and therefore the eggs are excreted in the urine and are often accompanied by hematuria or blood, as well as pus, in the urine.

Diagnosis of Schistosomiasis.

The adults of the blood flukes are not recovered from the stool or the urine as they remain in the small veins that supply the intestines and the bladder. Male and female adult blood flukes differ morphologically. The males, which range in size (length) from 0.6 to 2.2 cm, have the typical leaf shape of trematodes and are flattened below the ventral sucker. Under a dissecting scope they appear to be cylindrical because they curve in ventrally to form a circular depression called the gynecophoral canal where the female is found until she leaves to deposit her eggs.

Females range in size (length) from 1.2 to 2.6 cm and do not exhibit the typical leaf-shaped characteristic of other trematodes. Instead, they are long, slender, and nearly cylindrical in shape so they can fit "snugly" in a perpetual embrace in the gynecophoral canal formed by the body of the male.

Specific diagnosis of schistosomiasis relies on the recovery of characteristic eggs in the stool or urine. *S. japonicum* and *S. mansoni* eggs can be recovered in the stool of infected patients or may be seen in material from rectal biopsies. The eggs of *S. japonicum* are oval or spherical in shape, range in size from 55 to 85 microns, have a thin shell, are a light yellowish-brown color, and occasionally may possess a minute, rudimentary lateral spine. The eggs are embryonated when passed but nonoperculated (Figure 30-60 ■). The eggs of *S. mansoni* are elongate and ovoid in shape and light yellowish-brown in color. They have a thin shell, range in size (length) from 114 to 180 microns, and are embryonated but do not have an operculum. The most distinguishing characteristic is the presence of a large lateral spine (Figure 30-61 ■).

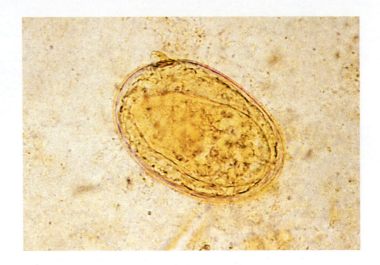

■ FIGURE 30-60 Egg of *Schistosoma japonicum* in a stool direct wet mount preparation (400× magnification).
CDC/Dr. Moore

The eggs of *S. haematobium* are frequently recovered from centrifuged urine but may also be seen in a bladder biopsy. They are elongate, ovoid, light yellowish-brown, and have a thin shell. They range in size (length) from 112 to 170 microns and, although they are embryonated, they do not have an operculum. The distinguishing characteristic of *S. haemotobium* eggs is the presence of a large terminal spine that looks like a bee stinger (Figure 30-62 ■).

℮ REAL WORLD TIP

The *Schistosoma* spp. eggs are lost using the zinc-sulfate concentration method because they rupture and sink.

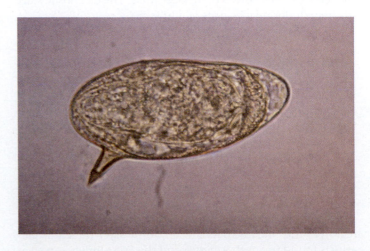

■ FIGURE 30-61 Egg of *Schistosoma mansoni* in a stool direct wet mount preparation (400× magnification).
CDC

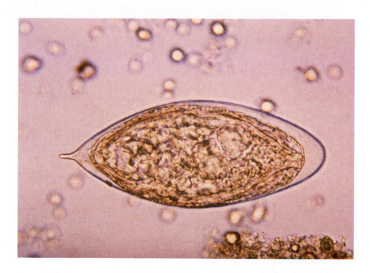

■ **FIGURE 30-62** Egg of *Schistosoma haematobium* in a urine direct wet mount preparation.
From Public Health Image Library (PHIL), CDC.

Checkpoint! 30–27 (Chapter Objective 3)

Eggs that are round to oval, range in size from 55 to 85 microns, and light yellowish-brown in color are discovered in the stool of a patient suffering from profuse watery diarrhea. The eggs have a rudimentary lateral spine, are fully embryonated, but do not possess an operculum. What is the most likely cause of the patient's symptoms?

A. *Schistosoma mansoni*
B. *S. haematobium*
C. *S. japonicum*

Checkpoint! 30–28 (Chapter Objective 4)

What is the best specimen to diagnose S. haematobium infection?

A. *Stool specimen*
B. *Rectal biopsy*
C. *Blood smear*
D. *Urine*
E. *Sputum*

The Intestinal Flukes

The intestinal flukes are flat and leaf shaped and distributed throughout the Far East, principally China, Japan, Korea, the Philippines, Vietnam, Thailand, Indonesia, Malaysia, and the Indian subcontinent. Infection also occurs in Spain, Israel, and Egypt.

The hermaphroditic adult flukes are found in the small intestines and it logically follows that the eggs would then be passed in the feces. These eggs are fully embryonated and if they reach a source of water, the miracidium is released. In all three of the intestinal flukes the miracidium must undergo multiplication and development in the first intermediate host, a mollusk. There are only slight differences in the way in which the larvae gain entrance into the snail's tissues in the life cycle of the three human intestinal flukes.

Heterophyid Intestinal Flukes. The life cycle of the heterophyid intestinal flukes, *Heterophyes heterophyes* and *Metagonimus yokogawai,* begins with ingestion of embryonated eggs by an aquatic snail. For many other trematode species the miracidium hatches when the stool containing the eggs are deposited in water but with the heterophyid intestinal flukes the first larval form only hatches when ingested by the appropriate host species. Within the first intermediate host the miracidium develops into cercariae that emerge from the snail and must find the second intermediate host, a fish. Having found and infected a fish, the cercariae encyst in the tissues or under the scales and develop into metacercariae, which may then be ingested in raw, pickled, or poorly cooked fish eaten by humans. The metacercariae become adults in the intestines of man, the definitive host, and produce eggs that are passed in the feces. When these eggs reach a source of water the life cycle will have been completed. The life cycle is visually represented on the Companion Website.

Fasciolopsis buski. When the eggs of *Fasciolopsis buski,* the "giant intestinal fluke," are deposited into water, the miracidium hatches and swims off to find and infect the first intermediate host, a snail, in which multiplication and development take place. The cercariae, which develop within the tissues of the snail, eventually emerge and must find a third intermediate host to undergo further development. The cercariae, which encyst on water vegetation such as bamboo shoots, water chestnuts, or lotus roots, develop into metacercariae. This third stage larva, which is the infective stage, may then be ingested along with the raw roots, stems, bulbs, or pods of aquatic vegetation, a major part of the diet in areas where the parasite is endemic. A flow chart of the life cycle is available on the Companion Website.

Infection by the intestinal flukes can easily be avoided because the metacercariae of *F. buski* and the heterophyid intestinal flukes are all killed by thoroughly cooking fish or vegetables.

Diagnosis of Intestinal Flukes. Intestinal fluke infection may be diagnosed by recovering either adults or eggs from the gastrointestinal tract. It is far easier to obtain eggs that are passed in the feces than attempting to recover adults that have oral and ventral suckers for attachment to the intestinal mucosa. *Fasciola hepatica,* the sheep liver fluke, and *Fasciolopsis buski* adults are of sufficient size and have such large suckers they are able to cause mechanical damage to the infected organs. Because the adult flukes have suckers for attachment they are usually only recovered after treatment that kills the worms so they are eventually expelled in the feces.

F. buski adults are large, fleshy worms that range in size from 2 to 7.5 cm in length, 0.8 to 2 cm in width, and 0.5 to 3 mm in thickness. They are broadly oval in shape and lack the cephalic cone that characterizes *F. hepatica*. The eggs of *F. buski* are very large and ellipsoid in shape. They are yellowish-brown in color, operculated (with a lid), and unembryonated when passed in the feces. They measure 130–140 microns in length and 80–85 microns in width and have a thin, transparent shell and resemble those of *Fasciola hepatica*.

REAL WORLD TIP

The eggs of *Fasciolopsis buski* and *Fasciola hepatica* are very similar and are difficult to differentiate. These eggs can also resemble that of *Diphylobothrium latum* but they are at least twice the size of *D. latum*.

Both *H. heterophyes* and *M. yokogawai* adults are small, leaf-shaped flukes that have a size range of 26.5–30 microns by 15–17 microns. *M. yokogawai* possesses the oral and ventral sucker normally found with human trematodes. Although *Heterophyes* adults very closely resembles *Metagonimus* adult flukes, the two can be differentiated from each other because, in addition to the oral and ventral suckers trematode adults usually possess, *Heterophyes heterophyes* has a third sucker surrounding the genital pore.

In contrast to the adult stage, the eggs of *H. heterophyes* and *M. yokogawai* are virtually indistiguishable and any differences that occur are not consistent enough to reliably differentiate the eggs of the two species. The eggs of both species are typically 26–30 microns by 15–17 microns. They are light brown in color and contain a fully developed miracidium when deposited in the feces. The minute eggs are ellipsoid in shape, have a thin shell, are operculated, and possess prominent opercular shoulders. They are very similar to the eggs of *Clonorchis sinensis*. If eggs are recovered they can be reported as heterophyid eggs with differential diagnosis being based on recovery of adult worms.

Checkpoint! 30–29
(Chapter Objective 3)

Unembryonated, yellowish-brown eggs, which possess the following morphological characteristics, are recovered from a freshly passed stool specimen: a length ranging from 130–140 μm, thin, transparent shell, barely perceptible operculum, and ellipsoidal shape. What parasitic species produces eggs fitting this description?

A. *Schistosoma mansoni*

B. *Heterophyes heterophyes*

C. *Metagonimus yokogawai*

D. *Clonorchis sinensis*

E. *Fasciolpsis buski*

The Liver Flukes
Clonorchis sinensis

Clonorchiasis.   *Clonorchis sinensis,* the "Chinese liver fluke," is found primarily in the Far East, particularly China, Korea, Taiwan, Vietnam, and Japan. Dogs and cats are naturally infected. Humans acquire the infection through the consumption of raw, smoked, poorly cooked, dried, or pickled fish. In areas outside of the Far East, infection may be acquired by eating fish shipped from areas where the parasite is endemic. Adult flukes live in the bile ducts and produce eggs that are expelled into the intestinal tract and out of the body through the feces. In heavy infections adults may be found in the gallbladder and the pancreatic ducts.

When the embryonated egg reaches water it must be ingested by a species of aquatic snail and once it is within the host's intestinal tract the miracidium hatches. The miracidium bores into the tissues of the snail and, after multiplying and passing through developmental stages, becomes a cercaria, which eventually emerges from the tissues and escapes into the water. The cercaria must then be ingested by a fresh water fish where it develops into a metacercaria. When man eats improperly cooked fish, the metacercaria is freed within the duodenum and the immature fluke migrates up into the common bile duct where it matures into the adult stage. A flow chart of the life cycle is available on the Companion Website.

While light infections may be asymptomatic, heavy infections may be accompanied by chills and fever, anorexia, diarrhea, edema, and hepatomegaly. Severe infections may lead to portal cirrhosis as well as cancer of the bile duct.

Diagnosis of Clonorchiasis.   Diagnosis of clonorchiasis is based on recovery of eggs and much less commonly the adult stage. The recommended specimen is either stool or a duodenal aspirate. *C. sinensis* adults are flat and slender with a rounded posterior end and an attenuated or tapered anterior end.

The eggs of the Chinese liver fluke very closely resemble those of the heterophyid liver flukes. They are minute, broadly ovoid, have a moderately thick shell, and are a light yellowish-brown in color. Eggs may range in size from 27 to 35 microns in length and 12 to about 20 microns in width. They are fully embryonated when passed, and possess a dome-shaped operculum with prominent opercular shoulders. At the aboper-cular end (opposite the operculum) there is often a small comma-shaped knob but this feature is not consistent enough to be a distinguishing characteristic. *C. sinesis* eggs that lack the aopercular knob may be indistinguishable from those of *H. heterophyes* and *M. yokogawai* (Figure 30-63 ■). In such cases it may be necessary to report the parasites as generic heterophyid eggs unless the source can be identified as coming from the bile duct or unless an adult can be recovered.

Fasciola hepatica Infection

Sheep Liver Rot.   *Fasciola hepatica*, which is also known as the "sheep liver fluke," is found in Mediterranean countries,

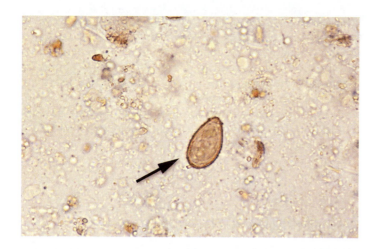

the Far East, Africa, and Central and South America. In the southern, eastern, and midwestern United States the sheep liver fluke are well established because, in addition to humans, herbivores such as sheep, cattle, goats, pigs, bison, deer, and rabbits are susceptible to infection.

If feces containing the eggs are deposited in water, a miracidium will develop over a period of 9–15 days. After hatching from the egg, the miracidium swims off to find a suitable intermediate snail host and after gaining entrance develops into cercariae within the tissues. The cercariae emerge from the snail and encyst on water vegetation, becoming metacercariae that must then be ingested by any number of mammalian herbivore hosts. The encysted infective stage larvae excyst in the intestines, burrow through the wall of the duodenum, and migrate across the peritoneal cavity and into the liver where they pass through liver tissue until they arrive at the bile duct. In the biliary passages the immature larvae settle down and mature into adults that deposit eggs into the bile duct. From the bile duct the eggs are carried into the intestinal lumen and pass out of the host's body with the feces. The life cycle is visually represented on the Companion Website.

Even with light infections, the adult sheep liver flukes are large and produce a severe inflammatory reaction with fibrosis and biliary obstruction. Fever, chills, coughing, vomiting, diarrhea, right upper quadrant pain, jaundice, and hepatomegaly can also accompany the infection. Migrating larval forms may miss the target organ and lodge in other tissues where abscesses or fibrotic lesions may develop.

Diagnosis of *Fascioliasis hepatica* Infection or Sheep Liver Rot.   Diagnosis of *Fasciola hepatica* infection relies primarily upon recovery of eggs in the stool. These eggs are indistinguishable from those of *Fasciolopsis buski,* the giant intestinal

fluke that was discussed previously (Figure 30-64 ■). A differential diagnosis can only be made upon recovery of the adult fluke. *F. hepatica* adults are moderately large, fleshy worms that may be up to 30 mm in length and 13 mm across. They have the characteristic flat, leaf-shaped body associated with flukes but also have a distinctive anteriorly located "cephalic cone."

Paragonimus westermani

Paragonimiasis.   *Paragonimus westermani,* also known as the "lung fluke," is endemic to the Far East, Pacific Islands, New Guinea, India, Africa, Central and South America, and in the eastern and midwestern United States. Dogs, cats, and other wild animals serve as reservoirs of infection for humans.

Adult lung flukes are found, usually in pairs, in fibrous, cyst-like structures in the lung tissues, as the name implies. If these fibrous structures, often near bronchioles, rupture, the eggs may be released and carried up the trachea to be coughed and spit out or swallowed where they end up in the gastrointestinal tract to be expelled with the feces. Once the unembryonated eggs are outside the body of the host they require 2 weeks or more for the miracidium to develop and hatch. Miracidia infect a snail and become cercariae, which erupt from the tissues of the snail to infect the second intermediate host, which may be either crabs or crayfish. Metacercariae develop in the crustaceans, and eaten raw or pickled the parasite excysts in the duodenum, penetrates its wall, and migrates across the peritoneal cavity, through the diaphragm, and into the lungs. Within the parenchyma of the lungs the metacercariae mature into adult worms, which produce eggs that may be expelled in the sputum or feces. A flow chart of the life cycle is available on the Companion Website.

The initial infection of the lung fluke may asymptomatic or may be characterized by fever and chills. The course of the disease is usually chronic with dilation of the bronchi, fibrosis,

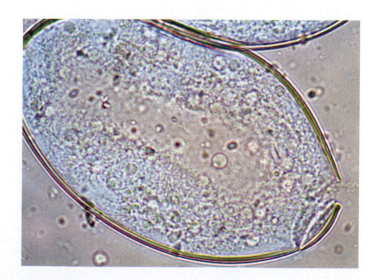

■ **FIGURE 30-64** Direct wet mount preparation containing a *Fasciola hepatica* egg. This egg is indistinguishable from that of *Fasciolopsis buskii* (400× magnification).

pseudopneumonia, and tuberculosis-like abscesses. Symptoms also include night sweats, chest pain, and persistent productive cough. Hemoptysis with viscous sputum containing dark, golden brown flecks would help in the differential diagnosis of lung fluke infection as opposed to viral or bacterial bronchopneumonia. Fatal cases have been reported.

Diagnosis of Paragonimiasis.   *Paragonimus westermani* adults range in size from 8 to 16 mm in length and 4 to 6 mm in breadth. They are reddish-brown in color and ovoid in shape, with the anterior end being abruptly rounded and the posterior end being somewhat tapered.

The eggs of *P. westermani* are 80–120 microns (length) by 48–60 microns (breadth), ovoid in shape, and operculated. They are a dark, golden brown color (hence the dark, golden

REAL WORLD TIP

The eggs of *Paragonimus westermani* and *Diphyllobothrium latum* may be confused. *P. westermani* has small, projecting shoulders at its lid end and a thickened opposite end. *D. latum* has no shoulders at its lid and a small knob at its opposite end.

✔ **Checkpoint! 30–30 (Chapter Objective 4)**

What is the infective stage for Paragonimus westermani?
  A. *Ingestion of metacercariae encysted in the flesh of crustaceans (such as crabs or crayfish)*
  B. *Ingestion of metacercariae encysted on water plants (such as bamboo shoots of water chestnuts)*
  C. *Ingestion of metacercariae encysted in the flesh of fish*
  D. *Penetration of the skin by cercariae*

✔ **Checkpoint! 30–31 (Chapter Objective 3)**

A formalin preserved stool specimen is sent to the laboratory for the identification of ova and parasites. Examination of a wet mount preparation from the sediment obtained using the formalin-ethyl acetate technique revealed the presence of broadly oval, embryonated eggs with a moderately thick shell. They are a light yellowish-brown color and the average size is 32 microns. A dome-shaped operculum and prominent opercular shoulders are clearly visible. A small commashaped abopercular knob is present. What is the most likely identification of the parasite producing these eggs?
  A. *Heterophyes heterophyes*
  B. *Metagonimus yokogawai*
  C. *Clonorchis sinensis*
  D. *Fasciolpsis buski*
  E. *Fasciola hepatica*

brown–flecked sputum), the operculum (lid) is flattened rather than domed, and the eggs possess distinct, raised opercular shoulders. The shell is moderately thick with an even thicker end opposite the operculum (Figure 30-65 ■). Eggs may be recovered from the sputum or the stool using the direct wet mount technique or a concentration procedure to demonstrate eggs that may be few in number. Distinguishing characteristics of trematode eggs are tabulated in Table 30-13.

▶ **ARTHROPODS AND HUMAN DISEASE**

THE PHYLUM *ARTHROPODA*

The phylum Arthropoda is divided into five classes. Most of the medically important arthropods are found in three of those classes: Insecta, Arachnia, and Crustacea. The phylum Arthropoda contains 80% of all animal life. Species within this group of invertebrates cause or transmit 80% of all diseases. They are also of major importance to agriculture where they play both beneficial and destructive roles. Due to the volume of material, this textbook is unable to attempt to discuss all medically significant arthropods. The Companion Website provides discussion of individual arthropods, their recognition, and their role in human disease.

SUMMARY

Developed countries with temperate climates have been spared much of the morbidity and mortality attributed to parasitic infections. For most parasites the harsh winter temperatures are a serious impediment to the completion of their life cycles, particularly those that require development outside the body of the host. Additionally, these countries lack intermediate hosts, reservoir hosts, and arthropod vectors vital to the per-

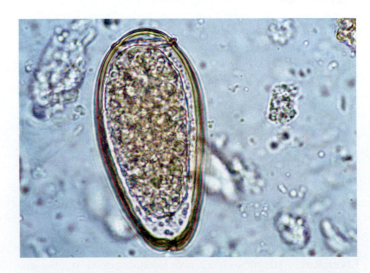

■ **FIGURE 30-65** Egg of *Paragonimus westermani,* the lung fluke, in a stool direct wet mount preparation (400× magnification).

✪ TABLE 30-13

Distinguishing Characteristics of Trematode Eggs

Parasite	Shape	Size (microns)	Color	State of Development (when passed)	Key Characteristics
Clonorchis sinensis	Egg-shaped	26–30 × 11–20	Brownish-yellow	Embryonated (miracidium)	Convex operculum with prominent opercular shoulders and in some cases a small abopercular knob is present
Fasciola hepatica	Ellipsoid	130–140 × 63–90	Yellowish-brown	Unembryonated	Very large, unembryonated eggs with thin, colorless shell
Fasciolopsis buskii	Very nearly indistinguishable from those of *Fasciola hepatica*				
Heterophyes heterophyes	Very closely resemble those of *Clonorchis sinensis*				
Metagonimus yokogawai	Very closely resemble those of *Clonorchis sinensis*				
Paragonimus westermani	Ovoid	80–120 × 39–67	Dark golden brown	Unembryonated	Flattened operculum with raised opercular shoulders and a thickening of the shell opposite the lid
Schistosoma haematobium	Elongated and ovoid	112–170 × 40–73	Light yellowish-brown	Embryonated (miracidium)	Large, nonoperculated eggs with a terminal (bee stinger) spine
Schistosoma japonicum	Spherical to ovoid	55–85	Light yellowish-brown	Embryonated (miracidium)	Oval embryonated egg with a small knob-like projection
Schistosoma mansoni	Elongated and ovoid	114–180 × 45–73	Light yellowish-brown	Embryonated (miracidium)	Large, nonoperculated eggs with a large, lateral (man-like) spine

petuation of many parasitic species. In spite of these facts some parasitic species have been able to enjoy a worldwide distribution, possibly a result of the ability to produce forms, such as cysts, which are resistant to environmental extremes.

Most individuals who live in developed countries have little knowledge of the threat that parasites pose unless they travel to countries where parasites are endemic. Without an understanding of the manner in which parasitic infections are spread they may come to harbor parasitic forms and may not be aware of the infection until the incubation period has passed and they have returned to their native country. When the symptoms appear their clinicians may be confronted with a disease for which they are not familiar. This is especially true in this day of jet travel where humans travel with great speed into and out of areas where parasites are endemic. Furthermore, with trade barriers being relaxed, foodstuffs that may harbor parasites may find their way into the markets and homes of those living in temperate climates. This has resulted in outbreaks of diarrheal diseases such as cryptosporidiosis or *Cyclospora cayetanensis* infection being reported with greater frequency.

Individuals who are immunocompromised have a much lower resistance to infection, which has made parasitic diseases of greater importance. Increases in this population have led to increases in infections not seen in immunocompetent individuals. They can also acquire infections that are more severe (hyperinfection). Additionally organisms are developing resistance to some of the drugs that have been used to combat parasitic infections. Man's ability to radically change his environment along with the failure of environmental con-

trol measures are additional factors and the importance of parasitology to the modern world has increased.

Parasites, organisms that live in close association with another organism deriving benefit from that relationship, have interacted with humans and other animals and in the process have developed life cycles that may involve humans, reservoir hosts, intermediate hosts, and arthropod vectors. Some of these parasites can infect the host without causing due harm and have been labeled commensal parasites. The shear numbers of parasites, their migration through and destruction of host tissue, and the elaboration of toxins allow them to cause various degrees of harm to the host and therefore this group is referred to as pathogenic parasites.

In some cases objects that are of plant, animal, or host origin very closely resemble true parasitic forms and these pseudoparasites may prove to be a source of confusion for the novice parasitologist. Mislabeling pseudoparasites and commensal parasites as pathogenic parasites or failing to recognize the presence of truly pathogenic parasites are two pitfalls that can only be avoided if laboratory workers have a thorough knowledge of the distinguishing morphological characteristics of parasitic species. For this reason, the diagnostic stages of parasites, their morphological characteristics, and those of pseudoparasites have been described in detail. In order to decrease the risk of acquiring parasitic diseases or to know when to administer drugs used to treat parasitic disease at a time when they will be most effective, one needs a knowledge of the life cycles of common and lesser known parasitic species and this text has sought to address that issue.

LEARNING OPPORTUNITIES

1. (Chapter Objective 3)
   Match the pseudoparasite with the distinguishing characteristics.

   1. _____ Leukocytes
   2. _____ Yeast
   3. _____ Plant parenchymal cells
   4. _____ Starch granules
   5. _____ Plant root hairs
   6. _____ Oil droplets
   7. _____ Pollen grains, diatoms, fungal spores
   8. _____ Vegetable spirals
   9. _____ Muscle fibers

   a. Presence of striations
   b. Stain blue to black with iodine solution
   c. Spiral configuration
   d. Increased nuclear to cytoplasmic ration
   e. Size variation and staining with fat stains
   f. Presence of solid nuclei and budding
   g. Highly refractile with no internal organs
   h. Variation in size and shape and hyaline cell walls
   i. Small and uniform in size and shape

2. (Chapter Objective 4)
   Match the parasitic infection with the correct diagnostic stage.

   1. _____ *Cryptosporidium parvum*
   2. _____ *Sarcocystis hominis*
   3. _____ *Isospora belli*
   4. _____ *Blastocystis hominis*
   5. _____ *Cyclospora cayetanensis*
   6. _____ *Sarcocystis tenella* (parasite of sheep)

   a. Ellipsoidal oöcysts measuring 30×12 μm
   b. Ovoidal sporocyst measuring 11×17 μm
   c. Sarcocyst with radial striations in the limiting membrane
   d. Spherical cysts 5–30 μm in diameter
   e. Spherical oöcysts 4–5 μm in diameter
   f. Spherical oöcysts 8–10 μm in diameter

3. (Chapter Objective 3) Describe how the following morphological characteristics
   of the trypomastigote will distinguish *Trypansoma rangeli* from *T. cruzi*.

Distinguishing Characteristics	*T. rangeli*	*T. cruzi*
Size of trypomastigote		
Kinetoplast		
Nucleus		
Other		

4. (Chapter Objective 4)
   Matching:

   Parasite

   _____ *Dracunculus medinensis*

   _____ *Toxoplasma gondii*

   _____ *Trichinella spiralis*

   _____ Visceral larval migrans

   Route of transmission to humans is through ingestion of:

   a. Food or water contaminated with cat feces
   b. Copepods
   c. Poorly cooked pork
   d. Embryonated eggs

CASE STUDY 30-1   (CHAPTER OBJECTIVES 3, 4, 5, AND 6)

A 48-year-old male with a history of hypertension and diabetes goes to his physician for his yearly physical. Although he claims to be in relatively good health he does have a complaint of slight transient abdominal discomfort. He assures his physician he has not experienced weight loss, vomiting, diarrhea, or constipation but has been feeling "tired, run-down, and has little stamina." The physician queries him further and learns the patient returned from a visit to Lima, Peru, some 6 months earlier and the abdominal discomfort began a short time later. He didn't recall receiving any insect bites but admitted trying out some of the local cuisine including "cerviche," a Peruvian delicacy consisting of vegetables (onions, peppers, tomatoes, and avocado) and freshly filleted fish, all of which is marinated with freshly squeezed lime juice.

Tests including a complete blood count, chemistry profile, urinalysis, and stool cultures are ordered. Serum chemistries and urinalysis results were normal. The stool cultures yeilded normal stool flora; no *Samonella*, *Shigella*, *Campylobacter*, or *Aeromonas* species were isolated. The blood tests revealed a normal white cell count but a reduced red cell count, low hemoglobin and hematocrit, macrocytosis, anisocytosis, and polychromatophilia. Initial diagnosis: anemia of unknown etiology. Occult blood and examination for ova and parasites were performed next. The occult blood test (guiac) was negative but numerous eggs with the following morphological characteristics were seen on the saline direct wet mount and a saline wet mount made using the sediment from the formalin-ethyl acetate concentration procedure:

Size: 65 × 49 microns, operculated, smooth shell of moderate thickness, yellowish-brown color, and unembryonated. The presence of a knob opposite the operculum is noted.

1. What should the final diagnosis be for this patient?
2. What is the most likely source of this parasitic infection?
3. What is the relationship of this organism to the patient's abnormal blood test results?
4. How might this infection have been avoided?
5. What are the diagnostic stages for this parasite?

CASE STUDY 30-2   (CHAPTER OBJECTIVES 3, 4, 5, AND 6)

A 25-year-old female is seen in the emergency room with the following complaints: dysuria, intense vulvar and vaginal pruritis, increased vaginal secretions, and dysmenorrhea. In addition to being copious, the vaginal discharge is characterized as greenish-colored, frothy, and foul-smelling. A small amount of discharge is collected during a speculum examination and is sent to the laboratory for a direct saline wet mount preparation. In addition, a urine specimen is sent for urinalysis. Examination of a wet mount from the urinary sediment and vaginal secretions identified the presence of a protozoan parasite with the following morphological char-acteristics: pear-shaped organisms with a single nucleus, four anteriorly located flagella, and an undulating membrane that extends halfway down the length of the organism. The average size of the parasite is approximately 20 microns in length. Jerky, nondirectional motility is also noted.

1. What is the identity of this parasite? Provide the genus-species name and stages present.
2. Is culture and sensitivity of this organism possible or warranted in this case?
3. How is this organism usually spread?

CASE STUDY 30-3   (CHAPTER OBJECTIVES 3, 4, 5, AND 6)

A father–son duo who enjoyed the "great outdoors" and who were hiking, camping, fishing, and hunting enthusiasts were suddenly stricken with diarrhea after returning from a hunting expedition in the Colorado Rockies. The 56-year-old father was the first to feel abdominal distress consisting of anorexia, severe abdominal pain, flatulence, and frequent episodes of watery diarrhea with mucus present but no blood. Two days later the 28-year-old son began to experience identical symptoms but with less intensity. After 6 days of "toughing it out" and the use of over-the-counter antidiarrhetics, the diarrhea abated but the abdominal dis-comfort persisted so the two males sought the assistance of their family physicians to alleviate their remaining symptoms. Stool samples (times 3) were collected and submitted to the laboratory for routine bacterial culture and susceptibility testing and, because of their recent history of travel, examination for ova and parasites.

Routine cultures failed to yield the presence of any pathogenic bacteria. Examination of both direct wet mounts and trichrome-stained permanent smears performed on stool samples from both patients revealed the presence of the same parasitic organism. Stool specimens collected on the first day revealed the presence of an occasional protozoan parasite with the following microscopic morphology: a size range of 9–21 microns in length, a tear-shape, bilateral symmetry with two nuclei, a sucking disc, and four pairs of flagella, giving the parasite a falling-leaf motility. The remaining specimens collected on days 2 and 3 revealed the presence of elliptical-shaped objects whose size range was 8–24 × 7–10 microns. On the trichrome-stained smears, four nuclei, four axonemes, and four median bodies were clearly evident inside small each oval object.

1. What should the final report from the parasitology section say? Provide the genus-species name and stages present.
2. How is this parasite transmitted?

PEARSON
myhealthprofessionskit

Use this address to access the interactive Companion Website created for this textbook. Simply select "Clinical Laboratory Science" from the choice of disciplines. Find this book and log in using your user name and password.

REFERENCES

Go to myhealthprofessionskit.com to view this chapter's references.

31

Intracellular Microorganisms

William C. Payne and Masih Shokrani

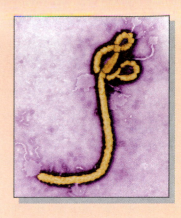

■ LEARNING OBJECTIVES

Upon completion of this chapter, the learner should be able to:

1. Correlate the pathogenic intracellular organisms with the diseases they cause.
2. Summarize the immunological response to infection by intracellular organisms.
3. Describe the physical and biochemical characteristics that differentiate intracellular organisms from other infectious agents.
4. Explain the importance of intracellular organisms as causes of human disease, including factors that predispose individuals to infections (risk factors).
5. Relate viral structures that are important in classifying different families of viruses.
6. Differentiate the reproduction cycles of chlamydiae and viruses.
7. Discuss the etiology, epidemiology, clinical manifestations, laboratory diagnosis, and treatment of the following intracellular organisms:
   a. *Chlamydiaceae*
   b. *Rickettsia, Orientia, Coxiella, Neorickettsia, Ehrlichia,* and *Anaplasma* species
   c. Viruses
8. Given pertinent patient demographics and clinical manifestations, choose testing procedures that aid in the diagnosis of infections caused by intracellular organisms.
9. Given the results of laboratory tests, provide a probable diagnosis and suggest further tests that might be necessary to confirm the diagnosis of an infection caused by an intracellular organism.

KEY TERMS

capsid

cell culture

cytopathic effect

ehrlichiosis

elementary body

hepatotropic viruses

intracytoplasmic

inclusions

lymphogranuloma

venereum

morulae

nucleocapsid

obligate intracellular

organisms

psittacosis

reticulate body

trachoma

virion

TAXONOMY

Family *Chlamydiaceae*
 Chlamydia trachomatis (klă-mid′-ee-ah tra-kō′-mah-tis)
 Chylamydophila psittaci (klă-mid′-o-fĭl-ah sit′ta-see)
 C. pneumoniae (new-mō-nee-eye)

Family *Rickettsiaceae* and Other Related Organisms
 Rickettsia rickettsii (rick-ett-sēa rĭ′-ket-sē-eye)
 R. akari (ah-kar′-ee)
 R. prowazekii (prō-ah-zee′-kee-eye)
 R. typhi (tī′-fee)
 Orientia tsutsugamushi (o-ree-ěn′tē-ah tsoo-tsoo-gah-mew-shee)
 Coxiella burnetii (kox-ee′-el-ah burn-ět-ee-eye)
 Ehrlichia chaffeensis (ěr-lick′-ee-ah chaff-ee′-ěn-sis)
 Anaplasma phagocytophilum (ăn-uh-plăs′-mah fă-gō-sītō-fĭl-ŭm)
 Neorickettsia sennetsu (nee-ōh-rĭ-ket′-sĭ-ah sěn-ěh-tsoo)

DNA viruses
 Herpes simplex viruses (her′-peez sĭm-plěx)
 Varicella zoster virus (văr′-ĭ-sěl′-ah zŏs-těr)
 Epstein–Barr virus (ěp-stīn băr)
 Cytomegalovirus (sī-tō-meg′-ă-lō –vīr-us)
 Human Herpesvirus 6 (her′-peez-vīr-us)
 Human Herpesvirus 7
 Human Herpesvirus 8

Smallpox virus (small-pocks)
Papilloma virus (pă-pĭl″-ō-mah)
Adenoviruses (ăd-ě-nō-vīr-us)
Hepatitis B virus (hěp′-ă-tī′-tĭs)

RNA Viruses
 Hepatitis A virus
 Hepatitis C virus
 Hepatitis D virus
 Hepatitis E virus
 Hepatitis G virus
 Poliomyelitis virus (pō′-lee-ō-my′-ě-lī-tĭs)
 Coxsackie viruses (kŏk-săk-ee)
 Rhinoviruses (rī′-nō-vīr′-us)
 Coronaviruses (kōr-ō-năh-vīr-us)
 Influenza viruses (ĭn-flū′-ěn-zah)
 Parainfluenza viruses (păr′-ah- ĭn-flū′-ěn-zah)
 Respiratory Syncytial virus (sĭn-sĭsh-ăl)
 Measles virus (mee′-zlz)
 Mumps virus (mŭm-ps)
 Rubella virus (roo′-běll-ah)
 Noroviruses (nor-ō-vīr-us)
 Rotaviruses (rōt′-ah-vīr-us)
 Rabies virus (ray-bees)
 Retroviruses (ret′-rō-vīr-us)

▶ INTRODUCTION

Obligate intracellular organisms are microorganisms that are incapable of replication outside a living host cell. They have no means of self-locomotion and are therefore completely dependent on physical forces from outside themselves to spread and infect susceptible host cells. Because these organisms cannot grow outside a living cell they cannot be cultured on artificial media such as solid agar plates, semi-solid media, or broths, even if they are supplemented with serum or whole blood. Isolation techniques involving animal inoculation or the use of embryonated chicken eggs have been employed in the past, but have largely been supplanted by the use of **cell cultures.** Cell cultures are monolayers of eukaryotic cells, most of which are of animal or human origin such as fibroblasts, neuroblastoma, monkey kidney, hamster ovary, and other cell types. ∞ Chapter 16, "Viral, Chlamydial, and Rickettsial Specimens," provides detailed information on specimen collection and detection methods.

Since they do not grow on solid agar they cannot form discrete colonies that can be seen with the naked eye. Most of these microbes are of such small size they are even difficult to visualize using light microscopy. The organisms may be observed as an inclusion body or mass within a cell or the by-products produced by cells infected with intracellular microorganisms, such as viruses, may be seen. Inclusion bodies may be seen inside the nucleus as intranuclear inclusions or within the cytoplasm of infected cells as **intracytoplasmic inclusions.** Diagnosis of infections caused by members of the family *Chlamydiaceae* is often based on the clinical symptoms experienced by the patient as well as laboratory findings, which include the presence of inclusion bodies within infected cells. **Trachoma**, a disease of the eye caused by the intracellular organism, *Chlamydia trachomatis,* is characterized by tiny, discrete, acidophilic intracytoplasmic forms called Prowazek-Greeff bodies. These inclusions are found in epithelial cells obtained by collecting conjunctival scrapings or swabs.

Rickettsiae and several related bacteria are also intracellular organisms. They are responsible for a number of febrile illnesses carried by arthropods such as ticks, lice, and fleas. Rickettsiae enter the body of the host through the bite and feeding of blood-sucking arthropods, spreading through the bloodstream to infect the vascular endothelium, which often leads to a rash, a symptom associated with infection. Rickettsial diseases occur worldwide with domestic and wild animals serving as important reservoirs of infection for humans.

Viruses are among the smallest of the known infectious agents, and can only be photographed using an electron microscope. These intracellular organisms cause a wide variety of illnesses, some asymptomatic, some mild, and some fatal. A single type of virus can be responsible for many different syndromes. Adenoviruses, for example, may cause pharyngitis, conjunctivitis, laryngitis, pneumonia, cystitis, and diarrhea, as well as systemic infection such as hepatitis. Conversely the same symptoms may be associated with different viruses. Viral pharyngitis, the most common cause of sore throat, may be associated with infections caused by herpes simplex viruses, the Epstein–Barr virus, rhinoviruses, coronaviruses, the parainfluenza virus, influenza viruses, coxsackie viruses, the respiratory syncytial virus, and measles viruses. This complicates the diagnosis of viral illnesses but identifying a specific viral agent allows for more precise treatment.

▶ THE FAMILY *CHLAMYDIACEAE*

The *Chlamydiaceae* family includes two genera: *Chlamydia* and *Chlamydophila*. They are pleomorphic, gram-negative bacteria that can only exist as obligate intracellular organisms because they are unable to make their own ATP (a source of energy). Infected cells contain intracytoplasmic inclusions around the nucleus of the host cell. The name of these infectious agents is derived from the Greek word, χλαμυσ (chlamys), meaning "cloak."

Members of the family *Chlamydiaceae* have a unique reproductive cycle. The infectious form of the bacterium, known

as the **elementary body** (EB), is not metabolically active but allows the organism limited existence outside the host cell. The EB is taken into the host cell by phagocytosis, a process whereby the cell engulfs the microbe and is taken into the cytoplasm. During the next 6–8 hours the EB reorganizes into the **reticulate body** (RB), a metabolically active form that is able to replicate within the cytoplasm of the host cell. This form is not infectious because it is too fragile to exist outside the host cell. The RB divides by binary fission over the next 18–24 hours before reorganizing once again to become an EB. Eventually the host cell lyses, releasing the elementary bodies, which are free to infect other cells.

Direct microscopic examination of clinical specimens is a means of rapid diagnosis but suffers from a lack of sensitivity, which is about 60%. Iodine and Giemsa staining has been used in the past to detect the intracytoplasmic inclusions. *Chlamydia trachomatis* produces compact inclusions containing glycogen, which stain with iodine as seen in Figure 31-1 ■. *Chlamydophila psittaci* and *Chlamydophila pneumoniae* produce diffuse inclusions, which do not stain with iodine due to the lack of glycogen. All three species can be stained with the Giemsa stain. With the Giemsa stain, elementary bodies stain a reddish purple, while the reticulate bodies stain a bluish color.

Even greater sensitivity can be achieved with the use of a fluorescent antibody technique. The direct antibody technique utilizes fluorescein-labeled monoclonal antibodies that attach to the EB so they are visible with an apple-green fluorescence. This technique can be used to detect the organisms in smears made from clinical specimens such as conjuctival scrapings, sputum, throat specimens, pleural fluid, urethral and cervical scrapings, rectal swabs, and lymph node aspirates.

Cell cultures, such as HeLa, McCoy, and monkey kidney cells, can be used to cultivate these microorganisms. The

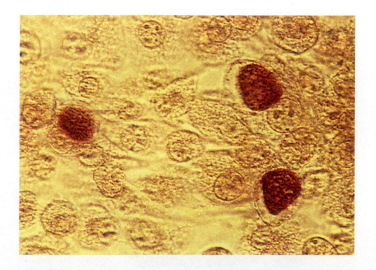

■ **FIGURE 31-1** Iodine-stained intracellular inclusions of *Chlamydia trachomatis* in a monolayer of McCoy cells. Magnification 200×.
Courtesy of CDC/Dr. E. Arum, Dr. N. Jacobs.

monolayer of the cell culture can then be stained and examined for perinuclear cytoplasmic inclusions. Iodine, Giemsa, and immunofluorescent stains can be used to visualize the organisms, as seen in Figure 31-1. Nucleic acid amplification and DNA probes increase the sensitivity and specificity of detection.

 REAL WORLD TIP

The key to detection of *Chlamydia* spp. is the quality of the specimen. The more epithelial cells present, the more organisms present, which in turn leads to better sensitivity for the test method used.

CHLAMYDIA TRACHOMATIS

C. trachomatis is an important cause of blindness throughout the world. Trachoma occurs mainly among the poor in areas such as the Middle East, North Africa, northern India, and in Native Americans of the southwestern United States. Infection is transmitted from person to person. Scarring, ulceration, and vascularization of the cornea eventually lead to blindness. The conjunctiva scars causing the eyelashes to turn in toward the eye. The friction of the lashes causes corneal damage.

C. trachomatis causes other diseases such as:

- Nongonococcal and postgonococcal urethritis has replaced gonorrhea as the most common sexually transmitted disease. Figure 31-2 ■ demonstrates a cervical infection due to *Chlamydia trachomatis*. If untreated, the organism can spread into the fallopian tubes and eventually into the peritoneal cavity causing pelvic inflammatory disease as well as ectopic pregnancies due to scarring, and infertility.

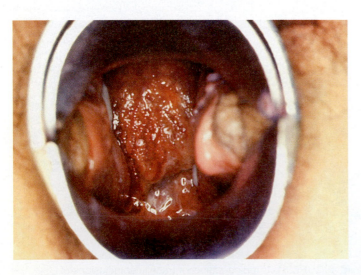

■ **FIGURE 31-2** Chlamydial infection of the cervix exhibiting erosive lesions and erythema.
Courtesy of CDC/Dr. Lourdes Fraw, Jim Pledger.

- **Lymphogranuloma venereum** is another sexually transmitted disease found in Africa, Asia, and South America. The initial lesion is a small, painless, vesicular lesion. This lesion and the resulting draining ulcer heal spontaneously. After a period of 2–6 weeks the patient experiences chills, fever, and lymphadenopathy or swollen painful lymph nodes.
- Inclusion conjunctivitis is a disease seen in newborns who acquire the organism as they pass through the birth canal of infected mothers. This infection differs from trachoma because there is no corneal scarring. Newborns may also develop a form of pneumonia via the same route of infection. Adults can acquire conjunctivitis through hand-to-eye contact with urogenital secretions containing the organism.

The organism can be detected by culture, antigen detection such as immunofluorescence, or nucleic acid assays. Often individuals are coinfected with *Neisseria gonorrhoeae* and *Chlamydia trachomatis*. Individuals are usually treated for both organisms. Azithromycin and doxycylcine are recommended.

 REAL WORLD TIP

In cases of sexual abuse and other situations that require the results to be used in a court of law, *Chlamydia trachomatis* culture is the gold standard.

CHLAMYDOPHILA PSITTACI

C. psittaci is primarily associated with animal infections. This organism infects birds, such as parrots, parakeets, canaries, turkeys, pigeons and ducks, and other mammals to cause **psittacosis**, a disease that may be mild or severe. The organism can be found in the feathers, tissues, and feces of infected birds. These infected animals may or may not be symptomatic. Humans acquire psittacosis by inhalation. Psittacosis is considered a zoonotic disease. Often those affected are those individuals, such as zoo workers, pet shop employees, poultry farmers, and veterinarians, who have prolonged exposure to birds.

 REAL WORLD TIP

Most cases of psittacosis are due to pet birds. The disease is also known as "parrot fever."

After inhalation, the organism enters the blood then the reticuloendothelial system and eventually reaches the lungs. Symptoms include fever, chills, fatigue, headache, and a nonproductive cough. Human infection may range from asymptomatic, to mild, to fatal cases of pneumonia. Often individuals present with pneumonia or a fever of unknown origin.

REAL WORLD TIP

Isolation of *Chlamydophila psittaci* should not be attempted in most laboratories. It is easily aerosolized and associated with lab-acquired infections.

CHLAMYDOPHILA PNEUMONIAE

C. pneumoniae is associated with an acute respiratory illness and can occur worldwide. Adolescents, young adults, and older adults are at greatest risk for infection. Transmission is person to person. As yet no animal reservoir has been found. This organism is responsible for respiratory illnesses such as pneumonia, bronchitis, pharyngitis, sinusitis, and a flu-like illness. The primary patient complaint is a persistent cough. The specimen of choice is collection of the epithelial cells in the nasopharynx. Sputum is not a satisfactory specimen for detection.

 REAL WORLD TIP

C. pneumoniae has also been linked to atherosclerosis or hardening of the arteries and coronary heart disease.

Both *C. psittaci* and *C. pneumoniae* can be diagnosed with cell culturing, immunofluorescence, or through serological procedures such as complement fixation (CF). In the CF test, the EB provides the antigen source and infected individuals demonstrate a fourfold rise in titer. Other *Chlamydia* spp. can cross-react in the complement fixation test. There is also a delay in diagnosis due to the need to wait for the appearance of antibodies.

Treatment for both organisms requires the use of tetracycline or doxycycline. Erythromycin is effective for individuals, such as children and pregnant females, who cannot be prescribed tetracycline.

✓ **Checkpoint! 31–1 (Chapter Objective 4)**

The infectious form of chlamydiae, which is actively taken into the host cell by phagocytosis, is known as a/an
  A. *Donvan body.*
  B. *Döhle body.*
  C. *reticulate body.*
  D. *elementary body.*

RICKETTSIA AND OTHER RELATED SPECIES

The *Rickettsia* species, *Coxiella burnetti,* and *Orientia tsutsugamushi,* are another group of intracellular organisms that require a host cell in order to reproduce. For the most part they are zoonotic agents whose native hosts are animal species but they do occasionally cause human infection. These organisms appear to be gram negative with cell walls containing lipopolysaccharide, lipoprotein, and peptidoglycan.

Rickettsiae and related species are of very small size, and, because they stain poorly with Gram stain reagents, there is a lack of contrast, with host tissues making these organisms hard to visualize. Visualization is much better with Giemsa stain.

Like most intracellular organisms, these organisms are very fragile, and, with the exception of *Coxiella burnetii,* are susceptible to heat, desiccation, and sunlight. All, except *C. burnetti,* are transmitted from animals by arthropod vectors such as ticks, lice, and mites. Figure 31-3 ■ demonstrates a feeding louse. Infections are associated with symptoms such as fever, headache, myalgia, and in some cases a rash, which is seen primarily in the rickettsial infections. Rocky Mountain spotted fever, rickettsialpox, and typhus fevers are all rickettsial illnesses, and many occur worldwide.

Coxiella burnetii is the causative agent of Q fever, a zoonotic disease. It can be found in cattle, sheep, and goats. Humans acquire the organisms from inhalation of or contact with the milk, urine, feces, and birth products of infected animals. High fevers, severe headache, chills, diarrhea, and eventual pneumonia are seen. There is no rash as noted with rickettsial infections. Because its signs and symptoms mimic other infections, accurate testing is necessary for detection.

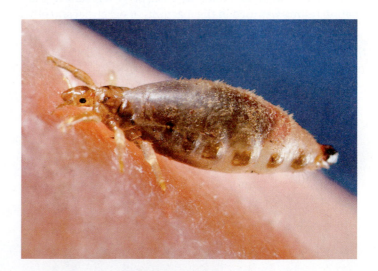

■ **FIGURE 31-3** Lateral view of a female body louse feeding on a human. Body lice, *Pediculus humanus ss corporis,* are known carriers of the etiological agent of epidemic typhus and Brill-Zinser disease, *Rickettsia prowazeckii.*
From Public Health Image Library (PHIL), CDC/Frank Collins, Ph.D.

Rickettsia and *Orientia* enter the endothelial cells of blood vessels. Damage occurs due to lesions throughout the body's vascular system. Figure 31-4 ■ demonstrates the small organisms inside a capillary endothelial cell.

Rickettsia rickettsii is best known for Rocky Mountain spotted fever (RMSF). It is endemic to the United States and is primarily a disease of children. RMSF presents as a triad of symptoms: fever, headache, and rash. In addition, there is usually a history of a tick bite. Figure 31-5 ■ shows the characteristic rash associated with RMSF. Most infections occur during the warm months of the year when hard ticks, as seen in Figure 31-6 ■, are most active. While the name Rocky Mountain spotted fever implies a disease that might be confined to the western United States, the disease is seen most often in the western and southeastern states including Arkansas, Oklahoma, Georgia, North and South Carolina, and Virginia. Other diseases caused by *Rickettsia* and *Orientia* are listed in Table 31-1 ✪.

Diagnosis of these organisms is through the use of cell culture techniques and serological tests such as indirect immunofluorescence assays, enzyme immunoassays, and immunoblotting techniques. In times past Weil-Felix agglutination testing was used in the diagnosis of rickettsial and other

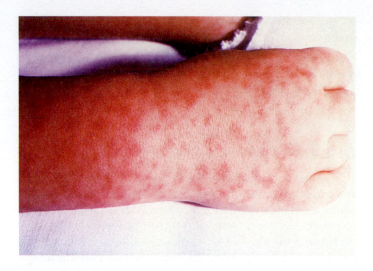

■ **FIGURE 31-5** The characteristic rash of Rocky Mountain spotted fever is small, flat, pink and non-itchy.
From Public Health Image Library (PHIL), CDC.

febrile illnesses but due to a lack of specificity are of limited clinical value.

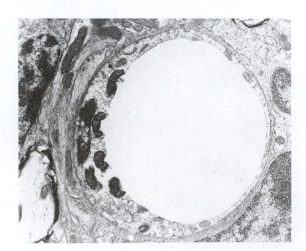

■ **FIGURE 31-4** The five rickettsial organisms present in this capillary endothelial cell are small compared to the cell's nucleus to their left.
From Public Health Image Library (PHIL), CDC/Dr. Edwin P. Ewing, Jr.

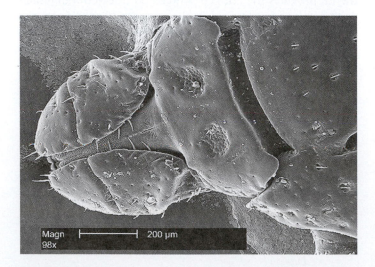

■ **FIGURE 31-6** Dorsal view of the American dog tick, *Dermacentor variabilis*, a known carrier of *Rickettsia rickettsii*, the cause of Rocky Mountain spotted fever.
From Public Health Image Library (PHIL), CDC.

⭐ TABLE 31-1

Rickettsiae and Related Organisms

Disease	Etiological Agent	Arthropod Vector
Rocky Mountain spotted fever	*Rickettsia rickettsii*	Wood tick (*Dermacentor andersoni*) and dog tick (*D. variabilis*)
Rickettsialpox	*R. akari*	House mouse mites (*Liponyssides sanguineous*)
Epidemic typhus	*R. prowazekii*	Human body louse (*Pediculus humanus corporis*)
Brill-Zinser disease		Squirrel flea and louse
Murine typhus	*R. typhi*	Rat flea (*Xenopsylla cheopis*)
Scrub typhus	*Orientia tsutsugamushi*	Trombiculid (chigger) mites (*Leptotrombidium akamushi*, *L. deliense, L. fletcheri*)
Q fever	*Coxiella burnetii*	None (spread by inhalation)
Trench fever	*Bartonella quintana*	Human body louse
Cat-scratch disease	*B. henselae*	Cat flea (*Ctenocephalides felis*)
Oroya fever	*B. bacilliformis*	Sandflies (*Lutzomyia* species)
Human monocytic ehrlichiosis	*Ehrlichia chaffeensis*	Lone star tick (*Amblyomma americanum*)
Human granulocytic anaplasmosis	*Anaplasma phagocytophilum*	Deer tick (*Ixodes scapularis*)
Sennetsu fever	*Neorickettsia sennetsu*	None (ingestion of fish)

NEORICKETTSIA, EHRLICHIA, AND ANAPLASMA SPECIES

This group of related species causes disease in wild and domestic animals, especially dogs, as well as humans. An infected tick is the vector. These organisms parasitize macrophages or granulocytes, as seen in Figure 31-7 ■, causing **ehrlichiosis**, a disease characterized by leukopenia and thrombocytopenia. Upon entry into the white blood cells, the organisms develop into a cluster, called a **morulae**, which can resemble a mul-

berry or blackberry. The disease and symptoms depend on the species and the white blood cell it infects.

Human monocytic ehrlichiosis, caused by *Ehrlichia chaffeensis* and *E. equi,* is a disease transmitted by the bite and feeding of *Amblyomma americanum,* the lone star tick, as seen in Figure 31-8 ■. Human granulocytic anaplasmosis or ehrlichiosis is caused by *Ehrlichia ewingii* and *Anaplasma phagocytophilum.* Symptoms are similar to those of Rocky Mountain spotted fever: high fever, headache, malaise, and myalgia, but a rash is rare. Incidence for *Ehrlichia* and *Anaplasma* is highest

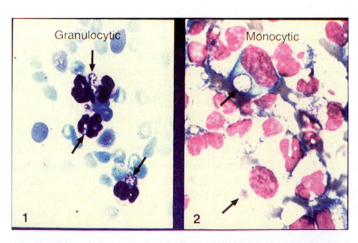

■ **FIGURE 31-7** Ehrlichiosis. Human white blood cells infected with the etiological agent of human granulocytic ehrlichiosis, *Anaplasma phagocytophilum* (Figure 1). Human white blood cells infected with the etiological agent of human monocytic ehrlichiosis, *Ehrlichia chafeensis* (Figure 2). *Courtesy of CDC.*

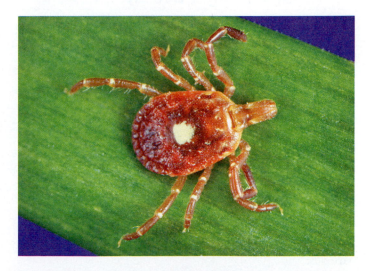

■ **FIGURE 31-8** Photomicrograph of the dorsal view of a female "lone star tick," *Amblyomma americanum,* a known carrier of *Ehrlichia chafeensis* and *E. ewingii,* agents of human disease. *From Public Health Image Library (PHIL), CDC/Michael L. Levin, Ph.D.*

in the southeastern and south central areas of the United States, including Oklahoma, Texas, Arkansas, Georgia, Missouri, and South Carolina. *Neorickettsia sennetsu* is an agent of a mononucleosis-like illness found in Japan and Malaysia. It infects the monocytes and macrophages.

Serological tests, such as indirect immunofluorescent assays demonstrating a fourfold rise in titer, are frequently used for diagnostic purposes. Molecular techniques such as the polymerase chain reaction, are effective but for the time being are cost-prohibitive for most clinical laboratories. Examination of Wright-stained blood smears may be attempted but is probably the least sensitive method for diagnosing ehrlichiosis. Smears are examined for the presence of morulae, cytoplasmic vacuoles in which *Ehrlichia* species grow, in peripheral white blood cells. *N. sennetsu* detection requires intraperitoneal inoculation of the blood in laboratory mice.

 REAL WORLD TIP

The presence of morulae is more common with human granulocytic anaplasmosis than in human monocytic ehrlichiosis. The hematologist may observe the morulae on review of the stained blood film of an infected individual.

Doxycycline is the drug of choice for treatment. Healthy individuals can make a full recovery. Ehrlichiosis can be fatal in those who are immunosuppressed.

 Checkpoint! 31–2 (Chapter Objective 5)

Rickettsiae are transmitted most often by
  A. *inhalation.*
  B. *arthropod vectors.*
  C. *ingestion.*
  D. *sexual intercourse.*

▶ **VIROLOGY**

Viruses, another group of obligate intracellular organisms, are among the smallest infectious agents known and range in size from about 20 nanometers (nm) to about 300 nm in diameter. They are incapable of growth or replication outside of a living cell and are considered by some to be inert biochemical particles.

Virologists are called upon to isolate and identify viruses from a variety of specimens. Specialized methods and a high level of expertise are required for the interpretation of results and identification of viruses. Laboratory diagnosis is impor-

tant because different viruses may cause diseases that have similar signs and symptoms. **Hepatotropic viruses**, for example, cause diseases of the liver, which have essentially the same signs and symptoms but represent viruses from markedly different families of viruses. Gastrointestinal viruses also cause similar symptoms such as nausea, vomiting, cramps, and diarrhea. Respiratory viruses exhibit fever, coryza or a head cold, and cough. Determining the etiological agent of a disease based purely on a particular clinical presentation is certainly not reliable. In order to determine the identity of the organism causing a particular viral illness it is often necessary to propagate the virus or use serological tests to show exposure to the virus in question.

Some of the procedures used in virology, such as complement fixation, viral neutralization, hemagglutination inhibition, and many of the molecular techniques are very complicated and difficult to perform or may require a significant investment of time and money. Such procedures are usually not incorporated into the workflow of routine clinical laboratories and are performed primarily at large institutions such as research centers, reference laboratories, and large medical centers that have a large enough workload to justify the expense. Recently diagnostic techniques have been developed that are simple to perform, rapid, sensitive, and reliable. Latex agglutination and enzyme immunoassay tests are good examples of techniques that can be performed in the routine clinical laboratory.

GENERAL PROPERTIES OF VIRUSES

Viruses are broadly classified on the basis of their genomic nucleic acid. The viral genome consists of only one kind of nucleic acid, either RNA or DNA, but not both. The viral nucleic acid can be single- or double-stranded, linear or circular, and positive or negative sense. It must carry the necessary genetic information to synthesize the proteins and nucleic acids necessary for replication. The viral genome codes for the outer protein coat and other proteins required for viral production that are not provided by the host cell. Some proteins are structural, meaning they become incorporated into the makeup of the virus particle. Some proteins are nonstructural, such as the viral polymerase enzymes.

Retroviruses are a special group of RNA viruses that carry a reverse transcriptase enzyme as part of their genetic makeup. Retroviruses are capable of transcribing their RNA into DNA and then integrating that DNA into the host cell genome in order for replication to take place. This is opposite the normal flow of genetic information, which is for DNA to be transcribed into RNA and for the RNA to be translated into proteins.

An outer protein shell of a virus that surrounds and provides protection of the viral genetic material is called the **capsid.** The viral capsid may be a spherical shape called icosahedral or helical in shape. The protein capsid and the viral nucleic acid comprise the **nucleocapsid.**

A virus particle, known as a **virion**, may consist of the viral genome and its capsid only or may have an additional component, an envelope that surrounds the nucleocapsid. The envelope consists of phospholipids as well as virus-encoded proteins and glycoproteins. Viral envelopes are of host cell origin and are acquired as the nucleocapsid buds out of the host cell, acquiring the bilipid-layered membrane of the host cell. Viruses that possess this host-derived bilipid layer are called enveloped viruses and those that lack this outer layer are known as unenveloped (naked) viruses.

Because viruses lack the cellular machinery for metabolism they are dependent upon the host cell to reproduce. The method by which they reproduce is known as viral replication and is unique to viruses.

VIRAL REPLICATION

Viruses infect unicellular organisms such as protozoa, bacteria, and algae, as well as multicellular organisms such as plants and animals. The viral nucleic acid or genome contains the information necessary for directing the infected host cell to synthesize specific macro-molecules necessary for the production of viral progeny. The viral genome must be inserted into the host cell in order for replication to take place. In order to reproduce, a virus must first attach to, and gain entrance into, a living host cell. Table 31-2 ✪ summarizes the life cycle of a virus. Figure 31-29, later in this chapter, depicts the life cycle of the human immunodeficiency virus.

There are several steps involved in the process of viral replication:

- Attachment and absorption. Complementary receptors on the surface of the host cell and the virus allow attachment and absorption.
- Penetration. After attachment to a susceptible host cell, the virus enters the cell by phagocytosis or endocytosis, or as is usually the case for enveloped viruses, fusion of the viral membrane and cell membrane.

✪ TABLE 31-2

The Life Cycle of Viruses

Sequence of steps in the life cycle of a virus	
Step	**Process**
Attachment	The virus attaches to the host cell
Penetration	The virus enters the host cell through fusion or endocytosis
Uncoating	The viral capsid is removed, releasing the nucleic acid strand(s)
Eclipse	The virus induces the host cell machinery to synthesize components for viral replication
Maturation	Newly synthesized viral components are assembled into a new virion; this assembly may occur in the nucleus (as in herpes viruses) or in the cytoplasm (as in polio viruses)
Release	The new virions are released from the host cell to infect other cells through lysis or budding

- Uncoating. Once the virus has gained entrance into the host cell the viral capsid is removed, probably by host enzymes, and the nucleic acid is released to do its work. The viral genome must be able to direct the host cell to make the required nucleic acid component and the proteins needed by the virus.
- Eclipse period. Many copies of the viral nucleic acid are produced during the replication cycle as well as enzymes required for further synthesis (early proteins) and structural proteins, which make up the viral capsid (late proteins). During this time of intracellular viral synthesis, there is no visible evidence of the presence of the virus within the cell.
- Maturation. During this period the viral capsid is assembled and the viral genome is inserted, forming the nucleocapsid. All the work being conducted—nucleic acid synthesis, protein synthesis, and the random assembly of the components into the nucleocapsid—is occurring at the molecular level.
- Release. Finally, the new viruses produced leave the host cell through cell lysis or through budding and exocytosis. For enveloped viruses the nucleocapsid migrates to the nuclear or cytoplasmic membrane. The membrane surrounds the nucleocapsid to form the envelope and the virus is released in a process that might approximate the reverse of penetration.

IMMUNITY TO VIRUSES

Many viruses use highly sophisticated mechanisms for cellular invasion into the host cell and evasion of the immune system. Virus latency and antigenic variation are the most effective mechanisms. Another escape mechanism is the production of cytokine analogs and cytokine receptor analogs. To counteract these invasive maneuvers the immune system of the host utilizes several mechanisms, including innate and adaptive immune responses. For a thorough discussion of the immune system the reader is invited to explore its various components, as addressed in ∞ Chapter 10, "Immunological Tests."

One of the first mechanisms employed by the host involves components of innate immunity. This involves the production of antiviral proteins such as interferons (IFN) and complement. IFN-α and IFN-β activate natural killer (NK) cells, which limit viral production by recognizing and killing virally infected cells by a process of antibody-dependent cell-mediated cytotoxicity (ADCC). In addition, IFN-γ that is secreted by NK cells activates macrophages, thereby priming the immune system for an adaptive immune response. A set of plasma proteins called complement are able to protect against viral infection by damaging the outermost layer of enveloped viruses or coating the receptors of unenveloped viruses.

The adaptive immune response involves the production of antibodies (humoral immunity), a defense mechanism designed to protect host cells from viral invasion. Antibodies are able to act on viruses by inhibiting the action of viral enzymes, activating complement, viral neutralization (coating viral particles), opsonization (enhancing phagocytosis), and ADCC of virally infected cells.

Among the classes of antibody produced to ward off viral infection are immunoglobulins (Ig) A, G, and M.

- IgA can prevent the virus from binding to the epithelial host cells that line the mucous membranes of the respiratory tract, the gastrointestinal tract, and the urogenital tract.

- IgG is the most potent antibody against viruses and is considered a neutralizing antibody because it is able to coat viruses and prevent them from infecting host cells. This class of antibody is a primary force in the development of lifelong immunity to certain viral infections such as chickenpox or measles. Furthermore, the presence of IgG on the surface of a virus enhances phagocytosis by polymorphonuclear white blood cells such as neutrophils, and

mononuclear cells such as macrophages. IgG is also capable of activating complement, whose ability to damage enveloped viruses and coat unenveloped viruses has been mentioned previously.

- IgM class antibodies are produced during the early stages of the immune response, the primary response. IgM, along with IgG class antibodies, provide a strong defense against invasion of the blood and is particularly effective during the viremic stage of viral infection. The protective mechanisms provided by IgM are similar to those of IgG. IgM class molecules are able to bind to a microbial surface and act as opsonins and are even more effective than IgG at activating complement.

If these innate and humoral reponses are not able to eliminate an established viral infection, cell-mediated immunity may provide assistance by recruiting cytotoxic T lymphocytes, which can kill virally infected cells (Figure 31-9 ■).

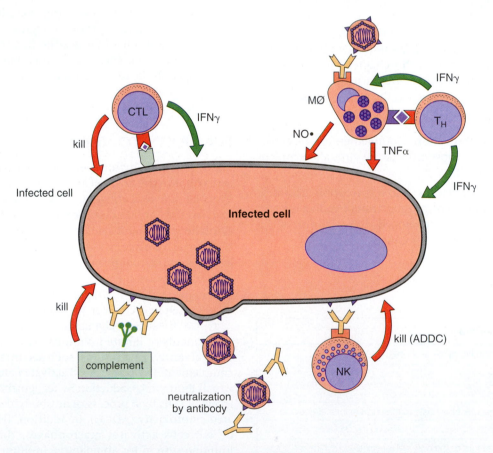

■ **FIGURE 31-9** Immune system mechanisms against virally infected cells. Entry of virus at mucosal surfaces is inhibited by IgA. Following the initial infection, the virus may spread to other tissues via the bloodstream. Interferons produced by the innate (IFNα and IFNβ) and adaptive (IFNγ) immune responses make neighboring cells resistant to virus infection. Antibodies are important in controlling free virus, whereas T cells and NK cells are effective at killing infected cells.
Reprinted from Male et al. (2006). Clinical Laboratory Immunology (7th ed.). Copyright 2006 with permission from Elsevier.

CLASSIFICATION OF VIRUSES

The taxonomy of viruses is as follows: Order (virales), Family (viridae), Subfamily (virinae), Genus (virus), and Species. Viruses are classified in different ways, such as the nature of their genetic material, which is either DNA or RNA, by their envelope, the mode of transmission, antigenic properties, type of the disease they cause and symptomatology, or identification of the infected host cell. David Baltimore originally proposed the classification of viruses based on the type of nucleic acid the virus contains. Furthermore, physical properties of virions such as pH stability, susceptibility to chemical agents especially ether and detergents, physical agent and thermal stability, and molecular mass may also be used to classify viruses. Classification may be based on viral genome properties including strandedness (single- or double-stranded), the size of the viral genome (measured in kilobases), whether or not the DNA/RNA is linear or circular, and sense, which determines if the viral RNA genome is copied directly (positive) or must be translated first by RNA polymerase (negative). Classification also includes the number and size of viral segments, nucleic acid sequence, special features such as 5'-terminal cap or 3'-terminal poly[A] tract, the position of the open reading frame, and the pattern of transcription and translation. Viral protein properties such as characteristics of structural and nonstructural proteins, amino acid sequence, and protein modification (phosphorylation, glycosylation, myristylation), and special functional activities such as fusion activities, reverse transcriptase, and neuraminidase have also contributed to our ability to group various viruses. See Tables 31-3 and 31-4 for examples of virus classification.

DIAGNOSIS OF VIRAL DISEASES

In many ways the complex nature of working with intracellular organisms such as viruses justifies the fact that highly trained individuals and specialized equipment are a vital part of the detection and isolation of viruses from patients, something usually available at large medical institutions better able to afford such an investment in manpower and equipment. A number of methodologies are utilized in the laboratory setting for the diagnosis of viral diseases. Viruses are obligate intracellular organisms and they need living cells in order to proliferate. Methods that have been used to isolate viruses from clinical specimens include:

- The use of embryonated eggs:
  - the isolation of influenza virus is augmented by the use of embryonated eggs.
- The use of animal inoculation:
  - certain coxsackie viruses need suckling mice for isolation purposes.
- The use of cell cultures:
  - living cells maintained *in vitro* for the isolation of intracellular organisms.

Once inoculated with a specimen, cell cultures are incubated for a period of 1–4 weeks. Examination of the cell culture for the presence of a virus is accomplished using a microscope to detect signs of cellular degeneration, known as **cytopathic effect** (CPE). CPE may be exhibited as any of several pathologies including necrosis (an area of dead or dying cells), the

TABLE 31-3

DNA Viruses

Family	Genus	Nucleic Acid	Virion	Capsid Aymmetry
Herpesviridae	Herpes Simplex virus • 1 and 2 Varicella Zoster virus Epstein–Barr Cytomegalovirus Human herpes virus 6 Human herpes virus 7 Human herpes virus 8	Double-stranded	Enveloped	Icosahedral
Hepadnaviridae	Hepatitis B virus	Double-stranded	Enveloped	Icosahedral
Poxviridae	Variola virus Vaccinia virus	Double-stranded	Enveloped	Complex
Adenoviridae	Adenovirus	Double-stranded	Naked	Icosahedral
Papillomaviridae	Papillomavirus	Double-stranded	Naked	Icosahedral
Parvoviridae	Parvovirus B-19	Single-stranded	Naked	Icosahedral

⭐ TABLE 31-4

RNA Viruses

Family	Genus	Nucleic Acid	Virion	Capsid Symmetry
Picornaviridae	Enterovirus Rhinovirus Hepatovirus	Single-stranded	Naked	Icosahedral
Caliciviridae	Norovirus Hepatitis E virus	Single-stranded	Naked	Icosahedral
Reoviridae	Rotavirus	Double-stranded	Naked	Icosahedral
Togaviridae	Alphavirus • Equine encephalitis viruses Rubivirus • Rubella	Single-stranded	Enveloped	Icosahedral
Orthomyxoviridae	Influenza A virus Influenza B virus Influenza C virus	Single-stranded	Enveloped	Helical
Paramyxoviridae	Respirovirus • Parainfluenza virus Pneumovirus • Respiratory syncytial virus • Human metapneumovirus Morbillivirus • Measles virus Rubulavirus • Mumps virus	Single-stranded	Enveloped	Helical
Filoviridae	Marburg virus Ebola virus	Single-stranded	Enveloped	Helical
Arenaviridae	Lassa virus	Single-stranded	Enveloped	Helical
Rhabdoviridae	Rabies virus	Single-stranded	Enveloped	Helical
Bunyaviridae	Hanta virus	Single-stranded	Enveloped	Helical
Flaviviridae	Flavivirus (Arbovirus) • Yellow fever virus • Dengue fever virus • West Nile virus • St. Louis encephalitis virus Hepacivirus • Hepatitis C virus	Single –stranded	Enveloped	Icosahedral
Coronaviridae	Corona virus • SARS	Single-stranded	Enveloped	Helical
Retroviridae	HIV-1 HIV-2 HTLV-1	Single-stranded	Enveloped	Icosahedral

formation of characteristic intracellular structures, called inclusion bodies, in infected cells. Rabies, for instance, may be diagnosed by the detection of eosinophilic cytoplasmic inclusions called Negri bodies, found within neurons. Other examples of CPE include the formation of multinucleate "giant cells" called syncytia, cytoplasmic modifications, or vacuolization.

Different types of cell cultures are used to isolate viruses. Once a cell culture has been subcultured and maintained *in vitro,* it becomes a cell line. The three commonly used cell lines or cell culture types utilized in virology labs include (1) primary cell cultures such as primary monkey kidney cells; (2) low passage or diploid cell cultures, such as human neonatal lung, where propagation is normally limited to about 50 generations; and (3) continuous cell cultures that can be propagated indefinitely. Vero cells derived from the epithelial cells of an African green monkey kidney is an example of a continuous or heteroploid cell culture. Availability, cost, and viral sensitivity as well as the type of virus to be isolated determine what type of cell culture should be used in a virology lab. Figure 31-10 ■ provides examples of uninfected cell lines and the cytopathic effect of two different strains of vaccinia virus.

 REAL WORLD TIP

The HeLa cell line is one of the oldest continuous human cell lines in use today for viral cultures. It originally came from a 31-year-old female in 1951. Her name was **He**nrietta **La**cks, hence the cell line name. The cells were cultured from her cervical cancer.

Direct Detection of the Virus

Direct detection of viruses in the clinical specimen can be used for noncultivable viruses or for rapid diagnosis. Immunostaining, nucleic acid probes, gene amplification methods, electron microscopy, and light microscopy, used to detect the cytopathic effect of certain viruses, are among the available methods of virus detection. The disadvantage of some of these methods is that they are labor-intensive and/or costly.

Molecular Diagnostics

The use of molecular techniques to identify viruses and to monitor the progression and response of specific viral diseases is becoming increasing more important. With the introduction of many of the techniques used in molecular biology, such as gene amplification, the laboratory's ability to diagnose viral infections is much more precise. Both qualitative and quantitative polymerase chain reaction (PCR) testing for viral disease, particularly for bloodborne pathogens such as human immunodeficiency virus-1 (HIV-1), hepatitis B virus (HBV), and hepatitis C virus (HCV), allow monitoring of the viral load of infected patients. Many of the viral agents that cause viral or aseptic meningitis can be diagnosed more rapidly using these techniques. In addition to PCR, other gene amplification methods such as nucleic acid sequence-based amplification (NASBA) can be also be used for viral identification of HIV, cytomegalovirus (CMV), human papillomavirus (HPV), the measles virus, and many more. The branched DNA (bDNA) method, which amplifies an electric signal, can also be used for the identification of viruses such as HIV or heptitis C virus. Refer to ∞ Chapter 9, "Final Identification," for a more complete discussion of molecular methods.

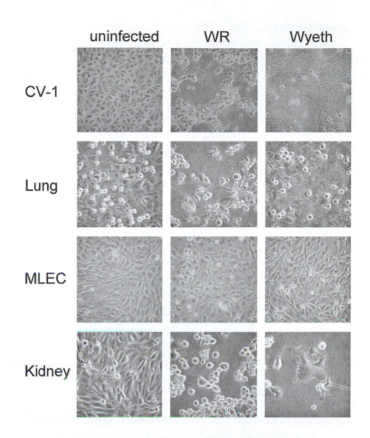

■ **FIGURE 31-10** Each uninfected cells line (CV-1, Lung, MLEC, and Kidney), in the left column, demonstrates smooth and even monolayer of cells. Note the cytopathic changes, as seen in the middle and right columns, when the cells are infected with one of two different strains (WR and Wyeth) of vaccinia virus. The CPE produced by some viruses is very characteristic and can help with identification.
From Hayasaka et al. (2007). Pathogeneses of respiratory infections with virulent and attenuated vaccinia viruses. Virology Journal, 4, 22.

Viral Serology

The use, detection, or measurement of antibodies in the diagnosis of disease (serology) has been of major importance in virology for decades. Serological assays can be used to measure a host's humoral response to a particular viral pathogen. These methods have been used to determine the immune status in viral diseases such as measles, rubella, or hepatitis infections. Transplant patients or those subjected to immunosuppressive therapy are monitored through the use of serological tests.

Two of the most commonly used serological tests for measuring antibody to viral antigen are radioimmunoassay (RIA) and enzyme imunoassay (EIA) procedures. Antibody titers, a semiquantitative measure of antibody levels, may be used to determine if the presence of antibody reflects an acute infection, a prior infection, or passively acquired antibody.

Other serological tests used to diagnose various viral infections include complement fixation, latex agglutination, immunofluorescent assays, and viral hemagglutination inhibition assays. The production of specific antibodies at detectable levels as a result of infection or immunization is termed seroconversion. Individuals with detectable antibody levels are said to be seropositive. Generally, a positive result or the presence of type-specific antibody is considered to be a good indication of seroconversion. A fourfold rise in antibody titer, between acute (early stage) and convalescent (recovery or late stage) sera run consecutively, is necessary to establish a diagnosis of recent infection. The acute-phase serum needs to be taken as soon as possible and the convalescence serum between 2 and 4 weeks later. The presence of IgM class antibodies, which are produced during the early acute stage of infection and evidence of the primary response, is a sign of current infections. The presence of IgG class antibodies could suggest a trend toward recovery, a late stage of infection, or possibly a past infection or immunization.

There are problems inherent in serological methods, including passive transfer of antibodies through transfusion or transplacental transmission, detection of cross-reactive or non-specific antibodies produced by the host, and antibody levels, which do not always correlate with the activity level or acute state of an infection.

VIRAL PATHOGENESIS

The methods in which viruses are able to inflict damage to the host organism are varied. Viral replication may result in cytolysis and subsequent release of virus particles. This could account for areas of tissue necrosis. The expression of viral antigen on host cells, which have been infected by the virus, can lead to an immune response in which those infected cells are destroyed by cytotoxic antibodies, complement activation, or cell-mediated destruction by natural killer cells, ADCC cells, or cytotoxic T lymphocytes. In such cases it is the host's immune response that is responsible for the signs and symptoms of disease and not a direct effect of the virus itself.

Checkpoint! 31–3 (Chapter Objective 2)

A component of the immune system that protects the host from viral infection by damaging the outermost layer of enveloped viruses or coating the receptors of unenveloped viruses is known as

A. *complement.*
B. *interferon.*
C. *lymphokines.*
D. *haptoglobin.*

▶ DNA VIRUSES

According to the classification system devised by the International Committee on the Taxonomy of Viruses (ICTV), there are six families of DNA viruses:

- *Herpesviridae*
- *Poxviridae*
- *Adenoviridae*
- *Papillomaviridae*
- *Parvoviridae* (a group designation, picodna, meaning "small" DNA viruses, was at one time proposed)
- *Hepadnaviridae* (<u>hepa</u>titis <u>DNA</u> virus, hence the family name)

The six families are divided into two groups. Group I contains those viruses whose genome is composed of double-stranded DNA, which includes the herpesviruses, adenoviruses, poxviruses, and others. Group II contains those viruses whose genome is composed of single-stranded DNA, the parvoviruses. The hepadnavirus and the herpesviruses are enveloped whereas the others are nonenveloped. The poxviruses have a more complicated morphology and although they may be considered to be one of the enveloped viruses, they have a complex outer coat. All of these families contain one or more virus species that are of medical importance.

THE HERPES VIRUSES

The human herpesviruses (HHV) are taxonomically grouped from one to eight. Included in the *Herpesviridae* family are herpes simplex viruses (HSV-1 and HSV-2, also known as HHV1 and HHV2), varicella zoster virus (VZV, or HHV-3), Epstein–Barr virus (EBV, or HHV-4), cytomegalovirus (CMV, or HHV-5), and the remaining human herpesviruses (HHV-6, HHV-7, and HHV-8). Human herpesviruses have a linear dsDNA genome, which is surrounded by a capsid and an outer envelope. Infection with human herpes viruses is marked by latency and life-long persistence.

Herpes Simplex Viruses (HSV-1 and HSV-2)

HSV maintains latency (an inactive infection) in cells of the nervous system. HSV-1 affects the mouth and lips, in particular, and causes an orofacial infection, herpes labial (lip). Symptoms associated with primary oral infections include rhinitis, pharyngitis, tonsillitis, and in young children an acute gingivostomatitis. The lip lesions associated with HSV-1 are often referred to as fever blisters or cold sores. HSV-2, on the other hand, generally causes genital infection or herpes genitalis. Most lesions in women are vulvar but in some cases they may

---

 REAL WORLD TIP

Herpes infection of the finger is called herpetic whitlow. It can be seen in children who suck their thumb, healthcare workers who deal with the oropharyngeal secretions of their patients, dentists, and dental hygienists.

occur on the cervix where they may pass unnoticed. Even though patients are asymptomatic the virus may be shed in urogenital secretions. To avoid neonatal infection it is recommended the newborn be delivered by cesarean section if lesions are present.

HSV-1, which is normally associated with the oral cavity, may also be recovered from the genitalia as well as the oropharyngeal regions. Vice versa, HSV-2 infections, which are normally expected to involve the urogenital tract, may also be responsible for lesions in the oropharyngeal region. HSV infections are very common and it is estimated that in the United States approximately 80% of the population has been infected with HSV type 1 and as much as 20% has been infected with HSV type 2. Among the factors that have been reported to activate HSV and stimulate herpes outbreak are stress, foods rich in arginine content such as chocolate and peanuts, exposure to sunlight, upper respiratory infections, and allergic reactions. The latent phase of these viruses occurs in the sensory neurons and reactivation is associated with the reappearance of the blister-like lesions or mucocutaneous lesions of the oral cavity and urogenital tract associated with primary herpes simplex infections. Tingling, burning, and pruritis (itching) are the prodromes or early symptoms associated with recurrences. Figure 31-11 ■ demonstrates the typical lip blister associated with herpes infection.

Neonatal herpes simplex infection through vertical transfer from mother to child is a rare but serious condition that can result in death of the newborn from disseminated HSV infection. Other forms of HSV infection include HSV encephalitis and ocular herpes. HSV encephalitis, caused by HSV-1 in adults and by HSV-2 in neonates, is rare but often extremely serious and may result in death. HSV-1 herpes encephalitis has a mortality rate of 60–80% if untreated. Ocular herpes affects the conjunctiva and can result in corneal perforation.

Acyclovir is an antiviral drug that is used to prevent transmission of HSV to the neonate. Besides acyclovir, a host of other medications, such as docosanol (Abreva), vavacyclovir, tromantadine, and lysine supplementation, has been used for the treatment of HSV infection. Currently, clinical trials are underway to develop a vaccine against HSV infection. An HSV-2 glycoprotein-D-subunit vaccine has shown certain efficacy against HSV-2 in clinical trials (Stanberry et al., 2002).

Diagnosis of HSV infection may be made through the use of virus cultures or direct detection of the virus. Figure 31-12a ■ and b ■ demonstrates the cytopathic effect of HSV-1 in a Vero cell culture. It causes the cells to enlarge and round up. Often the cells lyse and the monolayer disintegrates. CPE develops rapidly, often within 1 to 3 days. Tzank or Papanicoalaou (Pap) preparations may be employed for the direct detection of the virus in clinical specimens where giant cells with intranuclear inclusions may be seen. Figure 31-13 ■ demonstrates a Tzanck smear with the giant multinucleated cells seen in herpes lesions.

Detection of antibodies to G1 or G2 glycoprotein by enzyme immunoassay (EIA) is a specific method that may be used to differentiate HSV-1 from HSV-2. Additionally, a direct fluorescent antibody technique can be used to identify the presence of HSV antigens in material taken from the vesicular lesions, which is placed on slides specifically designed for this purpose. Antisera containing monoclonal antibodies specific for HSV-1 and HSV-2 can differentiate the two strains.

ⓔ **REAL WORLD TIP**

HSV is able to grow in A-549 (a human lung cancer), RK (rabbit kidney), WI-38 (human fibroblast), ML (mink lung), and MRC-5 (human fibroblast) cells. Immunofluorescence, using type-specific monoclonal antibodies, is often used to confirm the identification.

Varicella Zoster Virus (VZV)

VZV or HHV-3 is a double-stranded, enveloped DNA virus. VZV is the causative agent of the chicken pox (varicella) in children. It is more prevalent in the late winter and spring. In children, a characteristic presentation of vesicular rash as well as fever aids in clinical diagnosis. It can disseminate to cause pneumonia and encephalitis. The lesions are also prone to secondary bacterial infections. Figure 31-14 ■ demonstrates the characteristic pus-filled blisters associated with varicella infection. The virus is spread via aerosols and enters the respiratory mucosa to cause disease.

Once an individual is infected, VZV can remain dormant in the nervous system of the host in the trigeminal and dorsal root ganglia. In adults age 50 and older, reactivation of the

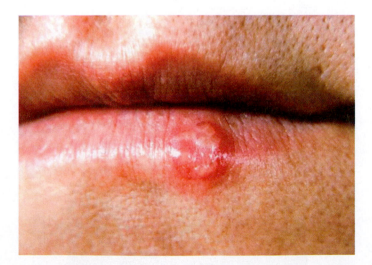

■ **FIGURE 31-11** This lip blister is characteristic for infection with herpes. Individuals usually note a tingling sensation prior to eruption of the blisters.
From Public Health Image Library (PHIL), CDC/Dr. Herrmann.

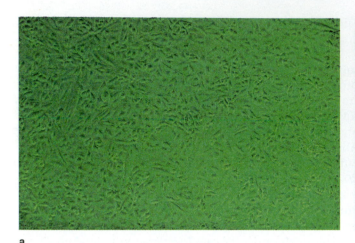

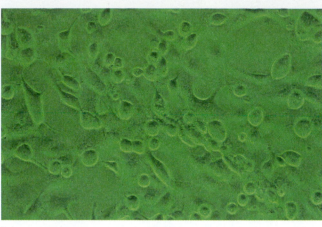

a

b

■ **FIGURE 31-12** a. an uninfected Vero cell line. b. Vero cells that have enlarged and rounded up due to the presence of HSV-1. With time the cells lyse and the entire monolayer is destroyed. Phase contrast microscopy, ×200.
From Athmanathan, Bandlapally, and Rao (2002). Comparison of the sensitivity of a 24 h-shell vial assay, and conventional tube culture, in the isolation of Herpes simplex virus–1 from corneal scrapings. BMC Clinical Pathology, 2, 1.

virus causes shingles (herpes zoster), which is evidenced by a rash spreading along the involved sensory ganglion. The rash, similar to that of HSV, usually appears on one side of the body such as the torso, neck, or face. Figure 31-15 ■ illustrates a zoster rash. Shingles can result in zoster multiplex, myelitis, and postherpetic neuralgia, which is associated with excruciating neuropathic nerve pain. It is estimated that more than 90% of adults possess antibodies to VZV.

Antiviral drugs such as acyclovir, vidarabine, and zoster immunoglobulin constitute therapeutic methods for the treatment of VZV infections. The shingles vaccine is recommended

for those 60 years and older to prevent the long-term pain associated with shingles.

Diagnosis of VZV infection is generally made on the basis of characteristic clinical findings. Culture of the virus is done using human embryonic lung fibroblast cells such as MRC-5 and WI-38 and A-549, a lung cancer cell. Its presence appears as clusters of large, rounded cells within 1 week of culture. A Tzank

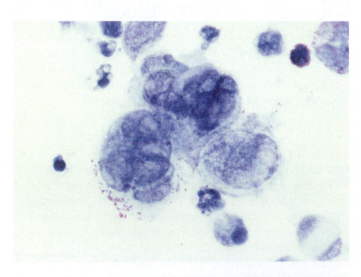

■ **FIGURE 31-13** The Tzank smear is used to diagnose herpes simplex, herpes zoster, and varicella. The large multinucleated cells can be observed in lesions due to these viruses. The presence of these cells and the lesions present help in the diagnosis.
From Public Health Image Library (PHIL), CDC/Joe Miller.

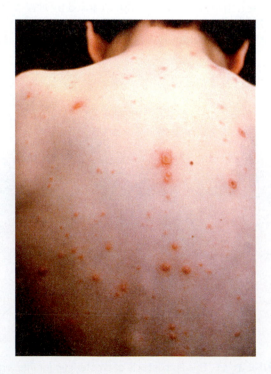

■ **FIGURE 31-14** Chickenpox or varicella usually appears as pus-filled blisters on the face, scalp, and trunk of children.
From Public Health Image Library (PHIL), CDC.

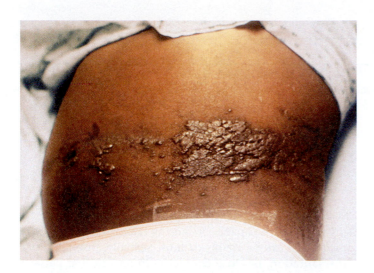

FIGURE 31-15 The zoster rash appears with blisters that tend to wrap around one side of the torso, neck, or face. The rash is often very painful and the pain can remain long after the rash is gone.
From Public Health Image Library (PHIL), CDC.

smear of a lesion demonstrates giant multinucleated cells. Immunofluorescence, performed on a positive cell culture, is highly specific when monoclonal antibodies are used. It can also be performed directly on cells from lesions. Additionally, latex agglutination methods provide another sensitive method that may be employed in the diagnosis of VZV infection.

 REAL WORLD TIP

VZV is usually only able to be cultured from the rash lesions for 1–2 days after they appear. The CPE can appear very similar to that of HSV but takes longer to appear.

Epstein–Barr Virus (EBV)

EBV or human herpes virus 4 (HHV-4) is an enveloped, double-stranded DNA virus and one of the most common viruses in humans. EBV infections are generally asymptomatic or exhibit mild symptoms. The mode of transmission of EBV is generally thought to be through oral contact but bloodborne and perinatal infections can occur as well. EBV targets epithelial cells in the oropharynx and B-lymphocytes by binding to the CD21 receptor on lymphocytes. Infected B cells die, releasing the virus to spread through the lymphatic system. This leads to polyclonal activation of B cells, as well as the production of EBV-specific antibodies, heterophile antibodies, and auto antibodies, all of which aid in the diagnosis of EBV infections.

EBV causes infectious mononucleosis or glandular fever in adults. Symptoms of infectious mono (IM) include fever, sore throat, lymphadenopathy, and less commonly, hepato-

splenomegaly. EBV has been associated with several cancers such as Burkitt's lymphoma as well as nasopharyngeal carcinoma, Hodgkin's lymphoma, and gastric carcinoma. An increase in one specific antibody can be associated with reactivation of EBV or a sign of Burkitt's lymphoma. On the other hand, increase in another specific IgA and viral capsid antibodies (VCA) are seen in the early stages of nasopharyngeal carcinoma.

Laboratory diagnosis of EBV infection is based on a high white blood cell count, lymphocytosis, including the presence of atypical lymphocytes or Downey cells, heterophile antibodies as evidenced by a positive monospot test, and an increase in EBV-specific antibodies.

 REAL WORLD TIP

Heterophile antibodies are those that are produced due to exposure to an organism such as a bacteria or virus. The antibody is able to cross-react with antigens other than those that originally caused its production.

The production of heterophile antibodies is the earliest antibody response to EBV infection. These antibodies are detected in over 80% of IM cases. The monospot heterophile antibody test is based on the Davidson differential test. This test looks for agglutination of sheep red blood cells after treatment with guinea pig kidney (GPK) cells and beef (ox) cells. Heterophile antibodies cross react with antigens other than those that originally caused their production. Heterophile antibodies produced due to IM agglutinate sheep red blood cells and can be absorbed by beef cells but not guinea pig kidney cells.

Forssman antibodies are also heterophile antibodies but are not the same as those produced during IM. They are usually created with exposure to animal tissue, agglutinate sheep red blood cells, and are absorbed by guinea pig kidney cells. Forssman antibodies can be produced naturally or due to serum sickness (a hypersensitivity reaction), antibiotics, the use of horse serum antitoxin, and in reaction to certain diseases such as rheumatoid arthritis.

In the Davidson differential test, an individual's serum is divided and one sample is allowed to react with guinea pig kidney cells while the other reacts with beef cells. Each specimen is then added to sheep red blood cells and observed for agglutination. The antibodies of an individual with IM are not absorbed by the GPK cells and so are left in the serum and cause agglutination when added to sheep red blood cells. The same individual's antibodies are absorbed by the beef cells and are not available when added to sheep red blood cells so agglutination does not occur.

Forssman antibodies are absorbed by the GPK cells and there is no agglutination when added to sheep red blood cells. The same serum may or may not be absorbed by beef cells. Those with serum sickness have heterophile antibodies that are absorbed by beef cells and no agglutination occurs when

✪ TABLE 31-5

Davidsohn Differential Absorption Test				
Heterophile Antibody	Absorbed by Guinea Pig Antigen	Agglutination of Sheep RBCs by Absorbed Serum	Absorbed by Beef Cell Antigen	Agglutination of Sheep RBCs by Absorbed Serum
Infectious mononucleosis	No	Yes	Yes	No
Serum sickness	Yes	No	Yes	No
Forsmann	Yes	No	No	Yes

added to sheep blood cells. Those possessing other Forssman heterophile antibodies are not absorbed by beef cells and cause agglutination of sheep red blood cells. False positive reactions can occur with some cancers, lupus, hepatitis, and infections due to some other viruses (CMV, influenza, rubella, and varicella). Table 31-5 ✪ provides a summary of the reactions of the Davidson differential absorption test.

Detection of EBV-specific antibody testing is accomplished using EIA, immunoblot, and indirect immunoflourescence tests. Among the EBV antigens that induce an antibody response are early antigens, produced in the early stages of viral replication, and late antigens, which are produced following viral replication. Early antigen diffuse (EA-D) and early antigen restricted (EA-R), viral capsid antigen (VCA), and Epstein–Barr nuclear antigen (EBNA) all induce immunoglobulin production. Figure 31-16 ■ illustrates the antibody response to EBV infection. After a sharp increase in anti-VCA IgM and anti-VCA IgG early in the infection, the VCA IgM begins to decrease. This usually occurs after the onset of clinical symptoms. VCA IgG, on the other hand, remains at detectable levels for life. EA antibody shows a slow rise after the clinical illness but begins to decline to low levels by 1 year. EBNA antibodies develop gradually after the clinical illness has resolved and remains at low levels for life. Table 31-6 ✪ provides the diagnosis of EBV infections based on the production of specific antigens and antibodies.

Cytomegalovirus (CMV)

CMV or human herpes virus-5 (HHV-5) is a double-stranded DNA virus that is capable of causing latent infections. CMV transmission can be via breast milk, sexually, through organ transplantation, or close contact with an infected patient. CMV is considered to be the most common cause of congenital infection in the United States. Most infections are asymptomatic intra-uterine infections in immune mothers who have had previous infection and have produced protective antibody. Primary infection of a nonimmune mother can lead to transplacental tranmission resulting in cytomegalic inclusion disease, a syndome that is associated with jaundice, hepatosplenomegaly, ophthalmic disorders, hearing loss, and mental retardation. Some cases may be fatal to the fetus.

Almost all cases of perinatal, early childhood, and adult CMV infection are asymptomatic but many individuals who have been infected with this virus maintain a latent infection with the virus being shed in saliva, urine, vaginal secretions, semen, and the nasopharynx in very low numbers. Transfusion-associated CMV infections are evidenced as a mononucleosis-like syndrome with prolonged fever, pharyngitis, lymphadenitis, atypical lymphocytosis, and hepatitis. In immunocompromised patients, such as HIV patients or transplant recipients, CMV may trigger disseminated and even life-threatening disease.

Testing for CMV includes the use of PCR and the detection of viral nucleic acid in whole blood or plasma by EIA. A posi-

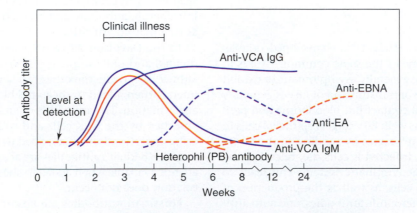

■ **FIGURE 31-16** A serological profile of detectable antibodies to EBV infection.
From Mahon et al. (2006). Clinical Laboratory Immunology. Prentice Hall, 2006, with permission.

⊗ TABLE 31-6

Diagnosis of Epstein–Barr Virus Infection Using EBV-Specific Antigens and Antibodies Produced

Phase of Infection	Antibodies to EBV-Specific Antigens
Early acute infection (infectious mononucleosis)	VCA–Ig M only
Acute infection (infectious mononucleosis)	Both VCA–IgG and EA-D are present
	VCA–IgG is present but anti-EBNA is absent
Past infection (infectious mononucleosis)	VCA–IgG and anti-EBNA only
Burkitts lymphoma	Anti-VCA, anti-EBNA, and anti-EA-R
Nasopharyngeal carcinoma	Anti-VCA, anti-EBNA, and anti-EA-D

VCA–IgM (IgM class antibodies to viral capsid antigen are transient); VCA–IgG (IgG class antibodies to viral capsid antigen persist for life); EA-D (antibodies to early antigen–diffuse are transient and disappear within 2 months); EA-R (antibodies to early antigen–restricted may be associated with reactivation of the latent viral carrier state); EBNA (antibodies to Epstein–Barr nuclear antigen persist for life)

tive PCR result allows monitoring of the viral load in the CMV-infected patient. Furthermore, isolation of the virus from human body tissue is one of the best confirmatory methods. The presence of the virus, in cultured lung fibroblast cells, displays cytopathic effect exhibiting large, basophilic, intranuclear inclusions, referred to as having an "owl eye" appearance. CPE may take 2–3 weeks to appear. It is used to aid in the diagnosis of the CMV. Figure 31-17 demonstrates the characteristic "owl eye" inclusion in a cell.

As with herpes simplex virus infections, serological methods have not proven as promising as other methods used in the diagnosis. False-positive results may be the result of seropositivity caused by infection with another virus, resulting in cross-reactions and other underlying diseases, such as autoimmune disorders. Serological testing does not always indicate current infection and may only demonstrate past exposure.

Treatment of CMV includes use of antiviral drugs such as ganciclovir and valganciclovir. An intensive effort aimed at the development of an effective vaccine against CMV is currently underway.

⊚ REAL WORLD TIP

Because there is a high prevalence of CMV-positive individuals, finding blood donors who are negative may be difficult. CMV is often found in leukocytes in peripheral blood. Blood banks now use leukoreduction to eliminate the white blood cells if CMV-negative blood units are not available. CMV-negative blood units should always be used for fetal and neonatal transfusions.

Human Herpesvirus 6 (HHV-6)

HHV-6 is a very common pathogen, being found worldwide and in the saliva of over 90% of adults. It is one of two etiological agents of roseola infantum, also known as exanthum subitum, sixth disease, or roseola, a disease of early childhood. Roseola is an acute, self-limiting disease associated with an incubation period of 14 days followed by the rapid onset of fever for 3–4 days. When the fever subsides a maculopapular rash appears and lasts for 1–2 days. Latent infection is established in T lymphocytes. HHV-6 may also cause a mononucleosis-like syndrome and lymphadenopathy. There may be evidence to support its role in multiple sclerosis (Carrigan, Harrington, & Knox, 1996). Infection with HHV-6 causes seroconversion in young children, with almost 50% of children demonstrating the presence of the antibody.

The virus can reactivate in immunosuppressed individuals such as those with AIDS or receiving a transplant. It can cause encephalitis, rash, fever, hepatitis, and bone marrow suppression.

It is seldom detected by culture. Detection of antibodies is through enzyme immunoassay but diagnosis of the HHV-6 is generally made clinically. Viral load testing and PCR also aids

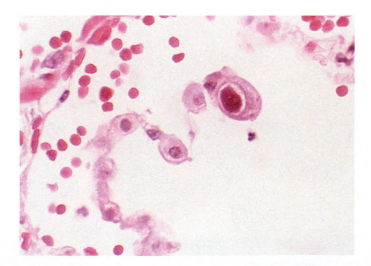

■ **FIGURE 31-17** This stained lung tissue, from an individual with AIDS, demonstrates the characteristic "owl eye" inclusion associated with infection with cytomegalovirus.
From Public Health Image Library (PHIL), CDC/Dr. Edwin P. Ewing, Jr.

in the diagnosis of infected patients. Currently, there is no vaccine available for sixth disease and treatment is generally supportive. The virus has been shown to be susceptible to antiviral drugs such as foscarnet or ganciclovir.

Human Herpesvirus 7 (HHV-7)

HHV-7 is very closely related to HHV-6 and is another cause of roseola infantum. Like HHV-6 it is contracted during childhood, with shedding of the virus in the saliva of the majority of adults. The virus replicates in CD4-positive lymphocytes in which it maintains a latent infection.

Human Herpesvirus 8 (HHV-8)

HHV-8 is a double-stranded DNA virus with a icosahedral capsid and a typical herpes virus envelope and tegument. In 1994 scientists isolated a previously unknown virus in patients with Kaposi's sarcoma, a rare form of skin cancer. HHV-8 is now considered by many to be the etiological agent for Kaposi's sarcoma and has been called the Kaposi sarcoma–associated herpesvirus (KSHV). Kaposi's sarcoma is seen primarily in immunocompromised individuals such as AIDS patients. It is rarely found in immunocompetent individuals. In addition to Kaposi's sarcoma, HHV-8 causes primary effusion lymphoma, a malignancy of B-cells. The virus has also been found in endothelial cells and tumor-infiltrating leukocytes. HHV-8 infection is less common than HHV-6 or HHV-7 infections.

The virus can remain in a latent state following infection. When the virus enters the lytic phase of replication, it uses the cellular machinery for self-replication. Virus particles make thousands of copies and cause cell death.

Currently, PCR is the only reliable test that can detect the virus in tissue or other various specimens. Antiviral drugs such as cidofovir, ganciclovir, and foscarnet are used in the treatment of HHV-8 infections. In HIV-infected patients, the use of anti-HIV medications have been more effective in controlling Kaposi's sarcoma.

 Checkpoint! 31–4 (Chapter Objective 1)

The virus responsible for infectious mononucleosis is
   A. *Herpes simplex virus (HSV) type 1.*
   B. *HSV type 2.*
   C. *Epstein–Barr virus.*
   D. *human herpesvirus 6.*

POX VIRUSES

Pox viruses are enveloped, double-stranded DNA viruses that belong to the *Poxviridae* family. Smallpox is considered to be the most important disease caused by members of this family. The original grouping of pox viruses was associated with their ability to cause the appearance of pox, vesicular or blister-like lesions, in the skin. It is believed the variola virus, which causes smallpox, the cowpox virus, and the vaccinia virus, were all derived from a common viral ancestry.

The vaccinia virus is well known for its contribution as a vaccine for the eradication of smallpox disease. Although the vaccinia virus has been used in gene therapy, recently concerns have been raised about its potential use in germ warfare. Nevertheless, novel vaccine strategies are currently under development against the smallpox virus using vaccinia virus. Diluted vaccinia has been used successfully to vaccinate individuals and protocols have been established to extend the limited stocks of smallpox vaccine through the use of diluted vaccinia.

The Smallpox Virus

Smallpox, also known as variola, is a double-stranded DNA virus that attacks skin cells and causes the characteristic lesions, as seen in Figure 31-18 , associated with this highly contagious viral disease. Those that survive may be left blind in one or both eyes, and have persistent skin scarring or pockmarks. Smallpox exists in two forms: variola major, with its 30% mortality rate, and variola minor, with a mortality rate less than 1%.

> Ⓔ **REAL WORLD TIP**
>
> The rash of smallpox forms first on the face then spreads to the arms and legs. The rash of chickenpox affects the face, neck, and torso.

English physician Edward Jenner was the first to observe that individuals who recovered from cowpox, a mild disease, were immune to the deadly smallpox. This observation led to the first successful vaccination in 1796, where Dr. Jenner innoculated material from cowpox lesions taken from a milkmaid, Sara Nelms, into the arms of a young boy named James Phipps. The boy suffered no serious effects from the innoculation and when challenged with the smallpox virus he proved

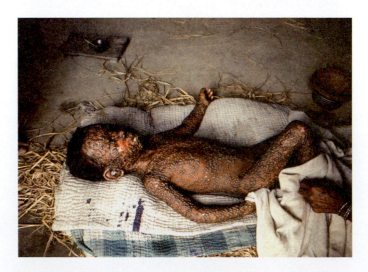

■ **FIGURE 31-18** A severe case of smallpox in a Bangladesh child (1975) exhibiting the typical maculopapular rash and pustules.
From Public Health Image Library (PHIL), CDC/Jean Roy.

to be immune. In time, his success led Jenner to immunize other patients in a similar manner. Eventually vaccination became an accepted practice. Immunity developed as a result of immune responses generated from infection with the cowpox virus. These immune responses had a protective effect against lethal infection with the smallpox virus.

Innumerable deaths have been attributed to smallpox infection. With the widespread use of vaccination against smallpox, eradication of the infection was accomplished in 1979. When the World Health Organization (WHO) certified eradication of the disease, smallpox vaccination was discontinued. In recent years, interest in reestablishing an effective vaccine has been aroused in an attempt to be prepared for possible future attacks where the smallpox virus may be used as a bioterrorism agent.

Smallpox is a reportable disease that requires notification of state and local health departments. Once the health departments determine there is a high risk for smallpox, CDC must be notified. Electron microscopy is used to visualize the pox virus. Figure 31-19 ■ demonstrates the smallpox virus as seen by electron microscopy. There are other species in the pox family and they cannot be differentiated from variola by morphology alone. Serology or nucleic acid assays are used to confirm the diagnosis.

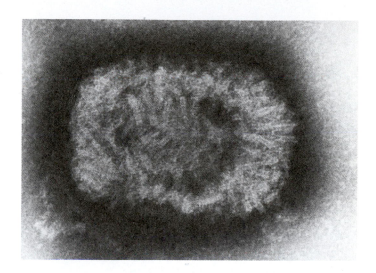

■ **FIGURE 31-19** A negative stained electron micrograph is used to visualize the variola virus as seen here magnified at 310,000×.
From Public Health Image Library (PHIL), CDC/J. Nakano.

 REAL WORLD TIP

- Vaccinia is a poxvirus used as a live suspension for vaccination against smallpox. It cross-protects against other poxviruses.

- Human monkeypox is a poxvirus that displays as a milder version of smallpox in humans. It originated in African monkeys, mice, rats, and squirrels. In 2003 it was isolated in the United States from infected pet prairie dogs. The smallpox virus may provide protection against the virus. The virus should be suspected in those who have contact with exotic animals such as zoo workers and research scientists.

HUMAN PAPILLOMA VIRUS

The human papilloma virus (HPV) is a double-stranded DNA virus that belongs to the *Papillomaviridae* family. HPV infection is considered to be the most prevalent sexually transmitted disease. Many types of HPV have been identified and they have been implicated as the cause of papillomas or benign skin warts such as plantar warts on the soles of the feet, flat warts on the face, and warts around the fingernails as well as anal and genital warts. HPV has also been identified as the cause of malignant cancers such as cervical cancer.

Types 6 and 11 are associated with the development of genital warts or condyloma acuminata while types 16 and 18 have been implicated as the etiological agent of cervical cancer. These two types are responsible for about 70% of HPV-related cervical cancers. Besides cervical cancer, strains of HPV have

been implicated in vulvar cancer, nonmelanoma cancer, laryngeal papillomatosis, and head and neck cancers. The E6 protein of HPV functions as an oncoprotein and contributes to the immortalization and transformation of cells by mechanisms such as degradation of p53, a tumor suppressor protein that controls DNA mutations. The HPV E6 protein binds to p53, facilitating cancer development. Worldwide an estimated 270,000 women died of cervical cancer, the second most common cancer in women in 2002.

According to the Centers for Disease Control and Prevention (CDC), at least 50% of sexually active males and females will acquire HPV infection sometime during their lifetime. The incidence of HPV infection is high among female adults and by age 50 as many as 80% will have acquired HPV infection, even though most may never fall under a high-risk disease category.

Detection of HPV is usually established through cytology, by the use of Pap smears where cervical cells are stained and examined. Gene amplification techniques, such as PCR, have also been used for identification.

Development of an effective vaccine against HPV is under intense study and recently a new vaccine called Gardasil has been approved by the Food and Drug Administration (FDA) and introduced to the market. Results from several clinical trials have shown Gardasil is effective against strains 16 and 18 of HPV. It is safe and has a 100% vaccine efficacy in prevention of persistent HPV infection and HPV-associated cervical cancer. The vaccine also blocks infection by other strains that are responsible for 90% of genital warts.

ADENOVIRUSES

Adenoviruses are nonenveloped, icosahedral, double-stranded DNA viruses in the *Adenoviridae* family. They are associated with self-limited respiratory, ocular, and gastrointestinal diseases.

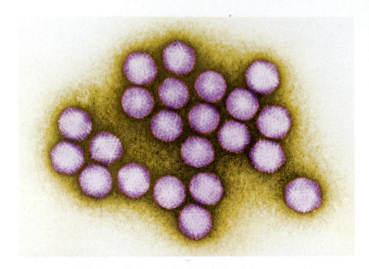

■ FIGURE 31-20 Transmission electron micrograph of adenoviruses (colorized).
From Public Health Image Library (PHIL), CDC/Dr. G. William Gary, Jr.

Adenovirus infections may be very common since 75% of the population has demonstrable levels of antibody by the age of 5.

In infants and children less than 4 years old, the virus is transmitted by the fecal–oral route. Using electron microscopy noncultivable adenoviruses have been observed in the feces of infants suffering from diarrhea, as demonstrated in Figure 31-20 ■. In adults, the virus is transmitted by respiratory aerosols, causing infections such as pharyngitis, colds, and other acute respiratory illnesses, most of which are not severe. Respiratory illness, due to adenovirus, is most often seen in winter, spring, and early summer. It is believed most infections are asymptomatic.

Outbreaks can occur in settings such as day care centers and schools with large numbers of susceptible individuals. Severe, disseminated disease may be seen in neonates, transplant patients, and with co-infection with EBV and HIV (human immunodeficiency virus) infections.

Diagnosis is often based on the use of immunofluorescence, electron microscopy, virus cultures, PCR, and serology. Specimens of choice depend on the symptoms of disease. Upper and lower respiratory symptoms often utilize nasopharyngeal aspirates or swabs as well as throat swabs and bronchial alveolar lavage. Gastrointestinal involvement requires a stool specimen. Prevention has been attempted through the use of inactivated vaccines.

HEPATITIS B VIRUS (HBV)

HBV belongs to the family *Hepadnaviridae* and, unlike the other hepatotropic viruses, its viral genome is composed of DNA. HBV is an icosahedral virus that has an outer envelope surface protein (HBsAg), core proteins (HBcAg and HBeAg), and DNA polymerase. This enveloped DNA virus is very hardy. It is able to survive at room temperature for up to 6 months, temperatures as high as 60°C for up to 4 hours, and the toxic effects of most disinfectants. Infectivity is rapidly destroyed by sodium hypochlorite or bleach and for this reason dilute sodium hypochlorite solutions are very popular as disinfectants in the health care setting.

Three distinct morphological forms can be found in the blood of individuals infected with the HBV: a small spherical particle, 22 nanometers in diameter, composed of HBsAg only; long filamentous forms of varying length, 22 nm in diameter and also composed of HBsAg (neither of these forms is infectious); and the infectious Dane particle (an intact hepatitis B particle), 42 nm in diameter, and the actual HBV virion.

The presence of HBsAg in the serum of a patient may indicate one of several conditions: the patient has active HBV infection, the patient is an acute carrier of the HBV, or the patient is in the incubation period. The hepatitis B core antigen (HBcAg) is part of the capsid (inner core), which lies beneath the envelope and surrounds the viral genome. HBeAg, a soluble protein that is also part of the core or capsid of the hepatitis B virus, is detectable 1 or 2 weeks into the infection and peaks at 4–8 weeks, followed by a decline at 14 weeks. The presence of HBeAg is a marker of acute replication and infectivity for HbsAg-positive serum.

The diagnosis of HBV infection relies primarily on the serological detection of antibodies against HBV antigens. Various serological methods, including RIA and EIA, are used in the detection of:

- IgM anti-HBcAg, which appears 2 weeks after HBsAg can be detected in the serum of infected individuals.
- IgG anti-HBcAg, which appears during the eighth week and remains for life.
- Anti-HBeAg, which appears at 5 months and declines at 10 months.
- Anti HBsAg, which appears at 6 months and persists for years (possibly for life). Anti-HBsAg is protective against infection and confers immunity to infection. The HBV vaccine contains HBsAg produced by recombinant (genetically engineered yeast). It induces the production of anti-HBsAg, the antibody that protects uninfected individuals exposed to the HBV virus.

Table 31-7✪ provides interpretation of Hepatitis B antigens and antibodies results to determine disease status.

REAL WORLD TIP

- Adenovirus CPE can be detected on HNK (human neonatal kidney) and A-549 (human lung cancer) cell lines. CPE appears as large, rounded cells in clusters like grapes within 1 week. Immunofluorescence is used to confirm its identification
- Adenovirus is excreted for long periods of time after disease. Detection of the virus may not mean active disease.

✪ TABLE 31-7

Hepatitis B Panel Interpretation

HBV DNA	HBsAg	Anti-HBs	Anti-HBc IgM	Total Anti-HBc	HBeAg	Anti HBe	Interpretation
−	−	−	−	−	−	−	Never infected
+	−	−	−	−	−	−	Early incubation; transient after vaccination
+	+	−	−	−	V	−	Late incubation
+	+	−	+	+	+	−	Acute infection
V	−	−	+	+	V	+	Acute resolving infection
−	−	+	−	+	−	+	Recovered and immune
+	+	−	−	+	V	+	Chronic infection
−	−	+	−	−	−	−	Immune after vaccination*

*Concentration of Anti-HBs of 10 mIU/ml or greater indicates immunity in the United States.
HBV DNA, Hepatitis B viral DNA; HBsAg, Hepatitis B surface antigen; Anti-HBs, antibody against Hepatis B surface antigen; Anti-HBc IgM, IgM antibody directed against Hepatitis B core antigen; Total Anti-HBc, Total antibody directed against Hepatitis B core antigen; HBeAg, Hepatitis B e antigen; Anti HBe, antibody directed against Hepatitis B e antigen; −, negative; +, positive; V, variable.

The mode of transmission is via blood, blood products, body fluids, vertical transmission from mother to unborn child, at birth through vaginal secretions, or afterward through breast milk. This mode of transmission is referred to as parenteral meaning outside the gastrointestinal tract because it is not transmitted by ingestion since the virus is not known to survive conditions found within the GI tract. The virus may be transmitted by activities such as tattooing, body piercing, intravenous drug abuse, needle sticks, dialysis, blood transfusions, and even shaving or manicures where bleeding occurs. In addition to blood the virus may be shed in saliva, urine, tears, cerebrospinal fluid, semen, and, as previously suggested, vaginal secretions and breast milk.

Unlike hepatitis A virus, hepatitis B virus infection is either acute and self-limiting or chronic and long-lasting. Ninety percent of patients have the acute form, which is rapidly developing and characterized by increasing severity. The clinical course of HBV infection starts with an incubation period, generally 2–3 months, followed by acute illness of 1–4 weeks and recovery at about 6 months. These patients usually clear the infection through the production of protective antibodies against HBV. Other patients may develop encephalopathy as a result of liver damage or icterus. This may eventually lead to coma and death.

About 10% of infected patients develop chronic hepatitis, a condition in which symptoms or elevated enzymes persist for more than 6 months. Because of the complicated nature of chronic HBV infection two terms are used to describe it:

- Chronic persistent hepatitis is a benign disease in which liver enzyme levels eventually return to normal but the individual continues to carry the virus.
- Chronic active hepatitis is a serious liver disease that can lead to the replacement of healthy liver tissue with fibrous tissue (cirrhosis), hepatic failure, and hepatocellular carcinoma.

HBV infection is endemic in some areas of the world, particularly in Southeast Asia, and is responsible for about 1 million deaths each year worldwide. The mortality is attributed to the complications found in HBV infection such as hepatocellular carcinoma, chronic hepatitis, and cirrhosis.

Detection of hepatitis B virus infection involves the use of blood tests that detect either viral antigens or antibodies produced by the host (Figure 31-21 ■). PCR tests measure the amount of viral nucleic acid in clinical specimens and are useful to assess a person's infection status and to monitor treatment. Hepatitis B surface antigen (HBsAg) is detected within 2–4 weeks and peaks at about 8 to 12 weeks, followed by a decline at about 20 weeks.

A vaccine providing lifelong immunity against HBV is available and should be provided to all clinical laboratory workers. A host of drugs such as alpha-interferon and antiviral drugs such as lamivudine and adefovir are available for treatment of HBV. Very recently, a new anti-HBV drug called entecavir has been introduced, which is designed to selectively inhibit the HBV replication process.

✓ Checkpoint! 31–5 (Chapter Objective 1)

Recent epidemiological, clinical, and diagnostic evidence has linked _____ with cervical carcinoma.

A. Epstein–Barr virus
B. adenoviruses
C. human papilloma viruses
D. the hepadnavirus

▶ RNA VIRUSES

RNA viruses have ribonucleic acid (RNA) as their genetic material. The genome may be single-stranded or double-stranded RNA. The majority of the known RNA viruses are single-

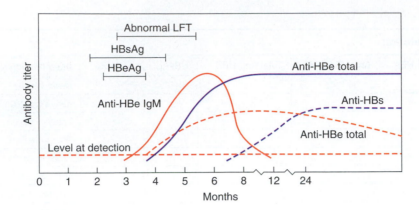

stranded RNA (ssRNA) viruses. Some medically important RNA viruses include hepatotropic viruses, influenza viruses, retroviruses, such as the AIDS virus, HIV, and filoviruses such as Marburg and Ebola viruses.

HEPATOTROPIC VIRUSES

Hepatitis refers to an inflammatory condition of the liver. Causes of hepatitis include infection caused by microorganisms such as viruses (viral hepatitis), bacteria, and organisms, exposure to chemicals, certain drugs and toxins, and autoimmunity. Signs and symptoms of hepatitis include fatigue, malaise, fever, joint and abdominal pain, occasional vomiting, anorexia (loss of appetite), dark urine, enlarged liver or hepatomegaly, and jaundice or icterus. Liver function tests (such as liver enzyme levels) can be indicative of hepatitis.

Six types of viral hepatitis have been identified. Hepatitis A virus (HAV), hepatitis B virus (HBV), hepatitis C virus (HCV), hepatitis D virus (HDV), hepatitis E virus (HEV), and hepatitis G virus (HGV). A virus referred to as hepatitis F virus was reportedly discovered in the 1990s, but existence of the virus has never been confirmed, and it was discredited as a viral cause for hepatitis. Although other viruses such as the Epstein–Barr virus, cytomegalovirus, and herpes simplex viruses can cause viral hepatitis, the six viruses mentioned above are called hepatotropic viruses because they specifically target liver cells or hepatocytes.

Hepatitis A Virus (HAV)

HAV is an enterovirus belonging to the family *Picornaviridae*. The viral genome of enteroviruses is composed of RNA. The term picorna virus is a combination of the prefix "pico," which means "small," and RNA, referring to the viral genome. Hence picornavirus literally translates into "small RNA" virus.

The mode of transmission is the fecal–oral route and occasionally through parenteral transmission. Parenteral transmis-

sion occurs by any means other than the gastrointestinal tract. Person-to-person contact, ingestion of food or water contaminated with the feces of individuals shedding the virus, contamination of water supplies with sewage, and ingestion of contaminated shellfish are all a means of virus transmission to uninfected individuals. Poor hygiene and overcrowding can all contribute to the spread of HAV infection so hand washing is an effective means to reduce the risk of person-to-person transmission. Because HAV infection can occur in outbreaks and often affects large numbers of people, it has been referred to as infectious hepatitis.

HAV can cause acute infections, chronic infections, or asymptomatic infections. In asymptomatic infections there are no clinical symptoms but liver enzymes are elevated and antibodies to the virus are detectable. The clinical course of HAV infection starts with an incubation period that can last anywhere from 2 to 6 weeks but generally extends over a period of 28 days. This is followed by acute illness lasting about a week. Symptoms include those of a flu-like illness (fever, anorexia, and vomiting) as well as pain in the right upper quadrant of the abdomen (the area of the liver). Viral shedding may occur for a period of 10–30 days with decreasing numbers after the onset of symptoms. Resolution of the infection is evidenced by a return of normal levels of liver enzymes within 6 months.

Anti-HAV antibodies emerge at about 10 days, with IgM class antibodies peaking at 30 days, followed by a drop in antibodies to undetectable serum levels at 6 months. IgG antibodies emerge after 14 days and peak at 30 days, as noted in Figure 31-22 ■. IgG antibodies may remain at detectable levels for more than 10 years. The most widely used method of diagnosing HAV infection is by demonstrating a significant rise in titer between acute and convalescent sera using RIA or EIA.

There is no specific treatment for Hepatitis A. Rest is recommended during the acute phase of the disease when the symptoms are most severe. Immunity, protection against future infections, is conferred by the production of antibodies directed against the hepatitis A virus. There is an HAV vaccine,

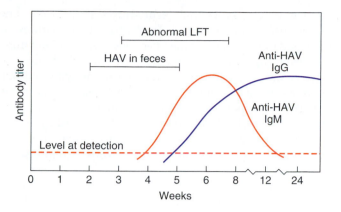

■ FIGURE 31-22 A serological profile of detectable antibodies to HAV infection. LFT, liver function tests.
Reprinted from Mahon and Tice (2006). Clinical Laboratory Immunology. *Prentice Hall, 2006, with permission.*

which can be administered to prevent infection in uninfected individuals exposed to HAV.

Hepatitis C Virus (HCV)

HCV is a single-stranded RNA virus and belongs to the family *Flaviviridae*. Prior to isolation of the actual virus in 1989, Hepatic C was known as non-A, non-B hepatitis and was associated with a transfusion-related hepatitis. The mode of transmission for HCV is parenterally, although perinatal and sexual transmission can also occur. The incubation period for HCV is from 2 weeks to 6 months and antibodies against HCV usually appear during this period. Twenty percent of HCV infections are acute while 80% of the cases of HCV can result in chronic infection. HCV is a lethal virus that can cause liver cirrhosis and cancer. Because both HIV and HCV are bloodborne and are present in similar populations, about 40% of patients infected with HIV are also coinfected with HCV. More than 170 million people worldwide have been infected with the potentially fatal liver disease caused by the hepatitis C virus, making the illness it causes the leading cause of liver transplants.

HCV structural proteins are C, E1, and E2 and its nonstructural proteins include NS1, NS2, NS3, NS4, and NS5. HCV has a high mutation rate, which makes vaccine production more difficult. One of the strategies for developing a vaccine is taking advantage of the fact HCV E1 and E2, noninfectious virus antigens, can trick the body into believing HCV is present, triggering an immune system defense. It is this antigen-induced false alarm that would make a vaccine effective. Once the body encounters actual HCV and is able to eradicate it from the body, the immune system remembers the attack and reacts with greater speed and potency when subsequent exposure to the virus occurs.

The diagnosis of HCV infection was previously based on the presence of elevated liver enzymes, such as alanine amino-transferse (ALT), and subsequent exclusion of the known viral etiological agents, in other words, negative serological tests for HAV, HBV, CMV, EBV, and other viruses known to be asso-

ciated with hepatitis. The symptoms of viral hepatitis for which no specific viral infectious agent could be found was known as non-A, non-B hepatitis. In 1990 the Federal Drug Administration approved a RIA procedure and more recently an EIA procedure to screen donor blood for anti-HCV antibodies, providing a means of diagnosis. Table 31-8 ✪ differentiates the diagnosis of hepatitis due to HAV, HBV, and HCV.

The treatment for HCV includes the use of antiviral drugs such as ribavirin and immunomodulatory drugs such as interferon-alpha.

Hepatitis D Virus (HDV)

The hepatitis D virus (HDV) is a single-stranded RNA virus whose genome lacks certain essential genes, making it a defective virus. The taxonomy of HDV is in question as some have suggested it not even be referred to as a virus but as a subviral agent because of its requirement of a helper virus. For this reason the microbe has often been referred to as the delta agent.

The hepatitis B virus acts as a helper virus to the HDV virus, and therefore, HDV infection can only occur in patients with hepatitis B virus infection. As a consequence of its inability to proliferate without the aid of the hepatitis B virus it must be transmitted simultaneously with the HBV (a co-infection) or as a superinfection of individuals already infected with HBV. Because HDV infection is so intertwined with that of HBV it is also transmitted parenterally. Unfortunately, coinfection or superinfection with HBV increases the risk of chronic or fulminant hepatitis, causing cirrhosis or liver cancer.

IgM class anti-HDV antibodies appear approximately 6–7 weeks after exposure and decline after the acute phase. IgG class antibodies against HDV appear shortly thereafter, during the acute phase, and decline within a few months. Both IgM and IgG are elevated during cases of chronic infection with HDV. Diagnosis of HDV infection relies upon the detection of antibody to HDV (delta) antigen.

Hepatitis E Virus (HEV)

HEV is a single-stranded RNA virus discovered in 1990, which was originally placed in the family *Caliciviridea;* however, more recently a new virus family, *Hepeviridae,* has been created for its inclusion due to the similarity of its genome to that of the rubella virus, a member of the family *Togaviridae.* Its mode of

✪ TABLE 31-8

Viral Hepatitis Panel Interpretation

Anti-HAV IgM	HBsAg	Anti-HBc IgM	Anti-HCV	Interpretation
+	−	−	−	Acute HAV infection
−	+	+	−	Acute HBV infection
−	−	−	+	Acute HCV infection

Anti-HAV IgM, IgM antibody against Hepatitis A virus (HAV); HBsAg, Hepatitis B surface antigen; Anti-HBc IgM, IgM antibody against Hepatitis B virus (HBV); Anti-HCV, Antibody against Hepatis C virus (HCV).

transmission is the oral–fecal route, a reflection of the fact the virus is excreted in feces and acquired through ingestion of contaminated food and water. Its clinical course is that of an acute, self-limiting illness with no chronic phase. The symptoms are similar to those of HAV infection; however, the mortality rate is particularly high in pregnant women. HEV is more prevalent in tropical and subtropical countries with a low standard of sanitation such as those in Asia (including the Indian subcontinent) and Africa. There is currently no vaccine available for HEV and the best means of prevention is through proper hygiene and good sanitation.

Diagnosis of HEV infection is through the detection of IgM class anti-HEV antibodies during the acute stage. These antibodies decline after the recovery phase. IgG class anti-HEV antibodies also rise during the acute phase and remain for a number of years.

Hepatitis G Virus (HGV)

HGV is a single-stranded RNA virus belonging to the *Flaviviridae* family. It was discovered in 1995 and occurs in both acute and chronic cases of hepatitis. It has been found in 1–2% of blood donors and is transmitted by the parenteral route (i.e., blood transfusions and intravenous drug abuse). Diagnosis is through the use of EIA, PCR, and Western blot (WB) techniques.

 Checkpoint! 31–6 (Chapter Objective 3)

Which hepatotropic virus is a single-stranded RNA virus that lacks certain essential genes, making it a defective virus?

   A. *Hepatitis A virus*
   B. *Hepatitis B virus*
   C. *Hepatitis C virus*
   D. *Hepatitis D virus*

PICORNAVIRUSES

The *Picornaviridae* family includes the following medically important genera:

- Enterovirus, which includes the coxsackie viruses and the polioviruses.
- Rhinovirus are a major cause of the common cold.
- Hepatovirus, which includes the hepatitis A virus.

Picornaviruses are very hardy and resistant to many disinfectants. Members of this family cause a wide variety of diseases both asymptomatic and symptomatic. Aseptic meningitis, a disease seen in infants less than a year old, may be fatal.

Enteroviruses

Enteroviruses are single stranded RNA viruses containing 72 different serotypes that have been divided into five groups: polioviruses types 1–3, coxsackie A viruses types 1–24, cox-

sackie B viruses types 1–6, echoviruses types 1–34, and enteroviruses serotypes 68–71. In humans, enteroviruses are the second most common viral infectious agents. Enteroviruses have been implicated in the emergence of specific diseases such as pandemic acute hemorrhagic conjunctivitis and outbreaks of other infectious diseases of major public health concern. The diseases range from asymptomatic to fatal. These viruses cause febrile illness, respiratory illness, rashes, aseptic meningitis, and paralysis. In Southeast Asia enterovirus 71 is a recognized cause of severe central nervous system diseases such as viral or aseptic meningitis.

Enteroviruses are very hardy and resistant to most commonly used disinfectants such as detergents, 70% alcohol, and phenolic compounds. Halides compounds such as iodine solutions and sodium hypochlorite or bleach are able to inactivate the viruses and are usually quite effective as disinfectants.

Children tend to be most commonly afflicted with enterovirus during the summer, fall, and winter. Transmission is often fecal–oral but these viruses can also be spread via respiratory aerosols. Cerebrospinal fluid is the specimen of choice for aseptic meningitis. Nucleic acid assays provide rapid results compared to the 2–5 days required for traditional cell culture.

 REAL WORLD TIP

At least four different cell lines are needed to detect enteroviruses. There are so many serotypes and no one cell line grows all of them well. Cell lines used include human monkey kidney cells, human lung cancer, and rhabdomyosarcoma. Enterovirus produce round, refractile cells in 2–5 days but the CPE can vary depending on the serotype. Immunofluorescence is used for identification.

The Poliomyelitis Viruses.   The poliomyelitis virus is a single-stranded RNA virus that causes polio, a paralytic disease, particularly in children. Infection is transmitted by the oral–fecal route through ingestion of contaminated food or water. The virus multiplies in the gastrointestinal tract before entering the bloodstream and finally invades the central nervous system where it may cause irreversible paralysis. More than 95% of polio infections are asymptomatic or mild febrile illnesses, a small percentage cause serious neurological illnesses, and less than 1% cause paralysis. In developing countries, mass vaccination using the oral vaccine, an attenuated live vaccine developed by Albert Sabin in 1961, has led to the eradication of the poliovirus but in third-world countries it remains a significant threat to human health.

Coxsackie Viruses.   Coxsackie viruses are single stranded RNA viruses that belong to the genus *Enterovirus*. The name of these viruses is derived from the fact they were originally identified in Coxsackie, New York. Coxsackie viruses known to cause pathology in humans include the coxsackie A and coxsackie B viruses. Coxsackie A16 is the cause of a common childhood illness called hand, foot, and mouth disease. Hand, foot, and mouth disease presents with fever, mouth blisters, and rash. Coxsackie A24 is the viral agent for hemorrhagic conjunctivitis. The diseases associated with coxsackie B virus include infectious pericarditis, myocarditis, and Bornholm disease or pleurodynia. In addition, both coxsackie A and coxsackie B viruses have been implicated in aseptic meningitis. Additionally, the coxsackie B24 virus has been identified as one of the agents responsible for triggering type 1 diabetes, an autoimmune disorder.

Rhinoviruses

Rhinoviruses only cause lower respiratory tract infections such as bronchitis and pneumonia on rare occasions, but they are a major cause of upper respiratory tract infections such as the common cold. They are responsible for 40% of all colds, principally those occurring during fall and spring, and are therefore partially responsible for the creation of a $4 billion cold remedy market in the United States alone.

Contrary to popular belief, and with no disrespect to mothers everywhere, children do not "catch" colds as a result of exposure to cold temperatures. While it can be demonstrated most colds occur during the fall, winter, and spring months when temperatures are at their lowest, the increase is more likely to be attributed to the fact more people are confined indoors and in close proximity to each other. These factors clearly increase the likelihood of transmission for reasons that will be explained below. Another misconception is that sneezing and coughing is the route in which rhinoviruses are transmitted. This also is not likely to be the case because sneezing and coughing expel saliva while rhinoviruses are shed in nasal secretions.

Similar to other viruses in the *Picornaviridae* family, rhinoviruses are very hardy, being heat stable and resistant to the effects of desiccation. The hands of infected individuals are implements for the transfer of rhinoviruses because symptoms such as coryza or runny nose permit nasal secretions to spread onto the skin, covering the hands. The virus is transferred directly to the hands of uninfected persons or surfaces such as doorknobs, tabletops, and elevator buttons. Uninfected persons then inoculate themselves with the virus when they perform normal human behaviors such as rubbing their eyes or nose.

Another factor that facilitates this transfer is the fact viral shedding begins a few days before symptoms appear and the infected person is not aware he or she has a cold. Additionally, viral shedding persists several days after symptoms have ceased and infected individuals feel they have recovered and are no longer infective. The fact that nearly half of rhinovirus infections are asymptomatic, yet virus particles are still shed in nasal secretions, also factors into the ease in which the common cold is spread.

Attempts have been made to develop a vaccine against the common cold but because there are over 100 different rhinovirus serotypes and antigenic shift (recombination of the viral genome) makes the task exceedingly difficult if not insurmountable. Consequently, the best means of controlling the spread of viruses is through frequent hand washing and avoiding contact between the hands, eyes, and nose.

Laboratory diagnosis of rhinovirus infection is rarely attempted because of the mild nature of the common cold. In spite of the misery that must be endured with cold symptoms, fatal cases of rhinovirus infection are rare and immunity to specific serotypes is good. Complications of a common cold can include sinusitis, otitis media, and lung problems for those with chronic lung disease, immunosuppression, or heart disease.

> ### REAL WORLD TIP
>
> Rhinovirus can be detected on cell culture. It grows in MRC-5 and WI-38 (both human lung fibroblasts) and PMK (primary monkey kidney). It produces CPE similar to that of enteroviruses within 1 week. Cell cultures should be incubated at 33°C rather than the traditional 35–37°C.

CORONAVIRUSES

Coronaviruses are enveloped, single-stranded RNA viruses in the family *Coronaviridae*. They are known to cause pharyngitis and most of the cases of the common cold that occur during the winter months. The route of transmission is similar to that of rhinoviruses: contact with respiratory secretions containing the virus. Coronaviruses gained their name due to the crown or halo effect seen on electron microscopy in Figure 31-23 ■.

Coronaviruses were also the cause of a global outbreak of severe acute respiratory syndrome or SARS, which emerged in the Far East in March 2003. This illness, which has an incubation period of 2–7 days, begins with symptoms including chills, fever,

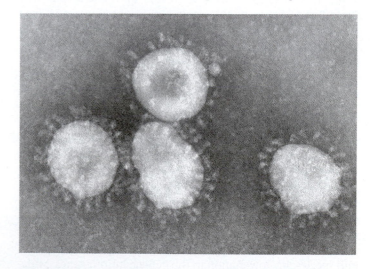

■ **FIGURE 31-23** Cornaviruses are so named due to the crown or halo surrounding them as seen in this electron micrograph. This virus is the causative agent of SARS.
From Public Health Image Library (PHIL), CDC/Dr. Fred Murphy.

myalgia, headache, pharyngitis, rhinorrhea (runny nose), and even diarrhea. Lower respiratory symptoms include cough, shortness of breath, and difficulty in breathing. A history of travel to areas where the SARS-Corona virus (SARS-CoV) is known to be endemic (China, Taiwan, Hong Kong, etc.), exposure to known cases of SARS, symptomology, and radiographic evidence of pneumonia all help to confirm a diagnosis of SARS. An acute serum sample, sputum, virus cultures, and ruling out other causes of pneumonia (bacteria, influenza virus, RSV, etc.) will also contribute to the diagnosis.

Prevention of SARS transmission involves early recognition of infected patients, hospitalization when necessary, adhering to contact and airborne infection isolation precautions, access to and instruction and training in the use of personal protective equipment, respirator fit testing, and cough etiquette (www.cdc.gov).

Specimens used for detection include nasopharyngeal, oropharyngeal, and lower respiratory such as bronchial alveolar lavage and lung tissue. Immunofluorescence, nucleic acid assays, and serology can be used for detection. This virus is difficult to grow in cell culture. While there is no treatment for SARS, researchers are investigating the development of treatment options and possible vaccines.

INFLUENZA VIRUSES

Influenza viruses, type A, B, and C belong to the *Orthomyxoviridae* family. Orthomyxoviruses are enveloped, single-stranded, segmented, negative-sense RNA viruses. Innumerable projections that resemble spikes can be found embedded into and projecting from the surface of the lipoprotein viral envelope. These glycoprotein viral antigens determine the subtype of the virus. The subtypes of type A influenza occur through specific combinations of the 19 hemagglutinin and 9 neuraminidase antigens such as H1N1, H2N2, H3N2, H5N1, and so on. Only types A and B cause life-threatening infections in humans. Even though the flu is self-limiting in most cases, complications such as bronchitis and pneumonia can be very serious in infants, older adults, and chronically ill patients.

Hemagglutinin (HA) is a major glycoprotein of the influenza virus and is responsible for the ability of the virus to attach to cells. Neuraminidase, a glycoprotein enzyme on the surface of the influenza virus, is responsible for release of viral progeny from infected cells. The first step in the initiation of the influenza virus infection is attachment of the virus to cells lining the mucous membranes of the upper respiratory tract using sialic acid as the receptor on host cells. Once replication has taken place within infected cells, the neuraminidase enzyme cleaves sialic acid residues from carbohydrate, promoting the release of the viral progeny.

Influenza strains have the ability to show selectivity for certain species due to variation in the hemagglutinin genes. Mutations in the hemagglutinin genes enable the viral proteins to bind to receptors on the surface of host cells. These mutations can allow the influenza virus to easily pass from animals to humans and lead to a pandemic. Influenza virus has a high

mutation rate that is a characteristic of many RNA viruses because they lack DNA polymerases that can find, fix, and repair DNA. It is able to escape the host defense through a mechanism called antigenic variation. Influenza virus has a segmented genome that can be resorted to yield new viral particles expressing a new combination of the surface antigens.

Influenza A is the virus most often implicated in pandemics or worldwide epidemics. The Spanish flu (1918–1919, H1N1 strain), Asian flu (1957–1958, H2N2 strain), and Hong Kong flu (1968–1969, H3N2 strain) represent three pandemics (worldwide outbreaks) caused by influenza A in the last century. In 2009, a new strain of influenza A, H1N1, called novel or swine flu, has been implicated in the most recent pandemic. In the past pandemics have tended to occur about every 10 years (H1N1 in 1947, H2N2 in 1957, H3N2 in 1968, and H1N1 in 1978). Pandemics are associated with antigenic shift that occurs when the virus undergoes a change from one hemagglutinin or neuraminidase to another, which results in the emergence of a new virus particle (Figure 31-24 ■).

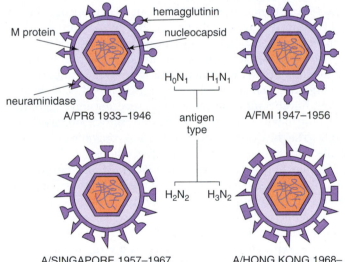

strains of influenza A

A/PR8 1933–1946

A/FMI 1947–1956

A/SINGAPORE 1957–1967

A/HONG KONG 1968–

■ **FIGURE 31-24** Antigenic shift in influenza virus. The major surface antigens of influenza virus are hemagglutinin and neuraminidase. Hemagglutinin is involved in attachment to cells, and antibodies to hemagglutinin are protective. Antibodies to neuraminidase are much less effective. The influenza virus can change its antigenic properties slightly (antigenic drift) or radically (antigenic shift). Alterations in the structure of the hemagglutinin antigen render earlier antibodies ineffective and new virus epidemics therefore break out. The diagram shows strains that have emerged by antigenic shift since 1933. The official influenza antigen nomenclature is based on the type of hemagglutinin (H_1, H_2, etc.) and neuraminidase (N_1, N_2, etc.) expressed on the surface of the virion. Note that, although new strains replace old strains, the internal antigens remain largely unchanged.

Reprinted from Male et al. (2006). Clinical Laboratory Immunology (7th ed.). Copyright 2006 with permission from Elsevier.

With an antigenic drift there are only minor changes (point mutations) in the amino acid sequences of the hemagglutinin or neuraminidase. With antigenic drift the subtype remains the same. Even these small changes give the virus a selective advantage. It is now believed that the Asian flu and Hong Kong flu were caused by strains that were the result of reassortment of human and avian viruses. Influenza A has also been found to infect swine, horses, birds, and other animals. H5N1 strains are able to merge their genes with the strains that are found in hosts such as humans, birds, and so on. Wild birds are the only animals that have all subtypes of influenza A.

H5N1 is a subtype of influenza A virus and is the etiological agent of the avian or bird flu. Some strains of avian influenza can be very virulent. In 2003 the H5N1 strain of the avain strain of influenza A was responsible for an outbreak in southeast Asian countries, which continues at the present time to be a major source of concern. The increased virulence seen in humans infected with this strain is the cause of this concern. At this point no cases of human-to-human transfer have been documented. Infection has been acquired by individuals in close contact with infected fowls.

Influenza A virus infection is often asymptomatic or mild. Symptoms include fever, chills, myalgia, sore throat, and cough. Fatalities are seen when viral pneumonia is contracted or if a secondary bacterial pneumonia follows. Influenza vaccination is the most effective method for preventing influenza virus infection and its potentially severe complications. The live, attenuated vaccine is made from weakened viruses and does not cause influenza. However, individuals who have severe allergies to chicken eggs should not be vaccinated as the virus is propagated using chicken eggs as a growth medium (http://www.cdc.gov/flu/professionals/vaccination/vax-summary.htm).

The influenza B virus usually causes a milder upper respiratory disease in young children. Complications such as pneumonia are rare. Reyes syndrome, a serious, often fatal, encephalopathy, has been associated with influenza B virus and much less often with the influenza A virus. Because this syndrome is often seen with the use of salicylates, it is recommended that children not be given aspirin to reduce fever. The influenza C virus is associated with a common mild illness in early childhood.

The influenza viruses are known for their appearance in November to December and lingering through March or April. Transmission is through respiratory aerosols. Because the viruses infect the respiratory mucosa, nasal washings or aspirates are the specimens of choice. Throat swabs can be used but contain less virus. During "flu" season, microbiology laboratories are inundated with specimens for testing using rapid immunoassay methods. Monoclonal antibodies are used to detect either influenza A or B or both. These methods have a sensitivity rate of about 80%. Often the lack of sensitivity is due to a poor-quality specimen with a low number of viruses present.

For immunoassays that test as negative, cell culture or direct immunofluorescence can be used as a backup. Primary monkey kidney and A-549 (human lung carcinoma) cells can be used for culture. In 3–5 days, the cells may display rounded cells, vacuoles in the cell lawn, or little effect. Immunofluoresence using monoclonal antibodies will identify A and B. Influenza virus–infected cells are able to adsorb guinea pig red blood cells onto their surface. This is due to the ability of the viral hemagglutinin to bind to the sialic receptor on the blood cells. Other respiratory viruses also have this ability so further testing is necessary. Hemagglutination inhibition can be performed.

 REAL WORLD TIP

Influenza, mumps, and parainfluenza viruses have the ability to adsorb and agglutinate red blood cells.

The flu vaccine confers immunity to specific strains or subtypes in general. Abrupt major changes in influenza virus can occur, such as with the 2009 H1N1 strain, and because the surface antigens of flu viruses can change over time, immunity to one strain does not prevent susceptibility to another strain. Those who are at risk of complications and health care workers are advised to be vaccinated against influenza virus. However, a new vaccine against influenza virus needs to be reformulated each year because each epidemic is antigenically different.

Several antiviral drugs have been used in the treatment and prophylaxis of flu. Neuraminidase inhibitors, such as zanamivir, are used in the prophylaxis and treatment of Influenza A and B. Antiviral drugs such as amantadine and rimantadine are effective against influenza A, while zanamivir is effective against both A and B. This makes their differentiation very important.

 REAL WORLD TIP

The 2009 pandemic of swine flu is due to a unique or novel H1N1 strain of the influenza A virus (see ∞ Chapter 42, "Global Threats"). The current rapid detection kits in place may be able to detect this strain but are only able to detect it as an influenza A virus and not specifically as the H1N1 strain. There have been reports of both false positive and false negatives with the rapid influenza detection kits. A positive rapid test may indicate the virus present is H1N1, a traditional seasonal influenza A strain or a false-positive reaction. Reverse transcription PCR or viral culture is necessary to confirm H1N1.

✓ **Checkpoint! 31–7 (Chapter Objective 1)**

The strain of influenza responsible for the avian or "bird" flu, an enzootic illness creating considerable concern in the first decade of the 21st century, is caused by subtype
A. H2N3.
B. H1N1.
C. H2N2.
D. H5N1.

THE PARAMYXOVIRUSES

Members of the *Paramyxoviridae* family are enveloped, helical RNA viruses that are large in size. The genera that contain viruses of medical importance are:

- The *Respirovirus* genus, which includes the parainfluenza virus.
- The *Pneumovirus* genus containing the respiratory syncytial virus and metapneumonia virus.
- The *Morbillivirus* genus, which includes the measles virus and canine distemper virus, which is not a human pathogen.
- The *Rubulavirus* genus, which includes the mumps virus.

The Parainfluenza Viruses

The parainfluenza viruses (1 and 3) cause acute respiratory illnesses seen primarily in children. Croup is an upper respiratory infection causing laryngitis, inflammation of the larynx, and is associated with a characteristic, hoarse cough like the bark of a seal. Parainfluenza viruses may also cause lower respiratory tract infections such as pneumonia or bronchitis in infants. These respiratory illnesses are spread by inhalation of droplets expelled by infected individuals or person to person by direct contact with respiratory secretions shed by infected persons. There is no vaccine available nor is there an effective treatment regimen for the illnesses caused by paramyxoviruses.

Diagnosis may be made by examining material obtained with throat swabs or nasopharyngeal washings. A direct fluorescent antibody stain can be used to demonstrate the presence of the virus in respiratory secretions. Cell culture using primary monkey kidney, human neonatal kidney, or human lung cancer can be performed. CPE may take up to 14 days and displays round, granular cells and syncytia or large cells with multiple fused nuclei. Eventually there is disintegration of the cell lawn. Immunofluorescence using monoclonal antibodies or hemadsorption with guinea pig red cells is performed on cells exhibiting CPE. Serological testing for the presence of antibodies is difficult because of frequent reinfection. There are currently no approved antiviral therapies available.

REAL WORLD TIP

Laboratories now use a pool of monoclonal antibodies either as a direct or indirect fluorescence method. The pool tests for the most common respiratory viruses, which include adenovirus, influenza A and B, and respiratory syncytial virus, the three most common types of parainfluenza viruses.

The Respiratory Syncytial Virus

The respiratory syncytial virus (RSV) is so named because of a characteristic cytopathic effect of extensive syncytia formation in cell cultures. Syncytia are created when the cells merge together to create large, multinucleated cells. RSV is a major cause of a number of upper respiratory diseases in infants, ranging from a mild upper respiratory disease, to bronchiolitis and pneumonia, to severe respiratory distress and death. Infants born prematurely or with congenital heart defects or chronic lung disease are at increased risk for RSV pneumonia. Infants with RSV pneumonia are at risk for developing asthma later in childhood. Most infections occur in late winter and early spring, with its peak in February and March, and may be seen as nursery outbreaks associated with high infection rates and some fatalities. Disease is spread by direct contact with respiratory secretions, making hand washing an important control measure. Infection of adults is normally seen as an acute, febrile, upper respiratory infection that may be chronic and more severe in older adults. Infection can lead to bronchiolitis and pneumonia. While no vaccine is available, ribavirin is an effective antiviral drug that can be administered.

Diagnosis of RSV infection can be made using nasal washings or aspirates subjected to a direct fluorescent antibody stain. Direct immunoassay tests are used in most laboratories. Overall most have a sensitivity and specificity over 80%. Direct fluorescence antibody or viral cultures should be performed on negative direct tests. HEp-2 (human larynx cancer) and H292 and A-549 (human lung cancers) are used for cell culture. RSV demonstrates syncytia or large merged cells in 3–5 days.

REAL WORLD TIP

RSV is a very fragile virus. It is extremely susceptible to changes in temperature such as heating or freezing. It does not survive in the environment without humidity. Crowded settings such as schools and day care centers are the perfect places for person-to-person transmission.

REAL WORLD TIP

Human metapneumovirus is a member of the same subfamily as RSV. It is a common cause of bronchiolitis and croup and appears at the same time of the year as RSV. It does not grow well in cell culture so reverse transcription PCR is currently the only means of identification. It should be suspected when CPE is detected but cannot be identified by fluorescent antibodies used for the most common respiratory viruses.

The Measles Virus

The rubeola or measles virus is an enveloped, single-stranded RNA virus in the *Paramyxoviridae* family. Measles is a highly infectious disease spread by respiratory aerosols containing the virus. After an incubation period of about 10 days, the symptoms of infection appear, including a fever of at least 3 days, coughing, coryza or runny nose, conjunctivitis or red, irritated eyes sensitive to light, cough, and a generalized erythematous rash. The rash erupts some days after the start of fever and spreads from the head to other parts of the body. Bright red spots with white centers, called Koplik's spots, appear on the oral mucosa and precede the characteristic skin rash. The skin rash and Koplik's spots are diagnostic of measles infection and, if apparent, laboratory diagnosis is unnecessary.

When laboratory diagnosis is required it is possible to identify the presence of the virus using a nasopharyngeal swab or urine specimen. The virus can be cultured on human kidney cells showing distinctive multinucleated cells. Additionally, serological tests may demonstrate the presence of IgM antibodies that appear during the acute phase of infection. Measles-specific IgM antibodies are also diagnostic of measles infection. Enzyme immunoassay and serum neutralization assays are commonly used as a means of obtaining antibody titers.

The best means of protection against measles virus infection is through vaccination. Prior to the advent of the measles vaccine, as much as 95% of the population were infected with the measles virus at some time during their lives. The measles vaccine available is being given to children at the age of 18 months as part of the measles, mumps, rubella (MMR) vaccine, with a booster being administered sometime before the child reaches the age of 5.

The Mumps Virus

The mumps virus is an enveloped, single-stranded RNA virus belonging to the *Paramyxoviridae* family. The virus causes mumps or epidemic parotitis, a self-limiting systemic viral disease, spread by droplets of infected saliva. In adolescence, it can cause severe symptoms such as a painful swelling of the parotid glands, which are responsible for the production of saliva, as well as fever, headache, and sore throat. The characteristic neck swelling associated with mumps can be seen in Figure 31-25 ■. In some cases the pancreas, ovaries, and testes can be

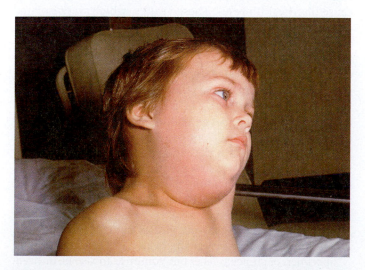

■ **FIGURE 31-25** Mumps is due to infection of the parotid or salivary glands by the virus. The resulting neck swelling is easily recognized.
From Public Health Image Library (PHIL), CDC/NIP/Barbara Rice.

affected. Orchitis, or inflammation of the testes, can lead to cases of infertility.

The virus can be isolated from saliva and the urine of infected persons. Direct detection of the mumps virus can be accomplished through immunofluorescence but diagnosis of mumps is most commonly made through serological testing using enzyme immunoassays, which measure IgG and IgM antibodies against mumps. A fourfold rise in titer is considered to be diagnostic. Other serological tests include hemagglutination inhibition and complement fixation.

As mentioned above, immunization against mumps is through the MMR vaccine, which is given to children.

THE RUBELLA VIRUS

The rubella virus, the causative agent for rubella or German measles, is an enveloped single-stranded RNA virus that belongs to the *Togaviridae* family. Rubella has also been called the 3-day measles or epidemic roseola. The infection can be transmitted by inhalation of respiratory droplets containing the virus. Rubella infection in young children is a mild disease and in most cases is asymptomatic. In adults, infection is often more severe. Symptomatic infection is associated with fever, a rash on the face and trunk or limbs, red papules on the soft palate, inflammation of the eyes, and lymphadenopathy.

It can be passed from infected mother to the baby transplacentally to cause congenital infection. When the mother contracts a primary infection on first contact with the virus, she does not possess a protective antibody that can cross the placenta and protect the fetus. Congenital infection acquired during the first trimester of pregnancy can result in severe developmental defects in the fetus, such as cataracts, glaucoma, deafness, congenital heart disease, and mental retardation, as well as spontaneous abortion, premature birth, or fetal death. Intrauterine infection after the first trimester poses little danger to the fetus. The virus can also be transmitted through breast milk, leading to postnatal rubella infection, which is usually a mild disease.

The rubella virus is shed in saliva, nasopharyngeal secretions, and the urine of infected individuals. It can be cultured in cell lines such as African green monkey kidney but this method is not used because it does not produce CPE. Additional testing such as PCR and immunofluorescence antibodies is necessary to confirm its presence.

Serological testing may include passive hemagglutination using viral antigen-coated red blood cells or agglutination of antigen-coated latex beads. Solid phase capture enzyme immune assay for IgM and IgG class antibodies are used to detect acute infection or to demonstrate immunity against rubella. The presence of IgM class antibodies to the virus aids in the diagnosis of the congenital disease since maternal IgM class antibodies are not able to cross the placenta. IgM class antibodies produced by the fetus or newborn will decline within 6 months after birth, afterward levels of IgG start to increase. In general, IgM antirubella detection is an indicator of acute illness and IgG antirubella antibody is an indication of a patient's immune status.

An effective attenuated vaccine against rubella is available for children around 1 year of age. It is given via injection as part of measles, mumps, and rubella vaccine (MMR vaccine). The MMR vaccine is given as a booster again in children before starting school.

ARBOVIRUS INFECTIONS

Arbovirus infections are often severe or fatal. In many cases, humans are the native host and therefore have no inherent resistance to infection. In addition to humans, monkeys, horses, birds, reptiles, and amphibians may also serve as hosts and additional sources of human infection.

The term arbovirus is derived from the fact these illnesses are arthropod-born virus infections. The insect vector for many arbovirus infections is the female mosquito, which transmits the virus when she obtains the high-protein blood meal she requires to produce a greater quantity of eggs. Because mosquitoes and other arthropods, such as ticks, are most prevalent in late spring, summer, and early fall, most infections are seen in these same seasons. The encephalitis viruses cause infections associated with symptoms such as fever, nausea, headaches, stiff neck and back, photosensitivity, confusion, and in severe cases, coma and death. Even in nonfatal cases neurological sequelae such as mental deficiencies, deafness, blindness, and paralysis may occur.

Arboviruses include alphaviruses such as:

- Eastern equine encephalitis virus (EEE)
- Western equine encephalitis virus (WEE)

- Venezuelan equine encephalitis virus (VEE) of North, Central, and South America

And flaviviruses including:

- St. Louis encephalitis virus (SLE) of North America
- West Nile virus (WNV), originating in Africa, the virus appeared in the United States in 1999
- Yellow fever virus of Africa and South America, which is known to cause degeneration of the liver (leading to jaundice, hence the name yellow fever), kidneys, and heart
- Dengue fever virus, which is found worldwide, especially in the tropics; Dengue hemorrhagic fever is associated with internal bleeding, loss of plasma, and shock.

Most laboratories should not attempt isolation of the arboviruses due to the potential for infection of laboratory workers. Serology, on blood and CSF, remains the mainstay for determination of infection with the arboviruses. PCR can provide faster results.

GASTROENTERITIS VIRUSES

Gastroenteritis viruses cause illnesses associated with vomiting, diarrhea, or both. These gastrointestinal diseases are often referred to as the "stomach flu," although influenza and parainfluenza viruses are not responsible. Viruses known to cause gastroenteritis include adenoviruses, noroviruses, and rotaviruses. They are spread via the fecal–oral route or person to person. Since adenoviruses have already been discussed they will only be referred to briefly in this discussion.

Noroviruses

Noroviruses, which were originally investigated in the 1940s, cause diarrheal illnesses. These viruses, which were isolated during an outbreak in Norwalk, Ohio, in 1968, are single-stranded, nonenveloped RNA viruses in the *Calciviridae* family. They are transmitted by the fecal–oral route through contaminated food and water or direct contact with feces containing the organism. These viruses are very hardy and are not inactivated by pH or heat. The gastrointestinal illness is associated with low-grade fever, abdominal pain, vomiting, and diarrhea. Symptoms last from 1 to 5 days after which recovery is usually complete. It is now thought that nearly 50% or all foodborne outbreaks of gastroenteritis are caused by noroviruses (www.cdc.gov). In older adults this viral infection can be more serious and sometimes fatal. Traveler's diarrhea (TD) is the most frequent health problem in travelers to developing countries. Besides bacteria and organisms, viruses such as Norwalk virus, rotavirus, and adenovirus are implicated in TD.

Specimen of choice is feces but vomitus can also be utilized. Diagnosis is accomplished through molecular techniques such as real-time PCR. Electron microscopy can be used to identify the small, rounded virus. This method may not be practical for most laboratories.

Rotaviruses

Rotaviruses were discovered in 1973 during an investigation of several cases of infant gastroenteritis. "Rota" is the Latin word for "wheel" and describes its morphology. These small, nonenveloped, double-stranded RNA viruses are in the *Reoviridae* family. Because these viruses possess a double capsid, the morphology observed with an electron microscope is described as resembling a wheel with a wide hub and short spokes radiating out from the hub to the rim of the wheel (Figure 31-26 ■).

Transmission is through the fecal–oral route by ingestion of contaminated food and water. Rotavirus infection may be asymptomatic, mild, or a severely dehydrating diarrheal illness that can be fatal. Symptoms, which may last from 3 to 8 days, include fever, vomiting, diarrhea, and dehydration due to water loss. Most cases occur in infants 16–24 months of age. Rotavirus infection is the most common cause of severe diarrhea and a leading cause of mortality in children. In developing countries hundreds of thousands of children succumb to the complications of this viral disease every year.

The route of transmission for this virus is through contaminated water and foods such as oysters, clams, and raw shellfish. Treatment for rotavirus infection, like other viral agents causing gastroenteritis, is through oral rehydration to prevent severe loss of fluids. Frequent hand washing can greatly reduce the chance of new infections with this virus. New vaccines have been licensed for rotavirus to protect against severe diarrhea and were shown to be effective and safe.

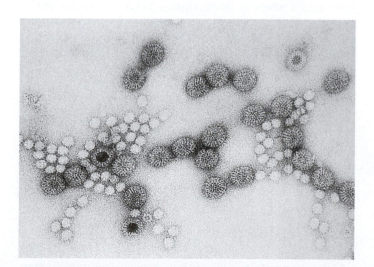

■ **FIGURE 31-26** Electron microphotograph showing a number of rotavirus virions and a number of unidentified smaller virion particles. Note the "wheel"-like appearance of the virions from which the virus name is derived (rota is Latin for "wheel").
From Public Health Image Library (PHIL), CDC/E. L. Palmer.

Diagnosis of rotavirus infection can be made using an enzyme immunoassay (EIA) technique to detect antigen in fecal specimens. Although molecular techniques, such as PCR, are available, EIA is rapid and relatively easy to perform. While rotavirus can grow in cell lines, it takes many passages and supplemented medium to achieve CPE.

RABIES VIRUS

The virus that causes rabies is a single-stranded RNA virus belonging to the *Rhabdoviridae* family. Transmission of rabies virus is through the bite of infected animals and possibly through transplant surgery. The virus is present in the saliva of infected animals such as dogs, cats, foxes, raccoons, and bats. Upon entering the host, the virus enters peripheral nerves and travels to the central nervous system. Once it is in the brain, the virus causes encephalitis (acute inflammation of the brain) and myelitis (swelling of the spinal cord).

Rabies is always fatal once the symptoms appear. The disease starts with pain in the site of the bite and progresses to flulike symptoms, which can take weeks to months to show. Next, symptoms progress to those involving the central nervous system, such as insomnia, anxiety, confusion, hallucinations, and hydrophobia. Eventually the host succumbs to coma and death.

Rabies can be prevented by vaccination in humans and infected animals. The rabies virus must travel from the site of exposure to the brain and spinal cord to cause serious damage. Because this route of travel is extremely slow, postexposure treatment consisting of vigorous cleaning of the wound site, administration of rabies vaccine, and immunoglobulin is extremely effective in providing protection from the lethal effects of the virus.

Diagnosis can be made through biopsy of the brain of infected patients. Infection with the rabies virus can be demonstrated by the presence of Negri bodies, which are characteristic of rabies and seen in 70–80% of rabies cases. Negri bodies are eosinophilic inclusion bodies in the cytoplasm of certain infected neurons (nerve cells), as seen in Figure 31-27 ■.

The diagnosis of rabies may also be accomplished through enzyme immunoassay testing to detect antibodies to the rabies virus. The rapid fluorescent-focus inhibition test (RFFIT) for rabies antibodies has been used recently for the identification of the virus. In addition, flow cytometry could be used to detect rabies virus antigen in infected cells with the potential advantages of automation and speed.

EMERGING VIRUSES

Emerging viruses are discussed more fully in ∞ Chapter 42, "Global Threats." These include:

- Hantavirus is an RNA virus in the family *Bunyaviridae*. It produces two distinct diseases: hemorrhagic fever as well as severe pulmonary disease. Aerosolized urine and feces of infected rodents are the source of infection. It first

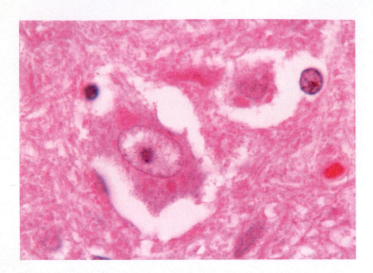

■ **FIGURE 31-27** Negri bodies, as seen in the neural cell in the center, is characteristic for rabies.
From Public Health Image Library (PHIL), CDC.

✓ **Checkpoint! 31–8
(Chapter Objectives 1 and 7)**

A small, nonenveloped, double-stranded RNA virus with a double capsule, and a member of the Reoviridae family, is said to have a microscopic morphology resembling a wheel with a wide hub and short spokes. This virus is an important cause of gastroenteritis and is particularly dangerous to infants. What is this group of viruses called?

A. *Adenoviruses*

B. *Stomach flu viruses*

C. *Noroviruses*

D. *Rotaviruses*

---

appeared in 1993 in the four corners area of the United States where Arizona, Colorado, Utah, and New Mexico meet. The pulmonary syndrome fills the infected individual's lungs with fluid so they literally drown. It has the potential to be used as a bioterrorism agent.

■ Rift valley fever virus is a member of the family *Bunyaviridae*. It is primarily found in cattle in Africa. Transmission is via mosquitoes or contact with infected animals. The virus can cause ocular infections, meningoencephalitis, or hemorrhagic fever.

■ The RNA filoviruses, of the family *Filoviridae*, include the Marburg and Ebola viruses. Potential sources for the viruses may be African monkeys and fruit bats but this has not been proven to date. They are known for causing hemorrhagic fever, which is usually fatal. These RNA viruses require a BSL 4 laboratory for testing. The filoviruses have the potential to be used as bioterrorism agents.

■ The RNA arenaviruses, of the family *Arenaviridae*, are found in rodents in Africa and South America. Diseases range from nonfatal lymphocytic choriomeningitis to the potentially fatal Lassa fever. A BSL 4 laboratory is necessary for handling specimens suspected of containing arenavirus. The arenaviruses have the potential to be used as bioterrorism agents.

RETROVIRUSES

Retroviruses are RNA viruses that use the enzyme reverse transcriptase (RT) to produce a DNA copy of their RNA genome. This DNA can then be incorporated into the host cell's nuclear DNA through another enzyme called integrase. Once the retroviral genome has been integrated into the host DNA, it is called a provirus. After being passively replicated along with the host genome, the provirus will eventually be activated and start transcription of its viral genome using the cellular machinery of the host cell. This finally leads to destruction of the host cell.

The three genes that human retroviruses use for the production of mature viruses are group-specific antigen (gag), polymerase (pol), and envelope (env). *Gag* genes code for the retroviral core and structural proteins. *Pol* codes for the retroviral enzymes reverse transcriptase, integrase, and protease. *Env* codes for the retroviral coat proteins. Retroviruses mutate more frequently because these viruses do not possess the proofreading seen with DNA replication (the error-correcting processes involved in transcription of a genetic code). It is the mutation capability of the retrovirus that enables the virus to grow resistant to antiviral medications rapidly, and is the cause of difficulty in the development of an effective vaccine against HIV-1 infection.

Human retroviruses, known as human T cell leukemia/lymphoma virus (HTLV-1 and HTLV-2) and HIV-1, have been isolated from patients with mature T cell malignancies. The exact mechanism whereby these viruses induce leukemia (malignancy of blood leukocytes) is still not clear, however, it is strongly believed that incorporation of retroviral genome into DNA of the host may lead to activation of proto-oncogenes, which have been implicated in initiating leukemia.

HIV and AIDS

The human immunodeficiency virus (HIV) is an enveloped RNA virus and a member of the *Retroviridae* family (genus, *Lentivirus*). The clinical manifestations of HIV were first reported in 1981. In 1986, the virus that causes acquired immunodeficiency syndrome (AIDS) was named HIV. According to the estimates of the World Health Organization (WHO), some 37–45 million people were living with the HIV by the end of 2005. HIV infection can be spread through several routes:

■ Percutaneous injuries, such as needlesticks, broken glass, and improper disposal of sharps

■ Intravenous drug abuse with contaminated needles

■ Mucous membrane exposure (splashes into the eyes, nasal passages, or oral cavity)

- Sexual intercourse with infected persons
- Intrauterine infection in babies born to infected mothers
- Blood transfusions

While AIDS was once considered to be a disease spread primarily through homosexual or bisexual practices, most new cases now appear among heterosexuals. Factors associated with the spread of HIV through intimate contact include multiple sexual partners; the type of sexual practices, especially those that result in mucosal trauma such as anal intercourse; and the use of recreational drugs such as cocaine, marijuana, and nitrate inhalants.

 REAL WORLD TIP

Health care workers have the risk of acquiring HBV, HCV, and HIV due to the nature of their work. The risk of infection, after exposure, for HBV is up to 30%, for HCV about 2%, and for HIV about 0.3%. It is strongly recommended that health care workers receive the HBV vaccine due to the high risk for acquiring the disease.

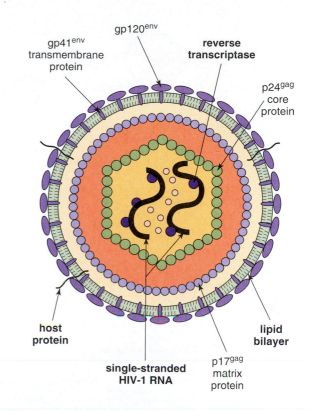

■ **FIGURE 31-28** Human immunodeficieney virus (HIV).
Reprinted from Male et al. (2006). Clinical Laboratory Immunology (7th ed.). Copyright 2006 with permission from Elsevier.

The HIV genome consists of two identical single-stranded RNA strands. The virion also carries three enzymes: reverse transcriptase, integrase, and protease. The two species of HIV that infect humans are HIV-1 and HIV-2. HIV-1 is seen throughout the world and is more virulent, while HIV-2 is more prevalent in West Africa. Like other retroviruses, HIV has *gag, pol,* and *env* genes. *Gag* codes for core and matrix proteins such as p24, p17, and p7/p9. *Pol* codes for the three HIV enzymes: reverse transcriptase, protease, and integrase. *Env* codes for envelope glycoproteins gp120 and gp41. The viral protease enzyme cleaves the product of the *env* gene, gp160, to produce gp120 and gp41. Viral reverse transcriptase is able to convert the RNA of HIV to double-stranded DNA, which is integrated into the host genome (Figure 31-28 ■).

HIV replication starts with the virus binding to its receptor on the host cell. After binding to its receptor, CD4 and a chemokine co-receptor, the outer membrane of HIV fuses with the host's cell membrane to gain entry into the cell. After internalization and uncoating, HIV enters the cytoplasm of the host cell where reverse transcriptase transcribes its single-stranded RNA into double-stranded DNA. The next step is for the newly transcribed viral cDNA to be transported into the nucleus where it is integrated into the host genome, creating the latent HIV provirus. This is accomplished by another viral enzyme called integrase. Eventually the provirus will be activated and begin transcription of massive quantities of its viral genome. This results in the production of viral mRNA inside the host nucleus. Next, the viral mRNA exits the nucleus of the

host cell. Once the RNA is transported into the cytoplasm, translation of viral proteins starts. Structural proteins for the new HIV nucleocaopsid and virion are produced and assembled in the cytoplasm. The final step is assembly of the new virions and maturation of HIV by viral proteases that cleave the viral poly proteins into functional HIV enzymes and proteins. This process occurs at the site of the cell membrane of the host cell. The viral *Env* protein (gp 160) is cleaved by the viral enzyme protease and processed into two HIV envelope glycoproteins gp 41 and gp 120. These two proteins allow newly formed viruses to infect new cells. Mature virus particles exit the host cell membrane through the process of budding and free HIV viruses are released. The newly created viruses go on to infect additional cells that have HIV receptors CD4 and chemokine co-receptor (Figure 31-29 ■).

Diagnosis, Therapy, and Prevention of HIV.
Enzyme immunoassay (EIA) is the method of choice for the detection of antibodies to HIV (Figure 31-30 ■). Western blot (immunoblot) is used as the confirmatory test to establish the diagnosis of HIV infection. In the immunoblot procedure, the patient's serum is added to nitrocellulose sheets on which HIV-antigens are bound. The serum of HIV-infected patients should contain antibodies that will attach to the HIV antigens on the nitrocellulose. A labeled antihuman antibody binds to the patient's antibody, producing specific bands upon completion

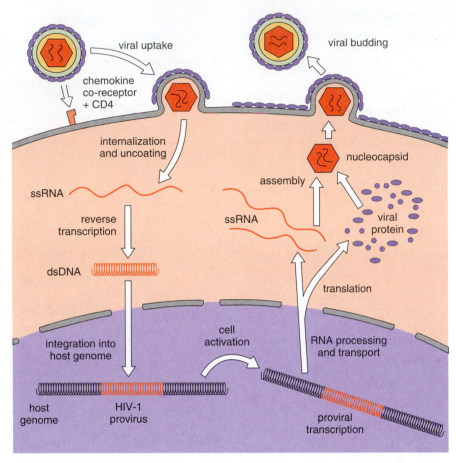

■ **FIGURE 31-29** HIV life cycle.
Reprinted from Male et al. (2006). Clinical Laboratory Immunology (7th ed.). Copyright 2006 with permission from Elsevier.

of the Western blot. This is very strong evidence of HIV infection (Figure 31-31 ■).

Viral load testing is the most commonly used molecular technique used in the diagnosis of HIV infection in clinical laboratories. The viral load methods used in clinical laboratories include HIV reverse transcriptase PCR (HIV RT-PCR), nucleic acid sequence-based amplification (NASBA), and branched chain DNA (bDNA). The lower limit viral detection for all three methods is at 40–50 copies/mol. Because a single measurement of viral load does not provide clinically desired information, a change in viral load over time must be observed to arrive at a conclusion regarding the success of treatment. In determining the viral load the number of HIV nucleic acid copies per milliliter of blood is calculated. This measurement is used to monitor therapy during chronic viral infections and to measure the severity of HIV infection. Highly active antiretroviral therapy (HAART) has been effective in reducing the emergence of mutant strains and in reducing the viral load.

On the basis of differences in the *env* gene, three groups of HIV isolates M, N, and O in humans have been identified, with group M being the most prevalent group. HIV vaccine development has encountered many obstacles because of the genetic properties and cellular effects of the virus. Besides the existence of different HIV strains, HIV envelope proteins recognized by the immune cells vary widely, particularly the viral envelope component gp120, which can be masked by conformational changes and by glycosylation (addition of a sugar molecule), making it difficult for the virus to be blocked with neutralizing antibodies. Viral tropism, which denotes the cell type the virus infects and replicates in, has become another obstacle in the development of an HIV vaccine. HIV attacks the very cells of the immune system that are designed to fight the infectious process in the first place. The macaque monkey has been used as the typical animal model of vaccine development. While some vaccines showed satisfactory results in macaques, humans that were immunized with similar constructs became infected later after exposure to HIV-1.

The FDA has approved a number of drugs to fight HIV infection. Reverse transcriptase inhibitors were the first type of drug used to treat HIV-infected individuals. As the name implies,

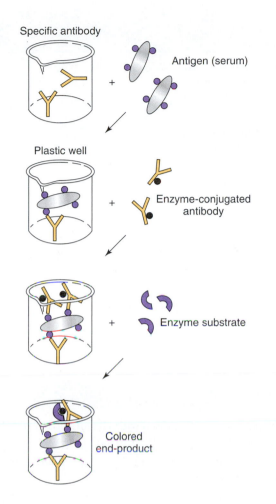

Specific antibody

Antigen (serum)

Plastic well

Enzyme-conjugated antibody

Enzyme substrate

Colored end-product

■ **FIGURE 31-30** Schematic flow diagram indirect sandwich immunoassay used in ELISA for the detection of antibodies in the serum of the HIV patients.
Modified from Mahon et al. (2006). Clinical Laboratory Immunology. Prentice Hall, 2006, with permission.

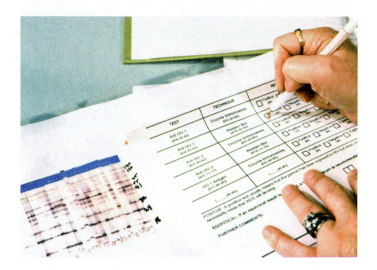

■ **FIGURE 31-31** CDC laboratory technician reporting a positive western blot result for HIV-1. The dark bands represent molecular size and indicate the presence of antibodies against the HIV envelope (P160, p120, and p41) and core protein (p24) antigens.

these drugs inhibit the reverse transcriptase enzymes, interfering with viral replication. Nucleoside/nucleotide analogues, another class of antiviral drugs, are compounds that are structurally similar to nucleotides. When they are incorporated into the HIV cDNA molecule, nonfunctional strands are created, once again inhibiting replication of the virus. A third class of drugs is the protease inhibitors. These drugs inhibit the enzymes that cleave the viral poly proteins into functional HIV proteins required for final assembly of the virus particle. The newest class of drugs approved to treat HIV infection is fusion inhibitors, which block merging of the virus envelope with the cell membrane. This interferes with the ability of HIV to enter into the host cell, denying the virus access to the machinery needed for viral replication.

SUMMARY

Intracellular microorganisms are small organisms that are larger than viruses but still too small to visualize. They share characteristics with bacteria but require living cells to grow and replicate. They live in epithelial cells or white blood cells.

Chlamydia and *Chlamydophila* cause infections ranging from sexually transmitted diseases to pneumonia depending on the species. Culture, serology, and cytology are used for detection. Ticks and lice are the vectors for *Rickettsia, Ehrlichia, Coxiella,* and others in this group. Rocky Mountain spotted fever, caused by *R. rickettsii,* is the most recognized disease in this group of intracellular microorganisms. Microscopy, PCR, culture, and serology are used for detection.

Viruses are completely dependent on living cells for their survival. They take over the cell and turn it into a living virus factory. Viral diseases range from the common cold to the always fatal hemorrhagic fever. The respiratory and gastrointestinal viruses are among the most commonly encountered.

Most laboratories do not have the resources to provide a full service virology laboratory but every laboratory can provide rapid direct testing for common viruses such as influenza A and B as well as respiratory syncytial virus. Many methods are available for the detection of viruses to include electron microscopy, cell culture, immunofluorescence, enzyme immunoassay, PCR, and serology. Often multiple methods must be used to detect a virus.

Antiviral agents are few and far between and resistance is developing. Many infections, due to viruses, may not have any treatment other than to relieve the signs and symptoms of the disease. Vaccination can be used to control some viruses.

LEARNING OPPORTUNITIES

1. Provide the (a) etiological agent, (b) scientific name, and (c) common name for the vectors of the following diseases: Rocky Mountain spotted fever, rickettsial pox, epidemic typhus, Q fever, and human monocytic ehrlichiosis. (Chapter Objectives 1 and 7)

2. Provide the etiological agents of the following diseases: trachoma, lymphogranuloma venereum, inclusion conjunctivitis, nongonococcal and postgonococcal urethritis, and psittacosis. (Chapter Objectives 1 and 7)

3. What are the five families of DNA viruses that cause disease in humans? (Chapter Objectives 1, 5, and 7)

4. What genus includes the hepatitis A virus? (Chapter Objectives 1 and 7)

5. What retrovirus is the etiological agent of acquired immunodeficiency syndrome (AIDS)? (Chapter Objectives 1 and 7)

6. What virus is the etiological agent of the German measles? (Chapter Objectives 1 and 7)

7. How does the reproductive cycle of chlamydiae differ from viruses? How is it the same? (Chapter Objective 6)

CASE STUDY 31-1 (CHAPTER OBJECTIVES 7, 8, AND 9)

A 40-year-old white male is seen in the emergency room complaining of shortness of breath, chills, fever, bloody cough, and fatigue. Over the last 30 months he has lost over 50 pounds. He complains that he started coughing about 1 month ago and his condition has been worsening. The fever began a week ago and his medical records show that he has been treated for a number of lower respiratory infections including influenza, bronchitis, and pneumonia. He has also contracted a number of urinary infections over the last 3 years. The patient was diagnosed to have contracted HIV and was treated with a combination of antiretroviral drugs.

1. The patient was diagnosed with HIV infection. List three common means of contracting HIV.

2. What are the two most common tests performed to diagnose HIV infection?

3. What lab test can be performed to evaluate the progression of HIV infection?

4. What are some of the antiretroviral drugs used to treated AIDS patients?

CASE STUDY 31-2 (CHAPTER OBJECTIVES 7 AND 9)

A 23-year-old female was seen by her gynecologist complaining of symptoms that included dysuria (pain and burning accompanying urination), polyuria (an increased frequency of urination) and an increased amount of cloudy discharge. Physical examination of the pelvic area disclosed no evidence of a foreign body or recent trauma. The patient had no significant history of allergies or any autoimmune diseases. She had not experienced any symptoms evident of a systemic disease (chills, fever, or malaise). She admitted to being sexually active over the past few years. Her current boyfriend had never admitted to having had any symptoms related to a sexually transmitted disease.

Her physician sent a cervical smear and vaginal swabs to the clinical laboratory for analysis. Her cervical smear was negative for the presence of abnormal cells suggestive of any malignant condition of the urogenital tract. A smear made from one of the vaginal swabs was Gram stained but no gram-negative diplococci were seen nor were gonococci isolated on the GC culture. A direct fluorescent antibody stain was performed on material from an urethral swab and the presence of intracellular and extracellular bodies exhibiting an apple-green fluorescence were noted.

1. What organism is the most likely cause of this patient's urogenital infection?

Use this address to access the interactive Companion Website created for this textbook. Simply select "Clinical Laboratory Science" from the choice of disciplines. Find this book and log in using your user name and password.

REFERENCES

Go to myhealthprofessionskit.com to view this chapter's references.

32

Cardiovascular System

Hassan Aziz

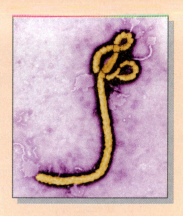

■ LEARNING OBJECTIVES

Upon completion of this chapter, the learner should be able to:

1. Describe the anatomy of the cardiovascular system.

   a. Describe the structure of the heart.

   b. Name the three types of blood vessels and explain their structure and functions.

   c. Outline the circulation of blood through the body.

2. Differentiate intravascular and extravascular infections.

3. Summarize the signs and symptoms associated with cardiovascular infections.

4. Identify factors that predispose an individual to bacteremia.

5. Differentiate bacteremia, sepsis, and septic shock.

   a. Determine potential sources of organisms for each.

   b. Correlate with the most common causative organisms.

6. Differentiate the two types of bacterial endocarditis

   a. Correlate with causative microorganisms.

7. Discuss the significance of catheter-related infections.

   a. Determine the source of potential pathogens.

   b. Correlate with the most common causative organisms.

8. Correlate patient history, signs and symptoms, identification testing results, and suscepti-bility testing results to determine the type of cardiovascular infection present, identify microor-ganisms, and assess their clinical significance.

9. Outline the blood culture collection procedure.

   a. Assess the importance of broth formulation, volume, timing, and additives when col-lecting a blood culture.

   b. Identify potential sources of errors.

10. Summarize methods used to process blood cultures.

    a. Note advantages, disadvantages, and limitations of each.

■ **LEARNING OBJECTIVES** (*continued*)

11. Summarize culture methods available for determining catheter-related infections.

12. Outline the handling of a positive blood culture.

13. Discuss criteria used to determine the significance of a blood culture isolate.

14. Describe special procedures used for detection, isolation, and identification of the following organisms in blood cultures:

    a. *Leptospira interrogans*

    b. *Brucella* spp.

    c. Nutritionally variant *Streptococcus*

    d. *Bartonella henselae*

    e. Fungi

    f. *Mycobacterium* spp.

    g. HACEK

KEY TERMS

acute bacterial
  endocarditis

bacteremia

biofilm

disseminated
  intravascular
  coagulation

emboli

endocarditis

extravascular infection

hemodynamics

intermittent bacteremia

intravascular infection

sepsis

septicemia

septic shock

subacute bacterial
  endocarditis (SBE)

transient bacteremia

▶ INTRODUCTION

The cardiovascular system consists of the heart and a network of vessels that circulates blood throughout the body. Its main function is to deliver nutrients to cells in the tissues and to remove metabolic waste. This function is carried out by the capillaries. Because the cardiovascular system circulates blood throughout the body, it can serve as a vehicle for the spread of infection. The blood is considered a sterile environment. Microorganisms recovered from blood usually indicate an infection. Their presence may be because of trauma, surgical wounds, burns, or secondary to other infections in the body. Microorganisms in the blood is one of the most serious infections encountered in the clinical microbiology laboratory. Timely detection and identification are key to positive patient outcomes. The purpose of this chapter is to describe the types of bloodstream infections and methods for detection and identification of the most common isolates capable of producing such infections.

▶ REVIEW OF ANATOMY AND PHYSIOLOGY

A review of the anatomy and physiology of the cardiovascular system is important to understand the function of each component and its potential for developing an infectious disease. Because the cardiovascular system circulates blood to all parts of the body, it can pick up or deliver potential pathogens at any point of the process.

ANATOMY

The cardiovascular system includes the heart and the blood vessels. The heart sits slightly left of center in the chest cavity behind the sternum bone. It is about the size of a man's fist. Three distinct layers of tissue make up the heart wall: epicardium, the outer layer of the wall of the heart; myocardium, the muscle of the heart; and endocardium, the inner layer of the heart. The heart is a four-chambered muscular organ (Figure 32-1 ■). Two chambers are on each side of the heart. One chamber is on the top, and one on the bottom. Each top chamber is called an atrium (plural: atria). The atria are the top chambers which receive the blood returning to the heart from the body and lungs. The two chambers on the bottom are called the ventricles. Their job is to send out the blood from the heart to the body and lungs. Separating the left side and the right side of the heart is a thick wall of muscle called the septum. Inside the heart are valves that regulate the flow of the blood. Two of the heart valves are the mitral or bicuspid valve and the tricuspid valve. They let blood flow from the atria to the ventricles. The other two are called the aortic valve and pulmonary valve, and they are in charge of controlling the flow as the blood leaves the ventricles. All the valves work to keep the blood flowing forward in one direction. Myocardial cells receive their blood by way of the coronary arteries, which wrap around the heart. The heart is encapsulated in a loose-fitting inflexible sac called the pericardium. Figure 32-1 shows the heart's anatomy and blood flow to and from the heart as well as inside the heart.

The blood leaves the heart through blood vessels, which channel and deliver it throughout the body. The blood vessels are formed by arteries, which lead to smaller arterioles and even smaller capillaries. The smaller capillaries connect with the small venules, which then lead to the veins. Arteries and veins have the same three tissue layers, but the proportions of these layers differ. The innermost layer is the tunica intima, next comes the tunica media; and the outermost is the tunica adventitia. Arteries pulse, in rhythm with the heart, to carry blood filled with nutrients away from the heart to all parts of the body. Veins, on the other hand, carry blood from the tissues toward the heart. The microscopic capillaries carry blood from the arterioles to the venules, where the vital functions of delivery and collection of essential materials and oxygen to and from the cells and tissues take place.

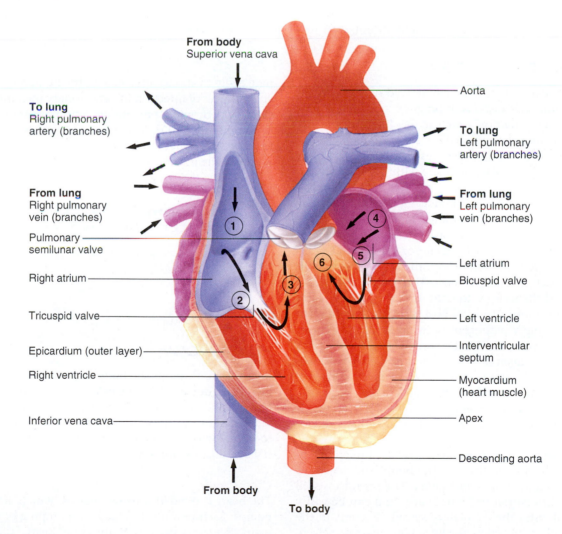

■ FIGURE 32-1 This illustration of the heart displays its external and internal anatomy. The pattern of blood flow to the heart, through it, and away from it is diagrammed.

**Checkpoint! 32–1
(Chapter Objectives 1, 1b, and 1c)**

*Which of the following statements is **correct** in regard to human blood vessels?*

A. *Arteries and veins have the same four tissue layers but with different proportions.*

B. *The inner most layer of an artery is the tunica media.*

C. *Veins carry blood away from the heart.*

D. *Capillaries carry blood from arterioles to venules, where the vital functions of delivery of oxygen transport and waste removal take place.*

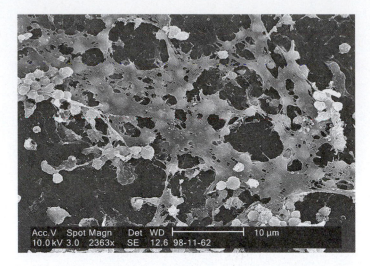

| Acc.V | Spot | Magn | Det | WD | | 10 μm |
| 10.0 kV | 3.0 | 2363x | SE | 12.6 | 98-11-62 | |

■ **FIGURE 32-2** This photograph is an electron microscope image of the interior of a catheter. The individual cells of *Staphylococcus aureus* are held tightly together and to the surface of the catheter with a sticky mesh the bacteria secrete. The organisms are protected by the biofilm from antibiotics as well as the host defenses.
From CDC, Rodney M. Dolan, PhD, and Janice Carr.

The lymphatic system is an integral part of the circulation of blood. Its two main functions are maintenance of fluid balance and immunity. Plasma, from the capillary blood, filters into interstitial or tissue spaces. Most of the fluid is absorbed by the surrounding tissue or reabsorbed by the blood. The remaining fluid is collected by lymphatic vessels and returned to the blood before it enters the heart right atrium.

SOURCES OF INFECTION

The cardiovascular system is usually devoid of microorganisms (sterile) unless a disease is in progress. Infection is considered a serious situation and can be life threatening. Organisms can enter the enclosed system by different methods. There are two major categories of blood infections. **Intravascular infections** originate within the cardiovascular system. Organisms can be directly introduced to the bloodstream by the use of intravenous catheters, artificial heart valves, a pacemaker, and arterial lines. Many patients in the hospital are critically ill and often have at least one intravenous line for the administration of fluids and/or antibiotics. Organisms are able to grow and flourish on the artificial surface of a device. The bacteria build up a **biofilm**, or a web of sticky material around themselves, to hold onto the surface better and prevent antibiotics and the host immune system from reaching them. Many pathogens of intravascular infections are those usually considered to be normal skin flora, such as *Staphylococcus* not *Staphylococcus aureus* and *Corynebacterium* spp. *Staphylococcus aureus*, members of the *Enterobacteriaceae*, *Pseudomonas aeruginosa*, and *Candida* spp. are also frequently isolated. Figure 32-2 ■ illustrates the sticky biofilm mass, which can help the organisms remain attached to the catheter surface as well as protect them from antibiotics.

Extravascular infections are the result of microorganisms entering the system through the lymphatic system or other routes such as surgery or trauma. The organisms spill over into the interstitial or tissue spaces and can be easily picked up and enter the circulatory system. Bacteria in the blood are usually removed by the liver, bone marrow, spleen, or circulating white blood cells. If the number of bacteria present overwhelms the body's defenses then they can dissemi-

nate easily to almost anywhere in the human body. Extravascular sources of infection include urinary tract infection, pericarditis, peritonitis, pneumonia, and pressure sores (Mahon & Manuselis, 2000). The potential pathogens that cause extravascular infections vary and depend on the original source of the infection.

 **Checkpoint! 32–2
(Chapter Objective 2)**

Extravascular infections are the result of microorganisms originating within the cardiovascular system.

A. *True*

B. *False*

PHYSIOLOGY

Blood flows through the body to provide fresh oxygenated blood and nutrients for the cells and removes waste and carbon dioxide from them. Knowledge of the flow of blood provides a better understanding of the importance of proper specimen selection and collection for venipuncture and arterial blood gases samples.

Circulation

The heart is divided into two halves, which act as separate pumps. Each pump is in charge of pumping blood into two main circulatory systems. In the "right heart," the pulmonary circulation delivers blood to and from the lungs. The pulmonary artery carries oxygen-poor blood from the "right heart" to the lungs, where oxygenation and carbon dioxide removal occur. Pulmonary veins carry oxygen-rich blood from the lungs back to the "left heart." Systemic circulation, driven by the "left heart," carries blood to the rest of the body. The aorta is the main artery for systemic circulation. Blood ultimately return to the "right heart" via the inferior and superior vena cavae. The atria and ventricles work as a team—the atria fill with blood and deliver it into the ventricles. The ventricles then squeeze, pumping blood out of the heart. While the ventricles are squeezing, the atria refill and get ready for the next contraction (Figure 32-3 ■).

Disease Processes

Cardiovascular infections range from being asymptomatic, which resolve without treatment, to serious and life threatening. Healthy individuals rarely develop life-threatening cardiovascular infections. However, when microorganisms are introduced directly into the cardiovascular system of immuno-compromised individuals, serious medical complications may develop.

Symptoms

The typical signs and symptoms of systemic cardiovascular infection include tachypnea, or rapid breathing, shaking chills, fever, abdominal pain, nausea, vomiting, and diarrhea (Beers, 2003). Some patients may exhibit diminished mental alertness and hypotension, or a drop in blood pressure. **Hemodynamics** is the force by which the heart pumps blood through the body. Hemodynamic instability occurs in 25% to 40% of infected patients and increases the risk of developing **septic shock**, which is a potentially fatal systemic response to a bloodstream infection. Septic shock symptoms include

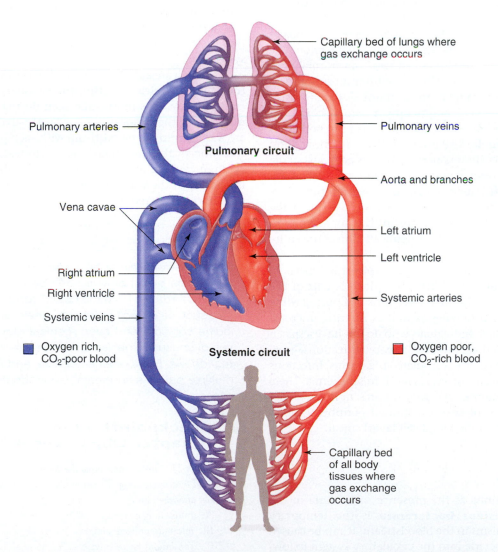

Capillary bed of lungs where gas exchange occurs

Pulmonary arteries

Pulmonary veins

Pulmonary circuit

Aorta and branches

Vena cavae

Left atrium

Left ventricle

Right atrium

Right ventricle

Systemic arteries

Systemic veins

■ Oxygen rich, CO$_2$-poor blood

■ Oxygen poor, CO$_2$-rich blood

Systemic circuit

Capillary bed of all body tissues where gas exchange occurs

■ **FIGURE 32-3** This illustrates the blood flow through the heart and the body. The arteries, in red, deliver the blood's oxygen and nutrients to the cells, whereas the capillaries of the veins, in blue, pick up carbon dioxide and waste.

low blood pressure, decreased consciousness, rapid heart and breathing rates, and multiple organ failures (Beers, 2003).

 Checkpoint! 32–3 (Chapter Objective 3)

The most dangerous symptom of cardiovascular infections is
  A. *chills.*
  B. *abdominal pain.*
  C. *vomiting.*
  D. *hemodynamic instability.*

▶ SPECIFIC DISEASES

Hospitalized individuals who are at the age extremes, such as the elderly, and those with progressive diseases, such as cancer, are at risk for infection. Many procedures used in today's medical settings can predispose an individual to infection. The use of broad-spectrum antibiotics can wipe out normal flora and promote resistant strains. The use of immunosuppressive agents such as steroids dampens the immune system. Invasive procedures such as surgery, endoscopy or colonoscopy, and dental extraction can introduce microorganisms to body sites that are normally sterile. The use of indwelling urinary and intravenous catheters allows microorganisms access to sterile environments. Extension of underlying infections such as urinary tract infections, meningitis, and pneumonia allow microorganisms to travel to other body sites through the bloodstream. All provide microorganisms the opportunity to reach beyond a local infection to systemically infect the entire body.

An individual who does not have a spleen is especially prone to bloodstream infections. The spleen is part of the immunity system and helps fight infections by housing white blood cells, creating antibodies as well as filtering microorganisms from the blood. Individuals who do not have a spleen are called asplenic and are prone to massive infections, especially with those caused by encapsulated organisms. Infections in an asplenic patient almost always result in septicemia. There is often such a large number of organisms present in the bloodstream that they can be seen on stained peripheral blood smears or buffy coat (white blood cell layer) smear.

BACTEREMIA

Bacteremia is defined as the presence of bacteria in the bloodstream. **Transient bacteremia** is the temporary appearance of organisms in the bloodstream. It can be caused by inoculation of bacteria into the circulatory system following dental procedures, insertion of a urinary catheter, incision and drainage of an abscess, and colonization of indwelling devices such as an intravenous catheter. Even the simple act of brushing your teeth can introduce bacteria into the bloodstream. In most instances, bacteria are usually present for only about 30 to 45 minutes. The immune system of healthy individuals removes the transient organisms easily. The liver and spleen help filter them out of the blood. Transient bacteremia is important because it can lead to **endocarditis**, infection of the endocardium or heart valves, in individuals with previously damaged heart valves or artificial heart valves. The organisms are able to latch onto the damaged or artificial surface and begin to grow.

In **intermittent bacteremia**, bacteria are released periodically from a site of infection and may have little effect on a healthy person, but it may be seriously important in immunocompromised patients with debilitating underlying conditions. The primary site of infection is usually in the lungs, genitourinary or gastrointestinal tracts, or tissue infections such as a decubitus ulcer (Beers, 2003). Organisms spill over into the bloodstream and are then cleared by the body's natural defenses. The process repeats itself until the original infection is cleared or the bacteria are able overcome the immune system.

If bacteria are able to overcome the host's immune system, then they are released within the vascular system at a fairly constant rate. It is most often seen during endocarditis, an infection of the endocardium or heart valves. The organisms are washed into the bloodstream with each pump of the heart. Infection of the meninges; the peritoneal, pleural, or pericardium cavities; and the reticuloendothelial system, which is made up of the bone marrow, spleen, and liver, can result in continuous bacteremia

 REAL WORLD TIP

Pseudobacteremia or false bacteremia is contamination of the blood after it has been collected from a patient. It results from the use of contaminated materials such as collection tubes or their rubber stoppers, iodine solution, and even medical gloves. The isolation of unusual organisms such as *Stenotrophomonas maltophilia*, *Burkholderia cepacia*, and *Bacillus* spp. in multiple patients suggests pseudobacteremia.

 Checkpoint! 32–4 (Chapter Objectives 4 and 5)

A healthy 21-year-old male visits the dentist for his annual examination and routine cleaning. The most likely type of bacteremia he could display after the visit is
  A. *transient bacteremia.*
  B. *intermittent bacteremia.*
  C. *continuous bacteremia.*
  D. *septic shock.*

SEPSIS

The terms **sepsis** and **septicemia** are often used interchangeably to describe the presence of actively dividing bacteria in the blood, their harmful by-products and the subsequent activation of the body's inflammation and immune response (Forbes & Weissfeld, 2002). It is a serious, rapidly progressing, life-threatening infection that can arise from infections throughout the body such as the lungs, abdomen, urinary tract, bones, central nervous system (CNS), or other tissues.

The process of sepsis is complex and results from the effects of circulating bacterial products on the host's cells and immune system and the subsequent cytokine release from neighboring cells. Sepsis usually occurs as a result of continuous bacteremia (Warren, 1997). The septic patient displays an increased body temperature, increased heart and respiratory rates, and a high white blood cell count. Although sepsis can affect a person of any age, it is more prevalent in young infants and people whose immune systems are compromised, such as the elderly and those with chronic illnesses. Sepsis can escalate to septic shock.

SEPTIC SHOCK

Septic shock results from the action of by-products of actively dividing organisms on the body and the body's reaction to these bacterial by-products. The most serious cases of septic shock are usually because of gram-negative rods, but it can also be caused by a variety of microorganisms. Bacterial endotoxins, such as lipopolysaccharide (LPS) found in the cell wall of gram-negative organisms, as well as exotoxins and other by-products, can cause damage to the endothelium of the blood vessels, trigger a massive attack by the body's immune system, and disrupt several body functions. The patient's blood pressure drops, and blood flow to the organs is decreased. The bacterial by-products inflame the body's cells, disrupt temperature regulation, deplete plasma complement, cause the blood vessels to leak and upset the metabolism of the body's cells so they become hypercatabolic. **Disseminated intravascular coagulation** (DIC) is a potentially fatal coagulation complication caused by sepsis. It begins with the development of clots in the blood vessels through out the body initiated by the by-products of the microorganisms and damaged cells. The body recognizes the clotting as an abnormal situation, so it begins to lyse them. This clot–lyse pattern continues until all the clotting factors are eventually used up. With all this chaos, the body can't move fluids and oxygen to the tissues, which leads to oxygen depletion, electrolyte and acid–base imbalance, and eventually complete organ failure. Once the cascade of events begins, it is difficult to stop, and a high mortality rate is associated with septic shock.

ENDOCARDITIS

Bacterial endocarditis is an infection of the heart's inner lining (endocardium) or the heart valves (American Heart Association, 2005). It occurs when bacteria, present in the blood, become lodged on abnormal, damaged, or artificial heart valves. Those with a history of rheumatic fever are at high risk because of the damage caused to the heart valves by previously untreated throat infections caused by *Streptococcus pyogenes* (group A beta *Streptococcus*). Intravenous drug use also puts an individual at risk for endocarditis.

Although several different microorganisms can cause endocarditis, it is usually caused by bacteria. As the bacteria grow on the damaged valvular area, they cause turbulence or a change in the force of the blood flow within the heart. With turbulence, there is often more tissue damage, after which platelets and fibrin deposits move in to repair the damage. The bacteria become embedded in the platelet–fibrin web, which now protects them from the host's immune system as well as antibiotics. As they continue to grow more turbulence is created, and eventually pieces of the mass break off to travel to blood vessels to cause blocks in the vessels know as emboli. If **emboli** (singular: embolus), or tiny clots of blood, fibrin, and organisms, lodge in the brain or lung, it can prove to be fatal. Figure 32-4 ■ shows the splinter fingernail hemorrhages characteristic of a patient with endocarditis. These thin streaklike hemorrhages are caused by tiny clots of organisms, fibrin, and platelets that have traveled from the heart to the small capillaries. Once blocked, the capillaries begin to leak and bleed under the skin. Figure 32-5 ■ shows the left ventricle of a heart at autopsy. The mitral valve has been opened to reveal masses because of the growth of bacteria as seen with endocarditis.

Bacterial endocarditis can be classified as either **subacute bacterial endocarditis (SBE)**, which progresses gradually with time, or **acute bacterial endocarditis**, which progresses rapidly. In cases of subacute bacterial endocarditis, infection is often because of less virulent organisms such as the *Streptococcus* viridans group. The *Streptococcus* viridans group are gram-positive cocci that are part of the normal oral flora. They account for up to 60% of cases of SBE in individuals with abnormal or damaged heart valves. SBE takes a more chronic course and develops slowly over weeks to months. More invasive and virulent bacteria such as *Staphylococcus*

ⓔ REAL WORLD TIP

Biological markers can assist with the rapid diagnosis of sepsis. Markers such as pro-atrial natriuretic peptide (ANP), procalcitonin (PCT), C-reactive protein (CRP), calcineurin B homologous protein (CHP) and interleukin (IL-6) increase with severe sepsis and septic shock. Earlier detection of sepsis means the physician can begin therapy, even before blood cultures grow.

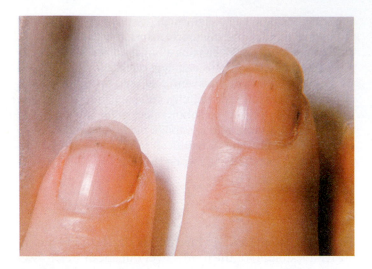

■ **FIGURE 32-4** This photograph shows a patient with splinter hemorrhages under her fingernails. Endocarditis causes tiny clots to be thrown into the bloodstream. The clots damage the small capillaries and cause bleeding under the skin. Although associated with endocarditis, splinter hemorrhages can also be because of trauma to the fingernail.
From CDC and Dr. Thomas F. Sellers from Emory University.

aureus result in a more fulminate, faster developing, or acute bacterial endocarditis (American Heart Association, 2005).

Patients with endocarditis often have heart murmurs because of the turbulence created by the masses and the subsequent damage to the heart and valves. The murmur can

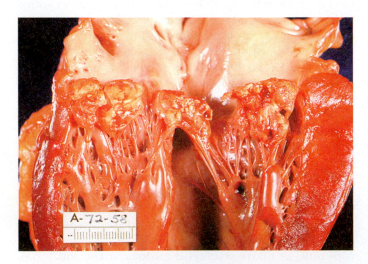

■ **FIGURE 32-5** This is the heart of a patient who died because of endocarditis. The left ventricle has been opened to reveal the mitral valve. The yellow masses, on the mitral valve, are made up of fibrin, platelets, and microorganisms. These masses disrupt the blood flow to cause damage to the heart as well as continuously seed organisms into the blood and throughout the body.
From CDC and Dr. Edwin P. Ewing, Jr.

become more pronounced as the disease progresses. Untreated, endocarditis permanently damages the endocardium and causes heart valve malfunction, which leads to congestive heart failure. Infection spreads via the bloodstream, usually as a continuous bacteremia and eventually to other parts of the body.

 Checkpoint! 32–5 (Chapter Objective 6)

The Streptococcus viridans *group, the most common cause of subacute bacterial endocarditis, originates as part of the normal _____ flora.*

   A. *skin*
   B. *gastrointestinal*
   C. *oral*
   D. *genital*

CATHETER-RELATED INFECTIONS

Catheters are used daily in hospitals to provide acute and long-term patients with fluids, drugs, and blood products as well as drain fluids such as urine from the patient. These plastic medical devices, although essential for care, put patients at risk for intravascular catheter-related infections. Intravenous and urinary catheters provide a highway for microorganisms to migrate from the skin surface to the blood or urine.

Intravenous catheters tend to be the most common source of bacteremia in patients in the intensive care units. The organisms colonize the device by creating a slime layer to help them attach to the device and protect them from antibiotics. They eventually reach the tip of the catheter and can then reach the interior of the device. Organisms can also reach the interior of the catheter through the hub, where the catheter attaches to the bag of fluids being given or removed. Once microorganisms are established, the catheter becomes a constant source of infection. Catheter-related infections increase the likelihood a patient will expire while in the hospital as well as add to the patient's length of stay, antibiotic use, and hospital costs.

The most common organisms associated with catheter-related infections are those found as part of the normal skin flora. They include *Staphylococcus* not *Staphylococcus aureus*, *Staphylococcus aureus*, *Corynebacterium* spp., especially *C. jeikeium*, and *Candida* spp. Bacteremia in a patient with an intravascular catheter may be difficult to diagnose. A physician should suspect a catheter-related infection when the patient exhibits fever and chills but there is no apparent source of infection. Blood cultures and culture of the catheter tip are required to make the diagnosis. A catheter-related infection is confirmed by the isolation of the same species of organism with the same susceptibility results from both cultures.

There have been reported cases of nosocomial bacteremia and sepsis because of the use of contaminated commercial intravenous fluid. Gram-negative bacteria such as *Enterobacter* spp. and *Klebsiella* spp. have been implicated. The organisms are able to reproduce at room temperature, and it is their by-products that cause the signs and symptoms of septicemia. The organisms' by-products are introduced into the vein of the patient with the fluid. Often the use of antibiotics has no effect because organisms may not be present, and antibiotics have no effect on their by-products. The patient improves when the contaminated fluid is discontinued.

TREATMENT

Antibiotics are usually effective against bacteremia. Close observation is required to guard against progression of bacteremia to septic shock. Because bacteremia is usually associated with an existing infection elsewhere in the body, finding and treating the initial source of infection is an important part of treatment. In some cases, such as gangrene of the intestine or gallbladder, surgery is mandatory. Large abscesses must be incised and drained and necrotic tissue removed (Beers, 2003). Transient bacteremia is often undetected and requires no therapy, except in patients especially at risk for infection, such as those with heart valve defects or whose immune systems are suppressed (Fauci, 1997). Individuals with damaged or artificial valves can receive antibiotics prior to procedures, such as teeth cleaning, to reduce the risk of endocarditis. One issue that has risen from this practice is the potential for increased antibiotic resistance. Catheter-related infections require the removal of the device in addition to antibiotics. Antibiotics alone will not resolve a catheter infection. They cannot penetrate the biofilm created by the organisms on the intravenous catheter. Removal of the device is necessary to remove the source of organisms.

REAL WORLD TIP

Effective October 1, 2008, Medicare no longer reimburses most hospitals for vascular catheter-associated infections on inpatients. If the infection is not present at the time of admission, Medicare will only reimburse for the original admitting diagnosis but not the complication of acquiring a vascular catheter-associated infection. Many of the conditions implemented for payment adjustments, as well as others being considered, are related to hospital-acquired infections. Most private insurance companies follow the lead of Medicare for reimbursement.

Prompt antibiotic therapy usually succeeds in clearing bacteria from the bloodstream. Recurrence may indicate an undiscovered site of infection. Untreated bacteria in the blood may spread, causing infection of the heart (endocarditis or pericarditis) or infection of the covering of the central nervous system (meningitis).

COMMON ISOLATES

Bacteremia can be caused by a variety of organisms; however, gram-positive organisms tend to be more frequently isolated. It is rare for bacteremia to be polymicrobic or caused by multiple organisms. It is usually caused by the presence of a single organism. Bacteria such as *Staphylococcus* not *Staphylococcus aureus*, *Staphylococcus aureus*, *Enterococcus* spp., *Streptococcus viridans* group, *Streptococcus pneumoniae*, and the beta-hemolytic *Streptococcus* are the most frequently isolated. The *Enterobacteriaceae* such as *E. coli*, *Enterobacter* spp., *Klebsiella* spp., and *Proteus* spp., as well as *Pseudomonas aeruginosa*, tend to cause bacteremia as the result of distant infections such as a urinary tract infection, pneumonia, and peritonitis, which allow bacteria to enter the bloodstream. *Pasteurella multocida*, *Staphylococcus intermedius*, and *Capnocytophaga canimorsus* can be found in the blood after animal bites. Anaerobes, especially *Bacteroides* spp. and *Clostridium* spp. can cause septicemia because of an infection such as appendicitis or abdominal surgery.

REAL WORLD TIP

Because of the integrity of the gastrointestinal (GI) tract, microorganisms rarely escape unless there is a lesion such as seen with colon cancer. The presence of certain GI organisms in the blood often indicates undiagnosed cancer of the colon. Organisms rarely seen in blood but associated with colon cancer include *Streptococcus gallolyticus* (formerly *S. bovis*), *Clostridium septicum*, *Campylobacter* spp., *Aeromonas hydrophila*, and *Plesiomonas shigelloides*.

Candida spp. and other fungi are usually found in the blood of immunocompromised patients or those with serious underlying illness. One yeast, *Malassezia furfur*, is known for its love of lipids. It is part of the skin flora and has been recovered from the blood cultures of patients especially neonates, receiving intravenous lipid-based nutrition. Oil must be added to agar plates to ensure its growth. The presence of any fungi in the blood should direct the physician to look for an infection somewhere else in the body as the source.

About 60% of cases of infective endocarditis of abnormal or damaged heart valves are because of the *Streptococcus* viridans group, which are members of the normal oral flora. One unique member of the *Streptococcus* viridans group of organisms is nutritionally variant *Streptococcus* (NVS). Two species within the NVS are *Abiotrophia* spp. and *Granulicatella* spp. The NVS are fastidious and very difficult to isolate from blood cultures. Culture techniques for these organisms will be discussed later in this chapter. Endocarditis immediately after insertion of artificial heart valves is usually caused by *Staphylococcus* spp., gram-negative rods, and *Candida* spp. Intravenous drug users are known to develop endocarditis because of *Staphylococcus aureus*.

Other organisms associated with endocarditis include *Enterococcus* spp., *Streptococcus gallolyticus*, *Pseudomonas aeruginosa*, and the HACEK (*Haemophilus parainfluenzae*, *Aggregatibacter aphrophilus*, *Aggregatibacter actinomycetemcomitans* [formerly known as *Actinobacillus actinomycetemcomitans*], *Cardiobacterium hominis*, *Eikenella corrodens*, and *Kingella* spp.) group. Members of the HACEK group are normal oral flora that can be released into the blood with dental procedures, tongue piercings, periodontal disease and injuries associated with human bites or fistfights. These organisms are slow growing and may be missed on culture if the agar plates are not incubated for at least 1 to 2 weeks in CO_2. Special culture procedures are discussed later in this chapter.

REAL WORLD TIP

There have been increasing reports of endocarditis associated with body piercings. *Staphylococcus* spp. endocarditis after nasal piercing, *Neisseria mucosa* and *Aggregatibacter aphrophilus* (formerly known as *Haemophilus aphrophilus*) endocarditis after tongue piercing, and *Staphylococcus epidermidis* endocarditis after nipple piercing have been reported (Akhondi & Rahimi, 2002).

Catheters used to deliver fluids and antibiotics can also deliver microorganisms directly to the bloodstream. Often the potential pathogens of catheter-related infections are members of the normal skin flora or organisms associated with being in a hospital environment. Gram-positive organisms are much more common than gram-negative in catheter-related infections. Potential pathogens include *Staphylococcus* not *Staphylococcus aureus*, *Staphylococcus aureus*, *Enterococcus* spp. *Corynebacterium* spp., especially *C. jeikeium*, *Candida albicans*, and gram-negative rods such as *E. coli* and *Pseudomonas aeruginosa*. Box 32-1 ✪ summarizes the most commonly encountered bacteria associated with cardiovascular infections.

Some parasites are able to thrive in the bloodstream. They are usually visualized on stained smears of the peripheral blood. *Plasmodium* spp. and *Babesia* spp. infect the red blood cells. *Trypanosoma* spp. and microfilariae can be seen swimming among the red blood cells in the peripheral blood. Viruses need living cells to survive. Although they do not infect red blood cells, they do have the ability to infect the white

blood cells. The human immunodeficiency virus (HIV) is known for its ability to attack and destroy T lymphocytes.

✪ BOX 32-1

The Most Common Organisms Associated with Bacteremia

- *Staphylococcus aureus*
- *Staphylococcus* not *Staphylococcus aureus*
- *Streptococcus pneumoniae*
- *Enterococcus* spp.
- *Streptococcus viridans* group
- Beta-hemolytic *Streptococcus*
- Enterobacteriaceae
  - *Escherichia coli*
  - *Klebsiella* spp.
  - *Enterobacter* spp.
- *Pseudomonas* spp.
- Anaerobes
  - *Bacteroides* spp.
  - *Clostridium* spp.
- *Candida* spp.

✓ Checkpoint! 32–6 (Chapter Objectives 5 and 5b)

Bacteremia can be caused by a variety of organisms. Which of the following tends to be the most frequently isolated?

    A. *gram-positive cocci*
    B. *gram-negative rods*
    C. *gram-positive rods*
    D. *gram-negative cocci*

▶ SPECIMEN COLLECTION AND INOCULATION

Virtually any organism may cause bacteremia. The isolation of any organism from a blood culture should be considered significant. Clinical laboratories consider positive blood cultures as a critical value and call the results as soon as detected. The physician must correlate the laboratory results with the patient's clinical picture to determine if septicemia exists. The ideal specimen for a blood culture is one that is obtained immediately before a rise in temperature, which is the time of the highest concentration of circulating organism. Blood cultures should be drawn prior to starting antibiotics whenever possible. In an emergency, blood cultures should still be drawn as soon as possible after institution of antibiotics. Most blood culture broths have added substances that absorb antibiotics, so any organism present can grow easier.

Fever is the classic sign of bacterial infection. When bacteria are released into the bloodstream, the body has a slightly delayed reaction, and it takes about 45 minutes for a fever to appear. If a physician wants blood cultures drawn based on a patient's fever, they should be monitored and drawn about 30 minutes prior to the development of the next fever.

A patient exhibits a fever about 45 minutes after the appearance of bacteria in the blood, so predicting the presence of bacteria in the blood during intermittent bacteremia can be very difficult. It is recommended that two to three blood culture sets be obtained from different venipuncture sites at no less than hourly intervals within a 24-hour period to achieve optimum blood culture sensitivity. A blood culture set traditionally consists of an aerobic bottle for the isolation of aerobic and facultative anaerobic organisms and an anaerobic bottle for the isolation of obligate anaerobes. It is generally agreed that obtaining more than three blood culture sets within a 24-hour period does not result in a significant increase in positive results. In the absence of antibiotic administration, 99.6% culture positivity can be seen with the collection of three blood culture sets (Mahon, 2000). Following an initial response to therapy, collection of additional blood cultures may be indicated if the patient fails to respond to appropriate antimicrobial therapy or develops a new episode of fever or sepsis. Endocarditis can usually be detected with a single blood culture because of the continuous bacteremia present. A single blood culture will be positive in 90 to 95% of cases. A second blood culture will establish the diagnosis in >98% of patients with endocarditis.

REAL WORLD TIP

- Many laboratory information systems have the ability to limit the number of cultures ordered within a 24-hour period. Only tests that are medically necessary should be ordered to support the diagnosis. Because collecting more than three blood cultures within a 24-hour period is usually not considered medically necessary, they may not be reimbursed by insurance companies.

- Since the 1970s, it has been long been held as true that almost all bloodstream infections can be detected with two to three blood cultures sets. Recent studies have shown that as many as four sets over a 24-hour period may be necessary to achieve a detection rate of >99% (Lee, Mirrett, Reller, & Weinstein, 2007).

Blood should be obtained from peripheral venous or arterial sites. Obtaining blood cultures from central venous catheters, arterial lines, and inguinal vessels increases the likelihood of obtaining a false-positive blood culture. The practice of drawing blood for culture from catheters or the groin should not be performed when a peripheral (i.e., noncatheterized) site is available. It is very difficult to ensure a catheter is disinfected adequately to ensure blood collected from it will not be contaminated. If a limb with an intravenous catheter is used for blood culture collection, blood should be drawn above the catheter to ensure the blood collected is not diluted with the fluid being infused. The procedure for obtaining a suitable specimen for blood culture is a two-step process—preparation of the site for the collection of the blood specimen and the collection itself. The procedure for collecting the optimal blood culture specimen is detailed in Box 32-2 .

REAL WORLD TIP

Always check expiration dates of the blood culture bottles before collecting specimens and before loading them into the instrument.

✪ BOX 32-2

Blood Culture Collection Procedure

1. Prepare the venipuncture site as follows: Phlebotomist must wear gloves and can choose to use a face shield.
   - Cleanse the skin with 70% alcohol to defat the skin.
   - Apply tincture of iodine in a circular fashion away from the venipuncture site, or use chlorhexidine to kill surface and subsurface bacteria.
      - If povidone-iodine is used, It is critical that the iodine remain on the skin surface for 1.5 to 2 minutes.
   - Remove the iodine with 70% alcohol and allow to air-dry.
      - Some individuals are sensitive to the iodine used so it is very important to clean it off completely.
   - After preparing the venipuncture site, DO NOT palpate the site unless a sterile glove is used.
2. While waiting for the site to dry, the plastic cap covering each blood culture bottle should be removed, and the rubber stoppers should be decontaminated with 70% alcohol. Allow to air-dry.
   - Iodine solutions will disintegrate the rubber stopper of blood culture bottles and should not be used.
3. Apply a tourniquet above the venipuncture site.
4. Draw 5 to 10 mL of blood, depending on the type of container used. In infants and young children, 1 to 2 mL of blood is acceptable.
5. Mix the bottles by gently inverting.
6. Transport specimens at room temperature.

REAL WORLD TIP

To ensure confidentiality and privacy of the patient, collect the correct amount and label all containers accurately prior to leaving the patient's side.

 REAL WORLD TIP

Blood cultures may be collected by nonlaboratory personnel in some clinical facilities. It is essential to provide the proper training to these individuals to ensure a reduced rate of contamination.

Skin antisepsis is extremely important at the time of collection of a blood culture sample to avoid contamination. Tincture of iodine (1% to 2%) left in contact with skin for 30 seconds, povidone-iodine (10%) left in contact with skin for 1.5 to 2 minutes, and chlorhexidine (0.5% in 70% alcohol) left in contact with skin for 30 seconds are ideal agents (Isenberg, 2003; Hall & Lyman, 2006). However, some individuals may be hypersensitive to iodine present in some of these agents.

The medium used in blood culture bottles is multipurpose and nutritionally enriched. Tryptic or trypticase soy, supplemented peptone broth, brain heart infusion, and Columbia broth are commonly used. All are commercially available. While blood culture broth is enriched to encourage the multiplication of most organisms, it must be remembered that it will also allow the multiplication of contaminating skin bacteria. Careful skin decontamination is essential to reduce contaminating bacteria.

 REAL WORLD TIP

After the conclusion of the blood collection procedure, remove all the iodine solution from the skin with alcohol to minimize the possibility of developing hypersensitivity.

Blood must be collected during the early stages of disease because the number of bacteria in blood is higher in the acute stage of disease. During a fever, the number of bacteria is also greater at high temperatures in patients. There is a direct relationship between the volume of blood collected and the yield of bacteria. The volume of blood collected is much more important than the timing of blood culture collection. The more blood collected, the better the chance of isolating microorganisms present. Because the volume of blood for culture is critical, the dilution ratio of blood to broth is also crit-

ical. The ideal ratio of blood to broth is between 1:5 (1 part blood to 5 parts broth) and 1:10 (1 part blood to 10 parts broth). The key is to draw the largest amount of blood into the smallest volume of broth to ensure the growth of bacteria while still inactivating white blood cells and complement (Auckenthaler, Listrup, & Washington, 1982).

Adults, with bacteremia, typically possess low numbers of organisms per milliliter (mL) of blood. They usually have less than 30 colonies per mL of blood. The collection of 10 to 20 mL is strongly recommended. The absolute minimum volume for most blood culture bottles is 10 mL. Forty to 60 mL of blood should be obtained per episode of fever. This means collecting two to three blood culture sets with 10 mL per bottle or 20 mL per set. Children and infants do not have a large enough blood volume to collect 40 to 60 mL, but they do have a tendency to have more organisms present per mL of blood. One to 5 mL is usually drawn with a minimum volume of 1 mL. For children, an easy rule of thumb is 1 mL of blood can be drawn for every year of age. Table 32-1 ✪ depicts the age–volume protocol recommended for the collection of a blood culture set. Some facilities collect blood culture volumes based on weight rather than age. Between the weight of 30 to 80 pounds, 10 to 20 mL can be safely drawn, and over 80 pounds 30 to 40 mL can be collected. Specimens should be transported to the laboratory and incubated as soon as possible. If a delay in transport or processing is anticipated, bottles should be kept at room temperature and not refrigerated.

Most commercially available blood culture media contain the anticoagulant sodium polyanethol sulfonate (SPS) in concentrations varying from 0.025% to 0.05%. Heparin, EDTA and citrate cannot be used because each inhibits the growth of bacteria. In addition to its anticoagulant properties, SPS also inactivates neutrophils and certain antibiotics, including streptomycin, kanamycin, gentamicin, and polymyxin, precipitates fibrinogen and lipoproteins, and counteracts the natural antibacterial components of serum complement. SPS may also inhibit the growth of certain bacteria, including *Peptostreptococcus anaerobius, Neisseria gonorrhoeae, Neisseria meningitidis, Streptobacillus moniliformis, Gardnerella vaginalis*, and *Moraxella catarrhalis*. The inhibitory effect of SPS can be neutralized by adding gelatin to a final concentration of 1% to the medium. Using the correct ratio of between one part blood to five parts

✪ **TABLE 32-1**

Recommended Volume of Blood to Be Collected Based on Age

Age	Volume of Blood Per Blood Culture Set
<2 years	2 mL
2–5 years	8 mL
6–10 years	12 mL
>10 years	20 mL

broth and one part blood to 10 parts broth will also overcome some of the inhibitory effect of SPS.

Blood culture bottles with special broth formulations may be used in specific circumstances. Hypertonic sucrose in a concentration of 10% has been advocated to improve the recovery of certain bacteria from patients receiving penicillin or cephalosporins. These antibiotics injure the cell walls of some organisms. The sucrose creates a hyperosmotic solution that allows cell wall–injured organisms to grow. It also promotes the growth of cell wall–deficient organisms such as *Mycoplasma* spp.

Inoculated blood culture bottles should be inspected for optimal volume after receipt in the microbiology laboratory. Fastidious organisms supplement (FOS) may be added to blood cultures with less-than-optimal volumes. FOS contains nutrients that may help the limited numbers of organisms present in a suboptimal sample grow better. Additives such as resin beads, activated charcoal, and Fuller's earth are used by some commercial blood culture bottle manufacturers. Resin beads enhance the recovery of *Staphylococcus* spp., especially when patients are on antimicrobial therapy. The gram-positive cocci are able to survive within the white blood cells. The resin beads

 REAL WORLD TIP

Blood culture broths containing resin beads or charcoal can make creating a slide for a Gram stain more difficult. The beads and charcoal particles can make the surface of the stained slide uneven and more difficult to read. The resin beads and charcoal can also mask organisms. To overcome the effect or resin beads and charcoal, place a drop of the blood culture broth to the left or right of center on a glass slide. Tip the slide slightly to allow the liquid to run to the center of the slide without going over the edge. Allow to the liquid to air-dry and then Gram stain. As long as the slide is not tipped too much, the resin beads or charcoal will stay to the edge of the slide and out of the way of the microscope objective.

 Checkpoint! 32–7 (Chapter Objectives 9 and 9a)

Match the age of the patient from Column A to the minimum acceptable blood volume in one blood culture bottle from Column B.

Column A	Column B
1. Age <2 years	A. 10 mL in each bottle
2. 6–10 years	B. 6 mL in each bottle
3. 2–5 years	C. 4 mL in each bottle
4. >10 years	D. 1 mL in each bottle

provide a surface for the organisms to grow on as well as absorbing antibiotics present. Activated charcoal and Fuller's earth absorb antimicrobial agents present in the patient's blood.

 REAL WORLD TIP

Body fluids (e.g., pleural and pericardial fluids) can be inoculated directly into blood culture bottles either at the bedside or once the specimen reaches the laboratory. Studies that have looked at body fluids have found recovery of organisms to be better when they are inoculated into blood culture bottles, but they differ on whether bedside inoculation is superior to laboratory inoculation (Chapin & Lauderdale, 1996).

 REAL WORLD TIP

Blood and platelet units, for transfusion, can become contaminated with bacteria at the time of collection or through a septic donor. If a patient has a transfusion reaction, the microbiology department receives a portion of the unit for culture and Gram stain. Recent regulations now require the blood bank department to culture all platelet units prior to use. Platelets are held at room temperature, increasing the risk of contaminated units growing bacteria, which can create toxins. Platelet cultures are performed using the same continuous monitoring blood culture systems used in most microbiology departments.

▶ SPECIMEN PROCESSING

Bacteria are the most common microorganisms found in blood infections. Laboratory analysis of a bacterial blood culture differs slightly from a fungal culture and significantly from a viral culture. Several types of systems, both manual and automated, are available to laboratories to carry out these processes.

CONVENTIONAL, MANUAL BLOOD CULTURE SYSTEMS

The first blood culture method developed was a manual two-bottle system used for the isolation of both aerobic and anaerobic organisms (Reller, Murray, & MacLowry, 1982). It is still in use today, but continuous monitoring blood culture systems have replaced it in most clinical microbiology laboratories.

In the conventional manual system, blood is drawn into a blood culture bottle containing nutritional broth medium. The broth in the blood culture bottle is the first step in creating an environment in which bacteria will grow. It contains all the nutrients that bacteria need to grow. Blood cultures are traditionally drawn as a set with one aerobic bottle and one anaerobic bottle. For anaerobic bacteria to grow, oxygen is kept out of one of the blood culture bottles, and if aerobes are expected, oxygen is allowed into one of the bottles by means of a vent. The vent typically consists of a sterile needle with a sterile cotton plug. The use of a vent on the aerobic blood culture bottle ensures growth of oxygen-dependent organisms such as yeast and *Pseudomonas aeruginosa*.

> ### ℮ REAL WORLD TIP
>
> Because of the decline in anaerobic bloodstream infections, some facilities have eliminated the use of anaerobic blood culture bottles and substituted two aerobic bottles instead. They reserve the use of anaerobic bottles for those patients with infections most likely caused by anaerobes. Examples of patient types who should have anaerobic blood cultures collected include those who have had surgery, are hospitalized in the ICU, or have a complicated labor and delivery.

The bottles are placed in an incubator and kept at body temperature (35°C to 37°C). Mechanical agitation of the aerobic blood culture bottle during incubation increases the recovery of yeast and *Staphylococcus* spp. The bottles are watched daily for signs of growth, including cloudiness or a color change in the broth, hemolysis, gas bubbles, or colonies growing on the broth or red cell surface. When a visual change is detected, an aliquot is removed, and the microbiologist performs a Gram stain and subcultures the blood–broth mixture to appropriate media.

If there is no immediate visible evidence of growth in the bottles, the microbiologist continues to visually monitor the blood culture bottles daily for up to 7 days. Traditionally visually negative blood culture bottles are blind subbed to chocolate agar and/or stained (Gram stain or acridine orange stain) no sooner than within 6 hours of incubation but within 72 hours of incubation (Dunne, Nolte, & Wilson, 1997). Blind subbing is performing a subculture when there is no visible indication of the presence of bacteria. Not all organisms are able to cause a visual change in the blood culture broth, so blind subbing is necessary in the conventional manual blood culture method. The use of chocolate agar will ensure the isolation of most fastidious organisms such as *Haemophilus* spp. Anaerobes usually cause a visual change in the broth, so anaerobic blind subcultures are not necessary.

The conventional two-bottle culture method is very time consuming, requiring many staff hours and several days for blind subcultures at 2 days and 5 days of incubation, and plate reading as well as microbial recovery, biochemical identification of the bacterial isolate, and determination of antimicrobial susceptibility (Reisner et al., 1999). Often it takes 48 hours for an organism to cause a visual change in the blood culture

broth, so there is a significant delay in the time to detection of positive blood cultures. The delay can lead to negative patient outcomes.

Other limitations of this system include the need for carefully timed blind subcultures and microscopic stains for the detection of fastidious or slow-growing organisms (Silva & Washington, 1980). The vent needle can be a potential safety hazard for the microbiologist during subculturing.

> ### ℮ REAL WORLD TIP
>
> *Streptococcus pneumoniae* is a fragile organism that easily autolyses in liquid medium. The faster the time to detection in blood culture broth, the better the recovery of the organism.

Three other manual blood culture methods now available include a biphasic system (Septi-Chek, Becton-Dickinson, Franklin Lakes, NJ; Figure 32-6 ■), a signal system (Oxoid Signal, Thermo Fisher Scientific, Waltham, MA; Figure 32-7 ■), and a lysis-centrifugation system (Isolator, Wampole Laboratories, Cranbury, NJ). The biphasic and signal systems provide the benefit of a self contained, standardized detection of growth (Henry et al., 1983; Waller et al., 1982) without the need for additional instrumentation. The lysis-centrifugation system requires minimal additional equipment for its use.

A chamber containing a paddle coated with media replaces the cap of the aerobic broth bottle of the two-bottle biphasic system once it is received in the laboratory. Often the paddle media includes chocolate, MacConkey, and fungal agars. The use of solid and broth media concurrently is called biphasic because two different phases of medium are used to cultivate potential organisms. The anaerobic bottle does not have a media paddle. Anaerobic organisms are detected by visual

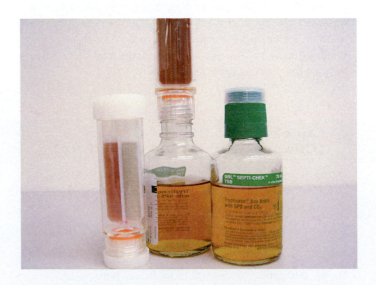

■ FIGURE 32-6 Septi-Check (biphasic) System (Becton-Dickinson, Franklin Lakes, NJ).

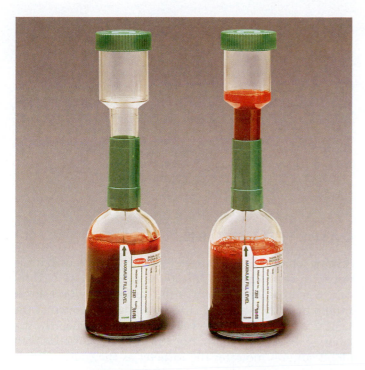

■ **FIGURE 32-7** Oxoid Signal System (Thermo Fisher Scientific, Waltham, MA).

changes in the broth. Both bottles are incubated at 35°C for 7 days. The aerobic bottles can be agitated during incubation if desired. The aerobic bottle is inverted twice on day 1 to inoculate the agar surfaces and then daily thereafter.

The use of a biphasic blood culture system has been shown to improve the sensitivity of organism recovery over traditional broth media. After the blood culture bottles are inoculated with blood and incubated, the agar surfaces on the slide allows the growth of colonies of aerobic, facultative anaerobic, and capnophilic microorganisms. The time to isolation for bacteria and yeast is faster than with the conventional manual method because they are detected as colonies on the media.

The signal manual system detects CO_2 production by microorganisms (Sawhney, Hinder, Swaine, & Bridson, 1986; Thombley & Anderson, 1987; Weinstein, Mirrett, & Reller, 1988). It is a one-bottle system in which both aerobic and anaerobic organisms can be recovered. A chamber with a plastic locking sleeve is attached to the top of the bottle. The chamber consists of a long needle and a clear plastic compartment with a narrow cylinder at the bottom and a larger upper reservoir. The chamber needle is inserted through the rubber stopper and positioned below the surface of the culture medium. As organisms grow in the bottle, gas is produced. The increased pressure in the air space above the broth forces the broth through the needle and into the chamber, signaling a positive culture. After the chamber is attached, the bottle is placed in a 35°C incubator on a mechanical agitator for 7 days. All bottles are inspected twice on day 1 and then daily thereafter. A positive appears as blood broth in the chamber, which is easily recognized. Recovery of organisms requires

subculture of the broth to media. The signal system, although making it easier to recognize a positive blood culture, still delays results by requiring subculture before colonies are available for workup.

The lysis-centrifugation manual method is unique because it does not use broth for culture medium. Blood is placed in a tube that contains a soaplike red and white blood cell lysing agent, an anticoagulant, and a fluorocarbon, which acts as a cushion during centrifugation. After centrifugation, the rubber stopper is removed, and the supernatant is removed via aspiration. The remaining pellet contains lysed red and white blood cells and microorganisms. The pellet is used to inoculate media. The lysis-centrifugation system requires more hands-on time and special equipment than the other two systems. There is the potential for aerosols, so the use of a laminar flow hood is necessary when processing the tubes. A twofold to eightfold increase in contamination rates over conventional systems is a significant problem in the use of the lysis-centrifugation system (Kim, Gottschall, Schwabe, & Randall, 1987). The system provides better recovery of fragile organisms such as *Streptococcus pneumoniae*, which tend to autolyse when grown in liquid medium. It is reported that this system also shows improved recovery of intracellular pathogens such as mycobacteria, yeast, and fungi because it lyses the cells present. It reduces the time to detection of the intracellular organism *Brucella* spp. to 2 to 5 days (Hawkins, Peterson, & de la Maza, 1986).

AUTOMATED BLOOD CULTURE SYSTEMS

Many remarkable improvements have been made in an attempt to reduce the time required to identify pathogens in blood, and over the last several decades, a variety of automated systems have been developed for detecting or identifying pathogenic microorganisms as well as for determining antimicrobial susceptibility. Continuous-monitoring blood culture systems (CMBCS) have emerged as the new standard in blood culture technology, enabling detection of a positive blood culture within 6 to 24 hours of initial incubation (Evangelista, Truant, & Bourbeau, 2002; Ferraro & Jorgensen, 1999). The systems automatically monitor the bottles containing the patient blood for evidence of microorganisms about every 10 minutes. Many data points are collected daily for each bottle and fed into a computer for analysis. Sophisticated mathematical calculations can determine when microorganisms have grown. Organisms are detected much faster then with manual methods. Because automated systems are much better at detecting organisms, most bottles need only to be held for 5 days rather than the 7-day incubation used for manual systems. In addition, all CMBCS instruments have the detection system, incubator, and agitation components combined into one unit. Although definitely more expensive than manual methods, the cost is outweighed by the faster detection of organisms, which can lead to better patient outcomes.

The BACTEC 9000 series of blood culture instruments (Becton-Dickinson, Franklin Lakes, NJ) is designed for the rapid detection of microorganisms in clinical specimens. The sample to be tested is inoculated into the broth vial, which is entered into the BACTEC instrument for incubation and periodic reading. Each vial contains a sensor that responds to the concentration of CO_2 produced by the metabolism of microorganisms or the consumption of oxygen needed for the growth of microorganisms. The sensor is monitored by the instrument every 10 minutes for an increase in fluorescence. With increasing amount of CO_2 or a decreasing amount of O_2 present in the vial, fluorescence increases. A positive reading indicates the presumptive presence of viable microorganisms in the vial (Becton, Dickinson and Company, 2005).

The BacT/Alert Microbial detection system (bioMérieux, Inc., Durham, NC) is a fully automated colorimetric blood culture system consisting of an instrument that incubates, agitates, and scans the bottles for positivity, and a computerized database management system to record and report results (Figure 32-8 ■). The carbon dioxide produced by bacterial growth changes the color of the colorimetric sensor at the base of each broth bottle for immediate detection of positive cultures. Activated charcoal present in the BacT/ALERT FAN bottles improves microorganism detection in samples especially from patients receiving antibiotic therapy (bioMérieux Inc., 2005). Continuous monitoring gives immediate notification of results with instant visual and audible alerts. Each bottle cell is equipped with a unique identifier ensuring instant bottle recognition and automated quality control.

The ESP (Accumed, West Lake, OH) is a manometric system that is based on monitoring headspace pressure changes in the space above the liquid because of gas production by bacteria. The blood culture bottle is attached to a pressure transducer.

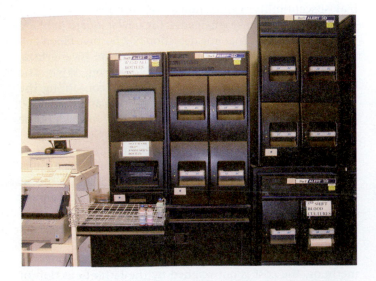

■ **FIGURE 32-8** BacT/Alert instrument and blood culture bottles.

✓ Checkpoint! 32–8 (Chapter Objective 10)

The principle of operation of the BacT/Alert blood culture system is
   A. *monitoring fluorescence production that is proportional to the amount of CO_2 in the bottle.*
   B. *CO_2 production that changes the color of the colorimetric sensor of the bottle.*
   C. *monitoring headspace pressure changes because of gas production by bacteria.*
   D. *lyses of both the red and the white blood cells.*

CATHETER CULTURE METHODS

Because some patients do not exhibit the typical signs of infection with catheter-related infections, diagnosis can be difficult. If an exudate is present at the catheter insertion site, it should be cultured. Blood cultures should be drawn at the same time from a vein as well as through the catheter. The isolation of the same organism from the exudates as well as both blood cultures indicates the catheter as the source of bacteremia.

A more commonly used culture method requires the removal of the catheter. A semiquantitative culture is done using the catheter tip rolled across a sheep blood agar plate. As the same time of removal of the catheter, blood cultures are drawn. The growth of more than 15 colonies on the catheter culture and the isolation of the same organism from the blood cultures indicates a catheter-related infection. This method will not detect organisms that may only be present in the lumen of the catheter. It will also not detect fastidious organisms that may not be able to grow on sheep blood agar. Because most catheter-related infections are because of normal skin flora, this is not a major drawback for the method.

HANDLING POSITIVE BLOOD CULTURES

Positive blood cultures are considered critical values. All suspected positive bottles are Gram stained and then subcultured onto the appropriate media. The Gram stain result of a positive blood culture needs to be reported in as much detail as possible. Based on the Gram stain, the physician will select an antibiotic for therapy. With a detailed Gram stain, the physician can select a specific antibiotic based on the organism seen,

 REAL WORLD TIP

Review Gram stained blood culture smears carefully. The red blood cells present usually lyse during the staining process. Gram-negative coccobacilli such as *Haemophilus* spp. and *Brucella* spp. can easily be hidden in the pink cellular debris.

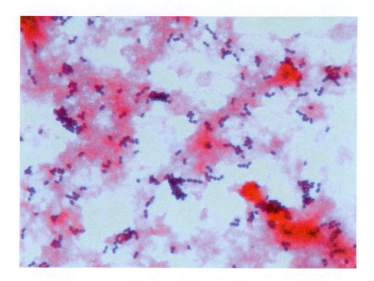

■ **FIGURE 32-9** Providing as much detail as possible from a blood culture Gram stain can help the physician tailor the treatment to a specific organism rather than using broad-spectrum antibiotics. In this Gram stain, reporting gram-positive cocci in pairs and short chains leads the physician to consider *Streptococcus pneumoniae* as the possible pathogen. A report of gram-positive cocci requires the physician to consider a much longer list of possible organisms.

rather than one that is broad spectrum. Figure 32-9 ■ demonstrates the need to provide as much detail as possible when reporting. Reporting gram-positive cocci in pairs versus gram-positive cocci provides the physician with information to indicate *Streptococcus pneumoniae* rather than *Staphylococcus* spp. or *Enterococcus* spp.

The media used for subculture should be selected based on the blood–broth Gram stain results. Table 32-2 ✪ illustrates the typical media used for positive blood cultures. Sheep blood and chocolate agars are routinely used for aerobic isolation. If gram-negative rods are observed, a MacConkey agar should be added. If yeast is observed on a Gram stain then fungal media is added. Organisms observed in the anaerobic blood culture bottle require subculture to aerobic media as well as reducible blood agar. Aerobic media is incubated for a minimum of 48 hours in either an ambient air or CO_2 incubator, whereas anaerobic media is held for up to 5 days in an anaerobic environment.

✪ TABLE 32-2

Media and Incubation Conditions

Media	Incubation Conditions
Blood agar (BAP)	CO_2 35°C × 48 hours
Chocolate agar (CHOC)	CO_2 35°C × 48 hours
MacConkey agar (MAC)	Ambient air, 35°C × 48 hours
Anaerobic agar	Anaerobic 35°C × 5 days

Rapid identification results and antimicrobial susceptibility tests are essential for guiding clinicians in the selection of the most appropriate treatment for patients with bloodstream infections (Doern, Vautour, Gaudet, & Levy, 1994). Identification and susceptibility testing should be attempted as soon as there is adequate growth on a subcultured plate. Organisms must be identified per laboratory policies and procedures.

Often multiple sets of bottles are drawn from a patient in a 24-hour period. Because each set of bottles is drawn at different time intervals, it is necessary to perform identification and susceptibility testing on each isolate from each set. This ensures each organism isolated is one and the same.

Rapid identification of organisms in the blood–broth mixture can be accomplished by directly inoculating identification tests. About 10 mL is removed from the positive blood culture bottle. First it is centrifuged slowly to remove the red blood cells, which can interfere with some tests, and then again at 1500 X *g* for 15 minutes to concentrate the organisms present. The remaining organism pellet can be used to perform testing such as identification strips or tube biochemical tests and even direct susceptibility testing. The microbiologist must review the manufacturer's literature to ensure the test method used has been validated to perform appropriately using an organism pellet directly from a blood culture. If it has not been shown to be validated using an organism pellet, then the microbiology laboratory can perform their own validation to prove the results achieved are reliable

Molecular methods can also be used to rapidly identify organisms directly from the blood culture broth. Peptide nucleic acid

(PNA) fluorescent in situ hybridization (FISH) has been shown to reduce the time to identification of *Staphylococcus aureus* and *Candida albicans* in blood cultures. The 2.5-hour procedure uses nucleic acid probes that target for specific species of organisms. Fluorescing cells indicates the presence of an organism that can be identified based on the specific probe used. The results take hours rather than days compared to traditional subcultures and testing. It can quickly tell the physician if gram-positive cocci in the blood are *Staphylococcus aureus* or not. *Staphylococcus aureus* is typically considered a significant organism in the blood, whereas a negative test would point toward a possible contaminant. The use of PNA FISH can save costs by eliminating unnecessary antibiotics when the blood culture indicates potential false bacteremia because of normal skin flora.

Elevated false-positive blood culture rates are associated with substantial health care costs. False-positive blood cultures lead to additional laboratory tests, unnecessary antibiotic use, and longer hospitalizations, which increase patient care costs. Assessing the clinical significance of blood culture isolates can be difficult, but actions ensuring the accurate determination of contaminants may minimize the associated costs and lower future contaminant rates (Richter et al., 2002).

Microbiologists traditionally cannot assess the clinical significance to blood culture isolates; only the physician can perform that role. The physician uses the patient history, signs and symptoms, as well as laboratory test results to confirm a diagnosis. Box 32-3✪ lists criteria often used to determine if an organism isolated from a blood culture is a potential contaminant or pathogen.

✪ REAL WORLD TIP

- A contaminant isolated from a blood culture can add to a patient's hospital bill by up to 39% because of the increased use of antibiotics and length of stay.

- The use of quality assurance is essential to ensure quality processes in the clinical laboratory. Many microbiology laboratories monitor their blood culture contamination rate to ensure the quality of the phlebotomy process. Most clinical laboratories set a threshold contamination rate of 3%. If more than 3% of blood cultures within a specified time period demonstrate contaminating skin organisms such as *Staphylococcus* not *Staphylococcus aureus*, then action must be taken to ensure the quality of the phlebotomy process. Often it is necessary to re-educate those performing phlebotomy on proper skin preparation. A dedicated phlebotomy team is less likely to collect blood cultures with skin contaminants than other health care workers.

Blood culture isolates may suggest an underlying disease process. The isolation of *Bacteroides fragilis* suggests an intestinal or pelvic source of infection, whereas *Klebsiella* spp. or

---

✪ BOX 32-3

Criteria Useful in the Determination of the Significance of a Blood Culture Isolate

Possible Contaminant
- Growth of organisms associated with normal skin flora or dust
  - *Staphylococcus* not *Staphylococcus aureus*
  - *Propionibacterium acnes*
  - *Corynebacterium* spp. (Diphtheroids)
  - *Bacillus* spp.
- Growth of multiple organisms from one bottle
  - Polymicrobic bacteremia is uncommon
- Patient's clinical signs and symptoms are not consistent with septicemia
- Organism isolated from blood is not consistent with organism isolated from primary site of infection
- Isolation of unusual organisms such as *Stenotrophomonas maltophilia* and *Burkholderia cepacia*. Although they can be significant gram-negative rods, they are associated with contaminated materials that could have been used during the blood culture collection procedure. Their isolation from the blood cultures of several patients suggests pseudobacteremia.

Potential Pathogen
- Growth of the same organism in repeated blood cultures obtained either at different times or from different sites
- Growth of certain organisms such as *Enterobacteriaceae*, *Streptococcus pneumoniae*, *Staphylococcus aureus*, gram-negative anaerobes, and *Streptococcus pyogenes*
- Growth of gram-negative rods in patients suspected of septic shock
- Growth of *Streptococcus* viridans group or *Enterococcus* spp. in patients suspected of endocarditis
- Isolation of any organism in blood from immunosuppressed patients or those with prosthetic devices

---

Enterococcus spp. suggest a gallbladder or urinary tract source more frequently than an intra-abdominal source. The blood isolate *Streptococcus gallolyticus* (formerly *S. bovis*) is associated with colon cancer. This organism is rarely seen in the blood and is usually only present with lesions in the intestine. Blood isolates can also indicate potential bioterrorism attacks. *Bacillus anthracis*, *Francisella tularensis*, *Brucella* spp., and *Yersinia pestis* are potential bioterrorism agents. Their isolation from a blood culture should alert the clinical microbiologist to notify the infectious disease specialist and infection control department immediately.

▶ SPECIAL PROCEDURES

Occasionally, some organisms require special conditions for successful isolation from blood culture specimens. Clinical findings and patient history prove to be extremely helpful in dealing with these organisms. The laboratory should be notified when one of these organisms is suspected.

LEPTOSPIRA INTERROGANS

Leptospira interrogans causes leptospirosis with resulting septicemia, meningitis, or kidney disease after exposure to infected animals or their urine and blood. The spirochete is found in the blood in the first 10 days of infection and later in the urine. Isolating the organism by culture provides definitive diagnosis. Culture must be done on specialized media containing rabbit serum and held for up to 8 weeks at 30°C in the dark. Routine blood cultures should not be used to isolate this organism. Most laboratories do not have the resources to isolate this organism. A reference laboratory should be used.

BRUCELLA SPECIES

Brucella spp is a slow-growing gram-negative coccobacillus that likes to hide within white blood cells. The organism is often acquired after contact with animals or their unpasteurized products such as milk. Signs and symptoms are often vague, with a fever that tends to come and go, chills, fatigue, and weight loss. Often the initial diagnosis is fever of unknown origin (FUO). A physician usually orders blood cultures when a fever is present with no apparent source of infection. Blood cultures are positive in 70% to 90% of patients but are not particularly helpful in initial diagnosis of the disease (Forbes & Weissfeld, 2002). Blood culture bottles should be kept for 3 weeks to 1 month and subcultured onto sheep blood and chocolate agars every week. Subcultures must be held a minimum of 3 weeks in a humidified, capnophilic atmosphere. Automated commercial blood culture systems can usually detect this organism within 7 days. Because many laboratories only hold blood cultures for 5 to 7 days, the physician must notify the laboratory if this organism is suspected. The commercial systems can be reprogrammed to hold the blood cultures longer. Because of the ease of aerosol transmission, any potential *Brucella* spp. specimens should be handled under a biohazard hood.

NUTRITIONALLY VARIANT STREPTOCOCCUS (NVS)

Nutritionally variant *Streptococcus* (NVS) should be suspected when gram-positive cocci in pairs and chains are observed on a Gram stain smear from a positive blood culture bottle but the organisms do not grow on routine subculture. The enriched broth media and human blood provide adequate amounts of vitamin B_6 required by the organism. Vitamin B_6 is also known as pyroxidal or thiol. Routine media may not contain adequate amounts of vitamin B_6 to allow the growth of this organism. One unique method to grow the organism is to spread a lawn of the blood culture onto a sheep blood agar plate. A streak of *Staphylococcus aureus* is placed down the center of the agar plate. After incubation, very small satelliting colonies of the NVS will appear next to the *Staphylococcus aureus* streak. *S. aureus* produces the vitamin B_6 required by the organism. It diffuses into the agar, and the NVS will grow wherever it is present. Figure 32-10 ■ displays the satelliting colonies of NVS around the *Staphylococcus aureus* colonies.

BARTONELLA SPECIES

Bartonella spp. are intracellular gram-negative coccobacilli that cause bacteremia and endocarditis. Reservoirs for the organism include cats and rodents, so humans acquire the organism via bites, scratches, and fleas. *Bartonella* infection is difficult to diagnose in the laboratory. The laboratory must be informed about suspicion of *Bartonella* infection, so laboratory personnel can perform the special culture methods required for isolation. The use of the lysis-centrifugation manual method improves its blood culture yield. Bottles of automated blood culture systems should be held at least 2 weeks because the organism is slow growing. Bottles should be examined and stained after 1 week of incubation with acridine orange to look for organisms that can easily be lost in the cellular debris of a blood Gram stain. If organisms are present, the bottles are subcultured onto blood or fresh chocolate agar that is less than 2 weeks old. Fresh media has more water present in it, which helps the organism grow. Plates are incubated at 37°C in 5% CO_2 and high humidity for up to 4 weeks.

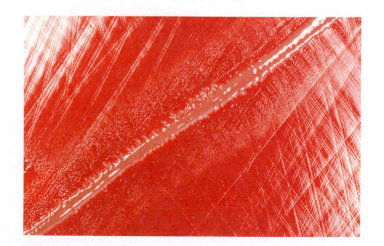

■ **FIGURE 32-10** The satelliting colonies of nutritionally variant *Streptococcus* (NVS) can be seen growing around the white colonies of *Staphylococcus aureus*. *S. aureus* provides the vitamin B_6 needed by the NVS to grow. The satelliting colonies of NVS are very similar to those seen with *Haemophilus influenzae* using the same method. A Gram stain will easily differentiate NVS (gram-positive cocci in pairs and chains) from *H. influenzae* (gram-negative coccobacilli).
From CDC and Dr. Mike Miller.

FUNGI

Fungemia can be a complication of venous or arterial catheterization, hyperalimentation, acquired immunodeficiency syndrome (AIDS), and therapy with steroids, antineoplastic drugs, radiation, or broad-spectrum antimicrobial agents. Intravenous drug abusers are prone to *Candida* spp. endocarditis. Although many fungal species, including *Histoplasma capsulatum*, *Coccidioides immitis*, and *Cryptococcus neoformans*, are recoverable from blood cultures, the most common cause of fungemia is *Candida albicans* followed by other *Candida* spp., including *Candida glabrata*.

Rarely blastospores or budding yeast structures and pseudohyphae can be seen by examination of Wright's stained venous peripheral blood smears. This technique may allow early diagnosis and therapy before culture results are available (Kates, Phair, Yungbluth, & Weil, 1988).

The laboratory should be informed by the physician if fungal septicemia is suspected because special media are often necessary for the optimum recovery of fungi. Numerous blood culture systems are available; however, all systems must be vented to atmospheric air, agitated, and incubated at 30°C to maximize the rate and time of recovery of fungal organisms. Cultures should be maintained for 4 weeks.

The recovery of fungi from blood may be enhanced by using a biphasic bottle containing a slant of brain heart infusion agar and 60 to 100 mL of BHI broth. A ratio of 1:10 to 1:20 (blood to broth) is recommended, a minimum of 5 mL of blood is required for each culture bottle. The biphasic culture bottle is kept vented and is tilted daily to allow broth to flow over the agar surface. These cultures must be carefully checked daily for growth. Because fungi will not turn the broth very cloudy, it is imperative to frequently Gram stain the bottle contents to detect fungal elements. The biphasic bottles should be incubated at 30°C and maintained for 4 weeks (Murray, Baron, Jorgensen, Pfaller, & Yolken, 2003).

The lysis-centrifugation system has been found to significantly improve the recovery of fungi from blood and is strongly recommend by Koneman, Allen, Janda, Schreckenberger, and Winn (1997) as the method of choice for processing blood cultures from patients with suspected fungal septicemia. Cultures should be incubated at 30°C and maintained for 4 weeks.

BACTEC has produced a special fungal media for enhanced fungal blood culture using their nonradiometric instruments. The white and red blood cells are lysed by the medium to enhance recovery of fungi. Antimicrobials have also been added to limit the growth of bacteria.

MYCOBACTERIUM SPECIES

Human immunodeficiency virus (HIV)-positive patients can present with positive blood cultures caused by *Mycobacterium avium* complex. When culturing blood for *Mycobacterium* spp., special media must be used. Automated and manual systems, such as the lysis-centrifugation method, can recover these organisms from blood. The average time for cultures to turn positive is about 10 days. Early in the course of infection, bacteremia may be low level or intermittent, in which case blood cultures may not be positive. Later in the course of infection, blood cultures are invariably positive. A culture is held for 6 weeks before negative results are reported. Organisms are identified by conventional biochemicals and/or high-pressure liquid chromatography (HPLC). Newer technologies, including ribosomal RNA probes or polymerase chain reaction, allow identification within 24 hours. Susceptibility tests are done by broth-based and conventional methods. (See ∞ Chapter 11.)

Checkpoint! 32–9 (Chapter Objective 14)

When brucellosis is suspected, blood cultures should be kept incubated and examined for

A. *5 days.*
B. *2 weeks.*
C. *1 month.*
D. *until it turns positive.*

HACEK

HACEK is an acronym that comes from the first letter of each genus included in this group of organisms. Members of the HACEK group include *Haemophilus parainfluenzae, Aggregatibacter aphrophilus, Aggregatibacter actinomycemcomitans, Cardiobacterium hominis, Eikenella corrodens,* and *Kingella kingae.* These organisms are fastidious gram-negative coccobacilli, which can be found as part of the normal oral flora. They are usually considered nonvirulent. They enter the bloodstream with manipulations of the oral cavity such as dental procedures, periodontal disease, piercings, or human bites. Individuals with previously damaged heart valves and poor dental

REAL WORLD TIP

A patient with endocarditis may have negative blood cultures. Individuals on previous antibiotic therapy may have injured organisms that will not grow. Endocarditis because of fungi may cause the organisms to become entrapped in the fibrin and platelet web because of the hyphae or tubelike branches produced. The most common cause for negative blood cultures in cases of endocarditis is fastidious organisms. Unusual organisms such as nutritionally-variant *Streptococcus, Campylobacter* spp., *Brucella* spp., *Bartonella* spp., and *Chlamydia* or *Chlamydiophila* spp. may require special media and atmosphere or prolonged incubation to recover.

hygiene are at higher risk for infection with these organisms. Because they are slow growing, the physician should notify the laboratory so blood cultures can be held for at least 2 weeks. Automated blood culture systems have been shown to detect the HACEK within 5 days. Chocolate agar should be used for subculture because these are fastidious organisms.

SUMMARY

The main function of the circulatory system is transport of oxygen and nutrients needed for metabolic processes in the tissues and removal of waste products. The circulatory system plays an important role in the body's defense mechanism. Once breached either by intravascular or extravascular sources, it can circulate and transport infectious organisms. Cardiovascular infections range from being asymptomatic and transient, to serious and life-threatening conditions. The volume of blood collected is the single most important factor in the detection of cardiovascular infections. Automated blood culture detection methods have dramatically reduced the time to detection of microorganisms in the blood. Gram-positive organisms are the most frequently isolated organisms. Once isolated, criteria may be used to determine the clinical significance of the organism present. The isolation of skin contaminants can result in unnecessary antibiotics and increased length of stay for the patient. Microbiologists play a vital role in the detection, isolation, and identification of potential pathogens in the septic patient.

LEARNING OPPORTUNITIES

1. Which of the following situations poses the greatest risk for development of an intravascular blood infection? (Chapter Objective 2)

    a. Presence of a decubitus ulcer

    b. Presence of an intravenous catheter

    c. Meningitis because of *Neisseria meningitidits*

    d. Surgery to repair a ruptured appendix

2. Which of the following individuals is most likely to be predisposed to developing bacteremia? (Chapter Objective 4)

    a. 17-year-old male who was injured in an all-terrain vehicle accident

    b. 33-year-old female delivering her first baby

    c. 52-year-old male in the hospital for hernia repair

    d. 77-year-old female in the ICU for pneumonia

3. Which of the following organisms is most likely to escalate a case of sepsis to septic shock? (Chapter Objective 5a)

    a. A lactose-fermenting gram-negative rod that is beta-hemolytic and indole positive

    b. A gram-positive cocci that is catalase positive and coagulase positive

    c. A gram-positive cocci that is catalase negative, esculin positive, and PYR positive

    d. A yeast that produces chlamydospores

4. The *Streptococcus* viridans group is most often associated with: (Chapter Objective 6a)

    a. septicemia

    b. septic shock

    c. subacute bacterial endocarditis

    d. acute bacterial endocarditis

5. All three sets of blood cultures from a patient in the intensive care unit were positive with *Staphylococcus* not *Staphylococcus aureus* (SNA). What additional culture should be performed? (Chapter Objectives 7, 7a, and 11)

    a. Nasal culture for colonization of SNA

    b. Intravenous catheter culture

    c. Urine culture

    d. Another set of blood cultures

6. A 39-year-old male was hospitalized for the removal of a brain abscess. After surgery, a culture of the abscess grew heavy growth of *Peptostreptococcus anaerobius*. The patient was placed on antibiotics, yet continued to exhibit a fever after surgery. Blood cultures were ordered. At 48 hours the blood cultures were negative. The physician calls to insist that there is something wrong with the blood cultures because he is sure the patient has septicemia because of his invasive surgery. Which of the following situations is the most likely explanation for the negative blood cultures? (Chapter Objectives 9a and 9 b)

   a. The SPS present has inhibited the growth of the organism.

   b. The organism is dead because of previous antibiotic therapy.

   c. The organism is fastidious and needs longer to grow.

   d. The fever is not because of a bloodstream infection.

7. A 64-year-old female was admitted for removal of a ruptured appendix. Her medical history was unremarkable except for a case of rheumatic fever as a child, which left her with a heart murmur. Two months after her surgery, she sees her physician complaining of fever, chills, fatigue, and dizziness. Her heart murmur is now more pronounced. Three sets of blood cultures are drawn. All six bottles grow *Enterococcus* spp. (Chapter Objectives 6, 6a, and 8)

   a. What infectious disease state do you suspect in this patient?

      a. Septic shock

      b. Subacute bacterial endocarditis

      c. Acute bacterial endocarditis

      d. Transient bacteremia

   b. Why was the patient predisposed to acquiring this infectious disease state?

      a. Previously damaged heart valves because of rheumatic fever

      b. Invasive surgery with the potential for the release of enteric organisms

      c. A 2-month delay before treatment was sought.

      d. a and b

      e. b and c

8. A patient has three sets of blood cultures drawn within a 24-hour period. One bottle drawn is positive at 24 hours. The Gram stain of the positive blood culture is shown in the photo. (Chapter Objectives 8, 12, and 13)

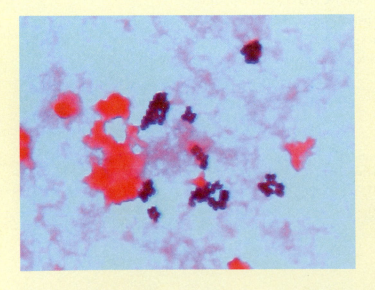

a. How would you report this positive blood culture based on the Gram stain provided?

    a. Gram-positive cocci seen

    b. Gram-positive cocci in clusters seen

    c. Gram-positive cocci seen in one bottle

    d. Gram-positive cocci in clusters seen in one bottle out of six total

b. Based on the Gram stain and number of positive blood cultures, how would you interpret the significance of this organism?

    a. Possible contaminant because it is present in only one bottle out of six total

    b. Probable pathogen because the Gram stain suggests *Staphylococcus aureus*

    c. Possible catheter-related infection

    d. Need to draw additional blood cultures to assess its significance

9. Which of the following conventional blood culture systems has the highest rate of contamination when compared to the other systems? (Chapter Objectives 10 and 10a)

    a. Signal method

    b. Biphasic method

    c. Lysis-centrifugation method

    d. Two-bottle manual method

10. An intravenous catheter tip is removed from a patient and submitted for culture. Two sets of blood cultures are also drawn at the time of the removal of the catheter. The catheter is rolled across a sheep blood agar and incubated overnight at 35°C in CO_2. The next day, 25 colonies of white, nonhemolytic, gram-positive cocci, which are catalase positive and coagulase negative, were isolated.

    Three of the four bottles of the blood culture drawn are positive at 12 hours. All three blood cultures produce the same Gram stain (see photo).

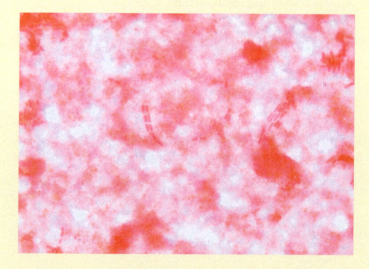

These results indicate: (Chapter Objectives 7a and 11)

a. no catheter-related infection because there are not enough colonies to be considered significant on the catheter culture

b. no catheter-related infection because different organisms were isolated from the catheter culture compared to the blood culture

c. a catheter-related infection because there were a significant number of colonies on the catheter culture

d. a catheter-related infection because both the catheter culture and the blood cultures grew organisms

11. Which of the following situations would be considered a significant isolate from blood cultures? (Chapter Objectives 8 and 13)

a. Growth of *Propionibacterium acnes* from two blood culture bottles out of six total from a patient with pneumonia because of *Streptococcus pneumoniae*

b. Growth of *Staphylococcus* not *Staphylococcus aureus* from three blood culture bottles out of four total from a patient on chemotherapy for leukemia

c. Growth of *Corynebacterium* spp. and *Staphylococcus* not *Staphylococcus aureus* from one blood culture bottle out of two total from an 11-month-old child with fever

d. Growth of *Bacillus* spp. from one blood culture bottle out of four total from a trauma patient

12. Gram-positive cocci in pairs and short chains are observed on the Gram stain of a positive blood culture broth. The blood broth is plated to sheep blood and chocolate agars and incubated at 35°C in CO_2 overnight. Both agar plates display no growth the next day. All but one of the following situations may explain these results. Select the one statement that is *unlikely*. (Chapter Objectives 8 and 14)

a. It could be a member of the HACEK group and needs longer to grow.

b. It may be dead because of previous antibiotic therapy.

c. It is possibly a nutritionally variant *Streptococcus* (NVS) and needs vitamin B_6 to grow.

d. It may be an obligate anaerobe and needs an anaerobic environment to grow.

PEARSON
myhealthprofessionskit™

Use this address to access the interactive Companion Website created for this textbook. Simply select "Clinical Laboratory Science" from the choice of disciplines. Find this book and log in using your user name and password.

REFERENCES

Go to myhealthprofessionskit.com to view this chapter's references.

33

Respiratory System

Ruth Masterson

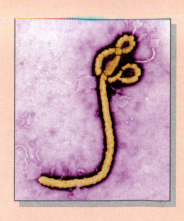

■ LEARNING OBJECTIVES

Upon completion of this chapter, the learner should be able to:

1. Review the anatomy and physiology of the respiratory system.
2. Summarize natural defense mechanisms used by the body.
3. Correlate physical signs and symptoms and disease states with potential pathogens.
4. Evaluate the acceptability of a clinical specimen.
5. Predict potential pathogens based on specimen type/body site and/or direct Gram stain results.
6. Select media for isolation of potential respiratory pathogens from clinical specimens.
7. Summarize the interpretation of respiratory cultures.
   a. Define the normal flora given the body site/specimen type and/or patient population.
8. Correlate patient history, specimen type/body site, direct Gram stain results, colony morphology, identification, and/or susceptibility test results to identify a microorganism, assess its clinical significance, and determine sources of errors.
9. Recommend testing procedures to detect or identify potential pathogens.

KEY TERMS

bacteriocins

bronchiolitis

bronchitis

community-acquired
  pneumonia

empyema

epiglottis

expectorated

hospital-acquired
  pneumonia

influenza

laryngitis

pharyngitis

phlegm

pneumonia

sinusitis

sputum

ventilator-associated
  pneumonia

▶ INTRODUCTION

The respiratory system provides the body oxygen, which the cells require to sustain life. This system is one of the few in the body that depends on the external environment to function. The body relies on air from the environment to carry oxygen down into the lungs. Unfortunately, the mechanism for getting oxygen into the lungs also provides a means for foreign substances and microorganisms to enter, colonize, and cause disease that, if left untreated, could cause death.

The microorganisms which attempt to invade and cause damage to the body will be explored. The collection and specimen processing necessary to cultivate and identify these pathogenic intruders will be discussed also. Testing methods will be described to help the microbiologist determine the best method for the patient populations served.

▶ ANATOMY AND PHYSIOLOGY OF THE RESPIRATORY SYSTEM

Oxygen must make its way to the lungs and then to the capillaries, where the red blood cells carry it throughout the body. The journey begins in the nose or mouth as a breath of air is pulled into the body with the help of the diaphragm. The diaphragm is a thin muscle that lies below the lungs and functions both voluntarily and involuntarily. Humans have the ability to voluntarily take a breath of air, but the body involuntarily makes this happen around the clock such as during sleep. As the diaphragm contracts, the rib cage rises, and negative pressure is created in the chest cavity. This causes the lungs to expand and draw in air. Oxygen is exchanged for carbon dioxide in the capillaries deep in the lungs. As the diaphragm relaxes, carbon dioxide is exhaled from the lungs. Figure 33-1 ■ depicts the basic anatomy of the respiratory system and its location within the body.

Cilia are small hairlike projections on the epithelial cells that line the nose and upper respiratory tract. They function to filter out microorganisms and any foreign substances in the air. As air is taken in, it is warmed by the blood in capillaries and provided with humidity as it passes over the mucus produced by goblet cells in the nasal and sinus cavities. The next structure encountered is the pharynx, or throat. It is lined with mucous membrane and acts as a passageway for air to the trachea as well as food to the esophagus. The nasopharynx is located at the back of the nose, where it connects with the throat. The oropharynx includes the mouth and the area located at the back of tongue. The tonsils are located in the throat and assist with removal of bacteria. The

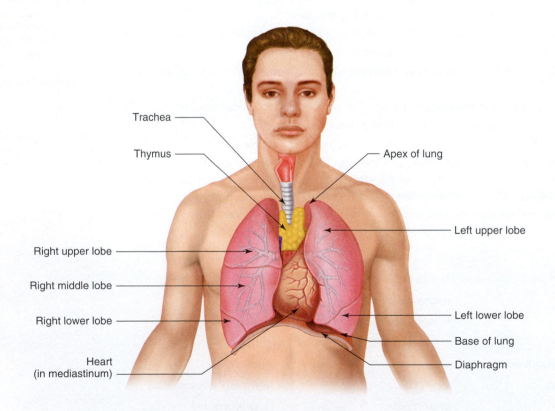

■ **FIGURE 33-1** This illustration demonstrates the basic anatomy of the respiratory system and its location within the thoracic cavity of the body.

nasopharynx also connects the eustachian tubes of the ears to the throat.

The larynx is located at the base of the pharynx, where it splits into the trachea leading to the lungs and the esophagus leading to the stomach. As air passes over the larynx, sound is produced. Common terms for the larynx are the voice box, vocal chords, or Adam's apple. Just in front of the larynx is the epiglottis, a leaf-shaped cartilage flap, found at the root of the tongue. It covers the entrance of the larynx after swallowing so food and liquid do not enter the lungs. The area from the epiglottis to the larynx is called the laryngopharynx. Collectively, the nose, oral cavity, pharynx, epiglottis, and lar-

ynx make up the upper respiratory tract system. Figure 33-2 ■ illustrates the anatomy of the upper respiratory system.

The trachea, or windpipe, is the beginning of the lower respiratory tract. It is a tube of cartilage and muscle that extends from the larynx down to the lungs. It is lined with ciliated epithelial cells that function to propel debris and foreign material up and out of the lower respiratory system. Smoking destroys the cilia, but they can regenerate once an individual stops.

The trachea divides at the bottom into two bronchial tubes so there is one bronchus (plural: bronchi) for each lung. The trachea and bronchi are lined with goblet cells, which produce

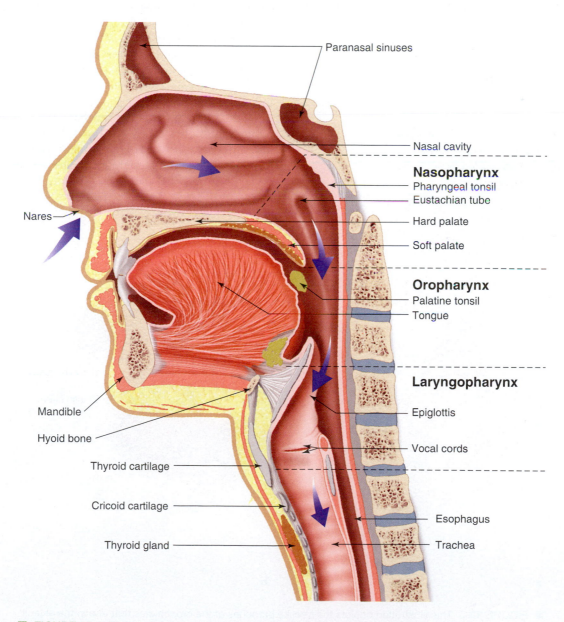

■ **FIGURE 33-2** The anatomy and structures of the upper respiratory system are illustrated.

mucus. Mucus helps trap dust particles and microorganisms so they don't reach the delicate lung tissue. The main bronchi of the left and right lungs branch into smaller and smaller further segments like the limbs of a tree. The smallest branches are called bronchioles. The right and left lungs are not the same size in the body because the heart is in the center of the chest cavity and leans to the left. The right lung has three lobes, but the left lung only has two lobes.

The bronchioles end in the alveoli (singular: alveolus), or tiny air sacs. They look like a cluster of grapes. They are lined with thin squamous epithelial cells and surrounded by capillaries (minute blood vessels). The exchange of oxygen and carbon dioxide is essential for the body to survive and is accomplished by diffusion through the very thin alveoli and capillary cell walls. Carbon dioxide is a waste product of the cells and is released into the alveoli and then expelled by the

body through the respiratory system. The respiratory system is ultimately responsible for gas exchange, which in turn maintains the acid–base balance of the body. Figure 33-3 ■ illustrates the alveoli and capillary system, where the exchange of gases occurs in the lung.

NATURAL DEFENSE MECHANISMS

The mucous membranes and cilia function by trapping and propelling foreign particles and microorganisms out of the respiratory system. The sticky material produced by the goblet cells along the respiratory tract is called **phlegm.** The body uses a variety of mechanisms such as sneezing, coughing, and swallowing to remove phlegm and trapped particles from the body.

Normal bacterial flora resides in the nasopharynx to prevent colonization of the upper respiratory tract by potentially pathogenic organisms. Colonization of the upper respiratory tract by potential pathogens usually requires interaction of the microbial surface and receptors on the host cells. If the potential pathogens cannot reach the tissues because of the vast numbers of normal flora organisms, then they cannot adhere to initiate infection.

Normal flora microorganisms have the ability to produce natural antibiotics called **bacteriocins**, which are toxic to invading organisms. The organisms can also prime the immune system just enough so they are not attacked by antibodies, but potential pathogens are immediately recognized as foreign. Antibodies are then created and remove the

 Checkpoint! 33–1 (Chapter Objective 1)

Select the proper order of the anatomy of the respiratory system, which allows oxygen to reach the body's red blood cells.

   A. *Pharynx, epiglottis, trachea, alveoli, bronchi*
   B. *Epiglottis, trachea, pharynx, bronchi, alveoli*
   C. *Pharynx, epiglottis, trachea, bronchi, alveoli*
   D. *Trachea, alveoli, bronchi, epiglottis, pharynx*

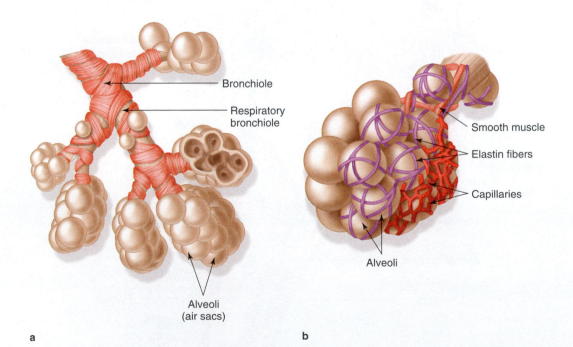

a   b

■ **FIGURE 33-3** This illustration depicts the treelike branches of the bronchioles that end in the alveoli (a). Gases transfer back and forth between the alveoli and the capillaries (b).

invaders quickly. Some antibodies, produced at low levels against some normal organisms, can cross react and act against pathogenic organisms. One well-known example is the ability of antibodies against *Escherichia coli* serotype K1 to cross react against the capsule of some serotypes of *Neisseria meningitidis*. This can help prevent *Neisseria meningitidis* from colonizing the upper respiratory tract system.

Potential pathogens have defenses of their own to evade the body's immune system such as possessing a capsule that covers the surface of the organism so the immune system cannot reach it. They produce toxins that can alter metabolism in the host cells with the potential for damage to the tissue. Once the host tissue is damaged, the pathogenic organisms can invade.

> ✓ **Checkpoint! 33–2**
> **(Chapter Objective 2)**
>
> *Which of the following is **not** a protective function of the normal flora of the upper respiratory tract?*
>
>   A. *Prevent colonization by their vast numbers*
>   B. *Produce natural antibiotics*
>   C. *Prime the immune system*
>   D. *Produce toxins*

▶ INFECTIOUS DISEASES ASSOCIATED WITH THE RESPIRATORY SYSTEM

All the structures of the upper and lower respiratory tract may be infected by viruses, bacteria, fungi, and even parasites. The upper respiratory tract is the beginning of the route that pathogens can attack to cause infections. Table 33-1 summarizes the potential pathogens of the upper respiratory tract.

UPPER RESPIRATORY TRACT INFECTIONS

Nasopharyngitis

The common cold is caused by any one of more than 200 different viruses that lead to inflammation of the nasal passages and pharynx, as well as the sinuses and middle ear. The most common virus implicated is the rhinovirus. Other viruses include coronavirus, the second-most-common cause, as well as parainfluenza virus, respiratory syncytial virus, influenza virus, and adenovirus. There are hundreds of viral serotypes, which accounts for the lack of a vaccine for the common cold.

Symptoms include scratchy throat, sneezing, a clear nasal discharge, and nasal obstruction. A cold is self-limiting but may last 1 to 2 weeks. The virus is passed via droplets in the air or on the hands. Adults and children are both prone to colds, especially during the winter months. Children are the main reservoirs because of their less-than-ideal hygiene habits. Adults experience 3 to 4 colds per year, whereas children average 8 to 10 per year.

✪ TABLE 33-1

Most Common Potential Pathogen of the Upper Respiratory Tract

Infectious Disease State	Common Potential Pathogens
Nasopharyngitis	■ Rhinovirus ■ Coronavirus ■ Other viruses
Pharyngitis	■ *Streptococcus pyogenes* (group A beta *Streptococcus*) ■ *Streptococcus* groups C and G ■ *Arcanobacterium haemolyticum* ■ *Corynebacterium diphtheriae* ■ Rhinovirus ■ Influenza virus ■ Other viruses
Sinusitis	■ *Streptococcus pneumoniae* ■ *Haemophilus influenzae* ■ *Staphylococcus aureus* ■ *Streptococcus pyogenes* ■ *Moraxella catarrhalis* ■ Anaerobes ■ *Aspergillus fumigatus* ■ Viruses
Epiglottitis	■ *Haemophilus influenzae* serotype b and non-type b ■ *Streptococcus pneumoniae* ■ *Streptococcus pyogenes* ■ *Staphylococcus aureus* ■ *Moraxella catarrhalis* ■ *Neisseria meningitidis* ■ *Pseudomonas aeruginosa* ■ *Candida albicans* ■ Viruses
Laryngitis	■ Viruses ■ *Streptococcus pyogenes* ■ *Bordetella pertussis* ■ *Moraxella catarrhalis* ■ *Corynebacterium diphtheriae* ■ *Mycoplasma pneumoniae* ■ *Chlamydophila pneumoniae*

A cold creates a change in the normal flora of the upper respiratory tract, which can lead to secondary bacterial infections. Nose blowing can push bacteria into the sinuses and middle ear, which can lead to infection. If the individual has a history of herpes simplex virus of the lips or nose, the constant friction created from wiping and blowing a runny nose may cause the virus to activate and erupt into blisters.

- The nasopharynx is the carrier site for *Staphylococcus aureus* and *Neisseria meningitides*.

- *Bordetella pertussis* specifically binds to respiratory ciliated epithelial cells and paralyzes them with toxin. A deep nasopharyngeal swab or nasopharyngeal wash will ensure collection of these cells and the detection of the organism.

Influenza, or the "flu," is infection and inflammation of the nose, throat, bronchi, and sometimes the lungs because of the influenza virus. This common disease state will be discussed in the pneumonia section of this chapter because pneumonia is the most common complication.

Pharyngitis

One of the most common upper respiratory tract complaints is a sore throat or **pharyngitis**. The most frequent bacterial causative agent is *Streptococcus pyogenes* (group A *Streptococcus*). After the organism colonizes, the throat's mucous membranes become inflamed, causing red and swollen oropharynx tissue accompanied by pain or difficulty in swallowing. A fever and headache are frequent. White exudate containing dead organisms, fibrin, and white blood cells can appear on the surface of the oropharynx, especially on the tonsils. The cervical lymph nodes of the neck become swollen. Figure 33-4 ■ demonstrates the swollen, red oropharynx and white exudate associated with pharyngitis. Strep throat, as it is commonly

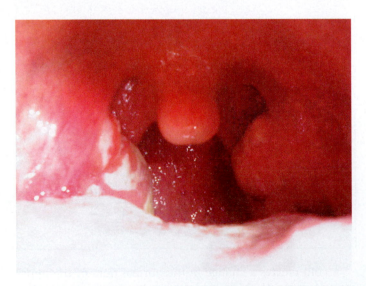

■ **FIGURE 33-4** This child displays the typical swollen, red throat associated with pharyngitis. White exudate, made up of white blood cells, organisms, and fibrin, is often observed on the tonsils and oropharynx in infection with *Streptococcus pyogenes*. *From http://commons.wikimedia.org/wiki/Image:Streptococcal_pharyngitis_1.jpg*

known, occurs mainly in school-age children, especially during the winter months, but all ages are susceptible. It passes person to person via respiratory droplets.

S. pyogenes produces many enzymes and toxins that are responsible for the disease it causes. Its virulence factors include a capsule as well as streptolysins S and O, deoxyribonucleases, hyaluronidase, streptokinase, and other toxins. Its major virulence factor is the M protein, which allows it to evade phagocytosis. There are more than 100 different M protein serotypes, so it is possible to develop immunity to one serotype but still be susceptible to the others. The wide range of serotypes explains the lack of a vaccine for *Streptococcus pyogenes*.

Streptococcus pyogenes produces streptolysins S and O, which can kill red and white blood cells as well as tissue. Streptolysin S is oxygen stable and causes the beta-hemolysis observed on the surface of the sheep blood agar plate. Streptolysin O is oxygen labile and produces beta-hemolysis under anaerobic conditions. When culturing for *S. pyogenes*, after streaking the sheep blood agar plate, stab the inoculation needle deep into the primary area of the plate two to three times. This creates mini anaerobic chambers, which allow the detection of the beta-hemolysis of streptolysin O.

Although most strains of *S. pyogenes* typically produce streptolysin S, there may be strains that only produce streptolysin O. Without the stab marks in the agar plate, their detection will be more difficult. Microbiologists should always practice the habit of stabbing the primary area of any sheep blood agar plate after inoculation.

Strep throat constitutes only about 12% of all sore throat cases seen by doctors (Simon, 2003). It possesses a specific cell wall carbohydrate ("C" or carbohydrate substance), which can be detected either after culture using a colony or with a direct commercially produced rapid test. The pros and cons of culture versus direct rapid testing are discussed later in this chapter under specimen processing. Because the rapid test detects only *S. pyogenes,* the microbiologist must keep in mind that other bacteria and viruses can also be the actual causative agent.

It is important to differentiate pharyngitis caused by *S. pyogenes* from other possible pathogens. *S. pyogenes* pharyngitis can be self-limiting but should be treated with antibiotics because of the potential for poststreptococcal nonsuppurative (without the formation of pus) sequelae. Poststreptococcal nonsuppurative sequelae are complications that can arise after untreated group A *Streptococcus* pharyngitis. The antibodies made against the organism's M protein can turn on its host to cause acute rheumatic fever and acute glomerulonephritis. It is possible for an individual to be an asymptomatic carrier of *S. pyogenes*. The strain is usually a-virulent because of decreased amounts of protein M. Carriers are not usually contagious.

REAL WORLD TIP

An individual with *Streptococcus pyogenes* pharyngitis is not infectious after receiving 24 hours of antibiotic therapy. Group A *Streptococcus* pharyngitis is responsible for many missed schooldays for children and many missed workdays for their parents. The faster the microbiology department can provide results for the patient, the faster they can receive appropriate therapy and return to school or work.

Several other pathogens must be considered if *S. pyogenes* is not the causative agent of pharyngitis. Beta-hemolytic *Streptococcus* groups C and G are associated with pharyngitis along with *Arcanobacterium haemolyticum. A. haemolyticum* is isolated primarily in adolescents and young adults. *Neisseria gonorrhoeae* should also be considered if the patient engages in risky sexual behavior. Other rare causes of bacterial pharyngitis include *Francisella tularensis, Yersinia enterocolitica, Mycoplasma pneumoniae,* and *Chlamydophila pneumoniae.* Bacterial infections of the tonsils, epiglottis, and adenoids may also cause pharyngitis.

REAL WORLD TIP

When working up a throat culture with a beta-hemolytic colony, perform the streptococcal serotyping for the most common cell wall antigens, A, C, and G. If they are all negative, perform a gram stain. *Arcanobacterium haemolyticum* is a catalase-negative, gram-positive rod whose colony resembles that of beta-hemolytic *Streptococcus* spp. after 48 hours.

Corynebacterium diphtheriae causes diphtheria, which can produce a tonsillar and oropharyngeal membrane that can reach down to the larynx. The membrane produced can mimic the white exudate observed in strep throat, so the two diseases must be differentiated with laboratory testing. This infectious disease is rare but can be seen in individuals who are unimmunized or have not received booster immunizations. Its virulence is because of an exotoxin produced. The organism can only produce the exotoxin after it has been infected with a specific bacteriophage or virus. The toxin enters the bloodstream to damage the heart, nerves, and kidneys.

REAL WORLD TIP

Haemophilus influenzae, Streptococcus pneumoniae, and *Staphylococcus aureus* are not causative agents of pharyngitis. Although the organisms can be isolated from the throat, they should not be worked up as potential pathogens. They may be present as the result of a viral infection. The viruses reduce the normal flora present, allowing these three organisms to take advantage of the situation. They may also be present as the result of postnasal drainage. A sinus infection cannot be diagnosed using a throat culture.

Viruses are the most common causes of pharyngitis. They include rhinovirus, coronavirus, adenovirus, influenza virus, and parainfluenza virus. Most infections caused by the rhinoviruses or the influenza (flu) virus and are self-limiting. Because viruses are not affected by antibiotics, they should not be used unless a bacterial pathogen has been identified as a secondary infection.

REAL WORLD TIP

Colds and influenza or flu are normally seen during the same time of year usually starting in late October and running through April. Because both of these conditions are caused by viruses, they are easily spread by direct contact from hand to mouth or by inhaling droplets from a cough or sneeze of an infected person. It is important to differentiate the two conditions because the flu can be treated with antiviral drugs if detected early but only supportive treatment is available for the common cold.

Sinusitis

Four pairs of sinus cavities are found in the skull. They open into the nose to warm and humidify the air breathed in before it enters the lungs. Another function may be to reduce the weight of the skull. The sinuses include the maxillary located inside each cheekbone, the ethmoid behind the bridge of the nose and between the eyes, the frontal over the eyes in the brow area, and the sphenoid behind the ethmoid sinuses and eyes. Each is lined with columnar epithelial cells and contains mucus-producing goblet cells.

The sinuses are normally sterile. **Sinusitis** is a condition in which the sinuses are inflamed or infected usually after a viral upper respiratory tract infection or allergies. The condition can be acute or chronic. Health experts estimate that 37 million Americans are affected by sinusitis every year and spend $5.8 billion each year on health care costs related to it (National Institute of Allergy and Infectious Diseases [NIAID], 2006).

Symptoms of sinusitis include coughing, sneezing, feeling tired and achy, nasal congestion, nasal discharge, and headache. Pressure and pain over the eyes in the brow area, under and behind the eyes, and in the cheekbone area are common. Individuals often experience jaw and tooth pain because of the pressure, caused by fluid retention, on the nerves. They may also experience a sore throat because of postnasal drip caused by mucus leaving the sinuses. The location of pressure and pain associated with sinusitis is dependent on the location where the blockage occurs.

Because of the close physical communication, microorganisms present in the nasopharynx can reach and cause infection in the sinuses. Organisms usually enter the sinuses secondary to another bacterial or viral infection such as a cold or allergies. Nose blowing creates pressure, which pushes organisms from the nasopharynx into the sinuses.

Microorganisms most commonly associated with acute sinusitis in adults include *Streptococcus pneumoniae, Haemophilus influenzae, Staphylococcus aureus*, and *Streptococcus pyogenes*. *Moraxella catarrhalis* is associated with sinusitis in children. Anaerobes, such as *Porphyromonas* spp., *Fusobacterium* spp., *Prevotella* spp., and *Peptostreptococcus* spp., are associated with chronic sinusitis and usually originate from the roots of abscessed teeth. The presence of *Enterobacteriaceae* usually indicates colonization from the throat rather than a true sinus infection.

Rhinoviruses and other upper respiratory viruses cause colds, which can damage the membranes and allow the sinuses to become colonized and then secondarily infected to cause sinusitis. Fungal sinusitis is usually the result of a compromised immune system or the presence of an underlying condition such as diabetes mellitus. *Aspergillus* spp. is the most common fungal pathogen. Nosocomial sinusitis can occur in critically ill patients with a nasal tube or on mechanical ventilation. *Streptococcus pyogenes, Staphylococcus aureus, Pseudomonas aeruginosa*, and the *Enterobacteriaceae* are common nosocomial pathogens.

Sinusitis can lead to serious complications. The microorganisms can extend beyond the sinuses to cause osteomyelitis of the skull. They can also reach the central nervous system to cause meningitis or a brain abscess. Orbital infections are another complication that can arise. Sinusitis caused by fungi can cause bone erosion and systemic infection.

Epiglottitis

Epiglottitis is caused by swelling and inflammation of the epiglottis and adjacent structures, which sit above the larynx. Visually, the infected epiglottis appears cherry red because of the massive inflammation. The infection is usually observed in young children between the ages of 3 to 7 years. It is more frequent during respiratory season, which are the winter months. It rarely occurs in adults. Symptoms appear abruptly and include drooling because of swelling, which leads to difficulty swallowing, loss of the voice, sore throat, difficulty breathing, fever, and mild cough.

Prior to 1985, most cases of epiglottis were caused by *Haemophilus influenzae* type b (Hib). The use of the Hib vaccine has reduced its incidence dramatically in children. Because the vaccine has only been available since 1985, most adults are not vaccinated. Adults may now present more frequently with infection caused by Hib than children.

Epiglottitis is still present today because of the wide variety of upper respiratory microorganisms that can initiate infection. These include *Haemophilus influenzae* serotypes other than b, *Streptococcus pneumoniae, Streptococcus pyogenes, Staphylococcus aureus, Moraxella catarrhalis, Haemophilus parainfluenzae, Neisseria meningitidis, Pseudomonas aeruginosa*, and *Candida albicans*. Although viruses do not cause epiglottitis, a previous viral upper respiratory infection can predispose the individual for a secondary bacterial infection.

Most individuals with epiglottitis caused by Hib also have bacteremia, which accounts for the fever present. Epiglottitis is considered a medical emergency. The airway can become so swollen that it leads to complete respiratory obstruction.

Laryngitis

Laryngitis is inflammation of the larynx or voice box. This condition usually comes on quickly, lasts for up to 2 weeks and then resolves on its own. The swelling caused by the inflammation affects the vibrations created by the larynx and therefore the voice. The affected individual usually exhibits fever, dry cough, runny nose, and a hoarse voice. Most cases accompany a viral upper respiratory infection.

Viruses associated with laryngitis include rhinovirus, influenza virus, parainfluenza virus, respiratory syncytial virus, and adenovirus. Bacteria can also cause infection of the larynx but are not as common. They include *Streptococcus pyogenes, Bordetella pertussis, Moraxella catarrhalis, Corynebacterium diphtheriae, Mycoplasma pneumoniae*, and *Chlamydophila pneumoniae*. Noninfectious inflammation of the larynx can occur with straining or overuse of the voice, such as singing, yelling, or cheering, allergies, or exposure to smoke.

> ✓ **Checkpoint! 33–3 (Chapter Objective 3)**
>
> *A 32-year-old female loses her voice 1 week after experiencing a cold. The most likely causative agent is*
>
>   A. *Corynebacterium diphtheriae.*
>   B. *Mycoplasma pneumoniae.*
>   C. *rhinovirus.*
>   D. *enterovirus.*

LOWER RESPIRATORY INFECTIONS

According to the World Health Organization, 3.9 million deaths occurred because of lower respiratory infections in 2004 (World Health Report, 2004). This section will review the organisms that cause bronchitis, bronchiolitis, pneumonia, and pleural effusion. Table 33-2 summarizes the potential pathogens associated with the lower respiratory tract.

✪ TABLE 33-2

Infectious Disease of the Lower Respiratory Tract and the Common Potential Pathogens

Infectious Disease	Common Potential Pathogens	
Bronchitis	■ Influenza virus ■ Respiratory syncytial virus ■ Other viruses ■ *Bordetella pertussis* ■ *Streptococcus pneumoniae*	■ *Haemophilus influenzae* ■ *Moraxella catarrhalis* ■ *Chlamydiophila pneumoniae* ■ *Mycoplasma pneumoniae*
Bronchiolitis	■ Respiratory syncytial virus	■ Adenovirus
Bronchiolitis in individual with cystic fibrosis	■ *Pseudomonas aeruginosa* ■ *Staphylococcus aureus* ■ *Burkholderia cepacia*	■ Other *Burkholderia* spp. ■ Fungi ■ Atypical *Mycobacterium* spp.
Community-acquired pneumonia	■ *Streptococcus pneumoniae* ■ *Haemophilus influenzae* ■ *Staphylococcus aureus* ■ *Legionella pneumophila* ■ *Moraxella catarrhalis* ■ *Mycoplasma pneumoniae* ■ *Chlamydophila pneumoniae*	■ Influenza virus ■ Adenovirus ■ Parainfluenza virus ■ Respiratory syncytial virus ■ Other viruses ■ *Mycobacterium tuberculosis* ■ Fungi
Hospital-acquired pneumonia	■ *Staphylococcus aureus* ■ *Enterobacteriaceae* ■ *Pseudomonas aeruginosa*	■ *Acinetobacter* spp. ■ *Legionella* spp.
Ventilator-associated pneumonia	■ *Enterobacteriaceae* ■ *Pseudomonas aeruginosa*	■ *Staphylococcus aureus* ■ *Haemophilus influenzae*
Aspiration pneumonia	■ Anaerobes ■ *Staphylococcus aureus*	■ *Enterobacteriaceae* ■ *Pseudomonas aeruginosa*
Pleural effusion	■ *Streptococcus pneumoniae* ■ *Staphylococcus aureus* ■ *Haemophilus influenzae*	■ *Enterobacteriaceae* ■ *Pseudomonas aeruginosa*

Bronchitis

Bronchitis is often a self-limiting condition causing inflammation of the bronchial tubes or bronchi. The mucous membrane of the bronchial tubes becomes irritated and inflamed and enlarges or thickens, which in turn narrows the airway. Add an increase in mucus and phlegm to the tubes and coughing, wheezing, and shortness of breath occur. The major symptom is a persistent cough, which can last for weeks after its appearance. Other symptoms include mild fever, fatigue, shortness of breath, wheezing, and production of clear, yellow, or green mucus. The first stage of symptoms lasts 1 to 5 days with fever, malaise, and muscle aches, which is similar to many other upper respiratory infections. The second stage usually lasts 1 to 3 weeks with persistent cough, phlegm production, and wheezing.

The two types of bronchitis are acute, which is often short lived, lasting only a few weeks, and chronic, which can last several months. Acute bronchitis is associated with both viral and bacterial pathogens. Chronic bronchitis is associated more often with cigarette smoking and pollutants in the environment.

Most cases of acute bronchitis seem to be of a nonbacterial etiology (Aagaard & Gonzales, 2004). The agents causing bronchitis are usually viral in origin, such as influenza virus, respiratory syncytial virus, rhinovirus, coronavirus, and adenovirus. They occur primarily during the winter months and usually in young children.

Three bacteria that are known to cause bronchitis are *Bordetella pertussis, Chlamydophila pneumoniae,* and *Mycoplasma pneumoniae.* The atypical bacteria *Chlamydophila pneumoniae* and *Mycoplasma pneumoniae* are discussed later in this chapter as causes of pneumonia. Other bacteria such as *Streptococcus pneumoniae, Haemophilus influenzae,* and *Moraxella catarrhalis* have been isolated in cases of bronchitis, but they may be present because of underlying lung disease, so it is hard to attribute their presence to the disease.

Bordetella pertussis is the causative agent of pertussis, or whooping cough. This gram-negative coccobacillus attaches to and damages the ciliated respiratory epithelium cells. The organism is spread in aerosolized droplets produced during coughing. Humans are the only known reservoir. Pertussis follows a 6-week course characterized by fits of intense coughing. The classic whoop is because of the intake of air through the narrowed bronchi. Vomiting can immediately follow coughing fits. Most cases occur in infants, children, and adolescents. Adults are a major reservoir source because of their waning immunity as they often do not receive the booster immunizations.

> ### REAL WORLD TIP
>
> Unvaccinated children with whooping cough often have a very high white blood cell count, with up to 75% lymphocytes. The organism's toxin, which is responsible for damage to the ciliated epithelial cells, also attracts lymphocytes.

Bronchiolitis. **Bronchiolitis** is inflammation of the smaller bronchioles. It is primarily an infection in infants and young children and usually occurs because of a viral infection. It is spread via respiratory droplets. Because the bronchioles are narrow, mucus produced can obstruct them and cause labored breathing. Most children have a cough and wheezing similar to asthma. Bronchiolitis can eventually cause infection of the entire lower respiratory tract.

Most cases are caused by viruses, with respiratory syncytial virus as the most common agent. The appearance of the disease correlates with respiratory season in late fall to early spring. Adenovirus is responsible for most of the remainder of cases.

One unique patient population extremely prone to infection of the bronchioles is children and young adults with the genetic disease cystic fibrosis (CF). Their respiratory signs and symptoms are not because of pneumonia, which is infection of the alveoli, but actually inflammation of the bronchioles. CF is caused by a faulty transport in the cells of the gastrointestinal, pulmonary, and endocrine systems. Sodium and chloride move out of the cells. Water follows the movement of these electrolytes, and the body's secretions become very thick and viscous. The increased viscosity of the mucus in the lungs leads to colonization by multiple microorganisms and, in turn, frequent infections, which can eventually destroy the airways.

Cystic fibrosis is associated with very specific pathogens. An extremely mucoid strain of *Pseudomonas aeruginosa* is frequently isolated in this patient population. It is so characteristic that its presence should warrant testing for cystic fibrosis if there is no previous diagnosis. Once established, this organism is extremely difficult to eradicate.

Other organisms associated with CF include *Staphylococcus aureus, Burkholderia cepacia,* other *Burkholderia* spp., fungi, and atypical *Mycobacterium* spp. The microbiologist must be extremely diligent in the recovery and proper identification of *Burkholderia cepacia* in a respiratory culture of a CF patient. Lung transplants are often used for treatment of CF. A CF individual harboring *B. cepacia* can be excluded from the lung transplant listing because of the high mortality rate associated with the presence of this organism.

> ### REAL WORLD TIP
>
> ■ The extremely mucoid strain of *Pseudomonas aeruginosa* observed in cystic fibrosis patients is because of its polysaccharide alginate capsule. This wet and viscous colony can also be observed in adult patients with chronic obstructive pulmonary disease (COPD). This unique colony morphology should be reported to the physician when observed.
>
> ■ The isolation of *Burkholderia cepacia* in the respiratory secretions of an individual with cystic fibrosis (CF) is often considered a death sentence. There is a high mortality rate in CF patients once they are colonized with the organism. *B. cepacia* is extremely difficult to eradicate because of its multidrug resistance. Selective medium is necessary to ensure its recovery in respiratory secretions. Once isolated, its identification must be verified by two methodologies. Once identified, the CF patient should no longer associate with other CF patients to prevent its spread.

Pneumonia

Pneumonia is the inflammation of the lungs caused primarily by bacteria, viruses, and chemical irritants. It is the sixth-most-common cause of death in the United States. From 1979 through 1994, the overall rate of death because of pneumonia and influenza increased by 59% in the United States (Bartlett et al., 2000). Symptoms include cough, fever, chills, shortness of breath, chest pain, and **sputum** (material from the respiratory tract) production. The sputum produced may be green and purulent because of the organisms and white blood cells present. Blood may be present because of capillaries breaking during coughing or invasive organisms.

The inflammation in the lungs actually occurs in the alveoli. They fill with fluid as the bacteria reproduce. Crackles and wheezing can be heard. The body attempts to fight off the infection, resulting in inflammation. With inflammation, less oxygen is being taken into the blood, and carbon dioxide is not removed as efficiently. The lungs have to work harder to get oxygen the body needs, which results in shortness of breath.

A chest x-ray is critical for the diagnosis of pneumonia and to distinguish it from bronchitis (Bartlett et al., 2000). Pneumonia appears as areas of white patches on x-rays because of the fluid-filled alveoli.

Older adults are prone to pneumonia. Their weakened immune state, less-effective ciliated epithelial cell function, and underlying conditions such diabetes mellitus create opportunities for microorganisms to reach the alveoli. Infants and children under the age of two can progress to pneumonia quickly because of their immature immune system. Certain conditions such as alcoholism, drug abuse, diabetes, infection with human immunodeficiency virus, and history of an upper respiratory tract infection can predispose an individual to the development of pneumonia.

Community-acquired pneumonia (CAP) describes the development of pneumonia in an individual who has not been hospitalized or resided in a long-term care facility more than 14 days before onset of symptoms. **Hospital-acquired pneumonia (HAP)** is also known as nosocomial pneumonia. HAP develops 48 hours or longer after a patient has been admitted to the hospital. **Ventilator-associated pneumonia (VAP)** develops 48 hours or more after the use of mechanical ventilation in a patient. Aspiration pneumonia results from inhalation of foreign material such as stomach contents or upper respiratory secretions. This can occur during sleep, during intoxication, and while under anesthesia.

REAL WORLD TIP

The Centers for Medicare and Medicaid Services (CMS) has identified ventilator-acquired pneumonia and Legionnaire's disease as hospital-acquired conditions that will no longer qualify for higher reimbursement rates. CMS will now only reimburse the hospital for the patient's original diagnosis.

Bacterial Pneumonia.   The most common organism found in two-thirds of all cases of community-acquired bacterial pneumonia is *Streptococcus pneumoniae*. This football- or lancet-shaped gram-positive diplococci is isolated more frequently during the winter respiratory season than any other time of the year. During the winter, it can colonize the nasopharynx. Its capsule makes it especially virulent. More than 90 different serotypes are based on its capsule. Disease can occur because of exposure to a serotype that an individual has not encountered previously or been vaccinated against. Those with sickle cell anemia or who do not possess a spleen are especially susceptible to this organism.

Haemophilus influenzae is the second most common causative agent of adult pneumonia. Although the b serotype has been virtually eliminated with the Hib vaccine, other serotypes and nontypeable strains can cause disease, given the right circumstances. Individuals infected often have underlying conditions.

Pneumonia caused by *Staphylococcus aureus* is most often seen secondary to viral respiratory infections such as influenza. Viruses destroy the respiratory epithelium, and colonizing *S. aureus* are able to cause a secondary infection. Methicillin-resistant *S. aureus* is known to cause infections primarily in hospitalized patients, but it is now being seen more often as a causative agent of community-acquired pneumonia.

Pseudomonas aeruginosa is the most common gram-negative rod followed by *Escherichia coli* and *Klebsiella pneumoniae*, especially in hospitalized patients. Most of the *Enterobacteriaceae* can be encountered in patients who have an underlying disease process such as cardiac disease, pulmonary illness, liver disease, and diabetes that has been active in the past year (Mandell, 2004). For most infectious agents, inhalation of infected aerosols is the usual route of entry, but aerobic gram-negative rods can use aspiration of oropharyngeal secretions as their route of entry.

REAL WORLD TIP

- If a predominance of lancet-shaped gram-positive diplococci (pairs) and neutrophils are observed on a direct Gram stain of a lower respiratory specimen, the microbiologist should report "gram-positive cocci suggestive of pneumococcus" in the preliminary report. This will provide the physician valuable information for treatment a full 18 to 24 hours before the culture results are available.

- If the direct Gram stain of a lower respiratory specimen shows a predominance of tiny gram-negative rods/coccobacilli and numerous neutrophils, the microbiologist should consider *Haemophilus* spp. as the potential causative agent. The organism will display no growth on the blood agar at 24 hours but growth on the chocolate or *Haemophilus* isolation agars.

A few organisms are considered "atypical" pneumonia pathogens. These include *Mycoplasma pneumoniae*, *Chlamydophila pneumoniae*, and *C. psittaci*. They are called atypical because they can infect healthy individuals, and the presentation of pneumonia tends be milder than other forms of pneumonia. The presence of either *C. pneumoniae* or *M. pneumoniae* may worsen the symptoms of asthma (Johnston & Martin, 2005).

Legionella pneumophila is a fastidious gram-negative rod that can cause both serious and milder forms of pneumonia. It is considered a strict pathogen. It can be missed because it will not grow on the routine media used to diagnose pneumonia.

Cases of *Mycoplasma pneumoniae* pneumonia can be observed singly or in small outbreaks in families or facilities such as boarding schools or barracks. It typically is seen in healthy individuals such as adolescents, young adults, and adults up to the age of 40. *Mycoplasma pneumoniae* can also cause bronchitis in those older than 5 years. After recovery, a cough may remain for weeks. Transmission is via human to human by droplets generated by coughing. It is commonly known as "walking" pneumonia because the infected individual is ill but not enough to require bed rest or hospitalization.

Chlamydophila pneumoniae is spread by respiratory secretions, especially among school-age children. Infections tend to be chronic with a slow recovery. A cough can last for weeks to months. *Chlamydophila psittaci* is spread via aerosols from infected birds such as chickens and turkeys. Both organisms are too difficult for most laboratories to grow. Serology can be used for diagnosis.

Legionella pneumophila, the most common species of the genus, is an environmental gram-negative rod associated with water. Water sources include freshwater, manmade water systems such as fountains, grocery store misters, and air conditioning towers of large buildings. The organism likes warmer temperatures (25°C to 42°C), stagnant water, and biofilms in the water. It was first isolated in 1976 in Philadelphia, Pennsylvania, from individuals who became ill while attending a national American Legion convention. The resulting disease has been named Legionnaire's disease, or legionellosis.

The organism is transmitted in water droplets that are inhaled or aspirated by the host. Its presence in humidifiers, respiratory therapy equipment, showers, and whirlpools makes it an ever-present potential nosocomial pathogen. Most individuals who present with Legionnaire's disease are elderly, smoke, and have underlying conditions such as heart or lung disease or are immunocompromised or immunosuppressed because of steroids.

REAL WORLD TIP

Pneumonia because of *Legionella pneumophila* produces sputum different from that produced because of other bacterial pneumonia pathogens. The sputum of an individual with legionellosis tends to be thin and watery with little purulent material.

Checkpoint! 33–4
(Chapter Objective 5)

You receive a sputum specimen for routine culture. The direct Gram stain shows a predominance of small gram-negative coccobacilli. The next day there is no growth on the blood agar plate but growth on the chocolate agar. What potential pathogen do you suspect?

    A. *Legionella pneumophila*
    B. *Haemophilus influenzae*
    C. *Mycoplasma pneumoniae*
    D. *Escherichia coli*

Viral Pneumonia.   Because of better detection methods, including molecular diagnostics, and the ability to treat some viruses with antiviral agents, the diagnosis of viral pneumonia has increased. The influenza viruses A and B are the most common cause of viral pneumonia in adults. Other viruses include adenovirus, parainfluenza viruses, and respiratory syncytial virus (RSV). The same viruses can affect children, but RSV is most common in this age group. Immunocompromised individuals, such as pregnant females and transplant recipients, tend to develop viral pneumonia because of cytomegalovirus, varicella zoster virus, herpes simplex virus, and adenovirus. Pneumonia can also occur as a complication of measles and chicken pox.

The influenza viruses and RSV are known for their appearance during the winter months. Transmission is person to person by means of airborne respiratory droplets, and once infected, individuals can shed the virus for up to 10 days. Each year the elderly, the very young, and those with weakened immune systems can develop severe signs and symptoms and acquire secondary bacterial infections, which often require hospitalization. All three of these patient populations have a potentially high rate of mortality with viral pneumonia. Healthy individuals tend to exhibit mild symptoms and recover.

The most common contagious airborne viral infectious disease is often called the "flu." It is caused by influenza A and B viruses and presents abruptly with fever, chills, headache, muscle and joint pain, cough, sore throat, and runny nose. Once the lungs are infected, the individual can suffer from respiratory distress. Secondary bacterial infections can occur because of the cell damage caused by replication of the viruses. *Staphylococcus aureus, Streptococcus pneumoniae,* and *Haemophilus influenzae* are common secondary bacterial invaders.

People often confuse the common cold for influenza and vice versa. Table 33-3✪ compares the signs and symptoms of the common cold against those of influenza or the common "flu." While the flu may be treatable with antiviral agents, the common cold is not affected.

There are several strains of the influenza virus, which are differentiated by their surface antigens. Influenza A usually causes more severe disease than the B strain. Influenza A is the major cause of worldwide epidemics or pandemics. During the 20th century there have been three pandemics, which killed millions of people. The first occurred in 1918 and was known as the Spanish flu. The second occurred in 1957 and was known as the Asian flu. The third took place in 1968 and was known as the Hong Kong flu. All three strains produced very high mortality rates. In 2009, a swine flu pandemic due to a novel H1N1 virus was declared by the World Health Organization (WHO). ∞ Chapter 42, "Global Threats," provides more detail about this recent outbreak.

One strain of influenza virus that is worrying experts is H5N1. It originated in birds and can now infect humans. It appeared in humans in 1997 and is known as the "avian flu" or "bird flu." Although there have only be a few cases in China, it has shown the potential for mutations that could change it

TABLE 33-3

Differentiation of the Common Cold and the "Flu"

Symptom	Cold	Flu
Fever	Rare	High (100°C–102°C) for 3–4 days
Headache	Rare	Predominant
General aches and pains	Slight	Usually severe
Fatigue/weakness	Quite mild	Lasts up to 2–3 weeks
Extreme exhaustion	Never	Early and prominent
Stuffy nose	Common	Sometimes
Sneezing	Usual	Sometimes
Sore throat	Common	Sometimes
Chest discomfort/cough	Mild to moderate	Common and can be severe
Complications	Sinus congestion and earache	Bronchitis Pneumonia (can be life threatening)
Prevention	None	Annual vaccine
Treatment	Relief of symptoms	Amantadine (resistance has now developed) Rimantadine (resistance has now developed) Oseltamivir (novel H1N1 resistance has developed) Zanamivir

into a new strain of virus that can be easily transmitted from person to person. Once a virus mutates, the body's immune system is unable to recognize it and is not prepared to fight it. This strain has a very high mortality rate because of its severe symptoms such as fluid-filled lungs and resistance to most current antiviral therapies.

Hantavirus is a rodent virus that can infect humans to cause pneumonia. It was discovered in the Four Corners area (Arizona, Colorado, New Mexico, and Utah) of the United States. The virus reaches the lungs after exposure to aerosolized rodent urine and feces. Disease develops rapidly because of fluid-filled lungs, which can lead to respiratory failure. Although the numbers of cases has been low, this is another example of the ability of viruses to jump from animals to humans to cause disease.

Fungal Pneumonia.   Fungi are considered opportunistic pathogens that take advantage of a compromised immune system. They can also be endemic to certain geographic regions, which allow them the opportunity to infect both healthy and compromised individuals. Infection can occur because of inhalation of the conidia or hyphae or because of hematogenous (blood route) spread from another body site.

Leukemia and the accompanying chemotherapy, transplantations, steroid therapy, acquired immunodeficiency syndrome, and neutropenia can predispose individuals to fungal infections. Symptoms of fungal pneumonia are often chronic and may begin 1 to 2 months prior to diagnosis. Signs and symptoms include fever, cough, chest pain, trouble breathing, and possible blood in the sputum because of the invasive nature of some fungi. A chest x-ray may show areas of consolidation or cavities similar to tuberculosis.

Fungi associated with pneumonia include the endemic fungi, *Histoplasma capsulatum*, *Coccidioides immitis*, *Blastomyces dermatitidis*, and *Paracoccidioides brasiliensis*, as well as *Cryptococcus neoformans*, *Candida* spp., *Aspergillus fumigatus*, *Rhizopus* spp., and *Mucor* spp. Fungi can disseminate to cause other infections such as meningitis. There is a high mortality rate because of fungal pneumonia when associated with a suppressed immune state.

Pneumocystis jiroveci (previously *P. carinii*) was initially thought to be a protozoan parasite, but has now been reclassified as a fungus. It is most commonly found in HIV-positive individuals with low CD4+ levels. Its presence often indicates the advancement of the disease status to full-blown acquired immunodeficiency syndrome (AIDS). The organism is inhaled and causes difficulty breathing, fever and chills, cough, and weight loss. Most HIV-positive individuals are maintained on preventive therapy to avoid infection.

Mycobacterial Pneumonia.   *Mycobacterium tuberculosis* (Mtb*)* is a rod-shaped bacterium that does not appear well on Gram stain because of an atypical cell wall. Special stains are needed to visually see the bacteria. The organisms have a lipophilic cell wall and are acid fast. Once stained with an acid-fast stain, they cannot be easily overdecolorized with acid alcohol. This is unlike a Gram stain, where microorganisms can be easily overdecolorized with acetone and appear gram-negative. This is unique characteristics has gained them the name "acid-fast bacilli (AFB)."

REAL WORLD TIP

Rapid-growing mycobacteria may not stain with carbol fuchsin acid-fast stains or fluoresce with fluorochrome stains.

Tuberculosis can originate after inhaling aerosols containing the organism, *Mycobacterium tuberculosis*. The organisms are engulfed by macrophages in the alveoli, where they are either killed, proliferate, or become dormant. Dormant organisms, which hide within cavities formed in the lungs, can reactivate with age or a compromised immune system, especially in human immunodeficiency virus (HIV) infected individuals.

Symptoms commonly associated with active tuberculosis include fever, night sweats, bloody sputum, weight loss, and cough. Individuals exhibiting these symptoms are extremely infectious. A chest x-ray will display an area of consolidation similar to a mass where the Mtb have created cavity like lesions in the lungs. The organism requires high oxygen content so it is very content in the lungs but can spread systemically if left untreated.

Although the infection can be eradicated with a cocktail of multiple antibiotics, multi-drug-resistant cases are increasing and have shown an increased mortality rate. *Mycobacterium tuberculosis* is discussed in detail in ∞ Chapters 13 and 26.

Parasitic Pneumonia.   Some parasites have a lung phase as part of their life cycle, which requires the larvae to enter the lung, work their way up the trachea, and then enter the esophagus to reach the gastrointestinal tract. *Ascaris lumbricoides, Strongyloides stercoralis,* and *Paragonimus westermani* are recognized for the lung phase present in their life cycle. Symptoms include fever, chest pain, cough, and difficulty breathing. One clue to the presence of a parasitic infection is an increased eosinophil count in the peripheral blood. Other parasites associated with pneumonia in immunocompromised hosts include *Toxoplasma gondii, Cryptosporidium parvum* and the microsporidium.

 Checkpoint! 33–5 (Chapter Objective 8)

A patient presents with a cough, fever, and flulike symptoms. His chest x-ray shows an area of consolidation in the right lung. Which two organisms should be suspected based on this information?

   A. Streptococcus pneumoniae and influenza virus

   B. Mycobacterium tuberculosis and Histoplasma capsulatum

   C. Blastomyces dermatidis and Staphylococcus aureus

   D. Staphylococcus aureus and Streptococcus pneumoniae

Nosocomial, or Hospital-Acquired, Pneumonia.
Admission to the hospital can lead to exposure to organisms that can colonize the upper respiratory system. These colonizers can then reach the lungs with aspiration, inhalation, or through the bloodstream. Extremes in ages and the presence of other conditions such as diabetes increase the risk for development of pneumonia. Nosocomial, or hospital-acquired, pneumonia (HAP) is most common in patients in intensive care units and those on mechanical ventilators.

Most often the organisms responsible for HAP are members of the family *Enterobacteriaceae* with *Klebsiella pneumoniae, E. coli, Enterobacter* spp., and *Serratia marcescens* as the most common isolates. *Pseudomonas aeruginosa* and *Staphylococcus aureus* can also cause HAP. *Acinetobacter* spp. and *Legionella* spp. are associated with outbreaks among multiple patients in the hospital setting.

Ventilator-Associated Pneumonia.   Ventilator-associated pneumonia (VAP) can develop 48 hours or longer after insertion of an endotracheal tube or tracheostomy for mechanical ventilation. The tracheal tube allows microorganisms to reach the lower respiratory system. Most cases of VAP are caused by aerobic gram-negative rods such as the *Enterobacteriaceae*, which include *Enterobacter* spp., *Klebsiella* spp., and *E. coli*, as well as *Pseudomonas aeruginosa, Staphylococcus*

aureus, and *Haemophilus influenzae.* These organisms are able to colonize the oropharynx. The presence of biofilm on the tracheal tube adds to the potential for infection.

Aspiration Pneumonia.   Aspiration of foreign material into the lungs can lead to infection. Unconsciousness because of alcohol or drug abuse, trouble swallowing because of a stroke, and being under anesthesia can depress the normal gag and cough reflexes, allowing oropharyngeal secretions and stomach contents to reach the lungs. Upper respiratory secretions can also reach the lungs during sleep. The presence of periodontal disease or poor oral hygiene can increase the number and variety of organisms aspirated. Intubated (ventilation or feeding) individuals are prone to aspiration of organisms, which build biofilm on the tubing. Infection occurs if the individual's immune status or respiratory defense mechanisms are impaired. The volume of material aspirated is also a factor in the initiation of infection.

Signs and symptoms of aspiration pneumonia can mimic that of traditionally acquired bacterial pneumonia. Periodontal disease or poor oral hygiene can shift the organism balance in the upper respiratory tract in favor of anaerobes. With anaerobic pneumonia, the sputum produced can have a putrid odor because of the metabolic by-products produced by the organisms.

Anaerobic pneumonia is usually caused by multiple organisms such as *Bacteroides* spp., *Porphyromonas* spp., *Prevotella* spp., *Fusobacterium* spp., and *Peptostreptococcus* spp. *Staphylococcus aureus,* the *Enterobacteriaceae,* and *Pseudomonas* spp. can also be among the causative agents if the aspiration occurs in the hospital setting.

Pleural Effusion and Empyema.   The pleural space is the area between the two thin membranes that cover the lungs. It contains about 1 mL of sterile fluid for lubrication when the lungs expand and contract. Fluid can accumulate in the space because of trauma, congestive heart failure, malignancy, pneumonia, or septicemia.

During pneumonia, fluid from the lungs moves into the pleural space. The fluid can remain sterile or become infected and lead to pus production. The collection of pus within a naturally existing body cavity such as the pleural space is known as **empyema.**

Because most cases of pleural effusion are associated with concurrent pneumonia, the signs and symptoms are those associated with pneumonia. Infected pleural fluid is thick with an increase in neutrophils. It may be foul smelling if it is the result of an anaerobic infection. Removal of the fluid may be necessary via thoracentesis (pleural fluid aspiration) if it continues to accumulate. As the fluid accumulates, it can cause pressure on the lungs and make breathing difficult. Chest pain may also be present.

Organisms associated with pleural effusion include those also associated with pneumonia. *Streptococcus pneumoniae* and *Staphylococcus aureus* are the most common pathogens.

Klebsiella spp., *Pseudomonas* spp., and *Haemophilus* spp. are the most common gram-negative isolates. The accumulation of pus in the pleural space can also be associated with the presence of multiple aerobic and anaerobic organisms.

▶ SPECIMEN COLLECTION

Appropriate specimen collection is very important for the microbiology lab to produce accurate and specific information to aid in the diagnosis and treatment of respiratory infections. The specimen collected should be one that will accurately assess the area where the infection is occurring. For the respiratory system, several types of specimens will be discussed in this section.

The nasopharyngeal swab consists of a calcium alginate-tipped swab on the end of a flexible wire shaft that can easily be inserted deep in the nasal passage to reach the back of the nasopharynx, where the swab is rotated a few times to pick up the microorganism residing there. Figure 33-5 ■ demonstrates an example of a nasopharyngeal swab.

The nasopharyngeal swab is required when testing for *Neisseria meningitidis, Bordetella pertussis,* influenza virus, and respiratory syncytial virus. The patient's head is tilted back to make it more comfortable for the swab to reach deep in the nasopharynx. Testing can be done directly on the swab using rapid kit testing or placed in saline, viral transport media, or bacterial transport media or used to inoculate agar plates based on the order from the physician. Although easy to use, swabs are not as productive in the recovery of viruses as nasopharyngeal washing and aspiration.

The swab routinely used for specimen collection for bacterial culture of the throat and nares consists of Dacron material wound onto a plastic shaft. Figure 33-6 ■ demonstrates a swab used in most laboratories for collection of samples for bacterial cultures. A calcium alginate swab can be used, but may be

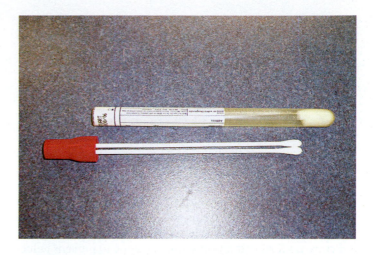

■ **FIGURE 33-6** This bacterial collection system provides two swabs. One can be used for a direct Gram stain, whereas the other can be used to inoculate the appropriate agar plates.

inhibitory to some organisms such as *Neisseria gonorrhoeae.* There may be one or two swabs within the plastic sheath, depending on the manufacturer. A bacterial transport medium is included in the plastic sheath to ensure the bacteria remain viable but static prior to culture. The transport media will keep the bacteria alive for quite some time, but if the swabs dry out or there are several days delay coming from a physician's office, the quality of the specimen and accuracy of the results can be greatly reduced. Viruses do not survive on bacterial collection swabs without special transport medium.

℮ REAL WORLD TIP

- *Streptococcus pyogenes* can survive up to 3 days on a dry collection swab. It is one of the few organisms that is very resistant to dessication.

- Cotton swabs, especially those with wooden shafts, are available but are not recommended for the collection of some organisms. Cotton and wood can be inhibitory to *Bordetella pertussis* and *Neisseria gonorrhoeae.* Calcium alginate swabs can inhibit the detection of *B. pertussis* by polymerase chain reaction.

During collection of a throat culture, the tongue is depressed gently with a tongue depressor so the back of the pharynx wall can be accessed with the swab. A swab is used to sample the tonsils as well as the area immediately behind the uvula (posterior pharynx). Care must be taken not to touch the cheeks, tongue, uvula, or lips to avoid excessive normal oral flora. Collection may trigger the gag reflex in some individuals when done properly.

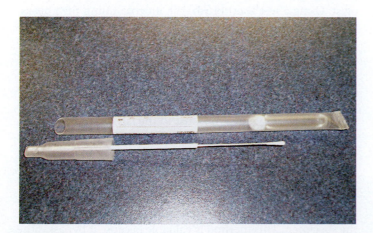

■ **FIGURE 33-5** The thin flexible shaft of this swab allows it to be inserted deeply into the nasopharynx to collect a sample for culture.

REAL WORLD TIP

Viral pharyngitis is rarely confirmed by culture. A throat specimen can be used to recover enterovirus when aseptic meningitis is suspected.

Nasal washing and aspiration is another method used to collect samples from the nasopharynx. Approximately 5 mL of sterile 0.85% saline or sodium chloride (NaCl) solution is instilled into the nostril while the patient's head is held back at a 70 degree angle. The fluid is then suctioned out with a bulb syringe or allowed to run out of the nostril into a sterile container. If testing for influenza virus or respiratory syncytial virus, no further dilution should be done to prevent reduction of the amount of virus present. An equal volume of viral transport media is added if submitted for other viral testing. Collection kits on the market include everything required to collect a nasal washing. These kits are more convenient for the physician or nurse who then does not have to assemble several items to collect the sample.

REAL WORLD TIP

Viruses are intracellular organisms that require living cells to replicate. Viral cultures require the collection of human cells to ensure the presence of virus for detection.

Sinus aspirates are obtained to aid in the diagnosis of sinusitis. The specimen must be collected without contamination by the upper respiratory normal flora. The physician may use an endoscope and swab to collect drainage. The best specimen is collected using a syringe puncture and aspiration technique and should be performed only by specially trained physicians such as otolaryngologists (ear, nose and throat [ENT] specialists). Because sinusitis can be caused by anaerobes, the specimen collected should be placed into an anaerobic transport system or the needle removed from the syringe, capped off, and sent immediately to the microbiology lab for processing.

Acute epiglottitis may require the establishment of an airway prior to collection of a specimen for culture. The infection creates a narrowed airway, which can spasm shut when cultured and prevent the passage of air. Blood cultures are usually collected at the same time as culture of the epiglottis.

Sputum specimens are used to aid in diagnosis of lower respiratory tract infections. The most common lower respiratory specimen collected is expectorated sputum. **Expectorated** sputum is voluntarily coughed up by an individual. Collection of this specimen requires specific instructions so an adequate and acceptable sample is obtained.

Many individuals think sputum is just "spit" or the saliva in their mouth. The public must be educated that sputum comes from down deep in the lungs. The best method of obtaining an acceptable sputum sample is to have the individual rinse their mouth and gargle with water prior to collection to remove excess saliva, which contains normal flora. They then need to cough deeply and try to bring up phlegm or mucus that may be present.

An acceptable sputum visually appears as thick mucus and may be yellow, green, or clear. Any blood that appears in the sputum should be used to inoculate culture media because the presence of blood can indicate invasive bacterial infection. If the sample is watery in consistency and contains bubbles, it is not likely to be good sputum. The specimen should be collected in a sterile container and labeled with patient information, date, time, initials of the person collecting the sample, specimen source, and test requested prior to submission to the lab.

REAL WORLD TIP

The sputum produced because of infection with *Legionella* spp. tends to be clear, thin, and watery. It may not contain white blood cells, which usually accompany bacterial infection.

Only one respiratory specimen per day should be submitted to the laboratory for testing. Mycobacterial or fungal infections may require multiple specimens to increase the chance of recovery of these pathogens. Even in these instances, it is still recommended that only one sputum per day be collected but over multiple days. The best sputum specimen is collected first thing in the morning when the individual rises. Phlegm collects during the night in the lungs, and the body's response is to cough it up and get it out of the lungs.

If an individual cannot produce sputum easily, it may be necessary to induce or stimulate a sample. This procedure is normally performed by a trained respiratory therapy technologist. Using a wet toothbrush, the mucosa lining the cheeks, tongue, and gums is brushed prior to the procedure. This is followed by rinsing the mouth with water, and then an ultrasonic nebulizer is used to allow the patient to inhale approximately 20 to 30 mL of aerosolized 0.85% NaCl. The finely misted saline enters deep into the lungs and triggers the cough reflex. The sputum collected from the induction is placed in a properly labeled sterile cup and submitted to the lab for testing.

A transtracheal specimen can be collected if an individual cannot provide acceptable expectorated sputum and cannot be induced because of other health reasons such as asthma or chronic obstructive pulmonary disease. A catheter is inserted through the skin over the trachea and threaded into the bronchioles. Sterile saline is introduced and reaspirated to provide the specimen. This method is valuable because it bypasses the normal upper respiratory flora, so any organism isolated is often significant. This method has been replaced by the use of a bronchoscope.

Tracheostomy and endotracheal aspirations (TA) are used when an individual is on a mechanical ventilator or has been removed from the ventilator but still has the endotracheal tube in place in the trachea. These aspirates are collected by a respiratory therapist or nurse in a Lukens or sputum trap, which uses suction to obtain the specimen. Figure 33-7 ■ shows an example of a Lukens or sputum trap.

The tracheostomy site and endotracheal tube become colonized with microorganisms, especially gram-negative rods, within 24 hours of insertion, so bacterial cultures must be evaluated carefully. Culture results must be correlated with significant clinical findings such as fever, high white blood cell count, or infiltration on a chest x-ray. These two specimens can be good specimens for culture if the patient exhibits the signs and symptoms of pneumonia because the mouth has been bypassed, and normal upper respiratory flora is not normally present.

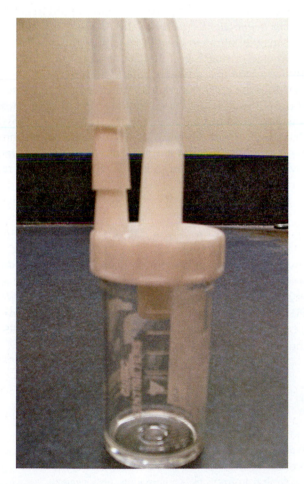

■ **FIGURE 33-7** A sputum or Lukens trap is used to a collect lower respiratory secretion via a tracheostomy site, endotracheal tube, or bronchoscopy procedure. Because using a sterile catheter and suction to obtain lower respiratory secretions is considered an invasive procedure, most microbiology laboratories accept specimens collected via these methods, even if squamous epithelial cells are present.
Photo credit: Ruth Masterson.

In the case of an infant in the neonatal intensive care unit (NICU), a tracheal aspirate is the only method used to obtain lower respiratory secretions for testing. These specimens tend to be collected in very small volumes. Cultures are usually performed for bacteria and viruses. Molecular techniques such as real-time polymerase chain reaction (RT-PCR) play a large and important role in rapid detection and identification of viral infections in NICU infants.

A bronchoscopy specimen is collected using a bronchoscope inserted through the nose or mouth in nonintubated patients or via the endotracheal tube if intubated. The bronchoscope is a long flexible fiber optic tube that allows the physician to view the bronchi, bronchioles, and alveoli and collect tissues and secretions. It is guided into position by the physician using an x-ray machine. To obtain a bronchial wash or bronchoalveolar lavage (BAL), sterile nonbacteriostatic 0.85% NaCl is injected into the inner lumen of the bronchoscope. Gentle suction is applied, and the specimen is collected into a sputum or Lukens trap.

The physician can submit specimens from the various lobes of the lung as well as cell samples or a tissue biopsy of the area while using the bronchoscope. A cell collection brush or biopsy instrument is encased in a catheter, which can be inserted through the lumen of the bronchoscope. The brush or biopsy instrument is extended out of the catheter once in the area to be sampled and then pulled back into the catheter once completed. The brush or tissue is then sent for culture and cytology examination.

Lung tissue can be collected as a needle biopsy through the chest wall or in surgery. The tissue can be submitted for culture of lung abscesses or invasive infections such as tuberculosis or fungi. The tissue should be transported to the laboratory under anaerobic conditions to ensure recovery of anaerobes.

Pleural fluid is usually collected via needle and syringe. Prior to transportation to the laboratory, the needle must be removed and the syringe capped. If a large volume of fluid has accumulated around the lungs, then sterile drainage tubing and a collection bottle may be necessary for collection. Ten mL of pleural fluid can be injected in each bottle of a blood culture set. The bottles should be held for 5 days.

@ **REAL WORLD TIP**

A swab should not be used to transport pleural fluid. It absorbs too little specimen to ensure recovery of possibly small numbers of organisms. Submission of as much fluid as possible is ideal.

▶ **SPECIMEN PROCESSING FOR CULTIVATION OR DETECTION**

Once a specimen has been collected and received in microbiology, it must be processed for the test(s) that have been ordered by the physician. Depending on the orders received, the microbiology laboratory may be looking for routine bacteria, fungi, mycobacteria, or viruses. The media required can be specific for each type of organism being cultured, and the incubation time and temperature can vary.

NASOPHARYNGEAL

A nasopharyngeal (NP) swab or nasal aspirate is usually used for detection of respiratory syncytial virus (RSV) and influenza viruses. The specimen should be collected as soon as possible after the onset of symptoms and no more than 4 days after onset. The specimen must contain cellular material because viruses are intracellular microorganisms. Rapid detection tests for RSV and influenza are routinely used rather than traditional culture. The NP swab or nasal washing is processed as defined by the manufacturer for the specific kit.

The manufacturers' kits for RSV and influenza viruses detect antigen specific for each virus using a solid phase or membrane enzyme immunoassay. Most use a substrate and conjugate to complete the reaction. Reactions are read visually as a colored dot or line. Each kit also contains a control to confirm that the procedure is performed correctly. If the control line or dot does not appear, then the result is invalid. Many tests on the market today use a flow-through technology in which the specimen migrates through a membrane so the reaction can occur. Most rapid tests are completed within 15 to 20 minutes.

REAL WORLD TIP

There are three types of influenza viruses—A, B, and C. Most infections are caused by types A and B. Type C is rarely associated with epidemic infections and is not routinely tested for in the laboratory. The microbiologist must be aware that not all rapid detection kits detect both A and B types.

The NP swab can also be used for pertussis testing. Most labs that perform pertussis testing usually request submission of two NP swabs. One swab is put in sterile 0.85% saline to be used for molecular testing for *Bordetella pertussis* and *Bordetella parapertussis*. The second swab is inoculated onto Regan-Lowe medium for transport to a reference laboratory if the culture is not performed on site.

If the culture is performed on site, the swab can be plated onto selective media such as Bordet-Gengou. A positive result from either culture or PCR is a reportable disease that requires notification of the public health department so appropriate measures can be initiated to prevent further spread of the disease.

Nasal carriers of *Staphylococcus aureus* and methicillin-resistant *Staphylococcus aureus* (MRSA) can also be identified with a nasopharyngeal culture swab. Molecular testing as well as selective and differential agars is helpful in its detection and

isolation. Chromogenic (color producing) agars can impart MRSA with a unique color to make its detection easier and much faster than traditional culture.

REAL WORLD TIP

Bordetella pertussis is very susceptible to azithromycin, which is the drug of choice for treating pertussis, or whooping cough. If the nasopharyngeal swabs are collected after treatment has been started, the organism will not be viable for culture and will not grow on culture but will still give a positive result by PCR.

Nasopharyngeal and throat swabs can be used to confirm the diagnosis of diphtheria. Selective and differential medium such as cystine tellurite or potassium tellurite can help isolate *Corynebacterium diphtheriae* from the normal flora present in these two body sites. On Loeffler's medium, the organism produces metachromatic granules, which are observed using methylene blue dye. Metachromatic granules stain as dark areas within the cells. The granules function as energy reserves.

If the NP swab is to be used for detection of other viruses, it must be placed in viral transport media as soon as possible so that the virus will survive until it is inoculated onto the cell lines or processed for other testing. A variety of transport media are available. The specimen should be refrigerated until ready for processing for culture.

REAL WORLD TIP

Enveloped viruses do not survive the freeze–thaw process well. Respiratory syncytial virus (RSV) is an enveloped RNA virus that is very sensitive to temperature changes. It can survive at room temperature and 4°C but not being slowly frozen. Specimens for RSV should never be frozen prior to processing.

✔ Checkpoint! 33–6 (Chapter Objective 4)

A throat swab is received in microbiology with a request for culture for pertussis. Is this an appropriate specimen for this request?

   A. *It is an acceptable specimen for pertussis culture.*

   B. *It is not an acceptable specimen. A culture of the epiglottis is required.*

   C. *It is not an acceptable specimen. Two nasopharyngeal swabs are necessary.*

   D. *It is not an acceptable specimen. A sputum specimen is required.*

THROAT

Streptococcus pyogenes is the most common throat pathogen, and a swab is used for specimen collection. The swab may be used for rapid group A *Streptococcus* testing, culture, or both. If rapid antigen testing is ordered, then one swab of a double swab set should be used, with the second swab saved for possible culture. The swab used for antigen testing is not appropriate for culture because the antigen extraction process inactivates the bacteria, and it will not grow on culture. The rapid group A *Streptococcus* antigen test can be completed in 10 to 20 minutes.

Keep in mind that the sensitivity of the rapid group A *Streptococcus* screen procedure is not 100% for every kit available on the market at this time. The sensitivity of the procedure decreases as the number of organisms present decreases. The screening kits are almost 100% sensitive when there are 50 to 100 organisms present but can be as low as 80% when there are 1 to 9 organisms present. Low numbers of organisms may be because of collection early in the infection or treatment prior to specimen collection. The current recommendation is that a negative rapid beta strep test must be backed up with a culture. With a double collection swab system, the second swab is still available for plating. If only one swab is collected, a sheep blood agar plate or group A streptococcus selective agar can be inoculated prior to rapid antigen testing on the swab. The medium is incubated in ambient air or anaerobically at 35° to 37°C.

REAL WORLD TIP

Many laboratories perform organism-specific rather than routine throat cultures except on special requests. This prevents the unnecessary workup and reporting of colonizing organisms such as *Streptococcus pneumoniae* and *Haemophilus influenzae*.

After 24 hours of incubation, the typical wide zone beta-hemolytic small gray colony of *Streptococcus pyogenes* is easily

REAL WORLD TIP

- A negative rapid group A *Streptococcus* screen does not necessarily mean the patient does not have pharyngitis. Other organisms such as group C and G *Streptococcus*, *Arcanobacterium haemolyticum*, and viruses can cause pharyngitis. More than 50% of pharyngitis cases are caused by viruses.

- *Streptococcus pneumoniae* and *Haemophilus influenzae* are not considered pharyngitis pathogens. These organisms can be normal upper respiratory flora, especially during the winter months. Both organisms may also be present because of drainage down the back of the throat, which can occur with sinusitis. In this instance, a throat culture cannot be used to diagnose sinusitis.

recognized on the sheep blood agar. A positive PYR and group A antigen test identify the isolate as group A beta-hemolytic streptococci. The microbiologist must remember that the colony of *Arcanobacterium haemolyticum,* a catalase negative gram-positive rod, which also causes pharyngitis, mimics that of *S. pyogenes*. It appears as a tiny colony at 24 hours and larger after 48 hours of incubation. A Gram stain is essential to differentiate the two organisms. The identification of these two organisms, as well as two other pharyngitis pathogens, groups C and G *Streptococcus,* are discussed in ∞ Chapters 17 and 19.

If the physician suspects *Neisseria gonorrhoeae* pharyngitis, the swab must be inoculated to media that will support the growth of this organism, such as chocolate agar, because it will not grow on blood agar. A Thayer-Martin agar is best for isolation of this organism from the throat. The agar will selectively isolate *Neisseria gonorrhoeae* from the normal upper respiratory flora present. The media needs to be incubated in 5% CO_2 and may require 2 to 4 days to grow. There are a number of biochemical kits and panels for automated systems to identify the organism. The identification of *N. gonorrhoeae* can be found in ∞ Chapter 18.

REAL WORLD TIP

Other *Neisseria* spp. can grow on Thayer-Martin agar. *Neisseria meningitidis*, *N. lactamica*, *N cinerea*, and *Moraxella catarrhalis* can be normal upper respiratory flora and able to grow on Thayer-Martin agar. Any oxidase-positive gram-negative diplococcus that grows on Thayer-Martin cannot be assumed to be *N. gonorrhoeae* or *N. meningitidis* and must be identified.

A throat swab may also be used in the detection of the causative agent of epiglottitis. Collecting the specimen may require immediate intubation of the patient because the epiglottis can spasm and close the airway. Blood cultures may reveal the causative agent as well.

SINUS ASPIRATES

A sinus aspirate is normally submitted in a syringe with requests for routine, fungal, or viral cultures. Routine and fungal cultures are the more common physician orders. Media for a routine culture needs to cover all the pathogens that are common to the sinuses, including *Streptococcus pneumoniae, Haemophilus influenzae, Staphylococcus aureus, Pseudomonas* species, *Moraxella catarrhalis,* and anaerobic organisms. The most common media used include sheep blood agar, chocolate agar, MacConkey agar, reducible blood agar, and LKV (laked blood, kanamycin, and vancomycin) agar. The last two media will aid in recovery of anaerobes. A direct Gram stain will provide the physician important information on which antibiotic therapy can be initiated.

Fungal cultures require specialized media incubated at 30°C for incubation up to 2 weeks. *Aspergillus fumigatus* is the most common pathogenic mould isolated, but others can cause sinusitis as well. Viruses can also be recovered in sinus aspirates. They require transport medium to maintain the viability of the virus before inoculation onto cell lines. Molecular methods can provide a rapid turnaround time versus culture, which can take up for 14 days for results.

SPUTUM, TRACHEAL ASPIRATE, BRONCHIAL WASHING, BRONCHIAL ALVEOLAR LAVAGE, AND LUNG TISSUE

Expectorated (deep cough) sputum specimen must pass through the upper respiratory tract during collection and so has the potential for contamination with normal upper respiratory flora. This can make the interpretation of a lower respiratory culture more difficult. The microbiologist must determine if a potential pathogen present in culture represents a true pathogen or a colonizer of the oropharynx.

Because of the possibility for contamination of the sputum specimen with normal upper respiratory flora, evaluation of a sputum specimen for acceptability is necessary. This ensures its quality so the culture results are an accurate picture of what is occurring in the lower respiratory system versus the upper respiratory system. A tracheal aspirate, bronchial washing, and bronchial alveolar lavage are usually always considered acceptable for culture because they are collected via invasive procedures that bypass normal upper respiratory flora.

Direct Gram stain of expectorated sputum is very important to determine its quality. Squamous epithelial cells (SECs) line the upper respiratory tract, and their presence in sputum indicates the potential presence of normal upper respiratory flora. The entire stained slide is scanned on 10× magnification (low objective) for SECs. An average SEC count is determined for the entire slide. The greater the number of SECs present per low power field (LPF), the more chance that the sample represents oropharyngeal contamination and a specimen of poor quality. Culturing a poor-quality specimen will produce poor results and lead to inappropriate or unnecessary treatment.

A second indicator, often used in conjunction with the review of expectorated sputum for SEC, is the presence of white blood cells (WBCs), specifically neutrophils. The more white blood cells present, the more likely the specimen indicates an active site of infection.

There are several methods, described in the literature, that can be used to evaluate the quality or acceptability of expectorated sputum for culture. One method uses a ratio of SECs to WBCs. Sputum with less than 10 SECs/low power field (LPF) is considered an acceptable specimen. One with greater than 10 to 25 SECs/LPF is considered unacceptable for culture. The presence of 10 to 25 WBCs per LPF indicates potential infection if there is also a low number of SECs present. If greater than 25 WBCs per LPF, the specimen is usually considered acceptable, even if there are greater than 10 SECs per LPF present. The large numbers of WBCs indicate a potential infection. Figure 33-8 ■ demonstrates an unacceptable expectorated sputum Gram stained specimen at 25× magnification. Figure 33-9 ■ shows an acceptable sputum Gram stain with many neutrophils but no SECs present at 1000× magnification.

⊚ REAL WORLD TIP

- Expectorated sputum of a neutropenic patient with pneumonia may not reveal greater than 25 WBCs per LPF. The number of SECs per LPF should still be used to determine the quality of the sputum specimen from this patient population.

- Do not reject sputum and endotracheal specimens for *Legionella* spp., *Mycobacterium* spp., and those from cystic fibrosis patients. *Legionella* spp. is a strict pathogen that grows only on selective medium that inhibits normal upper respiratory flora. Respiratory specimens for *Mycobacterium* spp. are decontaminated, prior to plating, to remove upper respiratory flora. Cystic fibrosis patients have lung disease because of a limited number of unique pathogens that are usually not present in normal upper respiratory flora.

Once a sputum specimen is determined to be unacceptable, the culture is not to be performed. The nurse in charge of the patient should be notified. The physician must determine if

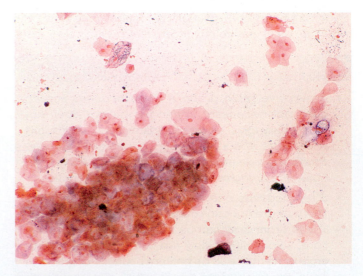

■ FIGURE 33-8 This Gram stained slide of sputum, at 25× magnification, illustrates a poor-quality specimen because of the presence of >10 to 25 SECs/LPF.

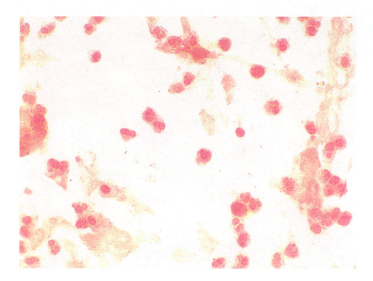

■ **FIGURE 33-9** This Gram stained slide of sputum, at 1000× magnification, demonstrates an acceptable specimen because of the absence of SECs and a predominance of neutrophils indicating a potential infection.

the specimen should be recollected and if sputum induction is necessary.

Once a Gram stained sputum specimen is determined to be acceptable, it can be reviewed for potential lower respiratory pathogens. The Gram stain of expectorated sputum from a pneumonia patient will reveal a predominance of neutrophils as well as a single potential pathogen because most cases of lower respiratory infections are usually caused by a single organism. Rather than reporting all organisms present, it makes sense to report only the predominant potential pathogen. An organism is considered predominant if it is present in a ratio of 10:1 when compared to other organisms present in the Gram stain smear. Reporting only the predominant organism provides the physician the information needed to direct specific therapy rather than initiating broad-spectrum antibiotics.

The most easily recognized pathogens associated with bacterial pneumonia include *Streptococcus pneumoniae* (lancet gram-positive diplococci), *Haemophilus influenzae* (gram-negative coccobacilli), the *Enterobacteriaceae* and *Pseudomonas aeruginosa* (gram-negative rods), *Moraxella catarrhalis* (intracellular gram-negative diplococci), *Candida albicans* (gram-positive budding yeast), and *Staphylococcus aureus* (gram-positive cocci in clusters). These organisms can be reported as patterns rather than listing all organisms present to help guide the physician. When there is no one predominant organism on the Gram stained smear or no organisms present, it can be reported as a "nondiagnostic" pattern. Figures 33-10a ■– 33-10d ■ demonstrate examples of Gram stained sputum specimens reported as bacterial patterns because of the predominance of a single organism.

REAL WORLD TIP

- A sputum Gram stain with a predominance of white blood cells and no organisms observed should be examined very carefully. *Haemophilus* spp. and *Pseudomonas* spp. can be small and become lost in the debris and mucus background. Perform an acridine orange stain on sputum samples with a predominance of WBCs and no organisms present.

- A sputum Gram stain can be used for quality assurance and personnel competency. The sputum Gram stain results should be compared to the culture results to ensure they correlate. If they do not correlate, the original sputum Gram stain should be reviewed again to resolve any discrepancies. If discrepancies are repeatedly documented, then re-education in Gram stain interpretation may be necessary.

Sputum, tracheal aspirates, and bronchial alveolar lavages are routinely cultured on sheep blood, chocolate, and MacConkey agars. These three agars grow all of the most common causative bacterial agents of pneumonia. If aspiration pneumonia is suspected, media for the recovery of anaerobes should be included.

REAL WORLD TIP

Blood cultures are recommended for hospitalized patients with pneumonia. Sputum cultures can have low specificity because of the potential for contamination with upper respiratory flora, and blood cultures may reveal the causative agent. Early detection can ensure appropriate antibiotic therapy is used. A urine antigen detection test is now available for *Streptococcus pneumoniae*, the most common cause of community-acquired pneumonia, and may replace blood cultures.

Quantitative culture of a bronchial alveolar lavage (BAL) can provide a more sensitive means of diagnosis of ventilator associated pneumonia. The presence of an endotracheal tube provides a surface for colonizing microorganisms, especially gram-negative rods. A BAL and protected bronchial brushing (PBB) can provide a deep specimen with minimal contamination from upper respiratory flora and colonizing organisms. A chocolate agar is the one best medium for processing quantitative respiratory cultures. The bronchial brush is vortexed in its diluent to provide the liquid for sampling. The BAL is plated onto two separate chocolate agar plates using a 0.01 mL (1 colony present on the agar plate equals 100 organisms/mL)

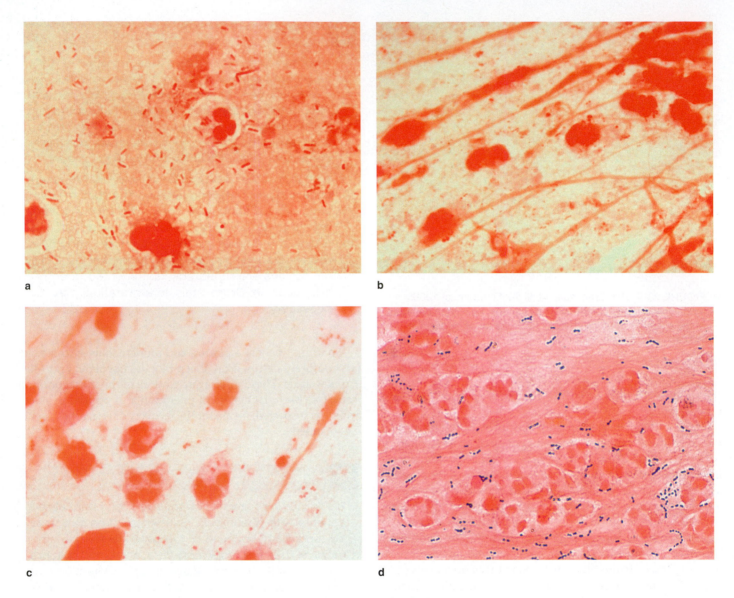

a

b

c

d

■ **FIGURE 33-10** These four expectorated sputum Gram stains at 1000× magnification illustrate some of the bacterial patterns associated with pneumonia. **a.** Shows a gram-negative rod pattern. Note the halo effect because of the presence of a capsule around the organism. **b.** Displays a predominance of gram-negative coccobacilli consistent with a *Haemophilus* pattern. Note how the tiny gram-negative coccobacilli of *H. influenzae* tend to blend into the background material. **c.** Demonstrates a gram-negative diplococci pattern. The organisms have been engulfed by the white blood cells, indicating a true infection with *Moraxella catarrhalis* rather than the presence of normal flora *Neisseria* spp. **d.** Displays lancet gram-positive cocci in pairs and chains associated with a pneumococcus pattern. Note the halo effect around *Streptococcus pneumoniae* because of capsule production.

and 0.001 mL (1 colony = 1000/mL) micropipette or loop. The PBB is usually plated onto two separate chocolate agar plates using 0.1 mL (1 colony = 10 CFU/mL) and 0.01 mL (1 colony = 100 CFU/mL) micropipette or loop. The concept behind quantitative cultures is that there should be low numbers of contaminating normal upper respiratory flora and colonizing organisms and higher numbers of the potential pathogen.

Cystic fibrosis (CF) patients can present the microbiologist with problems because the potential pathogens are different from those of other patient populations. The extremely mucoid *Pseudomonas aeruginosa* colonies can overgrow other potential pathogens present. Mannitol salt agar or a chromogenic agar can be added to selectively isolate *Staphylococcus aureus.*

The presence of *Burkholderia cepacia* in the CF patient can prevent their interaction with other CF patients and put an end to the possibility of receiving a lung transplant. The presence of this organism correlates with a high mortality rate. To ensure the isolation of *Burkholderia cepacia,* the addition of selective and differential media is essential. *Burkholderia cepacia* selective agar (BCSA) and *Pseudomonas cepacia* (PC) agar are available. Commercial identifications systems present with problems when identifying *B. cepacia*. Molecular techniques are highly recommended to ensure correct identification of this potentially lethal pathogen.

Legionella pneumophila has the potential to cause pneumonia in compromised individuals. The sputum produced often is very thin and watery. This is unlike the purulent sputum associated with bacterial pneumonia. Because the organism is fastidious, routine media cannot be used for its isolation, and the physician must specifically request a culture for *Legionella* spp. Buffered charcoal yeast extract (BCYE) agar provides the iron salts and cysteine the organism needs for growth. The organism also requires high humidity. Because the culture may take up to 7 days for final results, a direct fluorescent antibody (DFA) test should be used, in conjunction with culture, for more rapid results. There is the potential for cross reaction with other organisms, so DFA cannot replace culture. A more promising test is the detection of *Legionella* antigen in the urine.

REAL WORLD TIP

BCYE agar provides the cysteine required by *Legionella* spp. for growth. *Francisella tularensis* is another cysteine-requiring organism that can be isolated from sputum during the pneumonic form of tularemia. The microbiologist should examine BCYE agar plates under a laminar flow hood to reduce potential exposure to *F. tularensis*.

Chlamydophila pneumoniae and *Mycoplasma pneumoniae* produce mild forms of pneumonia. *C. pneumoniae* is an intracellular pathogen, so sputum is not a good specimen for its isolation. An oropharyngeal swab is better specimen choice. It must be placed in transport medium and refrigerated to ensure recovery of the organism. Cell lines such as McCoy or Hep-2 can be used to grow the organism. Details on this organism and its detection and identification can be found ∞ Chapters 16 and 31.

Mycoplasma pneumoniae has no cell wall, grows slowly, and requires special medium for isolation. The organism can be recovered from bronchial alveolar lavage, but a nasopharyngeal or throat swab is less invasive. Because the organism does not contain a cell wall, it is very susceptible to drying, and swabs must sent in special transport medium to ensure its recovery. Because the organism can be difficult to isolate and slow to grow, PCR assays may be beneficial. Serology testing is also available to detect the organism. ∞ Chapter 28 provides further details on its recovery and identification.

Three early morning sputum specimens over 3 days are recommended for detection of *Mycobacterium* spp. Culturing expectorated sputum requires a mucolytic and decontamination procedure because of the mucus present, which can trap

organisms, and the potential for oropharyngeal flora to be present in the specimen. The lower respiratory specimen must be digested to break up the mucus present and decontaminated to remove any normal flora present. It is then concentrated and used to prepare a smear for acid-fast stains such as the fluorochrome stain, rhodamine-auramine, or carbol fuchsin stains, Kinyoun, and Ziehl-Neelsen. The acid-fast stain is a rapid method to detect the slow-growing *Mycobacterium* spp., but because of its low sensitivity, it cannot replace culture.

The concentrate is used to plate special solid nonselective and selective media such as Lowenstein-Jensen and Middlebrook. Traditional cultures must be held for 6 to 8 weeks to ensure recovery of the slow-growing organisms. Liquid media is also available and is incubated in a continuously monitored system to speed up detection of *Mycobacterium* spp. Molecular diagnostic testing is available and reduces the time to detection dramatically compared to traditional culture. Rapid detection is essential to identify active cases of *M. tuberculosis* so they can be contained to prevent spread of the disease in the general population.

Lower respiratory specimens from immunocompromised individuals can be examined directly for the fungus *Pneumocystis jiroveci* (previously *P. carinii*). *P. jiroveci* can be visualized using calcofluor white, silver stain, or Giemsa stain. This microorganism cannot be grown in culture and is usually identified on stained smears of induced sputum or bronchial alveolar lavage.

Respiratory specimens for fungal culture should not be screened for SECs like a specimen for bacterial culture, and multiple specimens should be processed. Liquefaction of respiratory specimens will increase the recovery of fungi. Calcofluor can be used to visualize fungi in direct specimens. Fungi require special media. The use of selective, such as inhibitory mould agar, and nonselective media, such as sabouraud dextrose agar, is necessary to ensure the isolation of yeast and mould from the potential normal flora present. Fungal cultures are incubated at 30°C for at least 4 weeks.

REAL WORLD TIP

Any fluffy white mould colony should be examined under a laminar flow hood. *Blastomyces dermitidis*, *Coccidioides immitis*, and *Histoplasma capsulatum* produce fluffy white colonies and are potential fungal pathogens that can infect microbiologists who are exposed to their spores.

Parasites can be found in the sputum. Direct wet mounts will detect the ova produced by *Paragonimus westermani*. Sputum may also harbor the filariform larvae of *Strongyloides stercoralis* during hyperinfection or disseminated infection in immunocompromised individuals. *Entamoeba histolytica* can appear in the sputum when amoebic abscesses in the liver spread to the base of the lung. Trichrome stained smears of

Checkpoint! 33–7
(Chapter Objective 6)

The physician submits a bronchial alveolar lavage and requests the addition of a BCYE agar plate to the routine culture. What organisms is the physician suspecting?

   A. *Bordetella pertussis*
   B. *Burkholderia cepacia*
   C. Methicillin-resistant *Staphylococcus aureus*
   D. *Legionella pneumophila*

 REAL WORLD TIP

Strongyloides stercoralis can be found in the sputum both in the Gram stained smear as well as the culture. The filariform larvae are motile. After incubation of the sputum culture agar plates, the larvae move through the bacterial colonies. As they travel, they leave wandering trails or tracks of bacteria outside the normal streak lines. The microbiologist must learn to recognize this important clue to their presence in sputum. Hyperinfection or disseminated infection has an extremely high mortality rate.

the sputum will reveal the cysts and trophozoites of *E. histolytica.*

Lung tissue can be used to create touch preps on sterile glass slides for staining. The tissue is minced with sterile scissors or scalpel. One side of the exposed tissue is then touched to the slide surface multiple times. The procedure can be used for direct detection of *Pneumocystis jiroveci* and *Mycobacterium* spp. The minced tissue is then ground and used to inoculate appropriate media.

 REAL WORLD TIP

Lung tissue for fungal culture should be minced but not ground. The Zygomycetes, such as *Rhizopus* and *Mucor,* are delicate, and grinding destroys their fragile hyphae.

Pleural fluid requires Gram stain and culture using sheep blood, chocolate, and MacConkey agars. The direct Gram stain of pleural fluid should be made using a cytocentrifuge rather than a drop of fluid dried on a glass slide. The use of the cytocentrifuge increases the sensitivity of detection of organisms on the Gram stain.

The specimen should be centrifuged to concentrate any organisms present and the sediment used for inoculation. The same organisms responsible for pneumonia are often those

also found in pleural fluid. Because pleural fluid is located deep in the body, there is a potential for infection by anaerobes. The addition of anaerobic media should be considered if the routine aerobic cultures do not grow but organisms are visualized on the direct Gram stain.

▶ INTERPRETATION OF CULTURES

To interpret respiratory cultures appropriately, one must be able to identify the microorganisms that make up normal upper respiratory flora. Box 33-1 summarizes the organisms usually considered normal upper respiratory flora. Box 33-2✪ summarizes organisms that can colonize the upper respiratory tract. These organisms can be normal flora in many healthy individuals but can cause disease, given the right circumstances.

 REAL WORLD TIP

Small alpha-hemolytic colonies isolated above the waist are usually viridans *Streptococcus,* whereas those isolated below the waist are usually *Lactobacillus* spp.

Nasal, nasopharyngeal, and throat specimens are often heavily contaminated with normal upper respiratory flora and colonizing microorganisms. The colonizing organisms can be potential pathogens under the right conditions. This makes interpretation of these upper respiratory cultures challenging. These specimens should be examined for specific bacterial pathogens rather than as a "routine" culture. Table 33-4✪ pro-

✪ BOX 33-1

Microorganisms Usually Considered Normal Upper Respiratory Flora

Alpha- and gamma-hemolytic *Streptococcus* spp.
Beta-hemolytic *Streptococcus* spp. not group A, C, or G
Staphylococcus spp.
Corynebacterium spp. not *C. diphtheriae*
Neisseria spp. not *N. gonorrhoeae*
Haemophilus spp.
Eikenella spp.
Capnocytophaga spp.
Rothia spp.
Actinomyces spp.
Mycobacterium spp.
Mycoplasma spp.
Anaerobes
Spirochetes

Microorganisms That Can Colonize the Upper Respiratory Tract of Healthy Individuals

Enterobacteriaceae
Pseudomonas aeruginosa
Acinetobacter spp.
Stenotrophomonas maltophilia
Other nonfermenting gram-negative rods
Staphylococcus aureus
Streptococcus pneumoniae
Beta-hemolytic Streptococcus
Haemophilus influenzae
Neisseria meningitidis
Moraxella catarrhalis
Candida albicans
Other yeasts

✪ REAL WORLD TIP

- *Corynebacterium diphtheriae* will grow on sheep blood agar and can be beta-hemolytic. A Gram stain and catalase test is essential to differentiate *C. diphtheriae* from *Streptococcus pyogenes*. *C. diphtheriae* is a palisading gram-positive rod that is catalase positive.

- Always perform a Gram stain on any beta-hemolytic colony that is being worked up on any culture. A Gram stain is a cheap and easy means to begin the identification of any organism. It can save a lot of time, wasted media, and identification tests.

vides information related to the presumptive identification of commonly isolated respiratory system pathogens.

Nasal and nasopharyngeal cultures are usually requested and examined for carrier states of *Staphylococcus aureus*, methicillin-resistant *S. aureus*, and *Neisseria meningitidis*. They can be colonizers in healthy individuals and should only be worked up at the request of the physician. *Streptococcus pyogenes* and *Bordetella pertussis* are considered strict pathogens and should always be identified when isolated. Isolation of *Corynebacterium diphtheriae* is only considered diagnostic for diphtheria when it has been proven to be a toxigenic strain using the Elek test. Diphtheria is a reportable disease to the public health department.

Pharyngitis is usually caused by viruses, *Streptococcus pyogenes*, *Streptococcus* groups C and G, or *Arcanobacterium haemolyticum*. A rapid screen will rule in or rule out infection with *S. pyogenes* quickly. A negative group A *Streptococcus* screen is routinely plated to a sheep blood agar or group A selective agar and incubated in ambient air or anaerobically at 35° to 37°C. The agar plate is examined for any beta-hemolytic colonies resembling *Streptococcus pyogenes* at 24 and 48 hours. Any amount of any of the four most common bacterial pathogens is considered significant in a throat culture.

Neisseria gonorrhoeae is also considered a strict pathogen in a throat culture. Any other organisms, such as *Haemophilus influenzae* or *Streptococcus pneumoniae*, should only be worked up at the special request of the physician. These two organisms are colonizers, especially during the winter respiratory season.

✪ TABLE 33-4

Identification of Selected Respiratory System Pathogens

Pathogen	Microscopic Morphology	Colony Morphology			Identification Tests
		BA	CA	MAC	
Moraxella catarrhalis	gram-negative diplococci	Small gray to white, convex, "hockey puck"	Growth is often better than on BA	NG	GS, oxidase, butyrate esterase, growth at room temperature
Candida spp.	gram-positive, budding yeast	Creamy, white, may have "feet"	*	NG	GS, urease to rule out Cryptococcus
Beta-hemolytic streptococci	gram-positive cocci in chains	Small, gray, beta-hemolytic	*	NG	GS, catalase, PYR, group A, C, G antigen typing
Streptococcus pneumoniae	lancet- or football-shaped, gram-positive diplococci	Small, gray, alpha-hemolytic	*	NG	GS, catalase, bile solubility, optochin
Enteric and non-fermenting GNR	gram-negative bacilli	Large wet gray	*	LF or NLF	Oxidase, gram negative identification panel
Staphylococcus aureus	gram-positive cocci in clusters	Large, yellow or white, usually beta-hemolytic	*	NG	GS, catalase, slide latex or coagulase
Haemophilus influenzae	gram-negative coccobacilli (pleomorphic)	NG or satelliting colonies	Small, gray	NG	GS, catalase, ALA (porphyrin) test, horse blood agar

BA, blood agar; CA, chocolate agar; MAC, MacConkey agar; *, growth same as BA; NG, no growth; LF, lactose fermenting; NLF, nonlactose fermenting; GNR, gram-negative rods; GS, Gram stain; PYR, pyrrolidonyl arylamidase; ALA, amino-levulinic acid.

A deep nasal swab cannot diagnose sinusitis. An invasive procedure is usually needed to confirm the diagnosis and will avoid normal upper respiratory flora. Any organism encountered in a maxillary sinus puncture should be considered significant.

Cultures of the epiglottis and larynx are rarely performed. Laryngitis is usually caused by viruses, whereas epiglottitis is usually caused by bacteria. Cultures of the epiglottis may contain normal upper respiratory flora. The agar plates are examined for the potential pathogens associated with disease. Because each of those organisms can also be found in the upper respiratory flora, the microbiologist must be careful in the interpretation of an epiglottis culture. Typically the "true" pathogen is found in amounts greater than the normal flora present.

The direct Gram stain pattern of the lower respiratory sample will provide the microbiologist a clue to the potential pathogen. Pneumonia is usually caused by a single organism. A predominant potential pathogen will usually appear in amounts that comprise 25% or more of the organisms present on culture. Yeast is considered a potential pathogen when it comprises 50% or more compared to the normal flora. Once the culture is complete, the microbiologist should report the quantity of potential pathogen and normal flora. If there is an absence of normal flora, it should also be noted in the report.

When reading respiratory culture agar plates, it is easy to be overwhelmed by the number and variety of organisms present as normal flora. Focus on recognizing the common possible pathogens, and the normal flora will be easier to overlook. When reading the agar plates, first examine the sheep blood agar plate (SBA) for a predominance of the two distinct morphologies of *Streptococcus pneumoniae*. One colony morphology is alpha-hemolytic with a crater in the middle; the other is also alpha-hemolytic but is very mucoid. The SBA is then examined for a predominance of beta-hemolytic colonies consistent with *Staphylococcus aureus* and *Streptococcus* spp. *Candida albicans* appear as white, creamy colonies with fringed edges. It should only be worked up when found in amounts of 50% or more compared to the normal flora present.

Significant amounts of *Moraxella catarrhalis* appear as yellowish to white colonies that can be pushed around the agar surface like a hockey puck on both the SBA and chocolate agars. It usually grows better on chocolate agar then SBA. It may be possible to observe satelliting colonies of *Haemophilus* spp. around those of *S. aureus* and other hemolytic or NAD producing colonies on SBA.

REAL WORLD TIP

Laboratories may limit their identification of *Candida* species in respiratory specimens. A urease test is performed and if negative the isolate is reported as yeast, not *Cryptococcus*. Additional testing is performed on the isolate if urease positive or on special request (Barenfanger et al., 2003).

It is best to work with significant *Haemophilus* spp. from the chocolate agar. Compare the colonies of the chocolate agar to those on the SBA. *Haemophilus* spp. are gray, slightly wet, flat colonies that appear on chocolate agar but not on SBA. Last, the MacConkey is examined for a significant amount of gram-negative rods. Gram-negative rods will appear as large, gray wet colonies on both the SBA and chocolate agar.

Other organisms that appear in a significant amount on any agar plate should be identified and assessed for clinical significance. If there is more than one colony morphology of gram-negative rods, they should be reported as generic gram-negative rods rather than each individual identification. The presence of multiple gram-negative rods often indicates colonization rather than infection. Any mould present should be worked up because it is not considered normal flora.

A quantitative culture of a bronchial brush or bronchial alveolar lavage requires counting the colonies present to determine its significance. Normal flora should also be quantitated and reported. More than 10 colonies of an organism on a 0.01 mL culture of a bronchial brush or on a 0.001 mL culture of a BAL represents a significant amount.

Lower respiratory cultures from a CF patient are interpreted differently than other patient populations. The pathogenic organisms present in a CF patient tend to be limited to a few organisms. Almost every CF lower respiratory specimen will grow at least one pathogen. Mould, *Staphylococcus aureus*, *Pseudomonas aeruginosa*, *Burkholderia cepacia*, and other nonglucose fermenters are considered significant in any amount. *Haemophilus influenzae*, *Streptococcus pneumoniae*, and *Enterobacteriaceae* are considered significant when predominant compared to normal flora present. The use of selective agars such as *Burkholderia cepacia* selective agar and mannitol salt agar is essential to ensure the recovery of other potential pathogens that can be buried beneath the extremely mucoid *P. aeruginosa* that infects most CF patients.

Pleural fluid is considered sterile. Any organism isolated should be considered significant and reported. The presence of *Staphylococcus not S. aureus* is probably because of inadequate skin decontamination but should still be reported. The physician must determine its significance.

 Checkpoint! 33–8 (Chapter Objective 7)

A routine throat culture, taken from a 28-year-old male experiencing pharyngitis, reveals

> *Heavy growth of Haemophilus influenzae*
> *Heavy growth of normal upper respiratory flora*

The culture should be reported as

> A. *heavy growth of normal flora.*
> B. *heavy growth of H. influenzae and heavy growth of normal flora.*
> C. *organisms suggestive of sinusitis isolated.*
> D. *no pathogens isolated.*

SUMMARY

The respiratory system is a unique system that is crucial for the body to obtain oxygen for the red blood cells. It is also crucial in ridding the body of the waste product, carbon dioxide. Pathogenic organisms and environmental agents constantly challenge the respiratory system. The immune system and respiratory tract fight to prevent organisms from colonizing and initiating disease. Organisms that are able to reach the lungs have a good chance of causing serious disease. If left untreated or unchecked, the diseases they cause can lead to death.

Viruses play a large role in initiating respiratory infections. They invade the cells of the respiratory tract and cause damage, which allows bacteria to secondarily infect. The influenza virus has the potential to produce pandemics, so physicians and microbiologists need to have all the tools ready to deal with the massive numbers of patients that will contract the disease. Rapid testing and making information available for diagnosis is more important now than ever. Microbiology laboratories need to stay in tune with new technology and try to incorporate those that best suit the needs of their facility and community.

Pneumonia remains an illness that can result in death. This makes the microbiologist a key member of the health care team in the diagnosis and successful treatment of infectious diseases. As emerging resistance becomes more common for more and more bacteria, it is important that the overuse of antibiotics be monitored closely. May the air which we breath be not be polluted with organisms and substances that contaminate our unique and wonderful organs called the lungs.

LEARNING OPPORTUNITIES

1. An 83-year-old female is hospitalized for pneumonia. Which of the following rapid tests may help determine the most likely causative agent sooner than traditional culture results? (Chapter Objective 9)

    a. *Legionella pneumophila* urine antigen

    b. *Streptococcus pneumoniae* urine antigen

    c. Respiratory syncytial virus enzyme immunoassay

    d. Group A *Streptococcus* enzyme immunoassay

2. A throat swab is submitted for group A *Streptococcus*. The rapid screen is negative. After 24 hours, the sheep blood agar displays:

    No beta-hemolytic colonies present

    Heavy growth of an oxidase-positive, gram-negative diplococci, which ferments glucose and maltose but not lactose and sucrose

    Light growth of normal upper respiratory flora

    The next step in the process is to report the culture results as: (Chapter Objective 8)

    a. no group A *Streptococcus* isolated

    b. heavy growth of normal flora

    c. heavy growth of *Neisseria meningitidis* and light growth of normal flora

    d. light growth of normal flora

3. Which of the following structures is *not* considered part of the upper respiratory tract? (Chapter Objective 1)

    a. Epiglottis

    b. Larynx

    c. Trachea

    d. Voice box

4. Which of the following organisms can be considered normal upper respiratory flora but can also be a colonizer that may cause disease given the right circumstances? (Chapter Objective 7)

    a. Viridans *Streptococcus*

    b. Diphtheroids

    c. *Neisseria lactamica*

    d. *Staphylococcus aureus*

5. You are examining a Regan-Lowe agar plate. Which of the following is the most likely specimen used to inoculate this agar plate? (Chapter Objective 6)

   a. Nasopharyngeal aspiration

   b. Sputum

   c. Bronchial washing

   d. Bronchial alveolar lavage

6. A 3-year-old female with repeated respiratory problems is admitted with bronchiolitis. A bronchial washing is submitted for bacterial culture. The culture reveals an extremely mucoid, oxidase-positive gram-negative rod that produces pyoverdin and pyocyanin.

   a. Which of the following conditions accounts for the presence of this organism? (Chapter Objective 3)

      a. Diabetes

      b. Cystic fibrosis

      c. Immunosuppression

      d. Parasitic infestation

   b. What additional organism(s) is this little girl at risk for acquiring? (Chapter Objective 3)

      a. *Mycoplasma pneumoniae*

      b. *Legionella pneumophila*

      c. *Burkholderia cepacia*

      d. Anaerobes

7. A pleural fluid culture grows catalase-positive, coagulase-negative, gram-positive cocci in clusters. This organism is probably (Chapter Objective 7)

   a. normal flora

   b. a skin contaminant

   c. a potential pathogen

   d. a strict pathogen

8. Expectorated sputum from a 72-year-old hospitalized male was submitted for bacterial culture. He developed shortness of breath after suffering from the flu. A screen of the sputum Gram stain at 100× magnification revealed no squamous epithelial cells and many white blood cells. A Gram stain of the sputum at 1,000× magnification is provided in the photo.

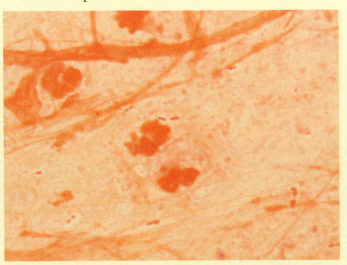

The bacterial sputum culture revealed:

   Moderate growth of normal upper respiratory flora

   Heavy growth of a very mucoid alpha hemolytic colony

The identification results of the mucoid alpha hemolytic colony revealed:

   Gram stain—gram-positive cocci in pairs and short chains

   Catalase—no bubbles

   Optochin—zone of inhibition = 17 mm

   Bile solubility—lysis of the organism

Which of the following statements would *not* explain the discrepancy between the direct sputum Gram stain result and the identification of the potential pathogen? (Chapter Objectives 5 and 8)

   a. The sputum Gram stain was overdecolorized.

   b. The patient was started on antibiotic therapy prior to the sputum collection, and the organism's cell wall was injured.

   c. The sputum sat at room temperature too long before it was processed, and the organism began to autolyse.

   d. The true pathogen was the influenza virus, and the mucoid alpha hemolytic colony is normal flora and should not have been identified.

9. A 58-year-old male has been hospitalized in the intensive care for unit for 3 days because of a motor vehicle crash. He is intubated, and a tracheal aspirate is submitted for bacterial culture. The tracheal aspirate direct Gram stain reveals a nondiagnostic pattern with rare white blood cells. His chest x-ray is clear with no lung infiltrates. He has no fever and is not on antibiotics at the time of the endotracheal culture collection.

   The bacterial culture shows moderate growth of *Klebsiella pneumoniae, Acinetobacter baumannii,* and *Stenotrophomonas maltophilia.* What does the isolation of these three organisms mean for this patient? (Chapter Objectives 5 and 8)

   a. He has pneumonia.

   b. His endotracheal tube is colonized with gram-negative rods.

   c. A repeat culture should be performed.

   d. His endotracheal tube must be replaced.

10. Review the direct Gram stain of a 33-year-old hospitalized male's expectorated sputum shown at 100× magnification in the photo. Determine the next step necessary for processing the specimen. (Chapter Objective 4)

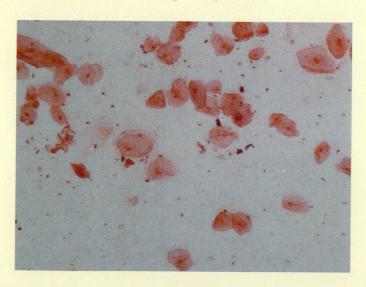

a. Reject the specimen and call the patient's floor for a recollect.

b. Reject the specimen and call the respiratory therapist for an induced sputum collection.

c. Read the gram stain pattern at 1,000× then inoculate to the appropriate media.

d. Request a *Legionella pneumophila* urine antigen.

PEARSON
myhealthprofessionskit™

Use this address to access the interactive Companion Website created for this textbook. Simply select "Clinical Laboratory Science" from the choice of disciplines. Find this book and log in using your user name and password.

REFERENCES

Go to myhealthprofessionskit.com to view this chapter's references.

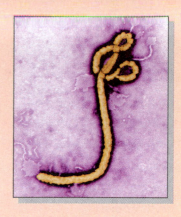

34

Urinary System

Mona Gleysteen

■ LEARNING OBJECTIVES

Upon completion of this chapter the learner should be able to:

1. List risk factors that contribute to increased incidence of urinary tract infections.

2. Describe and differentiate the pathogenesis and clinical symptoms of cystitis, pyelonephritis, ureteritis, urethritis, and acute urethral syndrome.

3. Assess whether a bacteruria is clinically significant.

4. Judge if a urine specimen is acceptable given a description of the collection process and the manner in which the specimen was handled prior to culturing it.

5. Select the appropriate media, inoculation procedures, and incubation conditions for a urine culture.

6. Correlate the results of the following screening methods with a positive urine culture:

   a. Routine urine culture with microscopic evaluation

   b. Gram stain

   c. Nitrate reduction and leukocyte esterase by dipstick

   d. Automated methods

7. Given the number and type of colonies and the size of the loop used to inoculate a urine culture, calculate the colony count and interpret culture results; determine the extent of identification and susceptibility testing.

8. Identify organisms associated with urinary tract infections and correlate to Gram stain morphology, colony morphology, spot and rapid test results, confirmatory test results, and antibiogram prior to reporting results.

KEY TERMS

acute urethral syndrome	fimbriae	perineum
bacteriuria	glomerulus	pyuria
CFU (colony forming unit)	hematogenous	pyelonephritis
cystitis	hematuria	ureteritis
dysuria	nephron	urethritis
erythropoiesis		

▶ INTRODUCTION

Approximately 10% of people will experience a urinary tract infection (UTI) at some point in their lifetimes (Forbes, Sahm, & Weissfeld, 2002). In the United States there are over 8 million urinary tract infections each year (http://kidney.niddk .nih.gov/kudiseases/pubs/kustats). Forty percent of all women have at least one episode of a UTI in their lifetime (Mahon & Manuselis, 2000; http://www.atsu.edu/faculty/chamberlain/ Website/lectures/lecture/uti.htm). Urinary tract infections are one of the most common bacterial infections in adults and are the second most common cause for visits to a health care practitioner for a prescription of antibiotics (Berkley et al., 1999). Urinary tract infections can occur at any age but there is an increased incidence in older populations and women.

▶ FUNCTION AND STRUCTURES OF THE URINARY SYSTEM

The urinary system is a large filter for the blood. Substances important to the body should be retained in the blood, but waste products plus a solvent (water) need to be excreted to maintain the health of the body. The urinary system is one of the body's waste treatment centers. It performs selective filtering, if it is working properly. Blood enters the kidney through the renal artery and is carried through the **glomerulus** into the capillaries of the **nephron.** The glomerulus is a structure composed of blood vessels that function as a filter; the nephron is the functional unit of the kidney. In the nephron, the processes of filtration, absorption, and secretion form urine. There are approximately 1 million nephrons per kidney. Once urine is produced in the kidney, it is carried and stored in the remaining components of the urinary system.

The urinary system (Figure 34-1 ■) consists of two kidneys, two ureters, a bladder, and a urethra in most individuals. Men have a prostate gland as well. The kidneys and ureters comprise what is known as the upper urinary system. The lower urinary system is the bladder, urethra, and prostate for males.

Additional functions of the kidney are production of hormones needed for **erythropoiesis** (the production of red blood cells) and bone formation, blood pressure maintenance including fluid and electrolyte balance, and acid-base regulation.

The **perineum** (Figure 34-2 ■) is an area that can be thought of as two triangles bounded by the buttocks and the thighs. One triangle (a urogenital triangle) contains the external genitals, urethral orifice (in females), and surrounding tissue. The other triangle (an anal triangle) contains the anus and surrounding tissue. This area contains the resident microflora that may infect the urinary tract (especially in females). The anatomy of the female urinary tract, most notably the short urethra in women and the close proximity of the vaginal and rectal regions, is of particular importance in

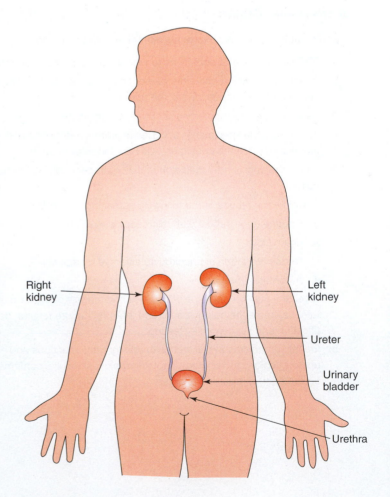

Right kidney

Left kidney

Ureter

Urinary bladder

Urethra

■ FIGURE 34-1 The urinary system.

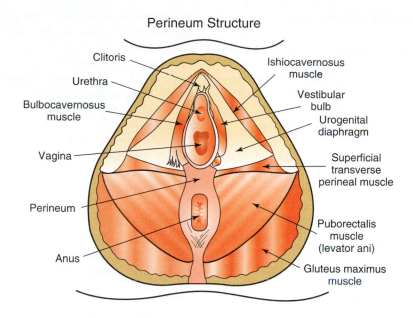

Perineum Structure

Clitoris
Urethra
Bulbocavernosus muscle
Vagina
Perineum
Anus

Ishiocavernosus muscle
Vestibular bulb
Urogenital diaphragm
Superficial transverse perineal muscle
Puborectalis muscle (levator ani)
Gluteus maximus muscle

■ **FIGURE 34-2** The female perineum.

the pathogenesis of UTIs in females. ∞ Chapter 36, "Genital System," provides figures (Figures 36-1 and 36-2) depicting the male and female genital systems, including the urinary systems.

► STERILITY OF URINARY SYSTEM

The normal genitourinary tract is sterile (except for the distal urethra). The structure of the urinary system helps prevent infections. The ureters and bladder normally prevent urine from backing up toward the kidneys. The continual flushing action of the urinary system is considered a defense mechanism against urinary tract infections (UTIs). This defense mechanism depends on urine flow rate, frequency of voiding, and residual bladder volume. A change in flow rate, voiding frequency, or bladder volume is likely to be responsible for higher rates of infection. The composition of urine is also inhibitory to many bacteria (gonococci, anaerobes, and urethral commensals) but is a good growth medium for others (facultative anaerobes). Extremes of pH (normal = 4.6 to 8), high urea (normal = 12 to 20 grams per 24 hours), and organic acid concentrations of urine may inhibit the aerobes. Bacteria that infect the urinary system generally have specialized virulence factors, such as adherence factors, **fimbriae** (short hair-like structures that adhere to epithelial cells), or pili. Visit ∞ Chapter 4 to review information related to the host's encounter with microbes.

The distal urethra contains resident microflora. There may also be transient colonizers that can include potential urinary pathogens. Urine must pass through this area of microflora, therefore necessitating a procedure for determining a true infection from contamination.

► INFECTIONS

Infections of the urinary tract may result in a totally asymptomatic individual to a very seriously ill hospitalized patient with bacteremia, or bacteria in the blood. Urinary tract abnormalities including kidney stones, instrumentation such as catheterization, and underlying medical conditions (e.g., diabetes mellitus) are predisposing factors. Women have more urinary tract infections due to a combination of factors: short urethra, hormonal changes, sexual activity, and close proximity of the gastrointestinal (GI) and vaginal tracts.

@ **REAL WORLD TIP**

Vesiculoureteral reflux can be the cause of recurrent UTIs in children. Due to an abnormality, obstruction, or previous UTI, urine backs up into the ureters and eventually the kidneys.

Infections of the urinary tract usually start as **cystitis** (bladder infection). This is referred to as an ascending route of infection. Bacteria travel up the urethra and infect the bladder. This is a common method of infection in women, as the urethra in women is shorter than the urethra in men. This is also a common route of infection in hospitalized patients that have had a foreign body introduced into the urinary tract such as a catheter. Lower UTIs include infection of the urethra (**urethritis**) and cystitis. If the infection is not treated or is treated inadequately, the infection may move up the ureters to the kidneys. Infection of the kidney (renal pelvis) is called

pyelonephritis. An upper UTI includes infection of the ureter (**ureteritis**) and pyelonephritis.

It may be difficult to determine the site of infection. In general, the presence of white blood cell casts in a urine sample from the patient indicates that the patient has pyelonephritis. White blood cell casts form in the tubules of the kidneys. They are made up of protein excreted by the tubules. The white blood cells become glued to the protein and the mass takes on the shape of the tubule.

Another inflammatory condition of the genito-urinary tract in males is prostatitis, infection of the prostate. Urethritis is often due to sexually transmitted disease, however, women with clinical urethritis may also have a condition called **acute urethral syndrome.** It has the symptoms of a UTI but without a significant number of organism in the urine. An infection can also reach the kidneys secondarily from the blood. The kidneys become infected as they filter the blood, but this is less common. Since the organism is transported in the blood, this is called **hematogenous** or descending route of infection.

Checkpoint! 34–1 (Chapter Objective 1)

Of the following, which contribute to women having more urinary tract infections than men?
  A. *Longer urethra in women*
  B. *Women drink more water*
  C. *Women have increased frequency of urination*
  D. *The urethral opening in women is in close proximity to the GI and vaginal tracts*

Bacteremia may develop in 10–65% of patients with acute pyelonephritis. Because the kidney is so vascular, the organisms spill over into the blood stream. Systemic complications occurring in patients with bacteremia due to pyelonephritis with gram-negative organisms include septic shock, disseminated intravascular coagulation, and the acute respiratory distress syndrome (ARDS). ∞ Chapter 32 provides additional information on infections of the cardiovascular system.

Acute urethral syndrome is a term describing adult women with acute symptoms of UTIs without significant (>10^5 organisms/mL) numbers of bacteria in their urine. This can be observed in about half of adult women with acute symptoms. Many of these women have periurethral colonization with uropathogenic organisms and low numbers of *E. coli, S. saprophyticus*, and enteric gram-negative organisms present in their urine. Often these patients respond to antibiotics so even a low count of bacteria (>10^2 organisms/mL) plus symptoms in these women constitutes a treatable situation. In females with symptoms of acute cystitis (acute urethral syndrome), the organism cutoff point of 10^2 (with white blood cells present) is utilized by many laboratories/physicians (Warren et al., 1999).

Most UTIs are caused by endogenous organisms (organisms that come from the patient's own flora). Colonization of the periurethral area in females with enteric organisms increases the incidence of infection. Bacteria that attach to urethelial cells with fimbriae are important in initiating colonization of the bladder. This promotes an inflammatory response and symptoms in the patient. Asymptomatic **bacteriuria** (bacteria in the urine) is usually caused by organisms that do not possess fimbriae and do not excite an inflammatory response.

There are single-episode UTIs that do not recur, but many patients experience recurrent infections. There are also uncomplicated infections due to a single organism, which is susceptible to antibiotics. People with structural genitourinary abnormalities, neurological problems such as spinal cord injury, or institutionalized or hospitalized older adults experience more complicated infections (more than one organism or antibiotic-resistant organisms).

Checkpoint! 34–2 (Chapter Objective 2)

Which of the following is an example of a urinary tract infection from a descending (hematogenous) route?
  A. *An initial bladder infection in a young woman that developed into a kidney infection*
  B. *A recurrent pyelonephritis caused by a drug-resistant organism in a nursing home patient*
  C. *A septic patient develops pyelonephritis*
  D. *A bladder infection in a pregnant woman*

Checkpoint! 34–3 (Chapter Objective 2)

Which of the following best describes cystitis?
  A. *Flank pain, tenderness, fever*
  B. *Vomiting, nausea, fatigue*
  C. *Dysuria, frequency*
  D. *Frothy vaginal discharge*

Checkpoint! 34–4 (Chapter Objective 2)

Which term matches this definition: Symptoms of a urinary tract infection without significant numbers of bacteria in the urine (found especially in women)?
  A. *Cystitis*
  B. *Pyelonephritis*
  C. *Hematogenous infection*
  D. *Acute urethral syndrome*

SYMPTOMS

Symptoms of UTIs depend on what part of the urinary system is infected. Pyelonephritis is usually accompanied by flank pain (pain in one side of the body between the upper abdomen and the back), tenderness, and fever. Vomiting, nausea, fatigue, malaise, **dysuria** (painful urination), frequency, nocturia (excessive urination at night), and urine changes (color and odor) may also be present. Cystitis has symptoms of dysuria, occasionally suprapubic tenderness, and increased frequency/urgency of urination. Low-grade fever may occur but is generally absent. The urine sample is often cloudy (due to presence of white blood cells, red blood cells, and/or bacteria) with a strong odor. **Hematuria** (presence of blood in the urine) may also be visible.

 REAL WORLD TIP

The presence of white blood cells in urine does not always mean the individual has a urinary tract infection. Some antibiotics, glomerulonephritis, autoimmune disease, and sexually transmitted diseases can cause the appearance of white blood cells in the urine.

Bacteriuria (bacteria in the urine) may or may not signify an infection. Bacteria are present on the skin and can be washed into the urine. Most bacteria enter a structurally normal bladder through massage of the female urethra, sexual intercourse, or instrumentation procedures. A definition of asymptomatic bacteriuria is the presence of more than 100,000 colony forming units (**CFU**) per mL of voided urine in patients with no symptoms. This may also be written 100,000 organisms/mL or 10^5 CFU/mL. The Infectious Diseases Society of America (IDSA) uses the following definition for asymptomatic bacteriuria:

- In women: two consecutive clean-catch voided urine specimens with isolation of the same bacterial strain in counts greater than or equal to 100,000 or $>10^5$ CFU/mL.

- In men: a single clean catch voided urine specimen with isolation of one bacterial species isolated in count greater than or equal to 100,000 or $>10^5$ CFU/mL.

- For any patient: a single catheterized urine specimen with one bacterial species isolated in counts greater than or equal to 1000 or $>10^3$ CFU/mL (Wegner, 2003).

Many patients may have asymptomatic infections, especially older adults. There can be very vague symptoms such as poor appetite, fatigue, and urinary incontinence in these individuals. Elderly individuals may also experience mental changes and/or confusion. Treatment of these patients has not been found to reduce either infectious complications or mortality (Berkley et al., 1999).

 Checkpoint! 34–5 (Chapter Objective 3)

Which of the following groups of patients with asymptomatic bacteriuria may not benefit from treatment?

A. Pregnant women
B. Patients with renal transplants
C. Patients who are about to undergo genitourinary tract procedures
D. Older adults

The treatment of three groups of patients with asymptomatic bacteriuria has shown benefit. These groups are: (1) pregnant women, (2) individuals with renal transplants, and (3) those who are about to undergo genitourinary tract procedures (http://www.atsu.edu/faculty/chamberlain/Website/lectures/lecture/uti.htm).

▶ SPECIMEN COLLECTION

Proper collection and processing of a urine specimen is crucial for reliable results from the microbiology laboratory. Acceptable methods of collection include midstream clean catch, catheterization, and suprapubic aspiration. Foley catheter tips should not be accepted as they are invariably contaminated with urethral flora. The midstream clean catch is the most common specimen submitted. ∞ Chapter 6 provides additional information on specimen collection. The following is a summary of the collection methods.

MIDSTREAM CLEAN CATCH

This is the least invasive and can yield valuable information if properly collected. Patient education is extremely important to ensure a clean, voided specimen. Detailed instructions must be provided. Briefly, the instructions for collection are:

- Clean urethra area with soap and water. Females are instructed to wipe from front to back.
- Rinse with wet gauze.
- Hold labia apart on female and retract foreskin on male. Begin voiding.
- After several milliliters have passed, collect a portion in a sterile container.

Studies exist that indicate the cleansing step may not be necessary to prevent contamination of the urine sample (Wilson & Gaido, 2004).

CATHETERIZATION

Straight Catheter (In and Out) Specimen

- Clean urethral area with soap and water.
- Rinse with wet gauze.
- Aseptically insert catheter into bladder.
- Allow 10–15 milliliters to pass and collect in a sterile container.
- Remove catheter.

Indwelling Catheter

- Disinfect catheter collection port with 70% alcohol.
- Use sterile needle and syringe to collect.
- Do not sample from the collection bag.

Indwelling catheters, in place for 4 days or more, frequently become colonized with biofilms of bacteria and yield positive cultures regardless of whether the patient has a urinary tract infection. Biofilms are complex associations that arise from a mixture of microorganisms growing together on the surface of a catheter. These specimens are only of use in evaluating epidemiological problems in an institution. In all other situations, the best time to collect a specimen from a chronically catheterized patient is 12–24 hours after a regularly scheduled catheter change. Go to ∞ Chapters 4, "The Host's Encounter with Microbes," and 41, "Nosocomial Infections," to review biofilms and their role in infectious disease.

SUPRAPUBIC ASPIRATION

- These specimens are collected by insertion of a needle through the lower abdominal wall into the bladder by qualified medical personnel using aseptic technique.
- Bladder must be full before performing.
- Acceptable for anaerobic culture because collection avoids the normal urethral flora.
- Used in situations when urine is difficult to obtain.

CYSTOSCOPY SPECIMENS

- Collected with a cystoscope (an instrument that passes through the urethra into the bladder).

SPECIAL CULTURES

Urine specimens can be cultured for fungus other then *Candida* and *Mycobacterium*. These specimens are processed differently than those submitted for routine urine culture. Mycology culture information can be found in ∞ Chapter 14, "Fungal Cultures." Mycobacterial culture information can be found in ∞ Chapter 13, "Acid-Fast Bacilli Cultures." The ideal mycobacterial urine specimen is first morning voided urine. It contains the highest concentration of organisms.

 REAL WORLD TIP

- Infants often require bagged collection of urine. A sterile plastic bag is taped over the genitalia. These specimens are often contaminated.

- Urine should not be collected from a urostomy bag but via a catheter inserted into the urostomy opening.

- Older adults and children have a difficult time obtaining clean voided urine and tend to have contaminated urine specimens.

 REAL WORLD TIP

Requests for a urine culture should be limited to one per patient per 24 hours.

TRANSPORTATION

Since most bacteria that cause urinary tract infections multiply quite rapidly, transport of specimens to the lab in a timely manner is important. Specimens should be transported and processed within 2 hours of collection. If this time is delayed, then the specimen should be refrigerated until it can be delivered to the laboratory. A urine can be refrigerated for up to 24 hours after collection and still be acceptable for culture.

In addition to refrigeration, there are commercial products available that contain boric acid. They preserve the urine specimen for up to 24 hours without refrigeration if the numbers of bacteria are greater than 10^5 CFU/mL (e.g., B-D Urine Culture Kit—Becton Dickinson Vacutainer Kits, Rutherford, NJ). Some organisms may be inhibited by this system and it must be used with at least 3 mL of urine. There is conflicting information as to the acceptability of boric acid as a urine preservative.

Unacceptable Specimens
- Urine catheter tips
- Pooled urine samples (i.e., 24-hour collections)
- Urine sample over 2 hours old that has not been refrigerated/preserved

PRECULTURE SCREENING

Up to 80% of urine cultures are negative for significant organisms. Rapid elimination of negative urine cultures saves media, time, and resources as well as providing same day results for the physician and patient. Screening of the urine specimen for bacteriuria and/or **pyuria** (presence of white blood cells) can yield significant information rapidly and assist in interpreting the culture results. These screening methods are relatively insensitive at levels below 10^5 CFU/mL. Screening is not useful for specimens obtained by suprapubic aspiration, catheterization, or cystoscopy for that reason. Some methods of screening are:

- Routine urinalysis with microscopic evaluation that may reveal significant numbers of bacteria and white blood cells.
- Gram stain—It has been determined that one or more organisms per OIF (oil immersion field) in a Gram stain (Figure 34-3 ■) translates into a positive urine culture (>10^5 CFU/mL). This is a method of screening that is low cost in reagents, but labor and time consuming.

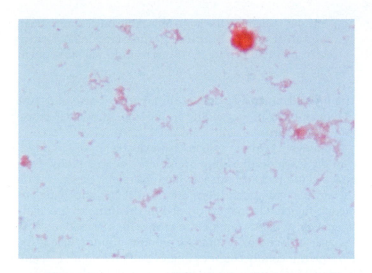

■ **FIGURE 34-3** Gram stain of midstream urine with a white blood cell and gram-negative rod visible. The patient's urine culture report was >100,000 CFU/mL of *E. coli*.

Checkpoint! 34–6 (Chapter Objective 4)

Determine which of the following specimens is acceptable:

- A. *A routine urine sample, submitted within 2 hours of collection, collected in a sterile container for a urine culture.*
- B. *A Foley catheter tip submitted for a culture.*
- C. *A pooled 24-hour collection of urine submitted for urine culture.*
- D. *A clean-catch midstream sample, collected in an unsterile container 20 hours ago and refrigerated until received in the laboratory, for a urine culture.*

- ■ Nitrate reductase and leukocyte esterase determined by dipstick. This is a quick method of screening, but has a low sensitivity and specificity. Organisms which do not produce nitrate, such as *Staphylococcus saprophyticus*, will be missed unless white blood cells are present.

- ■ Urine catalase determined by a commercial enzyme tube test that measures catalase produced by leukocytes, erythrocytes, and bacteria using hydrogen peroxide. The test kit (Uriscreen—J&S Medical Associates, Framingham, MA, and AccuTest—Jant Pharmacal Corp., Encino, CA) contains tubes with dehydrated colored reagent. Urine and hydrogen peroxide are added to the tube and examined for bubbles, a positive reaction. This method is used to screen asymptomatic patients. This method has been shown to be sensitive, with a high negative predictive value (Waisman, Zeren, Amir, & Mimouni, 1999). A negative result may rule out the need for urine culture.

- ■ Automated methods include methods for the presence of bacterial adenosine triphosphate (ATP). An example is the bioluminescence model, which uses light to measure the amount of bacterial ATP, which then correlates to the number of bacteria present.

► SETUP AND INCUBATION OF CULTURES

Routine urine cultures are inoculated onto appropriate culture media in a manner so quantitation of bacteria can be performed.

The media routinely used is blood agar plate (BA) and MacConkey agar (MAC). The BA will grow most significant bacteria—both gram positive and gram negative. MAC is a

differential and selective media that is used primarily for *Enterobacteriacae* (and some of the other gram-negative rods). Sometimes phenylethyl alcohol agar (PEA) or Columbia nalidixic acid agar (CNA) is added for selecting the gram-positive bacteria and should always be added to urostomy specimens. If *Haemophilus*, *Gardnerella*, or *Neisseria gonorrhoeae* is a possibility, chocolate agar should be inoculated with a 0.01 mL loop. The entire surface of the chocolate plate must be streaked and incubate at 35–37°C in carbon dioxide for 3 days. The physician must communicate with the laboratory to insure the addition of chocolate agar to a urine culture.

Suprapubic aspirates are considered acceptable specimens for anaerobic cultures. Chromogenic media is available for detecting common urine pathogens on the basis of their "unique and differential color" (D'Souza, Campbell, & Baron, 2004). Mixed cultures are more easily seen, reducing the need for workup, and results can be reported faster.

A calibrated wire or plastic loop is used to inoculate the media. A 0.001 mL loop is used for most urine specimens. Specimens from females with acute urethral syndrome or urines collected by catheterization or suprapubic aspiration may have bacterial concentrations as low as 100 CFU/mL. A 0.01 mL loop should be used since the lowest bacterial concentration that can be detected is 100 CFU/mL. To inoculate the media, the calibrated loop is inserted vertically into a well-mixed urine specimen and then inoculated in a perpendicular line onto the center of each media. The loop is then streaked horizontally across the initial inoculum (Figure 34-4 ■).

REAL WORLD TIP

The urine loop must be re-dipped into the urine specimen for each agar plate inoculated. If not, the colony counts will decrease on each subsequent agar plate inoculated.

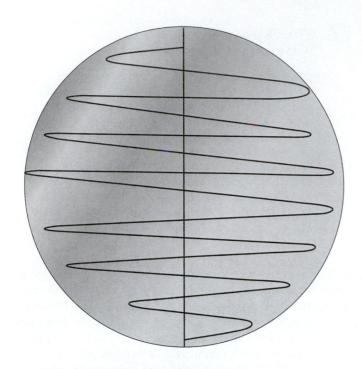

■ **FIGURE 34-4** Urine culture streak for colony count.

 **Checkpoint! 34–7
(Chapter Objective 4)**

Which of the following is an acceptable specimen for anaerobic culture?
  A. *Midstream clean catch specimen*
  B. *Specimen from a catheterized patient*
  C. *Suprapubic aspiration specimen*
  D. *Culture of a Foley catheter tip*

 REAL WORLD TIP

If the urine loop is not held vertically on insertion into the urine specimen, it will pick up a larger sample, increase the CFU present, and potentially lead to a false diagnosis of a UTI based on colony count. A urine loop held at a 45° angle rather than the accepted 90° angle will deliver 150% of the desired volume.

PROCEDURE FOR INOCULATION OF ROUTINE URINE CULTURES

1. Using well-mixed urine, take a flamed or sterile calibrated loop and, holding it vertically, immerse it just below the surface of the uncentrifuged urine specimen.

2. Spread the loopful of urine on the blood agar plate as described (one streak down the center of the plate). Without redipping or sterilizing, draw the loop back and forth across the entire surface of the agar plate perpendicular to the primary streak.

3. Without re-flaming the loop, repeat the procedure with an additional loopful of urine on the MacConkey agar or eosin methylene blue (EMB) agar and each subsequent agar plate used.

The media is incubated at 35°C in an atmosphere of 5–10% CO_2 or ambient air (depending on the laboratory's preference) for 24–48 hours.

Commercial culture systems are available for use in physician offices and other sites. Media may be in a plastic case, attached to a paddle, or in a divided agar plate. Depending on the system, calibrated loops may be used to inoculate the media, the paddle may be dipped in the urine to inoculate the media, or plastic samplers or prongs may be used to streak the agar surface with a standard amount of urine. These systems permit colony count estimates and presumptive identification of common urinary system bacterial pathogens.

 REAL WORLD TIP

Because the colony count defines a urinary tract infection, urine inoculation loops must be calibrated to ensure each delivers the desired volume. Most laboratories use plastic urine loops, calibrated by the manufacturer, which are used for one sample and discarded. Those who still use platinum loops must calibrate each periodically. Calibration methods available include measuring the density of a dye, collected by the loop, using a spectrophotometer, weighing the volume picked up by the loop, and using a gauge that verifies the loop diameter and thickness.

 **Checkpoint! 34–8
(Chapter Objective 5)**

A routine urine sample for a voided urine culture should be inoculated to which of the following media?
  A. *Blood agar and MAC or EMB*
  B. *MAC or EMB only*
  C. *Chocolate agar only*
  D. *Anaerobic blood agar and aerobic blood agar*

▶ INTERPRETATION OF CULTURES

After incubation, the colony count is determined by counting the numbers and types of colonies and multiplying by the dilution factor, which is determined by the size of loop used. For example, using the 0.001 mL loop, one colony of growth is equal to 1,000 colony forming units/mL of the organism. Therefore, if there are 10 colonies of one type of organism growth on the BA or MAC plate, $10 \times 1,000 =$ a colony count of 10,000 CFU/mL of organism. In another example, if the 0.01 mL loop is being used, one colony of growth equals 100

CFU/mL of organism. Ten colonies growing in this example provides a colony count of 1,000 CFU/mL of organism.

For many years the classic definition of a urinary tract infection (UTI) was >10^5 CFU/mL of a single organism. The organism was identified and susceptibility testing performed (if appropriate). Diagnosis of a urinary tract infection has become much more complicated. A colony count of 100,000 (10^5 CFU/mL) is no longer the magic number indicating infection. Counts of 10^3 (1000) CFU/mL of a single isolate of bacteria, or 10^2 (100) CFU/mL of an *Enterobacteriaceae* isolate, are now considered an indication of significant infection by many laboratories, especially if pyuria is present and if the specimen was collected by suprapubic aspiration, cystoscopy, or from a straight (in and out) catheter. Colony counts as low as 100 CFU/mL may be significant in individuals:

- with urinary frequency
- drinking high volumes of fluid
- with partially treated UTIs
- with dysuria or urethral syndrome.

There are many differing views of what constitutes a "positive" urine culture. The age and sex of the patient, whether the patient had symptoms, and the patient's medical history are all aids in diagnosis and the laboratory may not have access to this information. In general, results of a urine culture include:

- No growth is reported as "no growth" or "less than 1,000 CFU/mL (<10^3 CFU/mL)" or "less than 100 CFU/mL (<10^2 CFU/mL)" depending on the calibrated loop used.
- Colony counts of >10^2 CFU/mL of one organism from an asymptomatic woman, or a freshly catheterized urine specimen, or a urine obtained by suprapubic aspiration should be identified and susceptibility testing performed.
- Colony counts of >10^5 CFU/mL of one organism from a clean-catch midstream urine should be identified and susceptibility testing performed.
- Three or more organisms, with no predominance of any one organism, and a colony count of <10^3 CFU/mL should not be worked up. Report as "contaminated specimen" or "growth consistent with urethral flora" and hold the culture plates for one week.

Guidelines to aid the laboratory in interpretation of colony counts is found in Table 34-1. These guidelines should be viewed as an example and each laboratory should determine the criteria to be used based on the patient population served.

Often, physicians do not require a urine culture to diagnose a UTI in women with acute uncomplicated cystitis. These patients may be diagnosed and treated without a urine culture and sensitivity testing or laboratory work-up if clinical signs and symptoms characteristic of UTI exist (Guay, 2008). Up to 95% of uncomplicated cases of cystitis are due to one organism, *Escherichia coli*. This approach does not apply to males, pregnant females, or individuals at high risk for developing urinary tract infections such as those with catheters, diabetes, or immunosuppression. Urine cultures may be needed for recurrent UTI and treatment failures.

Sensitivity testing is often done on pathogens comprising 80% of the total growth with a colony count of 10^2 CFU/mL or more. The exception to this rule is found in cases where the patient has had a catheter in place for over 4–5 days (http://www.atsu.edu/faculty/chamberlain/Website/lectures/lecture/uti.htm). ∞ Chapter 11, "Susceptibility Testing," reviews susceptibility testing procedures.

 REAL WORLD TIP

A UTI is generally diagnosed with a combination of a urinalysis (UA) and a culture. UA results seen with an infection include bacteriuria and pyuria.

✓ **Checkpoint! 34–9 (Chapter Objective 6)**

A urine sample gave the following results during screening:

Macroscopic and Dipstick Results	Microscopic Examination
Color: dark brown (yellow)	
Transparency: cloudy (clear)	WBC: packed with clumps (0-5/HPF)
Specific Gravity: 1.024 (1.002–1.030)	RBC: TNTC (0–3/HPF)
pH 6.0 (4.5–7.5)	Epithelial cells: negative (few)
Leukocyte Esterase: positive (negative)	Bacteria: 3+ (none)
Nitrites: positive (negative)	Casts: 2–3 WBC casts/HPF (0/HPF)
Protein: marked (negative)	Crystals: none (0/HPF)
Glucose: negative (negative)	Mucus: trace (occasional)
Ketones: moderate (negative)	
Urobilinogen: 0.2 (0.2–1.0 mg/dl)	
Bilirubin: negative (negative)	
Blood: 3+ (negative)	

TNTC, too numerous to count; HPF, high power field; WBC, white blood cells; RBC, red blood cells; ( ) normal values

What do the urinalysis findings for this woman patient suggest?

A. Cystitis
B. Acute urethral syndrome
C. Glomerulonephritis
D. Pyelonephritis

⊛ TABLE 34-1

Guidelines for Laboratory Interpretation of Colony Counts

No. of Isolates from Specimen	Density of Isolates (CFU/mL)	Type of Specimen[a]	Significant Clinical Information Influencing Work-up[b]	Extent of Identification[c]	Suscept. Testing	Example of Report[d]	Reasonable Laboratory Interpretation
1	$>10^5$	CC, FC, SC, IL, SP, CYS	None	Definitive	Yes	>100,000 CFU/mL, genus, species	Probable UTI (urinary tract infection)
1	10^4–10^5	CC, FC, SC, IL, SP, CYS	None	Definitive	Yes	50,000 CFU/mL, genus, species	Possible UTI; patient evaluation necessary
1	10^2–10^5	SP, CYS, (SC)	None	Definitive	Yes	300 CFU/mL, genus, species	Probable UTI
1	10^3–10^4	CC, FC, SC, IL	Symptomatic female, or male with prostatitis, or WBC present	Definitive (if gram-negative rod or possible S. saprophyticus	Yes	5,000 CFU/mL, genus, species	Possible UTI; patient evaluation necessary
1	Any number (no.)	CC, FC, SC, IL, SP, CYS	Physician specifies specific organism (N. gonorrhoeae) or syndrome (urethritis) or systemic disease (cryptococcosis)	Definitive; specific organism if present	Yes	100 CFU/mL, N. gonorrhoeae; or 1,000 CFU/mL, H. influenzae; or 3,000 CFU/mL, Cryptococcus neoformans	Possible UTI or evidence of disseminated infection
2	Each $>10^3$	SP, CYS, (SC)	None	Definitive	Yes	>100,000 CFU/mL, genus, species and 50,000 CFU/mL, genus, species	Probable UTI
2	$>10^5$ and $>10^5$, or $>10^5$ and $>10^4$, or $>10^4$ and $>10^4$ (if possible pathogens)	CC, IL, (SC)	None	Definitive	Yes	>100,000 CFU/mL, genus, species and 50,000 CFU/mL, genus, species	Possible UTI; consider faulty collection or transportation or colonization
2	$>10^5$ and $>10^5$, or $>10^5$ and $>10^4$, or $>10^4$ and $>10^4$ (if possible pathogens)	FC, (IL)	Patient with neurogenic bladder or indwelling catheter	Descriptive	No; hold plate (5-7 days) for tests in case patient becomes septic	>100,000 CFU/mL, NLF, and >100,000 CFU/mL, LF	Doubtful UTI; colonization likely
2	One organism $>10^4$ and clearly predominant (ie, at least tenfold more than other)	CC, IL, FC, (SC)	None	Definitive; predominant organism	Yes; the predominant organism	>100,000 CFU/mL, genus, species, and 5,000 CFU/mL, GPC	Probable UTI caused by predominant species; the other is probably urethral or collection contaminant
2	Both $<10^4$, or one 10^4–10^5, but not predominant	CC, IC, FC, (SC)	None	Descriptive	No	30,000 CFU/mL, GPR, and 40,000 CFU/mL, GPC	

No. of colony types	Culture result	Specimen source[a]	Clinical information[b]	Report[c]	Work-up	Example	Interpretation
2 or more	A possible pathogen such as E. coli or S. saprophyticus at 10^3 and others at about the same level	CC, FC, SC, IL, SP, CYS	Symptomatic female, or male with prostatitis, or WBC present	Definitive; possible pathogens	Yes	8,000 CFU/mL, E. coli, with 10,000 CFU/mL, GPR	Possible UTI; patient evaluation necessary
3 or more	One organism >10^4 and clearly predominant	SP, CYS	None	Definitive; predominant organism	Yes; the predominant organism	30,000 CFU/mL, genus, species; 1,000 CFU/mL, GPC; and 1,000 CFU/mL, GPR	Probable UTI
3 or more	One organism >10^4 and clearly predominant	CC, IC, FC, SC	None	Definitive; predominant organism	Yes; the predominant organism	30,000 CFU/mL, genus, species; 1,000 CFU/mL, GPC; and 1,000 CFU/mL, GPR	Probable UTI caused by predominant species; the other is probably urethral or collection contaminant
3 or more	Mix of any no. with none predominant	CC, IC, FC, SC	None	Descriptive	No	Mixed growth of >100,000 CFU/mL, GNR (3 kinds)	Faulty collection or transportation
3 or more	Any combination of >10^5 and >10^4	FC, (IL)	Patient with neurogenic bladder or indwelling catheter	Descriptive	No; hold plate (5–7 days) for tests in case patient becomes septic	>100,000 CFU/mL, NLF (2 kinds), and >10,000 CFU/mL, GPC (2 kinds)	Colonization
No growth	<10^3 if 0.001-mL loop is used; <10^2 if 0.01-mL loop is used	CC, IC, FC, SC, SP, CYS	None or asymptomatic			No growth (<10^3 CFU/mL), or No growth (<10^2 CFU/mL)	No UTI
No growth	<10^3 if 0.001-mL loop is used; <10^2 if 0.01-mL loop is used	CC, IC, FC, SC, SP, CYS	Symptomatic			No growth (<10^3 CFU/mL), or No growth (<10^2 CFU/mL)	Patient on antibiotics?; check Gram stain for pyuria; consider AFB, chlamydiae, mycoplasmas, viruses

[a]CC = clean-catch (midstream) specimen; FC = specimen from indwelling catheter; SC = specimen from straight (in and out) catheter; IL = specimen from ileal conduit; SP = suprapubic aspirate specimen; CYS = cystoscopy specimen

[b]WBC, leukocytes

[c]Definitive = complete ID to species; Descriptive = ID can be determined from plates or Gram stain; i.e., lactose fermenter or gram-positive cocci

[d]GPC = gram-positive cocci; NLF = nonlactose-fermenting gram-negative rod; LF = lactose-fermenting gram-negative rod; GNR = gram-negative rod; GPR = gram-positive rod; AFB = acid-fast bacilli

Checkpoint! 34–10 (Chapter Objective 7)

A urine culture grew up a mixture of gram-positive and gram-negative organisms with no one organism predominant. The culture had been inoculated with a 0.001 ml loop and five colonies of the gram-positive cocci and five colonies of the gram-negative rod grew. What are the colony counts?

   A. 5,000 CFU/mL gram-positive cocci and 5,000 CFU/mL gram-negative rods

   B. 20,000 CFU/mL mixed organisms

   C. 500 CFU/mL gram-positive cocci and 500 CFU/mL gram-negative rods

   D. Over 100,000 CFU/mL mixed organisms

▶ TREATMENT

Treatment is often initiated before the culture report is completed. A treatment that is directed toward gram-negative bacilli and gram-positive organisms is recommended. Drug-resistant gram-negative organisms must also be suspected. Trimethoprim-sulfamethoxazole (Septra or Bactrim) is used for most cases of cystitis. Quinolone antibiotics or ampicillin are used in cases of cystitis if drug resistance is encountered. Pyelonephritis is more serious and treatment may begin with intravenous, extended-term administration of a broad-spectrum antibiotic often second- or third-generation cephalosporins.

In patients with acute pyelonephritis the treatment plan must be individualized to the patient. Some patients may require hospitalization and intravenous antimicrobial therapy; some patients will respond to outpatient oral therapy. The severity of illness, the patient's underlying status and reliability level, and the availability of a support system must be considered.

 REAL WORLD TIP

Cranberry juice may help prevent and treat urinary tract infections by inhibiting bacterial adherence to the bladder epithelium.

▶ MICROBES ASSOCIATED WITH URINARY TRACT INFECTIONS (UTIs)

Most cases of uncomplicated cystitis are caused by *Escherichia coli* (80–90% of cases) (Berkley et al., 1999). A predominant cause of UTIs in young, sexually active women is *Staphylococcus saprophyticus.* Complicated infections are more often polymicrobial. Organisms that cause these infections are often antibiotic resistant *E. coli, Klebsiella* spp., *Enterobacter* spp., *Proteus*

spp., group B and D streptococci, and *Enterococcus,* as well as *Pseudomonas aeruginosa* and coagulase-negative staphylococci. A listing of common and not-so-common etiological agents follows, but does not include every possible organism. Remember to correlate the growth pattern on media, Gram stain, colony morphology, testing results, and antibiogram to the final identification before issuing a final result. Question and investigate reactions and suspect antibiograms that do not match the identity.

COMMON ISOLATES

Enterobacteriaceae

Not all *E. coli* are equal in causing urinary tract infections, especially acute pyelonephritis. Six O-serotype groups of *E. coli* cause the majority of UTIs. O-serogroups denote the somatic antigens of the bacteria. Infecting strains have been found to have several virulence factors including siderophores, K antigen, hemolysins, and the presence of adhesions for uroepithelial cells. The siderophores probably are involved in iron acquisition for bacterial growth. The K (capsular) antigen has been shown to protect the organism from antibodies and/or complement and phagocytosis. Some strains have fimbriae (P fimbriae or pyelonephritis-associated pili) with terminal receptors for the "P" antigen. The "P" antigen is a blood group marker also found on the surface of cells lining the perineum and urinary tract. The majority (approximately 75%) of people express the "P" antigen. About 80% of *E. coli* strains from patients with pyelonephritis produce P fimbriae that is six times that of fecal strains.

Nosocomial infections in patients with indwelling bladder instruments are often due to multiple antibiotic-resistant members of *Enterobacteriaceae* and nonfermenting bacilli from the hands of hospital personnel, the environment, and contaminated solutions. These organisms include *Pseudomonas, Proteus, Klebsiella,* and *Enterobacter* species. *P. mirabilis* preferentially infects patients with urinary tracts having functional, anatomical, or other abnormalities, including indwelling urinary catheters. Infections with urease-positive organisms, such as *Proteus, Providencia,* or *Morganella,* may cause kidney stone formation. These stones are called struvite or apatite stones, which consist of magnesium ammonium phosphate (apatite). The urease enzyme, produced by the organism, breaks down urea in the urine to catalyze production of these stones.

Many of the commonly encountered aerobic gram-negative rods can be rapidly presumptively identified using colony morphology and very basic tests. The spot indole reagent will presumptively differentiate *E. coli* from other lactose-fermenters. *Citrobacter koseri* can be mistaken for *E. coli* as it may be a lactose-fermenter and indole positive. A citrate test would differentiate between the two. *Citrobacter* is citrate positive. The swarming *Enterobacteriaceae* can be differentiated by indole. *Proteus mirabilis* is negative whereas *Proteus vulgaris* is indole positive. The spot indole test should utilize the paradimethyl–amino–cinnamaldehyde spot indole reagent and be done on colonies growing on blood or chocolate agars. EMB or MacConkey agars lack the reactive substrate and will give erroneous reactions.

REAL WORLD TIP

Because *E. coli* is the most common isolate in urine cultures, the use of rapid identification criteria can save the laboratory time, energy, and resources. *E. coli* can be presumptively identified if it is: (1) beta hemolytic on BA, (2) a dark lactose fermenter on MAC, and (3) spot indole positive.

Rapid urea broth is a quick method for detecting urease activity. Most *Klebsiella* strains will be urease positive, indole negative, and lactose positive with the exception of *K. oxytoca*, which is indole positive. *Proteus, Providencia,* and *Morganella* (nonlactose-fermenting, gram-negative rods) will have a positive rapid phenylalanine deaminase (PAD) test and the urease test will be positive for all but some strains of *Providencia*.

A susceptible result for ampicillin, cefazolin, or cephalothin for organisms identified as *C. freundii, Enterobacter* species, or *S. marcescens* is suspicious. Be skeptical of an ampicillin-sensitive result for *Klebsiella, Providencia,* and *P. vulgaris.* Doubt any intermediate or resistant result for carbapenems when evaluating results for the *Enterobacteriaceae.*

∞ Chapter 8, "Presumptive Identification," and ∞ Chapter 9, "Final Identification," provide additional information on these rapid tests. Visit ∞ Chapter 21 to review information on the *Enterobacteriaceae.* ∞ Chapter 11, "Susceptibility Testing," discusses other unusual resistance profiles, which require evaluation.

Checkpoint! 34–11 (Chapter Objectives 7)

A urine culture grew up a pure culture of a beta hemolytic, dark lactose fermenter that is spot indole positive. A 0.001 mL loop was used to set up the culture. One hundred and ten colonies were counted on the plates. What would the colony count/identification be and would this be considered as significant for a UTI using the guidelines given in this chapter?

    A. Colony count 110,000 CFU/mL of E. coli; yes
    B. Colony count 110,000 CFU/mL of Proteus vulgaris; yes
    C. Colony count 11,000 CFU/mL of E. coli; no
    D. Colony count 11,000 CFU/mL of Proteus vulgaris; no

Enterococcus (Including Vancomycin-Resistant *Enterococcus*) and Other *Streptococcus*

One of the most commonly encountered gram-positive infective agents, *Enterococcus,* causes UTIs primarily in older men (over 50 years), particularly in association with urinary tract manipula-

tion or instrumentation or prostatic hypertrophy. Most clinical studies suggest that patients with normal host defenses are resistant to enterococcal infections. Susceptibility testing should be performed when *Enterococcus* is isolated, as many are notoriously resistant to many antibiotics especially vancomycin. An esculin and PYR test should be performed on alpha or gamma hemolytic streptococci if isolated in significant numbers. If the organism is PYR and esculin positive, *Enterococcus* should be reported. If the organism is esculin positive and PYR negative, the isolate is *Streptococcus gallolyticus,* formerly known as *S. bovis.* If both results are negative, then the organism is probably viridans streptococci. These last two organisms are very sensitive to penicillins and cephalosporins. There is often no need to differentiate or perform susceptibility testing.

REAL WORLD TIP

If an *Enterococcus* spp. is vancomycin resistant, it should be speciated. *E. faecalis* and *E. faecium* can pass on their vancomycin resistance genes. *E. casseliflavus* and *E. gallinarum*, which are intrinsically vancomycin resistant, are unable to transfer their resistance genes.

Beta-hemolytic streptococci could be *Streptococcus agalactiae,* a rare strain of *Enterococcus,* or rarely *S. pyogenes.* A pathogenic gram-positive cocci that can cause problems in nearly any body site, *S. pyogenes,* will grow on BA as a small, translucent colony with beta hemolysis. After obtaining a negative catalase test on a gram-positive cocci, beta-hemolytic isolate, a latex agglutination test, or PYR test can be performed. *S. pyogenes,* also known as a group A streptococci, are typically PYR positive. Latex grouping will indicate the various Lancefield groups of Streptococcus. Group A streptococci are the only commonly isolated beta-hemolytic streptococci that give a positive PYR reaction. Care must be taken, however, since very young colonies of *Staphylococcus aureus* may test PYR positive.

S. agalactiae (group B streptococci) (GBS) may be isolated from urine collected from both pregnant and nonpregnant women. Any amount of GBS isolated from urine collected from a pregnant woman should be reported to a physician (Schrag, Gorwitz, Fultz-Butts, & Schuchat, 2002). A large grayish-white colony with a narrow zone of beta-hemolysis that is catalase negative is characteristic of this organism. Occasional nonhemolytic strains occur and could be misidentified. Group B streptococci are PYR negative, CAMP positive, and hippurate hydrolysis positive. The latex agglutination test provides rapid results and is used in most laboratories for GBS identification.

Beta-hemolytic streptococci are expected to be sensitive to ampicillin, penicillin, and third-generation cephalosporins. Verify any unusual results to confirm identity and rule out technical error. ∞ Chapter 17 reviews information pertinent to gram-positive cocci.

Pseudomonas species

Most *Pseudomonas* urinary tract infections are hospital acquired and associated with either catheterization or surgery or with any cause of obstruction or persistent site of infections. Patients infected with *Pseudomonas* tend to have frequent recurrences and chronic presentations because of the organisms' natural resistance to antibiotics. These gram-negative rods are strictly aerobic, opportunistic bacilli. They can grow in environments with limited nutrients. Rapid identification of *Pseudomonas aeruginosa* includes a nonlactose fermenting colony on MAC, observation of a blue-green pigment, a unique odor (grape-like), and a positive oxidase test. The oxidase test must be performed on an isolate from a blood agar plate. Isolates from MacConkey agar can give false-negative reactions. ∞ Chapter 22 will provide additional information on *Pseudomonas* and other nonfermenting bacilli.

Staphylococcus (Including *S. saprophyticus*, *S. epidermidis*, and *S. aureus*)

One of the most common gram-positive causative UTI agents, *S. saprophyticus,* is found predominantly in symptomatic sexually active women younger than 40 years of age. It is unique in that the organism prefers to adhere to the epithelial cells of the urogenital system. Most patients (90%) are symptomatic and the symptoms are indistinguishable from UTIs caused by *E. coli*. These infections respond readily to traditional urinary tract antibiotics except nalidixic acid. *S. saprophyticus* is a gram-positive cocci that is catalase positive, coagulase negative, and resistant to novobiocin.

Staphylococcus epidermidis is found in hospitalized patients older than 50 years of age and in children. These individuals most often have had recent urinary tract surgery, indwelling urinary catheters, or chronic urinary tract disease. Most of these patients are asymptomatic. *S. epidermidis* is often resistant to multiple drugs and bacteriuria often persists after therapy. *S. epidermidis* is a gram-positive cocci, catalase positive, coagulase negative, and susceptible to novobiocin.

A particularly invasive organism associated with catheterized patients, *S. aureus* will grow on BA as a large, white to cream-colored colony that is often beta hemolytic. A catalase positive, gram-positive cocci should be tested using a latex agglutination test. The staphylococcal latex agglutination reagent methods react to clumping factor (bound coagulase) and also have antibodies reactive to *S. aureus* cell wall protein A. This organism is often acquired via hematogenous spread (the descending route of infection). Information related to staphylococci can be found in ∞ Chapter 17, "Aerobic Gram-Positive Cocci."

UNUSUAL ISOLATES

Corynebacterium urealyticum

This aerobic gram-positive bacillus forms nonhemolytic, tiny colonies on BA after 24-48 hours of incubation, requires lipid to grow, is unable to reduce nitrate, hydrolyzes urea, and possesses a multiple antibiotic resistance profile. It is only sus-

ceptible to vancomycin. It is recognized by its multiresistance, rapidly positive urease reaction, and inability to ferment carbohydrates. It is a common cause of alkaline-encrusted cystitis, which demonstrates ammonium magnesium phosphate crystals that may precipitate out in the walls of the already damaged bladder and cause ulcerations. The organism is also associated with kidney infections and struvite kidney stone production in renal transplant recipients. All immunosuppressed, urological, or renal transplant patients (especially with repeated urinary tract infections) should be considered at increased risk for this organism. These are slow growers due to a requirement for lipids, so BA plates should not be discarded prior to 48 hours. Vancomycin is the drug of choice to treat this infection. ∞ Chapter 17, "Aerobic Gram-Positive Rods," provides additional information about this organism.

Candida species

The major yeast commonly associated with UTIs is *Candida*. This organism may cause pyelonephritis via a hematogenous or bloodborne route. On agar medium, young colonies of *C. albicans* can resemble colonies of coagulase-negative staphylococci and may be misidentified if Gram-stained smears are not examined. *Candida* spp. is often recovered from hospitalized patients with indwelling catheters. Candiduria may be an indication of bladder or renal parenchymal infection, a urinary tract fungus ball, or disseminated candidiasis. Predisposing factors include diabetes mellitus, antibiotic and corticosteroid therapy, female gender, and disturbance of urine flow.

C. albicans will usually grow within 2 days. A Gram stain of the colonies (or a wet mount) can assist in providing an accurate identification. Creamy white colonies that appear star-like or "feet," with oval budding yeast observed microscopically and a positive germ tube result can be presumptively identified as *C. albicans*. Go to ∞ Chapter 14, "Fungal Cultures," and ∞ Chapter 29, "Medical Mycology," to review information pertinent to the identification of yeast.

> **ⓔ REAL WORLD TIP**
>
> *Candida glabrata* is another common urinary yeast pathogen. Its colony is pinpoint and may not appear until 48 hours. It is essential that urine BA culture plates be held a minimum of 48 hours to ensure recovery of this yeast. The pinpoint colony and production of blastoconidia only presumptively identify the organism as *C. glabrata*.

Aerococcus species

There are three species of *Aerococcus* associated with urinary system infections: *A. urinae, A. sanguinicola,* and *A. urinaehominis*. Most infections occur in older adults with predisposing conditions or catheters. The alpha-hemolytic, catalase-negative colony of *Aerococcus* resembles the enterococci and can be misidentified unless careful examination of a Gram stain is conducted. The three species of *Aerococcus* primarily associated with UTIs are catalase-negative, gram-positive cocci in clusters. PYR and LAP tests can be used to presumptively identify these organisms, although identification to species may not be clinically relevant (Facklam, Lovgren, Shewmaker, & Tyrrell, 2003). *A. urinae* is PYR negative and LAP positive; *A. sanguinicola* is PYR and LAP positive; and *A. urinaehominis* is PYR and LAP negative. These *Aerococcus* species are hippurate hydrolysis positive, which can distinguish them from the other catalase-negative, salt-tolerant, "staphylococcal" gram-positive cocci that are hippurate negative. Clinical and Laboratory Standards Institute (CLSI) does not have sensitivity testing standards or interpretive criteria for the *Aerococcus*. Visit ∞ Chapter 17 to read more about the catalase-negative gram-positive cocci.

Gardnerella vaginalis

Gardnerella vaginalis is considered an emerging urinary tract pathogen. The natural habitat is the human vagina. This organism is a facultative aerobe, gram-variable rod that requires enriched medium for growth. *G. vaginalis* is susceptible to penicillin, clindamycin, and relatively susceptible to metabolites of metronidazole. A patient with a *Gardnerella* infection is symptomatic, often experiencing trimethoprim/sulfamethoxazole failures. The urine sample usually exhibits high colony counts. The pure culture has tiny, pin-point colonies. If this type of colony is seen, Gram stain, and perform a catalase test. If the organism is catalase negative and is a gram-negative to gram-variable bacillus resembling diphtheroids, subculture to McCarthy starch agar and incubate in CO_2. Report as *Gardnerella* those isolates that produce zones of starch hydrolysis (clearing) around the colonies. *G. vaginalis* is susceptible to metronidazole (50 g disk), trimethoprim (5 g), and sulfonamide (1 mg). Susceptibility testing is not performed because there are no CLSI guidelines. *Gardnerella* may also be identified by commercial identification systems or by other biochemical reactions.

Lactobacillus species

This organism may be significant if it grows as a pure culture and the patient is symptomatic. It typically exhibits as long, thin, filamentous gram-positive bacilli with alpha-hemolytic or nonhemolytic small gray colonies that are catalase negative. Some *Lactobacillus* are microaerophilic. Do not speciate these organisms. The Gram stain reaction, microscopic morphology, catalase reaction, and characteristic colony are adequate for presumptive identification. There are no CLSI susceptibility testing guidelines.

Haemophilus species

Haemophilus usually causes UTIs in children with urinary tract abnormalities, but can affect all ages. Its true incidence may be unknown because chocolate agar is not used routinely for urine cultures. Additional information from the physician can ensure the organism is not missed. They may be identified by means of a commercial system after growing the culture on chocolate agar. If *Haemophilus* is identified, perform and report beta-lactamase test results. Inoculate chocolate agar plate with 0.01 mL urine loop to grow these and other low colony count positives. ∞ Chapter 20 provides additional information about fastidious gram-negative rods.

SALMONELLA SPECIES

These organisms are very invasive and have been known to cause pyelonephritis during a systemic infection, including bacteremia (hematogenous route). In addition, *Salmonella* spp. may be found in the urine during the early stages of typhoid fever. These gram-negative rods will grow as colorless colonies on EMB or MacConkey agar. They may be identified with commercial identification systems. Remember to report the isolation of any *Salmonella* to the state health department.

PATHOGENS THAT REQUIRE SPECIAL CULTURE OR RECOVERY TECHNIQUES

Leptospira interrogans is a thin, motile, helical spirochete that produces a zoonotic infection worldwide. Animals most often involved with transmission are rats, dogs, livestock, rodents, wild mammals, and cats. The peak incidence is summer and early autumn when young adult men often become infected, for example, after recreational exposure to contaminated water. Occupational exposure by farmers or veterinarians via urine-contaminated water or soil is the main avenue of transmission. The organism penetrates intact mucous membranes or abraded skin, enters the bloodstream, and spreads to all parts of the body. *L. interrogans* frequently localizes in the kidneys and can cause renal failure due to a direct toxic effect of the organism on the tubules. The organism may be isolated from the urine after the second week of infection. Tween 80-albumin (Fletcher's medium) or a media enriched with rabbit serum is viewed as the best available medium. Cultures should be maintained in the dark for up to 6 weeks at 28–30°C in the dark. The infection is usually diagnosed with a serological procedure. ∞ Chapter 25, "Spirochetes," provides information related to leptospirosis.

Mycobacterium spp. have been occasionally associated with UTIs, especially in patients infected with the human immunodeficiency virus (HIV) or other immunocompromised patients. Pyelonephritis due to *Mycobacterium tuberculosis* indicates hematogenous spread of the organism.

If *Mycobacterium* spp. are suspected, the specimen should be decontaminated prior to inoculation to media appropriate for isolation of these organisms. ∞ Chapter 13 provides information on decontamination procedures for acid-fast bacilli.

There are two viruses that have been associated as causative agents of cystitis. They are adenovirus (types 11 and 21) and herpes simplex virus. ∞ Chapter 31, "Intracellular Microorganisms," provides a review of these viruses.

Human schistosomes are parasitic trematodes found in the venous bloodstream of the intestine and bladder. The life cycle of this parasite must include a snail host. The cercariae stage of the parasite is released from the snail and penetrates the skin of the victim. The larval schistosome migrates to the lungs and then to the mesenteric and urinary bladder veins of the victim. *Schistosoma hematobium* releases eggs in the bladder blood vessels, which then burrow into the bladder tissue and cause granulomas to develop.

Features of *S. haematobium* infection are dysuria, urinary frequency, and hematuria. Examination of the urine sediment for eggs of this parasite aid in diagnosis. The trematode should respond to praziquantel. For a review of the schistosomes and their recovery, refer to ∞ Chapters 15 and 30.

Other organisms such as *Mycoplasma, Ureaplasma,* and *Chlamydia trachomatis* may be associated with pyuria but cannot be grown using routine culture media. ∞ Chapter 28 provides information on the cultivation of *Mycoplasma* and *Ureaplasma.* ∞ Chapter 31 discusses cultivation of *C. trachomatis.*

Checkpoint! 34–12 (Chapter Objective 8)

The organism most often implicated in UTIs of young, sexually active women is

  A. *E. coli.*
  B. *Staphylococcus saprophyticus.*
  C. *Enterococcus faecalis.*
  D. *Gardnerella vaginalis.*

▶ NORMAL CONTAMINANTS OF URINE

The key to the recognition of contaminants is that they are often present in low numbers and there are usually multiple genera or species present. Characteristic colonies and Gram stain reactions and microscopic morphology are usually adequate for identification. If the organisms are considered contaminants, they are often reported collectively as normal urethral flora rather than individual genus and species.

DIPHTHEROIDS

These organisms probably originate from the skin, are urease negative, and susceptible to antibiotics used to treat gram-positive organisms. They appear as opaque, white, or gray, strongly catalase-positive colonies. They should be urease negative. A Gram stain will reveal palisading, gram-positive rods. Diphtheroids colonies can resemble those of coagulase negative staphylococci so Gram stain is very important in their identification.

LACTOBACILLUS SPECIES

Lactobacilli usually represents normal vaginal flora. As previously described, the colony will be alpha hemolytic and small white or gray in color. The Gram stain demonstrates long, thin gram-positive bacilli that are chaining. The catalase reaction is negative.

VIRIDIANS *STREPTOCOCCUS*

The colonies of the viridians streptococci usually look like lactobacilli, but are often smoother and more convex. The Gram stain will show small gram-positive cocci that are usually in pairs or chains. These bacteria are catalase negative, LAP positive and PYR negative.

SUMMMARY

The urinary system is comprised of the kidneys, the ureters, bladder, and urethra. The urinary tract produces urine through the filtering of blood.

Proper specimen collection, handling, and transport are very important for reliable culture results. Acceptable collection techniques include midstream clean catch, catheterization, and suprapubic aspiration. Unacceptable specimens are urine catheter tips, pooled urine samples, and old urine specimens.

Normally the urine in the urinary tract is sterile but may acquire commensal bacteria from the distal portion of the urethra when collected. Therefore, the importance of a clean catch midstream urine collection cannot be overemphasized. If the patient does not receive proper instructions or fails to follow the instructions, the urine culture may grow commensals from the distal portion of the urethra, complicating the interpretation of the culture results.

Infection of the bladder (cystitis) can occur when bacteria move up the urethra—an ascending infection. If this condition persists, the infection may travel up the ureters to infect the kidney (pyelonephritis). The kidneys may be infected less commonly by organisms in the blood—hematogenous infection. Patients with symptomatic cystitis experience dysuria, frequency, and urine changes (smell, pyruria). Symptoms of pyelonephritis are flank pain, tenderness, and fever. UTIs in older adults may be asymptomatic or the symptoms may be vague—mental confusion, poor appetite, fatigue, or incontinence.

Cultures are performed by using a calibrated loop (0.001 or 0.01 mL) and plated on blood agar, MacConkey agar (or EMB), PEA or CNA (in cases of potentially mixed organisms), and chocolate (if isolation and identification of *Haemophilus* or *Gardnerella* is necessary).

Colony counts as low as 10^2 organisms/milliliter may indicate infection depending on the specimen, the patient (asymptomatic females), and the organism isolated. Isolates considered clinically significant are identified and tested for susceptibility.

Many organisms may cause a UTI, but *E. coli* is the most commonly implicated organism in the general population. *Staphylococcus saprophyticus* is often implicated in sexually active women younger than 40 years of age. *Corynebacterium* *urealyticum* is a common cause of alkaline-encrusted cystitis in the immunosuppressed. *Candida* spp. is the major yeast associated with UTIs.

LEARNING OPPORTUNITIES

1. Define the following terms: (Chapter Objective 2)

    a. UTI

    b. cystitis

    c. pyelonephritis

    d. urethritis

    e. pyuria

    f. hematuria

    g. dysuria

2. List three risk factors that contribute to increased incidence of UTIs. (Chapter Objective 1)

3. When is a symptomatic bacteruria of greater than or equal to 10^2 CFU/mL clinically significant? (Chapter Objective 3)

4. List two samples that would be unacceptable for urine culture. (Chapter Objective 4)

5. What is the appropriate media for a routine urine culture? (Chapter Objective 5)

6. What are the appropriate incubation conditions for a routine urine culture? (Chapter Objective 5)

7. For each of the following screening methods, indicate the expected result if that patient has cystitis and the causative agent of the infection is *Escherichia coli*: (Chapter Objective 6)

    a. Routine urine with microscopic evaluation

    b. Gram stain

    c. Nitrate reduction and leukocyte esterase by dipstick

8. Which organism is the most common cause of uncomplicated cystitis? (Chapter Objective 8)

CASE STUDY 34-1   (CHAPTER OBJECTIVES 6, 7, AND 8)

Patient: 83-year-old female

Background: The patient was admitted to the emergency room complaining of abdominal pain and tenderness. The patient has a history of interstitial cystitis and recurrent urinary tract infections. The patient was unable to void upon admission. She was catheterized by the emergency room nursing personnel and several hundred milliliters of urine were collected.

The urinalysis report on the collected urine was:

Color: dark brown (yellow)
Transparency: cloudy (clear)

Specific Gravity: 1.024 (1.002–1.030)
pH 6.0 (4.5–7.5)
Leukocyte Esterase: positive (negative)
Nitrites: positive (negative)
Protein: marked (negative)
Glucose: negative (negative)
Ketones: moderate (negative)
Urobilinogen: 0.2 (0.2–1.0 mg/dl)
Bilirubin: negative (negative)
Blood: 3+ (negative)

Microscopic examination

WBC: packed with clumps (0–5/HPF)
RBC: TNTC (0–3/HPF)
Epithelial cells: negative (few)
Bacteruria: 3+
Casts: none
Crystals: none
Mucus: trace (occasional)

A culture of the urine collected was performed. The following day the report showed a colony count of >100,000

CFU/mL of a beta hemolytic gram-negative rod that is also a lactose fermenter. The spot indole test was positive.

1. What did the urinalysis findings indicate?
2. How would you interpret the culture results?
3. What is the presumptive identity of the isolate?
4. Can you determine if this woman has cystitis or pyelonephritis?
5. What are some virulence factors produced by the organism implicated?

CASE STUDY 34-2   (CHAPTER OBJECTIVES 7, 8, AND 9)

Patient: 89-year-old male

Background: The patient has a diagnosis of prostatic hypertrophy. He had been living alone with minimal problems. Recently he has been feeling very tired and his family has noticed some slight confusion. He made a doctor's appointment and the physician had a battery of laboratory tests performed, including a urine sample.

The urinalysis report on the collected urine was:

Color: yellow (yellow)
Transparency: cloudy (clear)
Specific Gravity: 1.020 (1.002–1.030)
pH 6.5 (4.5–7.5)
Leukocyte esterase: positive (negative)
Nitrites: positive (negative)
Protein: marked (negative)
Glucose: negative (negative)
Ketones: moderate (negative)
Urobilinogen: 0.2 (0.2–1.0 mg/dl)
Bilirubin: negative (negative)
Blood: 1+ (negative)

Microscopic examination

WBC: 30–40 per HPF (0–5/HPF)
RBC: 5–8 per HPF (0–3/HPF)
Epithelial cells: negative (few)
Bacteruria: 3+
Casts: none
Crystals: none
Mucus: trace (occasional)

Another urine sample was collected clean-catch midstream for culture. The culture report was >100,000 CFU per mL of a gram-positive cocci. The organism was subsequently identified as *Enterococcus faecalis*.

1. What factor(s) related to this individual increases his chances of experiencing a urinary tract infection?
2. Why should susceptibility testing be performed on the organism identified?
3. What test(s) in the microbiology laboratory would help to identify a gram-positive cocci that is catalase negative as an enterococci?

CASE STUDY 34-3   (CHAPTER OBJECTIVES 3 AND 7)

Patient: 35-year-old female

Background: The urine culture grows mixed gram-negative rods (lactose and nonlactose fermenters) and gram-positive cocci. No one organism is 80% dominant with a colony count of >10,000 cfu/mL. The doctor requests identifications and susceptibilities on the isolated organisms.

1. Are the identifications and susceptibility tests needed?

2. How should the laboratory proceed with the physician's request?
3. How important is urine collection to the culturing process?
4. What will probably happen if the laboratory proceeds to identify and perform susceptibilities on each isolate?
5. What possible problems can arise from inappropriate antibiotic usage?

CASE STUDY 34-4   (CHAPTER OBJECTIVES 3 AND 4)

Patient: 87-year-old male with indwelling catheter

Background: The urine culture grows pure culture of *Enterococcus faecalis* antibiotic resistant, colony count of >100,000 CFU/mL. The laboratory requests information on the duration of current catheter. The current catheter has been in place for 1 week.

1. What is the significance of the *E. faecalis* in this specimen?

2. Why should the physician be cautioned regarding taking action (prescribing treatment) based on this urine culture?

3. What recommendation should be given to the nursing staff regarding collection of samples from patients with indwelling catheters?

PEARSON
myhealthprofessionskit™

Use this address to access the interactive Companion Website created for this textbook. Simply select "Clinical Laboratory Science" from the choice of disciplines. Find this book and log in using your user name and password.

REFERENCES

Go to myhealthprofessionskit.com to view this chapter's references.

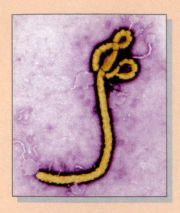

35

Gastrointestinal System

William C. Payne

■ LEARNING OBJECTIVES

Upon completion of this chapter, the learner should be able to:

1. Discuss the basic structure and function of the organs that make up the gastrointestinal system.

2. Discuss microbes that are normally present in nonsterile areas of the gastrointestinal tract including their role in maintaining health.

3. Discuss the pathogenesis, clinical manifestations, epidemiology, etiology, and laboratory diagnosis of diseases encountered in the gastrointestinal tract including bacterial, viral, parasitic, and toxigenic causes.

4. Evaluate the patient history, clinical signs and symptoms, and laboratory results in order to arrive at a laboratory diagnosis of gastrointestinal illnesses.

5. Presumptively identify an organism based on the Gram stain, description of macroscopic colony morphology, results of spot or rapid tests and other testing such as serotyping.

   a. Assess its clinical significance.

6. Correlate the colony morphologies of organisms on media used to isolate pathogenic organisms.

7. Select confirmatory tests necessary and evaluate the test results.

8. Describe toxigenic and nontoxigenic disease mechanisms responsible for systemic disease or localized pathology of the gastrointestinal tract.

9. Distinguish the pathogenic, invasive, toxigenic, and hemorrhagic strains of *Escherichia coli*.

10. Advise the most appropriate antimicrobial therapy and other forms of treatment as well as prevention of foodborne illness.

KEY TERMS

catabolism	exotoxin	microbiota
cytotoxin	fomite	neurotoxin
diarrhea	gastroenteritis	peristalsis
dysentery	hemolytic uremic	probiotics
enterotoxin	syndrome	rice water stool

▶ INTRODUCTION

Gastroenteritis, inflammation of the stomach and intestine, may include vomiting, nausea, **diarrhea** (loose, liquid stools with or without blood and mucus), fever, abdominal distension and pain and anorexia. Potential causes include microorganisms, medications, food intolerance, and food allergies. Because many cases are self-limiting, most do not seek treatment. Most individuals have experienced some form of food poisoning or "stomach flu" in their lifetime. This chapter focuses on gastroenteritis due to microorganisms.

ⓔ REAL WORLD TIP

The "stomach flu" is a viral gastroenteritis, but it is not caused by the influenza virus.

▶ ANATOMY AND PHYSIOLOGY OF THE GASTROINTESTINAL SYSTEM

FUNCTION OF THE GASTROINTESTINAL TRACT

The gastrointestinal (GI) tract or alimentary canal, along with its accessory organs, forms the digestive tract. The primary function of the gastrointestinal tract is the intake of food and breakdown of large food molecules to smaller molecules that can be absorbed. The process of food **catabolism** involves six basic processes:

1. Ingestion: taking food into the mouth
2. Secretion: cells of the gastrointestinal tract secrete acid, buffers, and enzymes involved in catabolism
3. Mixing and propulsion: accomplished through alternating contraction and relaxation of smooth muscle
4. Digestion: mechanical and chemical breakdown of food
   a. The mechanical process involves the cutting and grinding of food by the teeth with the aid of the tongue and cheeks. The smooth muscles of the stomach and small intestines mix the food with secretions.
   b. The chemical process involves the enzymatic breakdown of macromolecules such as complex lipids, protein, complex carbohydrates, and nucleic acids into triglycerides and fatty acids, sugars, amino acids, and nucleotides, respectively.
5. Absorption: passage of food into blood and lymph
6. Defecation: elimination of undigestible substances and bacteria through the anus

ANATOMICAL STRUCTURES OF THE GASTROINTESTINAL TRACT

The gastrointestinal tract is a continuous tube extending from the mouth to the anus and includes the following areas and organs: the mouth, oropharynx, esophagus, stomach, small intestine, and large intestine. Accessory organs include the teeth, salivary glands, liver, gallbladder, and pancreas. The small intestine can be subdivided into the duodenum, jejunum, and the ileum, including the ileocecal valve. The large intestine can also be subdivided into the cecum including the appendix, ascending colon, transverse colon, descending colon, sigmoid colon, rectum, and anus.

The mouth is formed by the lips, tongue, hard and soft palate, and the cheeks, all of which contribute to mechanical digestion and mixing of food with saliva (Figure 35-1 ■). Saliva lubricates the food as it is formed into a bolus or soft mass and begins the digestive process. Salivary amylase converts starches into maltose (a simple sugar) and lingual lipase acts on triglycerides.

The esophagus, a muscular tube that extends from the pharynx to the stomach, propels the bolus of food down into the stomach through the action of **peristalsis** or wave-like muscle contraction.

The stomach (Figure 35-2 ■), which extends from the esophagus to the duodenum, continues the process of mechanical digestion by muscular contraction and relaxation. Glands in the stomach produce mucus, hydrochloric acid, pepsin, and gastric lipase. Chemical digestion continues through the action of enzymes, such as pepsin, a protease that catabolizes dietary proteins into peptides. Water, certain ions, drugs, and alcohol are absorbed in the stomach.

More extensive chemical digestion takes place in the small intestine (Figure 35-3 ■) where cells secrete mucus and enzymes such as pancreatic amylase, trypsin, lipases, and nucleosidases. Starches are broken down into sugars, peptides

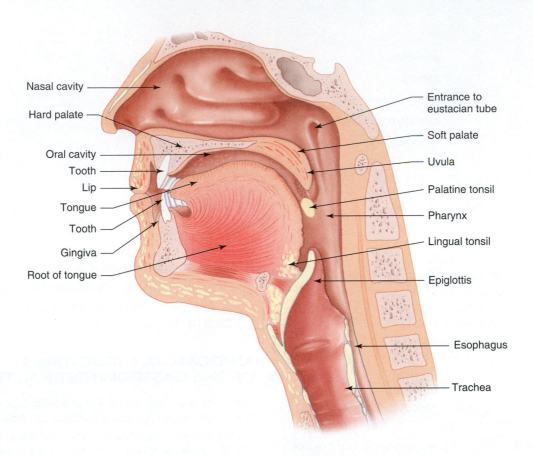

Nasal cavity

Hard palate

Oral cavity

Tooth

Lip

Tongue

Tooth

Gingiva

Root of tongue

Entrance to
eustacian tube

Soft palate

Uvula

Palatine tonsil

Pharynx

Lingual tonsil

Epiglottis

Esophagus

Trachea

■ **FIGURE 35-1** Sagittal view of the head and neck illustrating important anatomical structures of the gastrointestinal tract (lips, tongue, hard palate, soft palate, and the esophagus).

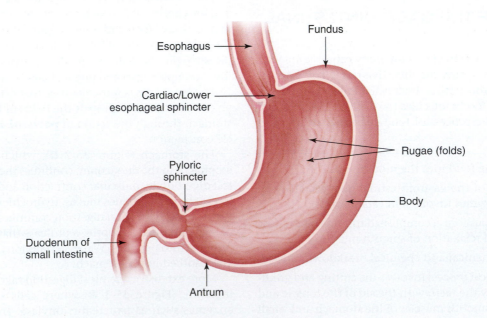

Esophagus

Fundus

Cardiac/Lower
esophageal sphincter

Pyloric
sphincter

Rugae (folds)

Body

Duodenum of
small intestine

Antrum

■ **FIGURE 35-2** Anatomical structures of the stomach.

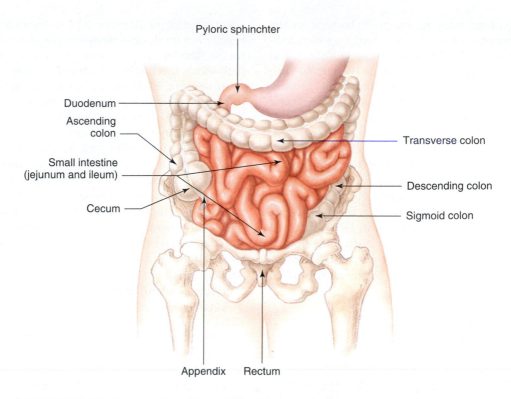

Pyloric sphinchter

Duodenum

Ascending
colon

Small intestine
(jejunum and ileum)

Cecum

Transverse colon

Descending colon

Sigmoid colon

Appendix   Rectum

■ **FIGURE 35-3** Anatomical structures of the large and small intestine.

into amino acids, fats into triglycerides and fatty acids, and nucleotides into pentoses and nitrogenous bases. Folds, villi, and microvilli increase the surface area of the small intestine, which facilitates the absorption of water, amino acids, short-chain fatty acids, monosaccharides, electrolytes, and vitamins.

In the large intestine (Figure 35-3), the last stage of the digestive process and the production of some vitamins occurs through bacterial action. Water, electrolytes, and vitamins are absorbed and feces, which consist of water, inorganic salts, epithelial cells, bacteria, and undigested foods, is expelled from the body by defecation. Bacteria can make up to 80% of the dry weight of feces.

While the appendix, located off the cecum, is often thought to no longer have a function in modern man, it may be a source of normal intestinal flora and replenish the large intestine with good bacteria after diarrheal episodes.

NORMAL BIODIVERSITY OF THE GASTROINTESTINAL TRACT

Unlike body systems such as the cardiovascular or nervous system, which are sterile, the gastrointestinal tract is colonized by microbes that play a beneficial role in good health. Commensal or nonpathogenic microbes, which reside in the mucous membranes of the GI tract and make up the **microbiota** (microbial organisms which colonize a specific region) of this body system compete with each other for space and nutrients and in the process inhibit the proliferation of path-

ogenic microbes. Additionally, nonpathogens stimulate the immune system, keeping it primed to repel invasion by more pathogenic organisms. The importance of this is seen with long-term use of broad-spectrum antibiotics, which may create an imbalance by eradicating susceptible species, allowing an overgrowth of normally harmless microbes or pathogens that are resistant to the antimicrobial agent. This can set the stage for an infectious process to begin.

Gram-positive cocci, such as the staphylococci and streptococci, including anaerobic gram-positive cocci as well as gram-negative cocci (*Neisseria* and *Veillonella* species), gram-positive rods (*Actinomyces, Lactobacillus, Bifidobacterium, Propionibacterium,* and *Arachnia* species), gram-negative rods (*Prevotella, Porphyromonas,* and *Fusobacterium* species), and spirochetes, are included among the large variety of bacteria that colonize the oral cavity.

The high acidity of the stomach prevents most microbes from becoming established, so the stomach is essentially sterile. There are some species that can survive passage through the stomach and these eventually colonize the small and large intestine. The same is true of some pathogenic microorganisms, which, in sufficient numbers, may cause disease through a variety of mechanisms including invasion of the tissues, toxin production, or damage to villi and microvilli, causing malabsorption. A full meal and drinking milk may buffer the stomach acid enough to allow organisms to survive passage.

The small intestine usually has small numbers of organisms present, most commonly lactobacilli, enterococci, and diphtheroids. In the large intestine anaerobic bacteria are the predominant organisms, including *Bacteroides* species, bifidobacteria, clostridia, lactobacilli, anaerobic streptococci, and *Eubacterium* species. There are 300 times as many anaerobic bacteria as facultative aerobic bacteria. Aerobic bacteria include members of the family *Enterobacteriaceae* (other than *Salmonella* and *Shigella*), such as *Escherichia coli,* enterococci, and streptococci.

In a small percentage of the population (3–11%), *Pseudomonas aeruginosa* may be isolated and 15–30% of the population can carry *Candida albicans.* Opportunists, such as *P. aeruginosa* and *C. albicans,* which are resistant to many antibiotics and normally present in numbers too small to pose a significant danger, may increase to such a degree they are able to cause overt disease. The elimination or reduction of the normal microbiota of the mucosa can disturb the normal balance that competition for space and nutrients provides. This allows organisms that are resistant to the antimicrobial agent to proliferate.

 ### Checkpoint! 35–1 (Chapter Objective 1)

Which of the following enzymes is a protease that catabolizes dietary proteins into peptides? It is produced by glands in the stomach and is active at an acid pH.

    A. *Pepsin*
    B. *Amylase*
    C. *Trypsin*
    D. *Catalase*

 ### Checkpoint! 35–2 (Chapter Objective 2)

Under normal circumstances, what is the predominant type of microorganism found in the large intestine?

    A. *Aerobic organisms, such as staphylococci and enterococci*
    B. *Anaerobic organisms, such as Bacteroides species and bifidobacteria*
    C. *Nonfermenting gram-negative rods such as Pseudomonas aeruginosa*
    D. *Members of the Enterobacteriaceae family (other than Salmonella and Shigella species)*

PATHOGENIC MECHANISMS

Diarrhea is the passage of liquid feces that can result from increased propulsion of intestinal contents by the intestinal muscles, resulting in less time for the bowel to reabsorb water or an increase in the amount of fluid held or produced in the intestine. Diarrheal illnesses caused by microbes usually occur because the organism: (1) adheres and grows on the surface of the intestinal epithelial cells, (2) invades or penetrates the intestinal mucosa, (3) produces an **enterotoxin** (a toxin excreted by a microorganism (**exotoxin**) in the intestine), (4) produces a **cytotoxin** (a substance which has a destructive

effect on cells), or (5) makes a preformed exotoxin that is then ingested or produces a **neurotoxin**, which acts on the autonomic nervous system. Some organisms may use multiple pathogenic mechanisms during infection.

Adherence is the first step in colonization. Once the organism can attach to the intestinal mucosa, it can begin to grow and cause infection. Diarrhea is produced because the cells lose their ability to absorb. An example of adherence is shown by enteropathogenic *E. coli.* Once an organism is attached to the epithelial cells, it can then go on to create toxins or invade cells. Invasive organisms penetrate and destroy the intestinal epithelial cells. *Shigella* spp. demonstrates the ability to invade cells. The diarrhea produced is bloody and contains many white blood cells. Some organisms can be engulfed by the epithelial cells and transported to the lymphatic system and blood vessels as seen with *Salmonella typhi.* Signs and symptoms often mimic those of septicemia including high fever.

Enterotoxins act on intestinal epithelial cells and cause them to secrete electrolytes, such as sodium and chloride. When sodium leaves the cells, water follows. Diarrhea due to enterotoxin is profuse and watery, and blood and leukocytes are usually not present. *Vibrio cholerae* is known for enterotoxin production. Cytotoxin damages intestinal mucosal cells. The diarrhea produced contains leukocytes and blood. Often there is fever, pain, cramps, and tenesmus (straining). *Campylobacter jejuni* produces cytotoxin. Neurotoxins can be created by organisms as they grow in food. Once ingested, the toxin causes the symptoms, which often include diarrhea and vomiting. *Clostridium botulinum* is known for its neurotoxin.

When an individual has prolonged diarrhea, other body systems can be affected. There may be an increased white blood cell count indicating an infectious disease process. The serum electrolytes can be affected. With dehydration, sodium and chloride levels can increase and potassium levels can decrease. Blood urea nitrogen (BUN) and creatinine can be elevated. Blood pH can show a metabolic acidosis. Box 35-1 details signs of diarrheal illness that require medical attention.

REAL WORLD TIP

Red and white blood cells are usually seen in the stool specimen of those diarrheal illnesses associated with invasive organisms.

✪ BOX 35-1

Signs of Diarrheal Illnesses Requiring Medical Attention

1. High fever: Body temperature over 101.5°F (38.6°C)
2. Presence of blood in the stools
3. Inability to keep liquids down due to prolonged vomiting
4. Diarrheal illness beyond 3 days duration
5. Dehydration

▶ THE MOST COMMON GASTROINTESTINAL DISEASES

Gastroenteritis or enterocolitis, of an abrupt onset, in a healthy individual is most often an infectious process. Potential pathogens include bacteria, viruses, parasites, and fungi. The route of transmission usually involves the five F's: flies, food, fingers, feces, or **fomites** (inanimate objects such as cutting boards, knives, or serving spoons). Most cases are self-limiting and do not require specific therapy. Those at risk for complications consist of older individuals, children under the age of 5 years and those with underlying diseases or compromised or suppressed immune systems.

CAMPYLOBACTER DIARRHEAL ILLNESS

Campylobacter jejuni is the most commonly identified bacterial cause of diarrheal illness in the world. This organism is found in the intestinal tract of healthy birds, and most raw poultry quickly become colonized with *Campylobacter*. As a result, the most frequent means of acquiring this infection is through the consumption of undercooked chicken or other foods that may become contaminated with the juices from raw chicken. Wild and domesticated animals such as cattle, sheep, swine, dogs, and cats can also carry the organism as intestinal flora.

A large dose of about 10,000 organisms is usually needed for infection. The illness typically has an incubation period of 2–10 days. Symptoms include abdominal cramps, bloody diarrhea, chills, and fever, yet nausea and vomiting are uncommon. The disease, in most cases, lasts for 3–6 days but untreated patients may excrete the organism for several months. Epidemics have been linked to contaminated unpasteurized milk, meat, and water, with the highest incidence occurring during the summer and fall months. The organism may even be transmitted sexually through anal intercourse.

Campylobacter jejuni causes inflammatory enteritis due to the release of enterotoxin and cytotoxin. The organism is motile, which enhances its ability to adhere to and penetrate intestinal cells. It can survive within vacuoles in the intestinal cell. The organism is able to produce a lethal cytotoxin that causes cell death. This explains the presence of blood and white blood cells with infection. The organism may also produce a cholera-like toxin that leads to excessive release of water into the intestine lumen.

A selective agar medium is required for the isolation of *C. jejuni*. Campy blood agar, is commercially available, as well as a liquid medium, Campy thioglycolate broth. The antibiotics trimethoprim, vancomycin, amphotericin B, polymyxin B, and cephalothin are incorporated into Campy blood agar medium to inhibit the growth of organisms that are part of the normal microbiota of the large intestine such as members of the family *Enterobacteriaceae*, staphylococci, and yeast. Incubation for 3 days at 42°C in a microaerophilic and capnophilic atmosphere (5% O_2, 10% CO_2, and 85% N_2) provides the best growth. The use of this temperature, atmosphere, and selective agar inhibits growth of normal enteric flora.

Campylobacter jejuni is unique in that it will also grow at 4°C. Cold enrichment can be used to enhance its growth and inhibit the growth of normal enteric flora. The Campy broth is inoculated with stool about 1 inch below its surface. This ensures the microaerophilic atmosphere for *Campylobacter* spp. After incubation overnight in the refrigerator, a few drops of the inoculated area of the broth is subcultured to a Campy blood agar. The Campy blood agar is then inoculated as previously described. Some facilities have eliminated the use of Campy thio due to the delay in results and lack of significant increased recovery compared to direct inoculation of a Campy blood agar. *C. jejuni* can be presumptively identified by its characteristic Gram stain (gram-negative spiral rods), positive catalase and oxidase reactions, and inability to grow on routine media at 35–37°C. ∞ Chapter 23 provides more information on *Campylobacter jejuni* and other *Campylobacter* species.

SALMONELLOSIS

Salmonella species are members of the family *Enterobacteriaceae* and are widespread in the intestine of birds, reptiles, and mammals. Raw or undercooked meat or poultry, eggs, and milk usually serve as the source of the organism. Humans are the only source for *S. typhi*, the causative agent of typhoid or enteric fever.

A high dose of the organism is usually needed to initiate infection. The symptoms typically include fever, diarrhea (the "runs" or a high volume of fluid), and abdominal cramps. Symptoms last for about one week but the organism can be shed in the stool for several weeks. In patients with underlying health issues or weakened immune systems, the bacteria may invade the blood and cause life-threatening infections. Most cases are due to *S. enteritidis*.

Typhoid fever, due to *S. typhi* and *S.* serotype Paratyphi, results in penetration of the intestinal cells and spread through the blood stream. After an incubation period of 8–14 days, the individual experiences fever, headache, myalgia, and gastrointestinal distress. The illness becomes progressively worse during the latter stages of the illness, with high fever, lethargy, prostration, and delirium. The word "typhoid" is derived from the Greek *typhos*, which means "smoke" or "cloud," referring to the stage of delirium that may develop. After invasion of the blood stream, the organism can cause infection that leads to deep intestinal ulcers and bloody stools. Surprisingly, the organism can also cause constipation rather than diarrhea. By the end of the third week the fever usually subsides, and the patient begins to improve.

Most *Salmonella* species cause disease by production of enterotoxin, which causes the intestinal cell to lose water and electrolytes. Some strains can also produce a cytotoxin that results in the presence of blood in the stool. *S. typhi* is able to move across the intestinal cells to reach the blood stream, be taken up by the lymphatic system, and infect the reticuloendothelial system (bone marrow, lymph nodes, liver, and spleen).

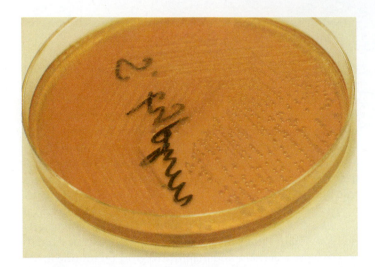

■ **FIGURE 35-4** *Salmonella* species growing on a MacConkey (MAC) agar plate. Because these organisms are nonlactose-fermenting, enteric Gram-negative rods, they produce colorless colonies after 18–24 hours of incubation at 35–37°C.

Media selective for enteric gram-negative rods is essential for the isolation and differentiation of *Salmonella* in stool cultures. *Salmonella* species will appear as nonlactose fermenters on agar of low selectivity such as MacConkey (Figure 35-4 ■) or eosin-methylene blue agars. The appearance of colorless colonies with black centers on moderately selective media such as Salmonella-Shigella (Figure 35-5 ■), red colonies with black centers (Figure 35-5) on xylose–lysine–deoxycholate (XLD), and blue-green colonies with black centers (Figure 35-6 ■) on hektoen enteric (HE) agars suggests *Salmonella* species.

For *Salmonella* species, identification is done using biochemical tests. In addition, serological testing is required to determine the serogroup of the isolate based on the somatic (O) and flagella (H) antigens. *S. typhi* characteristically exhibits

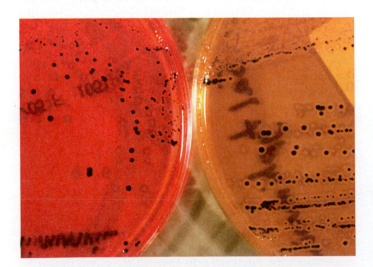

■ **FIGURE 35-5** Colonies of *Salmonella* growing on XLD (left) and SS (right). The black centers are due to hydrogen sulfide production.

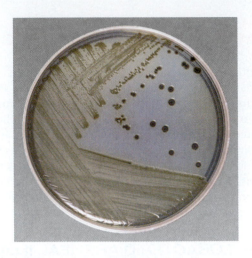

■ **FIGURE 35-6** Colonies of *Salmonella* growing on HE.
Photo courtesy of Remel, part of Thermo Fisher Scientific.

a capsular (Vi or virulent) antigen, which must be boiled away to reveal its group specific D somatic antigen. Isolation of *Salmonella* is reportable to the public health agencies. More information on *Salmonella* can be found in ∞ Chapter 21, "*Enterobacteriaceae.*"

 REAL WORLD TIP

If *S. typhi* cannot be detected by culture, the Widal test, a serological test to detect a rise in titer of antibodies to somatic and flagellar antigens, may be employed.

✓ **Checkpoint! 35–3 (Chapter Objective 3)**

The most commonly identified bacterial cause of diarrheal illness in the world is _____. This organism is found in the intestinal tract of healthy birds and is commonly transmitted through the ingestion of poorly cooked poultry.
    A. *Salmonella typhi*
    B. *Shigella dysenteriae*
    C. *Campylobacter jejuni*
    D. *Citrobacter freundii*

✓ **Checkpoint! 35–4 (Chapter Objective 3)**

The etiological agent of typhoid fever is
    A. *Salmonella typhimurium.*
    B. *Salmonella typhi.*
    C. *Campylobacter jejuni.*
    D. *Campylobacter coli.*

BACILLARY DYSENTERY

Shigella species are the etiological agents of **dysentery**, a gastrointestinal disease that has an incubation period of 1–7 days and is characterized by fever, cramping, abdominal pain, vomiting, and diarrhea ("squirts" or frequent elimination of a small volume of stool) containing blood, leukocytes, and mucus. Poor sanitation, overcrowding, and poor hygiene are important factors in the spread of the disease. Ingestion of contaminated food and water is the usual route of transmission and as few as 10 organisms may constitute an infective dose. *S. dysenteriae* is most common species in developing countries while *S. sonnei* most commonly occurs in the United States.

Shigella organisms are capable of elaborating cytotoxin. The shiga toxin produced by some strains of *Shigella* is the third most virulent toxin in the world after tetanus and botulism toxin. Pathogenesis is also attributed to the invasiveness of this bacterium. The organisms are able to penetrate the intestinal mucosa, invade epithelial cells, and multiply intracellularly. As the organism spreads laterally to adjacent cells, ulceration of the mucosa occurs. It rarely enters the bloodstream.

Shigella species can be recovered on media of low selectivity such as MacConkey and eosin–methylene blue agars, or moderately selective media such as XLD and HE agars. *Shigella* produces colorless colonies on MAC, Salmonella-Shigella (SS) (Figure 35-7 ■), and EMB agars as these organisms fail to ferment lactose. *Shigella* produces red or colorless colonies on

XLD (Figure 35-7) and blue-green colonies on HE. SS agar may not grow *S. dysenteriae* serotype 1 (Bopp et al., 1999). In addition to the use of biochemical tests to identify the organism, serological testing is required to determine the serogroup (A, B, C, or D) of the isolate. Shigellosis is reportable to the public health agencies. ∞ Chapter 21, "*Enterobacteriaceae*" provides more information on *Shigella*.

ESCHERICHIA COLI ASSOCIATED GASTROENTERITIS

E. coli is a gram-negative bacillus that is a normal constituent of the microbiota of the intestinal tract of both vertebrate and invertebrate animals. Most strains are harmless but there are several distinct serotypes that are associated with gastrointestinal distress. On MacConkey agar plates, a mildly selective, differential medium used to isolate enteric gram-negative rods, most strains of *E. coli* produce pink to red colonies because they are lactose fermenters. *E. coli* produce blue-black colonies with a green metallic sheen on EMB. Photos of *E. coli* growing on MAC and EMB can be found in ∞ Chapter 8, "Presumptive Identification," and ∞ Chapter 21, "*Enterobacteriaceae*."

Enterotoxigenic *E. coli* (ETEC) are the etiological agents of diarrhea in infants and "traveler's diarrhea" in developing countries. Gastrointestinal illness is characterized by diarrhea, vomiting, chills, headache, and fever following an incubation period of 1–2 days. Symptoms may last anywhere from 5 to 10 days. The route of transmission is through ingestion of food or water contaminated with the organism.

Strains of enterotoxigenic *E. coli* possess surface adhesions known as colonization factors and, in addition, are capable of producing enterotoxins, which function very similar to those of *Vibrio cholerae*. These enterotoxins induce secretion of chloride and water and produce a severe, watery disease that resembles cholera. Colonies of enterotoxigenic *E.coli* are indistinguishable from normal intestinal *E. coli* and therefore characterization of ETEC strains has relied on serological determination of lipopolysaccharide (O) and flagellar (H) serogroups. In addition, the ability to produce toxin must be established before the diagnosis is confirmed; with the use of DNA amplification techniques, molecular diagnostics may be valuable in the future.

Enteroinvasive *E. coli* (EIEC) invade the intestinal mucosa in a manner nearly identical to that of *Shigella* species and therefore produce symptoms that closely resemble those of shigellosis, including fever, tenesmus (an urgent desire to evacuate the bowels with only a small amount of feces being passed), abdominal cramps, and diarrhea with blood and pus. The incubation period is 12–24 hours. This organism is capable of invading and multiplying in the epithelial cells, which line the intestinal mucosa and resemble *Shigella* species not only biochemically and but also serologically.

Enteropathogenic *E. coli* (EPEC) are associated with outbreaks of hospital-acquired infantile diarrhea, which is characterized by diarrhea without blood or mucus. The greatest danger from this disease is the risk that it may lead to dehydration, shock, and death if supportive treatment is not initiated. The organism adheres to epithelial cells that comprise

---

> ### ⊘ REAL WORLD TIP
>
> To remember the serogroup of each of the *Shigella* species, use the mnemonic, dead flies on boy scouts. The first letter of each word tells you the species in order of serogroups. *S. dysenteriae* is group A (dead), *S. flexneri* is group B (flies), *S. boydii* is group C (boy), and *S. sonnei* is group D (scouts).

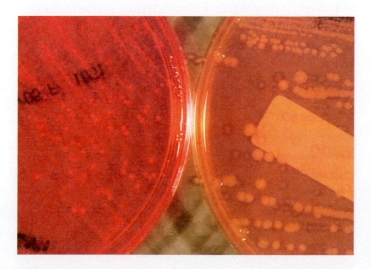

■ **FIGURE 35-7** Colonies of *Shigella* growing on XLD (left) and SS (right).

the microvilli. The aggregates of microorganisms lead to diarrhea due to the loss of the epithelial cells' ability to absorb.

Enterohemorrhagic *E. coli* (EHEC) produce an illness that is most often characterized by severe bloody diarrhea and painful abdominal cramps, known as hemorrhagic colitis, without generating a high fever. The damage to the mucosal epithelial cells is due to cytotoxins called "shiga-like toxins" (shiga toxin 1 and shiga toxin 2) that are structurally and biologically very much like shiga toxin from *Shigella dysenteriae* type 1. These organisms are also known as shiga-toxin-producing *E. coli* (STEC) or verotoxin *E. coli* (VTEC).

Cattle and other animals carry the organism in their intestine. This organism has a low infectious dose, and as few as 100 organisms may be capable of producing disease. In the United States these organisms were first associated with an outbreak of gastrointestinal illness following consumption of undercooked ground beef which had become contaminated with the organism. Hemorrhagic colitis is due to the effect of the toxins acting locally, damaging the intestinal mucosa and the blood vessels that supply it. When the toxins are absorbed, they enter the bloodstream and are carried to different sites such as the kidneys and the brain. The disease becomes systemic and complications such as thrombocytopenia, hemolytic anemia, and renal failure may occur. The temporary anemia, profuse bleeding, and kidney failure characterize a disease referred to as **hemolytic uremic syndrome** (HUS), a disease that strikes 3–5% of individuals infected with the etiological agent. HUS can occur several weeks after initial symptoms.

E. coli O157:H7 was once the serotype most commonly associated with hemorrhagic colitis and HUS. It is now known that other serotypes, referred to as non-O157 STEC, can also be associated with outbreaks of hemorrhagic colitis and HUS in many parts of the world.

SMAC (sorbitol MacConkey agar plates) is one of the most widely used methods. SMAC is designed to isolate and differentiate *E. coli* O157:H7 from stool samples. This medium contains sorbitol, in place of lactose, as the sole carbohydrate source. The majority of strains of *E. coli* ferment sorbitol and produce pink colonies, while *E. coli* O157:H7 does not ferment sorbitol and remains clear (Figure 35-8 ■) on this medium. Many facilities have eliminated the use of SMAC because serotypes other than O157:H7 are able to cause HUS. Polymerase chain reaction (PCR), cytotoxicity assays, or commercially available enzyme immunoassays should be performed to detect the presence of shiga toxins in stool samples. Isolation of shiga-toxin-producing *E. coli* should be reported to the public health agencies.

Enteroaggregative *E. coli* (EAEC) may cause chronic diarrhea in HIV-infected patients, travelers, and children in underdeveloped countries. The organisms arrange themselves like stacks of bricks on the cell surface. Aggregative adhesion appears to affect the microvilli of the small intestine, causing a decrease in fluid absorption and resulting diarrhea (Murray et al., 2002; Nataro & Kaper, 1998). Most clinical laboratories cannot detect these strains of *E. coli*.

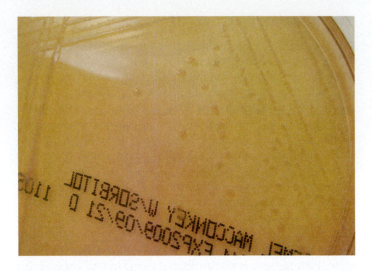

■ **FIGURE 35-8** Colorless colonies of *E. coli* O157:H7 growing on MacConkey with sorbitol.

CHOLERA

Vibrio cholerae is a curved, gram-negative rod that can be isolated from fresh or marine water and is the etiological agent of cholera. Most cases are asymptomatic or mild but there is a severe form that is characterized by a massive loss of fluid and electrolytes due to the production of large quantities of liquid feces. These stools are colorless, odorless, free of protein, and speckled with flecks of mucus. Because of the appearance of the watery stools, they are often referred to as **"rice water stools."** As much as 5 gallons of fluid a day may be lost in the severe form and this may lead to shock, acidosis, cardiovascular collapse, and death within a few hours.

The source of *V. cholerae* infection is food, usually seafood, or contaminated drinking water. The organism requires a large inoculum dose to initiate disease. Two to three days after ingestion patients may experience the abrupt onset of vomiting and severe, watery diarrhea. Pathogenicity is due to the production of a cholera toxin that binds to intestinal cells, inducing them to excrete water. Serogroups O1 and O139 are associated with epidemics. Persons with type O blood are more likely to develop severe cholera than those with other blood types (Bopp, Ries, & Wells, 1999).

 ⓔ **REAL WORLD TIP**

Vibrio parahaemolyticus is another oxidase positive, halophilic gram-negative rod that can cause diarrhea. It produces both cytotoxin and enterotoxin. This non-lactose fermenter (NLF) does not ferment sucrose so it produces a blue-green colony on TCBS. It will grow in 6.0% salt broth while *V. cholerae* will not.

This organism is not fastidious and grows well on routine culture media. Thiosulfate–citrate–bile salts–sucrose (TCBS) media is used to isolate the organism from stool because it is selective for *Vibrio* spp. and differentiates sucrose fermenters (such as *V. cholerae*), which form yellow colonies, from non-sucrose fermenters (such as *V. parahaemolyticus*), which form green colonies. Suspect colonies can be tested with O1 and O139 antisera. ∞ Chapter 23 provides additional information on *Vibrio* species.

CLOSTRIDIUM DIFFICILE

Clostridium difficile is an extremely important nosocomial pathogen. This anaerobic spore-forming gram-positive rod is the causative agent of antibiotic-associated diarrhea and pseudomembranous colitis. Individuals, within 1 to 2 weeks after starting antibiotic therapy, have disrupted colon flora and become colonized with spores in the hospital environment, usually from a previous patient. The organism produces two powerful toxins which cause the disease. Toxin A causes the lost of fluids and electrolytes from the intestinal cells while toxin B damages the cells and causes the formation of a membrane on the intestinal wall.

Watery diarrhea, fever, abdominal cramps, and the presence of white blood cells during or after antibiotic therapy is characteristic. Diagnosis is made by detection of the toxins by PCR, enzyme immunoassay (EIA), or tissue culture cytotoxicity, in stool. Because individuals can carry this organism as normal flora, culture of stool is not recommended. ∞ Chapter 24, "Anaerobic Bacteria," provides more information on *C. difficile*.

ROTAVIRUS

Rotavirus infection is very common in infants between 6 and 24 months and follows a characteristic seasonal pattern with the highest incidence occurring during the winter months. Nearly 50% of all pediatric gastroenteritis cases occurring during this time are caused by the rotaviruses.

Rotavirus infection is spread primarily by the fecal–oral route, with cold temperatures inducing individuals to remain inside where crowding may be a major factor facilitating the spread of the organism from person to person. It takes very few viral particles to initiate disease. The population at greatest risk is premature infants of low birth weight and malnourished infants. This organism can be a particular problem in hospital nurseries if strict infection control measures are not undertaken.

Infection is associated with an incubation period of 1–2 days followed by the sudden onset of symptoms, which include vomiting, diarrhea, fever, and occasionally abdominal pain. The virus infects and destroys intestinal cells. Vomiting and diarrhea can result in a substantial loss of water and electrolytes that may lead to dehydration and electrolyte imbalance, which can be fatal if supportive treatment is not initiated.

Commercially available enzyme immunoassays are used to diagnose rotavirus infection because they are simple to perform, easy to read, and are very useful in processing a large number of specimens. Latex agglutination (LA) tests are also easy to perform, require very little equipment, and provide results in a short time. Several PCR techniques have been developed to detect and type rotaviruses, but their use is restricted to research rather than being widely available for use in the clinical laboratory. ∞ Chapter 31, "Intracellular Organisms," provides additional information on rotavirus.

 REAL WORLD TIP

Adenovirus also causes diarrhea and vomiting in young children and immunocompromised individuals.

NOROVIRUS

Caliciviruses were the first viruses to be associated with gastroenteritis. Included in this group are the noroviruses, which cause an acute, infectious, nonbacterial gastroenteritis, and an extremely common cause of foodborne illness, second only to the common cold as a frequent cause of viral disease. The "Norwalk agent" was responsible for an outbreak of "winter vomiting disease," which occurred in Norwalk, Ohio, in 1968 and hence the name of this important group of viruses. Since that time a number of morphologically similar viruses have been discovered and are referred to as noroviruses.

These gastrointestinal pathogens cause an acute illness characterized by an incubation period of 16–48 hours followed by symptoms such as nausea, vomiting, diarrhea, abdominal cramps, headache, and low-grade fever, usually with more vomiting than diarrhea. The illness tends to be resolved in a few days. Unlike many foodborne pathogens that have animal reservoirs, Noroviruses spread primarily from person to person and often associated with cruise ships, restaurants, and the family setting. In some cases illness has been traced to contaminated food and water.

 REAL WORLD TIP

Adenoviruses and noroviruses are probably most often responsible for the "stomach flu."

 Checkpoint! 35–5 (Chapter Objective 6)

Sorbitol MacConkey (SMAC) agar plates are used in the isolation of
  A. *enterotoxigenic E. coli (ETEC).*
  B. *enteroinvasive E. coli (EIEC).*
  C. *enteropathogenic E. coli (EPEC).*
  D. *Shiga-toxin-producing E. coli (STEC).*

Diagnosis may be established by direct examination of the virus in stool specimens using electron microscopy since the viruses can be recognized by their distinct morphology, but this is not practical for most clinical laboratories. Attempts to cultivate the noroviruses have not been successful. The application of polymerase chain reaction technology has successfully been applied to the detection of most gastroenteritis viruses including the noroviruses but is usually only performed by state public health laboratories. For a review of intracellular organisms, refer to ∞ Chapter 31.

 Checkpoint! 35–6 (Chapter Objective 4)

The production of large quantities of liquid stools, which are colorless, odorless, free of protein, and speckled with flecks of mucus, and which have been referred to as "rice water stools" are characteristic of _____ infection.

 A. *Vibrio cholerae.*
 B. *Vibrio parahaemolyticus.*
 C. *Shiga-toxin producing E. coli.*
 D. *Shigella boydii.*

► LESS COMMON ETIOLOGICAL AGENTS OF GASTROINTESTINAL ILLNESSES

YERSINIA ENTEROCOLITICA

Yersinia enterocolitica, known to cause enterocolitis in infants and young children, is a diarrheal illness that may last as long as 2 weeks. The organism is not only invasive, but also produces a heat-stable toxin similar to the shiga toxin of *E. coli.* In adults this organism may cause an acute mesenteric lymphadenopathy, which involves the ileum, appendix, and right colon. The disease mimics the symptoms of appendicitis. This infection is transmitted through the consumption of contaminated food including dairy products.

Cefsulodin–irgasan–novobiocin (CIN) medium is a selective and differential medium for the isolation of *Yersinia enterocolitica* from clinical specimens. While most other bacteria are inhibited by the addition of antibiotics (cefsulodin, irgasan, and novobiocin) and other inhibitory substances such as bile salts and crystal violet, *Y. enterocolitica* produces colonies with red centers and thin colorless edges often referred to as a "bull's-eye" appearance (Figure 35-9 ■). Because this organism grows at low temperatures, cold enrichment at 4°C can facilitate isolation of this organism when they occur in small numbers. Growth at 4°C means the organism will continue to grow in refrigerated foods.

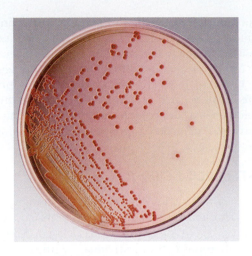

■ **FIGURE 35-9** Colonies of *Yersinia enterocolitica* growing on CIN agar.
Photo courtesy of Remel, part of Thermo Fisher Scientific.

PLESIOMONAS SHIGELLOIDES

Plesiomonas shigelloides causes diarrheal illness in humans and is seen primarily in tropical and subtropical countries but is occasionally seen in the United States and Europe. Infection is associated with both cold- and warm-blooded animals, which serve as reservoirs. While its exact mechanism of pathogencity is still unknown, it does produce enterotoxin but may also be invasive. This organism grows well on selective media such as MacConkey and SS agars and usually does not ferment lactose or sucrose. It does not grow on TCBS. While *P. shigelloides* may resemble nonlactose-fermenting members of the family *Enterobacteriaceae,* it is oxidase positive. Unlike *Vibrio* and *Aeromonas,* two additional enteric oxidase-positive gram-negative rods, this organism is DNase and gelatinase negative.

 REAL WORLD TIP

Plesiomonas shigelloides was once a member of the family *Vibrionaceae.* Based on studies of its genome, it has been placed in the family *Enterobacteriaceae,* even though it is oxidase positive.

AEROMONAS HYDROPHILA

Aeromonas hydrophila is found in fresh water and is associated with cold-blooded animals such as reptiles, amphibians, and fish, which not only serve as reservoirs but may also be infected. Humans acquire the disease from water sources and may also suffer wound, urinary, and respiratory infections

 REAL WORLD TIP

Yersinia enterocolitica is carried by pigs. There are reported outbreaks of disease due to *Y. enterocolitica* during the winter holidays. The handling and consumption of chitterlings (pig intestines) can be a source of infection.

caused by this organism, in addition to diarrheal disease. It has been implicated as a cause of traveler's diarrhea. It may cause disease due to enterotoxin and cytotoxin.

On blood agar and media selective for gram-negative rods, this organism resembles other enteric gram-negative rods, especially *E. coli*. It can ferment lactose and be beta hemolytic similar to some strains of *E. coli* on initial isolation. Fortunately this organism is oxidase positive whereas the *Enterobacteriaceae* are not. While most strains do not ferment lactose they usually are sucrose fermenters. CIN agar can be used to isolate *Aeromonas* as well as *Yersinia*. The colony is similar to that of *Yersinia*, with a "bull's-eye" appearance (colorless edge with a red center). *Yersinia* is oxidase negative whereas *Aeromonas* is oxidase positive. Other helpful biochemical characteristics include its ability to hydrolyze gelatin and the production of a DNase. Unlike *Vibrio*, another enteric oxidase-positive gram-negative rod, this organism is arginine positive but will not grow on TCBS.

LISTERIA MONOCYTOGENES

Listeria monocytogenes is a non-spore-forming, gram-positive bacillus that may occur singly or in short chains. This organism has been isolated from the gastrointestinal tract of healthy animals but is capable of causing systemic fatal diseases, such as meningoencephalitis and abortion, in ruminants and humans. Some cases occurring in humans are asymptomatic, acting as carriers, with the organism being found in the gastrointestinal or urogenital tract of 2–20% of the population. Pregnant females can pass the organism to the fetus to cause meningitis, septicemia, and death.

Humans are most likely to come in contact with *L. monocytogenes* through ingestion of contaminated food or contact with infected animals. Infection with *L. monocytogenes* has been associated with gastroenteritis with watery diarrhea, and vomiting accompanied by fever. The organism can penetrate the intestinal wall to cause systemic infection in immunocompromised individuals. Implicated food includes raw and pasteurized milk as well as soft cheese and raw vegetables.

Most hospital clinical laboratories do not routinely look for *Listeria* in stool samples. It is advisable to use a selective medium such as phenylethyl alcohol (PEA) agar or colistin-nalidixic acid (CNA) agar supplemented with sheep blood to insure its isolation. ∞ Chapter 19, "Aerobic Gram-Positive Rods," provides additional information on *L. monocytogenes*. Table 35-1 ✪ summarizes bacteria-associated diarrheal illnesses.

✓ Checkpoint! 35–7 (Chapter Objective 3)

Which of the following organisms causes an acute mesenteric lymphadenitis in adults that closely mimics the symptoms of appendicitis?

A. *Salmonella typhimurium*
B. *Plesiomonas shigelloides*
C. *Yersinia enterocolitica*
D. *Listeria monocytogenes*

✓ Checkpoint! 35–8 (Chapter Objective 8)

Which microorganism is associated with diarrhea after antibiotic use?

A. *Clostridium difficile*
B. *Listeria monocytogenes*
C. *Clostridium botulinum*
D. *Staphylococcus aureus*

AMOEBIC DYSENTERY

The etiological agent of amoebic dysentery is *Entamoeba histolytica*, a protozoan (single-celled) parasite that is associated with poor hygiene and poor sanitation. While the organism is found worldwide, clinical disease is most often encountered in tropical and subtropical countries where the standard of living is low. This intestinal parasite is transmitted by the fecal–oral route and often involves ingestion of contaminated food or water.

This organism produces disease by invading the lining of the intestinal tract, the intestinal mucosa and submucosa, which leads to the formation of ulcerative lesions along the colon and the presence of blood and mucus in the stool. Symptoms include abdominal pain, nausea, vomiting, anorexia, and occasionally a low-grade fever.

Diagnosis of amoebic dysentery can be accomplished by microscopic examination of a fresh stool specimen where actively motile trophozoites exhibiting rapid, progressive motility can be observed. Stained preparations can provide a more detailed picture where the presence of a characteristic, single nucleus may be observed. Ingested red blood cells contained within the cytoplasm serve to distinguish this pathogenic parasite from harmless commensal protozoans. Trophozoites can range in size from 20 to 30 microns. In cases of chronic infection, cysts, 10–20 microns in size, may be seen. ∞ Chapter 30, "Parasitology," provides further information on parasites and their identification.

GIARDIASIS

The etiological agent of giardiasis is *Giardia lamblia*, a flagellated protozoan parasite. This microbe, which is found worldwide, is carried by animals that thrive in a watery habitat, such as beavers, muskrats, and water voles. Transmission of the organism is associated with the same factors as those facilitating the spread of *E. histolytica*. Outbreaks of giardiasis have occurred in the United States, Russia, and other countries when water supplies have been contaminated with sewage.

The organism attaches to the microvilli and causes death of the intestinal cells. Eventually the organism coats the intestinal mucosal surface leading to malabsorption. Giardiasis has an incubation period of 1–3 weeks, after which the patient exhibits symptoms such as frequent, watery, foul-smelling

✪ TABLE 35-1

Bacterial Diarrheal Illnesses

Organism	Disease	Special Media	Appearance
Campylobacter jejuni	Gastroenteritis or enterocolitis	Campy agar or broth ■ microaerophilic and capnophilic atmosphere at 42° C	Round and convex or flat, spreading colonies, nonhemolytic, tan or pink color
Nontyphoid *Salmonella* species	Salmonellosis	MacConkey (MAC) agar Salmonella-Shigella (SS) agar Xylose–lysine–deoxycholate (XLD) agar Hektoen-enteric (HE) agar	Colorless colony Colorless colonies with black centers Red (clear) colonies with black centers Blue-green (clear) colonies with black centers
Salmonella typhi	Typhoid fever	MAC agar SS agar XLD agar HE agar	Colorless colony Colorless colonies with black centers Red (clear) colonies with black centers Blue-green (clear) colonies with black centers
Enterotoxigenic *Escherichia coli* (ETEC)	Traveler's diarrhea	MAC agar Sorbitol MacConkey (SMAC) agar EMB agar XLD agar HE agar	Pink to red colonies Pink colonies Green metallic sheen Orange to yellow colonies Orange to yellow colonies
Enteroinvasive *Escherichia coli* (EIEC)	Gastroenteritis or enterocolitis	MAC agar SMAC agar EMB agar XLD agar HE agar	Pink to red colonies Pink colonies Green metallic sheen Orange to yellow colonies Orange to yellow colonies
Enteropathogenic *Escherichia coli* (EPEC)	Hospital-acquired infantile diarrhea	MAC agar SMAC agar EMB agar XLD agar HE agar	Pink to red colonies Pink colonies Green metallic sheen Orange to yellow colonies Orange to yellow colonies
Shiga-toxin producing *Escherichia coli* (STEC)	Hemolytic–uremic syndrome (HUS) and Hemorrhagic colitis	Sorbitol-MacConkey (SMAC) agar (used for serotype O157:H7 only) MAC agar EMB agar XLD agar HE agar	Colorless colonies Pink to red colonies Green metallic sheen Orange to yellow colonies Orange to yellow colonies
Vibrio cholerae	Cholera (rice water stools)	Thiosulfate–citrate–bile salts–sucrose (TCBS) agar MAC agar XLD HE	Yellow colonies Colorless colonies Orange to yellow colonies Orange to yellow colonies
Vibrio parahaemolyticus	Gastroenteritis or enterocolitis	TCBS agar MAC XLD HE	Green (clear) colonies Colorless colonies Red colonies Green colonies

✪ TABLE 35-1

Bacterial Diarrheal Illnesses (continued)

Organism	Disease	Special Media	Appearance
Shigella species	Shigellosis, bacillary dysentery	MAC	Colorless colonies
		SS agar	Colorless colonies
		XLD agar	Red colonies
		HE agar	Green colonies
Yersinia enterocolitica	Gastroenteritis or enterocolitis	Cefsulodin–irgasan–novobiocin (CIN) agar	Colorless colonies with red centers
		MAC	Colorless colonies
		XLD	Yellow to orange colonies
		HE	Yellow to orange colonies
Aeromonas hydrophila	Gastroenteritis or enterocolitis	MAC	Colorless colonies much more common than pink colonies
		HE	Yellow colonies
		XLD	Yellow colonies
		TCBS	No growth
Plesiomonas shigelloides	Gastroenteritis or enterocolitis	MAC	Colorless or pink colonies
		XLD	Colorless or yellow to orange colonies
		HE	Colorless or yellow to orange colonies
		TCBS	No growth
Listeria monocytogenes	Listeriosis	Sheep blood agar	Translucent, gray-white, convex, subtle beta hemolytic colonies
		Phenylethyl alcohol (PEA) agar and Columbia–colistin–nalidixic acid (CNA) agar	Translucent, gray-white, convex colonies

stools that are pale yellow and fatty. The individual may also experience flatulence, abdominal pain, nausea, anorexia, and less often, fever and vomiting. Blood or mucus is rarely found in the stool. Symptoms may persist for 5–7 days and, in some patients, acute illness may extend over a period of 1–2 months.

Diagnosis is established by demonstrating the presence of actively motile microorganisms that move with a back and forth type of motility referred to as "falling-leaf" motility in freshly passed stool specimens. Stained smears should reveal the presence of pear-shaped trophozoites with two nuclei, a prominent sucking disc, intracytoplasmic flagella, and two median bodies. The cyst contains double the number of cytoplasmic inclusions enclosed within a cyst wall. Giardiasis is a nationally reportable infectious disease.

CRYPTOSPORIDIOSIS

Cryptosporidiosis, another diarrheal illness, is caused by a coccidian protozoan. This parasite may be transmitted from human to human and possibly from animal to human. Individuals who work with animals, particularly farmers and veterinarians, are at increased risk to acquire infection. Ingestion of contaminated food and water is a common route of transmission. As few as ten organisms are needed to initiate infection.

Cryptosporidiosis is caused by *Cryptosporidium parvum,* an organism that is very resistant to disinfectants including chlorination of waste water. The organism adheres to the epithelial cells and becomes engulfed. This causes chloride and water secretion. The illness has an incubation period of 2–14 days after which the patient suffers a profuse, watery diarrheal illness characterized by stools that lack blood and mucus. Patients may also experience a low-grade fever and abdominal cramps. Only supportive therapy is currently available but in most cases symptoms are resolved within 2 weeks. In immunocompromised hosts, such as AIDS patients, the illness may be prolonged, severe, and deadly.

Diagnosis is made by a modified acid-fast stain (Kinyoun's stain) is used to increase visibility of öocysts in the stool. The organism stains a bright red color, whereas other organisms and the background are blue in color.

CYCLOSPORA CAYETANENSIS

Cyclospora cayetanensis is another coccidian parasite that causes a self-limiting, prolonged, watery diarrheal illness that may last 3 or more weeks. A wide range of vertebrate animals are known to carry the organism, including reptiles, rodents, and insectivores. The route of transmission is through ingestion

✪ TABLE 35-2

Parasitic Diseases Commonly Associated with the Diarrheal Illness

Parasite	Disease	Microscopic Examination
Entamoeba histolytica	Amoebic dysentery	■ Trophozoites, with one nucleus and ingested red blood cells, ranging in size from 20 to 30 microns ■ Spherical cysts, with up to 4 nuclei, ranging in size from 10 to 20 microns
Giardia lamblia	Beaver fever or giardiasis	■ Pear-shaped trophozoites, measuring 9–21 microns, with 2 nuclei, a prominent sucking disc, intracytoplasmic flagella, and two median bodies ■ Ellipsoidal cysts with four nuclei, intracytoplasmic flagella, and four median bodies and measuring 8–12 microns
Cryptosporidium parvum	Cryptosporidiosis	Spherical oöcysts, 4–6 microns in diameter, that stain bright red with the modified Ziehl-Nielsen acid-fast stain
Cyclospora cayetanensis	*C. cayentanensis* infection	The presence of spherical oöcysts, 8–10 microns in diameter, that stain bright red with the modified acid-fast stain

of contaminated food and water and the life cycle involves the production of merozoites in cells that line the intestinal mucosa and the passage of infective oöcysts in the feces. Symptoms include abdominal cramping, nausea, vomiting, anorexia, weight loss, and low-grade fever.

Examination of a suspension of saline and fresh fecal material may reveal the presence of spherical oöcysts that are 8–10 microns in diameter. The modified acid-fast stain may be useful in visualizing the organism in a dried smear made from stool previously placed in a fixative such as formalin. A more detailed discussion of parasites can be found in ∞ Chapter 30. Table 35-2✪ summarizes microscopic detection of the most common parasites associated with diarrhea.

▶ TOXIGENIC GASTROINTESTINAL ILLNESSES

Some foodborne diseases are caused by the presence of toxic substances produced by microbes that have contaminated food. Some organisms produce exotoxins as they grow in food and are able to produce intestinal illness even if the microbes are no longer present.

In this case, the exotoxin is also an enterotoxin because, once secreted, it acts on the intestinal tract. Others can produce neurotoxins that cause intestinal symptoms because they act on the autonomic nervous system that directly controls the gastrointestinal system. Some neurotoxins also induce vomiting because they trigger the vomiting center located in the medulla of the brain.

BACTERIAL AGENTS ASSOCIATED WITH FOOD POISONING

Staphylococcus aureus

Staphylococcus aureus is usually associated with skin and wound infections but this organism is also associated with gastrointestinal illness because it produces an enterotoxin, which causes

intense vomiting. In a relatively short period of time, as little as 2 hours, the organism growing in contaminated, unrefrigerated food can produce enough toxins to produce symptoms.

Many foodstuffs have been implicated, including those containing mayonnaise, eggs, or dairy products (such as salad dressings, whipped cream, and pastries), canned foods, frozen foods, warmed-over foods, and processed meats, any of which can become contaminated with the bacterium. Ham is a common source because staphylococci are salt tolerant whereas most other organisms are not.

In 1–6 hours after consumption of contaminated food, symptoms such as nausea, vomiting, abdominal cramps, and watery diarrhea may begin. Asymptomatic carriers whose nasal passages (anterior nares) are colonized with the organism are often the source of food contamination. When these individuals contaminate their hands with nasal secretions and then handle food without washing their hands, they contaminate foodstuffs. The contaminated food provides the nutrients that allow the organism to grow and produce the enterotoxin. Often multiple people are affected due to eating the same food. The illness is self-limiting, usually resolving in one day, so most individuals do not seek treatment. Molecular methods are available for detection of the enterotoxin, but most clinical laboratories do not offer the testing. State public health laboratories are able to test for the presence of the toxin.

S. aureus is also a rare cause of antibiotic-associated diarrhea. Antibiotics can wipe out the normal enteric flora leaving methicillin resistant *S. aureus* (MRSA). The organism produces enterotoxin in the intestine, causing diarrhea. The organism should be considered significant when isolated as the predominant isolate in diarrheal stool of hospitalized patients. Visit ∞ Chapter 17, "Aerobic Gram-Positive Cocci," to review the identification of *S. aureus*.

Clostridium botulinum

Clostridium botulinum, an anaerobic, spore-forming gram-positive bacillus, is a normal inhabitant of soil and water. This organism may contaminate food and, under the right conditions, can grow and produce a powerful paralytic toxin. The botulism toxin is the most powerful neurotoxin known, more than a thousand times more powerful than rattlesnake venom. One pint of this toxin could kill the entire population of the world and as little as one ounce could kill the entire population of the United States. Home prepared foods implicated include sausage, mushrooms, olives, salami, and improperly canned foods (green beans, peppers, corn, beets, potatoes, onions, tomatoes, and garlic). Neurological symptoms occur 18–36 hours after consumption.

The botulism toxin causes paralysis by blocking the release of the neurotransmitter acetylcholine. Acetylcholine carries the nerve impulse across the neuromuscular synapse, causing the muscle to contract. Because the toxin blocks the release of the neurotransmitter, there is no muscle contraction and the end result is muscle weakness or paralysis. The descending paralysis first affects the ocular muscles, causing visual disturbances. Next, the pharyngeal muscles may be affected, leading to dysphagia (difficulty in swallowing) and hoarseness.

Paralysis of the respiratory muscles usually results in death unless antitoxin, a substance that counteracts the botulinum toxin, is administered. Fever is usually absent. Botulism should be suspected when diarrhea, vomiting, and nausea are accompanied by neurological problems. Only public health laboratories are equipped to test stool, gastric fluid, vomitus, and the implicated food for the presence of the botulism toxin.

Another type of botulism poisoning is possible in infants less than 1 year of age and is referred to as infant botulism. It is associated with ingestion of food containing the spores of *C. botulinum* and not food contaminated with botulism toxin. The source of the spores is usually food given to the infant or the immediate environment, which may be contaminated with spores.

In infants, the gastrointestinal microbiota has not been firmly established and there is not a sufficient number of commensal organisms to compete with pathogenic organisms and prevent their colonization of the gut. Once ingested, the spores germinate in the intestinal tract and, with little or no competition from the normal microbiota of the gastrointestinal tract,

the vegetative bacteria proliferate and produce the botulinum toxin. The toxin is absorbed in the GI tract and is carried throughout the body, leading to the symptoms of botulism poisoning. The foodstuff most commonly implicated is unpasteurized honey and for this reason honey should not be fed to children less than 2 years of age. Botulism is reportable to the Centers for Disease Control and Prevention (CDC). For a review of anaerobic bacteria, refer to ∞ Chapter 24.

Bacillus cereus

Bacillus cereus is an aerobic, spore-forming, gram-positive bacillus. The spores produced by this organism may contaminate food, germinate, and then the vegetative cells can produce an enterotoxin that is ingested along with the food. Two types of food poisoning have been documented: a diarrheal syndrome that is characterized by abdominal pain and diarrhea and an emetic syndrome which is characterized by profuse vomiting. In both cases the foods that have been implicated are those made with grains, especially fried rice that is allowed to cool, sit for a long period of time, and is then served. Table 35-3✪ summarizes toxigenic diarrheal illnesses.

**Checkpoint! 35–9
(Chapter Objective 8)**

What foods are most often implicated in food poisonings caused by Bacillus cereus?

    A. *Home canned green beans*
    B. *Grains such as rice*
    C. *Milk and milk products*
    D. *Poultry*

▶ SPECIMEN COLLECTION

Ideally a stool specimen should be collected within 4 days of the onset of diarrhea and before treatment. The specimen should be collected into a clean but not necessarily sterile, dry container,

✪ TABLE 35-3

Toxigenic Diarrheal Illnesses				
Etiological Agent	**Source of Contamination**	**Toxin**	**Foods Implicated**	**Pathology**
Staphylococcus aureus	Nasal passages of asymptomatic carriers	Staphylococcal enterotoxin	Foods containing mayonnaise, eggs, or dairy products, canned food, frozen foods, processed meats	Enterotoxin causes intense vomiting and is also a rare cause of antibiotic-associated diarrhea
Clostridium botulinum	Soil and water	Botulism neurotoxin	Home prepared sausage, mushrooms, olives, salami, improperly canned foods	Blocks release of the neurotransmitter acetyl choline, causing paralysis
Bacillus cereus	Environmental contaminant	Heat-labile enterotoxin	Grains, especially rice	Diarrheal syndrome (abdominal pain and diarrhea)
		Heat-stable enterotoxin		Emetic syndrome (profuse vomiting)

with a tight, leakproof lid. Bed pans should not be used for collection because they may contain disinfectants, urine, or other contaminants. If *Shigella* is suspected and the specimen cannot be processed within 30 minutes, it should be placed in transport medium. *Shigella* is very sensitive to changes in pH and begins to die rapidly once it leaves the body. A minimum of 1 teaspoon or a pea-sized specimen is necessary. A rectal swab should only be used as a last resort such as in the case of a child who may not be able to evacuate the bowels on demand.

The stool specimen can be refrigerated for up to 2 hours prior to processing. If the sample cannot be processed within 2 hours, it should be placed in transport medium and refrigerated at 4°C. Organisms are shed intermittently, but no more than two stools total, each collected on different days, should be submitted. Feces submitted for culture on patients hospitalized for more than 3 days should be rejected (Isenberg, 2004). Hospitalized patients usually have diarrhea due to antibiotic use and not the expected routine enteric pathogens. The antibiotics wipe out the normal stool flora and select for the growth of *Staphylococcus aureus* and *Clostridium difficile*. Detection of *C. difficile* requires diarrheal stool to test for the presence of toxins. Culture should not be performed. Refer to ∞ Chapter 6 for more information on specimen collection.

 REAL WORLD TIP

Diarrheal stool assumes the shape of the container.

 ### Checkpoint! 35–10 (Chapter Objective 8)

_____ *is an organism usually associated with skin and wound infections and is also associated with a gastrointestinal illness caused by the production of an enterotoxin. If the toxin is ingested in contaminated food, it produces intense vomiting in 1–6 hours following consumption.*

   A. *Clostridium botulinum*
   B. *Yersinia enterocolitica*
   C. *Staphylococcus aureus*
   D. *Listeria monocytogenes*

▶ MICROSCOPIC EXAMINATION OF SPECIMEN

Direct microscopic examination of the specimen can detect parasites, the darting motility of *Campylobacter,* white blood cells due to invasive organisms, or red blood cells that are the result of the action of a cytotoxin or invasion.

A wet preparation using one drop of saline or one drop of methylene blue can be used to examine the specimen for fecal leukocytes. White blood cells are commonly observed in infections associated with *Campylobacter* spp., *Shigella,* and *Salmonella.* They may also be seen with *Clostridium difficile, Yersinia enterocolitica, Vibrio parahaemolyticus, Aeromonas hydrophila,* EIEC, and EHEC. Observation of fecal leukocytes should not be performed

on inpatients, but may be diagnostic for outpatients (Savola, Baron, Tompkins, & Passaro, 2001). Red blood cells can be observed with *Campylobacter, C. difficile,* EHEC, EIEC, and *Salmonella* (Isenberg, 2004). White blood cells can be recognized on Gram stain, but it is not often performed. *Campylobacter* spp. is the one enteric pathogen (gram-negative spiral rods) that is microscopically characteristic enough to be recognized on Gram stain.

▶ SETUP AND INCUBATION OF CULTURES

Stool specimens should be inoculated as soon as possible after receipt in the laboratory. A drop of liquid feces can be placed on the surface of the first quadrant of the medium. A swab with fecal material can also be used to inoculate an area approximately 1 inch in diameter in the first quadrant of the medium. The media is struck for isolation, with many overlapping streaks, using the entire surface of the plate to ensure well-isolated colonies.

Each microbiology laboratory determines which diarrheal pathogen to look for and the appropriate media for their recovery. Most clinical laboratories routinely look for *Salmonella, Shigella,* and *Campylobacter* spp. A selective and differential medium such as MAC or EMB will distinguish the non-lactose fermenting colonies of *Salmonella* and *Shigella* spp. *Vibrio, Aeromonas,* and *Plesiomonas* spp. are also non-lactose fermenters (NLF). HE or XLD is considered moderately selective as well as differential for *Salmonella* and *Shigella* spp. Campy blood agar promotes the growth of *Campylobacter* spp.

A blood agar may be included to perform oxidase testing for detection of *Vibrio, Aeromonas,* or *Plesiomonas.* PEA or CNA may be added to examine for a predominance of *Staphylococcus aureus.* SMAC can be added to detect the shiga-toxin-producing *E. coli* serotype O157:H7. It should routinely be added to any grossly bloody stool specimen. It is now considered best practice to perform testing for the presence of shiga toxin since serotypes other than O157:H7 can cause HUS. CIN is added to isolate *Yersinia,* as well as *Aeromonas.* Laboratories in coastal states may routinely add TCBS agar to ensure recovery and differentiation of *Vibrio cholerae* and *V. parahaemolyticus.*

Enrichment broth such as gram-negative (GN) broth can be inoculated with a small amount of feces in order to increase the yield of *Salmonella* or *Shigella.* Subculture of the broth must be performed after 6–8 hours of incubation to prevent overgrowth of enteric pathogens by commensal flora. Most facilities no longer routinely use enrichment broth. Studies have shown it does not significantly increase the recovery of *Salmonella* and *Shigella* spp. GN broth can also be used to detect the shiga toxin of EHEC.

Patients hospitalized for more than 3 days do not have diarrhea due to the traditional enteric pathogens. They are often on multiple drugs and antibiotics that eliminate the normal enteric flora and allow resistant organisms such as *Clostridium difficile, Staphylococcus aureus, Pseudomonas areuginosa,* and yeast to overgrow. Routine enteric media is not used for culture. Often only sheep blood agar and PEA or CNA are necessary.

All media, except for CIN agar and Campy agar, is incubated in ambient air at 35–37°C for 48 hours. CIN agar is incubated in ambient air at room temperature (25°C), for 48 hours, to isolate *Yersinia*. Campy agar is incubated in a microaerophilic, capnophilic atmosphere at 42°C for 3 days.

Physicians must be informed of the organisms that are routinely cultured for in a stool culture. A thorough patient history including foods ingested, exposure to marine or fresh water, travel history, and exposure to animals can help the physician narrow down the possible agents of diarrhea. Communication of such information between the physician and the laboratory ensures the appropriate media and testing are used to detect the organisms suspected.

▶ INTERPRETATION OF CULTURES

Just as you look at a flower bed and distinguish the flowers from the weeds, you must be able to examine the growth on the stool culture media and differentiate the potential pathogens from the commensal flora. To be successful, it is critical to know what each bacterial pathogen colony looks like on each medium inoculated. It is far too expensive and time consuming to workup every isolate. Only the potential pathogens should be screened or tested biochemically.

EXAMINATION OF GROWTH

As with any culture, no one agar plate is the best for recovery of a potential pathogen. All of the media used for a stool culture work together to ensure the recovery of potential pathogens. Each agar must be examined. The microbiologist must learn to correlate an organism's colony on different agars to prevent duplicate and unnecessary testing.

Sheep Blood Agar

A predominance of colonies resembling *Staphylococcus aureus*, in a hospitalized patient, may be due to antibiotic use and may cause antibiotic associated enterocolitis. Predominance is defined as a colony which makes up 50% or more of the all of the colonies present.

The blood agar plate can also be used to screen for the presence of *Vibrio*, *Aeromonas*, and *Plesiomonas* spp. even if a special request was not made. A swipe of the large, wet gray colonies in the first quadrant of growth can be tested for oxidase. If positive then a search can be made for the individual oxidase positive colony. Most oxidase positive colonies end up being *Pseudomonas aeruginosa*. *P. aeruginosa* can be significant if it is the predominant organism. With the suppression of the normal enteric flora due to antibiotics, it can go systemic in an immunocompromised patient.

MacConkey Agar

Most enteric pathogens are non-lactose fermenters on MAC. When examining this agar plate, it can usually be assumed that any lactose fermenter present is part of the normal enteric flora. If a NLF is present, it should be screened with oxidase.

Those that are positive include *Vibrio*, *Aeromonas*, and *Plesiomonas* spp. Those that are negative include *Salmonella* and *Shigella* spp. Identification should be performed on both oxidase-positive and oxidase-negative NLF.

HE and XLD Agars

Hektoen enteric (HE) agar is moderately selective so normal enteric gram-negative rods are slightly inhibited but *Salmonella* and *Shigella* spp. grow better. If normal enteric flora is able to grow, they are usually able to ferment either lactose, sucrose, or salicin and appear yellow or orange. *Salmonella* and *Shigella* spp. are unable to ferment any of the three carbohydrates and so appear as clear or green (the color of the agar) colonies. HE can also detect hydrogen sulfide production (H_2S). Salmonella is a hydrogen sulfide producer and appears as a clear or green colony with a black center. Identification should be performed on any clear, green or clear, black centered colony. Suspect colonies should be screened with oxidase if possible. The production of H_2S may mask a positive reaction.

Xylose-lysine-deoxycholate (XLD) agar is also moderately selective and inhibits most normal enteric gram-negative rods. Lactose, sucrose and xylose are present as carbohydrates. Normal enteric flora that grow are usually able to ferment at least one of the them to create yellow or orange colonies. *Shigella* spp. appears as a clear, red (the color of the agar) colony. *Salmonella* can ferment xylose so the medium also has lysine incorporated. *Salmonella* is lysine positive. The basic pH reaction from the breakdown of lysine neutralizes the acid produced from xylose so the colony reverts back to red. The medium is also able to detect hydrogen sulfide production so *Salmonella* colonies are clear or red with a black center. Suspect colonies should be screened with oxidase if possible. The production of H_2S may mask a positive reaction. Most laboratories choose to use either HE or XLD but usually not both to save costs.

PEA or CNA Agar

PEA and CNA agars can be used to selectively isolate *Staphylococcus aureus*. If it is considered a predominant organism compared to the normal enteric flora, then it may be significant. These are useful agars when the sheep blood agar is swarmed over with *Proteus* spp., a common member of the normal enteric flora.

Campy Blood Agar

The atmosphere, incubation temperature, and inhibitory agar prevent the growth of most enteric flora other than *Campylobacter* spp. Suspicious colonies are gray to tan, wet, and tend to follow the streak line rather than forming individual colonies. Gram stain reaction and microscopic morphology, positive catalase and oxidase tests can be used to presumptively identify *C. jejuni*.

SMAC

This agar is a MacConkey agar with sorbitol substituted for lactose. EHEC, serotype O157:H7, is unique among other strains of *E. coli*. It is unable to ferment sorbitol. On SMAC, suspicious colonies remain clear. An oxidase test should be performed and, if negative, the colony identified. If the organism is *E. coli* then it must be tested with O157 and H7 antisera. If negative for either, the organism should be sent to a public health laboratory for further serotyping.

CIN

CIN is very important for the isolation of *Yersinia enterocolitica*. This organism will be missed on the other stool isolation media. This organism grows better at room temperature than 35–37°C and so appears pinpoint on these agars and is easily overlooked. *Y. enterocolitica* is able to ferment sucrose on HE and XLD and appears yellow if it is able to grow adequately.

On CIN, *Y. enterocolitica* produces a target or bulls-eye colony which is red centered with a clear edge. This occurs due to the fermentation of mannitol. Other organisms, such as *Citrobacter freundii* (a non-pathogen) and *Aeromonas hydrophila* (a potential pathogen), can create the same colony morphology. Suspicious colonies must be screened with oxidase and identified if negative.

SCREENING AND PRESUMPTIVE IDENTIFICATION TESTS

Suspect colonies can be minimally screened with oxidase, triple sugar iron (TSI), and urea. Figure 35-10 ■ demonstrates the screening results for a potential *Salmonella* spp. using TSI,

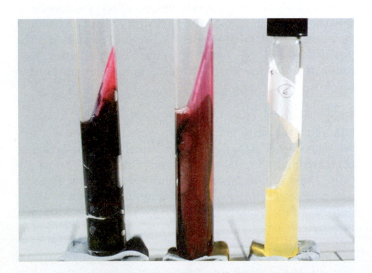

■ **FIGURE 35-10** TSI, screening results for red colonies with black centers from an XLD agar. The TSI slant on the left indicates an alkaline slant over a yellow deep/butt with H$_2$S production. The LIA slant in the center demonstrates a red slant due to peptone deamination over a purple deep/butt that is due to lysine decarboxylation. H$_2$S can be seen as a black precipitate at the apex of the slant where it meets the deep of the tube. The urea tube on the far right is negative. Lysine and H$_2$S production are suggestive of *Salmonella* spp. This isolate should be serotyped and biochemically confirmed.

lysine iron agar (LIA), and urea slants. Some laboratories add a rapid phenylalanine deaminase (PDA) test. A positive phenylalanine deaminase result rules out a pathogen because only *Proteus, Providencia,* and *Morganella* spp. are positive. Entero-Screen 4 is commercially available (Hardy Diagnostics) and provides screening results for lysine decarboxylation or deamination, H$_2$S, and urea. Screening results that indicate a potential pathogen can be presumptively identified with spot indole, pyrrolidonyl arylamidase (PYR), and motility.

The PYR and 4-methylumbelliferyl-beta-D-glucuronide (MUG) tests can be used to screen for *E. coli* serotype O157. The PYR result should be negative. Most strains of *E. coli* are able to break down the MUG substrate and are positive as indicated by fluorescence (Figure 35-11a ■). *E. coli* O157 is MUG negative (Figure 35-11b ■). A PYR-negative, MUG-negative colony should be serotyped with O157 antisera. Table 35-4✪ demonstrates how screening and presumptive identification tests can be used to determine potential pathogens.

Serotype

Isolates, which are presumptively identified as possible *Salmonella* or *Shigella* spp., should be confirmed biochemically and serotyped with the appropriate antisera. Possible *Salmonella* species should be typed with polyvalent and *Vi* (virulent capsule) antisera. If the polyvalent reaction is positive, then group-specific typing should be done, if the antiserum is available. The isolate should be submitted to a local public health laboratory for flagellar typing and epidemiology studies. Possible *Shigella* species should be typed with Group A, B, C, and D antisera. A positive result should be correlated to the final identification prior to reporting.

For both *Salmonella* and *Shigella* spp., if a negative serotyping result is obtained, the suspension should be boiled for 10 minutes and retested. This will destroy any capsule present that may be masking the somatic antigen. CDC may be notified if the isolate is nationally reportable. State regulation may require notification of local public health laboratories. Table 35-4 summarizes results of screening, presumptive, and serological tests for suspicious colonies isolated on enteric agar.

Reported Results

Reported results should reflect exactly what the physician ordered and what specific organisms are examined for in the stool culture. For example, if a clinical laboratory is only looking for *Salmonella, Shigella,* and *Campylobacter,* a negative culture result should be reported as "No *Salmonella, Shigella,* or *Campylobacter* isolated." If a potential enteric pathogen is isolated, the reported result should include the presumptive identity, serotype, if appropriate, and inform the physician if the isolate should be submitted to a public health laboratory for further testing. Enteric pathogens are not quantified as are most cultures. The presence of an enteric pathogen is significant regardless of the amount present. Isolates such as *Salmonella typhi, S.* serotype Paratyphi, *S.* serotype Choleraesuis, and *Vibrio cholerae* are life-threatening and of great epidemio-

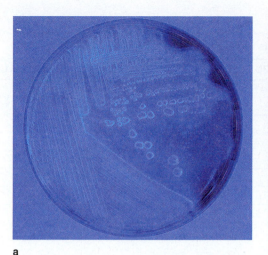
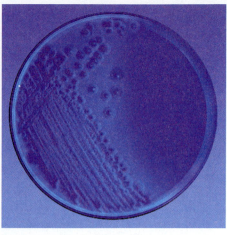

a   b

■ FIGURE 35-11 **a.** Colonies of *E. coli* growing on MacConkey agar with MUG. Exposing the growth to ultraviolet light reveals fluorescence, a positive MUG reaction. **b.** Colonies of *E. coli* O157:H7 growing on MacConkey agar with MUG. Exposing the growth to ultraviolet light reveals no fluorescence, a negative MUG reaction.
Photos courtesy of Remel, part of Thermo Fisher Scientific.

logical importance. The physician, infectious disease team, and public health should be immediately notified (Isenberg, 2004).

Predominant growth of yeast, *Pseudomonas aeruginosa*, *Staphylococcus aureus*, or *Bacillus cereus* should be noted. The lack of growth of gram-negative rods should also be reported to the physician to indicate the absence of commensal bowel flora.

REAL WORLD TIP

An oxidase positive, nonlactose fermenter that will not identify could potentially be a halophilic *Vibrio* spp. 1.0–2.0% NaCl must be added to each biochemical to ensure the growth and reactivity of the organism.

REAL WORLD TIP

It may be more cost-effective for smaller laboratories, which do not receive a large number of stool specimens for culture, to go directly to final biochemical identification rather than using screening or presumptive testing.

Susceptibility Testing

Susceptibility testing should not be performed on nontyphoid *Salmonella* because treatment will cause the organism to retreat and hide in the gallbladder. The individual then becomes a carrier such as in the case of typhoid Mary. Antibiotic therapy

increases the potential for hemolytic uremic syndrome with shiga-toxin-producing *E. coli*. Susceptibility tests should be performed on the other potential pathogens or systemic organisms due to their unpredictable susceptibility to antimicrobials. Usually only ampicillin, trimethoprim-sulfamethoxazole, and quinolone are reported for the gram-negative rods. Third-generation cephalosporin results may be reported if the isolate is resistant. Doxycycline or tetracycline should be reported if the isolate is identified as *V. cholerae* (Isenberg, 2004).

▶ TREATMENT OF GASTROINTESTINAL ILLNESSES

Different treatments may be required depending on the symptoms present. Diarrhea and vomiting can lead to dehydration if the person loses too much water and electrolytes. Replacing fluids and electrolytes is important and oral rehydration solutions can help prevent dehydration. Sports drinks should not be used to treat diarrheal illness. While they contain electrolytes, their high sugar content can prolong diarrhea.

Preparations of bismuth subsalicylate can reduce the duration and severity of simple diarrhea but these medications can also make the illness worse and should be avoided if the

REAL WORLD TIP

The use of bismuth subsalicylate can create black stools. Bismuth subsalicylate reacts with sulfur to cause the color change. The color is temporary and harmless.

⊙ TABLE 35-4

Screening Results for Potential Fecal Pathogens Isolated on Enteric Agar

Screening Tests	Possible Pathogen	Presumptive ID Tests	Serotype	Reportable to CDC
TSI: K/AG or K/A	Salmonella	Spot IND: –, PYR: –	Yes	Yes
H2S: +				
Ur: –				
Ox: –				
PDA: –				
TSI: K/A	Salmonella	Spot IND: –, PYR: –, MOT: +	Yes	Yes
H2S: –	Shigella	Spot IND: V, PYR: –, MOT: –	Yes	Yes
Ur: –				
Ox: –				
PDA: –				
TSI: K/A or A/A	Yersinia enterocolitica	Spot IND: V, PYR: +, MOT: – (35°C),	No	No
H2S: –		MOT: + (25°C), VP: +		
Ur: +				
Ox: –				
PDA: –				
Ox: +	Campylobacter jejuni	Hipp: +, Indoxyl acetate: +	No	No
Cat: mostly +				
GS: curved GNR	C. coli	Hipp: –, Indoxyl acetate: +		
MOT: + (darting)				
Ox: –	E. coli O157	PYR: –, MUG: –	Yes	Yes
Spot IND: +				(also STEC)
Ox: +	Aeromonas	String Test: –, O129: R, 6.5% NaCl: NG	No	No
TSI: K/A or A/A	Plesiomonas	String Test: –, O129: S, 6.5% NaCl: NG	No	No
IND: +	Vibrio cholerae	String Test: +, O129: S, 6.5% NaCl: NG	Yes	Yes
	Other Vibrio	String Test: +, O129: S, 6.5% NaCl: GW	Yes	Yes

TSI, triple sugar iron agar; H₂S, hydrogen sulfide; Ur, rapid urease; Ox, oxidase; PDA, rapid phenylalanine deaminase; IND, spot indole; PYR, L-pyrrolidonyl peptidase; MOT, wet mount motility; CAT, catalase; GS, Gram stain; Hipp, rapid hippurate; MUG, 4-methyl-umbelliferyl B-D-glucuronide; NG, no growth; GW, growth; +, positive; –, negative; V, variable; K, alkaline; A, acid; G, gas; S, sensitive; R, resistant; O129, 150 μg; VP, rapid Voges-Proskauer.

patient experiences a high fever or if blood is found in the stools.

Some gastrointestinal illnesses are caused by the use of antibiotic drugs that disrupt the digestive ecology enough to let antibiotic-resistant organisms gain a foothold, leading to diarrhea. A new area of bacteriology currently being investigated may prove to be therapeutic. **Probiotics** are species of bacteria that help to maintain health in humans and animals and that are part of the microbiota of mucous membranes. It has been proposed that, in the gut they not only exist in harmony with the body, but also aid digestion and may even act as a first line of defense against invading pathogens by competing for nutrients, energy, and habitats, and in so doing, deter invasion by harmful species. Some researchers believe they may even help to keep the immune system primed, increasing circulating specific and natural antibodies. Probiotics have been used to restore intestinal flora after antibiotic treatment, may reduce the duration of rotaviral diarrhea and gastroenteritis in infants, and may prevent traveler's diarrhea.

Checkpoint! 35–11 (Chapter Objectives 5 and 7)

A stool culture demonstrates a non-lactose fermenter that is also a clear colony on XLD. The organism provides the following results:

Oxidase = no color change
TSI = red slant over yellow deep/butt
Urea = no color change
PDA = no color change
Motility = no haziness along the stab line

What additional testing is necessary to confirm the identification of this organism?

A. *Salmonella serotyping*
B. *Shigella serotyping*
C. *E. coli O157 serotyping*
D. *No additional testing is needed because it is a nonpathogen.*

SUMMARY

The gastrointestinal tract is responsible for the intake and breakdown (catabolism) of food. This involves six basic processes: ingestion, secretion, mixing and propulsion, digestion, absorption, and defecation.

Organs and areas that make up the gastrointestinal tract include the mouth, esophagus, stomach, and the large and small intestines. Mechanical breakup, involving the teeth, tongue, hard and soft palate, and the cheeks, along with the mixing of food with saliva, begins the digestive process. Salivary amylase and lingual lipase begins the chemical digestion of food, which continues in the stomach through the action of pepsin and in the small intestines with pancreatic amylase, trypsin, lipases, and nucleotidases. The villi and microvilli of the small intestine facilitate absorption of water, amino acids, fatty acids, monosaccharides, electrolytes, and vitamins. In the large intestine vitamins can be produced through bacterial action, which, along with water and electrolytes, are subsequently absorbed. Waste products, in the form of feces, are expelled from the body through defecation.

Ingestion of food and water quickly allows the gastrointestinal tract to be colonized by bacteria after birth. These commensal or nonpathogenic microbes can inhibit the growth of pathogenic microorganisms and in so doing contribute to our good health. Eliminating these organisms through the long-term administration of antimicrobial drugs can disturb this balance and actually lower an individual's ability to stave off infection caused by organisms that are not affected by these inhibitory substances. Circumstances such as this have lead to gastrointestinal infections by yeast such as *Candida albicans,* and bacteria such as *Staphylococcus aureus, Pseudomonas aeruginosa,* and *Clostridium difficile,* an anaerobe.

Most foodborne illnesses result from the consumption of food and water contaminated with microbes or toxic chemicals. Clinical microbiologists are involved with the isolation and identification of bacteria, fungi, viruses, and parasites that cause disease including gastrointestinal illnesses. Symptoms such as nausea, vomiting, abdominal cramps, and diarrhea, along with a history of the foods consumed, can launch the investigative process of determining the cause of the patient's illness. Once the cause has been discovered, microbiologists are instrumental in choosing the most appropriate treatment options to bring about the patient's recovery and notifying public health authorities.

The most common bacterial cause of gastrointestinal disease is *Campylobacter jejuni,* which is found in the intestines of healthy birds. Eating undercooked chicken or other foods contaminated with the juices from raw chicken is frequently the route of infection for humans. However, epidemics have been attributed to contaminated milk, meat, and water.

Salmonella species are widespread in nature, having been isolated from the intestines of reptiles, birds, and mammals. Poultry serve as the primary source of human infection but spread of the infection has also been associated with the consumption of beef, pork, and contaminated water.

Salmonella typhi, the etiological agent of typhoid fever, only infects humans. There is no animal reservoir so the route of transmission is through ingestion of food or water contaminated with fecal material from humans. Individuals who are carriers of *S. typhi* have no symptoms of disease and because the organism is excreted in the stool, they are able to pass the infection to others. Diagnosis of *Salmonella* species, including *S. typhi,* requires the use of selective and differential media. Suspicious colonies are screened or identified biochemically. Serotyping must be employed to confirm the organism truly is a serotype belonging to the *Salmonella* genus. In cases where the numbers in the stool are too low to be detected by this means, the Widal test, a serological test demonstrating the presence of antibodies to the organism in the serum of infected patients, can be employed.

Escherichia coli is an organism that is commonly found in the intestinal tract of both invertebrates and vertebrate animals, where, in most cases, the organism is harmless. However, there are certain strains or serotypes of *E. coli* that are responsible for disease and death in humans. This includes the enterotoxigenic *E. coli,* which are responsible for "traveler's diarrhea," enteroinvasive *E. coli,* which produce a disease almost identical to shigellosis, enteropathogenic *E. coli,* which are responsible for outbreaks of hospital-acquired infantile diarrhea, and the shiga-toxin-producing strains of *E. coli,* which are responsible for hemorrhagic colitis and hemolytic uremic syndrome (HUS). Because these organisms resemble nonpathogenic strains of *E. coli* on laboratory media that are commonly used to isolate pathogenic species such as *Salmonella* and *Shigella* species, proof of an organism's ability to produce an enterotoxin or serological tests must be employed to demonstrate their virulence. One strain, known as *E. coli* O157:H7, can be presumptively identified using sorbitol MacConkey (SMAC) agar plates. This strain normally does not ferment sorbitol and will appear as colorless colonies.

Vibrio cholerae, the etiological agent of cholera, can be isolated from fresh and marine water sources. The severe form, associated with the production of "rice water stools," may be fatal but most cases are either mild or asymptomatic. Meat, fish, seafood, milk, and contaminated water have all been implicated in the transmission of the bacterium. Isolation of the organism from the stool of infected individuals can be accomplished through the use of thiosulfate–citrate–bile salts–sucrose (TCBS) agar, a selective and differential medium. Suspect colonies are serotyped with O1 and O139 antisera.

Shigella species, which are very closely related to *E. coli,* are responsible for bacillary dysentery. Poor sanitation and hygiene, resulting in the ingestion of contaminated food and water, are responsible for the spread of this pathogen. The organism is very virulent and as few as 10 organisms may bring about disease. In addition to the identification of the bacterium through the means of biochemical tests, serological tests are required to identify the serogroup to which it belongs.

Noroviruses and rotaviruses are also agents of acute gastrointestinal disease. They are spread primarily through person-to-person transmission and occasionally through contaminated food and water. Electron microscopy, immunoassays, and molecular diagnostics can be employed in order to elucidate the cause of the illness.

Less common causes of gastrointestinal illnesses include bacteria such as *Yersinia enterocolitica, Listeria monocytogenes, Plesiomonas shigelloides,* and *Aeromonas hydrophila.* Parasites including *Entamoeba histolytica,* the etiological agent of amoebic dysentery, *Giardia lamblia, Cryptosporidium parvum, Cyclospora cayetanensis,* and helminths such as roundworms, tapeworms, and flukes are also known to cause diarrheal illnesses.

Toxigenic gastrointestinal illness or food poisoning is another cause of gastrointestinal upset. In these cases the organism contaminates a foodstuff and, given a sufficient incubation period, produces sufficient quantities of exotoxin to cause symptoms. While many of these exotoxins affect the gastointestinal tract (and are referred to as enterotoxins), some may affect other organ systems, as occurs with botulism toxin.

Carriers of *Staphylococcus aureus* may contaminate foods when they don't practice good hygiene. Foods such as salad dressings, pastries, canned foods, frozen foods, and processed meats such as ham provide a rich source of nutrients for the bacterium. As the organism grows it produces the enterotoxin, which is consumed along with the contaminated food. One to six hours later the hapless individual experiences nausea, vomiting, cramps, and diarrhea.

Clostridium botulinum, an anaerobic organism that can be isolated from soil and water, can also contaminate food producing a paralytic toxin. This toxin, which blocks the neuromuscular transmitter acetyl choline, prevents the nerve impulse from triggering muscle contraction. Patients then experience muscle weakness or paralysis, which can be fatal if the muscles of the diaphragm are paralyzed and the patient can no longer breathe unassisted. Improperly canned foods, sausage, mushrooms, and olives have been implicated. Antitoxin must be administered early on to prevent death.

Bacillus cereus is another bacterium associated with food poisoning, contaminating foods made with grains such as rice. Diarrhea or vomiting may then ensue.

LEARNING OPPORTUNITIES

On the Web:

Visit The Foodborne Diseases Active Surveillance Network (FoodNet) at URL: http://www.cdc.gov/foodnet/index.htm, to see the location of FoodNet laboratories, get FoodNet News, and surveillance reports by year.

1. What function do the folds, villi, and microvilli of the small intestine serve? (Chapter Objective 1)

2. What useful role does the microbiota of the gastrointestinal tract, especially of the intestines, play in maintaining good health? (Chapter Objective 2)

3. What important phenotypic characteristics distinguish *Campylobacter jejuni* from other agents of diarrheal illness in the *Enterobacteriaceae* and *Vibrionaceae* families? (Chapter Objectives 3, 5, and 6)

4. List common routes of transmission for salmonellosis. (Chapter Objective 3)

5. A patient with a history of consumption of undercooked hamburger is experiencing severe abdominal pain, initially watery diarrhea, followed by grossly bloody diarrhea with little or no fever. A stool sample is collected and sent to the laboratory for culture and susceptibility testing. Some material from the stool sample is plated onto a sorbitol-MacConkey (SMAC) agar plate. After 18–24 hours of incubation, clear to tan colonies are observed to be the predominant organism. What is this most likely potential pathogen? (Chapter Objectives 3, 4, and 6)

6. The predominant organism observed on the MacConkey and xylose–lysine–deoxycholate plates of a stool culture are colorless. Biochemical testing reveals the isolate is oxidase positive, indole positive, string test negative, O129 resistant, does not ferment lactose, able to ferment sucrose, hydrolyzes gelatin, and produces DNase. Growth is inhibited in media containing an increased concentration of salt (NaCl). What is the most likely identification of this organism? (Chapter Objectives 4, 5, and 6)

7. Describe three ways fresh fruits and vegetables may be the source of gastrointestinal illness. (Chapter Objective 3)

8. What appropriate treatment should be administered to counteract the harmful effects diarrhea and vomiting have on the body? (Chapter Objective 10)

CASE STUDY 35-1   (CHAPTER OBJECTIVES 3, 4, 5, 7, AND 10)

Patient: 2-year-old female

Admitting diagnosis: gastrointestinal upset with diarrhea and vomiting

The pediatrician admitted this female to the pediatric unit after her initial visit to the children's clinic. The symptoms prompting the visit included 2 days of passing five to six watery stools and several episodes of emesis. The child's temperature on admission was 99.3°F. Her abdomen was not tender. Neither her parents nor her older sister, who was 6-years-old and attending grade school, were ill at the time. Because both parents were employed outside the home, the 2-year-old female was attending day care. At a later date it was discovered that four other children at the day care had also experienced diarrhea and vomiting.

A complete blood count (CBC), chemistry profile, fecal leukocytes, stool cultures times three, and blood cultures times three were performed with the following results:

CBC	Reference Ranges	Chemistry Profile	Reference Ranges
WBC 9.8×10^9/L	5.5–15.5 (early childhood)	Sodium 150 mEq/L	135–150 mEq/L
RBC 3.9×10^{12}/L	3.9–5.3 (early childhood)	Potassium 3.6 mEq/L	3.4–5.0 mEq/L
Hgb 96 g/L	115–135 (early childhood)	Chloride 97 mEq/L	98–107 mEq/L
Hct .34 L/L	.34–.40 (early childhood)	CO_2 25.5 mMol/L	22–29 mMol/L
MCV 87 fL	75–87 (early childhood)	Calcium 11.0 mg/dL	8.6–10.6 (child)
MCH 24.6 g/dL	24–30 (early childhood)	Glucose 120 mg/dL	70–110 (fasting)
MCHC 28.2 %	31–37 (early childhood)	BUN 19 mg/dL	7–18 mg/dL
Plt 112×10^9/L	150–400	Uric Acid 5.0 mg/dL	2.6–6.0 mg/dL
Differential:		Creatinine 1.1 mg/dL	0.5–1.1 mg/dL
Neutrophils 35%	25–60%	Total protein 8.5 mg/dL	6.5–8.3 mg/dL
Bands 5%	0–10%	Albumin 5.2 mg/dL	3.5–5.5 mg/Dl
Lymphocytes 55%	20–50%		
Monocytes 5%	0–8%		

Stool smears evaluated for fecal leukocytes revealed only a few white blood cells were present

Stool culture #1 = no *Shigella, Salmonella*, or *Campylobacter* isolated

Stool culture #2 = no *Shigella, Salmonella*, or *Campylobacter* isolated

Stool culture #3 = no *Shigella, Salmonella*, or *Campylobacter* isolated

Blood cultures (all three) = no growth after 7 days

Since this case occurred during early winter, an enzyme immunoassay test for a virus was performed with positive results

1. What is the most likely diagnosis for this patient?
2. What is the most likely source of the etiological agent?
3. What other tests can be used to diagnose this type of infection?
4. What serious consequences may arise if this disease is not diagnosed and treated properly?
5. What treatment options are available for this infection?

CASE STUDY 35-2   (CHAPTER OBJECTIVES 3, 4, 5, 6, 7, AND 10)

Four family members in a small New England town became ill after attending a family reunion picnic. A 4-year-old child became ill 3 days after the picnic, a 59-year-old female and her 64-year-old husband both became ill 4 days after the picnic, and a 29-year-old male became ill on day 6. All experienced fever, abdominal cramps, and diarrhea of several days duration. The 4-year-old female experienced a fever of 104°F (40°C) and was hospitalized while the others experienced only low-grade fevers and did not require hospitalization. Stool specimens from all four individuals were submitted for cultures and, in addition to normal stool flora, non-lactose fermenting gram-negative rods were isolated on the MacConkey, xylose–lysine–deoxycholate (XLD), and hektoen-enteric (HE) agar plates. The colonies on the XLD and HE plates had black centers indicating the production of H_2S. Additional biochemical characteristics are listed below.

Triple sugar iron agar slant = K/AG, H_2S
Indole production = negative
Citrate utilization = positive

Mucate utilization = positive
Urease production = negative
Lactose fermentation = negative
Ornithine decarboxylase = positive
Lysine decarboxylase = positive
Arginine dihydrolase = positive
Sorbitol = acid and gas production
Dulcitol = acid and gas production
o-nitrophenyl-β-D-galactopyranoside = negative

The results of the biochemical tests are consistent with non-typhoid *Salmonella* spp. No *Shigella* or *Campylobacter* species were isolated.

1. What additional testing, if any, should now be performed?
2. What are some possible sources of the microorganism responsible for the gastrointestinal distress experienced by the four patients?
3. What measures could have been taken to prevent this unfortunate occurrence?

PEARSON
myhealthprofessionskit™

Use this address to access the interactive Companion Website created for this textbook. Simply select "Clinical Laboratory Science" from the choice of disciplines. Find this book and log in using your user name and password.

REFERENCES

Go to myhealthprofessionskit.com to view this chapter's references.

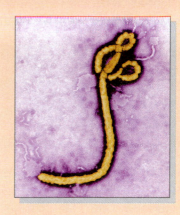

36

Genital System

Karen M. Kiser

■ LEARNING OBJECTIVES

Upon completion of this chapter, the learner should be able to:

1. Identify genital tract structures that can be infected, the routes of infection, innate defenses, and consequences of infection.

2. Identify microbes that are normally present in nonsterile areas of the genital system.

3. Correlate infectious disease(s) with etiological agent(s).

4. Describe the pathogenesis, clinical manifestations, and epidemiology of diseases associated with the genital tract to include bacterial, viral, fungal, parasitic, and toxigenic causes.

5. Select the best approach to identifying the presence of genital pathogens that are not routinely cultured.

6. Describe the processing of genital specimens to include specimen collection and selection, inoculation, and incubation of primary media.

7. Differentiate pathogenic and commensal colonies, correlate each on various media, and provide presumptive identification of potential pathogens using spot or rapid test results.

8. Determine alternative or confirmatory tests necessary and evaluate the test results.

9. Identify genital tract pathogens and correlate to Gram stain morphology, colony morphology, test outcomes, and antibiogram prior to reporting results.

10. Recognize genital pathogens that are reportable to the Centers for Disease Control and Prevention or other authorities for epidemiological or legal reasons.

11. Interpret Gram stain results of vaginal secretions diagnostic for bacterial vaginosis.

12. Discuss the extent of susceptibility testing required for isolated organisms.

KEY TERMS

empirically	mucopurulent	proctocolitis
endometritis	natal	salpingitis
epididymitis	neonate	transudate
fetus	postnatal	vaginitis
hepatosplenomegaly	prenatal	vaginosis
jaundice		

▶ INTRODUCTION

Genital tract infections include sexually transmitted diseases that affect males and females as well as infections that can be transmitted to a fetus or newborn and cause serious life-threatening disease. The culprits include bacteria, parasites, viruses, and fungi. This chapter begins with a review of the genital tract anatomy and physiology with a focus on microbial points of entry and exit as well as the system's innate defenses. Microorganisms that normally reside in the area or cause disease are described. Finally, information on specimen collection and processing is presented.

▶ FUNCTION AND STRUCTURE OF THE GENITAL SYSTEM

The genital system consists of the reproductive structures of the male and female. Each sex has unique structures that can interact to produce a baby. These unique structures also provide different entry points for microbes and defend against infectious disease. Symptoms of infectious diseases may differ depending on the sex of the patient. Female genital infections may be transmitted to a **fetus**, a baby still in the uterus or **neonate**, a newborn infant, and cause problems during pregnancy or after birth.

FUNCTION

The function of the genital system is to reproduce the human species. The male reproductive system is designed to produce sperm and insert them into the female. The male also determines the sex of the child. The function of the female is to produce eggs and nourish fertilized eggs, resulting in a fetus.

STRUCTURE

Male Reproductive System

The male reproductive system consists of the scrotum, testes or testicles, epididymis (a tightly coiled tube on each teste), and penis. See Figure 36-1 ■ for a detailed depiction of the male reproductive system. The male's contribution to the reproductive process is the sperm. Sites of infection in the male include the urethra, prostate, and epididymis.

Scrotum and Testes.   The male testes are a pair of organs responsible for producing sperm. Each teste contains tubules where sperm are produced. Sperm mature and enter the epididymis where they develop motility. Sperm are stored in the epididymis and the vas deferens. The testes are contained in a sac-like extension of the abdominal wall called the scrotum. Muscles and tendons can raise the scrotum up closer to the body to warm or lower the scrotum to cool, maintaining the temperature that sperm require to remain viable.

Penis.   The penis is a shaft of tissue that consists of a tube, the urethra, and connects to the vas deferens and seminal vesicle via the ejaculatory duct located near the base of the bladder. The penis is covered by loose skin that extends to the tip and folds down, forming a cuff called the foreskin. This foreskin can be removed by circumcision. If a male is uncircumcised, there is a higher risk for infection and inflammation. Underneath the skin of the penis lie nerves and erectile tissue consisting of blood sinusoids covered by connective tissue. Stimulation results in an erection. When sexual excitement peaks, ejaculation of semen occurs.

Intact skin provides a mechanical barrier to invading organisms. Commensal flora compete for space and nutrients as well as creating inhibitory by-products. Low pH of urine and the flushing action of urination helps to control microbial entry into the urethra. Breaks in the skin and the urethral opening provide an entry and exit point for microorganisms associated with sexually transmitted diseases (STDs) and urinary tract infections (Ryan, 1994). See ∞ Chapters 4 and 34 for more information on interactions of man versus microbe and urinary tract infections.

Semen.   Semen consists of sperm, fluid, and mucus. The fluids help to nourish the sperm and neutralize acidic vaginal secretions that can decrease sperm motility. Sperm is released from the epydidimis and vas deferens and are mixed with seminal and prostate fluid as well as mucus from the bulbourethral gland prior to ejaculation. Microbes associated with genital infections can be transmitted to sexual partners in the sperm.

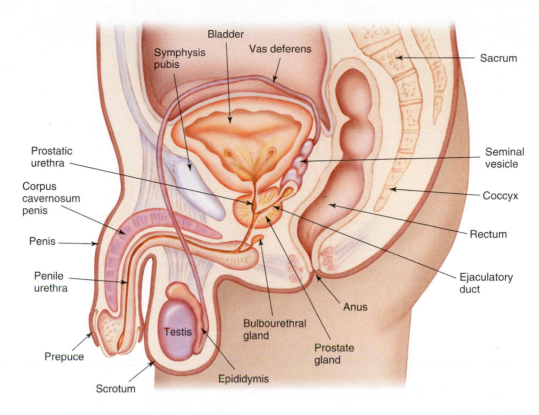

FIGURE 36-1 Male reproductive system.

 Checkpoint! 36–1 (Chapter Objective 1)

A portal of entrance for those organisms causing sexually transmitted disease such as gonorrhea or syphilis is:

1. *Breaks in the skin or mucous membrane*
2. *The urethral opening*
3. *The testes*
   A. *1 and 2*
   B. *2 and 3*
   C. *1 and 3*
   D. *1, 2, and 3*

Female Reproductive System

The female reproductive system consists of the ovaries, fallopian tubes, uterus, and vagina. See Figure 36-2 ■ to identify the female reproductive structures. The female's contribution to the reproductive process is the egg or ovum and a site for fetal development, the uterus. Sites of infection located in the female lower genital tract include the vagina, cervix, and vulva. Sites of infection in the female upper genital tract include the ovaries, fallopian tubes, and uterus.

Ovaries.   There are two ovaries attached to the end of the fallopian tubes by ligaments. Thousands of eggs are contained in the ovaries. When the ovary produces and releases an egg, projections on the ends of the fallopian tubes sweep it into the tube opening. Ovulation causes hormones to stimulate the preparation of the uterine lining for implantation and nurturing of a fertilized egg.

Fallopian Tubes.   The fallopian tubes are structures that extend out of each side of the uterus. The end opens into the peritoneal cavity, near the ovary. The open end receives the ova from the ovaries. Fimbria (plural fimbriae), a fringe of tissue, push the egg down the tube. The tube is lined with a ciliated mucous membrane that creates a current that moves the egg down the tube (Solomon, Schmidt, & Adragna, 1990). If the egg encounters a sperm, fertilization may occur.

Uterus and Cervix.   The uterus is a pear-shaped, muscular organ about the size of a small fist. The uterus is lined with a mucous membrane called the endometrium. The uterus responds to hormones each month preparing for a possible pregnancy by increasing the endometrial blood supply and storing nutrients. If no pregnancy occurs, the endometrial lining is shed during menstruation. If pregnancy occurs, the placenta and embryo tissue develop and burrow into the endometrial lining. The uterus narrows toward the bottom, forming an opening called the cervix.

Vagina and Vulva.   The vagina is a tube that connects to the lowest part of the uterus, the cervix, to the outside of the

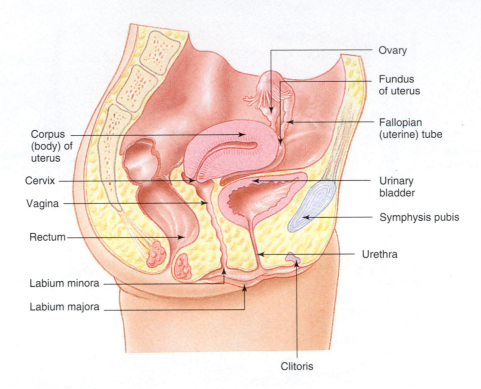

Ovary

Fundus
of uterus

Fallopian
(uterine) tube

Corpus
(body) of
uterus

Urinary
bladder

Cervix

Symphysis pubis

Vagina

Rectum

Urethra

Labium minora

Labium majora

Clitoris

■ **FIGURE 36-2** Female reproductive system.

body. The vagina is lined with mucosa consisting of transitional, columnar, and squamous epithelial cells (Forbes, Sahn, & Weissfeld, 2007). An intact mucous lining is the first line of defense against clinically significant microorganisms. Commensal flora reside on the vaginal mucous membrane, competing for nutrients and producing toxic by-products that helps control the adherence of and colonization by potential pathogens. IgA is also present on the surface of the vaginal mucous membrane to help provide immunity (Ryan, 1994).

The vagina enables the male to deposit sperm, provides an exit for the endometrial lining during menstruation, and enables the neonate to leave the uterus during the birthing process. The vagina is a major entry and exit point for organisms that cause genital tract infections.

The vulva is the external genitalia. The vulva consists of the labia major, labia minor, vaginal opening, mons pubis, and clitoris. The mons pubis is the pubic mound of fatty tissue that becomes covered with hair at puberty. The labia major are large folds of skin that typically meet in the middle, protecting the genital structures located beneath them. They are also covered with hair at puberty. The labia minor are small folds of hairless tissue located within the labia major. Hair follicles can be an entry point for infectious agents. The clitoris is located at the top juncture of the labia minor. It is erectile tissue that responds to sexual stimulation. The urethra is located near the clitoris and provides another entry point for sexually transmitted microorganisms and fecal organisms that

contaminate the perineum. Urination helps to flush potential pathogens out of the urethra. Glands near the vagina secrete mucus, providing lubrication during sexual intercourse. (Solomon et al., 1990). This mucus flow also helps to defend against invasion by microbes. Refer to ∞ Chapter 4 for more information about microbial defense.

 **Checkpoint! 36–2
(Chapter Objective 1)**

Vaginal defenses against potential pathogens include:
1. *Normal flora*
2. *Intact mucosa*
3. *IgA*
   A. *1 and 2*
   B. *1 and 3*
   C. *2 and 3*
   D. *1, 2, and 3*

▶ **STERILITY OF THE GENITAL SYSTEM**

Some of the genital system structures contain a resident commensal flora. The number and kind depend on the location of the structure and hormonal balance in the individual. The normal flora is more abundant on the moist, mucous membrane surfaces of the female genital tract. The flora found on the male and female external genitalia resembles that found on skin. The perineum, the area from the anus to the female vulva or male scrotum, may be contaminated with fecal microbes. The structures located deeper in the body are sterile.

Commensal flora of the urethra includes coagulase-negative staphylococci, corynebacteria, and obligate anaerobes. The external genitalia's resident flora consists of gram-positive bacteria and *Mycobacterium smegmatis*. The normal flora for prepubescent and postmenopausal females differs from that of reproductive females. Prepubescent and postmenopausal female flora consists of coagulase-negative staphylococci and corynebacteria while the commensal flora of reproductive females include *Enterobacteriaceae,* streptococci, staphylococci, lactobacilli, and anaerobes. Group B streptococci and yeast may be present. See Table 36-1✪ for more specific information on genital tract resident flora.

Commensal flora plays a key role in the defense against infectious disease. Their presence and associated metabolic by-products help to control growth of potential pathogens. In the female, production of estrogen causes glycogen to be deposited in the epithelial cells of the vagina. This in turn favors the growth of beneficial *Lactobacillus* spp. Lactobacilli utilize glycogen, producing lactic acid as a by-product. This acidity reduces the pH in the vagina, maintaining the predominance of lactobacilli associated with a healthy vagina (Murray, Baron, Jorgensen, Pfaller, & Yolken, 2003). Lactobacilli may also produce hydrogen peroxide, which is toxic to catalase negative bacteria (Eschenbach et al., 1989; Mandell, Dolin, & Bennett, 2005). Colonization of both the vagina and rectum help to maintain the healthy vagina's commensal flora (Antonio, Rabe, & Hillier, 2005).

Checkpoint! 36–3 (Chapter Objective 2)

Which of the following microorganisms can make up normal vagina flora?
1. *Lactobacilli*
2. *Coagulase-negative staphylococci*
3. *Corynebacteria*
   A. *1 only*
   B. *1 and 2*
   C. *2 only*
   D. *1, 2, and 3*

► INFECTIONS OF THE GENITAL SYSTEM

Genital system infections include sexually transmitted diseases, infections associated with pregnancy, and opportunistic infections. Infecting organisms enter via the urethra, vagina, or other entry points and can be transmitted to others via direct contact with the agent, the discharge, or blood and semen (Ryan, 1994). Most genital infections begin in the physical structures closer to the outside environment and can ascend, causing infections deeper in the body. Genital infections may cause premature delivery, stillbirth, or newborn infections; cervical cancer; or sterility. Sexual practices, birth control methods, hormonal levels, and a patient's health play a role in susceptibility to infectious agents.

SEXUALLY TRANSMITTED DISEASES

A sexually transmitted disease (STD) is an infection transmitted from the genitalia of one person to the genitalia or mucous membrane of another person during sexual activity (Ryan, 1994). Sexual practices, such as genital-anal intercourse, can result in infections in other body sites such as the anus, rectum, and throat (Forbes et al., 2007).

The most common reportable sexually transmitted disease in the United States is chlamydiae, followed by gonorrhea, syphilis, and chancroid (CDC, 2006c). Not all STDs are reportable, so the incidence of some may not be truly known. This includes the etiological agent of genital warts and herpes. Partners of an individual diagnosed with a sexually transmitted disease should be encouraged to seek medical advice and treatment.

Isolation of agents of sexually transmitted disease from infants or children may indicate child abuse. Transfer from the mother during birth must be ruled out. Diagnosis of gonorrhea, chlamydiae, syphilis, or HIV, once confirmed by appropriate laboratory tests, must be reported to the appropriate

✪ TABLE 36-1

Main Commensal Flora of the Genital Tract

Specimen Source	Commenal Flora
Urethra	Coagulase-negative staphylococci
	Corynebacteria
	Obligate anaerobes
External genitalia	Gram-positive bacteria
	Mycobacterium smegmatis
Prepubescent and postmenopausal females	Coagulase-negative staphylococci
	Corynebacteria
Reproductive females	*Enterobacteriaceae*
	Streptococci
	Staphylococci
	Lactobacilli
	Anaerobes
	Corynebacteria
	Gardnerella vaginalis
	Yeasts

authorities. Care must be taken to ensure reliability of diagnostic test results.

Enzyme immunoassays and nucleic acid tests for gonorrhea and chlamydiae may yield false positives due to cross-reaction with other organisms normally present in the genital flora. Culture is considered the gold standard for diagnosis of gonorrhoeae, but nucleic acid amplification tests are more sensitive for the detection of chlamydia (CDC, 2006c).

Diseases with Genital Ulcers

STDs that present with genital ulcers include genital herpes, chancroid, syphilis, lymphogranuloma venereum, and granuloma inguinale. More then one sexually transmitted disease may be present. Genital ulcers start out as a pustule then progress to an ulcer. The presence of ulcers creates an entrance for the human immunodeficiency virus (HIV), increasing the risk of HIV infection and making this sexually transmitted disease more communicable. The type of ulcer and the presence or absence of pain can be key distinguishing characteristics that the physician uses to make a presumptive diagnosis (Ryan, 1994). Diagnosis based only on signs and symptoms is often difficult and unreliable. Testing is required for accurate diagnosis and treatment. Testing for HIV should always be per-

formed with the diagnosis of any STD (CDC, 2006b). See Table 36-2✪ for specific information on diagnostic testing for sexually transmitted diseases.

Ulcers on the male can appear on the penis, scrotum, perianal tissue, inner thighs, and rectum. Ulcers on the female appear on the mons pubis, labia, vagina, cervix, inner thighs, or perianal tissue. Oral-genital sex can result in lesions on the lips of the mouth. Chancroid can be spread to nongenital sites via autoinoculation (Mandell et al., 2005). Painful ulcers typically occur with herpes and chancroid, while those associated with syphilis, lymphogranuloma venereum, and granuloma inguinale are painless. Regional lymph nodes are usually swollen.

Genital herpes (Figure 36-3 ■) is a chronic, lifelong infection. Herpes simplex virus (HSV) infects the epithelial cells then replicates and remains in the host's nervous system. The virus travels along the peripheral nervous system to establish chronic latent infections in the sensory ganglia. Table 36-3✪ provides an overview of herpes simplex virus and other sexually transmitted viruses including transmission, incubation, and potential for chronic infections. There are 2 types of HSV. HSV-1 is usually associated with oral lesions while HSV-2 is commonly associated with genital herpes. The location of the

---

✪ TABLE 36-2

Diagnostic Testing for Sexually Transmitted Diseases (STD)

Sign/Symptom	Disease	Pathogen	Laboratory Test
Genital ulcer	Genital herpes	HSV	Cell culture or direct fluorescent or immunoperoxidase antibody stains
	Syphilis	*Treponema pallidum*	Serology or darkfield exam or direct immunofluorescence
	Chancroid	*Haemophilus ducreyi*	Culture
	Granuloma inguinale	*Klebsiella granulomatis*	Observing Donovan bodies in tissue
	Lymphogranuloma venereum	*Chlamydia trachomatis*	Culture, direct immunofluorescence, nucleic acid detection
Urethritis/cervicitis	Gonorrhea	*Neisseria gonorrhoeae*	Culture, nucleic acid tests (Gram stain – males only)
	Chlamydia	*C. trachomatis*	Culture, nucleic acid tests
Vaginal discharge	Trichomoniasis	*Trichomonas vaginalis*	Microscopic exam (saline/KOH), culture, DNA probe
Vaginitis	Bacterial vaginosis	Mixed anaerobic GNR	Gram stain, DNA probe
	Candidiasis	*Candida albicans*	Microscopic exam (KOH), culture, DNA probe
Cervical cell dysplasia	HPV infection	HPV	Nucleic acid detection, PAP smear
Genital warts	HPV infection	HPV	Clinical diagnosis
	Syphilis	*T. pallidum*	Serology, darkfield, or direct immunofluorescence
Inflammation	Pelvic inflammatory disease	Numerous	Clinical diagnosis; R/O STD
Pain, swelling, inflammation	Epididymitis	*N. gonorrhoeae*	Gram stain, urine leukocyte esterase, or microscopic exam for WBC
		C. trachomatis	Culture, nucleic acid tests
		Enteric bacteria	Culture
Malaise, skin rash, lymphadenopathy, fever	HIV infection or AIDS	HIV	Antibody test, nucleic acid detection
Nausea, vomiting	Hepatitis	HAV, HBV, HCV	Serology, ALT

HSV, herpes simplex virus; GNR, gram-negative rod; HPV, human papilloma virus; Numerous, organisms associated with STD, vaginal flora, and bacterial vaginosis; HIV, human immunodeficiency virus; R/O, rule out; STD, sexually transmitted disease; HAV, Hepatitis A virus; HBV, Hepatitis B virus; HCV, Hepatitis C virus; ALT, alanine aminotransferase.

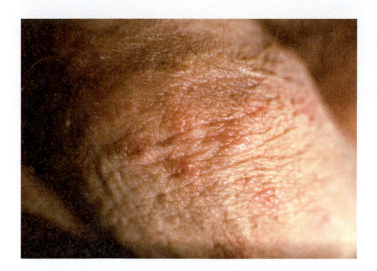

■ **FIGURE 36-3** Genital herpes outbreak on the shaft of the penis due to HSV-2.
From Public Image Library (PHIL), CDC/Susan Lindsley.

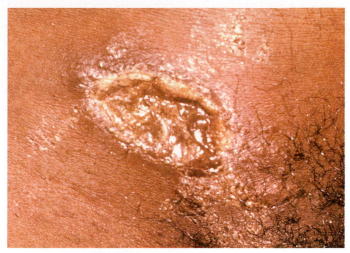

■ **FIGURE 36-4** A necrotic bubo in the inguinal region resulting from chancroid. The first sign of infection is usually the appearance of one or more sores or raised bumps on the genital organs. Sores are surrounded by a narrow red border. It soon becomes filled with pus and eventually ruptures, leaving a painful open wound.
From Public Image Library (PHIL), CDC/J. Pledger.

lesion can no longer diagnose the HSV strain present because both viruses can be found in either location.

Infections with HSV-1 are acquired during childhood, after exposure to oral secretions, in 50% of individuals (CDC, 2006c). HSV-2 infections tend to reactivate and shed viruses more commonly than HSV-1. It is important for prognostic reasons to identify which herpes virus is causing the infection. Many individuals with genital herpes are asymptomatic and unaware they are infected. Transmission to unaware sexual partners occurs due to sporadic viral shedding in the genital tract. Use of hormonal contraceptives, bacterial vaginosis, and large numbers of colonizing group B streptococci may increase HSV-2 shedding in women (Cherpes et al., 2005). To review the herpes simplex virus refer to ∞ Chapter 31, "Intracellular Microorganisms."

Chancroid (Figure 36-4 ■) is a local infection of the genitalia that can occur in the United States as isolated outbreaks. Asia, Africa, and Latin America have a higher incidence of this infectious disease (Murray et al., 2003). Chancroid is caused by *Haemophilus ducreyi.* Coinfection with syphilis or herpes sim-

plex virus occurs in 10% of patients that acquire the disease in the United States. Incidence of coinfection is higher when acquired outside the United States (CDC, 2006c). Refer to ∞ Chapter 20, "Fastidious Gram Negative Rods," to read more about *Haemophilus.*

Syphilis is a chronic, systemic disease that presents with ulcers (Figure 36-5 ■) during the primary infection. The organism is acquired by direct contact with an infectious lesion. The primary phase of syphilis may go unnoticed (Forbes et al., 2007). A secondary phase of infection is characterized by a skin rash that covers the entire body including the palms of the hands and soles of the feet (Figure 36-6 ■). There may also be lesions and swollen lymph nodes. Later stages of syphilis do not involve the genital tract (Baron et al., 1993). Latent infections are often asymptomatic. Tertiary infections affect the heart, eyes, and hearing. Syphilis is caused by the spirochete *Treponema pallidum.* The central nervous system can be

✪ TABLE 36-3

Sexually Transmitted Virus Overview

	Hepatitis A	Hepatitis B	Hepatitis C	HSV	HPV	HIV
Transmission	Fecal–oral	Percutaneous, permucosal	Percutaneous, permucosal	Oral, percutaneous, permucosal	Percutaneous, permucosal	Percutaneous, permucosal
Incubation	15–50 days	45–180 days	14–182 days	1–26 days	2–3 months	4–11 days
Chronic infection	No	Yes	Yes	Yes	Yes	Yes

HSV, herpes simplex virus; HPV, human papilloma virus; HIV, human immunodeficiency virus.

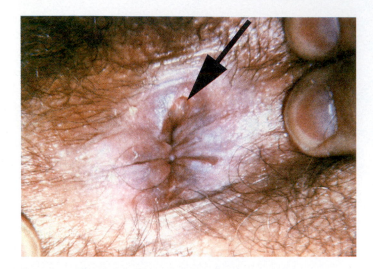

■ **FIGURE 36-5** A primary anorectal syphilitic ulcer or chancre during the primary stage of the disease. Primary syphilis usually presents itself as a genital ulcer or chancre that is usually firm, round, small, and painless, and appears at the spot where *Treponema pallidum* spirochetes entered the recipient's body.
From Public Image Library (PHIL), CDC/Susan Lindsley, VD.

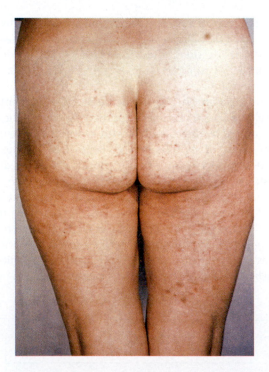

■ **FIGURE 36-6** A "roseola rash," similar to that of viral eczema, on the buttocks and legs during the secondary stage of syphilis. Secondary syphilis is the most contagious of all the stages, and is characterized by a systemic spread of the spirochete, *Treponema pallidum*. The secondary rash usually does not cause itching. It can appear as the primary chancre of syphilis is healing or even several weeks after the primary chancre has healed.
From Public Image Library (PHIL), CDC/J. Pledger, BSS/VD.

invaded at any time, causing neurosyphilis. There has been an increase in the cases of syphilis, particularly among men who have sex with men. An increase in high-risk behaviors appear to correlate with this increase in syphilis (LaFond & Lukehart, 2006). ∞ Chapter 25 provides additional information on spirochetes.

Lymphogranuloma venereum (LGV) is an STD caused by specific serovars of *Chlamydia trachomatis*. The lesion can be self-limited and disappear prior to a physician's exam. Swollen lymph nodes may be the only symptom. LGV is rare in the United States and is most commonly found in men who have sex with men. **Proctocolitis** or inflammation of the rectum may result from anal sex and often accompanies the lesion. Lympogranuloma venereum can be an invasive systemic disease if not treated early. Coinfection with other STD microorganisms or secondary infections can occur.

Granuloma inguinale, or donovanosis, is another STD that is rare. Most cases are acquired outside the United States. *Klebsiella granulomatis* (formerly known as *Calymmatobacterium granulomatis*) causes this disease. It is characterized by intracellular organism inclusions called Donovan bodies. Granuloma inguinale is endemic in some tropical and developing countries such as New Guinea, India, Papua, and southern Africa (CDC, 2006c).

> ✓ **Checkpoint! 36–4 (Chapter Objective 3)**
>
> *The etiological agent of chancroid is:*
>   A. *Candida albicans.*
>   B. *Klebsiella granulomatis.*
>   C. *Haemophilus ducreyi.*
>   D. *Treponema pallidum.*

Diseases with Cervicitis or Urethritis

Inflammation of the urethra with a purulent discharge (Figure 36-7) and painful urination is suspicious for urethritis. The most common cause is *Neisseria gonorrhoeae* or *Chlamydia trachomatis*. *Ureaplasma urealyticum* and *Mycoplasma genitalium* have also been implicated but are difficult to detect in the clinical laboratory. *Trichomonas vaginalis,* HSV, and adenovirus may also cause nongonococcal urethritis.

The signs and symptoms of cervicitis include purulent discharge and/or bleeding not associated with the menstrual cycle. The most likely cause is *N. gonorrhoeae* or *C. trachomatis*. Females infected with chlamydiae and gonorrhea may be asymptomatic or have mild symptoms. If untreated, they are a source of infection to sexual partners. They may also develop infertility or pelvic inflammatory disease (PID) (Forbes et al., 2007). PID is discussed later in this chapter.

Women with cervicitis should also be evaluated for *Trichomonas* and bacterial vaginosis. *Mycoplasma genitalium* may also cause cervicitis but is difficult to detect. Nonmicrobial causes of cervicitis exist such as excessive douching and exposure to chemicals.

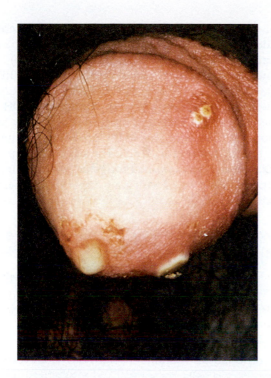

■ **FIGURE 36-7** A purulent penile discharge due to gonorrhea. *From Public Image Library (PHIL), CDC.*

infertility. In a small percentage of cases the organism disseminates and becomes systemic to cause sepsis or arthritis. The U.S. Preventative Health Task Force recommends routine screening of high-risk populations. Women under the age of 25, those with previously diagnosed STDs, new or multiple sex partners, drug use, and prostitutes should be screened. Refer to ∞ Chapter 18, "Aerobic Gram-Negative Cocci," for more information on *N. gonorrhoeae*.

Many gonorrhea infections are coinfected with chlamydiae. The task force recommends treatment for both gonorrhea and chlamydiae be prescribed (CDC, 2006c).

> ✓ **Checkpoint! 36–5 (Chapter Objective 4)**
>
> *Which organism(s) associated with urethritis or cervicitis can result in an asymptomatic infection in male or females?*
> 1. *Neisseria gonorrhoeae*
> 2. *Chlamydia trachomatis*
> 3. *Treponema pallidum*
>   A. 1 only
>   B. 2 only
>   C. 2 and 3
>   D. 1, 2, and 3

CHLAMYDIOSIS

Chlamydiosis is the most frequently reported sexually transmitted disease in the United States, especially in those less than 25 years of age. This disease is caused by an intracellular microbe, *Chlamydia trachomatis*. Both males and females can be asymptomatic, resulting in potential transmission to unsuspecting sexual partners, reinfection, and complications due to lack of treatment.

Epididymitis, prostatitis, and Reiter's syndrome (a reactive arthritis, conjunctivitis, and urethritis that follows gastrointestinal or genitourinary infection) can be complications in men infected with chlamydiae. Complication in females includes pelvic inflammatory disease (PID), ectopic pregnancy (a pregnancy located outside the uterus), and infertility. For a review of chlamydiae, refer to ∞ Chapter 31, "Intracellular Microorganisms."

GONORRHEA

Gonorrhea is the second most common sexually transmitted disease reported in the United States. *Neisseria gonorrhoeae* attaches to the epithelial cells and invades the mucosa. Men are symptomatic and seek treatment to relieve their symptoms. Women are frequently asymptomatic and risk not only exposing their partners but also developing complications associated with an untreated infection. Infection and complications of gonorrhea are similar to those of chlamydiosis, including PID and scarring of fallopian tubes that result in

Diseases with Vaginal Discharge

Vaginal infections or **vaginitis** (Figure 36-8 ■) usually result in a discharge, vaginal itching, and sometimes an odor. The two STDs associated with vaginal discharge include bacterial **vaginosis** and trichomoniasis. *Candida* infections may also cause a vaginal discharge but is not considered a sexually transmitted disease. *Candida* vaginitis is discussed later in this chapter.

During the pelvic exam the physician may collect vaginal secretions and perform some bedside tests and a microscopic exam. These bedside tests include a pH test, whiff test, and saline/potassium hydroxide (KOH) wet prep exam. They are described later. Specimens may also be collected and submitted to the laboratory for diagnostic testing. Gonorrhea and chlamydiae should also be ruled out.

Trichomoniasis is caused by the parasite *Trichomonas vaginalis*. *Trichomonas* infections are frequently found with other sexually transmitted diseases, especially gonorrhea and bacterial vaginosis (Schwebke & Burgess, 2004). The abundant discharge is greenish and foamy with a strong, foul odor (Murray et al., 2003). Signs of vulvar irritation are present. Symptoms include painful urination or sexual intercourse. Twenty-five percent of women with trichomoniasis are asymptomatic (Forbes et al., 2007). Vaginal secretions usually have a pH of greater than 5 (normal pH is 3.8–4.5) (Ryan, 1994). An examination of a saline wet prep (Figure 36-9 ■) may detect the twitching motility characteristic of the flagellated parasite.

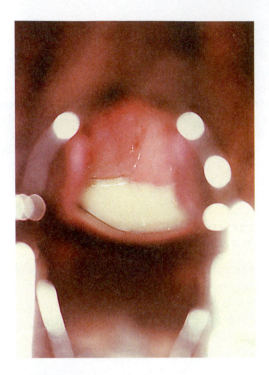

■ **FIGURE 36-8** A case of *Trichomonas* vaginitis revealing a copious purulent cervical discharge.
From Public Image Library (PHIL), CDC.

Bacterial vaginosis (BV) occurs when the commensal flora, primarily lactobacilli, is replaced by a mixture of anaerobic gram-negative rods, *Mycoplasma hominis,* and *Gardnerella vaginalis.* Occurrence of BV is also linked with douching and new or multiple sex partners. The discharge is homogeneous and yellow with a fishy odor. The discharge typically coats the vaginal wall. Bacterial vaginosis during pregnancy can lead to low birth weight, premature delivery, or fetal loss. Bacterial vagi-

nosis also appears to stimulate HIV-infected cells to enhance replication of the virus, increasing the risk of HIV transmission during sexual intercourse (Zarriffard et al., 2005).

Bedside diagnostic tests include pH and the "whiff" test. Vaginal secretions usually have a pH of 5 and a positive "whiff" test. The "whiff" test is performed by adding 10% KOH to the specimen saline wet prep and smelling for a fishy aroma. Detection of a fishy odor, due to the presence of amines, is a positive result (Murray et al., 2003). The saline wet prep (Figure 36-10 ■) can also be examined for "clue" cells. "Clue" cells are epithelial cells covered with gram-negative and gram-variable rods.

✆ REAL WORLD TIP

- *G. vaginalis* typically adhere more on the edges of the epithelial "clue" cell (Murray et al., 2003). Lactobacilli tend to be sparse and more uniformly distributed across the surface.

- Bacterial vaginosis is not characterized by a polymorphonuclear response. There are often very few white blood cells present.

- Many females carry *G. vaginalis* as part of normal vaginal flora so a culture cannot be used to diagnose bacterial vaginosis.

Vaginal secretions should be submitted to the laboratory for a Gram stain. A Gram stain of the vaginal discharge is diagnostic and preferred to culture. Criteria used in the examination of the Gram stain are discussed later in this chapter. Table 36-2 lists the diagnostic tests for vaginitis.

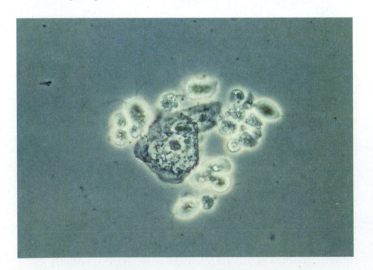

■ **FIGURE 36-9** Two large epithelial cells and multiple *Trichomonas vaginalis* protozoa observed in a wet mount of vaginal discharge using phase contrast microscopy.
From Public Image Library (PHIL), CDC.

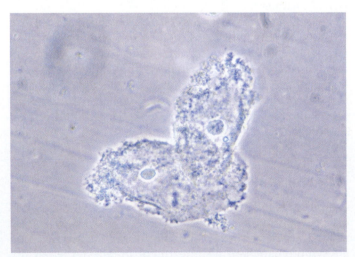

■ **FIGURE 36-10** Wet mount of vaginal discharge showing bacteria adhering to vaginal epithelial cells known as "clue cells." The presence of such clue cells is a sign that the patient has bacterial vaginosis.
From Public Image Library (PHIL), CDC/M. Rein.

✓ Checkpoint! 36–6 (Chapter Objective 5)

Bacterial vaginosis is best diagnosed with:
  A. *culture.*
  B. *"sneeze" test.*
  C. *Gram stain.*
  D. *serology.*

✓ Checkpoint! 36–7 (Chapter Objective 3)

The organism associated with genital warts is:
  A. *Human papilloma virus*
  B. *Human immunodeficiency virus*
  C. *Herpes simplex virus*
  D. *Human cervical virus*

Diseases with Genital Warts

Genital warts (Figure 36-11 ■) occur with human papilloma virus (HPV) and syphilis. Syphilis has already been discussed in a previous section describing diseases with genital ulcers.

Human papilloma virus infection is thought to be the most common STD in the United States, but it is not reportable to the CDC. Transmission is via skin-to-skin contact. See Table 36-3 to compare HPV with other sexually transmitted viruses. The more sexual partners one has and their sexual history increases the risk of acquiring this virus. The majority of genital infections associated with HPV are asymptomatic and self-limited. Some types of HPV can cause genital warts and cervical cell dysplasia. Persistent infections with these high-risk HPV types are associated with cervical cancer (CDC, 2006c). Vaccination may prevent HPV infection and cervical cancer in the future.

The presence of genital warts is sufficient evidence of HPV infection. No laboratory tests are required. Recurrence of genital warts may occur during the first few months after treatment. Not everyone exposed to the HPV virus develop genital warts. The immune system function of individuals is assumed to play a role (CDC, 2006c).

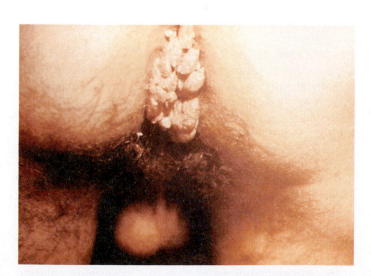

■ **FIGURE 36-11** Venereal or genital warts in the anal region of the perineum. Genital warts is a sexually transmitted disease caused by the human papilloma virus (HPV), which appears as bumps or warts on the genitalia or within the perineal region. *From Public Image Library (PHIL), CDC/Dr. Wiesner Phil.*

Pelvic Inflammatory Disease (PID)

Inflammation of the upper reproductive structures of women is called pelvic inflammatory disease, or PID. PID may result in **endometritis** or inflammation of the uterine lining, and **salpingitis** or inflammation of the uterine tubes, and/or pelvic abscess (Forbes et al., 2007). The main symptom of PID is abdominal pain. A **mucopurulent** discharge consisting of pus and mucus and microscopic observation of white blood cells is common in the majority of cases. An aspirate taken via an abdominal laparoscopy may be necessary.

N. gonorrhoeae and *C. trachomatis* can cause salpingitis. Cytomegalovirus (CMV), *Mycoplasma hominis, Ureaplasma urealyticum,* and *M. genitalium* have also been implicated in pelvic inflammatory disease (CDC, 2006c). Other organisms that may be members of the commensal flora can also be associated with this disease. *Enterobacteriaceae,* groups A and B streptococci, enterococci, and mixed anaerobes are associated with endometritis. Mixed aerobic and anaerobic flora can be isolated from a pelvic abscess. *Actinomyces* spp. can cause PID in women with intrauterine devices (IUDs) (Murray et al., 2003). See ∞ Chapter 24 to review *Actinomyces*.

Laboratory tests to rule out sexually transmitted organisms are recommended. In the absence of a STD, pelvic inflammatory disease is diagnosed clinically. The IUD may be submitted for anaerobic culture. Predominant growth or a pure culture of an anaerobe is usually clinically significant (Koneman, Allen, Janda, Schreckenberger, & Winn, 1997).

Epididymitis

Epididymitis or inflammation of the epididymis can be a chronic or acute condition. Sexually transmitted disease typically results in acute epididymitis. Acute epididymitis is characterized by symptoms of scrotal pain, inflammation, and swelling of less than 6 weeks duration (CDC, 2006c). *N. gonorrheae* and *C. trachomatis* are the most common culprits. Enteric bacteria such as *E. coli* and intestinal protozoa may be transmitted to the epididymis as a result of anal sex. Oral–genital sex may result in colonization or infection by *N. meningitidis.* Viruses, such as CMV, HIV and hepatitis, found in blood or secretions may be transmitted through sexual contact (Forbes et al., 2007). Laboratory tests to identify the presence of *N. gonorrheae, C. trachomatis,* and enteric bacteria are performed to identify the causative agent and guide treatment decisions.

HIV Infection or Acquired Immune Deficiency Syndrome

HIV infections or acquired immune deficiency syndrome (AIDS) is a systemic illness caused by the human immunodeficiency virus (HIV). Early HIV infections are asymptomatic but can progress to AIDS within months or up to 17 years if untreated (CDC, 2006b). The presence of lesions on the genitalia increases the risk of acquiring the virus from a HIV-infected sexual partner (Mandell et al., 2005). Individuals being evaluated for sexually transmitted diseases should be tested for HIV.

Transmission of the virus is through sexual contact and exposure to blood and other body fluids. Table 36-3 provides an overview of sexually transmitted viruses. HIV infection results in severe immunodeficiency that makes the individual more susceptible to opportunistic infections and rare cancers. The virus attacks a specific kind of lymphocyte, the CD4-positive, helper T lymphocyte. As the numbers of the CD4 T lymphocyte declines, immune system function declines, the viral load rises, and an individual's risk of acquiring an opportunistic infection or malignancy increases. Other CD4 positive cells such as macrophages and dendritic cells may be attacked as well (Scosyrev, 2006). Review the role that T lymphocytes play in defending the host from foreign invaders in ∞ Chapter 4, "The Host's Encounter with Microbes."

The disease process can vary from asymptomatic to severe, life-threatening infections or cancers. The acute or primary infection can be asymptomatic, present with persistent enlarged lymph nodes, or present with flu-like symptoms. During this stage the number of viruses in the blood or viral load increase as the CD4 lymphocyte counts decrease. When the patient's antibody response begins to control the HIV virus, CD4 lymphocyte counts increase and the viral load decreases. This results in a period of clinical latency where the virus is present in the body, but the patient is asymptomatic. This period of clinical latency or chronic HIV infection can last several years and is accompanied by a gradual decrease in the CD4 T lymphocyte count and an increase in the viral load (Scosyrev, 2006). Without treatment, most individuals will progress to AIDS. Even with treatment a patient may develop resistance to the drugs or their immune system function may decline, resulting in an increase in viral load and a decrease in the CD4 lymphocyte count. Acquired immune deficiency syndrome (AIDS) occurs when the patient develops one or more AIDS-defining conditions (rare cancer or infection) or the CD4 lymphocyte level is too low, less than 200 cells/μL. The consequence is recurring infections, debilitating illness, and ultimately death (CDC, 1992).

Signs and symptoms include fever, malaise, lymphadenopathy, and skin rash (CDC, 2006). Laboratory evaluation begins with an HIV antibody test. HIV-1 is the most common culprit, but HIV-2 should be evaluated if the patient's history includes travel to West Africa, blood transfusion or injection while in this country, or intimate contact with someone from West Africa (CDC, 2006b). If the HIV-1 antibody test is positive, supplemental testing by Western blot or immunofluorescence assay must be performed to confirm the positive result. If the HIV-1 antibody test is negative, nucleic acid tests for viral RNA should be performed to detect an early infection. Confirmatory testing should be performed 2–4 months after the initial negative antibody result (Department of Health and Human Services, 2007).

If a patient is HIV positive, additional testing is recommended. The patient should be screened for other sexually transmitted diseases such as syphilis, gonorrhea, and chlamydiae. Tests to detect antibodies against *Toxoplasma gondii,* an opportunistic parasite, should be performed. The patient's CD4 T-lymphocyte count and HIV viral load should be documented. Tests for the presence of antibodies to Hepatitis A, B, and C are recommended if contemplating vaccination for Hepatitis A and B. Other laboratory tests include a complete blood count (CBC), chemistry profile, and urinalysis. Additional diagnostic procedures usually include a PPD tuberculin skin test for exposure to *Mycobacterium tuberculosis* and chest X-ray (CDC, 2006). ∞ Chapter 31, "Intracellular Microorganisms," provides additional information on HIV.

Checkpoint! 36–8 (Chapter Objective 4)

Human immunodeficiency virus is transmitted:

1. *Percutaneous*
2. *Permucosal*
3. *Fecal–oral*
    A. *1 only*
    B. *2 only*
    C. *3 only*
    D. *1 and 2*

Hepatitis A, B, and C

Hepatitis, the inflammation of the liver, can be caused by the sexually acquired hepatitis viruses A, B, and C. Hepatitis A virus (HAV) is acquired by oral–anal contact. Men who have sex with men are at higher risk of acquiring HAV. The symptoms include jaundice, fatigue, abdominal pain, loss of appetite, nausea, diarrhea, and fever (CDC, 2007a). The age of the patient correlates with the appearance of clinical symptoms. Children under the age of 6 are usually asymptomatic. Older children and adults have symptoms and jaundice. Most cases are self-limited with a small percentage of patients developing fulminant hepatitis (Nainan, Xia, Vaughan, & Margolis, 2006).

Hepatitis B virus (HBV) results in **jaundice**, or a yellowing of the skin and conjunctiva; "flu-like" symptoms; enlarged liver; dark urine; and clay-colored stool. Hepatitis C virus (HCV) can be transmitted via sexual contact, but not as well as A or B. Exposure to infected blood is the most effective route (CDC, 2006a). Most patients (80%) infected with HCV are asymptomatic. Those with symptoms display jaundice, fatigue, dark urine, abdominal pain, loss of appetite, and nausea (CDC, 2005a). It is important for an HIV-infected person to know whether they are also infected with hepatitis C. Hepatitis C infections are usually worse in HIV-positive patients, quickly leading to liver damage. Highly active antiretroviral therapy (HAART) may also be affected by coinfection with HAV (CDC, 2005a). Table 36-3 provides an overview of sexually transmitted viruses.

Sexually transmitted disease due to Hepatitis A or B can be prevented by vaccination. Anyone evaluated or treated for an STD should receive a Hepatitis B vaccination. Those who are illicit drug users or men who have sex with men should be vaccinated for Hepatitis A (CDC, 2006a). Hepatitis C may be transmitted sexually. The risk is higher among illicit drug users (CDC, 2006a). There is no vaccine currently available for Hepatitis C.

Serological tests are used to diagnose hepatitis. See ∞ Chapter 31, "Intracellular Microorganisms," for a detailed explanation of a viral hepatitis panel. The presence of IgM antibodies to HAV indicates infection. Serological testing for HBV surface antigen (HBsAG) and core antibody (HBc) are necessary. The presence of Hepatitis B surface antigen and IgM core antibody is characteristic of an acute infection. A positive result for HBV surface antigen and total antibody but a negative result for IgM antibody is indicative of a chronic infection. Other reactions indicate recovery or false-positive results that need to be investigated further. Positive HCV antibody tests would be diagnostic of HCV infection. Those patients positive for chronic HBV or HAV should be evaluated for chronic liver disease. An elevated value for alanine aminotransferase (ALT), a chemistry analyte, is associated with chronic liver disease (CDC, 2006a).

 ## Checkpoint! 36–9 (Chapter Objective 9)

A male homosexual visits a clinic complaining of "flu-like" symptoms. His physician notices his patient's conjunctiva is yellow in color. Laboratory tests reveal a positive anti-HAV IgM and negative HBsAG, anti-HBc IgM, and anti-HCV. This patient has:

A. HIV.
B. HAV.
C. HBV.
D. HCV.

INFECTIONS ASSOCIATED WITH PREGNANCY

Infections associated with pregnancy include infectious or colonizing organisms of the mother that can be passed on to the baby. Infections of the baby can occur during the gestation period, birthing, or after birth. Susceptibility to infection is due to the fetal immune system not being fully developed.

The primary defenses of the fetus include the physical barrier provided by the amniotic membrane and maternal immunity shared via the placenta. The mother's cell mediated immunity is suppressed during pregnancy to avoid rejection of the fetus (Ryan, 1994).

Prenatal infections occur in the womb prior to birth. The organisms may infect the placenta via the bloodstream or cross the placenta, infecting the amniotic fluid that is normally swallowed and inhaled by the fetus. *Listeria monocytogenes,* syphilis, *Toxoplasma gondii,* and viruses such as HIV, HSV, cytomegalovirus (CMV), and rubella virus have this route of infection (Forbes et al., 2007). Organisms may also ascend or climb up from the mother's genital tract to infect the fetus. Torn or ruptured membranes can facilitate this invasion. Group B streptococci, *E. coli, L. monocytogenes, Chlamydia trachomatis, Mycoplasma* spp., *Ureaplasma urealyticum,* and viruses like herpes simplex virus or CMV invade in this way (Murray et al., 2003).

Natal infections are infections that occur as a result of exposure to organisms during the birthing process. The baby picks up the microbes from the mother's vagina. The pathogens enter the baby through their eyes, nose, mouth, and ears. These pathogens include group B streptococci, *E. coli, L. monocytogenes, Chlamydia trachomatis, N. gonorrheae,* and viruses such as herpes simplex virus, HIV, HBV, or CMV. The term congenital is used for infections that occur before or at birth (Ryan, 1994).

Postnatal infections are those that occur after birth. If the infection in the infant occurs during the first 4 weeks of life, it is called a neonatal infection. The pathogens may be acquired through the placenta by upward movement from the mother's genital tract or at birth from the vaginal canal. Pathogens may also be obtained from the nursery environment such as medical devices and water, health care workers, and visitors. In addition to the microbes previously mentioned, *Elizabethkingia meningoseptica* (previously known as *Chryseobacterium meningosepticum*), other gram-negative rods, and viruses such as respiratory syncytial virus can be etiological agents. *Trichomonas vaginalis* has caused neonatal pneumonia (Murray et al., 2003). Refer to ∞ Chapter 22, "Nonfermenting Gram-Negative Rods," to review the characteristics of *E. meningoseptica.*

Infection of the baby can result in birth defects, stillbirth, or a chronic lifelong infection such as seen with HIV or herpes simplex. The infection in the baby can also result in an immediate life-threatening illness. The agents of neonatal sepsis enter the baby via the body openings during birth and establish a focal infection in the sinuses, middle ear, lungs, and gastrointestinal tract. The microbes typically spread to the bloodstream, infecting meninges, kidneys, bones and joints, peritoneum, and skin. Infectious diseases include pneumonia, arthritis, osteomyelitis, septicemia, and meningitis. The infectious agent is often isolated from blood, cerebrospinal fluid, and urine. The baby exhibits nonspecific symptoms such as decreased sucking and activity; respiratory distress, jaundice, vomiting, or diarrhea; abdominal distension; and hyper- or hypothermia. Refer to ∞ Chapter 7, "Cultivation of Microorganisms," for more information on processing samples from these body sites.

The baby can acquire cutaneous and subcutaneous skin infections. Of greatest concern is *S. aureus*. Its exotoxin can cause scalded skin syndrome. Occasionally gram-negative rods are implicated (Ryan, 1994). Refer to ∞ Chapter 37 for more information on infections of the integumentary system.

Listeriosis is caused by *Listeria monocytogenes*. It is associated with ingestion of contaminated food. The mother eats food containing *Listeria,* usually found in soft cheeses, smoked fish, salad, or sausage. The organism crosses the intestinal wall, enters the bloodstream, and multiplies in the liver. The normal immune system suppression associated with pregnancy plays a role in the organism's ability to survive, gain access to the bloodstream, and cross the placenta, causing infection of the fetal membranes and amniotic fluid. The mother is asymptomatic or exhibits mild "flu-like" symptoms. The baby can be stillborn, or develop an acute, life-threatening neonatal infection such as meningitis, gastroenteritis, or pneumonia. The organism can be isolated from cultures of the mother's placenta and specimens collected from the baby (Vazoquez-Boland et al., 2001). More information on *Listeria* can be found in ∞ Chapter 19, "Aerobic Gram-Positive Rods."

Overall morbidity and mortality associated with group B streptococci (GBS) infections have declined as a result of the implementation of screening pregnant women for this organism, except among black infants (CDC, 2007b). GBS can colonize the vagina of women and about 5% of pregnant women are heavily colonized (Baron et al., 1993). At 35–37 weeks gestation, rectal and vaginal swabs are collected from the mother and screened for *S. agalactiae* using enrichment media. Molecular testing is now available to ensure rapid results due to the potential for harm to the baby with the organism's presence. Women with positive culture results receive antibiotics during labor to prevent perinatal disease (Baron, 2003). This offers antibiotic coverage to the baby due to the shared blood supply. Refer to ∞ Chapter 17 for more information on the virulence factors and laboratory tests used to identify *S. agalactiae.*

Once a physician rules out bacteria, chlamydiae, and syphilis as etiological agents of the baby's infection, testing should include those for the TORCH organisms. TORCH stands for **T**oxoplasmosis, **O**ther (usually Hepatitis B, HIV, enterovirus, coxsackie virus, human parvovirus, and varicella zoster virus [VZV]), **R**ubella, **C**ytomegalovirus (CMV), and **H**erpes simplex virus. Infections by these organisms are especially dangerous if acquired while in the womb. The baby may present with low birth weight, rash, jaundice, and **hepatosplenomegaly** or an enlarged liver and spleen. Clinical signs may not appear for weeks to years. Congenital infections may result in mental deterioration or retardation, hearing loss, or other birth defects (Ryan, 1994).

Serological or immunofluorescence tests, viral culture, or nucleic acid tests for the TORCH agents are performed on specimens from the pregnant woman or newborn. Physicians should request the specific viral analysis rather than an entire "TORCH" panel (Forbes et al., 2007). Tests for HSV, HIV, and hepatitis have been described in a previous section. See ∞ Chapter 31, "Intracellular Microorganisms," for specific testing information to detect rubella, CMV, VSV, enterovirus, cosackie virus, and human parvovirus.

Puerperal or postpartum infections occur in females during childbirth or immediately after birth of the baby. Bacterial vaginosis at the time of birth, premature rupture of the membranes, prolonged labor, and retained products of conception can increase the risk for infection. Endometritis, perineal cellulitis, and episiotomy (an incision in the perineum to enlarge the vagina for childbirth) infection can be serious. Infection is often noted by fever and chills, abdominal tenderness, and foul smelling lochia (postpartum vaginal discharge). Infection can be polymicrobic and include both aerobes, such as *Staphylococcus* spp., groups A and B streptococci, and *Enterobacteriaceae,* and anaerobes, such as *Bacteroides* spp.

✓ **Checkpoint! 36–10 (Chapter Objective 3)**

Elizabethkingia meningoseptica is associated with sepsis in patients located in:

    A. *the cardiac intensive care unit.*
    B. *the operating room.*
    C. *the newborn nursery.*
    D. *central supply.*

OPPORTUNISTIC INFECTIONS

Certain commensal organisms take advantage of a change in the host to cause an infection. The host change may be compromised immune function or result from antibiotic therapy or chemical exposure that upsets the ecological microbial balance in the genital system.

Candida albicans is the yeast most commonly associated with vaginal infections. Non–*C. albicans* species may also be isolated from genital specimens of symptomatic women and lead to treatment failure (Pirotta & Garland. 2006). Excessive douching or antibiotic therapy decreases the numbers of commensal flora and creates the right conditions for overgrowth by yeast. Symptoms are typical of vaginitis and include itching and discharge characteristic of vaginitis. Detection of budding yeast or pseudohyphae on a wet mount (Figure 36-12) of the vaginal secretions is diagnostic for *Candida* (Koneman et al., 1997). A fungal culture can also be performed. ∞ Chapter 14 presents information on processing fungal cultures. ∞ Chapter 29, "Medical Mycology," provides more information on *Candida* species.

Toxic shock syndrome (TSS) is caused by a toxigenic *S. aureus* or *S. pyogenes*. This infection in menstruating females is connected with tampon use. Continuous use of tampons has a higher risk than alternating tampons with pads. Patients

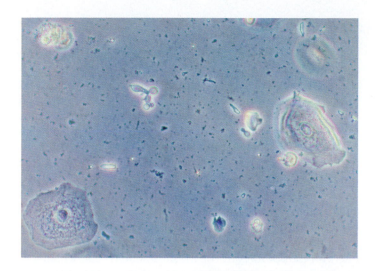

■ **FIGURE 36-12** Wet mount showing epithelial cells and *Candida albicans.*
From Public Image Library (PHIL), CDC/Dr. Stuart Brown.

in the original cases used highly absorbent tampons that are no longer available on the market. The current composition of tampons has changed to help prevent TSS. Packages are now labeled and package inserts contain a warning about TSS and encourage users to select lower absorbancy products. Cases of nonmenstrual toxic shock syndrome continue to occur (CDC, 1990). Men can develop toxic shock syndrome if infected by the toxic shock syndrome toxin (TSST) secreting *Staphylococcus aureus* or *Streptococcus pyogenes.*

▶ SPECIMEN COLLECTION

Specimen sources for sexually transmitted disease include the cervix, urethra, vagina, throat, or anus. Excess secretions should be removed and fresh discharge collected using a swab. Specimens collected for chlamydiae analysis require swab rotation so that the epithelial cell containing chlamydiae are in the sample (Koneman et al., 1997). HIV and hepatitis viruses are best detected using blood (Murray et al., 2003).

A variety of swabs need to be available for collection of specimens for sexually transmitted disease. Dacron and rayon swabs are less toxic to potential pathogens than cotton or calcium alginate swabs. Plastic shafts are less toxic than wooden shafts to potential pathogens. Smaller swabs or flexible shafts facilitate collection from pediatric patients and the urethra. Transport media should be used for specimens submitted for testing for viral, gonococcus (GC), *Chlamydia, Mycoplasma,* and *Ureaplasma* genital pathogens. GC specimens should not be refrigerated. Specimens should be collected in a manner that avoids contamination with vaginal normal flora (Murray et al., 2003).

Certain specimens should include culture for anaerobes. These include the placenta, amniotic fluid, culdocentesis fluid (fluid aspirated from the floor of the peritoneal cavity via the vagina), endometrial tissue or lochia, and an IUD. These specimen types should be submitted in anaerobic transport media. Cervical, urethral, and vaginal secretions should not be cultured anaerobically due to the presence of normal flora (Murray et al., 2003).

 REAL WORLD TIP

Swabbing the surface of a placenta for culture demonstrates a high level of vaginal flora contamination. Culture of the subchorionic fibrin layer, located just below the fetal membrane of the placenta, eliminates vaginal flora contamination and detects potential pathogens.

Lesions are rinsed with sterile saline prior to specimen collection. Any scabs present should be removed, and the **transudate**, a fluid that accumulates as a result of osmotic forces, is collected on a swab or slide. Slides examined for the causative agent of syphilis, *T. pallidum,* should be cover-slipped and transported to the laboratory in a petri dish with damp gauze.

Screening pregnant women for group B streptococci requires collection of vaginal and rectal swabs at 35–37 weeks' gestation (CDC, 2007b). See ∞ Chapter 6 for more information on specimen collection.

REAL WORLD TIP

Individuals with PID, endometritis, and disseminated gonorrhea should have blood cultures done in addition to culture of the origin of infection.

▶ DIRECT GRAM STAIN OF SPECIMEN

Urethral specimens from symptomatic males suspected of having gonorrhea should have a direct Gram stain performed on the exudate. Observation of polymorphonuclear leukocytes and intracellular, gram-negative "kidney bean"–shaped diplococci is diagnostic for gonorrhea in males. Go to ∞ Chapter 18, "Aerobic Gram-Negative Cocci," to view a positive Gram stain for gonorrhea. The direct Gram stain is not as sensitive for symptomatic females, due to the presence of other organisms that can mimic *N. gonorrhoeae,* and should be confirmed by culture. The direct Gram stain has very low sensitivity and specificity for asymptomatic females. Other genital specimens, other than those for group B streptococci, submitted for culture should have a direct Gram stain of the specimen performed (Murray et al., 2003).

▶ SETUP AND INCUBATION OF CULTURES

There are two approaches to processing genital cultures. The first approach is to process by specimen source as a routine culture. The second approach is by specific organism. An organism-specific culture request is a more focused and cost-effective approach to achieving diagnosis.

A routine vaginal culture should be performed if the individual is a premenstrual female. For an adult, a list of potentially pathogenic organisms should be provided to the physician for selection. *Listeria* should not be included on the list or routinely looked for in an adult vaginal culture (Schreckenberger, 2003). Specimens appropriate for culture of *Listeria monocytogenes* include the placenta or amniotic fluid.

It is important to distinguish vaginal pathogens from endocervical pathogens. Vaginal pathogens include *Trichomonas vaginalis,* group B streptococci, *Staphylococcus aureus, Candida,* and agents of bacterial vaginosis. Endocervical pathogens include *N. gonorrhoeae* and *C. trachomatis* (Schreckenberger, 2003). *S. aureus* should be cultured when toxic shock syndrome is suspected. Not all potential pathogens are diagnosed by culture. See Table 36-2 for a list of the diagnostic tests used to detect sexually transmitted diseases. Nucleic acid testing, immunological tests, Gram stain, and microscopic examination of wet preps may be better choices than culture to detect certain viruses, *Chlamydia,* syphilis, *Trichomonas,* and bacterial vaginosis.

CULTIVATION

The primary culture medium selected for each specimen source takes into account the presence of commensal flora and the potential pathogen. Vaginal or cervical specimens are inoculated onto sheep blood agar (BA) and a selective agar for gonorrhea such as Thayer-Martin (TM). Specimens collected from the urethra or penis are inoculated onto Thayer-Martin. Other genital tract specimens are inoculated onto sheep blood agar, MacConkey (MAC), chocolate agar (CA), and selective agar for gonorrhea and anaerobic culture media. Tissue submitted for culture should be inoculated using thioglycolate broth, BA, MAC, CA, and anaerobic culture media (Murray et al., 2003). Blood agar and chocolate agar must be incubated in carbon dioxide (CO_2) at 35–37°C. MacConkey can be incubated in ambient air at 35–37°C.

If the targeted or specified organism approach is used, the appropriate medium for recovery of the pathogen is inoculated. *N. gonorrhoeae* can be detected by culture or nucleic acid testing. Nucleic acid testing has the advantage of enabling the detection of chlamydiae as well as gonorrhea. If gonorrhea is suspected in a child or culture for GC is requested, then selective medium for *N. gonorrhoeae* such as Thayer-Martin should be inoculated with the specimen. Best results are obtained by inoculating the specimen on media at the patient's bedside and immediately incubate. Transgrow bottles (Figure 36-13 ■) and the JEMBEC system (Figure 36-14 ■) are available for use in doctor's offices and clinics. These systems contain selective media for gonorrhea and provide the required CO_2 atmosphere for transportation. The medium should be inoculated in a "Z" or "M" pattern to ensure adequate transfer of the specimen and increase the amount of inoculum on the agar surface. Finally, the medium is struck for isolation, transported to the clinical laboratory, and incubated at 35–37°C.

Screening for group B streptococci colonization is accomplished by inoculating the specimen into selective broth medium such as LIM or carrot broth. After incubation, the broth is subcultured to sheep blood agar for further examination (CDC, 2007). More information on screening for GBS can be found in ∞ Chapter 17, "Aerobic Gram-Positive Cocci."

Culture for *H. ducreyi* is accomplished by inoculating the specimen onto chocolate agar with 3 µg/mL of vancomycin.

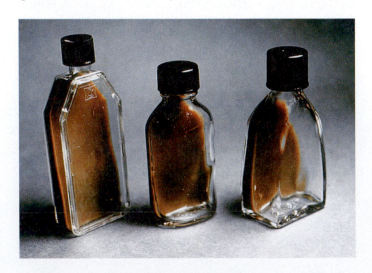

■ **FIGURE 36-13** Transgrow medium used to transport a specimen for *N. gonorrhoeae* to the laboratory for testing.
From Public Image Library (PHIL), CDC/Dr. A. Schroeter.

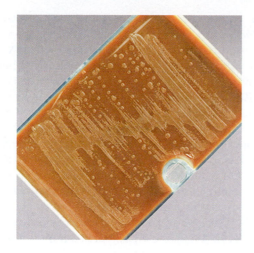

■ **FIGURE 36-14** JEMBEC transport system with Thayer-Martin media growing *N. gonorrhoeae*.
Photo courtesy of Remel, part of Thermo Fisher Scientific.

✓ **Checkpoint! 36–11 (Chapter Objective 6)**

It is recommended that swab specimens for GC only should be struck on the surface of the medium in a Z pattern in order to:

A. *honor the discoverer of gonorrhea.*
B. *indicate the presence of the specimen.*
C. *increase the inoculum.*
D. *zero in on specimen placement.*

Vancomycin disks can also be placed on the surface of the chocolate agar medium in different quadrants (Koneman et al., 1997). Incubation of the media is in CO_2 at 37°C. A Gram-stained direct smear of the specimen (Figure 36-15 ■) should be examined for tiny gram-negative rods that look like a "school of fish" (Murray et al., 2003).

Fungal media such as sabouraud's or CHROMagar Candida (CAC) can be used to grow *Candida* if the KOH preparation is negative. *Candida* will grow on blood agar but may require 48 hours incubation.

Specimens collected for targeted viral pathogens should be processed for culture, nucleic acid testing and immunofluo-rescent or serological testing as appropriate. See Table 36-2 for specific information on testing for each virus.

▶ **INTERPRETATION OF CULTURES**

A routine genital culture, processed for clinically significant pathogens, is a more challenging task than analyzing growth for a physician-specified organism. *H. ducreyi, N. gonorrheae,* group B streptococci (in pregnant females), *T. vaginalis, T. pallidum,* and *C. trachomatis* are always considered pathogens. In certain situations *S. aureus,* beta-hemolytic streptococci, yeast, *Enterobacteriaceae,* and anaerobes may be clinically significant when isolated as the predominant organism. *L. monocytogenes* should be considered when processing tissue obtained from a stillborn fetus or placenta (Murray et al., 2003).

One must use the Gram stain results, source of specimen, and amount of growth compared to the commensal flora to aid in determining the clinical significance. Input from the patient's physician may also be needed. Usually an organism isolated from a sterile specimen source or a predominant growth accompanied by the presence of segmented neu-trophils should be identified and reported (Murray et al., 2003). Some of the genital system pathogens are designated as reportable diseases at a national level. Each individual state may also require notification when detected in a patient specimen. See Box 36-1✪ for a more specific list of national reportable genital system disease.

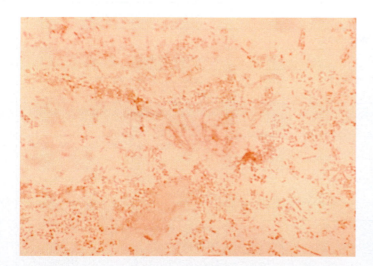

■ **FIGURE 36-15** *Haemophilus ducreyi* in a direct smear indicating a chancroid infection.
From Public Image Library (PHIL), CDC/Joe Miller, Dr. N. J. Fiumara.

✪ **BOX 36-1**

National-Level Reportable Genital Diseases

Acquired immunodeficiency syndrome (AIDS)
Chancroid
Chlamydia trachomatis
Gonorrhea
Hepatitis A
Hepatitis B
Hepatitis C
Human immunodeficiency virus (HIV)
Listeriosis
Streptococcal toxic shock syndrome
Toxic shock syndrome (not streptococcal)

EXAMINATION OF GROWTH

When analyzing a routine genital culture, the pattern of growth on the media is an important clue to the identity of the organism. Gram stain morphology, colony morphology, and screening tests enable a presumptive identification. Additional biochemical tests are performed to identify the isolate. See Table 36-4✪ for a summary of key observations and results.

If growth occurs only on the chocolate agar (CA), one would suspect a more fastidious organism such as *N. gonorrheae* or *H. ducreyi*. *N. gonorrhoeae* will also grow on media selective for pathogenic *Neisseria* spp. such as Thayer-Martin. Grayish, translucent colonies should be screened with oxidase. An oxidase-positive colony should be Gram stained to confirm the presence of gram-negative diplococci characteristic of gonorrhea. Testing for sugar utilization, enzyme production, or a nucleic acid probe will confirm the identity of *N. gonorrhoeae*. *N. gonorrhoeae* is glucose positive only and positive for the prolylaminopeptidase enzyme. If the specimen source is a throat, a nutrient agar incubated at 35–37°C in CO_2 and a CA at room temperature should be used to rule out *Neisseria* that are commensal flora in the upper respiratory tract. Commensal flora should grow while gonococcus will not. See ∞ Chapter 19 for more information on *N. gonorrhoeae*.

REAL WORLD TIP

One cannot assume growth on Thayer-Martin agar is *Neisseria gonorrhoeae. N. meningitidis, N. lactamica,* and *Neisseria lactamica* can also grow on TM.

If the colony Gram stain reveals gram-negative rods, *Haemophilus ducreyi* is a rare possibility. Small, adherent, gray, yellow, or tan colonies after 2–4 days are typical (Murray et al., 2003; Koneman et al., 1997). Observation of hemolysis requires use of human blood Tween agar. *H. ducreyi* is also oxidase positive but only with tetramethyl-p-phenylenediamine (Murray et al., 2003). The catalase test will be negative for this organism. Identification is confirmed with a porphyrin test, carbohydrate fermentation, nitrate test, or commercial identification kits. *H. ducreyi* is fastidious so the porphyrin test is preferred over X and V strips. This microbe is also negative for most biochemical tests except nitrate. A negative nitrate result may be observed in commercial kits (Murray et al., 2003). *H. ducreyi* is sensitive to sodium polyanethol sulfonate (SPS) (Koneman et al., 1997). See ∞ Chapter 20 for more information on *H. ducreyi.*

If a white or yellow hemolytic colony grows on blood and chocolate agars, but not MacConkey agar, suspect *Staphylococcus* spp. *Staphylococcus* is a gram-positive coccus in clusters that is catalase positive. A slide or latex agglutination coagulase test should be performed. The potential pathogen *S. aureus* is coagulase positive. Consult a physician to determine whether toxic shock syndrome is a possible diagnosis and sensitivity testing is warranted. See ∞ Chapter 17 for more information on *Staphylococcus aureus.*

If a small, gray colony with or without a narrow zone of beta-hemolysis grows on blood agar and chocolate agar but not MacConkey agar, one should consider a possible group B streptococci or *Listeria monocytogenes*. A catalase test and Gram stain will differentiate the two organisms. Group B streptococci are catalase-negative, gram-positive cocci. *Listeria* is a

✪ TABLE 36-4

Identification of Cultivated Bacterial Genital Tract Pathogens

Pathogen	Microscopic Morphology	Colony Morphology			Identification Tests
		BA	CA	MAC	
Neisseria gonorrhoeae	Gram-negative diplococci	NG	Small gray, translucent, convex, "sticky"	NG	Oxidase, GS, sugars, enzyme, or nucleic acid probe
Candida albicans	Gram-positive, budding yeast	Creamy, white, "feet"	*	NG	Germ tube and chlamydoconidia production, morphology on agar
Streptococcus agalactiae	Gram-positive cocci in chains	Small, gray-white, subtle beta hemolysis	*	NG	GS, catalase, B serotyping, hippurate, CAMP
Haemophilus ducreyi	Tiny, gram-negative bacilli, "school of fish"	NG	Tiny grayish	NG	GS, oxidase, catalase, porphyrin, commercial identification systems
Enterobacteriaceae	Gram-negative bacilli	Large, wet, gray	*	LF or NLF	Oxidase, gram-negative identification panel
Staphylococcus aureus	Gram-positive cocci, clusters	Large, yellow or white, beta hemolysis	*	NG	Catalase, slide or latex agglutination, coagulase
Listeria monocytogenes	Small, gram-positive rod	Small, gray, subtle beta hemolysis	*	NG	GS, catalase, esculin hydrolysis, RT motility

*, growth same as BA; NG, no growth; GS, Gram stain; LF, lactose fermenting; NLF, nonlactose fermenting; RT, room temperature.

catalase-positive, gram-positive rod. Group B streptococci are positive for the group B antigen whereas *Listeria* can react with groups B and G antisera. Both organisms are positive with hippurate and CAMP. The positive CAMP reaction for each organism has a different appearance. Group B streptococci have an arrow-shaped area of enhanced hemolysis whereas *Listeria* looks like a shovel. If *Listeria* is isolated, the physician should be consulted to determine significance and whether further testing is necessary. The tumbling motility of *Listeria monocytogenes* can be demonstrated by wet mount or inoculating motility medium and incubating at room temperature. An open umbrella or Christmas tree pattern appears in the motility medium if positive. See ∞ Chapters 17 and 19 to review group B streptococci and *Listeria monocytogenes*.

Enterobacteriaceae can be normal flora in the female genital tract but may be significant when isolated from male specimens. These gram-negative rods will grow as large, gray beta or nonhemolytic colonies on blood agar and chocolate agar. Growth on MacConkey agar will be lactose or nonlactose fermenting depending on the species. An oxidase test and gram-negative identification panel will provide the genus and species. Refer to ∞ Chapters 21 and 22 for more information on the identification of gram-negative rods.

If a creamy white or tan colony grows on BA or SAB after 24–48 hours incubation, one would suspect yeast. Sometimes the colony will have tiny extensions around the margin of the colony, giving an appearance of "feet" or "fringe." These "feet" indicate the presence of pseudohyphae and should not be used for germ tube testing (Murray et al., 2003). CHROMagar, a chromogenic agar, differentiates yeast species by color and colony characteristics. *C. albicans* appears green with smooth colonies on CHROMagar. Consult the manufacturer for specific colony appearances associated with *Candida* species on their medium.

Microscopically yeast appears as an oval, budding cell. Yeast usually stains gram positive. The presence of germ tubes presumptively identifies *Candida albicans*. *Candida albicans* also has pseudohyphae and single chlamydoconidia. *C. dubliniensis* is also germ tube, pseudohyphae, and chlamydoconidia positive but will not grow at 45°C whereas *C. albicans* will grow at this temperature. *C. glabrata* appear as small, budding yeast without pseudohyphae. *C. glabrata* is a germ tube negative, rapid trehalose positive yeast (Fenn, 2007). See ∞ Chapter 14, "Fungal Cultures," and ∞ Chapter 29, "Medical Mycology," for more information on the identification of yeast.

 REAL WORLD TIP

Candida tropicalis produce pseudohyphae so it is important to not call the germ tube test positive unless the typical morphology is observed. A germ tube will not have an indentation prior to the thin, narrow tube. Pseudohyphae are thicker, with an indentation.

An anaerobic microorganism should be suspected if the direct Gram stain of the specimen reveals an organism that does not grow on the primary media incubated in air or carbon dioxide. See ∞ Chapter 24 for more information about anaerobic bacteria associated with genital tract infections.

Mycoplasma, Ureaplasma, and viral pathogens require special culture techniques for isolation. They do not usually grow on the primary media under the conditions and time constraints routinely used to cultivate bacterial pathogens. See ∞ Chapter 28 for more information on the cultivation and identification of *Mycoplasma* and *Ureaplasma*.

 REAL WORLD TIP

If *Neisseria gonorrhoeae* is isolated from a child, the organism must be identified by two different methodologies. The isolation of *N. gonorrhoeae* from a child suggests sexual abuse and the results could potentially be used in court.

Serological testing results for hepatitis are described in this chapter and ∞ Chapter 31. See ∞ Chapter 10 for more information on the application of serological testing to diagnose infectious disease.

SUSCEPTIBILITY TESTS

Most sexually transmitted diseases are treated **empirically**, based on practical knowledge rather then scientific evidence. Susceptibility testing should be performed if treatment fails or a clinically significant isolate does not have a predictable sensitivity pattern. Gram negative rods and *S. aureus* require routine susceptibility testing. Some potential pathogens, like *N. gonorrhoeae*, require special conditions and media for accurate testing. Some cannot be tested using standardized procedures due to the lack of Clinical Laboratory Standards Institute (CLSI) interpretation guidelines.

Antibiograms are another clue as to the identity of the isolate. The following antibiogram pattern is suspect and the isolate should

✓ Checkpoint! 36–12 (Chapter Objective 7)

Mrs. Smith visited her physician complaining of "flu-like" symptoms. Upon physical examination, her fetus appeared to be "in distress." An amniotic fluid specimen was collected and submitted to the lab for culture. The culture grew gray colonies with a narrow zone of beta hemolysis after overnight incubation. One should perform a ____ on this colony.

   A. *Gram stain*

   B. *CAMP test*

   C. *Taxo A test*

   D. *Coagulase test*

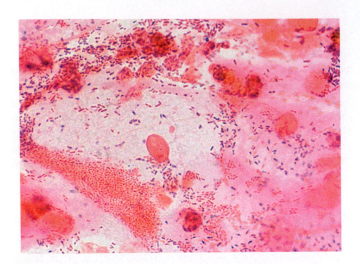

■ **FIGURE 36-16** This Gram stain of vaginal secretions is characteristic for bacterial vaginosis. There is a shift from the healthy vaginal flora, with a predominance of *Lactobacillus* spp., to anaerobic flora, with a predominance of gram-variable and gram-negative rods. Note the presence of "clue" cells in the Gram stain.
http://www.biomedcentral.com/1471-2180/5/61

be retested in-house or referred to a reference lab: (1) if the susceptibility result for group B streptococci is resistant to penicillin, vancomycin, teicoplanin, or linezolid; (2) if an isolate identified as *N. gonorrhoeae* is resistant to any third-generation cephalosporin; (3) any *S. aureus* resistant to vancomycin, teicoplanin, linezolid, or quinupristin-dalfopristin. *Listeria* is intrinsically resistant to broad-spectrum cephalosporins and fluoroquinolones. Do not report cephalosporins as susceptible (Miller, 2007). See ∞ Chapter 11 for additional susceptibility test information.

OTHER DIAGNOSTIC PROCEDURES

Bacterial vaginosis is best diagnosed by examination of a Gram stain and not by culture. Several oil immersion fields are examined and the average number of each morphotype per oil immersion field is determined. The observation of a predominance of gram-negative and gram-variable rods rather than long thin gram-positive rods is diagnostic. Figure 36-16 ■ illustrates a Gram stain of vaginal discharge that is characteristic for bacterial vaginosis. "Clue" cells are evident and can be recognized by the oval nucleus in the center. See Table 36-5✿ for a suggested Gram stain score sheet for the laboratory diagnosis of bacterial vaginosis. A score greater than or equal to 7 is considered consistent with bacterial vaginosis.

Saline wet mounts of vaginal fluid are examined for clue cells, budding yeast, pseudohyphae, or trichomonads. KOH prep can also be used to observe yeast. Clue cell morphology and trichomonas motility was described previously in the section on diseases with vaginal discharge.

Diamonds media can be used to culture for *Trichomonas*. It is more sensitive than microscopic exams of a wet mount (Schreckenberger, 2003). See ∞ Chapter 30 for more information on *Trichomonas*.

Treponema pallidum can be observed in darkfield examinations (Figure 36-17 ■) of tissue, exudates, and chancre specimen as motile spirochetes. Regular tight spirals and a "corkscrew" motility is typical of this organism (Murray et al., 2003). Syphilis can also be diagnosed with serology tests (EIA, RPR and VDRL).

Some organisms are better identified using molecular or immunological tests. These include chlamydiae, syphilis, and viral pathogens. Nucleic acid amplification and probes are commercially available to detect *N. gonorrhoeae* in endocervical,

✿ TABLE 36-5

Suggested Bacterial Vaginosis Gram Stain Score Sheet

Morphotype	Gram-positive rods with parallel sides suggestive of *Lactobacillus* spp.					Regular or coccobacillary gram-negative/variable rods suggestive of *Gardnerella vaginalis* and *Bacteroides* spp.					Curved gram-negative rods suggestive of *Mobiluncus* spp.					Total Score
Number/OIF	>30	6–30	1–5	<1	NOS	>30	6–30	1–5	<1	NOS	>30	6–30	1–5	<1	NOS	
Quantitation	4+	3+	2+	1+	0	4+	3+	2+	1+	0	4+	3+	2+	1+	0	
Score	0	1	2	3	4	4	3	2	1	0	2	2	1	1	0	
Interpretation									Date:						Tech:	

Directions: Circle score for each morphotype; add up the score for each morphotype and record as total score; interpret according to criteria listed below.
Interpretation Criteria: Total Score
Negative for Bacterial Vaginosis = 0–3
Inconclusive = 4–6
Bacterial Vaginosis = 7–10
OIF, oil immersion field; NOS, no organisms seen.

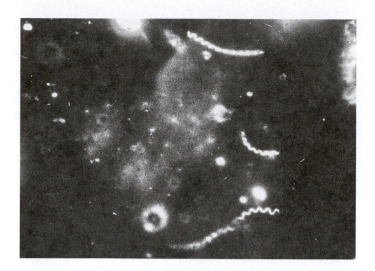

■ **FIGURE 36-17** *Treponema pallidum* in a darkfield preparation.
From Public Image Library (PHIL), CDC/Susan Lindsley.

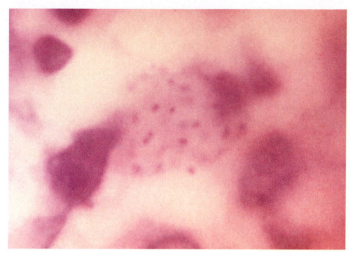

■ **FIGURE 36-18** A tissue sample showing Donovan bodies, or intracellular pathogens (specifically *Klebsiella granulomatis*, a gram-negative bacillus) confirming the diagnosis of granuloma inguinale.
From Public Image Library (PHIL), CDC/Susan Lindsley.

urethral, and urine specimens. Manufacturer's instructions regarding specimen collection and test procedures must be followed. False positives may occur with certain kits, so a positive may need to be confirmed by culture (Murrary et al., 2003). Molecular methods detecting both chlamydiae and gonorrhea are available. More testing to confirm a positive result for chlamydiae is recommended (Schachtear et al., 2006; CDC, 2002b). See Table 36-2 for more information on recommended lab tests. To review molecular testing refer to ∞ Chapter 9, "Final Identification."

Mycoplasma and *Ureaplasma* can grow as pin-point, translucent colonies on blood agar and chocolate agar but require 4 days of incubation (Murray et al., 2003). This is not standard practice in most clinical laboratories. These organisms lack a cell wall and will not stain. No tests are recommended to identify genital *Mycoplasma* or *Ureaplasma* (Miller, 2007). These organisms can be cultured on special media. Refer to ∞ Chapter 28 for more information on cultivating and identifying *Mycoplasma* and *Ureaplasma*. A positive genital *Mycoplasma* culture is usually associated with bacterial vaginosis (Murray et al., 2003).

 Checkpoint! 36–13 (Chapter Objectives 4 and 11)

A patient complains of vaginal itching, discharge, and a fishy odor. A Gram stain is examined and results recorded as follows: gram-positive rods = 3/OIF; regular gram-negative rods = 15/OIF, and curved gram-negative rods = 45/OIF. This Gram stain interpretation indicates:

  A. *negative for bacterial vaginosis.*
  B. *inconclusive.*
  C. *bacterial vaginosis.*
  D. *negative for gonorrhea.*

Klebsiella granulomatis, formerly known as *Calymmatobacterium granulomatis,* is a gram-negative rod that cannot be cultured (Murray et al., 2003) Tissue or subsurface scrapings should be transported to the laboratory and stained with Wright's or Giemsa stain (Murray et al., 2003). Observation of Donovan bodies (Figure 36-18 ■) or mononuclear cells with blue-black chromatin in tissue infected by this organism is diagnostic.

▶ TREATMENT

Treatment will be determined by the agent of disease, the age of the patient, and whether a female is pregnant or not. The sexually transmitted disease diagnosed will determine whether the sexual partner is treated or not. Sexual partners of patients diagnosed with chancroid and syphilis should be examined and treated. Sexual partners of patients with genital herpes should be offered testing if asymptomatic and treated if symptomatic (CDC, 2006c). Sexual partners of patients diagnosed with gonorrhea should be treated (Miller, 2007). Sexual partners of those with *Trichomonas* should be treated as well. Treatment of male sexual partners of women with bacterial vaginosis is not effective in preventing reoccurrence (CDC, 2006c; Murray et al., 2003). A patient may wish to skip treatment for genital warts and wait for the disease to disappear.

Treatment for PID should be with a broad-spectrum antibiotic effective against anaerobes, gonorrhea, and chlamydiae. Treating sexual partners for genital warts is not recommended (CDC, 2006c). Treatment for epididymitis is designed not only to eliminate the infecting organism but also to prevent complications such as sterility. Recommended antibiotic therapy is determined by the causative agent. Treatment for HIV includes highly active antiretroviral therapy (HAART) and behavioral and psychosocial counseling (CDC, 2006c). Prophylactic antimicrobials are administered to decrease the occurrence of opportunistic infections (CDC, 2006c). Pregnant women positive for group B streptococci are treated during labor with penicillin. If the patient is allergic to penicillin, erythromycin or clindamycin are alternative therapies (Baron, 2003).

As of 2006 there are five classes and more then 20 FDA antiretroviral approved drugs. The five classes include nucleoside/nucleotide reverse transcriptase inhibitors (NNRTI), non-nucleoside reverse transcriptase inhibitors (NRTI), protease inhibitors (PI), entry inhibitors (EI), and integrase inhibitors. Initial combination treatment usually includes one NNRTI and two NRTIs or a single or ritonavir-boosted PI and two NRTIs (Department of Health and Human Services [DHHS], 2007).

The CD4 T-lymphocyte count reflects the degree of immunosuppression and is used to guide treatment of individuals with HIV. HAART and antimicrobials work best within certain immune dysfunction parameters. According to the DHHS guidelines, persons with CD4 T-cell counts of less than 350/μL and an AIDS-defining illness should receive antiretroviral therapy. Pregnant patients and patients with HIV-associated nephropathy and coinfection with Hepatitis B should also receive HAART. Patients with CD4 T-cell counts of less than 200/μL should receive prophylaxis to prevent *Pneumocystis jiroveci* pneumonia (CDC, 1992). Genotypic drug resistance testing should be performed on all newly diagnosed patients, whether treatment is started or not. Repeat testing for drug resistance is recommended when beginning HAART therapy or with treatment failure (Department of Health and Human Services, 2007). See ∞ Chapter 31, "Intracellular Microorganisms," for more information on human immunodeficiency virus.

Vaccination can prevent hepatitis A, B, and human papilloma virus. Immune globulin can be given after exposure to a HAV-positive partner. Treatment for HBV-positive individuals includes interferon and antiviral drugs such as adefovir dipivoxil, lamivudine, entecavir, and telbivudine (CDC, 2007a). The treatment of choice for hepatitis C–positive individuals is combination therapy with interferon and ribavirin (CDC, 2005b). Reportable diseases may result in follow-up of the patient's contacts for epidemiological reasons. Counseling may be suggested to provide education on safe practices and psychological support. Table 36-6 provides information on the CDC suggested treatment for these infections as of 2007.

✪ TABLE 36-6

CDC Treatment Recommendation as of 2007

Disease	Treatment
Chancroid	Azithromycin, ceftriaxone, ciprofloxacin, or erythromycin
Genital herpes	Acyclovir, famciclovir, or valacyclovir
Syphilis	Penicillin G
Urethritis	Erythromycin, ofloxacin or levofloxacin
Cervicitis	Azithromycin or doxycycline
Trichomonas vaginalis	Metronidazole
Candidiasis	Oral fluconazole, topical azoles, or topical nystatin
Genital warts	■ Cryotherapy, trichloroacetic acid, or bichloroacetic acid, podophyllin resin, or surgical removal. ■ Patients may apply podofilox solution or gel or imiquimod cream.
Pelvic inflammatory disease	■ Cefotetan or cefoxitin plus doxycycline or clindamycin plus gentamicin ■ Levofloxacin or ofloxacin with or without metronidazole is recommended for oral treatment unless the patient or their partner has a history of foreign travel or acquired the infection in Hawaii or California. ■ Acquiring infection in a foreign countries, Hawaii, or California increases the risk of exposure to a quinolone resistant *N. gonorrhoeae*. ■ An alternative therapy includes a cephalosporin (e.g., ceftriaxone or cefoxitin) plus doxycycline with or without metronidazole.
Gonorrhea or chlamydiae	■ Ceftriaxone plus doxycycline ■ Allergies to these antibiotics or the causative agent is an enteric bacterium then ofloxacin or levofloxacin is recommended.
Bacterial vaginosis	■ Metronidazole or clindamycin

SUMMARY

This chapter reviewed the function and structure of the male and female genital systems with an emphasis on those sites frequently infected by genital pathogens. Commensal flora of the genital system is delineated and innate defenses against infection are described. See Table 36-1 to review the commensal flora of the genital tract. Genital infections can ascend, causing sterility, abdominal infections, and fetal disease or death. Infections can become systemic, causing arthritis, meningitis, and septicemia.

Microorganisms can also be passed on to an infant, causing neonatal sepsis, meningitis, or pneumonia. Information on sexually transmitted diseases is presented by symptom and etiological agent. See Table 36-2 to review these STDs. Isolation of sexually transmitted agents from children may indicate sexual assault and should be reported to authorities for investigation. Conventional tests rather than nucleic acid tests need to be performed in these cases.

The laboratory's role in processing specimens, performing sensitivity tests, and recognizing reportable results is outlined. Targeted genital cultures are now recommended rather than routine cultures. Most diseases are treated empirically and susceptibility testing is not routinely performed except with treatment failure. *S. aureus* and gram-negative rods do not have predictable sensitivity to antibiotics and are routinely tested. It is important to follow CLSI guidelines, so interpretation criteria are available for susceptibility testing results. Some organisms require special media and procedures for accurate results. Information on current treatment guidelines is presented in Table 36-6.

LEARNING OPPORTUNITIES

1. Why is it not acceptable to diagnose gonorrhea only from a Gram stain on females? (Chapter Objectives 8 and 9)

2. What virus is associated with cervical cancer? (Chapter Objective 4)

3. What is the advantage of nucleic acid testing (NAT) for gonorrhea rather than culture? When should culture be performed rather than NAT? (Chapter Objectives 5, 8 and 10)

CASE STUDY 36-1 FLUOROQUINOLONE-RESISTANT *NEISSERIA GONORRHOEAE*, SAN DIEGO, 1997 (CHAPTER OBJECTIVES 9, 10, AND 12)

Patient: James, a 25-year-old man

Patient history: Eddie sought help from a STD clinic after developing a purulent urethral discharge that lasted for 2 days. He admitted to having had sexual intercourse with a commercial sex worker while visiting Las Vegas. He was treated with ofloxacin and doxycycline, but his discharge persisted. He went to his primary physician for additional care. After the culture results were received he was placed on ceftriaxone and he recovered (CDC, 1998).

Clinical Laboratory Results: Gram stain (urethra): gram-negative intracellular diplococci

1. What was the initial diagnosis?

2. Is a culture required in this case?

3. Is this a national reportable disease?

CASE STUDY 36-2 HIV TRANSMISSION IN THE ADULT FILM INDUSTRY, LOS ANGELES, 2004 (CHAPTER OBJECTIVES 4, 5, AND 10)

Patient: Kirk, a 40-year-old man

Patient history: Kirk received regular monthly testing of blood samples for HIV. He tested positive in April, after negative results the previous 2 months. During the time between his two negative tests, he performed unprotected sex acts in a film produced in Brazil. He experienced a "flu-like" illness in March prior to returning to the United States. Upon his return, he engaged in unprotected sex with 13 female partners during filming. Three of the 13 became positive for HIV (CDC, 2005c).

1. What tests are performed to detect HIV?

2. How could HIV be transmitted in spite of negative test results?

3. What additional testing is performed on HIV-positive individuals?

4. What disease can HIV-positive patients progress to with time?

5. Is this a national reportable disease?

CASE STUDY 36-3   OUTBREAK OF LISTERIOSIS, 2002 (CHAPTER OBJECTIVES 3, 4, 6, 9, AND 10)

Patient: Elena, 3 months pregnant female

Patient history: Elena miscarried after exhibiting "flu-like" symptoms

Clinical Laboratory Results: Routine culture grew a beta-hemolytic, gray colony that was catalase negative and demonstrated a tumbling motility (CDC, 2002a).

1. What is the possible etiological agent?

2. What specimens and primary media should be used for culture?

3. What is the potential source of the microbe causing the infectious disease?

4. Is this a reportable disease?

PEARSON
myhealthprofessionskit™

Use this address to access the interactive Companion Website created for this textbook. Simply select "Clinical Laboratory Science" from the choice of disciplines. Find this book and log in using your user name and password.

REFERENCES

Go to myhealthprofessionskit.com to view this chapter's references.

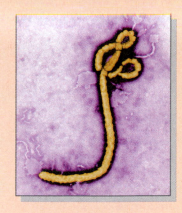

37

The Integumentary System

Joy T. Henderson

■ LEARNING OBJECTIVES

Upon completion of this chapter the learner should be able to:

1. Discuss the basic structure and function of the integumentary system to include structures that can be infected, the routes of infection, and innate defenses.

2. Discuss microbes that are normally present in nonsterile areas of the integumentary system, including their role in maintaining health.

3. Discuss the pathogenesis, clinical manifestations, epidemiology, etiology, and laboratory diagnosis of diseases associated with the integumentary system including bacterial and fungal causes.

4. Describe the processing of routinely cultured integumentary system specimens to include specimen collection and selection, inoculation, and incubation of primary media.

5. Evaluate specimen quality and presumptively identify an organism based on the Gram stain results of clinical material obtained from the integumentary system.

6. Examine colonies for potential pathogens, choose the most important potential pathogen, and provide presumptive identification of potential pathogens using Gram stain results, growth pattern, colony morphology, and spot or rapid test results.

7. Determine what confirmatory tests to perform and evaluate the test results.

8. Identify integumentary system pathogens and correlate to diagnosis, Gram stain morphology, colony morphology, test outcomes, and antibiogram prior to reporting results.

KEY TERMS

carbuncle	furuncle (boil)	perionychium
cellulitis	hidradenitis suppurativa	pilonidal cyst
crepitus	impetigo	root sheath
cutaneous	keratinocytes	stratum basale
dermis	Langerhans cells	(stratum geminativum)
epidermis	necrotizing fasciitis	stratum corneum
folliculitis	onychocyte	subcutaneous tissue

▶ INTRODUCTION

The integumentary system is the external covering of the body, comprised of the skin, hair, nails, sweat glands, and their products (i.e., sweat and mucus). It is the largest organ system by surface area, covering the entire outer body. This chapter reviews the structure and function as well as the infectious diseases associated with the integumentary system. In addition, this chapter intends to cover the role of a microbiology laboratory in the diagnosis of certain skin conditions. The integumentary system is complex and fascinating. This particular area of interest will reward success with a thorough understanding of the way in which the integumentary system works and protects itself.

▶ FUNCTION AND STRUCTURE OF THE INTEGUMENTARY SYSTEM

As mentioned previously, the integumentary system is composed of the skin, nails and sweat glands and their products (i.e., sweat and mucus). The name is derived from the Latin *integumentum,* which means a "covering." Its main function is to distinguish, separate, protect, and inform the animal with regard to its surroundings. Some animals actually use the outer layer (i.e., integument) to respire. This gas exchange system, called integumentary exchange, is where gases simply diffuse into and out of the interstitial fluid.

The **cutaneous** membrane (skin or cutis) (Figure 37-1) and its accessory structures make up the integumentary system. There are three layers of the skin: **epidermis**, **dermis**, and **subcutaneous tissue.** Below the dermis, the subcutaneous tissue acts to protect underlying muscles, tissues, and other organs. Hair on the surface of the skin helps maintain body temperature and filter out harmful particles including microbes. The cutaneous glands include the sweat glands (also known as sudoriferous glands), which act to excrete sweat to regulate temperature; the sebaceous glands, which produce oil, keeping the skin and hair moist and soft; the ceruminous glands of the ear canal, which produce the earwax; and finally, the mammary glands, which are the milk-producing glands located in the breasts.

✓ Checkpoint! 37–1 (Chapter Objective 1)

Which of the following make up the three layers of the skin?
   A.   *Epidermis*
   B.   *Dermis*
   C.   *Subcutaneous tissue*
   D.   *All of the above*
   E.   *None of the above*

THE EPIDERMIS: ITS COMPONENTS AND FUNCTIONS

The epidermis is the thin outer layer of the skin whose makeup consists mostly of stratified squamous epithelium and contains four principle types of cells. About 90% of the epidermal cells are **keratinocytes**, protein cells that harden the epidermal tissue to form fingernails as well as aid in waterproofing and protecting the skin and its underlying tissues. Another component that makes up about 8% of the epidermal cells is melanocytes, which provide the skin coloration. Melanin is the primary determinant of human skin color and allows for the absorption of ultraviolet (UV) light. Another type of cell in the epidermis is known as the **Langerhans cells.** These cells are formed in the bone marrow and migrate

✓ Checkpoint! 37–2 (Chapter Objective 1)

What is the difference between keratinocytes and melanocytes?
   A.   *Keratinocytes – provide skin coloration;*
        melanocytes – participate in fingernail formation
   B.   *Keratinocytes – participate in fingernail formation;*
        melanocytes – provide skin coloration
   C.   *Keratinocytes – participate in sweat gland formation;*
        melanocytes – provide skin coloration
   D.   *Keratinocytes – provide skin coloration;*
        melanocytes – participate in sweat gland formation

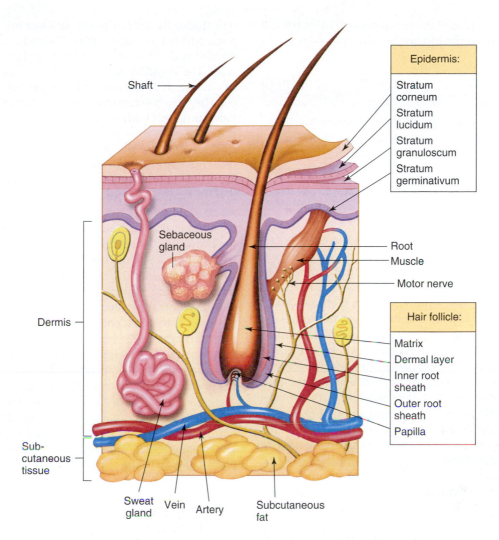

FIGURE 37-1 The integumentary system. This diagram of the skin shows its epithelial layers, dermal layers, and accessory structures.

to the epidermis. They interact with white blood cells and work to fight infections but are easily damaged by UV radiation. The final cell type found in the epidermis is called a Merkel cell. These are located in the deepest layer (**stratum basale**, also known as **stratum germinativum**) of the epi-

dermis of hairless skin, where they are attached to the keratinocytes. Merkel cells make contact with the flattened portion of the ending of a sensory neuron (nerve cell), called a tactile (Merkel) disc, and are thought to function in the sensation of touch. There are no blood vessels in the epidermidis. It relies on diffusion of needed nutrients from the dermis. The lack of blood circulation limits the ability of a microbe to move deeper into the body without the aid of spreading factors.

Additionally, the epidermis is further divided into five sublayers: the stratum germinativum (also called stratum basale), stratum spinosum, stratum granulosum, stratum lucidum, and **stratum corneum.** The deepest is the stratum germinativum or stratum basale. This single cuboidal to columnar layer of cells consists of stem cells, which participate in continued cell division, and melanocytes. The stem cells multiply, producing keratinocytes, which then push up toward the surface and become part of the more superficial layers. The nuclei of the

---

✓ Checkpoint! 37–3 (Chapter Objective 1)

Which of the following cells in the epidermis originate in the bone marrow?

  A. *Merkel cells*
  B. *Keratinocytes*
  C. *Melanocytes*
  D. *Langerhans cells*

keratinocytes degenerate, and the cells die. Eventually, the cell remnants are shed from the top layer of the epidermis.

 REAL WORLD TIP

Any microorganisms residing on the surface of the skin are sloughed off when the dead cells are shed from the skin. Of course, these organisms can be a source of infection if transferred to another site, inanimate object, or if picked up by a susceptible host.

Other stem cells in the stratum basale migrate into the dermis and give rise to sweat and oil glands, and hair follicles. The stratum basale is also referred to as stratum germinativum to indicate its role in germinating new cells, which replaces the epidermis. In addition, it also contains tactile (Merkel) discs that are sensitive to touch. The stratum granulosum is the layer of the epidermis that has three to five rows of flattened cells that develop the precursor to keratin. Keratin forms a tough barrier that protects deeper layers from injury, microbial invasion, and it waterproofs the skin. The nuclei of the cells in this area are in various stages of degeneration. As their nuclei break down, the cells can no longer carry on vital metabolic reactions, and they die. Stratum lucidum is usually found only on the thick skin of the palms and soles. It consists of three to five rows of clear, flat, dead cells that contain droplets of an intermediated substance that is eventually transformed to keratin. Finally, the most superficial layer is the stratum corneum. This layer consists of 25–30 rows of flat, dead cells completely filled with keratin. These cells are continuously shed and replaced by cells from deeper strata. An intact stratum corneum serves as an effective barrier against light, heat waves, bacteria, and many chemicals.

 Checkpoint! 37–4 (Chapter Objective 1)

Which of the following is the deepest layer of the epidermis?
A. Stratum geminativum
B. Stratum basale
C. Stratum corneum
D. A and B
E. B and C

THE DERMIS: ITS COMPONENTS AND FUNCTIONS

The dermis is the thick layer of connective tissue to which the epidermis is attached. It also consists of blood vessels, nerves that provide the main senses for touch and heat, as well as lymph vessels, sweat glands, sebaceous glands, receptors, and hair shafts. Its deepest part continues into the subcutaneous tissue without a definite defined boundary. The dermis may be divided into two sublayers: the papillary layer and reticular layer. The papillary layer consists of loose, cell-rich connective tissue. It is named for its finger-like projections called papillae, which extend toward the epidermis. The papillae provide the dermis with a rough surface that communicates with the epidermis, thus strengthening the connection between the two layers of the skin. In the palms, fingers, soles, and toes, the papillae projections form the contours in the skin surface. These contours are called friction ridges because they help the hand and foot grasp by increasing friction. Friction ridges occur in patterns (i.e., fingerprints) that are genetically determined and are therefore unique to every individual, making it possible to use fingerprints or footprints as a means of identification. The papillary area also contains receptors that communicate with the central nervous system, thus providing touch, pressure, and hot, cold, and pain receptors. The reticular layer, on the other hand, appears denser and contains fewer cells. Its thick collagen fiber composition often aggregate into bundles. It is worth mentioning that the collagen fibers form an interlacing network, and the predominant direction is parallel to the surface of the skin. The reticular layer lies deep in the papillary region. Its name is derived from the dense concentration of collagenous, elastic, and reticular fibers that weave throughout it. These protein fibers, in turn, give the dermis its properties of strength, extensibility, and elasticity. The main function of the dense elastic fibers found in the reticular layer is to house the hair follicles, nerves, and glands.

 Checkpoint! 37–5 (Chapter Objective 1)

Which are the two sublayers of the dermis?
A. Stratum lucidum, stratum spinosum
B. Stratum basale, stratum germinativum
C. Papillary layer, reticular layer
D. Keratinocytes, melanocytes

APPENDAGES OF THE SKIN AND THEIR FUNCTIONS

Hair

A common belief is that human skin lacks hair or pili on most of the body surface; however, this is a misconception. Actually most of the skin is haired, but it is short, fine, and only lightly colored. The truly hairless area of the body are the palms of hands, soles of feet, the distal phalanges, sides of fingers and toes, and parts of the external genitalia. The free part of each hair is called the shaft. The root of each hair is anchored in a tubular invagination of the epidermis, the hair follicle, which extends down into the dermis, and usually a short distance into the hypodermis. The deepest end of the hair follicle forms a bulb that contains cells that are mitotically active. Their progeny or offspring differentiates into the cell types that form the hair and the cells that surround its root and this is called the **root sheath.** Hair cells keratinize within the lower one-third of the hair follicle. Above this level it is not possible to identify individual cells within the hair. Each hair follicle has an associated bundle of smooth muscle. This muscle inserts with one end to the papillary layer of the dermis and with the other end to the dermal sheath of the hair follicle. Moreover, hair growth is discontinuous. Hairs are lost and replaced by new ones. The hair follicle goes through different stages that reflect the discontinuous hair growth. The length of the growth phase is variable in different regions of the body, lasting only a few months for the eyebrow and eyelashes area, but 2–5 years for the scalp area. It is important to note that hair growth is controlled by a number of hormonal and hereditary factors and their interactions. The hair mainly functions to augment the insulation the skin provides, but can also serve as a secondary sexual characteristic or as camouflage.

Nails

The fingernail (Figure 37-2 ■) is an important structure made of keratin, which has two purposes: (1) it acts as a protective plate and (2) it enhances sensation of the fingertip. The fingernail aids the ability of the hand to manipulate and grasp fine objects. The protection function of the fingernail is commonly known, but the sensation function is equally important. The fingertip has many nerve endings in it, which allows receipt of volumes of information about objects. The nail acts as a counterforce to the fingertip, providing even more sensory input when an object is touched. The nail plate is approximately 0.5 mm thick in females and 0.6 mm thick in males, and it tends to increase with age. Fingernails grow faster than toenails, and it takes about 6 months for a nail to grow from the root to the free edge. There are a number of factors that can affect the rate of nail growth. Stress or illness can inhibit growth, while biting or short trimming of the nail can accentuate growth. The hardness of the nail is dependent on the **onychocyte** bands, matrix proteins, and the hydration level of the nail (Neumeister & Danikas, 2004). The nail structure is divided into six specific parts: the root, nail bed, nail plate, eponychium (cuticle), **perionychium** (tissue surrounding the nail), and hyponychium (at the junction of the fingertip and the free edge of the nail). The root of the fingernail is actually under the skin behind the fingernail and extends into the finger. The fingernail root produces most of the volume of the nail and the nail bed. The edge of the nail root is seen as a white, crescent-shaped structure called the lunula. The nail bed extends from the edge of the lunula to the free edge of the nail. The nail bed consists of blood vessels, nerves, and melanocytes. The nail bed produces a semi-rigid keratin. This semi-rigid keratin, sometimes referred to as the horny solehorn, increases the overall thickness of the nail and also acts as superglue adhesive for the nail plate to maintain its adherence to the nail bed (Neumeister & Danikas, 2004). The nail plate is a multilayered stacked sheet of cornified cells derived from anucleate onychocytes that arise from the epithelium of the nail bed (Neumeister & Danikas, 2004). The nail plate is the actual fingernail made of translucent keratin. The pink appearance of the nail comes from the blood vessels underneath the nail. The underneath surface of the nail plate has grooves along the length of the nail that help anchor it to the nail bed. The cuticle or eponychium is situated between the skin of the finger and the nail plate fusing these structures together, providing a waterproof barrier. The perionychium is the skin that overlies the nail plate on its sides. It is also known as the paronychial edge. The perionychium is the site of hangnails, ingrown nails, and an infection of the skin called paronychia. Finally the hyponychium, at the junction of the fingertip and the free edge of the nail, functions as a waterproof barrier.

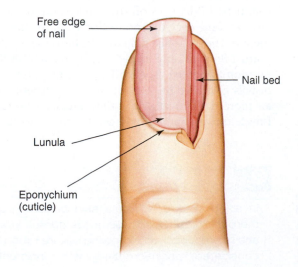
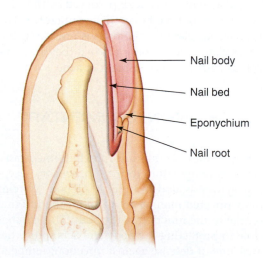

■ **FIGURE 37-2** The fingernail.

Sweat Glands

There are two types of sweat glands that are present in humans: merocrine sweat glands and apocrine sweat glands. They are distinguished by their secretory mechanisms as well as in the composition of the sweat they secret. Merocrine sweat glands are the only glands of the skin with a clearly defined biological function. They are of critical importance for the regulation of body temperature. The skin contains approximately 3 million sweat glands, which are found all over the body with the exception of the external genitalia. The sweat glands of the merocrine are simple tubular glands that open to the skin surface via a pore. The secretory tubulus and initial part of the excretory duct are coiled into a roughly round ball at the border between the dermis and subcutaneous tissue. The apocrine sweat glands occur in the axilla or armpit. They are stimulated by sexual hormones and are not fully developed or functional before puberty. Apocrine sweat is a milky, proteinaceous, and odorless secretion. Underarm odor is a result of bacterial decomposition. The excretory duct of apocrine sweat glands does not open directly onto the surface of the skin; instead, the duct empties the sweat into the upper part of the hair follicle. The sweat from these glands provides the high humidity and nutrients needed by certain colonizing microbes. Lysozyme in sweat can defend against infection.

Sebaceous Glands

Sebaceous glands empty their secretory product into the upper parts of the hair follicles. They are found in parts of the skin where hair is present. In addition, sebaceous glands are found in some of the areas where no hair is present such as the lips, oral surfaces of the cheeks, and external genitalia. Sebaceous glands are branched and the secretory portion consists of alveoli. The secretory cells will gradually accumulate lipids and grow in size. Then the nuclei will disintegrate and the cells will rupture. The lipid secretion of the sebaceous glands has no softening effect on the skin, and it has only limited antibacterial and antifungal activity. Fatty acids produced by the sebaceous glands can by metabolized be colonizing microbes. The importance of sebaceous glands in humans is unclear. Clinically, the sebaceous glands are important in that they are liable to infection such as with the development of acne.

FUNCTIONS OF THE INTEGUMENTARY SYSTEM

The integumentary system has multiple roles in homeostasis, including protection, temperature regulation, sensory reception, biochemical synthesis, and absorption. All body systems work in an interconnected manner to maintain the internal conditions essential to the function of the body. The skin has an important role in protecting the body and acts somewhat as the body's first line of defense against infection, temperature variation, and other challenges to homeostasis. The following is a list of the numerous roles the integumentary system plays in the human body: it protects the body's internal living tissues and organs against infectious organisms. This way it acts as an anatomical barrier between the internal and external environment. The Langerhans cells in the skin, for example, are part of the adaptive immune system that contributes to the body's defense. Furthermore, it protects the body from dehydration. The skin contains a blood supply far greater than its requirement, which allows precise control of energy loss by radiation, convection, conducting blood flow, and conserving heat, thus providing protection against abrupt changes in the temperature. It helps excrete waste material through perspiration, which at most adds to temperature regulation. Since it contains a variety of nerve endings the skin acts as a receptor for touch, pressure, pain, heat, and cold. Additionally, the skin acts as a storage facility for lipids and water as well as a means of synthesis of vitamin D and B by action of UV on certain parts of it. This synthesis is linked to pigmentation, with darker skin producing more vitamin B than D, and vice versa. Moreover, it is involved in evaporation control. Dilated blood vessels increase blood flow and promote heat loss and sweating while constricted vessels greatly reduce heat and fluid loss, making it a relatively dry and impermeable barrier. Loss of this function contributes to the massive fluid loss in burns. Also, the skin functions in absorption. It absorbs oxygen, nitrogen, and carbon dioxide, which diffuse into the epidermis in small amounts. Finally, the skin adds on aesthetics and communication, meaning it can assess mood, physical state, and attractiveness of an individual. Certain clinical symptoms such as jaundice (yellowish skin color) due to liver disease, for example, or cyanosis (bluish skin color) due to reduced blood blow can be observed on the skin.

▶ COMMENSAL FLORA OF THE INTEGUMENTARY SYSTEM

The skin is a harsh, dry environment for microbes. The resident commensal flora lives on the surface and in the follicles that provide some degree of protection from the ultraviolet rays of the sun. The microbial flora may be transient or temporary. The normal flora residing in the follicles reestablish the skin colonization as needed. The axilla, perineum, and scalp are more heavily colonized by microorganisms. Nutrients and humidity are more readily available in these areas, enabling microorganisms to thrive. Diphtheroids (aerobic and anaerobic), coagulase-

 REAL WORLD TIP

In a lab setting, when a skin culture grows diphtheroids, *Staphylococcus* not *S. aureus*, and/or viridians streptococci, the following culture report should be considered: "polymicrobial growth consistent with normal skin flora."

positive and -negative staphylococci, *Micrococcus* spp., and viridans streptococci represent the usual normal flora of skin. Gramnegative rods and yeast may be present in moister areas such as between the toes.

▶ INFECTIOUS DISEASES ASSOCIATED WITH THE INTEGUMENTARY SYSTEM

Microorganisms such as *Staphylococcus epidermidis* colonize the skin surface. The density of the skin flora depends on the region of the skin. The disinfected skin surface gets recolonized from bacteria residing in the deeper areas of the hair follicle, gut, and urogenital openings. Dirty skin favors the development of pathogenic organisms. The unclean skin is a combination of dead cells that continually slough off of the epidermis combined with the secretions of the sweat and sebaceous glands plus the dust found on the skin to form a filthy layer on its surface. If not cleaned, the slurry of sweat and sebaceous secretions mixed with dirt and dead skin is decomposed by bacterial flora, producing a foul smell. The skin functions are disturbed when it is excessively dirty, thus making the skin more susceptible to damage, and in turn decreases the release of antibacterial compounds, therefore increasing the chances of skin infections. The skin supports its own niche of microorganisms, including yeasts and bacteria, which cannot be removed by any amount of cleaning. It is estimated that the individual bacteria on the surface of one square inch of human skin is about 50 million. Oily surfaces, such as the face, may contain over 500 million bacteria per square inch. Despite these vast quantities, all of the bacteria found on the skin's surface would fit into a volume the size of a pea. In general, the microorganisms keep one another in check and are part of healthy skin. When the balance is disturbed, there may be an overgrowth and infection, as, for example, when antibiotics kill microbes, the result is an overgrowth of yeast. The skin is continous with the inner epithelial lining of the body at the orifices, each of which supports its own complement of microbes. It is worth noting that as skin ages, it becomes thinner and more easily damaged. Intensifying this effect is the decreasing ability of the skin to heal itself. Sagging skin is caused by a loss of elasticity and as aging continues the skin receives less blood flow and consequently gland activity dramatically decreases.

INFECTIONS IN OR AROUND HAIR FOLLICLES

Folliculitis

Folliculitis is the minor infection of hair follicles. In simple terms it is described as a papular or pustular inflammation of hair follicles (Figure 37-3 ■). Folliculitis occurs as a result of various infections or secondary to follicular trauma or occlusion (blockage) (Satter & Cyr, 2006).

The most common form is superficial folliculitis that manifests as a tender or painless pustule that heals without scar-

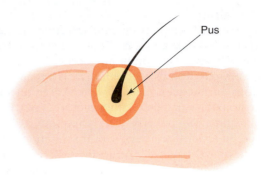

■ **FIGURE 37-3** Folliculitis (a pustule). The reddish area depicts inflammation.

ring. The hair shaft will freequently be seen in the center of the pustule. Multiple or single lesions may appear on any skin with hair, including the head, neck, trunk, buttocks, and extremities (Stulberg, Penrod, & Blatny, 2002). *Staphylococcus aureus* is the most likely pathogen; however, commensal organisms such as yeasts and fungi occasionally appear, especially in immunocompromised patients (Stulberg et al., 2002; Tolan, Baorto, & Baorto, 2007). Acne is a form of folliculitis and is caused by the anaerobic gram-positive rod *Propionibacterium acnes*. Topical therapy with erthromycin, clindamycin, mupirocin, or benzoyl peroxide can be administered to accelerate the healing process. Deep folliculitis occurs when staphylococci invade the deeper portion of the follicle, causing swelling and erythema with or without pustule at the skin surface. These lesions are painful and may scar. Oral antibiotics such as first-generation cephalosporins, penicillinase-resistant penicillins, macrolides, and fluoroquinolones are usually necessary to treat this kind of infection (Stulberg et al., 2002).

Folliculitis caused by gram-negative rods may also occur. Usually the organisms involved include *Klebsiella, Enterobacter,* and *Proteus* species. These kinds of infections are found in the face and affects patients with a history of long-term antibiotic therapy for acne (Stulberg et al., 2002). In addition, "hot tub" folliculitis caused by *Pseudomonas aeruginosa* occurs as a result of poorly maintained hot tubs or spas, but can also be spread by swimming in a contaminated pool or lake. The skin becomes itchy and progresses to a bumpy red rash and pus-filled blisters are usually found surrounding the hair follicle. *Pseudomonas aeruginosa* is ubiquitous in nature and can cause various mild to severe symptoms. The occurrence of dermatitis and otitis externa outbreaks associated with swimming pools, hot tubs, and water slides have been described (CDC, 1983, 2000). In order to avoid such infections in hot tubs and spas, it is important to note that they have warmer water than pools, so chlorine or other disinfectants break down faster. Ensuring frequent testing, control of disinfectant levels, and pH control are likely to prevent the spread of dermatitis (CDC, 1983, 2000). *Pseudomonas aeruginosa* is described in more detail in ∞ Chapter 22.

Furuncle (Boil)

A **furuncle** or **boil** begins as a painful infection of single hair follicles (Figure 37-4a ■ and b ■). Boils can grow to be larger than a golf ball, and they commonly occur on the buttocks, face, neck, armpits, and groin. A furuncle is a tender, erythematous, firm, or fluctuant mass of walled-off purulent material arising from the hair follicle (Stulbert et al., 2002). Furuncles rarely appear before puberty. The common pathogen is *Staphylococcus aureus*. For a review of information related to *S. aureus*, go to ∞ Chapter 17. Furuncles or boils are the hallmarks of community-acquired methicillin-resistant *Staphylococcus aureus* (CA-MRSA), associated especially in sports-related (e.g., football) activities (Nguyen et al., 2005; Tolan et al., 2007). It was found that the spread of infection was due to sharing of bars of soap, players having preexisting cuts or abrasions, sharing of towels, and living on campus with an associated nasal carrier person (Nguyen et al., 2005). There has been an increase in what the public believe to be an infected spider bite but is actually a boil due to MRSA. Furuncles also began to appear after spa pedicures beginning in 2000. The culprit, *Mycobacterium fortuitum* complex, was isolated from the screens and filters of the circulating footbaths and 34 of 110 patients with furuncles. Most of the patients had shaved their legs either the day of or the night before the pedicure (Trevino & Weissfeld, 2008). Eventually, the furuncle opens to the skin surface, allowing the purulent material to drain, either spontaneously or following incision. Patients with recurrent furunculosis should be treated for predisposing factors such as obesity, diabetes,

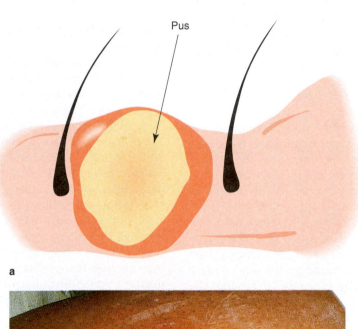

Pus

a

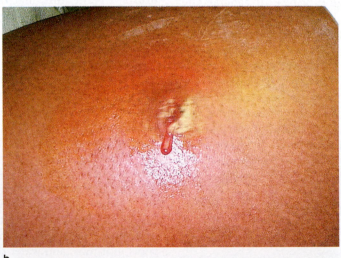

b

■ **FIGURE 37-4** **a.** A furuncle (an abscess). The reddish area depicts inflammation. **b.** Cutaneous abscess located on the hip of a prison inmate, which had begun to spontaneously drain, releasing its purulent contents. The abscess was caused by methicillin-resistant *Staphylococcus aureus* (MRSA).
From Public Health Image Library (PHIL), CDC/ Bruno Coignard, M.D., Jeff Hageman, M.H.S.

occupational or industrial exposure to inciting factors, and nasal carriage of *Staphylococcus aureus* (Merck, 2005).

Carbuncle

A **carbuncle** is a deeper skin infection that involves a group of infected hair follicles in one skin location (Figure 37-5a ■ and b ■). People with diabetes or other underlying conditions are more likely to develop this kind of infection. Fever and malaise are commonly associated with carbuncles but are rarely found in furuncles. Gentle incision and drainage is necessary when lesions "point" (fluctuant or boggy with a thin, shiny appearance of the overlying skin) (Stulberg et al., 2002). If the site is not drained then the antibiotics cannot penetrate

the pus to act on the organisms. In severe cases, parenteral antibiotics such as cloxacillin or first-generation cephalosporin such as cefazolin are required.

> ✓ **Checkpoint! 37–6**
> **(Chapter Objective 3)**
>
> *Which of the following is an infection of the hair follicles?*
>   A. *Folliculitis*
>   B. *Furuncle*
>   C. *Carbuncle*
>   D. *None of the above*
>   E. *All of the above*

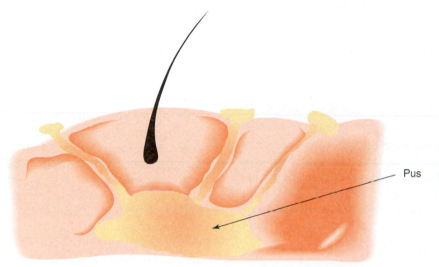

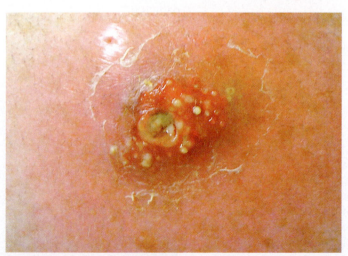

Pus

a

b

■ **FIGURE 37-5 a.** A carbuncle (often with multiple abscesses). The reddish area depicts inflammation. **b.** A cutaneous abscess located on the back, which had been caused by methicillin-resistant *Staphylococcus aureus* (MRSA).
Photo courtesy of Gregory Moran, M.D., http://www.cdc.gov/mrsa/mrsa_initiative/skin_infection/mrsa_photo_010.html.

INFECTIONS IN THE KERATINIZED LAYER OF THE EPIDERMIS

Dermatophytes

Dermatophytes generally grow only in keratinized tissues such as hair, nails, and the outer layer of the skin. The fungus usually stops spreading when it comes in contact with living cells or areas of inflammation. The mucous membranes are not affected. The clincial signs may vary depending on the affected region. Dermatophytosis is caused by one of the three genera of fungi collectively called dermatophytes: *Epidermophyton* species, *Microsporum* species, and *Trichophyton* species. The genus *Epidermophyton* involves the skin and nails, the genus *Microsporum* involves only the hair and skin, whereas the genus *Trichophyton* is capable of invading the hair, skin, and nails. Go to ∞ Chapters 14 and 29 to review the culture and identification of fungi. Cutaneous mycoses are perhaps the most common fungal infections in humans and are referred to as tinea or ringworm (Figure 37-6 ■). The gross appearance of the lesion is that of an outer ring of the active, progressing infection, with central healing within the ring.

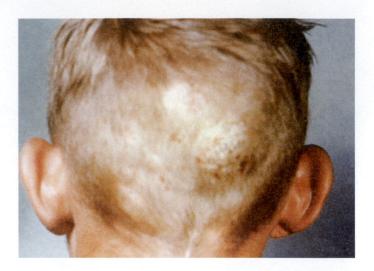

■ **FIGURE 37-6** This image shows a child with ringworm of the scalp, called "tinea capitis," caused by *Microsporum* spp.
From the Public Health Image Library (PHIL), CDC.

 REAL WORLD TIP

When a tissue is submitted to the laboratory for a fungus culture, it is best to mince the tissue and not grind it. Grinding would destroy the hyphae and decrease the viability of the organisms, especially for the "lid lifters" such as the Zygomycetes. The term "lid lifters" is used to describe moulds that grow quickly and reach the lid of the petri dish.

✓ **Checkpoint! 37–7 (Chapter Objective 8)**

What common fungal family causes dermatophytosis?
  A. *Zygomycetes*
  B. *Dermatophytes*
  C. *Opportunist moulds*
  D. *Systemic moulds*

 REAL WORLD TIP

When 10% potassium hydroxide (KOH) preparation is requested on skin, hair, and nails to rule out dermatophytes, it is best not to use a cotton swab to inoculate the slide because the cotton filaments may be confused as hyphal elements when read under a microscope.

INFECTIONS IN THE DEEPER LAYERS OF THE EPIDERMIS AND THE DERMIS

Erysipelas

Erysipelas, also known as St. Anthony's fire, is a skin infection typically caused by group A beta-hemolytic streptococci (Stulberg et al., 2002; Nochimson, 2006). It is presented as an intense erythematous infection with dermal lymphatic involvement (Figure 37-7 ■). It is characterized by a shiny, raised, indurated, and tender plaque-like lesion with distinct margins. It occurs most frequently on the legs and face and is accompanied by high fever, chills, and malaise (Merck, 2005; Nochimson, 2006). The incidence of erysipelas is rising, especially in young children, older adults, diabetics, alcoholics, and immunocompromised patients. A defect in skin barrier allows the infection to occur and since it is almost exclusively caused by group A beta-hemolytic streptococci, it can be treated with standard dosages of oral or intavenous penicillin.

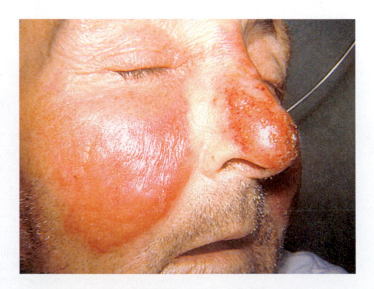

■ **FIGURE 37-7** Facial erysipelas manifested as severe cheek and nasal erythema and swelling.
From the Public Health Image Library (PHIL), CDC.

Erythrasma

Erythrasma is an infection with *Corynebacterium minutissimum,* a gram-positive rod that is most common in patients with diabetes. Erythrasma looks like tinea or a rash. It can be found in areas where the skin overlaps such as under the breast. It is most common in the foot, between the toes, where it presents as superficial scaling and in the groin, where it presents as irregular but sharply marginated pink or brown patches with fine scaling. Erythrasma flouoresces a characteristic red color under Wood's (ultraviolet) lamp and it may be distinguished from tinea by the absence of hyphae on skin scrapings. Treatment with erythromycin or tetracyline is effective (Merck, 2005).

Erysipeloid

Erysipeloid is an acute bacterial infection of traumatized skin and other organs. It is caused by a thin, hydrogen sulfide (H_2S)–positive, gram-positive bacillus called *Erysipelothrix rhusiopathiae,* which has long been known to cause animal and human infections. Direct contact between meat infected with this organism and traumatized human skin results in erysipeloid. Erysipeloid is an occupational zoonotic disease. Humans acquire the infection after direct contact with infected animals. The disease is more common among farmers, butchers, cooks, and homemakers (Merck, 2005).

Erysipelothrix rhusiopathiae is highly resistant to environmental factors and it enters the skin through scratches or pricks. In the skin, the organism is capable of producing enzymes that help it invade the tissues. It has been recently discovered that only pathogenic strains of *E. rhusiopathiae* are capable of producing the neuraminidase enzyme. This enzyme is speculated to help the microorganism invade tissues. The host's immune system is activated to start fighting against this foreign bacterium but the organism may escape immune surveillance and may spread in the body via the vascular system to the joints, heart, brain, CNS, and lungs. The organ most commonly affected other than the skin is the heart (Ghorayeb & Muallem, 2007).

Erysipeloid is an acute, self-limiting infection of the skin that can resolve without sequelae. Individuals with systemic infection may die of sepsis if the proper diagnosis is not made and treatment is not initiated early on. Erysipeloid comes in three clinical forms: the localized cutaneous form occurs on the affected hands and the lesions consist of bright to red to purple plaques with a smooth, shiny surface. The lesions leave a brownish discoloration on the skin when resolving and sometimes vesicles may be present. The diffuse form is where multiple lesions appear on various parts of the body and usually these are well demarcated and plaques are seen. Finally, the systemic form is presented as the skin lesions appear as localized areas of swelling surrounding a necrotic center. The skin lesion may also present as several follicular, erythematous papules. The antibiotic of choice for the three forms of erysipeloid is penicillin. The microorganism is resistant to vancomycin, which is important to consider in patients with endocarditis caused by *E. rhusiopathiae.* Also, it has been shown that this organism can be eradicated from surfaces by the use of simple home disinfectants. Spraying surfaces may aid in infection prevention (Ghorayeb

& Muallem, 2007). ∞ Chapter 19 provides additional information on this and other gram-positive rods.

 REAL WORLD TIP

The diagnosis of erysipelas is made clinically. Gram stain and culture are not helpful. Blood cultures are rarely positive. Erysipeloid can be diagnosed by culture of skin scraping or biopsy. Blood cultures can be positive if the individual has a systemic infection.

Impetigo

Impetigo is most commonly seen in children age 2–5 years and is classified as bullous (blister) or nonbullous (Figure 37-8 ■). The nonbullous type predominates and is characterized by erosive (ulcerative) lesions (sores), clusters of ulcerative lesions, or small vesicles or pustules that have an adherent or oozing honey-colored crust (Stulberg et al., 2002; Tolan et al., 2007). The predilection for the very young can be remembered by the common lay misnomer "infant tigo" (Stulberg et al., 2002).

Impetigo usually appears when there is a break in the skin. The bullous form presents as a large, thin-walled blisters containing serous yellow fluid. It often ruptures, leaving an area with a ring or arc of remaining bulla. It was previously thought that the nonbullous form was caused mainly by group A streptococcus, whereas the bullous form was caused by

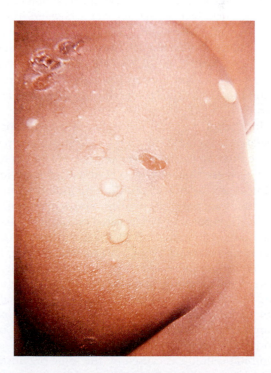

■ **FIGURE 37-8** This patient presented with these gluteal lesions that proved to be impetigo, but was first thought to be syphilis. *From the Public Health Image Library (PHIL), CDC.*

Staphylococcus aureus, but recent studies indicate that both forms are primarily caused by the latter organism mentioned, with streptoccoccus usually only involved in the nonbullous form. Impetigo can spread by direct person-to-person contact, so appropriate hygiene is warranted (Stulberg et al., 2002; Tolan et al., 2007).

A study was concluded indicating topical mupirocin (Bactroban) ointment is as effective as oral erythromcyin in treating impetigo. However, because of the developing resistance, erythromycin is no longer the drug of choice. Azithromycin (Zithromax) for 5 days and cephalexin (Keflex) for 10 days have been shown to be effective and well tolerated. In addition, broad-spectrum fluoroquinolones have also been shown to be effective and are known to have excellent skin penetration and good bioavailability. No generic floroquinolones are currently available, and they are only approved for use in adults.

Cellulitis

Cellulitis is an acute infection of the skin and soft tissues characterized by localized pain, swelling, tenderness, erythema, and warmth. It is generally a localized infection. Patients with lymphatic obstruction, venous insufficiency, pressure ulcers, and obesity are particularly vulnerable to recurrent episodes of cellulitis (Micali, Dhawan, & Nasca, 2006). Organisms on the skin gain entrance to the dermis and multiply to cause cellulitis. The vast majority of cases are caused by *Streptococcus pyogenes* or *Staphylococcus aureus.* Most patients that are treated appropriately recover completely. Mortality is rare but may occur in neglected cases or where cellulitis is due to a highly virulent organism such as *Pseudomonas aeruginosa.* The factors involved that may increase the risk of death include congestive heart failure, morbid obesity, hypoalbuminemia, and renal insufficiency (Micali et al., 2006). Cellulitis has no racial, gender, or age predilection; however, a higher incidence among males and those individuals older than 45 years old have been reported.

The incubation period is somewhat organism dependent. Postoperative cellulitis at the surgical site due to group A beta-hemolytic streptococci may develop more rapidly. On the contrary, cellulitis due to staphylococci is usually delayed in onset. The clinical appearance of cellulitis include the following: involved sites are red, hot, swollen, and tender and, unlike erysipelas, the borders are not elevated or sharply demarcated. Lymphangitis (inflammation of the lymphatic channels), regional lymphadenopathy, or both may be present, fever is common in severe cases, and patients may develop hypotension. The most commonly involved site is the leg. For diabetic patients with cellulitis, empiric treatment with penicillinase-resistant penicillin, first-generation cephalosporin, amoxicillin-clavulanate, macrolide, or fluoroquinolone (adults only) is appropriate.

Periorbital cellulitis is caused by the same organisms that cause other forms of cellulitis and is treated with warm soaks, oral antibiotics, and close follow-up. Children often have underlying sinusitis. *Haemophilus influenzae* type b (Hib) in young children was a significant concern until the widespread use of the Hib vaccine. Antibiotic coverage requires a parenteral third-generation cephalosporin (Stulberg et al., 2002).

Orbital cellulitis, on the other hand, occurs when the infection passes the orbital septum and is manifested by proptosis (abnormal bulging outward of the eye), orbital pain, restricted eye movement, visual disturbances, and sinusitis (Stulberg et al., 2002; Micali et al., 2006) (Figure 37-9 ■). Complications include abscess formation, persistent blindness, limited eye movement, and rarely meningitis. This kind of ocular problem requires intravenous antibiotics.

Perianal cellulitis is caused by group A beta-hemolytic streptococci and occurs most often in children. Ninety percent of patients experienced dermatitis, 78% itching, 52% rectal pain, and 35% had blood-streaked stools. Despite 10 days of oral antibiotics, primarily penicillin or erythromycin, the recurrence rate was high at 39%. If recurrence occurs, the presence of an abscess should be considered. Needle aspiration of the site for culture is more accurate than a skin swab (Stulberg et al., 2002; Micali et al., 2006; Curtis, 2007).

As mentioned earlier, *Staphylococcus aureus* and *Streptococcus pyogenes* represents the vast majority of cases of cellulitis, but less common causes include *Streptococcus agalactiae* (group B streptococci) in older patients with diabetes, gram-negative bacilli such as *Haemophilus influenzae* in children, and *Pseudomonas aeruginosa* in patients with diabetes, neutropenia, hot tub or spa users, and hospitalized patients (Merck, 2005; CDC, 1983, 2000). It is imperative to remember that

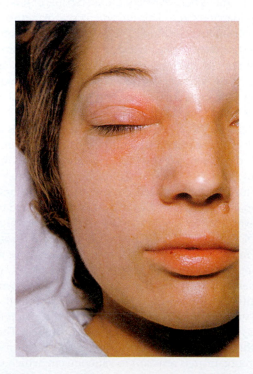

■ **FIGURE 37-9** This patient presented with staphylococcal orbital cellulitis. Note the periorbital swelling and erythema. *From the Public Health Image Library (PHIL), CDC.*

animal bites may also cause cellulitis due to *Pasteurella multocida* from cats and dogs and *Capnocytophaga* species from dogs. Injuries immersed in fresh water may result in cellulitis due to *Aeromonas hydrophila* and in warm salt water by *Vibrio vulnificus* (Merck, 2005; Micali et al., 2006; Curtis, 2007). More information on *Vibrio* and *Aeromonas* can be found in ∞ Chapter 23.

Dermatophytosis

Refer to the previous Dermatophytes discussion under "Infections in the Keratinized Layer of the Epidermis" in this chapter.

Hidradenitis Suppurativa

Hidradenitis suppurativa is a chronic, scarring inflammation of the apocrine (sweat) glands of the axillae, groin, around the nipples, and anus (Merck, 2005; Fite, 2006). The condition occurs when apocrine gland outlets become blocked by perspiration or are unable to drain normally because of incomplete gland development. Secretions trapped in the glands force perspiration and bacteria into surrounding tissue, causing subcutaneous induration, inflammation, and infection. Hidradenitis suppurativa is painful and can be disabling but is rarely fatal unless it progresses to overwhelming systemic infection in an immunocompromised patient. Extensive disease can prevent patients from performing normal work functions and from engaging in normal social activities. In some patients, especially those with severe disease, the condition creates significant psychological problems, particularly regarding sexual relationships. There is no real cause of this infection, but it is known to be more common in women and African Americans. It usually begins after the teen years and before the age of 40. It may run in the family, but it is not contagious (Shah, 2005). Ingrown hairs are a predisposing factor, thus an increased incidence of the disease occurs in patients with tightly curled hair (Fite, 2006). *Staphylococcus aureus* is almost always implicated in acute cases, but gram-negative organisms such as *Proteus* may predominate in chronic cases (Merck, 2005). Tight-fitting clothing and shaving the affected areas are to be strictly avoided. Treatment regimen may include a high dose of oral tetracycline or erythromycin. Incision, drainage, or surgical excision may be necessary for an abscess of the affected area if the disease persists (Merck, 2005; http://aocd.org/skin)

Infected Pilonidal Tuft Cyst or Hairs

A **pilonidal cyst** is found at the bottom of a tailbone, which can become infected and filled with pus. When this occurs, it is technically named pilonidal abscess and looks like a large pimple. It is more common in men than in women and usually happens in young people up into their 30s. Most physicians believe that these kinds of cysts are caused by ingrown hairs. Pilonidal means "nest of hair." It is common to find hair follicles inside the cyst. Another theory is that pilonidal cysts are acquired through trauma to the sacroccocygeal region. During World War II, more than 80,000 soldiers developed pilonidal cysts that required a hospital stay. People thought the cysts were due to irritation from riding in bumpy jeeps, thus it was called "Jeep disease" for a long time (Chatlin & Barton, 2003; Ringelheim, Silverberg, & Johnson-Villanueva, 2006). The most common bacteria reported depends upon the populations sampled and the evidence obtained by the investigator. In one study, anaerobic cocci were present 77% of the time, aerobic organisms account for 4%, and a mixure of aerobic and anaerobic is about 17%. Other studies quote *Staphylococcus aureus* as being the most common bacterial pathogen (Ringelheim et al., 2006). Pilonidal cyst infections are commonly red, swollen, and painful. Sitting in a warm tub may decrease the pain and may decrease the chance of cyst development, but it is important to note that this is still an abscess or a boil. It needs to be drained or lanced to resolve. Like other boils, it does not get better with antibiotics alone. The treatment regimen in regards to pilonidal cysts usually involves incision and drainage, removing of the hair follicles, and packing the cavity with gauze (Chatlin et al., 2003; Ringelheim et al., 2006).

Checkpoint! 37–8 (Chapter Objective 3)

The organisms(s) most frequently associated with impetigo is/are:
1. *Group B Streptococcus*
2. *Staphylococcus aureus*
3. *Group A Streptococcus*
   A. *1 and 2*
   B. *1 and 3*
   C. *2 and 3*
   D. *1, 2, and 3*

Checkpoint! 37–9 (Chapter Objective 3)

Which of the epidermal/dermal infections flouresce a red color under Wood's lamp?
   A. *Erythrasma*
   B. *Cellulitis*
   C. *Erysipelas*
   D. *Erysipeloid*

INFECTIONS OF THE MUSCLE FASCIA AND MUSCLES

Necrotizing Fasciitis

Necrotizing fasciitis is a progressive, rapidly spreading, inflammatory infection located in the deep fascia (connective tissue that permeates the body). Because of gas-forming organisms, the presence of subcutaneous gases is classically described in necrotizing fasciitis (Maynor, 2006). The primary symptom is intense pain. Affected tissues are red, hot, and swollen and rapidly become discolored. Bullae (large blisters), **crepitus** (crackling sound due to gas in the soft tissue), and gangrene (tissue necrosis) (Figure 37-10) may develop. Subcutaneous tissues die, with widespread undermining of surrounding tissue. Muscles are spared initially but eventually become necrotic. Patients are acutely ill, with high fever, tachycardia, altered mental status, and hypotension. Patients may be bacteremic or septic, and may require aggressive hemodynamic support (Merck, 2005; Maynor, 2006). Necrotizing fasciitis is typically caused by a mixture of aerobic and anaerobic organisms that cause necrosis of subcutaneous tissue and the infection commonly affects the extremities and perineum. Group A streptococci (*Streptococcus pyogenes*), *Clostridium,* MRSA, or a mixture of aerobic and anaerobic bacteria such as *Bacteroides* species typically cause the infection. These organisms extend to the subcutaneous tissue from a contiguous ulcer, infection, or after trauma (penetrating or nonpenetrating). Streptococci and the potential bioterror agent *Yersinia pestis* can arrive from a remote site of infection via the bloodstream. Perineal involvement, also called Fournier's gangrene, is usually a complication of recent surgery. Necrotizing fasciitis produces tissue ischemia by widespread blockage of small subcutaneous vessels. These result in skin necrosis, which facilitates the growth of obligate anaerobes while promoting anaerobic metabolism by facultative organisms such as *Escherichia coli,* resulting in gangrene. Anaerobic metabolism produces hydrogen and nitrogen, relatively insoluble gases that may accumulate in subcutaneous tissues (Merck, 2005; Maynor, 2006). The overall morbidity and mortality is 70–80%. Old age, underlying medical problems, delayed diagnosis and therapy, and insufficient surgical debridement worsen prognosis. Usually the treatment regimen is primarily surgical and IV antibiotics. Amputation of an extremity may be necessary in severe cases. Antibiotic choices are usually reviewed based on Gram stain and culture results of tissues obtained during surgery (Merck, 2005; Maynor, 2006).

> ### REAL WORLD TIP
>
> It is important to remember that necrotizing fascitis progresses so quickly that the necrosis may outpace the body's inflammatory response. Some pathogens may produce toxins that lyse phagocytes. Direct Gram stains may not show polymorphonuclear leukocytes but should show the morphotype of the infecting bacteria.

BURN WOUND INFECTION

Burns are one of the most common and devastating forms of trauma. Patients with serious thermal injury require immediate specialized care in order to minimize morbidity and mortality. The breached skin barrier is the hallmark of thermal injury. There are two ways in which burn injury can occur: thermal and chemical injury. Thermal injury involves the direct contact with a flame, hot surface, hot liquid, or a source of heat conduction, convection, or radiation, which causes a degree of cellular damage to the skin that varies with the temperature and duration of exposure. As the temperature rises, there is an increase in molecular damage that leads to cell membrane dysfunction as ion channels are disrupted, resulting in sodium and water intake. As the temperature keeps rising further, protein denaturation occurs, oxygen radicals are liberated, and eventually cells die with the formation of the burn eschar (Church, Elsayed, Reid, Winston, & Lindsay, 2006).

Chemical injuries are those caused by acidic as well as alkaline materials, which add to coagulation necrosis by denaturing proteins. The long-term effect of caustic dermal burns is scarring, and depending on the site of the burn, it can be significant. If the eyes are involved, ocular burns can result in a complete loss of vision (Cox & Brooks, 2005).

Local inflammation following injury is essential for wound healing and host defense against infection. However, large burns can cause a systemic inflammatory response, leading to organ failure and death. In addition, septic shock causes significant cellular and organ damage. An anti-inflammatory response is necessary in an effort to maintain homeostasis and restore normal physiology. Cytokines and cellular responses help regulate such an initial massive inflammatory response so it does not get out of control. For a review of cytokines and their actions, go to ∞ Chapter 4.

Although burn wound surfaces are sterile immediately following injury, these wounds eventually become colonized with

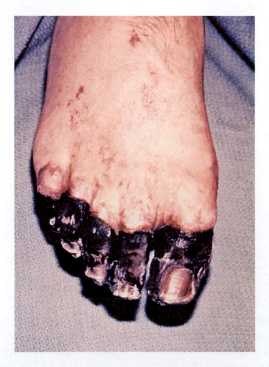

■ **FIGURE 37-10** Gangrene caused by *Yersinia pestis* (septicemic plague).
From Public Health Image Library (PHIL), CDC/William Archibald.

microorganisms. The nature and extent of the thermal injury along with the types and amounts of microorganisms colonizing the burn wound appear to influence the future risk of an invasive wound infection. Gram-positive bacteria that survive the thermal insult, such as staphylococci located deep within sweat glands and hair follicles, heavily colonize the wound surface within the first 48 hours unless treated with topical antimicrobial. Eventually, after 5–7 days, these wounds are subsequently colonized with other microbes such as gram-positive and gram-negative bacteria and yeast, which are derived from the host's normal gastrointestinal or upper respiratory flora or from the hospital environment or those transferred from health care workers. Over the last decades, gram-negative organisms have emerged as the most common etiologic agents of invasive infection due to their varied virulence factors and ability to demonstrate antimicrobial resistance.

Prior to the antibiotic era, *Streptococcus pyogenes* was the predominant pathogen implicated in burn wound infections and was a major cause of death in severely burned patients. Then shortly after the introduction of penicillin, *Staphylococcus aureus* became the principal pathogen in burn wound infections. Other gram-positive organisms involved in causing invasive burn wound infection include methicillin-resistant *Staphylococcus aureus,* coagulase-negative staphylococci, and *Enterococcus* species, including VRE. In addition to the above organisms, *Pseudomonas aeruginosa,* from the patient's endogenous gastrointestinal flora and environmental sources, is the most common cause of burn infections in many medical centers. The gram-negative organisms include *Escherichia coli, Klebsiella* species, *Enterobacter* species, and anaerobic bacteria (*Bacteroides* species, *Peptostreptococcus,* and *Proprianibacterium acnes*). It has become evident that viruses such as herpes simplex virus (HSV), cytomegalovirus, and varizella-zoster virus (VZV) can also cause burn wound infections. The fungi associated with infection include *Candida* species, *Aspergillus* species, *Fusarium* species, *Alternaria* species, *Rhizopus* species, and *Mucor* species (Bowler, Duerden, & Armstrong, 2001; Miller, 2007; Church et al., 2006; Weber & McManus, 2007; and Schwarz & Dulchaysky, 2005). Table 37-1 summarizes skin infections and potential pathogens of interest.

The emergence of antimicrobial resistance among a wide variety of human bacterial and fungal burn wound pathogens, particularly nosocomial isolates, limits the available therapeutic options for effective treatment of burn wound infections. Burn wound infections add to the delay in epidermal maturation and leads to additional scar tissue formation. Invasion of microorganisms into the tissue layers below the dermis may also result in bacteremia, sepsis, and multiple organ dysfunction syndrome. Clinical diagnosis of burn wound infection relies on regular monitoring of vital signs and inspection of the entire burn wound surface.

Burn wound infections invaded by bacteria or fungi are treated with surgical excision to the level of viable tissue. Wounds that can be excised completely should be covered with an allograft (donor skin) or autograft (the patient's own skin). If aggressive fungal infections occur particulary with

mucormycosis, radical debridement of muscle, including limb amputation, may be necessary to control infection. Antibiotics should be provided after injury to limit bacterial colonization. The established infection requires the use of topical agents that are able to penetrate the eschar to reduce microbial counts and prevent systemic dissemination (Schwarz & Dulchaysky, 2005).

> ### ✔ Checkpoint! 37–10 (Chapter Objective 3)
>
> *Which of the following is the primary gram-negative agent involved in burn wound infections in many medical centers?*
>   A. *MRSA*
>   B. *VRE*
>   C. *Escherichia coli*
>   D. *Pseudomonas aeruginosa*

POSTOPERATIVE SKIN INFECTIONS

In addition to breaks in the skin barrier, wound infections can occur as complications of surgery, trauma as in burns, and bites or diseases that interrrupt a mucosal or skin surface.

Surgery

Sources of surgical wound infections can further be evaluated by referring to ∞ Chapter 41, "Nosocomial Infection."

Bites

Human bite infections are potentially serious infections caused by a rapid growth of bacteria in broken skin. In adults, the most common form of human bite is the closed-fist injury, sometimes called the "fight bite." This type of injury results from forces sufficient enough to break the skin from striking an opponent's tooth and often inoculates the hand tendon and its sheath. As the hand is flexed at the time of impact, the bacterial load is transferred when the hand is opened and the tendon slides back to its relaxed state. Resulting contamination cannot be removed readily through normal cleansing and irrigation (McNamara, 2007). The infection itself can be caused by a number of bacteria that live in the human mouth. These include streptococci, particularly *Streptococcus anginosus* and *Streptococcus pyogenes, Staphylococcus aureus, Eikenella corrodens,* and oral anaerobes such as *Prevotella* species, *Fusobacterium* species, *Veilonella* species, and *Peptostreptococcus* species. Infections that begin less than 24 hours after the injury are usually produced by a mixture of organisms and can cause necrotizing infection resulting in death of a specific area of the tissue.

Microbiology of human bite wounds is fairly consistent, yet an untreated infected bite is cultured if purulence is present. Because of the deep nature of infected closed-fist injuries and relatively poor vascular supply to the tendons and other connective tissues, admitting patients for intravenous (IV) antibiotic therapy is best (McNamara, 2007). Debridement, the

Summary of Infectious Diseases of the Integumentary System

Infectious Disease	Usual Pathogen
Folliculitis	*Staphylococcus aureus*
	Candida
	Pseudomonas aeruginosa
	Malassezia
	Propionibacterium acnes (acne)
Furuncle (Boil)	*S. aureus*
	Mycobacterium fortuitum complex (pedicure related)
Carbuncle	*S. aureus*
Dermatophytosis	*Epidermophyton, Microsporum, Trichophyton*
Erysipelas	Group A beta-hemolytic streptococci
Erythrasma	*Corynebacterium minutissimum*
Erysipeloid	*Erysipelothrix rhusiopathiae*
Impetigo	*S. aureus*
	Group A beta-hemolytic streptococci
Cellulitis	*S. aureus*
	Beta-hemolytic streptococci, Group A, B, C, and G
	P. aeruginosa
	Rarely *Aeromonas, Vibrio vulnificus,* and others
	Haemophilus influenzae (periorbital in children)
Hidradenitis suppurativa	*S. aureus*
	gram-negative rods (e.g., *Proteus*)
Pilonidal abscess	Anaerobic cocci
	S. aureus
Necrotizing fasciitis	Beta-hemolytic streptococci groups A, C, and G
	Methicillin-resistant *S. aureus* (MRSA)
	Clostridium
	Mixed aerobic and anaerobic (e.g., *Bacteroides*)
Burn wound infection	*S. aureus*
	P. aeruginosa
	Group A beta-hemolytic streptococci
	Enterococci
	Coagulase-negative staphylococci
	Other gram-negative rods (*E. coli, Klebsiella, Enterobacter*)
	Anaerobic bacteria (*Bacteroides, Peptostreptococcus, Propionibacterium acnes*)
	Viruses (e.g., herpes simplex virus)
	Fungi (*Candida, Aspergillus, Fusarium, Alternaria, Rhizopus, Mucor*)
Bites	*Pasteurella multocida* and *P. canis* (animal)
	Capnocytophaga canimorsus (animal source)
	Eikenella corrodens (human and animal)
	Streptococci (human and animal)
	Staphylococci (human and animal)
	Anaerobic bacteria (*Bacteroides, Porphyromonas, Prevotella, Fusobacterium, Veillonella, Peptostreptococcus*) (human and animal)
	Less often *Moraxella, Neisseria weaveri, Corynebacterium,* and many others (human and animal)

removal of dead tissue and foreign objects from a wound, may also be necessary.

The most common problem following an animal bite is simple infection. The common animal bites usually are from dogs and cats. Dog bites are substantially more common than cat bites, but cat bites become infected more frequently than dog bites. Dog bites typically cause a crushing type wound because of their rounded teeth and strong jaws, whereas the sharp, pointed teeth of cats usually cause puncture wounds and lacerations that may inoculate bacteria into deep tissues. Bites of the hand generally have a high risk of infections because of the relatively poor blood supply (Stump, 2006).

Infections can be caused by nearly any group of pathogens. The most commonly isolated bacteria associated with dog bites include *Pasteurella* species (*Pasteurella multocida* and *Pasteurella canis*), *Streptococcus* species (*S. pyogenes* and viridans streptococci) and *Staphylococcus* species (*S. aureus, S. epidermidis,* and *S. intermedius*), and anaerobic bacteria (*Bacteroides* species, *Fusobacterium, Porphyromonas, Prevotella, Propionibacterium,* and *Peptostreptococcus*). The organisms most isolated in cat bites are: *Pasteurella multocida, Streptococcus* species, *Staphylococcus* (*S. epidermidis*), and the anaerobes described above. *Neisseria, Corynebacterium,* and *Moraxella* may also be isolated from infected bite sites. There are many other bacteria that have been implicated in bite infections. Microbes that are less frequently isolated from animal bites, but should be looked for, are *Capnocytophaga canimorsus* and *Eikenella corrodens* (Talan, Citron, Abrahamian, Moran, & Goldstein, 1999; Bowler et al., 2001; Miller, 2007). Table 37-1 provides a summary of important potential pathogens associated with bite wounds. Nearly all infections are mixed infections.

While local infection and cellulitis are the leading causes of morbidity, sepsis is a potential complication of bite wounds, particularly *Capnocytophaga canimorsus* sepsis in immunocompromised individuals. *Pasteurella multocida,* the cause of pasteurellosis, is the most common pathogen contracted from cat bites and may also be complicated by sepsis. Meningitis, osteomyelitis, and septic arthritis are additional concerns in bite wounds (Stump, 2006). Debridement, an effective means of preventing infection, should be performed and infected wounds should be cultured. In general, low-risk wounds do not need antibiotics, whereas high-risk wounds, such as cat

bites that are a true puncture, bites to the hand, and those in individuals with poor general health, require antibiotics. Visit ∞ Chapters 20 and 24 to review anaerobic bacteria and fastidious gram-negative rods.

▶ LABORATORY DIAGNOSTIC PROCEDURES

For many infections of the epidermis and dermis such as impetigo, folliculitis, furuncle, carbuncle, cellulitis, and erysipelas, diagnosis is generally made on a clincal basis. Superficial specimens from ulcers should not be cultured because they typically yield mixed aerobic and anaerobic isolates and the results cannot be used to guide therapy (Wilson & Winn, 2008). With each of the infections mentioned, it is important to have knowledge of the major bacterial pathogens involved.

SPECIMEN COLLECTION AND PROCESSING

If a dermatophyte infection is suspected, the lesion is cleaned and scrapings are obtained from the active border of the lesion. These scrapings should be examined for mycotic elements using 10% potassium hydroxide and fungal cultures should be done. In order to rule out erythrasma, use a Wood's lamp to detect the causative agent, which fluoresces with a characteristic coral-red color. *Corynebacterium minutissimum* produces porphyrin that accounts for the red flourescense. The absence of hyphae on skin scraping distinguishes erythrasma from tinea and in addition, this type of specimen should be cultured.

Since suspected lesions of cellulitis and erysipelas are generally diagnosed clinically, aspiration of the wound submitted for culture and Gram stain are of limited use. If the areas of infection form abscesses or bullae, then culture and Gram stain may be helpful. The aspirate should be plated onto a minimum of blood and chocolate agars along with liquid broth. Culture of any exudate obtained by aspiration or drainage of nodules is necessary and may require the addition of anaerobic media if collected properly.

With erysipeloid, a Gram stain may be performed on a skin scraping, which may show gram-positive rods; however, the stain is often negative because the infection is deep and the microorganism is not obtained with scraping. Culture of a biopsy may be necessary to reveal the organism. If systemic erysipeloid is suspected, blood cultures aid in the diagnosis.

For diagnosis of necrotizing fasciitis, it may be necessary to culture a blood specimen and tissues. It is important to note that a Gram stain in this case will usually show a mixture of polymicrobial flora with aerobic gram-negative rods and gram-positive cocci. Tissue biopsies are the best method to use when diagnosing this infection and can be performed from deeper tissues to obtain the proper isolation of the infecting microorganisms.

✓ Checkpoint! 37–11 (Chapter Objectives 6 and 8)

Carol was bitten by a dog. Several days later, a culture of the bite site grew an oxidase-positive, gram-negative rod on blood agar. The MacConkey agar showed no growth. The organism's probable identity is:

A. *Pseudomonas aeruginosa.*

B. *Pasteurella multocida.*

C. *Bacillus anthracis.*

D. *Neisseria spp.*

Media for the isolation of aerobes and anaerobes should be used for culture.

For burn patients, regular sampling of the burn wound either by surface swab or tissue biopsy for culture is done to monitor the presence of infection. Quantitative culture of tissue have been considered as the "gold standard" for confirming the presence of invasive burn wound infection; however, the value of laborious and costly quantitative burn wound tissue biopsy has been questioned. Many institutions have now shifted to the more convenient practice of obtaining burn wound surface swabs for qualitative or semiquantitative culture for infection. Burn wound surface swabs are a convenient and effective method for routinely collecting multiple superficial wound samples. In order to obtain enough cellular material for culture, the end of a sterile swab is moved over a minimum of one centimeter area of the open wound. Sufficient pressure should be applied to the tip of the swab to cause minimal bleeding in the underlying tissue. It has been shown that the recovery and reproducibility of organisms by using moistened swabs is far more superior than by using dry swabs.

It is important to consider the anaerobic organisms as potentially infecting organisms in burn wound infection when a specimen is collected. In order to isolate such organisms, an anaerobic transport system provides an optimal environment for the transport of inoculated surface swabs for culture. For viruses and fungi, tissue biopsy for culture and histology appear to be the most reliable diagnostic methods.

It is important to transport the swabs and tissue samples to the laboratory after collection to ensure optimal recovery of all types of microorganisms. If transport is delayed, the recovery of fastidious aerobes and anaerobes may be compromised. A direct Gram stain may provide information on the degree of microbial colonization. It is not considered to be suitable for diagnosing burn wound infection. Swabs submitted should be used to inoculate blood and MacConkey agars. Agar plates are inspected for growth after 24 and 48 hours of incubation at 35–37°C in ambient air. A qualitative microbiology report provides the identification of all potential pathogens regardless of amount and the results of antibiotic susceptibility testing by isolate (Church et al., 2006; Isenberg, 1992).

Superficial wounds should be inoculated onto blood, chocolate, and MacConkey agars, and thioglycolate broth (tissue only); media selective for gram-positive microbes such as PEA or CNA may be added. The BA and CA should be incubated in CO_2 at 35–37°C. MAC, Thio, and selective agar for gram-positives can be incubated in ambient air at 35–37°C. Abscesses and specimens collected from deeper wounds should have anaerobic media added to the above culture setup. A direct Gram stain can be helpful by revealing the presence of white blood cells, epithelial cells, and the predominant microbial morphology. If an abundance of epithelial cells are present, it may indicate an improperly collected specimen and anaerobic

Checkpoint! 37–12 (Chapter Objective 4)

Tommy developed a purulent abscess on his right toe. This material was aspirated and sent to the microbiology lab. This specimen should be inoculated on/in:

1. *Blood agar*
2. *Chocolate agar*
3. *MacConkey agar*
4. *Thioglycolate broth*
   A. *1, 2, and 3*
   B. *1, 3, and 4*
   C. *1, 2, and 4*
   D. *1, 2, 3, and 4*

culture should not be performed. Visit ∞ Chapter 7 to review the cultivation of specimens.

INTERPRETATION OF CULTURES

Plates are examined for growth after 24 hours of incubation. If no colonies are observed, the plates should be reincubated another 24 hours before the culture is reported as no growth.

 REAL WORLD TIP

In order to isolate the rapidly growing mycobacteria or aerobic actinomycetes the primary culture media should be held 3–5 days (Trevino & Weissfeld, 2008).

The direct Gram stain can be helpful in guiding the approach to the workup of the culture. If no growth occurs but bacteria are observed on the direct Gram stain, it could indicate an anaerobe, so the anaerobic cultures may reveal the pathogen. The thio should only be subcultured if the organisms are seen in the direct Gram stain, primary culture plates show no growth, and the thioglycolate shows growth. If the direct Gram stain reveals many epithelial cells, only minimal testing should be performed. Quality specimens will have few to no epithelial cells. Organisms such as coagulase-negative staphylococci, diptheroids, and viridans streptococci make up normal skin flora and should not be routinely worked up. Organisms that make up the normal skin flora may be significant when isolated from a sterile site, present in more than one culture, or present in the direct Gram stain as the predominant morphotype(s). All single isolates should be identified and susceptibility tested. If a culture shows mixed growth, only identify and perform susceptibility testing on a maximum of two organisms.

The most important organisms to report are beta-hemolytic streptococci, *Staphylococcus aureus*, *Pseudomonas aeruginosa*, and *Clostridium perfringens*. Beta-hemolytic streptococci are gram-positive cocci in chains that are catalase negative. Group-specific typing sera can be used to determine whether the isolate is group A, B, C, F, or G. Group A is also PYR positive.

S. aureus is seen as gram-positive cocci in clusters that are catalase and slide latex or coagulase positive. *P. aeruginosa* is a non-lactose fermenting gram-negative rod that can be presumptively identified with a positive oxidase result and the presence of a blue-green pigment and grape-like odor. *C. perfringens* is an anaerobic gram-positive rod (large boxcar shaped). It is catalase negative and can be presumptively identified based on its characteristic double zone hemolysis.

 REAL WORLD TIP

Remember to rule out *Staphylococcus intermedius* if a coagulase positive staphylococcus is isolated from a dog bite. *S. intermedius* is PYR positive whereas *S. aureus* is PYR negative.

If three or more organisms are present (rule of three) without a predominant organism, a report of mixed flora describing the number of gram-positive and gram-negative isolates can be sent to the physician. The plates should be held for one week to allow the physician the opportunity to request further workup (Isenberg, 2004).

The pattern of growth provides a clue as to the possible pathogen. If growth occurs on all plates (BA, CA, MAC) incubated aerobically, suspect a gram-negative rod such as *Pseudomonas* or one of the *Enterobacteriaceae*. Table 37-2✪ provides a guide for selecting identification tests to identify selected skin pathogens. If the colony growing on MAC is oxidase positive consider *Aeromonas* or *Vibrio* as well as other nonfermenters. A 6.5% NaCl will screen for a halophilic organism. *Vibrio* spp., other than *V. cholerae*, should be suspected if the 6.5% NaCl is positive. The string test is also helpful in differentiating *Aeromonas* (no string) from *Vibrio* (string of various lengths).

If growth occurs only on the BA and CA, suspect streptococci, enterococci, or staphylococci. If this pattern of growth occurs with a bite wound it could be an unusual isolate such as *Eikenella, Capnocytophaga*, or *Pasteurella*. *E. corrodens* is a gram-negative rod that may require 48 hours incubation for colonies to become visible. The colonies may pit the agar and display a distinct "bleach-like" odor. The organism is catalase, indole, and glucose negative but oxidase positive. *Capnocytophaga* is a fusiform-shaped gram-negative rod that may require 48–74

✪ TABLE 37-2

Identification of Selected Skin Pathogens

Pathogen	Microscopic Morphology	Colony Morphology			Identification Tests
		BA	CA	MAC	
Staphylococcus aureus	GPC, clusters	Large yellow or white, usually hemolytic	*	NG	CAT, slide latex, or coagulase
Beta-hemolytic streptococci	GPC in chains	Small gray, beta-hemolytic	*	NG	GS, CAT, PYR, Group A, B, C, G antigen typing
Pseudomonas aeruginosa	GNR	Large beta, aluminum foil sheen or blue-green pig, grape-like odor	*	NLF, Sheen, Green pig.	Ox, gram-negative identification panel if nonpigmented
Clostridium perfringens	Large "boxcar" GPR	Aerobic: NG Anaerobic: Large beta (double zone)	NG	NG	GS, CAT, Lecithinase
Aeromonas	GNR	Large gray, usually beta	*	LF or NLF	GS, Ox, String test, 6.5% NaCl, O129
Vibrio vulnificus	Curved GNR	Large gray	*	LF	GS, Ox, String test, 6.5% NaCl, O129
Haemophilus influenzae	Tiny, pleomorphic GNR	NG	Small, grayish	NG	GS, CAT, Porphyrin (ALA)
Candida albicans	Budding yeast	Creamy, white, "feet"	*	NG	Germ tube and chlamydoconidia, morphology agar
Eikenella corrodens	GNR	"Pitting," transparent, "bleach-like" odor	*	NG	GS, CAT, IND, Ox, GLU
Pasteurella	GNR (coccobacillary)	Large gray, musty odor	*	NG	GS, CAT, IND, Ox
Capnocytophaga	Fusiform GNR	Swarming, gray (48 hours)	*	NG	GS, CAT, IND, Ox
Enterobacteriaceae	GNR	Large gray	*	LF or NLF	Ox, gram-negative identification panel

GPC, gram-positive cocci; GPR, gram-positive rod; GNR, gram-negative rod; GNC, gram-negative cocci; *, growth same as BA; NG, no growth; LF, lactose fermenting; NLF, nonlactose fermenting; pig., pigment; GS, Gram stain; CAT, catalase; Coag, coagulase; PYR, pyrrolidonyl arylamidase; Ox, oxidase; Lecith, lecithinase; IND, indole; Glu, glucose; Arg, arginine; ALA, amino-levulinic acid.

hours for colonies to appear. They have a "gliding" motility, so a haze or swarming (like *Proteus*) may be observed around the colonies. *Capnocytophaga* is catalase and oxidase negative or weakly positive and indole negative. *Pasteurella* is a gram-negative coccobacillary microbe that is catalase, oxidase, and indole positive. ∞ Chapter 20, "Fastidious Gram-Negative Rods," provides more information on these organisms.

If growth occurs on the CA only, the isolate could be a fastidious organism like *Haemophilus* or *Neisseria*. Be aware that bioterror agents such as anthrax may manifest as a skin infection and should be reported to the local public health laboratory as soon as possible. Remember to correlate the Gram stain morphology, colony morphology, test results, identity and antibiogram prior to reporting the final results. Discrepancies must be resolved prior to generating the final report.

SUSCEPTIBILITY TESTING

Susceptibility testing should be performed on pure cultures and those with one or two predominant organisms when the Gram stain indicates a quality specimen or by doctor request. Susceptibility testing should not be performed on mixed cultures that do not have a predominant organism, normal skin flora, or isolates from poor specimens (i.e., many epithelial cells and no white blood cells observed in the Gram stain). ∞ Chapter 11 provides more information on susceptibility testing.

 ### Checkpoint! 37–13 (Chapter Objectives 6 and 8)

A gram-positive rod growing on blood agar anaerobically produces a double zone of beta-hemolysis. What is the presumptive identification?

  A. *Bacteroides ureolyticus*
  B. *Bacteroides fragilis*
  C. *Clostridium perfringens*
  D. *Clostridium difficile*

SUMMARY

The skin acts as a first line of defense against microbial infections. It physically blocks the entry of pathogens into the body, thus having an effective means in disease prevention. In summary, the skin is the body's largest and thinnest organ. It acts as a barrier between the external and internal environment. The skin along with its protective properties and components are able to serve and protect the human body from infectious organisms when subjected to trauma.

When a culture is requested by the physician, the specimen should be collected in such a way as to avoid contamination with normal skin flora. Aspirates and tissue are the preferred specimens. The direct Gram stain of the specimen can guide the extent of specimen workup. The presence of many epithelial cells in the direct specimen Gram stain may indicate a superficial or improperly collected specimen. Other microscopic procedures such as KOH preparations can also be performed. Aerobic culture usually includes BA, CA, MAC, and thioglycolate broth. Superficial specimens should not be cultured anaerobically. Single isolates or one or two predominant isolates should be identified and susceptibility tested. Mixed cultures should have minimal testing performed, but the plates should be held so physicians can request further workup. The most frequent and important organisms to workup are *S. aureus*, *Pseudomonas aeruginosa*, *Clostridium perfringens*, and beta-hemolytic streptococci. The clinical diagnosis can provide a clue as to the causative agent (Table 37-1). For example, a diagnosis of a boil or furuncle would lead to the expectation that *S. aureus* could be isolated. A diagnosis of "human bite" might result in the isolation of *Eikenella corrodens*. Remember to always correlate the Gram stain morphology, colony morphology, test results, identification, and antibiogram prior to reporting results. If the laboratory observations and results do not correlate to the identity then the discrepancy must be resolved prior to reporting. In this way, accurate and clinically relevant results will be received by the physician.

LEARNING OPPORTUNITIES

  1. Which of the following make up the integumentary system? (Chapter Objective 1)

  a. Skin

  b. Hair

  c. Nails

  d. Sweat glands

  e. All of the above

  f. None of the above

2. What is the main function of the integumentary system? (Chapter Objective 1)

   a. Distinguish

   b. Separate

   c. Protect

   d. Inform

   e. None of the above

   f. All of the above

3. Which of the following make up 90% of the epidermal cells? (Chapter Objective 1)

   a. Keratinocytes

   b. Melanocytes

   c. Langerhans cells

   d. Merkel cell

4. Which epidermal cells interact with white blood cells and work to fight infections but are easily damaged by UV radiation? (Chapter Objective 1)

   a. Merkel cells

   b. Langerhans cells

   c. Keratinocytes

   d. Melanocytes

5. A superficial wound specimen is submitted for culture and grows equal amounts of diphtheroids, alpha-hemolytic streptococci, and staphylococci. The next step is to: (Chapter Objectives 2 and 6)

   a. Report as normal skin flora

   b. Ask for a repeat specimen

   c. Identify the alpha-hemolytic *Streptococcus*

   d. Identify the staphylococci

6. Which disease is used to describe hair follicle infections? (Chapter Objective 3)

   a. Folliculitis

   b. Erysipelas

   c. Burn

   d. Cellulitis

7. Which fungus is associated with dermatophytosis? (Chapter Objective 3)

   a. *Trichophyton* species

   b. *Microsporum* species

   c. *Epidermophyton* species

   d. All of the above

   e. a and b only

8. Which epidermal/dermal infection is also known as "St. Anthony's fire"? (Chapter Objective 3)

   a. *Trichophyton* infection

   b. Erysipeloid

   c. Erysipelas

   d. Erythrasma

9. State the two ways in which burn injuries occur. (Chapter Objective 3)

   a. Thermal and chemical

   b. Physiological and social

   c. Inflammatory and thermal

   d. Mechanical and chemical

10. Prior to the antibiotic era, which of the following organisms was most predominant in burn wounds? (Chapter Objective 3)

    a. *Staphylococcus aureus*

    b. Vancomycin-resistant *Enterococcus* (VRE)

    c. *Streptococcus pyogenes*

    d. Coagulase negative staphylococci

11. A pustule drainage specimen from the right leg of a professional football player is submitted for culture and is plated onto primary media. After overnight incubation, the sheep blood agar and chocolate agar plate grows profuse white colonies with clear halos on sheep blood agar that bubble when tested with 3% hydrogen peroxide. The MacConkey shows no growth. The direct specimen Gram stain shows gram-positive cocci in clusters and polymorphonuclear leukocytes. (Chapter Objectives 1, 4, 5, 6, and 7)

    a. Is this a quality specimen?

    b. What is the possible genus?

    c. Should this organism be identified? (Explain your answer.)

    d. What would be the most appropriate test for additional identification of the isolate?

    e. What is the possible entry point for this microorganism?

CASE STUDY 37-1   (CHAPTER OBJECTIVES 3, 6, AND 8)

A 65-year-old retired woman helps her veterinarian son at his office. On a Monday morning, the son received a call about an injured horse and both of them drove to the farmer's home. A huge splinter had pierced the horse's leg, and the injury seemed infected and swollen, which left the horse in a lot of pain. The veterinarian and his mother were able to make an incision to remove the splinter and relieve the swelling. Days after surgery, she noticed a small cut on her finger that was swollen and tender. She thought nothing of it. Later in the week, the cut became bigger and it presented as a spreading cellulitis-like lesion on her hands and fingers. Upon examination she had a fever and noted pain. The patient's abscess was drained, aspirated, and the specimen collected was sent to the laboratory for culture. The organism that grew was a pleomorphic non-spore-forming, gram-positive rod. The organism grew barely on a blood agar plate showing alpha-hemolysis after prolonged incubation. The colonies are small, smooth, and translucent.

1. Which organism was isolated on the culture of the abscess?

2. What is the reservoir of this organism? How do humans commonly become infected by this organism?

3. How can infection with this organism be prevented?

4. Which other clinical syndromes can be caused by this organism?

5. Is the son's occupation significant to her case?

PEARSON myhealthprofessionskit™

Use this address to access the interactive Companion Website created for this textbook. Simply select "Clinical Laboratory Science" from the choice of disciplines. Find this book and log in using your user name and password.

REFERENCES

Go to myhealthprofessionskit.com to view this chapter's references.

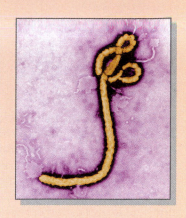

38

Central Nervous System

Teresa A. Taff

■ LEARNING OBJECTIVES

Upon completion of this chapter, the learner should be able to:

1. Locate the structures of the central nervous system, eye, and ear and describe their function(s).
2. Establish the source of microorganisms associated with infectious diseases of the central nervous system, eye, and ear and assess their clinical significance in culture.
3. Correlate patient history data and laboratory testing results in order to propose infectious disease states and their associated causative agents.
4. Determine patient populations at risk for infections by the microorganisms discussed.
5. Differentiate acute, chronic, and aseptic meningitis, brain abscess, and shunt infection based on laboratory testing results, physical appearance, and potential causative agents.
6. Select laboratory testing for and assess its value in the diagnosis of infectious disease processes.
7. Describe specimen collection and processing for all specimen types discussed.
8. Recognize discrepancies and propose potential source of errors with specimens and testing.
9. Select appropriate media for isolation of potential pathogens in patient clinical samples.
10. Recognize abnormal and critical values.

KEY TERMS

arachnoid membrane	encephalitis	pia mater
blood–brain barrier	endophthalmitis	pinkeye
brain abscess	keratitis	pleocytosis
cerebrospinal fluid	labyrinthitis	stye
conjunctiva	meninges	subarachnoid space
conjunctivitis	meningitis	trachoma
dacryocystitis	otitis media	tympanocentesis
dura mater		

▶ INTRODUCTION

Infections of the central nervous system can progress rapidly and lead to death if not diagnosed early. The role of the clinical microbiologist is critical for the detection and identification of pathogens that can cause disease. This chapter provides a review of the anatomy of the central nervous system, eye, and ear and a practical approach to the recognition, detection, and identification of the more common microorganisms that can cause infections.

▶ THE CENTRAL NERVOUS SYSTEM: REVIEW OF ANATOMY AND PHYSIOLOGY

The body's nervous system is composed of two major components: the central nervous system (CNS) and the peripheral nervous system. The central nervous system is made of the brain and spinal cord. The CNS is enclosed within bony structures for protection and is susceptible to infection by microorganisms.

The peripheral nervous system includes nerves that run from the brain and spinal cord to the rest of the body. They extend throughout the body much like a highway system. Many of these nerves are involved with sensations such as pain, temperature, and touch or voluntary and involuntary actions. They are not protected in bony structures such as the brain and spinal cord. This vulnerability can lead to damage due to trauma. The peripheral nervous system is prone to infectious agents such as human immunodeficiency virus (HIV), *Borrelia burgdorferi,* the causative agent of Lyme disease, herpes zoster, and hepatitis B and C. Refer to chapters related to these specific organisms for further details.

BRAIN AND CRANIAL NERVES

Principle Parts

Twelve pairs of cranial nerves connect to the underside of the brain and exit through the base of the skull through an opening called the foramen magnum. These nerves receive and send sensory and motor information for the head and neck area. The sense of smell, vision, hearing, and taste are all controlled by the cranial nerves. The rest of the body communicates with the central nervous system by means of the 31 spinal nerves originating in the spinal cord.

Protection and Coverings

The brain weighs about 3 pounds and is made of gray and white matter, which has a jelly-like appearance. The gray matter contains the brain's neurons and surrounds the white matter, which contains the nerve fibers. The brain is enclosed in a bony case called the skull. The skull serves to protect the brain from injury. Another protective measure provided by the body is the three layers of connective tissue that cover the

brain, spinal cord, and cranial nerves. The outermost layer is called the **dura mater.** This tough layer lies next to the skull. The middle layer is called the **arachnoid membrane.** Its name describes it structure. It is a thin, spongy spider web of connective tissue that lies just above the third layer, the **pia mater.** The pia mater is delicate and clings directly to the surface of the brain and spinal cord.

The space between the arachnoid membrane and the pia mater is called the **subarachnoid space.** It is filled with **cerebrospinal fluid** (CSF), a clear body fluid. The space allows the fluid to circulate from the interior ventricles of the brain, around the brain, and down the spinal cord. Nutrients are delivered and wastes removed via blood vessels that run through the subarachnoid space. The dura mater, arachnoid membrane, and pia mater are collectively referred to as the **meninges.** Figure 38-1 depicts the structure of the meninges.

✓ **Checkpoint! 38–1 (Chapter Objective 1)**

The meninges is/are comprised of the:
   A. *Dura mater*
   B. *Arachnoid membrane*
   C. *Pia mater*
   D. *A, B, and C*
   E. *B and C*

Cerebrospinal Fluid (CSF)

The cerebrospinal fluid is the bodily fluid that provides protection to the brain by acting as a cushion during sudden movement and trauma. It also carries nutrients and wastes within the central nervous system. The body contains a total volume of approximately 150 milliliters CSF. Each day the ventricles of the brain produce about 500 to 700 milliliters from the blood. As CSF is produced, it is also reabsorbed. This helps maintain the CSF's pressure level around the brain and within the spinal column. CSF differs from plasma by its slightly lower pH (7.33), very low levels of protein, and higher concentrations of glucose and chloride concentrations (Brandis, 2005). Protein levels are normally 15–45 mg/dl (milligrams per deciliter) while the glucose level is often 50–75 mg/dl. The glucose level of the CSF is usually two-thirds that of the blood glucose concentration. CSF is transparent in color and rarely contains red blood cells. It can contain 0–5 white blood cells/mm^3 (millimeters cubed) in the form of lymphocytes and/or monocytes. CSF is the specimen of choice for diagnosis of infection of the central nervous system.

Blood–Brain Barrier (BBB)

The **blood–brain barrier** is a physical structure formed by the tightly fused cells of the blood vessels of the brain. The blood vessel cells are surrounded by glial cells, which add structure to

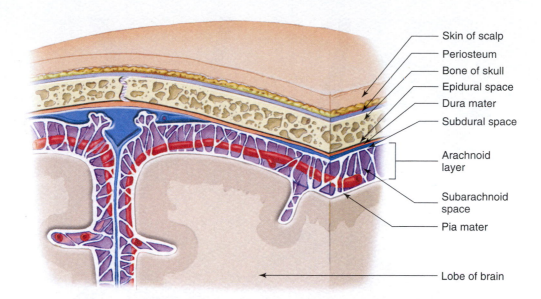

Skin of scalp
Periosteum
Bone of skull
Epidural space
Dura mater
Subdural space
Arachnoid layer
Subarachnoid space
Pia mater
Lobe of brain

■ **FIGURE 38-1** The three layers of the meninges, the dura mater, arachnoid membrane layer, and pia mater can be observed in this illustration of a cross-section of the brain. Note the spiderweb-like appearance of the arachnoid membrane within the subarachnoid space.

the vessels as well as hold the neurons of the brain. The unique structure of the BBB does not allow the exchange of substances that normally occurs in other blood vessels in the body. This can be a disadvantage when selecting drugs and antibiotics for delivery to the central nervous system. Some vital nutrients such as glucose are able to be transported to the brain by special mechanisms such as transporter molecules or absorption by the vessel cell membranes. The BBB can be weakened by inflammation due to infectious agents, trauma, or increased pressure. This allows it to be a potential route of infection for the central nervous system. Figure 38-2 ■ demonstrates the tight fusion of the blood vessel cells of the blood–brain barrier.

THE SPINAL CORD

Anatomy and Protective Coverings

The spinal cord is protected by the bony vertebrate of the neck and back. It is continuous with the brain and made up of gray and white matter. It is covered by the same three membranes—the dura mater, arachnoid membrane, and pia mater—as the brain. The spinal cord functions to relay sensory information from the body to the brain and motor commands from the brain. All of this is accomplished by means of the 31 pairs of spinal nerves.

Because the spinal cord is continuous with the brain, it is also surrounded and protected by CSF. The spinal cord runs about two-thirds of the way down the entire vertebral column. The point where the spinal cord ends can provide the physician easier access to the fluid for laboratory testing. CSF can be extracted by means of a needle puncture between two lower

back (lumbar) vertebrate. This procedure is referred to as a lumbar puncture or cerebrospinal tap. Sterility must be maintained to prevent microorganisms from entering the CSF during the procedure. Care must be taken to prevent damage to the spinal cord. Figure 38-3 ■ demonstrates a lumbar puncture or cerebrospinal tap.

▶ INFECTIOUS DISEASES OF THE CENTRAL NERVOUS SYSTEM

MENINGITIS

Bacterial **meningitis** is the term used to describe infection of the meninges. It is the most common presentation of infection of the central nervous system. It is a potentially life-threatening situation. Bacteria can cause inflammation of the meninges, infection of the CSF of the subarachnoid space, or both. The central nervous system is maintained as a sterile environment within the body. Microorganisms can gain access to the sterile setting by several mechanisms. The organisms may extend to the brain from infections of the nearby sinuses or middle ear. They may also start as an infection at another distant site such as the lung and travel to the brain through the bloodstream. Most infections begin with the individual acquiring an organism that they have not previously encountered. Without previous exposure, an individual does not usually have antibodies present to fight the organism.

For infection to begin, the organism initially colonizes the mucous membranes of the nasopharynx of the upper respiratory

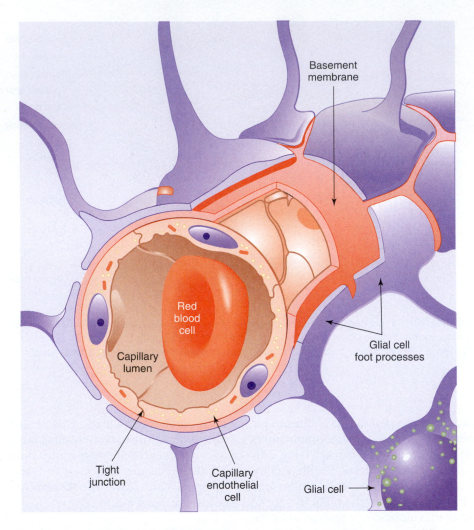

■ **FIGURE 38-2** The blood–brain barrier is effective in the prevention of the invasion of microorganisms due to the tightly fused endothelial cells of the blood vessels. The cells can weaken and allow particles to pass through the junctions due to inflammation, trauma, or increased pressure.

tract. Some possess surface structures such as fimbriae or pili, which allow them to adhere closely to the nasopharyngeal epithelial cells and escape detection by the body's immune system. Many organisms that invade the central nervous system possess a capsule that increases an organism's ability to invade normal tissue by preventing phagocytosis by white blood cells. The capsule antigens of some organisms can mimic the antigens of nonpathogenic organisms so the body does not recognize them as potentially dangerous.

Once the organism is able to colonize the mucosal membrane of the nasopharynx, it must invade the tissue and blood vessels and gain access to the bloodstream. In the bloodstream it must overcome the host's natural immune defenses such as antibodies, complement-mediated bactericidal activity, and neutrophil phagocytosis before it can invade the central nervous system. The presence of a capsule helps cloak the organisms so the host defenses do not see it as foreign. Many of the common bacterial meningitis pathogens possess capsules.

Once in the bloodstream, organisms must cross the blood–brain barrier. The presence of a capsule, lipopolysaccharide (LPS), or teichoic acid in the organism's cell wall, the production of toxins and other virulence factors, and the production of inflammatory host cytokines all play a role in increasing the BBB's permeability (Tunkel & Scheld, 1993). Increased permeability can also lead to brain swelling and increased intracranial pressure. The BBB's increased permeability can be an asset for treatment. It allows up to five times the normal amount of antibiotics to enter the CSF during infection (Cohen & Powderly, 2004).

Once the organisms gain access to the subarachnoid space they must proliferate to cause inflammation and infection. Cerebrospinal fluid has some innate disadvantages when it comes to fighting off organisms. Complement, a protein used in combination with antibodies to destroy foreign organisms, is normally absent and even inflammation within the central nervous system usually only leads to very low concentrations

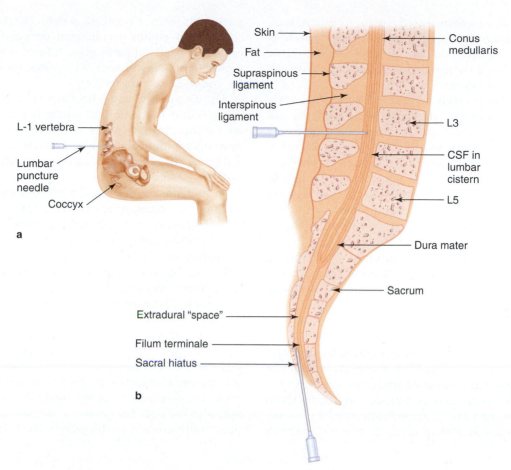

Skin

Fat

Supraspinous ligament

Interspinous ligament

Conus medullaris

L3

CSF in lumbar cistern

L5

Dura mater

Sacrum

L-1 vertebra

Lumbar puncture needle

Coccyx

a

Extradural "space"

Filum terminale

Sacral hiatus

b

■ **FIGURE 38-3** **a.** A lumbar puncture for the collection of CSF. The patient bends at the waist so the lumbar vertebrate separate for easier insertion of the collection needle. **b.** A detailed structure of the spinal column in the lower back. The needle is typically inserted between the third and fourth or fourth and fifth lumbar (back) verterbrate. The spinal column ends at about the first lumbar vertebrate so there is little chance of hitting it with the needle. CSF can be collected at the base of the spine as well but the procedure is rarely performed.

(Tunkel & Scheld, 1993). Immunoglobulin or antibody concentrations are very low in normal CSF. Immunoglobulin G does not appear in the CSF until late in the course of disease (Tunkel & Scheld, 1993). Normally there are only 0–5 white blood cells/mm^3 present in CSF and they are usually lymphocytes or monocytes. The presence of bacteria typically triggers the production of neutrophils as part of the body's immune defense mechanisms. The presence of 1,000 or more neutrophils/mm^3 in CSF is a classic sign of bacterial infection but they often lag behind the appearance of a microorganism. An increase in the number of white blood cells in a CSF is known as **pleocytosis.**

Most of the injury to the brain during meningitis occurs not due to direct invasion by microorganisms but due to the body's own immune response. As the body tries to attack the invading organism, it inadvertently hurts some of its own brain cells in the battle. Even after the organisms are eradi-cated with treatment, there is still potential for injury to the brain cells due to an overstimulated immune system.

The age, health status, and even genetic makeup of an individual can impact the ability of an organism to cause infection in the central nervous system. Extremes in age such as the very young and very old can render an individual more susceptible to meningitis. Both age groups are considered compromised immune states. The newborn acquires antibodies from the mother, which survive 3–9 months. Its immune system does not fully mature until about the age of 2 years. Prior to the *Haemophilus influenzae* type b (Hib) vaccine, children under the age of 2 were the most susceptible age group and accounted for most cases of bacterial meningitis (Cohen & Powderly, 2004). Older adults are prone to infection due to immune systems that can have reduced function. Anyone with an underlying condition such as neutropenia, alcoholism, diabetes mellitus, malignancies, loss of spleen function, and malnutrition can also be at increased risk for infection. Individuals can possess a genetic predisposition to infections with some meningitis pathogens due to deficiencies in the classic complement-mediated bactericidal pathway and other elements of the immune system.

Bacterial meningitis tends to peak in winter and early spring, which coincides with the incidence of bacterial and viral respiratory infections. Some meningitis pathogens are passed person-to-person whereas others begin as a local infection such as otitis media (middle ear infection) or pneumonia. Epidemic outbreaks can occur when groups of individuals spend time together in close proximity. Recruits in military barracks and students in university dormitories live in close proximity to each other for months. They encounter bacterial strains they have not been exposed to before and do not have circulating antibodies against. The physical and mental stress both groups experience can dampen their normal immune systems and make them more prone to developing infections.

Acute Meningitis

Acute meningitis in adults is often recognized by its major signs and symptoms: headache, fever, stiff neck, lethargy, or coma and an abnormal number of white blood cells in the cerebrospinal fluid. There may be a change in mental status such as confusion due to the increased intracranial pressure. Seizures occur in about 30% of patients who present with

meningitis (Betts, Chapman, & Penn, 2003). The disease usually develops rapidly over hours to days and is predominantly caused by bacterial pathogens. Infants may not exhibit the typical fever and stiff neck. They often present with irritability, vomiting, or poor feeding.

The diagnosis of acute bacterial meningitis requires laboratory testing of the CSF. All testing of CSF should be considered a top priority in the laboratory or STAT due to the necessity for immediate medical intervention. STAT is a medical term derived from the Latin word "statim," which means instantly or immediately.

In bacterial meningitis, the white blood count is usually elevated, at a count of greater than 1,000 per mm^3 and consists primarily of neutrophils. With an increase in white blood cells the fluid will often appear turbid or cloudy. Newborns, premature infants, and neutropenic patients may have low CSF white blood cell counts even in the presence of disease due to their compromised immune systems. The glucose level is typically decreased to less than 40 mg/dl (normal = 50–75 mg/dl). The protein level is usually increased to greater than 100 mg/dl (normal = 15–45 mg/dl). During meningitis, the brain and spinal tissues increase their use of glucose for energy. The circulating organisms and white blood cells present also use glucose to decrease its concentration even further. The increased permeability of the blood–brain barrier leaks protein into the CSF. The presence of the organisms and white blood cells also add to the protein level. Table 38-1✪ differ-

✪ TABLE 38-1

A Summary of Normal CSF Results Compared to those of Acute, Chronic and Aseptic Meningitis Based on Clinical Presentation, Cell Count, Predominant White Blood Cell Type, Glucose Level, and Protein Level

	Clinical Presentation	Cell Count as White Blood Cells/mm³	Predominant White Blood Cell	Glucose Level in mg/dl	Protein Level in mg/dl
Normal CSF	NA	0–5	Lymphocytes and/ or monocytes	50–75	15–45
Acute meningitis (bacterial)	■ Presents in hours to days ■ Stiff neck ■ Lethargy ■ Coma	>1,000	Neutrophils	↓ (0–40)	↑ (100–500)
Chronic meningitis	■ Presents in days, weeks, or months ■ Headache ■ Fever ■ Seizures	Fungal 10–200 Mycobacterial 200–500	Fungal ■ Lymphocytes Mycobacterial ■ Lymphocytes	Fungal N to slight ↓ Mycobacterial N to slight ↓	Fungal ↑ (50–200) Mycobacterial ↑ (50–300)
Aseptic meningitis (viral)	■ Presents in days to weeks ■ Headache ■ Fever ■ Photophobia ■ Malaise ■ Mental changes	100–500	Lymphocytes	N to slight ↓	N to ↑ (45–200)

N, normal; NA, not applicable; ↑, increased; ↓, decreased; >, greater than.

entiates acute, chronic, and aseptic meningitis from normal CSF based on clinical presentation and laboratory results.

> ✓ **Checkpoint! 38–2**
> **(Chapter Objective 5)**
>
> *Biochemically, acute bacterial meningitis is defined as:*
>
> | | Glucose Level | Protein Level | Predominant WBC Present |
> |---|---|---|---|
> | A. | normal | increased | lymphocyte |
> | B. | decreased | increased | neutrophil |
> | C. | decreased | increased | lymphocyte |
> | D. | increased | increased | neutrophil |

Microbes Associated with Acute Meningitis

Haemophilus influenzae. In the early 1980s *H. influenzae* caused about 50% of the bacterial meningitis cases in children under the age of 6 (Betts et al., 2003). The capsular serotype b was the most prevalent strain. Its invasiveness and virulence were attributed to the presence of its capsule. Underlying infections such as otitis media and sinusitis were often the initial source of the organism.

With the introduction of the *Haemophilus influenzae* b (Hib) conjugate vaccine in the mid-1980s, cases of bacterial meningitis due to serotype b dropped dramatically. The organism is rarely encountered in the clinical laboratory today due to the success of the vaccine. It now accounts for only about 7% of acute meningitis cases seen today (Betts et al., 2003). The key to prevention is ensuring all children are vaccinated.

> ⊙ **REAL WORLD TIP**
>
> ■ *Haemophilus influenzae* serotype b is invasive and always considered pathogenic in the CSF. An easy way to memorize the serotype is to remember b equals bad. It is rare for other capsular types to cause meningitis.
>
> ■ Most cases of *H. influenzae* type b meningitis occur in children who have not been vaccinated.

Neisseria meningitidis. *Neisseria meningitidis* is passed person to person by means of respiratory secretions. It can be highly contagious if an individual does not have antibodies to the strain of organism encountered. This organism accounts for about 25% of cases of acute meningitis in children and young adults and carries a high mortality rate (Betts et al., 2003). About 50–60% of infected individuals develop a characteristic rash due to the presence of the organism in the blood (Mandell, Bennett, & Dolin, 2000). The rash is due to lipopolysaccharide (LPS) present in the organism's cell wall. LPS is an endotoxin that damages the blood vessels and causes bleeding under the skin. Small dots of bleeding under the skin are called petechiae. As the petechiae enlarge and join together

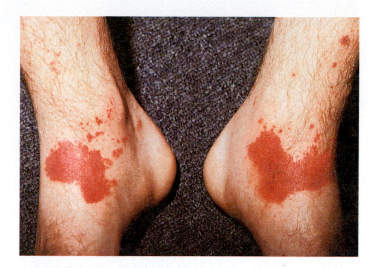

■ **FIGURE 38-4** This photograph demonstrates the characteristic rash associated with *Neisseria meningitidis* infection. The small petechiae are caused by blood vessels bleeding under the skin due to damage by lipopolysaccharide in the organism's cell wall. As the petechiae enlarge and join together they form purpura and begin to resemble bruises.
From http://en.wikipedia.org.

to form larger areas, they are called purpura. Figure 38-4 ■ demonstrates the characteristic rash associated with *Neisseria meningitidis* infection.

The disease can rapidly progress to death due to shock and multiple organ failure. LPS of the organism's cell wall creates problems in the body's coagulation system, which leads to massive tissue destruction of the extremities. Figure 38-5 ■

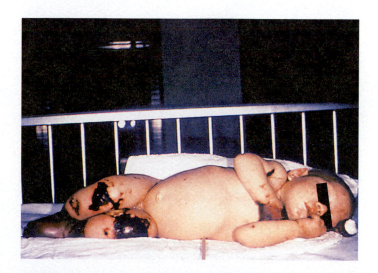

■ **FIGURE 38-5** This infant displays gangrene due to *Neisseria meningitidis.* The organism's capsule causes problems in the body's coagulation system. The blood vessels leak and are eventually destroyed so the tissues cannot be adequately oxygenated and die. The extremities are most often affected and can result in multiple amputations.
From Public Health Image Library (PHIL), CDC/Mr. Gust.

demonstrates the depth of the tissue damage which, can be caused by the presence of *Neiseseria meningitidis* in the blood.

A vaccine to *Neisseria meningitidis* capsular serotypes A, C, Y, and W135 is available and highly recommended for college-bound students and military recruits. The vaccine does not offer protection against serotype B. Serotype B does not elicit a good immune response in humans because its capsule antigens mimic an antigen present in human brain tissue. If antibodies were produced against this serotype, they would attack the host.

 REAL WORD TIP:

- *Neisseria meningitidis* seroptype B is extremely pathogenic for humans and there is no vaccine in use for protection against it. An easy way to memorize this serotype is to remember that b equals bad.

- A vaccine for *Neisseria meningitidis* serotype B has been developed and is currently in clinical trials. The current vaccine in use for serotypes A, C, W, and Y135 is directed against the capsule of these organisms to produce antibodies in humans. This method could prove to have harmful effects for humans if used for vaccine against serotype B. The research vaccine for serotype B is directed against the organism's outer membrane vesicles, which are subcapsular antigens (Findlow et al., 2006).

Checkpoint! 38–3 (Chapter Objective 4)

Which of the following individuals is most commonly associated with meningitis due to Neisseria meningitidis?

    A. *Infant born at 34 weeks gestation*
    B. *70-year-old male*
    C. *20-year-old college student*
    D. *Pregnant 27-year-old female*

Streptococcus pneumoniae. *Streptococcus pneumoniae* can infect all age groups, with the most severe disease encountered in the very young and very old. It accounts for about 47% of all cases of acute meningitis encountered and has a high mortality rate (Betts et al., 2003) Individuals often have underlying infections such as pneumonia, otitis media, and sinusitis, which act as a seeding site for the organism. Figure 38-6 illustrates the potentially lethal effect of *Streptococcus pneumoniae* meningitis. A vaccine against 23 of the most common capsular serotypes is available but does not cover all possible

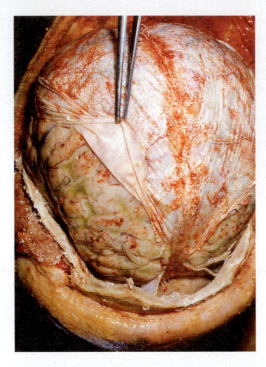

FIGURE 38-6 In this photograph taken at autopsy, the dura mater has been pulled back to reveal the collection of purulent (yellowish or greenish substance made up of organisms, white blood cells, fibrin, and cellular debris) material within the meninges. This individual died of bacterial meningitis due to *Streptococcus pneumoniae.*
From Public Health Image Library (PHIL), CDC/Dr. Edwin P. Ewing, Jr.

serotypes. The vaccine does not create a good immune response in children under the age of 2 years.

REAL WORLD TIP

Streptococcus pneumoniae is the leading cause of meningitis after head injury with resulting skull fracture (Plaisier et al., 2005). With head injury, a tear in the dura can occur which allows organisms from infected sinuses and middle ear to enter the CSF. If the skull fracture is not detected at the time of injury, the resulting meningitis may not appear for weeks to months after the event.

Streptococcus agalactiae. *Streptococcus agalactiae* (Group B *Streptococcus*) (GBS) is known for its affinity for neonates. This encapsulated organism can colonize the birth canal of the mother and be passed to the infant at birth. All pregnant women should be routinely screened for colonization with GBS at 35–37 weeks gestation. Antibiotics given to the mother at birth can lessen the neonate's chance of developing complications due to this organism.

- *Streptococcus agalactiae* is also known as Group B *Streptococcus* and is associated with infections in neonates. Its serotype is easy to memorize because b equals bad for babies.

- A pregnant woman can create antibodies against Group B *Streptococcus* and pass them on to her baby *in utero*. The presence of these antibodies protects the baby at birth against potential infection. A vaccine against Group B *Streptococcus* given to females would prove invaluable in preventing life-threatening infections in newborns. Investigations in creating a Group B *Streptococcus* vaccine have been ongoing since the 1980s. There does not appear to be one universal antigen that provides protection against the multiple strains of the organism. The organism also has the ability to vary its genes just like many other organisms. Both issues have slowed the progress of a vaccine for Group B *Streptococcus*.

Listeria monocytogenes.   *Listeria monocytogenes* is associated with acute meningitis in neonates and adults with underlying conditions such as malignancy, alcoholism, and transplant recipients on immunosuppressive therapy. Pregnant females can carry the organism in their genitourinary and gastrointestinal tracts with no signs or symptoms. The organism is transferred to the fetus *in utero* and can result in stillbirth. The organism can be acquired by adults through contaminated food such as unpasteurized milk, soft cheeses, or contact with domesticated animals such as cattle, sheep, and rabbits.

REAL WORLD TIP

- The colonies of *Listeria monocytogenes* and *Streptococcus agalactiae* (Group B *Streptococcus*) are so similar that they are hard to differentiate by physical characteristics only. Both appear as gray-white colonies that exhibit a soft (subtle) beta hemolysis. Gram stain and catalase are key reactions for differentiation of the organisms. *Listeria monocytogenes* is a small gram-positive rod that is catalase positive whereas *Streptococcus agalactiae* appears as gram-positive cocci in pairs and chains that is catalase negative.

- Hot dogs, cold cuts, and deli meats can be a potential source of *Listeria monocytogenes* for pregnant females and immunocompromised individuals. They should be thoroughly cooked before consumption.

Escherichia coli.   *E. coli* serotype K1 has an affinity for causing meningitis in neonates after birth. The K1 serotype is characterized by its capsule. The organism is probably acquired at birth from the mother as the baby passes through the birth canal or from individuals who come in contact with the baby after birth. Often babies that are affected have weakened immune responses at birth and therefore have a higher mortality rate with this organism. Adults with head trauma or with previous neurological surgery are prone to infection with this organism as well.

Naegleria fowleri.   While acute meningitis is most frequently caused by bacteria, one parasite is known for its ability to directly attack the CNS. *Naegleria fowleri,* an amoeba, lives in fresh water and swimming pools. Patients often have a history of swimming, water skiing, or diving in lakes. The organism enters through the nasal passage and travels up the olfactory lobes to the brain. The amoeba invades the brain cells to cause **encephalitis** or infection of the brain cells and meningitis. The disease it causes is known as primary amebic meningoencephalitis because the organism takes a direct route through the nose to attack the brain rather than reaching it through a secondary route such as the blood, sinuses, or middle ear. The patient experiences a sudden onset of symptoms with a high fever and severe headache. There is a rapid progression to coma and death in virtually all cases. Figure 38-7 ■ demonstrates the amoeba in brain tissue.

The CSF of primary amoebic meningoencephalitis is purulent or full of white blood cells just like that seen in acute bacterial meningitis. The white blood cells present can be neutrophils, lymphocytes, and eosinophils. The other CSF test results such

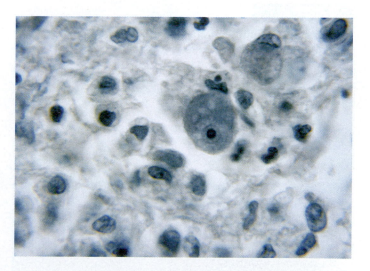

■ FIGURE 38-7 This stained section of brain tissue reveals the prominent single nucleus characteristic of the amoeba *Naegleria fowleri*. The rounded organism is located slightly above and to the right of the center of the picture. It is surrounded by inflammatory cells such as lymphocytes and neutrophils.
From Public Health Image Library (PHIL), CDC/Dr. Martin D. Hicklin.

as the glucose and protein levels also mimic a bacterial infection. The key difference is the lack of bacteria observed on a direct Gram stain examination of the CSF and negative cultures.

⊜ REAL WORLD TIP

■ While extremely rare, always consider *Naegleria fowleri* as a possible meningitis pathogen when the CSF is purulent but the Gram stain is negative for bacteria. Often the patient presents with an altered mental status and may not be able to provide the physician an adequate history.

■ *Naegleria fowleri* trophozoites can closely resemble white blood cells in CSF. In hematology, care must be taken not to misidentify the amoeba when examining the CSF in a hemocytometer or cell counting chamber. The amoeba has directional movement and internal structures such as a prominent single nucleus. Most clinical laboratories perform CSF cell counts on automated hematology analyzers. The amoeba will be misidentified as white blood cells using this method.

Acute Meningitis Outcomes. *Haemophilus influenzae, Neisseria meningitidis,* and *Streptococcus pneumoniae* are responsible for up to 80% of cases of acute bacterial meningitis (Corless et al., 2001). Box 38-1⊙ summarizes the most common bacterial pathogens of acute meningitis and correlates them with the most frequent patient population affected.

⊙ BOX 38-1

The Most Common Bacterial Meningitis Pathogens and the Patient Population(s) They Affect

■ *Haemophilus influenzae* type b
  • Children under the age of 6 years especially if not vaccinated
■ *Neisseria meningitis*
  • Children
  • Young adults
    ■ College-age students
    ■ Military recruits
■ *Streptococcus pneumoniae*
  • Older adults
  • Children under the age of 2 years
■ *Streptococcus agalactiae*
  • Neonates
■ *Listeria monocytogenes*
  • Neonates
  • Adults with underlying conditions such as malignancy, alcoholism, or on immunosuppressive therapy
■ *E. coli* K1
  • Neonates
  • Adults with head trauma or previous neurological surgery

Overall 10–15% of cases of acute meningitis are fatal. Even if the disease is treated early and aggressively, there may still be lasting effects down the road. Long-term effects include permanent hearing loss and mental retardation due to the damage caused by increased intracranial pressure and brain swelling. Acute meningitis with *Neisseria meningitidis* can result in loss of multiple limbs due to vessel damage triggered by the presence of the organism. Other complications include paralysis and seizures, which require lifelong care.

Chronic Meningitis

Chronic meningitis usually develops slowly over weeks to months and most often affects immunocompromised or immunosuppressed individuals. The typical patient has a diagnosis of AIDS or other malignancies or is on chemotherapy or long-term steroid use. An individual with a normal immune state may acquire chronic meningitis if they have an underlying condition such as tuberculosis.

Signs and symptoms of chronic meningitis may be similar to acute meningitis but usually vary greatly. Most individuals initially present with headache and fever. As the disease progresses, neurological signs such as seizures and mental status changes increase. A thorough physical and patient history will reveal the slow and gradual onset. Patient information such as previous exposure to animals, travel history, and even sexual history can assist the physician in narrowing down the etiological agent of chronic meningitis.

The causative agents of chronic meningitis cover the entire range of microorganisms—bacteria, viruses, fungi, and parasites. The white cell count of the cerebrospinal fluid is usually high but lower than that seen with bacterial meningitis. White blood cell counts are often in the range of 100–500 cells/mm^3. While this may seem similar to acute meningitis the type of white blood cell present will vary based on the causative agent. Chronic infections with bacteria usually present with neutrophils; viral and fungal infections elicit lymphocytes, whereas infestations with parasites may produce eosinophils. The CSF glucose level is most often decreased (<40 mg/dl) while the protein level is elevated (>45 mg/dl), but not as high as seen with acute meningitis. Because chronic meningitis usually affects those who are not able to produce a normal immune response to infection, the CSF laboratory test results can appear normal even with active disease.

Microbes Associated with Chronic Meningitis

Mycobacterium tuberculosis. Meningitis due to *M. tuberculosis* is often associated with untreated pulmonary tuberculosis that has spread outside the lungs. The organism reaches the subarachnoid space by spreading from a nearby infection site or through the bloodstream. Many cases are found in those with AIDS or underlying conditions such as alcohol or drug abuse and older adults. The patient develops a headache, nausea, and low-grade fever, which eventually progresses to drowsiness and coma. The cell count of the CSF is usually in the range of 200–500/mm^3 with a predominance of lymphocytes (Betts et al., 2003). The glucose and protein levels mimic those of acute meningitis.

Cryptococcus neoformans.   *Cryptococcus neoformans* is an encapsulated yeast that infects individuals with compromised or suppressed immune systems. Individuals with AIDS are highly susceptible. The organism is typically inhaled after contact with dried bird feces, especially those of pigeons. The organism spreads throughout the body with the central nervous system as the most common site of infection. CSF glucose is usually decreased but may be normal in two-thirds of AIDS patients. The protein concentration is increased while the white blood cell count is elevated, with a predominance of lymphocytes in the range of 10–200/mm^3 (Betts et al., 2003). Untreated infections are nearly always fatal.

Treponema pallidum.   The spirochete *T. pallidum* is transmitted by sexual contact or *in utero*. The causative agent of syphilis enters the CSF early in the infection but clinical CNS signs may not appear for months to years after initial infection. Chronic meningitis with *T. pallidum* is most often associated with individuals at risk for HIV infections such as intravenous drug users and prostitutes. Laboratory results include a predominance of lymphocytes with a mild decrease in the glucose concentration and elevated protein levels.

Toxoplasma gondii.   Parasites can invade the central nervous system. *Toxoplasma gondii* is an intracellular, single-celled parasite that infects many people but rarely causes significant disease except in fetuses, newborns, and immunosuppressed individuals. The organism can be passed to humans through the handling of the feces of an infected cat, ingestion of undercooked meat, or organ transplants. Fetuses and newborns acquire the organism from the mother during pregnancy either at birth or through the placenta. Physicians should advise pregnant females to avoid contact with cat feces.

Most individuals with intact immune systems are able to defend themselves against the organism. *T. gondii* retreats to form cysts in the muscles and organs, which remain for the life of the host. Once an individual becomes immunosuppressed, the organism is able to reactivate and break out of the cysts to cause many diseases including acute and chronic meningitis, encephalitis, or brain abscesses.

Most immunosuppressed patients display a chronic onset affecting the central nervous system. Signs and symptoms include fever, headache, confusion, and neurological weakness in the extremities. Diagnosis is usually made by observation of cysts in the brain using imaging studies as well as IgG and IgM antibody levels. The parasite is rarely found in the CSF. Brain biopsies are rarely done to confirm the diagnosis. CSF laboratory results mimic those of chronic or aseptic meningitis, with less than 100 lymphocytes/mm^3, normal to slightly decreased glucose levels, and normal to slightly increased protein levels.

Taenia solium.   *Taenia solium* is a pork tapeworm that is passed to humans through ingestion of undercooked meat.

This parasite is common in Mexico and Central and South America. The tapeworm larvae penetrate the intestine to form cysts in the tissues including the brain. Epilepsy in individuals with no previous history of seizures should lead the physician to suspect *T. solium*. While the parasite is not observed in the CSF, the fluid is often under increased pressure depending on the number of cysts and may display a predominance of eosinophils.

Chronic Meningitis Outcomes.   The prognosis of patients with chronic meningitis depends on their immune state. Those with competent immune states will respond to treatment with few long-range effects. Those with compromised or suppressed immune states may require long-term treatments. Those unable to mount a normal white blood cell and immune response will have a poor prognosis even with treatment. Box 38-2✪ summarizes causative agents of chronic meningitis. Not all possible causes are discussed in this chapter due to their rarity of isolation. Those not discussed here can be found in other chapters in this book.

Aseptic Meningitis
Aseptic diseases are characterized by the absence of bacteria on culture. The most common cause of aseptic meningitis is viruses. The signs and symptoms of viral meningitis can overlap those of bacterial meningitis but are usually milder, with

✪ BOX 38-2
Chronic Meningitis Agents

- Bacteria
  - *Mycobacterium tuberculosis*
  - *Nocardia* spp.
  - *Actinomyces* spp.
  - *Brucella* spp.
- Fungi
  - *Cryptococcus neoformans*
  - *Coccidioides immitis*
  - *Blastomyces dermititidis*
  - *Histoplasma capsulatum*
  - *Paracoccidioides brasiliensis*
  - *Candida* spp.
- Parasites
  - *Acanthamoeba* spp.
  - *Entamoeba histolytica*
  - *Taenia solium*
  - *Toxoplasma gondii*
  - *Trichenella spiralis*
- Others
  - *Treponema pallidum*
  - *Borrelia burgdorferi*
  - *Leptospira* spp.
  - *Ehrlichia* spp.
  - *Rickettsia* spp.

complete recovery in 7–10 days. Most cases probably go unreported or unrecognized. Viral meningitis displays a predominance of lymphocytes in the CSF but in the hundreds versus the thousands of neutrophils seen in bacterial meningitis. The protein level is often slightly elevated or normal whereas the glucose concentration is usually normal or slightly decreased. The cerebrospinal fluid is usually clear due to the decreased number of white blood cells present.

Viruses are able to enter the central nervous system through the bloodstream from a primary infection site or along a nerve root. They can cause inflammation of the meninges, brain, spinal cord, or nerve roots. Viral encephalitis, direct infection of the brain tissue, is a frequent and significant presentation of some viruses. Encephalitis can produce long-range complications for the patient. Severe headache, fever, photophobia or aversion to light, malaise, and mental status changes are common complaints. Those under the age of 1 are at greatest risk for infection due to an immature immune system. Their symptoms usually include lethargy and poor feeding. Older adults are also at risk due to their depressed immune system. Because most viral infections are self-limiting, mortality is usually very low and long-term effects of infection are rarely seen.

A thorough patient physical and history is essential in making the diagnosis of aseptic meningitis and differentiating the possible causative agents. The physician may be able to narrow the potential virus based on the current season of the year. Some viruses are transmitted by insects, such as mosquitoes and ticks, which are more prevalent in the summer and fall. Other viruses have unique presentations that may assist the physician in the diagnosis.

Partially treated bacterial meningitis may appear as aseptic meningitis on culture. The bacteria present are injured due to previous antibiotic therapy and may not grow.

Fastidious microorganisms such as *Borrelia burgdorferi* and *Leptospira* spp. are also potential causes of aseptic meningitis and will not grow in culture without special handling. A routine bacterial CSF culture should always be performed along with laboratory testing for viruses.

 **Checkpoint! 38–4
(Chapter Objective 5)**

Aseptic meningitis is most commonly caused by:
   A. *bacteria.*
   B. *fungi.*
   C. *viruses.*
   D. *parasites.*

Microbes Associated with Aseptic Meningitis

Enteroviruses.   The enteroviruses, the leading cause of aseptic meningitis, include echovirus, coxsackieviruses A and B, and poliovirus. These viruses are usually passed person to person by the oral–fecal route. Infants and young children are prone to infection, especially during the summer and fall months. Most infections are acquired in child-care facilities. Signs and complaints can be unremarkable and often present as flu-like symptoms. Neonates have the greatest potential for long-term complications and death. Overall most cases do not require hospitalization or lumbar puncture.

Arboviruses.   Mosquitoes and ticks are the primary means of transmission for aseptic meningitis due to the arthropod-borne virus. The name arbovirus comes from the first two letters of **ar**thropod and the first two letters of **bo**rne. The group is made up of several viral families. Animals and birds harbor these viruses and infections are spread to humans by the bite of the insect. There may be periodic epidemics when there is an increase in the number of mosquitoes or reservoir host animals. Young children and older adults are prone to infection due to their weakened immune systems.

Many of the viruses in this group cause encephalitis. Their disease name is often based on the geographic region where each occurs. St. Louis encephalitis is found in the Midwest and Texas while Eastern equine encephalitis occurs in the eastern United States. West Nile encephalitis, which is carried by birds, has been slowly moving across the United States since its appearance in 1999. Its victims are usually older adults due to their waning immune systems. Seizures are more common with the arboviruses than any other group because they primarily infect brain tissue rather than just the meninges (Vokshoor & Moore, 2004). Seizures may also be related to the fever produced by infections with these viruses.

Mumps Virus.   Mumps meningitis can follow the classic viral salivary gland infection. The initial infection often occurs in the winter and spring, with cases occurring primarily in children and young adults. The virus is spread person to person by respiratory droplets. Vaccination has dramatically decreased the incidence of mumps and its complications.

Herpes Simplex Virus (HSV).   HSV can cause aseptic meningitis or encephalitis. The virus can be passed to an infant born to an infected mother. Genital or mouth lesions can allow the virus to enter the bloodstream. The virus hides out in the trigeminal ganglion of the peripheral nervous system, which then reactivates. HSV tends to infect the temporal lobe of the brain. This lobe is located on the side of the brain and is associated with sensory input, language, and memory. Patients can present with loss of language, hallucinations, and personality changes. Complications and death from HSV infections of the central nervous system can reach 70% if left untreated (Betts et al., 2003).

Bacteria.   While aseptic meningitis is usually synonymous with viruses, occasionally other organisms can be the culprits. *Borrelia burgdorferi,* the causative agent of Lyme disease, is associated with meningitis weeks to months after initial infection. The spiral bacterium is transmitted by a tick bite so incidence is higher during warmer months. Infections are predominant in endemic regions such as the northeastern United States. A good physical and patient history will often reveal history of a previous tick bite or the appearance of the typical bull's-eye target lesion associated with the disease.

About 15% of patients with Lyme disease go on to develop central nervous system involvement (Betts et al., 2003). The organism enters the bloodstream and quickly enters the CSF. Most patients present with headache and malaise. Many experience cranial nerve involvement, especially the facial nerve. There may be tingling or numbness of the face. The CSF results often show an elevated white blood cell count with a predominance of lymphocytes and an elevated protein concentration and a normal to low glucose level. Special enriched media incubated for 6–8 weeks is required for culture. Diagnosis can be aided by serology.

Outcomes of Aseptic Meningitis.   Most cases of aseptic meningitis are self-limiting and resolve without further complications. The prognosis of the patient depends on the virulence of the organism encountered and the patient's immune state and age. Viruses, such as herpes simplex and arboviruses, can cause encephalitis. Encephalitis is associated with a much higher mortality rate and often results in long-term complications such as seizures, weakness, paralysis, and memory loss. Box 38-3✪ summarizes some of the viral agents associated with aseptic meningitis. Not all viruses listed in this box are discussed in this chapter. Please refer to ∞ Chapter 31 for more information on specific viruses.

✪ BOX 38-3

Viruses Associated with Aseptic Meningitis

- Arboviruses
  - St. Louis encephalitis virus
  - Equine encephalomyelitis viruses
  - Tick-borne encephalitis virus
  - West Nile virus
- Enteroviruses
  - Coxsackieviruses
  - Echoviruses
- Herpesviruses
  - Cytomegalovirus
  - Epstein–Barr virus
  - Herpes simplex virus type 1 and 2
  - Varicella-zoster virus
- Human immunodeficiency virus
- Measles virus
- Mumps virus
- Parvovirus
- Rabies virus
- Rubella virus

CSF Shunt Infection

Hydrocephalus is the abnormal buildup of CSF in the brain's ventricles. To relieve the increasing intracranial pressure a tube is implanted to detour the fluid to another part of the body such as the heart or peritoneal cavity. Figure 38-8 shows the placement of artificial shunt within the ventricles of the brain to allow drainage of excess CSF. Since the shunt is a foreign object in the body, it is prone to infection. Organisms are able to form biofilms on the shunt surface or interior, which hide them from the body's immune system and antibiotics. Up to 27% of cases become infected after shunt placement (Wang et al., 2004). Adults with CSF shunt infections display fever, changes in mental status, and seizures. Children tend to present with vague symptoms such as poor appetite, abdominal fullness, and mental status changes.

Laboratory testing results of the CSF will be similar to those of meningitis. An individual's normal skin flora is the most common source of infections. Organisms such as *Staphylococcus* not *S. aureus* and *Staphylococcus aureus* account for 80% of CSF shunt infections (Wang et al., 2004). The anaerobic gram-positive rod *Propionibacterium acnes* can also be a potential pathogen. Treatment requires early detection, removal of the infected shunt, and antibiotic therapy.

✪ REAL WORLD TIP

It is very important that fluid collected from a CSF ventricular shunt be labeled correctly. The organisms isolated from shunt infections are usually those considered to be normal skin flora. These organisms may be dismissed as contaminants, due to an inadequate skin cleaning prior to lumbar puncture, if the fluid is only identified as cerebrospinal fluid.

Brain Abscess

A **brain abscess** is a pocket of pus and cellular debris in a cavity within the brain tissue. It is a rare occurrence in the general population but an increased incidence has been

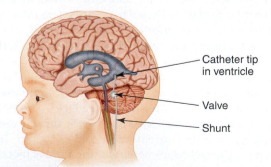

Catheter tip in ventricle

Valve

Shunt

■ **FIGURE 38-8** Hydrocephalus is the accumulation of CSF within the ventricles of the brain. Excess fluid must be continuously removed via an artificial shunt to prevent brain damage. The shunt can become contaminated with microorganisms and serve as a source of infection of the CSF.

observed in the immunocompromised, especially AIDS patients. A majority of the cases are due to infections of the sinuses, middle ear, or teeth, which spread directly to the brain to cause a localized infection. Microorganisms can also gain access from trauma or surgery with direct inoculation of the brain. A third route involves distant infections such as pneumonia or endocarditis. The organisms spill over into the bloodstream and are carried to the brain.

Signs and symptoms exhibited are often due to the pressure exerted by the growing mass rather than the infection itself. Headache, nausea, seizures, and mental status changes are frequently observed. A low-grade fever, a classic sign of infection, is only observed in about 50% of cases (Betts et al., 2003).

CSF testing rarely helps diagnose a brain abscess. There is a risk of brain herniation and the brain can slip into the spinal cord canal with a sudden change in pressure. This can occur during a lumbar puncture if the CSF pressure is too high. A lumbar puncture is usually done only to rule out other central nervous system diseases and infections. Magnetic resonance imaging (MRI) can be used to visualize the mass. A brain biopsy, performed at surgery, will provide the sample to reveal the causative agent. Microorganisms associated with brain abscess formation are most often part of the normal oral flora. Potential pathogens include aerobic and anaerobic *Streptococcus* spp., especially *S. anginosus, Staphylococcus aureus,* anaerobic gram-negative rods, *Actinomyces* spp., fungi, and *Entamoeba histolytica*. Infections can be polymicrobic due to the presence of several microorganisms. If the abscess ruptures into the ventricles or subarachnoid space, death occurs in about 80% of cases (Brook, 2005).

▶ SPECIMEN COLLECTION

Examination of CSF is required to diagnose most infections of the central nervous system. The physician, using aseptic technique, collects the fluid by lumbar puncture. The fluid should be taken prior to starting antibiotic therapy. Upon entering the spinal canal, the CSF pressure is measured. Increased pressure is often seen with central nervous system infection. If the pressure is too high, once the fluid is removed, it is believed that the brain can slip down into the spinal canal (herniate) and cause death.

Ideally at least three sterile tubes of CSF should be collected for testing. The first tube can be saved for additional testing, if required. Tube two is most often used for microbiology testing such as Gram stain, culture, etc. Tube three is used for the glucose and protein concentrations and cell count. Tube three is used for the cell count because if the fluid is bloody due to a traumatic tap, the red blood cells should clear by the last tube and not affect the test results. If only one tube is collected such as in infants or young children, the microbiology laboratory should have first access to ensure sterility.

> ✓ **Checkpoint! 38–5**
> **(Chapter Objective 8)**
>
> *A physician collects one tube of CSF from a premature infant. The laboratory's processing center receives the specimen and removes a portion for hematology and chemistry testing. The tube is then sent to the microbiology department for testing. A potential source of error in this situation includes:*
>
> A. *The physician did not collect enough CSF for all of the testing required.*
> B. *The specimen should have been centrifuged prior to aliquoting.*
> C. *The CSF tube was possibly contaminated by the processing department.*
> D. *The microbiology tests are in doubt due to the delay in receipt of the specimen.*

The volume of CSF collected will depend on the extent of testing requested by the physician. Microbiology testing often requires at least 10–15 milliliters of CSF if the physician wishes to process it for all possible microorganisms: bacteria, fungi, viruses, acid-fast bacilli, and parasites. If the volume received is less than required, the physician must prioritize the tests. If inadequate volumes of CSF are used for testing, the sensitivity of testing decreases and false-negative results are possible. It is better not to run the test than provide results that are inaccurate.

Blood cultures are often collected at the same time as the lumbar puncture. They will yield the causative agent in more than 69% of cases of acute bacterial meningitis (Cohen & Powderly, 2004). The blood cultures of patients with aseptic meningitis and chronic meningitis will rarely become positive.

Most virology laboratories are able to perform viral cultures of CSF for isolation of enteroviruses and herpes simplex virus. Detection of other viruses may require the use of a reference laboratory.

A brain biopsy is required to diagnose the causative agent(s) of a brain abscess. The specimen is taken at surgery and sent to the microbiology laboratory in an anaerobic transport system.

▶ SETUP AND INCUBATION OF CULTURES

The cerebrospinal fluid should arrive in the laboratory immediately or no longer than 1 hour after collection. The specimen must be labeled appropriately to ensure positive patient identification and physician orders must accompany it. Medical necessity requires the physician to order only tests that will support the patient diagnosis. Cerebrospinal fluid is rarely a recollectable specimen and is seldom rejected without valid criteria.

SPECIMEN PREPARATION

The specimen should be processed immediately. Meningitis is one disease state in which the clinical microbiologist can have an immediate positive impact on the patient's outcome. If there must be a delay in specimen processing, the fluid should be stored at room temperature or 35–37°C but not at 4°C. *Haemophilus influenzae, Neisseria meningitidis,* and *Streptococcus pneumoniae* are very susceptible to extremes in temperature. If viruses are suspected, a portion of the specimen should be removed and stored in the refrigerator until processed.

 REAL WORLD TIP

Due to the requirement for carbon dioxide and production of autolytic enzymes by *Streptococcus pneumoniae* and *Neisseria meningitidis,* the organisms may not be detected in CSF if there is a significant delay prior to processing.

The specimen is examined for color and turbidity. Normal CSF is colorless and clear. A turbid fluid indicates the presence of white blood cells, which correlates with infection. The CSF of chronic or aseptic meningitis patients may display a clear fluid because the number of white blood cells present is usually lower than seen in bacterial meningitis. A bloody fluid may be the result of a subarachnoid hemorrhage or a traumatic tap. A subarachnoid hemorrhage occurs when a brain blood vessel ruptures and bleeds into the subarachnoid space between the arachnoid membrane and pia mater. A traumatic

REAL WORLD TIP

- It is possible to initiate meningitis in a patient during a lumbar puncture when the infection is not present. If a patient has bacteremia or bacteria in the blood and the physician punctures a blood vessel as the spinal needle is introduced during a lumbar puncture, it is possible to introduce bacteria from the blood into the spinal column. The blood containing the bacteria enters the cerebrospinal fluid and could potentially set up the patient for meningitis.

- A traumatic tap will introduce white and red blood cells into the CSF. It will also cause a false increase in the protein level of the CSF. The effect of a traumatic tap can be roughly calculated so the results may still be of value. This may prevent the need to perform a repeat lumbar puncture. For every 1,000 red blood cells introduced through a traumatic tap, about one white blood cell and 1 mg/dl of protein is added.

tap occurs when the spinal needle hits a blood vessel as it is introduced into the spinal column during a lumbar puncture. If the blood is due to a traumatic tap, the CSF tubes will become clearer as the fluid is collected whereas those of a true hemorrhage will remain consistently bloody. A yellow color is due to the breakdown of red blood cells.

A Gram stain can be prepared from the sediment of centrifuged specimen or made prior to concentration by using a cytocentrifuge. More information on the CSF Gram stain can be found in the section "Direct Testing" later in this chapter.

Cerebrospinal fluid should be centrifuged at 2,500–3,000 rpm (1,500 × g) for 15 minutes. After concentration, all but about 0.5–1.0 milliliter of the supernatant is removed and saved. The remaining fluid and sediment is mixed using a sterile pipette and used to inoculate testing media. If less than 1 milliliter is available, the specimen should be plated directly without centrifugation.

CSF is usually not centrifuged prior to viral testing. A larger volume of fluid is required for viral culture due to the dilution of the number of cells present in the fluid. While some viruses can be isolated in cell culture, others can only be detected by molecular diagnostics or serology. A viral culture for enterovirus has a sensitivity of about 70% (Betts et al., 2003). An individual with aseptic meningitis due to enterovirus also sheds the virus in the stool and throat. A concurrent viral culture of the throat or stool may assist in the diagnosis if the CSF viral culture is negative. Refer to ∞ Chapter 31 for details on specific viral detection and confirmation methods.

The sensitivity of the culture for acid-fast bacilli is dependent on the volume of fluid and speed and duration of centrifugation. Processing at least 6 milliliters improves recovery (Thwaites, Chau, & Farrar, 2004). While CSF for mycobacteria culture does not require decontamination, it does require centrifugation at 3000 × g for at least 15 minutes prior to plating. Molecular detection methods have improved the time to detection of *Mycobacterium* spp. in CSF.

Detection of *Naegleria fowleri* requires either a wet mount examination of the CSF or a stained trichrome smear. On wet mount, the amoeba can resemble white blood cells and may be overlooked. Look for the directional movement of the amoeba compared to the white blood cells, which remain stationary.

 REAL WORLD TIP

A unique method for detection of *Naegleria fowleri* in CSF is by culture. A non-nutrient agar is covered with a lawn of *E. coli* bacteria. A drop of the suspected CSF is placed in the center of the agar plate. The inoculated agar plate is incubated at 35–37°C for 24–48 hours. The plate is examined, under a microscope using a 10× objective, for tracks. As the amoeba eat the bacteria they move and create visible tracks in the bacterial growth. Follow the track to its end to find the parasite.

DIRECT TESTING

Direct examination of the CSF by Gram stain provides rapid valuable information for the physician. Traditionally drops of fluid are dried on a glass slide prior to staining. This method is accurate as long as there were at least 10^5 organisms/milliliter of CSF (Shanholtzer, Schaper, & Peterson, 1982). While acute bacterial meningitis can reach these levels of organisms, chronic infections may not.

In order to increase the sensitivity of gram-stained smears, the specimen should be concentrated prior to staining. A cyto-

centrifuge concentrates a few drops of CSF onto a glass slide, which is then stained. It increases the sensitivity of detection of organisms on CSF gram-stained slides about 100 times versus using the sediment of a centrifuged specimen (Shanholtzer et al., 1982). This increase in sensitivity allows for rapid, simple, effective detection of causative agents as well as conservation of a valuable and limited specimen for additional testing. Figures 38-9a ■–38-9d ■ display examples of cytospun CSF gram-stained slides with bacteria present.

In the 1980s direct antigen testing (DAT) was introduced to the clinical laboratory. It was advertised as a rapid, easy-to-

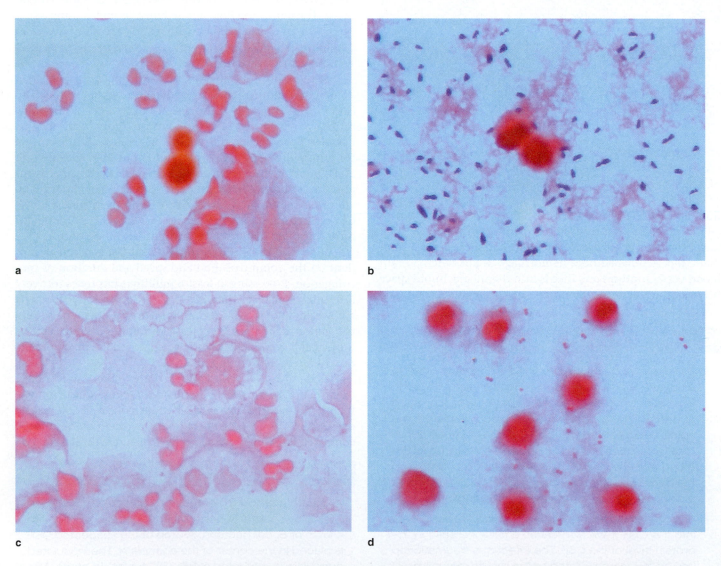

■ FIGURE 38-9 **a.** This CSF smear shows one large budding yeast in the center of a field of neutrophils. Yeast cells do not stain well on Gram stain and may be overlooked as an artifact on initial review. **b.** This Gram stain of CSF displays many gram-positive cocci in pairs with rare white blood cells. The cocci are more oval shaped with pointed or lancet ends rather than round, suggesting streptococci. The arrangement in pairs suggests specifically *Streptococcus pneumoniae.* **c.** *Haemophilus influenzae* can be difficult to see in a CSF Gram stain. Because they are small gram-negative coccobacilli, they tend to blend into the background of the cellular debris on a stained CSF smear. In liquid specimens such as CSF, *H. influenzae* can become very pleomorphic, displaying very short coccobacilli to very long rod shapes. **d.** The presence of gram-negative diplococci in this stained CSF suggests *Neisseria meningitidis* as the causative agent of meningitis in this patient. The large, pink round objects are neutrophils.

- The CSF Gram stain is very important in the diagnosis of meningitis. There have been documented cases of nonviable bacteria observed on CSF Gram stain, which were the result of contaminated tubes packaged in the commercial lumbar puncture kit used by physicians. A failure in the manufacturer's quality control is usually the reason for their presence. These nonviable organisms are often rare in number and there may be a cluster of patient cases exhibiting these false-positive results. A false-positive CSF Gram stain leads to unnecessary antibiotic therapy as well as an inaccurate diagnosis. The physician must ensure the patient's signs, symptoms, and other test results support a positive CSF Gram stain when making the diagnosis of meningitis

- If bacterial meningitis is suspected, but no organisms are seen (NOS) on the Gram stain of the CSF, an acridine orange stain can be performed. Acridine orange is a fluorescent stain that binds to nucleic acid. Human cells such as white blood cells also contain nucleic acid. If the CSF has a high white blood cell count, it may be difficult to differentiate the presence of microorganisms compared to the white blood cells. If bacteria are found, the stain will not differentiate between gram-positive and gram-negative organisms.

use test that displayed both high sensitivity and specificity. The agglutination test relied on the detection of the capsular antigens of the most common bacterial pathogens (*Haemophilus influenzae* type b; *Neisseria meningitidis* serogroups A, C, Y, and W135; *Streptococcus agalactiae* [group B *Streptococcus*]; *Streptococcus pneumoniae;* and *E. coli* serotype K1) by antibodies attached to latex beads. The test initially was meant to be used for patients who present with the characteristic physical signs and symptoms and display laboratory testing results consistent with meningitis. Physicians tended to use the test to screen all patients, even those with normal CSF laboratory tests. This proved to be a misuse of a valuable test (Kiska, Jones, Mangum, Orkiszewski, & Gilligan, 1995).

The DAT results can be affected by several factors. Many organisms can possess antigens that cross-react with the antibodies present. There is poorer detection of *Haemophilus influenzae* and *Streptococcus pneumoniae* than initially reported. Children recently vaccinated with the Hib vaccine, a routine practice today, present with false-positive DAT results due to the presence of circulating antigen (Perkins, Mirrett, & Reller, 1995). False-positive results can lengthen the hospital stay for the patient and may extend the use of unnecessary antibiotics. False-negative results can lead to poor patient outcomes due to the delay in treatment.

The cytocentrifuge has increased the sensitivity of CSF Gram stain so it is now an excellent and rapid indicator of disease. Many laboratories have reduced costs by eliminating or restricting the use of DAT without compromising patient outcomes (Perkins et al., 1995). Past CSF specimen data for an institution can be reviewed. If it is determined there are no examples of a positive CSF DAT without a positive Gram stain or culture, the use of the DAT test could be discontinued. The CSF DAT is an example of a once good test that now shows limited added value in the clinical laboratory today. Microbiologists must continuously assess laboratory testing to ensure each provides value-added results that assist the physician in the diagnosis and treatment of patients.

The DAT test is still useful in limited situations such as the detection of meningitis in immunosuppressed patients who may not exhibit the expected cell counts of bacterial meningitis. It is also helpful in detection of bacterial pathogens in patients with a history of antibiotic therapy prior to specimen collection. While the organisms may not be visualized or grow in culture, their capsular antigens will still be present. Most clinical laboratories have stopped performing DAT routinely but reference laboratories are available for the instances noted above.

Streptococcus pneumoniae is a fragile meningitis pathogen that can easily be lost due to autolysis or previous antibiotic treatment. The use of an immunochromatic assay can assist in the diagnosis of meningitis caused by this organism when it does not grow in blood and CSF cultures. A nitrocellulose membrane is coated with rabbit antibodies to *S. pneumoniae*. As the CSF mixes with the antibodies, if *S. pneumoniae* is present, a colored line appears. The test has proven to be highly sensitive and specific when detecting *S. pneumoniae* in CSF.

Cryptococcus neoformans, an encapsulated yeast, may be rapidly detected with the use of India ink. The CSF is mixed with a black dye, India ink, and examined for the presence of budding yeast surrounded by a capsule that appears as a clear halo against a dark background. While a positive test is diagnostic, a negative

Checkpoint! 38–6 (Chapter Objectives 6 and 8)

A physician requests a CSF direct antigen test for Haemophilus influenzae type b on a 2-year-old female suspected of having meningitis. The microbiology laboratory has discontinued the use of CSF direct antigen testsing (DAT). What explanation can you provide the physician to help him understand why the laboratory decided to eliminate the use of DAT?

   A. *The test has proven to be too expensive for use in the clinical setting.*

   B. *There is a potential for false-positive results due to recent Hib immunization.*

   C. *Haemophilus influenzae type b is not a likely potential pathogen for this patient.*

   D. *The test does not detect Haemophilus influenzae type b.*

result does not rule out disease. Only 25–50% of patients with cryptococcal meningitis display positive India ink preparations (King, Markanday, & Khan, 2004). Figure 38-10 ■ demonstrates a positive India ink CSF prep. It is much better to use a latex agglutination test for the detection of the yeast's capsular antigen in CSF. The antigen test is positive in about 90% of patients with cryptococcal meningitis (King et al., 2004). Cryptococcal antigen titers can be used to monitor the effectiveness of therapy.

Traditional CSF cultures may take 24–48 hours for detection of bacterial meningitis causative agents. It takes weeks for mycobacterial cultures. The use of polymerase chain reaction (PCR), a molecular biology detection method, can be used to screen CSF rapidly. The procedure targets a unique gene sequence for each organism screened. While the test has proven to be sensitive and provides same-day results, it is not cost-effective for most clinical laboratories at this time. The laboratory must weigh the benefit of positive patient outcomes versus costs in order to make a good decision for the inclusion of PCR in its test menu.

CULTIVATION

Because 80% of cases of acute bacterial meningitis are due to *Haemophilus influenzae, Neisseria meningitidis,* and *Streptococcus pneumoniae,* the clinical laboratory must select plating media that are able to grow all three organisms. *Streptococcus pneumoniae* will display its characteristic alpha-hemolytic, cratered or mucoid morphology on sheep blood agar and will grow on chocolate agar as well. *Neisseria meningitidis* will produce a gray-blue colony on both agars but slightly better growth is observed on chocolate agar. *Haemophilus influenzae* presents as a gray, wet colony that requires factors X (hemin) and V (NAD). These two factors are only present in chocolate agar. At

a minimum, a chocolate agar should be inoculated because these three organisms account for most cases of bacterial meningitis and are able to grow on this agar. If possible, a sheep blood agar should be added. MacConkey agar, which is selective for gram-negative rods, can be added if *Enterobacteriaceae* are suspected after reading the direct Gram stain. BA and CA agar plates should be incubated for 3 days at 35–37°C with CO_2, while MAC agar should be incubated in ambient air.

A thioglycolate broth is often added as a backup to the agar culture plates to ensure growth of minute numbers of organisms. The broth can easily become contaminated at inoculation and may grow skin organisms such as *Staphylococcus not S. aureus.* The physician must interpret the results of a culture-negative, broth-positive CSF culture carefully. Some facilities have eliminated the use of broth on a CSF culture as a cost-saving measure (Dunbar, Eason, Musher, & Clarridge, 1998). The broth is still useful in cases of patients with CSF shunts.

If chronic meningitis is suspected the physician may request CSF cultures for fungi and mycobacteria. Culture media for these organisms are addressed in specific chapters.

A specimen collected from a brain abscess should be cultured on sheep blood, chocolate, MacConkey, and selective agar for gram-positive organisms such as phenylethyl alcohol agar because the infection is usually polymicrobic due to the presence of several microorganisms. In addition to the aerobic media plates, appropriate anaerobic media and thioglycolate broth should be inoculated as well. There are several anaerobes known for their ability to cause brain abscesses. Refer to ∞ Chapter 7 for specific details on culture media and ∞ Chapter 24 for specific anaerobes associated with brain abscess formation. Aerobic agar plates are incubated for a minimum of 48 hours while the anaerobic plates and broth are incubated for a minimum of 5 days, with the first plate examination performed after 48 hours.

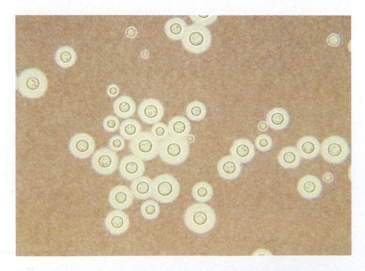

■ **FIGURE 38-10** The capsule of *Cryptococcus neoformans* appears as a clear halo around the yeast cell when the dark India ink is added to CSF. While characteristic for meningitis due to *C. neoformans,* less than 50% of patients exhibit this phenomenon.
From Public Health Image Library (PHIL), CDC/Dr. Leanor Haley.

> ✓ **Checkpoint! 38–7 (Chapter Objective 9)**
>
> *The microbiology laboratory receives five drops of CSF from a 5-year-old for bacterial culture. Assuming three drops were used for the cytocentrifuged Gram stain smear, select two medium that should be inoculated with the last two drops.*
>
> A. *Sheep blood and chocolate agars*
> B. *Chocolate and MacConkey agars*
> C. *Sheep blood and MacConkey agars*
> D. *Sheep blood agar and thioglycolate broth*

▶ INTERPRETATION OF CULTURES

ORGANISM WORKUP

All organisms isolated from the central nervous system should be identified as rapidly and completely as possible. Even organisms such as *Staphylococcus* not *S. aureus* can be clinically significant in patients with a CSF shunt. The laboratory alone is unable to determine if an organism is a true pathogen or a skin contaminant. A review of the CSF testing results (glucose and protein levels and white blood cell count and differential) and a discussion with the physician can assist the microbiologist in making the best decision in the extent of organism workup.

Serotyping of *Haemophilus influenzae* isolates is no longer performed in most microbiology laboratories. The use of the Hib vaccine has virtually eliminated the invasive serotype b. A reference laboratory can provide this service if needed.

SUSCEPTIBILITY TESTING

Once an organism is determined to be a potential pathogen, susceptibility testing should be performed if there is a valid, standardized method available for testing. If a method is not available, literature can provide valuable information for possible treatment.

The Clinical and Laboratory Standards Institute (CLSI) (formerly the National Committee for Clinical Laboratory Standards [NCCLS]) publishes guidelines that list antimicrobial agents appropriate for testing against specific organisms based on body site of isolation. It also provides best practices for valid, standardized methods for susceptibility testing. Only those antimicrobial agents that are able to pass through the blood–brain barrier should be tested and reported.

TREATMENT

Meningitis is a medical emergency and antibiotic therapy should begin within 60 minutes of the patient's arrival. The physician selects antibiotics based on the most likely pathogen, which is usually determined by the patient's signs and symptoms as well as their age and other factors. If the Gram stain reveals the specific pathogen then specific therapy is selected. If no pathogen is observed on the CSF Gram stain then the physician begins broad-spectrum therapy to cover the most common pathogens based on the patient's age. Ceftriaxone or cefotaxime plus vancomycin are often used for meningitis due to gram-positive cocci whereas penicillin G is used if gram-negative cocci are suspected. Gram-positive rods are often treated with ampicillin or penicillin G plus an aminoglycoside. Gram-negative rods are treated with ceftriaxone or cefotaxime plus an aminoglycoside. Corticosteroids are usually used in combination with antibiotics. The steroids reduce brain inflammation and so decrease patient mortality.

Close contacts of a patient with meningitis due to *H. influenzae* type b or *N. meningitidis* may be treated with rifampin to prevent nasopharyngeal colonization. Vaccines are recommended for those at high risk for infection such as the pneumococcal vaccine for older adults and the Hib vaccine for children.

Cryptococcal meningitis requires treatment with amphotericin B and flucytosine. Chronic meningitis due to

Mycobacterium tuberculosis requires a multiple drug approach to prevent the development of resistance. Often a combination of isoniazid, rifampin, ethambutol, and pyrazinamide is used.

Acyclovir is used as therapy for HSV meningoencephalitis. The other viruses that cause meningitis have no current therapies available. The only treatment options offered for the patient are for supportive care such as the relief of pain and fever.

Naegleria fowleri meningoencephalitis is usually rapidly fatal. There have been rare cases of survivors after treatment with amphotericin B, a fungal antibiotic.

OTHER

Organisms isolated from patients with confirmed cases of meningitis may need to be forwarded to the state public health laboratory for confirmation or epidemiology studies. Each state has specific regulations for organisms that must be monitored and reported to the public health department. Organisms isolated should be maintained for at least 1 year for further testing if needed. They may be frozen or lyophilized (freeze-dried).

▶ THE SPECIAL SENSES

THE EYE

The eye is the organ of sight. A patient with signs and symptoms of infection may elect to see a physician rather than an ophthalmologist. If left undiagnosed and untreated, infections of the eye can lead to loss of vision and the eye itself.

Anatomy of the Eye

The eyeball sits in the skeletal orbit for protection. It is held in place by muscles and ligaments. The sclera is a tough membrane that helps maintain its round shape. On the front surface of the eye the sclera is the white portion. In the rear of the eye, the optic nerve enters through the sclera.

The transparent cornea projects like a dome over the sclera in the front of the eye. It is analogous to the glass covering the face of a wristwatch. It acts like a window to allow light to enter the eye. The iris is a thin disk that supplies an individual's eye color. It lies between the cornea and lens. The pupil, the central opening in the iris, expands and contracts depending on how much light is needed to see. The translucent, biconvex lens sits behind the iris and provides the focusing mechanism for the eye, much like a camera lens.

There are two chambers within the eye. The front chamber consists of the small area from the cornea to the lens and is filled with aqueous humor. Aqueous humor is an alkaline fluid that is made up of primarily water and sodium chloride. It is continuously regenerated, which may make it less prone to the introduction of infection. The posterior chamber of the eye contains the vitreous fluid, which helps the eye retain its shape. It contains about 4 milliliters of clear gel, which is not regenerated. It is composed of mostly water with some salts and albumin. It can be removed for sampling but must be replaced with fluid similar in consistency and content.

The eyelids are movable flaps that cover the front of the eye. They provide a source of protection and help to keep moisture in and foreign objects out. Eyelashes line the free edge of both eyelids. The short, thick, curved hairs may be present in double or triple rows. Eyelashes protect the eye by capturing any objects that may float into the eye and scratch its surface. There are glands at the base of the eyelashes.

The **conjunctiva** is the mucous membrane of the eye. It is transparent and lines the inner surface of the eyelids and continues over the front sclera or white portion of the eye but does not cover the cornea. Each eye contains a lacrimal gland located in the upper eyelid and lacrimal ducts in the corner closest to the nose. Each gland has a structure similar to the salivary glands and secretes tears. Tears lubricate and moisten the eye as well as protect it by washing out objects that may scratch the conjunctiva. Tears contain antibacterial antibodies and provide nutrients and oxygen to the eye. The lacrimal ducts drain fluid from the eye into the nasal cavity. Figure 38-11 ■ illustrates the anatomy of the eye. Figure 38-12 ■ demonstrates the location of the lacrimal gland and ducts.

Infectious Diseases Associated with the Eye

While the surface of the eye may have transient microorganisms, the interior of the eye is considered sterile. The eye can become infected by microorganisms through multiple routes.

The most common route is hand-to-eye transmission. Children are most prone to infection this way. They touch an object carrying the infectious agent and then rub their eye. Another means of transmission is through penetration or ulceration of the sclera or cornea. Because the eye is fed by blood vessels, microorganisms can reach it through the bloodstream. Lastly, since the eye is situated close to the sinuses it can become secondarily infected. Table 38-2✪ summarizes the infections associated with the eye and the most commonly isolated pathogens.

Conjunctivitis.   Inflammation of the conjunctiva is called **pinkeye** or **conjunctivitis.** The blood vessels of the conjunctiva become congested with infection and the sclera of the eye appears red or pink. Conjunctivitis is the most common eye infection encountered. It accounts for 30% of all eye complaints seen by physicians (Silverman & Bessman, 2005). Since it is passed person to person, children are most commonly affected because they are not diligent in washing their hands. Figure 38-13 ■ shows the pink sclera associated with conjunctivitis.

It is important for the physician to distinguish conjunctivitis due to viruses versus bacteria. The treatments for each are very different. In general, conjunctivitis is not painful. Symptoms include a burning sensation or the feeling there is something caught in the eye plus a discharge. Viral infections typically produce a clear, watery discharge whereas the dis-

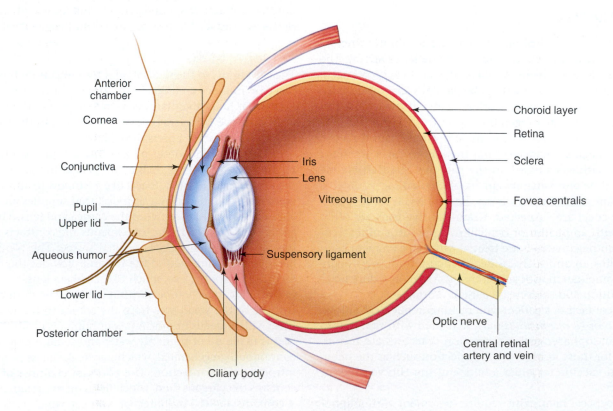

■ FIGURE 38-11 The internal and external structures of the eye.

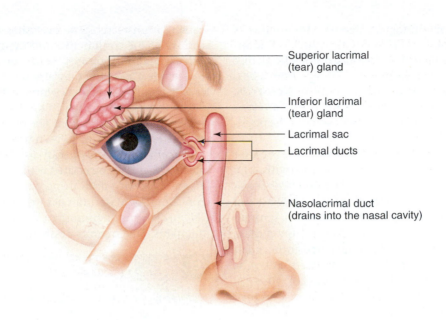

FIGURE 38-12 The location of the lacrimal gland and ducts.

| Superior lacrimal (tear) gland |
| Inferior lacrimal (tear) gland |
| Lacrimal sac |
| Lacrimal ducts |
| Nasolacrimal duct (drains into the nasal cavity) |

✪ TABLE 38-2

The Most Common Microorganisms Associated with Infectious Diseases of the Eye

Infectious Disease	Commonly Associated Microorganisms
Conjunctivitis	■ Viruses 　● Adenovirus 　● Herpes simplex virus ■ *Haemophilus aegyptius* (formerly *Haemophilus influenzae* biotype *aegyptius*) ■ *Streptococcus pneumoniae* ■ *Neisseria gonorrhoeae* ■ *Chlamydia trachomatis*
Keratitis	■ Herpes simplex virus ■ *Streptococcus* spp. ■ *Staphylococcus* spp. ■ Gram-negative rods 　● Enterobacteriaceae 　● *Pseudomonas aeruginosa* ■ *Acanthamoeba* spp.
Endophthalmitis	■ Gram-positive cocci 　● *Staphylococcus* not *Staphylococcus aureus* 　● *Staphylococcus aureus* ■ *Bacillus* spp. ■ *Candida albicans*
Stye	*Staphylococcus aureus*
Dacryocystitis	■ *Staphylococcus aureus* ■ *Haemophilus influenzae* ■ *Streptococcus pneumoniae* ■ Beta-hemolytic *Streptococcus*

charge of a bacterial infection is often thick and purulent. Conjunctivitis due to allergies produces a clear, mucoid discharge with itching.

The infection often begins in one eye and is easily transmitted to the other eye. Microorganisms can be transferred person to person with shared towels or makeup and the use of common computer keyboards, telephones, or microscopes. Conjunctivitis accounts for many missed school days for children and work days for their parents.

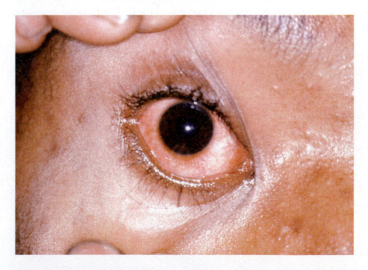

FIGURE 38-13 This individual displays the typical pink sclera seen with conjunctivitis or pinkeye. Bacteria or viruses cause the blood vessels of the conjunctiva to become congested and enlarged.
From Public Health Image Library (PHIL), CDC/Joe Miller, VD.

Viruses are common etiological agents. Adenovirus is responsible for most cases of conjunctivitis. While self-limiting, it is easily transferred to others to cause outbreaks. Herpes simplex virus (HSV) can be transferred to the eye from a blister at another body site to cause conjunctivitis or **keratitis**, which is inflammation of the cornea. A history of a recent upper respiratory infection or fever blisters can help the physician diagnose a viral causative agent.

A thick, purulent discharge that is able to seal the eye shut during sleep is a classic sign of bacterial conjunctivitis. The most common causative bacteria include *Haemophilus aegyptius* (formerly *Haemophilus influenzae* biogroup *aegyptius*) and *Streptococcus pneumoniae*. Genetic analysis supports a separate species designation for *H. aegyptius,* a relatively common cause of conjunctivitis. *H. aegyptius* is also implicated in Brazilian purpuric fever. It is a febrile hemorrhagic disease that begins with conjunctivitis and has a mortality rate of 40–90%. *H. aegyptius* is biochemically similar to *H. influenzae* so they are no longer differentiated in most laboratories. About 40% of patients exhibit conjunctivitis with concurrent otitis media or middle ear infection (Silverman & Bessman, 2005).

Neisseria gonorrhoeae is able to cause conjunctivitis in sexually active adults. Often it is transferred by contact such as rubbing the eye. The discharge tends to be very purulent. In newborns, *Neisseria gonorrhoeae* can cause a hyperpurulent conjunctivitis known as ophthalmia neonatorum. The organism is acquired at birth from the mother. The thick purulent discharge returns as soon as it is wiped away. Figure 38-14 ■ shows the thick purulent material associated with gonococcal ophthalmia neonatorum. Hospitals use eye ointment or drops at birth to prevent this infection.

Chlamydia trachomatis causes two types of diseases of the eye: **trachoma**, a chlamydial infection that can lead to blindness, and inclusion conjunctivitis, a milder infection. Trachoma begins as conjunctivitis, which eventually leads to

scarring if untreated. The eyelashes turn inward due to the scarring of the conjunctiva and then rub against the cornea with each blink. The constant friction against the cornea leads to ulceration. Scarring may also destroy tear function, which leads to more damage and eventually blindness. Inclusion conjunctivitis usually occurs in adults who have a concurrent chlamydia genital infection. The discharge is usually minimal and there is no scarring as seen with trachoma.

Chlamydia trachomatis can also be acquired at birth. The infection is usually associated with an acute purulent discharge but will heal with no scarring if untreated. The use of antimicrobial ointment or drops at birth prevents this eye infection. *Chlamydia* spp. pneumonia can occur in infants after conjunctivitis (Silverman & Bessman, 2005).

 REAL WORLD TIP

Chlamydia trachomatis in an intracellular bacterium that requires living cells to grow. The organism will not grow on routine agar plates. It is often detected with the use of cell cultures like those used to grow viruses.

Keratitis.   Keratitis is an infection of the cornea. Corneal infections produce pain, photophobia, ulceration, and decreased vision. There is usually no discharge present as seen in conjunctivitis. Keratitis is considered a medical emergency because it can lead to loss of vision due to perforation and extension into the sterile posterior chamber of the eye. Microorganisms gain entrance through trauma, abrasions in the cornea, as seen in tear deficiency, or the use of contact lenses, especially extended-wear lenses. Extended-wear contacts, especially soft lenses worn overnight, can cause trauma to the cornea and account for up to 42% of bacterial keratitis (Murillo-Lopez, 2004). Herpes simplex virus (HSV) is a common cause of corneal ulcers. HSV eye infections can reoccur for the rest of an individual's life because, once infected, the virus lives in the trigeminal nerve of the peripheral nervous system. Figure 38-15 ■ shows a corneal ulcer due to HSV.

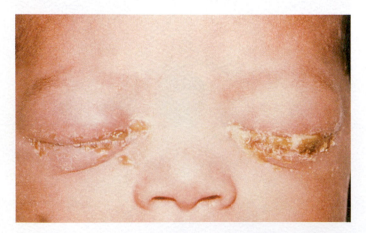

■ **FIGURE 38-14** The mother of this newborn had gonorrhea at the time of birth. This baby's eyes were inoculated with the organism to cause ophthalmia neonatorum. The thick purulent material is characteristic of conjunctivitis due to *Neisseria gonorrhoeae.*
From Public Health Image Library (PHIL), CDC/J. Pleger.

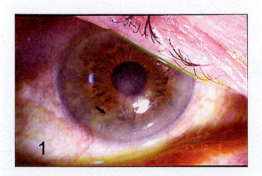

■ **FIGURE 38-15** The arrow in this photograph indicates a corneal ulcer due to herpes simplex virus.
From Cellini, Leonetti, and Campos (2007). Journal of Medical Care Reports, 1, 124. http://www.jmedicalcasereports.com/content/1/1/124.

Most bacterial cases of keratitis are due to gram-positive organisms such as *Streptococcus* and *Staphylococcus* spp. and gram-negative rods such as *Enterobacteriaceae* and *Pseudomonas* spp. Even normal flora organisms such as *Staphylococcus* not *S. aureus* are considered virulent when corneal trauma is present.

Acanthamoeba spp., an amoeba, can be present in tap water and may colonize the mouth and throat of individuals. It causes keratitis, characterized by severe pain and a red ring around the cornea. It is most often seen in patients who wear soft contact lenses or possess poor lens disinfection technique. The simple act of sitting the cap of the contact lens solution bottle on the sink countertop can potentially contaminate the entire bottle of solution with this organism. The infection caused is often confused with that caused by herpes simplex virus. Once established the infection is difficult to eradicate.

REAL WORLD TIP

- Contact lenses, especially extended-wear contact lenses, account for most cases of bacterial keratitis. The contact lens is a foreign body that rubs across the cornea with each eyeblink. Debris caught behind the lens can cause tiny scratches in the cornea, which allow bacteria to enter and cause infection.

- In early 2006, an outbreak of corneal fungal infections with *Fusarium* species occurred due to contaminated commercial contact lens solution.

Endophthalmitis.   When the interior of the eye becomes infected with microorganisms, it is called **endophthalmitis.** It can occur via the bloodstream from another infection site or from direct inoculation through trauma or surgery, especially after cataract surgery. Endophthalmitis is considered a medical emergency because it can lead to blindness and possible enucleation or removal of the eye. The disease process presents rapidly, often within 12–24 hours.

Cataract surgery can introduce microorganisms into the aqueous humor. Most cases are due to bacteria that temporarily colonize the surface of the conjunctiva. Nine out of 10 infections after cataract surgery are due to gram-positive organisms, especially *Staphylococcus aureus* and *Staphylococcus* not *S. aureus* (Betts et al., 2003). The use of antibiotics before and after surgery can reduce the incidence of infection.

REAL WORLD TIP

In recent years laser eye surgery has gained popularity due to its ability to correct most vision problems. Infections are a potential risk with the procedure but are a rare complication. The use of a laser rather than a microtome (cutting blade) to make the corneal flap has decreased infection rates.

Traumatic injury to the eye can introduce microorganisms to the sterile interior chambers. Metal objects have a greater chance of introducing an infectious agent versus glass (Betts et al., 2003). Accidents in a rural setting can lead to infection with multiple organisms due to the introduction of soil or organic matter (Peters & Peak, 2001). The introduction of foreign organic matter usually points toward *Bacillus* spp. as the causative agent (Peters & Peak, 2001). It accounts for up to 30% of posttraumatic endophthalmitis but any organism introduced through trauma should be considered clinically significant (Betts et al., 2003).

Intravenous drug users and the immunosuppressed are prone to endophthalmitis due to *Candida albicans*. The yeast enters the bloodstream from a distant infection site and then crosses the blood–eye barrier, which is similar to the blood–brain barrier. The right eye is twice as likely to become infected as the left eye because it is located very close to an artery (Peters & Peak, 2001).

✓ Checkpoint! 38–8 (Chapter Objectives 2, 3, and 4)

A 17-year-old male is the victim of a motor vehicle crash on a dark country road. He was not wearing a seat belt and was ejected at the crash site. He received massive facial trauma. The next day he developed endophthalmitis and required enucleation of his right eye. What microorganism is most likely the cause of his infection?

A. Staphylococcus not S. aureus
B. Bacillus spp.
C. Haemophilus influenzae
D. Adenovirus

Stye.   A **stye** is a localized infection in the hair follicle at the base of an eyelash. There is often a localized swelling, which is tender and painful. Most are self-limiting and spontaneously drain. A visit to the physician is usually not required unless the infection spreads. The most common causative agent is *Staphylococcus aureus*. Cultures are rarely required. Figure 38-16 ■ shows a stye with the characteristic collection of pus at the base on an eyelash.

Dacryocystitis.   **Dacryocystitis** is an infection of the nasolacrimal duct or tear duct located in the lower corner of the eye closest to the nose. The duct drains tears into the nasal cavity. The duct can become blocked and then infected due to organisms from the conjunctival surface or the nasal mucosa. Acute dacryocystitis appears, with sudden pain, swelling, and redness in the corner of the eye closest to the nose. Often there is concurrent conjunctivitis. Because of blockage of the duct there is increased tearing of the eye. Organisms associated with infection include *Staphylococcus aureus*, *Haemophilus influenzae*, *Streptococcus pneumoniae*, and beta-hemolytic *Streptococcus*.

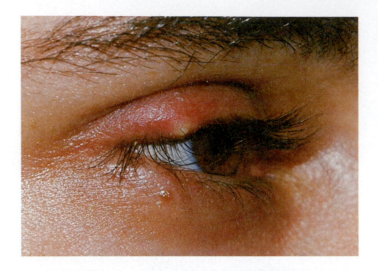

■ **FIGURE 38-16** This photograph shows a stye with the typical collection of pus at the base of an eyelash. The infection usually drains on its own without the need to see a physician.
From http://commons.wikimedia.org/wiki/Image:Stye02.jpg, Andre Riemann.

Specimen Collection

Due to the minute amounts of tissues and fluids collected, specimens from the eye are prone to drying out during transportation. The ophthalmologist usually elects to directly inoculate the agar plates after collection and prepare the smear for Gram stain. Ideally, sheep blood, chocolate, and MacConkey agars are inoculated. At a minimum a chocolate agar is used since it will grow most suspected pathogens. Conjunctivitis may be diagnosed with the collection of the drainage material using a sterile swab but conjunctival scrapings are better for detection of microorganisms. If *Chlamydia trachomatis* is suspected, a calcium alginate rather than a cotton swab should be used because cotton is inhibitory to the organism. Swabs with wooden shafts should also be avoided as well. *Chlamydia* spp. are sensitive to substances in the wood. It is important to remember that *Chlamydia trachomatis* is an intracellular organism. The physician must ensure cells are collected as part of the specimen for culture if this organism is suspected.

Conjunctival or corneal scrapings are collected using a sterile spatula or blade. Intraocular fluid is collected via needle aspiration. Excess air should be expelled from the syringe, the needle removed, and the syringe capped prior to transportation. The physician may elect to send the fluid to the laboratory in an anaerobic transportation system. Specimens for viral cultures need to be transferred in viral transport medium.

Setup and Incubation of Cultures

The microbiology laboratory may receive one to two swabs for cultures of conjunctivitis. Due to the fragility of some potential pathogens, the swabs should be stored at room temperature and processed as soon as possible. Specimens for keratitis and endophthalmitis should be processed immediately upon receipt due to the potential for loss of vision.

Specimen Preparation. Since conjunctival or corneal scrapings are usually inoculated directly by the physician, the agar plates must be transported immediately. Once in the laboratory, the plates are streaked for isolation and incubated in 5% CO_2 at 35–37°C.

When intraocular fluid is received, there is often only a tiny amount of fluid. About one milliliter of thioglycolate broth can be pulled up in the syringe to wash out the needle and interior. The broth-specimen mixture is used to inoculate the sheep blood, chocolate, and MacConkey agar plates and make the Gram stain smear. The remainder of the mixture is returned to the thioglycolate broth tube for incubation. A syringe should never be transported to the laboratory with a needle attached. Due to the very small volume of specimen, the laboratory should suggest sending a thioglycolate broth to the physician's office so the specimen may be processed immediately after collection.

Cultivation. A culture for bacteria causing eye infections should be plated to a minimum of a chocolate agar. A Thayer-Martin agar may be added if *Neisseria gonorrhoeae* is suspected but this organism will grow on chocolate agar so it may not be necessary in a routine culture. Fungal media is added if ordered by the physician. A reducible blood agar plate should be added if the specimen is intraocular fluid.

Chlamydia trachomatis, an intracellular organism, can be recovered on cell line culture just like viruses. The organism produces an inclusion in the cells that appears after staining with iodine. *Chlamydia* cultures can take up to 48–72 hours for detection. A direct fluorescent antibody stain can also be used for its detection.

Adenovirus and herpes simplex virus can be detected in cell cultures. The viruses cause changes in the cells that are recognized by an experienced microbiologist. Fluorescent antibody stains confirm the identification.

✓ **Checkpoint! 38–9 (Chapter Objective 7)**

An ophthalmologist calls the microbiology department for assistance. She wants to collect vitreous humor via a needle aspiration. She communicates there will be a very small amount of fluid removed and the specimen will probably remain in the needle rather than entering the syringe. How will you respond to her request for assistance?

  A. Instruct the physician to cap the needle and send the entire syringe to the laboratory immediately.

  B. Send an anaerobic thioglycolate broth to her office so she can wash the fluid out of the needle and transport the fluid–broth mixture immediately.

  C. Place the fluid onto a calcium alginate swab and transport it immediately.

  D. Refrigerate the specimen in the syringe until it can be transported to the laboratory.

Interpretation of Cultures

Organism Workup. All organisms isolated from the eye should be identified as rapidly and completely as possible. Even normal skin flora organisms such as *Staphylococcus* not *S. aureus* can be clinically significant in patients with keratitis.

Susceptibility Testing. Once an organism is determined to be a potential pathogen, susceptibility testing should be performed if a valid, standardized method available for testing exists. If a method is not available, literature can provide valuable information for recommended treatment.

Other. A rapid nucleic acid hybridization technique can be used to detect *Chlamydia trachomatis* in conjunctival swab specimens. When compared to cell culture methods with direct fluorescent antibody staining, nucleic acid hybridization shows a 99.0% agreement (Gen-Probe, Inc., 2001).

THE EAR

The ear, the organ of hearing, is prone to infection due to its close connection with the upper respiratory system. Ear infections can account for many sick days for children and missed work days for parents. Complications of infections can lead to hearing loss. Table 38-3✪ summarizes infectious diseases associated with the ear and the most common causative microorganisms.

Anatomy of the Ear

There are three parts to the ear: the external ear, the middle ear or tympanic space, and the internal ear or labyrinth. Each is prone to infection by microorganisms. The visible, fleshy portion of the ear is called the auricle. It acts as a funnel to collect vibrations that are converted into sound deep inside the ear. The auditory canal leads to the tympanic membrane, which is a stretched sheet that transmits vibrations that become sound.

The ear canal is lined with skin and contains glands that excrete ear wax. Ear wax serves to capture and move debris out of the auditory canal and away from the tympanic membrane.

The tympanic space or middle ear is contained within the temporal bone of the skull. It is filled with air and contains a chain of three tiny movable bones: malleus, incus, and stapes. The first bone in the link, the malleus, is attached to the tympanic membrane and transmits the vibrations received down the chain of bones. Vibrations are amplified and conducted to the internal ear. The tympanic space is connected to the nasopharynx through the auditory or eustachian tube. The eustachian tube is lined with mucosa similar to that of the respiratory tract as well as ciliated epithelial cells. When the cells and mucosa are damaged, such as during a viral upper respiratory infection, they provide an ideal site for upper respiratory bacteria to colonize and cause infection.

Beyond the tympanic space lies the inner ear, which contains the labyrinth. The labyrinth is a complex maze of canals and cavities filled with fluid and responsible for hearing and balance. It communicates with the auditory nerve of the brain. The stapes bone sends amplified vibrations to the labyrinth where sensory cells transmit them to the auditory nerve to become sound. Figure 38-17 ■ illustrates the anatomy of the ear.

Infectious Diseases Associated with the Ear

Otitis Externa. When the external ear or the canal becomes infected, it is known as otitis externa. Swimmers are most commonly afflicted with this type of infection. Excess moisture becomes trapped in the auditory canal and serves as the source of most infections. The external ear has several defenses to prevent infection: (1) ear wax, or cerumen, is acidic, preventing microorganisms from colonizing the skin; (2) ear wax is full of lipids and prevents water from reaching the skin; and (3) the dead skin cells, ear wax, and debris are carried away from the tympanic membrane to the outside. Once water is trapped in the canal, the skin lining is damaged or ear wax is overproduced or underproduced infection can occur.

Pseudomonas aeruginosa, a water-loving organism, is the most common causative agent but *Staphylococcus* spp., *Streptococcus* spp., and fungi such as *Aspergillus* spp. can cause infections as well. The disease process includes itching, swelling, a feeling of pressure in the ear, and a purulent discharge.

> **@ REAL WORLD TIP**
>
> The ear canal is the only dead-end opening in the body that is lined with skin. Trapped moisture plus its warm, dark environment makes it an ideal location for infection.

Otitis Media—Acute and Chronic. **Otitis media** or inflammation of the middle ear is a very common disease of children between the ages of 6 to 24 months. The inflammation can develop rapidly and persist for weeks or months.

✪ TABLE 38-3

Ear Infections and Most Common Potential Pathogens

Ear Infection	Most Common Potential Pathogen(s)
Otitis externa	*Pseudomonas aeruginosa*
	Staphylococcus spp.
	Streptococcus spp.
Acute otitis media	*Haemophilus influenzae*
	Moraxella catarrhalis
	Streptococcus pneumoniae
Chronic otitis media	*Pseudomonas aeruginosa*
	Staphylococcus aureus
Labyrinthitis	Viruses
	Bacteria

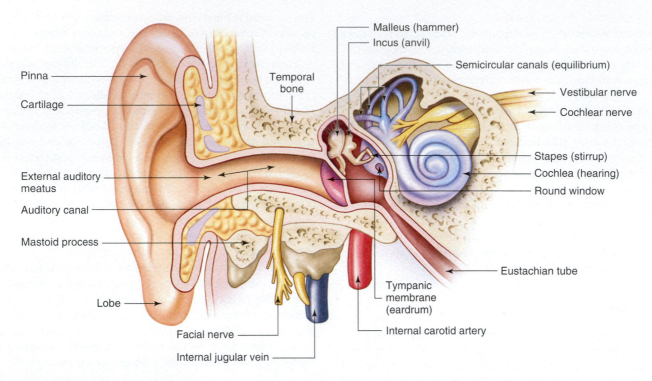

■ **FIGURE 38-17** The anatomy of the outer, middle, and inner ear.

Children under the age of 6 are primarily affected. The eustachian (auditory) tube of children sits at a lower angle and easily allows the backflow of upper respiratory secretions. Propping a milk bottle up for the child at bedtime can allow fluid to enter the eustachian tube. The fluid acts as culture medium for microorganisms from the upper respiratory tract. If otitis media is diagnosed before the age of 1, there is a tendency to develop recurrent acute disease and eventually chronic ear infections (Jones, Wilson, & Malis, 2004).

Several risk factors can lead to increased ear infections in children. Infants are prone due to their immature immune systems. The use of daycare exposes children to colonization with potential pathogens. Bottle-feeding does not provide the natural antibodies found in breast milk. Exposure to secondary smoke increases the incidence of respiratory infections. The increase in the incidence of respiratory infections in the winter and spring also causes an increase in ear infections. *Haemophilus influenzae, Moraxella catarrhalis,* and *Streptococcus pneumoniae* account for about 95% of all cases of acute otitis media (Jones et al., 2004). While viruses do not often cause ear infections, they do cause many upper respiratory infections (URI). Changes in the cells of the eustachian tube caused by the viral URI can allow bacteria to colonize and eventually cause secondary infections.

Often the child has a current respiratory infection or has had a recent one when the ear infection begins. Pain in the ear is one of the first signs of infection. If the child cannot verbalize, constant pulling at or brushing the ear is a common sign of pain. Most children exhibit fever.

Acute otitis media can progress to a chronic state if treatment is not adequate. With infection there is a buildup of serous fluid and pus in the tympanic space, which causes outward pressure against the tympanic membrane. The membrane can spontaneously rupture when the pressure becomes too great and pus and fluid drain into the ear canal. Once the tympanic membrane ruptures it can no longer transmit sound waves and hearing loss is a common complaint. Figure 38-18 ■ illustrates the anatomy of an ear with acute otitis media.

@ **REAL WORLD TIP**

A ruptured eardrum can heal in about 2 months, provided the hole is small. There may be scarring after healing, which can affect the individual's hearing.

Pseudomonas aeruginosa accounts for most cases of chronic otitis media. *Staphylococcus aureus* can also be a causative agent. Individuals with chronic disease complain of hearing loss and foul-smelling fluid leaking from the ear canal.

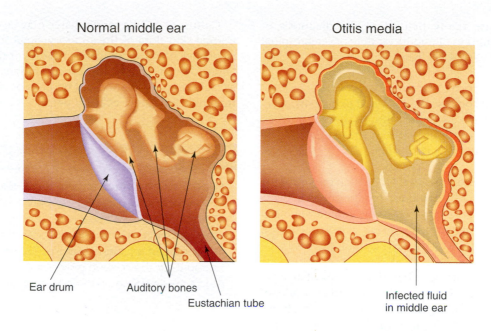

Normal middle ear   Otitis media

Ear drum   Auditory bones

Eustachian tube

Infected fluid
in middle ear

■ **FIGURE 38-18** On the right is a cross-section of the human ear that shows the buildup of purulent material in the tympanic space or middle ear due to acute otitis media. When compared to a normal middle ear on the left, it is easy to see the pressure caused by the infected fluid on the tympanic membrane. Looking through the external ear canal, the physician is able to view the inflamed, bulging tympanic membrane.

 REAL WORLD TIP

Otitis media with effusion (OME) is the buildup of clear fluid in the middle ear. It usually occurs after a viral infection such as a cold and it may take up to a month to disappear. It can also occur after a case of acute otitis media. It does not indicate infection. The patient is often asymptomatic and only complains of hearing problems due to the buildup of fluid. The best treatment for OME is a "wait and see" approach. It usually resolves on its own with time. Most antibiotic-resistant middle ear pathogens present today are due to the insistence of parents that their child receive antibiotics when they only have OME.

 Checkpoint! 38–10 (Chapter Objective 3)

Pseudomonas aeruginosa is the most common causative agent of:
- A. *otitis externa.*
- B. *acute otitis media.*
- C. *chronic otitis media.*
- D. *both A and C.*

Labyrinthitis.   Inflammation of the inner ear's labyrinth is called **labyrinthitis.** Patients complain of dizziness with accompanying nausea and vomiting. Often the signs and symptoms appear after a recent viral upper respiratory infection such as a common cold. Viral labyrinthitis, the most common form, has a sudden onset with hearing loss and dizziness. Most cases occur in adults. Viral labyrinthitis is usually self-limiting, lasting days to weeks.

Bacteria can also cause labyrinthitis but have a very low incidence. The same organisms that cause meningitis and otitis media are usually responsible. Bacterial labyrinthitis usually results in permanent hearing loss.

Specimen Collection

Otitis externa requires a thorough cleansing of the surface and a culture of the drainage, using a sterile swab, in order to assess the causative agent.

Otitis media is usually treated based on signs and symptoms alone. Due to the ability to predict the most common potential pathogens, no definitive laboratory testing is usually required. **Tympanocentesis**, a needle puncture of the tympanic membrane to collect the middle ear discharge, is rarely performed. The procedure can be performed if antibiotic therapy does not alleviate the source of infection. If the tympanic membrane has spontaneously ruptured, the exudate can be collected on a sterile swab.

Direct cultures are rarely helpful in the diagnosis of labyrinthitis. Often cultures of middle ear fluid or cerebrospinal fluid may reveal the etiological agent.

Setup and Incubation of Cultures

Due to the fragility of some of the potential pathogens, specimens collected on sterile swabs for cultures should be stored at room temperature. A syringe, without the needle, may be received if tympanocentesis is performed.

Specimen Preparation.
A direct Gram stain can reveal the etiological agent and guide the addition of supplemental media other than the routine agar plates. Due to the minute volume of specimen collected during tympanocentesis, direct inoculation of agar cultures can be done by the physician in the office.

Cultivation.
The use of sheep blood agar, chocolate agar, and MacConkey agar for a culture will recover the majority of the potential bacterial pathogens that cause ear infections. Since tympanocentesis is an invasive procedure, the addition of anaerobic media should be considered. Aerobic cultures (BA and CA) should be incubated at 35–37°C with CO_2 while MAC agar should be incubated in ambient air. All agar plates are examined at 24 and 48 hours before discarding.

Interpretation of Cultures

Organism Workup.
Streptococcus pneumoniae appears as alpha-hemolytic cratered or mucoid colonies on sheep blood and chocolate agar. *Haemophilus influenzae* displays a wet, gray colony, which grows only on the chocolate agar due to its requirement for X and V factors. *Moraxella catarrhalis* produces a gray-white opaque colony that has a tendency to move intact across the agar surface, like a hockey puck, when pushed with a sterile needle or stick. The organism grows on sheep blood agar but a little better on chocolate agar.

Cultures of the external ear may reveal normal skin flora due to inadequate cleansing prior to specimen collection. Often the potential pathogen is found in greater quantity when compared to the amount of normal flora present. The workup of normal flora organisms is not required. It is better to group organisms such as *Staphylococcus* not *S. aureus* and diphtheroids as normal skin flora rather listing each individually. Providing a normal skin organism a specific identification gives it more importance in the eye of the physician and may lead to unnecessary antibiotic treatment. These organisms should be kept for 1 week to allow the physician time to request further identification and susceptibility testing if the patient's clinical signs and symptoms warrant.

The use of flow charts or algorithms to determine the level of organism workup based on body site or specimen type may alleviate some of the gray areas of determining a potential pathogen in the presence of normal flora. A microbiologist should use common sense when working with flow charts and ensure the final outcome correlates with patient history and testing results.

Culture of middle ear discharge may be contaminated with normal skin flora of the auditory canal if the specimen was recovered after a spontaneous rupture of the tympanic membrane. Up to 50% of middle ear cultures may not grow bacteria because they are due to fluid buildup or effusion rather than true infection (Jones et al., 2004).

 REAL WORLD TIP

Recent studies have shown that *Helictobacter pylori* and *Alloiococcus otitidis* may play a role in otitis media effusion (OME) (Waseem & Aslam, 2007). Both are slow growing and would not appear after 48 hours incubation of a routine culture. These organisms may account for the reason why more than 50% of middle ear cultures do not grow an organism.

Susceptibility Testing.
Organisms determined to be clinically significant should be tested for susceptibility testing if valid, standardized methods exist. Drug-resistant *Streptococcus pneumoniae* (DRSP) has increased dramatically in the past 10 years. DRSP resistance includes penicillin, trimethoprim-sulfamethoxazole, and quinolone. About half of the strains of *H. influenzae* isolated are beta-lactamase positive, as are nearly 95% of strains of *M. catarrhalis*. Antibiotic-resistant strains of microorganisms account for many cases of treatment failures. It has made the management of ear infections a complex process for physicians. Many ear infections in children are treated without confirmation of the pathogen by culture. The physician often reserves tympanocentesis as a last resort if antibiotic therapy does not eliminate the source of the infection.

Other.
Tympanostomy tubes can be inserted to allow the release of discharge from the middle ear and prevent spontaneous rupture of the tympanic membrane. They are often inserted when antibiotic therapy fails to eliminate the infectious agent. Removal of the adenoids and tonsils may eliminate a potential source of ear pathogens (Jones et al., 2004).

SUMMARY

Meningitis is one of the few medical emergencies in which the clinical microbiologist can have an immediate positive impact on patient outcomes. Detection and identification of the potential pathogens of infections of the ear and eye can also prevent life-changing complications such as blindness and deafness.

Patient history such as age, immune state, signs and symptoms, and the results of other laboratory testing can help determine potential pathogens. Table 38-4✪ correlates physical and patient history clues with potential CSF, ear, and eye pathogens. While the microbiologist may not always receive

✪ TABLE 38-4

Patient Signs, Symptoms, or History Clues that Correlate with Specific Potential Pathogens of the CSF, Eye, or Ear

Clue	Associated Organism(s)
Infection of the Central Nervous System	
Age of patient	*Haemophilus influenzae*
■ Neonate to infant	■ Consider serotype b if there is no history of immunization
	Streptococcus agalactiae (Group B)
	Streptococcus pneumoniae
	Listeria monocytogenes
	Escherichia coli K1
	Toxoplasma gondii
■ 6 months to young adult	*Neisseria meningitidis*
	Haemophilus influenzae
	Streptococcus pneumoniae
■ Adult	*Neisseria meningitidis*
	Streptococcus pneumoniae
■ Older adults	*Streptococcus pneumoniae*
	Listeria monocytogenes
Military recruit or college student	*Neisseria meningitidis*
Suppressed or compromised immune state	*Listeria monocytogenes*
	Cryptococcus neoformans
	Mycobacterium tuberculosis
	Toxoplasma gondii
Rash with flu-like symptoms	*Neisseria meningitidis*
History of swimming, diving or skiing	*Naegleria fowleri*
Epilepsy with no previous history	*Taenia solium*
Presence of a CSF shunt	*Staphylococcus not Staphylococcus aureus*
	Staphylococcus aureus
	Propionibacterium acnes
Mosquito or tick bites	Mosquito
	■ Arboviruses
	Tick
	■ *Borrelia burgdorferi*
History of association with cats and their litter boxes	*Toxoplasma gondii*
Infection of the Eye	
Purulent discharge	Bacteria
Watery discharge	Virus
Presence of contact lenses	*Acanthamoeba spp.*
Trauma	*Bacillus* spp.
Intravenous drug user	*Candida albicans*
Infection of the Ear	
Swimmer	*Pseudomonas aeruginosa*

Note: This listing is not to be considered inclusive for all potential pathogens for each body site. It is a collection of patient clues correlated with the most predictable pathogen(s).

detailed patient history information, a physician who understands the value of the microbiologist and the depth of their knowledge base may provide these missing details. The ability to correlate patient history and laboratory testing with potential pathogens can ensure the appropriate media and methods are used for detection.

Because the central nervous system, eye, and ear are close in proximity, they can share common potential pathogens such as *Haemophilus influenzae* and *Streptococcus pneumoniae*. Once the most common causative agents have been ruled out then the hunt for uncommon pathogens can begin.

℮ REAL WORLD TIP

There is an old medical adage, "When you hear hoofbeats, think horses not zebras." It holds true in the clinical microbiology laboratory. When faced with the identification of an organism, always consider the most common potential pathogen(s) based on the body site and/or specimen source first. Once they have been ruled out then consider less frequently isolated or unusual organisms.

The clinical microbiologist must be knowledgeable of preanalytical components such as specimen collection and processing in order to ensure the specimen arrives in a state as close as possible to the time of collection and without the loss of potential pathogens. Direct detection methods such the polymerase chain reaction may provide a rapid alternative to traditional cultures.

Analysis of cultures should include the workup of only clinically significant organisms based on the body site or specimen type. Identifying normal flora such as *Staphylococcus* not *S. aureus* and diphtheroids in an external ear culture elevates them to a state of importance in the eye of the physician and provides the patient a disservice. On the other hand, the identification of *Staphylococcus* not *S. aureus* in a ventricular fluid represents a true potential pathogen. The microbiologist must use good judgment when determining the extent of organism identification based on the body site or specimen type. Many laboratories have created algorithms or flow charts for organism workup to ensure only potential pathogens are identified. Table 38-5 ✪ provides information on observations and tests that are helpful in the identification of selected CNS, eye, and ear pathogens.

Valid and standardized susceptibility methods must be employed on appropriate organisms. Antibiotics should be selected based on the specific pathogen and its isolation site for treatment. Not all antibiotics are able to achieve therapeutic levels in the CSF and other body sites. Some organisms do not require susceptibility testing if they have not exhibited any known resistance mechanisms but that list is becoming shorter and shorter each year.

✪ TABLE 38-5

Identification of Selected Central Nervous System Pathogens

Pathogen	Microscopic Morphology	Colony Morphology			Identification Tests
		BA	CA	MAC	
Staphylococcus aureus	Gram-positive cocci in clusters	Large yellow or white, usually beta-hemolytic	*	NG	GS, catalase, slide latex or coagulase
Staphylococcus not *S. aureus*	Gram-positive cocci in clusters	Large white, non-hemolytic	*	NG	GS, catalase, slide latex, or coagulase, trehalose-mannitol or polymyxin B, PYR, ORN
Streptococcus pneumoniae	Lancet or football shaped, gram-positive diplococci	Small gray, alpha-hemolytic	*	NG	GS, catalase, bile solubility, optochin
Neisseria meningitidis	Gram-negative diplococci	Small, cratered or mucoid, gray, may be alpha-hemolytic	*	NG	Oxidase, GS, sugars, enzyme, ONPG, polysaccharide from sucrose or BA/CA at 25°C, serology
Moraxella catarrhalis	Gram-negative diplococci	Small gray to white, convex, "hockey puck"	*	NG	Oxidase, GS, catalase, butyrate esterase, growth at room temperature
Pseudomonas aeruginosa	Gram-negative rod	Large beta, aluminum foil sheen or blue-green pigment, fruity odor	*	NLF, blue-green pigment	Oxidase, gram negative identification panel if non-pigmented
Enterobacteriaceae/ Nonfermenting bacilli	Gram-negative rod	Large gray, may be hemolytic, swarming or mucoid	*	LF or NLF	Oxidase, gram negative identification panel
Haemophilus influenzae or *H. aegypticus*	Tiny, gram-negative rod, pleomorphic or cocco-bacillary	NG	Small, gray	NG	GS, catalase, porphyrin (ALA), XV factor requirement, no hemolysis on HBA, xylose
Yeast	Gram-positive, budding yeast	Creamy, white, may have "feet"	*	NG	GS, India ink, urease, germ tube, morphology agar
Propionibacterium acnes	Palisading, gram-positive rod	Aerobic: usually NG Anaerobic: tiny gray-white	Usually NG	NG	GS, catalase, spot indole

BA, blood agar; CA, chocolate agar; MAC, MacConkey agar; *, Growth same as BA; NG, no growth; LF, lactose fermenting; NLF, non-lactose fermenting; GS, Gram stain; PYR, pyrrolidonyl arylamidase; ORN, ornithine decarboxylase; ONPG, beta-galactosidase; ALA, aminolevulinic acid; HBA, horse blood agar

LEARNING OPPORTUNITIES

1. In January, a previously healthy 73-year-old female awoke with a headache. As the day progressed, she complained the headache had worsened. By late afternoon, she became comatose and combative. On arrival in the emergency room, the physician suspected a stroke. In the process of working the patient up for the diagnosis of stroke, she developed a fever of 103°F. The physician drew blood cultures and performed a lumbar puncture, which revealed:

    CSF Glucose – 40 mg/dl

    CSF Protein – 272 mg/dl

    CSF Cell Count and Differential – 202 white blood cells/mm^3 with 78% neutrophils and 22% lymphocytes

    Bacterial CSF culture – No growth at 48 hours

    Blood culture – No growth at 5 days

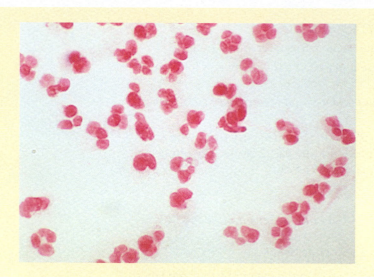

Gram stain of the CSF, prior to antibiotic therapy, of the 73-year-old female.
Public Health Image Library (PHIL)/CDC and Dr. Norman Jacobs

The patient was started on intravenous ceftriaxone, vancomycin, acyclovir, and steroids. She remained hospitalized comatose in the intensive care unit for 5 days. She regained consciousness on day 6 and was transferred to the neuroscience unit. After rehabilitation, she returned home with no deficits on day 12.

   a. With negative cultures, what additional testing can you suggest to the physician that can help him confirm the potential meningitis pathogen? (Chapter Objective 6)

     a. Viral throat culture

     b. Acridine Orange stain on CSF and blood

     c. Immunochromatic assay on CSF for *Streptococcus pneumoniae*

     d. Direct antigen testing on CSF for *Haemophilus influenzae* type b, *Neisseria meningitidis* serogroups A, C, Y, and W135, *Streptococcus agalactiae*, *Streptococcus pneumoniae*, and *E. coli* serotype K1

   b. Which microorganism do you suspect based on the patient history and laboratory results? (Chapter Objectives 3 and 4)

     a. *Listeria monocytogenes*

     b. *Streptococcus pneumoniae*

     c. Enterovirus

     d. *Haemophilus influenzae* type b

2. A cerebrospinal fluid was received in the laboratory at 4:15 A.M. with orders for Gram stain, routine bacterial culture, glucose and protein levels, and white blood cell count and differential. CSF tube #1 was saved for future testing. CSF tube #3 was used by the hematology and chemistry areas for the glucose and protein levels as well as the white blood cell count and differential. CSF tube #2 was stored at 4°C until the day microbiology shift arrived at 6:30 A.M. What is the effect of storage of tube #2 at 4°C prior to processing for CSF Gram stain and routine culture? (Chapter Objective 8)

   a. There will be no effect. Storage at 4°C is appropriate.

   b. The white blood cells will disintegrate in the refrigerator after 2 hours.

   c. The specimen may be used for culture if placed in a CO_2 incubator for 2 hours prior to processing.

   d. *Neisseria meningitidis* and *Streptococcus pneumoniae,* if present, may autolyse and be lost.

3. A 59-year-old male with advanced AIDS is seen in the emergency room with complaints of lethargy, headache, and slight fever for the past 2 weeks. The physician performs a lumbar puncture and the initial results reveal:

   Glucose – 48 mg/dl
   Protein – 93 mg/dl
   White blood cell count and differential – 40 white blood cells/mm^3 with 87% lymphocytes and 13% monocytes
   Gram stain – No organisms seen with a few white blood cells

   a. What microorganism(s) do you suspect based on the patient history and laboratory results? (Chapter Objectives 3 and 4)

      a. *Cryptococcus neoformans*

      b. *Mycobacterium tuberculosis*

      c. Both a and b

      d. Neither organism

   b. What additional testing should be recommended at this point? (Chapter Objective 6)

      a. India ink on the CSF

      b. Cryptococcal antigen test

      c. PCR for *Mycobacterium* spp.

      d. Both a and b

      e. Both b and c

4. In June, a child-care facility experienced an outbreak of flu-like symptoms among its young clients. One 4-year-old male developed a severe headache and fever. He was admitted to the hospital. A lumbar puncture revealed the following results for his CSF:

   Glucose – 53 mg/dl
   Protein – 75 mg/dl
   White blood cell count and differential – 120 cells/mm^3 with 100% lymphocytes
   Gram stain – No organisms seen with a few white blood cells
   Bacterial CSF culture – No growth at 48 hours

A viral culture of his CSF revealed the specific pathogen.

   a. What additional body site/specimen type could have been cultured if the CSF viral culture had proven negative for the pathogen? (Chapter Objective 2)

      a. Stool

      b. Urine

      c. Sputum

      d. Blood

b. What meningitis pathogen(s) do you suspect based on the patient history and results above? (Chapter Objectives 3, 4, and 5)

   a. Enterovirus

   b. Arbovirus

   c. Herpes simplex virus

   d. a and b

5. A physician notes her patient has ulceration of the right eye due to extensive scarring of the eyelid and inward rotation of the eyelashes. She calls you for information on specimen collection to ensure recovery of the suspected pathogen.

  a. What pathogen does the physician suspect? (Chapter Objective 3)

   a. *Haemophilus aegyptius*

   b. *Bacillus* spp.

   c. *Neisseria gonorrhoeae*

   d. *Chlamydia trachomatis*

   e. *Acanthamoeba* spp.

  b. What specimen collection technique will you advise the physician to use? (Chapter Objective 7)

   a. Eye discharge collected with a sterile cotton swab

   b. Eye discharge collected with a sterile calcium alginate swab with a wooden shaft

   c. Corneal scrapings using a sterile blade or spatula

   d. Vitreous fluid using a sterile syringe

6. Four CLS students develop conjunctivitis after each uses the same microscope to complete a blood differential practical examination. Each has pink conjunctiva and a thin, watery discharge in both eyes. What pathogen do you suspect caused their predicament? (Chapter Objectives 2, 3, and 4)

  a. Adenovirus

  b. Herpes simplex virus

  c. *Haemophilus influenzae*

  d. *Streptococcus pneumoniae*

7. A culture of middle ear drainage from a 6-year-old female with a ruptured tympanic membrane yielded:

Heavy growth of *Haemophilus influenzae*
Moderate growth of *Staphylococcus* not *S. aureus*
Light growth of Diphtheroids

How should this culture be reported on the patient's medical chart? (Chapter Objectives 2 and 3)

  a. Heavy growth of normal skin flora

  b. Heavy growth of *Haemophilus influenzae* and moderate growth of normal skin flora

  c. Heavy growth of *Haemophilus influenzae*, moderate growth of *Staphylococcus* not *S. aureus*, and light growth of Diphtheroids

  d. Moderate growth of *Staphylococcus* not *S. aureus* and heavy growth of normal skin flora

8. An oxidase-positive gray-white, opaque, hockey puck colony that grows a little better on chocolate than blood agar was isolated from a tympanocentesis fluid. Which of the following patients would you expect to be the owner of these results? (Chapter Objective 4)

   a. 88-year-old male smoker with a cold

   b. 18-month-old female in day care 5 days per week

   c. 10-year-old male with a history of recurrent strep throat

   d. 3-month-old female who is fed with breast milk

PEARSON
myhealthprofessionskit™

Use this address to access the interactive Companion Website created for this textbook. Simply select "Clinical Laboratory Science" from the choice of disciplines. Find this book and log in using your user name and password.

REFERENCES

Go to myhealthprofessionskit.com to view this chapter's references.

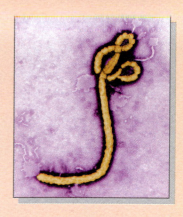

39

Skeletal System

Hassan Aziz

■ LEARNING OBJECTIVES

Upon completion of this chapter, the learner should be able to:

1. Review the basic anatomy and physiology of the skeletal system including the bone, synovial joint, and bone marrow.

2. Summarize the common microorganisms associated with infectious disease of bone, joint synovial fluid, and bone marrow and their origin.

   a. Indicate patient populations and underlying disease states at risk for infection.

   b. Review pathogenic mechanisms associated with each organism.

3. Determine specimen types/body sites for the culture and diagnosis of infectious diseases of bone, synovial joint fluid, or bone marrow.

4. Describe specimen collection and transportation requirements for bone, synovial joint fluid, and bone marrow.

5. Describe the steps in processing bone, synovial joint fluid, and bone marrow for culture.

6. Select appropriate routine and special media for culture of a bone biopsy, synovial joint fluid, and bone marrow.

7. Correlate patient history, body site or specimen type, colonial morphology, Gram stain reaction, identification test results, and/or susceptibility results to identify an organism and assess its clinical significance.

   a. Select additional or alternative testing needed.

KEY TERMS

cancellous bone tissue	hematopoiesis	osteocytes
contiguous	osteoarthritis	osteomyelitis
cortical bone tissue	osteoblasts	periosteum
hematogenous	osteoclasts	sinus tract

▶ INTRODUCTION

The skeletal system consists of bones, ligaments, joints, and bone marrow. These structures are responsible for locomotion, storage of calcium and other minerals, production of red and white blood cells and platelets, and protection of and support for many organs of the body such as the lungs, heart, and liver. There are 206 bones in the human body, which account for 14% of the body's total weight (Scanlon & Sanders, 1999). Infection of the skeletal system can occur because of surgery, penetrating injury, joint replacement, infection in adjacent tissues, or **hematogenous** (via the blood) spread.

▶ REVIEW OF SKELETAL ANATOMY AND PHYSIOLOGY

The bones of the skeletal system are classified as long bones, such as those in the arm and leg, short bones, such as in the wrist and foot, irregular bones, like the vertebrae, and flat bones, which include the skull and sternum (Thibodeau & Patton, 1999). Bone is made up of calcium hydroxyapatite, which gives it the necessary strength and hardness without adding a lot of weight. It also holds the body's store of calcium, phosphorus, sodium, and magnesium.

The bone's structure is made up of osteogenic (bone-generating) cells, an organic matrix, and minerals. Osteogenic cells consist of osteoblasts, osteocytes, and osteoclasts. These cells are responsible for the formation, repair, and resorption of bones throughout life. **Osteoblasts** are small bone cells that build bones. They secrete collagen, which is essential to the elasticity of the bones so they can give under pressure. **Osteocytes** are mature osteoblasts. They maintain the bone by regulating calcium and other minerals. **Osteoclasts** are larger and multicellular and absorb and remove worn bone. There is a check and balance system that regulates all three cells. The bone created is an organic substance composed of collagen fibers and a mixture of protein, polysaccharide, and minerals, which is hard and calcified (Thibodeau & Patton, 1999).

Two types of bone tissue are recognized: cancellous and cortical. **Cancellous bone tissue** is filled with many spaces and is often described as spongy or honeycomb. It is found on the interior of bone and is designed to bear stress from several directions. **Cortical bone tissue**, on the other hand, is compact and hard, like ivory, and makes up the exterior of most bones. Each bone is fed with blood vessels and supplied with nerves and lymphatic vessels, all of which lie within a thin tissue layer covering the bone called the **periosteum.** Up until the age of about 20, there are growth plates at the ends of long bones that lengthen the bone as a person grows. Infection in the bone can damage the growth plates, which can affect the height of an individual.

Two types of bone marrow exist: red and yellow. Red marrow is active in the production of red and white blood cells as well as platelets and fills the interior cancellous bone. The yellow marrow consists mainly of fat and connective tissue and fills the internal cavity of the long bones of adults. The bones of infants contain all red marrow. As a person ages, the red marrow becomes replaced by yellow marrow in the long bones. In adults, red marrow is found in certain bones such as the ribs, pelvis, vertebrae, skull, sternum, and the ends of the long bones. Figure 39-1 ■ depicts the structure of an adult long bone as well as the external and internal components that make up its anatomy.

Joints are found where bones meet. They are held in place between the long bones by short lengths of fibrous tissue called ligaments. Joints can be free moving, allow for limited movement, or remain immobile. Synovial joints are located at the ends of the long bones and contain a large space that allows for a wide range of motion. Lining the joint space is a membrane that secretes synovial fluid. The fluid contains hyaluronic acid, which lubricates and cushions movement, and mucin, which makes it viscous. Synovial fluid is a clear, colorless, thick liquid made from plasma and contains albumin, fat, and cells. A normal synovial fluid white blood cell count is usually less than 200 cells/µL, with only about 20 to 25% of those being neutrophils. Most of the white blood cells present are usually monocytes and histiocytes. The knee joint space contains about 2.5 to 3.5 mL of fluid.

Cartilage is a firm, dense type of connective tissue. It is more elastic and more compressible than bone and acts like a shock absorber. It holds bones together and allows for limited movement such as between the ribs and sternum. Articular cartilage covers the surface of the long bone ends, which are part of a synovial joint. Fibrous cartilage allows for little or no movement between bones and is found between the vertebrae and in the sutures of the skull (Scanlon & Sanders, 1999). Figure 39-2 ■ illustrates the structure of a synovial joint.

The skeletal system has five main functions: support, protection, movement, mineral storage, and **hematopoiesis** or blood cell production (Thibodeau & Patton, 1999). Bones act as the framework of the body, contributing to the shape and alignment of the body. They also protect many vital organs such as the brain and the heart. With the aid of joints and muscles, bones provide movement. They serve as an important reservoir for calcium, phosphorus, and other minerals, thus contributing to a balanced concentration of these minerals in the body. The bone marrow inside the bones plays a crucial role in the production of red and white blood cells and platelets in a process known as hematopoiesis.

Early in life, the skeletal system is made up of cartilage, which is later replaced by bones because of the activity of the osteoblasts and deposition of calcium and phosphorus around the cartilage. Throughout life, bone tissue is in a continuous breakdown and restoration process to maintain hemostasis, which is essential for healthy survival. When calcium is needed, osteoclasts break down bone, releasing calcium into the blood circulatory system. Likewise, when bone mass is required, such as after an injury, osteoblasts are activated to create new bone.

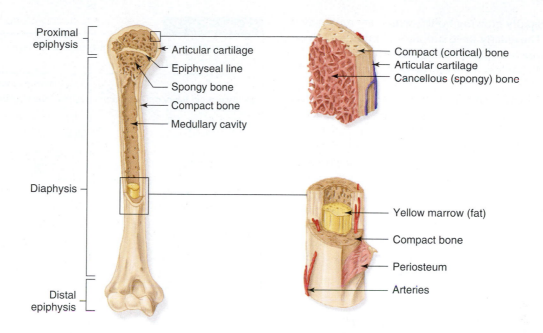

Proximal epiphysis

Articular cartilage
Epiphyseal line
Spongy bone
Compact bone
Medullary cavity

Compact (cortical) bone
Articular cartilage
Cancellous (spongy) bone

Diaphysis

Yellow marrow (fat)
Compact bone
Periosteum
Arteries

Distal epiphysis

■ **FIGURE 39-1** The structure of an adult long bone can be seen in this illustration. The two cross sections provide a view of its internal and external anatomy.

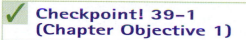

✓ Checkpoint! 39–1 (Chapter Objective 1)

The osteogenic cell responsible for building bones and for secreting collagen is the

A. osteoblast.
B. osteocyte.
C. osteoclast.
D. osteoerythrocyte.

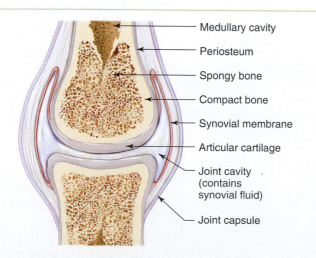

Medullary cavity
Periosteum
Spongy bone
Compact bone
Synovial membrane
Articular cartilage
Joint cavity (contains synovial fluid)
Joint capsule

■ **FIGURE 39-2** This image provides a cross-section view of a synovial joint and its internal structure.

▶ MICROORGANISMS ASSOCIATED WITH THE SKELETAL SYSTEM

BONES

Common bone diseases include osteoporosis (thinning of bone tissue); rickets, which causes bone deformities; tumors; and infections. Inflammation or infection of the bone is called **osteomyelitis** and is most often bacterial in nature. It can be further described as acute or chronic. Chronic osteomyelitis can smolder in the body and take weeks to present with visible signs and symptoms, whereas acute osteomyelitis has an abrupt onset. Osteomyelitis is most often caused by an organism reaching the bone through the bloodstream but can also be because of direct contamination such as trauma (e.g., open compound fracture).

The tibia, femur, humerus, vertebrae, and jaw are very vascular and especially prone to infection. Once infected, the bone marrow swells, which can decrease blood flow to the bone, which in turn accelerates the infection. White blood cells enter the infected area and release enzymes, which stimulate the osteoclasts to degrade bone. Lesions, visible on x-ray, can form where bone breakdown occurs. Pus accumulates and can spread to the surrounding tissues and joints. With time, a **sinus tract** (an abnormal opening from deep in the body to the skin surface) can form a tunnel from the bone to the skin surface, which allows the pus to drain.

The highest incidence of osteomyelitis occurs in children and the elderly, with more males than females affected.

Children have rapidly growing bones, which are more vascular than adults. The elderly have suppressed immune systems, making them more susceptible to any infection. Males tend to indulge in risky behaviors, which provide more opportunities for injury.

Symptoms of osteomyelitis include sudden and high fever, chills, tachycardia, redness and swelling, pain in the infected area, and reluctance to use the limb. Osteomyelitis may be classified as either hematogenous (originating in or distributed by the blood) or secondary to a **contiguous** (nearby or neighboring) source (Baron, 1996). Hematogenous spread usually results in osteomyelitis because of a single organism, whereas contiguous spread can result in infection with several organisms, depending on the site of origin. Osteomyelitis can be further differentiated based on its severity as acute, subacute or chronic. If an infection is left untreated or treated unsuccessfully, it becomes chronic, and necrosis (death) of the bone may occur.

Bacteria

Bacterial osteomyelitis may be caused by any pathogenic bacteria and occasionally by those not regarded as pathogenic. It is most commonly caused by *Staphylococcus aureus* and *Staphylococcus* not *S. aureus* (Forbes, Sahm, & Weissfeld, 2002) followed by *Streptococcus* spp., *Pseudomonas* spp., and the *Enterobacteriaceae* such as *Escherichia coli* and *Proteus* species. Literature suggests that the organisms associated with osteomyelitis can be divided into groups based on the age of the patient (Table 39-1✪), the mechanism of injury, and the presence of underlying conditions (Table 39-2✪; Carek, Dickerson, & Sack, 2001; Lew & Waldvogel, 1997).

Staphylococcus aureus is the most common cause of the disease in infants and is responsible for up to 90% of cases in otherwise healthy children (Cole, Dalziel, & Leitl, 1982). It is usually acquired during an episode of bacteremia. The organ-

✪ **TABLE 39-1**

Age-Related Osteomyelitis Organisms

Age	Organisms
Under 1 year	*Staphylococcus aureus*
	Streptococcus agalactiae (group B *Streptococcus*)
	Enterobacteriaceae
1 to 16 years	*Staphylococcus aureus*
	Streptococcus pyogenes (group A *Streptococcus*)
	Haemophilus influenzae type b
	Kingella kingae
Over 16 years	*Staphylococcus aureus*
	Staphylococcus epidermidis
	Pseudomonas aeruginosa
	Enterobacteriaceae
	Mycobacterium tuberculosis

✪ **TABLE 39-2**

Mechanism of Injury or Conditions and Related Osteomyelitis Organisms

Mechanism of Injury or Condition	Organisms Associated with Osteomyelitis
Nosocomial infection	Methicillin-resistant *Staphylococcus aureus* (MRSA)
	Pseudomonas aeruginosa
	Enterobacteriaceae
Human or animal bites or hand injuries due to fist fight	*Pasteurella multocida* (animal source)
	Eikenella corrodens (human source)
	Streptococcus spp.
	Anaerobes
	Staphylococcus aureus
Diabetes mellitus	*Staphylococcus aureus*
	Streptococcus spp.
	Anaerobes (e.g., *Bacteriodes* spp.)
Sickle cell anemia	*Streptococcus pneumoniae*
	Salmonella spp.
Human immunodeficiency virus (HIV)	*Mycobacterium tuberculosis*
	Mycobacterium avium-intracellulare
Immunocompromised state	*Mycobacterium tuberculosis*
	Candida albicans
	Other fungi
Prosthetic device	*Staphylococcus* not *S. aureus*
	Staphylococcus aureus
	Enterobacteriaceae
	Pseudomonas aeruginosa
	Propionibacterium spp.
	Corynebacterium spp.
Compound fracture	*Staphylococcus aureus*
	Staphylococcus not *S. aureus*
	Enterobacteriaceae
	Bacillus spp.
Intravenous drug use	*Staphylococcus aureus*
	Pseudomonas aeruginosa
	Candida spp.
	Eikenella corrodens
	Mycobacterium tuberculosis
Periodontal disease	*Actinomyces* spp.
	Aggregatibacter (previously *Actinobacillus*) *actinomycetemcomitans*
	Capnocytophaga spp.
	Eikenella corrodens
	Anaerobes

ism produces toxins and enzymes as well as possessing receptors that enable it to adhere to the smooth surfaces of bone. All these factors contribute to the pathogenicity of this organism (Forbes et al., 2002). Figure 39-3 ■ displays an advanced case of bacterial osteomyelitis.

Haemophilus influenzae type b has been virtually eliminated because of the development of a vaccine in the 1980s. It is rarely isolated in the clinical laboratory unless the child has been inadequately immunized or not immunized at all. If a child has no history of immunization, *Haemophilus influenzae* type b should be considered a potential causative agent. Neonates and infants are prone to *Streptococcus agalactiae* (group B *Streptococcus*) infections. Hospitalized patients and immunocompromised individuals are at higher risk of developing infection with nosocomial pathogens such as methicillin-resistant *S. aureus* (MRSA) and *Pseudomonas aeruginosa*.

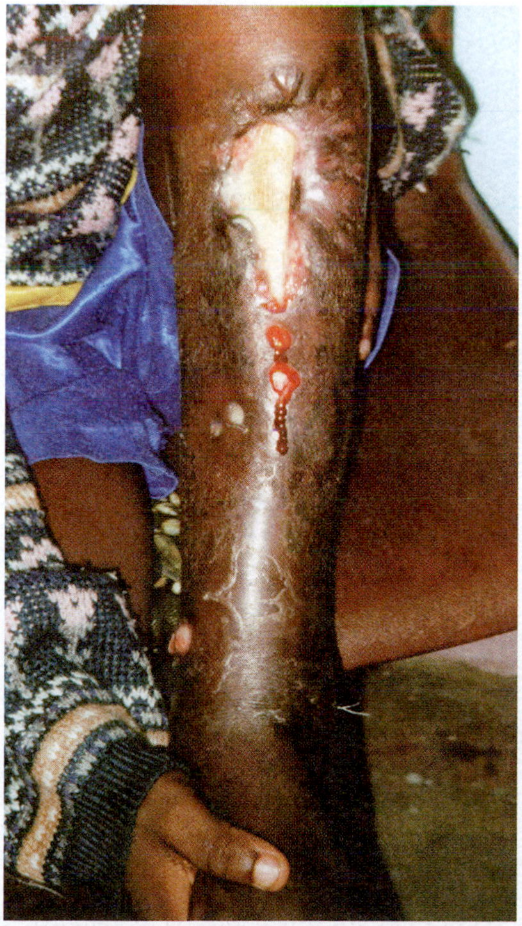

■ **FIGURE 39-3** This 6-year-old boy presented with an advanced case of bacterial osteomyelitis. The pus produced has tunneled to the skin surface, leaving multiple sinus tracts with exposed bone.
From Holtedahl, K., & Hurum, H. (2002). BMC international health and human rights, 2:2doi:10.1186/1472-698X-2-2. Retrieved August 7, 2008, from http://www.biomedcentral.com/1472-698X/2/2

Osteomyelitis caused by *Pasteurella multocida* is usually associated with animal bites. The presence of *Eikenella corrodens* is often related to human bites or intravenous drug use because of the habit of licking the needle prior to injection.

> Ⓔ **REAL WORLD TIP**
>
> Cats have needle teeth, which inject *Pasteurella multocida* deep into the tissue, bone, and joints. Dog bites tend to create crushing injuries of the tissue and bone, which can contain *Pasteurella multocida* but tend to have more *Staphylococcus aureus* and *S. intermedius* as well as *Streptococcus* spp.

Trauma and underlying conditions such as diabetes and sickle cell anemia are at risk for developing osteomyelitis with multiple isolates. Those with these two underlying conditions are prone to reduced blood flow to the extremities, which can lead to contiguous (in close proximity) infections because of several organisms, including normal skin organisms.

> Ⓔ **REAL WORLD TIP**
>
> ■ Children with sickle cell anemia are prone to osteomyelitis because of *Salmonella* spp. It is probably because of reduced blood flow to the intestines due to sickle cells blocking the vessels. The organisms are able to escape the intestine, enter the bloodstream, and reach the highly vascular bones.
>
> ■ Children are drawn to mud puddles. As they jump in the muddy water, their shoes absorb and hold the water. *Pseudomonas aeruginosa* loves water and can grow in wet shoes. If the child steps on a nail or other sharp pointed object, *Pseudomonas aeruginosa* can be pushed into the foot and reach the bone to cause osteomyelitis.

Oral organisms such as *Actinomyces* spp., *Aggregatibacter* (previously *Actinobacillus*) *actinomycetemcomitans*, *Capnocytophaga* spp., *Eikenella corrodens*, and anaerobes are associated with periodontitis, which can lead to osteomyelitis of the jaw. Other bones can be affected because of the ability of the organisms to spread via the bloodstream.

One organism, *Kingella kingae*, is unique in its preference for cardiac, heart valve, joint space, and skeletal tissue. This gram-negative rod is a member of the HACEK group of slightly fastidious, slow-growing organisms. Children under 2 years of age with a recent history of an upper respiratory tract infection are especially prone to septic arthritis and osteomyelitis with *K. kingae.*

> **REAL WORLD TIP**
>
> *Kingella kingae* is a fastidious gram-negative rod that grows slowly on sheep blood and chocolate agars but not on MacConkey agar. Because of its slow growth and fastidious nature, it is best isolated from the synovial fluid when incubated in blood culture broth bottles.

Skeletal tuberculosis is usually the result of hematogenous spread of *Mycobacterium tuberculosis* early in the course of a primary infection. The infection leads to the development of granulation tissue, which erodes and destroys the cartilage and cancellous bone, leading eventually to bone demineralization and necrosis (Baron, 1996). Osteomyelitis of the vertebrae of the spine is one of the most common forms of skeletal infection in individuals with tuberculosis.

> ## Checkpoint! 39–2
> ## (Chapter Objective 2)
>
> *The most common bacterial organism causing osteomyelitis in infants and children is a(n)*
>
> A. *oxidase-negative gram-negative rod.*
> B. *catalase-negative, CAMP-positive gram-positive cocci.*
> C. *catalase-positive, coagulase-positive gram-positive cocci.*
> D. *oxidase-positive gram-negative rod.*

Fungi

Bone infections because of fungi are extremely rare. When they do occur, they may be caused by a variety of fungal organisms, including *Coccidioides, Blastomyces,* and *Cryptococcus* species and moulds. The bone lesions produced are usually slow growing without the expected warmth, pain, or inflammation. Joint space extension may occur in coccidioidomycosis and blastomycosis (Baron, 1996).

Coccidioides immitis is a fungus that is endemic in the southwest United States. The infection usually begins as a respiratory disease and then spreads via the blood. Blastomycosis, caused by *Blastomyces dermatitidis,* is characterized by suppurative (pus forming) granulomatous (consisting of inflammatory cells) lesions, especially of the skin, lungs, and bone. This fungus usually enters the organism through the respiratory tract and may be disseminated throughout the body.

Cryptococcus neoformans represents another fungal pathogen that affects internal organs. The organism enters by way of the respiratory tract resulting in sinusitis and nasopharyngeal and pulmonary granulomas. Extension of the lesion from the respiratory system to the skeletal system is common. Other fungi that can cause osteomyelitis include *Candida* spp. and *Aspergillus* spp. Infection is usually spread through the blood in patients receiving antibiotics and immunosuppressive agents. Intravenous drug users are also prone to these two organisms.

Parasites

Hydatid cyst disease is caused by infestation with a dog tapeworm, *Echinococcus granulosus.* The dog is the definitive host, and a sheep is the intermediate host. If humans accidently ingest the eggs in food or water, they become the intermediate host in the life cycle of the organism. The cysts form in the bone and internal organs. The most common sites in the bone include the ilium of the pelvis, vertebrae, and occasionally long bones such as the femur and tibia. The only treatment is surgical removal of the cysts under very careful precautions to prevent spilling of the contents into the tissues. If the cyst ruptures, it can seed all exposed areas with tapeworm larvae.

It is important to remember that parasites are very rare causes of osteomyelitis. Others that have been associated with bone lesions include *Taenia solium, Toxoplasma gondii,* and *Trichinella spiralis.* Any parasite that has access to the blood has the potential to reach the bones and cause osteomyelitis.

Viruses

Viruses are rarely, if ever, etiologic agents of osteomyelitis. The viruses that cause chickenpox and smallpox have been found to cause osteomyelitis. Chickenpox, caused by varicella-zoster virus, is a common communicable childhood disease. It is characterized by skin lesions. In immunocompromised adults, the disease may be more severe, with a prolonged recovery rate and greater chance for more complications, such as osteomyelitis. Similarly, smallpox, though now eradicated, is capable of producing skin lesions that can progress to osteomyelitis and is often fatal.

JOINTS

The joints are prone to disease such as **osteoarthritis**, which is a chronic or acute inflammation with pain and potential permanent damage. Degenerative joint disease is the most common form seen. Rheumatoid arthritis is a damaging inflammatory disease because of an autoimmune response where the body's immune system turns on itself. It can lead to destruction of the joint. Infectious or suppurative or septic arthritis is caused by microorganisms that reach the joint either through the blood, the most common route, or spread from a contiguous site, such as osteomyelitis in an adjoining bone or direct inoculation with trauma or surgery.

Any joint is susceptible to infection with almost any microorganism. Previously damaged joints, such as those seen with rheumatoid arthritis, as well as individuals with underlying conditions, such as diabetes, are more susceptible to infection. Those with artificial joints are also prone to infection both during and after surgery. Septic arthritis is seen more commonly in children and those over 65 years old. The lower extremity joints, such as the knee and hip, are most often affected, followed by the shoulder, elbow, and wrist. Bacterial arthritis often has a much more rapid onset when compared to osteomyelitis.

Once an organism finds its way into the joint, it adheres and grows to cause damage to the synovial membrane and eventually damage to the bone's articular cartilage as well. White blood cells enter the fluid to fight the infection. The inflammatory process caused by the white blood cells and bacterial toxins and enzymes can create further damage. The more virulent the organism, the more damage produced. With damage and inflammation, the blood supply becomes compromised, and fluid builds to create pressure and swelling. An infected joint is usually painful, hot, and swollen.

Bacteria

Septic arthritis is designated as either gonococcal or nongonococcal. Gonococcal arthritis is caused by *Neisseria gonorrhoeae*, whereas nongonococcal is used to describe infectious arthritis caused by all other organisms. *Staphylococcus aureus* is the most common cause of nongonococcal septic arthritis. It is usually spread through the bloodstream and is most often present in only one joint, usually the knee. *Streptococcus* spp., including viridans *Streptococcus*, *S. pneumoniae*, and *S. agalactiae* are the next most common. Infections because of aerobic gram-negative rods can occur about as frequently as *Streptococcus* spp.

The infectious agent present in nongonococcal septic arthritis usually depends on the age and immune status of the individual and the presence of underlying conditions. *Pseudomonas aeruginosa* can be seen in intravenous drug users who use any water available to mix drugs prior to injection. Organisms associated with osteomyelitis are often the same ones responsible for nongonococcal septic arthritis because of the proximity of the joint to the bone. Table 39-3 ✪ lists the common organisms associated with septic arthritis based on the age of the patient or preexisting conditions.

Gonococcal arthritis is caused by *Neisseria gonorrhoeae* and usually results from disseminated gonorrhea infection (DGI) after colonization of the mucous membranes of the urogenital, gastrointestinal, or upper respiratory systems. It is most often seen in sexually active young adults. Females are more prone to DGI because they can harbor asymptomatic infections, which delay treatment and lead to seeding of the bloodstream. Individuals with specific complement deficiencies can be prone to systemic infection with *Neisseria gonorrhoeae*.

With DGI, an individual may exhibit a skin rash and a few purulent lesions on the extremities. The organism can infect multiple joints or settle in a single joint. The joints usually affected include the knees, elbows, wrists, ankles, fingers, and toes. The infective arthritis can travel from joint to joint and affect only one of two symmetrical joints, such as the knee.

✪ TABLE 39-3

Common Organisms Associated with Septic Arthritis

Age/Preexisting Condition	Associated Organism(s)
Neonates and children	*Staphylococcus aureus*
	Streptococcus spp.
	S. agalactiae (group B *Streptococcus*)
	S. pyogenes (group A *Streptococcus*)
	Enterobacteriaceae
	Haemophilus influenzae type b
	Kingella kingae
Adults	*Staphylococcus aureus*
	Streptococcus spp.
	Enterobacteriaceae
Sexually active	*Neisseria gonorrhoeae*
Artificial joint	*Staphylococcus aureus*
	Staphylococcus not *S. aureus*
	Propionibacterium spp.
Intravenous drug use	*Staphylococcus aureus*
	Pseudomonas aeruginosa
	Eikenella corrodens
Animal bite	*Pasteurella multocida*
Human bite or fistfight	*Eikenella corrodens*

Eventually it settles in one joint. An individual with gonococcal arthritis often complains of fever, lethargy, and hot, swollen joints with limited movement. Figure 39-4 ■ presents an individual with gonococcal arthritis of the hand.

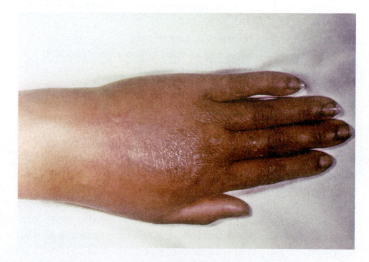

■ **FIGURE 39-4** This photograph reveals the swollen hand and wrist of an individual with gonococcal arthritis caused by *Neisseria gonorrhoeae.* The organism has the ability to disseminate throughout the body from an infection originating in the genital tract, mouth, or rectum.
Public Health Image Library, CDC and Susan Lindsley, VD.

REAL WORLD TIP

A chocolate agar must always be included when performing a joint fluid culture. The chocolate agar is necessary for the growth of *Neisseria gonorrhoeae*, which is a potential causative agent of septic arthritis, as well as other fastidious organisms.

Prosthetic or artificial joints are prone to infection with *Staphylococcus aureus*, *Staphylococcus* not *S. aureus* (SNA), and other skin organisms such as *Propionibacterium* spp. and *Corynebacterium* spp. These organisms are usually present at the time of implantation and cause infection within a few days and to up to 3 months after the procedure. Infections that occur more than 3 months after the procedure are usually because of organisms that gain access through the bloodstream. These include *Staphylococcus aureus*, *Streptococcus* spp., the *Enterobacteriaceae*, and anaerobes. The cement used to hold the prosthesis to the bone appears to inhibit phagocytosis and the immune process, which enhances an organism's ability to adhere and cause infection (Brause, 2005). *Staphylococcus* spp. is especially adapted to eluding the immune process because of the formation of biofilms on the artificial surface.

> ### ✓ Checkpoint! 39–3 (Chapter Objective 7)
>
> *A 22-year-old female presents to the emergency room with a hot, painful, swollen right elbow and no visible signs of injury. The physician suspects septic arthritis. Which of the following patient history questions may reveal valuable information that could lead to the potential pathogen?*
>
> *A. Have you been bitten by a cat recently?*
> *B. Have you had joint replacement surgery in the recent past?*
> *C. Have you been in a fistfight recently?*
> *D. Are you sexually active?*

Fungi

Immunosuppression often makes an individual prone to fungal infection. The same fungi that cause osteomyelitis also cause septic arthritis. The onset of fungal septic arthritis is usually more chronic versus bacteria's rapid presentation. *Candida* spp., *Cryptococcus* spp., and *Aspergillus* spp. are the most common pathogens. *Candida albicans* is most often associated with hospitalized patients, immunosuppression, and intravenous drug users and infects both natural and artificial joints. *Cryptococcus neoformans* is associated with severe immunosuppression, such as seen with AIDS.

Healthy individuals can develop fungal septic arthritis. Those who live in areas endemic with the dimorphic fungi, *Coccidioides immitis*, *Blastomyces dermatitidis*, and *Paracoccidioides brasiliensis* can develop infection after inhalation of their spores. Infection with *Aspergillus* spp. tends to occur because of penetrating injuries and contaminated compound (open) fractures.

Parasites

Arthritis because of parasites is rare. The inflammation present may be because of an immune response to the presence of organisms in the body rather than a true infection. The immune system reacts to the parasite and causes an inflammatory response in the joint. Parasites associated with arthritis include *Toxoplasmosis gondii*, *Entamoeba histolytica*, the filariae, and helminths, as well as *Giardia lamblia*.

Viruses

Viral arthritis is an acute or subacute process that may be because of the body's immune response rather than direct infection of the joint with a virus. Individuals present with fever and mild to moderate pain in multiple joints, especially the hands. Viruses reach the joint spaces during viremia. Most cases of viral arthritis are self-limiting with spontaneous resolution and little damage to the joint.

The most common virus associated with arthritis is the human parvovirus B19. It is the causative agent of "fifth" disease in children who have flulike symptoms and a rash. Other viruses associated with infective arthritis include herpes simplex, varicella zoster, Epstein-Barr, cytomegalovirus, hepatitis B and C, and human immunodeficiency virus (HIV). Infective arthritis because of rubella can occur because of infection or be vaccine related.

REACTIVE ARTHRITIS

Reactive arthritis is a self-limited, sterile arthritis because of an inflammatory reaction to an infection somewhere else in the body. It often appears 2 weeks to 2 months after the initial infection. It is commonly observed in individuals who possess the major histocompatibility complex antigen HLA-B27, but its significance in the disease process is unknown (Shirtliff & Mader, 2002). The organism's antigens probably trigger an autoimmune response in the joint. Organisms associated with reactive arthritis include the enteric pathogens, *Campylobacter* spp., *Salmonella* spp., *Shigella* spp., and *Yersinia* spp., as well as the sexually transmitted pathogens *Chlamydia trachomatis* and *Neisseria gonorrhoeae*. It can also occur as a poststreptococcal sequelae after an upper respiratory tract infection with *Streptococcus pyogenes*.

Borrelia burgdorferi, a spirochete, causes tick-borne Lyme disease. Chronic inflammation of the joints is one of the clinical features of the disease. A few weeks after infection, the organisms are present in the joints. After a few months without treatment, the organisms are no longer present in the joints, but a reactive arthritis is usually present in the knees.

Checkpoint! 39–4 (Chapter Objective 3)

The specimen of choice for detection of organisms causing reactive arthritis is

    A. *synovial joint fluid.*
    B. *bone biopsy.*
    C. *there is no specimen of choice.*
    D. *stool.*

BONE MARROW

The bone marrow is responsible for production of red and white blood cells as well as platelets. It is one of the primary organs of the reticuloendothelial system (RES). The RES also includes the lymph nodes, liver, and spleen. It becomes infected when organisms are able to survive the killing action of macrophages after ingestion. These intracellular organisms are able to travel to other tissues, including the bone marrow, protected within the macrophage. Once in the bone marrow, the organisms can flourish and create anemia and leukopenia. The infected cells take up valuable space, so there is less room to create new red and white blood cells.

Often the bone marrow is cultured when a patient presents with a fever of unknown origin (FUO) because the organism may be hiding in the reticuloendothelial system. One organism that often presents with FUO is *Brucella* spp. This gram-negative coccobacillus invades the macrophages, enters the RES, and lives hidden from the body's immune system. As it outgrows its macrophage home, it is released, and the body reacts with fever. Once it moves into another macrophage, the fever resolves. This explains why the disease *Brucella* spp. causes what is called undulant fever. The fever comes and goes, or undulates. Bone marrow and blood are valuable specimens for diagnosis of brucellosis.

Other organisms that can be found in the bone marrow include the bacteria: *Borrelia recurrentis, Ehrlichia* spp., *Legionella* spp., *Francisella tularensis, Salmonella typhi, Mycobacterium tuberculosis,* and *M. avium-intracellulare.* The fungi *Histoplasma* spp. and *Cryptococcus* spp. are also prone to infection of the bone marrow, especially in immunocompromised individuals. The human immunodeficiency virus and hepatitis viruses are well known for their ability to infiltrate the bone marrow. Parasites such as *Leishmania* spp., *Trypanosoma cruzi,* and *Plasmodium* spp. can also infect the bone marrow. Figure 39-5 ■ demonstrates the amastigote form of *Leishmania donovani* inside a macrophage in the bone marrow.

▶ SPECIMEN COLLECTION

The diagnosis of osteomyelitis is usually made by a bone scan, blood cultures, bone biopsy, histologic studies, and culture. The bone scan can reveal the lesions present in the bone

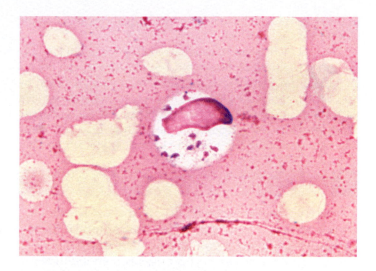

■ **FIGURE 39-5** This stained smear of bone marrow reveals the small amastigote forms of *Leishmania donovani* living within the cytoplasm of a macrophage.
Public Health Image Library, CDC and Dr. L.L. Moore, Jr.

because of the damage caused by the organism and activated osteoclasts. Either an aspiration of the painful area or a piece of the bone is collected via needle biopsy and sent to the laboratory for examination and culture. The bone biopsy is considered the gold standard for the diagnosis of osteomyelitis. The patient may require surgical intervention, depending on the extent of damage to the bone. The bone biopsy should be collected in a clean, sterile container. A small amount of sterile nonbacteriostatic saline may be added to prevent drying. If a delay in transport or processing is anticipated, the specimen should be kept at 4°C. Although formaldehyde is often used to preserve specimens for the histology laboratory, it cannot be used for specimens for microbiology culture. Any organisms present are killed by the presence of this preserving agent.

Joint fluid is usually collected via needle aspiration. The fluid is sent in a sterile tube as soon as possible because of the potential for the presence of the fastidious organism *Neisseria gonorrhoeae.* There is the potential for clotting of the fluid without an organism friendly anticoagulant such as sodium polyanetholsulfonate (SPS). The issue with using an anticoagulant is that some strains of *Neisseria* spp. can be inhibited by SPS. On the other hand, if an anticoagulant is not used for transportation, the fluid can clot, and organisms will be caught

 REAL WORLD TIP

Neisseria gonorrhoeae, Neisseria meningitidis, Streptobacillus moniliformis, and *Peptostreptococcus anaerobius* may be inhibited by SPS present in blood culture bottles. If the body fluid and blood culture broth are in appropriate proportions, then the inhibitory effect is diluted, and the organisms should grow.

in the clot. This can be remedied by manually breaking up the clot on receipt in the lab.

The best method for transportation of synovial fluid is inoculation into blood culture broth bottles. Ideally, the bottles should be inoculated with the same volumes as required by the bottle manufacturer. Because most septic joints are swollen with fluid, this should not be a problem. The blood culture broth provides the nutrients for fastidious organisms while preventing the fluid from clotting because of the SPS present.

 REAL WORLD TIP

A capped needle and syringe of fluid should never be transported to the laboratory. The potential for a needlestick is too great. The hospital's and laboratory's safety policies and procedures should never allow this practice.

Bone marrow aspiration is sometimes required to determine the etiology of an infection. The back of the iliac crest of the pelvis is usually used to perform this method, but the sternum may be used in some cases. The specimen is aspirated using a needle and syringe. Bone marrow is usually not processed for culture, as blood cultures can serve the same purpose clinically (Forbes et al., 2002). If a bone marrow culture is necessary to confirm a diagnosis, it can be collected in blood culture broth bottles.

 REAL WORLD TIP

Bone marrow culture is more sensitive then blood cultures for the isolation of *Brucella* spp. because of the increased concentration of organisms present in the reticuloendothelial system (Al-Nassir, 2006).

Diagnosis of infections related to prosthetic joints usually requires tissue samples from the area around the device. The tissue should be transported anaerobically and ground on receipt in the laboratory.

✓ **Checkpoint! 39–5 (Chapter Objective 4)**

Which of the following statements regarding bone or bone marrow specimens is not true?

A. *A bone biopsy is collected in a sterile container with a small amount of nonbacteriostatic saline.*

B. *Bone marrow is not usually processed for culture, as blood culture can serve the same purpose clinically.*

C. *If a delay in transport or processing is anticipated, the specimen should be kept at 4°C.*

D. *Formaldehyde is an acceptable preservative in specimens submitted for microbiological cultures.*

▶ SPECIMEN PROCESSING

The diagnosis of osteomyelitis rests on isolation of the agent from the bone or blood. Blood cultures are positive in up to one-half of children with acute osteomyelitis (Carek et al., 2001). In bacterial hematogenous osteomyelitis, positive blood cultures often avoid the need for a bone biopsy when there is radiographic evidence of lesions characteristic for osteomyelitis (Maguire, 1997). In chronic osteomyelitis, sinus tract cultures are not reliable for predicting which organism will be isolated from the infected bone. Often the sinus tract is contaminated with normal skin organisms as well as other colonizing microorganisms. In most instances, bone biopsy cultures are mandatory to guide specific antimicrobial therapy.

 REAL WORLD TIP

A swab of a sinus tract cannot reveal the causative agent of osteomyelitis. The sinus tract is usually contaminated with many colonizing organisms, making it nearly impossible to determine the true potential pathogen. A sinus tract swab is an unacceptable specimen and, if processed, provides inaccurate results. The laboratory, not the physician, is responsible if an unacceptable specimen is processed and those results are then used to treat the patient (Harty-Golder, 2004).

Bone biopsies and bone marrow are first homogenized (ground) to allow better recovery of organisms. This can be done either using a motorized tissue homogenizer or manually. A sterile scalpel can be used to chop or shave the bone into small pieces. Infected bones are usually soft and necrotic, making manual grinding the preferred method. A liquid joint fluid culture requires centrifugation and concentration. A minimum of 3 mL is required. If the fluid is clotted, it must be manually homogenized.

At least two slides are prepared: one for Gram stain and one for calcofluor white stain. Because of the presence of background material, calcofluor white will make organisms present visible under ultraviolet light. Joint fluid should be cytocentrifuged for Gram stain to concentrate the organisms. A cytocentrifuged Gram stain slide has an increased sensitivity of 100-fold for the detection of organisms compared to dropping the fluid on a slide.

 REAL WORLD TIP

Read a Gram stained smear of joint fluid carefully. The mucin present in the fluid is responsible for its thick consistency. It can precipitate out on the stained smear and make reading it more difficult. Ensure the entire slide is reviewed thoroughly.

Bones are very difficult to break. Always look for necrotic tissue, as it should be easier to scrape small shavings from it.

Bone marrow aspirates can be examined for parasites. The specimen should be collected in EDTA to prevent clotting. Thick and thin smears are made, stained with a Giemsa stain, and examined.

Once a bone biopsy is collected and processed, the appropriate media is inoculated as described in Table 39-4. Media for the recovering of anaerobes should always be included with bone and joint fluid cultures. Joint fluid and bone marrow culture should use the same media as a bone biopsy culture. The only exception for incubation of media is if *Brucella* spp. is suspected in the bone marrow. Cultures for *Brucella* spp. are held a minimum of 21 days because of the slow-growing nature of the organism. Special media should be considered when fastidious organisms or fungi are suspected.

Tissue for culture and histology is usually required for the diagnosis of skeletal tuberculosis. Cultures for *Mycobacterium tuberculosis* are positive in approximately 60% of the cases, but 6 weeks may be required for growth and identification of the organism (Baron, 1996). Histology showing granulomatous tissue compatible with tuberculosis and a positive tuberculin skin test are usually sufficient to begin tuberculosis therapy.

 Checkpoint! 39–6 (Chapter Objective 5)

Bone biopsies for culture should be processed by
A. bleaching.
B. centrifugation.
C. homogenization.
D. preservation in formaldehyde.

TABLE 39-4

Media and Incubation Conditions of Bone Cultures

Media	Incubation Conditions
Blood agar (BAP)	CO_2, 35°C × 48 hours
MacConkey agar (MAC)	O_2, 35°C × 48 hours
Chocolate agar (CHOC)	CO_2, 35°C × 48 hours
Anaerobic blood agar (ANA BAP)	AnO_2, 35°C × 5 days
Kanamycin/vancomycin laked blood agar (KVLB)	AnO_2, 35°C × 5 days
Fastidious anaerobic broth (ATHIO)	O_2, 35°C × 5 days

SPECIAL MEDIA

Routinely, bone, joint fluid, and bone marrow specimens are cultured on sheep blood agar plate (BAP), chocolate agar (CHOC), MacConkey (MAC), anaerobic thioglycolate broth (ATHIO), and anaerobic blood agar (ANA BAP). Examination for fungal and mycobacterial organisms is also performed on request.

Brucella spp. can grow on BAP, CHOC, modified Thayer Martin, and buffered charcoal yeast extract (BCYE). These culture plates should be held for at least 21 days in humidified CO_2. Traditional broth cultures for *Brucella* spp. should be incubated for up to 30 days, and the broth subculture plates should be held for at least 21 days in humidified CO_2.

REAL WORLD TIP

Continuous monitoring automated blood culture systems are very good at the recovery of *Brucella* spp. from blood and bone marrow. The organism is usually recovered within the 5-day incubation period suggested for most instruments. The incubation time can be extended to up to 30 days if the bottles are negative at 5 days.

Before automated blood culture systems, a traditional biphasic blood culture bottle, the Castañeda bottle, was used for recovery of *Brucella* spp. from blood or bone marrow. The biphasic bottle contains both liquid broth and solid culture medium. Every day the inoculated bottle is tilted to run the broth over the solid medium, which is attached up the side of the bottle. The bottle is held a minimum of 21 days to recover the slow-growing organism.

For fungal cultures, no single medium is ideal for recovery of all fungi. For fastidious dimorphic fungi, brain heart infusion (BHI) with 5% sheep blood agar should be used (Murray, Baron, Jorgensen, Pfaller, & Yolken, 2003). Routine fungal agar plates should be incubated at 30°C for up to 4 weeks. Cultures for the dimorphic fungi, *Histoplasma, Blastomyces,* and *Paracoccidioides,* should be incubated at 25°C as well as 35°C for up to 8 weeks. Media containing antimicrobial agents such as gentamicin can be used if contamination with microbial flora is expected. In addition, media containing substrates such as L-dopa can be used for the isolation of *Cryptococcus neoformans* (Murray et al., 2003). Extreme care must be exercised with specimens expected to contain *Coccidioides immitis.*

Shell vial culture is a technique used to enhance viral infectivity and to improve the chances of isolating the pathogenic virus. It takes advantage of using a living cell system and enhances viral recovery by centrifuging the clinical sample onto a monolayer. In this technique a small vial with a removable round glass coverslip is used to grow the cells as a monolayer on the coverslip (Wagner & Hewlett, 2004). Molecular testing such as polymerase chain reaction (PCR) has now proven to be a valuable procedure because of the difficulty of isolation of some viruses.

CULTIVATION

Aerobic culture plates are examined after 24 and 48 hours incubation and the anaerobic plates after 48 hours incubation. The ATHIO is examined daily for evidence of growth. If no growth is observed on the culture plates but there is evidence of growth in ATHIO, then Gram stain and subculture the ATHIO onto BAP, MAC, CHOC, and ANA-BAP. After 48 hours incubation, the ATHIO is kept for a total of 5 days before discarding. All isolates are to be identified as appropriate, and susceptibility testing is performed if medically indicated.

For *Mycobacterium* species, testing includes culture and acid-fast stain. A minimum of 3 to 10 mL of synovial fluid is needed for processing. If a mycobacterial species is isolated, the organism will be identified. Susceptibility testing will be performed depending on the isolate identification.

Checkpoint! 39–7 (Chapter Objective 6)

Which of the following media combinations is acceptable for a routine bone biopsy culture?
    A. *BAP, CHOC, MAC, ATHIO, and ANA BAP*
    B. *MAC, EMB, and HE*
    C. *BAP and MAC*
    D. *ANA BAP, KVLB, and ATHIO*

▶ OTHER LABORATORY TESTING

Additional laboratory testing may assist with the diagnosis of osteomyelitis. The white blood cell count can be elevated as well as the erythrocyte sedimentation rate (ESR). Another test result that may be useful is an elevated C-reactive protein (CRP). Both the ESR and CRP are nonspecific tests for inflammation that do not indicate a specific disease, only that an infection is possibly present in the body.

Individuals with septic arthritis can present with an elevated white count but only about half the time. The ESR as well as the CRP can also be elevated. Additional testing is usually requested on joint fluid to differentiate infection from other forms of noninfectious arthritis. A white cell count of the fluid indicates septic arthritis if it has more than 50,000 cells/μL with 75% or more neutrophils. A synovial fluid with over 50,000 cells/μL will appear turbid. The fluid is usually also examined for the presence of crystals such as uric acid to differentiate gout.

Culture of the throat, rectum, and genital tract may be done to determine the source of *Neisseria gonorrhoeae* in cases of gonococcal arthritis. Culture for the presence of *Borrelia*

burgdorferi in joint fluid is too difficult for most microbiology laboratories. Serology may help with the diagnosis, but PCR testing has shown to be the most promising.

▶ TREATMENT

Cases of osteomyelitis require antibiotic therapy and may necessitate surgical debridement, depending on the clinical response to antimicrobial therapy. A minimum of 3 to 6 weeks of intravenous antibiotic therapy is usually needed. Dead bone must be removed, and bone grafts may be necessary, depending on the extent of bone tissue removed. Amputation is used only as a last resort.

Septic arthritis requires aspiration of the infected joint and antimicrobial therapy. The joint may require multiple aspirations. Surgical drainage may be necessary if the infection is not responding to therapy. The downside of surgery is the potential for scar tissue formation and subsequent loss of mobility of the joint.

Infection of prosthetic devices may require removal and replacement of the device and debridement of the site. Six weeks of intravenous antimicrobial therapy is recommended. To prevent infection at surgery, antibiotics can be incorporated into the cement used to hold the joint in place. Infection of the bone marrow requires a minimum of 6 weeks of antimicrobial therapy to ensure all the intracellular organisms have been eliminated and to prevent relapse.

SUMMARY

Osteomyelitis can be a serious, life-threatening infection that is usually hematogenous in origin. *Staphylococcus aureus* accounts for most cases of osteomyelitis across all ages. Some disease states can predispose an individual to osteomyelitis. These include diabetes mellitus, sickle cell anemia, intravenous drug use, and immunosuppression. Bone biopsy remains the gold standard for confirmation of osteomyelitis. Inflammatory markers may help indicate whether or not there is an infection. The erythrocyte sedimentation rate (ESR) and the C-reactive protein (CRP) are two markers for inflammation. They are elevated in 80 to 90% of patients with osteomyelitis.

Septic arthritis is usually the result of microorganisms reaching the joint space through the blood. It is caused by two main classes of organisms: gonococcal, caused by *Neisseria gonorrhoeae*, and nongonococcal, which is usually caused by *Staphylococcus aureus*. *Staphylococcus aureus* is known for the significant damage caused in the joint space. The presence of prosthetic devices used for orthopedic surgery is also a risk factor, with *Staphylococcus aureus* and *Staphylococcus* not *S. aureus* as the two most common causative agents. Reactive arthritis is an immune response that attacks the joints after infection with some enteric pathogens. Most cases of septic arthritis occur in the knee. Culture of the synovial fluid provides the physician with valuable information for therapy.

Bone marrow is part of the reticuloendothelial system and is prone to microorganisms that infect this body system. *Brucella* spp. is known for its ability to hide in macrophages and infiltrate the bone marrow. Given the sensitivity of continuous monitoring automated blood culture systems, bone marrow should be collected and incubated in blood culture broth bottles.

LEARNING OPPORTUNITIES

1. Which of the following individuals is at greatest risk for osteomyelitis because of *Staphylococcus* not *S. aureus?* (Chapter Objective 2)

    a. A 3-month-old male with sickle cell anemia

    b. A 78-year-old female hospitalized after hip replacement

    c. A 27-year-old male with an untreated sexually transmitted disease

    d. A 58-year-old female with diabetes

2. A 48-year-old homeless male with AIDS presents with back pain. Bone scans reveal lesions on his vertebrae. The Ziehl-Neelsen stain of a vertebral bone biopsy is shown in the photo. Select the most likely causative agent of osteomyelitis in this case. (Chapter Objectives 2 and 7)

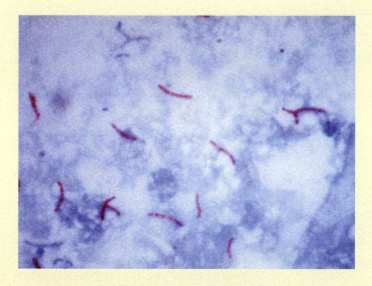

Public Health Image Library, CDC and Dr. George P. Kubica

    a. *Pseudomonas aeruginosa*

    b. *Candida albicans*

    c. *Pasteurella multocida*

    d. *Mycobacterium tuberculosis*

3. A resident asks for information on the collection and transportation of a bone marrow aspiration for *Brucella* spp. culture. You advise her to (Chapter Objective 4)

    a. draw blood cultures instead of submitting bone marrow

    b. place the bone marrow into an EDTA tube

    c. place the bone marrow into a blood culture bottle

    d. wait until the patient experiences a fever and then take the marrow sample

4. A synovial fluid is received in microbiology. The technologist notes that it is clotted on receipt. How should the specimen be processed for culture?
(Chapter Objective 5)

   a. Homogenize the specimen by manually breaking up the clot.

   b. Place the clot in a blood culture bottle.

   c. Place the clot into an EDTA tube to lyse it.

   d. Reject the specimen, and request a recollect.

5. The microbiology department receives a tube with only a few drops of synovial fluid. The technologist is able to perform a cytocentrifuged Gram stain, but only has enough fluid left to set up one bacterial culture medium. Select the most appropriate single medium for inoculation. (Chapter Objective 6)

   a. Sheep blood agar

   b. Chocolate agar

   c. Reducible blood agar

   d. MacConkey agar

6. A 57-year-old male presents with multiple draining abscesses on his jaw line. He had periodontal surgery 2 weeks earlier. His physician suspects he has osteomyelitis of the jaw. A bone biopsy and blood cultures all reveal the same gram-negative coccobacillus. At 24 hours, the colony appears to eat into the sheep blood agar and does not grow on MacConkey. The organism is oxidase positive and catalase negative with a distinctive bleachlike odor when the sheep blood agar plate is first opened. Based on these results, the most likely potential pathogen is (Chapter Objectives 2 and 7)

   a. *Haemophilus influenzae*

   b. *Aggregatibacter (Actinobacillus) actinomycetemcomitans*

   c. *Kingella kingae*

   d. *Eikenella corrodens*

CASE STUDY 39-1   THE PURPLE PATHOGEN STRIKES AGAIN (CHAPTER OBJECTIVES 2, 4, 5, 6, AND 7)

Patient: John W., a 64-year-old male, is in general good health but with a bad left knee.

Background: He is admitted to the hospital for a total knee replacement surgery. After few days, John returns to his surgeon complaining of fever, chills, redness and swelling, and pain in his left leg. The surgeon, in consultation with the primary care physician, decides to collect a bone biopsy. The specimen is sent to the laboratory. The microbiology laboratory receives the specimen in a dry, sterile container. Another specimen is sent to the anatomical laboratory for histologic studies. A Gram stain is performed, and many white blood cells and gram-positive cocci in clusters are observed under the microscope. The specimen is inoculated on BAP, MAC, and ATHIO.

Fungal and mycobacterial cultures are also inoculated. After 24 hours, growth is seen on BAP and in the ATHIO.

1. What is the most likely identification of the isolated organism? (Chapter Objective 7)

2. What additional tests should be done on the isolated organism to confirm its identity? (Chapter Objective 7)

3. What is the source of infection? (Chapter Objective 2)

4. Was the specimen transported to the microbiology laboratory properly? Explain. (Chapter Objective 4)

5. Was the specimen processed properly in the microbiology laboratory? Explain. (Chapter Objectives 5 and 6)

CASE STUDY 39-2   THAT DARN CAT (CHAPTER OBJECTIVES 1, 2, AND 7)

Patient: A 59-year-old female, with a history of rheumatoid arthritis.

Background: She is bitten on her right hand by her cat while feeding it at 5 p.m. She washes the wound with soap and water and applies an antiseptic cream. During the night she develops a fever, and her hand becomes swollen and hot with draining pus. She sees her physician the next day. He aspirates a sample and places her on antibiotics. The sample submitted grows a gram-negative coccobacillus on sheep blood and chocolate agars but not on MacConkey agar. Five days later, she returns to her physician with a fever and a swollen, red, hot left knee. A synovial fluid sample, aspirated by the physician, reveals 100,000 white blood cells/µL with 95% neutrophils. A culture of the fluid grows a gram-negative coccobacillus on sheep blood and chocolate agars with no growth on MacConkey agar. It appears to be the same organism as previously isolated from her hand wound.

1. What is the most likely pathogen isolated from her hand wound and knee synovial fluid? (Chapter Objectives 2 and 7)

2. What biochemical testing will presumptively identify this organism? (Chapter Objective 7)

3. What complication occurred as a result of her initial infection? (Chapter Objective 2)

4. How did the organism from her initial infection come to infect her knee? (Chapter Objectives 1 and 2)

5. Explain how her history of rheumatoid arthritis contributed to her knee infection. (Chapter Objective 2)

PEARSON
myhealthprofessionskit™

Use this address to access the interactive Companion Website created for this textbook. Simply select "Clinical Laboratory Science" from the choice of disciplines. Find this book and log in using your user name and password.

REFERENCES

Go to myhealthprofessionskit.com to view this chapter's references.

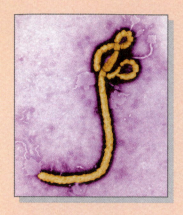

40

Opportunistic Infections

Teresa A. Taff

■ LEARNING OBJECTIVES

Upon completion of this chapter, the learner should be able to:

1. Explain the role of normal flora, mucous membranes, and other mechanisms in preventing infections.
2. Differentiate the components and their primary functions in the innate and adaptive immune systems.
   a. Visually recognize white blood cells, on a peripheral blood smear, associated with each immune system.
3. Discuss the clinical picture of defects to the innate and adaptive immune system.
   a. Visually recognize white blood cells defects, on a peripheral blood smear, associated with deficiencies in each immune system.
4. Discuss the potential causes and clinical picture of secondary immunodeficiencies.
5. Correlate patient history, clinical presentation, laboratory results, and infections and organisms present to deduce the potential immune deficiency and associated disease or syndrome.
6. Summarize potential treatments and supportive therapies for the immunodeficiencies discussed.

KEY TERMS

agammaglobulinemia	chemotaxis	immunodeficiency
albinism	complement	innate
antibody	cytokine	lysozymes
antigen	endogenous	opportunistic
asplenic	exogenous	opsonin
bacteriocins	granuloma	phagocytosis
buffy coat		

► INTRODUCTION

The human immune system is an amazingly effective yet still fragile network. Microorganisms can invade to cause infection when the immune system is altered because of inherited or spontaneous mutations in one or more of its components. Errors in the immune system can also be acquired through **exogenous** (outside the human body) sources. Defects can occur when a microorganism, malignancy, or drug attacks the immune system directly and renders it ineffective. An altered or defective immune system results in **immunodeficiency** (a reduced or absent immune response).

Once the immune system is weakened or breached, any microorganism, even those considered to be "normal flora," can cause infections. Organisms that cause infections in an individual with a weakened immune system but not in those with an intact immune system are called **opportunistic.** Immunocompromised individuals are often prone to frequent and lengthy infections with unusual microorganisms that do not typically cause infections in a person with an intact immune system. The chief complaint of an immunocompromised individual is often recurrent infections that do not respond to traditional treatment. The physician faces the daunting task of ensuring that the appropriate laboratory tests are used to identify and treat an individual with an immune deficiency. Visit the appropriate chapters in this textbook to review the characteristics and laboratory tests used to identify the microorganisms discussed in this chapter.

► INFECTIONS RELATED TO DEFECTIVE PHYSICAL BARRIERS OF THE IMMUNE SYSTEM

The human body has many physical barriers in place that act as the first line of defense against infection by microorganisms.

NORMAL FLORA

Normal flora plays a critical role in preventing potential pathogens from gaining a foothold in the human body and causing infection. They can number in the trillions (10^{12}), depending on the body site. They fill every crevice of each mucous membrane they inhabit. Normal organisms compete for the nutrients present so there are none left for the invading organisms. The potential pathogens cannot thrive when there is no room or food available. The production of natural **bacteriocins** (antibiotics) by normal organisms are toxic to the potential pathogens (Dieffenbach & Tramont, 2005).

Normal organisms prepare the immune system so that it is always at the ready for the potential invasion of pathogens. They stimulate it just enough so they are not harmed but potential pathogens would be immediately recognized as foreign. The **antibodies** (protective blood proteins produced when the body is exposed to foreign material) created because of the low-level stimulation of normal organisms may have the ability to cross react with potential pathogens. This ensures that the immune system is always on high alert status. Once a potential pathogen invades, the immune response is rapid. Examples of cross-reactive antibodies are those produced because of the presence of *Escherichia coli.* The polysaccharide capsule of some serotypes of *E. coli* acts as an **antigen** (substances that stimulate the production of antibodies) so the body produces low-level antibodies because of its presence. These natural antibodies have the ability to cross react with the polysaccharide capsule *Neisseria meningitidis.* This may prevent some serotypes of *Neisseria meningitidis* from being able to colonize the human host and therefore prevent the potential harmful effects to the central nervous system (VanAlphen, Arends, & Hopman, 1988).

Any disruption in the balance of normal flora can shift the odds in favor of potential pathogens. Broad-spectrum antibiotics can decrease the number of normal flora organisms present in the intestinal or female genital tract. The classic example of the shift from normal flora to potential pathogen is the overgrowth of intestinal *Clostridium difficile* when vancomycin is used as the antibiotic of choice for infection in another body site. Normal flora is eliminated because of the antibiotic, and the spores of *C. difficile* survive and germinate to produce toxin, which causes enterocolitis. Antibiotic use can also eliminate the normal flora of the female genital tract, allowing yeast such as *Candida albicans* to overgrow.

 Checkpoint! 40–1 (Chapter Objective 1)

Normal flora has the ability to fight invading pathogens by all of the following methods except:

    A. *production of bacteriocins (natural antibiotics).*
    B. *low-level stimulation of the immune system.*
    C. *production of antibodies.*
    D. *competition for nutrients and space.*

SKIN

The skin, the largest organ of the human body, covers about 1.5 to 2.0 square meters on the average adult (Church, Elsayed, Reid, Winston, & Lindsay, 2006). The outermost layer of skin is called the epidermis. It is made up of several layers of squamous epithelial cells that move outward to the surface as new cells are generated from below. As the cells age and move to the surface, they die, lose their nucleus, become filled with keratin, and dry out. Keratin is a water-repellant protein and is selective in the substances it allows to enter and leave the skin. The numerous layers of overlapping epithelial cells and the continuous shedding of cells provide an effective physical barrier against the entry of microorganisms.

The skin has a mildly acid pH, which is created by the breakdown of lipids into fatty acids by the countless number of normal skin microorganisms present on its surface (Dieffenbach & Tramont, 2005). The sheer number of normal skin microorganisms is also an effective shield against those causing infections. Invading organisms have trouble multiplying.

Most invading microorganisms are able to overcome the natural barrier of the skin when there is a physical break in its surface. All individuals, regardless of health status, are prone to infection when there are breaks in the skin. Trauma, even as simple as a paper cut, provides a gateway for organisms to enter the underlying vascular layers of the skin. Entry points for potential pathogens can also include bites, surgical incisions, and intravenous catheters. Any microorganism, even those considered to be normal flora such as *Staphylococcus epidermidis,* can initiate an infection once it is able to overcome the physical barrier of skin. *Staphylococcus epidermidis* is well known for its ability to leave the skin surface and enter the bloodstream via an intravenous catheter in hospitalized patients.

The most common infectious agent that takes advantage of breaks in the skin is *Staphylococcus aureus.* Its ability to produce enzymes such as hyaluronidase aid in its spread to deeper tissues once it enters the body.

There are instances of a few microorganisms that are able to penetrate intact skin. The dermatophyte fungi, such as *Epidermatophyton, Microsporum,* and *Trichophyton,* are able to digest the keratin present in the top layers of the skin. These classic agents of ringworm rarely invade beyond the epidermis layer. *Francisella tularensis, Treponema* species, and *Leptospira* species are thought to enter through intact skin, but they probably gain access through minute breaks in the skin that are not easily used by other organisms. Several parasites, such as *Strongyloides stercoralis, Hookworm* spp., and *Schistosoma* spp., are able to burrow through intact skin as part of their life cycle.

The burn patient is the classic example of a skin disruption that can lead to infection. Infection is the leading cause of death in hospitalized individuals with full-thickness burns

REAL WORLD TIP

Burn wound cultures can be qualitative or quantitative. A qualitative culture is performed using a sterile swab and determines whether organisms are present or absent. A quantitative culture requires a tissue biopsy, which is weighed prior to maceration and dilution for culture. A burn wound biopsy will indicate the number of organisms present per gram of tissue. A count of more than 10^5 organisms/gram of tissue correlates with a high mortality rate. In addition to culture, histologic analysis will determine the how deep the organisms have invaded the tissues.

(Schwarz & Dulchavsky, 2005). A full-thickness burn provides a moist environment with no blood supply, which is an ideal setting for invasion by microorganisms. Organisms, such as *Staphylococcus aureus, Enterococcus faecalis, Pseudomonas aeruginosa, Klebsiella pneumoniae, Candida albicans,* and other fungi, colonize the exposed area and eventually penetrate the tissues. Once in the tissues, the organisms reach the bloodstream to cause sepsis (the multiplication of microorganisms in the blood) and ultimately organ failure.

MUCOUS MEMBRANES

Moist mucous membranes line the oral cavity as well as the respiratory, gastrointestinal, and genitourinary tracts. The membranes secrete fluids that aid in various bodily functions. They also act as a physical barrier to invasion as well as physically move organisms out of the body as the secretions flow. The secretions contain many natural antibacterial agents such as **lysozymes** (bacteria-killing enzymes) and antibodies or immunoglobulins.

The respiratory tract has its own air filter in the form of cilia, which trap particles such as bacteria as they are breathed in through the nose. Any organisms that make it past the cilia become trapped in secretions as they land on the mucus-producing cells that line the respiratory tract. The cough reflex propels any organisms trapped in mucus out of the body. The intestinal tract uses acid as a defense mechanism against the invasion of organisms. The sheer number of normal bacteria in the intestine makes it difficult for potential pathogens, which make it past the acid test, to thrive. The urinary system also makes use of pH as a defense mechanism. Its slightly acidic pH prevents many organisms from growing in urine. The very act of urinating four to eight times per day flushes out any organisms that may have reached the bladder via the urethra. The female genital tract contains normal flora that maintain an acidic environment because of metabolic by-products. This creates a hostile environment for many invading organisms.

The mucous membranes of any individual can be overpowered by several ways. Smoking can kill the respiratory tract cilia, which then allow organisms to enter the lungs much easier. Alcohol use can dampen the cough reflex and allow organisms to remain in the respiratory tract and eventually reach the lungs. Milk, although it provides vital nutrients, can raise the pH of the stomach and allow intestinal pathogens to avoid being killed. Antibiotics, although necessary to treat some infections, may also kill the normal flora of the intestine or female genital tract. Without the protection of the normal flora, potential pathogens can attach, colonize the mucous membranes, and go on to cause infections. Every day our habits can unknowingly affect our first-line defenses against microorganisms.

Mucous membrane secretions can become abnormal as in the case of the cystic fibrosis (CF) patient. The natural secretions of an individual with CF become abnormally thick and are not easily cleared from the body. This thick mucus produced is the result of a recessive gene that leads to persistent lung infections. *Pseudomonas aeruginosa* has an affinity for causing lung infections in the CF patient. A unique colony morphology of *Pseudomonas aeruginosa* can be found in the sputum culture of an individual with CF. The colony is extremely mucoid or wet because of its ability to adapt and survive in the abnormal sections of the lung.

► INFECTIONS LINKED TO INNATE (NATURAL) IMMUNE SYSTEM DYSFUNCTION

The **innate** (natural) immune system is always present because an individual is born with it. It reacts the same way each time it is challenged by a microorganism, regardless of how many times it occurs. The innate immune system is made up of white blood cells and **complement** (a set of proteins that acts in sequence to enhance the immune system).

WHITE BLOOD CELLS

The white blood cells act as a defense line within the human body. They make up only about 1% of a tube of whole blood but are a powerful part of the immune system. If an infectious agent is able to survive the physical barriers and natural antimicrobial actions of the human body, then the white blood cells are standing guard ready to take action against the invader.

Granulocytes

The polymorphonuclear (PMN) white blood cells consist of the neutrophils, eosinophils and basophils. These three white blood cell lines contain a characteristic segmented nucleus and granules. The granules provide enzymes that are used to kill organisms.

Neutrophils.   The neutrophils are the most numerous of the three granule laden white blood cells. They make up 50 to 75% of all the white blood cells present. They are easily recognized by the multilobed nucleus and the presence of fine granules throughout the cytoplasm. Figure 40-1 ■ reveals the characteristic morphology of a neutrophil from a Wright-Giemsa stained peripheral blood smear at 1000× magnification (Girgis, Marler, & Siders, 2008). They circulate through the blood and are able to travel outside the blood vessels to areas of infection to phagocytize (engulf) the invading organisms. They envelop any foreign objects present. Organisms are then killed by enzymes present in their granules. After the bacteria are killed, the empty vacuoles remain in the neutrophil cytoplasm. Figure 40-2 ■ shows two vacuolated neutrophils in a Wright-Giemsa stained peripheral blood smear viewed at 1000× magnification (Girgis et al., 2008). They both contain clusters of cocci. The presence of empty vacuoles often indicates the presence of a bacterial infection.

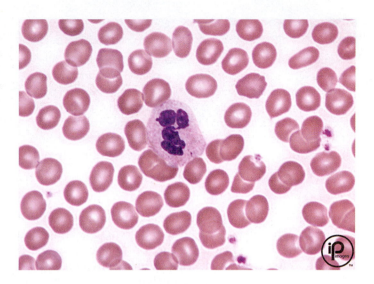

■ **FIGURE 40-1** This Wright-Giemsa stained blood smear reveals a characteristic neutrophil. Note its multilobed nucleus and fine cytoplasm granulation. (1000× magnification.)
From Girgis G, Marler LM, and Siders JA, *Hematology Image Atlas* CD-ROM, Indiana Pathology Images, 2008.

Neutrophils are drawn to the site of an infection by **chemotaxis** (deliberate movement because of attraction to a substance). Chemicals and compounds carried by the invading organisms and produced by infected or injured tissues provide the chemotactic substances.

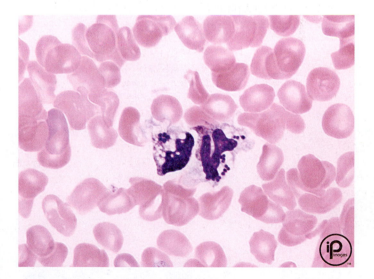

■ **FIGURE 40-2** This Wright-Giemsa stained blood smear demonstrates the vacuoles in the neutrophils associated with bacterial infection. Clusters of cocci can be seen within both white blood cells. Note the absence of the fine cytoplasm granules typical of neutrophils. After organisms are ingested, the granules fuse with the vacuole and empty their contents to kill the organisms, leaving only a hole in the neutrophil's cytoplasm. (1000× magnification.)
From Girgis G, Marler LM, and Siders JA, *Hematology Image Atlas* CD-ROM, Indiana Pathology Images, 2008.

Eosinophils.   Eosinophils contain prominent granules that take up red dye when stained using the Wright-Giemsa stain commonly used in hematology. They only make up about 3% of all the white cells present. Their primary function is to kill parasites. They can also engulf foreign objects and microorganisms once they have been attacked by antibodies. Figure 40-3 ■ displays a peripheral blood smear stained using the Wright-Giemsa stain at 1000× magnification (Girgis et al., 2008). In the center of the picture is a typical eosinophil with its multilobed nucleus and large red cytoplasm granules.

Basophils.   The basophils make up only about 1% of the white blood cells present. Their large granules tend to take up the purple-black portion of the Wright-Giemsa stain. They play a role in allergic reactions and hypersensitivity. Figure 40-4 ■ demonstrates the characteristic large black granules associated with basophils (Girgis et al., 2008). The nucleus is segmented into several lobes.

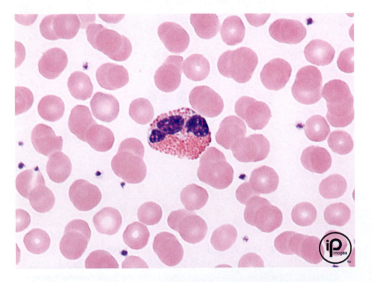

■ **FIGURE 40-3** Note the characteristic appearance of an eosinophil. It contains a multilobed nucleus and large red granules. These granules play a role in defense against parasites. (Wright-Giemsa stained peripheral blood smear at 1000× magnification.)
From Girgis G, Marler LM, and Siders JA, *Hematology Image Atlas* CD-ROM, Indiana Pathology Images, 2008.

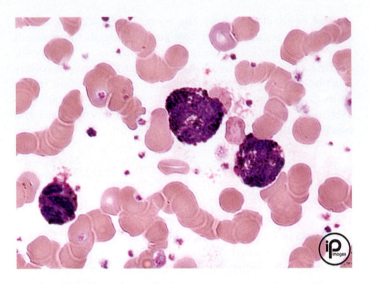

■ **FIGURE 40-4** This peripheral blood smear is stained using a Wright-Giemsa stain and viewed at 1000× magnification. Three basophils can be observed. The large basophil granules can take up the purple-black stain so well that they may obscure the segmented nucleus of the cell.
From Girgis G, Marler LM, and Siders JA, *Hematology Image Atlas* CD-ROM, Indiana Pathology Images, 2008.

Mononuclear Cells

The remaining white blood cells are called mononuclear cells. They have a nucleus that is in one piece rather than segmented and contain very fine granules that are not as prevalent as those in the PMNs.

Monocyte and Macrophage.   One mononuclear cell is the monocyte. It makes up about 3% of the white blood cells. It has the ability to migrate into tissues, where it is called a macrophage. The monocyte destroys microorganisms and cellular debris with enzymes. Once the debris has been digested, the process leaves vacuoles (clear bubbles) in its cytoplasm. It also helps the lymphocytes by presenting a piece of the offending organism to the T lymphocytes so they can process it for the B cells. The B cells then produce antibodies and remember

the organism quickly if it happens to invade again. The macrophage can remove organisms that have been coated with antibody (protective proteins produced by plasma cells) but not killed. The lymphocytes function differently than the other white blood cells and will be discussed later in this chapter as part of the acquired immune system. Figure 40-5 ■ demonstrates typical bean or horseshoe-shaped nucleus of a monocyte on a peripheral blood smear stained with Wright-Giemsa and at a magnification of 1000× (Girgis et al., 2008).

✓ Checkpoint! 40–2 (Chapter Objective 2)

The monocyte is a mononuclear white blood cell that can exist in two forms. Once it leaves the circulation and enters the tissues, it is called a

A. *phagocyte.*
B. *lymphocyte.*
C. *granulocyte.*
D. *macrophage.*

COMPLEMENT

The complement system is a set of circulating proteins that initiate biological functions such as inflammation once they are set into motion. The proteins react with each other in a specific sequence along several pathways. The pathways can be triggered by the appearance of microorganisms or their by-products such as lipopolysaccharides, chemicals released by injured human cells, and the presence of antigen–antibody complexes. Once activated, the pathways initiate the release of neutrophils from the bone marrow, chemotaxis of white blood cells, and enhancement of phagocytosis by white blood

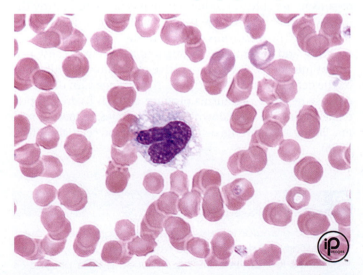

■ **FIGURE 40-5** The nucleus of a monocyte is often horseshoe- or bean shaped. Because they ingest bacteria, they can contain vacuoles as seen in this Wright-Giemsa stained peripheral blood smear at 1000× magnification.
From Girgis G, Marler LM, and Siders JA, *Hematology Image Atlas* CD-ROM, Indiana Pathology Images, 2008.

cells. The pathways also play a role in increasing vascular permeability, lysis of bacteria, virus-loaded cells, and malignant cells and other biological functions.

DEFECTS OF THE INNATE IMMUNE SYSTEM

Low White Blood Cell Count

A low white blood cell count can make the host, of any age, prone to infections. Genetic mutations can lead to a low white count early in childhood but are a rare occurrence. Most low cell counts are because of injury to the bone marrow, the source of red and white blood cells as well as platelets. Drugs such as cancer treatments as well as several antibiotics, such as chloramphenicol and sulfonamides, are the most common cause of a decreased production of neutrophils. Exposure to chemicals and radiation may also depress the bone marrow and deplete the white blood cells.

Once the white blood cell count drops below 500/μL (normal = 4500–11,000/μL), an individual is prone to infections with **endogenous** (from within the body) microorganisms such as *Staphylococcus aureus*, *Streptococcus* spp., and gram-negative rods such as *E. coli* and *Pseudomonas* spp., as well as anaerobes (Bagby, 2004). Fungal infections caused by *Candida albicans* are also common. When there are fewer than 100 white blood cells/μL, there is nearly a 100% chance of acquiring an infection (Distenfeld, 2006).

Someone with a low white count may appear normal even while fighting an active infection. Without an adequate number of white blood cells, the typical signs and symptoms of infection, such the presence of pus, do not exist. By the time the individual visits the doctor, infections can be massive and life threatening.

Often discontinuation of the offending drug may resolve the white blood cell deficiency. This may not be a practical solution if the drug is necessary to fight cancer cells, and no other alternative is available. Recombinant human granulopoietic factors that stimulate the bone marrow to produce white blood cells are now available. They have proven to be successful when given during cancer chemotherapy.

White Blood Cell Function

Most problems associated with the white blood cells are not because of their numbers but their function. Genetic mutations can cause defects in the structure and function of the white blood cells, which are more common than those causing low white blood cell counts but are still considered rare. Defects of the white blood cells account for about 15% of immune deficiencies (Cunningham-Rundles, 2004). Because genetic mutations exist from birth, most patients are identified early. Defects in the granulocytes (neutrophils, eosinophils, and basophils), as well as the monocytes and macrophages, should be suspected when patients experience recurrent, severe bacterial or fungal infections (Schumacher, Rosenzweig, Notarangelo, & Holland, 2004). Unusual organisms such as *Burkholderia cepacia* or infections in unusual body sites such as the liver can provide a hint that there is a white blood cell defect.

Leukocyte Adhesion Deficiency.

White blood cells are able to cross the endothelium of the blood vessels and enter the tissues to fight an infectious agent. To cross the endothelium, the cells must first adhere to the vessel wall. The white blood cells of some individuals lack this ability. Without adherence, the white blood cells are not able to cross the vessel wall and migrate to the site of an infection. The white blood cells function normally but cannot leave the bloodstream. These individuals often have an extremely high white blood cell counts. Counts greater than 15,000/µL are not unusual (Schumacher, 2004). The white blood cells cannot leave the bloodstream, so they continue to accumulate as new ones are produced. Because the white cells are unable to leave the bloodstream, there is a characteristic absence of pus formation with infection.

 REAL WORLD TIP

The inability to produce pus at the site of an infection is the first clue a patient may have a leukocyte function deficiency. The adhesive properties of the neutrophils can be tested in vitro (in the test tube). A substance that stimulates adhesion of the leukocytes is added to a sample of the patient's white blood cells. The mixture is then added to an artificial surface for attachment of the white blood cell. After a time, the surface is washed. The number of white blood cells remaining determines the strength of adhesion of the leukocytes.

A much more specific test employs flow cytometry using monoclonal antibodies. A deficiency in specific cell markers can diagnose leukocyte adhesion deficiency more effectively.

Affected individuals are prone to severe infections of the oral cavity, including gingivitis and periodontitis. *Staphylococcus aureus,* gram-negative rods, and fungi often cause recurrent infections and necrosis of the mouth, skin, respiratory, and intestinal tracts (Schumacher, 2004). The ulcers present are slow to heal and scar easily. There can be varying degrees of disease depending on the specific type of genetic defect. Those with a moderate form of disease are often diagnosed later in life because of fewer infections than those with the severe form of disease. Those with the most severe disease rarely live to the age of 10 (Rosen, Cooper, & Wedgewood, 1995). Necrosis may require surgery to remove dead tissue. Prophylactic (preventive) antibiotics are necessary to avoid infections. Bone marrow transplantation from a matched sibling or parent can restore the adhesive properties of the white blood cells (Boxer, 2004).

Chronic Granulomatous Disease.

Once the white blood cells have migrated to the site of an infectious agent, they phagocytize the microorganisms and destroy it with enzymes present in their granules. Genetic defects can occur that cause deficiencies in the function of the granules and their associated enzymes. The white blood cells are able to engulf the microorganisms but cannot kill them. Symptoms can appear any time from early infancy to young adulthood (Boxer, 2004).

White blood cells produce hydrogen peroxide (H_2O_2), which acts as an intracellular bleach to kill ingested microorganisms (Kamani, 2002). Normally the cells are able to produce enough hydrogen peroxide to kill even catalase-producing bacteria. Catalase-positive organisms such as *Staphylococcus* spp. are able to destroy hydrogen peroxide, which accumulates as a result of their aerobic breakdown of carbohydrates. Once they are engulfed in a normal white blood cell, they have the ability to produce enough catalase to allow them to survive within the cell. With time either the organisms are killed because they are overcome by other white blood cell killing mechanisms or they overtake the cell because of their many virulence factors produced.

Chronic granulomatous disease (CGD) is a genetic defect that limits the amount of hydrogen peroxide produced by white blood cells because of the deficiency of an essential enzyme. The disease can vary in severity so it can present any time from childhood to adulthood. Most patients are diagnosed before the age of 5 (Kamani, 2002). Recurrent, life-threatening infections are often because of catalase-positive organisms such as *Staphylococcus aureus, Nocardia* spp., gram-negative rods, both enteric and nonfermenters, as well as fungi such as *Aspergillus* spp. and *Candida* spp. (Dinauer, 2005). These organisms are able to produce enough catalase to destroy the limited hydrogen peroxide that may be present in the white blood cell. The organisms are able to survive within the cell, multiply, and disseminate throughout the body to cause persistent infections. Catalase-negative organisms are still killed by the defective white blood cells. In a strange turn of events, catalase-negative organisms produce enough hydrogen peroxide, during the breakdown of carbohydrates, to fuel the normal killing action of the deficient white blood cell (Distenfeld, 2006).

 REAL WORLD TIP

Chronic granulomatous disease is diagnosed by the reduction of a dye, nitroblue tetrazolium (NBT), by the patient's leukocytes. NBT is reduced by the production of hydrogen peroxide. With reduction, the NBT changes from a colorless substance to a blue precipitate. Patients with CGD cannot reduce NBT, and no blue is observed in the white blood cells under the microscope.

The typical patient develops inflammatory **granulomas** (masses that form because of constant inflammation) and abscesses in the organs and on the skin. These nodules form because of the continuous irritation of the infecting microorganisms. The granulomas and the subsequent characteristic scarring can cause obstructions in both the gastrointestinal and genitourinary tracts (Schumacher et al., 2004). Infections are common in the all body sites, especially on the skin, lymph nodes, bones, lungs, and deep organs such as the liver and spleen.

Continuous monitoring for infections and antibiotics, given on a daily basis, can improve the prognosis for CGD patients. Trimethoprim/sulfamethoxazole and dicloxacillin are effective prophylactic antibiotics. Antibiotics that are able to penetrate the white blood cells should be used for current infections. Treatment with interferon (proteins that enhance the immune system) may improve phagocyte function by killing the microorganisms present by other immune mechanisms (Dinauer, 2005). It has been shown that infections caused by bacteria and fungi can be reduced by up to 70% with interferon treatment (Lekstrom-Himes & Gallin, 2000).

Bone marrow (stem cell) transplantation is the only true cure for CGD but requires a matched sibling to avoid the problems associated with host versus graft disease (Kamani, 2002). Gene therapy is possible because this disease is caused by a genetic defect. Current studies have shown that gene correction of even 20% of the white blood cells, in the bone marrow, could provide protection against infection and granuloma production (Dinauer, 2005).

✓ Checkpoint! 40-3 (Chapter Objectives 2, 3, and 6)

Individuals with chronic granulomatous disease are prone to infections with catalase-positive organisms but not catalase-negative organisms. This is because

   A. *complement can use another pathway to kill catalase-negative organisms.*

   B. *catalase-positive organisms are able to destroy residual H_2O_2 present in the WBCs.*

   C. *catalase-positive organisms do not attract the WBCs via chemotaxis.*

   D. *there are only limited WBCs, so they attack the catalase-negative organisms first.*

Myeloperoxidase Deficiency. The granules of the white blood cells contain an enzyme, myeloperoxidase (MPO), which produces a microorganism killing acid from hydrogen peroxide and chlorine. MPO deficient white blood cells are able to phagocytize bacteria, but killing them takes longer (Sheikh, 2006). The white blood cells are still rich in hydrogen peroxide, which eventually kills the organisms present (Boxer, 2004). There seems to be a complete lack of ability to kill fungi such as *Candida* spp. and *Aspergillus* spp. (Sheikh, 2006).

MPO deficiency is the most common of the defects in neutrophils (Lekstrom-Himes & Gallin, 2000). The MPO deficiency can be present at birth because of a genetic defect or acquired through the onset of various leukemias or the use of cancer-killing drugs. Acquired MPO deficiency is usually transient and may only affect a portion of the white blood cells present (Sheikh, 2006).

Because the white cells are able to make up for an MPO deficiency, individuals are often asymptomatic and undiagnosed (Dinauer & Coates, 2005). Severe infections are rare. Infections present are usually because of *Candida* spp., especially in those with diabetes mellitus (Sheikh, 2006). Disseminated *Candida* spp. infections in an individual with diabetes mellitus or someone who presents with recurrent serious infections because of fungi should warrant evaluation of phagocyte function. The prognosis for individuals with an MPO deficiency is good. The white blood cells are able to compensate for the deficiency by killing bacteria with other mechanisms such as the accumulation of hydrogen peroxide. With underlying conditions such as diabetes mellitus and the use of steroids or chemotherapy, infections can be overwhelming and require aggressive antifungal therapy to resolve.

Chédiak-Higashi Disease. Chédiak-Higashi disease is characterized by white blood cells that have problems with chemotaxis, phagocytosis, and killing microorganisms once ingested. A rare inherited gene creates white blood cells with giant granules that do not function properly. Figure 40-6 ■ demonstrates the abnormal giant fused neutrophil granules associated with the disorder (Girgis et al., 2008).

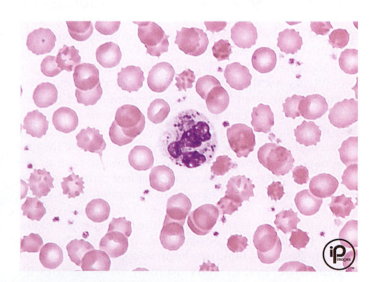

■ **FIGURE 40-6** This 1000× magnification of a Wright-Giemsa stained peripheral blood smear demonstrates the prominent granules of a neutrophil associated with Chédiak-Higashi disease. The giant granules can be present in all white blood cells. These cells are unable to kill ingested bacteria.

From Girgis G, Marler LM, and Siders JA, *Hematology Image Atlas* CD-ROM, Indiana Pathology Images, 2008.

Just as there are defects in the granules of the white blood cells, there are also defects in the granules of skin and hair cells that cause **albinism** (absence of pigment). The skin, hair, and eyes have less pigment then normal (Nowicki & Henryk, 2005). There are many hematological disorders such as bruising and bleeding.

From birth, affected individuals display severe neural problems as well as recurrent skin infections. *Staphylococcus aureus* and beta-hemolytic *Streptococcus* spp. are the most common causes of superficial and deep abscesses (Lekstrom-Himes & Gallin, 2000). Those affected usually perish because of infection before the age of 10. With time, infections because of viruses such as the Epstein-Barr virus can trigger a lymphoma-like illness that ultimately proves to be fatal (Nowicki & Henryk, 2005).

Prophylactic antibiotics can help prevent infections. A bone marrow transplant with a matched sibling can help with the hematological disorders that exist but not the neurological problems.

Complement Cascade

Complement is a set of soluble proteins that act in a specific sequence to defend its host against microorganisms. There are three different initiating pathways, classical, alternative, and mannose binding lectin, which eventually merge into one final terminal pathway. Complement can be attracted and activated by antibodies that bind to the surface of microorganisms (opsonization) or by the organisms themselves. It attacks bacteria and punches a hole in the organism's cell wall so its contents spill out. It also plays a role as an **opsonin** (white blood cell magnet). Once attached to the bacterial surface, it promotes phagocytosis by attracting white blood cells to the site of an infection. Deficiencies can occur in any step in the any of the multiple pathways.

Complement deficiencies are usually inherited. They are rare and may not always present with specific symptoms. They account for less than 2% of all of the immune deficiencies identified (Cunningham-Rundles, 2004). *Neisseria meningitidis* and other encapsulated organisms such as *Streptococcus pneumoniae* and *Haemophilus influenzae* type b tend to be the predominant pathogens. The capsules of these organisms are naturally antiphagocytic when complement cannot function properly to attract white blood cells via opsonization. Infections begin to develop early in life. At 3 to 6 months of age, the natural antibodies provided by the mother begin to disappear. The child is now susceptible to colonization by potential pathogens, and infections begin to appear.

Deficiencies in the classical pathway are associated with recurrent infections with encapsulated pyogenic organisms such as *Streptococcus pneumoniae* and *Haemophilus influenzae*. Deficiencies in the common terminal pathway result in recurrent potentially fatal infections because of *Neisseria* spp., especially *N. meningitidis*. The infections are often systemic, leading to meningococcemia, and may be caused by any of the serotypes. Individuals with a common terminal pathway defi-

ciency are at a 1,000 to 10,000 higher risk for meningococcal disease than the normal population (Kirschfink & Mollnes, 2003).

 REAL WORLD TIP

The total hemolytic complement assay (CH_{50}) analyzes the function of the classic pathway of the complement system. The classic pathway is triggered by the presence of antibodies bound to microorganisms or other antigens. Complement fixes to antigen–antibody complexes. If this occurs on red blood cells, the cells lyse. The CH_{50} test determines the ability of the patient's serum to lyse antibody coated sheep blood cells. With a defect in the classic pathway, the ability to lyse the cells is reduced or absent.

Treatments such as gene therapy or providing the missing pathway protein are not possible yet (Shigeoka, 2002). The physician must concentrate on recognizing the signs and symptoms of recurrent infections and prescribe appropriate antibiotics in a timely manner to avoid serious complications such as meningococcemia. Vaccines against *N. meningitidis*, *S. pneumoniae*, and *H. influenzae* are critical to prevent the organisms from colonizing and causing infections.

 Checkpoint! 40–4 (Chapter Objectives 2, 3, and 6)

A 20-year-old female patient presents to the emergency room with a petechial rash across her chest and extremities. She is lethargic and displays a stiff neck. The ER physician reviews her medical records and notes that this is the second time in the last year that she has presented with these signs and symptoms. What potential pathogen and immunodeficiency combination may explain this patient's presentation?

	Potential Pathogen	*Possible Immunodeficiency*
A.	*Neisseria meningitidis*	*Complement deficiency in common terminal pathway*
B.	*Streptococcus pneumoniae*	*Leukocyte adhesion deficiency*
C.	*Haemophilus influenzae*	*Myeloperoxidase deficiency*
D.	*Staphylococcus aureus*	*Hydrogen peroxide deficiency*

▶ INFECTIONS LINKED TO ACQUIRED (ADAPTIVE) IMMUNE SYSTEM DYSFUNCTION

The acquired (adaptive) immune system is unique because it remembers every encounter with a microorganism. It adapts to the situation at hand. Every time it meets a microorganism, it checks its memory banks to see if it has had a previous encounter. If the two have met before, then the organism is attacked rapidly with antibodies produced specifically against it.

COMPONENTS

The lymphocytes are key players in the acquired immune system. They make up about 30 to 40% of the white blood cells. They circulate in the blood, but they are also present in the lymph organs such as the spleen, lymph nodes, and tonsils. Lymphocytes serve as the memory cells for the immune system. There are two types of lymphocytes—the T cells and the B cells. The T lymphocytes outnumber the B cells about 7:1 in the circulation (Hagey & Sakamoto, 2002). Figure 40-7 ■ demonstrates a typical lymphocyte on a Wright-Giemsa stained peripheral blood at 1000× magnification (Girgis et al., 2008). Figure 40-8 ■ shows the transformation of a typical lymphocyte to a reactive lymphocyte once it has been stimulated by antigen (Girgis et al., 2008). Reactive lymphocytes are most commonly associated with viral infections such as infectious mononucleosis.

T LYMPHOCYTES

T cells migrate from the bone marrow to the thymus to mature and receive one of several specific job assignments. One type of T lymphocyte, called the T cytotoxic cell, releases toxic chemicals that kill cells infected with viruses and intracellular organisms. These cells carry a specific cell marker called $CD8^+$, which is a receptor for antigens. Another type of T cell releases **cytokines** (cellular chemicals), which help activate the B lym-

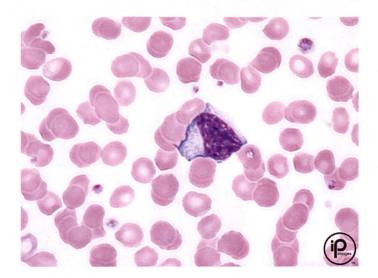

■ **FIGURE 40-8** This Wright stained peripheral blood smear magnified to 1000× displays the cellular changes of a lymphocyte once it has been stimulated by antigen. It enlarges, the cytoplasm becomes larger, and the nucleus stains lighter and less compact. The cell's cytoplasm may appear to hug nearby red blood cells. Reactive T and B lymphocytes cannot be differentiated visually.
From Girgis G, Marler LM, and Siders JA, Hematology Image Atlas CD-ROM, Indiana Pathology Images, 2008.

phocytes. Their ability to help the B cells has earned them the name "T helper cells." The T helper cells express a specific cell marker called $CD4^+$, which binds to antigen. One T lymphocyte remembers an offending organism so the antibody response is much more rapid the next time that specific organism appears in the human host. This earns them the name "T memory cells," and they carry the $CD4^+$ cell marker. The T lymphocytes can also act as an "off" switch to ensure the lymphocytes do not attack its human host and cause harm once the offending organism is eliminated. These cells have earned the name "T suppressor cell" for this function, and they also carry the $CD8^+$ cell marker. There are about 50% $CD4^+$ T lymphocytes and 20% $CD8^+$ T lymphocytes (Hagey & Sakamoto, 2002). A ratio of greater than 2 $CD4^+$ cells:1 $CD8^+$ cell is crucial for a competent immune system. If the ratio becomes reversed, immunity weakens.

B LYMPHOCYTES

The B lymphocytes originate in the liver in the fetus and eventually in the bone marrow in adults. Once stimulated by the T helper lymphocytes, the B lymphocytes eventually become the body's plasma cells, which produce antibodies. Some stimulated B cells go on to become memory cells, which allow the body to respond faster and produce a greater concentration of antibodies in the future. Figure 40-9 ■ demonstrates a plasma cell. Although rarely observed in the peripheral blood, they can be seen with intense stimulation as seen with certain infectious diseases and malignancies (Girgis et al., 2008).

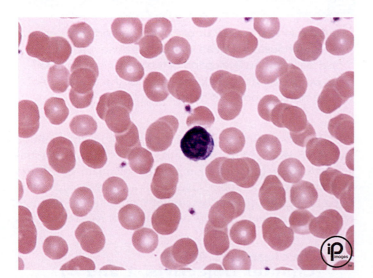

■ **FIGURE 40-7** The dense nucleus of a lymphocyte is approximately the size of a red blood cell. One cannot differentiate between T and B lymphocytes by visual morphology. Flow cytometry is needed to detect specific cell markers on each for differentiation. (Wright-Giemsa stain on peripheral blood at 1000× magnification.)
From Girgis G, Marler LM, and Siders JA, Hematology Image Atlas CD-ROM, Indiana Pathology Images, 2008.

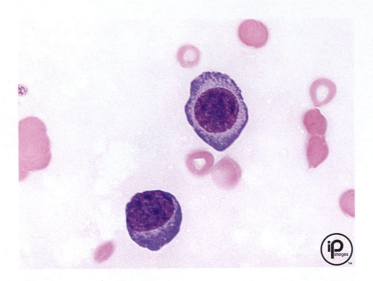

■ **FIGURE 40-9** The nucleus of the plasma cell stains darkly and is off center often placed to one side of the cell. Their function is to secrete antibodies. (Wright-Giemsa stain of peripheral blood magnified 1000×.)
From Girgis G, Marler LM, and Siders JA, *Hematology Image Atlas* CD-ROM, Indiana Pathology Images, 2008.

There are five types of antibodies or immunoglobulins (abbreviated Ig)—IgG, IgM, IgA, IgE, and IgD. IgG is the most prevalent antibody and is known for its ability to kill viruses and bacteria. IgM is the largest molecule and the first to appear with an infection. Secretory IgA is only found in bodily secretions such as milk, saliva, tears, and sweat. Another form of IgA, serum IgA, is found in the blood. IgE attacks parasites and is present in allergic reactions and hypersensitivity. IgD's function is unclear. It may act as an antibody to antibody on the surface of stimulated B cells and act like an "off" switch.

Each antibody produced will only react with one specific antigen. Once the antibody binds to the antigen or offending organism, then the white blood cells can attack and destroy it. Antibodies attached to an offending organism can also act as an opsonin (magnet) and activate the complement system to cause lysis of the cell wall.

DEFECTS OF THE ACQUIRED (ADAPTIVE) IMMUNE SYSTEM

Deficiencies in the acquired immune system can occur because of genetic disorders of the T cells, B cells, and a combination of both cell types. Deficiencies can also result because of the action of drugs, infection of the cells because of the human immunodeficiency virus (HIV), cancers of the bone marrow and the immune cells, and other causes. Pure T cell defects account for only about 5 to 10% of immune deficiencies, whereas B cell disorders account for up to 65% of most immune problems (Cunningham-Rundles, 2004). Combined T and B cell defects make up about 25% of all reported immune deficiencies (Cunningham-Rundles, 2004).

DiGeorge Syndrome

The thymus is the source of mature T lymphocytes for the body. Once mature, the cells leave to populate the spleen and lymph nodes. If the thymus is removed or diseased in an adult, eventually there is a deficiency of T cells because there is no source for new cells. If the thymus does not develop properly in the fetus, there can be an absence of mature T cells in the blood or lymph organs. DiGeorge syndrome (DGS) is because of a genetic defect that leads to an absent or underdeveloped thymus. There are varying degrees of defects that affect the development of the thymus. Those with the most severe form of the defect are diagnosed at birth. Most individuals with this syndrome have some residual thymus tissue present at birth. Initially they present with low T cell counts at birth but can show improvement in fighting infections with age (Cunningham-Rundles, 2004).

A child with DiGeorge syndrome is easily recognized at birth by facial and cardiac abnormalities (Chaganti, Moyer, & Kishiyama, 2006). Infections typically begin to appear in a child after the age of 3 to 6 months. This is the time frame when the mother's natural antibodies, acquired through the placenta, begin to decline. Recurrent infections can occur because of bacteria, fungi, viruses, and parasites.

One of the functions of the T cells is to help the B cells create antibodies by presenting pieces of microorganisms. Without T cells, B cells may not be able to properly respond to infections with antibody production. Individuals with DGS can have low levels of immunoglobulins.

REAL WORD TIP

The diagnosis of DGS at birth can be confirmed by a low lymphocyte count as well as the absence of a thymus on x-ray. An evaluation of the immunoglobulin levels will not be diagnostic because of the presence of maternal antibodies at birth.

A thymus transplant early in life can reboot the immune system (Hussain, Win, & Guduri, 2006). Intravenous immunoglobulin is given to maintain adequate IgG levels (Frattarelli & Bawle, 2002). Live virus vaccines should not be given to the DGS patient because of their defective immune systems. Household members should also not receive live virus

✓ Checkpoint! 40–5 (Chapter Objectives 2 and 4)

An individual diagnosed with DiGeorge syndrome displays a deficiency of T cells because of
   A. *the lack of a vital enzyme because of a genetic defect.*
   B. *the lack of plasma cells.*
   C. *an exposure to a drug.*
   D. *an absent or underdeveloped thymus.*

vaccines because of the risk of shedding live virus (Hussain et al., 2006). Trimethoprim-sulfamethoxazole is given on a daily basis to prevent infections.

Bruton's Agammaglobulinemia

Bruton's agammaglobulinemia is also known as X-linked agammaglobulinemia (XLA). It is called X-linked because the defective gene is present on the X chromosome. Males (and females who inherit two defective X chromosomes) are affected severely, whereas females who carry a normal X chromosome become carriers of the defect and possess normal immunity. The defective gene does not code for a vital enzyme, Bruton tyrosine kinase (BTK), which is responsible for the maturation and proliferation of the B cells. Without BTK, individuals do not produce any B cells or plasma cells. Without mature B cells and plasma cells, there are no immunoglobulins produced, and so the use of the term **agammaglobulinemia.**

Males with XLA present with infections as early as 3 to 6 months of age. The antibodies acquired from the mother are exhausted by that time. Typical infections are caused by encapsulated organisms such as *Streptococcus pneumoniae* and *Haemophilus influenzae*. The patient experiences recurrent infections such as otitis media, pneumonia, septicemia, and meningitis. *Staphylococcus aureus* and *Streptococcus pyogenes* (group A *Streptococcus*) cause skin infections such as abscesses and cellulitis. Diarrhea caused by *Campylobacter* spp., enterovirus, and *Giardia lamblia* is a common presentation (Granja Jander, Schwartz, & Desposito, 2005). The frequent pulmonary infections often cause chronic lung problems, which eventually lead to death in adulthood (Granja Jander et al., 2005).

REAL WORLD TIP

XLA is often diagnosed by the absence or reduced levels of all five immunoglobulin classes (IgA, IgD, IgE, IgM and IgG). Diagnosis in infants up to the age of 6 months is difficult because of the presence of maternal antibodies.

Treatment includes intravenous immunoglobulin infusions to replenish the missing antibodies. Patients can live into their 40s with antibody replacement therapy (Granja Jander et al., 2005). Antibiotics are critical for treatment of current infections. Patients with XLA should not receive live virus vaccines (Chin & Shigeoka, 2004).

Common Variable Immunodeficiency.

Common variable immunodeficiency (CVID) is the most common of the B cell defects (Park, 2004). Those afflicted have a normal number of B cells but lack the ability to differentiate into plasma cells. Without plasma cells, there are decreased levels of all or some of the immunoglobulins, a condition known as agammaglobulinemia. The cause of CVID is not entirely known (Park, 2004). There may be a genetic link or it may be associated with certain drugs (Schwartz & Modak, 2006). It can appear any time from infancy up to 40 years of age. Most individuals are diagnosed in their 20s (Schwartz & Modak, 2006). It is uncertain if the cause is genetic because both males and females can be affected.

CVID is characterized by recurrent upper and lower infections, the appearance of autoimmune diseases, and eventual malignancies (Park, 2004). Pathogens include *Streptococcus pneumoniae, Haemophilus influenzae,* and *Staphylococcus aureus.* Individuals experience recurrent episodes of sinusitis, pneumoniae, and otitis media. Unusual organisms such as *Pneumocystis jiroveci* (previously *Pneumocystis carinii*), *Mycoplasma* spp., and *Giardia lamblia* are frequent causes of infections (Schwartz & Modak, 2006).

REAL WORLD TIP

The inability to produce antibodies after immunization may establish the diagnosis of CVID. The individual may not possess the normal blood group antibodies (anti-A and anti-B). Live attenuated vaccines should not be used for immunizations.

Individuals with CVID are also prone to autoimmune disorders such as rheumatoid arthritis, thrombocytopenia, hemolytic anemia, and pernicious anemia (Rosen et al., 1995). There is a very high rate of lymphomas and gastrointestinal cancer, as well as other cancers (Park, 2004). Lymphoma is the most common cause of death in the female CVID patient (Schwartz & Modak, 2006).

Treatment requires regular immunoglobulin transfusions as well as antibiotics for current infections. Additional therapy is necessary for the autoimmune disorders and malignancies that can appear. Pregnant CVID females are not able to produce IgG, so the fetus does not acquire antibodies naturally in utero. Intravenous immunoglobulins for the mother are able to provide IgG for transport across the placenta, so the neonate is protected at birth (Park, 2004).

Severe Combined Immunodeficiency

Severe combined immunodeficiency (SCID) gained notoriety when it was the subject of the 1976 movie, *The Boy in the Plastic Bubble*. The plot of the movie followed a boy (portrayed by John Travolta) as he grew up and lived in a sterile environment because he lacked an intact immune system. In 1976, there were no viable treatments for SCID, and the movie portrayed the only known option for survival at the time.

SCID is the result of one of many genetic defects, all of which present with the same outcome. The genetic defects cause the loss of the thymus with the subsequent loss of T cells as well as the loss of B cells and the subsequent loss of immunoglobulins (agammaglobulinemia). Although SCID is extremely rare, more than 50% of cases occur in males because the genetic defect is located on the X chromosome (Secord, 2005).

Infections begin early in life, often within 2 to 3 months of birth. Infections tend to be more severe than those in individuals with an intact immune system. The SCID patient is susceptible to nearly any microorganism (bacteria, virus, fungi, and parasites). Continuous diarrhea either because of infectious agents or an autoimmune process leads to weight loss and malnutrition. Oral thrush, diaper rash, and skin infections because of *Candida albicans* are almost continuously present (Wong & Yang, 2006). *Pneumocystis jiroveci* (previously *Pneumocystis carinii*) pneumonia within the first 3 months of life often leads to the diagnosis of SCID (Shigeoka, 2003). Vaccinations with live viruses are lethal for the SCID patient.

 REAL WORLD TIP

Patients with SCID are susceptible to infection with nearly every known microorganism. Infections tend to be much more severe than those in immunocompetent individuals.

Without a bone marrow transplant, ideally from a matched sibling, the child will either die by the age of 2 because of infections or be destined to live in a sterile environment.

Other T and B Cell Disorders. Many other T and B cells deficiencies are beyond the scope of this chapter. They are rare and all are prone to recurrent infections. One example is Wiskott-Aldrich syndrome (WAS). WAS is an X-linked genetic defect, primarily seen in males, in which defective T cells cannot communicate properly with the B cells. The B cells can have selective deficiencies in the production of one or more immunoglobulins types. Most individuals die by the age of 8 (Dibbern & Routes, 2005). Infections are usually because of encapsulated organisms, *Pneumocysts jiroveci* (previously *Pneumocystis carinii*), and viruses. Treatment requires immunoglobulin transfusions and eventually a bone marrow transplant. There are many more additional potential disorders, but they are rare occurrences in the general population. A trusted immunology reference book can detail the rare T and B cell defects and their associated infections. Table 40-1✪ summarizes the defects of the innate and acquired immune systems discussed in this chapter as well as their effects and associated organisms.

> ✓ **Checkpoint! 40–6 (Chapter Objective 6)**
>
> *Severe combined immunodeficiency (SCID) is ultimately not compatible with life without*
>
> A. *intravenous immunoglobulin transfusions.*
> B. *a bone marrow transplant.*
> C. *antibiotics.*
> D. *vaccinations.*

▶ SECONDARY IMMUNODEFICIENCIES

Although many of the disorders of the immune system are because of defects of the primary components (white blood cells, complement, antibodies), it is possible to acquire immunodeficiencies secondarily because of drugs, other diseases, and microorganisms.

DRUGS

Corticosteroids are known for their powerful ability to suppress the immune system. They are used to treat inflammatory diseases such as asthma. Steroids affect both arms of the immune system (innate and adaptive). They inhibit the adhesion of white blood cells so they cannot migrate. They have the ability to reduce phagocytosis by the white blood cells as well as inhibit T cell function. Large doses of steroids eventually inhibit immunoglobulin production because of the close relationship between T and B cells. Infections because of steroid therapy often include intracellular bacteria such as *Listeria monocytogenes*, *Mycobacterium* spp., and *Legionella* spp., as well as viruses and fungi (Tolkoff-Rubin & Rubin, 2004).

Cyclosporine is a powerful immunosuppressive agent that is used to dampen the immune system so transplanted tissue is not rejected by the host. This drug affects T cell function, so the host is prone to viral infections, especially cytomegalovirus and Epstein-Barr virus (Tolkoff-Rubin & Rubin, 2004).

Chemotherapeutic agents, such as methotrexate, are cytotoxic for rapidly dividing cells such as cancer cells. Unfortunately normal cells such as the developing white bloods are also destroyed in the bone marrow. The drugs can also break down the mucous membranes to allow bacteria, viruses, and fungi free entry into the body. Both gram-positive and gram-negative bacteria are potential pathogens. Chemotherapeutic drugs also damage the phagocytes by causing decreased migration, phagocytosis and killing action All these increase the likelihood of infections. T cells are also affected. Potential infectious agents include bacteria, fungi, and viruses (Bart & Pantaleo, 2004).

SPLEEN

The spleen is one of the major organs for antibody production. It houses T and B cells as well as plasma cells and macrophages. As blood filters through the spleen, any organisms present are exposed to phagocytes and lymphocytes. Phagocytes have trouble engulfing encapsulated bacteria. A portion of the antibodies produced in the spleen attach to the surface of the invading encapsulated organism. The antibodies acts as opsonins (magnets) and help the phagocytes recognize the pathogen easier. The spleen macrophages can also remove the coated offenders if the white cells have not had time to complete their job. The spleen also functions as a strainer to remove damaged cells and foreign substances from the blood.

TABLE 40-1

A Summary of Defects of the Innate and Acquired Immune Systems

Disease/Syndrome	Deficiency	Signs/Symptoms	Associated Organisms
Myeloperoxidase deficiency	Neutrophil myeloperoxidase enzyme	■ Often asymptomatic ■ Recurrent fungal infections	■ *Candida* spp. ■ *Aspergillus* spp.
Chédiak–Higashi disease	Granulocyte granules	■ Recurrent skin infections ■ Albinism ■ Severe neural problems	■ *Staphylococcus aureus* ■ Beta-hemolytic *Streptococcus* spp.
Leukocyte adhesion disease	Leukocyte adhesion	■ WBC count >15,000/µL ■ Gingivitis ■ Periodontitis	■ *Staphylococcus aureus* ■ Gram-negative rods ■ Fungi
Chronic granulomatous disease	Leukocyte H_2O_2	■ Granulomas throughout the body	■ Catalase-positive organisms ● *Staphylococcus aureus* ■ *Nocardia* spp. ■ Gram-negative rods ■ *Aspergillus* spp. ■ *Candida* spp.

Complement deficiency	Classical pathway	■ Recurrent infections	■ Encapsulated organisms
			  ● *Streptococcus pneumoniae*
			  ● *Haemophilus influenzae*

Complement deficiency	Terminal pathway	■ Meningococcemia	■ *Neisseria meningitidis*
DiGeorge syndrome	T cell	■ Absent or underdeveloped thymus ■ Facial and cardiac abnormalities	■ All microorganisms

Bruton's agammaglobulinemia	Bruton tyrosine kinase	■ Recurrent infections	■ Encapsulated organisms
			  ● *Streptococcus pneumoniae*
			  ● *Haemophilus influenzae*
			■ Group A *Streptococcus*

Common variable immune deficiency	Antibody	■ Recurrent upper and lower infections
		■ Autoimmune diseases
		■ Malignancies
			■ *Streptococcus pneumoniae*
			■ *Haemophilus influenzae*
			■ *Staphylococcus aureus*
			■ Unusual organisms
			  ● *Pneumocystis jiroveci*
			  ● *Mycoplasma* spp.
			  ● *Giardia lamblia*

Severe combined immunodeficiency	T cell, B cell, and antibody	■ Oral thrush
		■ Skin infections
		■ Diarrhea
		■ Pneumonia
			■ All microorganisms
			  ● Encapsulated organisms
			  ● *Pneumocytis jiroveci*
			  ● Viruses
			  ● Fungi

Once the spleen is removed because of trauma or disease, the body loses a powerful line of defense. A person without a spleen is at risk for life-threatening infections, especially sepsis, which can kill in a matter of hours. The most common pathogen for the **asplenic** (without a spleen) patient is *Streptococcus pneumoniae.* Other common pathogens include *Haemophilus influenzae* type b and *Neisseria meningitidis.* One unusual pathogen, *Capnocytophaga canimorsus,* is a fastidious gram-negative rod that is associated with an overwhelming systemic infection in the asplenic individual following a dog bite (Lutwick, 2005).

Prophylactic antibiotics may be necessary for the life of the asplenic individual. Immunization with vaccines against *Streptococcus pneumoniae, Haemophilus influenzae,* and *Neisseria meningitidis* are absolutely essential to prevent infections.

REAL WORLD TIP

Asplenic patients can present with extremely high numbers of bacteria in the blood. The diagnosis of sepsis must be made quickly to prevent fatal outcomes. Routine blood cultures may require incubation of 6 to 24 hours to detect organisms. A Gram stain of the peripheral **buffy coat** (the white blood cell layer of centrifuged blood) or even the peripheral blood itself can rapidly reveal the causative agent.

BONE MARROW TRANSPLANT

Individuals undergoing a bone marrow transplant must have their immune system eliminated prior to receiving new bone marrow or peripheral blood stem cells. Until the new cells take and begin proliferating, the recipient is at high risk for infection with bacteria, fungi, and viruses. Laminar flow rooms with positive pressure are essential to remove organisms in the air. Once the new cells begin to proliferate, there is still a potential for infection until the neutropenia is resolved. After the white count and humoral immunity have risen to a protective level, the recipient is able to stop immunosuppressive medications. Infections should no longer be a concern.

✓ Checkpoint! 40–7 (Chapter Objective 5)

The loss of the spleen makes an individual extremely susceptible to a

  A. *catalase-negative, optochin-susceptible gram-positive cocci.*

  B. *catalase-positive, coagulase-positive gram-positive cocci.*

  C. *chlamydospore-producing yeast.*

  D. *catalase-negative, bacitracin-susceptible gram-positive cocci.*

ACQUIRED IMMUNODEFICIENCY SYNDROME (AIDS)

In the early 1980s, a new disease appeared that presented with many unusual opportunistic infections. The stricken individual seemed to have no immune system. The cause was determined to be a virus—the human immunodeficiency virus (HIV). The disease eventually became known as acquired immunodeficiency syndrome (AIDS). It is now the second leading cause of death in men between the ages of 25 and 44 (Abbas, 2005). For women of the same age group, AIDS is the third leading cause of death (Abbas, 2005). The disease is sweeping the world, and HIV has infected over 40 million people (Abbas, 2005).

HIV is a lentivirus that belongs to the retrovirus group. There are two forms of the virus, HIV-1 and HIV-2. Both types are serologically related and cause the same disease states but differ in the geographic locations in which they are prevalent. HIV-2 is found primarily in Africa and tends to be slower in weakening the immune system. It is naturally resistant to drugs used for treatment of HIV-1. The two forms can be differentiated by antibody, antigen, and polymerase chain reaction (PCR) tests. The virus can be contracted by sexual contact, exchange of blood and body fluids, and passage from mother to infant. The retrovirus group is known for its persistent viremia and incredible ability to weaken the immune system (Dubin, 2004).

 REAL WORLD TIP

Although HIV-1 is the most common serotype found in the United States, all blood donations are screened for HIV-1 and HIV-2.

HIV attacks lymphocytes and monocytes/macrophages as well as the central nervous system. The virus specifically attaches to the CD4$^+$ cell marker on T helper and T memory lymphocytes. It then enters to take over the cell to replicate itself. About 60% of the circulating lymphocytes can become infected. As the virus matures, the cells lyse, and more viruses are released to infect more cells. One to two billion T cells die each day, which in turn produces 100 billion new viruses (Abbas, 2005).

Initially the immune system tries to cope by producing antibodies against the invading virus. The number of T cells drops at first, but the body recovers by producing more. The immune system works very hard to contain the infection but cannot destroy the virus completely. Eventually the T cells become overwhelmed, and the ratio of CD4$^+$ and CD8$^+$ cells reverses so the CD4$^+$ cells are outnumbered. A normal immune system maintains a CD4$^+$:CD8$^+$ ratio of greater than 2:1. The CD4$^+$ count provides the best assessment of the health of the immune system in HIV-positive individuals.

Without viral treatment, after 7 to 10 years, the T cells are completely overwhelmed, and the number of viruses begins to rise exponentially. This is the point at which signs and symptoms of active infection begin to appear, and the patient is considered to have developed full-blown acquired immunodeficiency disease (AIDS). There is a complete breakdown of the immune system, and numerous opportunistic infections, malignancies, and central nervous system symptoms begin to appear. Death is usually because of secondary infections caused by organisms such as atypical *Mycobacterium* spp. or *Pneumocysts jiroveci* (previously *Pneumocystis carinii*).

Infections in an individual with AIDS run the gamut of microorganisms, and multiple infections can appear simultaneously. *Candida albicans* frequently causes infections of the mouth (thrush) and upper respiratory system. Herpes simplex virus can make the AIDS patient miserable. Varicella-zoster virus is often reactivated to cause painful shingles. Cytomegalovirus (CMV) attacks the eye to cause retinitis and potential vision loss. The AIDS patient is especially prone to infections with *M. tuberculosis* as well as atypical *Mycobacterium* spp. *Mycobacterium avium-intracellulare* complex is known to cause infections throughout the body. Diarrhea is commonly caused by *Cryptosporidium* spp., as well as other intestinal parasites such as *Isospora, Cyclospora,* and *Microsporidia. Cryptococcus* spp. and *Toxoplasma gondii* attack the central nervous system. Pneumonia because of *Pneumocystis jiroveci* (previously *Pneumocystis carinii*) is a common symptom in the AIDS patient. For some individuals, their positive HIV status and subsequent development of AIDS is unknown to them until they present with *Pneumocystis* pneumonia (PCP).

Highly active antiretroviral therapy (HAART) in HIV positive, but asymptomatic individuals have proven successful in preventing the infection of new T cells. The virus can never be eliminated but can be controlled at a level that extends the life of the HIV-positive individual. Prophylactic antibiotics can stem infections, which are the most common cause of death. The lack of a viable vaccine against the virus ensures it will remain in the human population.

SUMMARY

A competent immune system is essential to resist infectious agents. The human body has natural physicals barriers such as the skin, presence of normal flora, and the mucous membranes, which are present at birth and continuously on guard against potential pathogens. The innate immune system is composed of the white blood cells and complement. They function as the first line of immune defense once the physical barriers have been breached. The adaptive immune system develops as an individual is exposed to microorganisms. It needs to be primed by meeting an invading organism before it can attack. T and B lymphocytes work together to produce antibodies against organisms they encounter.

The immune system can be compromised when there is a defect in one or more of any of its components. Defects can be inherited or because of genetic mutations and become apparent early in life. These defects are rare but can present with severe problems when they occur. Defects in the immune system can also be caused secondarily because of drugs or microorganisms such as HIV. These are much more common.

A compromised immune system is prone to recurrent infections, which run the gamut of microorganisms. There are numerous organisms associated with each defect. The types of infections present and the causative agents may lead to the discovery of an underlying immune deficiency. The laboratory plays a key role in confirming or establishing the diagnosis of immunodeficiency.

LEARNING OPPORTUNITIES

1. Which of the following is prone to lung infections because of abnormal secretions of the respiratory tract? (Chapter Objective 1)

   a. A 68-year-old male alcoholic

   b. A 55-year-old female smoker

   c. A 12-year-old female with cystic fibrosis

   d. A 40-year-old male on vancomycin for pneumonia

2. Which white blood cell would you expect to find increased in the blood of an individual who presented with the microorganism shown in the photo? (Chapter Objective 2)

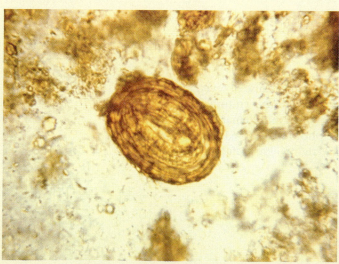

Public Health Image Library, CDC

   a. Neutrophils

   b. Lymphocytes

   c. Basophils

   d. Eosinophils

3. The cell pictured releases cytokines, which in turn activate a second type of cell to produce antibodies. The cell is a (Chapter Objective 2)

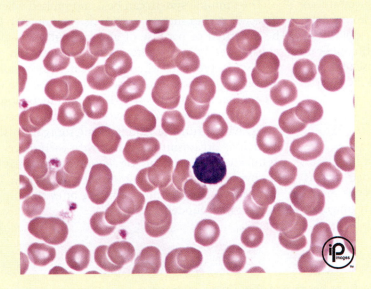

From Girgis G, Marler LM, and Siders JA, *Hematology Image Atlas* CD-ROM, Indiana Pathology Images, 2008.

   a. T lymphocyte

   b. B lymphocyte

   c. reactive lymphocyte

   d. plasma cell

4. Asplenic individuals are prone to infection with (Chapter Objective 4)

   a. viruses

   b. fungi

   c. catalase-positive organisms

   d. encapsulated organisms

5. A 1-month-old female was seen by her pediatrician because of fever, multiple skin lesions, and oral ulcers, which made feeding difficult. After culture, the skin lesions grew heavy growth of *Staphylococcus aureus*. An observant hematology technologist discovered the lymphocyte pictured in the photo (page 1051) on review of the baby's peripheral blood smear stained with Wright-Giemsa stain at 1000× magnification.

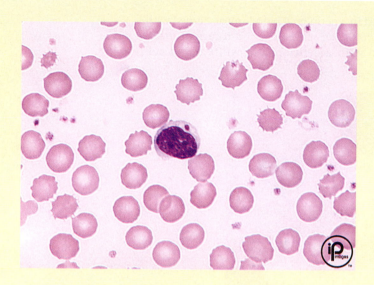

From Girgis G, Marler LM, and Siders JA, *Hematology Image Atlas* CD-ROM, Indiana Pathology Images, 2008.

You would also expect this child to also exhibit (Chapter Objectives 3 and 5)

a. albinism

b. an underdeveloped thymus

c. agammaglobulinemia

d. facial and cardiac abnormalities

6. A 27-year-old female presents with night sweats, unexplained weight loss, and pneumonia. The pneumonia was found to be caused by *Pneumocystis jiroveci*. Her complete blood count reveals low numbers of lymphocytes. The patient's history is significant for intravenous drug use from the ages of 17 to 21. Her immunodeficiency is potentially because of (Chapter Objectives 3 and 5)

a. an absent or underdeveloped thymus

b. a deficiency of Bruton tyrosine kinase

c. a lack of B cells because of her previous drug use

d. the loss of T cells because of human immunodeficiency virus

7. The neutrophils in the photo were observed in a peripheral blood smear stained with Wright-Giemsa stain and magnified at 1000×. Disseminated and recurrent infections with this organism are associated with a deficiency in white blood cell (Chapter Objective 5)

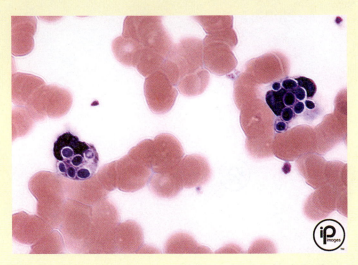

From Girgis G, Marler LM, and Siders JA, *Hematology Image Atlas* CD-ROM, Indiana Pathology Images, 2008.

   a. adhesion

   b. granules

   c. myeloperoxidase

   d. hydrogen peroxide

8. Which of the following deficiencies of the acquired immune system responds to a thymus transplant rather than relying on regular immunoglobulin transfusions? (Chapter Objective 6)

   a. DiGeorge syndrome

   b. Bruton's agammaglobulinemia

   c. Common variable immunodeficiency

   d. Severe combined immunodeficiency

PEARSON myhealthprofessionskit™

Use this address to access the interactive Companion Website created for this textbook. Simply select "Clinical Laboratory Science" from the choice of disciplines. Find this book and log in using your user name and password.

REFERENCES

Go to myhealthprofessionskit.com to view this chapter's references.

41

Nosocomial Infection

Joy T. Henderson

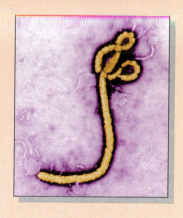

■ LEARNING OBJECTIVES

Upon completion of this chapter, the learner should be able to:

1. Identify a nosocomial infection.
2. Discuss the factors that play a role in the incidence of nosocomial infections.
3. Determine the most common types of bacterial, viral, fungal, and parasitic nosocomial infections.
4. Describe the epidemiology of each major type of nosocomial infection.
5. Correlate nosocomial infections discussed with the most common pathogens, their source(s), and mechanism(s) of pathogenicity.
6. Discuss the significance of medical devices in relation to nosocomial infections.
    a. Describe how a medical device is capable of causing an infection.
    b. Correlate potentially pathogenic organisms with medical device–related infections.
7. Determine control measures that are effective in the prevention and management of nosocomial infections.
8. Determine acceptable specimens for determination of nosocomial infections.
    a. Discuss unique specimen collection and processing and interpretation of culture results.
    b. Given an algorithm, determine the significance of organisms isolated.
9. Summarize emerging antimicrobial resistance for the organisms discussed and their significance in nosocomial infections.
10. Describe the role of an infection control program and the tools used.
11. Relate the role of the microbiologist as a member of the infection control team.

KEY TERMS

algorithm	epidemic	mortality
antibiogram	epidemiology	nosocomial
biofilm	exogenous	standard precautions
contact precautions	morbidity	surveillance
endogenous		

▶ INTRODUCTION

Nosocomial infections, also known as hospital-acquired infections (HAI), develop in patients during the course of their hospital stay. Infections are usually considered nosocomial if they first appear 48 hours or more after hospital admission or within 30 days after discharge. The word *nosocomial* comes from the Greek word *nosokomeion,* meaning hospital (*nosos* = disease, *komeo* = to take care of).

Nosocomial infections are a major source of **morbidity** (the state of being diseased) and **mortality** (death), affecting more than two million patients annually in the United States (Emori & Gaynes, 1993), costing more than $4.5 billion, and accounting for half of all major hospital complications (Ma, Tsui, Hogan, Wagner, & Ma, 2003). In 2008, the Centers for Medicare and Medicaid (CMS) selected hospital-acquired infections, such as catheter-associated urinary tract infections and vascular catheter-associated infection, as conditions that will no longer be paid for reimbursement. In 2009, they added Legionnaire's disease, ventilator-associated pneumonia, *Staphylococcus aureus* septicemia, and *Clostridium difficile* associated disease to the list of conditions. Hospitals will longer receive CMS payments for nosocomial infections in Medicare and Medicaid patients. Other insurance companies are sure to follow suit.

The discussions in this chapter will range from the types and distribution of nosocomial infection, the factors that increases patients' susceptibility to infection, the nosocomial culprits involved, and the emerging patterns of antimicrobial resistance that contribute to nosocomial infections, as well as the role of the laboratory and other health care professionals in the infection control program. Visit the appropriate chapter to review the characteristics and laboratory tests used to identify each microorganism mentioned in this chapter.

▶ EPIDEMIOLOGY OF NOSOCOMIAL INFECTIONS

HOST FACTORS

To understand nosocomial infections, one must possess knowledge of **epidemiology**, which is the study of the causes and transmission of diseases. Many host factors play a role in the prevention of disease. Once the natural and acquired defense mechanisms are breached, then organisms can cause infection. If the host defenses are disrupted while the individual is hospitalized, their own organisms as well as those present in the hospital environment are ready to take advantage of the opportunity. Other host factors that can increase the risk of invasion of organisms include the age of the patient, severity of the original illness, the presence of underlying conditions such as diabetes, and the length of hospital stay. ∞ Chapter 4 of this textbook discusses in detail the host factors that are present as part of the innate and acquired defense mechanisms of humans.

Immunocompromised Hosts

Individuals with an altered or defective immune system are known as immunodeficient, immunosuppressed, or immuno-compromised. Corticosteroids and chemotherapy agents dampen the immune system, making an individual more susceptible to nosocomial infection. Immunosuppression can also be acquired through genetic defects or the human immuno-deficiency virus (HIV). Once hospitalized, any organism encountered can rapidly become a potential pathogen for these individuals. ∞ Chapter 40 discusses in detail the effect of a compromised immune system and the organisms associated with infection in this unique patient population.

ENVIRONMENTAL FACTORS

The hospital environment provides many opportunities for microorganisms to hide in waiting for the chance to invade and cause infection. Because of the presence of organisms on the skin of every human being, the patient, visitors, as well as health care personnel can be a source of potential pathogens. The use of medical devices such as an intravenous or urinary catheter provides an artificial surface for organisms to colonize and initiate infections throughout the body.

Certain hospital locations, such as the intensive care unit, are prone to nosocomial infections. The ICU patient tends to be very ill, hospitalized longer than the average patient, on multiple drugs and antibiotics, and may have multiple catheters and an endotracheal tube. These hospital locations tend to harbor multi-drug-resistant strains of microorganisms that are difficult to completely eliminate.

℮ REAL WORLD TIP

Artificial nails and long natural nails were associated with an outbreak in a neonatal ICU caused by *Pseudomonas aeruginosa*. Health care workers wearing artifical nails have also been implicated in other outbreaks, including wound infections and osteomyelitis caused by gram-negative rods and yeast. Artificial nails or extenders should not be worn by those having direct contact with high risk patients (e.g., those patients in ICU and operating rooms). Natural nails should be kept trimmed to less than ¼ inch long (CDC, 2002a).

Many organisms are able to survive in water or damp areas. The plumbing may expose patients to organisms such as *Legionella* spp. Flowers brought to cheer up a patient can harbor water-loving organisms such as *Pseudomonas* spp. The air, water, and food of the hospital can provide a source of organisms. Although housekeeping measures normally reduce the presence of organisms, there can be breaks in procedures that allow their proliferation. Most environmental-related infections are because of contaminated instruments or equipment.

The nurse-to-patient ratio can also have an impact on the rate of nosocomial infection in an institution. An increased number of patients can result in breaks in hygiene for both the patient and staff. Patients placed together in the same room can provide exposure to organisms from each other as well as from visitors who enter the room. A health care worker assisting one patient can innocently touch the arm of the roommate on the way out and transfer organisms. Many hospitals have returned to using private rooms for patients to decrease the potential for nosocomial infections.

MICROORGANISM FACTORS

Microbes must colonize a body site before being able to cause infection. Organisms, such as gram-negative rods, are able to colonize the hospital patient's skin and respiratory and genitourinary tracts within hours of admission. The amount of organism inoculum can affect the ability to colonize. The more organisms present, the easier it is to overcome the protective nature of normal flora. The organism's use of enzymes and toxins can make colonization easier. An organism that produces spores can be transmitted easily on the skin and instruments.

Many hospitalized patients receive antibiotics. Antibiotics select for resistant strains or cause spontaneous mutations that promote resistance. Microbial antibiotic resistance has become a major threat in the hospital and now in the community as well. Because hospitals use large amounts of antibiotics, health care workers can spread the resulting resistant organisms from patient to patient. Antibiotic resistance and its contribution to nosocomial infection is discussed in detail later in this chapter.

Checkpoint! 41–1 (Chapter Objective 2)

An 89-year-old female is hospitalized in the intensive care unit. She is intubated and receiving intravenous ceftriaxone, vancomycin, acyclovir, and corticosteroids. She has a urinary catheter in place. She is allowed a dedicated nurse on each shift and is only allowed two visitors for 5 minutes at the top of each hour.

How many factors are present that could contribute to the development of a nosocomial infection in this individual?

    A. 3
    B. 5
    C. 7
    D. 9

▶ BACTERIAL NOSOCOMIAL INFECTIONS

EPIDEMIOLOGY

The incidence of nosocomial infections varies by body site and is determined to a large extent by underlying disease conditions in the patients and their exposure to high-risk med-

ical interventions, such as surgical operations and invasive devices. Five common types of infections account for more than 80% of all nosocomial infections and include catheter-related urinary tract infections, surgical and wound infections, bloodstream infections, especially when associated with use of an intravascular device, ventilator-assisted pneumonia, and gastrointestinal infections.

Checkpoint! 41–2 (Chapter Objective 3)

Which of the following common types of bacterial nosocomial infections is usually not caused by the presence of a medical device?

    A. *Gastrointestinal infection*
    B. *Bloodstream infection*
    C. *Pneumonia*
    D. *Urinary tract infection*

URINARY TRACT INFECTIONS (CATHETER-ASSOCIATED)

Epidemiology

A urinary tract infection (UTI) is a condition in which one or more structures of the urinary tract become infected after bacteria overcome its powerful natural defenses. Despite these defenses, infection of the urinary tract is the most common hospital-acquired infection in North America and is the most frequent nosocomial infections in critically ill patients (Johnson, Kuskowski, & Wilt, 2006; Laupland et al., 2005). Urinary tract infection in the hospital setting is most often caused by the insertion of a catheter into the urinary tract. Catheterization is necessary in cases where a sterile urine specimen needs to be obtained in a person who cannot voluntarily urinate, when an infection is suspected in the urinary tract, or when urine is retained. A single "in and out" urinary catheterization for the collection of a urine sample carries a relatively low risk for development of an infection. The possibility of acquiring infection depends on the method and duration of catheterization, the quality of catheter care, and host susceptibility. Individuals who are immobile or unconscious often require long-term indwelling urinary catheterization, which carries a higher risk of infection. The longer the catheter is left in place, the greater the chance for development of a urinary tract infection.

A Foley catheter is the thin flexible tubing used to drain urine from the bladder. It can be inserted, a urine specimen collected, and quickly removed. If it is left in place, it is called an indwelling catheter. Figure 41-1 ■ provides an example of an indwelling urinary catheter. The tubing is held in place by a balloon filled with sterile water after insertion. The tubing then leads to a collection bag.

Consider how a catheter is inserted into the bladder, and you can better understand how an infection can occur. The collection tubing must pass through the urethra to enter the

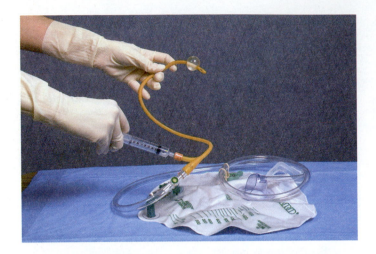

■ **FIGURE 41-1** This is an example of an indwelling urinary catheter. Once the flexible tubing is in the bladder, the balloon is filled with sterile water to hold the catheter tubing in place. The sampling port on the tubing allows for collection of free flowing urine from the bladder. The tubing leads to the collection bag, which has a drainage outlet so it can be emptied.

bladder. Trauma can occur as the tubing is forced over the delicate mucous membranes. Normal flora organisms colonize the urethra of both males and females. If the area is not cleaned adequately prior to catheterization, organisms can be pushed into the bladder by the tubing. Because a catheter is a foreign device, it can provide an artificial surface for organisms to create a biofilm. A **biofilm** is a polysaccharide slime layer that forms around organisms to allow them to adhere to an artificial surface and hide from antibiotics and the immune defense system. Biofilms are discussed in more detail later in this chapter under catheter-associated bloodstream infections.

Several guidelines can be followed to minimize the occurrence of catheter-related infection. These include avoiding unnecessary catheterizations, the use of a condom collection device for males or suprapubic catheter, removal of the catheter as soon as no longer needed, maintaining an uncompromised and closed drainage system (Maki & Tambyah, 2001), and perhaps the most important, insertion of the catheter by trained personnel who utilize strict aseptic (organism-free) technique (Gupta & Stamm, 2006).

Pathogenesis

Catheter-associated urinary tract infections (CAUTI) are caused by a variety of pathogens, such as the *Enterobacteriaceae,* which include *Escherichia coli, Klebsiella* spp., *Proteus* spp., *Enterobacter* spp., and *Serratia* spp., as well as *Pseudomonas* spp., *Enterococcus* spp., *Staphylococcus aureus,* and *Candida* spp. Most infections are caused by gram-negative organisms, which are part of the patient's **endogenous** (from within the body) bowel flora. Microorganisms can also be acquired by cross-contamination from other patients, hospital personnel, or by exposure to contaminated solutions or nonsterile equip-

ment. Although many microorganisms can cause UTIs, most catheter-associated cases are caused by only a few enteric organisms.

E. coli is the most common causative agent, but only a limited number of serogroups cause a significant proportion of UTIs. Numerous investigations indicate that these serotypes of *Escherichia coli* possess certain virulence factors that enhance their ability to colonize and invade the urinary tract. Some of these virulence factors include increased adherence to vaginal and uroepithelial cells by bacterial surface structures, alpha-hemolysin production, and resistance to serum killing activity. The chromosomes of some *Escherichia coli* strains have been shown to possess potential virulence factor genes associated with the acquisition and development of UTIs. These unique genes are encoded on a pathogenicity island, which is a cluster of genes only found in virulent strains and absent from avirulent or less virulent strains of the same species (Forbes, Sahm, & Weissfeld, 2007).

Urinary tract pathogens such as *Serratia marcescens* and *Burkholderia cepacia,* although rare, have special epidemiologic significance. These two organisms do not commonly reside in the gastrointestinal tract, and their isolation from catheterized patients suggests acquisition from an **exogenous** (from outside the body) source (Wong, 1981). They also tend to be resistant to multiple antibiotics.

 REAL WORLD TIP

The sampling port on the tubing of a urinary catheter must be used to collect a urine sample from a catheterized patient. Urine in the collection bag is not satisfactory for culture. Urine is a good culture medium for bacteria. The urine in the collection bag allows bacteria present to keep multiplying and will not provide an accurate colony count on culture or a true picture of the causative agent causing the infection.

Control Measures

Whether from endogenous or exogenous sources, infecting microorganisms gain access to the urinary tract by several routes. These include the catheter during insertion, its sampling port connecting the catheter to the drainage tubing, the urine flow through tubing, the collection bag, and the drainage outlet from the bag. Comprehensive infection control measures should address the risk of contamination via all possible routes. Several available products may address each potential route to prevent future infections.

For the microorganisms that inhabit the meatus or distal urethra, a Foley catheter with a silver alloy coating may be used to reduce bacterial adherence. Silver has an antimicrobial effect. For those pathogens that may enter the urine via sampling port in the drainage tubing, a seal and needleless safe sampling port may minimize the risk of contamination.

The seal functions as an indicator of the system opening and thus serves as a reminder to caregivers to keep the system closed.

To address the problem of microorganisms gaining access to the catheter lumen (interior), drainage tubing can be used that contains a unique antimicrobial agent that repels many common gram-positive and gram-negative bacteria as well as yeasts. For those bacteria that can migrate into the collection bag, a bacteriostatic (bacteria-inhibiting) collection bag can be used. The bag is impregnated with an antimicrobial agent that resists pathogens commonly associated with catheter-related urinary tract infection.

Finally, attention should also be directed to the bag's outflow spigot to reduce the chance of infection. A microbicidal outlet tube can be used to create a zone of inhibition against the most common organisms and protect against bacterial migration into the bag and up the tubing (Bard Medical, 2003).

Microbiology Laboratory and Urinary Tract Infections

Quantitative urine cultures for the diagnosis of UTI are used to discriminate between contamination, colonization, and infection. A culture determines whether an individual has a urinary tract (bladder or kidney) infection because the demonstration of bacteria is the only reliable means of making a specific diagnosis of bacteriuria (bacteria in the urine).

Specimen Collection

The avoidance of urethral flora is the most important criteria and is of clinical relevance when collecting urine for cultures. A catheterized urine specimen is usually collected by either a physician or professional health care worker. The collection process involves the acquisition of a urine sample by inserting a sterile thin rubber tube through the urethra into the bladder. Prior to insertion of the catheter, the nurse or physician washes the area thoroughly around the opening of the urethra. A well-lubricated catheter is then gently inserted and advanced until it enters the bladder. The urine drains into a sterile container, and the catheter is either removed or left in place, depending on the status of the patient.

If a urine sample cannot be obtained by conventional methods, a suprapubic bladder aspiration may be performed. This procedure entails the withdrawing of urine directly into a syringe through a percutaneously (through the skin situated over the bladder) inserted needle. This ensures a contamination-free specimen provided the skin was cleaned adequately. The bladder must be full before performing this procedure. It is suggested that suprapubic catheterization and aspiration is superior to clean-catch or transurethral (via catheterization) collection of bladder urine for bacteriologic study (Roth & Choi, 2006). Suprapubic collection is most often used for children and infants who cannot clean themselves appropriately prior to urine collection or are unable to urinate on demand. Refer to ∞ Chapter 34, "Urinary System," to review the processing of a urine sample.

 REAL WORLD TIP

A Foley catheter is not acceptable for culture. It is often colonized with multiple organisms. Urinary tract infections are usually because of a single organism. Free-flowing urine collected from the tubing provides the most accurate bacterial count on culture.

Catheterized Urine Culture Interpretation

Because most laboratories receive very little clinical patient information, urine culture interpretation can become complicated. Determining what is contamination and what is infection can become increasingly difficult. Many laboratories establish their own guidelines and interpretive criteria for urine cultures based on the type of urine submitted.

It is important to know that most UTIs are caused by a single pathogen in a predominant amount and there are usually a limited number of bacteria that cause UTIs. For example, the enteric gram-negative rods cause most urinary infections. In all urines, regardless of the extent of the final workup, all isolates should be enumerated (counted). A quantitative urine culture is used to determine bacterial counts indicative of "significant" bacteriuria. Significant counts can vary with the host and type of infection. For indwelling catheters, greater than 10^3 (1000) CFU (colony forming units) of potential pathogens/mL of urine should be considered significant.

Interpretation of a urine culture depends on the policies and procedures of a particular institution. Figure 41-2 ■ illustrates an **algorithm** or a flowchart that demonstrates the possible workup of a catheterized urine culture in a clinical microbiology laboratory setting. The use of an algorithm provides consistent workup of organisms from technologist to technologist. It eliminates subjective interpretation of policies and procedures and provides a more objective approach.

 REAL WORLD TIP

If a urine culture contains more than three organisms of mixed uropathogens and nonpathogens (i.e., diphtheroids, *Staphylococcus* not *S. aureus* (SNA), and streptococci), the laboratory should consider consolidating the report to state "polymicrobial growth consistent with normal urethral flora" and suggest specimen recollection. More than three organisms present in a catheterized urine culture indicates that the specimen was probably taken from the collection bag rather than free flowing in the tubing leading from the bladder to the bag.

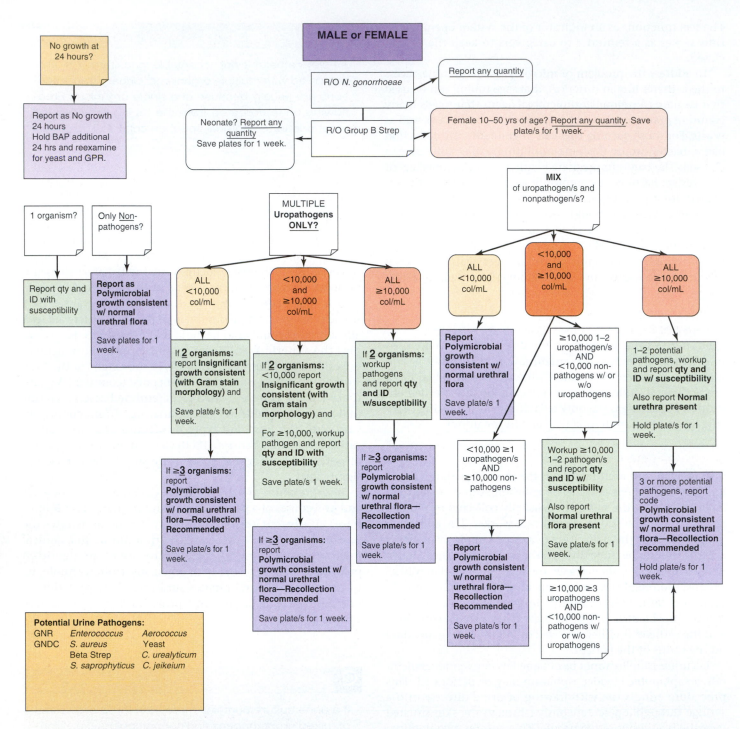

■ **FIGURE 41-2** Catheterized urine workup guidelines. The use of this flowchart eliminates the subjectivity that can occur with enumeration, level of workup and reporting of urine cultures with pure or mix growth of organisms.
Adapted from Isenberg, H. D. (1992). Clinical microbiology procedure handbook. *Washington, DC: American Society for Microbiology.*

Checkpoint! 41–3 (Chapter Objective 4)

Which of the following patients is most likely to develop a catheter-related urinary tract infection?

A. *An 11-month-old female, with a fever, requiring a suprapubic urine collection.*

B. *An 89-year-old male requiring an "in and out" catheterization because of urine retention.*

C. *A 27-year-old quadriplegic male with an indwelling catheter.*

D. *A 49-year-old female with a catheter during surgery for breast implants.*

SURGICAL AND WOUND NOSOCOMIAL INFECTIONS

Epidemiology

A wound is the result of physical disruption of the skin. The skin is the first line of defense against entry of organisms deeper into the body. Once bacteria are able to breach this barrier, infection can result.

The most common underlying event for all wounds is trauma. Trauma may be accidental or intentional such as surgery. Surgical infections can occur when (a) there is a break in surgical technique, (b) surgery involves a contaminated site such as the intestinal tract, (c) the surgery environment is not sterile, or (d) the surgical team sheds organisms.

One example of a hospital-acquired wound is a pressure sore or bedsore caused by local ischemia or decreased blood flow. It is also referred to as a decubitus ulcer because it is usually caused by lying down or remaining in a sitting position for long periods of time. With constant pressure over hard, bony areas such as the hip, tailbone, or heel, the skin and soft tissue can ulcerate because of the loss of blood supply. When the ulcer becomes infected, it is often colonized by multiple enteric bacterial species. Infections of hospital-acquired wounds are among the leading nosocomial causes of morbidity, mortality, and increasing medical expense, which adds between 10 to 20% to hospital costs (Giacometti et al., 2000; Nandi et al., 1999).

Pathogenesis

All surgical wounds are usually contaminated by bacteria, but only a minority actually go on to cause clinical infection (Fry, 2003). In most patients, infection does not develop because innate host defenses are quite efficient in the elimination of contaminants at the surgical site. Whether an infection occurs depends on several factors, with the most important being the number of bacteria entering the wound, type and virulence (ability to cause infection) of the bacteria, host defense mechanisms (i.e., effectiveness of inflammatory response and status of the immune system), and external factors, such as being in the hospital several days before surgery or the operation last-ing more than 4 hours. Two factors that can help minimize the number of organisms entering the wound are the skill and experience of the surgeon and the use of good surgical technique (Rubin, 2006).

Pathogens that infect surgical wounds can be acquired from an endogenous source of the patient or exogenous sources such as the hospital environment or personnel. Endogenous sources appear to be responsible for the most infections (Singhal, 2006). Sources of endogenous contamination include the gastrointestinal and genitourinary tract and the pathogens involved include gram-negative bacilli and gram-positive microbes, including *Enterococcus* spp. and anaerobes.

Exogenous contamination of a surgical incision is responsible for a substantial portion of infections in clean wounds. Exogenous contamination may come from any personnel or environmental source. Direct contact with the wound by the surgical team is probably the most common pathway for surgical wound infections. Most infections, endogenous or exogenous, appear as a result of contamination occurring in the operating room.

An **epidemic** is an outbreak of disease affecting a large number of individuals. Epidemics caused by *Staphylococcus aureus* and *Streptococcus pyogenes* (group A *Streptococcus*) suggest health care personnel carriers as a source (Topal, 2001). Epidemics caused by gram-negative microorganisms may be acquired from environmental sources, such as irrigating solutions and anesthesia or respiratory therapy equipment.

The most common group of bacteria responsible for surgical and wound infections include *Staphylococcus aureus* (including methicillin-resistant *S. aureus* [MRSA]), *Staphylococcus* not *S. aureus, Enterococcus* spp. (including vancomycin-resistant *Enterococcus* [VRE]), *Escherichia coli, Pseudomonas aeruginosa, Enterobacter* species, *Proteus mirabilis, Klebsiella pneumoniae,* other streptococci, *Candida albicans,* Group D *Streptococcus,* other gram-positive aerobes, and *Bacteroides fragilis* (Singhal, 2006). The emergence of resistant strains has considerably increased the mortality associated with wound infections.

Antibiotic use and abuse has pressured methicillin-resistant *Staphylococcus aureus* (MRSA) and vancomycin-resistant *Enterococcus* (VRE) to become the leading causes of hospital-acquired infections. Their multiresistance, ability to colonize debilitated individuals, and capacity to spread throughout the hospital environment has allowed them to exist in every health care facility on earth. MRSA has now escaped the hospital setting to become a challenge in the community as well. Go to ∞ Chapter 37, "Integumentary System," to review the collection and processing of wound-related specimens.

Control Measures

Reducing the pressure on the skin and tissue can prevent decubitus ulcers. Turning and repositioning the patient every 2 hours is essential in any health care environment. The use of foam or air-filled mattresses can also help relieve pressure. Frequent cleaning of the skin, to prevent urine and feces from contaminating the area, is also necessary. Once a decubitus

**Checkpoint! 41–4
(Chapter Objective 5)**

A 69-year-old female develops a decubitus ulcer while in the hospital for a broken hip. Which organism(s) would you expect to culture from this site?

   A. *E. coli*
   B. *Streptococcus pyogenes*
   C. *Enterococcus spp.*
   D. *A and C*
   E. *all the above*

ulcer is established, wound treatment requires careful cleaning, wound dressing, and antibiotic use. Depending on the extent of the wound, it may require surgery to remove necrotic tissue and reestablish blood flow to the infected area.

The most critical factors in the prevention of postoperative infections, although difficult to measure, are the sound judgment and proper technique of the surgeon and surgical team, as well as the general health and disease state of the patient (Nichols, 2001). There are several recommended guidelines for reducing the risk of surgical associated infections. For exogenous sources of infections, sterilization of instruments and suturing materials, positive pressure ventilation of operating theatres, laminar air flow in high-risk areas, and exclusion of staff with infections should be utilized.

To prevent infection originating from exogenous sources, the following should used: skin preparation, antibiotic prophylaxis, and good surgical technique. Preoperative skin preparation of a patient can reduce the infection rate in surgical site infection. The Centers for Disease Control and Prevention (CDC) advocates an antiseptic shower or bath provided the patient is ambulatory. The procedure requires the active participation of the surgical patient and should occur 6 to 12 hours before the time the surgical site is prepped. The preoperative antiseptic or bath has been shown to decrease skin microbial colony counts by ninefold (Seal & Paul-Cheadle, 2004). Preoperative surgical patient skin preparation has been shown to have a positive impact on surgical site infection rates and may eliminate some additional costs associated with this preventable event.

The skin preparation products currently used are compliant with the Food and Drug Administration (FDA) to ensure the presence of good chemistry between the patient's skin and the product used. In this manner, they are less likely to be irritating and more likely to be mutually enhancing so that there is additive effect when used with antimicrobics.

It has been long recognized that alcohol, either ethanol or isopropanol, is the most effective and rapid acting skin antiseptic. The use of scrubbing materials such as a bristled brush in conjunction with isopropyl alcohol may provide benefits on the skin preparation process prior to surgery (Keblish, Zurakowski, Wilson, & Chiodo, 2005). Because of alcohol's limited staying power, it may be mixed with iodophors, zinc pyrithione, and chlorhexidine gluconate (CHG). CHG has a slow antibacterial activity, but it remains active for 5 to 6 hours, which is longer than any other currently used preparation. In addition, CHG has one advantage over alcohols in that it retains antibacterial action in the presence of blood and other organic material. Combined, they can extend and provide a more powerful antimicrobial effect on surgical skin preparation than when used alone.

Another common practice performed prior to surgery is shaving the surgical site. Shaving can create minute cuts in the skin, providing entry sites for potential pathogens. The use of clippers just prior to surgery rather than a razor used the night before can reduce the risk for infection.

In addition to preoperative surgical skin preparation, patients who undergo colonic surgical procedures usually require a bowel preparation. This generally includes a mechanical bowel preparation and prophylactic antibiotics. The purpose of mechanical bowel preparation is to rid the colon of solid stool, thus reducing the bacterial load and minimizing the risk of infection and other complications. With improvements in surgical techniques and more effective prophylactic antibiotics, some practitioners believe that mechanical bowel preparation may no longer be necessary.

Another crucial factor in reducing exogenous sources in surgical site infection is the practice of a good surgical technique. This includes the scrubbing and disinfection techniques of surgeons prior to surgery. Proper hand washing is one of the most effective ways to reduce the spread of infection in health care settings, and it should be done before and after examining a patient, before putting on gloves for clinical procedures, and after removing gloves. Generally, aseptic techniques are performed just before or during a medical procedure and should include hand scrubbing as well as using physical barriers such as gloves, gowns, and surgical attires. Glove usage has been good in preventing infection, but gloves may give a false sense of security of protection against bacteria. They can provide an ideal environment for bacterial growth—moisture and warmth—so good hand-scrub technique is still valuable.

Perhaps the greatest area of interest in the prevention of surgical site infection has been the use of antibiotics. Ideally prophylactic (preventive) drugs should be directed against the most likely infecting organisms. For most procedures, an inexpensive first- or second-generation cephalosporin such as cefazolin, which has a moderately long half-life and is active against staphylococci and streptococci, has been effective when given intravenously. When methicillin-resistant *Staphylococcus aureus* (MRSA) are important postoperative pathogens, vancomycin can be used. Its routine use for prophylaxis should be avoided because it may promote the emergence of resistant organisms such as vancomycin-resistant *Enterococcus* (Infection Prevention Guidelines, n.d.b).

As the length of hospital stay after surgery continues to decline, a greater proportion of surgical site infections will occur after discharge; this presents challenges for the accurate monitoring of surgical infection rates. More research on methods to measure surgical site infection rates after hospital discharge is needed (Petherick, Dalton, Moore, & Cullum, 2006).

REAL WORLD TIP

Hyperglycemia can place surgical patients at increased risk for nosocomial infections. An increased serum glucose level tends to reduce the function of leukocytes. After surgery, if the patient's serum glucose is maintained at 80 to 120 mg/dL, there is a lower incidence of septicemia and surgical wound infections.

BLOODSTREAM INFECTIONS (INTRAVASCULAR DEVICE RELATED)

Epidemiology

Nosocomial bloodstream infection is defined by a positive blood culture obtained from patients who had been hospitalized for 48 hours or longer (Friedman et al., 2002), whereas a "bloodstream infection episode" is determined from the time the first positive blood cultures were obtained (Diekema et al., 2003). The use of intravascular devices, both venous and arterial, for delivery of sterile fluids, medications, and nutritional products, as well as for central monitoring of blood pressure and other hemodynamic functions, has dramatically increased (Best Practice, 1998). It is estimated that about 50% of all patients admitted to hospitals receive intravenous therapy, creating a large population at risk for local or systemic bloodstream infections.

Because catheters, inserted into the venous or arterial bloodstream, bypass normal skin defense mechanism, these devices provide a means for microorganisms to enter the bloodstream at the time of insertion, from subsequent contamination of the device or attachments (i.e., tubing connected to the blood monitoring apparatus) or the fluids being administered, or from the skin surrounding the insertion site.

Pathogenesis

A bloodstream infection is defined as the isolation of one or more recognized bacterial and fungal pathogens from one or more blood cultures (i.e., *Staphylococcus aureus, Streptococcus pneumoniae, Escherichia coli, Klebsiella* spp., *Proteus* spp., *Salmonella* spp., and *Candida albicans*). Other criteria used to define a bloodstream infection include the patient having at least one of the following signs and symptoms within 24 hours of a positive blood culture being collected: fever (>38°C), chills or rigors, or hypotension and the isolation of the same potential contaminant from two or more blood cultures drawn on separate occasions within a 48-hour period, where isolates are identified by suitable microbiological techniques (Australian Infection Control Association, 2006).

It is important to note that there has been a change in the distribution of pathogens reported to cause nosocomial bloodstream infections. Data from the National Nosocomial Infections Surveillance System (NNIS) from January 1990 to May 1999 indicates that *Staphylococcus* not *S. aureus* was isolated from bloodstream infections in patients in intensive care units more often than *Staphylococcus aureus*. *Staphylococcus* not *S. aureus* is found as part of the normal flora of human skin and mucous membranes; they have long been regarded as harmless skin commensals (Christensen, Simpson, Younger, & Baddour, 1985) and dismissed as culture contaminants. In recent years, however, their potentially important role as pathogens and their increasing incidence have been recognized.

One of the major challenges facing laboratories is distinguishing the clinically significant, pathogenic strains from contaminant strains. Infection is the major complication associated with the use of foreign bodies such as catheters. *Staphylococcus* not *S. aureus* is an important pathogen in bloodstream infections related to the use of vascular catheters, and *Staphylococcus epidermidis* is responsible for most catheter-related infections. About 50% of all hospitalized patients receive an intravascular device during their hospital stay.

REAL WORLD TIP

Staphylococcus haemolyticus and *S. lugdunensis* are coagulase-negative gram-positive cocci that can also cause infection because of medical devices. They can be presumptively identified using PYR and ornithine decarboxylase tests. Both are PYR positive, but *S. lugdunensis* is ornithine positive while *S. haemolyticus* is ornithine negative. Most microbiology laboratories do not routinely identify these two organisms to species because of the large battery of biochemical tests needed. A reference laboratory can perform the testing if needed.

Implanted, long-term catheters, such as a port-a-cath, have the lowest rates of bacteremia. The injection port is placed under the skin, which reduces potential skin contamination, provided the skin area is cleaned well prior to injection. Long-term Hickman or Broviac catheters are used for nutrition, medication, and fluids and to remove blood samples. They are placed under the skin of the chest wall and into the large vein leading to the heart. Peripherally inserted central catheters (PICC or PIC lines) are inserted into a peripheral vein and threaded into larger veins until it reaches the heart. Because of their prolonged use of these catheters and exposure to skin flora, as many as 30% of them become infected.

Medical devices, such as intravenous and urinary catheters, endotracheal tubes, artificial heart valves, and prosthetic joints, are used widely in acute care hospitals. *Staphylococcus* spp. are known for their affinity for artificial medical devices. Various virulence factors are involved in the ability of *Staphylococcus* spp. to cause medical device infections. The most important factor is the colonization of the foreign body's surface with organisms embedded in an extracellular matrix. The colonized bacteria and the extracellular material on a medical device are collectively referred to as a biofilm. The mass of microbial cells is irreversibly attached to a medical device surface and enclosed in a sticky matrix of primarily polysaccharide material (referred to as slime; Donlan, 2002; Souli & Giamarellou, 1998). Figure 41-3 ■ demonstrates the sticky mesh that makes up a biofilm on the interior of a catheter. The cocci are hidden under the material. It is easy to visualize why antibiotics and the body's natural immune defenses are not able to reach the organism.

Colonization of an intravenous catheter occurs quickly. The organisms travel from the skin surface and along the catheter's surface. With time they can also reach the interior surface or lumen of the catheter. As the biofilm grows, pieces can break off and travel through the blood. The organisms that reach damaged or artificial heart valves can attach and go on to cause endocarditis. There is a direct correlation between the number of organisms present on the catheter and the potential for bloodstream infection.

A number of factors can increase the risk of infection because of intravascular devices. For example, infection rates are higher among critically ill patients in large hospitals, those with burns or surgical wounds, or those who are malnourished or immunocompromised. Organisms usually reach the bloodstream by colonizing the catheter site, injection/sampling hub or through the fluid being infused. Contaminated equipment and solutions can provide microorganisms access to the bloodstream through cracks in the infusion bottles, punctures in plastic containers, nonsterile preparation of intravenous infusion fluid, and multiple changes of IV fluid containers while using the same IV administration set.

Checkpoint! 41–5 (Chapter Objective 6)

Which of the following gram-positive cocci is the most common causative agent of medical related device infections?
- A. *Catalase positive, coagulase positive, and oxacillin resistant*
- B. *Catalase negative, bile esculin, and 6.5% salt broth positive, vancomycin resistant*
- C. *Catalase negative, bile esculin, and 6.5% salt broth negative, optochin resistant*
- D. *Catalase positive, coagulase negative, thermonuclease negative*

Control Measures

To reduce the risk of nosocomial infection associated with all types of intravascular devices, one should use the following strategies: hand hygiene and gloves, site care and dressings, and site selection and rotation. The simple acts of washing one's hands and wearing clean examination gloves before touching an IV set will reduce the rate of nosocomial infections. With site care and dressing, the cleaning of the insertion site, especially if visibly dirty, with soap and clean water and drying it before applying the skin antiseptic should minimize the rate of infection. For adult intravenous catheter site selection and rotation, hand veins are preferred over arm veins, and arm veins over leg and foot veins. Rotating intravenous sites at 72 to 96 hours will reduce phlebitis or vein inflammation, which is an important complication associated with the use of peripheral venous catheters as well as local infection (Infection Prevention Guidelines, n.d.a).

Perhaps the most important recommendation for the prevention of nosocomial intravascular device related infection is education and training. Conducting ongoing education and training of health care workers regarding the management of intravascular devices and appropriate infection control measure is essential. In addition, both the surface and the lumen of the catheter can be impregnated with antibiotics to control colonization.

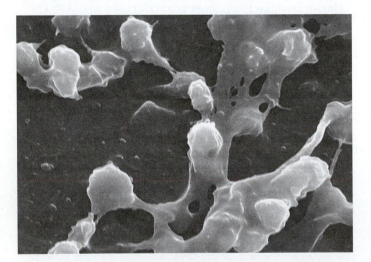

■ **FIGURE 41-3** This highly magnified electron micrograph depicted numbers of *Staphylococcus aureus* bacteria, which were found on the luminal surface of an indwelling catheter. Of importance is the sticky-looking substance woven between the round cocci bacteria, which was composed of polysaccharides and is known as "biofilm." This biofilm has been found to protect the bacteria that secrete the substance from attacks by antimicrobial agents such as antibiotics; magnified 2363×.
From the Centers for Disease Control and Prevention. Photo Credit: Janice Carr.

 REAL WORLD TIP

Antibiotics alone will not treat catheter-related infections. The biofilm present will always be a source of organisms as long as the infected catheter is in place. Removal and replacement of the medical device is often the only option.

Microbiology Laboratory and Bloodstream Infections (Intravascular Device Related)

The blood of healthy individuals is normally sterile, so the presence of microorganisms in the blood is of utmost diagnostic importance. When microorganisms multiply in the bloodstream at a rate faster than the reticuloendothelial system can remove them, the result is a state of bacteremia (Isenberg, 1992). The presence of microorganisms in a patient's bloodstream can be life threatening and associated with a significant mortality rate.

Specimen Collection

Blood for culture must be obtained using sterile methods. Refer to ∞ Chapter 6 ("Specimen Collection") and ∞ Chapter 32 ("Cardiovascular Systems") for more details.

Diagnosis of catheter-related bloodstream infections can be best made by culture of the catheter tip as well as concurrent blood cultures. A 2-inch piece, including the tip, of the catheter is aseptically removed and placed into a sterile container. Because of the potential for drying out, the catheter tip should be transported to the laboratory as soon as possible. Culture of the blood catheter is described in more detail in ∞ Chapter 32, "Cardiovascular Systems."

 REAL WORLD TIP

- If a patient has an intravenous catheter, blood cultures can be drawn from that arm provided they are collected below the IV site. If drawn above the IV line, the blood collected will be diluted with any fluids being infused.

- Blood cultures should not be drawn from the intravenous tubing or injection hub. These sites are difficult to clean and are easily contaminated with colonizing organisms.

BLOOD CULTURES INTERPRETATION

In general, each blood culture set includes a blood culture bottle designated for aerobic recovery and one for anaerobic recovery of bacteria. Because of the increasing incidence of organisms considered nonvirulent and part of indigenous microflora, the interpretation of blood culture has become more difficult.

Staphylococcus not *S. aureus* is a common inhabitant of the skin, and viridans *Streptococcus* is readily found as part of the normal upper respiratory tract flora. It can be difficult to determine the significance of these two organisms when they are isolated in blood cultures. They could be present because of contamination at collection or a true infection. The use of guidelines can assist with the culture workup of these two organisms. Figure 41-4 ■ provides a potential algorithm or work flow that can be used to distinguish probable pathogens from contaminants in adult blood cultures.

 REAL WORLD TIP

Although algorithms are valuable tools, one must remember they are not to be considered all inclusive and may not be accurate in every situation encountered. The microbiologist should use good, sound judgment when using algorithms. The algorithm should not replace a solid knowledge base, common sense, and lessons learned from experience. Always ask, "Does this result make sense in this situation?"

✓ Checkpoint! 41–6 (Chapter Objectives 6 and 8)

A 27-year-old female intravenous drug user is hospitalized for incision and drainage of several large abscesses on her arms. After surgery she receives antibiotics via a Hickman catheter. Two sets of blood cultures are drawn. At 24 hours the following results were obtained:

Blood culture set 1—aerobic bottle—gram-positive cocci in clusters seen; anaerobic bottle—no growth

Blood culture set 2—aerobic bottle—gram-positive cocci in clusters seen; anaerobic bottle—no growth

The positive bottles were plated to agar plates and incubated. After 24 hours incubation, the agar plates of both positive blood culture bottles revealed:

White, nonhemolytic colonies
Catalase positive
Coagulase negative

Using the algorithm in Figure 41-4, determine the significance of the organism isolated.

A. *Report Staphylococcus not S. aureus and results of susceptibility testing.*

B. *Report Staphylococcus aureus and results of susceptibility testing.*

C. *Report viridans Streptococcus and perform susceptibility testing on request only.*

D. *Report Staphylococcus not S. aureus and perform susceptibility testing on request only.*

Culture techniques can be used to diagnose catheter-related infections that quantitate the resulting bacterial growth and then determine its significance. Quantitative catheter cultures methods are used to attempt to differentiate colonization of the intravenous catheter from true infection. Each colony type is enumerated (counted) and presumptively identified by Gram stain and colonial morphology. Qualifying bacterial growth of 15 or greater colonies should be fully identified and tested for antimicrobial susceptibility and is considered as significant growth. On the other hand, qualifying bacterial growth of 14 or fewer colonies requires identification only and should be considered insignificant growth. There are, however, exceptions, such as *Staphylococcus aureus*, which is

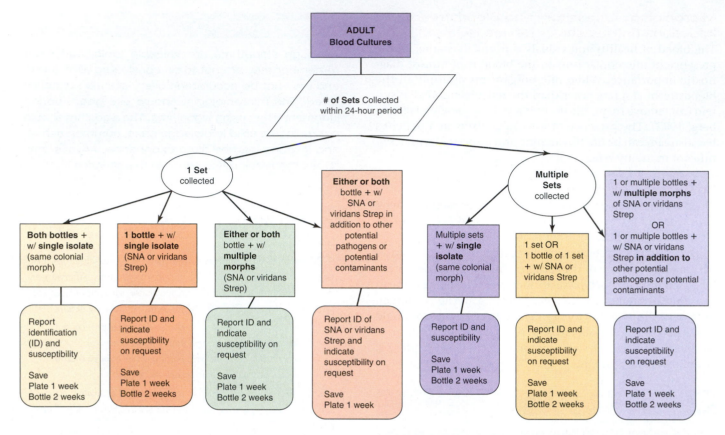

■ **FIGURE 41-4** Guidelines for reporting *Staphylococcus* not *S. aureus* (SNA) and viridans *Streptococcus* from blood cultures of adult patients. This algorithm/flowchart helps determine whether *Staphylococcus* not *S. aureus* and viridans *Streptococcus* should be considered significant or as a potential contaminant.
Adapted from Isenberg, H. D. (1992). Clinical microbiology procedure handbook. *Washington, DC: American Society for Microbiology.*

identified regardless of quantity. It should be screened for MRSA and the same concept applies for *Enterococcus* spp., which should be screened for VRE. These two organisms should always be considered true pathogens and significant in catheter-related bloodstream infections.

There are also various approaches taken in the diagnosis of catheter-related infection. One method is based on comparison of the blood cultures collected within 2 days prior to submission of the intravenous catheter and the catheter culture results. Figure 41-5 ■ provides an example of an algorithm for the interpretation and identification of significant or insignificant organisms found in blood cultures and the catheter tip culture.

VENTILATOR-ASSOCIATED PNEUMONIA

Epidemiology

Ventilator-associated pneumonia (VAP) is defined as nosocomial pneumonia in a patient on mechanical ventilatory support (by endotracheal tube or tracheostomy) for greater than or equal to 48 hours (Mayhall, 2001). Ventilator-associated pneumonia has a high mortality rate and has serious compli-

cations. Risk factors for ventilator-associated pneumonia include preexisting sinusitis and the administration of paralytic agent. Sinusitis allows organisms to drip down the back of the throat and potentially enter the lungs. Paralytic drugs depress the natural cough and gag reflexes.

The presence of an endotracheal tube is potentially the largest contributor. Most patients at risk for VAP are in the intensive care unit (ICU) or coronary care unit. There is a high rate of mortality for VAP because these patients are usually very ill.

Pathogenesis

Several factors affect the cause of ventilator-associated pneumonia. Such factors include severity of the patient's condition and level of consciousness, time of onset after hospitalization, stress-induced and antibiotic flora changes, quality of respiratory care, and exposure to contamination and colonization with nosocomial pathogens from personnel and the environment. Clinically pneumonia is difficult to diagnose in mechanically ventilated patients, and factors that complicate diagnosis include lack of respiratory symptoms in sedated patients on mechanical ventilation and the isolation of potential

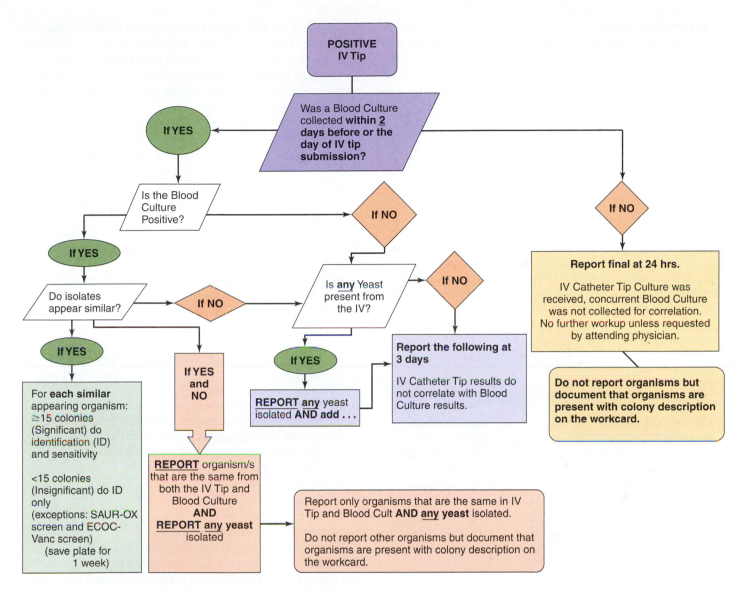

■ **FIGURE 41-5** IV tip culture guidelines for determining the significance of cultures of intravascular catheter tips. A culture of an intravascular catheter tip in combination with a patient's blood culture can determine the source of bacteremia. The culture of an intravascular catheter tip should be performed only when concurrent blood cultures are obtained.

pathogens from endotracheal secretions, which do not necessarily reflect the flora of the lower respiratory tract. Accurate data on the epidemiology of ventilator-associated pneumonia is limited because of the lack of standardized criteria for its diagnosis.

For microorganisms to cause VAP, they must first colonize the oropharynx and, with time, can enter the lower respiratory tract. Biofilms form on the endotracheal tube and can break free to enter the lungs. Pneumonia results from microbial invasion of the normally sterile lower respiratory tract and lung parenchyma because of a defect in host defenses, invasion by particular virulent microorganisms, or an overwhelming inoculum.

The normal human respiratory tract possesses a variety of defense mechanisms that protect the lung from infection, for example: anatomic barriers such as the glottis and larynx; cough reflexes; tracheobronchial secretions; mucociliary lining; cell-mediated and humoral immunity; and phagocytes, which include both alveolar macrophages and neutrophils. When these coordinated components function properly, invading microbes are eliminated, and clinical disease is avoided, but when these defenses are impaired or they are overcome by a high inoculum of organism or organisms of unusual virulence, pneumonitis results (Chastre & Fagon, 2002).

Another potential source of organisms is the presence of a feeding tube. The pH of the stomach is normally very acidic, which does not allow the growth of bacteria. With tube feeding, the pH can become elevated, allowing colonization by microorganisms especially gram-negative rods. These organisms can be regurgitated and aspirated into the lungs.

The microorganisms responsible for ventilator-associated pneumonia may differ according to the population of patients in the ICU and the duration of the hospital stay. The high rate of respiratory infections because of gram-negative bacilli has been repeatedly documented. The predominant gram-negative bacilli isolated on ventilator-associated pneumonia include *Pseudomonas aeruginosa* and *Acinetobacter* species, followed by the *Enterobacteriaceae* such as *Enterobacter* species, *Escherichia coli,* and *Klebsiella* species, as well as *Haemophilus influenzae.* More recently, gram-positive bacteria have been increasing, with *Staphylococcus aureus* (including MRSA) being the predominant gram-positive isolate. It is, however, important to note that underlying diseases may predispose patients to infection with specific organisms. For example, in a patient with chronic obstructive pulmonary disease (COPD), infections with *Haemophilus influenzae, Moraxella catarrhalis,* or *Streptococcus pneumoniae* are highly likely. Those suffering with cystic fibrosis have an increased risk for *Pseudomonas aeruginosa* and/or *Staphylococcus aureus* infection, whereas for those who have experienced trauma and neurological problems, *Staphylococcus aureus* is the most likely culprit.

 REAL WORLD TIP

Early onset ventilator-associated pneumonia usually appears within 4 to 5 days of intubation. It is associated with antibiotic sensitive organisms and has a better prognosis than late-onset VAP. Late-onset VAP appears after 5 days and is usually because of multi-antibiotic-resistant organisms such as *Pseudomonas aeruginosa, Klebsiella pneumoniae,* and *Acinetobacter baumannii.* Patients with late-onset VAP have a higher rate of mortality.

Control Measures

To help prevent ventilator-associated pneumonia, clinicians caring for patients who are receiving mechanical ventilation should participate in programs aimed at its prevention. These programs may be part of a general infection control effort directed at preventing nosocomial infections. In addition, nonpharmacologic strategies can be implemented to help prevent ventilator-associated pneumonia with simple yet effective efforts such as hand washing and the use of protective gowns and gloves. Hand washing is widely recognized as an important but underused measure to prevent nosocomial infections. If strict hand-washing techniques, combined with other measures of infection control, fail to control an outbreak of ventilator-associated pneumonia attributed to a specific high-risk pathogen, the respiratory therapy equipment or aerosol solutions are probably contaminated.

Pharmacologic preventions are also recommended in ventilator-associated pneumonia cases. These may include stress ulcer preventive treatment because patients receiving mechanical ventilation are at high risk for upper gastrointestinal (GI) hemorrhage. The downside to the use of GI ulcer prophylaxis is the neutralization of the stomach acid, which can allow colonization of organisms. The administration of aerosolized or topical prophylactic antibiotics has been shown to decrease oropharyngeal colonization.

Placing the ventilated patient in a semiupright position prevents the pooling of secretions, which can be a source of potential pathogens. It can also prevent aspiration from the gastric tube. Good oral hygiene such as brushing the teeth and swabbing the mouth is effective as a preventive measure. Frequent suctioning removes secretions that act as culture medium for microorganisms.

Microbiology Laboratory and Ventilator-Associated Pneumonia

A rapid determination of the etiologic agents involved in managing pneumonia is important. Diagnosis of this infection frequently is complicated by the contamination of specimens with upper respiratory tract secretions during collection. The upper respiratory tract may be colonized with potential pathogens not involved in the infection of the lower tract and may yield organisms capable of inhibiting the bacteria involved in lower tract pathology. The laboratory should ensure that an appropriate specimen is processed. The specimen must be microscopically examined both to assess its quality and to look for organisms associated with an inflammatory cell response (Isenberg, 1992).

An intubated patient cannot voluntarily provide an expectorated sputum specimen. Secretions of the tracheal tube can be suctioned and provided as a respiratory specimen. The use of tracheal secretions for diagnosis of VAP can be easily contaminated with colonizing organisms from the upper respiratory tract and biofilm on the ventilator and feeding tubings. This creates confusion for the microbiologist when interpreting these cultures. A bronchial alveolar lavage (BAL) may provide the most specific results because it bypasses contaminating flora. These are risks associated with this invasive procedure. The physician must weigh the risks with the value of the results provided. BAL specimens can be quantitated on culture because there is a correlation between the number of organisms present (10^3–10^4 organisms/mL) and the presence of pneumonia. Visit ∞ Chapter 33, "Respiratory System," to review the processing of specimens for respiratory pathogens.

 REAL WORLD TIP

Both *Acinetobacter* spp. and *Legionella* spp. are associated with nosocomial pneumonia but are uncommon compared to other gram-negative rods. Their isolation usually indicates an outbreak, which should trigger an investigation by the infection control team.

GASTROINTESTINAL INFECTIONS

Epidemiology

Hospital-acquired diarrhea is rarely caused by the traditional enteric bacterial pathogens such as *Salmonella* spp. and *Shigella* spp. However, food-borne illness, described in ∞ Chapter 35, can occur in the hospital setting. Many cases of diarrheal illness can be because of the side effects of antibiotics or other medications or stress related to being hospitalized.

The most common bacterial pathogen associated with diarrhea during hospitalization is *Clostridium difficile*. This spore-forming gram-positive anaerobic rod is found as normal flora in about 5% of adults and 30 to 50% of neonates. The spores produced can easily contaminate the hospital environment, the hands of health care workers, and instruments used on patients such as stethoscopes or blood pressure cuffs. The spores are very resistant to most commonly used cleaning disinfectants as well as alcohol, which makes them difficult to eradicate once established in the hospital environment.

Pathogenesis

Clostridium difficile is best known for antibiotic-associated diarrhea, which can appear up to 2 months after antibiotic use. The normal flora of the intestinal tract has the ability to prevent colonization by potential pathogens. Once the patient is exposed to and colonized with the spores of *C. difficile,* antibiotics, such as clindamycin and broad-spectrum cephalosporins, can inhibit the normal flora of the gastrointestinal tract. The spores regenerate and grow to produce toxins, which cause fluid secretion, inflammation, hemorrhage, and mucosal damage. The organism can cause a variety of diseases ranging from watery diarrhea to colitis to systemic infection. *Clostridium difficile,* its significance, and detection is discussed in detail in ∞ Chapter 24, "Anaerobic Bacteria."

REAL WORLD TIP

Other organisms are able to cause antibiotic-associated diarrhea. These include *Staphylococcus aureus*, *Candida* spp., and *Clostridium perfringens*. Once they are able to overgrow the normal flora of the gastrointestinal tract, *S. aureus* and *C. perfringens* produce enterotoxins that cause diarrhea. The pathogenicity mechanism of *C. albicans* is not fully understood.

Control Measures

Hand hygiene with traditional soap and water rather than alcohol-based cleansers and a clean environment are essential for controlling the spread of *C. difficile* spores. Closing patient rooms may be required when outbreaks occur. The careful use of antibiotics for absolutely no longer than necessary is also recommended. Although most disinfectants are not able to kill *C. difficile* spores, bleach has proven effective. The issue with bleach is that it cannot be used in all situations. Patient isolation and the use of specific, limited personnel in these areas can also be practiced but may not be practical.

Microbiology Laboratory and Gastrointestinal Infections

Because an individual can be colonized with *Clostridium difficile,* traditional culture is not effective for the diagnosis of *C. difficile* antibiotic-associated diarrhea. The presence of the organism does not correlate with disease. The presence of the toxin produced indicates disease. Detection of the toxin in stool is done by tissue culture assay or enzyme immunoassay. Only liquid stool specimens should be accepted for testing.

 ## Checkpoint! 41–7 (Chapter Objective 7)

A phlebotomist enters a patient's room to draw blood for a laboratory test. The patient is on isolation for Clostridium difficile. After completion of the blood draw and removal of her gloves, the phlebotomist should wash her hands with

   A. an alcohol-based cleanser.
   B. bleach.
   C. nothing. Her gloves protected her skin.
   D. old-fashioned soap and water.

▶ VIRAL NOSOCOMIAL INFECTIONS

EPIDEMIOLOGY

Viruses are capable of causing nosocomial infections. They are spread in the same manner as bacteria: endogenous and exogenous, including staff to patient, patient to patient, and visitor to staff or patient. Infants, children, and elderly tend to be more prone to viral infections, especially for those that have a seasonal cycle. Because viruses are so dependent on humans for transmission, the appearance of nosocomial viral infections are usually concurrent with viral infections in the community.

PATHOGENESIS

Respiratory syncytial virus, influenza A and B, parainfluenza virus, rhinovirus, and adenoviruses are the most common causative agents of nosocomial infections during the winter months. Infants and elderly are most prone to infection with these microorganisms. Infants are especially prone to respiratory syncytial virus. Transmission is via aerosol droplets.

Rotavirus and enterovirus are transmitted by the oral-fecal route. Rotavirus causes gastroenteritis in infants and children as well as the elderly during the winter to spring months. Enterovirus is a group of viruses that are shed by way of the oropharynx as well as the intestine. They are associated with febrile illness during the summer and fall.

Varicella-zoster virus (VZV) is known for causing chickenpox and shingles. It is transmitted by close direct contact. Although most cases of chickenpox occur in children and usually present with mild illness, adults can become very ill, with resulting pneumonitis and encephalitis. Shingles is a reactivated case of VZV that causes a painful skin rash in adults. VZV can be fatal for immunosuppressed individuals. Close contact is needed for transmission.

CONTROL MEASURES

Staff members as well as the patients and visitors can serve as the source of viral infections. The most important control measures have proven to be adequate hand washing and adherence to infection control policies such as the use of masks and gowns for staff and visitors for droplet containment. A hospital may choose to limit entry of visitors who exhibit signs and symptoms of viral illness, especially for immunosuppressed patients. Cohorting or cohabitation of individuals with the same viral illness can remove them as a source of infection for noninfected patients. Cohorting requires dedicated nursing staff who do not mix with the noninfected patient population. Vaccination of the staff is highly recommended. Health care workers who are exhibiting signs and symptoms of viral illness, such as a rash because of shingles, should avoid working with high-risk patients or may be placed on medical leave until no longer infectious.

MICROBIOLOGY LABORATORY AND VIRAL INFECTIONS

The laboratory can prove to be an asset for the containment of nosocomial viral infections. Many rapid viral stains and enzyme immunoassays now make the diagnosis much faster. Molecular methods have exploded on the scene and provide results for viruses that do not grow on routine culture. Key to ensuring the sensitivity and specificity of any microbiology test is education of health care workers on proper specimen collection. This is especially important for viruses. Remember that a properly collected specimen equals quality results. More details on viruses, their clinical significance, and testing can be reviewed in ∞ Chapters 16 ("Viral, Chlamydial, and Rickettsial Specimens") and 31 ("Intracellular Organisms").

REAL WORLD TIP

Rabies is usually not known to be present in the hospital environment. One thinks of the rabies virus being transmitted in an infected animal's saliva, but there have been cases of it being transmitted to patients who receive transplanted organs from an infected donor. Transplanted livers, kidneys, and corneas have passed the virus onto recipients, with their subsequent death.

▶ FUNGAL NOSOCOMIAL INFECTIONS

EPIDEMIOLOGY

Severely ill patients are living longer thanks to many advances in medicine. These patients are especially prone to fungal infections because of their immunocompromised state. There are certain patient groups at risk for fungal infections; these include individuals who are:

- On chemotherapy, steroids, or long-term antibiotics
- Neutropenic
- Immunosuppressed because of an organ transplant or other causes
- Diabetic or have other underlying medical and personal conditions such as drug use, malnourishment, extensive burns, or an indwelling catheter

Although most nosocomial infections are because of bacteria, fungi have now emerged as a potential nosocomial pathogen.

PATHOGENESIS

Candida spp. is well known in the hospital setting as a human pathogen. This organism can be part of the normal endogenous flora of the gastrointestinal, genitourinary, and respiratory tracts, as well as the skin. This makes this group of yeasts a potential nosocomial pathogen that can be transmitted to the patient via contaminated instruments or by direct contact. *Candida albicans* is the most common isolate, but *C. tropicalis, C. parapsilosis, C. krusei, C. lusitaniae,* and *C. glabrata* have emerged as pathogens. This may be because of the increased use of antifungal agents and the subsequent appearance of more resistant strains. Because of their presence on the skin, they can easily colonize indwelling catheters and go on to cause fungemia or fungus in the blood. They also cause oral infections such as thrush as well as antibiotic-associated diarrhea.

Malassezia spp. is a lipophilic (lipid-loving) yeast found on the oily areas of the skin. This organism is associated with bloodstream infections in newborns. Most patients who develop fungemia with *M. furfur* are receiving intravenous lipids and parenteral nutrition (nutrition provided to the individual via an intravenous line).

REAL WORLD TIP

A culture for *Malassezia furfur* requires that the agar plates be overlaid with sterile olive oil so this lipophilic organism will grow.

Aspergillus spp. infections in hospitalized patients are usually because of renovation, new construction, and contaminated air and ventilation systems. This mould is especially significant for infections in severely immunosuppressed patients such as those waiting for or receiving a transplant. It usually presents as pneumonia because of the inhalation of spores. It can also rapidly disseminate to cause a fatal systemic infection.

CONTROL MEASURES

Hand washing and adherence to infection control procedures are essential as control measures. Prophylaxis antibiotic therapy may inhibit normal flora and allow yeast to flourish. Physicians need to utilize antibiotics effectively to reach a balance between treating the patient and setting them up for infection. When yeast is implicated in catheter-related infections, the same control measures used for bacteria apply.

The use of routine environmental cultures for *Aspergillus* spp. is not practical as a preventive measure but may be necessary during outbreaks. Preventive maintenance and cleaning of the ventilation system is necessary, especially in areas in which patients are at high risk. Once the spores are in the environment, they can settle on inanimate objects such as the carpeting and be stirred up with each step.

MICROBIOLOGY LABORATORY AND FUNGAL INFECTIONS

Rapid testing for the detection of fungi has not materialized as quickly as it has for bacteria and viruses. Fungi are slow growing, which is frustrating for the physician who is trying to treat a severely ill patient. On culture, the presence of yeast or mould must be evaluated carefully by the microbiologist. Moulds are frequently contaminants in the laboratory and can randomly appear on culture plates. ∞ Chapters 14 ("Fungal Cultures") and 29 ("Medical Mycology") can provide detailed information on fungi and their isolation, significance, and identification.

 REAL WORLD TIP

A test using fluorescence in situ hybridization (FISH) with a peptide nucleic acid probe (PNA) has been developed for the detection of *Candida albicans* in blood cultures. Previously, traditional cultures could take up to 5 days to recover this organism. PNA FISH allows its detection directly from blood culture bottles in hours.

▶ PARASITIC NOSOCOMIAL INFECTIONS

Nosocomial infections because of parasites are usually rare. Intestinal parasites such as *Giardia lamblia* and *Cryptosporidium parvum* are common parasites, and individuals who are admitted to the hospital may harbor these organisms in their intestines. Nosocomial parasitic infections are possible with cross infection either via health care workers or the patients themselves. Proper hand washing techniques and maintaining a clean environment is necessary to prevent passing these organisms onto others.

Individuals may be admitted to the hospital infested with ectoparasites such as lice, mites, or fleas. These organisms require close contact for transfer to another individual. This allows for the potential for cross contamination with others.

Flies and cockroaches can be pests in the hospital environment. Flies are able to lay eggs in open wounds producing maggots. Cockroaches can spread organisms such as *Salmonella* spp. Maintaining a clean environment is essential to eliminate the presence of these insects.

REAL WORLD TIP

Maggots can be used to treat infected deep wounds when traditional methods fail. The maggots consume necrotic tissue, which restores blood flow to the site. They also kill microorganisms with their secretions.

▶ EMERGING ANTIMICROBIAL RESISTANCE

When the body's normal defenses cannot prevent or overcome a disease, the individual becomes ill. The physician then uses various treatments such as drugs to alleviate the patient's symptoms and to cure the patient of the disease. The term *chemotherapeutic agent* applies to any drug used for any medical condition. For many diseases, there are no treatments that eliminate the infectious agents. In these instances, the physician uses supportive therapies that rely on the body's immune defenses to fight off the infection. The simplest supportive therapies include rest and eating healthy foods. By following this advice, the body is best able to mount an immune response against the infection. The physician can also select drugs to maintain the comfort of the patient by limiting pain.

In contrast to supportive therapies, antimicrobial drugs are used to eliminate infecting agents. They act by killing microorganisms or by interfering with the growth of microorganisms. Numerous antimicrobial agents are available for treating diseases caused by microorganisms. Such drugs have become an essential part of modern medical practice.

The antimicrobial agents used in medical practice are aimed at eliminating infecting microorganisms. They can also act to prevent the establishment of an infection. Antibiotics, which are defined as antimicrobial substances produced by microorganisms, have been used in medicine only since the mid-1940s. Soon after the introduction of penicillin, it was recognized that bacteria could develop resistance to antibacterial agents (Emori & Gaynes, 1993). By 1948, most of the *Staphylococcus* spp. isolated were resistant to penicillin. As other antimicrobial agents were introduced, resistant organisms were isolated from infected patients or the environment. This has developed into a cycle of antimicrobial agent development, introduction to clinical use, and development of resistance, often to the point where the antimicrobial agent becomes quickly useless.

Multi-drug-resistant organisms (MDROs), including gram-positive cocci such as methicillin-resistant *Staphylococcus aureus* (MRSA) and vancomycin-resistant *Enterococcus* (VRE), gram-negative bacilli (GNB) such as carbapenem-resistant *Enterobacteriaceae* (CRE) and *Acinetobacter* spp. as well as *Mycobacterium tuberculosis* have important infection control implications that either have not been addressed or received only limited consideration in previous isolation guidelines. Increasing experience with these organisms is improving understanding of the routes of transmission and effective preventive measures. Transmission of MDROs is most frequently documented in health care facilities. All health care settings, including nursing homes and long-term care facilities, are affected by the emergence and transmission of antimicrobial-resistant microbes. The severity and extent of disease caused by these pathogens varies by the population affected and by the institution in which they are found.

MDRO, for epidemiologic purposes, are defined as microorganisms, predominantly bacteria, that are resistant to one or more classes of antimicrobial agents (Siegel et al., 2006). Although the names of certain MDROs describe resistance to only one agent such as MRSA and VRE, these pathogens are frequently resistant to most available antimicrobial agents. In addition to MRSA and VRE, certain gram-negative bacilli, including those producing extended spectrum beta-lactamase (ESBLs) such as *Escherichia coli* and *Klebsiella* species, strains of multi-drug-resistant *Acinetobacter baumannii* as well as the emergence of third-generation cephalosporin-resistant *Enterobacter* species have become prominent. Other resistant organisms such as *Streptococcus pneumoniae* resistant to penicillin and macrolides and strains of *Staphylococcus aureus* intermediate and resistant to vancomycin have emerged as well (Siegel et al., 2006). Information related to the detection of MDROs can be found in ∞ Chapter 11, "Susceptibility Testing."

GRAM-POSITIVE ORGANISMS

Nosocomial infections with multi-drug-resistant organisms are occurring with alarming frequency, and the number of cases caused by these organisms increases each year. The most common of all isolates include methicillin-resistant *Staphylococcus aureus* (MRSA) and vancomycin-resistant *Enterococcus* (VRE; Smith, Dushoff, Perencevich, Harris, & Levin, 2004).

MRSA appeared in 1961 only 1 year after the introduction of methicillin. It has now become one of the most prevalent pathogens causing nosocomial infections. *Staphylococcus aureus* has always relied on beta-lactamase to destroy the beta-lactam antibiotics such as penicillin and the cephalosporins. Oxacillin and methicillin are not susceptible to beta-lactamase. After methicillin's introduction, *S. aureus* began to produce a unique penicillin-binding protein called PBP2' or PBP2a. This protein does not allow oxacillin and methicillin to bind and inhibit cell wall synthesis. This results in methicillin and oxacillin resistance. PBP2' is encoded by the *mec*A gene (Katayama, Robinson, Enright, & Chambers, 2005; Katayama, Zhang, Hong, & Chambers, 2003; Kwon et al., 2005). The beta-lactam antibiotics, such as penicillin and cephalosporins, also cannot bind to PBP2a at therapeutic concentrations and therefore are ineffective against infections caused by methicillin-resistant *Staphylococcus* spp.

Recently, MRSA infections have increasingly been reported among groups of individuals with no apparent connection to hospitals. These community-acquired (CA)-MRSA strains are on the rise but not yet to the same level as the hospital strains. CA-MRSA is characteristically susceptible to many antibiotics and contains no other antibiotic resistance genes except *mec*A. In contrast to CA-MRSA, the majority of hospital-acquired MRSA (HA-MRSA) strains display characteristics of multidrug resistance. One theory is that CA-MRSA strains might have originated from hospital-acquired MRSA strains and have undergone deletions of some antibiotic-resistant genes because of low antibiotic selective pressure in the community (Kwon et al., 2005).

Nosocomial infections with MRSA are a major health care problem in most developed countries. Despite an increasing number of reports on infections caused by so-called CA-MRSA, the majority of MRSA infections are still hospital related. Asymptomatic carriage of MRSA is now endemic among hospitalized patients in many countries, such as the UK, Germany, and Belgium, with reported cases of staphylococci bloodstream infections caused by MRSA.

Scandinavian countries and the Netherlands, however, have maintained relatively low levels of nosocomial MRSA infections, presumably because of nationwide policies to identify MRSA carriage and specific infection control measures for managing colonized patients. This so-called search and destroy policy was implemented in the 1980s. Although successful, this strategy is not based on well-designed studies (Bootsma Diekmann, & Bonten, 2006).

There is, however, an important distinction made in the epidemiology of multi-drug-resistance organisms between infection and colonization. Infection is characterized by serious illness when MDROs contaminate wounds, the bloodstream, and other tissues. On the other hand, colonization with MDROs may occur in the gut, nasal cavities, or other body surfaces. Colonizing bacteria may exist for years without causing disease or harm, and such individuals are called carriers (Smith et al., 2004). These carriers increase colonization pressure, which in turn increases the risk of turning another patient into a carrier or acquiring a resistant infection.

It is important to note that MRSA may behave different from other MDROs. When patients with MRSA have been compared to patients with methicillin-susceptible *Staphylococcus aureus* (MSSA), MRSA-colonized patients more frequently develop symptomatic infections. Also, it has been observed that certain MRSA infections cause higher fatality rates. These outcomes may result in delays in the administration of vancomycin, the relative decrease in the bactericidal activity for vancomycin, or persistent bacteremia associated with certain MRSA strains (Siegel et al., 2006).

As a consequence of the rise in MRSA isolates, vancomycin use in many U.S. hospitals appears to be on the rise. The CDC has received confirmed reports of vancomycin-resistant *Staphylococcus aureus* among clinical isolates (Centers for Disease Control [CDC], 2002, 2004). The development of a vancomycin-resistant *Staphylococcus aureus* can have disastrous public health consequences because effective alternative antibiotic treatment may not be available in the United States (Emori et al., 1993).

With the increased use of vancomycin for treatment of MRSA, vancomycin-resistant *Enterococcus* spp. have now emerged. The prevalence of vancomycin-resistant *Enterococcus* (VRE) has been linked with increased mortality, length of hospital stay, admission to ICU, surgical procedures, and costs. VRE may serve as a reservoir of resistance genes that can be passed to other organisms via plasmids to create a more virulent strain. Methicillin-resistant *Staphylococcus aureus* has been shown capable of acquiring and expressing vancomycin resistance in the laboratory (Emori et al., 1993). In 2002, the first case of vancomycin-resistant *S. aureus* (VRSA) was documented in the United States.

Much like the disastrous appearance of a vancomycin-resistant *Staphylococcus aureus,* the appearance of linezolid-resistant, vancomycin-resistant *Enterococcus* (LR-VRE) has complicated the management of such organisms. Linezolid, the first drug in the oxazolidinone class, was approved for use in the United States in March of 2000 for the treatment of infections caused by gram-positive cocci including VRE. Studies have now reported cases of linezolid resistance in *Enterococcus* spp.

The clinical management of enterococcal infections has been greatly compromised by the emergence of vancomycin-resistant strains over the past two decades. Linezolid is one compound useful for treating these resistant organisms, but the advent of LR-VRE makes clinical management a bit more difficult to handle because it greatly limits available treatment options.

GRAM-NEGATIVE ORGANISMS

In recent years, several reports have emphasized the development of antibiotic resistance among gram-negative bacilli, especially *Pseudomonas aeruginosa, Acinetobacter* species, *Klebsiella pneumoniae,* and *Enterobacter* species. These organisms are increasing in incidence among nosocomial pathogens largely because of their ability to express certain resistance phenotypes (Emori et al., 1993).

Beta-lactam antibiotics are widely used in the treatment of bacterial infections. However, the production of extended-spectrum beta-lactamase (ESBLs), one of the resistance mechanisms encountered in some *Enterobacteriaceae,* has been associated with several treatment failures (Moubareck et al., 2005). With the use and availability of second- and third-generation cephalosporins and other extended-spectrum beta-lactam agents, the concern over resistance to these agents has been escalated. *Klebsiella* spp. are prime examples. *Klebsiella pneumoniae,* a gram-negative bacillus, is an important hos-

pital-acquired pathogen with the potential to cause severe morbidity and mortality in patients (Cartelle et al., 2004). Resistance to beta-lactam antimicrobial agents in gram-negative bacilli is primarily mediated by beta-lactamases. These beta-lactamases can extend their spectrum of enzyme activity to include penicillins, the extended-spectrum cephalosporins such as ceftazidime, and aztreonam and now include carbapenemases as well (Steward et al., 2001).

Other types of resistance among nosocomial gram-negative bacilli also have become apparent. Imipenem, the broadest-spectrum parenteral antimicrobial agent that is commercially available, has remained useful in treating gram-negative infection. Resistance has now developed because of a beta-lactamase (Emori et al., 1993). Imipenem resistance has been found to be common in *Enterobacter* isolates as well as in *Pseudomonas aeruginosa* in teaching hospitals. Most are isolates from respiratory tract versus bloodstream, urinary tract, or surgical wounds. In December 2003, aminoglycoside-resistant *Enterobacter cloacae* appeared. With the assistance of a classical surveillance (monitoring) system (CSS), it was found to be caused by the spread of a specific clone. Based on genotyping of clinical strains of *Enterobacter cloacae,* it was concluded that aminoglycoside-resistant *Enterobacter cloacae* has actually been present since April 2001 (Leverstein-van Hall et al., 2006).

The prevalence of MDROs varies widely based on geography and even individual hospitals. During the last several decades, the prevalence in U.S. hospitals and medical centers has increased steadily. It is important to understand that once MDROs are introduced into a health care setting, transmission and persistence of the resistant strain is determined by the variety and acuity of patients, selective pressure exerted by antimicrobial use, and increased potential for transmission from large numbers of colonized or infected patients. The impact of implementation and adherence of prevention efforts becomes very important.

 Checkpoint! 41–8 (Chapter Objective 9)

Which of the following are the two most common gram-positive MDROs encountered in a hospital environment?

  A. *MRSA and VRE*
  B. *MRSA and MSSA*
  C. *VRE and VSSA*
  D. *VRE and MSSA*

▶ INFECTION CONTROL AND ITS ROLE IN PREVENTING NOSOCOMIAL INFECTIONS

Preventing infections will reduce the burden caused by MDROs in health care settings. Prevention of antimicrobial resistance depends on appropriate clinical practices, which should be incorporated into all routine patient care. The success of the hospital's infection control efforts hinges to a large extent on the active involvement of the microbiology laboratory in all aspects of the infection control program.

Infection control refers to the policies and procedures used to minimize the risk of spreading infections, especially in hospitals and other health care facilities. The purpose of infection control is to reduce the occurrence of infectious diseases. In the 1940s and 1950s, severe *Staphylococcus aureus* pandemics (a disease that is prevalent over a large area) caused substantial morbidity and mortality in U.S. hospitals. In 1958, because of such pandemics, the Joint Commission recommended that hospitals appoint infection control committees.

Faced with growing numbers of drug-resistant pathogens, increasing use of high-risk medical interventions, and the introduction of more immunosuppressive agents and therapies, hospitals, along with regulatory and accrediting organizations, began to realize that a committee alone cannot adequately deal with the problem of nosocomial infections. In the 1960s, infection control programs began, and professionals, including physicians, registered nurses, clinical laboratory scientists, pharmacists, and respiratory therapists, became major members of hospitalwide infection control programs. The Joint Commission has had considerable influence on the hospital adoption of infection control programs.

CDC, through its guideline development, nosocomial infection surveillance (monitoring) methodology, outbreak investigations, and laboratory studies, has provided much of the scientific and epidemiologic basis for infection control in the United States. Its landmark study on the efficacy of nosocomial infection control (SENIC Project) demonstrated that to be effective, nosocomial infection programs must include the following components: organized surveillance (monitoring) and control activities, adequate number of trained infection control staff, and a system for reporting surgical site infections (SSI) to surgeons (Emori et al., 1993).

There are various types of interventions used to control or eradicate MDROs, and they can be grouped into seven categories. These include administrative support, careful use of antimicrobials, surveillance (monitoring), standard and contact precautions (detailed infection control practices used to prevent the spread of infectious agents), environmental measures, education, and decolonization.

With administrative support, interventions include implementing system changes to ensure prompt and effective communications in identifying patients previously known to be colonized or infected with MDROs, providing the necessary number and appropriate placement of hand washing sinks and alcohol-containing hand rub dispensers in the facility, maintaining staffing levels appropriate for the level of care required, and enforcing adherence to recommended infection control practices such as hand hygiene and standard and contact precautions (discussed later in this chapter).

For generations, hand washing with soap and water has been considered a measure of personal hygiene. Organisms are often acquired by hospital workers during direct contact with patients or contact with contaminated environmental surfaces within close proximity of the patient. The hands of health care workers may become persistently colonized with pathogenic flora such as *Staphylococcus aureus,* gram-negative bacilli, and yeasts. It has been documented that although the number of transient and resident flora varies considerably from person to person; it is often relatively constant for any specific person. There have been many discussions on which method of hand washing is ideal, whether it be cleaning by the use of plain old soap and water or by using alcohol-based solutions. Regardless of which is the preferred method, adherence to recommended hand hygiene practices in the prevention of nosocomial infection must become part of a culture of patient safety (CDC, 2002a).

℮ REAL WORLD TIP

While washing your hands, sing the "Happy Birthday" song or recite the "ABCs." It takes approximately 20 seconds from start to finish and will ensure adequate hand hygiene and limit the spread of infection. Singing or talking out loud is optional.

Another major intervention is education. Education campaigns to enhance adherence to hand hygiene practices in conjunction with other control measures have been associated with decreases in MDRO transmission in various health care settings. Attention to the careful use of antimicrobics has also become highly important. The CDC campaign to prevent antimicrobial resistance was launched in 2002. It provides evidence-based principles for the wise use of antimicrobials and tools for implementation. This effort targets all health care settings and focuses on effective antimicrobial treatment of infections, use of narrow-spectrum agents, treatment of infections and not contaminants, avoiding excessive length of therapy, and restricting use of broad-spectrum or more potent antimicrobials to treatment of serious infections when the pathogen is not known or when other effective agents are unavailable. Achieving these objectives will most likely diminish the proliferation of MDROs.

Surveillance is defined as the ongoing, systematic collection, analysis, and interpretation of health data essential to the planning, implementation, and the evaluation of public health care practice, closely integrated with the timely dissemination of these data to those who need to know (Emori et al., 1993). Surveillance allows the detection of newly emerging pathogens, monitoring epidemic trends, and measuring the effectiveness of interventions.

One method of MDRO surveillance is monitoring clinical microbiology isolates and their antibiotic resistance patterns and documenting the results. An **antibiogram** is a tool that compiles the antibiotic susceptibility results for specific organisms for a health care facility over the course of 1 year. The clinical microbiology laboratory maintains the antibiogram and shares it annually with the physicians and pharmacists. Figure 41-6 ■ provides an example of an antibiogram. It is use-

Organism (# tested)	Ampicillin	Ampicillin/ Sulbactam	Aztreonam	Cefazolin	Ceftazidime	Ceftriaxone	Clindamycin	Gentamicin	Levofloxacin	Nitrofurantoin	Rifampin	Tobramycin	Trimethoprim/ Sulfamethoxazole	Tetracycline	Vancomycin
MRSA (700)							46	98		100	98		95	95	100
SNA (550)							58	66		100	95		65	89	100
VRE (365)	24								99	44					
S. pneumoniae (170)						90	80		99				58		
E. coli (1020)	60	68	98	92	97	98		91	86	99			98	98	
K. pneumoniae (435)		78	93	91	93	93		98	92	74			94	92	
P. aeruginosa (425)			76		83			84	80			93			

The number in each column indicates % sensitive isolates.

■ FIGURE 41-6 An example of a hospital antibiogram. This simple antibiogram lists only some of the more common isolates and antibiotics used for treatment. Susceptibility data is compiled for 1 year and displayed as a table listing the most common isolates and antibiotics. Susceptibility is listed as a percentage against each appropriate antibiotic. The data can also be reported by unit in a large facility. Providing this data allows physicians to see how organisms isolated in the hospital react with certain antibiotics. It also allows infection control to look for patterns of emerging resistance. Pharmacy can use the data to better direct proper use of antibiotics by physicians.

ful to detect emergence of new MDROs not previously detected, either within an individual health institution or community wide. Results can be compared from year to year to look for trends in resistance and antibiotic use. It is also a good source of information that can prepare a facility for a specific prevalence of resistance among clinical isolates.

An antibiogram can guide the physician to a specific treatment before culture results are available. It can also be utilized by the pharmacy department to better direct the proper use of antibiotics by physicians. Realize that the infection control team does not depend only on the annual antibiogram for monitoring isolates. They also review the microbiology results on a daily basis.

Other kinds of surveillance programs include the use of clinical microbiology to calculate measures of incidence of MDRO isolates in specific patient populations. Clinical cultures can also be used to identify MDRO infection, but some require molecular typing of isolates to confirm clonal transmission. This provides a better understanding of MDRO transmission and the effect of interventions. Another use is the active surveillance cultures (ASC) to identify patients and coworkers who are colonized with an MDRO. More research is necessary to determine which ASCs are most beneficial. Their use should be considered in some areas, especially if other control measures have been ineffective.

Since 1996, the CDC has recommended the use of standard and contact precautions for MDROs. **Standard precautions** are specific practices that follow the rule that all bodily fluids and secretions can transmit infection agents. These practices include hand hygiene and use of gloves, gowns, and eye and mouth protection. Standard precautions are followed for all patients (infected and noninfected) and their body fluids and have an essential role in preventing MDRO transmission. **Contact precautions**, on the other hand, are practices intended to prevent transmission of infectious agents, which are transmitted by direct or indirect contact with patient or the patient's environment. These include transmission via droplets and airborne as well. A private room is preferred for patients who require contact precautions. Health care professionals should wear gown and gloves for interactions when dealing with contact precaution patients. A mask is required for airborne pathogens. Donning gown and gloves on room entry and discarding before exiting the patient room helps contain the pathogens.

The role of environmental reservoirs, such as surfaces and medical equipment, in the transmission of MDROs has been the subject of many reports. Although environmental cultures are not routinely recommended, they have been used in several studies to show contamination and thus leading to interventions and awareness of dedicated education of personnel as well as the cleaning of medical equipment and disinfection of frequently used surfaces.

Finally, decolonization involves treatment of patients and personnel colonized with specific MDROs, usually MRSA, to eradicate carriage of the organism. Up to 20% of health care workers can be asymptomatic carriers of MRSA. The decolonization of MRSA in the patient's nares (nose) has been proven possible with several regimens that include topical mupirocin alone or in combination with orally administered antibiotics such as rifampin in combination with trimethoprim-sulfamethoxazole or ciprofloxacin plus the use of antimicrobial soap for bathing (Boyce, 2001).

REAL WORLD TIP

Household pets, especially dogs, can carry and potentially pass MDROs such as methicillin-resistant *Staphylococcus aureus* to their owners. This may be an important piece of the puzzle when investigating the source of an infection.

The microbiology laboratory should be involved in all aspects in the management of reducing the emergence of organism resistance. Tracking infection rates is necessary to compare the hospital's infection experience with that of other hospitals or at its own hospital over time. Much has been learned in the past 30 years about how epidemiologic techniques can be used to prevent and control nosocomial infections (Emori et al., 1993). With selection of appropriate infection control measures, the reduction of MDRO burden can be overcome.

REAL WORLD TIP

Because of the dangling effect of a necktie, which is a traditional symbol of male medical authority, it should be considered for epidemiological reasons as a source of increased risk in passing infection from one patient to another.

Checkpoint! 41–9 (Chapter Objectives 8 and 11)

A 67-year-old male is hospitalized for left knee replacement. While receiving intravenous antibiotics, he develops diarrhea because of Clostridium difficile. What infection control practices should be used for this patient?

    A. Standard precautions
    B. Contact precautions
    C. No precautions are necessary
    D. Hand washing only is necessary

▶ THE MICROBIOLOGY LABORATORY AND ITS ROLE IN PREVENTING NOSOCOMIAL INFECTIONS

The microbiology laboratory must be an enthusiastic member of the infection control team. The data provided by the laboratory is invaluable for surveillance and epidemiologic studies.

Microbiologists review laboratory results every day. The data available in the microbiology lab is similar to a gold mine. A microbiologist can be compared to a gold miner. They are able to dig through the data and discover the unusual isolates and resistance trends. This "early-warning system" provides the infection control team with a valuable resource that can help prevent outbreaks and provide for early response once a trend is detected. The microbiology laboratory is also responsible for the compilation of data that makes up the health care facility's annual antibiogram.

Communication, between the infection control team and the microbiology laboratory is absolutely essential. It is very frustrating when requests for environmental and personnel cultures appear in the microbiology laboratory with little or no information on the reasoning behind them. Outbreak investigational, environmental, and personnel cultures must be coordinated between both parties to ensure the cultures are collected, processed, and interpreted correctly. Once organisms have been isolated and identified, the microbiology laboratory stores the organisms, either by freezing or lyophilization, for additional testing as needed.

Phenotypic testing of organisms has been the standard in the microbiology laboratory for many decades. This traditional method of testing using biochemical tubes, agar plates, reagents, and can sometimes take 1 to 2 days or even more to complete. Results are needed much quicker now to track and contain nosocomial pathogens. Microbiologists must remain informed of new technologies and incorporate them when the benefit of rapid results outweighs the cost of the technology.

Molecular diagnostics has risen to the challenge that nosocomial infections have thrown at health care facilities. Molecular typing or DNA fingerprinting can differentiate organisms at the genetic level within hours. This technology allows the laboratory to determine the strain relatedness between organisms to determine a transmission route.

Molecular testing can also be used to detect specific resistance, such as the *mec*A gene in MRSA, much quicker than traditional cultures and susceptibility testing. Many health care facilities are now screening incoming patients for MRSA colonization using real-time polymerase chain reaction. Results are available in about 2 hours. This rapid turnaround allows the infection control team to know in advance if a patient has MRSA or not and make decisions on their placement within the facility. A patient entering the facility with MRSA may require cohorting with another who is also colonized with the organism. If a previously colonized patient develops an MRSA infection, further molecular testing must be done to determine if it is the same strain as the one colonizing the patient. A patient who is not colonized with MRSA and later develops a MRSA infection must be investigated to determine the nosocomial source of the infectious agent.

An experienced microbiologist is an excellent candidate for employment in the hospital's infection control department. This area is usually exclusively staffed by nurses. The knowledge and skills brought by the microbiologist is a perfect complement to those of the nurses.

Checkpoint! 41–10 (Chapter Objectives 10 and 11)

The identification and susceptibility data provided by the microbiology laboratory is used in many ways. A physician suspects a hospitalized burn patient has developed an infection because of Pseudomonas aeruginosa. What can the physician do to narrow down the antibiotic choices for treatment of this organism before the patient's culture results are available?

A. *Request molecular typing for the presence of resistance genes.*

B. *Review the hospital's antibiogram.*

C. *Review past environmental cultures of the burn unit.*

D. *Wait until culture results are available for this patient.*

SUMMARY

Nosocomial infection represents an enormous patient safety and economic problem in today's health care. Many of these infections lead to the death of hospitalized patients or, at minimum, additional complications and antimicrobial chemotherapy. To minimize nosocomial infection, substantial efforts in infection control need to be made. Simple hand washing still represents the cornerstone of modern infection control programs today. The microbiology laboratory must step up and be actively involved in all elements of the infection control program.

LEARNING OPPORTUNITIES

1. When are infections considered nosocomial? (Chapter Objective 1)

   a. 48 hours or greater after hospital admission

   b. Within 30 days after discharge

   c. a and b

   d. none of the above

2. What is the most important factor in the initiation of infection because of medical devices? (Chapter Objective 6)

   a. Cross contamination

   b. Immunocompromised state

   c. Contaminated equipment

   d. Colonization of organisms because of formation of a biofilm

3. Extended-spectrum beta-lactamases are commonly associated with which of the following nosocomial organisms? (Chapter Objective 9)

   a. *Klebsiella pneumoniae*

   b. *Acinetobacter baumannii*

   c. Vancomycin-resistant *Enterococcus*

   d. Methicillin-resistant *Staphylococcus aureus*

4. A catheterized urine on a female is received in the microbiology department. After incubation, the culture reveals 5,000 colonies/mL of diphtheroids and 50,000 colonies/mL of *Enterococcus* spp. Based on the results and using the algorithm in Figure 41-2, the microbiologist will report (Chapter Objective 8)

   a. normal urethral flora for the diphtheroids and the quantity, identification, and susceptibility for the *Enterococcus* spp.

   b. the quantity, identification, and susceptibility for both organisms

   c. polymicrobial growth consistent with normal urethral flora

   d. the quantity, identification, and susceptibility for the diphtheroids and normal urethral flora for the *Enterococcus* spp.

CASE STUDY 41-1 (CHAPTER OBJECTIVES 5, 7, 9, AND 10)

A 50-year-old male traveling salesman was experiencing left arm discomfort. He ignored the pain and reasoned it away as being because of his heavy sample case and workload. Because of his many travels, his dietary history included coconut donuts, carrot cake, pizza, Chinese food, and beer. On his way home on a Saturday morning, the pain reoccurred as he complained about it to his wife on the phone. His wife asked him to pick a birthday gift for their future son-in-law, but the pain grew more intense. He finally drove himself to the emergency room and was diagnosed with a myocardial infarction. He underwent quadruple bypass surgery because of greater than 90% blockage of his arteries. Two days after surgery, an x-ray of his chest revealed a left lower infiltrate with pleural effusion. A chest tube was attached to drain the fluid. Pus was noted on his sternal wound. Blood cultures were collected along with fluid from his chest tube drainage, tracheal aspirates and pus from his sternal wound. The laboratory results revealed gram-positive cocci in clusters, which are yellow, β-hemolytic colonies on blood agar. The organism is catalase and coagulase positive.

1. What is the most likely organism causing his infection? (Chapter Objective 5)

2. The organism revealed the following Kirby-Bauer disk susceptibility results:

Penicillin—R	Oxacillin—R
Gentamicin—R	Vancomycin—S
Erythromycin—R	Clindamycin—R
Trimethoprim/Sulfamethoxazole—S	

   Key: S = susceptible, R = resistant

   How would you interpret these susceptibility results? (Chapter Objective 9)

3. Is this organism recovered more frequently as a nosocomial pathogen, a community-acquired pathogen, or equally in both settings? Explain your choice. (Chapter Objective 5)

4. If this organism was found to be strictly hospital acquired, what is the simplest infection control method an institution can implement to prevent this infection from spreading to others? (Chapter Objectives 7 and 10)

5. What additional infection control practices or programs can be used to limit the spread of this infection? (Chapter Objectives 7 and 10)

CASE STUDY 41-2 (CHAPTER OBJECTIVES 5, 6, 7, 8, AND 11)

A 6-year-old female has a Hickman catheter inserted for treatment of acute lymphocytic leukemia. While on chemotherapy, she develops a fever. Three sets of blood cultures are drawn that reveal gram-positive cocci in clusters that are catalase positive, coagulase negative, and thermonuclease negative in all six bottles. The catheter is then withdrawn and replaced. The catheter tip is sent to the laboratory for culture 24 hours after the blood cultures were drawn. The catheter tip reveals 27 colonies of the same organism present in the blood cultures. After replacement of the catheter and antibiotic treatment, her fever resolved.

1. What is the identification of the organism that caused her infection? (Chapter Objectives 5 and 6)

2. What is probably the source of the organism causing her infection? (Chapter Objective 5)

3. What is the reason for performing both the blood culture and catheter tip culture? (Chapter Objectives 6 and 8)

4. The organism proved to be susceptible to many antibiotics, including vancomycin. Why was the original catheter removed? (Chapter Objectives 6 and 7)

5. The infectious disease physician wants to verify whether this organism originated from the patient or her nurse. What can the microbiology department do to assist the physician? (Chapter Objective 11)

PEARSON
myhealthprofessionskit™

Use this address to access the interactive Companion Website created for this textbook. Simply select "Clinical Laboratory Science" from the choice of disciplines. Find this book and log in using your user name and password.

REFERENCES

Go to myhealthprofessionskit.com to view this chapter's references.

42

Global Threats

Marcia A. Firmani

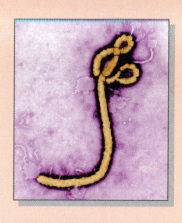

■ LEARNING OBJECTIVES

Upon completion of this chapter, the students should be able to:

1. Define emerging and reemerging infections and relate factors contributing to the emergence of infectious diseases

2. Select the bacterial, viral, and parasitic agents that cause emerging or reemerging diseases.

3. Correlate clinical characteristics to select emerging diseases to include:

    a. clinical manifestations

    b. epidemiology

    c. treatment

    d. prevention and control strategies

    e. pathogenic mechanisms

4. Assess risk factors for emerging and reemerging infections

5. Define drug resistance and select the organisms associated with multi-drug-resistant infections

6. Relate the key characteristics of bioterrorism agents and the categories of priority pathogens

KEY TERMS

antigenic drift	epidemic	prion
antigenic shift	hantavirus pulmonary	reemerging infection
Creutzfeldt–Jacob	syndrome	ribavirin
disease (CJD)	hemolytic uremic	scrapie
cross-resistance	syndrome (HUS)	severe acute respiratory
emerging infections	parasite resistance	syndrome (SARS)

▶ **INTRODUCTION**

Emerging infections are caused by microorganisms whose incidence in humans have increased within the past two decades or threaten to increase in the near future. Emergence may be due to the spread of a new agent, to the recognition of an infection that has been present in the population but has gone undetected, or to the realization that an established disease has an infectious origin. Emergence may also be used to describe the reappearance or reemergence of a known infection after a significant decline in incidence (Lederberg et al.,

1992). There are 29 pathogenic microbes that have been recognized since 1973 (Table 42-1 ✪) and in the last two decades over 20 diseases known as **reemerging infections** have resurfaced due to various factors (Table 42-2 ✪). Factors that contribute to the emergence or reemergence of infectious agents include climate change, ecosystem disturbance, increased movement of people and products, and the deterioration of public health infrastructures.

In addition to the emergence of new pathogens, the United States is vulnerable to biological agent release by rogue nations or terrorists, which may also result in the spread of infectious diseases. The use of microorganisms as agents of biological

✪ TABLE 42-1

Pathogenic Microbes and Infectious Diseases Recognized Since 1973

Microbe	Disease	Year Identified
Bacteria		
Legionella pneumophila	Legionnaire's disease	1977
Campylobacter jejuni	Enteric pathogen with global distribution	1977
Toxic strains of *Staphylococcus aureus*	Toxic shock syndrome	1981
Escherichia coli O157:H7	Hemorrhagic colitis; hemolytic uremic syndrome	1982
Borrelia burgdorferi	Lyme disease	1982
Helicobacter pylori	Peptic ulcer disease	1983
Ehrlichia chaffeensis	Human ehrlichiosis	1989
Vibrio cholera O139	Epidemic cholera	1992
Bartonella henselae	Cat-scratch disease; bacillary angiomatosis	1992
Virus		
Rotavirus	Infantile diarrhea	1973
Parvovirus B19	Aplastic crisis in chronic hemolytic anemia	1975
Ebola virus	Ebola hemorrhagic fever	1977
Hantavirus	Hemorrhagic fever with renal syndrome	1977
Human T-lymphotropic	T-cell leukemia virus I (HTLV-I)	1980
HTLV-II	Hairy cell leukemia	1982
Human immunodeficiency virus	Acquired immunodeficiency syndrome (AIDS)	1983
Human herpesvirus-6 (HHV-6)	Roseola subitum	1988
Hepatitis E	Enterically transmitted non-A, non-B hepatitis	1988
Hepatitis C	Parenterally transmitted non-A, non-B liver infection	1989
Guanarito virus	Venezuelan hemorrhagic fever	1991
Sin Nombre virus	Adult respiratory distress syndrome	1993
Sabia virus	Brazilian hemorrhagic fever	1994
HHV-8	Kaposi sarcoma in AIDS patients	1995
Parasite		
Cryptosporidium parvum	Acute and chronic diarrhea	1976
Enterocytozoon bieneusi	Persistent diarrhea	1985
Cyclospora cayetanensis	Persistent diarrhea	1986
Encephalitozoon hellem	Conjunctivitis	1991
New *Babesia* species	Atypical babesiosis	1991
Encephalitozoon cuniculi	Disseminated disease	1993

✪ TABLE 42-2

Reemerging Infections and Factors Contributing to Emergence

Disease or Pathogen	Contributing Factors in Reemergence
Bacteria	
Group A *Streptococcus*	Unclear
Trench fever	Breakdown of public health measures
Plague	Economic development; land use
Diphtheria	Interruption of immunization program
Tuberculosis	Human demographics and behavior; industry and technology; international commerce and travel; breakdown of public health measures; microbial adaptation
Pertussis	Refusal to vaccinate
Salmonella	Industry and technology; human demographics and behavior; microbial adaptation; food changes
E. coli O157	Food processing and shipment
Pneumococcus	Human demographics; microbial adaptation; international travel and commerce; misuse and overuse of antibiotics
Cholera	Travel; reduced water chlorination
Virus	
Rabies	Breakdown in public health measures; changes in land use; travel
Dengue hemorrhagic fever	Transportation; travel and migration; urbanization
Yellow Fever	Drug and insecticide resistance; civil strife; lack of economic resources
Parasite	
Schistosomiasis	Dam construction; improved irrigation; ecological changes favoring snail host
Neurocysticercosis	Immigration
Acanthamebiasis	Introduction of soft contact lenses
Visceral leishmaniasis	War; population displacement; immigration; habitat changes favorable to insect vector; increase in immunocompromised human hosts
Malaria	Favorable conditions for mosquito vector
Toxoplasmosis	Increase in immunocompromised human hosts
Giardiasis	Increased use of child-care facilities
Echinococcosis	Ecological changes that affect the habitats of the intermediate hosts

warfare is considered inevitable for several reasons, including ease of production and dispersion, delayed onset of symptoms, ability to cause high rates of morbidity and mortality, and difficulty in diagnosis. Table 42-3✪ lists the National Institute of Allergy and Infectious Diseases (NIAID) priority pathogens. Category A agents are those that can be easily disseminated or transmitted person to person, cause high mortality with potential for major public health impact, may cause public panic and social disruption, and require special action for public health preparedness. Category B agents are next in priority and include those that are relatively easy to disseminate, cause moderate morbidity and low mortality, and require specific enhancements of the Centers for Disease Control and Prevention's (CDC) diagnostic capacity and enhanced disease surveillance. Category C consists of emerging pathogens that could be engineered for mass dissemination because of their availability, ease of production and dissemination, and potential for high morbidity and mortality.

Some of the agents found in Tables 42-1, 42-2, and 42-3 are discussed in this chapter. Although all of these organisms have been previously described throughout the textbook, this chapter aims to emphasize the potential of these pathogens to cause significant global morbidity and mortality.

✓ Checkpoint! 42–1 (Chapter Objective 1)

Factors that contribute to the emergence or reemergence of infectious agents include
- A. *climate change.*
- B. *ecosystem disturbance.*
- C. *increased movement of people and products.*
- D. *all of the above.*

✪ TABLE 42-3

NIAID Priority Pathogens

Category A	Category B	Category C
Bacillus anthracis	*Burkholderia pseudomallei*	Tickborne Hemorrhagic fever viruses: Nairovirus (Crimean Congo hemorrhagic fever)
Clostridium botulinum	*Coxiella burnetii*	
Yersinia pestis	*Brucella* species	
Variola major (smallpox)	*Burkholderia mallei*	Tickborne encephalitis virus
Francisella tularensis	Epsilon toxins of *Clostridium perfringens*	Yellow fever virus
Viral hemorrhagic fevers:	*Staphylococcus* enterotoxin B	Multidrug resistant *Mycobacterium tuberculosis* (MDR-TB)
Arenaviruses	Typus fever	
Lymphocytic chori-omeningitis virus (LCM), Junin virus	Food and water pathogens:	Influenza virus
	Bacteria	*Rickettsia prowazekii*
	Diarrheagenic *E. coli*	Rabies virus
Machupo virus	Pathogenic *Vibrio* species	Nipah virus
Guanarito virus	*Shigella* species	Hantaviruses
Lassa Fever virus	*Salmonella*	
Bunyaviruses	*Listeria monocytogenes*	
Hantaviruses	*Campylobacter jejuni*	
Rift Valley fever virus	*Yersinia enterocolitica*	
Flaviviruses	Caliciviruses, Hepatitis A	
Dengue virus	*Cryptosporidium parvum*	
Filoviruses	*Cyclospora cyatanensis*	
Ebola virus	*Giardia lamblia*	
Marburg virus	*Entamoeba histolytica*	
	Toxoplasma gondii	
	Microsporidia	
	Additional encephalitis viruses:	
	West Nile virus	
	LaCrosse virus	
	California encephalitis virus	
	Venezuelan equine encephalitis (VEE) virus	
	Eastern equine encephalitis (EEE) virus	
	Western equine encephalitis (WEE) virus	
	Japanese encephalitis fever virus	
	Kyasanur Forest virus	

▶ EMERGING AND REEMERGING PATHOGENS AND DISEASES

Fifty years ago, it was believed that infectious diseases would no longer threaten the morbidity and mortality of the human population due to the identification and mass production of antibiotics. However, we recently have been forced to realize that our battle with infectious agents is far from over. At least 12 new diseases have been identified within the past 30 years, including AIDS and hantavirus pulmonary syndrome. Moreover, diseases that were declining to the point of potential eradication, such as tuberculosis, are resurging. Even more disturbing is the fact that many of the antimicrobial agents that we previously thought would save us from infectious diseases have become useless to treat certain infections due to the ability of the organisms to become resistant.

BACTERIA

There are five major types of infectious agents that cause disease: bacteria, viruses, fungi, parasites, and prions. In this section, bacteria that have recently emerged and reemerged after numerous years of decline are discussed.

Cholera

Cholera is a serious diarrheal disease that has been involved in recurring global pandemics since 1817. An ongoing pandemic of the El Tor biotype of *Vibrio cholerae* O1 began in 1961 and emerged in Indonesia. This pandemic spread through Asia and Africa and reached Latin America in 1991 (CDC, 1991). Cholera remains **epidemic** in Latin America, with a dramatic increase of disease incidence in a defined population at a specific time. In addition to *V. cholerae* O1, other strains have appeared in Latin America, with at least one strain being resistant to multiple antimicrobial drugs (Evins et al., 1995). *V. cholerae* O139 Bengal emerged in Asia in 1992, causing a new cholera epidemic (Ramamurthy et al., 1993). Serogroups O139 Bengal and O1 now coexist and continue to cause large cholera outbreaks in India and Bangladesh. Moreover, it has been hypothesized that the O139 serogroup will likely cause the next pandemic of cholera.

V. cholerae is able to cause diarrhea through two different mechanisms. The first is the production of cholera-toxin (CT), which is a potent stimulator of adenylate cyclase, and the second is decreased intestinal absorption due to tissue damage. CT-producing strains cause a highly secretory form of diarrhea in the absence of inflammation. In contrast, *V. cholerae* strains that do not produce CT cause milder cases of diarrhea but the disease may be more inflammatory (Silva et al., 1996).

Although the typical clinical symptom of cholera is severe diarrhea, many individuals infected with *V. cholerae* have mild diarrhea or no symptoms at all. The severity of infection depends on many factors, including previous exposure or vaccination, the inoculum size, the gastric-acid barrier level, and the patient's blood group. It has been demonstrated that individuals of blood group O are at much higher risk of developing severe cholera from the El Tor biotype than individuals of other blood groups (Barua & Paguio, 1977; Clemens et al., 1989; Glass et al., 1985). The case fatality rate for severe cholera without treatment is approximately 50% (Sack et al., 2004). Fluid replacement is the most effective and simplest treatment for this disease. Severely dehydrated patients require replacement of 10% of their body weight within 2–4 hours. The signs of dehydration can be found in Table 42-4✪.

Epidemiological investigations have identified various food and water sources of *V. cholerae*. For example, the El Tor biotype of *V. cholerae* O1 rapidly multiplies in moist foods of neutral acidity (Kolvin & Roberts, 1982). Understanding these transmission pathways is essential to the development of successful control strategies. A study by Tauxe and colleagues (1995) in Latin America demonstrated that cholera was being transmitted by several, distinct mechanisms. Waterborne transmission was identified in the majority of the investigations (Tauxe et al., 1995). In many cases, the implicated water came from municipal systems. Therefore, a major prevention strategy is to provide safe, uncontaminated drinking water. The second major route of cholera transmission is food contamination in markets or the home, including food sold by street vendors. Foods that are contaminated during preparation and stored at ambient temperatures allow the bacteria to multiply rapidly. Consequently, improving food handling is another key form of cholera prevention. A third major source of cholera infection is contaminated seafood. Marine creatures may harbor *V. cholerae* O1 before they are harvested. In addition, shellfish can become contaminated by infected seawater used in processing plants. *V. cholerae* can survive light cooking and will subsequently grow if seafood is held many hours before eating (Blake et al., 1980). Prevention of seafood-associated cholera relies on improving sanitation in processing plants and education to discourage consumption of raw or undercooked shellfish.

✪ **TABLE 42-4**

Assessment of Patients with Severe Diarrhea for Dehydration

	No Dehydration	Some Dehydration	Severe Dehydration**
General appearance	Alert	Restless, irritable	Lethargic or unconscious
Eyes	Normal	Sunken	Very sunken and dry
Tears*	Present	Absent	Absent
Mouth/tongue	Moist	Dry	Very dry
Thirst	Not thirsty	Thirsty	Not able to drink
Skin pinch	Goes back quickly	Goes back slowly	Goes back very slowly

*Tears are relevant only for infants and young children.
**In children >5 years and adults, absence of radial pulse and low blood pressure are additional signs of severe dehydration.
This table was published in Sack, D. A. (2004). Cholera. The Lancet, 363, 223. Copyright Elsevier.

The introduction of new *Vibrio* strains is difficult to prevent due to an increase in global travel as well as importation involving ships carrying contaminated ballast water. The key to controlling a cholera epidemic lies in limiting its spread using measures that prevent sustained transmission. See ∞ Chapter 23 for a review of the characteristics and identification of *Vibrio*.

Enterohemorrhagic *Escherichia coli* (EHEC)

Escherichia coli (*E. coli*) is a commensal organism that resides in the human intestine. However, *E. coli* can also be a pathogen and is best known for its ability to cause intestinal diseases. Currently, there are four recognized classes of enterovirulent *E. coli:* enterotoxigenic *E. coli* (ETEC), enteroinvasive *E. coli* (EIEC), enterohemorrhagic *E. coli* (EHEC), and enteropathogenic *E. coli* (EPEC). Each manifests distinct features in pathogenesis and can be differentiated by their unique serotypes defined by their somatic (O) and flagellar (H) antigens (Orskov et al., 1982). In addition, a new class of enterovirulent *E. coli* has been identified as enteroaggregative *E. coli* (EggEC); however, the pathogenesis of EggEC is not fully understood.

Of the enterovirulent *E. coli,* EHEC is the most common due to numerous, highly publicized outbreaks caused by this organism. To date, O157:H7 is the most frequently encountered EHEC strain isolated in stool specimens. However, there are at least 50 other EHEC serotypes reported as being associated with the development of hemorrhagic colitis or **hemolytic uremic syndrome** (HUS). One virulence trait of all EHEC strains is the ability to produce potent verotoxins (VT) (or shiga-like toxins) that cause severe damage to the lining of the intestine. These toxins are closely related or identical to the toxin produced by another enteric pathogen, *Shigella dysenteriae.* Greater verotoxin production per bacterium is associated with increasing severity of human disease (Pradel et al., 2001).

E. coli O157:H7 is usually a zoonotic infection. Cattle and other ruminants may be the natural reservoir for *E. coli* O157:H7 and other verotoxin-producing *E. coli* (VTEC). However, toxin-producing *E. coli* commonly present in cattle are not frequently isolated from human patients. This may be due to genetic phenotypic and pathogenic diversity among these pathogens (Kim et al., 1999; LeJeune, Takemura, Christie, & Sreevatsan, 2004; McNally et al., 2001). Transmission to humans can occur directly from person-to-person contact via a fecal–oral route or indirectly from cross-contamination or consumption of contaminated food or water (McClure & Hall, 2000). The major routes of infection include the consumption of undercooked ground beef or meat products, raw milk or dairy products, fruits, vegetables, and contaminated water. Animal-to-human transmission can also occur after contact with animals in public settings such as petting zoos, fairs, and schools.

E. coli O157:H7 has a low infectious dose of only 1–100 bacteria and can survive in a variety of food types. Clinical symptoms usually commence within 5 days following the ingestion of infected food products. Symptoms of EHEC infection include severe cramping (abdominal pain) and diarrhea that is initially watery but becomes grossly bloody within 48 hours.

Vomiting can occasionally occur and fever is either low-grade or absent. The illness is usually self-limited and lasts for an average of 8 days. However, severe life-threatening conditions such as hemorrhagic colitis and hemolytic uremic syndrome (HUS) may develop.

In the laboratory, *E. coli* O157:H7 can be isolated using sorbitol-MacConkey (SMAC) agar plates. SMAC plates differentiate between sorbitol fermenting and sorbitol nonfermenting gram-negative organisms but are not inhibitory to normal non–*E. coli* flora. If a possible *E. coli* O157 is isolated, the isolate must be confirmed for the presence of O157 antigen as well as pulse field gel electrophoresis (PFGE) strain typing. Testing for the presence of shiga-like toxins should also be performed. Other verotoxin producing serotypes of *E. coli* cannot be differentiated on SMAC like the O157:H7 serotype. It is now considered best practice to test for the presence of verotoxin rather than culture for these organisms.

Patients with *E. coli* O157:H7 infections are usually managed supportively. In addition, patients must be monitored for the development of HUS, especially in high-risk patients such as children less than age 5 years and older adults. Treatment with antimicrobial agents is highly controversial; hence, further studies are necessary to determine the appropriate therapeutic regimen. Antibiotics may increase the risk of development of HUS.

E. coli O157:H7 infections can be prevented through education about the risks of ingesting undercooked ground beef and unpasteurized dairy products and juices. Children should be discouraged from putting their fingers into their mouths while in an animal area. Hands should be washed when exiting animal areas in public places and before eating and drinking. In addition, infected children should be excluded from attending day-care centers until two consecutive stool cultures test negative for *E. coli* O157:H7. Any isolate identified with *E. coli* O157:H7 must be reported to the local public health authorities. See ∞ Chapters 21 and 35 for more information on identification and processing specimens for *E. coli* O157:H7 and other *E. coli* associated with diarrhea.

 Checkpoint! 42–2 (Chapter Objective 2)

Which enterovirulent Escherichia coli is most associated with causing hemolytic uremic syndrome (HUS), especially in children?

    A. *Enterohemmorhagic E. coli*
    B. *Enterotoxigenic E. coli*
    C. *Enteroinvasive E. coli*
    D. *Enteropathogenic E. coli*

Typhoid Fever

Typhoid fever is a systemic infection caused by the bacterium *Salmonella enterica* serotype Typhi. *Salmonella* is highly adapted to humans and has evolved numerous mechanisms that enable it to persist in the host to ensure its survival and transmission. Typhoid fever was a serious cause of illness and death in the

United States and Europe during the nineteenth century due to overcrowding and unsanitary conditions. However, the development of sewage systems and clean water decreased the incidence of typhoid dramatically in these regions. Today, most of the burden of the disease occurs in developing countries where sanitary conditions remain poor. The development of chloramphenicol in 1948 dramatically reduced the severity of this infection; however, the emergence of chloramphenicol resistance has caused a major setback (Mirza et al., 1996). Complications associated with typhoid fever can be found in Box 42-1 ✪.

S. enterica serotype Typhi is transmitted via the ingestion of contaminated water. Water usually becomes contaminated by individuals carrying the organism and excreting it in the feces or urine. In developed countries, typhoid fever is a sporadic disease occurring mainly in travelers returning from endemic areas. In endemic areas, risk factors include eating food prepared outside of the home, drinking contaminated water, close contact with an individual with recent typhoid fever, poor housing with inadequate facilities for personal hygiene, and recent use of antimicrobial agents (Parry et al.,

2002). The global distribution of *Salmonella typhi* can be found in Figure 42-1 ■.

In developing countries, reducing the incidence in the general population requires provision of safe drinking water, effective sewage disposal, and hygienic food preparation. Mass immunization has been successful in some areas. In developed countries, identification of chronic carriers can aid in the control. Since most cases in developed countries are a result of travel to endemic areas, it is important for these individuals to take precautions. For example, all drinking water must be bottled or boiled and food should be thoroughly cooked. In addition, fruits or vegetables washed with unknown water sources should be avoided. Vaccination is recommended for travelers to areas where typhoid is endemic, household contacts of typhoid carriers, and lab workers highly likely to handle the bacteria. In the event of a typhoid epidemic, mass immunization should be considered in combination with adequate provision of safe water and food.

✪ BOX 42-1

Important Complications of Typhoid Fever

Abdominal
Gastrointestinal perforation
Gastrointestinal hemorrhage
Hepatitis
Cholecystitis

Cardiovascular
Asymptomatic electrocardiographic changes
Myocarditis
Shock

Neuropsychiatric
Encephalopathy
Delirium
Psychotic states
Meningitis
Impairment of coordination

Respiratory
Bronchitis
Pneumonia

Hematological
Anemia
Disseminated intravascular coagulation

Other
Focal abscess
Pharyngitis
Miscarriage
Relapse
Chronic carrier state

✓ Checkpoint! 42–3 (Chapter Objective 3d)

Of the following choices, which is the best method for preventing typhoid fever when traveling to an endemic area?

   A. *Filter drinking water*
   B. *Do not eat fruits or vegetables washed with unknown water sources*
   C. *Vaccination*
   D. *Do not eat uncooked foods*

Plague

Plague is caused by infection with the bacteria *Yersinia pestis*. Pandemics of plague have occurred for centuries and were responsible for millions of casualties. Plaque remains an enzootic infection of rats, ground squirrels, prairie dogs, and other rodents. Bubonic plague (Figure 42-2 ■) most commonly occurs when plague-infected fleas (Figure 42-3 ■) bite humans. Pets, such as outside dogs and cats, can bring plague-infested fleas into the home and transmit the disease to their owners. During the Cold War, the U.S. and Soviet biological weapons programs developed techniques to directly aerosolize plague particles that cause pneumonic plague, a highly lethal and potentially contagious form. A biological attack of plague would most likely occur via aerosol dissemination of *Y. pestis*, resulting in an outbreak of pneumonic plague.

Pneumonic plague begins after an incubation period of 1–6 days, with symptoms such as high fever, chills, headache, and malaise, followed by cough with blood. The disease progresses rapidly to dyspnea, stridor, cyanosis, and death (Darling et al., 2004). Plague should be suspected whenever large numbers of previously healthy individuals develop fulminant gram-negative pneumonia, especially if hemoptysis is present. *Y. pestis* is commonly diagnosed based on its appearance and biochemical profile in a clinical microbiology laboratory. The bacteria

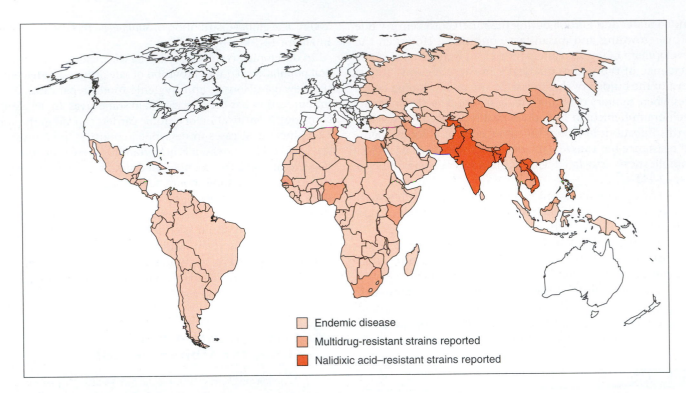

■ **FIGURE 42-1** Global distribution of resistance to *Salmonella enterica* serotype Typhi, 1990 through 2002. All shaded areas are areas of endemic disease.

From Parry, C. M., Hien, T. T., et al. (2002). Typhoid fever. *New England Journal of Medicine, 347*(22), 1770–1782.

demonstrate bipolar (safety pin) staining with Wright, Giemsa, or Wayson stain (Figure 42-4 ■). In addition, the organism is a non-lactose fermenter, urease and indole negative and colonies are initially much smaller than other *Enterobacteriaceae*. The organism prefers to grow at room temperature rather than 35–37°C. Observable growth on blood or Mac-

Conkey agar typically takes 48 hours. *Yersinia pestis* is a Category A bioterror pathogen, so state public health laboratories should be notified and the suspected plague isolate submitted for confirmation.

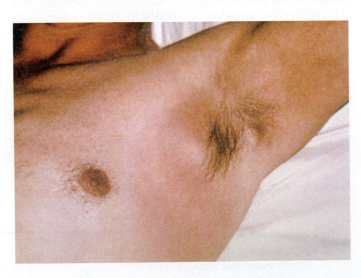

■ **FIGURE 42-2** An axillary swollen lymph node or bubo and edema exhibited by a plague patient.

From Public Health Image Library (PHIL), CDC/Margaret Parsons, Dr. Karl F. Meyer.

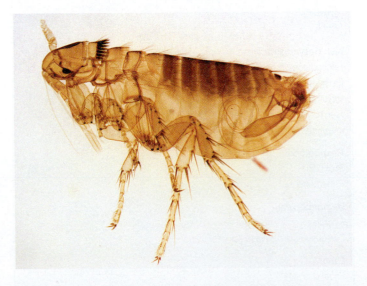

■ **FIGURE 42-3** This flea is a common ectoparasite of the rock squirrel and in the western United States is an important vector for *Yersinia pestis*, the pathogen responsible for causing plague.

From Public Health Image Library (PHIL), CDC/DVBID, BZB, Entomology and Ecology Activity, Vector Ecology & Control Laboratory, Fort Collins, CO.

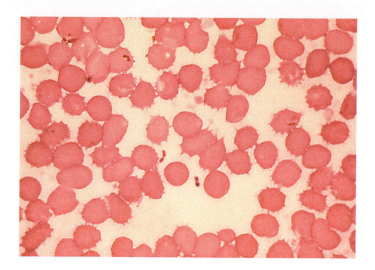

■ **FIGURE 42-4** Blood smear containing plague bacteria showing the characteristic bipolar, "safety-pin"–like appearance of *Yersinia pestis*.
From Public Health Image Library (PHIL), CDC/Dr. Jack Poland.

REAL WORLD TIP

Automated identification systems may identify *Y. pestis* as *Shigella*, H_2S negative *Salmonella*, *Acinetobacter*, or other non–*Y. pestis* species. Remember to correlate Gram stain morphology, growth characteristics, and biochemical results in order to avoid reporting erroneous results.

A 70 kbp virulence plasmid (pYV) enables *Y. pestis* to survive and multiply in the host. This plasmid encodes the Yop virulon, a system consisting of secreted proteins called Yops and their dedicated type III secretion apparatus called Ysc. This Yop virulon allows extracellular *Y. pestis* to inject the Yops that block production of pro-inflammatory cytokines and induce apoptosis of macrophages (Cornelis, 2000). Most strains of *Y. pestis* produce an F1-antigen *in vivo,* which can be detected in serum samples by immunoassay (Darling et al., 2004). Considering the dramatic increase in antibiotic resistance among a variety of bacteria as well as the threat of biological terrorism, a fluorescence resonance energy transfer (FRET)–based assay to detect *Y. pestis* mutants that are resistant to ciprofloxacin has recently been developed.

Pneumonic plague is invariably fatal if antibiotic therapy is delayed more than 1 day after the onset of symptoms. Recommended antibiotics are streptomycin, gentamicin, ciprofloxacin, or doxycycline for 10–14 days. Doxycycline is recommended for prophylactic treatment of asymptomatic exposed individuals. Alternative antibiotics include tetracycline and chloramphenicol. The U.S.-licensed formaldehyde-killed whole bacilli vaccine is effective against bubonic plague but not against pneumonic plague (Inglesby et al., 2000). How-

ever, this vaccine was discontinued for use in 1999. No vaccine is currently available for prophylaxis of plague.

VIRUSES

Viruses are capable of infecting all organisms, from plants to bacteria. Similar to bacteria, viruses cause disease by disrupting normal cellular function using a variety of mechanisms. This section discusses the viruses that have been recently identified within the past 30 years, such as the human immunodeficiency virus, which has caused enormous morbidity and mortality to the human population worldwide.

HIV/AIDS

Acquired immunodeficiency syndrome (AIDS) has had the most profound effect on human illness and death of all of the infectious diseases recognized in the twentieth century. AIDS is thought to be caused by the human immunodeficiency virus (HIV) and has close to a 100% fatality rate. AIDS was not recognized as a specific disease until 1980 and HIV was not identified as the causative agent until 1983. To date, an estimated 16 million people have died from AIDS worldwide, with 50 million currently infected with HIV (Levin et al., 2001). Although HIV was initially susceptible to a variety of antiviral agents, the virus is now resistant to these drugs due to the emergence of resistance mutations. Since HIV can mutate rapidly, developing an effective vaccine is extremely difficult.

The HIV pandemic has been largely restricted to subpopulations or risk groups that have a greater likelihood of infection. The risk groups include homosexual men with multiple sexual partners, injection drug users, and sex workers (including their patrons and spouses). There is ample evidence that HIV type-1 (HIV-1) was transferred to humans from the chimpanzee, which harbors a related virus, simian immunodeficiency virus (SIVcpz), and lives in central Africa (Gao et al., 1999; Santiago et al., 2002). HIV type 2 (HIV-2) is 40–60% homologous to HIV-1 and is thought to have originated from SIVsm harbored in the sooty mangabey monkeys of coastal West Africa (Hahn et al., 2000). In all known instances of infection of the natural primate host of SIV, neither a disease resembling AIDS nor a profound depletion of CD4+ T cells develops. However, SIV transmission to unnatural hosts, such as the rhesus macaque monkey, causes a progressive loss of CD4+ T cells and a high degree of susceptibility to infectious disease acquisition. Hence, HIV is considered a zoonotic infection. In the human host, HIV resides mainly in the CD4+ T cells. The loss of CD4+ T cells is attributed to be the cause of many of the disease manifestations of HIV (Douek et al., 2003).

Diagnosis of HIV infection is a crucial factor in preventing the spread of this epidemic. Following initial infection, there is a low rise in HIV-specific antibody titers. In the United States, HIV-1 is the causative agent for the majority of HIV infections. Since HIV-2 prevalence in the United States is low, testing is not required. However, HIV-2 is highly concentrated in West African countries such as Senegal, Ivory Coast, Cape Verde,

Gambia, Guinea-Bissau, Liberia, Ghana, and Nigeria (de Cock et al., 1993). Hence, HIV-2 testing would be recommended in certain situations, including individuals with known HIV-2-infected sex partners; individuals from HIV-2 endemic countries; individuals who received a blood transfusion or shared needles with an HIV-2-infected person; or children of women who have risk factors for HIV-2.

The standard HIV testing protocol is comprised of two assays. Serum or plasma is first screened for HIV antibodies using an enzyme-linked immunoassay (ELISA). Currently there are several ELISA test kits for HIV-1 antibody that are approved by the FDA. HIV antibodies are usually detectable within 6–12 weeks postinfection. A confirmatory test is performed on any sample that is positive with the ELISA test. The confirmatory test is either a Western Blot or an immunoflourescence assay (IFA). In addition to serum or plasma, alternative specimens such as oral fluid and urine can be used for HIV testing on individuals who dislike or cannot tolerate blood draws. However, the alternative specimens have decreased sensitivity and specificity compared to blood specimens. During the acute stage of HIV infection where viral loads are highest, virus can be detected in serum and plasma prior to the development of antibodies. Consequently, nucleic acid testing to detect viral load is a more recent approach to rapidly determine an individual's HIV status as well as to monitor disease progression. Studies have demonstrated that individuals who maintain elevated plasma viral loads during the first year of HIV infection have a higher risk of disease progression (Mellors et al., 1995, 1997). In addition, viral load can be used to determine antiretroviral treatment efficacy. For example, a study by Hecht et al. (2006) determined that initiating highly active antiretroviral therapy (HAART) within 2 weeks of antibody seroconversion was associated with viral load and CD4$^+$ T cell count benefits for 24 weeks after termination of HAART, which suggest that treatment given during acute HIV infection may modify the long-term course of disease. Consequently, early detection of HIV infection is instrumental for timely initiation of antiretroviral therapy and subsequent reduction in morbidity and mortality.

Hemorrhagic Fevers

Viral hemorrhagic fever (VHF) syndrome describes the disease processes caused by several RNA viruses from the *Filoviridae* (Ebola and Marburg), *Arenaviridae* (Junin, Lassa, Machupo, Guanarito), *Bunyaviridae* (Nairovirus, Phlebovirus, Hantavirus), and *Flaviviridae* (Yellow fever virus, Dengue viruses, Kyasanur Forest disease virus, Omsk hemorrhagic fever virus) families (Zaki & Goldsmith, 1999).

VHF syndrome is an acute febrile illness characterized by malaise, prostration, generalized signs of vascular permeability, and abnormalities of circulatory regulation. Shock, generalized mucous membrane hemorrhage, and organ involvement often follows, with each type having distinguishing clinical features. The incubation period of VHF ranges from 2 days for Ebola virus (Ndambi et al., 1999) and up to 3 weeks for Lassa

virus (McCormick et al., 1987). The viruses are typically transmitted to humans by contact with infected animal reservoirs or arthropod vectors (Franz et al., 1997). In endemic regions, human-to-human transmission of Ebola, Lassa, and Crimean-Congo hemorrhagic fever (CCHF) viruses has been observed. To date, a reservoir and vector of Ebola and Marburg virus has not been identified. The filoviruses (Ebola and Marburg) that cause the most tissue destruction and the highest fatality rates among the hemorrhagic fever viruses are further discussed here.

The filoviruses contain four subtypes of Ebola virus (Zaire, Sudan, Ivory Coast, and Reston) and a single species of Marburg virus. Filovirus virions have distinct bacilliform morphology. However, particles may also appear as circular, branched, filamentous, and U- or 6-shaped forms (Figure 42-5 ■). A lipid envelope derived from the host cell plasma membrane surrounds a dense central core formed by the ribonucleoprotein complex. The genomic RNA sequence has been determined for the Ebola Zaire subtype and two strains of Marburg. The genome contains approximately 19,000 base pairs with seven linearly arranged genes (Khan et al., 1998). The encoded proteins have been extensively studied but the complete pathogenic mechanism of the virus is yet unknown. The virion glycoprotein (GP) of Ebola Zaire encoded by gene 4 has been identified as the main viral determinant of vascular cell cytotoxicity and injury.

Due to the severity of the symptoms of VHF, the diagnosis is usually made based on the clinical features of the disease. Classical methods of viral diagnostics such as cell culture, electron microscopy, or serology for VHF require either specialized equipment or access to a Biosafety level–4 (BSL-4) laboratory. Consequently, the use of these diagnostic methods in most hospital-based clinical laboratories is not feasible. Other techniques to detect Ebola antigens include ELISA

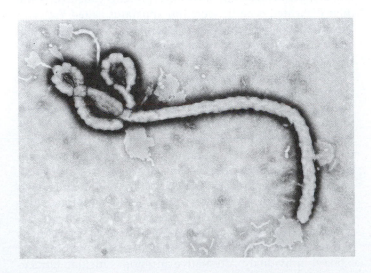

■ **FIGURE 42-5** Electron micrograph (TEM) of Ebola virus reveals some of the structural morphology displayed by the virion.
From Public Health Image Library (PHIL), CDC/Frederick A. Murphy.

(Peters & Khan, 1999). In addition, an immunohistochemical test using formalin-fixed skin biopsy specimens has been used for the diagnosis of Ebola hemorrhagic fever. Advantages of this technique are that the formalin-fixed biopsy samples are not infectious and can be easily collected, handled, and transported. In addition, polymerase chain reaction (PCR) techniques have been developed to rapidly identify VHF. Serum or plasma is the most common clinical material used for VHF PCR-based testing (Drosten, Kummerer, et al., 2003).

Management of infected patients consists primarily of contact isolation and supportive care. **Ribavirin**, a nonimmunosuppressive nucleoside analog with broad antiviral properties, has been shown to be somewhat effective for therapy of Lassa fever, Argentina hemorrhagic fever, Crimean-Congo hemorrhagic fever, Rift Valley fever, and Bolivian hemorrhagic fever but has poor activity against filoviruses and flaviviruses (Franz et al., 1997; Darling et al., 2004). Available vaccines include yellow fever vaccine and Argentine hemorrhagic fever vaccine.

Human Monkeypox

Monkeypox is an orthopoxvirus that was first recognized in 1970. The disease is most commonly a sporadic smallpox-like zoonotic infection in central and western Africa. However, in May 2003, the disease emerged in the United States, causing a monkeypox outbreak. Epidemiological investigations of this outbreak identified the source of infection as a shipment of African rodents that resulted in secondary infections to prairie dogs. The outbreak involved 37 human infections and included exotic pet dealers, pet owners, and veterinary care workers (CDC, 2003b). Pathological investigations suggested that direct mucocutaneous contact and respiratory routes played a role in transmission (Guarner et al., 2004).

Unlike smallpox, monkeypox does not have the high mortality rate usually associated with the more virulent viral diseases. To date, there is no cure for monkeypox and the clinical presentation is variable among individuals. The incubation period for monkeypox is approximately 5–21 days. The usual symptoms include fever, generalized aches and pains, headache, swollen lymph nodes, and rash (pocks). Pocks are cutaneous vesicles that become pustular and evolve over a period of 2–3 weeks. As the pock lesion dries, it forms a scab and frequently leaves a scar. Many poxviruses were named after the animal from which they were originally isolated (Frey & Belshe, 2004). Poxviruses, other than the etiological agent of smallpox (Variola), usually cause self-limited disease in immunocompetent human hosts.

Monkeypox is not readily transmitted from animals to humans or from humans to other humans without direct contact. Most cases of monkeypox that have occurred in the United States have reported direct contact with sick animals. Wild rodents are thought to be the principal reservoir for these viruses, however, many species act as incidental hosts that may expose and infect humans. As immunity to smallpox wanes in the general population and the popularity of exotic animal pets increases, the risk of human disease from animal orthopoxviruses may also increase (Figure 42-6a ■ and b ■).

Monkeypox virus can be isolated in tissue culture and observed daily for cytopathic effect (CPE). In addition, PCR may be used to confirm the presence of monkeypox virus in samples from infected humans or animals. The U.S. monkeypox virus outbreak demonstrated how new diseases can emerge due to the ease of movement of an infected species from one location to another (including illegal transportation of exotic animals).

Hantavirus Pulmonary Syndrome

New world hantaviruses belong to the family *Bunyaviridae* and were first recognized in 1993 when healthy young adults in the southwestern United States came down with a mysterious pulmonary illness resulting in death (Ksiazek et al., 1995). Investigations identified a novel hantavirus, Sin Nombre virus (SNV), as the cause of a new disease: **hantavirus pulmonary syndrome (HPS)** (Figure 42-7 ■). The earliest case of a serologically conformed SNV infection was in a person who developed an HPS-compatible illness in July 1959 and was found to have IgG antibodies in September 1994. Hence, although HPS is newly identified it is actually not a new disease.

Patients with HPS usually present in a nonspecific way with a relatively short febrile prodrome lasting 3–5 days. Early symptoms include fever, myalgias, headache, chills, dizziness, nonproductive cough, nausea, vomiting, and other gastrointestinal symptoms (CDC, 2002a). Cough and tachypnea generally do not develop until day seven. However, once the cardiopulmonary phase begins the disease progresses rapidly. At this phase patients usually require hospitalization and ventilation within 24 hours. A summary of the clinical presentation of HPC can be found in Table 42-5 ✪.

If hantavirus is suspected, a complete blood count (CBC) and blood chemistry should be performed every 8–12 hours. The white blood cell count tends to be raised with a marked left shift due to the release of immature white blood cells. In approximately 80% of HPS patients, the platelet count is less than 150,000 units. Severe cases of HPS develop disseminated intravenous coagulation (DIC); however, this is not a common complication. Proteinuria and mild elevations of transaminases, CPK, amylase, and creatinine may also be present. The prodromal (early) phase of HPS is indistinguishable from many other viral infections. However, the combination of atypical lymphocytes and thrombocytopenia in combination with pulmonary edema is strongly suggestive of hantavirus infection.

Treatment of patients with HPS is supportive. A positive serological test result, evidence of viral antigen in tissues by immunohistochemistry, or the presence of amplifiable viral RNA sequences in blood or tissue with a compatible clinical history is diagnostic for HPS. An IgG test can be used in conjunction with the IgM capture test. Serological tests include ELISA to detect IgM antibodies to SNV. Acute and convalescent sera reflecting a fourfold rise in IgG antibody titer or the presence of IgM in acute sera are diagnostic for hantavirus

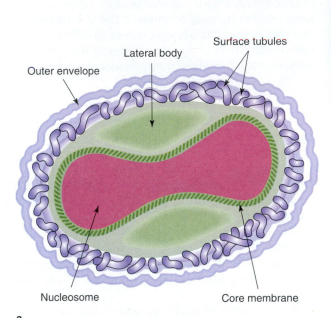

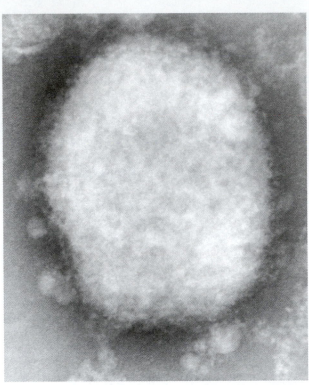

a

b

■ **FIGURE 42-6** **a.** Structure of the monkeypox virus. *From Frey, S. E., & Belshe, R. B. (2004). Poxvirus zoonoses—putting pocks into context. New England Journal of Medicine, 350(4), 324–327.* **b.** Electron micrograph of monkeypox that reveals an "M" (mulberry-type) virion in human vesicular fluid. The surface of "M," or "mulberry," virions are covered with short, whorled filaments, while "C," or "capsular," form virions penetrated by stain present as a sharply defined, dense core surrounded by several laminated zones of differing densities. *From Public Health Image Library (PHIL), CDC/Charles D. Humphrey, Tiara Morehead, and Russell Regnery.*

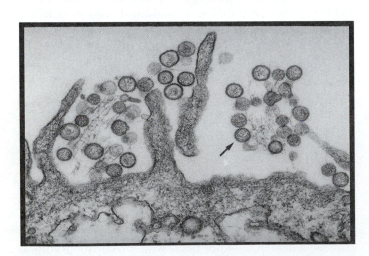

■ **FIGURE 42-7** Thin-section electron micrograph of a Sin Nombre virus isolate from the 1993 outbreak of HPS in the southwestern United States.
Image courtesy of Cynthia Goldsmith, Sherif Zaki, and Luanne Elliott.

infection. A Western Blot assay using recombinant antigens and isotype-specific conjugates for IgM–IgG differentiation has also been developed.

Aerosols from infected rodents are the main route of transmission to humans. Humans contact the virus when saliva or excreta (urine and feces) from infected rodents are inhaled as aerosols. Transmission may also occur when fresh or dried materials contaminated by rodent excreta are disturbed, directly introduced into broken skin or eyes, or via ingestion

✪ **TABLE 42-5**

HPS Clinical Presentation

Most Frequent	Frequent	Other
fever	headaches	shortness of breath
chills	nausea, vomiting	dizziness
myalgias	abdominal pain	arthralgia
	diarrhea	back or chest pain
	cough	sweats
	malaise	

of contaminated food or water. In addition, individuals have been infected after being bitten by infected rodents. Arthropods and biting insects such as ticks, fleas, and mosquitoes have not been implicated in the transmission of HPS. Nosocomial transmission of HPS has never been documented in the United States (Wells et al., 1997).

The major risk factor for HPS is an increased number of rodents in the household (Armstrong et al., 1995). Disruption or inhabitation of a closed, actively rodent-infested structure may also be an important risk factor for contracting HPS. However, travel to and within areas where hantavirus infection has been reported is not considered a risk factor for infection. Moreover, the risk of exposure to campers, hikers, and tourists is very small and is decreased as steps are taken to reduce rodent contact (CDC, 2002a).

The deer mouse (*Peromyscus maniculatus*) is the primary rodent reservoir (Figure 42-8 ■). However, HPS caused by similar hantaviruses have been identified with transmission via different rodent hosts. For example, an infection of HPS in Dade County, Florida (Rollin et al., 1995) was caused by the Black Creek Canal virus (BCCV) and is associated with the cotton rat (*Sigmodon hispidus*). In Louisiana and Texas, HPS is caused by the Bayou virus (Morzunov et al., 1995), which is associated with the rice rat (*Oryzomys palustris*). Furthermore, in the northeastern United States, a similar virus to SNV, New York–1 virus, is associated with the deer mouse as well as the white-footed mouse (*Peromyscus leucopus*). However, most HPS cases have been associated with SNV.

H5N1 and Novel H1N1 Influenza Viruses

Avian influenza viruses have been implicated in numerous outbreaks in a variety of mammals including seals, whales, pigs, and domestic poultry. Since the first human influenza virus was isolated in 1933, new subtypes of human type A influenza viruses have been identified. Of the three types of influenza viruses (A, B, and C), only A and B have been implicated as the cause of epidemic human disease. Hemagglutinin (HA) and neuraminidase (NA) proteins are the two surface antigens that induce protective antibody responses and are the basis for subtyping influenza A viruses. Influenza B viruses are not categorized into subtypes (Bridges et al., 2002).

Aquatic birds are the reservoirs of all 15 subtypes of influenza A viruses (Widjaja et al., 2004). In wild ducks, influenza viruses replicate in intestinal cells, cause no disease symptoms, and are excreted in high concentrations in feces (Webster et al., 1978). Avian influenza viruses have been isolated from freshly deposited fecal material and from unconcentrated lake water. Consequently, transmission by feces provides an efficient way for wild ducks to spread viruses to other domestic and feral birds as they migrate (Halvorson et al., 1983). Since all known influenza A virus subtypes are found in aquatic birds in nature, influenza is not an eradicable disease; hence prevention and control are essential. Agricultural authorities have recommended avoiding direct or indirect contact between domestic poultry and wild birds.

Current inactivated vaccines provide essential protection when the vaccine antigens and the circulating viruses share a high degree of similarity in the HA protein (Lee & Chen, 2004). However, influenza viruses undergo considerable antigenic variation. Influenza viruses undergo two types of antigenic variation: drift and shift. **Antigenic drift** involves minor changes in HA and NA proteins. **Antigenic shift** involves major changes resulting from replacement of gene segments (Webster, 1998). Genetic reassortment of influenza A viruses have been demonstrated *in vivo, in vitro,* and in nature. Hence, the influenza virus continues to evolve and new antigenic variants are constantly emerging, causing yearly epidemics. Moreover, when strains emerge for which humans have no immunity, the result can be catastrophic. For example, a highly pathogenic subtype, H5N1, caused disease in 18 patients, with six deaths in Hong Kong in 1997.

Initial transmission of avian influenza viruses to mammals, including pigs and horses, most likely occurs via fecal contamination of water. Both pigs and poultry are commonly raised on the same commercial farms, which may also facilitate interspecies transmission of influenza viruses (Webster,

 Checkpoint! 42–4 (Chapter Objective 4)

The main risk factor for contracting Sin Nombre virus (hantavirus) is:

   A. *travel to areas where hantavirus has been reported.*
   B. *hiking or camping in wooded areas.*
   C. *close contact with an infected individual.*
   D. *increased number of rodents in household.*

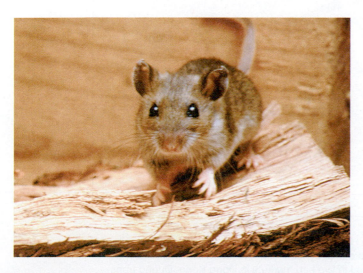

■ **FIGURE 42-8** This is a photo of a deer mouse, *Peromyscus maniculatus*, that can be a hantavirus carrier.
From Public Health Image Library (PHIL), CDC/James Gathany.

1998). Transmission of H5N1 is thought to have crossed the species barrier from poultry to humans (Figure 42-9 ■). In 2003, H5N1 influenza virus reemerged among poultry in eight Asian countries. This outbreak is the largest of avian influenza in poultry ever described (WHO, 2004). Since 2001, H5N1 influenza viruses have circulated throughout mainland China and have demonstrated a seasonal pattern, peaking from October to March, when the mean temperature is below 20°C (Figure 42-10 ■). H5N1 is now endemic in poultry throughout Asia. Consequently, the virus has gained an ecological niche, which generates a long-term pandemic threat to humans (Li et al., 2004).

"The world is now at the start of the 2009 influenza pandemic," said Dr. Margaret Chan, Director-General of the World Health Organization. In April 2009 a novel influenza A virus emerged and began to spread from person to person and country to country. As of November 22, 2009, there were over 622,000 confirmed cases in 207 countries and over 7820 deaths.

"In North America, the Caribbean islands and a limited number of European countries there are signs that disease activity has peaked. In the temperate regions of the southern hemisphere little pandemic activity has been reported" (WHO, November, 27, 2009). The earliest human case was a 5-year-old boy in La Gloria, Mexico. This swine influenza virus spread to Mexico City and San Luis Potosi as well as Southern California and Texas. Features associated with this novel H1N1 virus include serious disease in people less than 60 years of age and person-to-person transmission during the low season for circulating viruses. Some of the infections are aggressive, with pneumonia requiring ventilator support that progresses to acute respiratory distress syndrome. Some of the deaths occurred in previously healthy individuals (CDC, 2009c). Children, young adults, and pregnant women are particularly susceptible to a life-threatening infection caused by novel H1N1 influenza virus.

Since new antigenic variants frequently emerge, vaccine antigens need to be frequently updated. These updates are

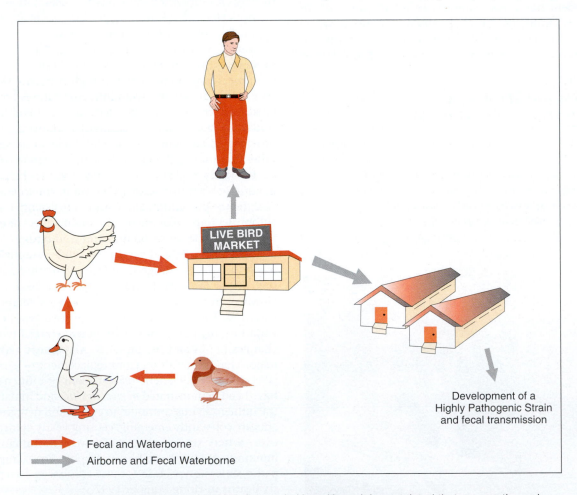

■ FIGURE 42-9 The emergence of H5N1 influenza in Hong Kong. It is postulated that a nonpathogenic H5N1 influenza spread from migrating shorebirds to ducks by fecal contamination of water. The virus was transmitted to chickens and became established in live bird markets in Hong Kong. During transmission between different species, the virus became highly pathogenic for chickens and occasionally was transmitted to humans from chickens in the markets. Despite high pathogenicity for chickens (and humans), H5N1 were nonpathogenic for ducks and geese.

From Webster, R. G. (1998). Influenza: An emerging disease. *Emerging Infectious Diseases, 4*(3), 436–441.

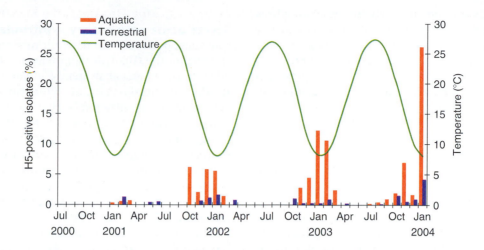

FIGURE 42-10 Seasonality of the isolation of avian H5N1 viruses from domestic poultry in mainland China during July 2000 to January 2004. The mean monthly temperature in southern China (approximated from the monthly average temperatures of the cities Changsha, Kunming, and Xiamen) is shown for reference.

Reprinted by permission from Macmillan Publishers Ltd: Li, K. S., Guan, Y., et al. (2004). Genesis of a highly pathogenic and potentially pandemic H5N1 influenza virus in eastern Asia. *Nature, 430,* 209–213.

based on results of global surveillance, including clinical, virological, and immunological studies (Bridges et al., 2002). Dr. Chan concluded her remarks on June 11, 2009, by saying "We are all in this together, and we will all get through this together" (WHO, 2009b). To review influenza outbreaks in history, see ∞ Chapter 1.

Rift Valley Fever

Rift Valley fever (RVF) is an undifferentiated febrile illness caused by Rift Valley fever virus (RVFV). RVFV is a member of the *Bunyaviridae* family and is widespread in sub-Saharan Africa and Egypt. In 2000, an outbreak of RVF occurred in the Arabian Peninsula and was the first recorded outbreak of RVF outside of Africa, which resulted in considerable human and animal fatalities (Ahmad, 2000; CDC, 2000).

The epidemiology of RVF consists of both epizootic and interepizootic cycles. During an epizootic cycle, virus circulates among infected arthropod vectors and mammalian hosts, particularly cattle and sheep (Nabeth et al., 2001). The interepizootic cycle involves transovarian transmission of the virus within the *Aedes* mosquitoes (Sidwell & Smee, 2003; Zeller & Bouloy, 2000). The incubation period of RVF is approximately 6 days, with a maximum of 13 days (Drosten, Minnak, et al., 2002). Onset of symptoms is sudden with fever, myalgia, dizziness, neck pain and stiffness, backache, headache, sore throat, and photophobia. Over a period of several days, infected individuals may experience sharp mood swings along with confusion and aggression (Drosten, Minnak, et al., 2002). After 2–4 days, agitation may be replaced by sleepiness and depression. Encephalitis and retinitis are severe complications of RVF that develop 1 or 2 weeks into the course of disease. However, severe and frequently fatal encephalitis is rare and develops in less than 1% of infected individuals.

Clinical signs include hepatomegaly, tachycardia, lymphadenopathy, and petechial rash on internal mucosal surfaces and the skin. A number of RFV infections in laboratory workers have been reported, which suggests that it can be easily transmitted by aerosol inhalation (Smithburn et al., 1949). The World Health Organization has estimated that if 50 kg of RFV were released from an aircraft along a 2 km line upwind of a population center of 500,000 persons, 400 would die and 35,000 would be incapacitated (Christopher et al., 1997). Consequently, diagnosis should be performed in specially equipped, high-biosafety-level laboratories. IgG and IgM antibodies may be detected in serum via ELISA from approximately day 6 of illness. IgM antibody remains detectable for up to 4 months and IgG levels are detectable for up to 5 years. Treatment is supportive with intensive monitoring. To date, there is no safe and effective vaccine widely available for human use. People in endemic areas should use personal protective measures that include avoidance of insect vectors.

Human Metapneumovirus

Avian metapneumovirus was originally an organism that infected poultry, specifically turkeys. This virus was first described in South Africa in the late 1970s as the etiological agent of turkey rhinotracheitis. However, in 2001, a novel human pneumovirinae virus was isolated from nasopharyngeal aspirates of children in the Netherlands. The infected children presented with symptoms similar to respiratory syncytial virus (RSV). The newly isolated virus was found to be phylogenically similar to human respiratory syncytial virus (hRSV) and was tentatively named human metapneumovirus (hMPV) due to its genetic and morphological similarities to avian metapneumovirus.

Seroprevalence studies from archived samples dating back to 1958 indicate that the prevalence of hMPV is approximately 100% by age 5 and that it has been present in the human population for nearly 50 years (van den Hoogen et al., 2001). Subsequent studies have indicated that hMPV is prevalent worldwide. In addition, it may be responsible for a large portion of respiratory tract disease in all age groups and may be a leading cause of severe respiratory tract infection in the very young and the very old (Boivin et al., 2002; Chan et al., 2003; Nissen et al., 2002; Stephenson, 2003).

Human metapneumovirus and hRSV are both classified in the family *Paramyxovirdae* and contain RSV. Analysis of the genomic sequence of hMPV demonstrates 56–88% homology to avian metapneumovirus and 20% homology to RSV (van den Hoogen et al., 2001, 2002). Sequence studies have identified two main lineages, which may co-circulate during the winter season in patients with acute respiratory illness in North America (Boivin et al., 2002).

Pathogenesis effects of hMPV are similar to hRSV. Cytopathic effects (CPE) begin approximately 10 to 14 days postinoculation in tertiary monkey kidney cells with the appearance of characteristic syncytia formation, followed by rapid internal disruption of the cells and subsequent detachment from culture media (van den Hoogen et al., 2001).

In children, presentation of hMPV is similar to hRSV, with symptoms ranging from mild respiratory problems to severe cough, bronchiolitis, and pneumonia with associated symptoms of high fever, myalgia, and vomiting (van den Hoogen et al., 2001). Adults infected with hMPV primarily present with cough and congestion, rhinorrhea (runny nose), hoarseness, sputum production, and wheezing. In contrast to children, fever is not a common symptom in infected adults (Falsey et al., 2003). Laboratory results commonly observed include decreased hemoglobin, decreased hematocrit, and thrombocytosis (van den Hoogen et al., 2003).

There are mainly two methods used to diagnose hMPV infection. The first method uses cell culture techniques to isolate the virus from clinical samples. However, hMPV is difficult to isolate in cell culture because it requires prolonged incubation and causes mild cytopathicity. The second method employs molecular techniques, specifically RT-PCR, using hMPV RNA. Both methods can successfully isolate hMPV from nasal aspirates, throat swabs, sputum, or bronchoalveolar samples. Another traditional method to diagnose viruses is electron microscopy.

Since transmission presumably occurs via direct contact or inhalation of contaminated respiratory droplet aerosols, it is important for health care workers and visitors to adhere to strict hand washing techniques as well as the use of barrier precautions and contact isolation when exposed to this organism. The treatment for hMPV infection is supportive care. The exact role of hMPV as a disease entity and as a co-pathogen with other respiratory viruses is emerging and is the focus of numerous studies.

Severe Acute Respiratory Syndrome

Severe acute respiratory syndrome (SARS) is a rapidly spreading, potentially fatal, febrile respiratory illness that first emerged in the Guangdong province of China in November 2002. It gained global awareness in late February 2003 when the disease spread outside of China. On March 13, 2003, the World Health Organization (WHO) issued a global health alert as reports of more than 150 cases of SARS emerged from Hong Kong, Canada, Vietnam, Singapore, and Taiwan. Within 6 weeks of the global outbreak, a concerted effort by the international scientific community resulted in the rapid isolation and identification of the causative agent, a novel coronavirus (Figure 42-11 ■). The virus was later named SARS-coronavirus (SARS-CoV) (Peiris et al., 2003).

The *Coronaviridae* are a family of enveloped, positive-stranded RNA viruses that cause common colds and other respiratory infections in humans and diverse illnesses in birds and mammals. In 2003, Peiris, Yuenn, Osterhaus, and Stöhr established the etiological link between coronavirus and SARS while investigating the outbreak in Hong Kong. Coronavirus was initially isolated from 2 of the 50 patients with respiratory symptoms. Later, using serological and RT-PCR assays specific for the virus, SARS-CoV was isolated from an additional 45 of the 50 patients. Within 1 month of a mid-March 2003 issuance of a global alert by the WHO, the entire genomic sequence of SARS-CoV was completed (Drosten, Gunther, et al., 2003; Ksiazek et al., 2003).

The SARS-CoV genome consists of 29,727 nucleotides (Rota et al., 2003). The proteins within the genus coronavirus consists of replicase (*rep*), spike (S), envelope (E), membrane (M), and nucleocapsid (N). The coronavirus S glycoprotein is involved in cellular membrane binding and fusion and is a major antigenic determinant. However, the SARS-CoV protein

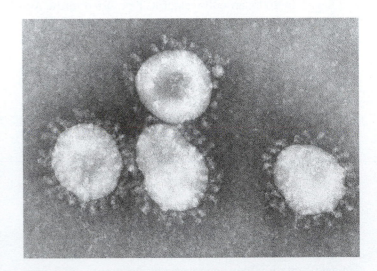

■ **FIGURE 42-11** SARS is caused by coronaviruses, a group of viruses that have a halo or crown-like (corona) appearance when viewed under an electron microscope.
From Public Health Image Library (PHIL), CDC/Dr. Fred Murphy.

S only has 20–27% pairwise amino acid similarity compared to other coronavirus S proteins (Rota et al., 2003). Vaccine research with components of SARS-CoV protein S is currently underway.

Due to its epidemic potential and possible spread by aerosolization, governments and international organizations are developing policies for vigilant surveillance and quarantining of suspected cases and carriers. The Council of State and Territorial Epidemiologists (CSTE) has added SARS-CoV disease to the National Notifiable Disease Surveillance System (CDC, 2003c). Laboratory cultures and samples must be rigorously handled with precaution. Unlike other coronaviruses, which require a biosafety level 2 laboratory for routine handling and testing of specimens, a biosafety level 3 is required for SARS-CoV culture or inoculation of animals (WHO, 2003a).

 REAL WORLD TIP

Other viruses discussed in previous sections are also nationally notifiable diseases. They include hantavirus, HIV, and novel H1N1 influenza A.

The SARS-CoV is transmitted primarily by airborne spread and possibly through contamination of surfaces. Recent data suggest that the virus remains viable for up to 24 hours on a dry surface; thus, fomite transmission may be a mechanism for infection (WHO, 2003a). The actual viral shedding phase of the illness is unclear. Studies have shown that there are asymptomatic carriers and "super spreaders" among infected individuals. Asymptomatic carriers show no symptoms or only mild febrile illness even when they test positive serologically. Super spreaders are patients who directly infect 10 or more individuals. Many super spreaders in the 2003 outbreak were health care workers (HCW), family members, social contacts, or visitors to an infected healthcare facility.

The WHO and CDC define a suspect SARS case as a person presenting with a high fever (temperature over 38°C or 100.4°F), lower respiratory symptoms of coughing or difficulty breathing, and prior exposure within 10 days of symptom onset. Prior exposure includes travel to an area with documented transmission of SARS, close contact with a person who is a suspect or a probable case of SARS, or residence in an affected area. A suspect case becomes a probable case when evidence of infiltrates consistent with pneumonia or acute respiratory distress syndrome is discovered without an identifiable explanation (CDC, 2003c).

Epidemiological analysis of 1,425 cases in Hong Kong revealed that the mean incubation period for infection was approximately 6.4 days (95% CI 5.2–7.7) and the mean time to symptom onset and hospitalization was three to five days. Estimated case fatality was 13.2% for patients less than 60 years old and 43.3% for patients older than 60. The mean viral load appears to peak around the 10th day of illness and decreases by the 15th day of illness.

Three clinical phases have been described in SARS infections. The initial phase consists of 2–4 days of fever and a dry, nonproductive cough. Phase two begins in the second week, with progressive shortness of breath. Clinically, patients often present with recurrent fever, hypoxemia, diarrhea, and an infiltrate on chest radiograph (Peiris et al., 2003). By week three or phase three, 20% of the infected patients develop acute respiratory distress syndrome (ARDS) and require ventilator support. The case fatality rate is 3–12% but may be as high as 45% in patients who have preexisting conditions or are over 60 years of age.

The diagnosis of SARS is difficult, and currently there is no single "gold standard" test recommended by the WHO. Laboratory confirmation for SARS includes PCR testing for SARS-CoV, seroconversion by ELISA or IFA (either fourfold increase in titer or positive convalescent titer), and virus isolation from cell culture with PCR confirmation. The utility of these tests is dictated by the stage of illness. For example, PCR does not identify the virus within the first couple of days of infection. A high clinical suspicion and working diagnosis based on the clinical definition for a suspect versus probable case are most important. The initial workup should exclude other potential causes of respiratory infection such as influenza, respiratory syncytial virus, *Legionella,* and other microorganisms. Sputum Gram stain and culture should be obtained along with paired sera for acute and convalescent serology (if greater than 21 days after onset of symptoms). Paired sera and other clinical specimens can be sent to the CDC for additional testing including viral culture and PCR. Seroconversion takes approximately 10 days to occur (WHO, 2003a).

Each hospital must have an emergency response plan, strict isolation policy, and mechanisms in place for surveillance and dissemination of findings via local and global networks. Surveillance monitoring includes daily screening of HCW, family members, and acquaintances exposed to SARS-infected persons within the previous 10 days. People with unprotected exposures that develop fever or respiratory symptoms should be isolated and their symptoms should be documented. HCW with high-risk, unprotected exposure, such as intubation, respiratory suction, or bronchoscopy should be quarantined for at least 10 days and closely monitored for symptoms (WHO, 2003a).

There is no specific treatment available for SARS. Management consists of supportive care and proper infection-control measures to prevent spread. Because the initial diagnosis is typically uncertain, empiric antibiotic therapy for community-acquired pneumonia should be administered, including coverage for atypical bacterial respiratory pathogens. Ribavirin, an antiviral agent, was used in most patients treated in Hong Kong and Toronto but without evidence of efficacy (Booth et al., 2003; Peiris et al., 2003).

Early recognition and isolation of patients with SARS are critical to limiting disease spread. Since viremia peaks during the second phase of the illness, transmission may occur after isolation of index cases. Patients need to be screened with targeted questions and triaged for the possibility of early SARS infection. The risk of exposure provides a vital clue and forms the epidemiological criterion for making a diagnosis. Identification of cases followed by proper isolation in negative pressure rooms is essential. HCW should follow strict contact and airborne isolation measures including frequent hand washing, wearing disposable gowns, changing gloves between patients, and wearing respiratory N-95 masks. Public health officials should be notified for confirmed cases (WHO, 2003a; CDC, 2003c).

PARASITES

Parasites are organisms that live by feeding upon another organism. Human parasites infect and reside within the human body. There are several types of parasites, including the protozoa, which are single-celled organisms, and helminths, which are multicelled worms. This section discusses the recently emerged parasitic diseases of humans.

Cyclosporiasis

The protozoan parasite *Cyclospora cayetanensis* was first recognized as a cause of human illness in 1979. *Cyclospora* is a coccidian parasite closely related to the genus *Eimeria* (Ortega et al., 1993; Relman et al., 1996). To be infectious, the spherical oocyst (8–10 μm) must sporulate in the environment, which may take several days depending on the conditions. The incubation period between infection and onset of symptoms averages 1 week (Figure 42-12 ■).

C. cayetanensis infects the small intestine and usually causes frequent bouts of watery diarrhea. Other symptoms include loss of appetite, weight loss, stomach cramps, vomiting, fatigue, increased flatus, and low-grade fever. Some infected individuals do not have any symptoms. The duration of symptoms is usually several weeks and can recur over a course of 1–2 months. Transmission occurs via water and food. The most common route of infection is through ingestion of contaminated raw fruits or vegetables. In endemic areas, transmission is seasonal, with outbreaks occurring most often in late spring to early summer. In May–June 1996, several outbreaks of cyclosporiasis were reported in the United States and Canada (CDC, 1996). Investigations of these outbreaks implicated the consumption of imported, fresh raspberries as the source of infection (Colley, 1996). *Cyclospora* species are highly resistant to disinfecting agents.

Cyclosporiasis has been reported in many countries, but is most common in tropical and subtropical environments. In endemic areas, transmission is seasonal, with outbreaks occurring most often in late spring to early summer. Diagnostic features of *Cyclospora* infection include characteristic morphology and size, positive staining with Kinyoun's acid-fast stain, positive autofluorescence under ultraviolet light, and sporulation of oocysts with formation of sporocysts after a 10-day incubation period (Garcia-Lopez et al., 1996). Cyclosporiasis can be treated with trimethoprim-sulfamethoxazole. Prevention includes avoiding food or water that may be contaminated with infected fecal matter.

Cryptosporidiosis

Cryptosporidium was reported as a human pathogen in 1976 (Nime et al., 1976). Infection with *Cryptosporidium* species results in a wide range of manifestations, from asymptomatic infections to severe, life-threatening illness. Watery diarrhea is the most frequent symptom, and can be accompanied by dehydration, weight loss, abdominal pain, fever, nausea, and vomiting. In immunocompetent persons, symptoms are usually short lived (1–2 weeks); however, they can be chronic and more severe in immunocompromised patients, especially those with CD4 counts <200/μl. While the small intestine is the site most commonly affected, symptomatic *Cryptosporidium* infections have also been found in other organs including other digestive tract organs, the lungs, and possibly conjunctiva.

Oocysts in stool specimens (fresh or in storage media) remain infective for extended periods. Thus stool specimens should be preserved in 10% buffered formalin or sodium acetate–acetic acid–formalin (SAF) to render oocysts nonviable. Contact time with formalin necessary to kill oocysts is not clear; at least 18–24 hours has been suggested. In addition, the usual safety measures for handling potentially infectious material should be adopted.

Stool specimens may be submitted fresh, preserved in 10% buffered formalin, or suspended in a storage medium composed of aqueous potassium dichromate (2.5% w/v, final concentration). The use of mercuric chloride-containing preservatives (e.g., polyvinyl alcohol, or PVA) is not recommended due to incompatibilities with some methodologies and the environmental hazards posed by the disposal of mercury-containing compounds. Oocyst numbers can be quite variable, even in liquid stools. Multiple stool samples should be tested before a negative diagnostic interpretation is reported. To maximize recovery of oocysts, stool samples should be concentrated prior to microscopic examination. Formalin-ethyl acetate sedimentation is the recommended stool concentration method for clinical laboratories.

Acid-fast staining methods, with or without stool concentration, are most frequently used in clinical laboratories. For greatest sensitivity and specificity, immunofluorescence microscopy is the method of choice (Kehl et al., 1995; Newman et al., 1993). Molecular methods may also be used, but are mainly a research tool. There are currently no commercially available serological assays for the detection of *Cryptosporidium*-specific antibodies. However, immunoblots for detecting the 17 and 27 kDa sporozoite antigens associated with recent infection may be useful for epidemiological investigations.

There is no established specific therapy for human cryptosporidiosis. Rapid loss of fluids because of diarrhea can be managed by fluid and electrolyte replacement. Infection in healthy, immunocompetent persons is self-limited. Nitazoxanide has provided some encouraging results in the management of cryptosporidial diarrhea in immunocompetent patients and has been FDA approved for treatment of

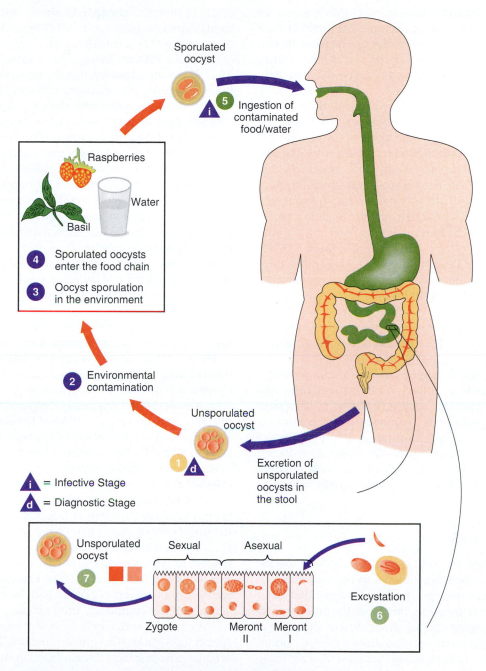

Sporulated
oocyst

5 Ingestion of
contaminated
food/water

i = Infective Stage

Raspberries

Water

Basil

4 Sporulated oocysts
enter the food chain

3 Oocyst sporulation
in the environment

2 Environmental
contamination

Unsporulated
oocyst

1 d

i = Infective Stage

d = Diagnostic Stage

Excretion of
unsporulated
oocysts in
the stool

Unsporulated
oocyst

7

Sexual   Asexual

Zygote   Meront   Meront
                II   I

Excystation

6

■ **FIGURE 42-12** *Cyclospora* life cycle. When freshly passed in stools, the oocyst is not infective ❶ (thus, direct fecal–oral transmission cannot occur; this differentiates *Cyclospora* from another important coccidian parasite, *Cryptosporidium*). In the environment ❷, sporulation occurs after days or weeks at temperatures between 22°C and 32°C, resulting in division of the sporont into two sporocysts, each containing two elongate sporozoites ❸. Fresh produce and water can serve as vehicles for transmission ❹ and the sporulated oocysts are ingested in contaminated food or water ❺. The oocysts excyst in the gastrointestinal tract, freeing the sporozoites, which invade the epithelial cells of the small intestine ❻. Inside the cells undergo asexual multiplication and sexual development to mature into oocysts, which will be shed in stools ❼. The potential mechanisms of contamination of food and water are still under investigation. Some of the elements in this figure were created based on an illustration by Ortega et al. (1998), pages 399–418.

cryptosporidiosis in immunocompetent children under 12 years old. Immunocompromised persons and those in poor health are at highest risk for severe illness. For persons with AIDS, antiretroviral therapy, which improves immune status, will also reduce oocyst excretion and decrease diarrhea associated with cryptosporidiosis.

Cryptosporidium parvum is considered a major threat to the U.S. water supply since only 30 oocysts are capable of causing an infection. The life cycle of *Cryptosporidium* can be found in Figure 42-13 ■. Cryptosporidium is found in untreated surface water, swimming and wade pools, day-care centers, and hospitals (Guerrant, 1997). The organism is resistant to chlorine, small (4–6 µm), difficult to filter, and ubiquitous in a variety of animals (Table 42-6✪). Hence, the organism would be difficult to eradicate. The best method to prevent the spread of cryptosporidiosis is to treat drinking water (heat 72°C for 1 min or use of a water filter that limit <1 µm) and to thoroughly wash all raw fruits and vegetables before ingestion (Addiss et al., 1996; Anderson, 1985). In 1993, a massive outbreak occurred in Milwaukee, WI, due to failure of the city's water treatment plant. The parasite caused diarrhea in 50% of the population of 800,000. Four thousand were hospitalized, and 100 immunocompromised individuals died.

Prevention is especially important for immunocompromised individuals where an infection can easily become life-threatening. In a stool sample, oocysts of *Cryptosporidium* must be differentiated from those of *Cyclospora*. This is commonly done by performing acid-fast staining on a suspected stool specimen and measuring the oocysts—*Cryptosporidium* oocysts are smaller than those of *Cyclospora* (Figure 42-14a ■ and b ■). Cryptosporidiosis and cyclosporiasis are nationally reportable diseases.

MISCELLANEOUS

There are several categories that do not fall under a specific infectious agent, thus have been placed in the miscellaneous section of the chapter. One type of infectious agent that is discussed in this section is the prion. Prions are the most recently identified infectious agent and are thought to be the cause of transmissible spongiform encephalopathies; however, prions are not the traditional microorganism that most of us are familiar with in the laboratory setting. In addition to the prion, bacteria that have recently become highly resistant to one or more antimicrobial agents have been placed in the miscellaneous category. Infections caused by prions and the resistant microbes are very difficult or impossible to treat and, unfortunately, the transmission and spread of all of these agents is on the rise.

TRANSMISSIBLE SPONGIFORM ENCEPHALOPATHIES

Transmissible spongiform encephalopathies (TSEs) are rare forms of progressive neurodegenerative disorders that affect both humans and animals (DeArmond & Prusiner, 1995). Some of the common TSEs are **Creutzfeldt–Jacob disease**

(CJD) in humans, **scrapie** in sheep and goats, and bovine spongiform encephalopathy (BSE) in cattle. However, the etiology of the TSEs is controversial.

All of the TSEs are thought to be caused by **prions** (Figure 42-15 ■), an altered protein that accumulates in brain tissue causing spongiform (vacuolation) changes. Prions are grouped together on the basis of similar clinical and pathological features. TSEs are characterized by the accumulation of an abnormal form of the normal host prion protein. The function of the normal prion protein is not yet known. Both the abnormal prion protein (PrP-res) and the normal prion protein (PrP-sen) differ mainly in their polypeptide fold. Prp-res is the only identified constituent of the infectious particle of the TSE agent and has been proposed to act as a protein-only agent (Prusiner, 1982). One major difference between Prp-res and PrP-sen is that the abnormal protein is partially resistant to proteolysis (Pan et al., 1993; Riek et al., 1996). PrP-res accumulation appears to be primarily restricted to the nervous system and, in some species, the lymphoreticular system of the infected host (Bolton et al., 1982; Kitamoto et al., 1991). A striking feature of prions is their high resistance to conventional sterilization procedures and their capacity to bind to metal and plastic surfaces without losing infectivity.

Human TSEs, more commonly known as CJD, can be divided into three groups: sporadic, genetic, and iatrogenic. Genetically inherited CJD is rare and includes Gertmann–Straussler–Scheinker syndrome (GSS) and fatal familial insomnia (FFI) (Kovacs et al., 2002). Most human CJD is categorized as sporadic. A small portion of sporadic CJD cases are iatrogenic (an unintentional effect of treatment), resulting from inadvertent inoculation with contaminated tissue derived from infected donors. Iatrogenic transmission includes the administration of contaminated pituitary-derived human growth hormone; transplantation of infected dural grafts or corneas; the use of contaminated neurosurgical instruments (Brown et al., 2000); and potentially through contaminated blood transfusions. In 1996, a new form of CJD, called variant CJD (vCJD), was identified (Will et al., 1996). Evidence suggests a causal relationship between vCJD and BSE; however, this is controversial and not completely understood.

BSE or mad cow disease is a TSE that affects cows and is widespread throughout the United Kingdom. BSE appears to have originated from scrapie disease found in sheep and goats. It has been hypothesized that carcasses of livestock (including sheep) were fed to ruminants in the form of meat and bone meal products and that this is how cattle became infected with the BSE agent. Consequently in 1988, the feeding of rendered livestock to ruminants was banned in an effort to eliminate infection to cattle. Although BSE is most prevalent in the United Kingdom, cases have occurred in many other countries, including the United States, as a result of imported live animals or livestock food supplements. BSE recently emerged in the United States in December 2004 from a cow that had been imported to a farm in the state of Washington from Canada (CDC, 2003a).

Epidemiological surveillance has suggested that vCJD is transmitted through ingestion of contaminated beef products derived from BSE-infected cattle. The vCJD differs from classic

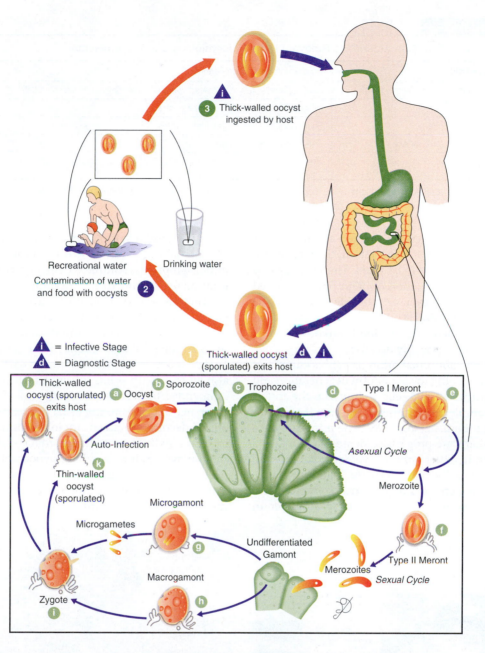

■ **FIGURE 42-13** Life cycle of *Cryptosporidium parvum* and *C. hominis.* Sporulated oocysts, containing four sporozoites, are excreted by the infected host through feces and possibly other routes such as respiratory secretions ❶. Transmission of *Cryptosporidium parvum* and *C. hominis* occurs mainly through contact with contaminated water (e.g., drinking or recreational water). Occasionally food sources, such as chicken salad, may serve as vehicles for transmission. Many outbreaks in the United States have occurred in water parks, community swimming pools, and day-care centers. Zoonotic transmission of *C. parvum* and *C. hominis* occur through exposure to infected animals or exposure to water contaminated by feces of infected animals ❷. Following ingestion (and possibly inhalation) by a suitable host ❸, excystation ⓐ occurs. The sporozoites are released and parasitize epithelial cells (ⓑ, ⓒ) of the gastrointestinal tract or other tissues such as the respiratory tract. In these cells, the parasites undergo asexual multiplication (schizogony or merogony) (ⓓ, ⓔ, ⓕ) and then sexual multiplication (gametogony), producing microgamonts (male) ⓖ and macrogamonts (female) ⓗ. Upon fertilization of the macrogamonts by the microgametes (ⓘ), oocysts (ⓙ, ⓚ) develop that sporulate in the infected host. Two different types of oocysts are produced, the thick-walled oocyst, which is commonly excreted from the host ⓙ, and the thin-walled oocyst ⓚ, which is primarily involved in autoinfection. Oocysts are infective upon excretion, thus permitting direct and immediate fecal–oral transmission.
From Juranek, D. D. Cryptosporidiosis. In G. T. Strickland (Ed.). (2000). Hunter's tropical medicine (8th ed., pp. 594–600). Philadelphia, PA: W. B. Saunders.

⊘ TABLE 42-6

Cryptosporidium Characteristics Relevant to Its Epidemiology and Transmission

Characteristic	Epidemiological Significance
Chlorine (and acid)-resistant oocysts	Easily spread in fully chlorinated water or swimming pools and acidic foods
Small size	Difficult to filter; threat to water industry
Low infectious dose	Easily acquired with high infection rates
Infectious when shed in feces	Person-to-person spread
Zoonotic potential	Transmission through animal contact

This table was published in Dillingham, R. A., Lima, A. A., & Guerrant, R. L. (2002). Cryptosporidiosis: Epidemiology and impact. Microbes and Infection, 4, 1059–1066. Copyright Elsevier.

CJD in several ways. For instance, the median age at death of patients with classic CJD is 68 years. In contrast, the median age at death of patients with vCJD is 28 years. The vCJD can be confirmed only though examination of brain tissue obtained by biopsy or at autopsy; however, a "probable case" of vCJD can be diagnosed based on clinical criteria. Since vCJD is a relatively new disease, the incubation period is unknown, but is most likely several years or possibly decades.

In prion diseases, the abnormal prion protein accumulates mainly in brain tissue leading to spongiform degeneration and is accompanied by activated glial cells. In humans, the abnormal protein can accumulate in a diffuse fashion or it can form amyloid-like plaques (Budka et al., 1995). The primary symptoms of TSEs in humans are progressive dementia and ataxia (lack of muscle control). Other symptoms observed in infected patients include personality changes, hallucinations, muscle twitching, nervousness, changes in gait, speech impairment, lack of coordination, memory loss, and anxiety. However, in vCJD, the initial symptoms usually manifest as personality changes and psychosis. Within 6 months after the onset of initial symptoms, complete dementia commonly occurs and is ultimately fatal within 7–12 months after diagnosis.

Prion diseases are difficult to diagnose and usually rely on behavioral and neurological symptoms as well as electroencephalography. The ultimate diagnostic procedure is a histopathological assessment of the central nervous system. To date, there is no known cure for CJD. Infection control is also an issue with prion infections. Disposable items are recommended to prevent iatrogenic infections, because of the resistance of prions to the usual physical and chemical methods of decontamination. Incineration is recommended for instruments that have had contact with tissues. Stringent sodium hydroxide and sodium hypochlorite decontamination procedures is recommended by the WHO for heat-resistant instruments that have come into contact with infected tissue (usually brain, spinal cord, CSF, and eye) (Finberg, 2004).

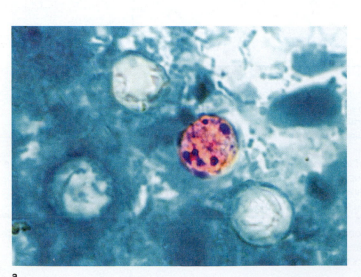

a

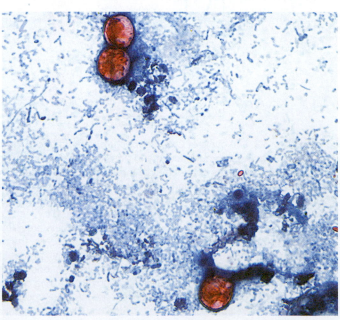

b

■ **FIGURE 42-14** Modified acid fast staining of **a.** *Cryptospordium,* and **b.** *Cyclospora* oocysts in stool.
From http://www.dpd.cdc.gov/dpdx/HTML/PDF_Files/Crypto_bench.pdf#search=%22cryptosporidium%20versus%20cyclospora%22.

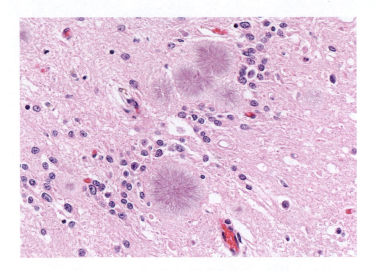

■ FIGURE 42-15 Magnified 158×, and stained with H&E (hematoxylin and eosin) staining technique, this light photomicrograph of brain tissue reveals the presence of typical amyloid plaques found in a case of variant Creutzfeldt–Jakob disease (vCJD). Note that the plaques vary in size, and consist of a hyaline eosinophilic core with a peripheral margin of radiating fibrils surrounded by a pale halo.
From Public Health Image Library (PHIL), CDC/Teresa Hammett.

HIGHLY RESISTANT ORGANISMS

The discovery of antibiotics is one of the greatest accomplishments of modern medicine. Antibiotics became widely used during the World War II era and since their inception have saved countless lives. However, after more than 50 years of widespread use, bacteria have evolved mechanisms that enable them to survive despite the use of these agents. For example, the *Enterobacteriaceae* swap resistance genes readily via conjugation and are rapidly evolving resistance to new antibiotics. Consequently, these newly resistant microorganisms make treatment very difficult and contribute to increased global morbidity and mortality. Diseases such as tuberculosis and malaria are currently more difficult to treat than they were decades ago. Drug resistance in the hospital setting is especially problematic due to the fact that hospitals harbor critically ill patients who are more susceptible to infections than the general population. Moreover, hospitalized patients require the use of more antibiotics, which increases the probability of mutations in bacteria that generate drug resistance. Antimicrobial resistance is increasing health care costs, the severity of disease, and death rates from certain infections. ∞ Chapter 11, "Susceptibility Testing," has more information on the resistance mechanisms and susceptibility testing of the *Enterobacteriaceae* and other microbes.

Vancomycin-Resistant Staphylococcus

Staphylococcus aureus is a major cause of community-acquired as well as nosocomial infections. Infection with *S. aureus* has been complicated due to the increasing numbers of strains exhibiting resistance to oxacillin (methicillin-resistant *S. aureus*, or MRSA). In 2003, a unique strain of MRSA emerged from an animal reservoir and entered the human population in the Netherlands. It is now responsible for more than 20% of MRSA cases in that country (Loo et al., 2007). Even more disturbing are the recent reports of infections caused by *S. aureus* exhibiting intermediate resistance to vancomycin (VISA). The Clinical and Laboratory Standards Institute (CLSI, 2009) defines *S. aureus* requiring concentrations of vancomycin of <4 µg/mL for growth inhibition as susceptible, those requiring concentrations of 4–8 µg/mL as intermediate, and those requiring concentrations of ≥16 µg/mL as resistant. The first clinical isolate of *S. aureus* with reduced or intermediate susceptibility to VISA was reported from Japan in 1996 (Hiramatsu et al., 1997). By June 2002, eight patients with clinical infections caused by VISA were confirmed in the United States (Fridkin, 2001; Smith et al., 1999).

The first documented case of vancomycin-resistant *S. aureus* (VRSA) in the United States occurred in 2002. The VRSA isolate was identified at a local hospital laboratory and was confirmed by the Michigan Department of Community Health and CDC. Identification methods used at CDC included traditional testing as well as DNA sequence analysis. The isolate contained the *vanA* vancomycin resistance gene (usually found in enterococci) and the oxacillin resistance gene *mecA*. The isolate was susceptible to chloramphenicol, linezolid, minocycline, quinupristin/dalfopristin, tetracycline, and trimethoprim/sulfamethoxazole (CDC, 2002b). Genetic analyses of VRSA isolates suggest that the vancomycin resistance gene from *Enterococcus faecalis* was transferred to a methicillin-resistant *S. aureus* strain by interspecies transfer of the mobile genetic element Tn1546 (Weigel et al., 2003).

Resistance to vancomycin was first reported in 1988 from an isolate of *Enterococcus faecium* (Leclercq et al., 1988). Vancomycin resistance is associated with one of several gene clusters that have been classified as *vanA* to *vanG*. High-level resistance to vancomycin via the acquisition of *vanA* is mediated by a mobile genetic element or transposon. To date, all of the individuals that developed VISA and VRSA infections had severe underlying health conditions, previous MRSA infection, catheters, recent hospitalization, and recent exposure to vancomycin and other antimicrobial agents. In addition, all VISA and VRSA isolates have been susceptible to

✓ Checkpoint! 42–5 (Chapter Objective 5)

The Clinical and Laboratory Standards Institute (CLSI) defines Staphylococcus aureus requiring concentrations of vancomycin of 4–8 µg/mL for growth inhibition as:

A. *susceptible.*

B. *intermediate.*

C. *resistant.*

several FDA-approved drugs. The best method to prevent the spread of these isolates is the use of appropriate infection control practices such as barrier protection before and after contact with infectious agents and hand hygiene. More information about *S. aureus* is in ∞ Chapter 17, "Aerobic Gram-Positive Cocci."

Multi-Drug-Resistant Tuberculosis

In 1993, the World Health Organization (WHO) declared tuberculosis (TB) a global emergency (WHO, 2002). Approximately one-third of the world's population is infected with TB, resulting in an estimated 2 million deaths per year. The current TB epidemic is due to multiple factors including the breakdown of health care infrastructure, the increase in HIV/AIDS, and the emergence of multi-drug-resistant TB (MDR-TB) (WHO, 2002).

Mycobacterium drug resistance was first noted in the 1940s shortly after the introduction of streptomycin for the treatment of TB (Canetti, 1965). MDR-TB is defined as *Mycobacterium tuberculosis* (Mtb) strains that are resistant to at least isoniazid (INH) and rifampin (RMP). Nosocomial and community outbreaks of MDR-TB began in the early 1990s and have become a significant problem in many parts of the world. Control and treatment of MDR-TB can be difficult not only due to the limited number of susceptible drugs, but also that these drugs are often less effective, more expensive, and may have more side effects due to increased toxicity.

Mtb drug resistance develops due to spontaneous chromosomal mutations. Mutations are more likely to occur in large cavitary lesions that contain high numbers of organisms. However, the use of combination therapy decreases the rate of acquired resistance during therapy (Iseman, 1999). MDR-TB is listed as a CDC category C bioterrorism agent. Bioterrorism potential of MDR-TB is derived from its ability to be disseminated by aerosolization as well as the difficulty in treatment. Although TB is a slow and progressive illness, its effects can be rapidly devastating, especially in the immunocompromised individual.

Mtb is transmitted primarily by inhalation of aerosolized respiratory droplet nuclei. Particles of 1–5 μm in diameter are produced via forced expiration during coughing. Multi-drug-resistant strains of Mtb are transmitted in the same manner as susceptible strains, resulting in an infection with a resistant organism. The initial focus of infection is usually in the lung. Alveolar macrophages infected with Mtb spread to regional lymph nodes and are carried hematogenously throughout the body. Rarely nonpulmonary infection can occur in the skin, intestine, oropharynx, genitalia, and lymph nodes (Small & Selcer, 2000).

Aside from primary infection, MDR-TB may also develop during treatment of active TB in a patient infected with a previously susceptible Mtb strain. This usually occurs due to a number of factors, including nonadherence to medication by the patient, incorrect prescription of medication by the health care provider, lack of second-line medications, or insufficient absorption of medication. Once resistance develops to one antimycobacterial drug, subsequent resistance to other agents may also develop due to inadequate therapy. Furthermore, these patients remain infectious and can transmit multi-drug-resistant Mtb to others.

The clinical presentation of MDR-TB infection is the same as for susceptible strains. Greater than 90% of individuals infected with *M. tuberculosis* harbor the organism without progression to active TB and are asymptomatic and not infectious. If latent TB infection is not diagnosed or patients fail to complete therapy for the treatment of latent TB infection, active TB can develop. Treatment of active TB includes three to four first-line agents including INH and RMP. However, if a patient is infected with MDR-TB, despite adherence to these first-line agents, persistent symptoms of fever, chills, night sweats, weight loss, worsening radiographic changes, and/or continued sputum positivity may occur due to the ineffective treatment regimen (McKenna et al., 1995).

Surveillance and detection is the most important strategy in the control of MDR-TB. Currently in the United States, drug susceptibility testing is recommended for all initial isolates and subsequently for persistently positive cultures and relapses. An increased understanding of molecular genetics has allowed for the development of rapid techniques for identifying regions containing mutations that confer high resistance. New diagnostic tools such as a molecular probe have improved the capability for rapid detection of Mtb from other *Mycobacterium* species. Improvements in the identification methods of resistant strains are necessary to make proper epidemiological links for rapid case detection, contact tracing, and management and control of an outbreak. Effective control and medical management of both MDR-TB and pan-sensitive cases is essential to the prevention of further MDR-TB transmission. Improved resistance testing with timely introduction of second-line agents is the most cost-effective and feasible strategy in the long-term care of MDR-TB patients (Dye et al., 2002).

MDR-TB treatment requires the use of second-line drugs that cost more, are more toxic, and are less effective than isoniazid and rifampin. In 2000 reports of cases of MDR-TB resistant to almost all of the second line drugs emerged (CDC, 2007). TB cases resistant to isoniazid and rifampin and at least three of the six second-line drugs (aminoglycosides, polypeptides, fluoroquinolones, thioamides, cycloserine, and para-aminosalicyclic acid) are called extensively drug-resistant tuberculosis (XDR-TB) (CDC, 2006). In the United States XDR-TB represents only 3% of MDR-TB. Cases were reported in nine states, with the largest number of cases in California and New York City. Although the highest mortality is associated with HIV-infected individuals, the proportion of cases in this population has decreased. The proportion of cases among foreign-born persons and Asians increased. Successful treatment depends on adherence to treatment and the function of the patient's immune system.

Drug-Resistant Malaria

Malaria is a highly prevalent and deadly parasitic disease of humans and is estimated to cause between 1 and 2 million deaths every year. Malaria is caused by one or more of four species of *Plasmodium* (*P. falciparum, P. vivax, P. ovale,* and *P. malariae*). To date, drug resistance has been documented in *P. falciparum* and *P. vivax. Plasmodium falciparum* accounts for the majority of morbidity and mortality associated with malaria in Africa, especially since the parasite has developed resistance to nearly all available antimalarials.

Quinine, extracted from the bark of the cinchona tree, was used as an antimalarial agent as early as 1632 (Baird et al., 1996). By the nineteenth century, quinine was still the only known antimalarial agent. Other antimalarial agents such as primaquine and quinacrine were produced after World War I. Chloroquine was produced in 1934 and became the drug of choice to treat malaria. The earliest anecdotal reports of resistance to an antimalarial agent are those for quinine in 1844 and 1910. Chloroquine resistance emerged in 1957 in Southeast Asia and from there it began to spread. Currently, resistance has emerged to all classes of antimalarial drugs except the artemisinins and has contributed to an increase in malaria-related mortality (White, 2004; WHO, 2001).

The genetic events leading to antimalarial drug resistance are spontaneous and include mutations in the copy number of genes associated with the organism's influx/efflux pumps that affect drug concentrations within the parasite (White, 2004). In experimental animal models, drug resistance mutations can be selected by exposing large numbers of malaria parasites to subtherapeutic concentrations of antimalarial drugs (Peters, 1987, 1990). Unlike most bacteria, transferable resistance genes are not involved in the emergence of drug-resistant malaria. In some instances, **cross-resistance** occurs when resistance to one drug is selected for by another drug where the mechanism of resistance is similar.

The term **parasite resistance** has been defined as the ability of a parasite strain to survive and/or multiply despite the administration and absorption of a drug in doses equal to or higher than those usually recommended but within the limits of tolerance of the subject (WHO, 1965). Moreover, the drug must gain access to the parasite or the infected red blood cell for the duration of the time necessary for the normal action of the drug (Bruce-Chwatt et al., 1986). The factors responsible for the emergence and rate of spread of parasite resistance are unclear.

Several methods for monitoring antimalarial drug resistance exist and include both *in vivo* and *in vitro* tests as well as molecular markers. *In vivo* testing is considered the gold standard since it is a more accurate reflection of the biological nature of the treatment response. *In vitro* tests are based on the inhibition of the growth and development of malaria parasites by different concentrations of a given drug relative to the drug-free controls.

There are two major efforts used to control malaria. The first is to control the mosquito vector and the second is effec-

TABLE 42-7

Factors Contributing to the Selection of Antimalarial Drug Resistance

1	The frequency with which the resistance mechanism arises
2	The cost to the fitness of the parasite because of the resistance mechanism present
3	The number of parasites in the human host that are exposed to the drug
4	Concentration of drug to which parasites are exposed
5	Pharmacodynamic properities of the drug or drugs
6	Degree of resistance resulting from genetic changes
7	Level of host defense
8	Simultaneous presence of other antimalarial drugs in the blood that will continue to kill the parasite if it develops resistance to one drug

Adapted from White, N. J. (2004). Antimalarial drug resistance. *Journal of Clinical Investigation, 113*(8), 1084–1092.

tive case management. Treating patients with antimalarial agents, such as chloroquine, is an efficient method to manage malaria cases. Unfortunately, misuse of these agents is widespread and has contributed to the selective pressure of the parasite to evolve resistance mechanisms (Table 42-7✪). See ∞ Chapters 15 and 30 to review specimen processing for and identification of parasites.

▶ BIOTERRORISM

Concerns about the use of chemical or biological agents by countries, terrorist groups, or individuals have dramatically increased following the 9/11/01 attack on the United States. Prior to 2001 there were two events in which microbes were used in domestic bioterror cases. In 1985 an Oregon cult sprayed a salad bar with *Salmonella,* causing an outbreak that affected 751 people (Török et al., 1997). In another report, a laboratory worker used a stock culture to spike pastries with *Shigella dysenteriae.* Twelve of the laboratory staff developed severe, acute diarrhea after eating muffins and donuts that were in the staff lounge (Kolavic et al., 1997). Biological warfare agents are easy to manufacture, generally don't require sophisticated delivery systems, have the ability to kill or injure large populations, cause illnesses that are unrecognized in their initial stages, and may affect large geographical areas. Hence, the Centers for Disease Control and Prevention Strategic Planning Workgroup recommends that preparedness efforts focus on agents with the potential for the greatest impact on health and security, especially those that are highly contagious or that can be engineered for widespread dissemination via aerosols, such as smallpox.

Depending on the intent of the person, group, or nation using biological agents the incident may be overt (announced) or covert (unannounced). In either case, rapid identification of the etiological agent is essential. In the case of a covert biological attack, clinicians and emergency response workers will most likely be the first to recognize a disease as an incident of bioterrorism based on the pattern and frequency of symptoms. In addition, clinical microbiologists will most likely make the initial identification of the organism. Consequently, it is imperative that the medical community is familiar with the characteristics of these agents and the technologies available for their detection and identification.

 Checkpoint! 42–6 (Chapter Objective 6)

The key characteristics associated with agents of bioterror include
  A. *Easy to manufacture*
  B. *Cause injury or death to a large number of individuals*
  C. *Cause symptoms that are unrecognizable due to their similarity with other illnesses*
  D. *All of the above*

SUMMARY

There are many questions yet to be answered regarding the emergence of novel pathogens, such as *E. coli* O157:H7 and HIV. These and other emerging infectious diseases present some of the most significant health and security challenges facing the global community. It is clear that many emerging organisms become capable of crossing the barrier from their natural reservoirs into human populations. Ecological changes, climate changes, ease of travel, and human behavior are believed to play a role in the emergence of novel pathogens and subsequent human-to-human transmission. In addition, genetic changes in the pathogen or in the population of the new host provide opportunities for the organism to adapt to new environments; hence, the emergence of a new or previously unidentified disease develops. Scientific breakthroughs such as recombinant DNA technology, immunology, genomics, and proteomics hold considerable promise against emerging infections and diseases of terrorism. These innovations are being applied to the challenge of protecting the American population by identifying new diagnostic techniques and treatments.

LEARNING OPPORTUNITIES

1. On the Web:
   Monitor outbreaks around the world at Pro-MED-mail, URL: www.promedmail.org
   More information on bioterror agents can be found at URL:
   http://www.asm.org/ php?option=com_content&view=article&id=520&title= Biodefense%20Resources%20Center and http://emergency.cdc.gov/bioterrorism

2. What is the current treatment for an individual with transmissible spongiform encephalopathy? (Chapter Objective 3)

3. Which of the following risk factors is associated with acquiring cholera? (Chapter Objective 4)
   a. mosquito resistance to insecticides
   b. misuse of antibiotics
   c. travel to a foreign country
   d. an immunocompromised state

4. Which of the following organisms is a category A pathogen that could be easily distributed due to its ability to produce spores? (Chapter Objective 6)
   a. *Francisella tularensis*
   b. *Bacillus anthracis*
   c. *Brucella* spp.
   d. *Yersinia pestis*

CASE STUDY 42-1   (CHAPTER OBJECTIVES 3 AND 4)

In June 2002, VRSA was isolated from a swab obtained from a catheter exit site from a Michigan resident age 40 years. The patient was suffering from diabetes, peripheral vascular disease and chronic renal failure. The patient received dialysis at an outpatient facility. Starting April 2001, the patient had been treated for chronic foot ulcerations with multiple courses of antibiotic therapy, including vancomycin. In April 2002 the patient underwent amputation of a gangrenous toe and subsequently developed MRSA bacteremia caused by an infected ateriovenous hemodialysis graft. The infection was treated with vancomycin, rifampin, and removal of the infected graft. In June, the patient developed a suspected catheter exit-site infection. Cultures of the infected area as well as the catheter tip grew *S. aureus* resistant to oxacillin and vancomycin. The patient responded to treatment con-

sisting of aggressive wound care and systemic antimicrobial therapy with trimethoprim/sulfamethoxazole.

1. Based on what you have read in this chapter, what is a likely factor that contributed to the development of vancomycin resistance in this patient's *S. aureus* isolate?

2. Discuss three methods that can be used to prevent the spread of antimicrobial resistance.

CASE STUDY 42-2   THE FIRST (INDEX) CASE OF SARS AND THE "SUPERSPREADING" EVENT THAT LED TO THE SARS OUTBREAK (CHAPTER OBJECTIVE 3)

In November 2002, a very contagious atypical pneumonia appeared in the Guangdong Province of the People's Republic of China. Despite public chaos in the province, the news of the outbreak was mainly reported within China. In addition, a concurrent fatal influenza A (H5N1 subtype) outbreak was occurring in the Fujian Province of China. On February 11, 2003, the Chinese health authorities reported to the WHO 305 cases of an unknown influenza-like illness that produced five fatalities. On February 21, 2003, a 65-year-old physician from Guangdong, who had cared for patients with this unknown respiratory illness and had been ill since February 15, traveled to Hong Kong and stayed on the ninth floor of a local hotel for one day. The next day, he was admitted to a hospital with fever and respiratory symptoms and subsequently died of respiratory failure. This index case infected at least 17 other hotel guests, health care workers (HCW), and visitors and set off clusters of outbreaks,

both locally and internationally, as infected individuals traveled to Singapore, Vietnam, Toronto, Canada, and the United States (Peiris et al., 2003). Over the next few months, increased recognition of the disease and mechanisms of its transmission assisted international scientists and local health officials in setting guidelines for infection control that eventually contained this outbreak. Aggressive and novel methods such as quarantine of thousands of people, travel restrictions, and temperature checks at airports were implemented. Military presence and monetary incentives, coupled with video and telephone monitoring systems, helped enforce quarantines in several countries. Hospital infection-control measures included temperature screening of all HCW, enforcement of no-visitation rules, and designating one hospital for SARS cases.

1. List the methods employed during this outbreak that reduced the spread of SARS.

CASE STUDY 42-3   THE INDEX CASE OF H5N1 INFLUENZA VIRUS IN HUMANS ADAPTED FROM WEBSTER (1998) (CHAPTER OBJECTIVE 2)

In May 1997 a 3-year-old boy from Hong Kong died in an ICU on day 5 of hospitalization from a respiratory illness of unknown origin. The child had no indication of other underlying disease, including immunodeficiency or cardiopulmonary disease. Studies of respiratory specimens from the child recovered an influenza virus; however, pathogenic bacteria were never isolated from any of the samples. In hemagglutination inhibition assays, the virus did not react with antisera to recent isolates of human and swine influenza subtypes. Further studies demonstrated that the

isolate was an H5 influenza A virus. Neuraminidase inhibition tests indicated that the neuraminidase was of the N1 subtype. Nucleotide sequence analyses of HA and NA gene segments confirmed that the virus was an H5N1 subtype. In addition, these studies confirmed that the virus was of avian origin and was highly pathogenic to chickens (Subbarao et al., 1998).

1. Why was the identification of the virus in this study so important?

CASE STUDY 42-4 A CASE STUDY DEMONSTRATING THE DIFFICULTY IN DIAGNOSING CYCLOSPORIASIS (ADAPTED FROM KRISHNA AND DAVIS [2004]) (CHAPTER OBJECTIVE 3)

On February 6–8, 2004, a conference was held in Irving, Texas. Approximately 40 individuals from 15 states attended this conference. One week after the conference, at least seven attendees developed gastrointestinal symptoms. On March 4, the CDC confirmed the diagnosis of *Cyclospora* infection by examining the stool specimen from the index-case patient. An epidemiological investigation was initiated. On February 12, one of the conference attendees developed fever, nausea, vomiting, and diarrhea. The individual was hospitalized from February 16–28 due to severe symptoms. Cyclosporiasis was considered but rejected based on a negative laboratory test. The patient was readmitted February 29–March 2 because of severe cellulitis. A stool sample from March 5 was positive for *Cyclospora*.

1. What are two potential shortcomings of oocyst concentration techniques?

CASE STUDY 42-5 THE FIRST CASE OF BSE IN THE UNITED STATES (CDC, 2003a) (CHAPTER OBJECTIVE 3)

A 6½-year-old cow was slaughtered on December 9. Before slaughter, the cow was nonambulatory. The condition of the cow was attributed to complications to calving (giving birth). A U.S. Department of Agriculture (USDA) Food Safety and Inspection Service (FSIS) veterinary medical officer examined the animal before and after slaughter. After examination, the carcass was released for use as food for human consumption. Tissues (e.g., brain, spinal cord, and small intestine) considered to be high risk for transmission of the BSE agent were removed from the cow and sent for inedible rendering (often used as nonruminant animal feed). Brain tissue samples were taken as part of the targeted surveillance for BSE. On December 23, 2003, the USDA made a preliminary diagnosis of BSE and the herd to which this cow belonged was placed under a state hold order. On December 24, FSIS recalled beef from cattle slaughtered in the same plant on the same day as the positive cow. Some of the beef had already been shipped to several establishments, which processed the meat further. On December 25, the BSE international reference laboratory in Weybridge, England, confirmed the diagnosis. The BSE-positive cow was traced back to a farm in Alberta, Canada, which was one of 81 cattle that were shipped to the United States on September 4, 2001. On December 30, the USDA announced additional safeguards to further minimize the risk for human exposure to BSE in the United States. The occurrence of BSE in the United States reinforces the need for health care workers to be aware of the clinical features of vCJD. Brain autopsies should be performed on all patients with suspected or probable CJD to assess the neuropathology of these patients.

1. How is the diagnosis of BSE made in humans?
2. Identify 3 ways to decontaminate instruments used for an autopsy of a patient identified with BSE.

PEARSON **myhealthprofessionskit**™

Use this address to access the interactive Companion Website created for this textbook. Simply select "Clinical Laboratory Science" from the choice of disciplines. Find this book and log in using your user name and password.

REFERENCES

Go to myhealthprofessionskit.com to view this chapter's references.

APPENDIX
Answers to Checkpoints

✓

Chapter 1

1-1	D	1-4	A
1-2	D	1-5	B
1-3	B		

Chapter 2

2-1	D	2-6	D
2-2	A	2-7	G
2-3	A, B, D, C	2-8	C
2-4	A	2-9	B
2-5	C		

Chapter 3

3-1	B	3-13	C
3-2	A	3-14	C
3-3	C	3-15	B
3-4	B	3-16	B
3-5	C	3-17	E
3-6	C	3-18	A
3-7	C	3-19	A
3-8	B		
3-9	A		
3-10	A		
3-11	A		

3-12 E; From masses given in Table I, the number of *E. coli* per human is: $(6.75 \times 10^4$ g per human$)/(2 \times 10^{-12}$ g per *E. coli*$) = 3.375 \times 10^{16}$ *E. coli* per human. From eq. 3-3, cell number $= 2^n = 3.375 \times 10^{16}$. To solve this, remember the tricks you learned for logarithms in high school algebra: $n \log 2 = \log 3.375 \times 10^{16}$; $n (0.301) = 16.53$; $n = 54.9$ generations. Since there are 3 generations per hour, $54.9/3 = 18.3$ h! Therefore in one long day, a single *E. coli* can match the weight of a 148.5-pound (67.5 Kg) person!

Chapter 4

4-1	B	4-4	D
4-2	B	4-5	C
4-3	A		

Chapter 5

5-1	A	5-7	D
5-2	B	5-8	B
5-3	B	5-9	A
5-4	B	5-10	C
5-5	C	5-11	A
5-6	B		

Chapter 6

6-1	D	6-5	B
6-2	C	6-6	B
6-3	C	6-7	B
6-4	A		

Chapter 7

7-1	A	7-6	B
7-2	B	7-7	C
7-3	B	7-8	D
7-4	C	7-9	A
7-5	D	7-10	D

Chapter 8

8-1	D	8-6	C
8-2	C	8-7	A
8-3	C	8-8	A
8-4	D	8-9	B
8-5	C	8-10	D

Chapter 9

9-1	C	9-7	A
9-2	A	9-8	B
9-3	A	9-9	A
9-4	D	9-10	C
9-5	B	9-11	D
9-6	B		

Chapter 10

10-1	C	10-4	B
10-2	A	10-5	D
10-3	B	10-6	E

Chapter 11

11-1	B	11-9	B
11-2	D	11-10	C
11-3	A	11-11	A
11-4	A	11-12	B
11-5	B	11-13	C
11-6	D	11-14	A
11-7	C	11-15	B
11-8	D	11-16	D

Chapter 12

12-1	C	12-3	B
12-2	D	12-4	D

Chapter 13

13-1	B	13-6	A
13-2	C	13-7	D
13-3	A	13-8	A
13-4	A	13-9	A
13-5	D	13-10	C

Chapter 14

14-1	C	14-6	E
14-2	B	14-7	C
14-3	B	14-8	D
14-4	E	14-9	B
14-5	A		

Chapter 15

15-1	D	15-7	D
15-2	C	15-8	A
15-3	C	15-9	B
15-4	A	15-10	D
15-5	B	15-11	A
15-6	C		

Chapter 16

16-1	C	16-6	B
16-2	B	16-7	A
16-3	D	16-8	C
16-4	B	16-9	A
16-5	C	16-10	A

Chapter 17

17-1	B	17-11	B
17-2	B	17-12	D
17-3	C	17-13	D
17-4	A	17-14	B
17-5	D	17-15	A
17-6	A	17-16	C
17-7	B	17-17	D
17-8	D	17-18	D
17-9	C	17-19	D
17-10	C		

Chapter 18

18-1	B	18-6	D
18-2	B	18-7	B
18-3	C	18-8	A
18-4	D	18-9	C
18-5	A	18-10	C

Chapter 19

19-1	C	19-10	A
19-2	D	19-11	A
19-3	D	19-12	C
19-4	B	19-13	B
19-5	A	19-14	A
19-6	C	19-15	C
19-7	D	19-16	A
19-8	B	19-17	D
19-9	B		

Chapter 20

20-1	B	20-4	A
20-2	E	20-5	C
20-3	C		

Chapter 21

21-1	E	21-6	A
21-2	B	21-7	C
21-3	B	21-8	D
21-4	B	21-9	B
21-5	E		

Chapter 22

22-1	A	22-6	B
22-2	C	22-7	B
22-3	B	22-8	C
22-4	D	22-9	D
22-5	D	22-10	A

Chapter 23

23-1	C	23-6	C
23-2	A	23-7	A
23-3	D	23-8	A
23-4	B	23-9	C
23-5	B	23-10	A

Chapter 24

24-1	A, B, C, D	24-11	A
24-2	D	24-12	A
24-3	B	24-13	B
24-4	C	24-14	D
24-5	D	24-15	A
24-6	D	24-16	C
24-7	B	24-17	D
24-8	D	24-18	A
24-9	A	24-19	B
24-10	D		

Chapter 25

25-1	D	25-3	B
25-2	C	25-4	C

Chapter 26

26-1	B	26-6	C
26-2	C	26-7	D
26-3	A	26-8	C
26-4	B	26-9	D
26-5	B	26-10	E

Chapter 27

27-1	D	27-3	C
27-2	B		

Chapter 28

28-1	B	28-5	A
28-2	C	28-6	C
28-3	B	28-7	D
28-4	D	28-8	C

Chapter 29

29-1	E	29-6	A
29-2	A	29-7	A
29-3	B	29-8	D
29-4	A	29-9	C
29-5	B		

Chapter 30

30-1	E	30-17	A
30-2	B	30-18	B
30-3	B	30-19	C
30-4	C	30-20	C
30-5	C	30-21	C
30-6	A	30-22	E
30-7	C	30-23	D
30-8	A	30-24	A
30-9	C	30-25	D
30-10	B	30-26	A
30-11	D	30-27	C
30-12	B	30-28	D
30-13	A	30-29	E
30-14	C	30-30	A
30-15	B	30-31	C
30-16	A		

Chapter 31

31-1	D	31-5	C
31-2	B	31-6	D
31-3	A	31-7	D
31-4	C	31-8	D

Chapter 32

32-1	D	32-7	1-D
32-2	B		2-B
32-3	D		3-C
32-4	A		4-A
32-5	C	32-8	B
32-6	A	32-9	C

Chapter 33

33-1	C	33-5	B
33-2	D	33-6	C
33-3	C	33-7	D
33-4	B	33-8	A

Chapter 34

34-1	D	34-7	C
34-2	C	34-8	A
34-3	C	34-9	D
34-4	D	34-10	A
34-5	D	34-11	A
34-6	A	34-12	B

Chapter 35

35-1	A	35-7	C
35-2	B	35-8	A
35-3	C	35-9	B
35-4	B	35-10	C
35-5	D	35-11	B
35-6	A		

Chapter 36

36-1	A	36-8	D
36-2	D	36-9	B
36-3	D	36-10	C
36-4	C	36-11	C
36-5	B	36-12	A
36-6	C	36-13	C
36-7	A		

Chapter 37

37-1	D	37-8	C
37-2	B	37-9	A
37-3	D	37-10	D
37-4	D	37-11	B
37-5	C	37-12	A
37-6	E	37-13	C
37-7	B		

Chapter 38

38-1	D	38-6	B
38-2	B	38-7	A
38-3	C	38-8	B
38-4	C	38-9	B
38-5	C	38-10	D

Chapter 39

39-1	A	39-5	D
39-2	C	39-6	C
39-3	D	39-7	A
39-4	C		

Chapter 40

40-1	C	40-5	D
40-2	D	40-6	B
40-3	B	40-7	A
40-4	A		

Chapter 41

41-1	C; older patient, ICU patient, intubated, receiving antibiotics, receiving steroids, urinary catheter present and visitors	41-4	D
		41-5	D
		41-6	A
		41-7	D
		41-8	A
41-2	A	41-9	B
42-3	C	41-10	B

Chapter 42

42-1	D	42-4	D
42-2	A	42-5	B
42-3	C	42-6	D

INDEX

Page numbers with b, f, or t indicate boxes, figures, or tables respectively.

▶ S